MW00845835

Fifth Edition

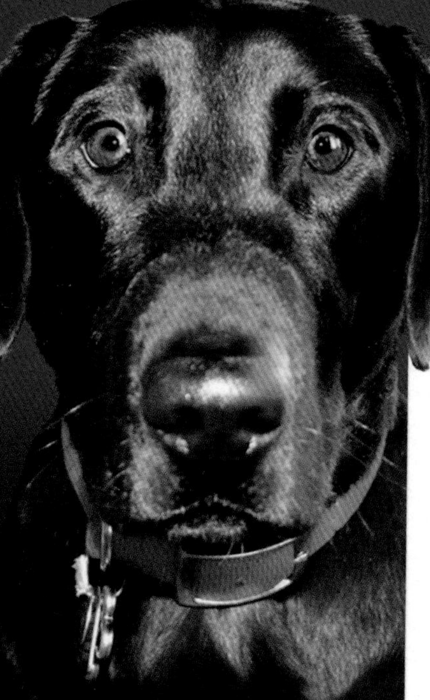

Dyce, Sack and Wensing's

Textbook of VETERINARY ANATOMY

BALJIT SINGH BVSc&AH, MVSc, PhD, FAAA

3M National Teaching Fellow
Professor and Dean
Faculty of Veterinary Medicine
University of Calgary
Calgary, Canada

ELSEVIER

ELSEVIER

3251 Riverport Lane
St. Louis, Missouri 63043

DYCE, SACK AND WENSING'S TEXTBOOK OF VETERINARY ANATOMY, FIFTH EDITION ISBN: 9780323442640

International Standard Book Number: 978-0-323442640

Content Strategy Director: Penny Rudolph
Content Development Manager: Ellen Wurm-Cutter
Content Development Specialist: Alexandra York
Publishing Services Manager: Deepthi Unni
Senior Project Manager: Kamatchi Madhavan
Designer: Patrick Ferguson

Printed in China

Last digit is the print number: 9 8 7 6 5 4 3 2 1

For
my dear wife, Sarbjit Kaur,
son, Pahul Singh,
and our dog, Boomrang

Dedicated to our parents,
Sardar Modan Singh and Sadarni Gurmail Kaur
Sardar Pritam Singh and Sardarni Mohinder Kaur

Contributors

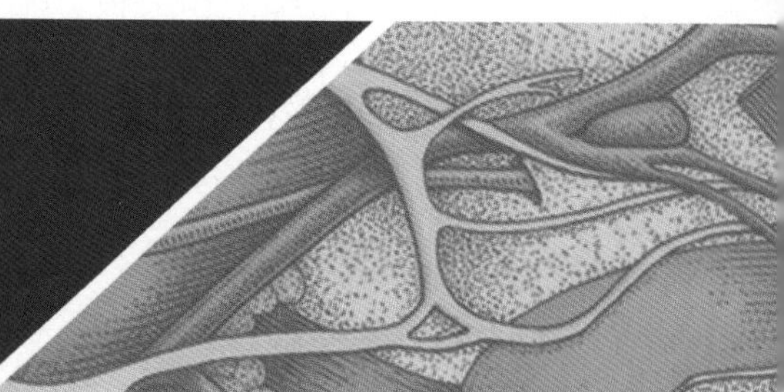

CHAPTER CONTRIBUTORS

Judy Klimek, DVM, MS

Associate Professor
Department of Anatomy and Physiology
Kansas State University College of Veterinary Medicine
Manhattan, KS

Emily J. Reppert, DVM, MS, DACVIM

Assistant Professor
Livestock Services
Department of Clinical Sciences
Kansas State University
Manhattan, KS

Gillian Muir, DVM, PhD

Professor and Head
Department of Veterinary Biomedical Sciences
Western College of Veterinary Medicine
University of Saskatchewan
Canada

FIGURE CONTRIBUTORS

Kalman Czeibert, DVM

Research Fellow
Justanatomy Ltd.
Hungary

Ors Petnehazy, DVM, PhD

Research Fellow
Institute of Diagnostic Imaging and Radiation Oncology
Kaposvár University
CEO, Justanatomy Ltd.
Hungary

Ram S. Sethi, BVSc&AH, MVSc, PhD

Professor
School of Animal Biotechnology
Guru Angad Dev Veterinary and Animal Sciences University
Ludhiana, Punjab

Jaswant Singh, BVSc&AH, MVSc, PhD

Professor
Department of Veterinary Biomedical Sciences
University of Saskatchewan
Saskatoon, Canada

Preface

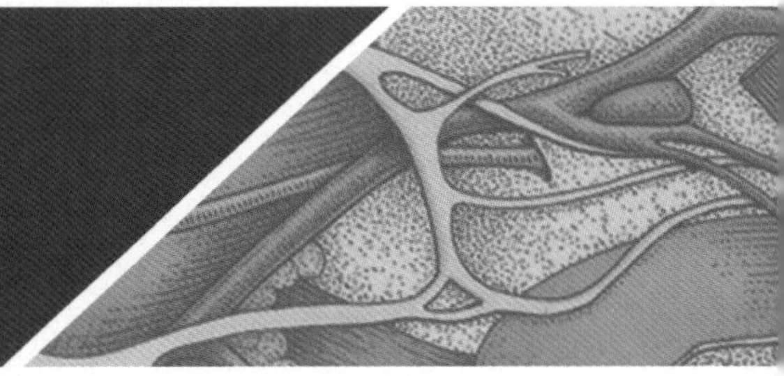

It is an honour and a true privilege to be entrusted with the task of preparing the 5th edition of *Textbook of Veterinary Anatomy* by Dyce, Sack and Wensing. When starting as a graduate teaching assistant in veterinary anatomy courses, I never did or could imagine such an opportunity. Of the three highly distinguished anatomists and original authors of this text, I met only Prof. Wolfgang Sack at the American Association of Veterinary Anatomists meeting in Knoxville in 1996, when I was a postdoctoral fellow. Naturally, I was in awe of him! But he was highly encouraging of my efforts to become a teacher of veterinary anatomy.

I have taken exceptional care to maintain the foundational integrity of the textbook as developed and nurtured by Profs. Dyce, Sack and Wensing. Students accept this text to be the "go-to" anatomy text for their foundational reading as well as a quick check-in. I have also found this book in large numbers of veterinary clinics, and veterinarians attest to its authoritative usefulness in their clinical practice of veterinary medicine. These observations underscore the established value of the text and its fundamental endurance.

There are many current trends that impact the teaching of veterinary anatomy. These trends, including an increase in the volume of veterinary clinical and biomedical information, have resulted in reduced allocation of time to educate students in veterinary anatomical sciences in general. Veterinary embryology has nearly been eliminated from the veterinary medical curricula. The time in veterinary curricula to teach histology has also been reduced significantly. There however is resurging realization that these trends are not fostering development of sufficient foundational knowledge of veterinary anatomy and an integrated set of concepts for the students. For example, the growth in the use of imaging modalities in veterinary medicine has created a need for better education in veterinary anatomy. Also, reduction in time devoted to the instruction of veterinary anatomy is stimulating interest in more integrated teaching of anatomy, histology, and embryology; the *Textbook of Veterinary Anatomy* has been at the forefront of such integrated instruction of veterinary anatomy.

The 5th edition of the *Textbook of Veterinary Anatomy* introduces many changes and makes a gentle pivot to indicate the future direction of the book. In preparing this edition, I have had many discussions with students, and some with fellow teachers. The major changes are as follows:

- significant editing of the text to remove many redundancies;
- removal of text that is not germane to the veterinary medical student;
- addition of nearly 100 new figures;
- addition of many figures at the sub-gross level to create a link between the gross anatomy and histology;
- addition of a new chapter on camelids;
- creation of more than 120 highlighted text boxes to make to easier to grasp important concepts and some clinical features;
- addition of new tables to summarize information;
- creation of a new box called Comprehension Check at the end of each chapter to facilitate group discussion and practice;
- introduction of new contributors: Dr. Gillian Muir has worked on chapters related to the nervous system, and Dr. Judy Klimek and Dr. Emily Reppert have contributed a new chapter on camelids. Dr. Jaswant Singh, Dr. Ors Petnehazy, Dr. Kalman Czeibert, and Dr. R. S. Sethi have contributed illustrations.

Taken together, these changes enable the textbook, while maintaining its rigorous content, to start to look toward a new phase of its life.

This work would not be possible without the exceptional support received from the Elsevier team. In particular, I express sincere thanks to Penny Rudolph, who engaged me in the creation of educational materials for learning veterinary anatomy. Having worked with her in creating Elsevier's *Veterinary Anatomy Flash Cards* and *Veterinary Anatomy Coloring Book,* I have enjoyed doing so again in preparing the 5th edition of the *Textbook of Veterinary Anatomy*. Throughout the preparation of this edition, I received high levels of support and encouragement from Alexandra York, Kamatchi Madhavan, Shelly Stringer, and Brian Loehr.

Finally, I thank many teachers and students who been instrumental in my development as a teacher. Special thanks to Dr. Alastair Summerlee, an exceptional teacher and scholar, who gave me my first opportunity to be a graduate teaching assistant in anatomy laboratories.

I look forward to receiving comments from students and my fellow anatomy teachers to make further improvements to the book and will welcome their opinions on the changes introduced in this edition.

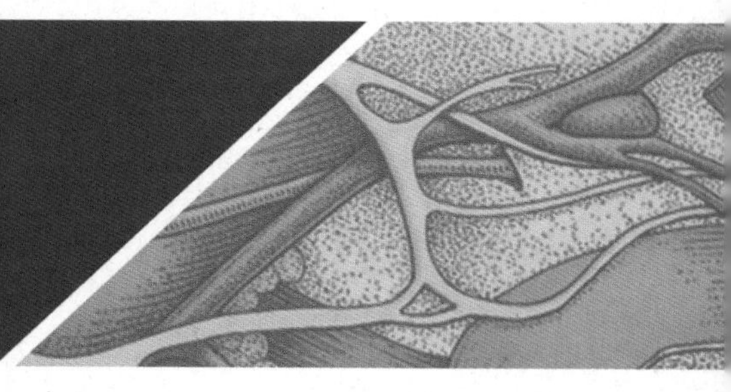

About the Author

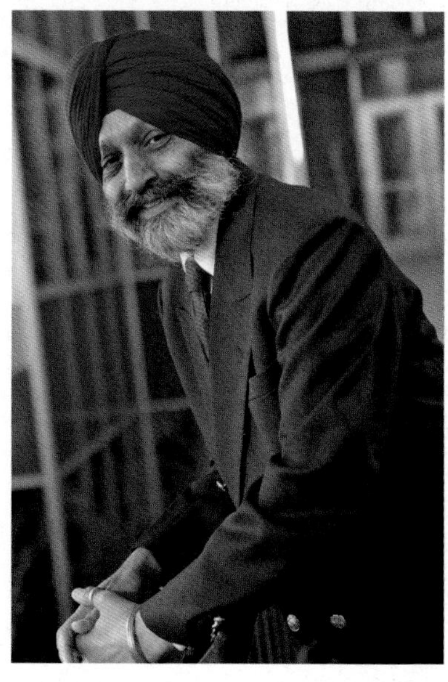

Baljit Singh is Dean and Professor of Veterinary Anatomy at Faculty of Veterinary Medicine, University of Calgary. Before this, he was Professor and Associate Dean (Research) at Western College of Veterinary Medicine, University of Saskatchewan. He obtained a BVSc&AH and an MVSc from Punjab Agricultural University and a PhD from the University of Guelph, and he completed postdoctoral training at Texas A&M University and Columbia University in New York. He is licensed as a Veterinarian in Canada.

Baljit is a recipient of many teaching awards, including Outstanding Veterinary Anatomist Award (2016) from the American Association of Veterinary Anatomists; 3M Canadian National Teaching Fellowship (2009), Canada's highest teaching honour; and Master Teacher Award of the University of Saskatchewan. He is a Fellow of the American Association of Anatomists. He has served as the President of the American Association of Veterinary Anatomists (2005-2008), as a member of the Canadian National Examining Board for Veterinary Medicine (2006-2013), and as a member of the Council on Education of the American-Canadian Veterinary Medical Associations.

Baljit's research program is in the areas of lung inflammation, infectious disease, and nanomedicines. He has trained more than 90 postgraduate, undergraduate, and postdoctoral students and published approximately 95 research papers. He is currently Section Editor (Immunology/Inflammation) of *Cell and Tissue Research* and an editor of *Advances in Anatomy, Embryology and Cell Biology*. He has received the Pfizer Research Excellence Award, Visiting Professorship at the Centre for Excellence in Immunology, Hannover, Germany, and has given many invited lectures.

Sources of Non-Original Illustrations

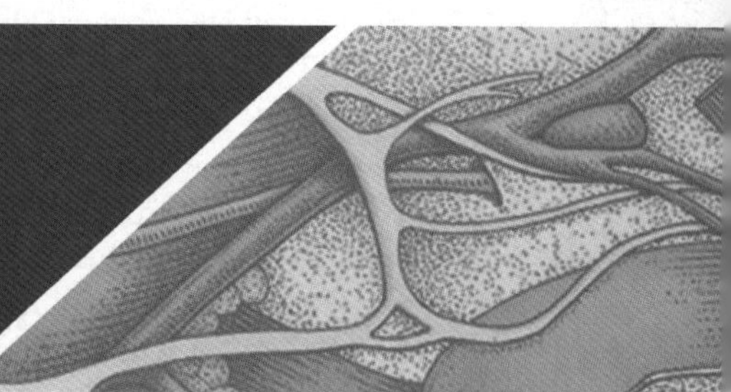

Figure 1.3: After Feeney DA, Fletcher TF, Hardy RM: *Atlas of correlative imaging anatomy of the normal dog,* Philadelphia, 1991, Saunders.

Figures 1.14, A; 1.20, A; 1.22, A; 2.1; 2.23; 2.24; 2.27; 2.53; 11.44, A; 12.9; 12.12; 15.13; 16.2; 16.5; 16.13; 17.3; 30.5: Drawn by DS Geary. Courtesy Dr. A Horowitz, Oregon State University; and from Horowitz A: *Guide for the laboratory examination of the anatomy of the horse,* Columbus, 1965, The University of Ohio, Dept. of Veterinary Anatomy [Published by the author]; and Horowitz A: *The fundamental principles of anatomy: dissection of the dog,* Saskatoon, 1970, University of Saskatchewan [Published by the author].

Figure 1.5, A: Courtesy Dr. JS Boyd, Glasgow University.

Figures 1.5, B; 22.16: Courtesy Dr. BA Ball, Cornell University.

Figure 1.12: After Dawkins MJR, Hull D: The production of heat by fat, *Scient Am* 213:62–67, 1965.

Figure 1.15: After Brookes M, Elkin AC, Harrison RG, Heald CB: A new concept of capillary circulation in bone cortex, *Lancet* 1:1078–1081, 1961.

Figures 2.15; 2.63; 17.5: After Taylor IA: *Regional and Applied Anatomy of the Domestic Animals,* Edinburgh, 1970, Oliver & Boyd.

Figures 2.25; 15.12: Courtesy Dr. A Rijnberk, Utrecht University.

Figure 2.26: After Bradley OC: *Topographic anatomy of the dog,* ed 6, Edinburgh, 1959, Oliver & Boyd.

Figures 2.37; 5.38; 18.3, B: Based on Nickel R, Schummer A, Seiferle E: *Lehrbuch der anatomie der haustiere,* Berlin, 1987, Paul Parey.

Figure 3.26: From Nickel R, Schummer A, Seiferle E: Lehrbuch der anatomie der haustiere, Berlin, 1987, Paul Parey.

Figures 3.37; 10.18; 10.19: Redrawn from Ellenberger W, Baum H: *Handbuch der vergleichenden anatomie der haustiere,* ed 18, Berlin, 1974, Springer.

Figure 3.45: Courtesy Dr. F Preuss, Berlin.

Figures 4.3, B; 11.10, B; 11.42; 11.45, B; 14.13, B; 14.27, B; 14.32, B; 23.22; 23.24, A: Courtesy Dr. PV Scrivani, Cornell University.

Figures 4.10; 4.18: After Nickel R, Schummer A, Seiferle E, Sack WO: *The viscera of the domestic animals,* ed 2, New York, 1978, Springer.

Figures 5.40; 5.62; 5.73, B; 15.9; 15.10; 34.3: Courtesy Dr. B Colenbrander, Utrecht University.

Figure 5.68: Courtesy Dr. DF Antczak, Cornell University.

Figures 5.72, A; 37.20: Courtesy Dr. JM Fentener van Vlissingen, Rotterdam.

Figures 5.73; 11.2; 11.3; 11.4; 15.26: Courtesy M Gaus, Lelystad.

Figure 7.2: Redrawn after Noden, DM, and de Lahunta A: *The embryology of domestic animals,* Baltimore, 1985, Williams & Wilkins.

Figure 7.26: Redrawn after Moore KL: *The developing human: clinically oriented embryology,* ed 5, Philadelphia, 1993, Saunders.

Figures 7.39: After Simoens P, de Vos NE: Angiology. In Schaller O, editor: *Illustrated veterinary anatomical nomenclature,* Kinderhook, NY, 1992, IBD Ltd.

Figure 7.41: Based on Evans HE, de Lahunta A: *Guide to the dissection of the dog,* ed 7, Philadelphia, 2010, Saunders.

Figures 7.42, 7.44: After Budras KD, Fricke W: *Atlas der anatomie des hundes, kompendium für tierärzte und studierende,* Hannover, 1993, Schlütersche Verlagsanstalt.

Figures 7.53; 7.54: Based on Frewein J, Vollmerhaus B, editors: *Anatomie von hund und katze,* Berlin, 1994, Blackwell.

Figures 7.55; 7.59: After Baum H: *Das lymphgefasssystem des hundes,* Berlin, 1918, Hirschwald.

Figure 7.60: Based on Vollmerhaus B: In Nickel R, Schummer A, Seiferle E, editors: *The anatomy of the domestic animals,* Vol. 3, Berlin, 1981, Paul Parey.

Figure 7.62: After Steger G: Zur biologie der milz der haussäugetiere, *Deutsch Tierärztl Wochenschr* 39:609–614, 1939.

Figures 8.12; 8.25: Based on Romer AS: *The vertebrate body,* ed 3, Philadelphia, Saunders, 1962.

Figures 8.20; 8.23; 8.58; 11.19; 11.20: Courtesy Dr. J Ruberte, Barcelona.

Figure 8.61: From de Lahunta A: *Veterinary neuroanatomy and clinical neurology,* ed 3, Philadelphia, 2009, Saunders.

Figure 8.77: Redrawn from Mizeres, NJ: The anatomy of the autonomic nervous system in the dog, *Am J Anat* 96:285–318, 1955.

Figures 9.4; 9.6; 9.14; 11.37, A-B: Courtesy Dr. F Stades and Dr. M Boeve, Utrecht University.

Figure 9.22: Courtesy Dr. P Simoens, Gent University.

Figures 11.7, B; 11.10, C; 16.10, E-F; 17.8, B: Courtesy Dr. C Poulsen Nautrup, Hannover.

Figures 11.17, B; 15.2; 16.3, C-D; 16.8, C-D; 16.9, C-D; 17.1, C-D; 18.6; 18.27; 23.7; 23.9; 23.13: Courtesy Dr. N Dykes, Cornell University.

Figures 11.18; 11.31, A-B; 11.43, A-B: Courtesy Dr. AJ Venker van Haagen, Utrecht University.

Figure 11.22: Redrawn from de Lahunta A, Habel RE: *Applied veterinary anatomy,* Philadelphia, 1998, Saunders.

Figures 11.23; 13.20; 15.23, B; 17.4, D; 17.7, C-D; 37.16, A: Courtesy Dr. BJ Smith, Virginia Technical and State University.

Figures 13.13, B; 14.2; 14.3: After Marthen G: Über die arterien der körperwand des hundes, *Morph Jahrb* 84:187–219, 1939.

Figure 15.20: Redrawn from Christensen GC: Angioarchitecture of the canine penis and the process of erection, *Am J Anat* 95:227–262, 1954.

Figures 16.12; 17.10: Courtesy Dr. RL Kitchell, University of California, Davis.

Figures 18.21; 18.22: Courtesy Dr. I Kassianoff, Hannover.

Figures 18.24; 18.25: Courtesy Dr. L de Schaepdrijver, Gent University.

Figure 18.33: Courtesy Dr. KE Baptiste, Copenhagen.

Figures 21.9; 21.15; 23.33; 23.38, A; 24.7, A: From (and based on) Schmaltz R: *Atlas der anatomie des pferdes,* Vol. 4, Die Eingeweide, Berlin, 1927, Paul Parey; and Schmaltz R: *Atlas der anatomie des pferdes,* ed 3, Vol. 1. Berlin und Hamburg, 1911, Paul Parey.

Figures 22.4: Modified from Hopkins GS: *Guide to the dissection and study of the blood vessels and nerves of the horse,* ed 3, Ithaca, NY, 1937, [Published by the author].

Figure 22.12: Dr. TAE Stout, Utrecht University.

Figure 23.1: After Blythe LL, Kitchell RL: Electrophysiologic studies of the thoracic limb of the horse, *Am J Vet Res* 43:1511–1524, 1982.

Figure 23.4: After Ellenberger W, Dittrich H, Baum H: *Atlas of animal anatomy for artists,* New York, 1956, Dover Publications.

Figure 23.14, B: Courtesy Dr. AJ Nixon, Cornell University.

Figures 23.16; 24.4; 24.11, A: After B Volmerhaus, München.

Figure 23.35, B: Courtesy Dr. N Crevier-Denoix, École National Vétérinaire Alfort.

Figure 23.37: Courtesy Dr. H Brugalla, Berlin.

Figure 24.19: After Pohlmeyer K, Redecker, R: Die für die klinik bedeutsamen nerven an den gliedmassen des pferdes einschliesslich möglicher varianten, *Deutsche Tierärztl Wschr* 81:501–505, 1974.

Figures 25.25; 30.14, A; 30.16; 31.9, A; 31.11: Courtesy Dr. JE Smallwood, North Carolina State University.

Figure 26.1, B: Courtesy Dr. A Meekma, The Netherlands.

Figure 27.1: Courtesy Dr. C Pavaux, Toulouse.

Figures 28.16, A; 28.17: Courtesy Dr. RR Hofmann, Berlin.

Figure 28.20: After Lagerlöf N: Investigations of the topography of the abdominal organs in cattle, and some clinical observations and remarks in connection with the subject, *Skand Vet* 19:1–96, 1929.

Figure 29.4: Redrawn from Habel RE: *Guide to the dissection of domestic ruminants,* ed 3, Ithaca, NY, 1983, [Published by the author].

Figure 29.38: Courtesy Dr. GH Wentink, Arnhem.

Figure 29.44: Courtesy J Peter, Zürich.

Figure 30.1: Courtesy Dr. AD McCauley and Dr. FH Fox, Cornell University.

Figure 31.3: Courtesy Dr. C Maala, University of the Philippines.

Figures 31.7: Courtesy Dr. GC van der Weyden, Utrecht.

Figures 32.3; 32.14: Drawn by Kramer B, Geary DS: From Sack WO, editor: *Horowitz/Kramer atlas of the musculoskeletal anatomy of the pig,* Ithaca, NY, 1982, Veterinary Textbooks.

Figure 32.13: After Saar LI, Getty R: The interrelationship of the lymph vessel connections of the lymph nodes of the head, neck, and shoulder regions of swine, *Am J Vet Res* 25:618–636, 1964.

Figure 35.9: After Mollerus FW: *Zur funktionellen anatomie des eberpenis,* Berlin (FU), 1967, Vet. Diss.

Figure 35.10: After Meyen J: Neue untersuchungen zur funktion des präputialbeutels des schweines, *Zentralbl Vet Med* 5:475–492, 1958.

Figures 37.2; 37.4: After Lucas AM, Stettenheim PR: *Avian anatomy: integument, parts I and II. Agriculture handbook 362,* Washington DC, 1972, US Government Printing Office.

Figure 37.3: Courtesy Dr. M Frankenhuis, Amsterdam Zoo.

Figure 37.22: After Komarek V: Die männliche kloake der entenvögel, *Anat Anz* 124:434–442, 1969.

Figure 38.1: Image by Richard Masoner; unmodified from original. Available at: https://commons.wikimedia.org/w/index.php?curid=3131886. This work is licensed under the Creative Commons Attribution-Share Alike 2.0 Generic license.

Figure 38.2: Image by Andy Farrington; modified from original (cropped). Available at: http://www.geograph.org.uk/reuse.php?id=2525996 This work is licensed under the Creative Commons Attribution-Share Alike 2.0 Generic license.

Figure 38.3: Image by Jaxxon; unmodified from original. Available at: https://commons.wikimedia.org/wiki/File:Andean_woman_with_alpaca.jpg. This work is licensed under the Creative Commons Attribution-Share Alike 3.0 Unported, 2.5 Generic, 2.0 Generic and 1.0 Generic license.

Figure 38.4A: A, Image by Johann Dréo, Wikimedia Commons. Unmodified from original. Available at: https://en.wikipedia.org/wiki/File:Unshorn_alpaca_grazing.jpg. This work is licensed under the Creative Commons Attribution-Share Alike 2.0 Generic license

Figure 38.4B: B, Alpaca at Little Durnford Manor, by Trish Steel; modified from original (cropped). Available at: https://commons.wikimedia.org/wiki/File:Alpaca_-_geograph.org.uk_-_511843.jpg. This work is licensed under the Creative Commons Attribution-Share Alike 2.0 Generic license.

Figure 38.10: Image by Arbutus Photography. Available at: https://www.flickr.com/photos/arbutusridge/8672528601/in/pool-1087584@n20. This work is licensed under the Creative Commons Attribution-Share Alike 2.0 Generic license.

Figure 38.12: Unmodified from original. Available at: https://www.flickr.com/photos/justinlindsay/91878991 This work is licensed under the Creative Commons Attribution-Share Alike 2.0 Generic license.

Figures 38.16, 38.21, 38.22, 38.25, 38.27, 38.31, 38.34, 38.37: From Cebra C, Anderson DE, Tibary A, et al: Llama and alpaca care: medicine, surgery reproduction, nutrition, and herd health, St. Louis, 2014, Elsevier, Fig. 38-11.

Figure 38.26: Drawn from Tibary A, and Vaughan J: Reproductive physiology and infertility in male South American camelids: a review and clinical observations, Small Ruminant Res 61:283–298, 2006.

Figure 38.30: From Cebra C, Anderson DE, Tibary A, et al: Llama and alpaca care: medicine, surgery reproduction, nutrition, and herd health, St. Louis, 2014, Elsevier.

Figure 38.41: Courtesy of Dr. Gheorghe M. Constantinescu, University of Missouri. IN Constantinescu GM, Reed SK, Constantinescu IA: The Suspensory Apparatus and Digital Flexor Muscles of the Llama (Llama glama) 1. The Pelvic Limb, Int J Morphol 26(3):551-556, 2008.

Contents

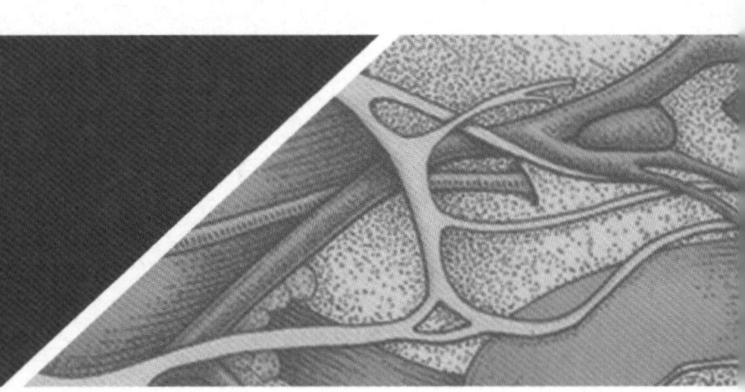

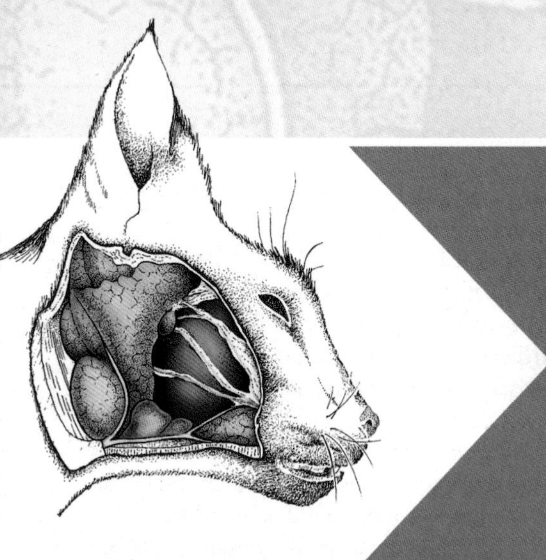

Part I

General Anatomy

Some Basic Facts and Concepts 1

THE SCOPE OF ANATOMY

Anatomy is the study of the form, arrangement, and structure of the tissues and organs that compose the body. It is fundamental to the art and practice of veterinary medicine. The word, of Greek origin, means "cutting apart," and the dissection of the dead is the traditional method used in anatomy. Anatomists do employ a host of other techniques to supplement the knowledge of gross anatomy obtained by use of the scalpel. The use of light microscopy and electron microscopy to study the structures invisible to the eye is a subdiscipline of anatomy known as *microscopic* anatomy. The discipline is also extended by the study of the stages through which the organism evolves from conception through birth, youth, and maturity to old age; this study, known as *developmental* anatomy, is rather broader in scope than classic embryology, which confines its attention to the unborn. The central focus of the anatomy now is to understand the relationships between structure and function, which can be described as *functional* anatomy.

This book is concerned mainly with gross anatomy because of the general practice of presenting microscopic anatomy and developmental anatomy in separate courses. Nonetheless, the book draws on microscopic and developmental aspects to promote an understanding of gross anatomy or as a means of enlivening what would otherwise be a rather dry account.

The information obtained by dissection can be arranged and organized in two principal and complementary ways. *Systematic* anatomy is the study of groups of organs that are closely related in their functions to constitute body systems—the digestive system, the cardiovascular system, and so forth. Systematic anatomy lends itself to a comparative approach; readily combines gross, microscopic, developmental, and functional aspects; and provides the basis for the study of the other medical sciences. Moreover, for the beginner, it is easier to understand than regional anatomy. It is the approach employed in Chapters 2 through 10.

The alternative approach, *regional* anatomy, is used in the second and larger part of this book. Regional (or topographic) anatomy is directly concerned with the form and relationships of all the organs present in particular parts or regions of the body. It pays less attention to function than systematic anatomy but has immediate application to clinical work. Because matters of detail that may lack theoretical interest are often relevant to the clinician, it is necessary to give separate consideration to the regional anatomy of the different species. Regional anatomy is one of the foundations of clinical practice, and different aspects pursued with particular aims are sometimes known as *surface, applied, surgical,* and *radiographic* anatomy—terms whose connotations overlap but hardly require definition.

THE LANGUAGE OF ANATOMY

Anatomic language must be precise and unambiguous. In an ideal world each term would have a single meaning, each structure a single name. Unhappily, there has long been an alarming superfluity of terms and much inconsistency in their use. In the hope of reducing this confusion, an internationally agreed-on vocabulary—*Nomina*

Anatomica Veterinaria (NAV)*—was introduced in 1968 and has since obtained wide acceptance. It was revised most recently in 2012, and we have tried to use it consistently throughout this work. Occasionally, we have included a second, older, and unofficial alternative when such a term appears to be so deeply rooted in clinical use that it is unlikely to be eliminated by edict. The terms of the NAV are in Latin, but it is permissible to translate them into vernacular equivalents. We have used translations that closely resemble the original Latin and give the Latin name only when the translation could be in doubt or there is no handy English equivalent. Because the names, whether in Latin or in English, are intended to be informative and an aid to comprehension, the reader should look terms up in a medical dictionary when their meaning is not self-evident.

The terms that indicate position and direction must be mastered at once. These official terms are more precise than the common alternatives because they retain their relevance regardless of the actual posture of the subject. They are defined in the following list, and their use is illustrated in Fig. 1.1. We have not used them pedantically when there is no reasonable prospect of misunderstanding. When we use common terms (above, behind, and so forth), we always have in mind a standard anatomic position, which, for a quadruped, is that in which the animal stands square and alert. It differs from the human anatomic position. Medical anatomists make much use of the terms *anterior* and *posterior* and *superior* and *inferior*, all of which have very different connotations when applied to quadrupeds. These terms are therefore best avoided,

*There is a separate but similar vocabulary (*Nomina Anatomica Avium*) that is concerned with the anatomy of birds.

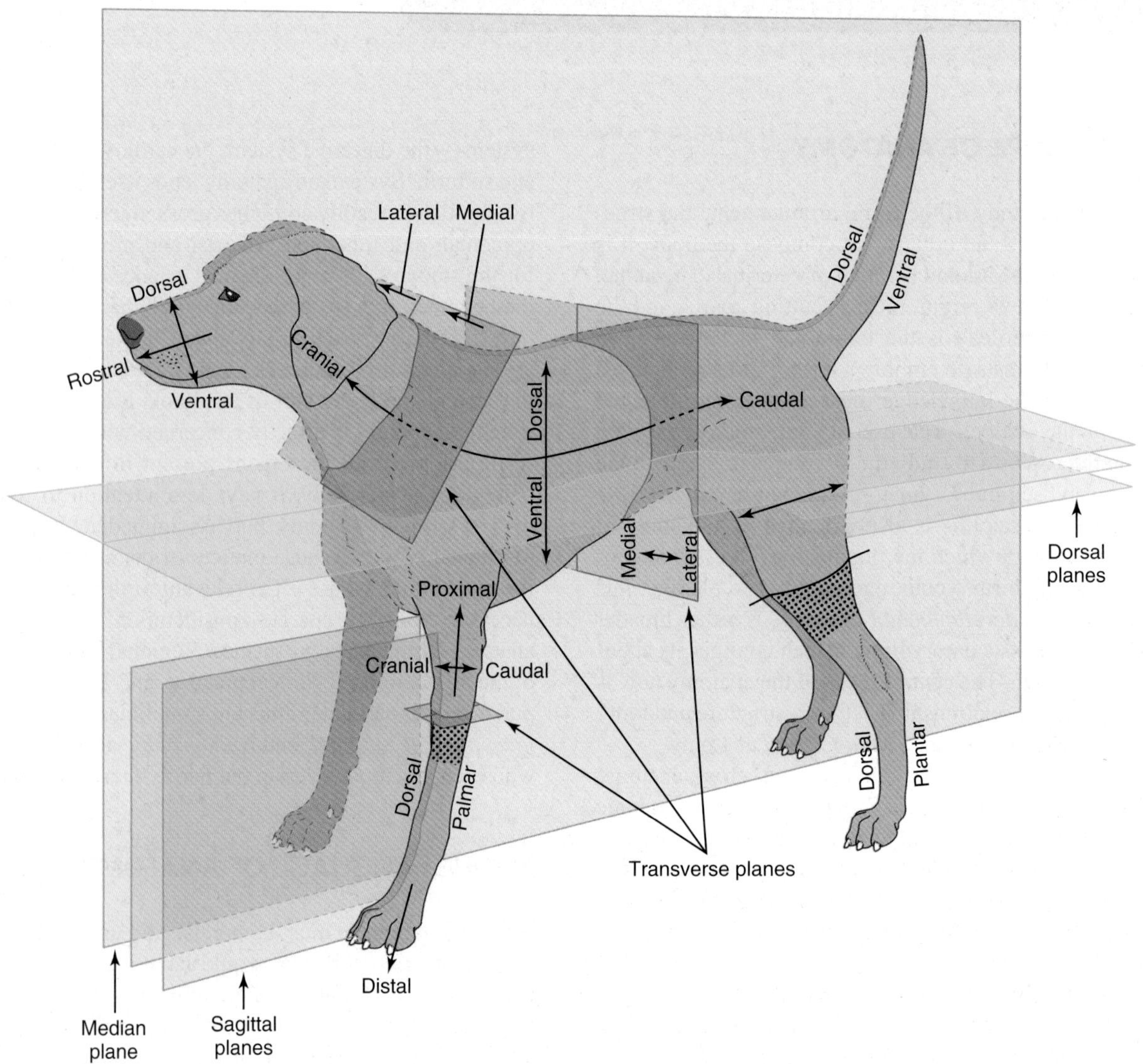

Fig. 1.1 Directional terms and planes of the animal body. The *stippled areas* represent the carpus and tarsus on forelimbs and hindlimbs, respectively.

except for a few specific applications to the anatomy of the head.

The principal recommended terms of position and direction are arranged in pairs, and it should be emphasized that they refer to relative, not absolute, positions. Most of these adjectives, which are listed here, form corresponding adverbs with the addition of the suffix *ly*.

Dorsal structures (or positions) lie toward the back (*dorsum*) of the trunk or, by extension, toward the corresponding surface of the head or tail.

Ventral structures lie toward the belly (*venter*) or the corresponding surface of the head or tail.

Cranial structures lie toward the head (*cranium*, literally skull), caudal ones toward the tail (*cauda*). Within the head, structures toward the muzzle (*rostrum*) are said to be rostral; caudal remains appropriate.

Medial structures lie toward the median plane (*medianus,* in the middle) that divides the body into symmetrical right and left "halves."

Lateral structures lie toward the side (*latus,* flank) of the animal.

Different conventions apply within the limbs. Structures that lie toward the junction with the body are proximal (*proximus,* near), whereas those at a greater distance are distal (*distantia,* distance). Within the proximal part of the limb (which is defined for this purpose as extending to the proximal limit of the *carpus* [wrist] or *tarsus* [hock, ankle]), structures that lie toward the "front" are said to be cranial, those that lie toward the "rear" caudal. Within the remaining distal part of the limb, structures toward the "front" are dorsal (*dorsum,* back of the hand), and those toward the "rear" are palmar (*palma,* palm of the hand) in the forelimb or plantar (*planta,* sole of the foot) in the hindlimb. Additional terms may be applied to the anatomy of the digits. Axial structures lie close to the axis of a central digit, close to the axis of the limb if this passes between two digits; abaxial (*ab,* away from) positions are at a distance from the reference axis.

The terms *external* and *internal, superficial,* and *deep* (*profundus*) hardly require explanation or definition.

Sometimes it is necessary to refer to a section through the body or a part of it (see Fig. 1.1). The *median* plane divides the body into symmetrical right and left halves. Any plane parallel to this is a *sagittal* plane, and those close to the median are sometimes termed *paramedian* planes. A *dorsal* plane sections the trunk or other part parallel to the dorsal surface. A *transverse* plane transects the trunk, head, limb, or other appendage perpendicular to its own long axis.

An Introduction to Regional Anatomy

Although the first nine chapters that follow deal with systematic anatomy, those readers who are about to begin a laboratory course will find that they require an elementary knowledge of several systems at once. It is the principal purpose of the remainder of this chapter to supply that background. However, devoting some attention to the live animal also has benefits.

Study of the Live Animal

Regional anatomy is conveniently studied by means of dissection, but this approach has obvious limitations if the goal is knowledge of the anatomy of the living. The embalmed organs are inert and greatly changed in color and consistency from their living state. The impressions gained in the dissection room or from prosection must therefore be modified and corrected by frequent reference to fresh material or radiographic images; by observation of surgical operations, whenever possible; and by application of the simpler methods of clinical examination to normal animals. We suggest that the student use many experiential learning opportunities to develop a strong foundation of anatomic knowledge.

The simplest method is *observation* of the contours, the proportions, and the posture of the body. Bony projections provide the clearest landmarks, but superficial muscles and blood vessels are also useful, if less striking; reference to these landmarks allows the positions of other structures to be deduced from their known relationships. Little experience is required to reveal the importance of breed, age, sex, and individual variation or to show that although some landmarks are fixed and reliable, others are prone to move. Some (e.g., the costal arch) move with each respiration, whereas other features change more gradually, for example, becoming more or less prominent or shifting in position with the deposition or depletion of fat or with the advance of pregnancy.

Structures that are not directly visible may be identified by *palpation*—that is, by gentle or firmer touch as circumstances require. Bones may be identified by their rigidity, muscles by their contraction, arteries by pulsation, veins by swelling when the blood flow is interrupted by pressure, and lymph nodes and internal organs by their size, configuration, and consistency. Nonetheless, variation is great and is affected by many factors. Palpation through the skin can be supplemented by digital or manual exploration per rectum and per vaginam.

Certain organs may be identified by *percussion* to elicit resonance when the overlying skin is struck a sharp blow (in a prescribed clinical fashion). Different materials produce different notes; a gas-filled organ is more resonant whereas a solid or fluid-filled emits duller notes. The normal activities of certain organs produce sounds continuously or intermittently. Although the lungs and heart (not forgetting the fetal heart) are the prime examples of organs whose positions can be determined by *auscultation,* the movement of blood within vessels or of gas or of ingesta within the stomach or intestines can also be a useful source of anatomic information. While applying these techniques one must remember that the vagaries of sound conduction through materials of different densities may provide a distorted indication of the position and dimensions of the source.

The study of the anatomy of the live animal can be enlarged by other methods whose exercise requires considerable training and more elaborate apparatus than the simple stethoscope. These additional procedures have provided a variety of new illustrations scattered through later chapters; some elementary knowledge of how these illustrations were obtained may assist their appreciation, but detailed consideration of the various technologies involved is clearly beyond the scope of this book.

Many parts and cavities that are normally out of sight can be brought into view with the use of various instruments. Perhaps the most familiar of these are the ophthalmoscope, used to study the fundus of the eye, and the otoscope, used to explore the external ear canal. Other instruments for which the generic title "endoscope" is available may be introduced into natural orifices and advanced to allow inspection of deeper parts, such as the nasal cavity, bronchial tree, or gastric lumen. These examples of endoscopy are noninvasive, but other examinations require preparatory surgery. Among these are arthroscopy, the inspection of the interior of synovial joints, and laparoscopy, the technique in which an endoscope is passed into the peritoneal cavity through a small opening in the abdominal wall. This latter technique may be employed for diagnostic purposes or for the visual control of ("keyhole") surgery with the use of instruments introduced through separate portals.

The rigidity of the early endoscopes limited their utility. The modern endoscopes use flexible fiberoptic systems and are remotely controlled. The essential components of the fiberoptic instrument are two bundles of glass fibers. One bundle is used to convey light distally, from an external source to the region to be viewed; the component fibers can be relatively coarse and randomly arranged. The second bundle conveys the image and is composed of finer fibers that maintain fixed positions in relation to one another. The image is composed of many tiny units, each corresponding to an individual fiber, and is presented to the eye (or to a camera or video system) at the proximal end of the instrument.

Radiographic anatomy has for some time been an indispensable component of every course of anatomy. X rays are produced by bombarding with electrons a tungsten target (focus) housed within a shielded tube. Only a narrow x-ray beam is permitted to escape, and this beam is directed toward the relevant region of the subject. The passage of the rays through the body is affected by the tissues they encounter; tissues substantially composed of elements of high atomic weight tend to scatter or absorb the rays, and tissues substantially composed of elements of low atomic weight have proportionately less effect. Because of its calcium content, bone clearly belongs to the first (radiopaque) category, whereas soft tissues generally belong to the second (radiolucent) category. Those rays that succeed in passing through the subject are allowed to impinge on a sensitive film (or other detector), which responds to the radiation received. When the film is developed, mostly as digital images these days, those areas that were overlain by soft tissues (or gas-filled spaces) appear dark, even black, and those areas that were overlain by bone (or other radiopaque material) appear lighter, even white. The distinction between tissues of similar radiodensity may be enhanced by introducing an appropriate contrast agent to coat a surface or fill a space. Specific methods utilizing various materials are available to depict such different features as the gastric lumen, urinary tract, and subarachnoid space.

Radiographic views are appropriately identified by reference to the direction taken by the x-ray beam in its passage through the subject. Thus a radiograph of a supine animal, presenting its belly to the x-ray source, is described as a *ventrodorsal* film; that obtained with the animal turned over, with its belly now facing the film, is described as a *dorsoventral* film. The convention provides little scope for confusion but occasionally produces an awkward term, such as *dorsolateral-plantaromedial,* which specifies a particular oblique view of the hock.

Awareness of certain general principles helps one avoid some common misinterpretations: the image of any structure is always magnified to the degree determined by the ratio between the distance from focus to film and distance from focus to object; the divergence of the x rays produces an apparent shift in position of any object not directly below the focus. Two simple diagrams (Fig. 1.2) will make these points clear. A less easily resolved difficulty results from the superimposition of the images of structures that lie over each other. An ingenious, only partly successful, solution to this problem was sought in the coordinated movement—in opposite directions—of tube and film during the period of the exposure (Fig. 1.3A). In this technique, known as *tomography,* the axis about which tube and film travel coincides with the plane of the horizontal slice of the subject that is of current interest. Structures contained within this slice remain more or less in focus throughout the exposure, whereas the images produced by structures at other levels are blurred or subsumed within the general background. Such tomograms never found much employment in veterinary radiology. The later developed and more sophisticated technique known as *computed tomography* (CT) has a different basis but retains the aim of clearly depicting the parts within one particular body slice while excluding extraneous images. Despite the considerable cost of the apparatus and its limited suitability for use with large animals, the technique is now widely offered by veterinary referral centers.

In the modern CT scanner, the x-ray source is moved in a circle that is centered on the longitudinal axis of the subject during the procedure, which takes from one to several

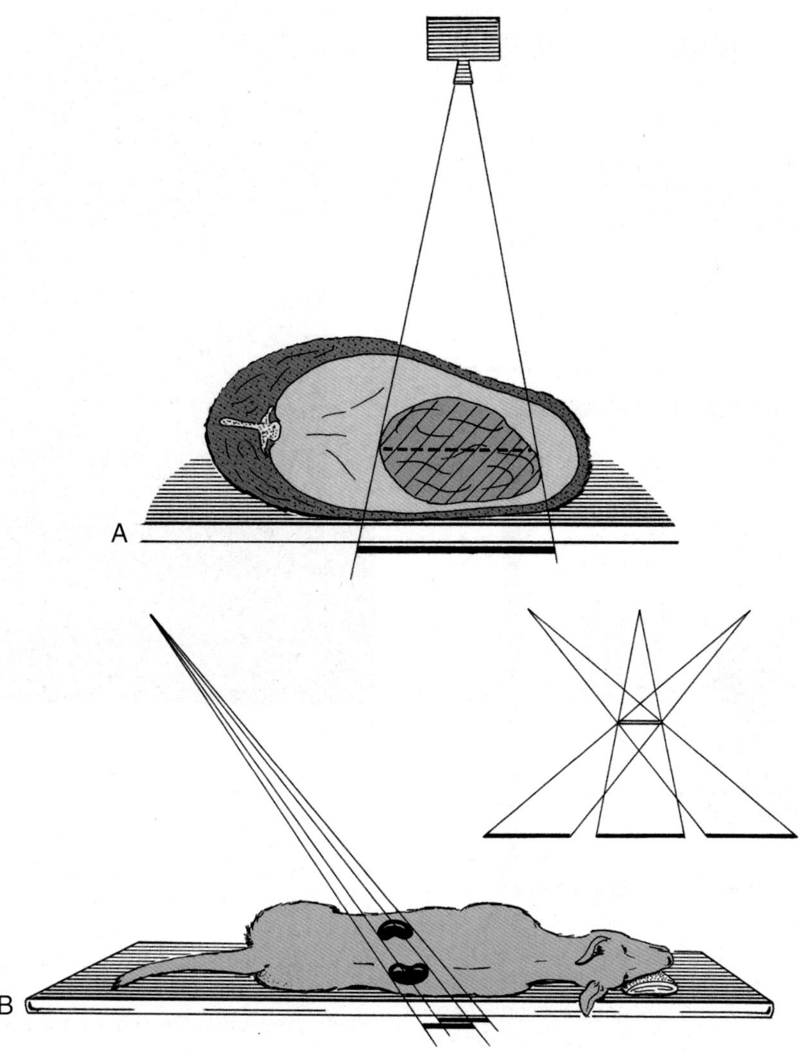

Fig. 1.2 (A) Schematic drawing illustrating the magnifying effect on radiographs caused by the divergence of x rays. (B) Schematic drawing illustrating the apparent shift in position on radiographs of an organ that is not directly below the focus.

seconds for its completion (see Fig. 1.3B). During this time the movement of the tube is repeatedly arrested for very short periods; during each of these, a burst of radiation is directed through the subject along a different radius. The beams that penetrate the selected, very narrow slice of the subject impinge on a series of discrete detectors or, in some designs, on portions of a continuous circumferential detector and are photomultiplied. After the procedure is completed, these records are analyzed, compared, and combined according to complex formulae (algorithms); from these computations, a single cross-sectional image is constructed in which the forms, locations, and comparative radiodensities of all the tissues within the selected body slice are represented (Fig. 1.4). In more complex settings, multiple overlapping or adjacent slices can be imaged in an extended, continuous process. With the amount of information the extended process supplies, it is possible by even more elaborate computation to construct images in other than transverse planes. The data may also be manipulated to enhance subtle differences in contrast presented by tissues of very similar radiodensity.

CT is, of course, not free of all drawbacks: subjects must be strictly immobilized during the exposure procedure; the total radiation dose may be quite considerable, even though individual exposures are very short, and the resulting images amplified; artifacts may produce deceptive images; and current apparatus designed for medical use is suitable for small animals but must be adapted for application with large animals and is then limited to the investigation of the head and limbs. One by-product of CT is the revival of interest in cross-sectional anatomy, an approach to the discipline that had been regarded as irretrievably passé but is now clearly indispensable to CT interpretation.

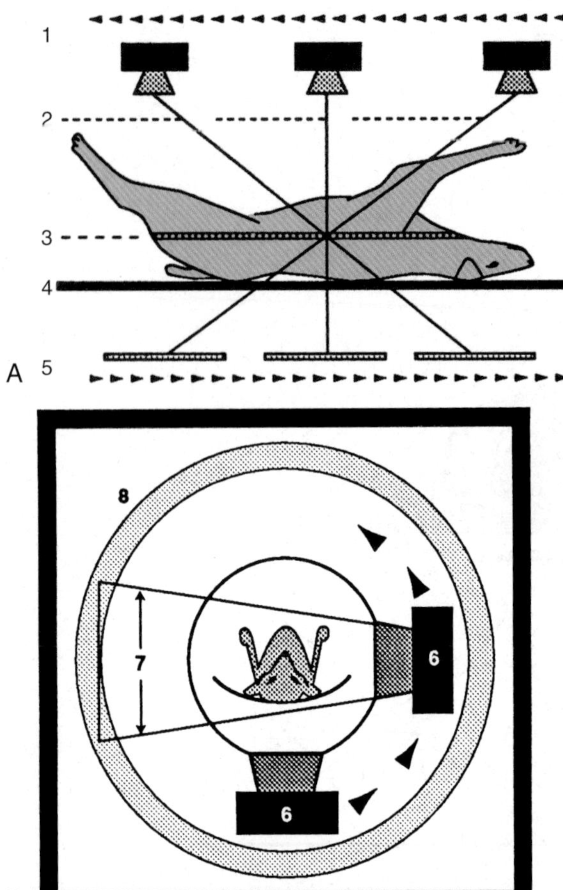

Fig. 1.3 Diagrams of a basic (noncomputed) x-ray tomographic apparatus (A) and of a fourth-generation computed tomography (CT) scanner (B). *1,* Movement of x-ray source during exposure; *2,* lines indicating mechanical connection between x-ray source and radiation detector (i.e., film); *3,* plane of focus; *4,* supine patient on stationary table; *5,* movement (in the opposite direction) of detector during exposure; *6,* movement of x-ray source around stationary patient; *7,* x-ray beam during exposure; *8,* ring of fixed detectors surrounding the rotating x-ray tube mechanism.

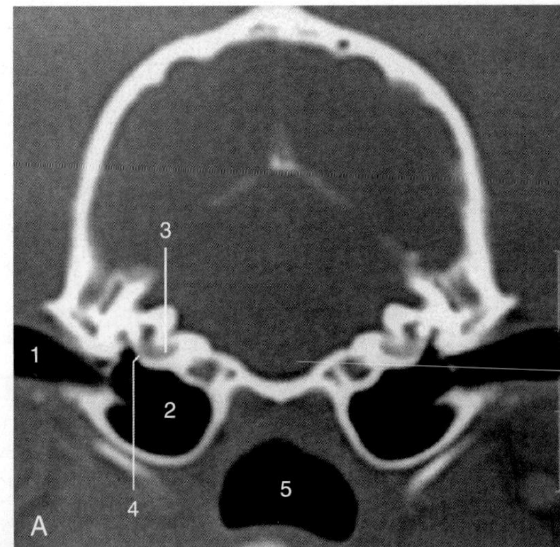

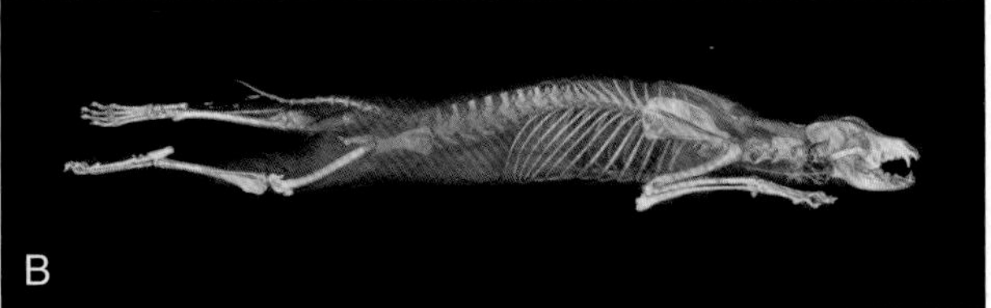

Fig. 1.4 A, Transverse image of a 2-mm-thick computed tomography slice of the canine tympanic bullae and petrous temporal bones. (Bone settings were used.) *1,* External acoustic meatus; *2,* tympanic bulla; *3,* cochlea; *4,* round window; *5,* nasopharynx. B, Three dimensional model generated from whole body computed tomography of a female dog.

Our knowledge of anatomy, especially the correlates of structure and function, will continue to grow through the implementation of new tools such as positron emission tomography–magnetic resonance imaging (PET-MRI), which exploits the high-resolution capability of MRI with the use of sophisticated imaging tracers in PET.

Familiarity with cross-sectional anatomy is also required for the practice of *ultrasonography*. This technique depends on the capacity of a piezoelectric crystal to convert electrical energy into sound waves and vice versa. When stimulated, a suitably housed crystal transducer, coupled to the appropriate area of skin, directs a narrow beam of sound waves of uniform frequency into the body. The waves are propagated through the tissues with decaying intensity, and a fraction is directed back toward the source at each encounter, with an interface between tissues offering different resistance (acoustic impedance). Reconverted into electrical energy, the echoes generate a visible image on a screen. This image, which can be "frozen" or recorded in various ways, represents the thin body slice directly below the transducer. The sound wave is produced not continuously but in very short bursts, perhaps lasting for no more than one-millionth part of a second. The longer silences that alternate with these bursts allow the time necessary for the receipt of echoes bounced back from interfaces at different depths.

The frequency and the wavelength of sound waves are inversely related. The first variable determines the depth to which waves will penetrate; the second, the resolution that may be obtained (i.e., the detail that may be distinguished). Because waves of high frequency penetrate less deeply but record more detail, a compromise is involved in the selection of the appropriate crystal to deploy for a specific examination: several crystals are normally at hand, and each has its own inherent and invariable oscillation frequency. The maximum depth from which it is possible to obtain useful images is about 25 cm, thus limiting the application of ultrasonography in horses and cattle. In these large species its use is more or less restricted to the examination of the distal parts of the limbs and of the reproductive system

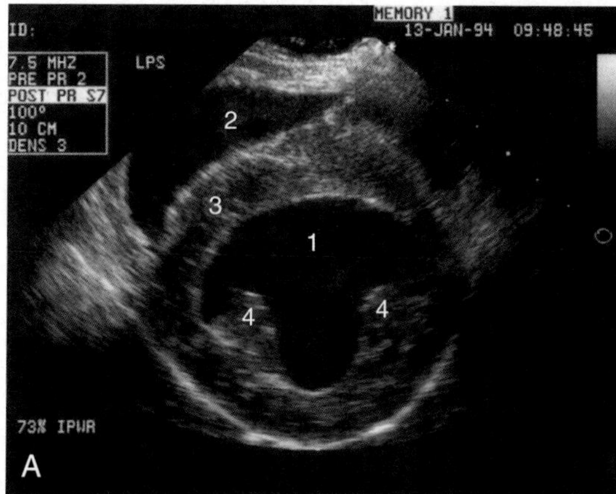

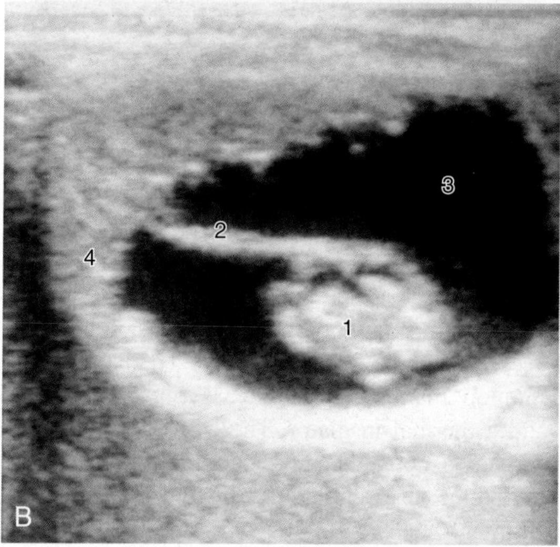

Fig. 1.5 (A) Ultrasonographic transverse (short-axis) view of the canine heart. *1,* Left ventricle; *2,* right ventricle; *3,* septum; *4,* papillary muscles. (B) Ultrasonographic view of a 42-day-old equine embryo. *1,* Embryo, about 2 cm in length; *2,* umbilical cord; *3,* allantoic fluid; *4,* uterine wall.

(for which the transducer may be applied to the rectal mucosa). Ultrasonography is also widely used in the diagnosis of pregnancy in sows (although here a transabdominal approach is employed).

Water, blood, and most soft tissues offer very similar acoustic impedance, and interfaces between these substances are, at best, only moderately reflective; they are hypoechoic in ultrasonographers' jargon. In contrast, the difference in impedance between soft tissue and bone, or between soft tissue and a gas-filled cavity, is very large, and the reflection of sound waves is almost total—the interface is *hyperechoic*. This feature makes it impossible to image tissues and organs that, like the brain within the skull, lie deep to bone; such parts are said to be within acoustic shadow. Conversely, a distended bladder, or other large volume of uniform impedance, may be used as a window through which deeper structures may be approached.

There are many differences in transducer design and usage. Some transducers contain multiple crystals arranged in line, which upon sequential activation create a rectangular image representing the thin slice of tissue situated deep to the transducer. More often a single crystal is employed but so arranged that the narrow beam that it generates swings repetitively in an arc, producing a wedge- or sector-shaped image (Fig. 1.5). In these B (or brightness) settings, the image represents a cross section through the field surveyed. In the alternative M (or motion) setting, the beam is emitted only at one fixed point in the crystal's oscillation, and the recording is therefore limited to the structures penetrated along a single axis. If the parts are moving, successive images reveal their changing shapes, and the changes are emphasized if successive images are recorded side by side. M-mode recordings are especially useful for demonstrating the movements of the walls of the heart chambers and valves.

Ultrasonograms are, in general, less easy for the novice to interpret than radiographs. Reverberations occur when the waves bounce back and forth, often because of defective coupling of the transducer to the skin, and may produce what appear to be multiple parallel interfaces within an organ. Small interfaces between the parenchyma and fibrous scaffolding of certain tissues produce diffuse scattering, or a stippled effect. Despite these (and other) drawbacks, ultrasonography possesses very considerable advantages, including absence of ionizing radiation.

Magnetic resonance imaging requires less extensive consideration because the expense of installation and operation of the equipment limits its current availability to only a few veterinary centers. The theoretical basis of MRI lies in changes in the structure of hydrogen atoms induced by strong magnetic fields and radio waves. Weak radio signals are subsequently produced when the subatomic structure returns to its normal configuration. These signals may be amplified, and their origins within the body may be precisely fixed in three dimensions. Because different tissues contain different concentrations of hydrogen atoms, their different responses can be used to distinguish them. Tissues such as fat that are rich in hydrogen produce bright images, in contrast to the black images of hydrogen-poor tissues such as bone (Fig. 1.6). Extremely high resolution is possible. There appear to be no health risks associated with the MRI scanner. Both CT and MRI are especially useful in the study of intracranial structures.

Skin

The skin covers the body and protects it against injury. Skin plays an important part in temperature control and enables the animal to respond to various external stimuli by virtue of its many nerve endings. There are numerous local modifications of skin (see Chapter 10), but at present, we are concerned only with its more general properties.

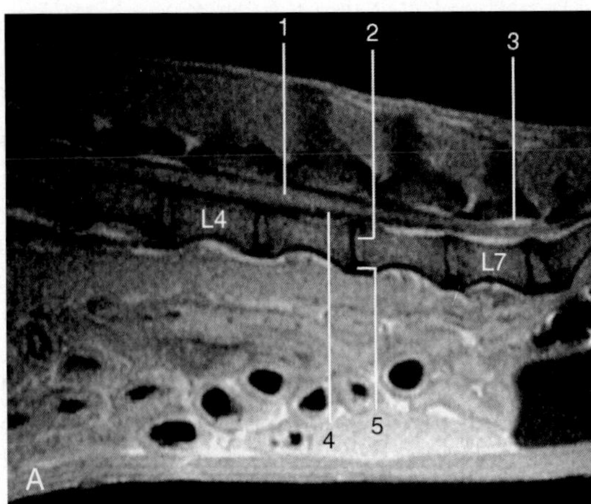

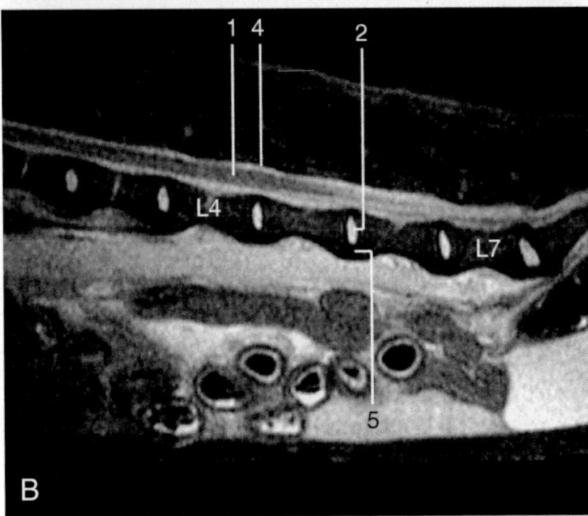

Fig. 1.6 Midsagittal images of 3-mm-thick spin-echo magnetic resonance slices of the canine lumbar vertebral column. (A) T1-weighted (fat appears white, fluids dark). (B) T2-weighted (fluids appear white, fat darker than on T1-weighted images). *1,* Spinal cord; *2,* nucleus pulposus; *3,* epidural fat; *4,* cerebrospinal fluid; *5,* annulus fibrosus.

The skin varies greatly in thickness and flexibility, both among species and within the same animal. It is naturally thicker in larger animals (though not in constant proportion to their size) and in more exposed areas. Although the skin is generally closely molded to the underlying structures, it forms folds and creases to increase surface area in certain areas to allow for change in posture, heat dissipation, and sometimes an expression of breeders' whims, grotesquely illustrated by the Shar-Pei breed of dog.

Skin consists of an outer epidermis and an inner dermis, and in most situations it rests on a looser connective tissue variously known as the *subcutis, hypodermis,* or *superficial fascia* (Fig. 1.7). The epidermis is a stratified squamous epithelium, and its thickness responds to rough usage, as exemplified by the footpads of dogs and cats. This layer is modified in many ways, including the occurrence of sweat and sebaceous glands, which are widely spread, and of hair. Sweat glands are most important as a provision for heat loss by surface evaporation but also play a subsidiary role in the excretion of waste. The sebaceous glands

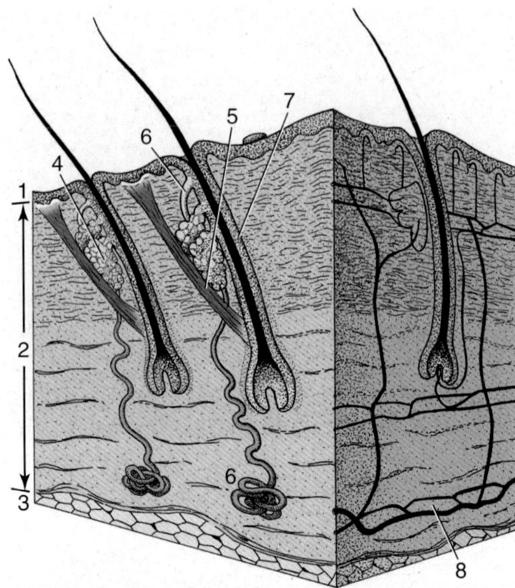

Fig. 1.7 A block of skin. *1,* Epidermis; *2,* dermis; *3,* subcutis; *4,* sebaceous gland; *5,* arrector pili muscle; *6,* sweat gland; *7,* hair follicle; *8,* arterial networks.

produce an oily secretion that waterproofs the surface and provides certain relatively naked areas, such as the groin of horses, with a characteristic sheen. The haircoat, which is a uniquely mammalian feature, is a mechanical protection and a thermal insulator. The haircoat is also usually widespread. Among the more familiar species, only the human and the pig are relatively devoid of extensive haircoat, although such conditions may appear in other species as occasional "sports," which is the origin, for example, of the Sphynx breed of cat. Some aquatic mammals, such as whales, are wholly naked.

The dermis, which consists essentially of felted connective tissue fibers, is the raw material of leather. It is secured to the epidermis by interlocking papillae, which are most pronounced where normal wear might risk separation. In most situations, the skin moves easily over the underlying tissues, and this looseness facilitates the flaying of a carcass. It is more tightly bound down in a few places where it grades into a tougher-than-usual underlying fascia; good examples of this binding are provided by the scrotum and the lips. Some risk of pressure injury is present where the dermis is molded over bony prominences, and synovial bursae (p. 22) often develop adventitiously in such sites. Unlike the epidermis, the dermis is well supplied with blood vessels (see Fig. 1.7) and cutaneous nerves.

The superficial fascia is considered in the following section.

Fascia and Fat

The connective tissue that separates and surrounds the more obviously important structures is generically known as *fascia;* many of its larger accumulations, particularly

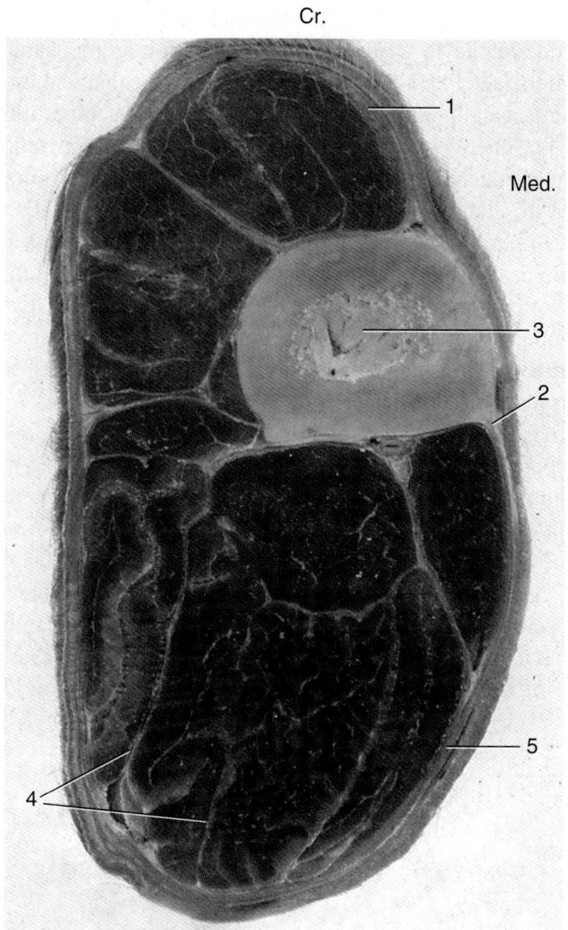

Fig. 1.8 Osteofascial compartments in the forearm of a horse. *1,* Superficial fascia; *2,* cephalic vein; *3,* radius; *4,* septa of deep fascia enclosing individual muscles or groups of muscles; *5,* deep fascia. (In transverse sections of the limbs, cranial *[Cr.]* and medial *[Med.]* are identified.)

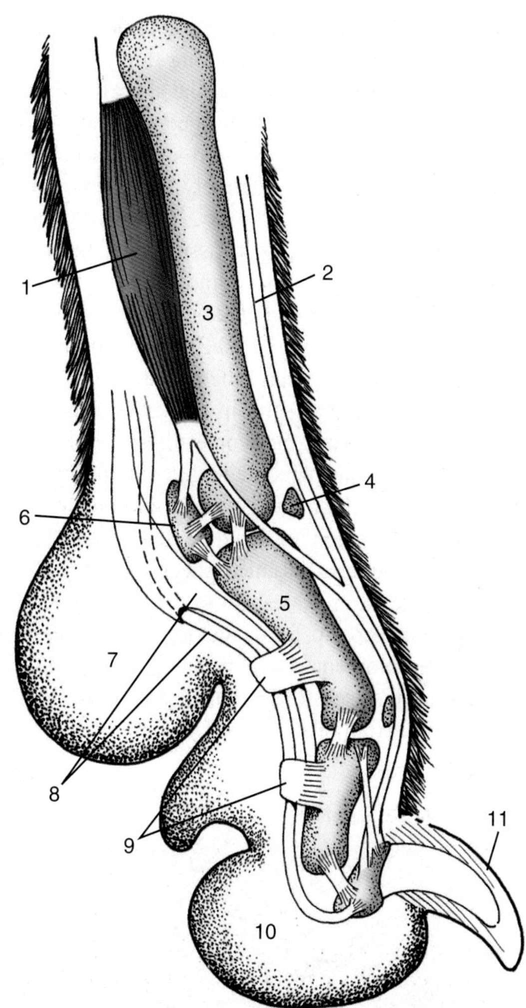

Fig. 1.9 Axial section of a dog's paw; the metacarpal pad *(7)* is in contact with the ground during standing. *1,* Interosseous muscle; *2,* extensor tendon; *3,* metacarpal bone; *4,* dorsal sesamoid bone; *5,* proximal phalanx; *6,* proximal sesamoid bone; *8,* flexor tendons; *9,* retinacula; *10,* digital pad; *11,* claw.

those of a sheetlike nature, have specific names. The fascia has important functions as it is encountered in surgery.

The *superficial fascia* (subcutis) is a loose (areolar) tissue extensively spread below the skin of animals that possess a hairy coat. A similar tissue surrounds many deeper organs, and in both situations, the loose fascia allows neighboring structures to change in shape and to move easily against each other. Its looseness varies with the amount of fluid it contains and may provide an indication of ill health. The superficial fascia is one of the principal sites for the storage of fat. In naked species, the fat forms a continuous layer, the *panniculus adiposus*.

The *deep fascia* is generally organized into much tougher fibrous sheets. A layer beneath the superficial fascia extends over most of the body and fuses to bony prominences. In many places it detaches septa that penetrate between the muscles, enclosing them individually or in groups (Fig. 1.8); sometimes the periosteum, the fibrous covering of the bones, participates in outlining the enclosures. This division into fascial or osteofascial compartments is very prominent in the forearm and leg and plays a part in the circulation, assisting the return of blood and lymph to the heart. The contraction of muscles presses the structures such as valved veins contained within their unyielding walls to return the blood toward the heart. For this reason, muscular paralysis or prolonged inactivity may lead to stasis of blood or lymph flow. Arteries and nerves whose functions would not be assisted by compression often travel in small tunnels within the septa.

More specific functions can be assigned to localized thickenings (e.g., *retinacula,* tethers) of deep fascia, which hold tendons in place and sometimes provide pulleys around which the tendons wind to change direction. Good examples are provided by the retinacula on the dorsal aspect of the hock and the palmar aspect of the digits (Fig. 1.9/*9*).

Because dense fascia is relatively impermeable, it determines the direction taken by spreading fluids such as pus, which sometimes tracks below a fascial sheet before breaking through far from its source. Surgeons exploit both the toughness of the deep fascia to hold sutures securely and its cleavage planes to gain relatively bloodless access to deeper parts during surgery.

Most deposits of *fat* (adipose tissue) may be regarded primarily as food reserves. Small amounts of fat are widely distributed, but the bulk is contained in three or four places: in the superficial fascia (Fig. 1.10/*2*); between and within muscles; below the peritoneum (the delicate membrane lining the abdominal cavity); and in the marrow cavities of long bones. Subcutaneous fat deposits help mold the body contours and often show specific and gender differences in localization and development. Animals that are adapted to hot habitats often develop localized fat depots (e.g., humped zebu cattle and camels, fat-tailed sheep), leaving the rest of the body surface to release heat to the environment. The onset of puberty leads to fat deposition in the breasts and over the hips in women. In many male animals, much fat is deposited in the tissues of the dorsal part of the neck: the thickened crest of stallions is a good example.

Some fat deposits, like that enclosed within a fibrous lattice in the footpad of the dog, function as mechanical buffers (see Fig. 1.9/*7* and *10*). Fat with a mechanical function is usually resistant to mobilization during starvation.

The chemical and physical differences in fat may reflect diet as much as specific genetic factors. The fat of horses and of Channel Island breeds of cattle is yellow, that of sheep hard and white, and that of pigs soft and grayish. It should also be remembered that fat at body temperature is softer (semifluid) than that exposed in a colder environment. Certain procedures employed by the cosmetic surgeon—liposuction and lipofixation—depend on this fortunate circumstance.

All these remarks refer to the common sort of fat. A second variety, *brown fat,* is of much more restricted distribution in time and place. Brown fat differs in structure (Fig. 1.11) and function as well as in color. In domestic species, it is found especially during the fetal and neonatal periods; in wild species, it is especially prominent in those that hibernate (Fig. 1.12). The brown adipocyte contains numerous smaller droplets and a much higher number of mitochondria. It is richly vascularized. It provides both groups in which it is especially found with a readily

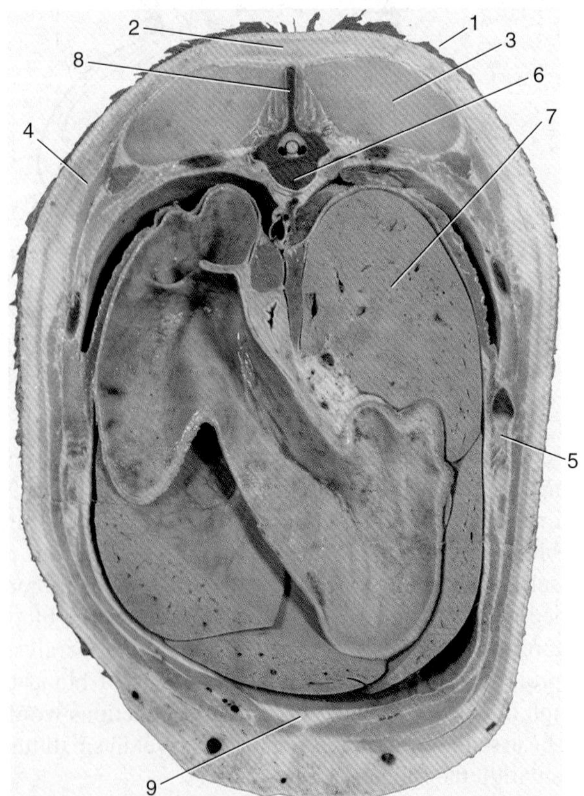

Fig. 1.10 Transverse section of the back of a pig. *1,* Skin; *2,* fat (panniculus adiposus) associated with the superficial fascia; *3,* back muscles; *4,* cutaneous muscle enclosed within superficial fascia; *5,* rib; *6,* thoracic vertebra; *7,* liver; *8,* spinous process of vertebra; *9,* additional fat deposited between muscles.

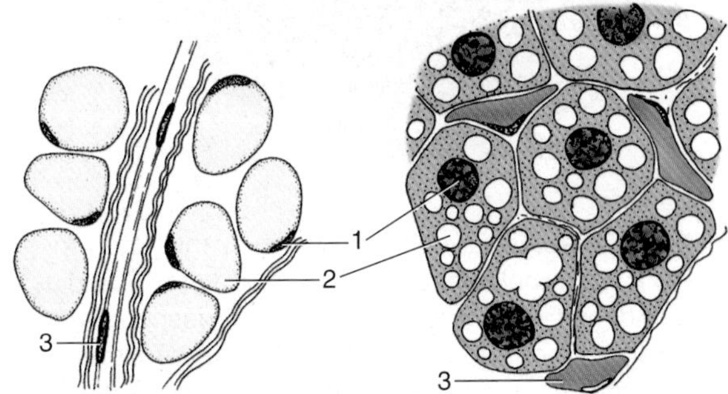

Fig. 1.11 Fat cells of white *(left)* and brown *(right)* fat. In white fat a single large fat vacuole displaces the cytoplasm and the nucleus to the periphery of the cell. The small fat vacuoles are evenly distributed in the cells of brown fat. *1,* Nuclei; *2,* fat vacuoles; *3,* capillaries.

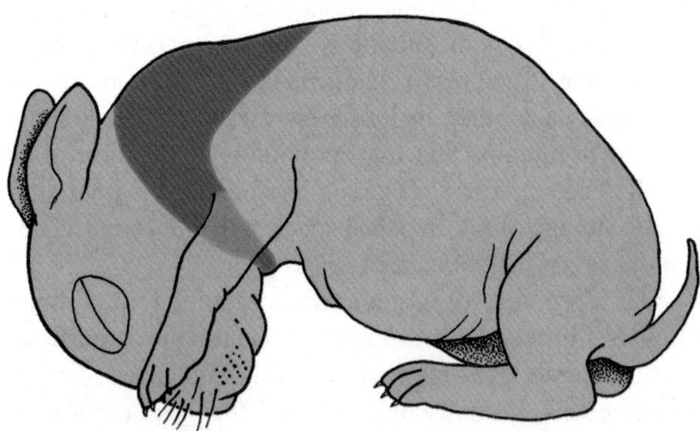

Fig. 1.12 The distribution of brown fat in the newborn rabbit, concentrated around the neck and between the shoulder- [Per Dorland's and other chapters.] blades.

available source of heat, which is equally useful in newborn animals with imperfect thermoregulation and in hibernators required to awaken rapidly from a deep winter sleep.

Bones

The primary functions of the skeleton are to support the body, to provide the system of levers used in locomotion, and to protect soft parts. Therefore, biomechanical factors are most important in shaping the bones and in determining their microscopic design. The major skeletal tissue, bone, has a secondary role in mineral homeostasis: being a reservoir for calcium, phosphate, and other ions.

The Classification of Bones

Bones may be classified in various ways. A topographic classification recognizes a cranial skeleton (of the head) and a postcranial skeleton consisting of two divisions: the axial skeleton of the trunk and the appendicular skeleton of the limbs. A second classification based on ontogeny distinguishes the somatic skeleton, formed in the body wall, from the visceral skeleton, derived from the pharyngeal (branchial) arches. A third system also based on development distinguishes parts preformed in cartilage (and later largely replaced by bone) from those that ossify directly in fibrous connective tissue. This classification reflects phylogeny, in that bones that develop in membrane are homologous with dermal bones of lower vertebrates.

Bones are also classified on the basis of shape (Fig. 1.13).

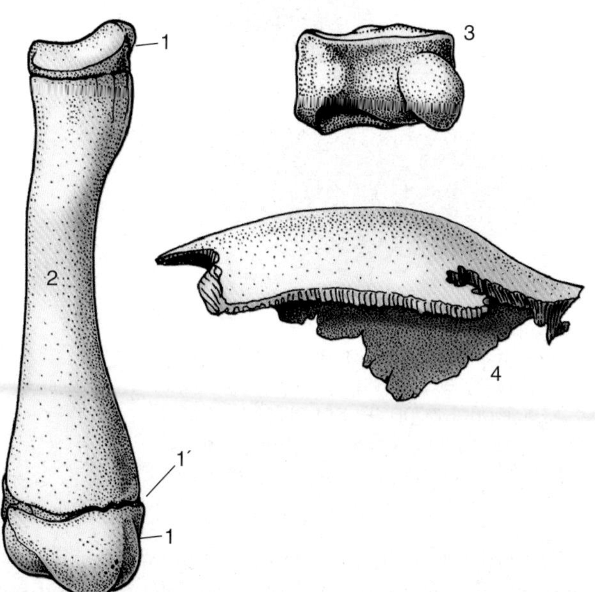

Fig. 1.13 Long *(left)*, short *(top right)*, and flat *(bottom right)* bones. *1*, Proximal and distal epiphyses; *1′*, epiphysial cartilage; *2*, diaphysis of a young dog's radius; *3*, carpal bone of a horse; *4*, parietal bone from the skull of a dog.

Long bones, as in the limbs, are broadly cylindrical and act as levers. They develop from at least three centers of ossification: one for the shaft (diaphysis) and one for each extremity (epiphysis) (p. 65).

Short bones have no dimension that greatly exceeds the others. Many such bones are grouped together at the carpus and tarsus to generate multiple articulations for facilitating complex movements and diminishing concussion. The majority of short bones develop from a single center of ossification; replication of centers generally indicates that the bone represents the fusion of elements distinct in ancestral forms.

Flat bones are expanded in two directions. The category includes the scapula, the bones of the pelvic girdle, and many of those of the skull. Their broad surfaces afford attachment to large muscle masses and protection to underlying soft parts.

The remaining bones are too irregular in form to be grouped in clearly defined categories. Neither flat nor irregular bones exhibit uniformity in development.

The Organization of a Long Bone

The longitudinal section of a long bone shows many features of its construction (Fig. 1.14A). The form of the bone is determined by a sheath or cortex of solid (compact) bone that is composed of thin lamellae arranged mainly in series of concentric tubes about small central canals. Each such system is known as an *osteone* (Fig. 1.14B). The cortex is thick toward the middle of the shaft but thins as it flares toward each end, over which it continues as a crust. The external surface is smooth except where irregularities serve as the attachment sites for muscles or ligaments; these irregularities may be raised or depressed and, in either case, permit a concentration of the attachment. These features are generally most pronounced in larger, older males. They are given a variety of descriptive names of conventional significance; most elevations are known as *lines, crests, tubercles, tuberosities,* or *spines;* most depressions are known as *fossae* or *grooves* (sulci).

The inner surface of the shaft bounds a central medullary (marrow) cavity and is rough; the irregularities are low and without apparent significance.

The extremities are occupied by cancellous or *spongy bone,* which forms a three-dimensional lattice of interlacing spicules, plates, and tubes of varying density.

The medullary cavity and the interstitial spaces of the spongy bone are occupied by bone marrow, which occurs in two intergrading forms. Red bone marrow is a richly vascularized, gelatinous tissue with hematopoietic properties; it produces the red and granular white corpuscles of the blood. Although all marrow is of this type in the young animal, most is later infiltrated with fat and converted into waxy yellow marrow whose hematopoietic potential is dormant. It is the marrow in the larger spaces that first

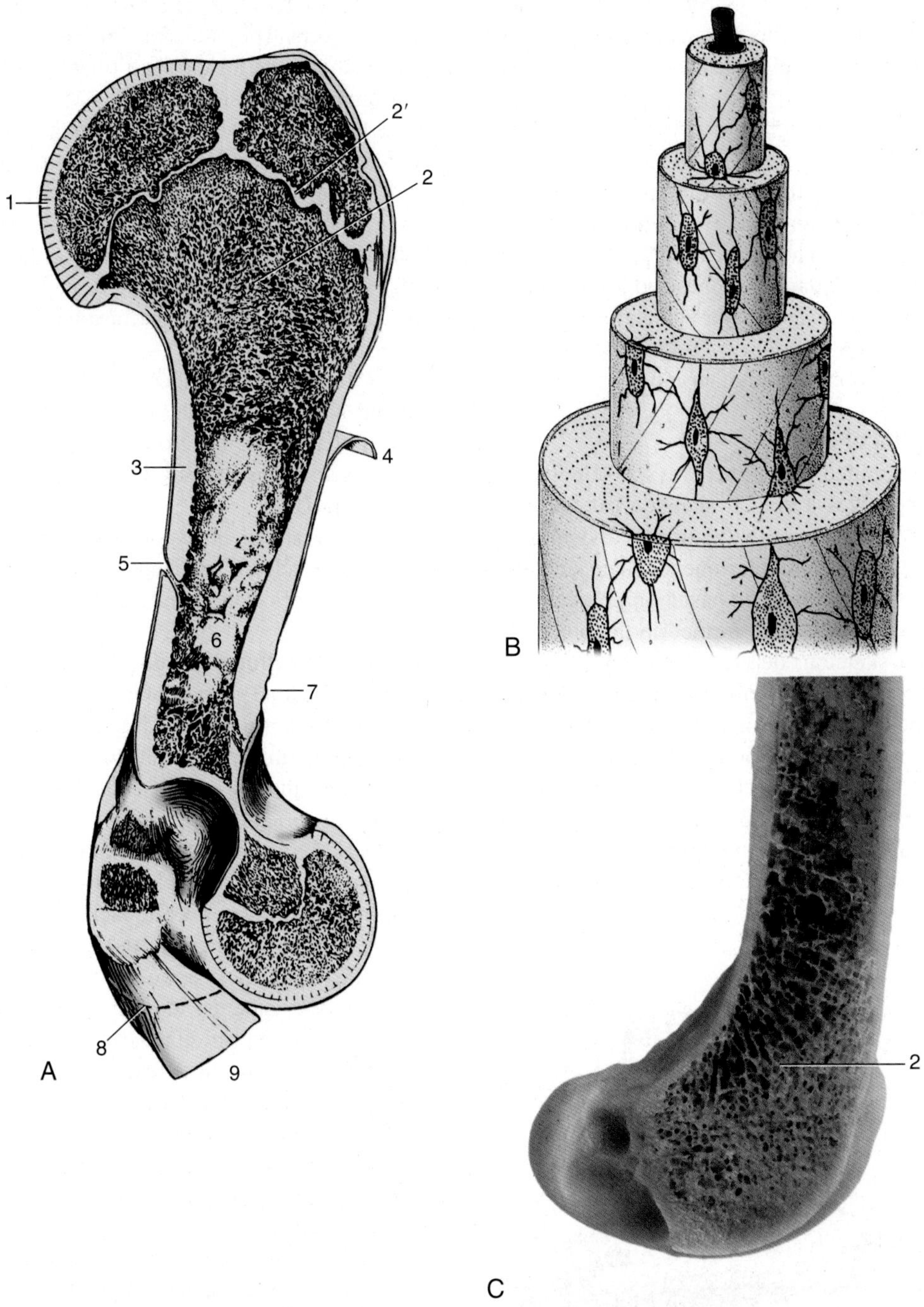

Fig. 1.14 (A) A schematic view of long bone (bovine humerus) sectioned longitudinally. (B) Osteone with central (haversian) canal. (C) Femur of dog sectioned sagitally. *1,* Articular cartilage; *2,* spongy bone; *2′,* epiphysial cartilage; *3,* compact bone; *4,* periosteum, partly reflected; *5,* nutrient foramen; *6,* medullary cavity; *7,* roughened area for attachment of muscle or ligament; *8,* distal extent of medial epicondyle; *9,* tendons of origin of carpal and digital flexors.

becomes inactive, followed by that of the spongy bone of the distal limb bones, until finally active marrow is confined to the proximal ends of the humerus and femur, the bones of the limb girdles, and those of the axial skeleton. The chronology of these events for domestic animals is uncertain.

The articular surfaces of bones are more extensive than the areas in contact in any position of the joint and provide a range of movement. They are smooth and clothed in hyaline *articular cartilage*. The cartilage is not uniform in structure; it is calcified in its deepest layer, which is firmly attached to the underlying cortex, and becomes fibrous

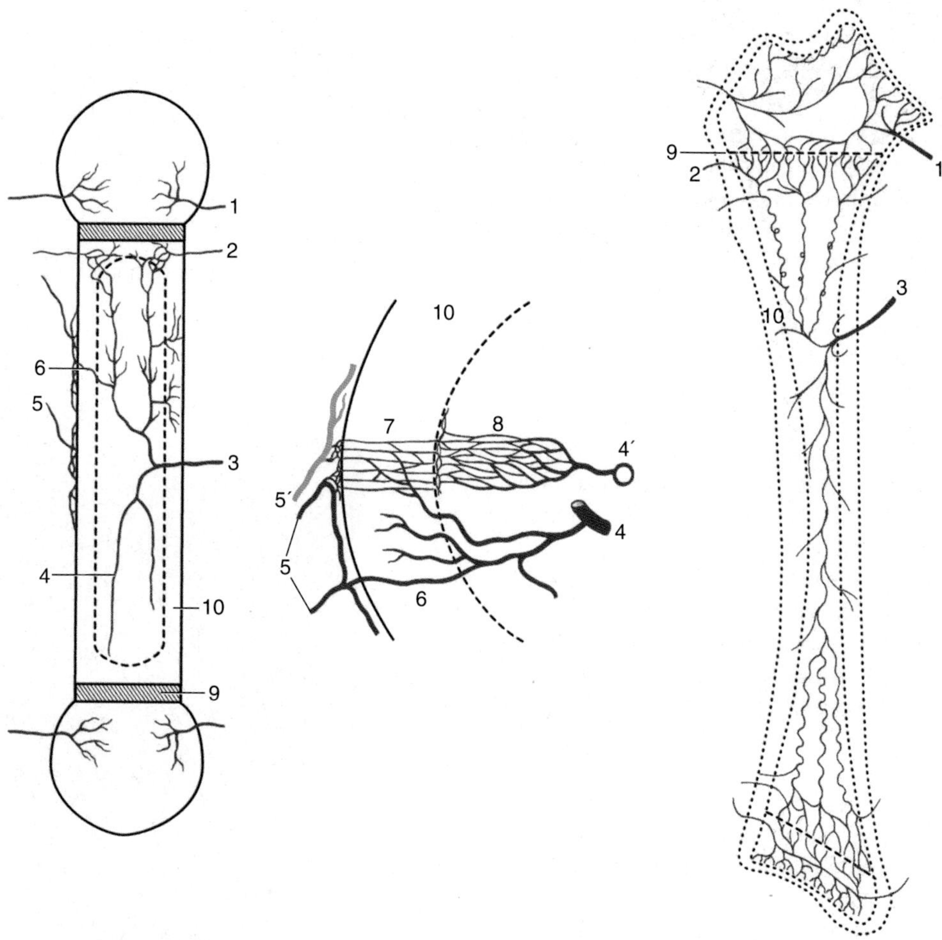

Fig. 1.15 The blood supply of a long bone, schematic. The supply of the cortex is shown (enlarged) in the center. *1,* Epiphysial arteries; *2,* metaphysial arteries; *3,* nutrient artery; *4, 4′,* artery and vein of the bone marrow, respectively; *5,* periosteal arteries; *5′,* periosteal vein; *6,* anastomosis between periosteal and bone marrow arteries; *7,* capillaries of the cortex; *8,* sinusoids in the bone marrow; *9,* growth cartilage; *10,* cortex.

toward the periphery, where it blends with the periosteum and joint capsule.

A tough fibrous membrane, the *periosteum,* ensheathes the remainder of the outer surface, from which it can be readily stripped, except where it is penetrated by tendons and ligaments to anchor in the compacta. Its appearance is rather misleading because the deeper layer is cellular and, even in adults, retains the bone-forming capacity that is exercised during development. This osteogenic function is reactivated in the healing of a fracture.

Bones have a generous *blood supply,* perhaps amounting to 5% to 10% of the cardiac output. Several sets of vessels exist; the so-called nutrient artery, though generally the largest single source, probably contributes less than the others in the aggregate. The nutrient artery penetrates toward the middle of the shaft in a position that is fairly constant for each bone. It is usually directed toward one end of the bone, and the foramen through which it passes may simulate an oblique fracture when depicted in radiographs. The two branches of the artery diverge and further branch within the marrow and pursue very tortuous courses, which may reduce the pressure within the vessels of the delicate marrow (Fig. 1.15). The smaller branches supply the sinusoids of the marrow tissue and also the arterioles and capillaries that permeate a system of tiny central channels (haversian canals) within the osteones of compact bone. A further supply to the cortex arises from the medullary sinusoids. Branches of the nutrient artery that reach the metaphyseal region (the part of the shaft adjacent to the epiphysis) anastomose there with branches of metaphyseal and epiphyseal vessels that enter the bone toward its extremity. The central region of this part of the shaft probably relies mainly on the nutrient artery, whereas the peripheral part relies on metaphyseal arteries. The collateral circulation is generally sufficient to allow a fractured bone to survive deprivation of part of its usual supply. One technique employed in fracture repair (intramedullary pinning) is possibly even more damaging to the vessels than the initial injury, and its success serves to emphasize the value of the anastomoses. There is some debate about additional blood supply to the cortex from small but numerous periosteal arteries.

The main drainage of the marrow is effected by large, thin-walled veins that accompany the major arteries and emerge through the nutrient, epiphyseal, and metaphyseal foramina. The capillaries within cortical tissue drain into venules within the periosteum. The normal cortical circulation is therefore centrifugal—from within outward. No lymphatic vessels are present within bone, although infections of bone may spread to the lymphatics that drain neighboring tissues.

One important difference is exhibited by the circulation in young growing bones. In them, the circulation within the epiphyses forms separate and independent compartments, because (with few exceptions) arteries do not penetrate the growth (epiphyseal) cartilage.

Nerves accompany the larger vessels, and their branches are to be found within the central canals of the osteones. Some (vasomotor) fibers pass to the vessels, some are sensory to the bone tissues (especially the periosteum), and the destination of others remains unclear. It is no longer believed that nerves exert a trophic influence on bone.

Biomechanical Aspects

It has long been the convention to explain the tubular construction of long bones by drawing the comparison with a loaded beam of some stiff, homogeneous material supported at both ends (Fig. 1.16). In this construction the tensile forces that tend to disrupt the material are concentrated toward the lower surface while the compressive forces that tend to crush and compact the material are concentrated toward the upper surface. These forces tend to neutralize each other along, and close to, the axis, and the material here is more or less redundant. It can be dispensed with or replaced by some weaker but lighter material, as in a long bone. The analogy is not exact—for a start, bone is a composite material—but it is useful as a first approach. The diagram in Fig. 1.16 shows that the lines of principal compressive and tensile stress intersect in orthogonal fashion toward the extremities of the model; the spongy architecture of a bone (Fig. 1.17) closely mimics the theoretical pattern.

Compact bone is a plastic, composite material of considerable strength, capable of sustaining and recovering from considerable deformation. When it is bent, the lamellae and osteones of which compact bone is constructed first shear past each other; if the bone is bent too far, a crack appears at right angles to the line of shear and then quickly spreads to create a brittle fracture. Most fractures are caused by excessive bending, which stresses both aspects of the bone approximately equally. The fact that the side under tensile stress generally fails first indicates that compact bone is better able to resist compression. However, spongy bone is commonly crushed and impacted by compression.

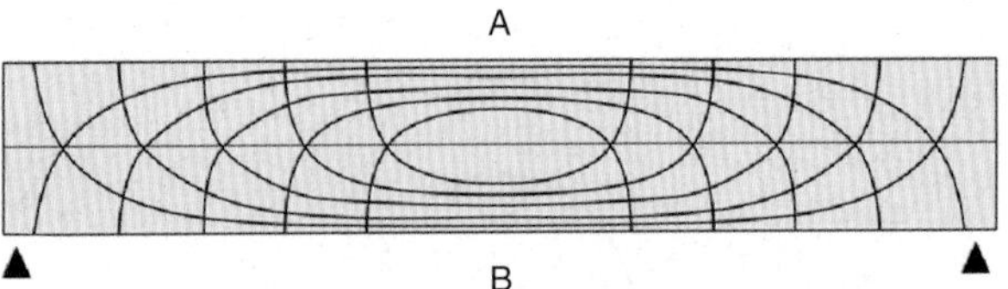

Fig. 1.16 Pattern of compressive (A) and tensile (B) stress lines in a beam supported at both ends. The greatest stresses (indicated by closeness of lines) occur in the middle of the beam toward the surfaces.

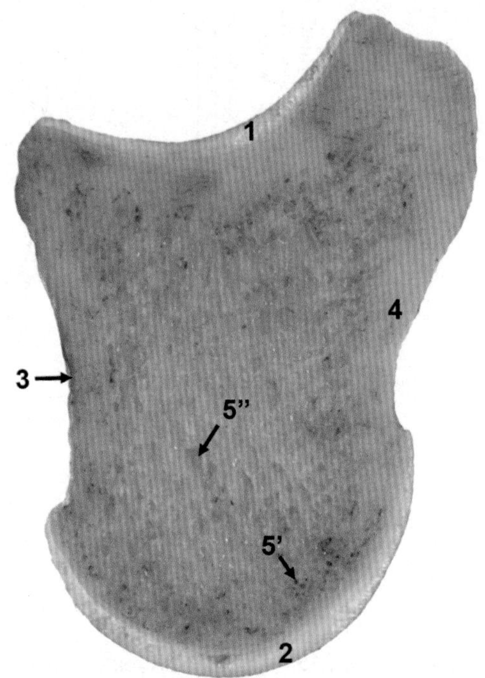

Fig. 1.17 Median section of the unfixed fresh specimen of the second phalanx of equine foot showing articular cartilage at the proximal extremity *(1)* and distal extremity *(2)*, thin layer of periosteum *(3)*. Notice the change in thickness of the articular cartilages. Cortical compact bone *(4)* forms the periphery of the bone, and central spongy bone *(5)* is filled with red *(5′)* and yellow *(5″)* bone marrow.

Some Specialized Varieties of Bones

Bones are often found within tendons (rarely within ligaments), where they change direction over prominences that would expose them to excessive pressure and friction. These bones, known as *sesamoid bones,* form regular synovial joints with the major bones with which they are in contact. In addition to preventing tendon wear, a sesamoid bone displaces the tendon farther from the axis of the adjacent joint and increases the leverage exerted by the muscle. The best known example is the patella (kneecap) in the principal extender of the stifle joint (see Figs. 2.63 and 17.3). In the dog, smaller sesamoids also develop in muscles behind the stifle, in the tendons passing behind the metacarpophalangeal joints (at the bases of the digits), and in the extensor tendons within the digits (see Fig. 1.9). These and other lesser sesamoids may be wrongly identified as chip fractures in radiographs. In large animals, one or more additional sesamoids form dorsal to the deep flexor tendon shortly before its insertion on the distal phalanx (or phalanges). In the dog the reaction is limited to the development of a nubbin of cartilage in each branch of the tendon.

The major sesamoids develop in the embryo before movement is possible, and their origin must therefore be genetically determined. They reform after extirpation only if movement is allowed to indicate their development in reaction to an appropriate stimulus in the lifetime of the animal.

Splanchnic bones develop in soft organs, remote from the rest of the skeleton. The most familiar, indeed the only significant, examples in veterinary anatomy are the os penis (and the female equivalent, os clitoridis) of the dog and cat and the ossa cordis found in the heart, especially in the hearts of ruminants.

Certain bones contain air spaces. In mammals, these *pneumatic bones* are confined to the skull and contain the paranasal sinuses, which communicate with the nasal cavities. The sinuses develop principally after birth, when outgrowths of the nasal mucosa invade certain skull bones and replace the *diploë,* the spongy bone between the outer and inner layers ("tables") of compacta. The separation of the tables can be very considerable and can lead to a remarkable postnatal remodeling of the skull, best exhibited by cattle and pigs. The postcranial skeleton of birds develops an extensive system of air-filled cavities in communication with the respiratory organs.

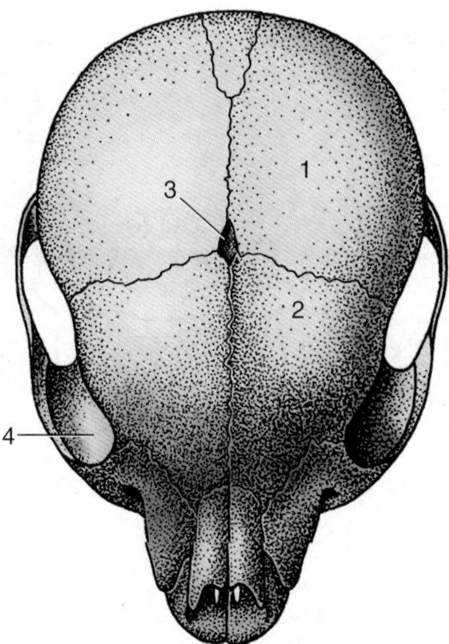

Fig. 1.18 Sutures between the bones of a puppy's skull. *1,* Parietal bone; *2,* frontal bone; *3,* fontanelle (fonticulus); *4,* orbit.

Joints

Bones form joints or articulations, of which some unite the bones firmly and others allow free movement. The many variations in joint shapes and structures do not permit an easy system of classification. Periodic revisions of terminology have seen new categories defined and former categories merged or renamed so that some confusion now exists and many superfluous terms circulate. The current official system recognizes three major categories—namely, the fibrous joint, in which the bones are united by dense connective tissues; the cartilaginous joint, in which the bones are united by cartilage; and the synovial joint, in which a fluid-filled cavity intervenes between the bones. It is obvious that most joints of the first and second categories must be relatively immovable or even rigid; these classes were formerly together known as *synarthroses*. In contrast, most joints of the third category are freely movable; they were formerly termed *diarthroses*. Both of these terms are obsolete.

Fibrous Joints

Most fibrous joints occur in the skull and are known as *sutures* (Fig. 1.18). The narrow strips of fibrous tissue that outline and unite the margins of the bones represent the surviving part of the originally continuous membrane in which the separate ossification centers appeared. Sutures play an important role in the young animal, allowing for the growth of the skull through the extension of individual bones at their margins while proliferation of the membrane continues. Sutures are gradually eliminated when ossification extends across the membrane after it has ceased to grow. This is a slow and uneven process that is not complete even in the aged. The gradual modification of the suture pattern is used in anthropology and forensic medicine as a not very reliable guide to the age of the individual. In comparison with sutures of the adult skull, the wider sutures of the fetal skull allow some useful passive deformation during birth in some species, including primates.

The *syndesmoses* are fibrous joints in which two bones are joined by connective tissue ligaments. In some syndesmoses, relatively broad areas of bone are united by short ligaments, allowing very restricted movement; examples are the joints between the major and minor bones of the horse's metacarpus. In others the ligaments are longer and their attachments narrower so that more appreciable movement is possible; an example is the joint between the shafts of the radius and ulna in the forearm of the dog.

The attachment of a tooth to the bone of its socket, or *gomphosis,* may be included among the fibrous joints.

Cartilaginous Joints

Most cartilaginous joints are known as *synchondroses*. They include the joints between the epiphyses and diaphyses of juvenile long bones and the corresponding joints of the base of the skull. These temporary joints disappear with ossification of the cartilage. The few permanent synchondroses include the joint between the skull and hyoid apparatus (p. 57), which allows appreciable movement in some species.

In the more complicated *symphysis* the articulating bones are divided by a succession of tissues; usually cartilage covers the bones, with fibrocartilage or fibrous tissue

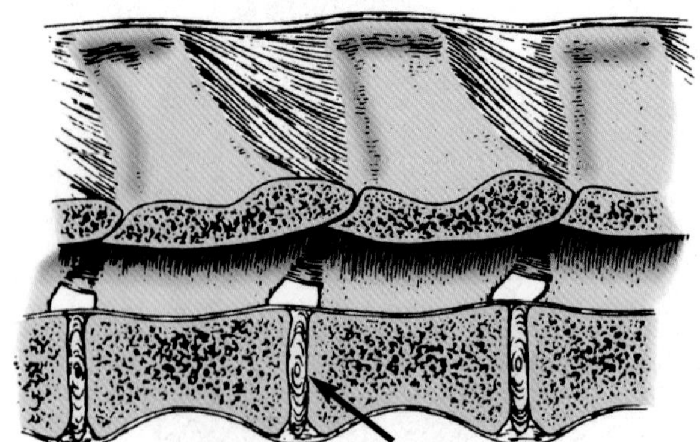

Fig. 1.19 Intervertebral disk *(arrow)* joining bodies of adjacent vertebrae.

in the middle. The category includes the joints between the symmetrical halves of the mandible (in species such as the dog, cat, and ruminants, in which fusion is not complete) and of the pelvic girdle and the joints between the bodies of successive vertebrae (Fig. 1.19). Each of these joints presents its own, sometimes specifically variable, features that are best considered later.

Synovial Joints

Structure. In synovial joints the articulating bones are separated by a fluid-filled space, the joint cavity (Fig. 1.20). The boundaries of the space are completed by a sleeve of delicate connective tissue, the synovial membrane. The membrane is attached around the periphery of the articular surfaces. However, in most synovial joints the synovial membrane is strengthened externally by a fibrous capsule, and additional fibrous bands (ligaments) are strategically placed to join the bones and to restrict movement to the required directions and extents. Synovial joint injuries are highly prevalent in domestic animals.

The *articular* surface is covered with articular cartilage that is generally of the hyaline variety, although fibrocartilage or even dense fibrous tissue is found in a few locations. The thickness of the cartilage ranges from about a millimeter in the joints of the dog to several millimeters in the larger joints of horses and cattle. It accentuates the curvature of the underlying bone, being thickest in the center of convex surfaces and about the periphery of concave ones. The cartilage is a pliant material that is translucent and glassy in appearance, and although generally white with a blue or pink tinge in young animals, it becomes yellowish and less elastic with age. The surface is smooth to the touch and to the naked eye but quite irregular when seen at low magnification.

The cartilage has a complex structure in which fine fibers within its matrix pass from the underlying bone to the surface, where they bend to lie close together. Because splitting of the cartilage, common in joint disease, tends to follow the fiber course, superficial lesions lead to tangential flaking, whereas lesions that extend more deeply create more or less vertical cracks.

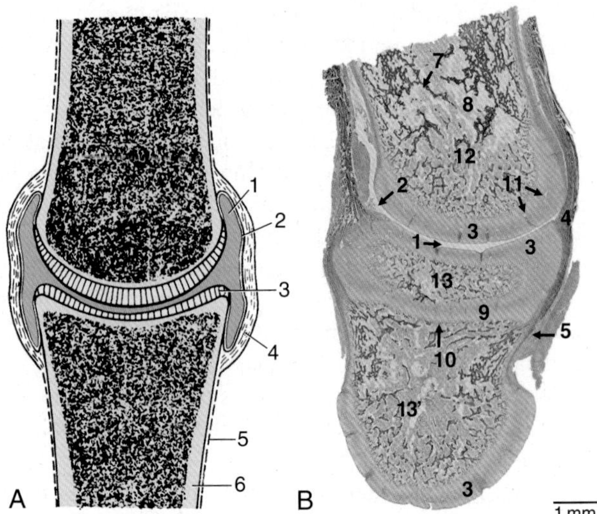

Fig. 1.20 (A) A synovial joint in section. (B) Sagittal section through the decalcified digit of a newborn lamb stained with Masson's trichrome. *1,* Joint cavity; *2,* synovial membrane; *3,* articular hyaline cartilage; *4,* fibrous layer of joint capsule; *4′,* joint capsule; *5,* periosteum; *6,* compact bone; *7,* trabeculae; *8,* hemopoietic tissue; *9,* shaft; *10,* growth plate; *11,* vascular channels in hyalline cartilage; *12,* proximal phalanx; *13,* middle phalanx.

Articular cartilage is insensitive and avascular. The insensitivity explains why joint lesions may progress far before the patient becomes aware of their existence. The oxygen and nutritive requirements are met by diffusion from three sources: fluid within the joint cavity, vessels in the tissues at the periphery of the cartilage, and vessels in the subjacent marrow spaces. Diffusion is assisted by the porosity of the cartilage matrix, which soaks up and releases fluid as the cartilage is alternately unloaded and compressed during movements of the joint.

Certain large articular cartilages are interrupted by depressed areas that may indent the periphery or appear as islands. These naked areas (synovial fossae) are clothed by a thin connective tissue resting on the underlying bone. Their significance is disputed but not the constancy of their occurrence nor their frequent coincidence in opposing bones in certain positions of the joint.*

The *synovial membrane,* which completes the lining of the joint, is a glistening pink connective tissue sheet. It may

*Among domestic mammals, horses and cattle have *synovial fossae.* Although not quite constant, synovial fossae appear in the majority of animals and are always bilateral in the limbs. They appear as early as 10 days after birth in foals. In the horse, opposing synovial fossae are found at the shoulder, elbow, carpal, tarsocrural, and talocalcaneal joints. A single fossa is present in the fetlock joints (of both forelimbs and hindlimbs), on the acetabulum, and on the atlantal surface of the atlanto- axial joint. In cattle, more or less distinct synovial fossae may be present in all limb joints, other than the shoulder and hip. They also may be present at the atlantooccipital and atlanto- axial joints be left entirely unsupported, may rest directly on a tough outer fibrous capsule, or may be separated from it by the interposition of pads of fat; all three arrangements may occur in different regions of the same joint. The membrane may pouch where it is unsupported, and these diverticula may extend quite far, a point of potential significance because it explains how joints may be entered by apparently remote wounds. The inner surface of the membrane carries many projections of various sizes and degrees of permanency that greatly increase its surface area (see Fig. 1.20B). Unlike mucous membranes, the synovial membrane has no continuous covering of cells. The more cellular parts, limited to relatively protected situations, are responsible for the production of the lubricant component (aminoglycans) of the synovial fluid. The other components are derived from the blood plasma. The membrane is both vascular and sensitive.

Synovia, the fluid within the cavity, obtains its name from its resemblance to egg white. It is a viscous, fluid whose color ranges from pale straw to medium brown. It is usually said to be present in very small amounts but is, in fact, quite copious in the larger joints; as much as 20 to 40 mL can sometimes be aspirated from limb joints of horses and cattle. The quantity is greatest in animals permitted free exercise.

Synovia has both lubricant and nutritive functions. The ways in which it acts as a lubricant are disputed, but it is certainly very efficient, the friction being such that virtually no wear occurs in healthy joints. The fluid helps nourish the articular cartilage, any intraarticular structures, and, possibly, the surface layer of the synovial membrane itself.

An outer *fibrous layer* usually completes the capsule. It attaches around the margins of the articular surfaces and contains local thickenings, which are named individually as *ligaments* when well developed and discrete. Some, of which the cruciate ligaments of the stifle are good examples, appear to run within the joint cavity from bone to bone. Such ligaments are sometimes designated *intracapsular* to distinguish them from the majority in peripheral and clearly extracapsular positions; however, they are actually excluded from the cavity by a covering of synovial membrane (Fig. 1.21). The fibrous layer and ligaments are supplied with proprioceptive nerve endings that register the position and the rate of change in position of the joint; other receptors register pain.

A few joints possess *disks* or *menisci* that are truly intracapsular (Fig. 1.22). A disk, such as occurs in the temporomandibular joint formed between the mandible and the skull, fuses with the synovial membrane around its periphery and so divides the cavity into upper and lower compartments. Paired menisci, which are semilunar as the name suggests, are found within the stifle joint. They are attached only around their convex borders and therefore divide the cavity incompletely. Both of these structures are composed of hyaline cartilage, fibrocartilage, and fibrous tissue in proportions that vary with the part, the species, and the age. Menisci and disks provide congruence of incompatible articulating surfaces, but this feature

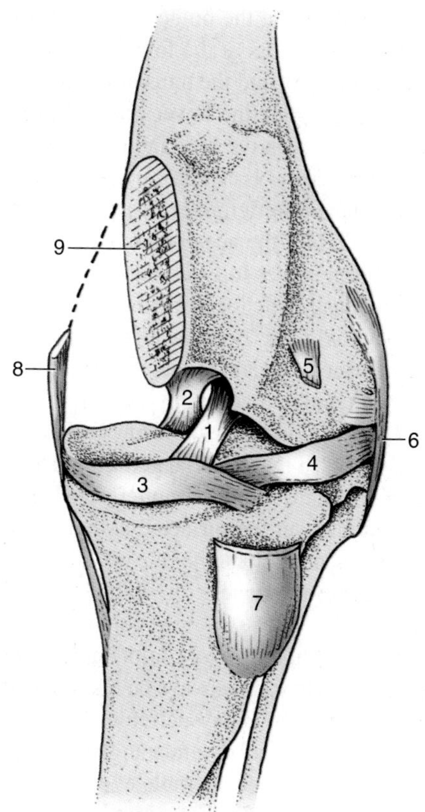

Fig. 1.21 Cranial view of left stifle joint of the dog, resected to show intracapsular *(1, 2)* and extracapsular *(6, 8)* ligaments. *1,* Cranial cruciate ligament; *2,* caudal cruciate ligament; *3,* medial meniscus; *4,* lateral meniscus; *5,* tendon of origin of long digital extensor; *6,* lateral collateral ligament; *7,* patellar ligament; *8,* medial collateral ligament; *9,* medial condyle, partly removed.

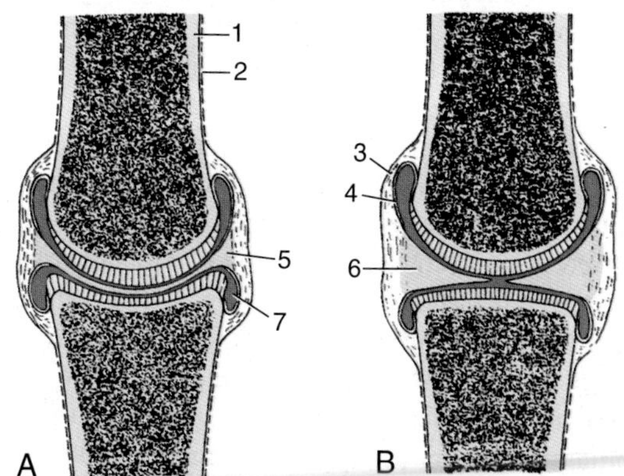

Fig. 1.22 (A) Synovial joint with articular disk. (B) Synovial joint with meniscus. *1,* Compact bone; *2,* periosteum; *3,* fibrous layer of joint capsule; *4,* synovial membrane; *5,* articular disk; *6,* meniscus; *7,* joint cavity.

can hardly explain their presence because congruence is achieved at other joints more simply. The most probable alternative explanation is that they are a means of resolving complicated movements into simpler components that are assigned to different levels of the articulation. Thus, in the temporomandibular joint the hinge movement involved in opening the mouth occurs at the lower level (between the disk and the mandible), and the translatory movements that protrude, retract, or slide the lower jaw sideways occur at the upper level (between the disk and the skull).

An *articular labrum* is a fibrocartilaginous lip or rim placed around the circumference of certain concave articular surfaces, including the acetabulum (the deep socket at the hip). A labrum serves to extend and deepen the articular surface, increasing the load-bearing area and helping to spread the synovial fluid. Because a labrum is deformable, it allows the surface to adapt to disparities in the curvature of the bone with which it comes in contact.

Synovial pads or cushions are formed where fat masses are included between the synovial and fibrous layers of the joint capsule. They are sometimes interpreted as swabs that spread the synovia over the surface, but their main purpose is to allow the synovial membrane to accommodate its shape to the part of the bone with which it is momentarily in contact.

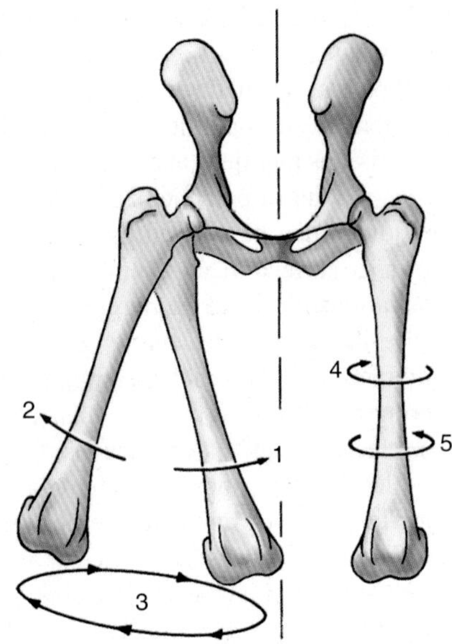

Fig. 1.23 Limb movements illustrated by the femurs of the dog, cranial view. *1,* Adduction; *2,* abduction; *3,* circumduction; *4,* inward rotation; *5,* outward rotation.

Movements. Although many joint movements appear to be complicated, they can always be resolved into simple components. Moreover, many activities are the result of coordinated movement at several neighboring joints; the sum of changes can be considerable even when the movement at each individual joint is modest.

The simplest type of movement is *translation*. In its pure form, translation consists of one flat surface sliding over another while the bodies to which the surfaces belong maintain their original orientation. True translatory movements probably never occur because the prerequisites are perfectly flat surfaces and the absence of spin. Nonetheless, a category of joint (plane joint) is defined in which movement is supposed to be of this kind. These joints have small articular surfaces that appear flat at first scrutiny; in reality, articular surfaces are always curved.

All other movements involve angular change. In some, the moving bone turns (spins) about an axis perpendicular to its articular surface, a movement called *rotation*. Rotation can always be reversed, so its direction must always be specified. According to convention, an internal rotation of a limb carries the cranial surface medially (Fig. 1.23/*4*); an external rotation carries this surface laterally (see Fig. 1.23/*5*).

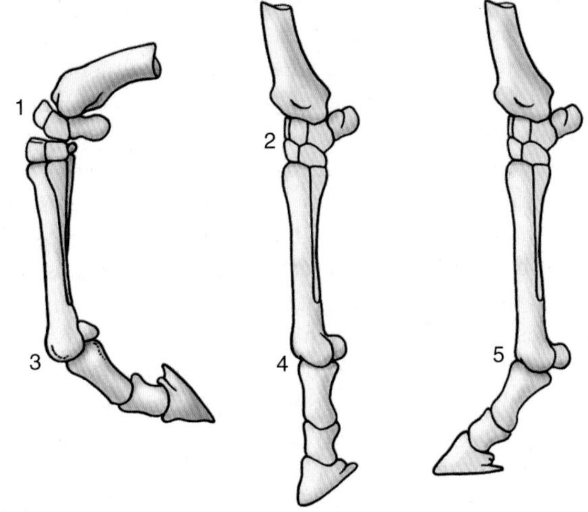

Fig. 1.24 Flexion, extension, and overextension illustrated by the distal part of the horse's forelimb. *1,* Flexed carpal joint; *2,* extended carpal joint; *3,* flexed fetlock joint; *4,* extended fetlock joint; *5,* overextended fetlock joint.

Other movements involve the moving bone turning about an axis parallel to its articular surface in a pendular or rolling movement (Fig. 1.24/*3*); this is a slide between curved surfaces and may be described as a swing. Most swings are accompanied by some rotation, although it often goes undetected.

Pendular movements in sagittal planes predominate in the joints of the limbs and are known as flexion and extension. *Flexion* reduces the angle between the two segments of the limb. The opposite movement, *extension,* opens the angle and brings the two segments more closely into alignment (see Fig. 1.24). However, the movement at some joints ranges from one flexed position through full extension (180 degrees) to a second flexed position at the other limit. The fetlock joint of the horse is a good example of a joint with such a wide range of movement. In such cases the two terminal positions may be distinguished as overextension (or dorsal flexion), the posture of the animal standing at rest, and (palmar) flexion, the posture when the foot is passively raised. Fig. 1.24 may make this rather confusing distinction plain.

Adduction and abduction are pendular movements in transverse planes (see Fig. 1.23/*1* and *2*). *Adduction* carries the moving part toward the median plane, and *abduction* carries it away from this plane. When applied to the digits, adduction and abduction describe movement with reference to the axis of the limb and indicate the convergence and the spread of the digits, respectively.

The combination of flexion and extension and adduction and abduction allows the extremity of the limb to describe a circle or ellipse, a movement known as *circumduction.*

Several limitations are placed on the movements of all joints. The shape of the articular surfaces is obviously relevant. A degree of incongruence is required to maintain a wedge of the lubricant synovia between the surfaces. This wedge is reduced when the radius of curvature of the convex surface increases toward its margin to approximate to the radius of curvature of the opposing concave surface. The surfaces thus become congruent in the closely packed terminal position, and further movement is checked by their being squeezed together.

Tension in extracapsular ligaments can certainly arrest movement, although it is uncertain whether this method of braking is required in normal circumstances. Some ligaments appear to be moderately taut throughout the normal range of movement, whereas others are generally slack and become taut only when movement threatens to go beyond the normal limit.

In some situations, contact between extra-articular structures may be of importance; the olecranon obviously prevents forceful overextension of the elbow, and apposition of the caudal muscles of the thigh and calf prevents overflexion of the human knee. Tension in muscles and other soft structures in the neighborhood of a joint may first decelerate and then arrest movement; inability of the muscles of the caudal aspect of the human thigh to stretch beyond a certain limit—passive insufficiency—prohibits many people from touching their toes. The contraction of muscles that oppose a given movement may be the most important factor; its significance is discussed in the following section.

Classification Synovial joints may be classified according to numerical and geometrical criteria. The numerical system distinguishes *simple* joints, with one pair of articular surfaces, and *composite* joints, in which more than two opposing surfaces are involved and movement occurs at more than one level within a shared capsule. The shoulder joint illustrates the first and the carpal joint the second variety.

There are seven categories in the current version of the geometrical system. One, the *plane joint* (Fig. 1.25A), has already been mentioned.

The *hinge joint* (ginglymus; Fig. 1.25B) has one articular surface shaped like a segment of a cylinder and the other excavated to receive it. Pendular movement is possible in one plane only. The other movements are prohibited by stout collateral (one to each side) ligaments and possibly by the development of matching ridges and grooves on the articular surfaces. The elbow joint between the humerus and bones of the forearm is an example.

The *pivot joint* (articulatio trochoidea; Fig. 1.25C) comprises a peg fitted within a ring. Movement takes place about the long axis of the peg. In some joints (e.g., the proximal radioulnar joint) the peg rotates within the fixed ring; in others (e.g., the atlantoaxial joint between the first two vertebrae) the ring rotates about the fixed peg.

The *condylar joint* (Fig. 1.25D) is formed by two knuckle-shaped condyles that engage with corresponding concave surfaces. The two complexes may be close together, as in the femorotibial joint, or widely separate and provided with independent joint capsules, as are the twin articulations of the mandible. In each case the whole arrangement is regarded as constituting a single condylar joint. Movement is primarily uniaxial, about a transverse axis common to the two condyles; certain amounts of rotation and slide are also permitted.

The *ellipsoidal joint* (Fig. 1.25E) consists of an ovoid convex surface that fits into a corresponding concavity. Movements occur principally in two planes at right angles to each other (flexion-extension; adduction-abduction), but a small amount of rotation may be possible. The radiocarpal joint of the dog is ellipsoidal.

The *saddle joint* (articulatio sellaris; Fig. 1.25F) combines two surfaces, each maximally convex in one direction and maximally concave in a second direction at right angles to the first. These are also biaxial joints, allowing flexion-extension and adduction-abduction but with a certain amount of rotation permitted or imposed by the geometry of the surfaces. An example is the distal interphalangeal joint of the dog.

The ball-and-socket or *spheroidal joint* (Fig. 1.25G) consists of a portion of a sphere received within a corresponding cup. This multiaxial joint enjoys the greatest versatility of movement. The hip joint is the best example; the human shoulder joint also conforms closely to the pattern, but the shoulder of domestic species largely restricts its movement to flexion and extension.

It must be emphasized that anatomic joints correspond very imperfectly to the theoretical models. Sometimes, the departure from the ideal can be sufficiently large to make it a matter of controversy as to which category best accommodates a particular articulation.

Muscles

Muscular contractions underlie most of the body movements that are grossly visible. Muscle is also used to prevent movement, stabilizing joints to prevent their collapse under a load and maintaining continence of bladder and bowel. A subsidiary function of the skeletal muscles is to generate heat by *shivering,* involuntary tremors initiated by exposure to cold.

There are three varieties of muscle tissue, but two, the specialized (cardiac) muscle that forms the bulk of the

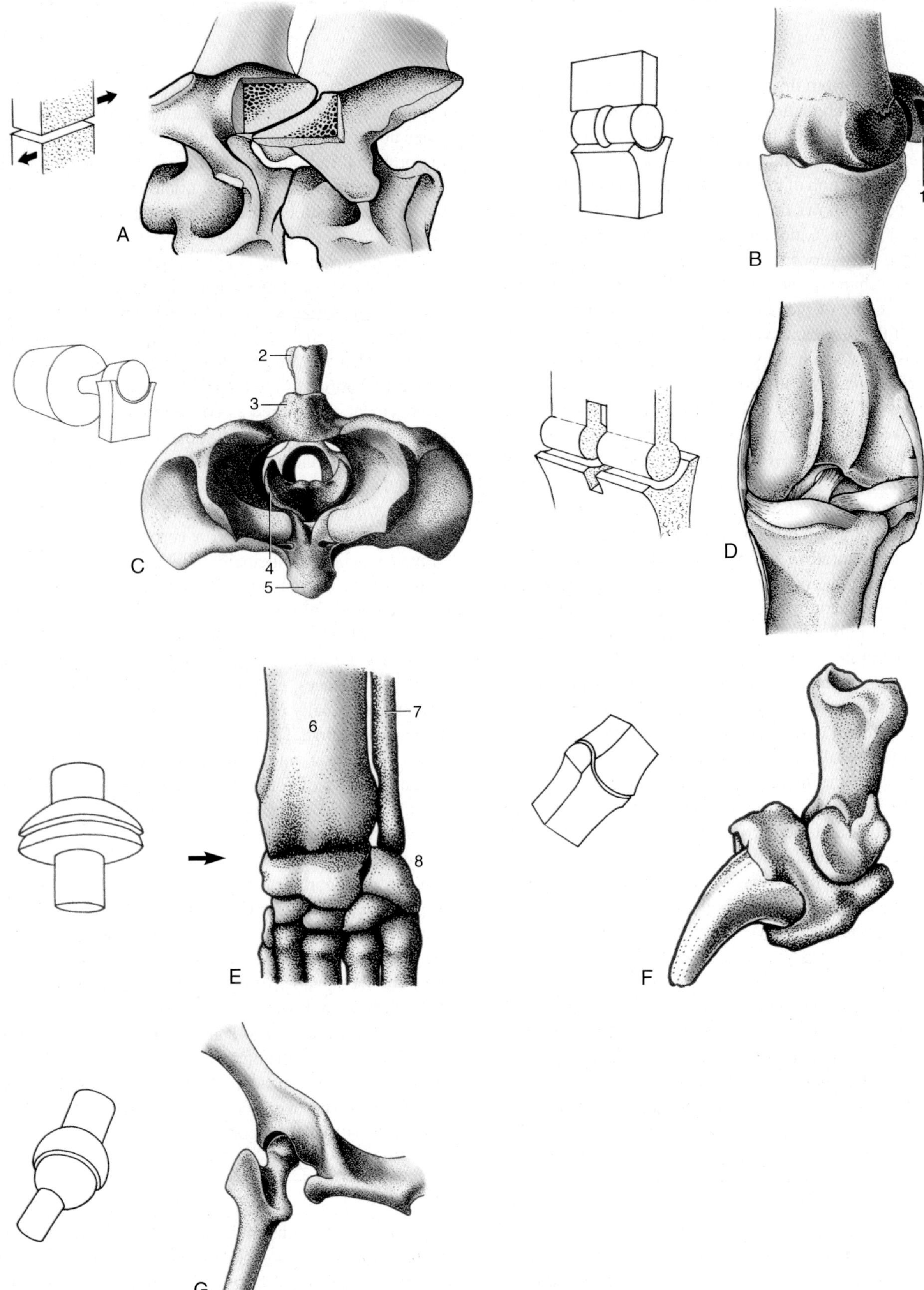

Fig. 1.25 The seven types of synovial joints, with examples. (A) Plane joint: articular processes of equine cervical vertebrae. (B) Hinge joint: equine fetlock (metacarpophalangeal) joint. (C) Pivot joint: bovine atlantoaxial joint (cranial view). (D) Condylar joint: canine femorotibial joint (stifle). (E) Ellipsoidal joint: canine carpus. (F) Saddle joint: canine distal interphalangeal joint. (G) Spheroidal joint: canine hip joint (caudodorsal view). *1,* Proximal sesamoid bone; *2,* spine of axis; *3,* dorsal arch of atlas; *4,* dens of axis; *5,* ventral arch of atlas; *6,* radius; *7,* ulna; *8,* proximal row of carpal bones.

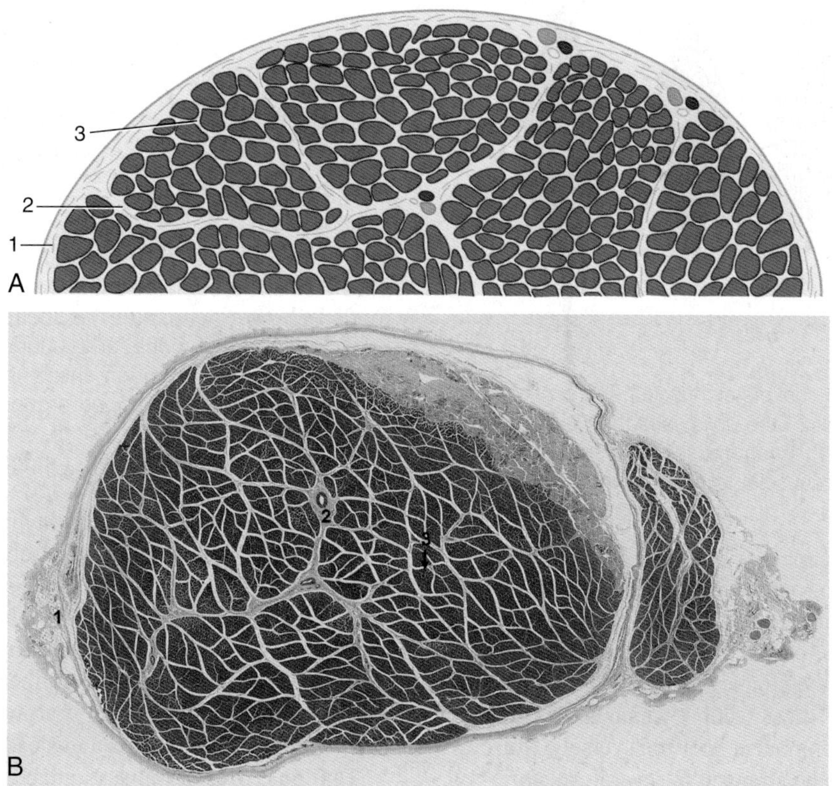

Fig. 1.26 (A) Schematic transection of a skeletal muscle; the fibrous tissue has been emphasized. (B) Cross-section of a skeletal muscle stained with Masson's trichrome stain that shows cellular elements as red and connective tissue as blue. *1,* Epimysium; *2,* perimysium; *3,* endomysium (lightly stained parts in the fascicle).

heart and the smooth (visceral) muscle of the blood vessels and viscera (internal organs), are not of present concern. The third variety is generally known as *skeletal muscle* because the muscles are mostly attached to the bones and induce their movement. Skeletal muscle is also known as *striated, somatic,* or *voluntary muscle,* but these terms are less acceptable for one reason or another.

The Organization of Skeletal Muscles

Skeletal muscle is butcher's meat and accounts for about half the weight of an animal carcass (the proportion varies with species, breed, age, sex, and method of husbandry). Each muscle is composed of many cells held together by connective tissue. In comparison with the common run of cell, these muscle cells are giants, varying from about 10 to 100 μm in diameter and being about 5 or 10 cm in length (some are probably much longer). They are visible to the naked eye when teased apart and are also called *muscle fibers* because of their size and shape. The whole muscle is covered by a dense connective tissue sheet, the *epimysium* (Fig. 1.26); below this, a looser layer, the *perimysium,* covers the small bundles (fasciculi) into which the fibers are grouped. Finally, each fiber is provided with its own delicate covering, the *endomysium.* These connective tissue components merge at each end of the muscle "belly" and continue as the tendons by which the muscle makes its attachment. The amount and quality of the connective tissue partly explain variations in the appearance and in the cooking and table qualities of different cuts of meat (another important factor is the amount of shortening that is allowed by hanging during postmortem rigor).

Variations in Muscle Architecture. There is great variety in the way in which the muscle fibers are arranged within the muscle belly, which can be explained by reference to two principles. The shortening that a muscle may demonstrate on contraction (about 50%) is a function of the length of the component fibers. The power that it may develop is a function of the aggregate of their cross-sectional areas. The greatest displacement, necessarily not the force, is therefore produced by the so-called strap muscle (Fig. 1.27), in which the fibers run parallel to the long axis and throughout the length of the muscle, which is completed by very short tendons of attachment.

Muscles in which the fibers join the tendons at an angle tend to be strong in relation to their bulk because more fibers and a greater total cross section can be accommodated. Although muscles of this sort are powerful, they waste a proportion of their strength and their potential

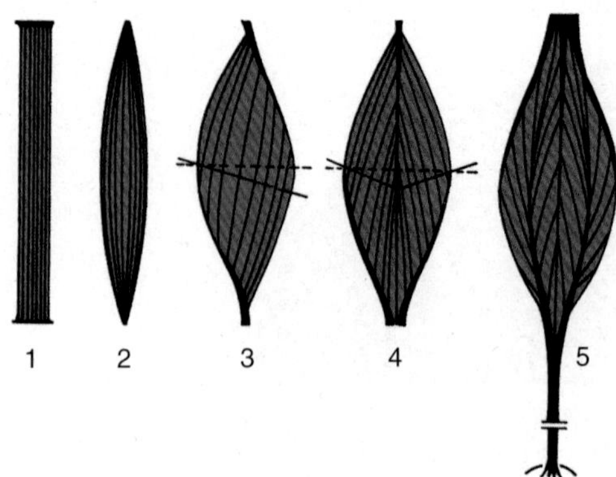

Fig. 1.27 Architecture of skeletal muscles. The *broken lines* represent the "anatomic," the *solid lines* the "physiologic" transverse sections. *1,* Strap muscle; *2,* spindle-shaped muscle; *3,* pennate muscle; *4,* bipennate muscle; *5,* multipennate muscle.

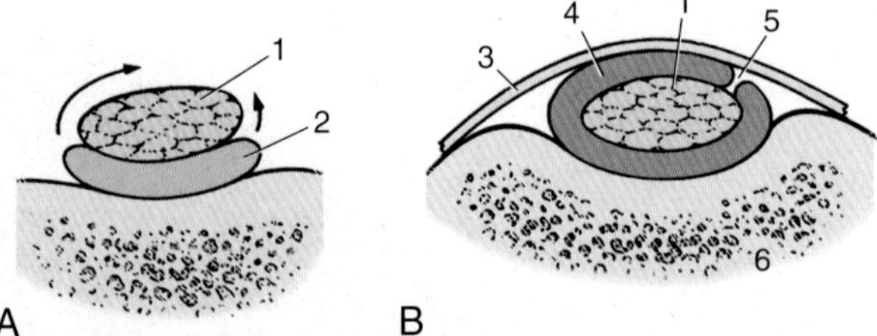

Fig. 1.28 Sections of a synovial bursa (A) and a tendon sheath (B). The bursa permits frictionless movement of a tendon *(1)* over bone, and the sheath permits movement of a tendon over bone and under a retinaculum. The *arrows* show that a tendon sheath may be regarded as a large bursa that has wrapped around a tendon. *2,* Bursa; *3,* retinaculum; *4,* tendon sheath; *5,* mesotendon, through which blood vessels reach the tendon; *6,* bone.

for displacement; only part, corresponding to the cosine of the angle of fiber insertion, is applied along the line of pull. In calculating the power that such muscles develop, one needs to replace the simple "anatomic" cross section with the "physiologic" cross section, which is the complex plane that cuts each component fiber transversely. Muscles with angled fibers can be arranged in several categories of increasing complexity of construction: pennate, bipennate, circumpennate, and multipennate (see Fig. 1.27).

Many limb muscles have a pennate form and, unlike the strap muscles, have long, cordlike tendons that permit the heavy bellies to be placed close to the trunk; because only the light tendons extend to the digits to operate the joints, less energy is required to swing the limb to and fro. Certain muscles of the body wall form thin flat layers that are continued by broad tendon sheets (distinguished as aponeuroses), an arrangement clearly adapted to supporting the abdominal organs. Other muscles arise by two, three, or four separate heads that join in a common tendon; these arrangements are indicated by inclusion of the descriptive term *biceps* (two-headed), *triceps,* or *quadriceps,* respectively, in the muscles' names.

In another less common variety, two or more fleshy units are separated by intermediate tendon-forming digastric (two-bellied) or polygastric units. Still other muscles are arranged in rings that surround natural orifices, such as the mouth or anus, and act as sphincters to constrict or close the opening. In all these examples the construction of the muscle is clearly adapted to its functions.

Paired muscles lying against, or originating from, the midline are separated by a connective tissue strip known as a *raphe*.

The color of muscles is a reflection of the amount of myoglobin in their fibers. The difference, well exemplified by the pale breast and dark leg muscles of the chicken, is generally regarded as reflecting a pale muscle's adaptation for rapid contraction over a short period and a darker muscle's adaptation for slower but sustained activity. Most muscles are actually composed of two fiber types in varying proportions: fast twitch fibers that rely on glycolytic metabolism predominate in dark (red) muscles, and slow twitch fibers that obtain their energy from aerobic metabolism in pale (white) muscles. There are many other structural and physiologic differences between fibers, and the suggestion that there are only these two, sharply distinguished varieties, although convenient, is a misleading simplification.

Tendons. Muscles always attach by means of connective tissue tendons. Sometimes the tendons may be so short as to create the illusion that a muscle directly attaches to the bone. Tendons consist almost entirely of collagen bundles in regular arrangement, and they possess great tensile strength. Indeed, excessive tension is more likely to rupture the muscle belly or to detach a fragment of bone at the insertion than to disrupt the tendon itself. The elastic nature of tendons allows them to absorb and store energy to generate recoil that aids in locomotion. Also, a good fraction of the metabolic work performed by many muscles is devoted to stretching tendons so that the stored energy can later be released.

Although they are tough, tendons may be damaged by excessive pressure or friction, particularly when they change direction over bony prominences or are shifted over hard tissues. One form of the protection that they develop in such places, local chondrification or ossification (sesamoid bones), has been mentioned. An alternative is provided by the development of fluid-filled cushions at the danger sites. If only one aspect of the tendon is at risk, a bag (bursa synovialis) may be interposed on that side (Fig. 1.28A); if a greater part of the circumference is vulnerable, the cushion wraps around the tendon, enclosing it within a tendon sheath (vagina synovialis; Fig. 1.28B). The walls of these bursae and sheaths and the fluid they contain resemble the similar components of synovial joints. When the tendon moves, it is the lubricated synovial layers that rub together.

Inflammation of synovial bursae and sheaths is common, and it is necessary to know their positions and extents; however, this is not difficult because they occur precisely where they can be seen to be required.

Blood and Nerve Supplies of Muscles. Muscles receive a relatively generous blood supply from neighboring arteries. Sometimes, a single artery enters the muscle belly, and then the well-being of the muscle clearly depends on the integrity of that artery. Often, two or more arteries enter separately and connect with each other within the muscle. Unfortunately, these connections (anastomoses) are not always sufficient to allow the muscle to survive unscathed an interruption to one of its sources of supply. The intramuscular arteries ramify within the perimysium to open into capillaries that follow the endomysial sheaths of individual fibers.

The veins are satellite to the arteries. Normal activity, during which only a fraction of the muscle fibers contract, probably promotes the circulation within the muscle by massaging the capillaries and smaller veins. Mass contractions squeeze these vessels from all sides, stopping the circulation, and are likely to be harmful if sustained.

Tendons have low metabolic needs, are poorly vascularized, and do not hemorrhage when cut. These features, initially apparent advantages, have their adverse side: damaged tendons are inevitably slow to heal. Lymphatic vessels are found within the larger connective tissue tracts of the muscle belly.

Most muscles are supplied by a single nerve, but those of the trunk that are formed from several somites (p. 28) retain multiple innervation. The nerve that enters a muscle, generally in company with the principal vessels, ramifies within the connective tissue septa. It consists of fibers of several types: large alpha motor fibers supply the muscle fibers of the main mass; smaller gamma motor fibers supply modified muscle cells within the muscle spindles buried in the muscle; nonmyelinated vasomotor fibers supply blood vessels; and sensory fibers supply the spindles, tendon organs, and other receptors. The ratio of motor to sensory fibers varies considerably and is one among many complications in the determination of motor unit size.

The motor neurons that supply a particular muscle are roughly grouped within the ventral horns of gray matter in the spinal cord (or within motor nuclei of the brainstem). The axon from each neuron branches repeatedly in its passage, both within the nerve trunk and within the intermuscular septa, and ultimately ends in the motor end plates of several or many muscle fibers. The single neuron, as well as the (alpha) fibers it supplies, is known as the *motor unit,* an important concept because it is the physiologic unit of muscular contraction. It is these groups and not individual fibers that are called up for or discharged from service when a muscle varies the force of its contraction. The muscle fibers belonging to a unit are intermingled with those of other units and do not correspond with any readily identifiable portion of the muscle—they do not correspond with the fasciculi, as one might suppose. The fibers constituting a motor unit are invariably of a uniform type.

In the human species, the numbers of fibers within a unit varies, numbering about 5 to 10 in the muscles that move the eyeball, around 200 in the muscles of the fingers, and approximately 2000 in the muscles of the limbs. The exact figures are not important, but the trend is: the muscles with the smallest units are those capable of the most delicate adjustment. Motor unit size is determined from the innervation ratio, the ratio between the numbers of fibers within a muscle and the numbers of motor neurons that supply it.

Muscle Actions

When a muscle is activated, its fibers attempt to shorten. When shortening occurs, the tension in the muscle may increase, stay the same, or decrease, according to circumstances. When external forces prevent the muscle from shortening, the tension within it increases; such activity is said to be isometric.

The usual activity of most muscles involves changes in the angle of the joint(s) bridged by that muscle. The musculoskeletal system thus operates as a system of levers in which the joints act as fulcrums. The mechanical advantages of the arrangement depend on the positions (relative to the fulcrum) of the muscle attachment and the application of the load (Fig. 1.29). Although a muscle attaching close to a fulcrum is less powerful than a comparable muscle attaching at a greater distance, it produces its effect more rapidly; the requirements of speed and power thus conflict. When several muscles are available to move a joint in a particular way, the attachments of some make them more suited to getting the movement started, whereas the attachments of others make them more suited to carrying the movement through to completion.

Biarticular or polyarticular muscles (those that cross two or several joints, respectively) may be incapable of shortening sufficiently to produce the full range of movement at both or all of the relevant joints at the same time. Such muscles are said to be actively insufficient.

Any muscle that produces a certain effect may be termed an *agonist* or *prime mover*; a muscle capable of actively opposing that movement is termed an *antagonist.* Clearly, these terms have force only in relation to a specified movement. Thus, in flexion of the elbow, the brachialis muscle that produces the movement is the agonist, and the triceps brachii that opposes the movement is the antagonist; in extension of the same joint, however, the triceps muscle is the agonist, and the brachialis muscle the antagonist. Other muscles may neither facilitate nor directly oppose a movement but may modify the action of the agonist, perhaps by eliminating an unwanted side effect. Such muscles are known as *synergists.* When muscles are employed to stabilize joints rather than to promote their movement, they are known as *fixators*. Fixation or stabilization of a joint often involves the co-contraction of muscles that oppose each other when the joint is moved.

The terms *origin* and *insertion* have been left undefined until now. Conventionally, *origin* denotes the more proximal

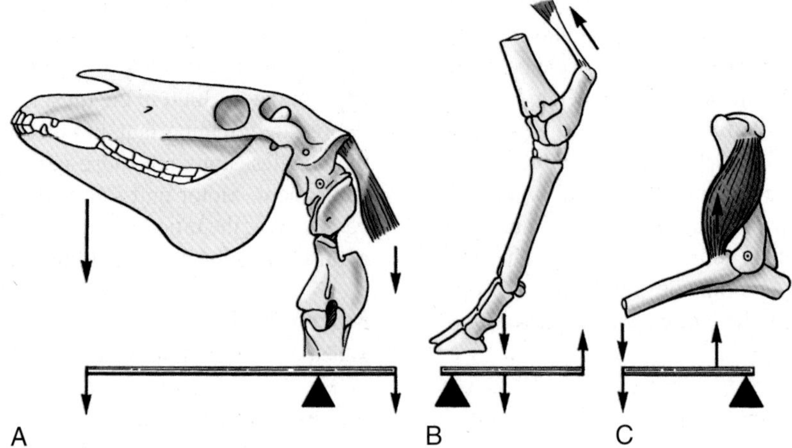

Fig. 1.29 The action of muscles on the skeleton can be compared to different lever systems. (A) Support of the head by dorsal neck muscles. (B) Extension of the hock joint. (C) Flexion of the elbow joint.

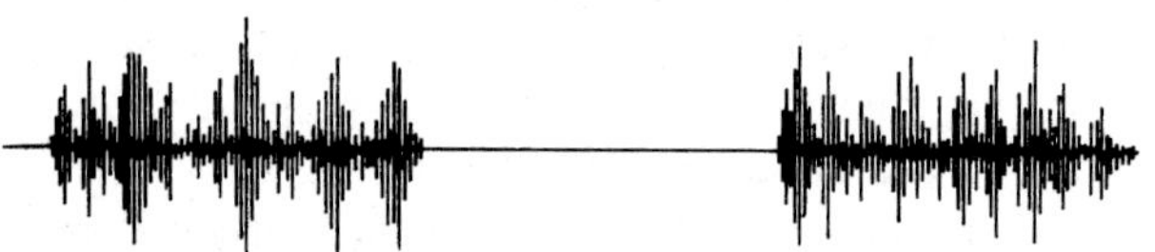

Fig. 1.30 Record (electromyogram) of electrical activity during muscle contraction.

or central attachment and *insertion* the more distal or peripheral attachment. Although it is true that in their common employment most muscles draw the insertion toward the origin, the vast majority are able to shorten toward either end. Which attachment will maintain its position and which will be drawn toward the other depend on external circumstances. These circumstances must always be taken into account when one is considering the possible actions of a muscle.

The attachments of muscles in relation to the axis (axes) of the joint(s) permit deductions about their functions. If these deductions are sound, they indicate what a muscle can do but not how it is habitually used in life. Direct stimulation of a muscle or of its nerve shows what that muscle can do when it acts alone. It does not, however, show how the muscle is used naturally, because often, several alternative muscles are available to perform a given movement but not all are normally used.

The most elegant technique for studying muscle actions is *electromyography,* the registration of the electrical activity that accompanies muscular contraction. In this method, electrodes are placed over or inserted into the muscles to time the activity and crudely quantify its intensity (Fig. 1.30). The use of this technique has upset many long-held beliefs concerning the actions and use of the muscles of humans; much remains to be investigated where domestic animals are concerned. Even this method demands that caution be used in interpretation of findings. It shows when a muscle is active but leaves the experimenter to interpret the activity as agonistic, antagonistic, or a mere adjustment to the alteration in joint angle brought about by other forces.

Peripheral Blood Vessels

The peripheral blood vessels comprise arteries that lead blood from the heart, veins that return blood to the heart, and capillaries that are the minute connections between the smallest arteries and the smallest veins within the tissues. These vessels are arranged to form two circuits (Fig. 1.31). One, the systemic circulation, arises from the left ventricle, conveys oxygenated (arterial) blood to all organs and parts of the body other than the exchange tissue of the lungs, and then transports the now deoxygenated (venous) blood back to the right atrium; the second, the pulmonary circulation, conveys deoxygenated blood from the right ventricle to the exchange tissue of the lungs, where it is reoxygenated before being returned to the left atrium by a special set of veins. The systemic and pulmonary circulations together with the chambers of the heart form a single complex course through which the blood circulates endlessly.

Arteries

In the dissection room, the arteries may be distinguished from other vessels by their white, thick, and relatively rigid walls and their empty lumina (unless filled with an injection mass for the convenience of the dissector). The larger arteries follow a rather constant pattern, but their smaller branches show much variation—so much that some patterns described in the textbooks, though the most common, may actually occur in only a minority of subjects. When arteries branch, the combined cross-sectional area of the daughter vessels always exceeds the cross-sectional area of the parent trunk (Fig. 1.32).

A general correspondence exists between the absolute and relative sizes of parent and daughter vessels and the angles at which the latter diverge from the main trunk. Although there are exceptions, larger branches diverge at more acute angles to minimize resistance. Hemodynamic factors are less important where small branches are

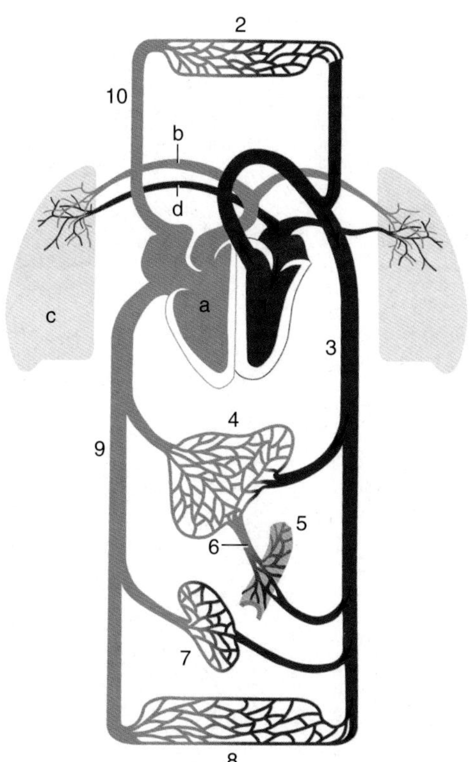

Fig. 1.31 Schema of the circulation; vessels carrying oxygenated blood are shown in *red,* those carrying deoxygenated blood in *blue.* Systemic circulation: *1,* Left side of the heart; *2,* vessels in the cranial part of the body; *3,* aorta; *4,* liver; *5,* intestines; *6,* portal vein; *7,* kidneys; *8,* vessels in the caudal part of the body; *9,* caudal vena cava; *10,* cranial vena cava. Pulmonary circulation: *a,* Right side of the heart; *b,* pulmonary artery; *c,* lung; *d,* pulmonary vein.

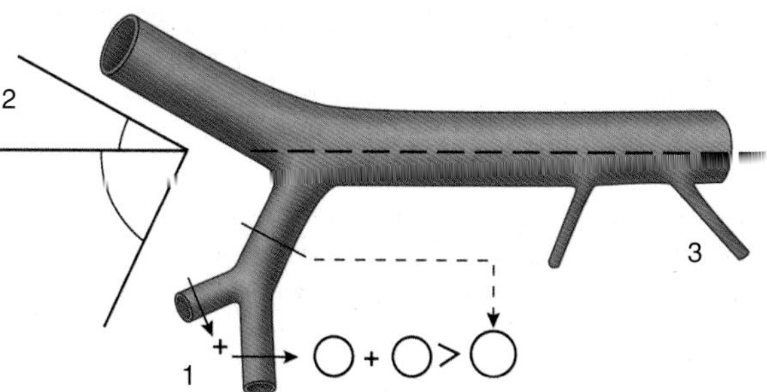

Fig. 1.32 The branching of the arteries. Note that *(1)* the sum of the cross-sectional areas of the branches always exceeds that of the parent trunk; *(2)* large branches leave the trunk at more acute angles than smaller branches; and *(3)* the smallest branches leave erratically.

concerned, and these often follow the shortest routes to their destinations (see Fig. 1.32).

Another factor influencing arterial course is a preference for protected situations; it is well illustrated in the limbs, where the major vessels tend to run medially and also tend to reorient themselves to cross the flexor aspects of successive joints. In comparable fashion, arteries that supply

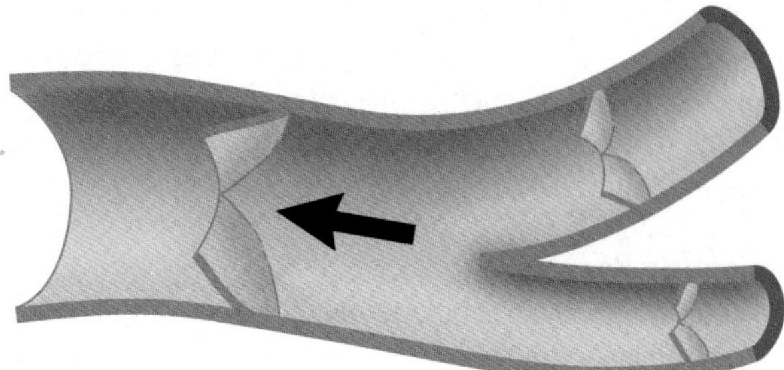

Fig. 1.33 A branching vein opened to expose valves. The *arrow* indicates the direction of blood flow.

organs that change much in size or position are protected against stretching by their meandering courses.

Although arteries ultimately discharge into capillary beds, most also have more proximal and more substantial connections with their neighbors. These interarterial connections (anastomoses) provide alternative, collateral pathways or bypasses by which circulation can be maintained when the more direct route is blocked. Collateral circulation operates as soon as a main trunk is obstructed and becomes more efficient with the passage of time.

The possibility of collateral circulation in different regions and organs has obvious importance to the clinician and the pathologist, and more attention is given to this topic later (p. 228). Meanwhile, this possibility suggests that it may be unnecessary to know the details of all the smaller vessels.

Veins

In the dissection room, veins are distinguished by their thinner walls, their frequently collapsed appearance, and their capacity, which is invariably greater than that of the associated arteries. They appear blue when filled with clotted blood. Most veins are also distinguished by the presence of valves, which are repeated at intervals along their length; the valves ensure a unidirectional flow and prevent reflux of blood when the circulation stagnates (Fig. 1.33). Each valve consists of two or three semilunar cusps facing each other. Valves are most numerous in veins that are exposed to intermittent changes in external pressure and are wholly lacking in those isolated from such influences. They are thus common in veins running between muscles and absent from those in the vertebral canal and cranial cavity; partly on this account, the veins in the last site are known by the special term *venous sinuses.*

The very largest arteries and veins run separately, but most veins of medium and lesser size accompany the corresponding arteries to which they are said to be satellite. However, they show even more variation than the arteries and are quite commonly duplicated, further replicated, or arranged in plexus formation.

Lymphatic Structures

The lymphatic system has two components. The first is a system of lymphatic capillaries and larger vessels that return interstitial fluid to the bloodstream. The second comprises a variety of widely scattered aggregations of lymphoid tissue, including the many lymph nodes; less discrete lymphoid aggregations, such as tonsils, are not considered until later (p. 241).

Lymphatic Vessels

A plexus of lymphatic capillaries that is spread through most tissues collects a fraction of the interstitial fluid. This fraction is disproportionately important because it includes the proteins and other large molecules that are unable to enter the less permeable blood vessels. The greater permeability of the lymphatic capillaries also allows them to take in particulate matter, including microorganisms, on occasion. The lymphatic capillaries commence blindly and form plexuses from which larger lymphatic vessels take origin. These larger vessels closely resemble veins in structure but are more delicate. Because the fluid (lymph) they contain is generally pale, they are rarely conspicuous; however, they are easily identified once seen, as closely spaced valves give them a distinctive beaded appearance when they are well filled. The largest vessels take independent courses, but many of smaller size accompany blood vessels and nerves. The lymphatic vascular tree eventually converges on two or three large trunks that open in a rather erratic fashion into major veins at the junction of the neck and thorax (Fig. 1.34).

Lymph Nodes

Lymph nodes, often incorrectly termed lymph glands, are placed along the lymph pathways in a pattern that shows considerable specific and some individual variation. Groups of neighboring nodes constitute lymphocenters, whose occurrence and drainage territories exhibit greater constancy than is shown by individual nodes. There are important interspecific differences in the lymphocenters: in domestic carnivores and ruminants, particularly in cattle, each center contains rather few but individually large nodes, and in pigs, and more especially horses, each contains a great many small nodes packed together.

Lymph nodes are firm, smooth surfaced, and generally ovoid or bean shaped. Some that are superficial can be identified on palpation through the skin. Naturally, they are more easily found when they are enlarged, and it is therefore a matter of importance to have a clear expectation of which nodes can usually be identified in the healthy animal. Each node is bounded by a capsule, below which runs an open space (subcapsular sinus) into which the afferent vessels open at scattered sites. Branches from the subcapsular sinus lead to a medullary sinus close to the generally indented hilus, where the few efferent vessels emerge (Fig. 1.35A; see also Fig. 7.50). The tissue of the node is divided into cortical and medullary regions. The cortex contains the germinal centers in which lymphocytes are continually produced; the medulla consists of looser branching cellular cords. Both are supported by a reticular framework containing many phagocytic cells. The organization of

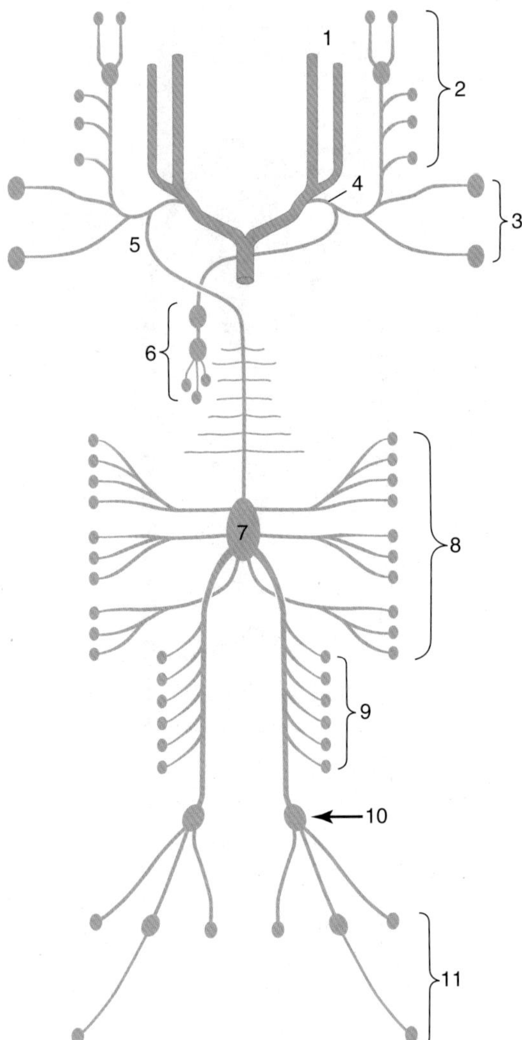

Fig. 1.34 Generalized schema of the lymph nodes and lymphatic vessels (dorsal view). The *top* of the diagram represents the neck region. *1,* External and internal jugular veins; *2,* lymph from the head; *3,* lymph from the shoulder and forelimb; *4,* tracheal duct; *5,* thoracic duct; *6,* lymph from the thoracic organs; *7,* cisterna chyli; *8,* lymph from the abdominal organs; *9,* lymph from the lumbar region and kidneys; *10,* lymph nodes of the pelvis; *11,* lymph from the hindlimb.

the lymph nodes of pigs (Fig. 1.35B) shows a reversal of the usual flow pattern: the afferent vessels enter together, whereas the efferent vessels have dispersed origins (Fig. 7.51A–B).

With very few exceptions (and these are disputed), all lymph passes through at least one node in its passage from the tissues to the bloodstream. As it percolates through the node, it receives a recruitment of lymphocytes and is also exposed to the activities of the phagocytes. These cells remove and destroy, or attempt to remove and destroy, particulate matter, including any microorganisms within the lymph. The lymph node thus provides a barrier to the spread of infection and tumors, some varieties of which

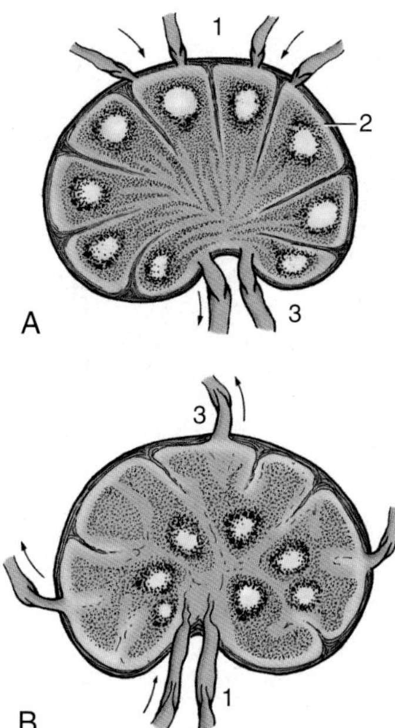

Fig. 1.35 (A) Structure of a lymph node in which the germinal centers (lymph nodules) occupy the cortical region. (B) In the pig the germinal centers lie centrally. The *arrows* indicate the direction of lymph flow. *1,* Afferent lymphatics; *2,* subcapsular sinus; *3,* efferent lymphatics.

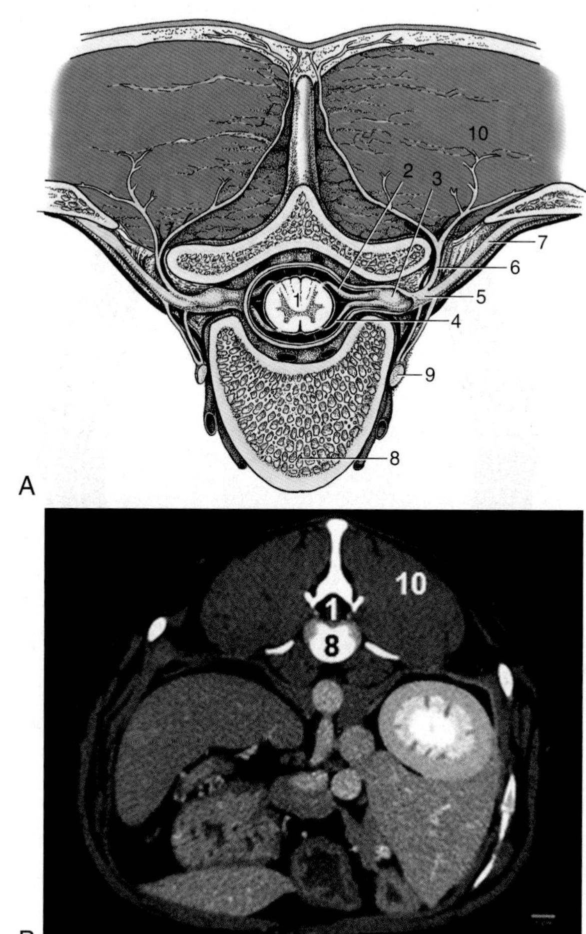

Fig. 1.36 Schematic (A) transection of the vertebral column to show the formation of a spinal nerve. B shows a CT of the abdomen of a female dog. *1,* Spinal cord; *2,* dorsal root; *3,* spinal ganglion; *4,* ventral root; *5,* spinal nerve; *6,* dorsal branch of spinal nerve; *7,* ventral branch of spinal nerve; *8,* body of vertebra; *9,* sympathetic trunk; *10,* epaxial muscles.

favor lymphatic pathways for their dissemination. Swelling of a lymph node frequently indicates the existence of a disease process in its drainage territory. It is clear that the role of the lymphatic system in disease is equivocal. On the one hand, lymph flow facilitates the spread of microorganisms or tumor cells; on the other, the intervention of the node provides an opportunity for their containment and destruction. There are obviously weighty reasons why the position, the accessibility, the drainage territory, and the destination of the efferent flow of all major nodes must be familiar to the clinician, the pathologist, and the veterinarian engaged in meat inspection.

Peripheral Nerves

The central nervous system, the brain and spinal cord, is in two-way communication with virtually all body tissues by means of a system of branching peripheral nerves. These are composed of *afferent* (sensory) fibers, which convey information to the central nervous system from peripheral receptors, and *efferent* (motor) fibers, which convey instructions from the central nervous system to peripheral effector organs. The peripheral nerves comprise the 12 pairs of cranial nerves and the considerably larger number of pairs of spinal nerves whose total varies with the vertebral formula. The dog has 8 cervical, 13 thoracic, 7 lumbar, 3 sacral, and about 5 caudal pairs. The present discussion is restricted to the rather uniform spinal nerves; the cranial nerves differ from these and from one another in many respects that are considered later (p. 301).

The orderly origin of the spinal nerves reveals the segmentation of the spinal cord. Each nerve is formed by the union of two roots (Fig. 1.36). The *dorsal root* is almost exclusively composed of afferent fibers whose cell bodies are clumped together to form a visible swelling, the spinal (dorsal root) ganglion. The central processes enter the cord along a dorsolateral furrow. The peripheral processes extend from the wide variety of exteroceptive, proprioceptive, and enteroceptive endings that respond to external stimuli, changes within the muscles and other locomotor organs, and changes in the internal organs, respectively. The *ventral root* is exclusively composed of efferent fibers emanating from motor neurons within the ventral horn of gray matter and leaving the cord along a ventrolateral strip; they are in passage to the effector organs—muscles and glands.

The dorsal and ventral roots join peripheral to the dorsal root ganglion to form the mixed *spinal nerve* (Fig. 1.36/5), which leaves the vertebral canal through

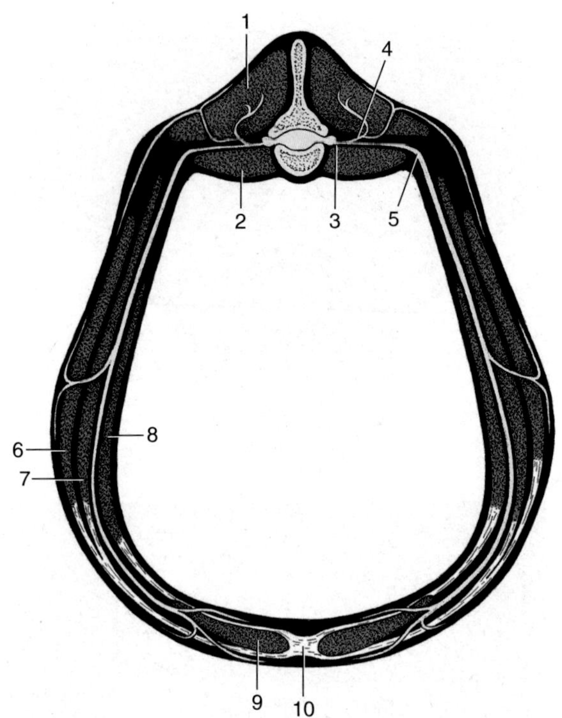

Fig. 1.37 The distribution of a (lumbar) spinal nerve. *1,* Epaxial muscles; *2,* sublumbar muscles; *3,* spinal nerve; *4,* dorsal branch of spinal nerve; *5,* ventral branch of spinal nerve; *6, 7,* external and internal abdominal oblique muscles; *8,* transversus abdominis muscle; *9,* rectus abdominis muscle; *10,* linea alba.

the appropriate intervertebral foramen. In the cervical region, each nerve emerges cranial to the vertebra of the same numerical designation as the nerve, except the eighth, which emerges between the last cervical and first thoracic vertebrae. In other regions, each nerve emerges caudal to the vertebra of the same numerical designation.

The mixed trunk formed by the union of dorsal and ventral roots divides almost at once into dorsal and ventral branches (rami). The *dorsal branch* is distributed to dorsal structures: epaxial muscles of the trunk (broadly, those that lie dorsal to the line of transverse processes) and the skin over the back (Fig. 1.37). The much larger *ventral branch* is distributed to hypaxial muscles of the trunk (broadly, those ventral to the transverse processes), the muscles of the limbs (with a few exceptions), and the remaining part of the skin, including that of the limbs. Both dorsal and ventral branches have connections with their neighbors that form continuous dorsal and ventral plexuses. These plexuses are generally neither obvious nor important, except for enlarged portions of the ventral plexus opposite the origins of the limbs. These, the brachial and lumbosacral plexuses, give rise to the nerves that are distributed to forelimb and hindlimb structures, respectively.

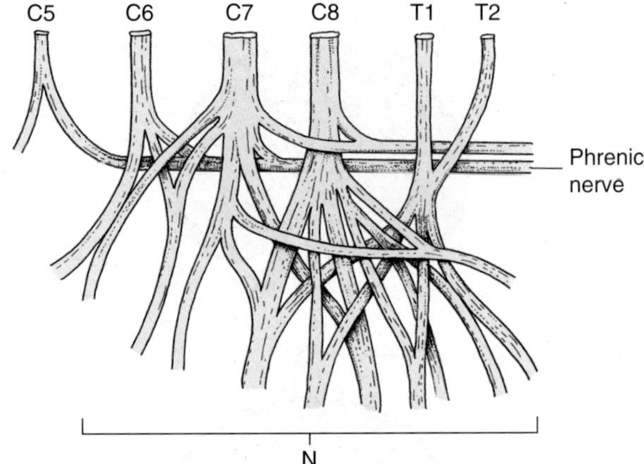

Fig. 1.38 The brachial plexus. The ventral divisions of the spinal nerves (*C6* through *T2*) contributing to the plexus are at the *top* of the schema, the peripheral branches *(N)* supplying the forelimb at the *bottom*. Contributions from C5, C6, and C7 form the phrenic nerve.

The *brachial plexus* (Fig. 1.38) is usually formed by contributions from the last three cervical and the first two thoracic nerves and the *lumbosacral plexus* by contributions from the last few lumbar and the first two sacral nerves. The limb plexuses allow for regrouping and reassociation of the constituent nerve fibers, and the nerve trunks that emerge distally are each composed of fibers derived from two or three spinal segments; thus the median nerve is composed of fibers from spinal nerves C8 and T1, the femoral nerve of fibers from L4 to L6.

The courses of the major peripheral nerve trunks must be known to avoid placing the nerves at unnecessary risk during surgery. Their central connections are important in two contexts. First, local anesthetic solutions injected near selected spinal nerves have predictable effects in paralyzing muscles and in depriving skin areas of sensation. Conversely, paralysis of particular muscles or absence or alteration of the sensibility of specific skin areas may point to the precise location of a central lesion.

So far, reference to nerve fibers concerned with the innervation of blood vessels, glands, and internal organs has been avoided. These structures are supplied by the autonomic division of the nervous system, which is described in Chapter 8. For the present, it is sufficient to state that although autonomic fibers are not present in the roots of every spinal nerve, arrangements exist that ensure that each peripheral nerve receives its necessary quota.

COMPREHENSION CHECK

Is a knowledge of anatomy critical for a person to become a competent veterinary medical professional? If so, list arguments to support your position.

The Locomotor Apparatus 2

The focus of this chapter is integrated study of systematic osteology, arthrology, and myology.* The description of bones, muscles, and joints is grouped into regions of the body—the trunk, the head, the forelimb, and the hindlimb—to make them manageable and suitable to accompany dissection. Here, the dog is used as the model species, with only the most salient comparative features noted. Many additional details, particularly those that have an applied value, are found in the regional chapters. The introduction to each section mentions those features of development that are likely to be immediately helpful in understanding adult anatomy.

THE TRUNK

Basic Plan and Development

The trunk is the large part of the carcass that remains after the removal of the head and neck, the tail, and the forelimbs and hindlimbs (Fig. 2.1). It consists of three segments—the thorax, abdomen, and pelvis—which are not clearly divided externally. Each is bounded by the body wall, and each contains a cavity, or a potential cavity, because in life, the space is more or less obliterated by the close apposition of the walls and contents. The thoracic cavity lies cranial to the diaphragm, a domed sheet of muscle and tendon with a peripheral attachment to the body wall and a free center that bulges cranially. The abdominal cavity lies caudal to the diaphragm and corresponds to the belly. It communicates freely with the pelvic cavity within the enclosure of the bony pelvis (Fig. 2.2).

The *dorsal part of the body wall* that roofs the thoracic, abdominal, and pelvic cavities is known as the back. It is formed by the vertebral column and associated muscles, which are structures that also extend through the neck and tail. It is therefore convenient, if not entirely appropriate, to consider the vertebrae and associated structures of the neck and tail in this section. The structures of the ventral part of the neck are included with the head.

The neck, back, and tail exhibit a serial repetition of like elements, most notably the vertebrae. This apparent segmentation is, as reference to a young embryo shows (Fig. 2.3), a legacy of the somites, the blocks into which the paraxial mesoderm is segregated to each side of the neural tube and notochord. The appearance in the adult is somewhat misleading; the vertebrae are, in fact, each formed by contributions from two somites of each side and are therefore more accurately described as intersegmental. Together with the ribs and sternum, they are produced from the medial portions of the somites known as *sclerotomes*. The muscles of the vertebral column are derived from the lateral portions of the somites, the myotomes. Many adult muscles are polysegmental and combine contributions from several or even many myotomes, but certain groups of deeper units retain the unisegmental pattern. Because the vertebrae are intersegmental, even the shortest muscles bridge, and thus can move, the joint between two successive bones.

Early on, each myotome attracts a single nerve (Fig. 2.3/8) that grows out from the adjacent neural tube; it follows that the motor innervation of the muscles is also segmental and that polysegmental muscles will have multiple innervation. A similar pattern is apparent in the sensory innervation of the skin. It was formerly believed that the connective tissue component of the skin, the dermis, derived exclusively from third portions of the somites, the dermatomes. Cells from these were supposed to migrate to underlie specific regions of the surface ectoderm. This ordered pattern of migration is now in question, and it is thought that the dermis may be in part produced through mesenchymal differentiation in situ. Be that as it may, a segmental innervation of skin (Fig. 2.4) exists in the adult that is very regular in some places and less so in others. The bands of skin that are supplied by particular pairs of spinal nerves are also known as *dermatomes*. Many overlap their neighbors. The associations between these bands and particular sensory nerves develop quite separately from those between the motor nerves and the muscles. The sensory component of the spinal nerve develops from a group of ganglion cells of neural crest origin; central branches of these cells form the dorsal root, which grows into the segment of the neural tube already defined by the outgrowth of the motor root. Together, the dorsal and ventral roots constitute the mixed spinal nerve.

In contrast to the segmental pattern of the nerves, the arteries to the body wall are branches of the aorta that initially pass intersegmentally between the somites (Fig. 2.3/5). Nevertheless, the arteries and nerves later associate in a way that fails to reflect the different patterns of their origins.

* *Osteology* derives from *osteon,* Greek (bone); arthrology from *arthron,* Greek (joint); and *myology* from *mys,* Greek (muscle). These terms, rather than the Latin equivalents, provide the stems for many medical terms: osteoma, arthrosis, myositis, and so forth. *Syndesmology* is sometimes used as an alternative term for the study of joints.

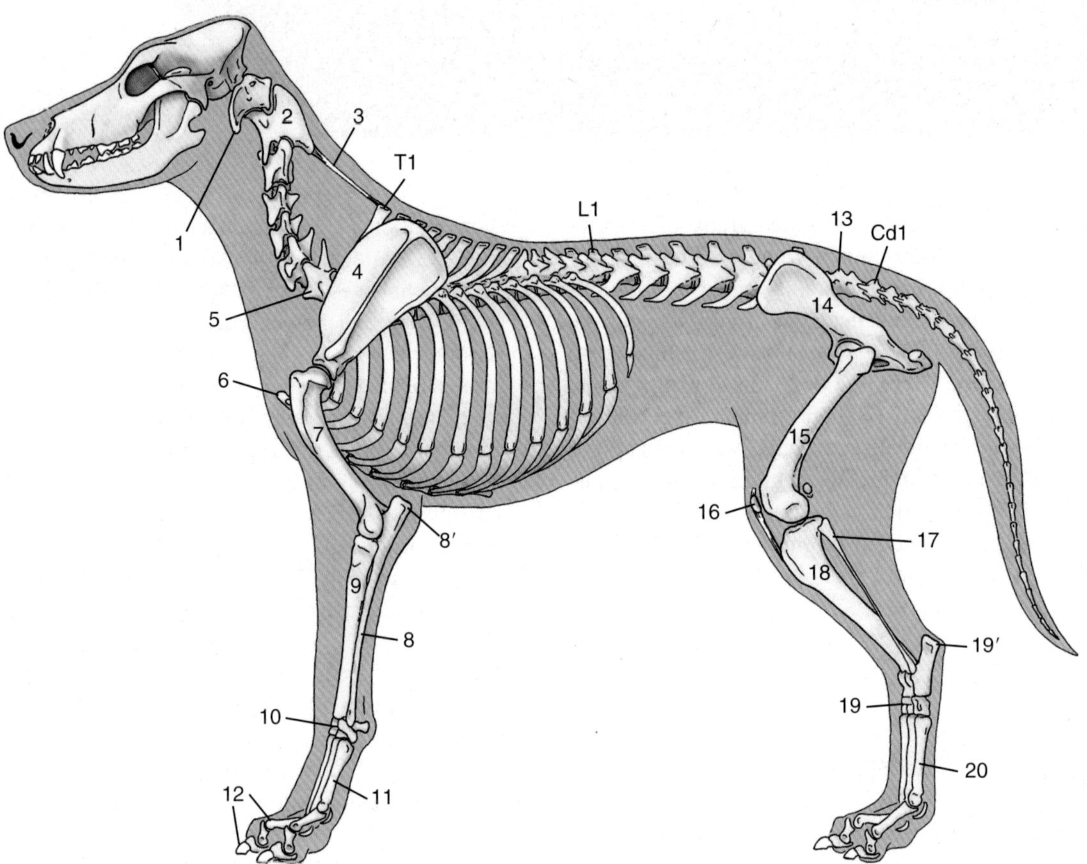

Fig. 2.1 The skeleton of the dog. *1,* Wing of atlas, first cervical vertebra (C1); *2,* spine of axis (C2); *3,* ligamentum nuchae; *4,* scapula; *5,* last cervical vertebra (C7); *6,* cranial end (manubrium) of sternum; *7,* humerus; *8,* ulna; *8′,* olecranon (point of elbow); *9,* radius; *10,* carpal bones; *11,* metacarpal bones; *12,* proximal, middle, and distal phalanges; *13,* sacrum; *14,* hip bone (os coxae); *15,* femur; *16,* patella; *17,* fibula; *18,* tibia; *19,* tarsal bones; *19′,* calcanean tuber (point of hock); *20,* metatarsal bones; *T1, L1,* and *Cd1,* first thoracic, first lumbar, and first caudal (tail) vertebrae.

The *lateral and ventral parts of the body wall* are initially unsegmented (see Fig. 2.3). The tissues of these parts develop in the somatopleure, which is formed by the association of the ectoderm and the outer of the two sheets into which the lateral plate mesoderm is split. The inner sheet of the lateral mesoderm is, of course, combined with the endoderm to constitute the splanchnopleure or gut wall. The separation of these sheets is achieved by the coalescence of initially scattered spaces to form a continuous cavity (Fig. 2.5/*9*). The cavity, known as the *celom*, is afterward divided to yield the pericardial and pleural spaces of the thorax and the peritoneal space of the abdomen and pelvis. The somatopleure is later invaded by cells that migrate ventrally from local somites. Cells that migrate from the sclerotomes of thoracic somites differentiate to form the ribs and sternum. Cells that migrate from the myotomes of both thoracic and abdominal somites differentiate to form the muscles of the thoracic and abdominal walls. The presence of the ribs ensures that the thoracic wall retains a segmental pattern, which is almost completely lost by the abdominal wall.

The embryo is still open ventrally while these events are proceeding. The ventral aspect of the body wall closes only in the final stage of the folding (reversal) process (p. 91) that converts the embryonic disk into a more or less cylindrical body. Ventral midline structures including the sternum and the linea alba—the median connective tissue strip of the abdominal floor—are therefore initially represented bilaterally. The umbilical scar, our "belly button," betrays the site of final closure of the body wall.

The clinician's chief interest in the umbilical scar relates to the prevalence of umbilical hernia, a congenital (possibly inherited) defect that frequently occurs in domestic species. Some delay in the closure of the ventral abdominal wall is always necessary to allow for the temporary physiologic herniation (p.136) of a part of the gut into the extraembryonic celom (within the umbilical cord). Normally the herniated loops of intestine are soon drawn back into the abdomen, and narrowing and eventually closure of the peritoneal ring at the junction of the intraembryonic and extraembryonic parts of the celom then follow. This closure

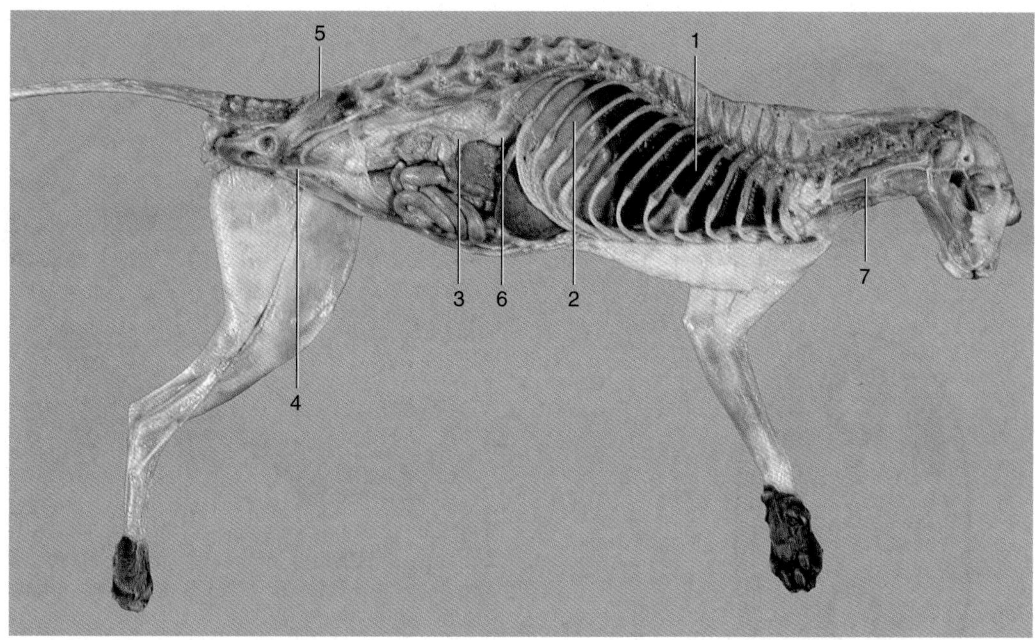

Fig. 2.2 The thoracic, abdominal, and pelvic cavities of a cat; viewed from the left. *1,* Thoracic cavity (with lung); *2,* diaphragm; *3,* abdominal cavity; *4,* pelvic cavity; *5,* sacrum; *6,* right kidney; *7,* esophagus.

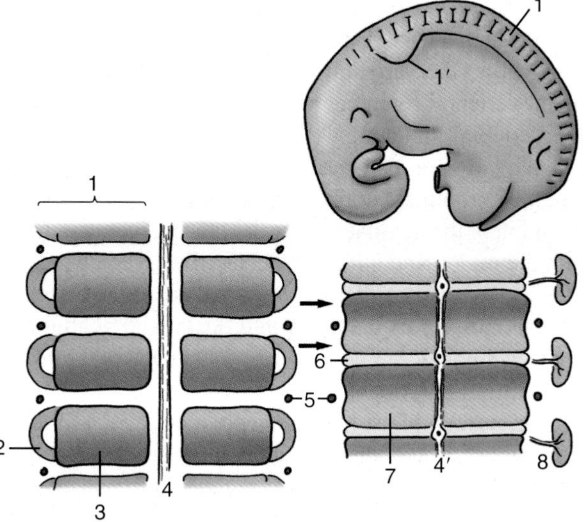

Fig. 2.3 Segmentation of the paraxial mesoderm shown in a 10-mm bovine embryo *(top)* together with two stages in the development of the vertebrae and related vessels and nerves *(bottom).* The *arrows* show the formation of each vertebra from two pairs of adjacent somites. *1,* Somite; *1′,* forelimb bud; *2,* myotome; *3,* sclerotome; *4,* notochord; *4′,* notochord giving rise to the nucleus pulposus in the center of the intervertebral disk (*6*); *5,* intersegmental artery; *6,* intervertebral disk; *7,* body of vertebra; *8,* myotome with segmental nerve.

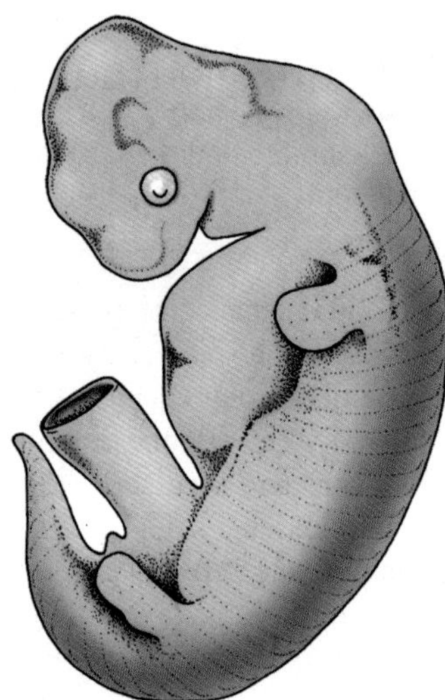

Fig. 2.4 Embryo with "dermatomes" indicating the segmental innervation of the skin.

in turn allows the closure of the defect in the mesodermal tissues, creating the umbilical scar. These processes may be faulty. The intestine may fail to complete its return to the abdomen or, once returned, may make a second escape into the umbilical cord through a persistent peritoneal ring and thus be exposed when the cord is ruptured at birth. More commonly, the peritoneal ring closes but the overlying tissues remain defective, and herniation occurs into a protuberant sac formed by stretching of the peritoneum and covering fasciae and skin. Fortunately, umbilical hernia is usually amenable to simple surgical correction.

The Skeleton and Joints of the Trunk

The Vertebral Column

The vertebral column (or spine) comprises vertebrae and extends from the skull to the tip of the tail. The vertebrae are firmly but not rigidly joined together. In addition to

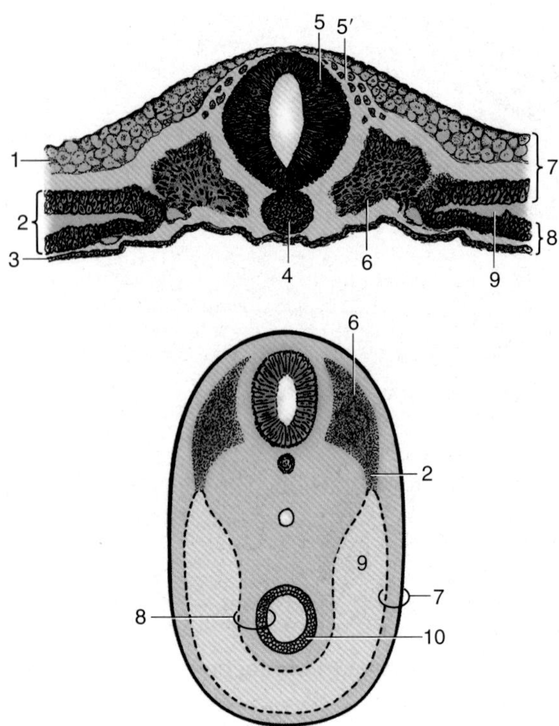

Fig. 2.5 Transections of an early discoidal embryo *(top)* and of an older ventrally closed one *(bottom)* to show the splitting of the lateral mesoderm and the development of the celom. *1,* Ectoderm; *2,* lateral plate of mesoderm; *3,* endoderm; *4,* notochord; *5,* neural tube; *5′,* neural crest cells; *6,* somite; *7,* somatopleure; *8,* splanchnopleure; *9,* celom; *10,* primitive gut.

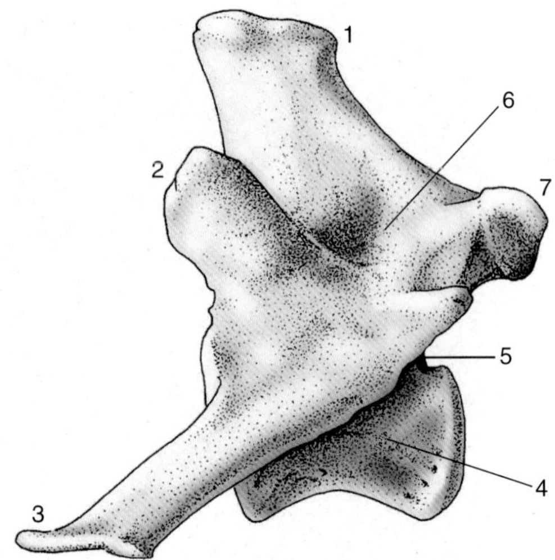

Fig. 2.6 Lumbar vertebra of the dog, left lateral view. *1,* Spinous process; *2,* cranial articular process; *3,* transverse process; *4,* body; *5,* caudal vertebral notch; *6,* arch; *7,* caudal articular process.

contributing to the maintenance of posture through stiffening of the body axis, the spine plays a part in progression and other activities through flexion and extension and sometimes by torsion. The vertebral column encloses and protects the spinal cord and accessory structures within a central canal in particular and shields the structures of the neck, thorax, abdomen, and pelvis in general (see Fig. 2.1).

Most vertebrae conform to a common pattern with superimposed features that distinguish the several regions: cervical (C; neck), thoracic (T; back, in the narrow sense), lumbar (L; loins), sacral (S; croup), and caudal (Cd; tail). The numbers of vertebrae that compose these regions vary among species and also, although to a much smaller extent, individually. They can be represented by a formula: that for the dog is C7, T13, L7, S3, Cd20–23.

A typical vertebra consists of a massive body surmounted by an arch that completes the enclosure of a vertebral foramen (Fig. 2.6). The foramina together constitute the vertebral canal. The body, broadly cylindrical, is somewhat flattened on its dorsal surface, which faces into the vertebral canal. It may carry a median crest ventrally. Its extremities are usually curved: the cranial one is convex, the caudal one concave. The arch consists of two upright pedicles, and from each of these a lamina projects medially to meet its fellow and thus complete the ring about the spinal cord. The bases of the pedicles are notched, and when successive bones articulate, these notches combine to outline intervertebral foramina, openings through which pass both the spinal nerves and the vessels that supply the structures within the vertebral canal. Sometimes an additional lateral vertebral foramen perforates the pedicle next to the intervertebral foramen.

Each vertebra also carries a number of processes. The generally prominent dorsal or spinous process springs from the union of the laminae, and its length and inclination vary with the region and with the species. Transverse processes arise at the level of the intervertebral foramina and separate the muscles of the trunk into dorsal and ventral divisions. Synovial joints connect restricted parts of the arches. Sometimes the articular facets hardly rise above the level of their surroundings, but elsewhere, and especially in the caudal thoracic and lumbar region, the facets are carried on articular processes that project cranially and caudally from the dorsal portions of the arches (Fig. 2.6/*2* and *7*).

In domestic as in almost all mammals there are seven *cervical vertebrae.* The first two, the atlas and the axis, are much modified to allow free movement of the head and require individual description. The remaining five are more typical.

The *atlas* is the most unusual of all the vertebrae because it appears to possess no body but to consist of two lateral masses joined by dorsal and ventral arches (Fig. 2.7A). This form results from the fusion (in early embryonic life) of a component of the atlantal body with the corresponding part of the following bone, the axis. This addition provides the axis with a cranial projection (dens; Fig. 2.7B/*5*), which fits into the vertebral foramen of the atlas and serves as a pivot around which the atlas (and the head) may be rotated.

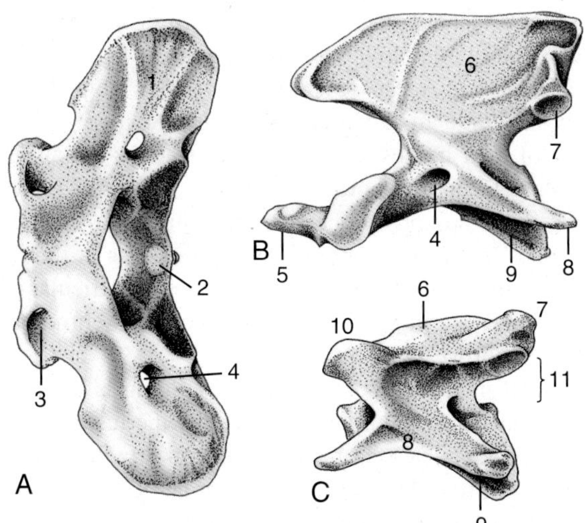

Fig. 2.7 Cervical vertebrae of the dog; cranial is to the *left.* (A) Atlas, dorsal view. (B) Axis, lateral view. (C) Fifth vertebra, lateral view. *1,* Wing of atlas; *2,* fovea dentis; *3,* lateral vertebral foramen; *4,* transverse foramen; *5,* dens; *6,* spinous process; *7,* caudal articular process; *8,* transverse process; *9,* body; *10,* cranial articular process; *11,* position of vertebral foramen.

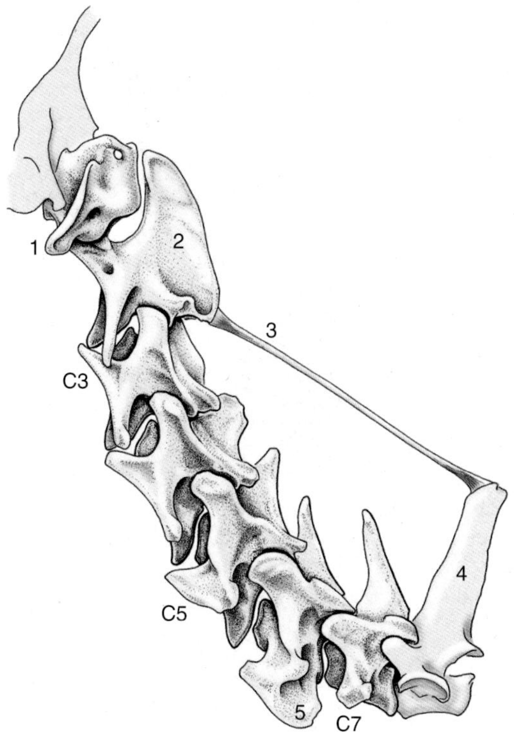

Fig. 2.8 Nuchal ligament of the dog. *1,* Wing of atlas; *2,* spinous process of axis; *3,* nuchal ligament; *4,* spinous process of first thoracic vertebra; *5,* platelike extension of transverse process.

A plate of bone, the wing of the atlas (ala atlantis, transverse process), projects laterally from each mass, constituting a landmark that is often visible and always palpable in the living animal. The cranial aspect of the ventral arch and the adjacent areas on the wings carry two deep excavations that receive the occipital condyles of the skull. These facets approach each other ventrally, and in some species they merge. The caudal aspect of the ventral arch is hollowed transversely to articulate with the cranial extremity of the axis. An extension (fovea dentis; Fig. 2.7A/*2*) of this facet onto the dorsal surface of the ventral arch accommodates the dens. The dorsal arch is perforated by openings that correspond with the transverse and intervertebral foramina of more typical cervical vertebrae; in some species a third (alar) foramen perforates the wing.

The *axis* is the longest vertebra. Its cranial extremity carries the dens, which is rodlike in carnivores and more spoutlike in some other species. The cranial extremity of the body and the ventral surface of the dens together form a single wide articular surface for the atlas. Dorsally the dens is roughened for the attachment of ligaments that hold it in place. The arch carries a very high (and in the dog, long) spinous process that bears articular facets at its caudal extremity that articulate with corresponding facets on the third cervical vertebra. The transverse processes are large, and each has a transverse foramen in its root to transmit the vertebral artery, vein, and nerve.

The remaining cervical vertebrae become progressively shorter as the series is followed toward its junction with the thorax. The extremities of the body are more strongly curved than in other regions and slope obliquely. The ventral surface carries a stout crest. The arch is strong and wide, but the spinous process is poorly developed except on the last (considerable variation, however, exists among species). The large transverse process (Fig. 2.7/*8*) branches into dorsal and ventral tubercles, the latter commonly developing a caudal platelike extension (Fig. 2.8/*5*). On the third to sixth bones the process is perforated by a transverse foramen for the passage of the vertebral vessels and nerve. The articular facets are large and flat but do not rise above the surrounding level. The seventh cervical vertebra, transitional to those of the thoracic region, is distinguished by its taller spinous process, its unperforated transverse process, and the presence of facets on the caudal extremity of its body for articulation with the first pair of ribs.

The *thoracic vertebrae* (Fig. 2.9) articulate with the ribs and correspond with them in number. Minor variations in number are not uncommon, but the compensation in the lumbar region leaves the thoracolumbar region unaffected. All thoracic vertebrae have common features, but serial changes also occur that gradually (and on some points abruptly) distinguish the more cranial from the more caudal bones. Common thoracic features are short bodies with flattened extremities; costal facets, on both extremities for the rib heads and on the transverse processes for the rib tubercles; short, stubby transverse processes; closely fitting

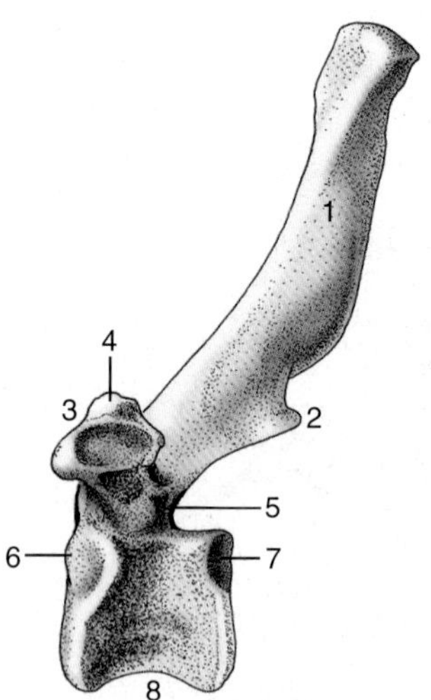

Fig. 2.9 Thoracic vertebra of the dog, left lateral view. *1,* Spinous process; *2,* caudal articular process; *3,* transverse process with costal fovea; *4,* mammillary process; *5,* caudal vertebral notch; *6* and *7,* costal foveae; *8,* body.

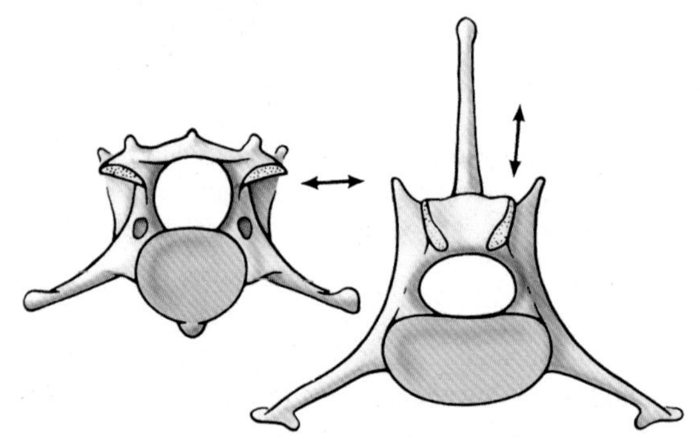

Fig. 2.10 Contrast the orientation *(arrows)* of the articular surfaces of a cervical vertebra *(left)* and a lumbar *(right)* vertebra of the dog, caudal view.

arches; very prominent spinous processes; and low articular processes.

Conspicuous serial features are a rapid increase in the height of the spinous processes, which reaches a maximum a few vertebrae behind the cervicothoracic junction, followed by gradual decline; progressive simplification of the costal facets (those on the transverse processes approach and finally merge with those on the cranial extremity); reduction (and eventual disappearance) of the caudal costal facets; and appearance of an additional (mammillary) process as a projection from the transverse process and its gradual migration to join the cranial articular process. More abrupt changes toward the end of the thoracic series include sudden alteration from a caudodorsal to a craniodorsal orientation of the spinous processes and a change in the character of the articular facets from the cervical to the lumbar pattern (Fig. 2.10). In some species, including the dog, the last members of the thoracic series possess yet other (accessory) processes that spring from the caudal part of the arch to overlap the following bone.

The *lumbar vertebrae* (Fig. 2.11) differ from the thoracic vertebrae in the greater length and more uniform shape of their bodies. Other regional features are absence of costal facets; a shorter height and generally forward slope of the spinous processes; long, flattened transverse processes that project laterally, sometimes (as in the dog) with a cranioventral inclination; interlocking articular processes; and prominent mammillary, and sometimes also accessory, processes.

Caudal to the loins the vertebral column is continued by the *sacrum,* a single bone formed by the fusion of several vertebrae. The sacrum forms a firm articulation with the pelvic girdle that transmits the thrust of the hindlimbs to the trunk. Usually only one or two of the constituent vertebrae directly participate in the articulation. The more caudal bones project behind it to furnish the greater part of the roof of the pelvic cavity. In some animals (especially pigs) one or more tail vertebrae may fuse with the sacrum in later life. In the dog the three sacral vertebrae form a short quadrilateral block (Fig. 2.12).

The sacrum commonly narrows from its cranial to its caudal extremity and is curved along its length to present a smooth, slightly concave face to the pelvic cavity. In most species the dorsal surface is marked by the appropriate number of spinous processes, although they may be much reduced or even absent (e.g., pig). They may preserve their independence (e.g., dog or horse) or fuse to form a continuous crest (e.g., ruminants). Lateral to this crest, a lower irregular crest usually marks the site of the redundant articular processes. The margin of the bone is formed by the fused transverse processes and carries toward its cranial extremity the articular surface for the ilium; this is often ear-shaped, hence the name *auricular surface* (Fig. 2.12/*2*).

The degree of fusion, least in the pig, of the sacral vertebrae varies among species. Even when fusion is total, the composition of the sacrum is betrayed by the number of foramina that mark both surfaces; the dorsal and the ventral branches of the sacral nerves issue separately through them. The junction of the ventral surface with the cranial extremity forms a lip known as the *promontory* (Fig. 2.12/*1*); though often inconspicuous, it is a reference point in obstetrics.

The number of *caudal vertebrae* varies greatly, even within a single species. These vertebrae show a progressive simplification in form, and although the first few resemble miniature lumbar vertebrae, the middle and later members of the series are reduced to simple rods. In addition to the usual features, the more cranial vertebrae of some species provide protection to the main artery of the tail in the form of ventral (hemal) arches, separate small chevron (V-shaped) bones connected to the undersurfaces of the bodies, or paired ventral (hemal) processes (Fig. 2.12E).

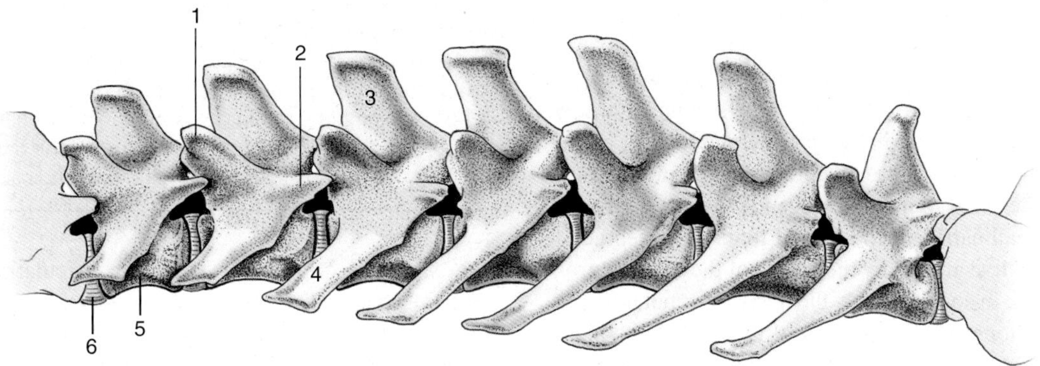

Fig. 2.11 Lumbar vertebrae of the dog, left lateral view. *1,* Mammillary process; *2,* accessory process; *3,* spinous process; *4,* transverse process; *5,* body; *6,* intervertebral disk.

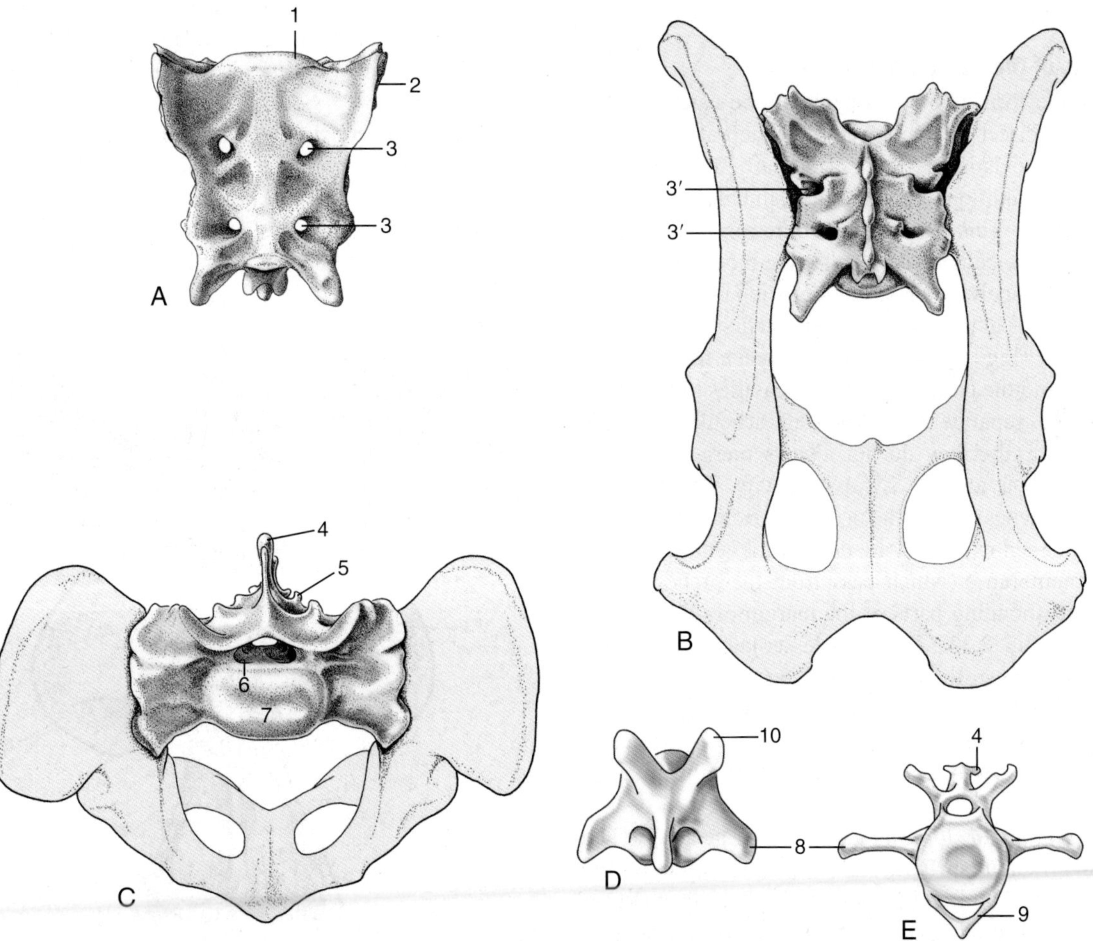

Fig. 2.12 Canine sacrum and caudal vertebrae. (A) Sacrum, ventral view. (B) Sacrum, dorsal view. (C) Sacrum, cranial view. (D) Caudal vertebra, dorsal view. (E) Caudal vertebra, cranial view. *1,* Promontory; *2,* auricular articular surface; *3,* ventral (*3′* dorsal) sacral foramina for ventral (*3′* dorsal) branches of sacral nerves; *4,* spinous process; *5,* rudimentary articular process; *6,* vertebral canal; *7,* body; *8,* transverse process; *9,* hemal arch, also called chevron; *10,* cranial articular process.

The *contours of the vertebral column* vary with the posture, the species, and the breed. In general, the vertebrae from the caudal thoracic region to the tail head follow a more or less horizontal line. The more cranial thoracic vertebrae slope downward to reach the lowest point at the entrance to the chest, where an abrupt change in direction puts the spine on a course that ascends toward the head. The ventral inclination of the cranial thoracic vertebrae is masked in the live animal by the height of the spinous processes; indeed, in some species, the horse most notably, the spines are so long that the contour of this part of the back is raised to constitute the withers. Except toward the poll, the cervical vertebrae run at some distance from the dorsal skin. This feature is not apparent in the live subject, and in larger animals it may not be easy to determine, even on palpation. The greater part of the tail hangs down in large animals, but its posture is more variable in dogs and cats, being an expression of emotion in both species and influenced by breed in the former.

The Joints of the Vertebral Column

The vertebrae form two sets of joints: one cartilaginous, involving the direct connection of the vertebral bodies, the other synovial, existing between facets carried on the vertebral arches. In addition, certain long ligaments extend over many vertebrae. This pattern is modified in two regions; cranially, allowance is made for the free movement of the head, and in the pelvic region, sacral fusion occurs.

The two joints of the atlas are described first. The *atlanto-occipital joint* (Fig. 2.13) is formed between the condyles of the skull and the corresponding concavities of the atlas. Although the separate right and left articular surfaces converge ventrally, they do not always merge, although generally there is a single synovial cavity. The synovial membrane attaches around the occipital and atlantal facets. It is strengthened externally by dorsal and ventral atlanto-occipital membranes, which pass from the arches of the atlas to corresponding parts of the margin of the foramen magnum (see Fig. 2.32/*12*), and by lesser lateral ligaments, which pass between the atlas and adjacent regions of the skull. Despite its odd character, the joint functions as a ginglymus: movement is virtually restricted to flexion and extension in the sagittal plane (the nodding movement in humans).

The *atlantoaxial joint* is even more peculiar. The extensive articular surfaces of the ventral arch of the atlas and of the body and dens of the axis face into a single synovial cavity. The surfaces are so formed that only limited areas are in contact in any position of the head. This limitation of contact, together with the roomy capsule, allows some versatility of movement, although mainly confined to rotation about a longitudinal axis (the head-shaking movement in humans). The dorsal atlanto-axial ligament that joins adjacent parts of these vertebrae imposes little restraint.

The Axis and Death: The dens of the axis is strapped by one or more ligaments to the adjacent part of the upper surface of the ventral atlantal arch and sometimes also to the occipital bone (as in the dog). In judicial hanging, the rupture of these ligaments—or fracture of the dens itself—allows the axis to strike against the cord and cause death.

A single description serves for the articulations of most other vertebrae. The *intervertebral articulations* combine symphyses between the bodies and synovial joints between the articular processes. The thick flexible pads, the intervertebral disks, connect the bodies of adjacent vertebrae and contribute to about 10%, 16%, and 25% of the vertebral length in ungulates, dogs, and humans, respectively. The disks are among the organs that most consistently show degenerative changes with advancing age and are a common source of back troubles long recognized in ourselves and in dogs, which are now also diagnosed in other domestic and even wild animals. But the nature of the medical conditions related to disks is not the same in humans as in quadrupeds.

Each disk consists of two parts, a *nucleus pulposus* and an *anulus fibrosus* (Fig. 2.14). The nucleus occupies a slightly eccentric position. In the young animal, it consists of an unusual semifluid tissue derived from the

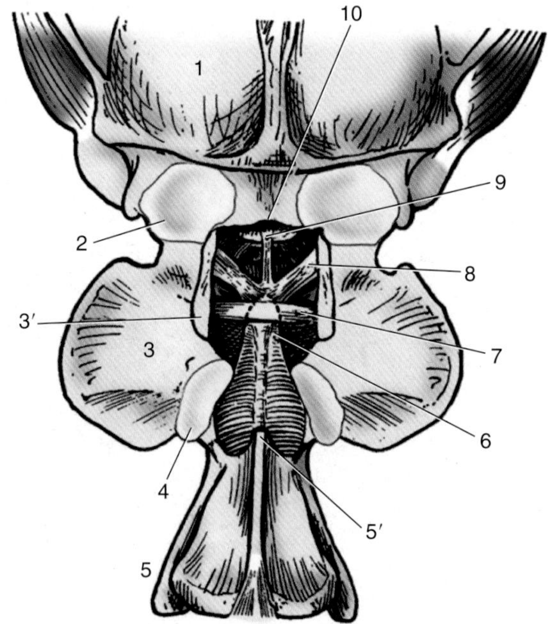

Fig. 2.13 Canine atlanto-occipital joint, dorsal view; the dorsal arch of the atlas has been removed. *1,* Skull; *2,* atlanto-occipital joint capsule; *3,* wing of atlas; *3′,* dorsal arch of atlas, resected; *4,* atlantoaxial joint capsule; *5,* axis; *5′,* spine of axis, its overhanging cranial portion having been removed; *6,* dens; *7,* transverse ligament of atlas; *8,* alar ligaments; *9,* apical ligament of dens; *10,* dorsal margin of foramen magnum.

embryonic notochord and retains some resemblance to it in structure. It is contained under pressure and escapes if afforded opportunity. The anulus fibrosus consists of encircling bundles of fibrous tissue that pass obliquely from one vertebra to the other, in most species merging with cartilage plates that cap the bones. The orientation of the fibers changes between about 20 successive lamellae. The distinction between anulus and nucleus is not always very clear, particularly in the larger species. Retention of the nucleus within the fibrous ring absorbs shock and spreads the compressive forces to which the column is subjected over a wider part of the vertebrae.

The Intervertebral Disk Pathology: Both nucleus and anulus start to change in a subtle manner rather early in life. For example, fragmentation of the ring leads to escape of the nucleus into the vertebral canal and subsequent pressure on the spinal cord. Age-related calcification of the nucleus reduces the normal resilience and flexibility of the spine. Degenerative changes may affect any disk, but the disks at the most mobile regions, such as the neck and, in large animals, the lumbosacral junction, are especially susceptible. Most thoracic disks are crossed dorsally by the intercapital ligaments that unite the heads of the right and left ribs (p. 39), and these ligaments are alleged to mitigate the effects of disk rupture at these levels.

The synovial joints are interposed between the vertebral arches, and the joint mobility varies with the spaciousness of the joint, the region, and to some extent the species. In the cervical and cranial thoracic regions the joint surfaces are arranged tangential to the circumference of a circle centered in the vertebral body (see Fig. 2.10), which allows rotation in addition to flexion and extension. The radial alignment of the articulating surfaces in the caudal thoracic and lumbar regions restricts the movement mostly to the median plane. Movement is most free in the neck, where the articular surfaces are largest and the capsules loosest. The elastic interarcuate ligaments fill the dorsal spaces between the arches of successive vertebrae, and their extent is inversely related to the width of the arches. In certain regions, interspinous and intertransverse ligaments also exist, but these are of less importance.

Three *long ligaments* extend along substantial portions of the column. A dorsal longitudinal ligament (Fig. 2.15/7) runs along the floor of the vertebral canal from the axis to the sacrum, narrowing over the middle of each vertebral body and widening where it crosses each intervertebral disk. A ventral longitudinal ligament follows the ventral aspect of the vertebrae from the midthoracic region to the sacrum; more cranially, its role is filled by the longus colli muscles. It also widens over and fuses with the intervertebral disks.

A third (supraspinous) common ligament runs over (or to each side of) the summits of the spinous processes of the thoracic and lumbar vertebrae. It merges with the tendons of the epaxial muscles so completely that some writers dispute its independent existence. Except in the pig and cat, a cranial continuation of this ligament leaves the highest spines of the withers and runs by the shortest route to attach to the nuchal surface of the skull or, as in the dog, the spinous process of the axis (see Fig. 2.8). This nuchal ligament runs close to the upper contour of the neck, and for most of its length, it is well separated from the more ventral course followed by the cervical vertebrae. Unlike the other long ligaments, this ligament is elastic and supports the burden of the head when it is held high without interfering with the animal's ability to lower the head to feed or drink from the ground. There is an obvious correlation between the strength of this ligament and the weight of the head and the length of the lever arm of the neck; the nuchal ligament is therefore much more powerfully developed, and more complicated, in the larger species (see Fig. 19.3).

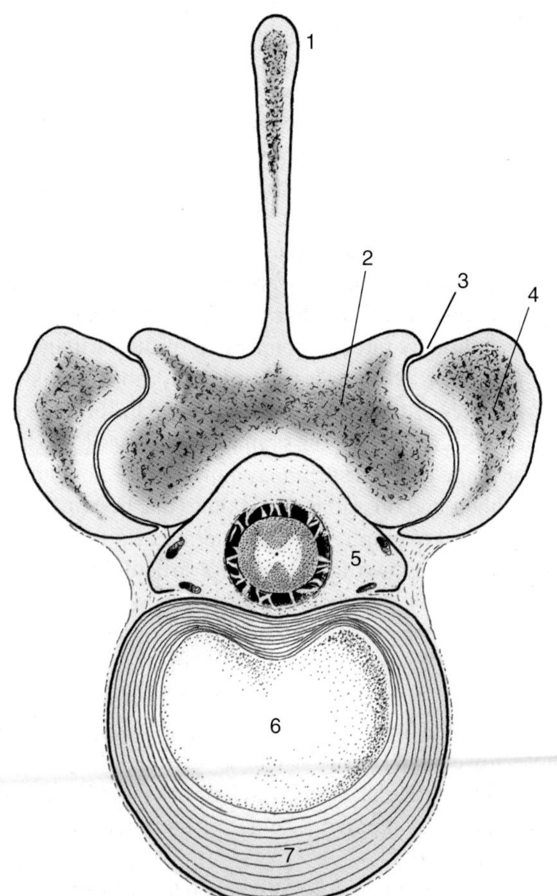

Fig. 2.14 Bovine lumbar intervertebral disk. *1,* Spinous process; *2,* lamina; *3,* synovial intervertebral joint; *4,* articular process of adjacent vertebra; *5,* vertebral canal with contents (spinal cord and meninges surrounded by epidural fat); *6,* nucleus pulposus; *7,* anulus fibrosus.

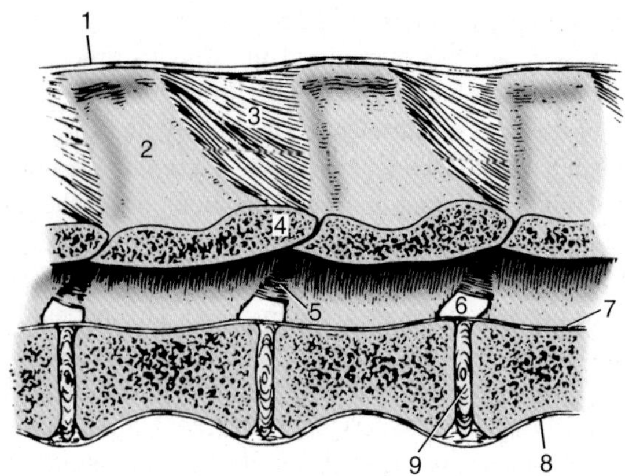

Fig. 2.15 Ligaments of the vertebral column. Paramedian section of lumbar vertebrae of a dog, viewed from the left. *1,* Supraspinous ligament; *2,* spinous process; *3,* interspinous ligament; *4,* arch of vertebra; *5,* interarcuate ligament; *6,* intervertebral foramen; *7,* dorsal longitudinal ligament; *8,* ventral longitudinal ligament; *9,* intervertebral disk.

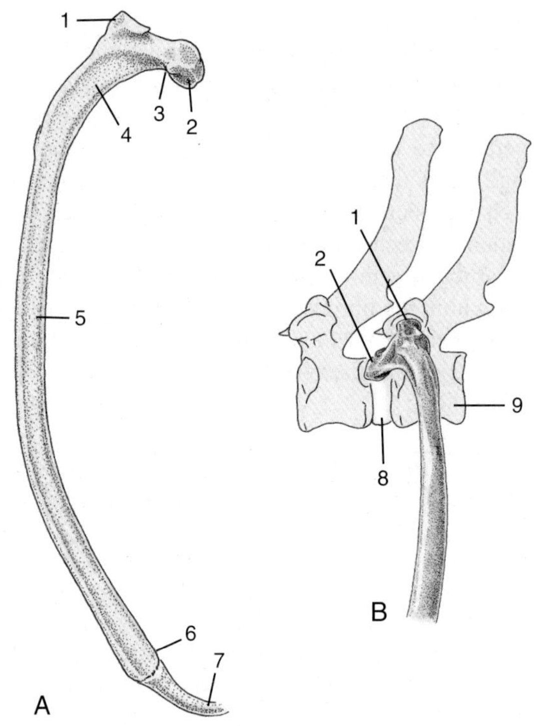

Fig. 2.16 (A) Left rib of a dog, caudal view. (B) Left rib of a dog articulating with two vertebrae, lateral view. *1,* Tubercle; *2,* head; *3,* neck; *4,* angle; *5,* body; *6,* costochondral junction; *7,* costal cartilage; *8,* intervertebral disk; *9,* vertebra of same number as rib.

The Ribs and Sternum

The thoracic skeleton is completed by the ribs and sternum. The *ribs* (costae) are arranged in pairs and generally articulate with two successive vertebrae: the caudal vertebra is the one with the same numerical designation as the rib. Each rib consists of a bony dorsal part, the rib proper, and a cartilaginous ventral part, the costal cartilage (Fig. 2.16A). The two parts meet at a costochondral junction. The dorsal part of the rib articulates with the vertebral column, whereas the cartilage articulates with the sternum either directly, as do the first eight or so sternal or "true" ribs, or indirectly through connection of the cartilage with that in front, as do the asternal or "false" ribs. In this way, the cartilages of the asternal ribs combine to form the costal arch (Fig. 2.17A/*6*), the cranial boundary of the flank. The cartilage of the last rib may fail to make contact with its neighbor, and this rib is then said to be "floating."

The dorsal extremity of the rib terminates in a rounded head that carries two facets, one for articulation with the body of each of the two vertebrae with which it is connected. These facets are separated by a rougher area (crest) that makes contact with the intervertebral disk and on most ribs also gives origin to the intercapital ligament. The head is joined to the body of the rib by a short constricted neck whose lower part carries a lateral tubercle. The tubercle bears a third articular facet, which meets that on the transverse process of the more caudal of the associated vertebrae (Fig. 2.16B).

The body of the rib begins beyond the tubercle. It is long, curved in its length, and usually laterally flattened, particularly in the larger species and toward the lower end. It is most strongly bent at a region known as the angle (Fig. 2.16/*4*), where the lateral surface is roughened for the attachment of the iliocostalis. The cranial and caudal margins of the body are often sharply defined and give attachment to the intercostal muscles that fill the space between successive ribs. The caudal margin may also be grooved to give protection to the neurovascular bundle of the intercostal space.

The costal cartilage is flexible in the young animal, especially if it is long and thin, as in the dog. It becomes more rigid as calcification develops and increases with age. The cartilage either meets the bony rib at an angle (knee, genu) or is itself flexed cranioventrally some way beyond the costochondral junction.

Serial changes are obvious. The first rib is always relatively strong, short, and straight. Its cartilage is also stumpy and articulates with the sternum at a tight joint that fixes the rib to create a firm base toward which the other ribs may be drawn on inspiration. The succeeding ribs increase in length, in curvature, and in caudoventral inclination, most markedly over the caudal part of the thoracic wall, although the very last two or three may be somewhat shorter. The three articular facets of the upper end approach and eventually merge on the ribs toward the end of the series. The cartilages of the sternal ribs are short and about as thick as the bony ribs; those of the asternal ribs are mostly slender and taper toward their ventral extremities.

The *sternum* is composed of three parts. The most cranial part, known as the manubrium (Fig. 2.17/*1*), generally projects in front of the first ribs and may be palpated at the root of the neck. It is rodlike in the dog and cat but

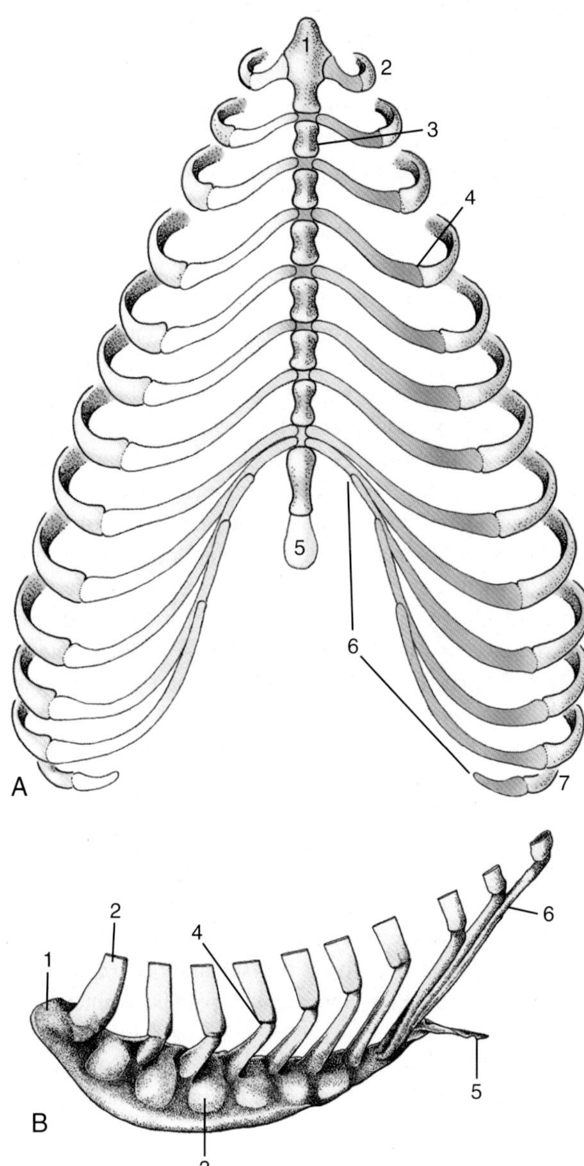

Fig. 2.17 (A) Canine and (B) equine sternum and costal cartilages, ventral and left lateral views. *1,* Manubrium; *2,* first rib; *3,* sternebra; *4,* costochondral junction; *5,* xiphoid cartilage; *6,* costal arch; *7,* floating rib.

is laterally compressed in the larger animals. The body of the bone is composed of several segments (sternebrae), in youth joined by cartilage that later ossifies. The sternum is cylindrical in the dog, is wide and flat in ruminants, and carries a ventral keel in the horse (Fig. 2.17B). Its dorsolateral margin bears a series of depressions that articulate with costal cartilages. The more cranial of these depressions alternate with the sternebrae, and each receives a single cartilage; the more caudal depressions are crowded more closely together and may receive more than one cartilage. The caudal part of the sternum consists of flat (xiphoid) cartilage (Fig. 2.17/*5*) that projects between the lower parts of the costal arches. It supports the most cranial part of the abdominal floor and gives attachment to the linea alba.

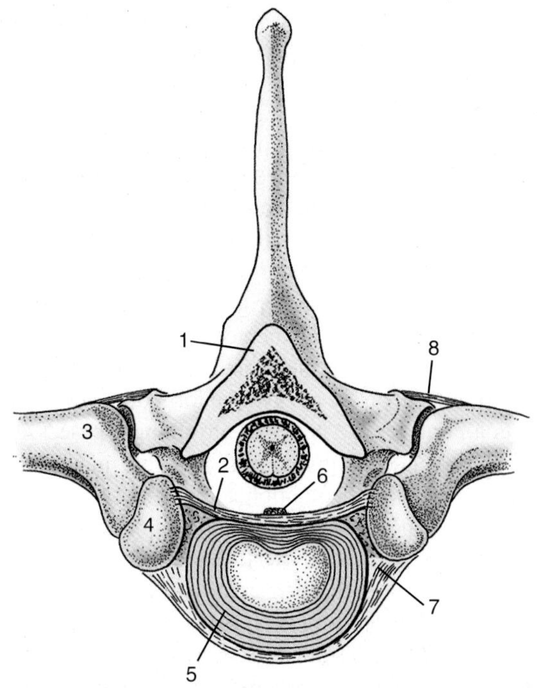

Fig. 2.18 Costovertebral articulations; transverse section of the vertebral column of the dog (about T8). *1,* Lamina of vertebra; *2,* intercapital ligament; *3,* tubercle of rib; *4,* head of rib; *5,* intervertebral disk; *6,* dorsal longitudinal ligament; *7,* costovertebral joint; *8,* costotransverse joint covered by costotransverse ligament.

The Joints of the Thoracic Wall

Most ribs make two separate articulations with the vertebral column. The head participates in a ball-and-socket *costovertebral joint* of unusually restricted mobility. The joint cavity is divided into two compartments by the intercapital ligament (Fig. 2.18/*2*), which arises from the interarticular crest. This ligament passes through the intervertebral foramen, crosses the floor of the vertebral canal, and ends by inserting on the corresponding region of the rib of the other side. In its passage, it detaches slips that anchor to the intervertebral disk and the adjacent parts of the vertebrae. It passes below the dorsal longitudinal ligament (Fig. 2.18/*6*) and offers some protection against nuclear material from protrusion of a ruptured disk into the vertebral canal. An intercapital ligament is not found at the first costovertebral joint or at the last few. Additional short and tight ligaments support the joint dorsally and ventrally.

The *costotransverse joint* in which the tubercle participates is of the sliding variety. It is supported by a ligament that passes between the neck of the rib and the transverse process of the vertebra (Fig. 2.18/*8*).

The *costosternal joints* are synovial joints of the pivot variety. The *interchondral joints* of the asternal ribs are syndesmoses of a rather elastic nature. The *intersternal joints* are mostly impermanent synchondroses, although in some species the manubrium articulates with the body at a synovial joint.

The movements possible at these joints are discussed with the actions of the muscles of the thoracic wall.

The Pelvic Girdle

Although the pelvic girdle is formally a part of the hindlimb skeleton, discussing it here seems more sensible because it is fully integrated into the construction of the trunk. The girdle consists of symmetrical halves, the hip bones (*ossa coxarum*), which meet at the pelvic symphysis ventrally and form firm, though not rigid, articulations with the sacrum dorsally. When augmented by the sacrum and first few tail vertebrae, the girdle forms a ring known as the *bony pelvis* around the pelvic cavity. The form of the bony pelvis reflects a compromise between physiologic processes, of which those related to giving birth are most important, and the requirements of locomotion and posture.

Each hip bone is composed of three bones that develop from separate ossifications within a single cartilage plate. The strips of cartilage that demarcate the boundaries between the bones to allow for growth disappear once growth is complete. It is therefore artificial to describe the three components—ilium, pubis, and ischium—as separate units. The ilium (Fig. 2.19/*1*) is the craniodorsal part that extends obliquely forward from the hip joint to articulate with the sacrum. The pubis (Fig. 2.19/*6*) extends medially from the joint to form the cranial part of the pelvic floor. The ischium (Fig. 2.19/*8*) is more caudal and forms the larger part of the floor, although it also sends a branch to the joint. Both pubis and ischium participate in the symphysial joint in domestic species, although only the pubis does so in the human pelvis.

The *ilium* consists of a cranial expansion or wing and a caudal shaft or body. The wing is oblong with a more or less sagittal orientation in the dog and cat but is triangular and almost vertical in the horse and ruminants (see Fig. 2.19). Its margin forms saliences, generally thickened, at certain points. Dorsally (dorsomedially in the larger species), it forms a sacral tuber that is reduced to two low (cranial and caudal dorsal iliac) spines in the dog and cat (Fig. 2.19/*3*) but is prominent in the large animals, in which it is close to the spinous processes of the vertebrae (Fig. 2.19/*3′*). Ventrally (ventrolaterally in the larger species), the ilium forms a coxal tuber (Fig. 2.19/*2′* and *2*) which is also reduced to low (cranial and caudal ventral iliac) spines in the carnivores but is prominent in large species, forming the point of the hip at the dorsocaudal corner of the flank (Fig. 2.20B/*8*). Including these projections, the margin of the wing is known as the *iliac crest*; thickened and convex in carnivores, it is thin and concave in large animals. Some of these features form important landmarks in the living animal.

The lateral (dorsolateral) surface is excavated and largely given over to the origin of the gluteus medius, whose attachment may raise one or more quite prominent ridges. The medial (ventromedial) surface faces toward the body cavity. The ventral part gives origin to the iliacus, whereas more dorsally it bears the roughened auricular articular surface for the sacrum (see Fig. 2.19B/*15*). The dorsal border of the wing at its junction with the shaft forms the greater sciatic notch (incisura; see Fig. 2.19/*4*), over which the sciatic nerve runs in passage to the hindlimb.

The shaft of the ilium is robust and columnar. Its caudal extremity contributes to the acetabulum, the deep cavity that receives the head of the femur. Its ventral border is marked by the low arcuate line that serves as part of the arbitrary boundary ("terminal line") between the abdominal and pelvic cavities. Except in the dog, the line carries the psoas tubercle midway along its length, where the psoas minor attaches.

The *pubis* (Fig. 2.19/*6*), essentially L-shaped, consists of cranial (acetabular) and caudal (symphysial) branches. The lateral end of the cranial branch contributes to the acetabulum and is known as the body. Its cranial edge, known as the pecten of the pubis, bears the iliopubic eminence and gives attachment to the abdominal muscles. Between them, the two branches account for about half the circumference of the obturator foramen (Fig. 2.19/*7*), the large opening in the pelvic floor through which the obturator nerve emerges. The foramen is closed by muscle and membrane in the fresh state.

The *ischium* (Fig. 2.19/*8*) is a horizontal plate extended cranially by symphysial and acetabular branches, one to each side of the obturator foramen. The extremity of the acetabular branch that contributes to the articular cup is known as the *body*. The body and the cranial part of this branch are surmounted by a crest, the ischial spine (Fig. 2.19/*5*), which also extends onto the caudal part of the ilium. Marked by the origin of the gluteus profundus, ischial spine is relatively low in the dog and particularly high in ruminants. The caudolateral corner of the plate forms the ischial tuber (Fig. 2.19/*9*); the border between this tuber and the spine is indented by the lesser sciatic notch (Fig. 2.19/*10*). The ischial tuber is a horizontal thickening in the dog and a conspicuously triangular swelling in cattle. In most species it is subcutaneous, and it may be a visible landmark. The remaining part of the caudal border forms with its fellow the ischial arch, a notch that is broad and, except in the horse, shallow.

The *acetabulum* is a deep articular cup to which all three bones contribute; an additional small acetabular bone may be found in young animals. The acetabulum is contained by a prominent rim that is interrupted by a notch caudoventrally. It carries a lunate articular surface internally, but the depth of the cup is nonarticular and rough.

The form of pelvic girdle differs among species. The larger and heavier species have a nearly vertical ilium that brings the sacroiliac joint, and therefore the weight of the trunk, more nearly above the hip joint (see Fig. 2.20B). In smaller species, the highly oblique ilium (see Fig. 2.1) displaces the pelvic floor caudally relative to the vertebral column and increases the effectiveness of the abdominal muscles that flex the column in bounding gaits. Caudal displacement of the ischial tuber also increases the leverage that may be exerted by the hamstring muscles that arise here.

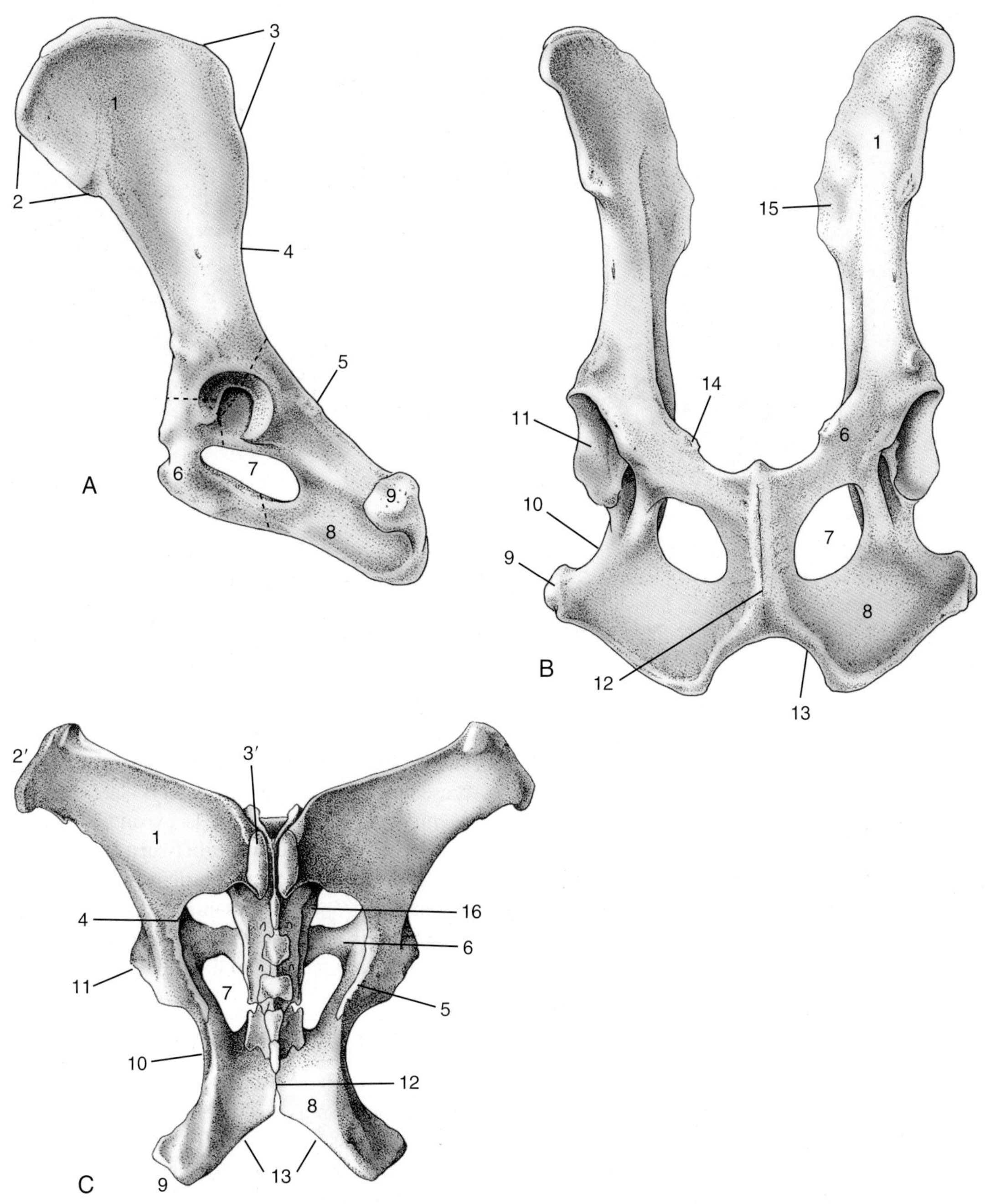

Fig. 2.19 Canine hip bones in left lateral (A) and ventral (B) views. (C) Dorsal view of equine pelvis. The broken lines give the approximate extents of ilium, pubis, and ischium. *1,* Wing of ilium; *2,* ventral iliac spines; *2′,* coxal tuber; *3,* dorsal iliac spines; *3′,* sacral tuber; *4,* greater sciatic notch; *5,* ischial spine; *6,* pubis; *7,* obturator foramen; *8,* ischium; *9,* ischial tuber; *10,* lesser sciatic notch; *11,* acetabulum; *12,* pelvic symphysis; *13,* ischial arch; *14,* iliopubic eminence; *15,* auricular articular surface; *16,* sacrum.

The dimensions of the girdle are most important in species that carry a single large offspring. They are of little significance in polytocous species (those that normally carry a litter), in which the full-term fetuses are relatively small. These aspects of pelvic conformation are discussed in later chapters.

The Joints and Ligaments of the Pelvic Girdle

The pelvic symphysis is a secondary cartilaginous joint that ossifies with advancing age. The process of ossification is irregular because it commences at different ages and advances at different rates, even in a single species. It usually starts earlier and is more advanced at any stage in the

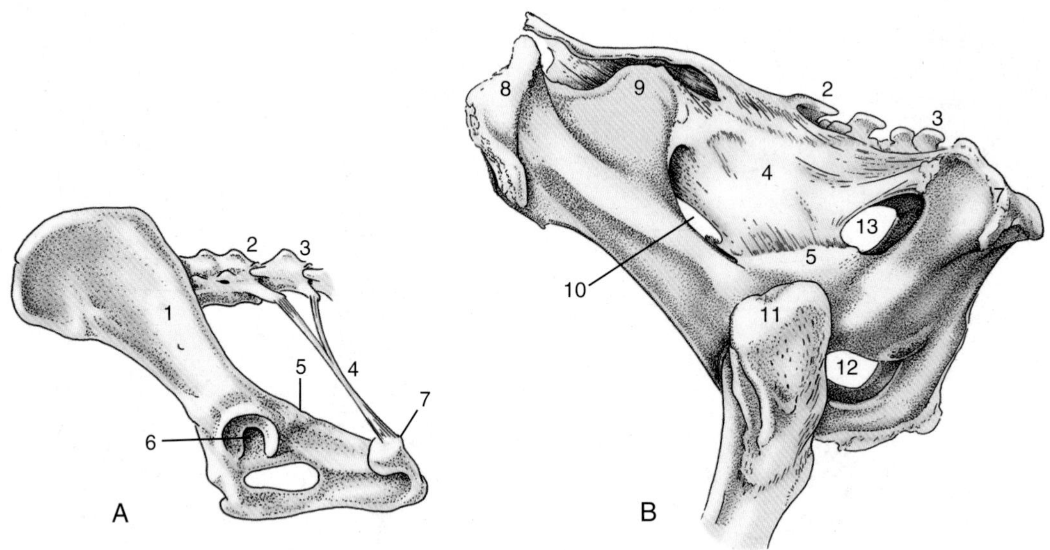

Fig. 2.20 Canine sacrotuberous ligament (A) and bovine sacrosciatic ligament (B), left lateral views. *1,* Ilium; *2,* sacrum; *3,* caudal vertebra(e); *4,* sacrotuberous ligament in A, sacrosciatic ligament in B; *5,* ischial spine; *6,* acetabulum; *7,* ischial tuber; *8,* coxal tuber; *9,* sacral tuber; *10,* greater sciatic foramen; *11,* greater trochanter; *12,* obturator foramen; *13,* lesser sciatic foramen.

pubic than in the ischial part. It is sometimes asserted that in certain domestic species changes can be detected in the tissues of the symphysis (and sacroiliac joint) in advance of parturition. These changes, if present, are minor in comparison with those that occur in guinea pigs and many other small animals at this time; in the latter animals, complete dissolution of the symphysis, which allows the two halves of the girdle to move apart to enlarge the birth passage, may occur.

The *sacroiliac joints* are curious in combining a synovial joint with an adjacent region of extensive fibrous union. The arrangement appears designed to combine firmness of attachment with some shock-absorbent capacity, because these joints are required to transmit the weight of the trunk to the hindlimbs during standing and the thrust of the limbs to the trunk during progression. The sacrum is wedged between the two halves of the pelvic girdle. Each sacral wing carries an articular surface that is broadly flat (but irregular in detail) to match the corresponding iliac surface. The joint capsule is tight and is surrounded and supported by short fascicles of connective tissue that join adjacent parts of the two bones. It is a matter of preference whether certain longer sacroiliac ligaments, at a greater distance from the synovial articulation, are to be regarded as components of that joint or as independent structures. They may include long and short dorsal ligaments passing between the wing of the ilium and the spinous processes and other features of the sacrum. A ventral ligament offers more immediate support to the joint.

The *sacrotuberous ligament* (Fig. 2.20/*4*) is of considerably greater interest. In the dog, it is a stout rounded cord extending between the caudolateral angle of the sacrum and the lateral part of the ischial tuber; no such ligament is present in the cat. In ungulates, it is better named the *sacrosciatic ligament* because it is expanded to a broad sheet that largely fills the space between the lateral border of the sacrum and the dorsal border of the ilium and ischium, which leaves open two foramina adjacent to the greater and lesser sciatic notches. The caudal edge is palpable in dogs and cattle (see p. 481 and p. 686).

The Muscles of the Trunk

The Cutaneous Muscle of the Trunk

The cutaneous muscle of the trunk (Fig. 2.21) varies in relative thickness and extent but generally covers the lateral aspect of the thorax and abdomen with fascicles with a predominately horizontal course. Contained with the superficial fascia, it tenses and twitches the skin. In some animals, detachments are associated with the prepuce, and in horses and cattle a separate lamella covers the shoulder and arm regions. The innervation comes from the brachial plexus.

The Muscles of the Vertebral Column

The muscles of the vertebral column can be separated into two divisions according to their position and innervation. The *epaxial division* (Fig. 2.22B/*12*) is dorsal to the line of the transverse processes of the vertebrae and receives its nerve supply from dorsal branches of the spinal nerves. The *hypaxial division* (Fig. 2.22/*14*), ventral to the transverse processes, is supplied by the ventral branches of these nerves. It includes the muscles of the thoracic and

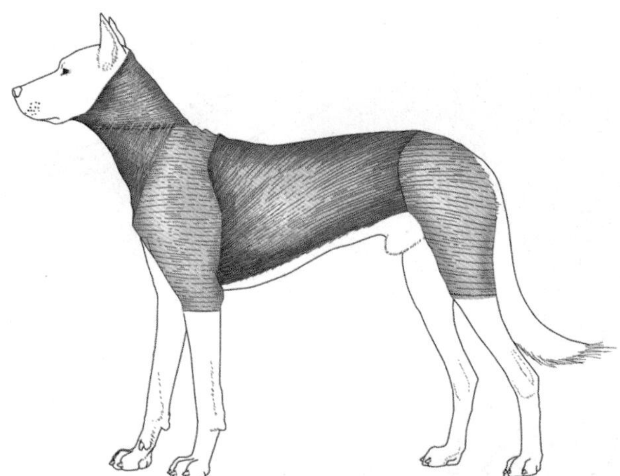

Fig. 2.21 The cutaneous muscle of the dog.

abdominal walls in addition to those placed closely on the vertebrae. The thoracic and abdominal muscles are considered in later sections.

The Epaxial Muscles. Although numerous and complicated, the epaxial muscles fortunately do not require detailed description because they are rarely of clinical importance, except in the dog (p. 398). The major muscles are arranged in three parallel columns (Fig. 2.22C/*19–21*), which show some tendency to fuse over the loins and to split into additional units in the neck. They are extensors of the vertebral column, locally or more generally according to their extent, and are relatively more powerful in animals that make use of a bounding gait when traveling at speed (e.g., the dog).

The *lateral column,* the *iliocostalis*, arises from the ilium and transverse processes of the lumbar vertebrae and inserts on the more cranial lumbar vertebrae and ribs with, in most species, a weaker continuation into the neck. It is composed of many fascicles that overlap and generally span about four vertebrae. Its lateral position also makes this column effective in bending the trunk to the side (Fig. 2.23B/*17*).

The *middle column,* the *longissimus* (Fig. 2.23/*16*), is strongest and can be followed into the neck and even to the head. Some of its more cranial parts are independent to a greater or lesser degree. The caudal attachments, which are the conventional origin, are from the ilium, the sacrum, and the mammillary processes, whereas the insertions are to the transverse processes and ribs. The fascicles thus pursue a cranial, lateral, and ventral course, and each bridges several vertebrae; the longest fascicles span the especially mobile thoracolumbar junction. Different parts may be designated longissimus lumborum, longissimus dorsi, longissimus cervicis, longissimus atlantis, and longissimus capitis, but usually the generic term is sufficient. The muscle tends to fuse with its medial and lateral neighbors in the lumbar region.

In addition to the more or less direct continuation, the cervical part of the longissimus is closely associated with

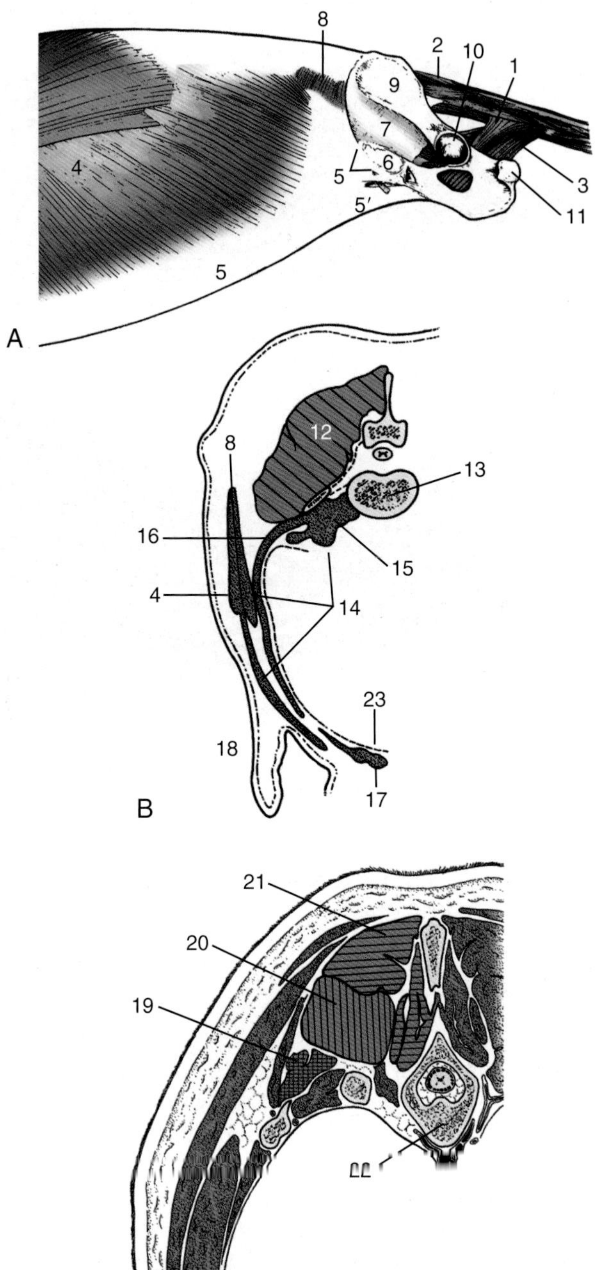

Fig. 2.22 (A) Trunk muscles of the dog, lateral view; the limbs have been removed. (B) Epaxial *(hatched)* and hypaxial *(stippled)* muscles shown in a transverse section of the lumbar region. (C) The three systems of epaxial muscles at the level of the thorax. *1,* Coccygeus; *2,* dorsal sacrocaudal; *3,* levator ani; *4,* external abdominal oblique; *5,* its aponeurosis, pelvic tendon, and inguinal ligament; *5′,* abdominal tendon; *6,* vascular lacuna; *7,* iliopsoas; *8,* internal abdominal oblique; *9,* wing of ilium; *10,* acetabulum; *11,* ischial tuber; *12,* epaxial muscles; *13,* lumbar vertebra—its transverse process appears as detached section; *14,* hypaxial muscles; *15,* psoas muscles; *16,* transverse abdominis; *17,* rectus abdominis; *18,* flank fold; *19,* iliocostalis system *(crosshatched)*; *20,* longissimus system *(vertically hatched)*; *21,* transversospinalis system *(horizontally hatched)*; *22,* thoracic vertebra and ribs; *23,* peritoneum.

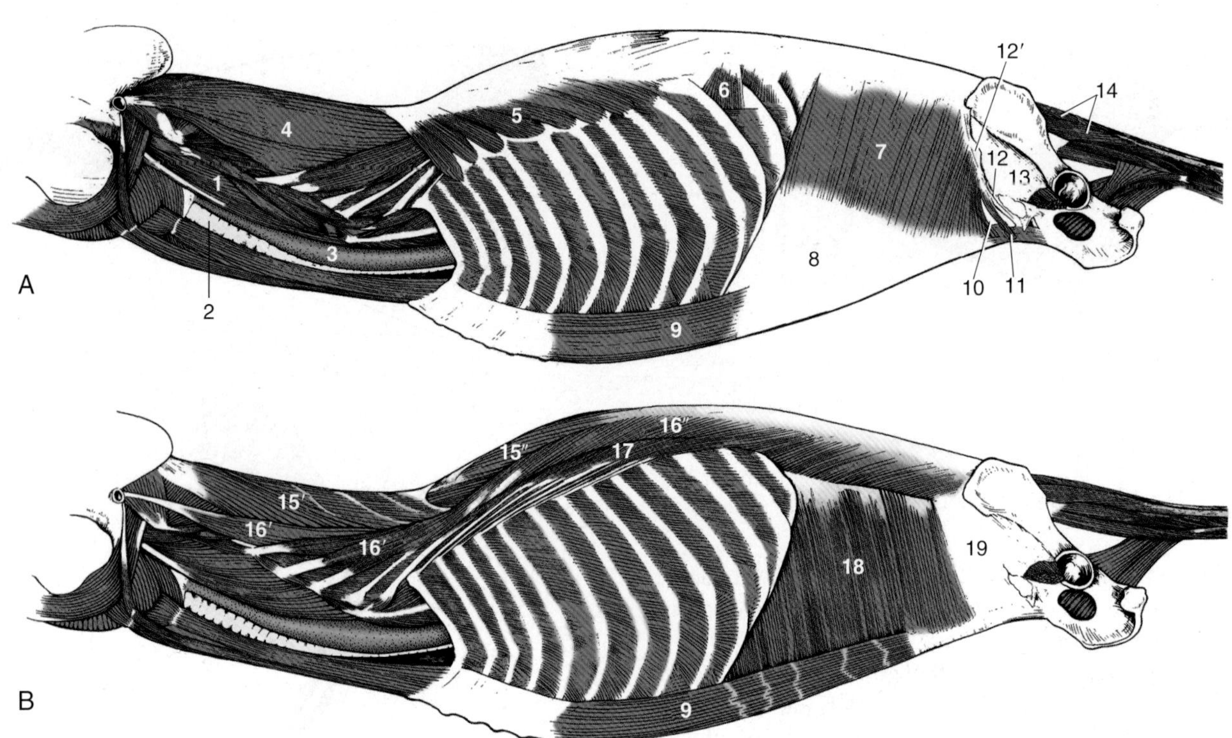

Fig. 2.23 (A) and (B) Trunk muscles of the dog, deeper layers. *1,* Longus capitis; *2,* trachea; *3,* esophagus; *4,* splenius; *5,* serratus dorsalis cranialis; *6,* serratus caudalis; *7,* internal abdominal oblique; *8,* its aponeurosis; *9,* rectus abdominis; *10,* caudal free border of internal abdominal oblique; *11,* cremaster; *12,* inguinal ligament; *12′,* external abdominal oblique aponeurosis, cut and reflected; *13,* fascia iliopsoas; *14,* dorsal sacrocaudal muscles; *15,* transversospinalis system; *15′,* semispinalis capitis; *15″,* spinalis et semispinalis; *16,* longissimus system; *16′,* longissimus capitis and longissimus cervicis; *16″,* longissimus thoracis; *17,* iliocostalis; *18,* transversus abdominis; *19,* transverse fascia.

the more superficial *splenius* (Fig. 2.23A/*4*). This muscle passes from the highest spines of the withers and thoracolumbar fascia to the occipitomastoid region of the skull. It is covered by certain muscles of the thoracic girdle, especially the trapezius and rhomboideus.

The longissimus complex also includes certain small muscles passing between adjacent transverse processes as well as the dorsal (sacrocaudal) muscles of the tail (Fig. 2.23/*14*); the latter are fleshy at their origin and are continued by tendons that run the length of the tail.

The *medial column,* the *transversospinalis system* (Fig. 2.24/*2*), is the most complex, and the number of discrete subunits varies among species. It lies on and between the medial parts of the vertebral arches and the spinous processes. Some fascicles run sagittally; others pursue a cranial, medial, and dorsal course from their caudal origin. The sagittal bundles include small units, often converted into ligaments, that pass between adjacent spinous processes as well as larger units that span several vertebrae. The oblique bundles run from mammillary to spinous processes and may be distinguished by name according to whether they span one, two, three, or more joints. The longest fascicles are again concentrated at the middle, most mobile region of the back.

A number of specialized units bridge the joints between the axis, the atlas, and the skull and are responsible for the special movements in this region. Those of the dog are briefly described later (p. 398).

The Hypaxial Muscles. The hypaxial muscles are flexor muscles of the neck or tail. The *longus colli* (Fig. 2.24/*9*) runs from the cranial thoracic region to the atlas, covering the ventral surfaces of the vertebral bodies. It has a complex organization, and most of its constituent bundles of varying orientation are relatively short and cross only a few joints. It is complemented by the *rectus capitis ventralis* (Fig. 2.24/*1*), which extends from the atlas to the ventral aspect of the skull, and the *longus capitis* (Fig. 2.24/*1*), which lies lateral to the longus colli and extends from the transverse processes of the midcervical vertebrae to the skull. The *scalenus* group occupies a similar position in relation to the caudal cervical vertebrae. It passes to the first one or few ribs, which it helps stabilize during inspiration. In some species the scalenus is readily divisible into dorsal, middle, and ventral parts.

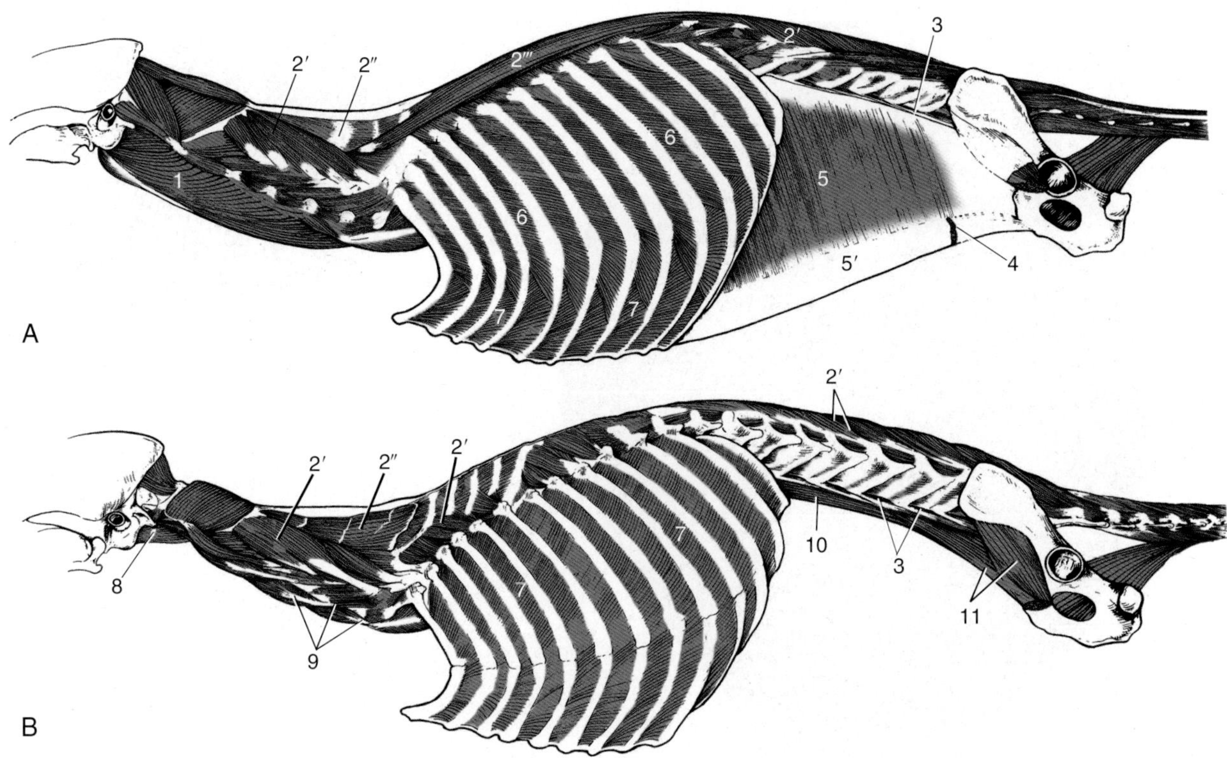

Fig. 2.24 (A) and (B) Trunk muscles of the dog, deepest layers. *1,* Longus capitis; *2,* transversospinalis system; 2′, multifidus; 2″, spinalis cervicis; *2‴,* spinalis et semispinalis; *3,* quadratus lumborum; *4,* rectus abdominis; *5,* transversus abdominis; *5′,* its aponeurosis; *6,* external intercostal muscles; *7,* internal intercostal muscles; *8,* rectus capitis ventralis; *9,* longus colli; *10,* psoas minor; *11,* iliopsoas (psoas major and iliacus).

The ventral muscles of the tail are close counterparts of the dorsal muscles.

The Muscles of the Thoracic Wall

The muscles of the thoracic wall are primarily concerned with respiration. Most are inspiratory and enlarge the thoracic cavity, causing air to flow into the lungs. Some are expiratory and diminish the cavity, expelling air. They comprise muscles that fill the spaces between the ribs, certain small units placed lateral to the ribs, and, by far the most important, the diaphragm.

The intercostal muscles are theoretically arranged in three layers that correspond to the layers of the abdominal wall. The *external intercostal* muscles are outermost (Fig. 2.24/*6*). Each of these muscles is confined to a single intercostal space in which its fibers run caudoventrally from one rib to the following rib. They fill the spaces from the upper ends to the costochondral junctions and sometimes beyond them but fail to reach the sternum. The parts between the cartilages are sometimes separately named. The *internal intercostal* muscles (Fig. 2.24/*7*) are placed more deeply within the intercostal spaces and run cranioventrally, approximately perpendicular to the course of the external muscles. They do not occupy the most dorsal parts of the spaces but do reach the margin of the sternum. The third (subcostal) layer is so weak and so inconsistently developed that it may be ignored. The *transversus thoracis* is a triangular sheet that arises from and covers the dorsal surface of the sternum. The apex points cranially, and the muscle splits into slips that run caudolaterally to insert on the sternal ribs close to the costochondral junctions. It is morphologically the equivalent of the ventral part of the transversus abdominis.

Two muscles lie on the lateral surface of the thoracic wall. The *rectus thoracis* is a small quadrilateral sheet placed over the lower ends of the first four ribs in apparent continuation of the rectus abdominis. The *serratus dorsalis* (Fig. 2.23A/*5* and *6*) lies over the dorsal parts of the ribs. It takes origin from the fascia of the back and inserts on the ribs by a series of slips. The slips of the cranial part of the muscle slope caudoventrally, and those of the caudal part slope cranioventrally, a difference that points to antagonistic functions. The two parts are sometimes quite widely separated. The *scalenus,* mentioned in the preceding section, has an attachment to the first rib; in some species it also passes quite extensively over the rib cage.

The *diaphragm* separates the thoracic and abdominal cavities. It is dome-shaped, being convex in all directions on its cranial surface, and bulges cranially under cover of the ribs to enlarge the abdomen at the expense of the

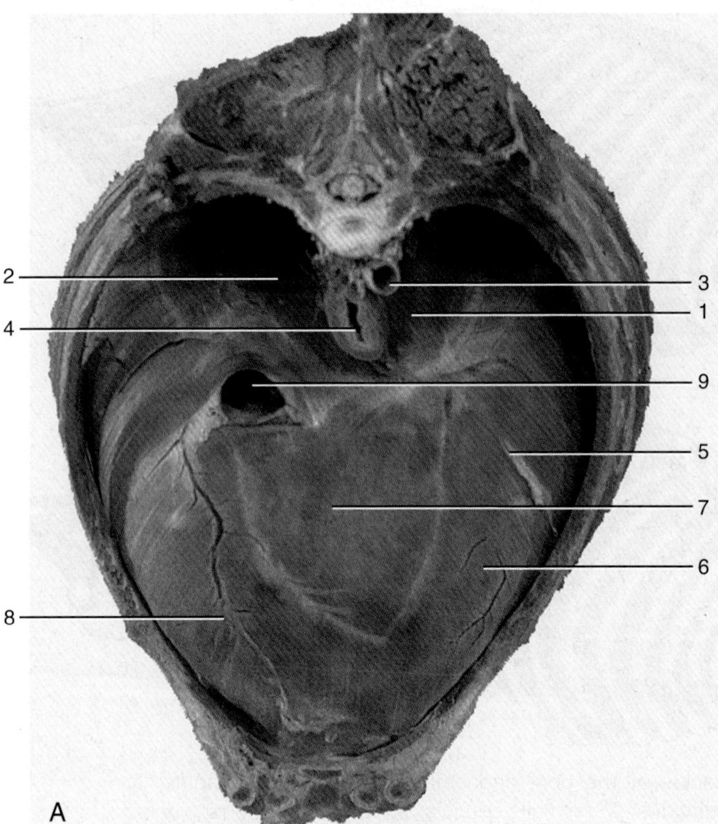

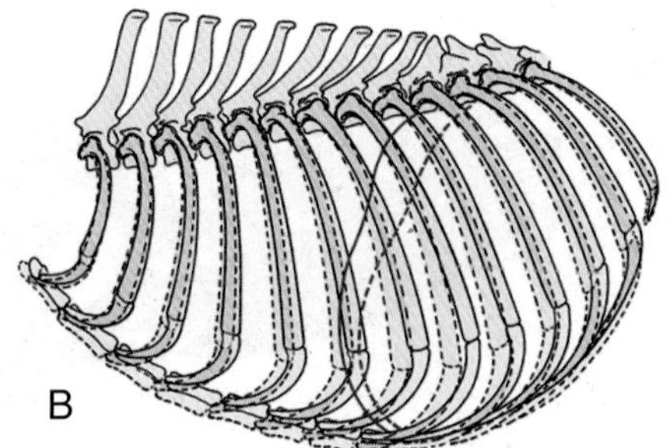

Fig. 2.25 A, Cranial view, preserved specimen, of the canine diaphragm. *1,* Left crus; *2,* right crus; *3,* aorta; *4,* esophagus; *5,* attachment of caudal mediastinum to diaphragm; *6,* sternal and costal parts of diaphragm; *7,* tendinous center; *8,* attachment of plica venae cavae; *9,* caudal vena cava. (B) Lateral view diagram of the canine thorax showing ribs and cranial extent of diaphragm in inspiration *(broken lines)* and expiration *(solid lines).*

thoracic cavity (Figs. 2.2 and 2.25A). It consists of a heart-shaped (trefoil-shaped in the dog) central tendon (Fig. 2.25/*7*) and a muscular periphery that is divisible into portions that arise from the lumbar vertebrae, the caudal ribs, and the sternum.

The central tendon, the most cranial part, forms the vertex. In the neutral position between full inspiration and full expiration, this tendon reaches the level of the lower part of the sixth rib (or following space) and is thus only a little behind the plane of the olecranon in an animal standing square. Knowledge of this fact and of the line of the costal attachment is indispensable in appreciating the extent of the thoracic cavity (Fig. 2.25B).

The powerful lumbar portion of the peripheral muscle consists of left and right crura (Fig. 2.25/*1* and *2*) that arise from the ventral aspect of the first three or four lumbar vertebrae by means of stout tendons. The right crus is considerably the larger, and it divides into three branches that radiate ventrally to join the central tendon. The left crus is undivided.

The origin of the thinner costal part is from the inner surfaces of the ribs and costal cartilages. Although the most caudal, also most dorsal slip, arises close to the dorsal end of the last rib, the cranial slips arise at successively more ventral levels with the last costal digitation following the cartilage of the eighth rib to the sternum. A final sternal slip arises from the dorsal surface of the sternum and runs dorsally to meet the tendon, which is thus bordered by muscle on all sides.

The diaphragm has three openings called the *aortic hiatus,* the *esophageal hiatus,* and the *caval foramen* (Fig. 2.25). These diaphragmatic openings transmit various structures.

The diaphragm is supplied by the *phrenic nerves* formed from contributions by ventral branches of caudal cervical nerves (usually C5–C7). Despite the apparently involuntary nature of breathing, the phrenic nerves are ordinary somatic nerves of mixed composition. The other muscles of the chest wall are supplied by intercostal nerves (ventral branches of thoracic spinal nerves).

Functional Considerations. The form and construction of the thorax represent a compromise between the requirements of posture and locomotion and the more specialized needs of respiration. In most domestic mammals the advantages of a barrel-shaped thorax for respiration are largely sacrificed to the easier movement allowed to the scapulae by flattening of the cranial part of the rib cage. The potential for movement of the cranial ribs is also reduced in favor of the more rigid construction that provides a stable origin for the muscles that pass between the trunk and the forelimbs.

Respiration causes changes in the form of the caudal part of the rib cage and abdomen. All species exhibit both costal and abdominal (i.e., diaphragmatic) modes of breathing, but their relative importance varies with the species, with the prevailing circumstances, and with the individual. It is certainly safe to conclude that normal respiration is always accompanied by contraction of the diaphragm, whereas involvement of the intercostal and other accessory respiratory muscles is less certain.

The diaphragm contracts against the resistance of the abdominal viscera, which must be displaced caudally into space provided by relaxation of the abdominal floor and flanks. In the course of this movement the central part of the dome of the diaphragm shifts backward, perhaps half a vertebral length in quiet breathing, while additional thoracic enlargement is obtained through flattening of diaphragm's peripheral parts. The attachment of liver to diaphragm also acts as a piston during fast locomotion to flatten parts of the caudal lobes of the lungs. Contraction of the sternocostal parts of the diaphragm, which attach to the last ribs, tends to pull these ribs inward in opposition to the outward and forward pull exerted on them by the intercostal muscles. It is a common observation (easily confirmed by watching a sleeping dog) that the last rib may actually be tucked inward during inspiration while its more cranial fellows move outward to broaden the thorax.

The actual movements undertaken by the ribs and the forces that produce them are controversial. The caudal inclination of the lower part of the rib (before it is turned forward by the cartilage) results in a movement by the rib that is compared to raising a bucket handle. Although there is dispute regarding the mechanisms of engagement of articular surfaces during rib movement, it is clear that the overall effect is to widen while shortening the rib cage. In humans and some quadrupeds (including the dog), a concurrent ventral displacement of the sternum occurs.

A considerable number of the muscles attaching to the ribs and sternum appear from their geometry to be capable of producing the necessary movements. However, human studies show that little of this potential is actually employed in quiet breathing. During inspiration the external intercostals and the interchondral parts of the internal intercostals are most consistently engaged. The scalenus (and possibly also muscles that pass forward from the manubrium) may assist in fixing the thoracic inlet. Expiration is mainly passive, and the elastic recoil of the lungs is the major force. The muscles of the abdominal wall may contract to reinforce the passive tension in the tendinous parts that raises the viscera and that indirectly helps to restore the diaphragm to its former position. Sometimes the deeper layer of intercostal muscle—the interosseous parts of the internal intercostals and the transversus thoracis—is also engaged.

Contrary to common belief, the diaphragm is not indispensable. Evidence obtained from experimental and clinical subjects (dogs and ruminants) shows that section or paralysis of both phrenic nerves caused little obvious loss of respiratory efficiency even under moderate stress. This evidence of course does not deny the diaphragm the major role in normal animals but does confirm both the presence of an ample reserve of inspiratory muscle and the role of the mechanical function of the abdominal viscera in respiration.

The Muscles of the Abdominal Wall

The muscles of the abdominal wall are conveniently divided into ventrolateral and dorsal (sublumbar) groups (Fig. 2.22B). The first comprises the muscles of the flanks and abdominal floor, which are important because they are incised in almost all surgical approaches to the abdomen. Most muscles of the second group properly belong to the girdle division of hindlimb musculature. They are included here because they constitute part of the body wall—namely, the roof of the abdomen to each side of the vertebral column.

The Ventrolateral Group. The intrinsic musculature of the flank comprises three broad fleshy sheets superimposed on each other with contrasting orientation of their fibers. Each is continued ventrally by an aponeurotic tendon that principally inserts within a fibrous cord, the linea alba, which runs in the ventral midline from the xiphoid cartilage to the cranial end of the pelvic symphysis (via the prepubic tendon). In so doing, the tendons ensheath the fourth muscle, the rectus abdominis, which pursues a sagittal course within the abdominal floor directly to the side of the linea alba. The following account is of the basic arrangement. The details vary among species and may have surgical importance, especially in the small species (Fig. 2.26; see also pp. 419–420).

The outermost *external abdominal oblique* muscle (Fig. 2.22/*4*) arises from the lateral surfaces of the ribs and from the lumbar fascia. The majority of its fibers runs caudoventrally, but the most dorsal bundles follow a more horizontal course. The aponeurosis (Fig. 2.22/*5*) that succeeds the fleshy part divides into two parts (tendons) before its insertion. The larger abdominal tendon terminates on the linea alba after passing ventral to the rectus muscle; the smaller pelvic tendon proceeds to attach on the fascia over the iliopsoas and on the pubic brim lateral to the insertion of the rectus (Fig. 2.27/*3′* and *4*).

The second muscle, the *internal abdominal oblique* (Fig. 2.23/*7*), arises mainly from the coxal tuber (or the equivalent region of the ilium) but to lesser extents from

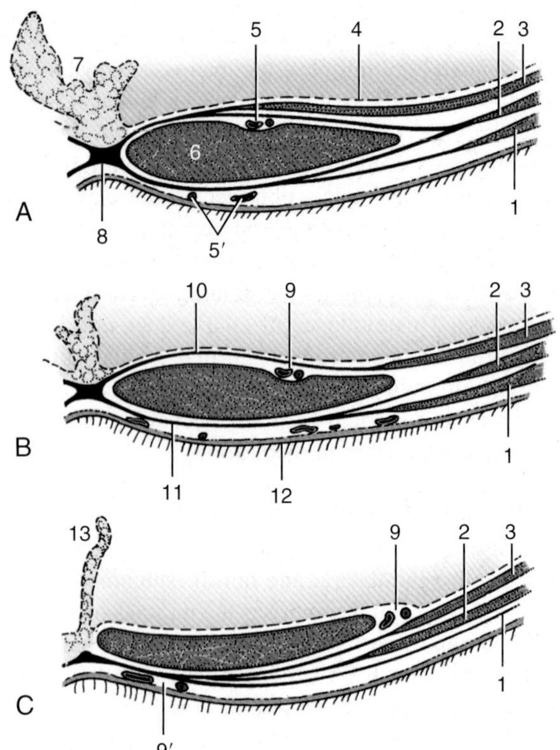

Fig. 2.26 Rectus sheath of the dog in transverse sections from (A) cranial and (B) caudal to the umbilicus and (C) near the pubis. *1,* External abdominal oblique; *2,* internal abdominal oblique; *3,* transversus abdominis; *4,* peritoneum; *5,* cranial epigastric vessels; *5′,* cranial superficial epigastric vessels; *6,* rectus abdominis; *7,* fat-filled falciform ligament; *8,* linea alba; *9,* caudal epigastric vessels; *9′,* caudal superficial epigastric vessels; *10,* internal lamina of rectus sheath; *11,* external lamina of rectus sheath; *12,* skin; *13,* median ligament of the bladder.

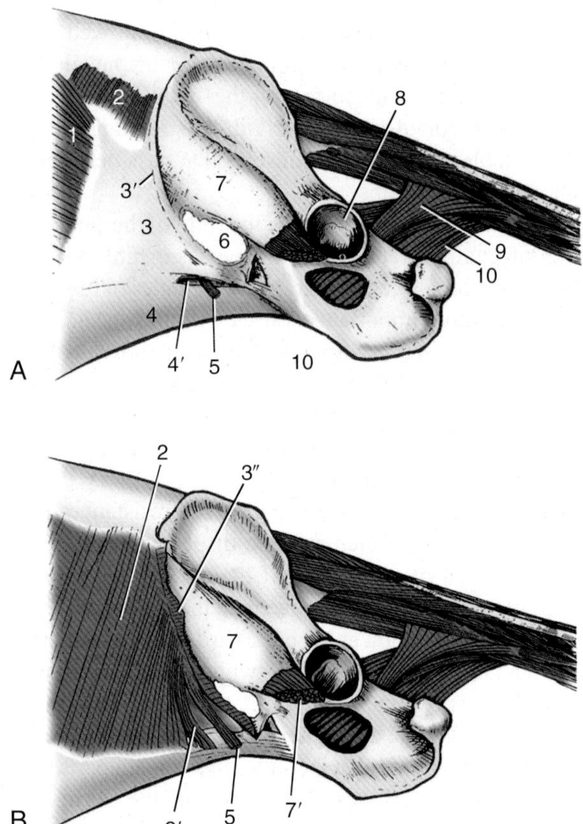

Fig. 2.27 Inguinal canal and pelvic diaphragm of the dog, left lateral view. The external abdominal oblique muscle, present in A, has been removed in B. *1,* External abdominal oblique; *2,* internal abdominal oblique; *2′,* free caudal edge of internal oblique, forming border of deep inguinal ring; *3,* pelvic tendon of external oblique aponeurosis; *3′,* caudal border of 3 (inguinal ligament) ending on 7; *3″,* stump of external oblique aponeurosis reflected caudally (B); *4,* abdominal tendon of external oblique aponeurosis; *4′,* superficial inguinal ring; *5,* cremaster derived from internal oblique; *6,* vascular lacuna; *7,* iliac fascia covering iliopsoas; *7′,* iliopsoas; *8,* acetabulum; *9,* coccygeus; *10,* levator ani.

the insertion of the pelvic tendon of the external oblique, the thoracolumbar fascia, and the tips of the lumbar transverse processes. This muscle fans out more obviously: its most caudal fascicles pass ventrocaudally, and although the next group runs more or less transversely in the plane of the coxal tuber, most pass ventrocranially. Some cranial fascicles insert directly on the last rib, but the bulk are continued by an aponeurosis (Fig. 2.23/*8*) that passes ventral to the rectus to reach the linea alba. Toward the midline some interchange of fibers between the aponeuroses of the two oblique muscles usually occurs. The origin from the pelvic tendon allows the muscle a free caudal edge (Fig. 2.23/*10*), which is mentioned again shortly in connection with the inguinal canal. A caudal slip (cremaster; Fig. 2.23/*11*) detached from the internal oblique passes onto the spermatic cord (p. 179).

The deepest muscle of the flank, the *transversus abdominis* (Fig. 2.24/*5*), arises from the inner surfaces of the last ribs and the transverse processes of the lumbar vertebrae. Its fibers run more or less transversely and are succeeded by an aponeurosis (Fig. 2.24/*5′*) that passes dorsal to the rectus abdominis before terminating on the linea alba. This muscle does not extend caudal to the coxal tuber. The caudal part of the tendon passes ventral to the rectus so that the most caudal part of that muscle is left uncovered dorsally.

The fourth muscle, the *rectus abdominis* (Fig. 2.23/*9*), forms a broad band to the side of the linea alba in the abdominal floor. It arises from the ventral surfaces of the rib cartilages and sternum and inserts on the pubic brim by means of a prepubic tendon. The fleshy part, which is widest about the middle of the abdomen, is divided into a series of segments by irregular transverse septa (tendinous intersections) that recall its polysegmental origin. The prepubic tendon serves as a common insertion for the abdominal muscles and the linea alba and may incorporate part of the tendons of origin of adductor (pectineus and gracilis) muscles of the thigh.

The *rectus sheath* (vagina musculi recti abdominis), the arrangement of the aponeurotic tendons of the flank muscles about the rectus abdominis, varies in detail among species. In the basic arrangement, the tendons of the two oblique muscles form a layer on the external (ventral) surface of the rectus, whereas that of the transversus lies against the internal surface; both layers merge with the linea alba to complete the enclosure (see Fig. 2.26 and p. 420).

The abdominal wall is perforated in the region of the groin by the inguinal canal (Figs. 2.27 and 21.5). Before or shortly after birth this canal transmits the testis in its descent toward the scrotum. In the adult male it contains the spermatic cord, consisting of the duct from the testis, and associated structures within an outpouching of the peritoneum. In both sexes, it also transmits the external pudendal artery and (usually) vein, efferent vessels from the superficial inguinal lymph nodes, and the genitofemoral nerve, all structures associated with the groin.

The term *canal* is misleading because it suggests a roomier passage than actually exists. The canal is a potential flat space between the fleshy part of the internal oblique on the one side and the pelvic tendon of the external oblique aponeurosis on the other (Fig. 2.27/*2* and *3*). The walls are apposed and joined by areolar tissue except where the transmitted structures hold them apart. The slitlike abdominal entrance to the canal (the deep inguinal ring) lies along the free caudal edge of the internal oblique muscle (Fig. 2.27/*2'*). The exit from the canal (the superficial inguinal ring; Fig. 2.27/*4'*) is contained between the two divisions of the external oblique tendon. (The edges of the superficial inguinal ring are known as medial and lateral crura.) Species differences are mentioned in later chapters and may be of great importance because some explain why the escape of organs into and through the canal (inguinal hernia) occurs more readily in certain animals. Other differences are of immediate relevance to surgery in this area, most obviously in connection with castration, whether of the normal male or of one in which the testis has failed to descend and remains hidden within the abdomen or within the canal itself (cryptorchidism).

Functional Considerations. Observation and palpation suggest that animals standing quietly make little active use of the abdominal muscles in support of the viscera; the support is obtained from passive tension. Some electromyographic studies have revealed slight though continuous activity in the internal oblique and sporadic bursts in other muscles of the flank. Greater, and more pronounced in labored breathing, activity of the abdominal muscles may occur toward the end of quiet expiration to assist the forward recovery of the diaphragm.

When the abdominal muscles are contracted against a fixed diaphragm, the animal is said to "strain." The resulting increase in intraabdominal pressure reinforces the efforts of visceral muscle to expel urine, feces, or a fetus. The use made of straining varies with the species and conditions. Those animals that adopt a squatting posture for micturition (e.g., goat) or defecation (e.g., dog) obviously make more use of the abdominal muscles to assist expulsion.

The rigidity of the abdominal wall produced by contraction of these muscles may be used to protect the viscera during palpation in an animal with abdominal visceral pain. This defense is used by a nervous dog when efforts, particularly if unskillful, are made to palpate its abdomen; gentle massage may be necessary to allay the fear before the muscles relax.

These muscles are also used in the adjustment of posture and in progression. Acting unilaterally, the muscles of the flank bend the trunk to that side. Acting bilaterally, they may assist in arching the back, which is a movement of great importance in bounding gaits.

The ventrolateral abdominal muscles are supplied by caudal intercostal nerves and the ventral branches of the lumbar nerves, particularly those more cranial in the series.

The Sublumbar Muscles. The *psoas minor* (Fig. 2.24/*10*) arises from the bodies of the thoracolumbar vertebrae and inserts on the psoas minor tubercle on the ilium. Much tendon is intermingled in the flesh, supporting the contention that the muscle is probably employed mainly to stabilize the vertebral column. It may also rotate the pelvis at the sacroiliac joint.

The *psoas major* and *iliacus* muscles may be regarded as vertebral and pelvic heads of a single muscle (iliopsoas; Fig. 2.24/*11*) that terminates on the lesser trochanter of the femur. The psoas major arises from the bodies and ventral surfaces of the transverse processes of the lumbar vertebrae lateral to the psoas minor. The iliacus arises from the ventral aspect of the wing and shaft of the ilium. The tendons of the two heads combine shortly before insertion. The iliopsoas is a flexor of the hip and an outward rotator of the thigh. The psoas head probably also contributes to the stability of the vertebral column.

The *quadratus lumborum* (Fig. 2.24/*3*) arises from the last ribs and from the transverse processes of the lumbar vertebrae and inserts on the wing of the sacrum (sometimes also on the ilium). It stabilizes the lumbar portion of the vertebral column.

These muscles are principally innervated by direct twigs from the ventral branches of the last few thoracic and the lumbar nerves. Other twigs detach from named branches of the lumbosacral plexus, principally the femoral nerve.

The Muscles of the Pelvic Outlet

The pelvic outlet is closed about the terminal parts of the digestive and urogenital tracts by a portion of the body wall known as the *perineum*. The projection of the perineum on the skin outlines the perineal region, the principal features of which are the anus and the vulva (in the female, to which we principally refer here). Because the ventral part of the vulva falls below the level of the pelvic floor, it is usual to enlarge the concept of the perineal region to embrace the whole vulva. Very often the dorsocaudal part of the udder (in animals such as the cow) is also included. Several muscles and fasciae interlace in a node between the anus and the vulva and vestibule, and this formation is properly known as the perineal body or center; however, in clinical, especially obstetric, literature the perineal body is frequently known simply, though incorrectly, as "the perineum." The three concepts—perineum, perineal region, and perineal body—should be kept distinct. Another potential source of confusion exists. In human anatomy, the structures that occupy the pelvic outlet are said to form a "floor" to the pelvic cavity. In quadrupeds, the "floor" is provided by the pelvic girdle. The difference in posture not only affects the appropriate use of vernacular terms but, more important, also modifies the function of homologous structures. The principal component of the dorsal part of the perineum is the *pelvic diaphragm*, an arrangement of striated muscles contained between fasciae, which closes about the anorectal junction. A similar but less conspicuous arrangement in the ventral part of the perineum, the urogenital diaphragm, closes about the vestibule.

The *pelvic diaphragm* attaches laterally to the pelvic wall and spreads caudomedially to close about the anal canal. The term *diaphragm* aptly describes the human arrangement, which forms a basin in which the pelvic organs rest. It is less appropriate in domestic species, in which the "halves" of the diaphragm have more sagittal courses and converge more gently on the anus, as a result of the relatively greater length of the pelvic girdle.

The more lateral of the two muscles of the diaphragm, the *coccygeus* (Fig. 2.27/*9*), is essentially a muscle of the tail. Rhomboidal in outline, it arises from the ischial spine, crosses the sacrotuberous ligament medially, and inserts on and about the transverse processes of the first few tail vertebrae.

The medial, thinner, and more extensive muscle, the *levator ani,* runs more obliquely in a dorsocaudal direction and is only partly covered by the coccygeus. The two muscles arise close together or by a common tendon in ungulates. In the dog, the levator has a more widely spread origin that continues from the iliac shaft over the cranial ramus of the pubis to follow the pelvic symphysis (Fig. 2.27/*10*). The insertion is divided between the fascia and vertebrae of the tail (extending distal to the insertion of the coccygeus) and the fascia about the anus and external anal sphincter. The tail attachment predominates in carnivores, the anal one in ungulates, in which considerable exchange of fascicles with the anal sphincter and constrictor vestibuli muscles occurs.

The coccygeus flexes the tail laterally or, when acting in concert with its fellow, draws the tail ventrally to cover the perineum, an attitude familiar in the nervous dog. The action of the levator is best known from an electromyographic study in the goat, and it is possible that important species differences exist. In the goat the muscle is active whenever the intra-abdominal pressure is raised, presumably to oppose the tendency to displace pelvic organs caudally. Although also involved in other visceral functions, it has a very definite relationship to defecation; it is active before the event (when it may fix the position of the anus against the contraction of the smooth muscle of the colon), becomes inactive during the event, and regains activity following the event (when it may restore the parts to their resting positions). The jerky movements of the dog's tail after defecation are probably evidence of levator activity in this species. Both muscles are supplied by ventral branches of the sacral nerves.

The smaller *urogenital diaphragm* (membrana perinei) contains more slender muscles, which are more appropriately described later with the reproductive organs. The fascia of the urogenital diaphragm attaches to the ischial arch and curves cranially, dorsally, and medially to blend with the ventral edge of the pelvic diaphragm and embrace the vestibule. It helps anchor the reproductive tract against a forward drag when the pregnant uterus sinks within the abdomen and against a backward displacement during parturition.

It may now be evident that to each side there is a space that is enclosed by the pelvic girdle but is excluded from the pelvic cavity by the pelvic diaphragm. This space is pyramidal and has a cranial apex, a lateral wall furnished by the ischial tuber and sacrotuberous ligament, a medial wall furnished by the pelvic diaphragm, a ventral wall furnished by the pelvic floor, and a base directed toward the skin. Appropriately known as the *ischiorectal fossa,* this space is normally occupied by fat (see Fig. 29.10/*12*). When this fat is depleted, a pronounced sinking of the skin to the side of the anus is apparent (except in the horse and pig, in which the vertebral head of the semimembranosus covers the region).

THE HEAD AND VENTRAL PART OF THE NECK

Basic Plan and Development

Even a cursory examination of the head, intact or in sagittal section, shows that it consists of two principal parts. One, the neural part, comprises the brain together with the encasing structures; the other, the facial part, is much larger in most adult mammals and is formed by the jaws and the initial parts of the respiratory and digestive systems. The distinction between neural and facial parts is already plain in embryos at the somite stage (Fig. 2.28).

At this stage of development the dorsal structures predominate, and the size and form of the head are largely determined by the brain.

The neural part (cranium) of the skull has its primordium in a series of cartilages that form ventral to the brain and are supplemented by cartilaginous capsules enclosing the primitive olfactory organs, eyeballs, and labyrinths of the ears. Later, "dermal bones" appear by ossification within the membrane that covers the brain to the sides and above; ultimately, all of these elements fuse with one another and with the bones of the face.

The ventral part of the head—the future face—is much smaller and at this stage blends smoothly with the neck, which is largely occupied by the heart. This ventral part exhibits a quite different pattern of segmentation imposed by the pharyngeal arches, which are serial thickenings of the unsplit mesoderm lateral and ventral to the rostral part of the foregut that becomes the pharynx.

The formation, significance, and detailed fate of these arches is not described here; at present it is sufficient to recall that a cartilaginous skeleton with associated musculature innervated by a specific cranial nerve develops within the core of each arch. Each arch is also supplied by an arterial loop connecting the ventral aorta to the dorsal aorta. The structures formed within the various pharyngeal arches are listed in Table 2.1; from this list it can be seen that the cartilaginous parts ultimately make only a small contribution to the skeleton of the face. The definitive facial skeleton is provided mainly by dermal bones formed in the connective tissue of the jaws, although certain elements for a time obtain support from cartilaginous precursors such as the cartilage of the first arch and the nasal capsule.

In most mammals the facial part enlarges disproportionately and comes to lie as much before as below the brain.

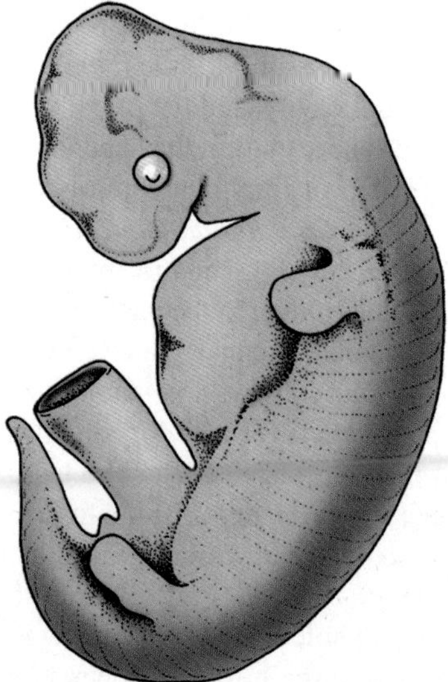

Fig. 2.28 Pig embryo (1.5 cm) to show dominance of the neural over the facial part of the head at this stage.

Despite many qualitative and quantitative differences the basic arrangement is the same in all species. The relationships and topography of the major organs and cavities of the head should be studied before one passes on to more detailed matters. Figs. 4.2 and 4.3 provide the necessary information.

The Skull

The complete skeleton of the head comprises the skull,* the mandible or lower jawbone, the hyoid apparatus, the ossicles of the middle ear, and the cartilages of the external ear, nose, and larynx.

The *skull* (in the narrower sense) is a mosaic of many bones, mostly paired but some median and unpaired, that fit closely together to form a single rigid construction. The separate elements, which are named individually, develop from independent centers of ossification and have, for the most part, well-established homologies. In the young animal they are separated from each other by narrow strips of fibrous tissue—cartilage in a few situations—and this pattern of joints or sutures provides for growth. Once growth has ceased, ossification extends into the connective tissue, finally welding the bones together. This process is drawn out, and it may never be completed; the outlines of most bones are therefore discernible, even in skulls of old animals. Acquaintance with the names, positions, and approximate extents of the individual bones (Fig. 2.29) is essential as it provides a useful system of reference to regions of the head, but a detailed knowledge of the disarticulated units has little practical value.

Conventional descriptions are based on the views obtained from various directions with the skull resting on a flat surface. In most views the two distinct portions of the skull are immediately apparent: the caudal part encasing the brain and the rostral part supporting the face. The orbits, the fossae containing the eyeballs, are part of the face but lie at the boundary. In most domestic animals the facial part of the skull is larger than the neural part and is situated mainly in front of this. However, the ratio varies among species and also with breed, age, and individual conformation. The many particular differences make it impossible to provide even a general description of the skull that is valid for all species.

The Skull of the Dog

This initial account is of the skull of an adult dog of average (mesaticephalic) conformation, neither short-headed (brachycephalic) like a Pekingese nor long-headed

*This term is sometimes used elsewhere in a wider sense to include the mandible and even the hyoid apparatus. Because contemporary practice is inconsistent, a writer's intention must often be deduced from the context.

TABLE 2.1 **DERIVATIVES OF THE PHARYNGEAL ARCHES**

Pharyngeal Arch	Skeleton	Muscles	Motor Innervation
First (mandibular)	Mandible (in part); certain ear ossicles (malleus and incus)	Muscles of mastication; mylohyoideus; digastricus (in part); tensor veli palatini; tensor tympani	Mandibular division of trigeminal nerve (V3)
Second (hyoid)	Hyoid apparatus (in part); ear ossicles (stapes)	Muscles of facial expression; digastricus (in part); stapedius	Facial nerve (VII)
Third	Hyoid apparatus (remaining part)	Stylopharyngeus caudalis; possibly other pharyngeal muscles	Glossopharyngeal nerve (IX)
Fourth (and subsequent arches)	Most laryngeal cartilages	Pharyngeal and laryngeal muscles; muscles of accessory nerve field	Vagus nerve (X); (medullary) part of accessory nerve (XI)

(dolichocephalic) like a Borzoi. Some salient breed differences are mentioned later (p. 359).

In the *dorsal view* (Fig. 2.30), the ovoid cranium meets the bones of the face where the zygomatic processes (Fig. 2.30/*4'*) of the frontal bones project laterally to form the dorsocaudal parts of the orbital walls. The caudal extremity of the cranium is marked by the external occipital protuberance in the midline, and its demarcation from the caudal (nuchal) surface is completed by the nuchal crests that extend laterally to each side. The median sagittal crest that extends forward from the occipital protuberance is most prominent in robust, well-muscled animals. All these features are easily palpated in life. The dorsal and lateral surfaces of each half of the cranium blend in a continuous and slightly roughened surface from which the temporalis muscle arises. Rostral to the zygomatic processes of the frontal bones the dorsal surface of the skull dips, sometimes quite markedly, before continuing as the straight and narrow dorsum of the nose. This ends at the wide nasal aperture, beyond which the bony skull is prolonged by pliant nasal cartilages.

The orbit is the most prominent feature of the *lateral view* (Fig. 2.31). Behind the orbit, the dorsolateral part of the braincase forms the wall of the temporal fossa (Fig. 2.31/*16*). The ventrolateral part is more complicated and presents the zygomatic arch and ear regions. The zygomatic arch (Fig. 2.31/*15*) springs free from the braincase and, bowing laterally, passes below the orbit to rejoin the facial part of the skull. It is formed by two bones, the squamous temporal and the zygomatic, which meet at an overlapping suture. The ventral surface of the caudal part of this arch is shaped like a transverse gutter for articulation with the mandible; the articular area continues caudal to the rostral surface of the retroarticular process (Fig. 2.31/*6*). The large, smooth dome of the tympanic bulla (Fig. 2.31/*9*) (enclosing part of the cavity of the middle ear) and the rough mastoid process lie behind the retroarticular process. Three openings are present in this region of the skull: the retroarticular foramen emits a major vein draining the cranial cavity; the stylomastoid foramen gives passage to the facial nerve; and the external acoustic meatus is, in the fresh state, closed by a membrane (eardrum) that separates the canal of the external ear from the cavity of the middle ear. The paracondylar process (Fig. 2.31/*11*) is conspicuous at the caudal limit of the skull.

The orbit is funnel shaped, and in the macerated state its walls are very incomplete. In life the orbital rim is completed by a ligament (Fig. 2.31/*1*) that connects the zygomatic process of the frontal bone to the zygomatic arch. Ventrally the orbital cavity is continuous with the pterygopalatine fossa (Fig. 2.31/*4*), but in the fresh state these regions are separated by the periorbita, a dense fascial sheet that completes the definition of the orbit. Two groups of foramina are visible in this region. The caudal group (Fig. 2.31/*5*) comprises the optic canal, orbital fissure, and rostral alar foramen. The optic opening, placed at the apex of the conical orbital cavity, is the portal of entry of the optic nerve. The more ventral orbital fissure transmits the nerves (ophthalmic, oculomotor, trochlear, and abducent) that supply ancillary structures of the eye and the external ophthalmic vein. Most ventrally the rostral alar foramen provides a common opening for the maxillary nerve, passing from the cranial cavity, and the maxillary artery, which traverses a canal (alar canal) in the sphenoid bone.

The rostral group of foramina comprises the *maxillary, sphenopalatine,* and *caudal palatine foramina.* The maxillary foramen (Fig. 2.30/*2'*) leads to the infraorbital canal, the sphenopalatine foramen to the nasal cavity, and the caudal palatine to the palatine canal, which emerges on the hard palate; each opening conveys like-named branches of the maxillary artery and nerve. More dorsally the rostral orbital wall contains the lacrimal fossa for the lacrimal sac (Fig. 2.30/*3*). An opening in the depth of the fossa leads to a passage that conveys the nasolacrimal (tear) duct to the nose.

The *infraorbital foramen* (Fig. 2.30/*2*), the most prominent and easily palpable feature of the lateral aspect of the face, provides exit to the infraorbital nerve, which continues from the maxillary nerve through the infraorbital canal. Toward the alveolar margin the facial skeleton is molded

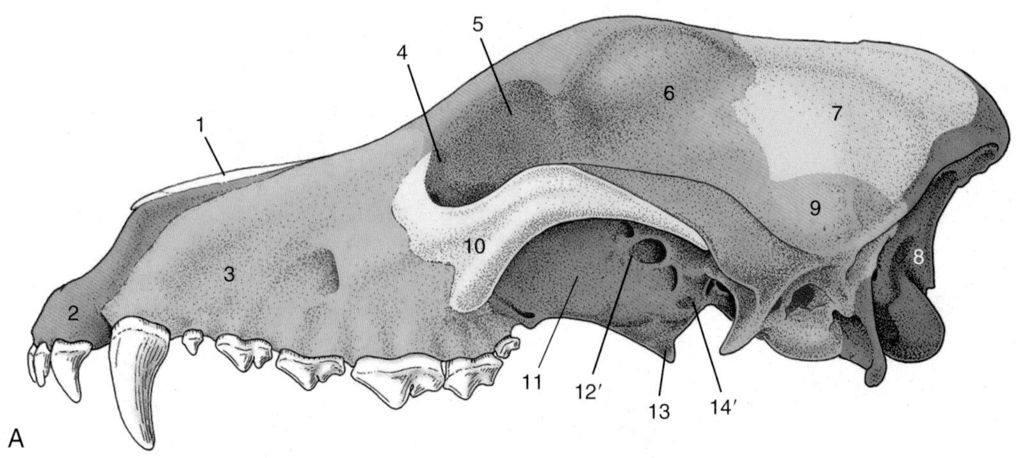

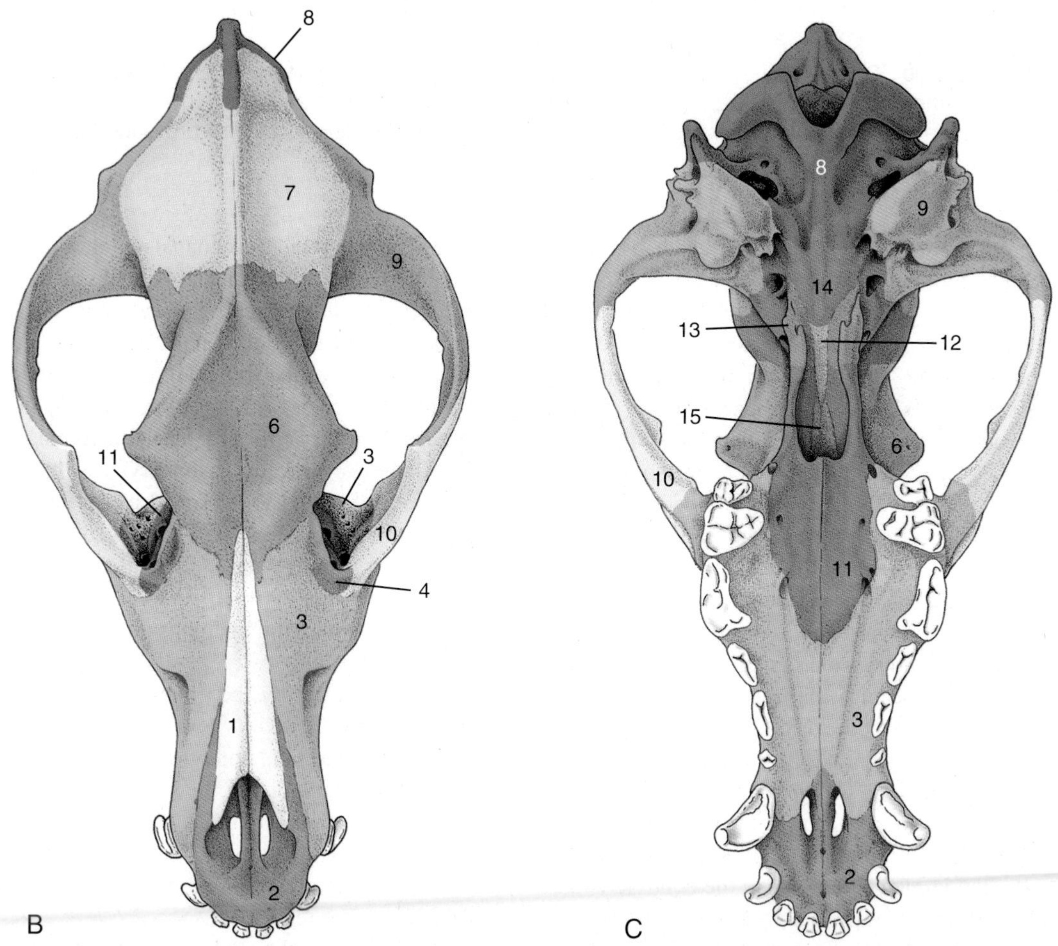

Fig. 2.29 (A) Lateral, (B) dorsal, and (C) ventral views of the canine skull to show the extents of the cranial bones. *1,* Nasal bone; *2,* incisive bone; *3,* maxilla; *4,* lacrimal bone; *5,* orbit; *6,* frontal bone; *7,* parietal bone; *8,* occipital bone; *9,* temporal bone; *10,* zygomatic bone; *11,* palatine bone; *12,* presphenoid; *12′,* wing of presphenoid; *13,* pterygoid bone; *14,* basisphenoid; *14′,* pterygoid process of basisphenoid; *15,* vomer.

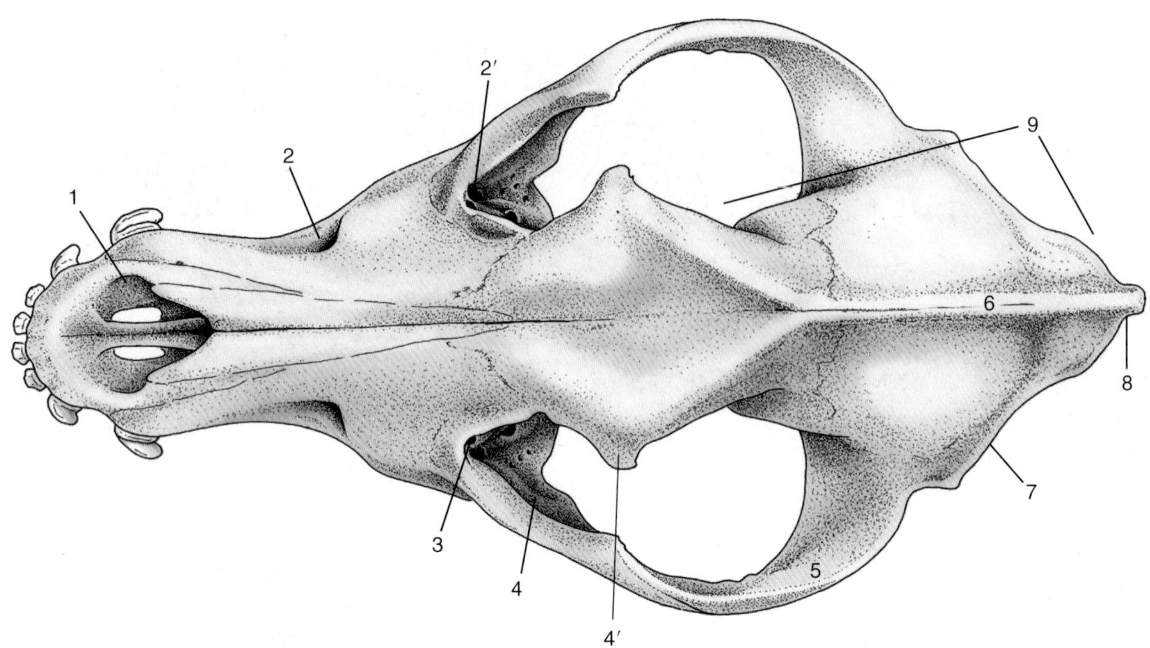

Fig. 2.30 Dorsal view of canine skull. *1,* Nasal aperture; *2,* infraorbital foramen; *2′,* maxillary foramen; *3,* fossa for lacrimal sac; *4,* orbit; *4′,* zygomatic process of frontal bone; *5,* zygomatic arch; *6,* external sagittal crest; *7,* nuchal crest; *8,* external occipital protuberance; *9,* cranium.

over the roots of the teeth, most especially over the large root of the canine tooth.

In the *ventral view* (Fig. 2.32), three regions of the skull are distinct: the base of the cranium, the choanal region where the nasal cavities open into the pharynx, and the hard palate. The first shows at its caudal limit the ovoid, obliquely oriented occipital condyles that flank the foramen magnum (Fig. 2.32/*12*), through which the spinal cord connects with the brain. Rostral to this the median area is generally flat, although midway along its length, tubercles are present for the attachment of muscles that flex the head on the neck. The tympanic bulla and paracondylar process occupy much space to each side. The medial aspect of the bulla (Fig. 2.32/*7*) meets the occipital bone, and this fusion separates two openings that are confluent in some other species (e.g., horse; see Fig. 2.37)—namely, the more caudal jugular foramen and the more rostral foramen lacerum (Fig. 2.32/*8* and *6*). The glossopharyngeal, vagus, and accessory nerves emerge through the jugular foramen together with a large vein draining the interior of the cranium. Between the jugular foramen and the condyle is the hypoglossal canal, which transmits the hypoglossal nerve.

Lateral to the foramen lacerum, small fissures exist for the exit of the chorda tympani (a branch of the facial nerve) and for the communication of the cartilaginous auditory tube with the cavity of the middle ear. Rostral to these is the prominent oval foramen (Fig. 2.32/*4*), through which the mandibular nerve emerges.

The openings (choanae) that lead from the nasal cavities to the nasopharynx are the main features of the middle part of the ventral aspect. The choanal region is bounded dorsally by the floor of the cranium and laterally by the thin plates of bone whose outer surfaces were earlier noted as forming the medial walls of the pterygopalatine fossae. The soft palate, which arises from the free margin of the hard palate, in life provides the floor of the space—essentially the first part of the nasopharynx—enclosed by these formations. The palate, which lies rostral to nasopharynx, is broad behind and narrower in front. It is margined by the alveoli or sockets in which the upper teeth are implanted. Toward its rostral extremity, it is perforated by the large bilateral palatine fissures. Several smaller foramina toward the caudal extremity of the palate are rostral openings of the palatine canal.

The *nuchal surface* (Fig. 2.31/*13*), broadly triangular, is limited dorsally by the external occipital protuberance and the nuchal crests. Its lower part presents the foramen magnum, the occipital condyles, and the paracondylar processes. The remainder of the surface is roughened for the attachment of dorsal muscles of the neck.

The *apex* of the skull is formed by the nasal aperture situated dorsal to the rostral extremities of the jaws that carry the incisor teeth.

The cavities of the skull are described with the respiratory system (Chapter 4), central nervous system (Chapter 8), and ear (Chapter 9).

The lower jaw or *mandible* comprises two parts (Fig. 2.33). In the dog these are firmly but not rigidly united by the connective tissues of the mandibular symphysis. Each half is divided between a body, or horizontal part, and a ramus, or vertical part. The body carries the alveoli of the

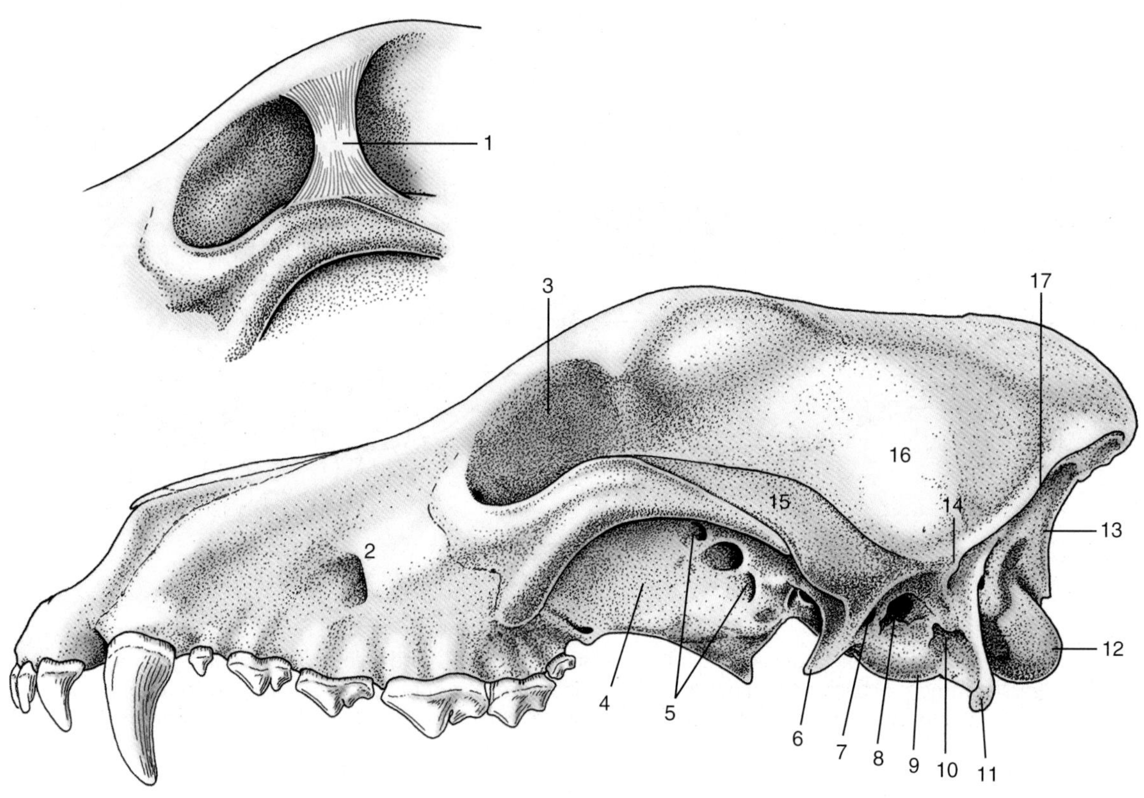

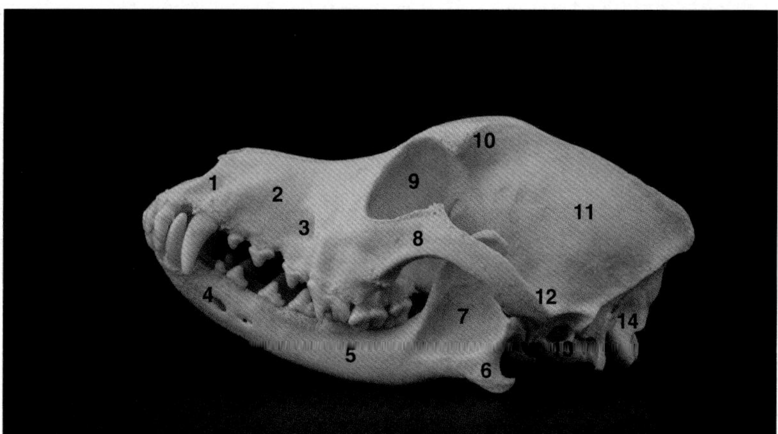

Fig. 2.31 Lateral view of canine skull. *1,* Orbital ligament *(inset)*; *2,* infraorbital foramen; *3,* orbit; *4,* pterygopalatine fossa; *5,* optic canal, orbital fissure, and rostral alar foramen; *6,* retroarticular process; *7,* retroarticular foramen; *8,* external acoustic meatus; *9,* tympanic bulla; *10,* stylomastoid foramen; *11,* paracondylar process; *12,* occipital condyle; *13,* nuchal surface; *14,* mastoid process; *15,* zygomatic arch; *16,* temporal fossa; *17,* nuchal crest.

lower teeth and is laterally compressed. Except at its rostral extremity, it diverges from its fellow to bound an intermandibular space. Toward its rostral extremity the lateral surface presents several mental foramina, one generally much larger than the rest; through these emerge the mental branches of the inferior alveolar nerve and vessels. The ramus (Fig. 2.33/*2*) is wider but less robust. Its dorsal extremity ends in the coronoid process, which projects into the temporal fossa and gives attachment to the temporalis muscle, and the lower and more caudal condylar process (Fig. 2.33/*3*), which carries an articular head shaped like a portion of a truncated cone. The lower part of the caudal margin of the ramus carries the projecting angular process that gives attachment to the masseter and medial pterygoid muscles. The lateral surface has a roughened depression where the masseter inserts. The medial surface gives insertion to the pterygoid muscles and also presents the large mandibular foramen (Fig. 2.33/*7*) for entry of the inferior alveolar vessels and nerve.

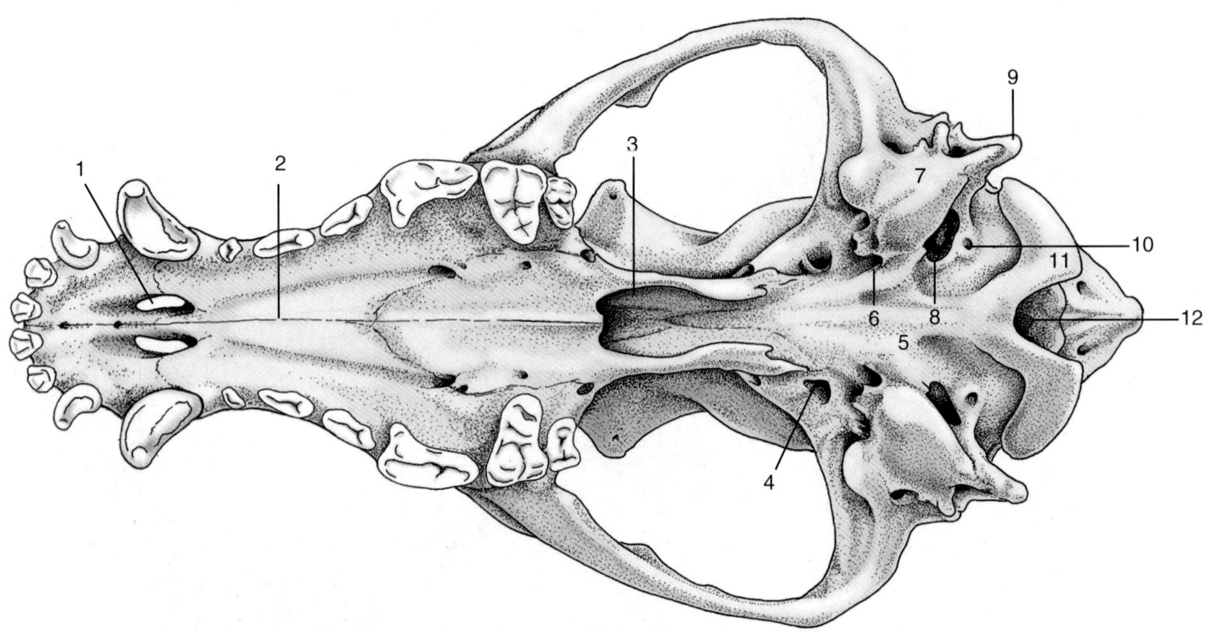

Fig. 2.32 Ventral view of canine skull. *1,* Palatine fissure; *2,* hard palate; *3,* choanal region; *4,* oval foramen; *5,* base of cranium; *6,* foramen lacerum; *7,* tympanic bulla; *8,* jugular foramen; *9,* paracondylar process; *10,* hypoglossal canal; *11,* occipital condyle; *12,* foramen magnum.

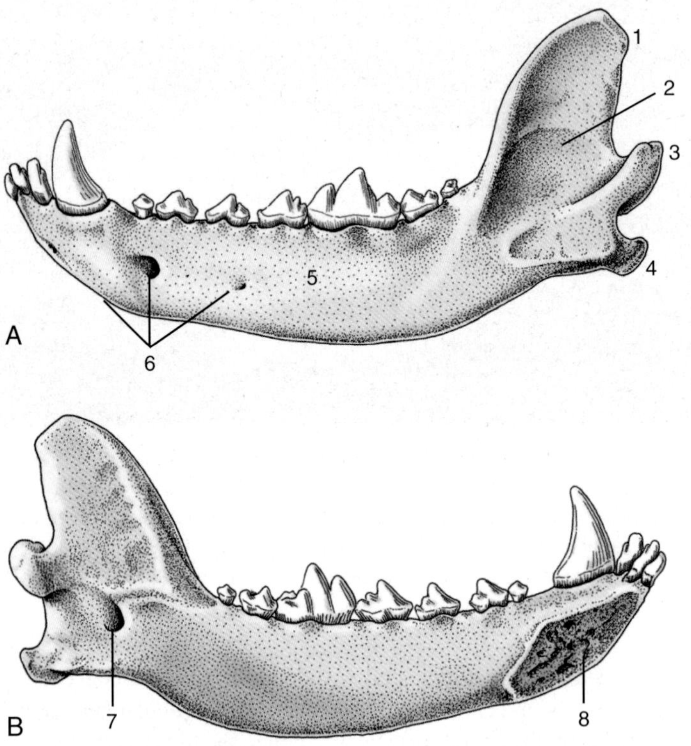

Fig. 2.33 (A) Lateral and (B) medial views of the left half of the canine mandible. *1,* Coronoid process; *2,* vertical part (ramus); *3,* condylar process; *4,* angular process; *5,* horizontal part (body); *6,* mental foramina; *7,* mandibular foramen; *8,* symphysial surface.

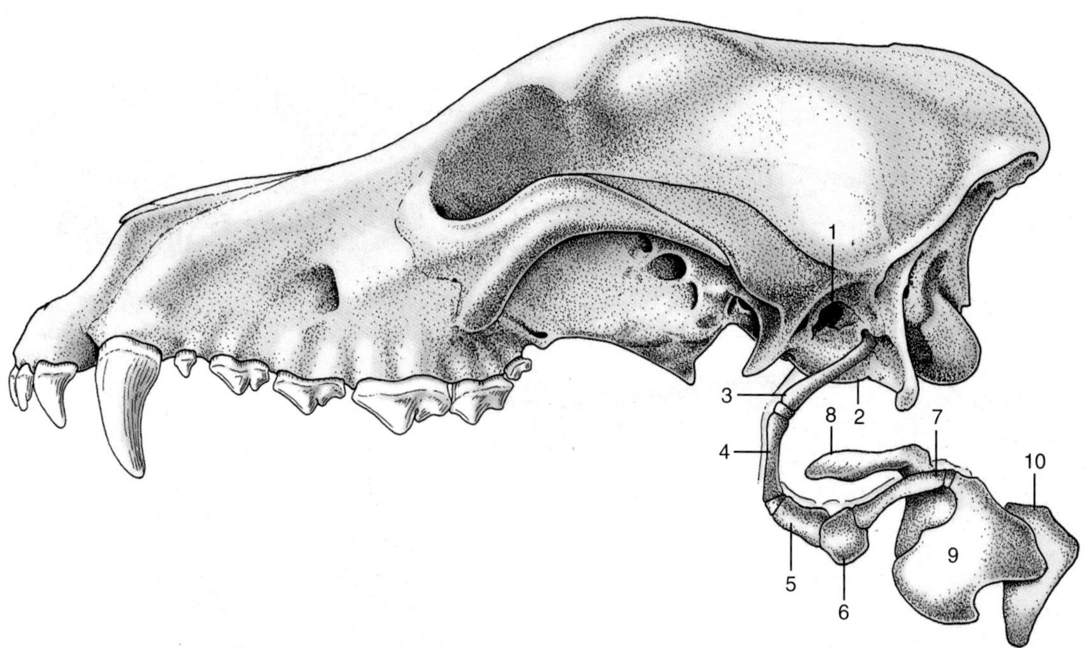

Fig. 2.34 Hyoid apparatus and larynx suspended from the temporal region of a canine skull. *1,* External acoustic meatus; *2,* tympanic bulla; *3,* stylohyoid; *4,* epihyoid; *5,* ceratohyoid; *6,* basihyoid; *7,* thyrohyoid; *8,* epiglottic cartilage; *9,* thyroid cartilage; *10,* cricoid cartilage.

The *hyoid apparatus* is a series of bony rods jointed together and forming a means of suspending the tongue and larynx from the skull. Fig. 2.34 shows the names of the several parts, their arrangement, and the attachment of the apparatus as a whole to the temporal region of the skull. The transversely placed basihyoid may be palpated within the intermandibular space; other parts are palpable—indeed their positions are visible—when the walls of the pharynx are inspected through the mouth.

Some Comparative Features of the Skull

When equipped with the mandible the *skull of the cat* (Fig. 2.35) appears globular. Several features combine to create this conformation:

- the rounded cranial capsule, surmounted by a short, often weak sagittal crest, and corresponding closely to the contours of the brain
- the very salient convex zygomatic arches
- the relative shortness of the face, which may account for as little as 20% of the total length

The orbital region is distinctive. The orbits are large, face more directly forward than in the dog, and have more complete bony margins. The frontal process of the zygomatic bone and the zygomatic process of the frontal bone leave only a small gap in the ovoid margin to be closed by the orbital ligament. The zygomatic arch is surprisingly strong where it contributes to the orbital rim. The infraorbital foramen is placed close to the rostroventral part of the orbit, where it may be palpated.

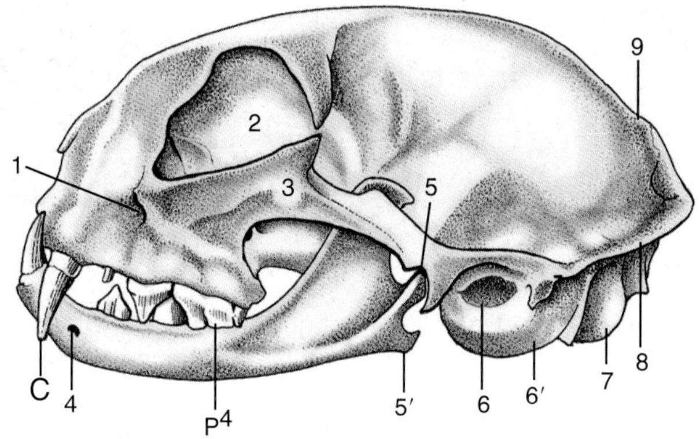

Fig. 2.35 Feline skull with mandible. *1,* Infraorbital foramen; *2,* orbit; *3,* zygomatic arch; *4,* mental foramen; *5,* temporomandibular joint; *5′,* angular process of mandible; *6,* external acoustic meatus; *6′,* tympanic bulla; *7,* occipital condyle; *8,* nuchal crest; *9,* sagittal crest; *C,* canine tooth; *p4,* upper fourth premolar.

On the ventral aspect, the hard palate is short and wide, and it carries alveoli for only four cheek teeth. That for the largest of these teeth (P4) is located dangerously close to the orbit, which may become involved in a spreading alveolar abscess. Caudally, the deep gutter of the temporomandibular articulation is bounded by a prominent retroarticular process. The very large tympanic bulla may be palpated between the caudal part of the zygomatic arch and the wing of the atlas.

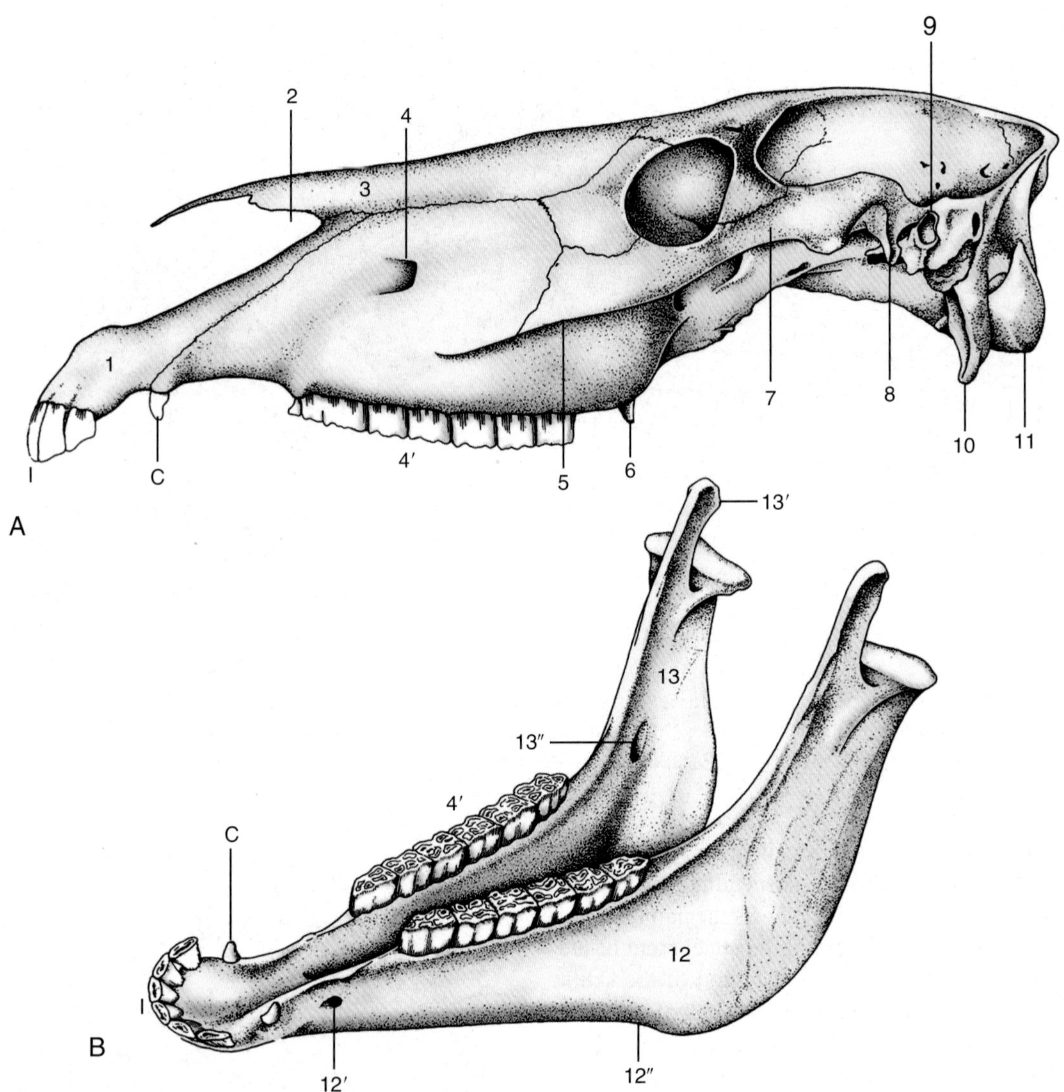

Fig. 2.36 (A) Equine skull and (B) equine mandible. *1,* Incisive bone; *2,* nasoincisive notch; *3,* nasal bone; *4,* infraorbital foramen; *4′,* cheek teeth; *5,* facial crest; *6,* hamulus of pterygoid bone; *7,* zygomatic arch; *8,* retroarticular process; *9,* external acoustic meatus; *10,* paracondylar process; *11,* occipital condyle; *12,* horizontal part (body) of mandible; *12′,* mental foramen; *12″,* vascular notch; *13,* vertical part (ramus) of mandible; *13′,* coronoid process; *13″,* mandibular foramen; I, incisors; *C,* canine tooth (present only in the male).

As in the dog, the halves of the mandible do not fuse, even in old age, and a small degree of movement is allowed at the mandibular symphysis. Each half carries sockets for only three cheek teeth.

Breed differences are more pronounced than sometimes supposed. The skulls of Siamese and similar cats have much longer faces, which often blend smoothly with the cranium without any break (stop) in the dorsal contour. In contrasting types—for example, the Persian—the face is short and shallow, and the stop is prominent.

The *equine skull* (Fig. 2.36) is characterized by a relatively long face, a feature that develops further with increasing size; it is therefore more pronounced in mature than in juvenile animals and in large than in small breeds. The cranium is relatively narrow and generally not unlike that of the dog. The external sagittal crest is weaker. The forehead is wide between the origins of the zygomatic processes of the frontal bones, which bend ventrally to join the zygomatic arches.

The zygomatic arch (Fig. 2.36/*7*) is conspicuously strong, even without the extra support it obtains from the zygomatic process connecting it with the frontal bone taken into account. It is not bowed laterally to any extent and carries a rather complicated articular surface on its caudoventral aspect; this comprises a rostral tuber, an intermediate fossa, and a salient retroarticular process (Fig. 2.36/*8*). The orbit faces almost laterally and has a complete bony rim. A large maxillary tuberosity appears to continue the alveolar

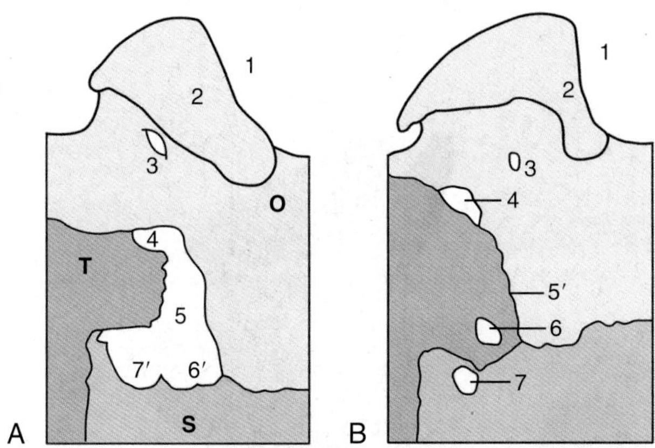

Fig. 2.37 Left caudolateral parts of the base of the (A) equine and (B) canine cranium, showing portions of the occipital *(O)*, sphenoid *(S)*, and temporal *(T)* bones; ventral view (schematic). *1*, Foramen magnum; *2*, occipital condyle; *3*, hypoglossal canal; *4*, jugular foramen; *5*, foramen lacerum; *5′*, petro-occipital suture; *6*, foramen lacerum; *6′*, carotid notches; *7*, oval foramen; *7′*, oval notch.

process directly. The zygomatic arch is continued rostrally, beyond the orbit, as a prominent ridge on the lateral surface of the face. This ridge, the facial crest (Fig. 2.36/*5*), runs parallel to the dorsal contour of the nose and ends above a septum between the alveoli of the third and fourth cheek teeth in the adult.

A deep (nasoincisive) notch separates the pointed nasal bone from the incisive bone (Fig. 2.36/*1–3*). This notch and the rostral end of the facial crest are both very easily identified landmarks; they are used as guides to the position of the infraorbital foramen, which lies a little caudal to the middle of the connecting line (Fig. 2.36/*4*).

The features visible on the ventral view lie more or less on one level. The caudal part of this surface is distinguished by the large and very salient paracondylar processes (Fig. 2.36/*10*) and the jagged outlines of the large openings to each side of the occipital bone. Each opening results from the failure of the temporal bone to reach the lateral margin of the occipital bone, which permits the confluence of several foramina that are distinct in the dog. The caudal part is the equivalent of the jugular foramen; the cranial part (foramen lacerum) combines the oval and carotid foramina (Fig. 2.37/*7* and *6*). In life the greater part of the large opening is occluded by membrane that leaves barely sufficient passage for the various nerves and vessels. The tympanic bulla is not prominent, but the styloid (for the hyoid apparatus) and muscular processes of the temporal bone are well developed.

The choanae lie almost in the plane of the hard palate. The vertical plate of bone that separates the choanal from the pterygopalatine region carries a prominent hamular process (Fig. 2.36/*6*). The greater part of the margin of flat and unremarkable palate is occupied by the alveoli of the incisor and cheek teeth. A well-marked external occipital protuberance is present on the nuchal surface, midway between the nuchal crest and the dorsal margin of the foramen magnum.

The mandible has the following features:

- It is massive, and its right and left halves diverge at a relatively small angle (Fig. 2.36B).
- Its symphysis becomes obliterated quite early, usually about 2 years after birth.
- Its lower margin carries a prominent vascular notch where the facial vessels wind onto the face (Fig. 2.36/*12‴*).
- Its ramus is high, the coronoid process projects far into the temporal fossa, and the articular process carries the ovoid articular surface well above the occlusal plane of the cheek teeth.

The parts of the hyoid apparatus (see Fig. 4.8) are of different proportions to their counterparts in the dog and are laterally compressed. A substantial lingual process projects from the basihyoid into the root of the tongue.

The *bovine skull* (Fig. 2.38) is relatively short and wide with a general pyramidal form. Cornual (horn) processes project from the frontal bones of horned breeds where the dorsal, lateral, and nuchal surfaces meet; their size and direction vary greatly with breed, age, and sex. The very wide and flat frontal region is bounded by a prominent temporal line that overhangs the deep temporal fossa and confines it to the lateral aspect of the skull.

The principal features of the lateral aspect are the confinement of the temporal fossa and the elevation of the orbital rim above its surroundings. The rim is complete and is formed by the meeting of processes from the zygomatic and frontal bones in its caudal part. There is no facial crest, only a discrete facial tuberosity from which the rostral part of the masseter arises. The infraorbital foramen is directly above the first cheek tooth, rather low toward the palate.

The ventral surface is very uneven, and the cranial base is located in a considerably more dorsal plane than the palate. The temporal and occipital bones are separated by a narrow fissure, which is an arrangement intermediate between the suture of the dog and the wide opening of the horse and pig. The tympanic bulla is prominent and laterally compressed. The choanae are separated by the caudal prolongation of the ventral part of the nasal septum and are enclosed laterally by very extensive plates of bone. The palate, long and narrow, is bounded by high alveolar processes. Of course, no alveoli are present for incisor or canine teeth, which are lacking in the upper jaws of ruminants.

The mandibular symphysis ossifies late, if at all, in ruminants. In general, the mandible is weaker than that of the horse, which is a feature very apparent in the body of the bone with its gently convex ventral border. The coronoid process is high and caudally inflected. The articular surface is concave and widened laterally.

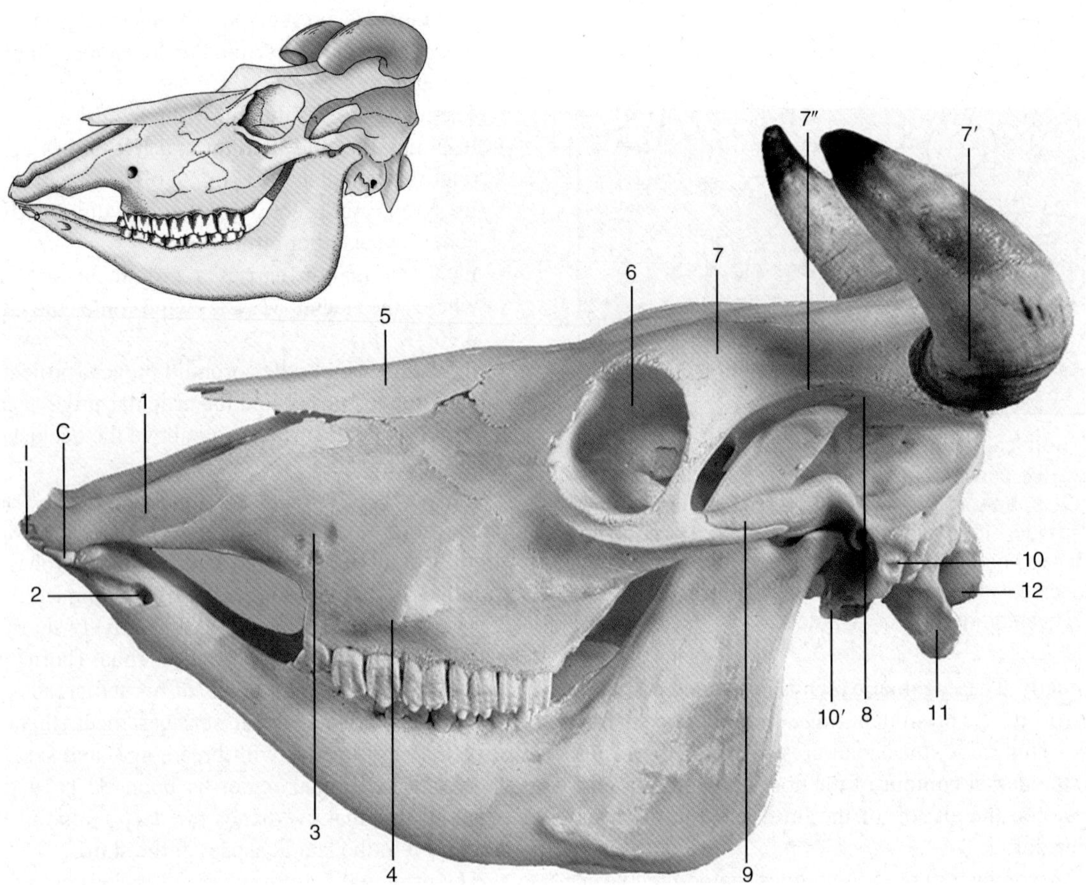

Fig. 2.38 Bovine skull with mandible. *1,* Incisive bone; *2,* mental foramen; *3,* infraorbital foramen; *4,* facial tuberosity; *5,* nasal bone; *6,* orbit; *7,* frontal bone; *7′,* horn surrounding cornual process of frontal bone; *7″,* temporal line; *8,* temporal fossa; *9,* zygomatic arch; *10,* external acoustic meatus; *10′,* tympanic bulla; *11,* paracondylar process; *12,* occipital condyle; *I,* incisors; *C,* canine tooth, incorporated in the row of incisors.

The few remarks necessary regarding the skulls of the small ruminants and the pig are found on pages 634 and 739, respectively.

The Joints of the Head

The articulations between the skull and mandible (temporomandibular joints) and between the halves of the mandible (mandibular symphysis) are appropriately considered in the following chapter (p. 104) because the teeth, the muscles of mastication, and the joints form a single functional complex.

The Muscles of the Head and Ventral Part of the Neck

The principal groups into which the muscles of the head may be divided are listed in Table 2.2, which draws attention to the correspondence between embryologic origin, innervation, and function. The functional associations are so well defined and specific that it is more convenient to include most of them in other chapters, with related organs.

The first four groups take origin in the unsplit mesoderm, which covers the lateral and ventral walls of the pharynx and condenses to form the cores of the pharyngeal arches.

In lower vertebrates the muscles equivalent to the last two groups in Table 2.2 are known to develop from somites that appear to each side of the hindbrain, some rostral to the otocyst, the primordium of the inner ear, and the others caudal to it. A similar origin may be assumed in mammals, although the evidence for the formation of these somites is unconvincing at least. They are of course somatic muscles with the appropriate type of innervation.

The Trigeminal Musculature

The muscles of mastication constitute the greater part of the musculature supplied by the mandibular division of the trigeminal nerve, the motor nerve to the first pharyngeal arch. They are described in the chapter on the digestive system (p. 105). The same chapter deals with the digastricus—a composite muscle to which the mandibular field makes a contribution; the mylohyoideus which slings the tongue

TABLE 2.2 SOURCE AND INNERVATION OF THE PRINCIPAL MUSCLE GROUPS OF THE HEAD

Muscle Group	Source	Innervation
Masticatory musculature	First pharyngeal arch	Mandibular division of trigeminal nerve (V3)
Mimetic musculature	Second pharyngeal arch	Facial nerve (VII)
Pharyngeal and palatine musculature	Third and fourth pharyngeal arches	Glossopharyngeal (IX) and vagus (X) nerves
Laryngeal musculature	Sixth pharyngeal arch	Vagus nerve (X)
External ocular musculature	Hypothetical preotic somites	Oculomotor (III), trochlear (IV), and abducent (VI) nerves
Lingual musculature	Hypothetical postotic somites	Hypoglossal nerve (XII)

between the lower jaws; and one of the muscles (tensor veli palatini) of the soft palate (p. 109). The tensor tympani is considered with the middle ear (p. 333).

The Facial Musculature

The musculature supplied by the facial nerve, the nerve of the second pharyngeal arch, is resolvable into two divisions. The superficial division comprises the cutaneous muscle of the head and neck in addition to many small units that control the posture of the lips, cheeks, nostrils, eyelids, and external ears. The deep division is rather scattered but includes some muscles associated with the hyoid apparatus, a contribution to the digastricus (p. 109), and the stapedius (p. 334) of the middle ear.

The Superficial Division. The muscles of the superficial division are conjectured to have their source in an ancestral deep sphincter muscle of the neck, which may be envisaged as arranged in three incomplete overlapping layers. The outermost layer, consisting of transversely disposed fascicles, is reduced to insignificance or is entirely lacking in domestic mammals. A remnant (sphincter colli) survives in the dog. A more substantial portion of the middle layer commonly persists as platysma organized as a sheet of longitudinally disposed fibers covering the ventral part of the face and extending onto the neck, even reaching the nape in the dog. Detached slips are believed to provide the small muscles that attach to the caudal aspect of the external ear.

The third and deepest layer is also transverse and is believed to be the origin of the many discrete muscles of the mammalian face. These are extremely variable among species, but very few require detailed notice. Because of their effect on the appearance of the face, they are collectively known as the *muscles of facial expression* or *mimetic musculature*.

The principal muscles of the lips and cheeks are the buccinator, orbicularis oris, caninus, levator nasolabialis, levator labii superioris, and depressor labii inferioris (Figs. 2.39 and 11.6). The *buccinator* (Fig. 2.39/*4*) passes between the margins of the upper and lower jaws and is partly covered by the masseter. It forms the basis of the cheek and opposes the tongue to prevent food from collecting in the vestibule by returning it to the central cavity of the mouth. The buccal salivary glands are scattered among its fascicles, and discharge of their secretion into the mouth may be assisted by contraction of the muscle. The *orbicularis oris* (Fig. 2.39/*1*) surrounds the mouth opening, where it is closely attached to the skin and mucosa of the lips. It closes the opening of the mouth by pursing the lips and is important in sucking. The *caninus* (Fig. 2.39/*2*) arises ventral to the infraorbital foramen and radiates into the wing of the nostril and the upper lip. It dilates the nostril and elevates the corner of the mouth in the snarling gesture, especially in the dog. The *levator nasolabialis* (Fig. 2.39/*5*) arises over the dorsum of the nose and inserts partly on the wing of the nostril and partly into the lateral part of the upper lip. It is able to dilate the nostril and to elevate and retract the upper lip. The medial part of the upper lip is elevated by the separate *levator labii superioris* (Fig. 2.39/*6*). This muscle arises on the lateral aspect of the face and runs dorsorostrally to form with its fellow a common tendon that descends into the lip between the nostrils. A special *depressor labii inferioris* is present in the lower lip of certain species (excluding the dog and cat). It appears to be a detachment from the buccinator muscle. Other muscles associated with the lips and nostrils do not merit specific mention, although some are identified in various illustrations.

The muscles of the eyelids include one, the *levator palpebrae superioris,* that is clearly foreign to the facial group because it arises within the orbit and is supplied by the oculomotor nerve (see p. 328). The muscles of the lids that are supplied by the facial nerve include a sphincter—*the orbicularis oculi* (Fig. 2.39/*7*)—that surrounds the palpebral fissure, the opening between the lids. It is anchored at the medial and lateral commissures and therefore narrows the opening to a horizontal slit when it contracts. Other muscles are present to raise the upper (levator anguli oculi) lid and to depress the lower (malaris) lid, enlarging the eye opening.

The muscles of the external ear are especially numerous but of little account individually. A caudal group has

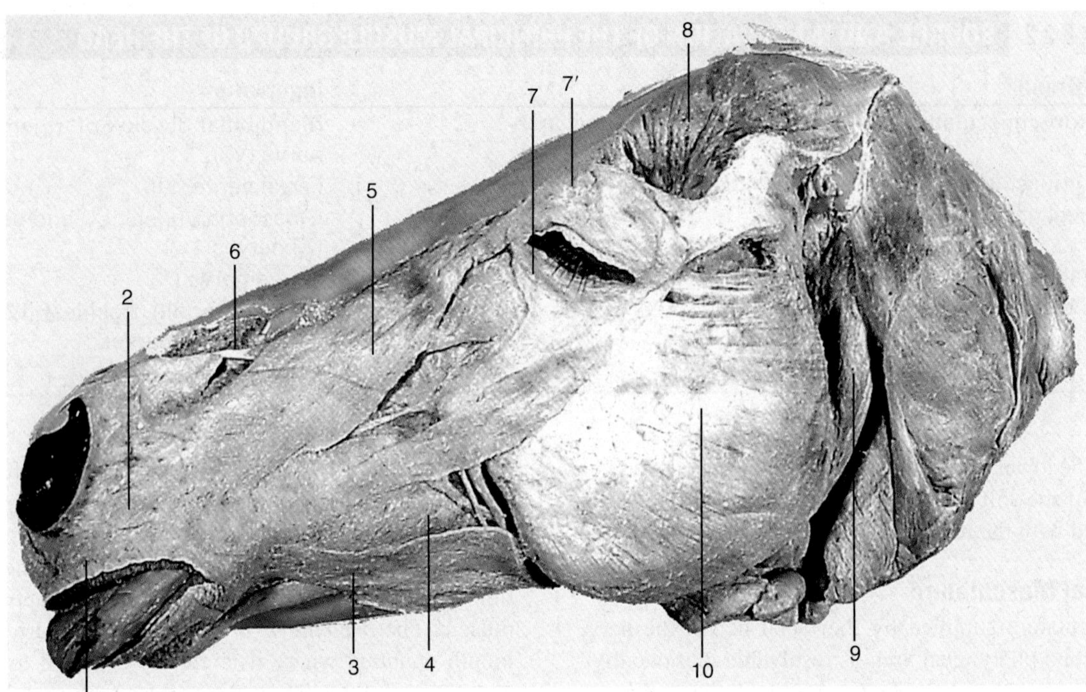

Fig. 2.39 Superficial muscles of the equine head. The cutaneous muscle has been removed. *1,* Orbicularis oris; *2,* caninus; *3,* depressor labii inferioris; *4,* buccinator; *5,* levator nasolabialis; *6,* levator labii superioris; *7,* orbicularis oculi; *7′,* levator anguli oculi medialis; *8,* temporalis; *9,* occipitomandibular part of digastricus; *10,* masseter.

already been mentioned. Others converge on the auricle—the skin-covered cartilaginous ear "trumpet"—from medial, rostral, and lateral directions; they lie between the skin and the temporalis muscle and skull and form a thin, incomplete sheet that includes a (scutiform) cartilage plate. The scattered origins and precisely located insertions provide for displacement and rotation of the ear in all directions. One, the *parotidoauricularis,* is of somewhat greater importance because it is encountered in the operation for drainage of infections of the external ear of the dog (p. 381). As its name suggests, it arises from the fascia over the parotid gland and approaches the auricle from the ventrolateral direction.

Besides the individual functions mentioned or implied in the preceding paragraphs, these muscles have a collective function in communication, mainly within the species but also between species. Human observers can intuitively, or as the result of experience, interpret many obvious facial gestures of animals: one need only recall the hangdog expression of submission, the evident threat conveyed by snarling or laying back the ears, or the quizzical look a dog may adopt.

Paralysis of these muscles is not uncommon after damage to the facial nerve. Because different groups are supplied by branches of the nerve that arise at different levels, the particular pattern of distortions can be a valuable pointer to the location of the nerve lesion (p. 305).

The Deep Division. The muscles attaching to the hyoid apparatus are a rather heterogeneous assemblage. Although certain small units supplied by the facial nerve elevate the hyoid, to draw the tongue backward to aid in swallowing, the muscles do not appear to merit description. The digastricus, in part derived from the facial musculature, is described on page 105; the stapedius of the middle ear is described on page 333.

The Muscles of the Pharynx and Soft Palate

The muscles of the pharynx and soft palate are considered beginning on page 107.

The Muscles of the Larynx

The laryngeal muscles are considered beginning on page 144.

The External Muscles of the Eyeball

The external muscles of the eyeball are considered beginning on page 327.

The Muscles of the Tongue

The tongue muscles are considered beginning on page 95.

The Muscles of the Ventral Part of the Neck

The neck connects the head with the trunk and is usually distinguished by its relatively slender construction—although

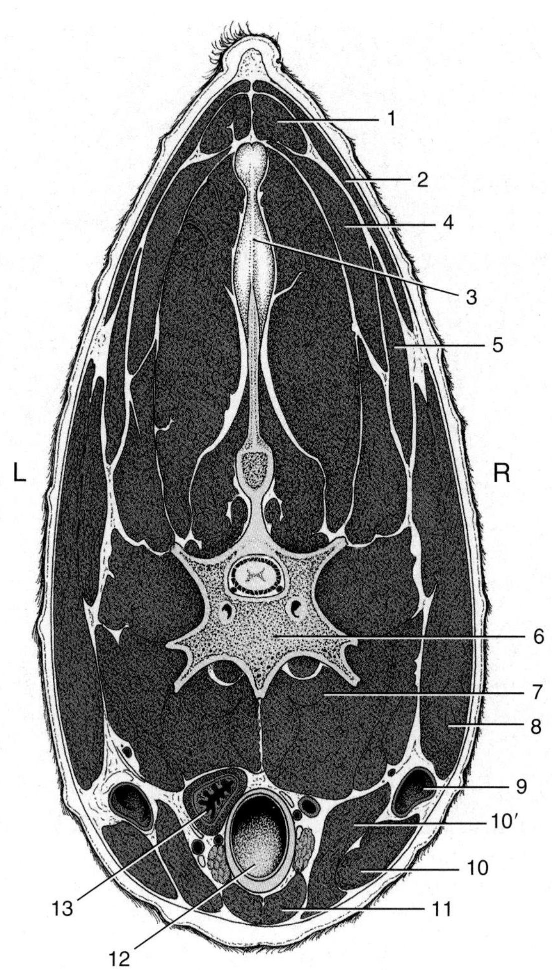

Fig. 2.40 Transverse section of the bovine neck. *1,* Rhomboideus; *2,* trapezius; *3,* nuchal ligament; *4,* splenius; *5,* omotransversarius; *6,* vertebra; *7,* longus colli; *8,* brachiocephalicus; *9,* external jugular vein in jugular groove; *10* and *10′,* sternocephalicus, mandibular and mastoid parts; *11,* combined sternohyoideus and sternothyroideus; *12,* trachea; *13,* esophagus (ventral to it, nerves, blood vessels, and thymus); *L,* left; *R,* right.

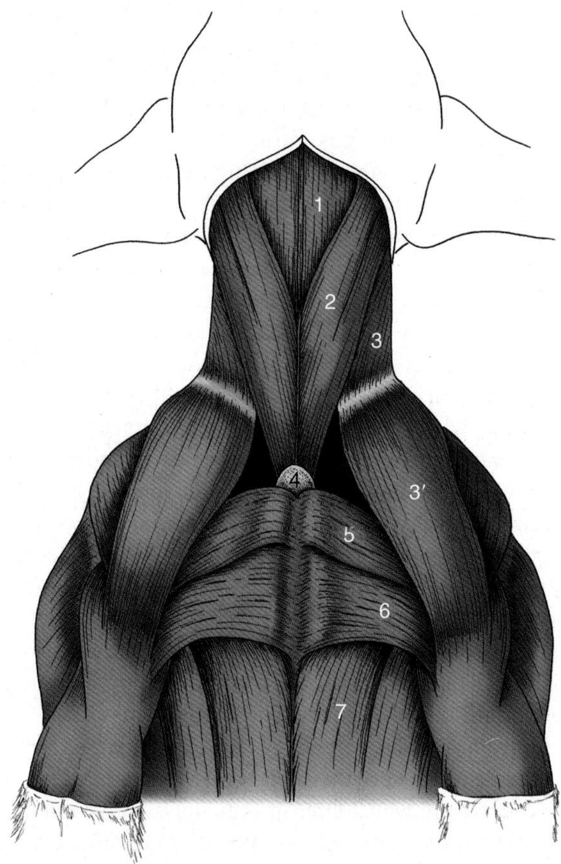

Fig. 2.41 Ventral muscles of the canine neck and thorax. *1,* Combined sternohyoideus and sternothyroideus; *2,* sternocephalicus; *3* and *3′,* brachiocephalicus: cleidocervicalis and cleidobrachialis; *4,* manubrium of sternum; *5,* pectoralis descendens; *6,* pectoralis transversus; *7,* pectoralis profundus.

this is hardly true of the pig. The neck has a generally cylindrical form in the dog and cat but is quite obviously compressed from side to side in the larger animals, in which it deepens considerably toward its junction with the thorax (Fig. 2.40). The core structures of the neck—the cervical vertebrae and the muscles closely applied to them—were described with the trunk (p. 42). Certain superficial muscles are considered under the heading of "Girdle Muscles of the Forelimb" (p. 75). The present section is therefore concerned only with the ventral part of the neck, a region of considerable clinical importance on account of the numerous visceral, vascular, and nervous structures that traverse it en route between the head and thorax.

These structures, with the important exception of the external jugular veins (Fig. 2.40/9), occupy a central visceral space. The roof of this space is provided by the muscles immediately ventral to the vertebrae—namely, the longus colli, longus capitis, rectus capitis ventralis, and scalenus (p. 44). The side and ventral walls blend together and are provided by thinner muscles disposed with a sagittal course and joined by stout fasciae.

The cervical part of the *cutaneous muscle* (m. cutaneous colli) is unimportant in the dog and cat. It is much better developed in the ungulates, in which it radiates from a stout origin on the manubrium of the sternum; it thins as it passes cranially and laterally and eventually fades away. In the horse, the cutaneous muscle provides a relatively thick cover to the caudal third or so of the jugular groove.

The straplike *sternocephalicus* (Fig. 2.41/2) is the most ventral of the other muscles. It also arises from the manubrium, ascends the neck, and diverges laterally toward its insertion, which varies among species but includes one or the other (or both) of the angle of the mandible and the mastoid process of the skull. The divergence of the right and left muscles leaves a very thin layer of the deeper muscle, enabling palpation of the trachea through the skin. The sternocephalicus is supplied by the ventral branch of the accessory nerve. Unilateral contraction draws the head and neck to that side. Bilateral contraction flexes the head and neck ventrally. In species with a mandibular insertion the sternocephalicus may assist in opening the mouth.

The sternocephalicus forms the ventral border of the jugular groove that houses the external jugular vein (Fig. 2.42). The dorsal border of the groove is furnished by the *brachiocephalicus,* described more fully elsewhere (p. 76). The groove is often visible in life, particularly toward the upper part of the neck.

The deeper infrahyoid group of muscles provides an incomplete cover to the lateral and ventral aspects of the trachea and inserts, directly or indirectly, on the hyoid apparatus, which they all stabilize and retract toward the thorax during swallowing. The obvious members of the group are the sternothyroideus, sternohyoideus, and omohyoideus; the thyrohyoideus on the lateral aspect of the larynx may be regarded as a detached member. The nerve supply is mainly, although possibly not entirely, from the first and second cervical nerves.

The *sternothyroideus* and *sternohyoideus* are very thin ribbonlike muscles that take a common origin from the manubrium of the sternum. The caudal parts of the right and left muscles are not always distinctly divided, and in the middle of the neck they may have a common intermediate tendon from which three or four slips diverge cranially. The sternothyroideus inclines laterally to terminate on the lateral aspect of the thyroid cartilage. The sternohyoideus, not always separable from its fellow, passes beside the midline to insert on the basihyoid.

The *omohyoideus,* lacking in carnivores, is also thin and straplike. Its absence is compensated by the relative enlargement of the other muscles. In the horse it arises from the subscapular fascia and in the ruminants from the deep fascia of the neck; thereafter it edges medially to join the lateral margin of the sternohyoideus beside which it inserts. In the horse the omohyoideus provides a floor to the caudal part of the jugular groove, separating the vein from the structures within the visceral space.

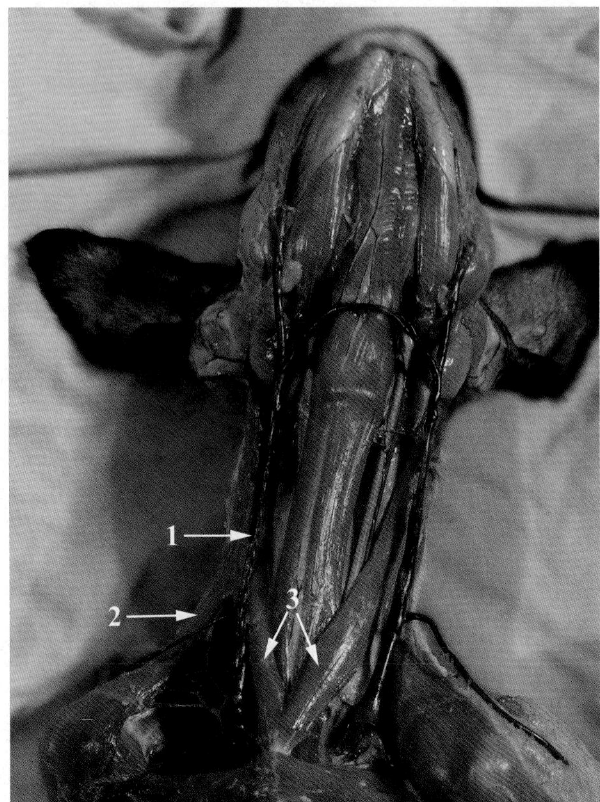

Fig. 2.42 The ventral part of the neck of a dog. Notice the external jugular vein *(1)* in the groove formed by the brachiocephalic muscle *(2)* dorsal, and the sternocephalicus muscle *(3)* ventrally.

THE LIMBS

Basic Plan and Development

Although the forelimbs and hindlimbs are not homologous, they are similar in organization and segmentation with a remarkably close correspondence of analogous parts. Each first appears as a bud that grows out from the ventrolateral surface of the body of the young embryo at a level corresponding to the origin of the nerves by which it will later be supplied. The bud of the forelimb appears before that of the hindlimb, and its development maintains this advantage for some time—indeed, until after birth in puppies and other animals born in a rather immature state. These animals initially confine their locomotor activities to dragging themselves, using the forelimbs only, toward their dam's teats.

When first formed, a limb bud consists of a mass of mesenchyme, the loose embryonic connective tissue, within an ectodermal covering. The ectoderm becomes the epidermis, including its derivatives; the mesenchyme differentiates to form skeletal tissues, muscles and tendons, fasciae, and blood vessels. Thus it is only the limb nerves that invade from outside; all other structures develop in situ. The limb bud lengthens, and its free distal part expands to form a flattened hand (foot) plate while the more proximal part acquires a more columnar form. Thickenings corresponding to the digital rays soon appear in the plate and are accentuated when the intervening tissues are reduced. The details of this development naturally vary with the species, for it is only some that retain the primitive pentadactyl (five-digit) pattern and only a few that show a complete separation of digits. It is interesting to note that five digits appear in most species; when evolution has reduced the complement to fewer, the adult condition is usually attained by fetal regression of some digits. Creases formed in the proximal part of the bud soon allow recognition of segments corresponding to the arm and forearm (or thigh and leg) regions of the adult.

The first indication of the future limb skeleton is provided by an axial condensation of the mesoderm to produce a denser core. In the early stages of development (but not always later) a definite proximodistal gradient of differentiation occurs. This gradient establishes and then maintains the girdle elements in advance of those of the arm or thigh and the latter in advance of more distal parts.

In the next stage of development, the mesoderm is locally transformed to create a series of cartilaginous models in the pattern of the adult bones. These precursors soon come to resemble the final forms in broad outline; they remain ensheathed by thin coverings of the unmodified mesoderm, now appropriately known as *perichondrium*. Dense mesoderm also remains between the cartilages where the joints will develop.

The cartilage models grow mainly by interstitial growth, in which each part expands more or less uniformly to maintain the general form. The next stage involves the replacement of the cartilage by bone tissue—not its transformation into bone, a distinction that deserves to be emphasized. The process does not occur identically or synchronously in different bones, and the remarks that follow concern that hypothetical concept, the "typical long bone."

The initial ossification involves two processes. In one, the perichondrium around the middle of the shaft lays bone down on the cartilage. This process of bone formation is known as intramembranous ossification because it occurs within the connective tissue membrane. Its details must be sought in textbooks of histology. A tubular bony sheath, the periosteal collar, is thus formed about the center of the shaft; it is gradually extended toward each extremity (Fig. 2.43). In the other process, the cartilage of the center of the shaft shows aging or degenerative changes; its cells hypertrophy, come to occupy enlarged lacunae (spaces) in the matrix, and then die, while the matrix becomes impregnated with calcium salts. This central patch of dead cartilage is now invaded by a connective tissue sprout that pushes in from the periosteum (as the perichondrium is now more appropriately known in the region of the collar). The progress of this sprout, which is rather cellular and well vascularized, is facilitated by the spongy texture given to the dead cartilage by the enlarged lacunae. Some of the cells that are carried inward have the capacity to engulf and remove calcified matrix, others have the capacity to lay bone down on the surviving framework, and a third group are precursors of marrow cells. The processes of construction and destruction continue in parallel and transform the whole middle portion of the shaft into a parcel of bone known as the primary or diaphysial center of ossification.

Later (much later in some species and mainly after birth in humans), similar sprouts from the perichondrium invade the centers of the two extremities to establish secondary or epiphysial centers of ossification. The secondary centers are not preceded by the formation of any equivalent to the periosteal collar of the shaft. The general stage of development of the long bone at this time is shown in Fig. 2.43/*8*. This drawing demonstrates that the original cartilage now survives only as two plates, the epiphysial or growth cartilages, that intervene between the primary and secondary centers. These have a special significance since they are responsible for the growth in length of the bone. They are clearly polarized, with cell division and matrix expansion confined to the epiphyseal aspect and degeneration, calcification, and replacement occurring at the central or diaphyseal side (Fig. 2.44). The replacement adds continuously to the length of the diaphysis, while the growth of the cartilage continues to shift the epiphyses away from it. The two processes are balanced until finally growth fails to keep pace with replacement. The

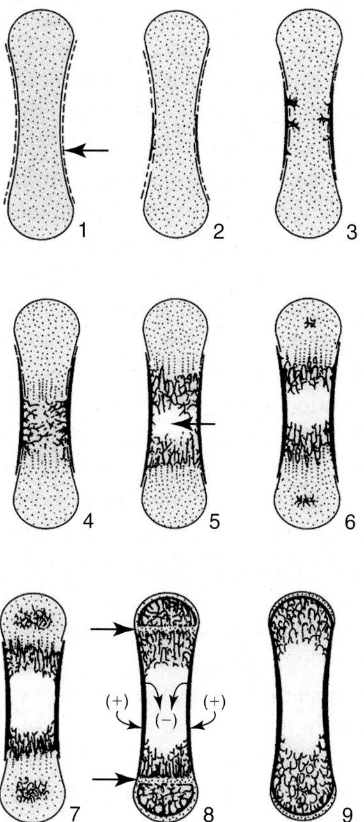

Fig. 2.43 Development of a long bone, schematic. *1*, Cartilage model with perichondral membrane *(arrow)*; *2*, intramembranous ossification of diaphysis; *3*, *4*, endochondral (primary) ossification of diaphysis, replaces cartilage; *5*, beginning of medullary cavity *(arrow)*; *6*, epiphysial ossification centers appear; *7*, endochondral (secondary) ossification of epiphyses; *8*, narrow epiphysial cartilages *(arrows)* separate the diaphysis from epiphyses: these and the articular cartilages are all that remain of the cartilage model *(1)*; note circumferential growth of diaphysis by removal *(–)* and addition *(+)* of compact bone; *9*, mature bone consisting of articular cartilage, spongy bone, and compact bone; the epiphysial cartilages have disappeared.

plate thins and ultimately is quite destroyed. The epiphysis and diaphysis have now fused as one, and further longitudinal growth is impossible. Neither the rates of growth nor the times of final disappearance are necessarily the same in the two growth cartilages of a long bone. Meanwhile, however, the bone has also been increasing in its girth, which is the result of further lamellae being laid in succession on the existing bone within the periosteal sheath. Some of the larger projections on long bones develop from independent centers of ossification and remain separated from the shaft by cartilage growth plates while growth continues. The projections distinguished in this way are known as *apophyses*.

Little reflection is necessary before one realizes that bone growth must be more complicated than the processes just described. The form established by the original model would not be maintained by continuous accretion. A simultaneous process of destruction maintains the shape of the metaphyses (the regions of the shaft adjoining the growth cartilages), keeps surface features in the same relationship to each other, and establishes and then enlarges the medullary cavity. The bone grows by apposition, the deposition of new material on that previously existing while the periosteum grows interstitially as though uniformly stretched. The periosteal sheath therefore shifts relative to the underlying bone, and the consequent drag on the nutrient vessels explains the generally oblique orientation of the adult nutrient foramina. By the time of birth, skeletal development has reached very different stages in different mammalian species. In the precocious ungulates, which are active immediately after birth, almost all epiphyses are well established at term. This characteristic contrasts sharply with the much less mature condition of the canine and, most especially, human neonates, in which many of the secondary ossification centers have yet to appear. The individual rate of skeletal development is affected by many factors—inherited, nutritional, and hormonal—the last covering a complex situation in which hormones of hypophyseal, thyroid, adrenal, and gonadal origin are involved. It is hardly surprising that abnormality of skeletal development is common.

The *development of joints* occurs through derivation of joint tissues from the mesoderm left between the cartilaginous primordia of the bones. Spaces that develop in this tissue coalesce to form a single synovial cavity bounded by articular cartilage and synovial membrane. The former is probably produced by delayed chondrification of the mesoderm bordering the cartilaginous models; structural differences suggest that it is not the outer shell of this model left over after completion of epiphyseal ossification. The synovial membrane is a more direct transformation of the mesoderm bordering the space. The fibrous part of the capsule and periarticular ligaments develop from more peripheral mesoderm.

It is now generally agreed that the limb muscles develop within the buds. The attractive notion that portions of myotomes migrate into these buds, pulling along the appropriate nerves, has been abandoned. Certain mesenchymal cells outside the denser axial core differentiate into precursor muscle cells (myoblasts), which then increase in number through

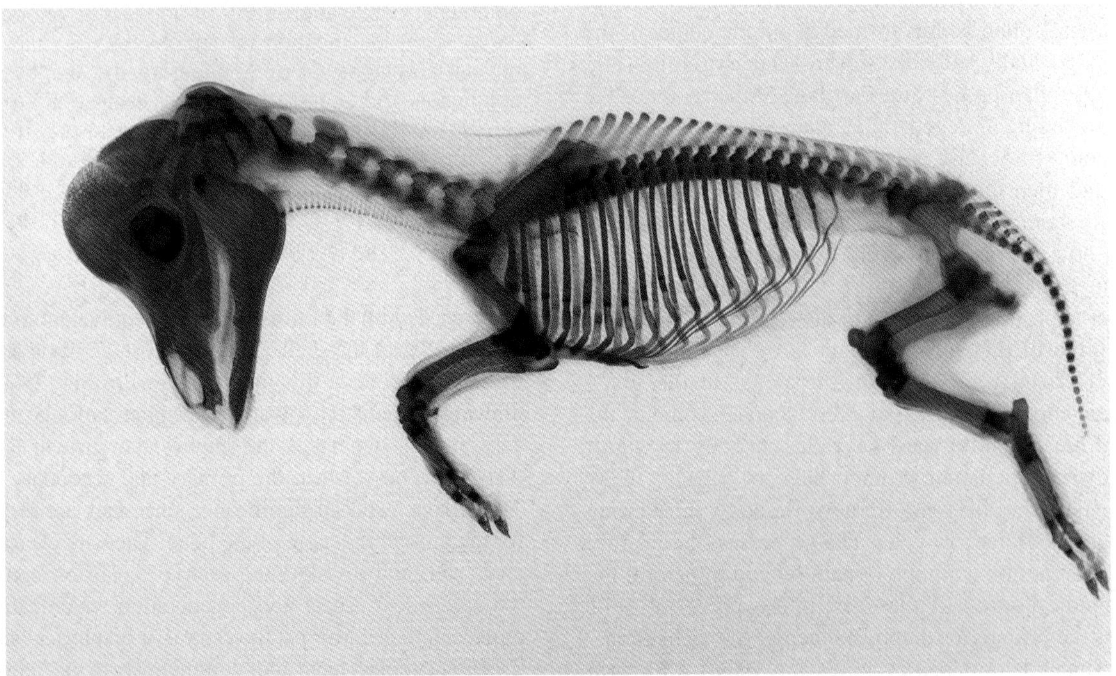

Fig. 2.44 Equine (pony) fetus 80 days. The developing skeleton has been colored with Alcian blue and Alizarin red. The calcified parts are *red* (Alizarin). The epiphyses have not begun to calcify; these cartilaginous parts are *blue*.

mitosis while recruitment from the mesenchyme continues. The myoblasts then form myocytes or muscle cells by a maturation in which the nuclei increase in number and migrate to the periphery of the cells. The final number of muscle cells seems, in most species, to be established before birth, perhaps well before birth. The later growth of muscles therefore depends on an increase in the size of existing elements.

The limb nerves grow in from the ventral rami of certain spinal nerves: generally C6–T2 for the forelimb and L4–S2 for the hindlimb. The segmental pattern becomes disturbed by the development of the limb plexuses, in which fibers from the several ventral rami reassort before combining as the named peripheral trunks. As a consequence, all but a few very small muscles are supplied by fibers that lead from neurons in more than one spinal segment. The sensory fibers to the skin arrange themselves so that specific regions are more or less the territory of particular spinal segments. The basis for this pattern has become more difficult to understand now that it is believed that the dermis of the limb skin develops from cells of local origin, not from cells that migrated from particular somites.

Table 2.3 lists, in parallel columns, the bones of the forelimb skeleton and the parts to which they give support; for comparison, columns for the corresponding bones and parts of the hindlimb (which, it will be recalled, are analogous and not homologous) are also included. A central column gives additional terms, more common in zoologic than in veterinary literature, that are common to both limbs; most are not used in this text but may be encountered elsewhere.

Some entries in the first and last columns may include three terms. Those printed in plain type are the technical words used in reference to domestic animals, the terms commonly employed by veterinarians; those *italicized* are the corresponding words used in human anatomy; and those in [brackets] are the more elevated Latin terms. Probably the most surprising feature of the table is the apparent absence of vernacular terms for certain regions of animals. The situation is in fact rather better, or rather worse according to one's point of view, than it appears. Many additional vernacular terms are restricted by custom to certain species; for example, the metacarpus of the horse is known as the cannon, but that of the dog is not. A particular difficulty is presented by the lack of handy equivalents to "paw" in description of farm animals: manus and pes are unacceptably pedantic (hence enclosed in brackets) and not employed in this book, and forefoot and hindfoot are usually (if not entirely logically) preferred; however, to the horse owner the foot generally means only the hoof and its contents. It is impossible to avoid all inconsistency.

It is of course more sensible to use the everyday terms in conversation with laypeople.

The Skeleton of the Forelimb

Pectoral Girdle

The *scapula,* or shoulder-blade (Fig. 2.45), is a flat bone that lies over the laterally compressed, craniodorsal part of the thorax, where it is held in place by an arrangement (synsarcosis) of muscles without forming a conventional articulation with the trunk. It is the basis of the *shoulder region,* a term that embraces much more than the immediate neighborhood of the shoulder joint. In

TABLE 2.3 TERMS IN USE FOR THE PARTS AND BONES OF THE LIMBS[a]

Forelimb			Hindlimb	
Body Part	**Skeleton**	**Terms Common to Both Limbs**	**Skeleton**	**Body Part**
Shoulder region, *shoulder*	Scapula and clavicle	Cingulum (girdle)	Os coxae (hip bone)	Pelvis
			Ilium	
			Pubis	
			Ischium	
Arm, *upper arm* (brachium)	Humerus	Stylopodium	Femur (properly os femoris)	Thigh (femur)
Forearm (antebrachium)	Radius and ulna	Zeugopodium	Tibia and fibula	Leg (crus)
[Manus]		[Autopodium]		[Pes]
Carpus, *wrist*	Carpal bones	Basipodium	Tarsal bones	Hock, *ankle* (tarsus)
Metacarpus	Metacarpal bones	Metapodium	Metatarsal bones	Metatarsus
Digit, *finger*	Proximal, middle, and distal phalanges	Acropodium	Proximal, middle, and distal phalanges	Digit, *toe*

[a]Terms printed in plain type are the technical words used when referring to parts and bones in domestic animals, the terms commonly employed by veterinarians; those *italicized* are the corresponding words used in human anatomy; and those in [brackets] are the more elevated Latin terms.

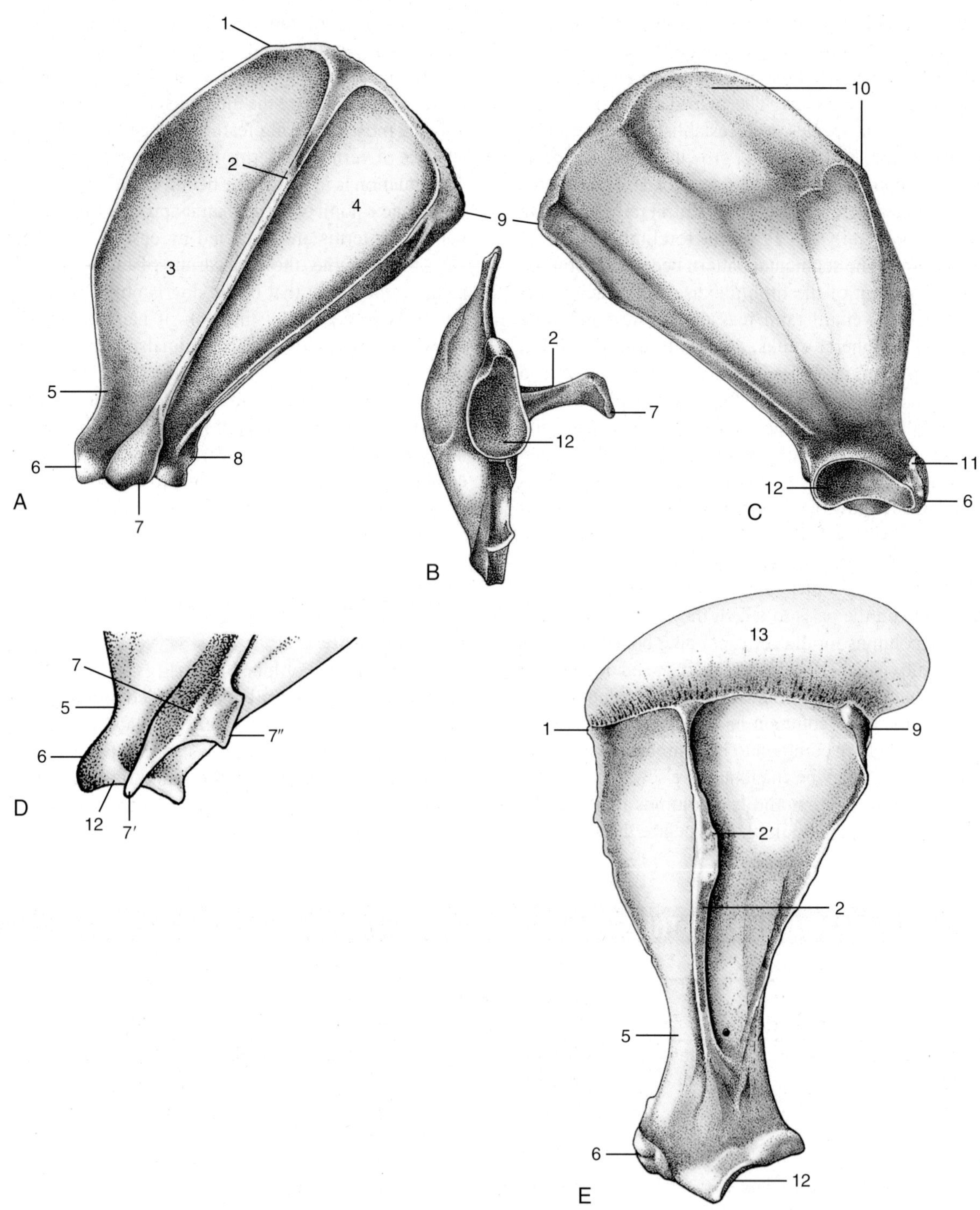

Fig. 2.45 Left scapula of the dog. (A) lateral, (B) ventral, and (C) medial views. (D) Distal end of left feline scapula. (E) Left equine scapula. *1,* Cranial angle; *2,* spine; *2′,* tuber of spine; *3,* supraspinous fossa; *4,* infraspinous fossa; *5,* neck; *6,* supraglenoid tubercle; *7,* acromion; *7′* and *7″,* hamate and suprahamate processes of acromion; *8,* infraglenoid tubercle; *9,* caudal angle; *10,* facies serrata; *11,* coracoid process; *12,* glenoid cavity; *13,* scapular cartilage.

ungulates, the scapula is extended dorsally by an unossified portion, the scapular cartilage (Fig. 2.45E/*13*), which enlarges the area for muscular attachment. The cartilage becomes increasingly calcified and thus more rigid with age.

The scapula is roughly triangular, though less so in the dog and cat than in the other domestic species. A prominent spine divides its lateral surface into supraspinous and infraspinous fossae, each occupied by the like-named muscle. The spine extends from the dorsal border almost to the articular angle and may bear palpable thickening for the insertion of the thoracic part of the trapezius. In all but the horse and pig, it ends in a prominent process (acromion), laterally flattened to form a hamate process in the carnivores (Fig. 2.45/*7′*) and furnished with an additional projection (suprahamate process; Fig. 2.45/*7″*) in the cat. The medial surface of the bone has a shallow fossa and it largely offers origin of the subscapularis; a more dorsal roughened area, where the serratus ventralis attaches, extends onto the cartilage in the larger species.

The caudal border is thickened and almost straight. The thinner and sinuous cranial border is notched toward its distal end for the passage of the suprascapular nerve. The dorsal border is also generally straight and extends between cranial and caudal angles; the latter is thickened and more easily identified on palpation. The ventral or articular angle is joined to the body of the bone by a slightly constricted neck. Its caudal part carries a shallow glenoid cavity (Fig. 2.45/*12*) for articulation with the head of the humerus. The cavity, which is somewhat extended in the sagittal direction, faces more or less ventrally. A large muscular process, the supraglenoid tubercle, projects in front of the cavity and gives origin to the biceps brachii.

The clavicle is reduced to a nubbin of bone in dog and a slender rodlet in the cat and lies at a fibrous intersection in the brachiocephalicus. These may be misinterpreted when viewed on radiographs.

Skeleton of the Free Appendage

The *humerus* (Fig. 2.46) forms the skeleton of the arm. It is a long bone that lies obliquely against the ventral part of the thorax, more horizontally in the large species than in the small. It is also relatively shorter and more robust in horses and cattle than in the small ruminants and carnivores. The proximal extremity carries a large spheroidal articular head (Fig. 2.46/*2*) that articulates with the relatively smaller glenoid cavity of the scapula and thus is offset in relation to the shaft to which it is joined by a neck. Two processes, the greater (lateral) and lesser (medial) tubercles, are placed in front and to the side of the articular area. They are separated by the intertubercular groove (Fig. 2.46/*13*), through which the biceps tendon passes. The processes are sometimes more or less equal, as in the horse. More often the lateral one, which forms the basis of the surface feature known as the point of the shoulder, is larger, as in the dog. In the horse and in cattle, both tubercles are divided into cranial and caudal parts (Fig. 2.46/*1′*, *1″*, and *3′*); the intertubercular groove is also molded by an intermediate tubercle in the horse (Fig. 2.46/*13′*). The medial and lateral tubercles give attachment to the muscles that brace and support the shoulder joint, substituting for collateral ligaments.

A twisted appearance is imparted to the shaft by a groove (Fig. 2.46/*12*) that spirals over the lateral aspect and carries the brachialis muscle and the radial nerve. Laterally, toward its upper end, the shaft carries the large, easily

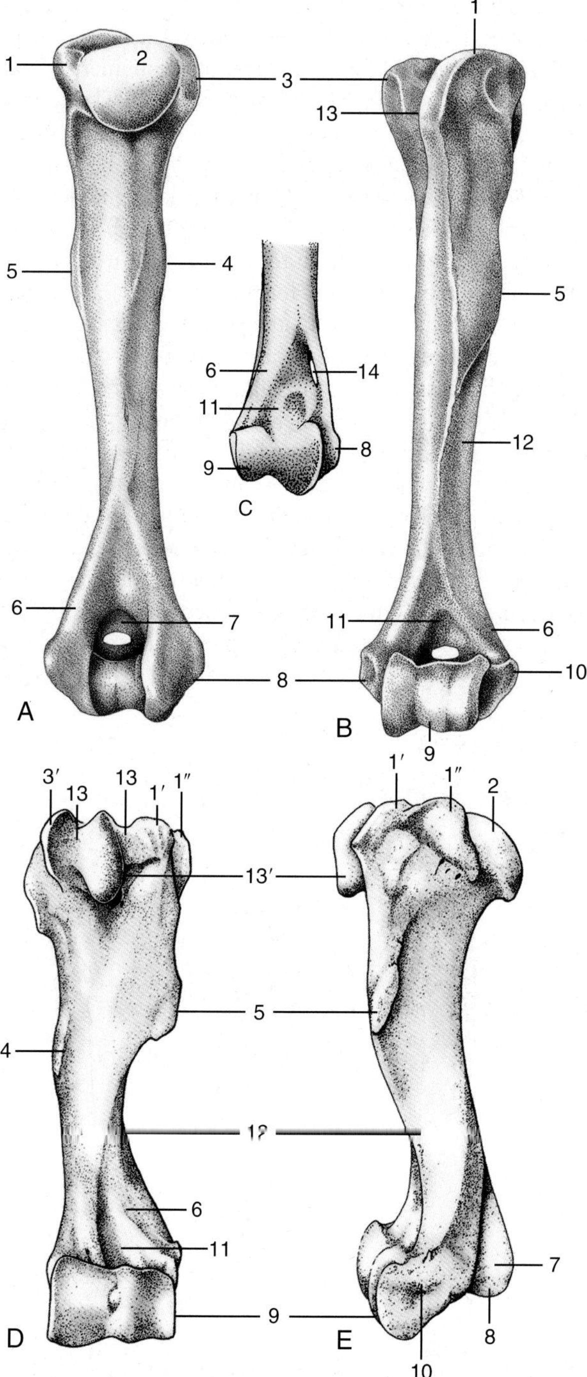

Fig. 2.46 Left humerus of the dog. (A) Caudal and (B) cranial views. (C) Distal end of right feline humerus: cranial view. (D) Cranial and (E) lateral views of left equine humerus. *1,* Greater tubercle; *1′* and *1″,* cranial and caudal parts of greater tubercle; *2,* head; *3,* lesser tubercle; *3′,* cranial part of lesser tubercle; *4,* teres (major) tuberosity; *5,* deltoid tuberosity; *6,* lateral supracondylar crest; *7,* olecranon fossa (with supratrochlear foramen in dog); *8,* medial epicondyle; *9,* condyle; *10,* lateral epicondyle; *11,* radial fossa; *12,* groove for brachialis; *13,* intertubercular groove; *13′,* intermediate tubercle; *14,* supracondylar foramen.

palpated deltoid tuberosity (Fig. 2.46/*5*), which is joined to the greater tubercle by a prominent ridge. A less prominent, gradually subsiding ridge, the crest of the humerus, continues distally beyond the deltoid tuberosity. The medial aspect of the shaft is marked by a much less salient roughening, the teres (major) tuberosity.

The distal extremity bears an articular condyle (Fig. 2.46/*9*) that in large animals has the form of a trochlea to engage with the radius. In the dog and cat it is divided into a medial area (trochlea) for the ulna and a lateral area (capitulum) for the radius. In all species the caudal part of the groove of the trochlea continues proximally into a deep (olecranon) fossa (Fig. 2.46/*7*) that receives the anconeal process of the ulna. Two saliences proximal to the articular surface are known as epicondyles. The more prominent medial epicondyle (Fig. 2.46/*8*) has a caudally directed projection that gives origin to the flexor muscles of the carpus and digit. The cranial aspect of the lateral epicondyle (Fig. 2.46/*10*) gives origin to the extensor muscles of the carpus and digit. To the side, each epicondyle gives origin to the corresponding collateral ligament of the elbow joint.

In the dog the floor of the olecranon fossa is perforated by a supratrochlear foramen that opens to a much shallower radial fossa on the cranial aspect of the shaft (Fig. 2.46/*7* and *11*). In the cat alone, a supracondylar foramen, located in the mediodistal part of the humerus (Fig. 2.46/*14*), gives passage to the median nerve and brachial artery.

The *skeleton of the forearm* is provided by two bones, the radius and the ulna (Fig. 2.47). In the standing position they are arranged with the ulna caudal to the radius in the upper part of the forearm but lateral in the lower part. In the primitive condition these bones articulate only at their extremities, leaving an interosseous space between their shafts. The two bones are held together by ligaments or by fusion as in domestic animals, resulting, respectively, in reduction or loss of the rotational movements of the human forearm (supination and pronation). When supination is possible, it consists of rotation of the upper extremity of the radius within the embrace of the ulna while the distal extremity is carried in an arc around the ulna.

In ungulates the bones are fused, and in the horse only the upper end of the ulna remains distinct (Fig. 2.47D/*1*).

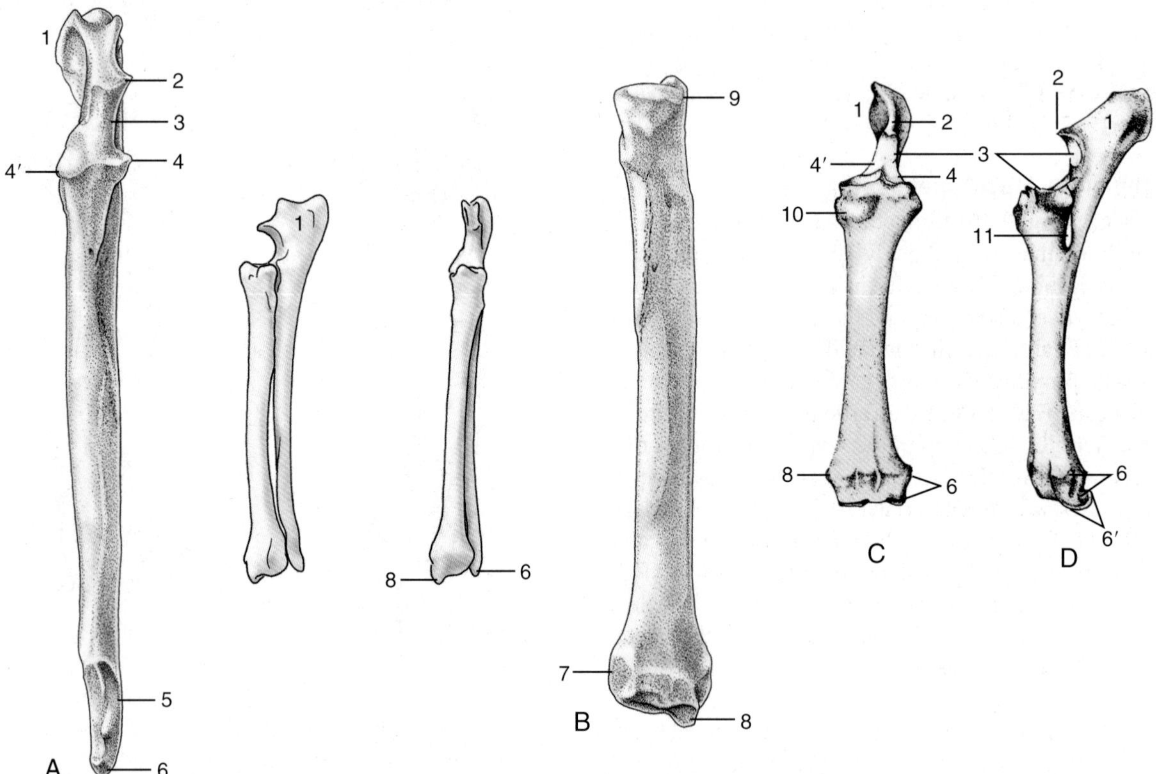

Fig. 2.47 (A) Left ulna and (B) left radius of the dog. In sequence from the *left:* cranial view of the ulna, craniolateral and cranial views of the radius and ulna, and caudal view of the radius alone. (C) Cranial and (D) lateral views of fused left radius and ulna of the horse. *1,* Olecranon; *2,* anconeal process; *3,* trochlear notch; *4* and *4′,* lateral and medial coronoid processes; *5,* distal articular facet for radius; *6,* lateral styloid process (with facet for the ulnar carpal bone in the dog); *6′,* distal end of ulna incorporated within radius; *7,* articular facet for ulna; *8,* medial styloid process; *9,* circumferential facet; *10,* radial tuberosity; *11,* interosseous space.

The ruminants and pig show intermediate conditions. About 45 degrees of supination is allowed in the dog and somewhat more in the cat. (Rotation at the carpus contributes a substantial extra component to the movement subjectively interpreted as supination.)

The radius is a rather simple rodlike bone, usually much stronger than the ulna in ungulates but less dominant in carnivores, in particular the cat. Its proximal extremity is transversely widened, though tending to a more circular plan in carnivores, in which some supinatory capacity remains. It articulates with the distal articular surface of the humerus. A circumferential facet (Fig. 2.47B/*9*) on the caudal part of the proximal extremity articulates with the ulna and is present even when no supination is possible. The shaft is craniocaudally compressed and slightly bowed in its length. The distal part of the cranial surface is grooved for the passage of the extensor tendons (Fig. 2.47C), whereas the caudal surface is roughened for muscular attachment. The medial border is subcutaneous and therefore palpable.

The distal extremity of the radius carries an articular surface that is concave in its cranial part and convex in its caudal part in ungulates; it has a slightly concave ovoid form in carnivores, in which some abduction, adduction, and rotation of the antebrachiocarpal joint are allowed in addition to the major movements of flexion and extension. Medial to the articulation, the radius is prolonged to form a styloid process (Fig. 2.47B/*8*). The corresponding lateral projection is furnished by the ulna and, in the horse, by the portion of the radius representing the incorporated ulna.

The shaft of the ulna is greatly reduced, and its proximal extremity is prolonged beyond the articular surface to form the high olecranon, the point of the elbow, which gives attachment to the triceps. The cranial margin of the olecranon carries the beaklike anconeal process (Fig. 2.47/*2*), which fits into the olecranon fossa of the humerus, above an articular notch that engages with the humeral trochlea; yet farther from the extremity, there is a facet for the circumferential articular area of the radius. In the dog the shaft, though slender, runs the full length of the radius, from which it is separated by an interosseous space that is bridged by membrane in life. The distal extremity carries a small articular facet for the radius and beyond this is continued as the lateral styloid process (Fig. 2.47/*6*), which makes contact with the ulnar carpal bone.

Reduction of the ulna is greatest in the horse, in which the shaft tapers to end at midforearm level (Fig. 2.47D). The distal part became incorporated within the radius in fetal life (Fig. 2.47/*6'*).

The short *carpal bones,* arranged in two rows in domestic animals, articulate in complex fashion (Fig. 2.48). The proximal row comprises (in mediolateral sequence) radial, intermediate, ulnar, and accessory bones; the last appears as an appendage projecting behind the carpus and is a prominent landmark in the live animal. The radial and intermediate carpals fuse in the dog and cat. The elements of the distal row are numbered from 1 to 5 (again in mediolateral sequence), although the fifth never appears as a separate bone but is either suppressed or fused with the fourth. The first is also often lacking whereas the second and third fuse in ruminants. Apart from the accessory carpal bone, which is probably a sesamoid by origin, a small sesamoid bone is embedded in the medial tissues of the joint of the dog. Intrinsically unimportant, it can confuse radiographic interpretation by wrongly suggesting a "chip" fracture.

Viewed as a whole, the carpus is convex from side to side on its cranial aspect and flat and very irregular caudally, although in life these irregularities are smoothed by thick ligaments. Most movement occurs at the antebrachiocarpal level, some at the intercarpal level, and virtually none at the carpometacarpal level or between neighboring bones in a row. The combined proximal articular surface is the reciprocal of that of the radius (see earlier) and in carnivores has a convex ovoid form.

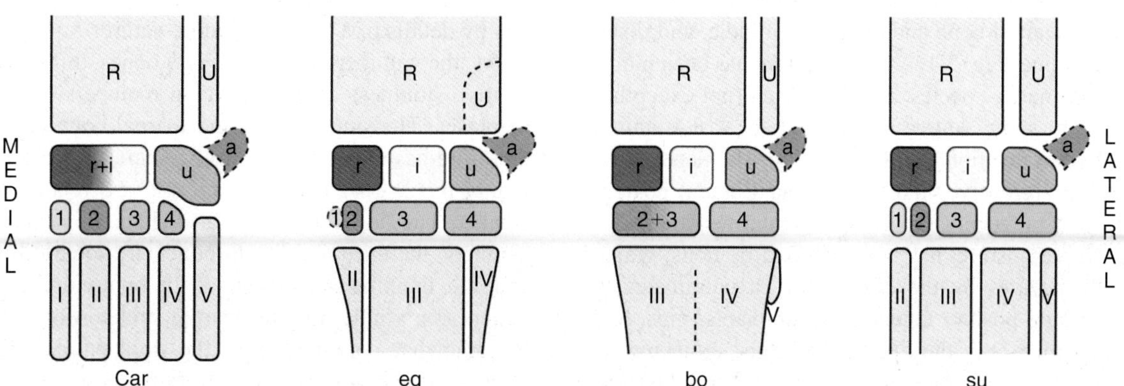

Fig. 2.48 The bones of the carpal skeleton in the carnivores *(Car),* horse *(eq),* cattle *(bo),* and pig *(su)* schematic. *Roman numerals* identify the metacarpal bones, *arabic numerals* the distal carpal bones. *A,* Accessory carpal bone; *i,* intermediate carpal bone; *R,* radius; *r,* radial carpal bone; *U,* ulna; *u,* ulnar carpal bone.

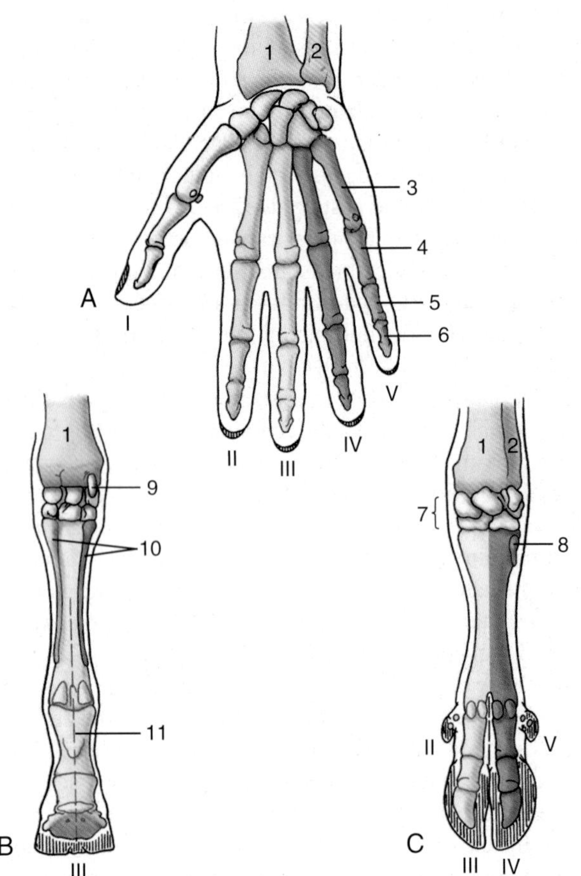

Fig. 2.49 Right manus of (A) human (hand), (B) horse, and (C) ruminant, palmar views. The *Roman numerals* number the rays. *1,* Radius; *2,* ulna; *3,* metacarpal; *4, 5,* and *6,* proximal, middle, and distal phalanges; *7,* carpal bones; *8,* rudimentary metacarpal V; *9,* accessory carpal bone; *10,* rudimentary metacarpals II and IV (medial and lateral splint bones); *11,* axis in line with ray III (mesaxonic), in C paraxonic.

The primitive pattern for the skeleton of the mammalian *manus* exhibits five more or less equal rays, each consisting of a metacarpal bone and proximal, middle, and distal phalanges in line (Fig. 2.49A). This pattern has been modified in all domestic species, each of which (not excepting the pig) is to some degree specialized for fast running. Cursorial specialization involves raising the manus (and pes) from the primitive "flatfooted" (plantigrade) posture demonstrated by bears (Fig. 2.50). An intermediate stage, the digitigrade posture, has been attained by dogs, which support themselves by the digits only; it culminates in the unguligrade posture attained by ruminants, pigs, and horses, in which only the tips of the digits, protected by hooves (ungulae), give support. As a result of this process, the abaxial digits first lose permanent contact with the ground, and the remaining digits develop compensatorily to carry an increased proportion of the weight. The process has not progressed very far in the dog and cat, in which only the most medial (first) digit has lost contact

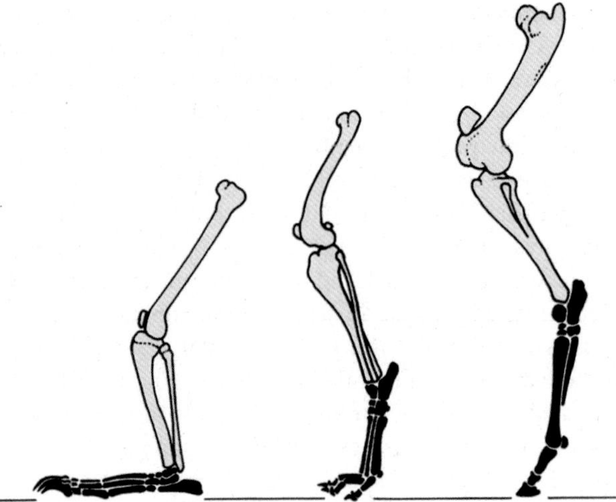

Fig. 2.50 Hindlimbs of bear, dog, and horse (from *left* to *right),* illustrating plantigrade, digitigrade, and unguligrade postures, respectively.

and is retained as a nonfunctional dewclaw (Fig. 2.51). The four functional digits are broadly equal, with the axis of the manus passing between the third and fourth digits (a paraxonic position). Pigs have entirely lost the first digit; the second and fifth digits are very much reduced, although each retains a complete skeleton. In ruminants the process has gone further, and although elements of four digits are present, those of the abaxial pair are vestigial; the metacarpal bones of the functional third and fourth digits are fused in a single bone that retains evidence of its composite origin (Fig. 2.49C).

In the horse (Fig. 2.49B), only the third ray survives in functional form, and its axis coincides with that of the limb; the manus is said to be mesaxonic. Remnants of the second and fourth metacarpal bones survive as the splint bones that flank the third metacarpal or cannon bone and end in nodules.

The differences in the metacarpal and digital skeleton are very striking as a consequence of these changes, and the short description that follows is amplified in later chapters by details of a species-specific nature.

As the number of *metacarpal* bones diminishes, the relative stoutness of the surviving members of the series increases. The single (third) metacarpal bone of the horse therefore has a particularly strong shaft, whereas the individual metacarpal bones of the dog are relatively much weaker. The dog's bones are also shaped by their mutual contacts; the third and fourth bones are square in section, and the flanking second and fifth bones are triangular. Taken as a whole, the metacarpal skeleton of all species is somewhat compressed in the dorsopalmar direction. Each bone has a proximal extremity (base), a shaft, and a distal extremity (caput). The base has a flattish articular surface for the distal row of carpal bones and may, according to its position in the metacarpal series, have medial and lateral facets where it makes contact with neighbors. The distal extremity articulates with the proximal phalanx

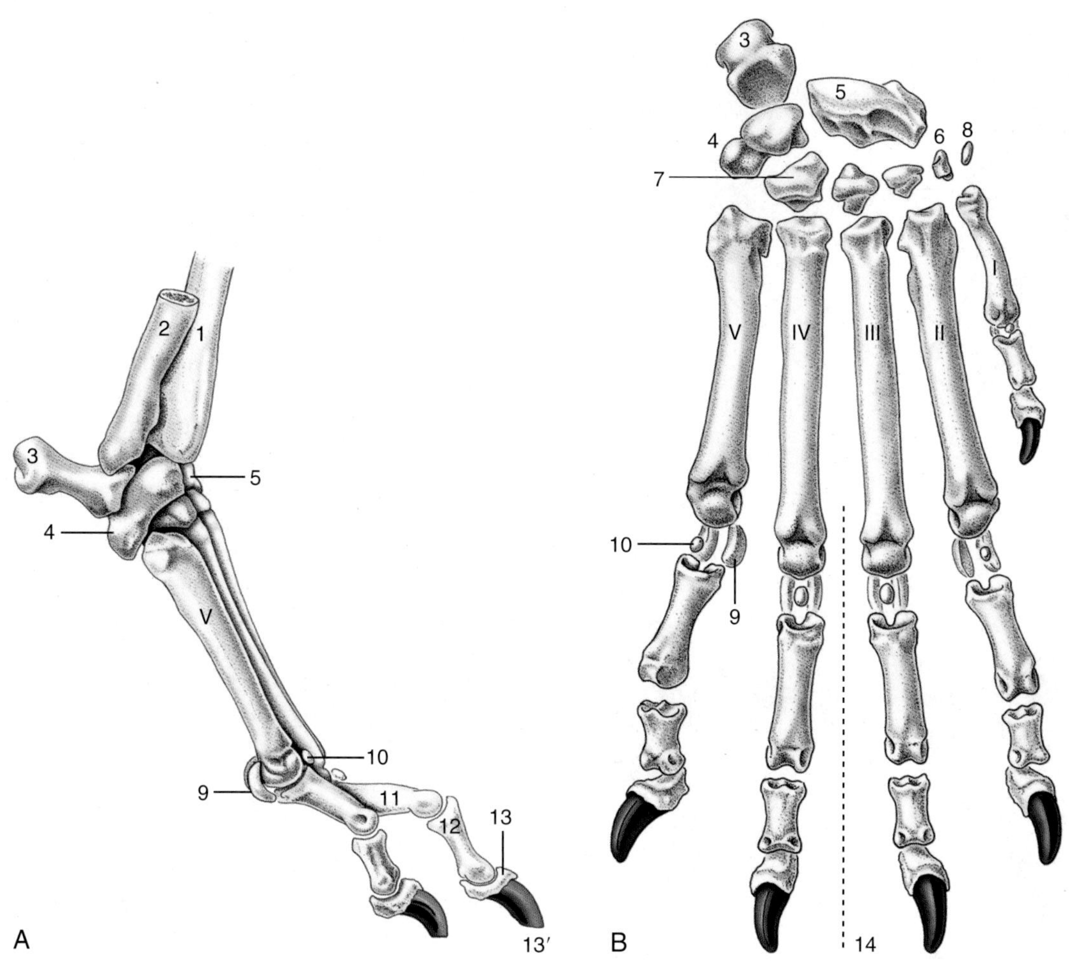

Fig. 2.51 Skeleton of the right manus of the dog. (A) Lateral and (B) dorsal views. The *Roman numerals* identify the metacarpal bones. *1,* Radius; *2,* ulna; *3,* accessory carpal; *4,* ulnar carpal; *5,* radial carpal (intermedioradial in the dog); *6, 7,* first and fourth of the distal row of carpal bones; *8,* sesamoid bone; *9,* proximal sesamoid bones; *10,* dorsal sesamoid bone; *11, 12,* and *13,* proximal, middle, and distal phalanges; *13′,* claw; *14,* axis of manus.

by a hemicylindrical surface with a central ridge. Various roughenings for ligamentous attachment are present at both extremities.

The *proximal phalanx* is a short cylindrical bone with a proximal extremity adapted to the caput of the metacarpal bone and a distal articulation in the form of a shallow trochlea. Again, the bone may be shaped by its position in the digital series.

The *middle phalanx* is shorter than, but basically very similar to, the first phalanx. The *distal phalanx* corresponds to the form of the hoof or claw in which it is wholly (hoof) or partly (claw) contained. The digital skeleton is completed by paired *proximal sesamoid bones* at the palmar aspect of the metacarpophalangeal joint and by a *distal sesamoid bone* (cartilage in the dog) at the palmar aspect of the distal interphalangeal joint. In the dog small sesamoids also exist within the extensor tendons over the dorsal aspect of the metacarpophalangeal joints.

The Joints of the Forelimb

The *shoulder joint* (Fig. 2.52A) links the scapula and humerus, and although it has attributes of the spheroidal variety, sagittal excursions predominate in practice. The glenoid cavity of the scapula is considerably smaller than the head of the humerus. In large animals, both surfaces may be indented peripherally by naked areas (synovial fossae) simulating, to the inexperienced eye, lesions of the cartilage. The joint capsule is roomy and is strengthened here and there through fusion with the tendons of the surrounding muscles, notably the subscapularis. The medial subscapularis and the lateral infraspinatus also brace the joint in the absence of the usual pericapsular ligaments. In all but the horse and ox the capsule forms a protective synovial sheath around the tendon of origin of the biceps brachii, where this origin lies within the intertubercular groove. The capsule is replaced by a discrete intertubercular bursa in the two large species.

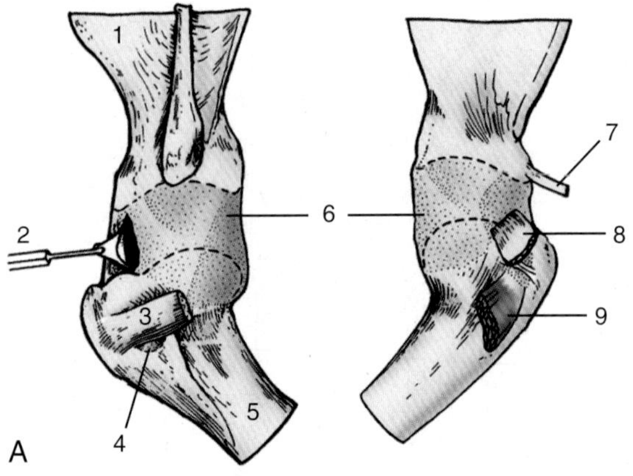

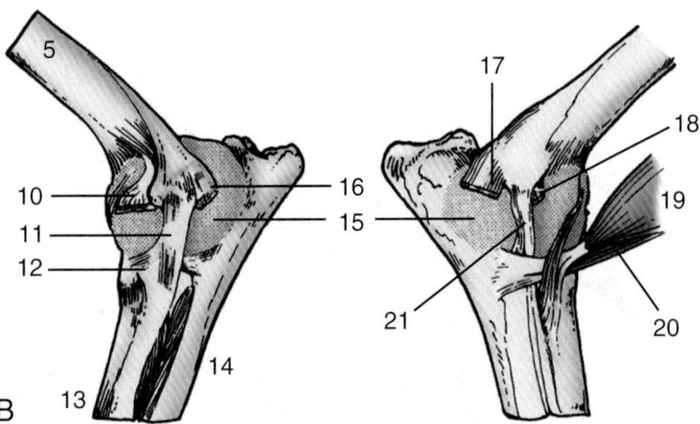

Fig. 2.52 (A) Left shoulder and (B) elbow joints of the dog. The drawings on the *left* are lateral views, those on the *right* medial. *1,* Scapula; *2,* joint capsule opened to expose biceps tendon; *3,* tendon of infraspinatus; *4,* infraspinatus bursa; *5,* humerus; *6,* joint capsule, stretched by pulling bones apart; *7,* tendon of coracobrachialis; *8,* tendon of subscapularis, reflected ventrally; *9,* biceps tendon emerging from intertubercular groove; *10,* stump of extensor carpi radialis and common digital extensor; *11,* lateral collateral ligament; *12,* annular ligament of radius; *13,* radius; *14,* ulna; *15,* joint capsule; *16,* stump of ulnaris lateralis; *17,* common stump of carpal and digital flexors; *18,* stump of pronator teres; *19,* biceps; *20,* brachialis; *21,* medial collateral ligament.

Movement is most free in the sagittal direction, but significant amounts of rotation, abduction, and adduction, and therefore also of circumduction, are possible, particularly in the dog and cat; in these animals a component of the movement interpreted as supination probably occurs at shoulder level.

The *elbow joint* (Fig. 2.52B) combines within a single capsule the hinge joint between the humerus and the radius and ulna and, at least in carnivores, the pivot joint between the proximal extremities of the radius and ulna. The humeral surface is broadly trochlear, and the lower surface, variously furnished by the radius and ulna, is its reciprocal. Ridging of the surfaces, most pronounced in the larger animals, impedes other than hinge movements. A proximal radioulnar articulation between a circumferential facet on the radius and a corresponding but smaller area on the ulna is present even when more distal fusion precludes the possibility of movement. The joint capsule is surprisingly roomy and, when distended, bulges to each side of the ulna within the olecranon fossa. The strongest ligaments are medial and lateral collateral ligaments for this joint, which is basically a hinge joint. The lateral of these ligaments is short and thick (Fig. 2.52/*11*), and the medial one is longer, more slender, and divisible into two parts (Fig. 2.52/*21*)—radial and ulnar in the dog and cat and superficial and deep in the larger animals. The dog and cat have an additional oblique ligament over the flexor aspect of the joint and also an annular ligament (Fig. 2.52/*12*) between the collateral ligaments to completely enclose the head of the radius within an osseoligamentous ring.

In the large species, most notably the horse, the curvature of the humeral surface is not uniform. This feature, combined with the eccentric proximal attachment of the collateral ligaments (see Fig. 2.10), makes the joint more stable in the normal standing position (which approaches but does not reach maximal extension); some effort is required to "unlock" the joint before it can be flexed.

The *carpal joint* includes antebrachiocarpal, midcarpal, and carpometacarpal levels of articulation and also a distal radioulnar joint. The antebrachiocarpal and radioulnar joints share a joint cavity. The midcarpal and carpometacarpal joint cavities are interconnected. In hoofed species the proximal joint may be regarded as being of the hinge variety (although the form of the surfaces introduces a certain obliquity of movement in ruminants), but in dogs and cats it is more versatile and can be regarded as an ellipsoidal joint, although a poor example of the type. The hinge movement is quite free at the antebrachiocarpal level (horse: ca. 90 degrees). Considerable movement is also possible at the midcarpal level (ca. 45 degrees), but virtually no movement is allowed at the carpometacarpal level. Medial and lateral collateral ligaments are well developed in ungulates but are necessarily much weaker in the dog and cat to allow for some adduction and abduction. On the dorsal aspect, a number of short ligaments join neighboring bones in the same row and those of the row distal to the metacarpus. More robust ligaments are found on the palmar aspect, where a deep ligament (Fig. 2.53/*6*) covers the entire palmar surface of the skeleton, burying the unevenness of the bones. A second, superficial, transverse ligament (flexor retinaculum) passes obliquely from the free extremity of the accessory carpal bone to the medial aspect of the carpus (Fig. 2.53/*7*), completing the carpal canal, behind the carpus, for passage of the flexor tendons and other structures into the foot from the forearm. Additional

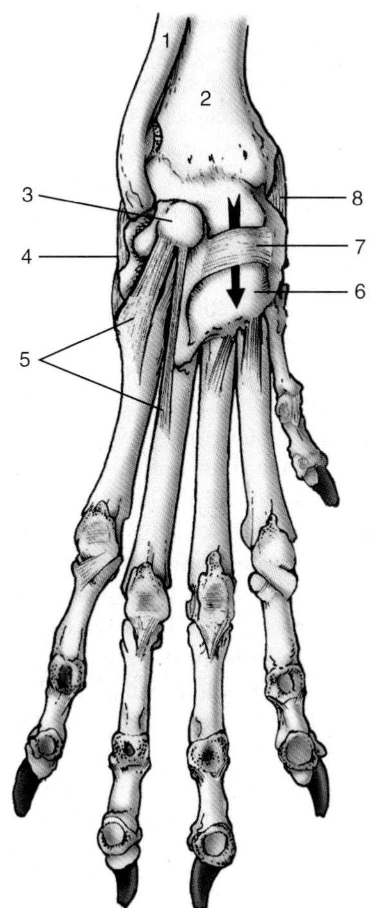

Fig. 2.53 Left carpal joint of the dog, palmar view, with ligaments shown in *blue*. *1,* Ulna; *2,* radius; *3,* accessory carpal; *4,* lateral collateral ligament; *5,* distal ligaments of accessory carpal; *6,* palmar carpal ligament; *7,* flexor retinaculum; *8,* medial collateral ligament; the *arrow* is in the carpal canal.

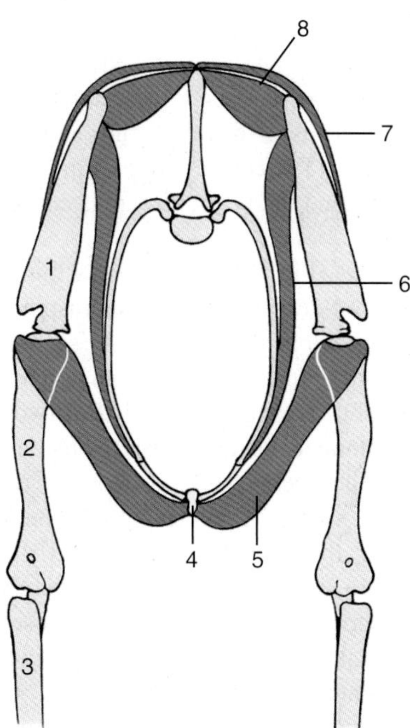

Fig. 2.54 Muscular suspension of the thorax between the forelimbs (dog). *1,* Scapula; *2,* humerus; *3,* radius and ulna; *4,* sternum; *5,* pectoralis profundus (ascendens); *6,* serratus ventralis; *7,* trapezius; *8,* rhomboideus.

small ligaments (Fig. 2.53/5) join the accessory bone to the adjacent carpal and metacarpal bones. These palmar ligaments do not interfere with flexion but assist in preventing overextension.

Description of the more distal joints is best deferred because of the marked interspecific variation. These joints are only important in the large species.

The Muscles of the Forelimb

The muscles of the forelimb comprise the girdle musculature, passing between the trunk and the limb, and the intrinsic musculature.

Girdle Muscles

The girdle muscles join the forelimb to the trunk, forming a connection known as a synsarcosis that substitutes for a conventional joint. When the animal is standing, some of the muscles of the synsarcosis (the serratus ventralis and pectoralis profundus) sling the body between the forelimbs to which they transmit the weight of the head, neck, and cranial part of the trunk (Fig. 2.54). These and other girdle muscles can also stabilize the scapula against external forces, preventing its displacement or rotation, as seen in a cat pouncing with forelimbs rigidly braced against the trunk. During progression the same muscles resolve into antagonistic groups that control the protraction or retraction of the limb. These actions are better understood if one knows that the scapula may be moved against the chest wall in two different ways. In one, the bone is rotated about a transverse axis located toward its upper end. The position of this imaginary axis is fixed by the balance of opposing muscles, chiefly the rhomboideus and serratus ventralis, attached on the dorsal part of the scapula. In the other movement, the whole bone is shifted on the thoracic wall. It is slid downward and forward as the limb is advanced and upward and backward in recovery during retraction. This movement of the scapula is permitted by the looseness of the connective tissue that intervenes between the limb and the trunk and creates a potential space, the axilla, corresponding to the human armpit. The axilla also gives passage to the nerves and vessels entering the limb from the trunk, and it contains the axillary lymph nodes.

For the purpose of description, the girdle muscles can be considered in two layers.

The Superficial Layer. The superficial layer of girdle muscles consists of a cranial group (trapezius, omotransversarius, and brachiocephalicus) that split from a single primordium in the embryo and are supplied mostly by the accessory nerve, except the caudal part of the brachiocephalius that is of deltoid origin and is supplied by the axillary nerve. The caudal group of muscles consists of latissimus dorsi and the ventral group is comprised of pectoral muscles.

The *trapezius* (Fig. 2.55/*5* and *5′*) is thin. It takes origin from the mid-dorsal raphe and supraspinous ligament, extending from about the level of the second cervical to that of the ninth thoracic vertebra, and converges to insert on the spine of the scapula. It consists of two fleshy parts, cervical and thoracic, usually separated by an intermediate aponeurosis. The fibers of the cervical part run caudoventrally to attach along the greater part of the length of the scapular spine; those of the thoracic part run cranioventrally to a more confined insertion on the tuberous thickening of the spine. The trapezius may raise the scapula against the trunk and swing the ventral angle of the bone cranially, thus advancing the limb.

The *omotransversarius* (Fig. 2.55/*3*) is a narrow muscle that extends between the transverse processes of the atlas (and possibly also the succeeding vertebrae) and the acromion and adjacent part of the scapula. It assists in advancement of the limb.

The *brachiocephalicus* (Fig. 2.55/*2* and *2′*) is more complex, being formed by the union of two elements that are separated by the much reduced clavicle. The caudal part (cleidobrachialis) passes between the clavicle and the humerus and is a component of the deltoideus muscle. The muscles supplied by the accessory nerve split from a single primordium in the embryo. However, the caudal part of the

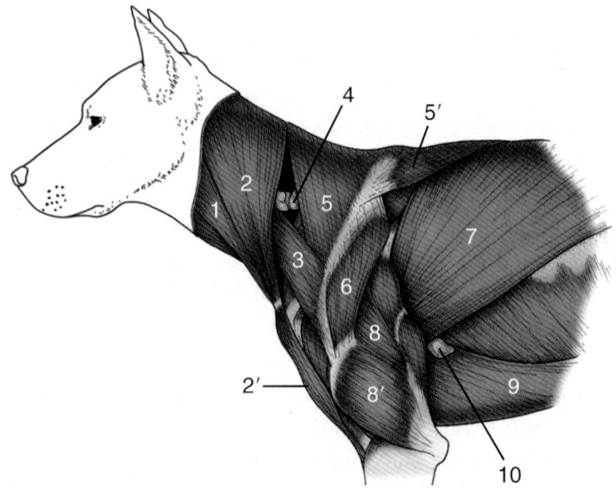

Fig. 2.55 Superficial muscles of the shoulder and arm. *1,* Sternocephalicus; *2* and *2′,* brachiocephalicus: cleidocervicalis and cleidobrachialis; *3,* omotransversarius; *4,* superficial cervical lymph node; *5* and *5′,* cervical and thoracic parts of trapezius; *6,* deltoideus; *7,* latissimus dorsi; *8* and *8′,* long and lateral heads of triceps; *9,* pectoralis profundus (ascendens); *10,* accessory axillary lymph node.

brachiocephalicus of deltoid origin retains the appropriate innervation by the axillary nerve. The cranial part passes cranially from the clavicle to several attachments in the head and neck. These attachments vary among species, and hence there is a rather bewildering array of names for particular units, cleido-occipitalis, cleidomastoideus, and so forth. In domestic species the two parts are in tandem, and the clavicle is generally reduced to a fibrous intersection in the combined muscle at the level of the shoulder joint, although vestigial ossifications are present in the dog and cat. *Brachiocephalicus* is a most appropriate name for the whole complex because it does not specify precise attachments. The brachiocephalicus advances the limb, possibly also extending the shoulder joint, when the cranial attachment is fixed and the limb is free to move; in contrast, when the limb is fixed and the head is free, this complex draws the head and neck ventrally when acting bilaterally and toward the side when acting unilaterally.

The *latissimus dorsi* (Fig. 2.55/*7*) has a very broad origin from the thoracolumbar fascia and converges to an insertion on the teres tuberosity of the humerus. The most cranial fibers cover the caudal angle of the scapula and strap it against the chest. The muscle retracts the free limb and may also flex the shoulder joint. On the other hand, when the limb is advanced and the foot firmly planted on the ground, the latissimus may draw the trunk forward. It may be regarded as antagonist to the brachiocephalicus. It is supplied by a local branch (thoracodorsal nerve) of the brachial plexus.

Two *superficial pectoral muscles* (see Fig. 2.41/*5* and *6*) arise, one behind the other, from the cranial part of the sternum. The cranial muscle (pectoralis descendens) terminates on the crest of the humerus, distal to the deltoid tuberosity. The caudal muscle (pectoralis transversus) descends over the medial aspect of the arm and in the larger species continues distally over the elbow joint, covering the median artery and nerve, to insert into the medial fascia of the forearm. Both muscles adduct the limb through the sideways shift of the trunk toward a previously abducted limb. The muscle may also assist protraction or retraction, depending on the initial position of the limb relative to the trunk. They are supplied by local branches (cranial pectoral nerves) from the brachial plexus.

The Deep Layer. The deep layer of girdle muscles comprises the rhomboideus dorsally, the serratus ventralis medially, and the pectoralis profundus ventrally.

The *rhomboideus* (Fig. 2.54/*8*) arises from median connective tissue structures extending from the poll to the withers and lies deep to the trapezius. In addition to cervical and thoracic parts, it has a capital part in carnivores. All attach to the dorsal border and adjacent area on the medial surface of the scapula. Most of the muscle draws the dorsal part of the scapula cranially, thereby retracting the limb. The muscle may also raise the limb and hold it firmly against the trunk. It is supplied from the brachial plexus in the dog, but in some species it is also supplied by *dorsal* branches of local spinal nerves, unusual for a limb muscle.

The *serratus ventralis* (Fig. 2.54/*6*) is a large fan-shaped muscle that takes an extensive origin via separate digitations from the fourth cervical vertebra to the tenth rib. The fibers run dorsally to terminate on a well-defined area on the medial aspect of the scapula and scapular cartilage. The direction of the fibers indicates that this muscle must play a large part in supporting the weight of the trunk, and in the larger species it is better adapted to this function by the presence of a strong fascial covering and intersections. The cervical portion of the muscle, which inserts craniodorsal to the axis of scapular rotation, can retract the limb; the caudal portion, which inserts caudodorsal to the axis, can advance the limb. When acting unilaterally, the cervical fibers may also draw the neck to that side; when acting bilaterally, they raise the neck. The thoracic part is a potential inspiratory muscle, although it is not normally used in that capacity. The innervation is mainly by a branch (long thoracic nerve) of the brachial plexus.

The *pectoralis profundus* (Fig. 2.55/*9*) may be regarded as having cranial and caudal parts. The cranial part, well-formed only in the horse and pig, probably corresponds to the subclavius of other mammals and is now so named officially. Both parts (or muscles) arise from the ventral aspect of the length of the sternum and adjacent cartilages, and the most caudal fibers extend beyond it onto the abdominal floor. In the horse and pig the subclavius passes dorsally along the leading edge of the scapula, attaching to the supraspinatus (see Fig. 23.5A/*2*). The larger caudal part, also known as the *pectoralis ascendens*, inserts on the lesser tubercle of the humerus. Both play a role, secondary to that of the serratus ventralis, in slinging the trunk between the forelimbs. They may also act as retractors of the forelimb when this is free. When the limb is advanced and fixed, they draw the trunk forward, toward the limb. The nerves are local branches (caudal pectoral nerves) of the brachial plexus.

Intrinsic Muscles of the Forelimb

The intrinsic muscles are conveniently grouped according to their common location, actions, and innervations.

Muscles Acting Primarily on the Shoulder Joint. The muscles acting on the shoulder joint are arranged in lateral, medial, and caudal groups.

The *lateral group* comprises the supraspinatus and infraspinatus, which arise from and fill the corresponding fossae of the scapula. The *supraspinatus* (Fig. 2.56/*3*) terminates on the summits of both tubercles of the humerus. The *infraspinatus* inserts by a tendon that splits into a shorter deep part, which attaches to the summit, and a longer superficial part, which attaches to the lateral face of the (caudal part of the) greater tubercle; *a bursa between the bone and the longer tendon may be the seat of a painful inflammation.* Both muscles brace the joint laterally. The supraspinatus tendon passes cranial to the axis of rotation and may therefore also extend the shoulder. It is sometimes asserted that the infraspinatus tendon passes cranial or caudal to the axis of rotation depending on the actual position of the joint and may then further extend the already extended joint or further flex the already flexed joint; clearly, it is unlikely to be very effective in either role. Both muscles are supplied by the suprascapular nerve from the brachial plexus.

The *medial group* consists of the subscapularis and coracobrachialis. The *subscapularis* (Fig. 2.56/*9*) arises over much of the deep surface of the scapula and inserts on the medial tubercle of the humerus, distal to the axis of the shoulder joint. It braces the medial aspect of the joint. It is also a potential adductor of the arm and, like the infraspinatus, has an equivocal relationship to flexion and extension of the shoulder. It is supplied by the subscapular nerve from the brachial plexus. The small *coracobrachialis* (Fig. 2.56/*10*) extends between the medial aspect of the supraglenoid tubercle and the proximal part of the shaft of the humerus. It is a fixator of the shoulder with the same equivocal relationship to shoulder flexion and extension. It is supplied by the proximal branch of the *musculocutaneous nerve* from the brachial plexus.

The *caudal* or *flexor* group comprises the deltoideus, teres major, and teres minor. The *deltoideus* has one head of origin in the horse and two in species possessing an acromion (Fig. 2.56/*4* and *4'*). The constant head arises from the caudal border and spine of the scapula; the inconstant second head arises from the acromion. Both insert on the deltoid tuberosity of the humerus. The *teres major* (Fig. 2.56/*2*) arises from the dorsal part of the caudal margin of the scapula and terminates on the teres tuberosity, midway down the humerus. The relatively insignificant *teres minor* lies over the caudolateral aspect of the joint between the deltoideus and infraspinatus. These three muscles are clearly primarily flexor, the deltoideus may also be an abductor and an outward rotator of the arm. The group is supplied by the axillary nerve from the brachial plexus.

In contrast to the well-defined group of flexors, it seems that no muscles are clearly established as primarily extensors of the shoulder. The potential candidates, brachiocephalicus, biceps brachii, supraspinatus, and pectoralis ascendens, have other, apparently more important, roles.

Muscles Acting Primarily on the Elbow Joint. There are extensor and flexor groups for the elbow joint. The *extensor group,* which largely fills the angle between the scapula and humerus, consists of the triceps brachii, tensor fasciae antebrachii, and anconeus. The large and powerful *triceps brachii* (Fig. 2.56/*6*, *6'*, and *6''*) possesses three (four in the dog) heads of origin. The long head, which arises from the caudal margin of the scapula, is potentially also a flexor of the shoulder. The lateral, medial, and (in the dog) accessory heads arise from the shaft of the humerus and act on the elbow. The heads combine to make a stout

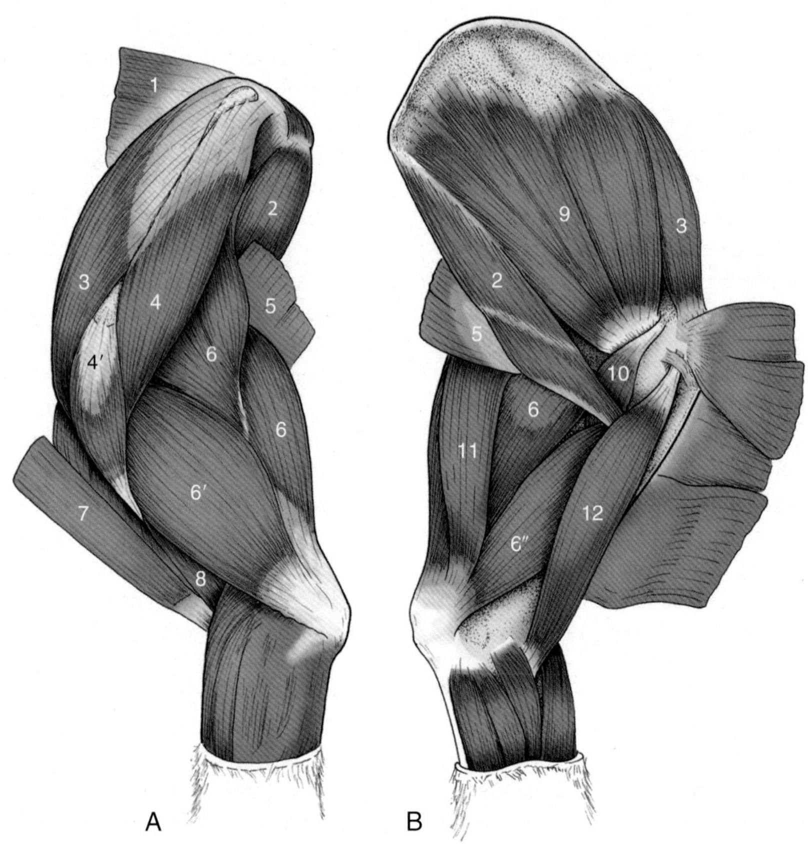

Fig. 2.56 Intrinsic muscles of the left shoulder and arm of the dog. (A) Lateral and (B) medial views. *1,* Rhomboideus; *2,* teres major; *3,* supraspinatus; *4* and *4′,* scapular and acromial parts of deltoideus; *5,* latissimus dorsi; *6, 6′,* and *6″,* long, lateral, and medial heads of triceps; *7,* brachiocephalicus; *8,* brachialis; *9,* subscapularis; *10,* coracobrachialis; *11,* tensor fasciae antebrachii; *12,* biceps.

tendon that inserts on the summit of the olecranon, where it is protected on its deep aspect—against the bone—by the tricipital bursa. A second, subcutaneous bursa often lies between the tendon and the skin.

The *tensor fasciae antebrachii* (Fig. 2.56/*11*) is a thin sheet, partly muscular, partly aponeurotic, that lies over the medial aspect of the long head of the triceps, extending from the scapula to the olecranon. The *anconeus* is much smaller and arises from the distal part of the humerus to insert on the lateral part of the olecranon; it is directly related to the elbow joint capsule and may have the additional function of tensing the capsule so that it is not pinched between the humerus and ulna. All parts of the extensor group are supplied by the radial nerve from the brachial plexus.

All of the extensors previously described are supplied by the **radial nerve.**

The *flexor group* comprises the biceps brachii and brachialis. The biarticular *biceps brachii* (Fig. 2.56/*12*) arises from the supraglenoid tubercle of the scapula and runs through the intertubercular groove of the humerus before continuing distally to insert on the medial tuberosity of the proximal extremity of the radius and on the adjacent part of the ulna. It is thus also a potential extensor of the shoulder. The *brachialis* (Fig. 2.56/*8*) arises from the proximocaudal part of the humerus and winds laterally in the spiral groove of this bone before inserting next to the biceps. Both are supplied by the *musculocutaneous nerve.*

Pronator and Supinator Muscles of the Forearm. Generalized mammals possess forearm muscles that have supination or pronation as a prime function, but these muscles tend to become vestigial or to disappear when the capacity for the movements is reduced or lost. Among domestic species significant movement is possible only in the dog and cat, in which there are two supinator muscles and two pronators. The *brachioradialis* or long supinator is a thin fleshy ribbon that extends from the lateral epicondyle of the humerus to the distal medial part of the forearm within the superficial fascia. It is quite prominent in the cat but is slight, often lost, in the dog. The short *supinator* muscle is more consistently developed. It is a small fusiform muscle, placed

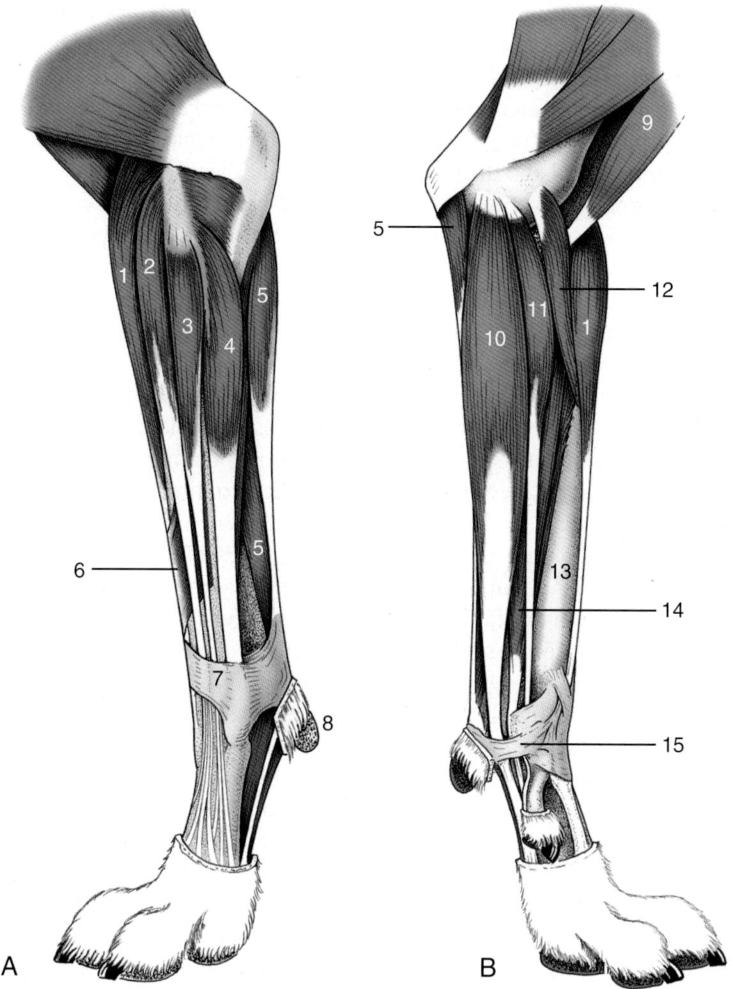

Fig. 2.57 Muscles of the left forearm of the dog. (A) Lateral and (B) medial views. *1,* Extensor carpi radialis; *2,* common digital extensor; *3,* lateral digital extensor; *4,* ulnaris lateralis; *5,* flexor carpi ulnaris; *6,* extensor carpi obliquus; *7,* extensor retinaculum; *8,* carpal pad; *9,* biceps; *10,* superficial digital flexor; *11,* flexor carpi radialis; *12,* pronator teres; *13,* radius; *14,* deep digital flexor; *15,* flexor retinaculum.

deep to the extensor muscles and passing obliquely over the flexor aspect of the elbow from the lateral humeral epicondyle to the upper quarter of the medial border of the radius. The supinator muscles are supplied by the radial nerve.

The *pronator teres* (Fig. 2.57/*12*) arises from the medial epicondyle of the humerus and converges on the insertion of the supinator on the radius. It is functional only in the dog and cat. The *pronator quadratus* is found only in carnivores. It passes from the shaft of the ulna to that of the radius, bridging the medial aspect of the interosseous space of the forearm. The pronator muscles are supplied by the median nerve.

The rotation from the neutral position that may be produced by these muscles is most free when the elbow is flexed. The movements are limited to about 40 degrees of pronation and about 45 degrees of supination in the dog, although the cat has a somewhat larger range.

Muscles Acting Primarily on the Carpal and Digital Joints. Muscles that act primarily on the carpal and digital joints are simply classified as flexor or extensor, although the action of one muscle is equivocal.

The Extensor Muscles of the Carpus and Digits. Extensor muscles of the carpus and digits include digital extensor muscles in addition to muscles whose action is confined to the carpus.

All carpal and digital extensors have an extensor action at the carpus, a craniolateral position in the forearm, a radial nerve supply, and, with one exception, an origin from the cranial aspect of the lateral epicondyle of the humerus.

The *extensor carpi radialis* (Fig. 2.57/*1*), the most medial member of the group, is situated directly cranial to the subcutaneous border of the radius. It inserts on the proximal extremity of the third (sometimes also second) metacarpal bone. The *ulnaris lateralis* (Fig. 2.57/*4*) (extensor carpi ulnaris) is the most lateral member and runs parallel to the ulnar flexor of the carpus on the outer aspect of the limb to insert on the accessory carpal and the upper end of the most lateral metacarpal bone. It may extend an already extended carpus but further flexes the joint when it is in a flexed position. This muscle may also deviate the paw laterally. Despite its equivocal character the ulnaris lateralis retains the extensor nerve supply. The *extensor carpi obliquus* (Fig. 2.57/*6*) (also known as the *abductor pollicis longus*) originates from the cranial surface of the radius and has an oblique mediodistal course to attach to the most medial metacarpal bone. It is an extensor of the carpus and potentially, in the dog and the cat, deviates the paw medially.

All species possess both a common and a lateral digital extensor muscle; however, the common one may be subdivided. Because the common digital extensor (Fig. 2.57/*2*) inserts on the extensor process of the distal phalanx of each functional digit, the number of branches corresponds to the number of digits. A subdivision of the common extensor, which is present in all species but the horse and cat, inserts on the most medial of the functional digits; it sends an oblique branch to the dewclaw in the dog. It is unofficially but usefully termed *medial digital extensor*. Running on the lateral edge of the common extensor is the *lateral digital extensor* (Fig. 2.57/*3*). The undivided tendon inserts on the dorsal surface of the proximal phalanx in the horse. The muscle also has one insertion tendon in ruminants, two in the pig, three in the dog, and four in the cat; in these species the insertion is in common with that of the branch of the common extensor to the distal phalanx of the most lateral one, two, three, or four functional digits. In the smaller species, separation of the digital divisions begins more proximally and is more complete.

The Flexor Muscles of the Carpus and Digits. The carpal flexor group includes digital flexor muscles in addition to muscles that act only at the carpus.

> **All carpal and digital flexors** have a caudal position in the forearm; arise, in part at least, from the caudal aspect of the medial epicondyle of the humerus; and are supplied by the median or ulnar nerve or from both these nerves.

Some have additional, even principal, origins in the forearm and also act on the digital joints. The *flexor carpi radialis* (Fig. 2.57/*11*) is most medial and runs directly caudal to the subcutaneous border of the radius. It ends on the upper end of the second (sometimes third) metacarpal bone. The *flexor carpi ulnaris* (Fig. 2.57/*5*) is lateral and ends on the accessory carpal bone. Both muscles are solely carpal flexors.

The *superficial digital flexor* (Fig. 2.57/*10*) sits in the caudomedial part of the forearm and is not enclosed in a synovial sheath where it passes the carpus. Later it divides into a branch for each functional digit and inserts in the region of the proximal interphalangeal joint. Each branch of the superficial flexor tendon splits into two diverging slips that create an arch to let through the deep digital flexor tendon to its more distal insertions. The *deep digital flexor* (Fig. 2.57/*14*) lies more deeply in the forearm and passes the carpus through the carpal canal before dividing into one to four digital branches; each perforates the corresponding branch of the superficial flexor tendon and then continues to its insertion on the palmar aspect of a distal phalanx.

Short Digital Muscles. *Interosseous muscles* support the metacarpophalangeal joints. They show marked species differences in number, structure (they are mostly tendinous in the large species), and function. These muscles arise from the palmar aspect of the proximal ends of the metacarpal bones and find initial insertion on the sesamoid bones at the metacarpophalangeal joints; from here they are continued by distal sesamoidean ligaments that attach to the phalanges and by extensor branches that wind around to the dorsal aspect of the digit to join the extensor tendons. They are considered in detail later for the species in which they are important.

In the carnivores and pig a number of small digital muscles assist in the extension, flexion, abduction, or adduction of the abaxial digits—one, two, and five in the dog and the cat and two and five in the pig. It is unnecessary to describe them.

The Skeleton of the Hindlimb

Pelvic Girdle

The pelvic girdle has been described with the trunk (p. 40) for the reason previously given.

Skeleton of the Free Appendage

The *femur* (os femoris; Fig. 2.58), the skeleton of the thigh, is the strongest of the long bones. The proximal end curves medially so that the proximal articular surface, the head, is offset in relation to the long axis of the shaft. The femoral head is hemispherical and is joined to the shaft by a neck, which is best defined in the smaller species. The articular surface has a nonarticular area (fovea) to which the intracapsular ligament(s) attach(es); the fovea is round and central in the dog and is wedge-shaped and extended to the medial periphery in the horse. A large process, the greater trochanter (Fig. 2.58/*3*), is lateral to the head and rises level with the head in small animals but projects high above it in larger species (Fig. 2.58/*3′* and *3″*). The greater trochanter gives attachment to the bulk of the gluteal muscles, providing these extensors of the hip with a long lever arm. The trochanteric fossa lies between the trochanter and the femoral neck (Fig. 2.58/*5*) and the site of insertion of the small rotator muscles of the hip.

The caudal aspect of the femoral shaft is flattened, but the other aspects combine in a continuous smooth surface. The borders between the flat and rounded areas are roughened for muscular attachments. Two processes mark the proximal half of the shaft. A low and rough lesser trochanter (Fig. 2.58/*4*) projects from the medial border and gives insertion to the iliopsoas muscle. The third trochanter located at the base of the greater trochanter (trochanter tertius; Fig. 2.58/*4′*) is salient only in the horse and gives attachment to the gluteus superficialis. In the large animals the caudodistal part of the shaft has a deep supracondylar fossa that increases the area of origin of the superficial digital flexor (Fig. 2.58/*7′*). The same function is fulfilled by tuberosities in the dog.

The distal extremity of the femur articulates with the tibia and the patella. The articulation with the tibia is accomplished by two condyles directed caudodistally and separated by a deep intercondylar fossa. The abaxial surfaces of the condyles are roughened and give attachment to the collateral ligaments of the stifle. The lateral condyle has a cranial depression called the *extensor fossa* (Fig. 2.58/*12*), which gives origin to the long digital extensor and peroneus tertius muscles, and a caudal depression (Fig. 2.58/*13*) for the popliteus. In the dog and cat the caudal aspect of each condyle is surmounted by a small flat facet for articulation with one of the small sesamoid bones (Fig. 2.58/*11*; formerly fabellae) in the origin of the gastrocnemius (see Fig. 17.3). A cranial trochlea (Fig. 2.58/*6*) articulates with the patella and extends proximally on the cranial surface. The bounding ridges are low and more or less equal in size in the dog and relatively larger and disparate in the horse and in cattle, in which the stouter medial ridge ends in a proximal enlargement (Fig. 2.58/*6′*).

The *patella,* the kneecap, is a sesamoid developed within the insertion of the quadriceps femoris, the main

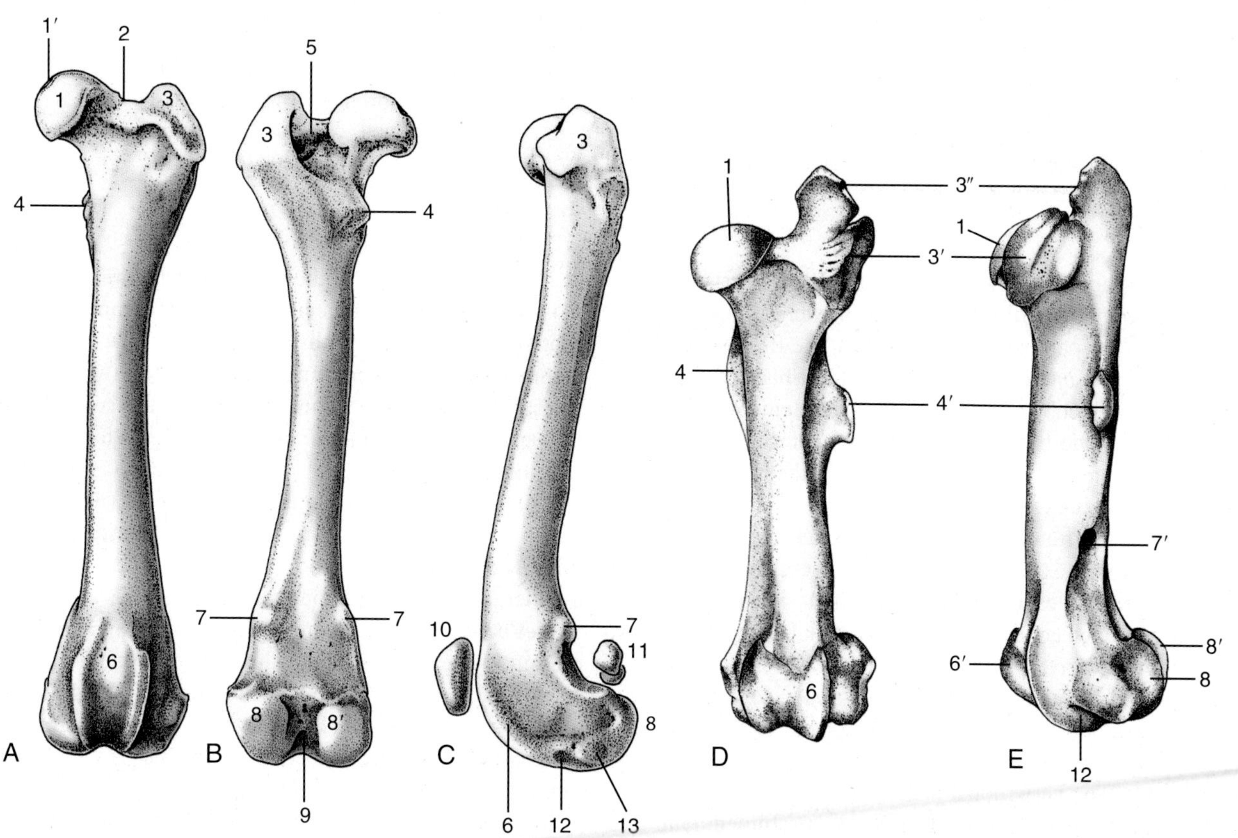

Fig. 2.58 Left femur of the dog. (A) Cranial, (B) caudal, and (C) lateral views. Left equine femur. (D) Cranial and (E) lateral views. *1,* Head; *1′,* fovea; *2,* neck; *3,* greater trochanter; *3′* and *3″*, cranial and caudal parts of greater trochanter; *4,* lesser trochanter; *4′,* third trochanter; *5,* trochanteric fossa; *6,* trochlea; *6′,* enlarged proximal end of medial trochlear ridge; *7,* supracondylar tuberosities; *7′,* supracondylar fossa; *8* and *8′,* lateral and medial condyles; *9,* intercondylar fossa; *10,* patella; *11,* sesamoid bones (in gastrocnemius); *12,* extensor fossa; *13,* fossa for popliteus.

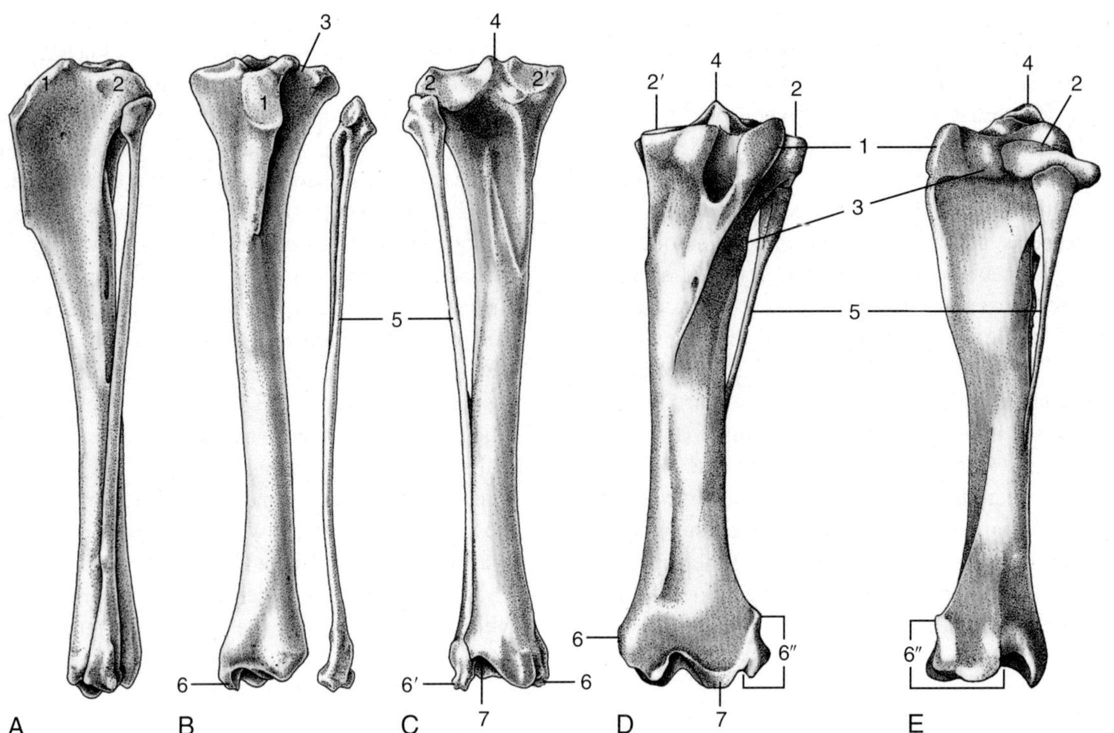

Fig. 2.59 Left tibia and fibula of the dog. (A) Lateral, (B) cranial, and (C) caudal views. Left equine tibia and fibula. (D) Cranial and (E) lateral views. *1*, Tibial tuberosity; *2* and *2′*, lateral and medial condyles; *3*, extensor groove; *4*, intercondylar eminence; *5*, fibula; *6* and *6′*, medial and lateral malleoli; *6″*, lateral malleolus in the horse (representing distal end of fibula), *7*, cochlea.

extensor of the stifle. It is ovoid in the dog but prismatic in the horse and in cattle. The patella is extended medially and laterally by parapatellar cartilages in the fresh state.

The *skeleton of the leg* consists of the tibia and fibula (Fig. 2.59), which, unlike the analogous elements of the forelimb, run side by side without any tendency to cross. The medial bone, the tibia, is always by far the larger of the two. The fibula is excluded from articulation with the femur and has only restricted contact with the hock skeleton.

The proximal extremity of the *tibia* presents two condyles divided by a caudal popliteal notch that has the *popliteal muscle*. Each condyle has a gently undulating articular surface for the corresponding condyle of the femur; a narrow intermediate nonarticular area carries a central eminence (Fig. 2.59/*4*). A depression of the eminence and less defined areas cranial and caudal to it indicate ligamentous attachments. The very robust tibial tuberosity (Fig. 2.59/*1*) on the cranial aspect of this extremity is a prominent landmark in life and is continued by a gradually subsiding crest. A groove (Fig. 2.59/*3*) lodging the tendons of certain muscles of the leg (crus) separates the tuberosity from the cranial aspect of the lateral condyle. Caudal to this groove, the edge of the condyle carries a small facet for articulation with the fibula, although in some species the joint space is obliterated by fusion.

The proximal part of the tibial shaft is three-sided, but more distally the bone is craniocaudally compressed. The change is brought about by the smooth surface that faces craniolaterally in its proximal part but then twists to face directly forward. The entire medial surface is subcutaneous and flat. The caudal surface is ridged for muscular attachment.

The distal extremity contains the cochlea (Fig. 2.59/*7*), which articulates with the trochlea of the talus. The central ridge and the flanking grooves of the cochlea have a craniolateral deflection, although the angle varies among species. A bony salience, the medial malleolus (Fig. 2.59/*6*), is present to the medial side of the cochlea. A similar lateral swelling found only in the horse represents the assimilated distal part of the fibula (Fig. 2.59/*6″*). In other species the corresponding feature (lateral malleolus) is provided by the fibula.

The *fibula* of the carnivores and the pig is reduced in robustness but not in length. It is separated from the tibia by an interosseous space that runs the whole length of the leg in the pig but is limited to the proximal half in the dog. The shaft of the fibula is reduced in the ruminants to a tear-shaped process fused to the lateral condyle of the tibia; the distal extremity is isolated as a small compact malleolar bone that forms an interlocking joint with the tibia, thus

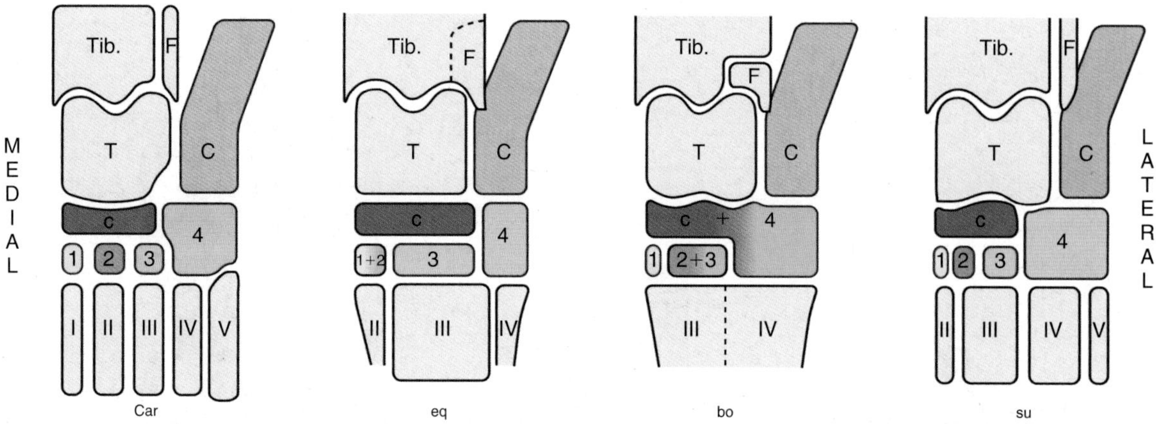

Fig. 2.60 The bones of the tarsal skeleton in the carnivores *(Car)*, horse *(eq)*, cattle *(bo)*, and pig *(su)* schematic. *Roman numerals* identify the metatarsal bones, *arabic numerals* the distal tarsal bones. *C*, calcaneus; *c*, central tarsal bone; *F*, fibula; *T*, talus; *Tib.*, tibia.

completing the articular surface for the talus. The flattened proximal head of the fibula of the horse is closely applied to the tibia, and the slender shaft that leads from it converges on the tibia but fades toward the middle of the leg.

The *tarsal bones* are arranged in three tiers. The proximal tier consists of two relatively large bones: the talus medially and the calcaneus laterally. The middle tier comprises only a single central tarsal bone, but the distal tier consists of up to four bones, which are numbered in mediolateral sequence. The lateral fourth tarsal bone is constantly present and, being much deeper than the others, intrudes into the middle tier (Fig. 2.60).

The talus (Fig. 2.61) has a proximal trochlear surface shaped to fit the tibia. The distal surface, which articulates with the central bone, is flattened in the horse and more rounded in other species. The calcaneus lies mainly lateral to the talus but extends a shelflike process (sustentaculum tali; Fig. 2.61/*3′*) that overlaps the talus on its plantar surface and supports the deep digital flexor tendon. The larger part of the bone projects proximally behind the tibia as a free lever arm to which the common calcanean tendon attaches. The talus ends in a thickening that is the basis of the point of the hock (Fig. 2.61/*3″*) and corresponds to the human heel. The distal extremity of the calcaneus rests on the fourth tarsal bone (Fig. 2.61/*6*). The central tarsal bone is interposed between the talus proximally and the first, second, and third tarsal bones distally; its proximal surface conforms to the talus and is concave in most animals but flat in the horse. Its distal articular surface is flattened. The central and fourth tarsal bones fuse in ruminants.

The distal tarsal bones are not always separate: the first and second are fused in the horse, and the second and third are fused in ruminants. Individually irregular, these bones together form a more or less flattened disk interposed between the central tarsal and the metatarsal bones. The cuboidal fourth tarsal bone is interposed between the calcaneus and the lateral metatarsal bones; in some species it also gives support to the talus.

The remaining bones of the hindlimb closely resemble those of the forelimb. The metatarsal bones are longer (by about 20%) than the metacarpals and are more rounded in cross section. The first metatarsal is rudimentary in the dog, of which only a few breeds consistently possess a dewclaw in the hindlimb.

The Joints of the Hindlimb

The *hip joint* (Fig. 2.62) is a spheroidal joint formed between the lunate surface of the acetabulum and the head of the femur. The acetabular surface is enlarged by an articular labrum (Fig. 2.62/*2′*) continuous with the transverse acetabular ligament (Fig. 2.62/*2″*) that bridges the notch interrupting the medial wall of the socket. The synovial membrane of the joint is supported externally by a fibrous covering, which is not uniformly strong. The head of the femur is joined to the depth of the acetabulum by the intracapsular ligament of the femoral head, which is covered by a reflection of the synovial membrane. In the horse a second (accessory) ligament inserts on the nonarticular area of the head (p. 612).

The hip does not enjoy the full range of movement expected of spheroidal joints. In the large animals movement is largely restricted to flexion and extension. In conformity with the dominance of sagittal movement, the articular area tends to extend onto the neck in ruminants. The restriction on movement is due to intraarticular ligament(s) and the massive medial muscles of the thigh. The joint has a more versatile range in the dog.

The *stifle joint* (Fig. 2.63), corresponding to the human knee, comprises femorotibial, femoropatellar, and proximal tibiofibular joints. The dog also has the joint between the femur and paired sesamoids in the origins of the

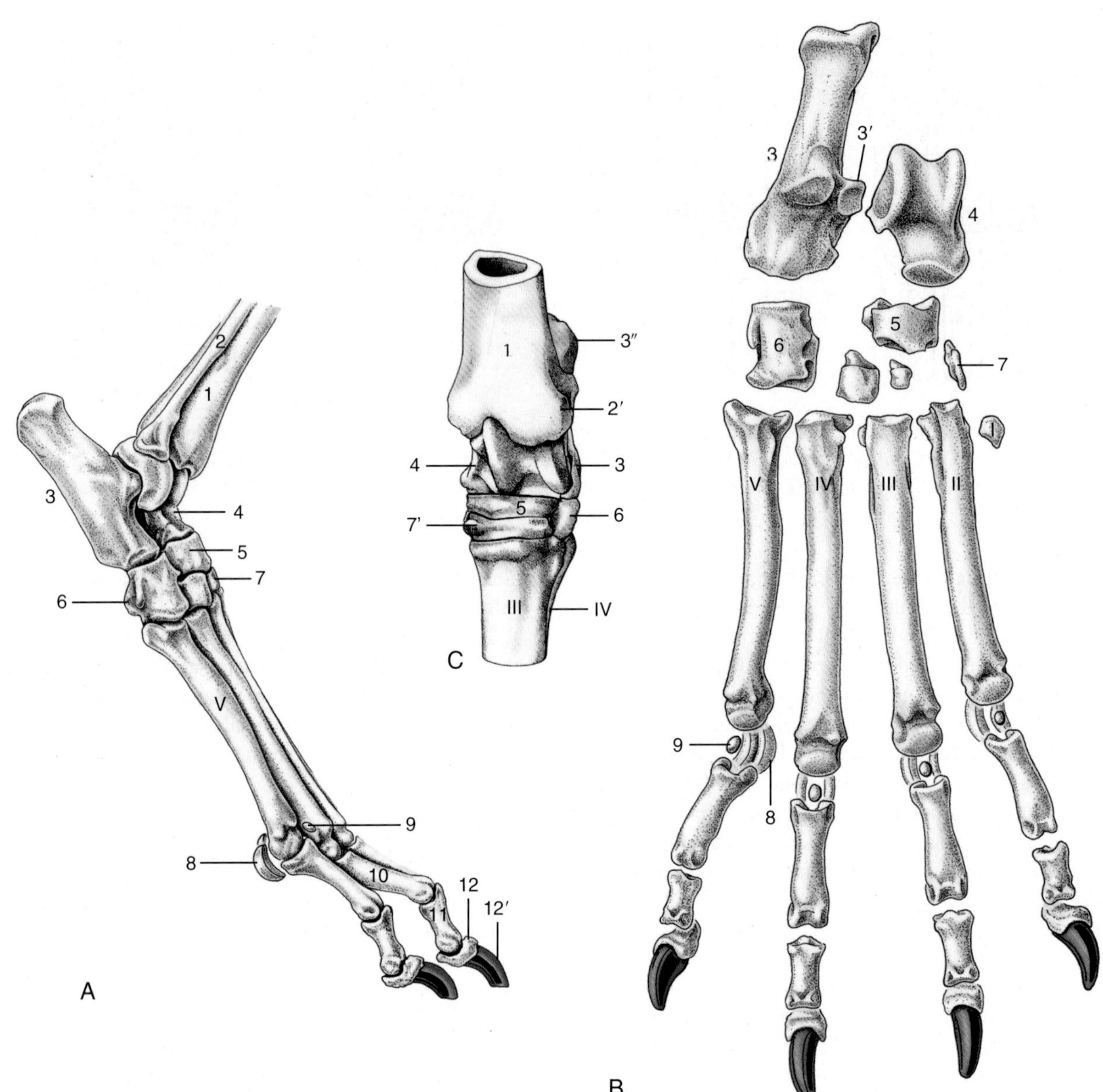

Fig. 2.61 Skeleton of right pes of the dog. (A) Lateral and (B) dorsal views. (C) Left equine tarsus, dorsal view. *Roman numerals* identify the metatarsal bones. *1,* Tibia; *2,* fibula; *2′,* lateral malleolus; *3,* calcaneus; *3′,* sustentaculum tali; *3″,* calcanean tuber (point of hock); *4,* talus; *5,* central tarsal; *6,* fourth tarsal; *7,* first, second, and third tarsal bones in distal row; *7′,* third tarsal in the horse; *8,* proximal sesamoid bones; *9,* dorsal sesamoid bones; *10, 11,* and *12,* proximal, middle, and distal phalanges; *12′,* claw.

gastrocnemius and the joint between the tibia and the sesamoid in the popliteus tendon. In the dog, all these articulations have a common synovial cavity, but in the large species the femoropatellar and the medial and lateral femorotibial compartments have more restricted communication with one another.

The femorotibial joint is unusual in having two fibrocartilaginous menisci (Fig. 2.63/*10* and *17*) interposed between the femoral and tibial condyles. The menisci, which compensate for the incongruence of the articular surfaces, are each semilunar in plan and wedge-shaped in section and have concave proximal and flattened distal surfaces. Each is secured by ligaments that extend between its cranial and caudal extremities and the central nonarticular area of the proximal extremity of the tibia; the lateral meniscus is also attached caudally to the intercondylar fossa of the femur.

Four ligaments join the femur to the bones of the leg. A medial collateral ligament passes between the femoral epicondyle and the proximal part of the tibia, toward the caudal part of the joint. The corresponding lateral ligament

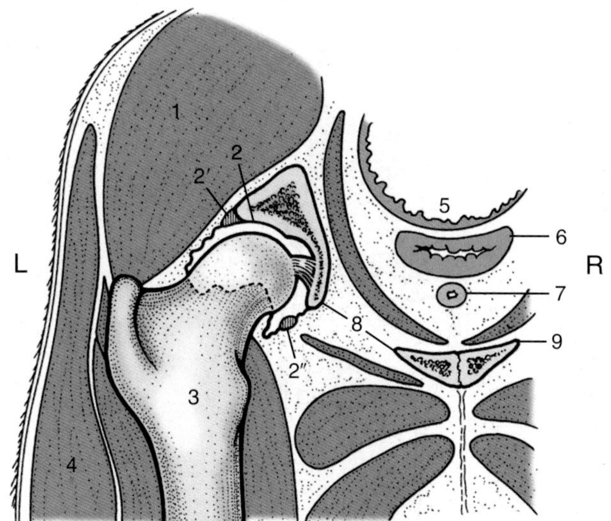

Fig. 2.62 Schematic transverse section through the left hip joint of a dog. The femur has been drawn in relief. *1,* Gluteus medius; *2,* acetabulum, connected to the femoral head by the ligament of the head of the femur; *2′,* fibrous rim (labrum) of acetabulum; *2″,* transverse acetabular ligament; *3,* femur; *4,* biceps; *5,* rectum; *6,* vagina; *7,* urethra; *8,* obturator foramen; *9,* pelvic floor; *L,* left; *R,* right.

has a similar disposition but attaches to the fibular head. The cruciate ligaments are centrally placed. The cranial (lateral) cruciate ligament (Fig. 2.63/*16*) arises from the lateral condyle of the femur within the intercondylar fossa and runs craniodistally to attach on the tibia. The caudal (medial) cruciate ligament (Fig. 2.63/*15*) runs at right angles to the cranial one and attaches far back on the tibia near the popliteal notch.

The femoropatellar joint is formed between the femoral trochlea and the patella and is extended by its parapatellar cartilages, the medial of which is especially well developed in the large animals. Relatively weak collateral femoropatellar ligaments (Fig. 2.63/*12*) run between the cartilages and the femur. Distally the patella is joined to the tibial tuberosity by a single patellar ligament, except in the horse and ox, in which three ligamentous thickenings are present—medial, intermediate, and lateral—connected by a fibrous sheet (see Fig. 24.4). The middle (or single) patellar ligament represents the insertion tendon of the quadriceps femoris; the others, when present, represent the continuation of other muscles inserting about the joint.

The synovial membrane attaches around the peripheries of the articular surfaces and the menisci. It covers the cruciate ligaments and here forms a partition, complete only in the horse, between the medial and lateral femorotibial joints. The femoropatellar portion of the cavity extends proximally between the femur and the quadriceps. In the horse it generally communicates only with the medial femorotibial compartment, but in other species it has free communication with both. Diverticula of the capsule embrace the lesser joints with the fibula and the sesamoid bones and extend along the tendons of origin of the long digital extensor and popliteus muscles.

Despite its complexity, the stifle functions as a hinge joint mainly entrusted with flexion and extension. The femoral condyles roll on the menisci, which in turn slide over the tibial plateau—cranially on extension, caudally on flexion. The travel between the femur and menisci is about three times that between the menisci and the tibia. The spiral configuration of the femoral condyles, when viewed from the side, tightens the ligaments and slows the movement when the joint moves toward the extended position. The stability of the articulation depends much on the cruciate ligaments. Rupture of one of these, which is not an uncommon misfortune, allows the tibia unusual mobility; it may slip forward when the cranial ligament is torn and backward when the caudal ligament is torn. Rotation imposed on the joint, particularly when the joint is extended, places great strain on the menisci and their attachments.

The *tarsal joint* of quadrupeds is usually known as the hock. Although it has four levels of articulation, in most species almost all movement occurs at the crurotarsal level. This is a hinge joint, but the obliquity of the interlocking ridges and grooves of the tibia and talus imposes a lateral deviation of the foot when it is carried forward on flexion. In ruminants and carnivores, limited flexion is also possible at the curved surfaces of the talocentral joint.

Among the many ligaments, the most important are the medial and lateral collateral ligaments, which extend, with intermediate attachments, from the tibia (and fibula) to the proximal extremity of the metatarsus. Each comprises a long superficial part of full extent and a shorter deeper part restricted to the proximal level of articulation. Another long ligament is found caudally, extending from the plantar surface of the calcaneus over the fourth tarsal bone to the metatarsus. The remaining smaller ligaments firmly hold the tarsal bones together.

There are several compartments to the joint. That between the tibia and talus is most capacious and may possess a number of local pouches, as the less supported parts of joint capsules are known. The other synovial sacs are much tighter and often communicate. The details are most important in the horse (p. 621).

The remaining joints of the hindlimb are considered in the regional chapters, insofar as they require to be differentiated from the corresponding forelimb joints.

The Muscles of the Hindlimb

The girdle musculature has been described (p. 49).

The Intrinsic Muscles of the Hindlimb

Muscles Acting Primarily on the Hip Joint. The muscles acting at the hip are arranged topographically in gluteal, medial, deep, and caudal (hamstring) groups.

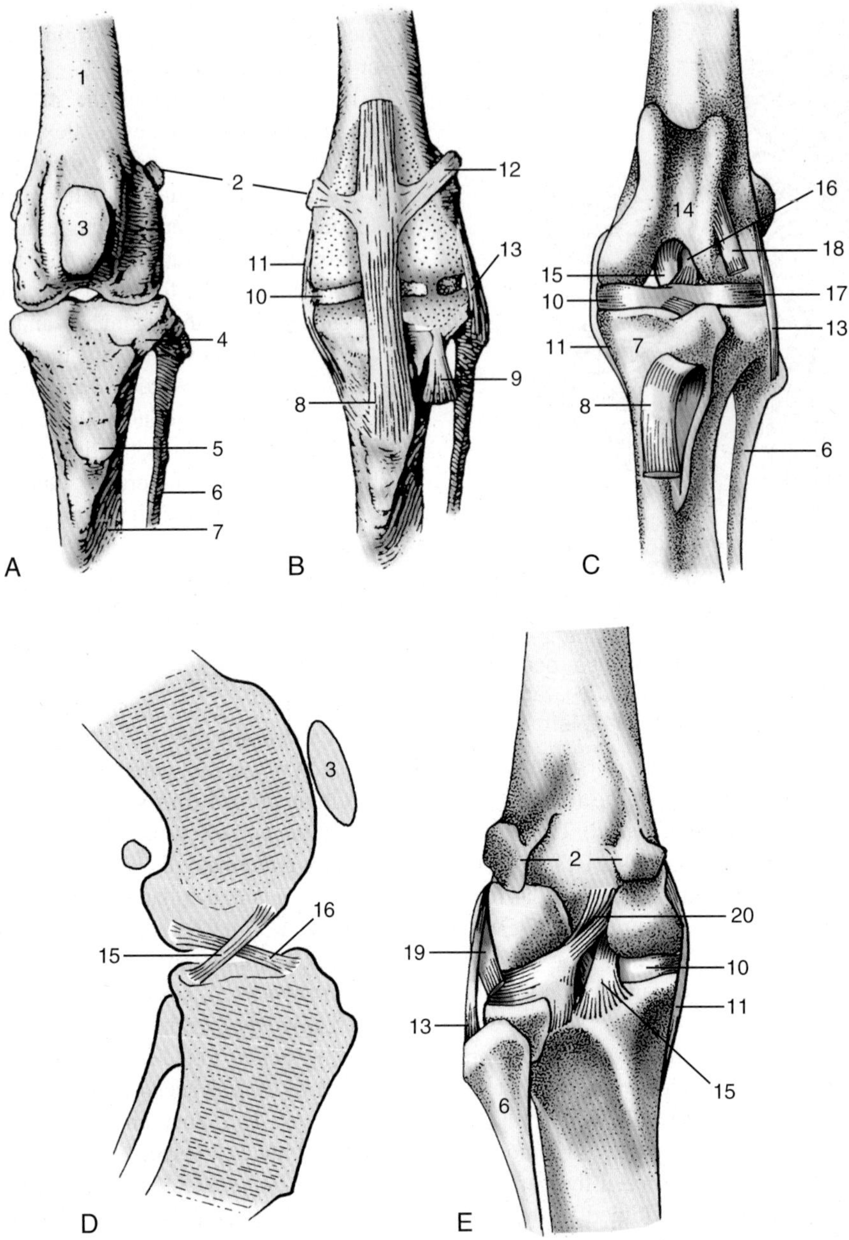

Fig. 2.63 (A to C) Left stifle joint of the dog, cranial views. (B) The extent of the joint capsule. (C) The patella has been removed. Crossing of the cruciate ligaments in (D) medial and (E) caudal views. *1,* Femur; *2,* sesamoids in the gastrocnemius; *3,* patella; *4,* extensor groove; *5,* tibial tuberosity; *6,* fibula; *7,* tibia; *8,* patellar ligament; *9,* tendon of long digital extensor passing through extensor groove; *10,* medial meniscus; *11,* medial collateral ligament; *12,* lateral femoropatellar ligament; *13,* lateral collateral ligament; *14,* trochlea; *15,* caudal cruciate ligament; *16,* cranial cruciate ligament; *17,* lateral meniscus; *18,* stump of 9; *19,* popliteus tendon; *20,* meniscofemoral ligament.

The *gluteal group* comprises superficial, middle, and deep gluteal muscles and the tensor fasciae latae. The gluteus superficialis in the dog is a relatively narrow muscle that covers the caudal part of the gluteus medius, extending from the gluteal and caudal fascia to the third trochanter of the femur (Fig. 2.64/*4*). In ungulates a part becomes incorporated within the biceps femoris, and sometimes also the semitendinosus, supplying them with vertebral heads of origin. The gluteus superficialis is an extensor of the hip and therefore a retractor of the limb. It is supplied by the caudal gluteal nerve.

The *gluteus medius* (Fig. 2.64/*3*) is by far the largest of the group. It arises from the outer surface of the ilium and the gluteal fascia and inserts on the greater

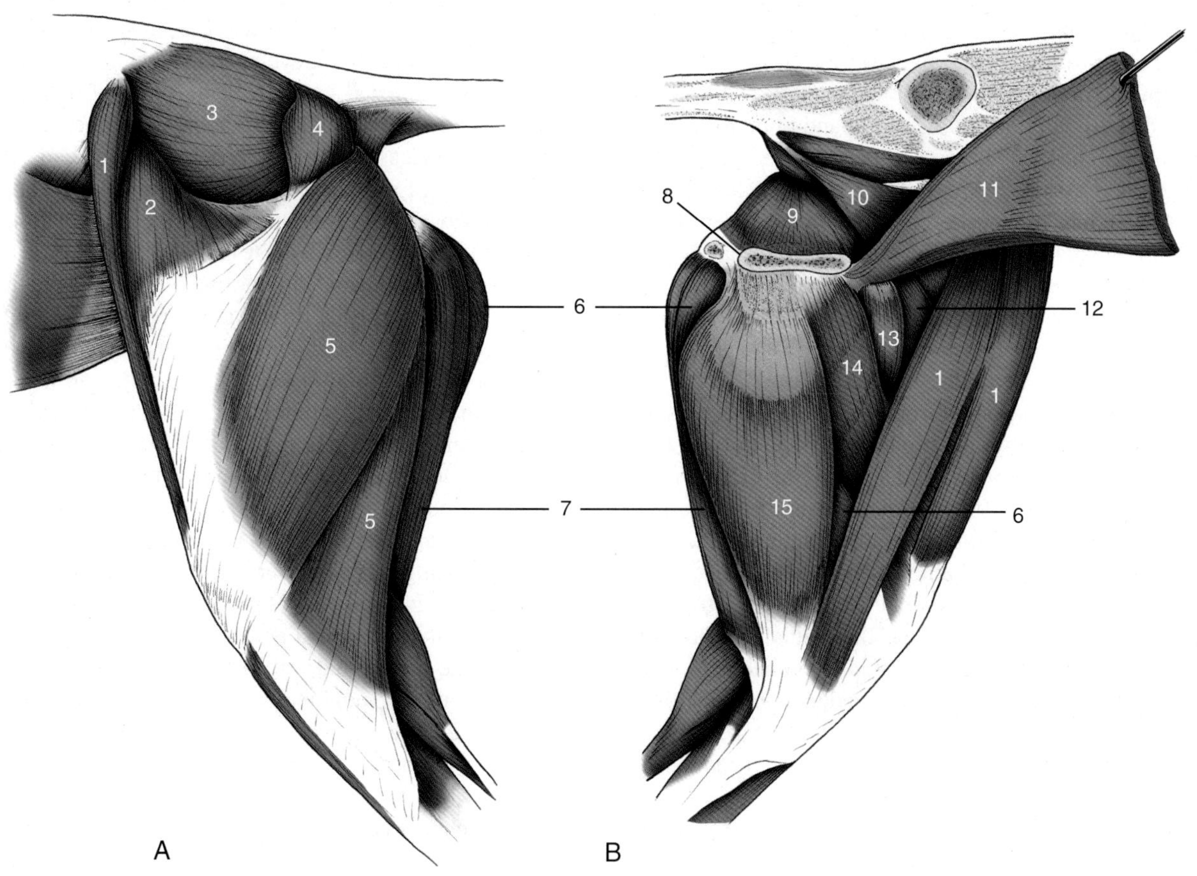

Fig. 2.64 Muscles of the canine hindquarter and thigh. (A) Lateral and (B) medial views. *1,* Sartorius; *2,* tensor fasciae latae; *3,* gluteus medius; *4,* gluteus superficialis; *5,* biceps; *6,* semimembranosus; *7,* semitendinosus; *8,* pelvic symphysis; *9,* internal obturator; *10,* levator ani; *11,* rectus abdominis; *12,* quadriceps; *13,* pectineus; *14,* adductor; *15,* gracilis.

trochanter. It is an exceptionally powerful extensor of the hip, with some abduction potential. The actions of deeper subdivisions, the gluteus accessorius and the more caudal piriformis, are similar to those of the main mass. The muscle is principally supplied by the cranial gluteal nerve.

The much smaller *gluteus profundus* is completely covered by the gluteus medius. It arises from the ischial spine and adjacent region of the os coxae and inserts on the cranial part of the greater trochanter. It may also extend the hip, but the transverse course of most of its fibers makes it a more useful abductor. It is also supplied by the cranial gluteal nerve. The *tensor fasciae latae* (Fig. 2.64/*2*) is the most cranial muscle of the group. It arises from the coxal tuber (or equivalent) and from the adjacent part of the ilium and extends down the cranial border of the thigh before inserting into the heavy lateral femoral fascia, which provides it with attachment to the patella and other structures of the stifle region. Supplied by the cranial gluteal nerve, the tensor fasciae latae is primarily a flexor of the hip. In the horse its most caudal part extends toward and fuses with a cranial slip of the gluteus superficialis.

The *medial group* is principally employed to adduct the hindlimb; *adduction* is, of course, a term that also embraces the prevention of unwanted abduction. Most muscles of this group are supplied by the obturator nerve and they—gracilis, pectineus, adductor, and external obturator—are sometimes specifically termed the *adductors*. The sartorius has a rather different origin and relationship.

The *gracilis,* a broad but thin muscle, takes an aponeurotic origin from the symphyseal region of the pelvis (Fig. 2.64/*15*). Its insertion, also aponeurotic, merges with the crural fascia through which it finds attachment to the tibial crest and other medial structures of the stifle region.

The *pectineus* is a small fusiform muscle, which in the dog forms a prominent surface feature of the proximal part of the thigh (Fig. 2.64/*13*). It arises from the cranial branch of the pubis and from the prepubic tendon and inserts on the proximal part of the medial "rough line" of the femur. In the larger species, but not in the dog, a considerable part of the tendon of origin decussates with its fellow within the prepubic tendon.

The *adductor* is often divided into several individually named parts, but these distinctions are unnecessary. The muscle arises over an extensive area of the ventral aspect of the pelvic floor and inserts along the distal two thirds of the medial "rough line" of the femur and to the fascia and ligaments of the medial aspect of the stifle (Fig. 2.64/*14*).

The *obturator externus* is conveniently included here, although it has obvious affinities with the deep group described next. It arises from the ventral surface of the pelvic floor, over and around the obturator foramen, and inserts within the ventral part of the trochanteric fossa. In addition to being an adductor, this muscle is potentially an outward rotator of the thigh.

The *sartorius* is set apart from the other medial muscles by its innervation from the saphenous branch of the femoral nerve. It is superficial and follows the craniomedial aspect of the thigh; in the dog it consists of two parallel bellies, one of which forms the cranial contour of the thigh (Fig. 2.64/*1*). Except in the horse (in which it arises from the iliac fascia on the abdominal roof), it arises from the iliac crest, and its insertion is to the medial structures of the stifle region. Flexion of the hip is probably its main action, but it has some capacity for adduction of the thigh and extension of the stifle. The superficial space between the caudal margin of the sartorius and the pectineus is often designated the *femoral canal.*

The *deep muscles of the hip* form a rather heterogeneous community of small and essentially trivial muscles: the obturator internus, gemelli, quadratus femoris, and articularis coxae. Most are supplied by the sciatic nerve.

The *obturator internus* (Fig. 2.64/*9*) is a thin muscle that arises from the dorsal surface of the femur in the vicinity of the obturator foramen; in carnivores and in the horse its tendon leaves the pelvis by passing over the ischium, caudal to the acetabulum, to end in the trochanteric fossa. In other species the tendon passes through the obturator foramen; in this arrangement, the muscle may have its origin as a detachment from the external obturator. The muscle is an external rotator of the thigh.

The *gemelli* are two small "twin" bundles that pass from the ischial spine to the trochanteric fossa. They are also external rotators.

The *quadratus femoris* passes from the ventral aspect of the ischium to end on the femoral shaft close to the trochanteric fossa. It is described as an extensor but can be of no significance in this role.

The *articularis coxae* lies on the capsule over the cranial aspect of the hip and protects it from being nipped between the femoral and acetabular surfaces.

The *muscles of the caudal (hamstring) group*—biceps femoris, semitendinosus, and semimembranosus—flesh the caudal part of the thigh. They extend from the ischial tuber and adjacent part of the sacrotuberous ligament to a broad insertion both proximal and distal to the joint space of the stifle; certain components continue within the common calcanean tendon to the calcaneus. In ungulates, one (or more) muscle(s) is also extended proximally through an origin (vertebral head) from the sacrocaudal vertebrae. The vertebral heads are best developed in the horse and account for the full, rounded contour of the rump of this animal, which contrasts with the more angular appearance in the ox or dog. At least part of the vertebral extension is due to assimilation of a superficial gluteal component. The term *gluteobiceps* may be encountered for the combination.

The *biceps femoris* is most lateral (Fig. 2.64/*5*). In the horse and in ruminants, but not in the dog, it has both vertebral and pelvic heads. In the lower part of the thigh the united muscle divides into insertions that attach, by way of the femoral and crural fascia, to the patella and ligaments of the stifle joint both proximal and distal to the joint space; an additional insertion to the point of the hock is achieved through a contribution (tarsal tendon) to the common calcanean tendon.

The *semitendinosus* (Fig. 2.64/*7*) forms the caudal contour of the thigh. It has a vertebral head only in the horse and pig. The insertion is to the medial aspect of the proximal extremity of the tibia and to the calcaneus. The insertions of the biceps and semitendinosus, one to each side of the depression (popliteal fossa) behind the stifle, can be palpated in life—they are the "strings of the ham" that give the group its name.

The *semimembranosus* (Fig. 2.64/*6*) is most medial and has a vertebral head only in the horse. The insertion is divided between a cranial part attaching to the medial femoral condyle and a caudal part attaching to the medial tibial condyle.

In the dog a ribbon-like and functionally insignificant abductor cruris caudalis lies on the deep face of the biceps and is probably derived from it.

The vertebral heads of these muscles are generally supplied by the caudal gluteal nerve, and the pelvic heads by the sciatic nerve (or its tibial division).

Collectively these muscles undoubtedly provide forceful extension of the hip joint that thrusts the trunk forward. In addition, the biceps has an abductor potential, and the semimembranosus an adductor potential, at the hip. When consideration is given to muscle action on the stifle, the points of insertion relative to the joint axis are more informative. it is probably more useful to divide the muscles into a cranial division inserting proximal to the joint axis and a caudal division inserting distal to this axis rather than to consider the named units. Those cranial to the axis extend the stifle when the foot is planted on the ground, whereas the caudal division has the same action when the foot is fixed but flexes the joint when the foot is free to move. The parts of the biceps and semitendinosus that insert on the calcaneus can obviously extend the hock. All these effects, however, cannot be accomplished simultaneously because of both the potential antagonism of the cranial and caudal divisions at the stifle and the undesirability of flexing the stifle while extending the hock. Indeed, in the horse in particular, the reciprocal apparatus precludes this combination of actions (p. 625). Different parts of these muscles must therefore be used at different times and in different combinations.

Muscles Acting Primarily on the Stifle Joint. There are extensor and flexor groups in the muscles acting on the stifle joint. The *quadriceps femoris,* the principal extensor of the stifle, forms the mass of muscle cranial to the femur (see Fig. 17.2/*9*). It originates as four parts but inserts as a single tendon distally. The rectus femoris originates from the shaft of the ilium immediately cranial to the acetabulum; the others, however—vastus medialis, intermedius, and lateralis—arise, respectively, from the medial, cranial, and lateral aspects of the femoral shaft. The common insertion appears to be on the patella but is actually on the tibial tuberosity because the muscle is continued distal to the patella by the patellar ligament(s). The rectus femoris has the potential secondary action of flexion of the hip. The quadriceps is supplied by the femoral nerve.

The small *popliteus* muscle lies directly over the caudal aspect of the joint. It takes a tendinous and confined origin from the lateral condyle of the femur and fans out to a broad fleshy insertion on the proximal third of the caudal surface of the tibia (Fig. 2.65/*15*). Its tendon of origin contains a sesamoid in the dog and cat. In addition to being a flexor of the stifle, the popliteus rotates the distal part of the limb. It is supplied by the tibial nerve.

Muscles Acting Primarily on the Tarsal and Digital Joints. The muscles acting on the tarsal and digital joints, which comprise extensors and flexors of the hock and the digits, are grouped in two masses: one craniolateral to the tibia and the other caudal to the tibia.

Craniolateral Muscles of the Leg. Some of the craniolateral group only flex the hock and others flex the hock and extend the digits. This arrangement contrasts with the digital extensors of the forelimb, which extend both carpal and distal joints. All of the craniolateral crural muscles are innervated through the peroneal* nerve (Fig. 2.65/*3*).

A full set of the muscles that are pure flexors of the hock are not found in any domestic species; it would consist of

* The adjective *fibular* has equivalent meaning to *peroneal* and is substituted for it by some writers. At present, peroneal (in its Latin form, *peroneus*) is official.

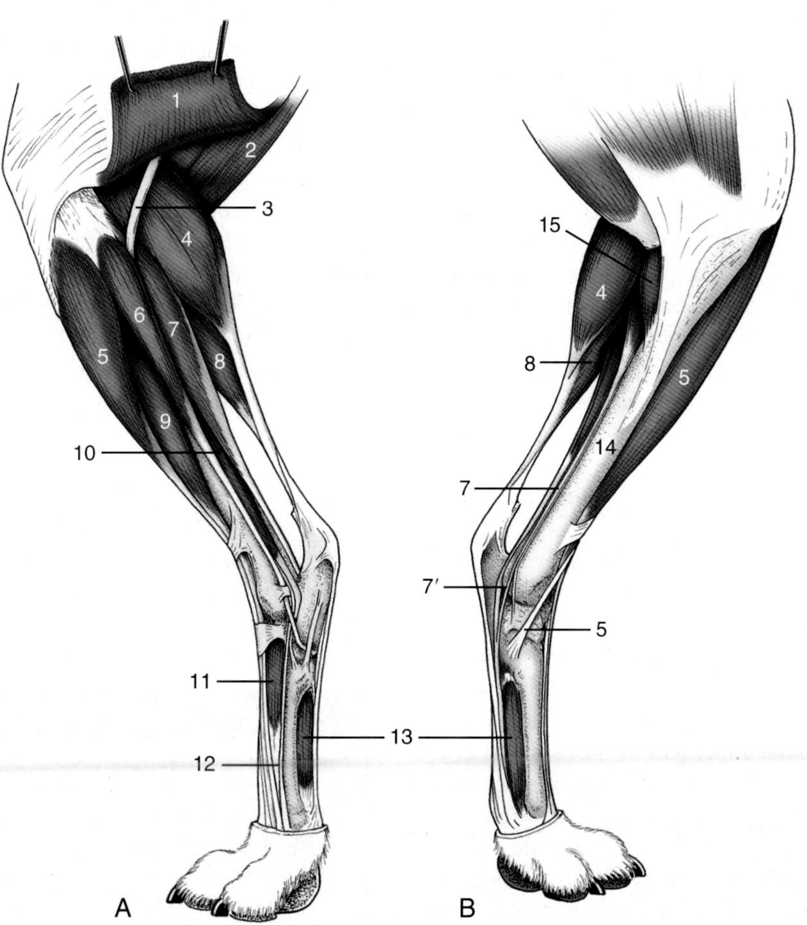

Fig. 2.65 Muscles of the left canine leg. (A) Lateral and (B) medial views. *1,* Biceps; *2,* semitendinosus; *3,* peroneal nerve; *4,* gastrocnemius; *5,* tibialis cranialis; *6,* peroneus longus; *7,* lateral deep digital flexor; *7′,* tendon of the smaller medial deep digital flexor; *8,* superficial digital flexor; *9,* long digital extensor; *10,* peroneus brevis; *11,* extensor brevis; *12,* tendon of lateral digital extensor; *13,* interossei; *14,* tibia; *15,* popliteus.

the tibialis cranialis, peroneus tertius, peroneus longus, and peroneus brevis.

The *tibialis cranialis,* always substantial, lies immediately cranial to the subcutaneous medial surface of the tibia (Fig. 2.65/*5*). After arising from the lateral condyle of the tibia, it inserts on the mediodistal tarsal and adjacent metatarsal skeleton. With hock flexion as its primary role, this muscle also is a supinator. The *peroneus tertius* is most important in the horse because of its critical role in the so-called reciprocal mechanism.

The weak *peroneus longus* arises from and around the distal part of the lateral collateral ligament of the stifle joint (Fig. 2.65/6). It crosses the lateral aspect of the tarsus before turning medially, over the plantar aspect, to end on the proximal parts of the medial metatarsal bone. It is primarily a pronator of the foot but may also flex the hock. The *peroneus brevis* is of no practical importance.

The number and the arrangement of the extensor muscles of the digits are naturally correlated with the digital pattern. A long digital extensor muscle (Fig. 2.65/*9*) arises from the distal extremity of the femur and follows the lateral border of the tibialis cranialis. Its tendon is held down by a retinaculum on the dorsal surface of the hock before it splits to send one branch for each functional digit. Each branch inserts on the extensor process of a distal phalanx. In the dog, the tendons develop small sesamoid bones similar to those in the forelimb.

A *lateral digital extensor* (Fig. 2.65/*12*) arises from the head of the fibula, crosses the lateral aspect of the hock, and enters the most lateral functional digit, where it terminates either on the proximal phalanx (dog) or by joining the long extensor tendon (horse). In certain species, including the dog, a small discrete *extensor hallucis longus* is associated with the medial digit; it arises on the cranial border of the fibula and inserts on the proximal part of the digit.

Caudal Muscles of the Leg. The caudal muscles of the leg are the twin-bellied gastrocnemius, the soleus, and the superficial and deep digital flexors. All are supplied by the tibial nerve.

The gastrocnemius and the soleus, the latter insignificant except in the cat and absent in the dog, are sometimes collectively known as the *triceps surae*. The two heads of the *gastrocnemius* (Fig. 2.65/*4*) spring from the caudal aspect of the femur proximal to the condyles; two sesamoid bones are included in their origins in carnivores. The heads combine in the upper part of the crus and give rise to a single stout tendon that inserts on the point of the hock. It is the principal component of the common calcanean (Achilles) tendon. Despite its inclusion among the extensors of the hock, the role of the gastrocnemius is enigmatic because its proximal attachment suggests that it is a potential flexor of the stifle; stifle and hock, however, normally move in unison. The apparent contradiction in these actions is not easily explained. It has been suggested that the prime function of the gastrocnemius is not to move either joint but to oppose bending of the tibia, ensuring that the strain is always directed along its long axis.

The *superficial digital flexor* (Fig. 2.65/*8*) arises from a supracondylar fossa or tubercle on the caudal aspect of the femur, close to the origin of the gastrocnemius. It first runs deeply, between the two parts of the latter muscle; its tendon later winds around the medial border of the gastrocnemius tendon to gain the more superficial position. It forms a broad cap over the point of the hock, where part finds attachment through medial and lateral slips, before continuing over the plantar aspect of the calcaneus to enter the foot; it is then disposed like the corresponding tendon of the forelimb. The muscle is heavily infiltrated by connective tissue, especially in the horse, in which it becomes almost entirely tendinous and forms the caudal component of the reciprocal mechanism.

There are three *deep digital flexor muscles* whose independence varies among species. The three—*lateral and medial flexors* and the *tibialis caudalis*—lie close together on the caudal surface of the tibia (and fibula), from which they take origin (Fig. 2.65/7). In the ungulates, the tendons of the lateral muscle and the tibialis caudalis unite above the tarsus and then run over the plantar aspect of the joint, medial to the calcaneus; this common tendon is then joined in the upper part of the metatarsus by that of the medial muscle, which descends over the medial malleolus. The combined deep flexor tendon ends as the corresponding tendon of the forelimb. In carnivores, only the lateral (Fig. 2.65/*7*) and medial (Fig. 2.65/*7′*) muscles unite. The rather small tibialis caudalis remains aloof and inserts separately on the hock; this truncated course transforms it into an extensor of the hock and a supinator of the foot.

The most important *short digital muscles* are the interossei (Fig. 2.65/*13*), which resemble those of the forelimb. A number of other small muscles that occur, especially in the dog, are of trivial significance.

COMPREHENSION CHECK

Develop a plan for integrated actions of bones and muscles of the limbs and the thorax that balance locomotion with respiration.

Develop a schematic view of musculoskeletal adaptations that facilitate quadrupeds to "carry" their heads.

What constitutes the carpal canal?

3 The Digestive Apparatus

The digestive apparatus* comprises the organs concerned with the reception, mechanical reduction, chemical digestion, and absorption of food and drink and with the elimination of unabsorbed residues. It consists of the alimentary tract, extending from the mouth to the anus, and certain glands—the salivary glands, pancreas, and liver—that drain into the tract. The parts of the alimentary tract in proper sequence are the mouth, pharynx, esophagus, stomach, small intestine, and large intestine (Fig. 3.1). Some of the digestive organs have other, sometimes just as vital functions that are quite distinct from the processing of food intake.

These organs are primarily formed of endoderm, the germ layer that lines the yolk sac, although the muscle and connective tissues that support the epithelium are of mesodermal origin, as elsewhere. The separation of the digestive tube from the yolk sac is achieved in the folding process that converts the flat embryonic disk into a more or less cylindrical body. The folding occurs because the disk grows more rapidly than the extraembryonic tissue with which it is continuous; as a consequence of the constraint exerted at the periphery, the disk buckles upward while its edges are folded or rolled under. Because growth is most rapid along the longitudinal axis, the folding is more pronounced at the head and tail extremities than along the lateral margins.

This process ensures that the part of the yolk sac taken into the body presents two horns extending cranially and caudally from a middle region that retains free communication with the larger part of the yolk sac remaining outside the embryo. The included part of the yolk sac is known as the *gut,* and its three regions are the *foregut, midgut,* and *hindgut.* The midgut joins the other regions through tapering parts known as the *cranial* and *caudal intestinal portals* (Fig. 3.2).

THE MOUTH

The term *mouth* (os, genitive form oris) designates the cavity, its walls, and also the accessory structures that project (teeth, tongue) and drain (salivary glands) into it. The mouth has as its main functions the prehension, mastication, and insalivation of food. It may also play a role in aggression and defense, whereas in ourselves it is important in the formulation of the sounds of speech. In most species it functions as an airway when flow through the nose is impaired.

The mouth (oral cavity) is entered between the lips and continues into the pharynx (Fig. 3.3) through a caudal narrowing at the level of the palatoglossal arches (see later). It is divided by the teeth and margins of the jaws into an outer vestibule, bounded by the lips and cheeks externally and the central oral cavity proper. When the mouth is closed, these divisions communicate through gaps behind and between the teeth. The vestibule extends caudally toward the ramus of the mandible and the masseter muscle. The proportion of its walls formed by the lips varies with feeding habits; a wide gape is necessary in species that feed greedily or use their teeth to seize prey or in fighting, whereas a smaller opening suffices in most herbivores and rodents.

Diet and feeding habits also determine the form of the *lips* (labia oris). In some species, such as the horse, the lips are sensitive and mobile to accomplish the task of food collection and its introduction into the mouth. When other parts are more important in prehension the lips can be less mobile and smaller (e.g., cat) or thickened and insensitive (e.g., ox). The lips of the dog are extensive but thin and can be posed to show aggressive intent or submission. In newborn animals the lips form the seal about the teat that is necessary for successful sucking. The mimetic muscles that encircle the mouth and raise, depress, and retract the lips are supplied by the facial nerve.

The lips are composed of skin, an intermediate layer of muscle, tendon, and glands, and the oral mucosa. The skin and mucosa usually meet along the margin of the lips, though the boundary can be displaced in either direction. Small salivary glands are scattered among the muscle bundles below the mucosa, especially toward the angles (commissures) where the two lips meet.

Compared with the upper lip, the lower lip is usually unremarkable. In the dog it is rather loose but fastened to the lower jaw at the level of the canine tooth and has a thin, serrated margin. The upper lip sometimes has a median naked area that continues with the modified skin around the nostrils. The extensive moist and glandular nasolabial plate of the ox and the rostral disk of the pig are good examples of this. The area of modified skin, referred to by

*The digestive, respiratory, urinary, and male and female reproductive organs constitute a series of systems or apparatuses whose study collectively is known as *splanchnology.* Most of the component parts are known as *viscera* (plural of *viscus,* Latin for organ).

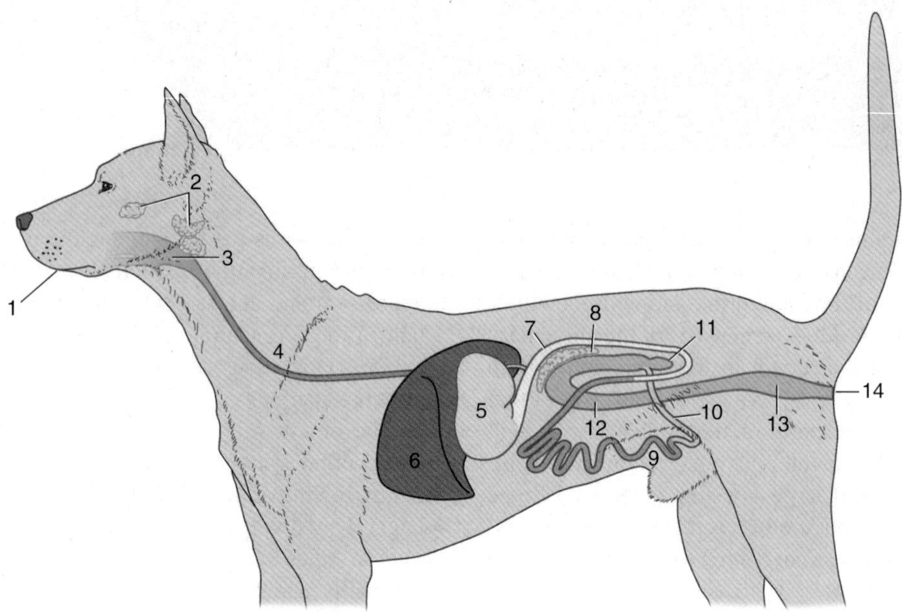

Fig. 3.1 Schematic representation of the digestive apparatus in the dog. *1,* Mouth; *2,* salivary glands; *3,* pharynx; *4,* esophagus; *5,* stomach; *6,* liver; *7,* duodenum; *8,* pancreas; *9,* jejunum; *10,* ileum; *11,* cecum; *12,* colon; *13,* rectum; *14,* anus.

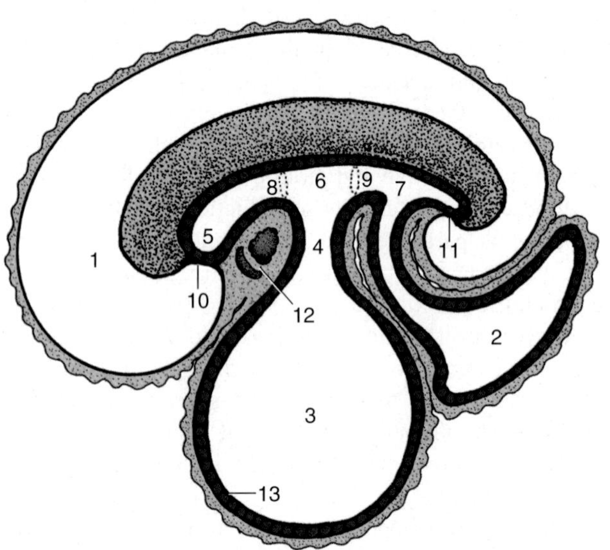

Fig. 3.2 Sagittal section of an early embryo. Part of the yolk sac is taken into the body in the folding process. *1,* Amniotic cavity; *2,* allantoic cavity; *3,* yolk sac; *4,* stalk of yolk sac; *5,* foregut; *6,* midgut; *7,* hindgut; *8,* cranial intestinal portal; *9,* caudal intestinal portal; *10,* oral plate; *11,* cloacal plate; *12,* heart and pericardial cavity; *13,* endoderm.

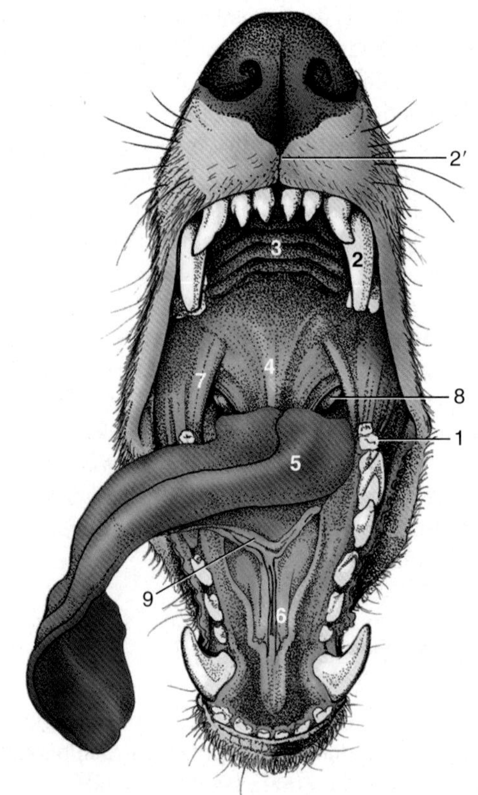

Fig. 3.3 General view of the oral cavity of the dog. *1,* Vestibule; *2,* canine tooth; *2′,* philtrum; *3,* hard palate; *4,* soft palate; *5,* tongue; *6,* sublingual caruncle; *7,* palatoglossal arch; *8,* palatine tonsil; *9,* frenulum.

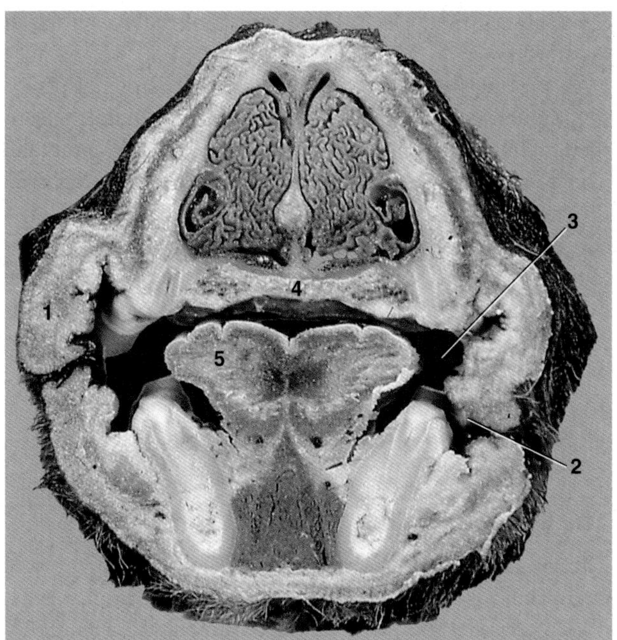

Fig. 3.4 Transverse section of the head of the dog at the level of P2. *1,* Cheek (with buccal folds); *2,* vestibule; *3,* oral cavity proper; *4,* hard palate (with venous plexus); *5,* tongue.

dog breeders as "nose leather," is often much narrower and may be divided by a median groove (philtrum) (see Fig. 3.3). In the human and in the horse a hairy integument extends across the entire upper lip.

The *cheeks* (buccae), which are most capacious in herbivores, are structurally similar to the lips. The principal support is the buccinator muscle, which functions to return to the central cavity any food that has escaped into the vestibule. Certain rodents and monkeys have diverticula of the oral vestibule (cheek pouches) to store rapidly harvested food for later mastication. The large cheek pouches in hamsters reach well into the thorax and have their own supporting musculature. There are additional salivary glands, sometimes aggregated in quite large masses: the zygomatic gland of the dog (see Fig. 3.12/*8*) that are concealed below the zygomatic arch. The buccal mucosa tends to be tightly anchored in some places such that it is sufficiently loose to allow the occasional maximal opening of the mouth while avoiding large folds that would get injured from the teeth (Fig. 3.4). In ruminants, whose food may be dry and rough, large, closely spaced, pointed papillae provide protection (see Fig. 3.7). A small papilla (in h easily found with the tongue tip) carries the opening of the duct of the parotid gland.

The cavity within the dental arcades—the *mouth cavity proper*—is roofed by the palate; bounded laterally by the teeth, gums, and margins of the jaws; and floored by the tongue and the small area of mucosa left uncovered by the tongue. Most of the walls are rigid, and when the

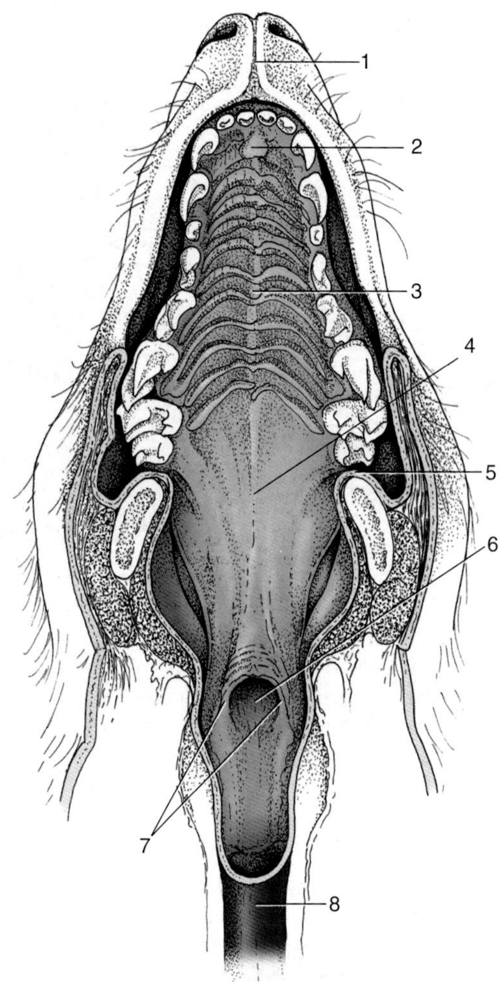

Fig. 3.5 The hard and soft palate of the dog. *1,* Philtrum; *2,* incisive papilla; *3,* hard palate with rugae; *4,* soft palate; *5,* palatoglossal arch; *6,* intrapharyngeal ostium; *7,* palatopharyngeal arches; *8,* esophagus.

mouth is closed, the size of the cavity can be altered only by raising or lowering the tongue and floor.

The larger, rostral part of the roof is based on a bony shelf formed of the palatine processes of the incisive, maxillary, and palatine bones and is known as the *hard palate* (palatum durum). This structure is continued caudally, without external demarcation, by the soft palate, in which a connective tissue aponeurosis replaces the bone.

The hard palate is usually flat (though vaulted in humans) and is covered by a thick mucosa fashioned into a series of more or less transverse ridges (rugae), which may guide the food backward (Fig. 3.5). In general, these ridges are most prominent and their covering epithelium most heavily keratinized in herbivores. A small median swelling, the incisive papilla, is commonly found behind the incisor teeth, flanked by the orifices of small (incisive) ducts that perforate the palate. These ducts branch and lead to the nasal cavity and to the vomeronasal organ (Fig. 3.6). They convey small amounts of the fluid from the mouth

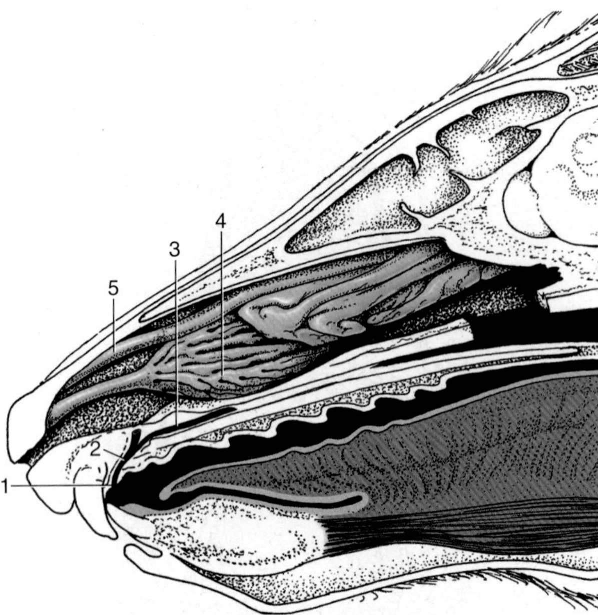

Fig. 3.6 Paramedian section of the rostral part of the head of the dog. The plane of section fails to demonstrate the opening of the incisive duct into the nasal cavity. *1,* Incisive papilla; *2,* incisive duct; *3,* vomeronasal organ; *4,* ventral nasal concha; *5,* dorsal nasal concha.

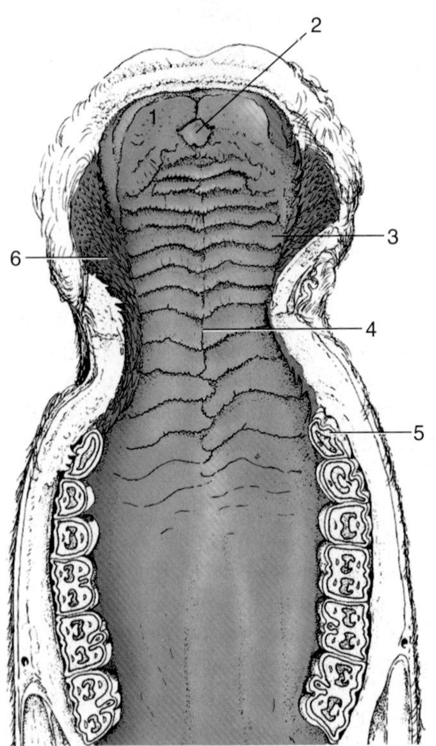

Fig. 3.7 The hard palate of a cow. *1,* Dental pad; *2,* incisive papilla; *3,* rugae of hard palate; *4,* palatine raphe; *5,* P2; *6,* buccal papillae.

for appraisal by the olfactory mucosa of the vomeronasal organ (p. 337).

A striking peculiarity in ruminants is the dental pad, a tough but yielding cushion in the position generally occupied by upper incisor teeth (lacking in these animals). The dental pad acts as a counterpart to the lower incisors in grazing (Fig. 3.7). A dense, richly vascularized tissue beneath the palatine epithelium functions both as the lamina propria of the mucosa and as the periosteum of the bone, attaching so tightly that not even the most vigorous mastication shifts it. Peripherally, the hard palate blends with the gums, the rather insensitive mucosa along the alveolar margins of the jaws.

The soft palate is described with the pharynx (p. 109).

The Tongue

The tongue (lingua) occupies the greater part of the oral cavity but also extends into the oropharynx (Fig. 3.8). It has an attached root and body and a free apex. The highly muscular construction makes the tongue capable of both vigorous and precise movements, as in prehension, lapping, grooming, and manipulating the food within the mouth on the one hand and speech articulation on the other. The mobility is achieved by restriction of the attachments to the more caudal part, which leaves the apex free to move both within and beyond the mouth. The attachment of the root is to the hyoid bone, and that of the body is to the symphyseal region of the mandible. The tongue is slung between the lower jaws by paired mylohyoideus muscles

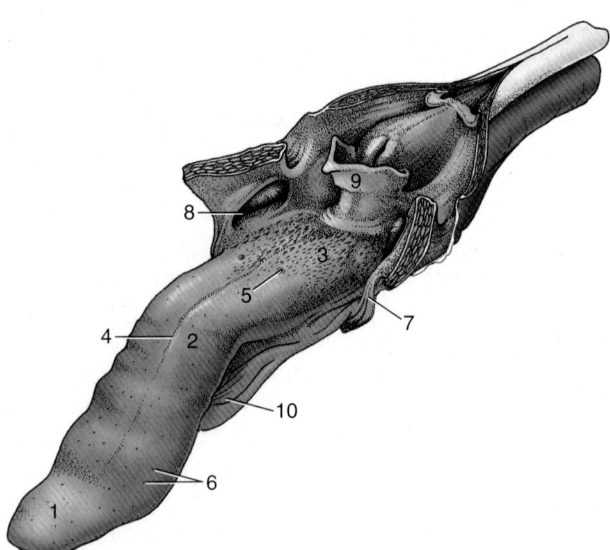

Fig. 3.8 The tongue of the dog. The soft palate and the esophagus are sectioned in the median plane. *1,* Apex; *2,* body; *3,* root, forming floor of oropharynx; *4,* median groove; *5,* vallate papilla; *6,* fungiform papillae; *7,* palatoglossal arch; *8,* palatine tonsil in tonsillar fossa; *9,* epiglottis; *10,* frenulum.

that originate from the medial aspect of the mandible and meet in a median raphe (see Fig. 3.21/*4*). Dogs also use their tongues for heat loss by panting, a process facilitated by the very generous supply of blood and the numerous arteriovenous anastomoses (p. 226).

In general shape, the tongue corresponds to the oral cavity. The apex is dorsoventrally compressed, the succeeding middle portion is somewhat triangular in section (being joined to the oral floor by a mucosal fold or frenulum), and the root is uniformly wide to allow entry to the muscles passing forward from the hyoid bone. Mucosal reflections (palatoglossal arches; Fig. 3.8/*7*) also pass from each side of the root to join the soft palate and demarcate the boundaries of the mouth.

The mucosa is tough and tightly adherent where repeated contact with abrasive food occurs but looser and less heavily keratinized where a softer diet or a more protected position allows. Much of the surface is covered by a variety of papillae. Some are soft and threadlike (filiform), scattered widely over the human tongue to provide additional protection, but the harsh conical papillae make the cat's tongue essentially function as a rasp. Other papillae carry taste buds and have a more restricted distribution, characteristic for each species (Fig. 3.9): their names—*fungiform, foliate,* and *vallate papillae*—give good indications of their shapes. A few small salivary glands lie below the epithelium.

The bulk of the tongue consists of muscle, usually divided into intrinsic and extrinsic groups. Four pairs of extrinsic muscles exist (Fig. 3.10). One, the *geniohyoideus,* lies somewhat apart and below the tongue and passes from the incisive part of the mandible to the body of the hyoid bone. It is able to draw the hyoid and thus the tongue forward. The *genioglossus* arises more dorsally than the geniohyoideus and first runs back below the floor of the mouth before dividing into bundles that fan upward in the sagittal plane. Those bundles going to the apex of the tongue retract this part while those to the root draw the whole tongue forward. The middle group passes toward the upper surface (dorsum), which it may depress. The other two muscles arise from the hyoid apparatus. The *hyoglossus* takes origin from the basihyoid and runs forward, lateral to the genioglossus; the *styloglossus* takes origin from the stylohyoid but farther to the side. Both draw the tongue back but in rather different fashions; the styloglossus also tends to elevate it. The bundles of intrinsic muscle run longitudinally, transversely, and vertically (see Fig. 4.2). Simultaneous contraction of the transverse and vertical bundles stiffens the tongue.

The muscle bundles are interspersed with considerable amounts of fat, which is an arrangement that imparts a unique consistency and flavor to the cooked tongue. This fat is very resistant to mobilization in starvation.

In the dog, alone among the domestic species, the ventral part of the tongue contains a prominent fibrous condensation, the lyssa, easily recognized on palpation. A fibrous septum that extends from this is responsible for the conspicuous median groove on the upper surface.

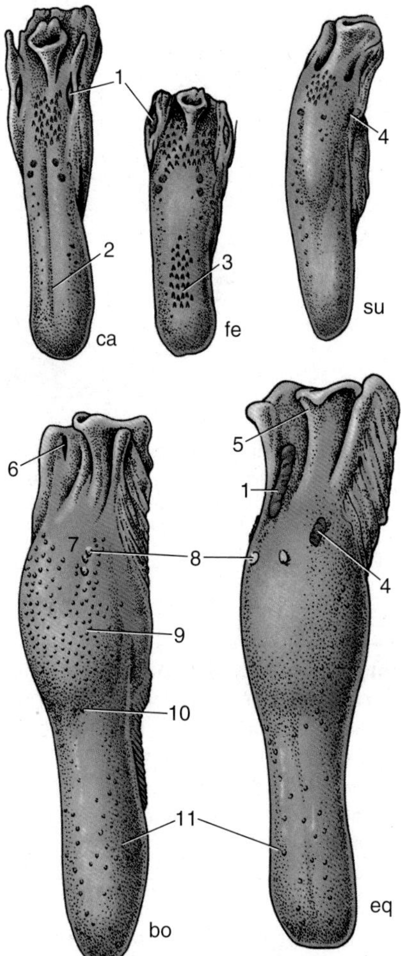

Fig. 3.9 Dorsal view of the tongue and epiglottis of the dog *(ca)*, cat *(fe)*, pig *(su)*, cattle *(bo)*, and horse *(eq)*. *1,* Palatine tonsil; *2,* median groove; *3,* filiform papillae; *4,* foliate papillae; *5,* epiglottis; *6,* tonsillar sinus; *7,* root of tongue; *8,* vallate papillae; *9,* torus linguae; *10,* fossa linguae; *11,* fungiform papillae.

The *innervation* accurately reflects the origin of the tongue as an unpaired swelling of the pharyngeal floor (see Fig. 3.58C) that is later extended by contributions from the ventral parts of the adjacent pharyngeal (branchial) arches. The mucosa retains a sensory innervation from the corresponding arch nerves. The lingual branch of the mandibular nerve is responsible for general sensation over the rostral two thirds of the tongue; the chorda tympani, a branch of the facial nerve, is responsible for the special sensation of taste in the same area. Both general and special sensations of the root region are the responsibility of the glossopharyngeal and, to a small extent, the vagus nerves.

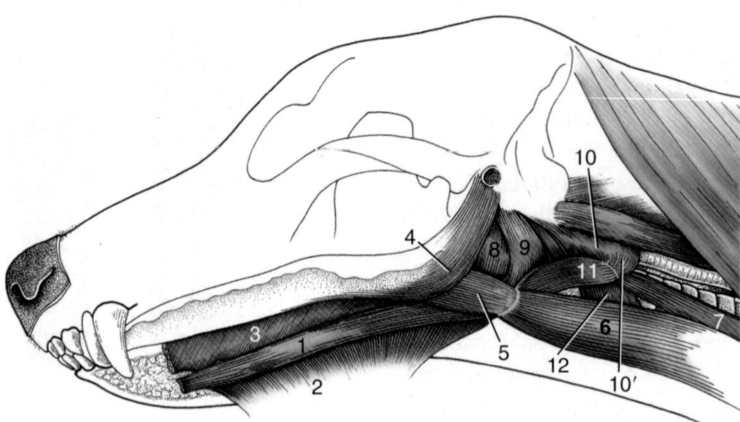

Fig. 3.10 Muscles of the tongue and pharynx of the dog. *1,* Geniohyoideus; *2,* mylohyoideus; *3,* genioglossus; *4,* styloglossus; *5,* hyoglossus; *6,* sternohyoideus; *7,* sternothyroideus; *8 and 9,* hyopharyngeus (two parts); *10,* thyropharyngeus; *10′,* cricopharyngeus; *11,* thyrohyoideus; *12,* cricothyroideus.

The extrinsic and intrinsic muscles are all supplied by the hypoglossal nerve, although it is probable that the sensory fibers emanating from spindles and other receptors in these muscles travel mainly in the lingual nerve. The mylohyoideus muscle is supplied by the mandibular nerve and plays an important part in initiating swallowing.

Relatively little of the *floor of the mouth* is left accessible rostral and lateral to the attachments of the tongue. The largest free area lies ventral to the apex, behind the incisor teeth. The mucosa here covers the incisive part of the mandible directly, but elsewhere it lies on muscle and the floor yields under pressure. The most prominent features are fleshy protuberances or caruncles behind the central incisors, and located in them are the common openings of the mandibular and major sublingual salivary ducts (see Fig. 3.3). In some species, much smaller serial elevations to each side of the frenulum mark the openings of the lesser ducts of the sublingual gland.

The Salivary Glands

Numerous salivary glands, small and large, drain into the oral cavity. Small salivary glands occur in the lips, cheeks, tongue, soft palate, pharynx, and esophagus. Although they are individually unimportant, their collective contribution must be considerable. However, certain larger glands contribute most of the saliva into the mouth cavity via secretory ducts (Fig. 3.11). Unlike the minor glands, which mostly produce a mucous secretion, some of these major glands produce a more watery (serous) fluid containing the enzyme ptyalin, which plays a minor role in carbohydrate digestion. The saliva keeps the mouth clean and moist, and upon mixing with food, it facilitates mastication and lubricates its passage. It may also contribute to deposition of tartar on teeth.

The *parotid gland,* which is purely serous in most species (though not in the dog), is molded around the ventral part of the auricular cartilage (Fig. 3.12). In the dog it is small and confined to the vicinity of the cartilage. In herbivores, the gland is large and extends rostrally onto the masseter muscle, ventrally toward the angle of the jaw, and caudally toward the atlantal fossa. It produces copious amounts of serous saliva to moisten and soften foods. In all species it is enclosed within a fascial covering that sends trabeculae inward to divide the gland into obvious lobules. The major collecting ducts run within these trabeculae and eventually join to form a single duct that leaves the cranial aspect. In the dog this duct takes the shortcut across the lateral surface of the masseter to open into the vestibule of the mouth opposite the fourth upper premolar tooth. In the large domestic animals the duct takes the longer but more protected route medial to the angle of the jaw and winds below the mandible to enter the face along the rostral margin of the masseter.

The *mandibular gland* (Fig. 3.11B) produces a mixed mucous and serous secretion. Generally smaller than the parotid, it is more compact and is placed close to the angle of the jaw. It is a moderately large, very regular ovoid structure in the dog. It too is much larger and deeper in herbivores. This gland also drains by a single large duct that runs ventral to the mucous membrane of the floor of the mouth, close to the frenulum of the tongue, to open on the sublingual caruncle.

The *sublingual gland* is also commonly mixed and sometimes consists of parts: one is compact (monostomatic) and

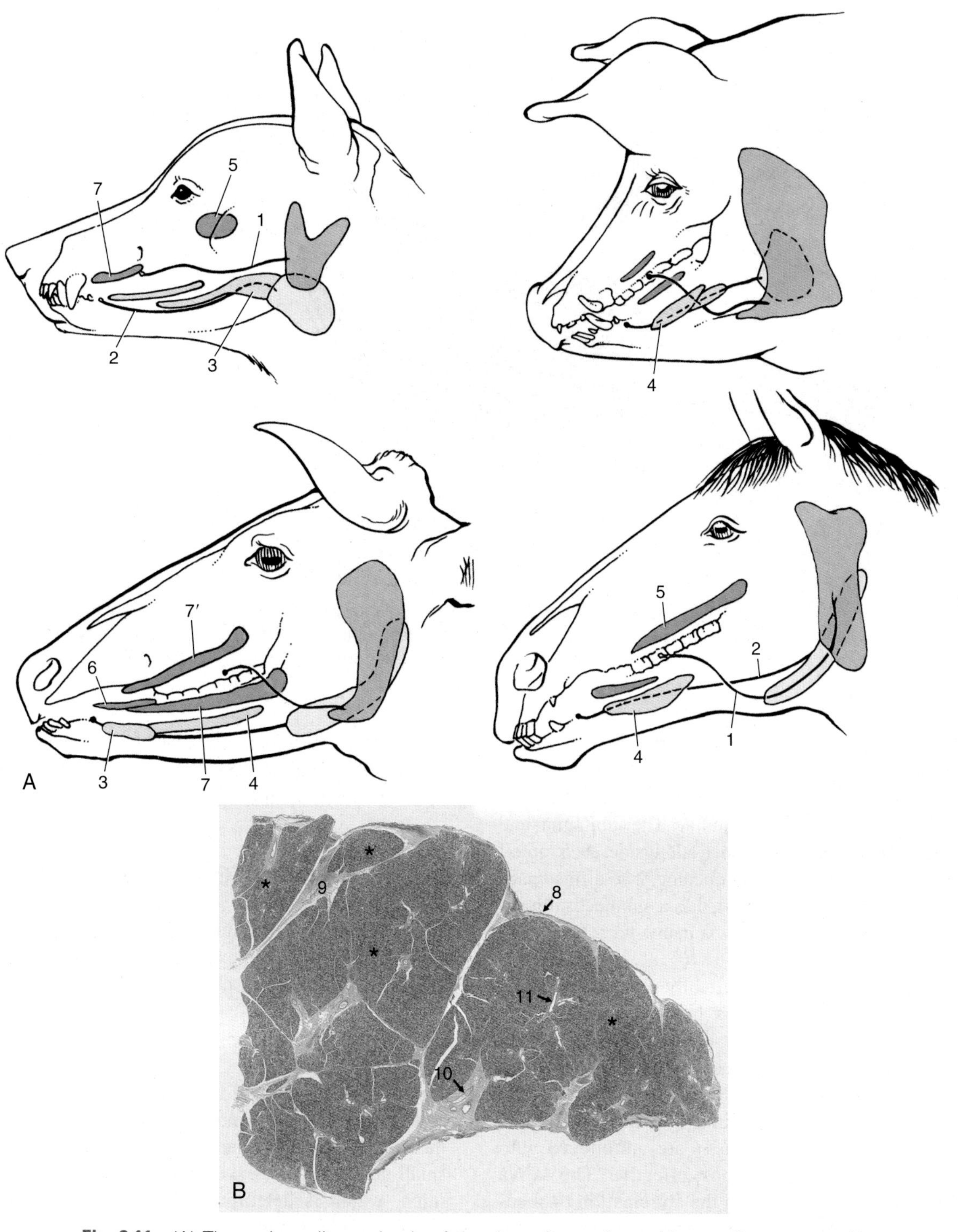

Fig. 3.11 (A) The major salivary glands of the dog, pig, cattle, and horse. *Orange,* parotid gland; *white,* mandibular gland; *yellow,* sublingual glands; *red,* buccal glands. *1,* Parotid duct; *2,* mandibular duct; *3,* compact (monostomatic) part of sublingual gland; *4,* diffuse (polystomatic) part of sublingual gland; *5,* dorsal buccal glands (zygomatic gland in the dog); *6,* middle buccal glands; *7,* ventral buccal glands; *7′,* middle buccal gland. (B) Mandibular salivary gland of horse. Hematoxylin and eosin stain. This small portion of gland illustrates the organization of the secretory units. Notice that the gland is surrounded by adventitial connective tissue *(8),* and many lobules (*) are separated by connective tissue septas *(9)* containing interlobular ducts *(10),* blood vessels, and nerve bundles. The mixed nature of the horse mandibular gland is evident by the serous (dark purple) and mucous (light pinkish) components present within the same lobule. Many intralobular or striated ducts *(11)* are visible among the secretory end-pieces within the lobules (hematoxylin and eosin stain).

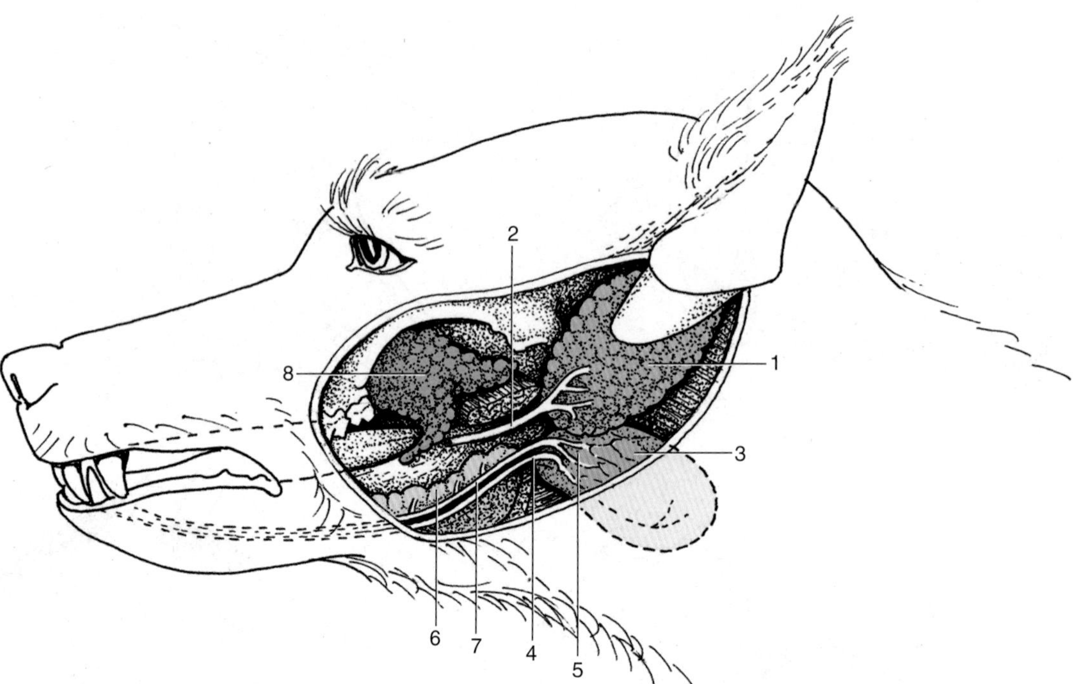

Fig. 3.12 The salivary glands of the dog. *1,* Parotid gland; *2,* parotid duct; *3,* mandibular gland; *4,* mandibular duct; *5,* caudal part of compact sublingual gland; *6,* rostral part of compact sublingual gland; *7,* major sublingual duct; *8,* zygomatic gland.

drains by a single duct, and the other is diffuse (polystomatic) and opens by several small ducts. In the dog the compact part fits over the rostral extremity of the mandibular gland, which it appears to continue. The sublingual and mandibular ducts travel and open alongside each other; they may even have a common opening. The diffuse part, the only part present in the horse, has a submucosal location in the oral floor and opens via many ducts beside the frenulum.

The flow of saliva is normally continuous, and although the rate is influenced by many factors it is under neural control. The flow is depressed by anxiety or fear and may be wholly suspended when the body is dehydrated: the resulting dryness of the mouth contributes to the sensation of thirst. It is increased when substances—even inedible ones—are introduced into the mouth, although food is most effective. The saliva production increases even with the anticipation of feeding. The salivary glands receive both sympathetic and parasympathetic supplies, the latter being vastly more important. The parasympathetic fibers come from the two salivatory nuclei of the brainstem and first travel in the facial and glossopharyngeal nerves; later the fibers are carried to their destination in various branches of the trigeminal nerve. The preganglionic fibers synapse close to the gland, and the postganglionic fibers terminate in direct contact with the secretory cells. The parasympathetic stimulation induces copious flow accompanied by vasodilation. Sympathetic stimulation produces vasoconstriction, which slows the rate of production and alters the composition of the saliva.

THE MASTICATORY APPARATUS

The masticatory apparatus comprises the teeth and gums, the temporomandibular and symphyseal joints of the jaws, and the masticatory muscles.

Dentition

The mammalian *dentition** possesses certain characters that in combination, if not individually, are diagnostic of the class. The complement of teeth is limited to a fairly small number, rarely exceeding 44 in the permanent dentition, which is determined for each species—although minor variations may occur. Unlike those of most other vertebrates, the teeth of mammals are very differently developed in different regions of the mouth for better performance of special tasks; this character, known as *heterodonty,* allows the recognition of incisor, canine, premolar, and molar groups. A single replacement of the teeth first

* Terms relating to the teeth—for example, *dentin, periodontium, orthodontics,* and so forth—are derived from the Latin (*dens*) or the Greek (*odous*).

erupted is provided by a second, stronger set that is better adapted to the larger jaws and to the more vigorous mastication of the adult. The sequence is known as *diphyodonty,* in contrast to the *polyphyodonty* (multiple succession) in most other vertebrates. Finally, the teeth are implanted in sockets set along the margins of the jaws, an arrangement described as *thecodont*.

The number and classification of the teeth in a particular species are conveniently represented by a formula in which *I* stands for incisor, *C* for canine, *P* for premolar, and *M* for molar. For the dog, the formula of the permanent dentition may be written

$$\frac{\text{I3 - C1 - P4 - M2}}{\text{I - C1 - P4 - M3}} = 42$$

or, more succinctly and no less clearly,

$$\frac{3\text{ - }1\text{ - }4\text{ - }2}{3\text{ - }1\text{ - }4\text{ - }3}$$

The temporary (milk or deciduous) dentition of the same animal may be represented

$$\frac{3\text{ - }1\text{ - }3}{3\text{ - }1\text{ - }3}$$

without risk of confusion, as molar teeth are always lacking in the milk set. There are various notations for the identification of individual teeth. The most convenient would use upper- and lowercase letters to denote the permanent and temporary, respectively, and superscript and subscript numerals to show the upper and lower teeth, respectively. For example, P^1 may stand for the first permanent upper premolar, i_2 for the secondary temporary lower incisor.

The term *diastema* is used for a considerable gap between teeth in the one jaw, most usually for that between the incisors and premolars.

The *description of a simple tooth* may be considered before the discussion returns to the features of the different types of teeth. A tooth (*dens*) consists of crown and root, and each is easily distinguished. The crown is encased in enamel, a very resistant, calcified, slightly opalescent, white material, whereas the root is encased in cement, a softer, less shiny, yellowish tissue. The part of the tooth between root and crown is termed the *neck* (Fig. 3.13). Certain variations in structure may occur at the neck: the cement and enamel commonly abut, but the cement may overlie the enamel or sometimes the two tissues fail to meet, exposing a narrow strip of dentin, the third calcified tissue of the tooth. The dentin, which is also known as ivory, provides the greater part of the substance of the tooth and contains a small central cavity that houses the connective tissue pulp. The pulp continues through a

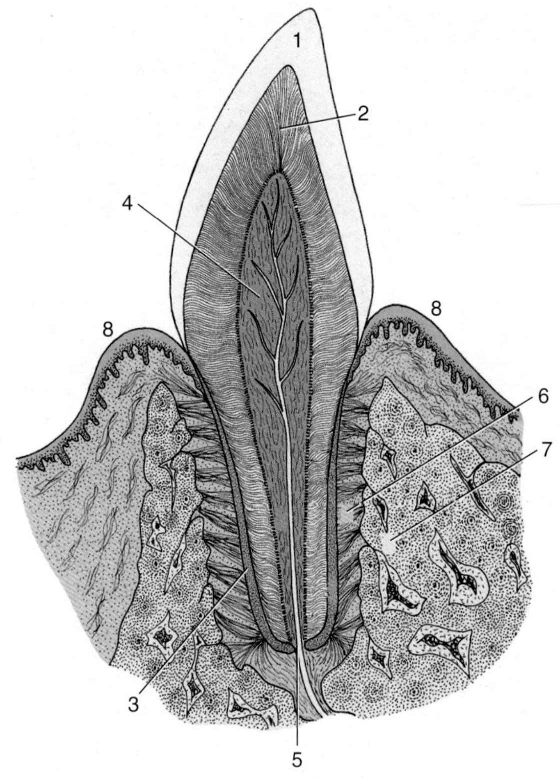

Fig. 3.13 Schematic longitudinal section of a simple tooth. *1,* Enamel; *2,* dentin; *3,* cement; *4,* pulp; *5,* apical foramen; *6,* periodontal ligament; *7,* socket (alveolus); *8,* gum.

canal in the root of the tooth to merge with the connective tissue in the depth of the tooth socket (*alveolus*).

Fig. 3.13 depicts the idealized condition in which both the gum (*gingiva*) embraces the neck and the crown corresponds to the exposed part of the tooth. The gums may recede with advancing age, exposing the cervical part of the root, a condition familiar in many older people who are said, on this account, to be "long in the tooth." In many mammals, especially the herbivores, part of the enamel-covered crown is concealed below the gum line, which is extruded gradually to compensate for the loss at the masticator surface. Such high-crowned teeth are called *hypsodont* (or hypseledont) and are characteristic of animals feeding on abrasive food. Even in species such as primates or dogs with low-crowned (*brachydont*) teeth suited to a softer diet that produces less wear, part of the enamel-covered region commonly lies below the gum during initial use of the tooth. For these reasons it is useful to distinguish the "clinical crown" from the anatomic crown: the first term specifies the exposed part of the tooth regardless of its structure, and the second specifies the enamel-covered part regardless of its location (Fig. 3.14).

The detailed description of the *crown* requires some system for indicating its various surfaces because the usual terms of relative position are inadequate, considering that

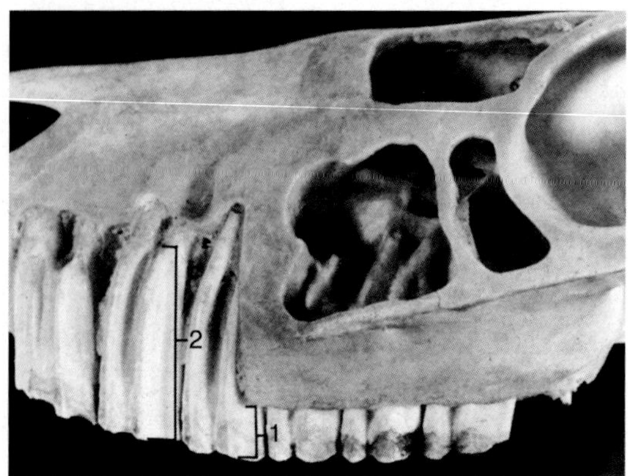

Fig. 3.14 Premolar teeth exposed in the upper jaw of a horse. The part protruding above the gum is the clinical crown *(1)*; the whole enamel-covered part is the anatomic crown or body *(2)* of the tooth.

the curved line followed by the tooth row (arcade) alters the orientation of equivalent surfaces of successive teeth in the series. Less ambiguous terms are *vestibular* (labial, buccal) and *lingual* and *mesial* and *distal;* their usage is indicated in Fig. 3.18. Where adjacent teeth touch, the appropriate mesial and distal surfaces may both be termed *contact surfaces*. The working area, if extensive and not a mere cutting edge, is known as the *occlusal* or *masticatory surface*.

Enamel is a densely calcified tissue of ectodermal origin. It is acellular and lacks regenerative capacity to patch a hole or repair a fracture. Because it is exposed to rough treatment, it is necessarily very hard. Nevertheless, the enamel casing may eventually be breached, and the softer dentin that wears away more rapidly would then be exposed. The thickness and the resistance of the enamel therefore largely determine the working life of the brachydont tooth. In species in which the tooth crown is high and only gradually passed above the gum line, the enamel may be folded in a very complicated fashion; this folding increases the efficiency of the masticatory surface, because the unequal resistance of the tissues exposed on opening of the enamel casing results in an irregular ridged arrangement (see Figs. 3.19 and 18.20).

Cement is the least hard of the calcified tissues of the tooth and resembles bone in structure, although it lacks so regular an organization. The initial deposit over the root is thin, but as deposition continues throughout life it may eventually form quite a thick crust. Collagen fibers extend from the cement into the periodontal ligament or membrane (*periodontium*), the specialized connective tissue that fastens the tooth in its socket. Although broadly comparable to bone in structure and development, cement differs in one important respect: it is relatively immune to pressure erosion. Orthodontists make use of this characteristic when they adjust the position of a tooth in the jaw by fitting an appliance that presses the tooth against the alveolar wall. If the adjustment is performed correctly, the pressure produces an erosion of the bone but leaves the tooth unaffected and free to shift into the space created. This lack of response to pressure is relative, not absolute, and excessive pressure causes resorption; indeed, the roots of the temporary teeth are resorbed under pressure from their permanent replacements thrusting against them.

Dentin is also similar to bone in having a calcified, collagen-rich matrix. In bone the osteoblasts become imprisoned in the matrix, but the dentin-producing cells (*odontoblasts*) recede from the newly formed dentin and remain as a continuous layer on the surface lining the dental (*pulp*) cavity. The odontoblasts retain their productive capacity throughout life, and a slow but continuous production of secondary dentin, with corresponding reduction of the dental cavity, continues into old age. This process may be accelerated when local damage or abrasion of the crown threatens to expose the pulp. Secondary dentin is easily recognized from its darker color. Although once disputed, it is generally believed that fine nerve processes enter a short distance into the dentin from the pulp.

The *dental cavity* reflects the external form of the tooth, sending a branch into each major elevation of the crown and through a narrow passage in the root where it opens at the apical foramen. There may be more than one root, with each joining the central cavity via a channel.

The *pulp* that fills this space is a very delicate connective tissue margined by the odontoblast layer and richly vascularized. A lymphatic plexus also exists, although it is difficult to demonstrate. Numerous nerves run within the pulp; some are vasomotor, although most are sensory and possess endings that can be stimulated in various ways. Whatever the stimulus, thermal, mechanical, or chemical, the sensation perceived is pain. Because the pulp is contained within unyielding walls, even a slight inflammatory swelling is quickly appreciated.

Each tooth is implanted in a separate socket in the margin of a jaw. The form of the socket corresponds to that of the root and is therefore often branched and irregular. Where the teeth lie close together the septa between adjacent sockets may be very delicate or even defective. Typically, the socket is lined by a thin lamina of compact bone perforated for the passage of the vessels and nerves supplying both the socket and the tooth. The outer surface of the lamina may be braced by trabeculae of spongy bone extending toward the surface of the jaw or radiating into surrounding parts. In the areas where the alveolar margin is narrow, however, the lamina merges with the external compacta of the jaw. The tooth is attached to the socket by means of the tough fibrous periodontal ligament made up of collagen fibers. The fibers are attached to both the cement and the alveolar bone and actually suspend the tooth in a sling. This

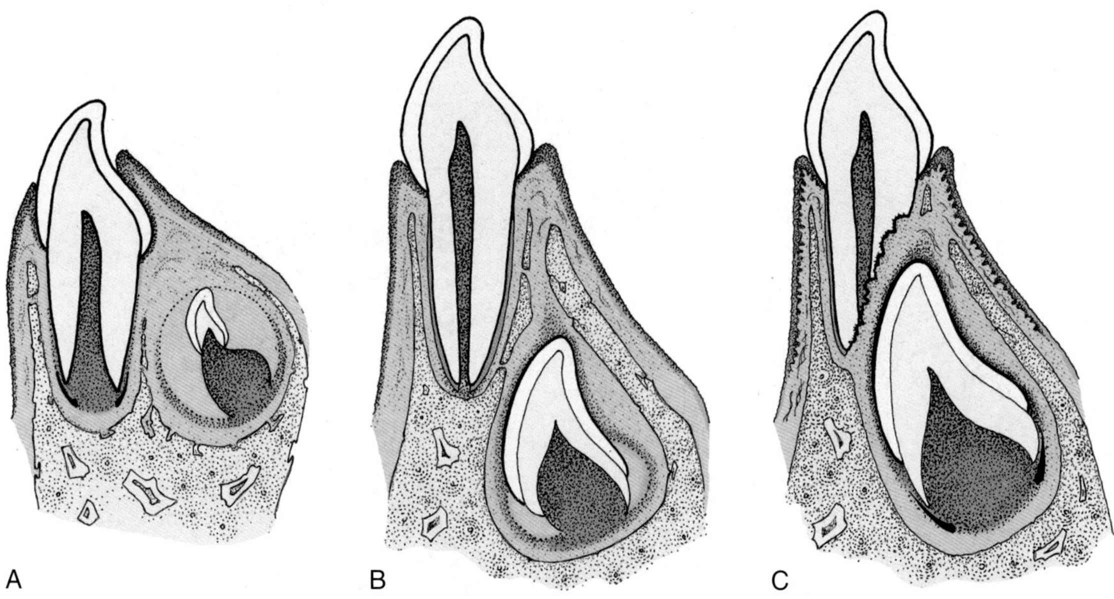

Fig. 3.15 Schematic drawings representing tooth eruption and replacement. (A) Eruption of a deciduous tooth. The primordium of the permanent tooth is located on the lingual side of the deciduous tooth. (B) The fully developed deciduous tooth within a bony alveolus. The crown of the permanent tooth has already formed. (C) The permanent tooth is ready to break through. The root of the deciduous tooth has been resorbed; formation of the root of the permanent tooth is in progress.

arrangement allows the tooth a certain (though usually very limited) mobility, resulting in slight rotation and tilting during mastication.

The vessels and nerves that supply the teeth are derived from the major trunks (*superior and inferior alveolar arteries, veins, and nerves*) that course through canals in the jaws.

Tooth *eruption* is a complicated and controversial process involving a number of factors: root growth, bone growth, pulpal proliferation, tissue pressure, and periodontal traction. Their relative importance is disputed, but the last factor is probably the most significant. The temporary teeth rise in the jaws after the crown is completed but before the root is formed; this process carries the tooth closer to the surface and provides the space necessary for the formation of the root. The movement of the crown is facilitated by a loosening of the connective tissue of the dental follicle and gum and by the presence of remnants of the epithelium of the dental lamina, which define the line of passage. However, if these remnants are large and cystic, as sometimes happens, they may obstruct rather than facilitate the movement of the tooth, divert it from its true path, and give rise to troublesome anomalies of site and spacing. The retention of an epithelial covering over the unerupted crown ensures that no breach of continuity occurs when the tooth breaks through to the surface, as this remnant of the enamel fuses with the epithelium of the gums embracing the tooth (Fig. 3.15).

The eruption of the permanent teeth is more complicated. They develop in bony crypts deep to the roots of the equivalent teeth of the temporary set. To erupt they must escape from this confinement and displace their predecessors. The erosion of the roof and the continuous adjustment of the walls of the embedded alveolus involve the usual processes of bone remodeling such that the permanent tooth and its alveolus migrate as a unit through the jaw to enter the alveolus of the temporary tooth. The replacement tooth then presses on the root of the temporary tooth, causing its resorption. The attachment of the temporary tooth is loosened, allowing it to shift and become increasingly mobile during mastication, followed by shedding and replacement by the permanent tooth. Proper eruption of the permanent teeth depends on places being held ready for them by the temporary teeth. If the decidual teeth are prematurely lost, the filling of the alveoli by bone may make it difficult for the permanent teeth to establish their proper occlusal relationships.

The *dentition of the dog*, although relatively simple, is well adapted to the feeding habits of the animal (Fig. 3.16). The incisor teeth are small and peglike and are crowded together in the rostral part of each jaw. On eruption, each upper incisor presents a trilobed crown with a labial cutting edge. The lower incisors are bilobed. These features are lost as wear reduces the tooth to a simple prismatic peg. The name *incisor* suggests that these teeth

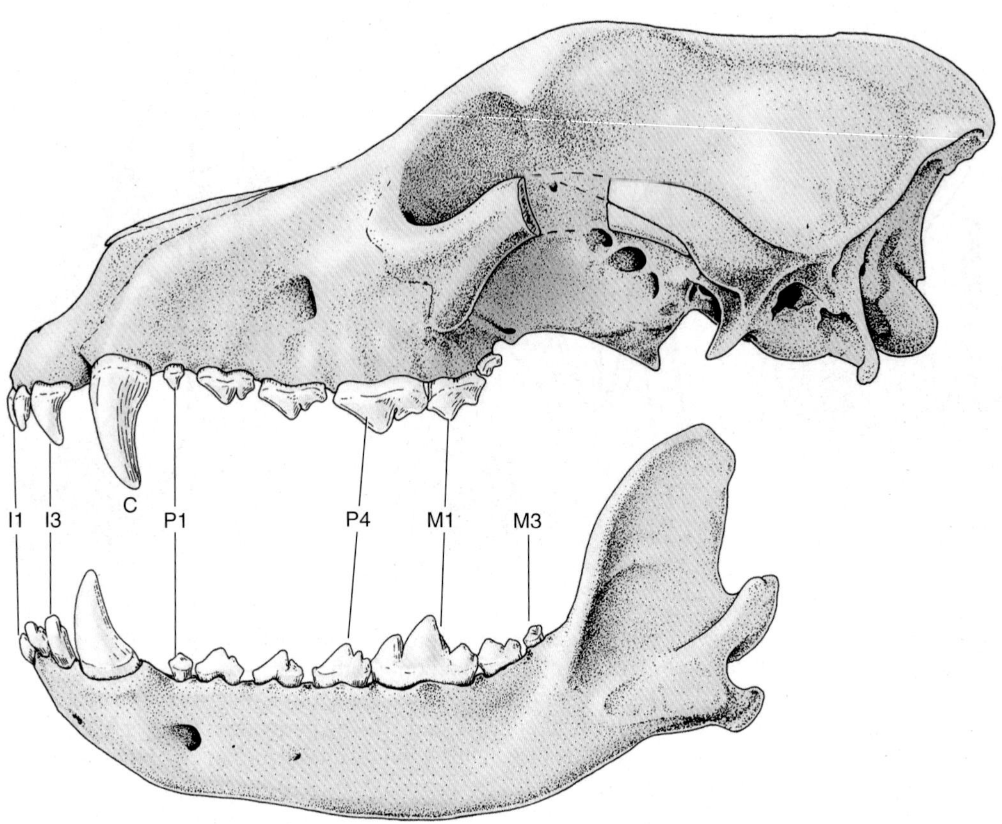

Fig. 3.16 Lateral view of the permanent dentition of the dog. *I*, incisor; *C*, canine; *P*, premolar; *M*, molar. *Numbers* indicate position of a tooth, with count beginning at the front.

are used for dividing food before it is taken into the mouth, but in this species a second and more efficient shear is provided by teeth farther back in the mouth. The incisors in the dog are employed mainly in nibbling and grooming.

The *canine teeth* are particularly well developed, so much so that the generic name (*Canis*) for doglike animals also is the term for similar teeth in all mammals. Canines are large, curved, and laterally compressed teeth of simple form capable of inflicting a deep wound that are used for aggressive and holding purposes. A large part of each canine tooth is implanted in the jaw. The bony ridge over the alveolus reveals the extent and position of the embedded part of the upper canine.

The premolar and molar teeth together constitute the *cheek teeth,* a term more common and more useful in describing the assimilation of these two groups of teeth into one in herbivorous species. In all mammals the first few (maximally four) cheek teeth are represented in both dentitions and are assigned to the premolar group; the remainder (maximally three) are represented only in the permanent dentition and are known as *molar teeth.* The *premolars* of the dog form an irregular but fairly closely spaced series of increasing size and complexity. The cusps or projections of the individual crowns are aligned one behind the other to form a discontinuous serrated cutting edge to enable a more rapid and cleaner division while the notches help hold the food in place. The more caudal *molars* also possess a cutting potential but are principally developed for crushing by their broader and more extensive masticatory surfaces. Their cusps or elevations are arranged in a pattern that is faithfully reproduced on the teeth of all members of the species; their homologues can be recognized, although sometimes only with great difficulty, in the teeth of other mammals.

Most of the cheek teeth, unlike the incisors and canines, have more than one root. Multiple roots, especially if divergent, provide firmer anchorage but make extraction difficult.

The *dentition of the cat* is reduced to

$$\frac{3\text{-}1\text{-}3\text{-}1}{3\text{-}1\text{-}2\text{-}1}$$

in the permanent set (Fig. 3.17). It is even more closely adapted to a fleshy diet, and crushing potential is largely eliminated with a reduced molar series. The cutting action of the cat's cheek teeth earns them the description *secodont;* the dual-purpose structure of the dog's molars is

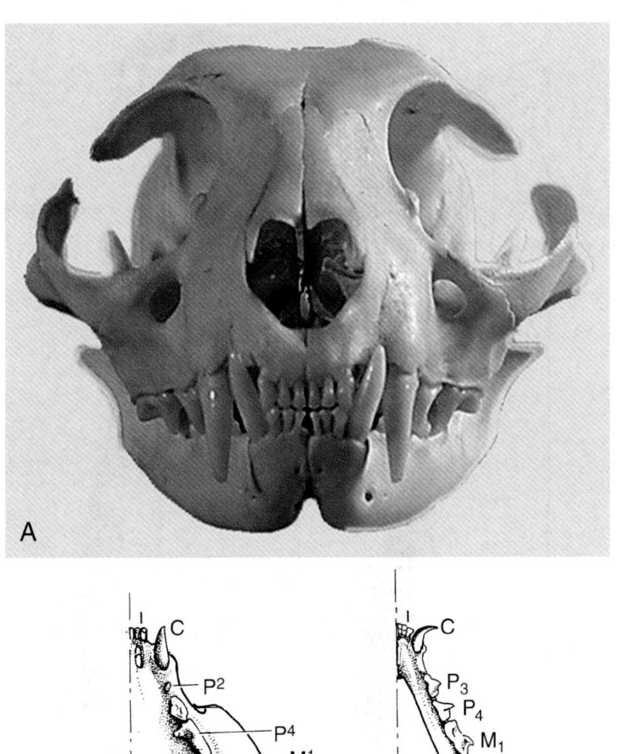

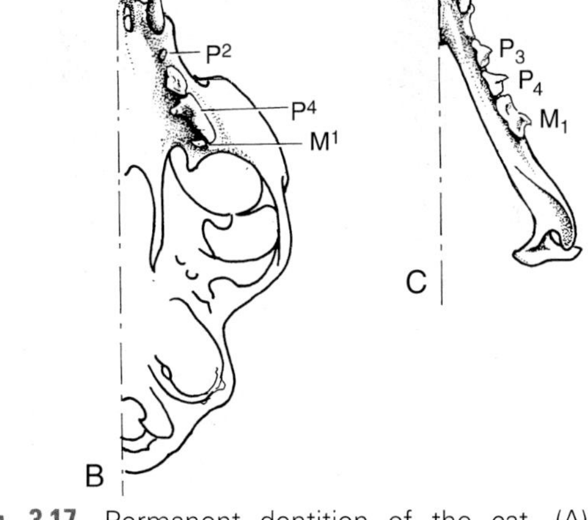

Fig. 3.17 Permanent dentition of the cat. (A) Rostral view. (B) Upper jaw. (C) Lower jaw. *I*, incisor; *C*, canine; *P*, premolar; *M*, molar. *Numbers* indicate position of a tooth, with count beginning at the front, with *superscript* indicating upper jaw and *subscript* lower jaw.

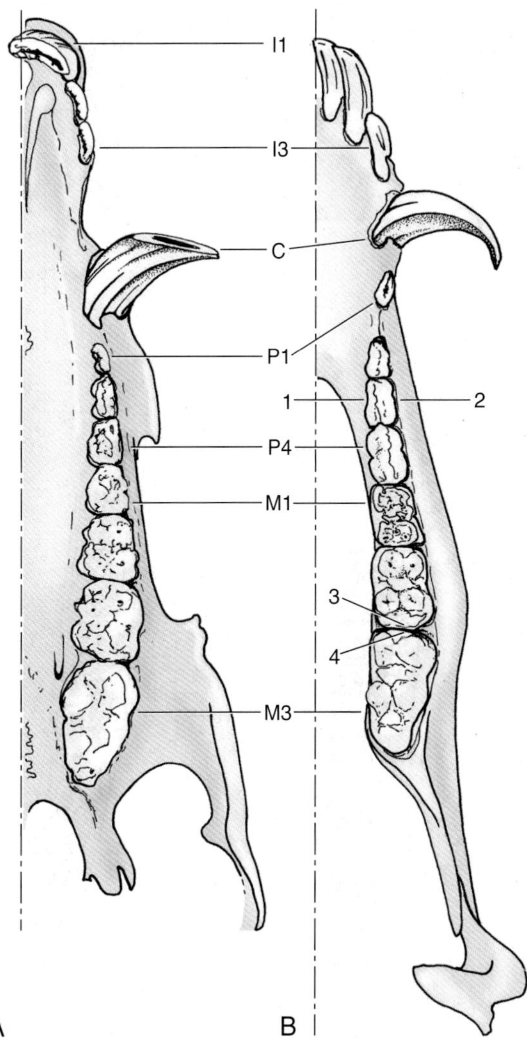

Fig. 3.18 Permanent dentition of the pig. (A) Upper and (B) lower jaws. *1*, Lingual surface; *2*, vestibular surface; *3*, distal surface; *4*, mesial surface. *I*, incisor; *C*, canine; *P*, premolar; *M*, molar. *Numbers* indicate position of a tooth, with count beginning at the front.

better described as *tuberculosectorial.* The incisors of cats are remarkably small and the canine teeth relatively large.

In other domestic species, the diet is much more abrasive and requires considerably more crushing and grinding. Only the most conspicuous features of the modified dentition are presented here (details in the later chapters). In the *dentition of the pig* the broad crowns of the cheek teeth carry an elaborate formation of blunt cusps that make them very effective crushing instruments, and these teeth are said to be *bunodont* (Fig. 3.18). The canine teeth of this species remain open at the embedded end (root) so that accretion of dental tissues continues throughout the animal's life. This persistent growth, coupled with their curved form, allows them to assume very striking forms in older individuals, particularly in boars.

The *dentition of horses and ruminants* that are restricted to herbivorous diet, in contrast to the diet of the omnivorous pig, must allow for continuous and considerable wear at the masticatory surfaces. This requirement is met by the enlargement of these surfaces, by the increase in height of the crowns, which are only gradually extruded (the delayed development of the roots allows growth to continue for some years after the teeth have come into wear), and, above all, by complicated folding of the enamel. This folding has two important consequences: there is an increased amount of the hardest and most durable component of the tooth that is exposed to reduce its attrition, and alternating harder and softer materials wear at different rates to produce an uneven and rasplike masticatory surface (Figs. 3.19 and 3.20).

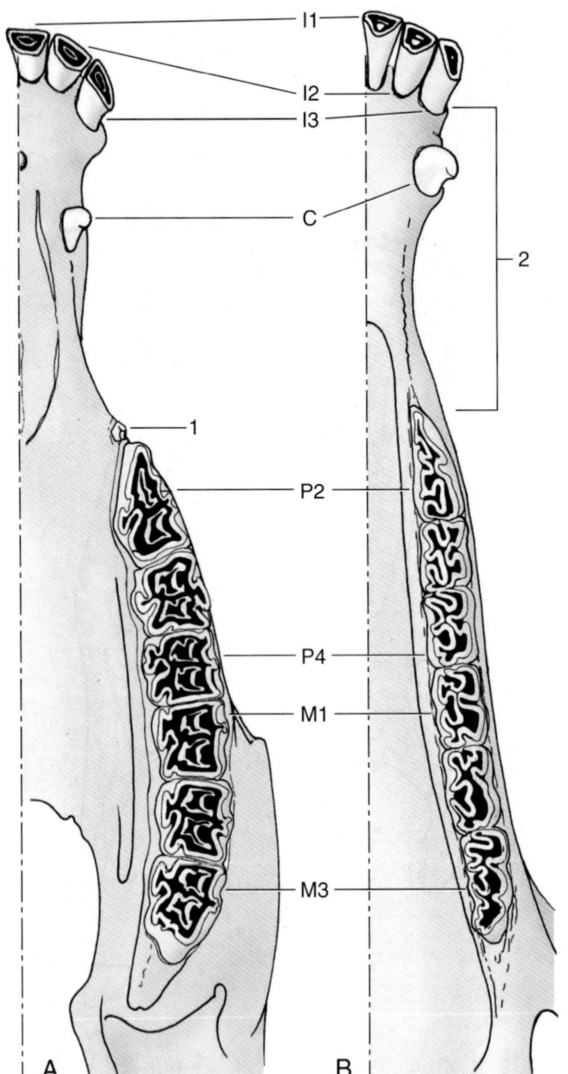

Fig. 3.19 Permanent dentition of the horse. (A) Upper and (B) lower jaws. *1,* Wolf tooth (P1); *2,* diastema. *I,* incisor; *C,* canine; *P,* premolar; *M,* molar. *Numbers* indicate position of a tooth, with count beginning at the front.

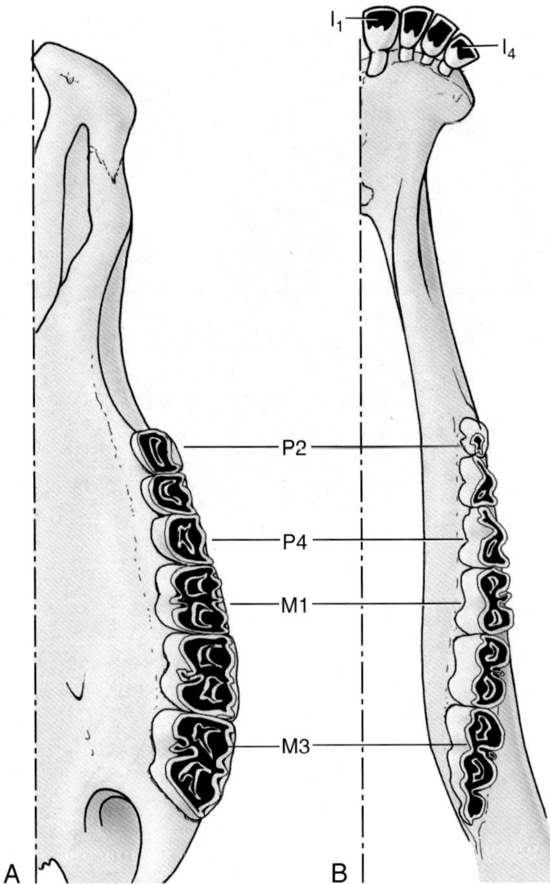

Fig. 3.20 Permanent dentition of cattle. (A) Upper and (B) lower jaws. *I,* incisor; *C,* canine; *P,* premolar; *M,* molar. *Numbers* indicate position of a tooth, with count beginning at the front.

The Articulations of the Jaws

Although it is customary to describe two *temporomandibular joints,* these may be regarded as the widely separated halves of a single condylar joint (p. 19). Clearly, movement at one side must be accompanied by a movement, not necessarily identical, at the other side.

The joint is between the condylar process of the mandible and the mandibular fossa of the skull, a facet mainly formed by the squamous temporal bone. The forms of the two surfaces reflect the feeding habits, and in species such as the dog, in which hingelike movements of the lower jaw predominate, the head takes the form of a transverse condyle to which the fossa provides a corresponding gutter. Backward dislocation of the jaw is opposed by the prominent retroarticular process placed directly behind the mandibular fossa. A peculiarity of the joint is the presence of a fibrous or fibrocartilaginous articular disk that divides the cavity into upper and lower compartments. Although the phylogenetic origin of this structure is disputed, it may resolve the complex movements of the joint into simpler components; a hinge movement occurs between the mandible and the disk, whereas gross sliding movements (translations) of the mandible relative to the skull occur at the upper level. The disk is rather thin and poorly developed in the dog. In species in which lateral grinding movements predominate, the mandibular head is larger, the surface more plateau-like, and the disk thicker, although the details differ considerably.

In most species the halves of the mandible are firmly fused together. In the dog (and in ruminants) the *symphysis joint* allows small movements that may be important in securing more precise adjustment of the upper and lower tooth rows and therefore a more effective cutting or crushing mechanism. Two types of movements appear to be possible: a spreading movement, altering the angle between the halves of the mandible, and one in which each half rotates about its own long axis so that the tooth cusps alter their inclination to the vertical. The dog appears to make use of these possibilities when adjusting the position of a bone between the teeth before attempting to crack it.

The temporomandibular joint or ramus of the mandible may need to be accessed to repair fractures. Repairs can be done from the ventral border of the zygomatic arch through incisions of the platysma and the masseter muscles with care taken to protect the dorsal and ventral buccal branches of the facial nerve and the parotid gland along with its duct.

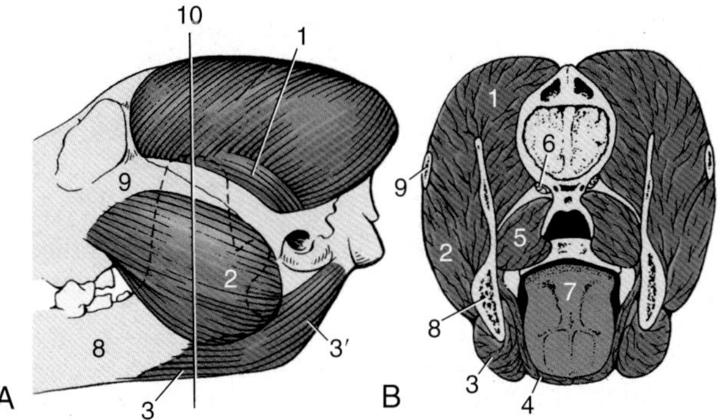

Fig. 3.21 The muscles of mastication of the dog. (A) Left lateral aspect and (B) in section. *1,* Temporalis; *2,* masseter; *3* and *3′,* rostral and caudal bellies of digastricus; *4,* mylohyoideus; *5,* medial pterygoid; *6,* origin of lateral pterygoid; *7,* tongue; *8,* mandible; *9,* zygomatic arch; *10,* level of transection of (B).

THE MUSCLES OF MASTICATION AND THEIR ACTIONS

The masticatory muscles (the temporalis, masseter, pterygoideus medialis, and pterygoideus lateralis) are derived from the first pharyngeal arch and, consequently, supplied by the mandibular nerve (Fig. 3.21). Other muscles that play some part in jaw movements, particularly in opening the mouth, are not normally included as muscles of mastication.

The *temporalis* arises from an extensive area on the lateral surface of the cranium and converges to an insertion on the coronoid process of the mandible. On contraction the muscle pulls the mandible mainly upward, although some fibers draw it forward and others pull the condyle against the retroarticular process. The muscle is especially large in species such as the dog and cat, which employ a scissor-like movement of their jaws. A measure of the development of the temporalis is provided by the salience of the zygomatic arch that provides more room for it.

The *masseter* lies lateral to the mandible. It takes its origin from the maxillary region of the skull and the zygomatic arch and has a wide insertion on the more caudal part of the mandible. It is frequently a multipennate muscle intersected by strong tendon plates. The different parts of the muscle may have contrasting functions. Some may protrude the mandible, and others may retract it; however, the general effect is to raise the mandible and draw it toward the active side, because mastication is restricted to one side at a time in domestic species. The masseter muscle is rather small in the dog but proportionately better developed in herbivorous species that make lateral and rotational movements when chewing.

The *pterygoid* mass of muscle lies medial to the mandible and passes to this bone from the pterygopalatine region of the skull. Generally the mass is clearly divided into a small lateral muscle and a larger medial muscle. Some fibers of the lateral pterygoid muscle attach to the articular disk and help to control its movements, but the principal function of the mass is to raise the mandible and draw it inward with some simultaneous protrusion. In species in which transverse movements are important the masseter and contralateral pterygoid muscles may form a functional pair.

In addition to gravity the digastricus and the sternocephalicus, in species where the latter has mandibular attachment, assist in opening the mouth. The *digastricus* passes from the skull, caudal to the temporomandibular joint, to the ventral margin of the mandible. The rostral and caudal parts of the muscle, arranged in tandem, are supplied by the mandibular and the facial nerves, respectively, to indicate a composite origin of the muscle in the mesoderm of the first two pharyngeal arches.

The resting position of the mouth in most mammals is closed. This position occurs through the tonic activity of the masticatory muscles and possibly the hermetic seal created by the application of the dorsum of the tongue to the palate. The jaws are symmetrically placed in relation to the median plane, and the upper and lower tooth rows are slightly separated or in gentle, interrupted contact. The arcade formed by the upper teeth is generally wider than its counterpart, and the tooth rows are superimposed for only part of their widths. In some species, such as the rat, simultaneous occlusion is impossible in both incisor and molar regions; in them, the lower jaw must be advanced and dropped to bring the incisor tips together and then withdrawn and raised for molar contact. Such animals generally favor an intermediate position of the lower jaw at rest.

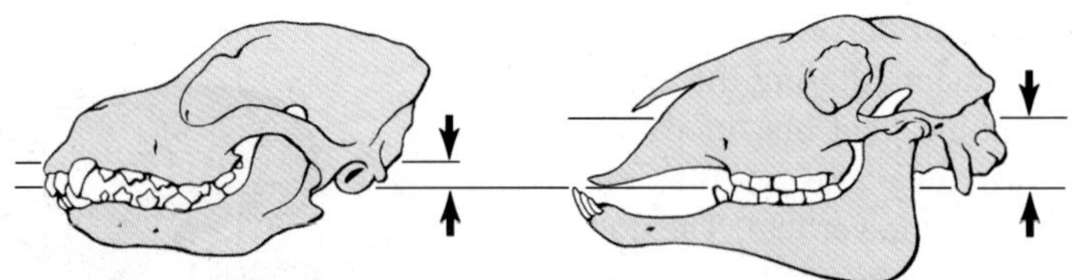

Fig. 3.22 The relationships of the articular and occlusal surfaces in the dog *(left)* and sheep *(right)* (indicated by the *upper* and *lower arrows,* respectively).

A slight increase in muscular activity brings the teeth into more extensive contact, which is known as *centric occlusion*. The relationships between the teeth in this position are variable, even in the same individual at different ages because the teeth come together in altered fashion as wear reduces the more salient projections (and in some species also by migration of teeth within the jaws). It is usual to find that each cheek tooth engages with two teeth of the opposite series, and the lower teeth are generally a little mesial to their upper counterparts. In the dog, the last upper premolar and the first lower molar are the largest teeth that bite together and constitute the sectorial (or carnassial) teeth (see Fig. 3.16). The teeth in front of the sectorials do not meet but instead leave open a carrying space, and the last cheek teeth make extensive contact. The lower canine engages in front of the upper canine, filling the space between this and the third incisor.

The relationship between the teeth is a dynamic one. A tooth deprived of normal support may drift under the influence of the masticatory forces. The pressures exerted by the lips, cheek, and tongue are also important in maintaining normal contact and alignment. Through the common control of the growth of the two jaws and the development of the teeth, there is normally a harmonious and dynamic relationship between the two at all stages of development. However, anomalies are not uncommon, and "undershot" and "overshot" jaws are well illustrated by Bulldogs and by many Afghan Hounds, respectively.

The simplest activity that is common to all species, regardless of their masticatory habits, is the *gaping* that occurs on depression of the lower jaw. Gaping is achieved by slackening or cessation of activity in the masticatory muscles, by contraction of their antagonists, and by gravity. As the jaw is lowered the mandibular head rolls on the articular disk while the disk itself slides forward in the mandibular fossa, probably assisted by those lateral pterygoid fibers that attach to it. Closure of the mouth requires the reversal of these processes and must at times be vigorous enough to detach a morsel. Sometimes the detachment is achieved by the incisors, and in certain species the hinge movement is complicated by a preliminary protrusion of the lower jaw to bring the incisor edges into alignment. When the cheek teeth are employed in biting, the action is unilateral. Herbivores employ the cheek teeth for grinding food already taken into the mouth, and the active (closing) movement is preceded by lateral displacement. The temporomandibular joint of these animals is situated high above the occlusal plane, and the lower teeth are drawn forward over their upper fellows as they approach. This arrangement contributes a grinding component that is absent when the joint and occlusal surfaces are more nearly level. The sheep and dog, typical examples of herbivore and carnivore, illustrate these differences in the position of the joint in relation to the teeth (Fig. 3.22).

THE PHARYNX AND SOFT PALATE

The pharynx lies behind the mouth and continues into the esophagus. It is a funnel-shaped chamber contained between the base of the skull and the first couple of cervical vertebrae dorsally, the larynx ventrally, and the pterygoid muscles, the mandible, and the dorsal part of the hyoid apparatus laterally. Because the pharynx communicates freely with other cavities in the head, forming a clear conception of its boundaries and extent is rather difficult (Figs. 3.23 and 4.2). Fig. 3.24 illustrates the crossing of the air and food pathways and is a reminder that the pharynx possesses a respiratory function as well as an alimentary function.

The key to understanding the pharynx is provided by the soft palate, already encountered as the continuation of the hard palate beyond the choanal margin. In repose the soft palate lies on the tongue, but when the animal swallows, the soft palate is raised into a more horizontal position and then more obviously divides the pharynx into dorsal and ventral parts. Two pairs of arches connect the soft palate to adjacent structures. The palatopharyngeal arches pass onto the lateral wall of the pharynx and may be long enough to meet above the entrance to the esophagus (see Fig. 3.23). Together with the free margin of the palate they circumscribe the constriction of the lumen—the intrapharyngeal ostium—that marks the separation of the pharynx into dorsal and ventral compartments. The dorsal compartment is known as the nasopharynx. The

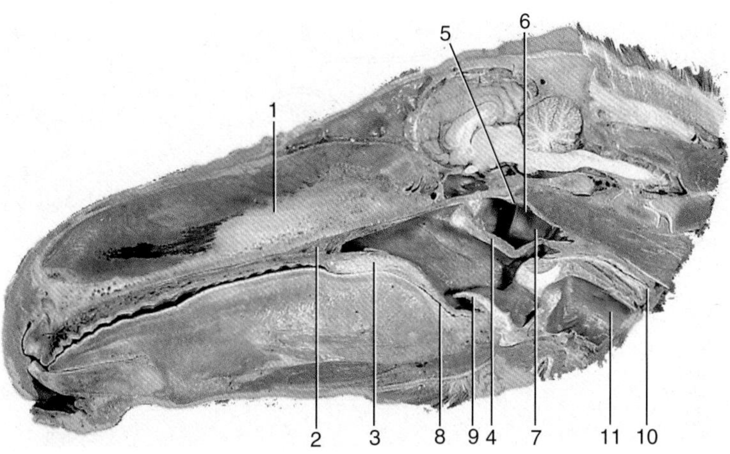

Fig. 3.23 Paramedian section through the equine head. *1,* Nasal septum; *2,* hard palate; *3,* soft palate; *4,* palatopharyngeal arch; *5,* roof of nasopharynx; *6,* nasopharynx; *7,* entrance to auditory tube; *8,* oropharynx; *9,* epiglottis; *10,* esophagus; *11,* trachea.

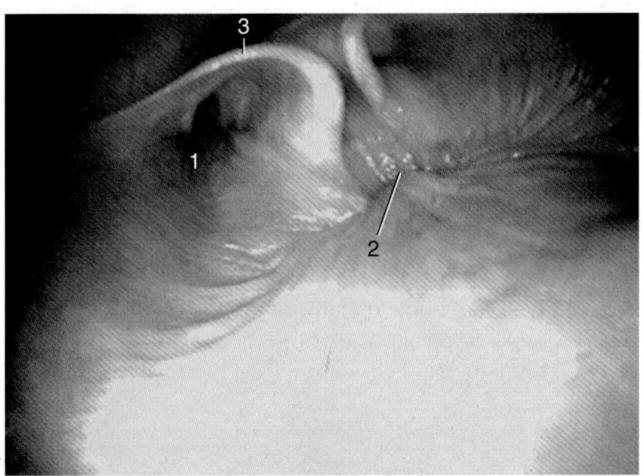

Fig. 3.24 Caudal part of nasopharynx (horse). *1,* Entrance to auditory tube; *2,* closure between the rostral and caudal parts of the nasopharynx (during swallowing); *3,* cartilage flange supporting the auditory tube.

more rostral palatoglossal arches pass onto the sides of the tongue at its root to demarcate the passage from the mouth to the oropharynx (see Fig. 3.3). The oropharynx is somewhat arbitrarily divided from the third subdivision, the laryngopharynx, at the level of the epiglottis. The laryngopharynx lies above the larynx and corresponds with it in extent.

Functionally the *nasopharynx* could well be regarded as a part of the nasal cavity because food does not enter it, it takes no part in the swallowing process, and it passively conveys air. The topography of the connection with the nasal cavity varies much among species; a single duct-like communication is present in the dog. In addition to the major connections, the nasopharynx communicates with the cavities of the middle ears through the auditory (eustachian) tubes. The paired tubal openings are placed on the summits of small pimple-like elevations in the dog. Small muscle bundles radiate over the pharyngeal wall from the opening and provide a mechanism for dilating the orifice, thus allowing air to pass to or from the middle ear so that the pressure on the two sides of the eardrum may be equalized (Fig. 3.25). Much of the wall of the nasopharynx is reduced to a thin mucosa that finds support by attaching to neighboring structures, mainly the base of the skull and the ventral straight muscles of the head. The mucosa possesses a typical respiratory epithelium and contains numerous mucous glands and much lymphoid tissue, of which some is scattered and some is massed. The lymphoid masses that form elevations visible to the naked eye are known as the *pharyngeal tonsils* (adenoids in humans) and form part of the ring of lymphoid tissue that guards the passage from the nose and mouth to the pharynx and beyond (Fig. 3.26A), like other lymphoid developments they are larger in infancy than later. The palatine tonsil of a cow (Fig. 3.26B) shows the organization of the lymphoid tissue and the active germinal center. Excessively enlarged tonsils impair the airflow.

The narrowness of the *oropharynx* limits the size of the morsels that can be swallowed. Its lateral walls are supported by a fascia and are the site of the palatine tonsils. These are very differently arranged in different species; in some (e.g., the horse) they are diffuse (though raised slightly), whereas in others they constitute a compact mass that may project away from or toward the lumen, as in the ox or dog, respectively (see Fig. 3.26). Tonsils that project into the lumen are overlain by flaps of mucosa that partly hide them from inspection through the open mouth (see Fig. 3.8/*8* and Fig. 3.27).

The *laryngopharynx* is the largest part of the pharynx. It is wide in front but narrows before joining the esophagus

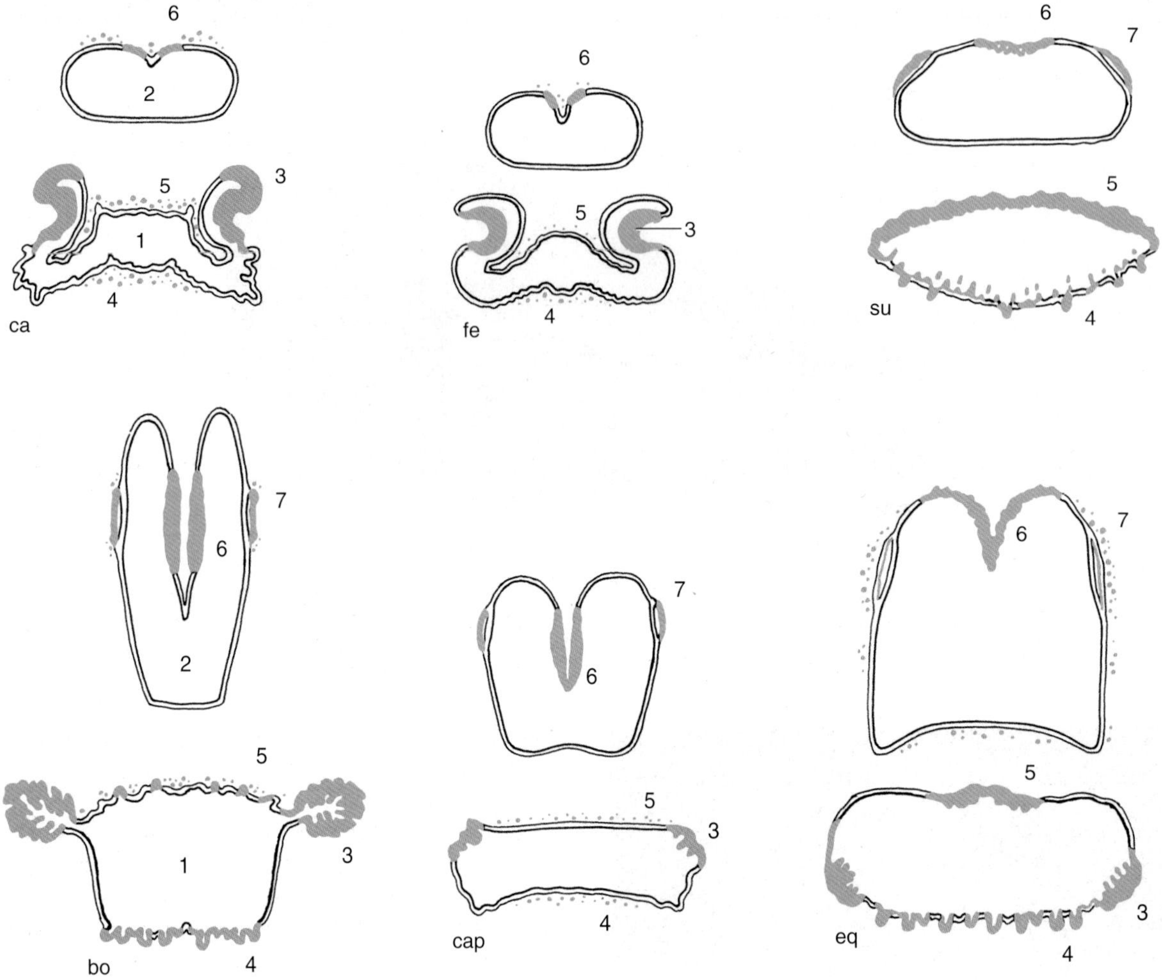

Fig. 3.25 Tonsils in the wall of oropharynx and nasopharynx; *ca,* dog; *fe,* cat; *su,* pig; *bo,* cattle; *cap,* goat; *eq,* horse. *1,* Oropharynx; *2,* nasopharynx; *3,* palatine tonsil; *4,* lingual tonsil; *5,* tonsil of the soft palate; *6,* pharyngeal tonsil; *7,* tubal tonsil.

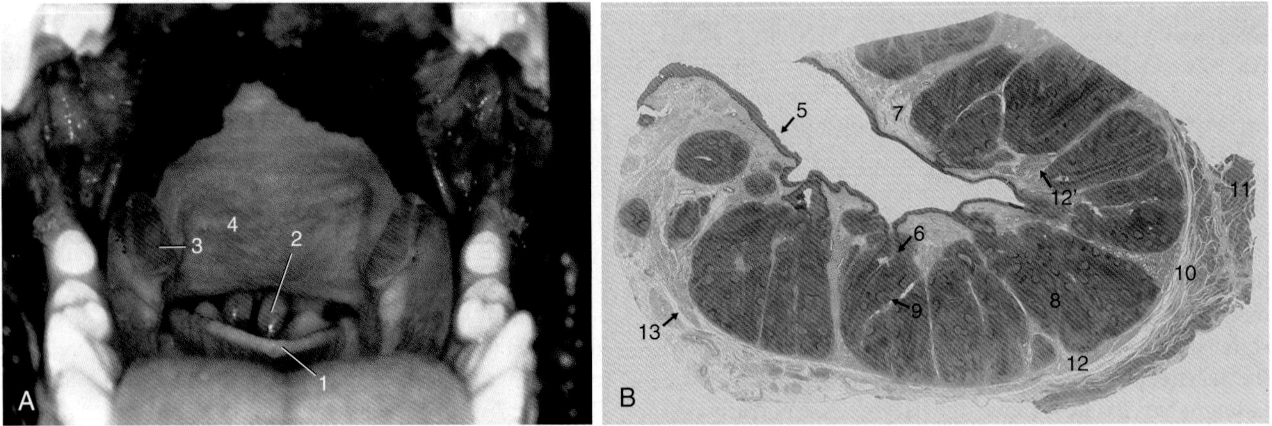

Fig. 3.26 (A) View into the oropharynx of a dog. *1,* Epiglottis; *2,* cuneiform process of arytenoid cartilages; *3,* palatine tonsils; *4,* soft palate. (B) Palatine tonsil of cow. Hematoxylin and eosin stain. The tonsils are regions of modified mucosa of soft palate covered by a stratified squamous epithelium (*5*) forming deep pits or tonsillary crypts (*6*) infiltrated by lymphocytes. The underlying lamina propria and tunica submucosa (*7*) is converted into scattered (*8*) and nodular lymphatic tissue. The lymphatic nodules (*9*) are very active as indicated by the well-developed germinal centers (central region) and mantle layer of small lymphocytes (peripheral darker cap region) that faces the epithelium of the crypts. The lymphatic tissue is separated by a capsule of connective tissue (*10*) from the underlying skeletal muscle (*11*) and lobules of the mucous glands (*12*). Mucous glands (*12'*) are also present in between the lymphatic tissue. Many lymphatic vessels (*13*) are located in deep tissue surrounding the lymphatic tissue (hematoxylin and eosin stain).

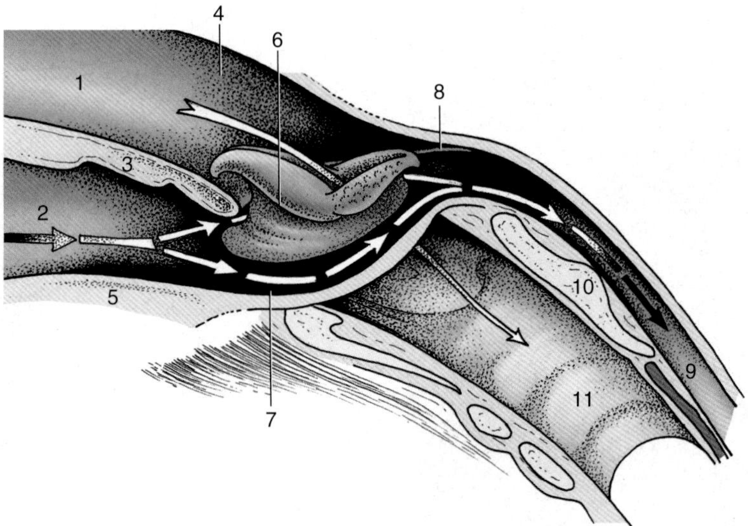

Fig. 3.27 Schematic drawing of the pharynx showing its rostral connection with the nasal and oral cavities and caudal connection with the esophagus and larynx. Broken arrow indicates passage of the food and the single arrow shows passage of the air. *1,* Nasal cavity; *2,* oral cavity; *3,* soft palate; *4,* nasopharynx; *5,* root of tongue; *6,* larynx (protruding through pharyngeal floor); *7,* laryngopharynx (piriform recess); *8,* caudal end of palatopharyngeal arch; *9,* esophagus; *10,* lamina of cricoid cartilage; *11,* trachea.

at a boundary that is well defined by a mucosal fold in the dog but more difficult to recognize in most other species. At rest, the lumen of the caudal part of the laryngopharynx is closed by the apposition of the lateral walls and roof to the floor. The floor is largely occupied by the entrance to the larynx, which contains the epiglottis, the arytenoid cartilages, and the aryepiglottic folds. The epiglottis serves as a breakwater to deflect fluids to the side, into gutters (piriform recesses) that run beside the projection of the larynx (see Fig. 3.24).

Below an external fascia, the greater part of the pharyngeal wall is covered by a set of striated muscles. These fall into three groups—constrictor, dilator, and shortener—although no individual muscle has an action quite so simple as these terms suggest (Fig. 3.28). The constrictor muscles arise from certain fixed points conveniently placed to each side and run onto the roof of the pharynx; with their fellows they form a series of arches that enclose the lumen on its lateral and dorsal aspects. For most purposes it is sufficient to recognize rostral, middle, and caudal constrictor muscles, although each may be divided into lesser units. The *rostral constrictor* arises from the pterygoid region of the skull (pterygopharyngeus) and the aponeurosis of the soft palate (palatopharyngeus) and embraces the pharynx at the level of the palatopharyngeal arch. Many of their fibers take an almost longitudinal course and thus also assist in shortening the pharynx, drawing it onto and over a bolus received from the mouth. The *middle constrictor* (hyopharyngeus) arises from neighboring parts of the hyoid bone. The *caudal constrictor* arises in two parts, from the thyroid (thyropharyngeus) and cricoid (cricopharyngeus) cartilages. When the three constrictors contract in succession, they hurry the bolus distally into the esophagus. The *dilator muscle* (stylopharyngeus caudalis) arises from the hyoid apparatus, runs more transversely to fan out in the pharyngeal wall, and widens the rostral part of the pharynx to enable acceptance of the bolus more easily.

The mucosa is supported by a fibroelastic aponeurosis in the muscles. The aponeurosis also provides insertion for many fibers of the paired muscles, which continue to the skull and fix the whole organ in position. The mucous membrane of the oral and laryngeal parts of the pharynx is covered by a stratified squamous epithelium and possesses many small salivary glands that provide additional lubrication to the passage of food.

The *soft palate* (velum palatinum) is bounded by a respiratory mucosa on its dorsal surface and an oral mucosa ventrally. It is braced by a stout aponeurosis below the dorsal mucosa. The part ventral to the aponeurosis consists mainly of close-packed salivary glands, interrupted toward the midline by the longitudinally disposed palatinus muscle, which shortens the palate. The tensor veli palatini and the levator veli palatini arise from the muscular process of the temporal bone, insert into the lateral part of the aponeurosis tense or, and raise the soft palate, respectively. The mucous membrane of the pharynx and soft palate and the muscles, except the tensor, which is supplied by the mandibular nerve, obtain their innervation from a plexus to which the vagus nerve makes the chief contribution and the glossopharyngeal nerve a minor contribution.

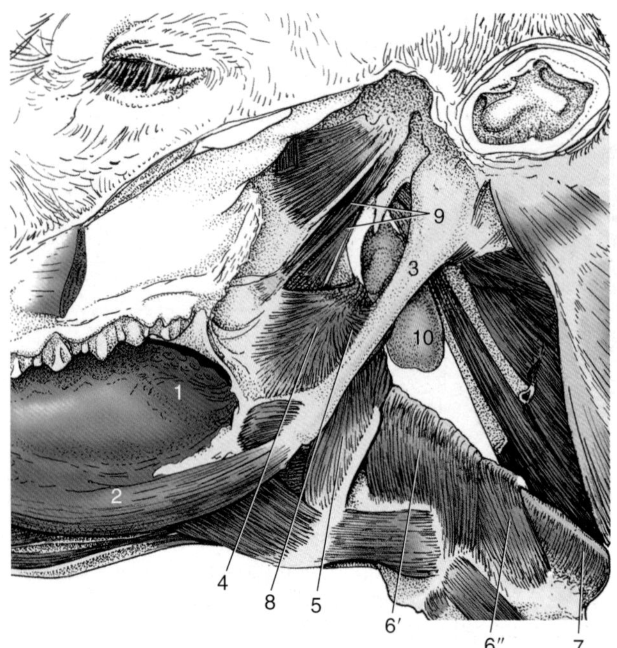

Fig. 3.28 Lateral view of the connection of the pharynx with the base of the bovine skull. *1,* Root of tongue; *2,* styloglossus; *3,* stylohyoid; *4,* rostral pharyngeal constrictor; *5,* middle pharyngeal constrictor; *6,* caudal pharyngeal constrictor *(6′,* thyropharyngeus; *6″,* cricopharyngeus); *7,* esophagus; *8,* pharyngeal dilator (stylopharyngeus caudalis); *9,* tensor and levator veli palatini; *10,* medial retropharyngeal lymph node.

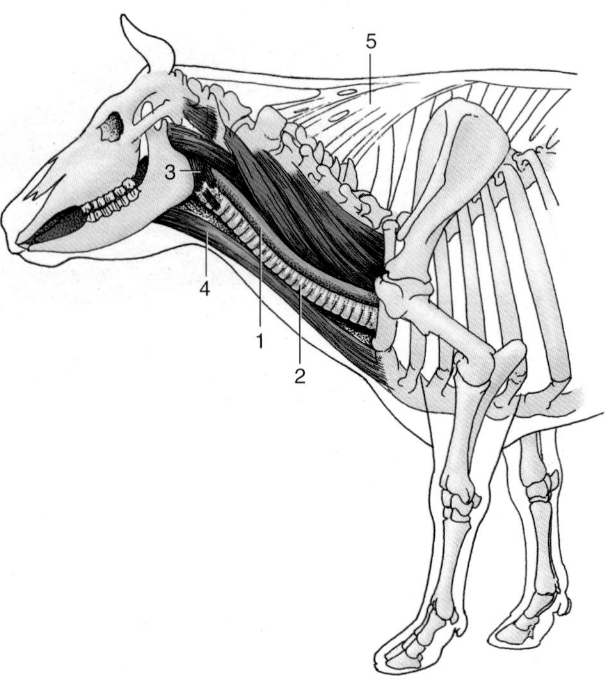

Fig. 3.29 Lateral view of the bovine neck. In the midneck the esophagus lies on the left dorsolateral aspect of the trachea. *1,* Esophagus; *2,* trachea; *3,* pharyngeal musculature; *4,* sternocephalicus muscle; *5,* nuchal ligament.

THE ESOPHAGUS

The esophagus (or gullet) conveys food from the pharynx to the stomach. This relatively narrow tube begins dorsal to the cricoid cartilage of the larynx and follows the trachea down the neck, at first inclining to the left but regaining a median position above the trachea before or shortly after entering the thorax (Fig. 3.29). Within the thorax it runs in the mediastinum (p. 147); continuing beyond the tracheal bifurcation, it passes over the heart before penetrating the esophageal hiatus of the diaphragm. It then makes its way over the dorsal border of the liver to join the stomach at the cardia. It thus has cervical, thoracic, and abdominal portions, although the last is very short.

The cervical part of the esophagus runs within the visceral space of the neck, related to the subvertebral muscles dorsally and the left side of the trachea medioventrally (see Fig. 3.29) and accompanied by the left common carotid artery and vagosympathetic and recurrent laryngeal nerves.

The thoracic part crosses to the right of the aortic arch. Caudally, its dorsal and ventral borders are followed by the respective vagal trunks into which fibers of the right and left vagus nerves are regrouped.

The structural pattern of the esophagus is similar to that of the rest of the alimentary canal. The outer coat is a loose connective tissue (adventitia) in the neck, but this is largely replaced by serosa* in the thorax and abdomen. The muscle is striated at the origin of the esophagus, but in some species (e.g., cat, pig, and horse) the striated muscle is replaced by smooth muscle at some point within the thorax. Both layers of the muscles are spiral, and they wind in opposite directions in the first part of the esophagus. Closer to the stomach the outer coat becomes more longitudinal and the inner one more circular (Fig. 3.30). There is considerable interlacing of muscle bundles between the two layers. Although not proven morphologically, a number of esophageal sphincters are suggested by functional studies. They include a cranial sphincter, probably provided by fibers of the cricopharyngeus muscle and possibly others within the thorax, where the passage of food tends to be delayed. Although a thickening suggestive of a sphincter occurs at the junction of the esophagus with the stomach, the flow of food is actually more impeded immediately in front of the diaphragm.

*Most organs contained within the body cavities (divisions of the embryonic celom) are protected by "serous membranes" (serosae). These coverings, which extend to line the walls of the body cavities, consist of a layer of flat mesothelial cells supported by a delicate connective tissue. A small amount of watery (serous) fluid keeps the membranes moist and minimizes friction when opposing surfaces move against each other.

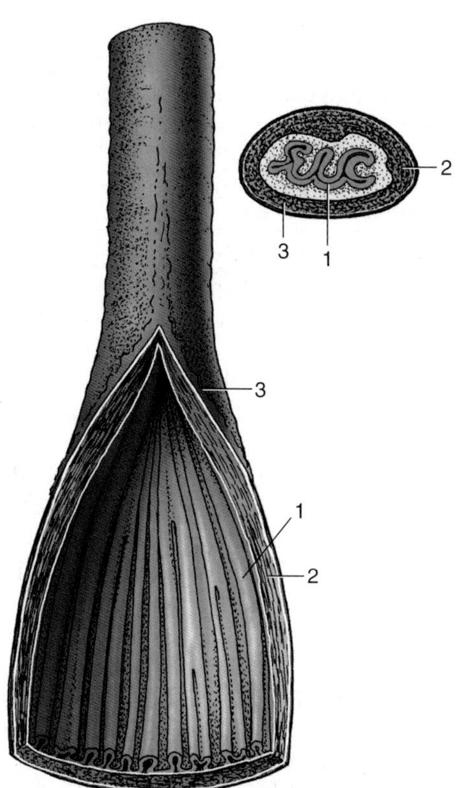

Fig. 3.30 Semischematic drawing of the structure of the esophagus, sectioned longitudinally and transversely. *1*, Mucosa; *2*, muscular layer (longitudinal and circular); *3*, adventitia.

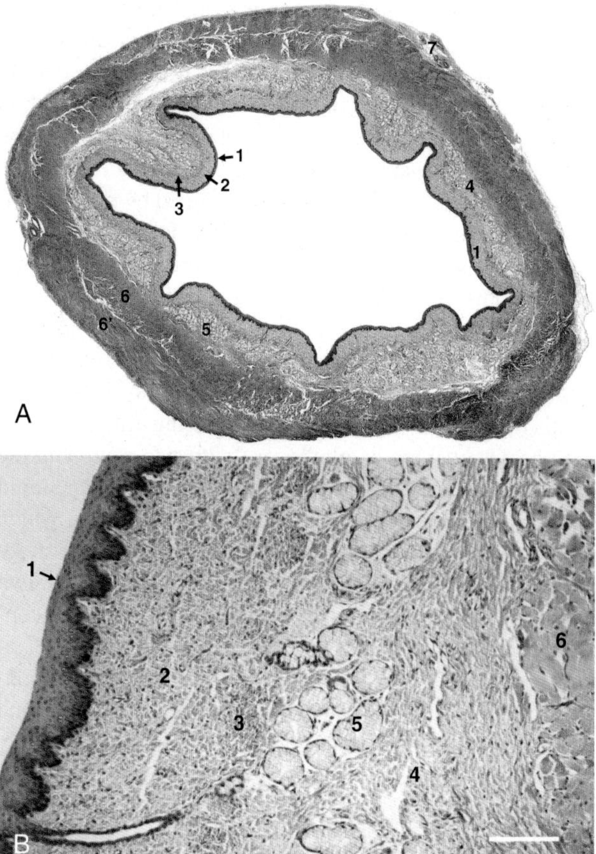

Fig. 3.31 Esophagus, in the dog (A) stained with Masson's trichrome showing collagen as green and cellular components as purple red and goat (B) stained with hematoxylin and eosin (70×) showing four main tunics: *1*, mucosa; *2*, submucosa; *3*, muscular layer and *4*, adventitia. Mucosal layer is composed of *1′*, stratified squamous epithelium; *1″*, lamina propria (connective tissue); and *1‴*, lamina muscularis mucosae (smooth muscles). Submucosa contains *5*, mucus-secreting tubuloacinar glands in the connective tissue and the muscle layer is arranged in *3′*, inner layer; and *3″*, outer layer.

The inner part of the wall is divided between submucosa and mucosa by a fenestrated muscularis mucosae, usually more prominent in the thoracic esophagus (Fig. 3.31B). It helps throw the lining of the empty organ into longitudinal folds. The surface epithelium is generally stratified squamous, and the degree of keratinization and thickness reflects the diet of the species, as illustrated in Fig. 3.31. In comparison with the goat esophagus, the canine esophagus has many submucosal mucus-secreting tubuloacinar glands. The boundary between esophageal and gastric epithelia is sharp and may be displaced to either side of the cardia. In humans, prolonged or repeated exposure to gastric juice (e.g., heartburn) may provoke transformation of the stratified epithelium of the lower esophagus into the columnar gastric variety.

The esophagus receives its *innervation* from the sympathetic and vagus nerves, including the recurrent laryngeal branches. The vagal supply is the more important. The striated muscle arises from the mesoderm of the pharyngeal arches and is under control of the general visceral motor neurons of the vagus, whereas the smooth muscle portions are under direct control of the intrinsic nervous system and indirect control of the autonomic nervous system. A myenteric plexus extends the length of the esophagus.

The blood supply from various local arteries presents no features of special interest.

DEGLUTITION

The first stage of deglutition is a voluntary act, but once the food has left the mouth its progress is not under control of the will.

Food that has been sufficiently prepared by mastication and insalivation is collected in a recess formed when the dorsal surface of the tongue is cupped; it is then isolated when the apex of the tongue is pressed against the palate. The jaws are closed, and brisk contraction of the mylohyoid, hyoglossal, and styloglossal muscles raises the tongue and impels the bolus into the oropharynx. Inevitably the food touches the pharyngeal mucosa, and this contact initiates the reflex that completes the act. The afferent nerves include branches of the mandibular, glossopharyngeal, and vagal trunks. As the food passes caudally, the soft palate is raised, and its free margin is drawn toward the dorsocaudal pharyngeal wall. Closure of the intrapharyngeal ostium prevents dissipation of the pressure generated in the mouth and ensures that the food is carried toward the esophagus by denying escape into the nasopharynx. This stage is accompanied by brief inhibition of breathing, with the glottis closed. The hyoid apparatus and the larynx are simultaneously drawn forward, and the epiglottis, meeting the tongue, is tilted back to provide some cover to the laryngeal entrance; however, no question of its fitting into the opening (as is often assumed) exists, and it is known that surgical resection of most of the human epiglottis does not seriously impair swallowing efficiency. The food passes over the epiglottis, or to the side of it, with the impetus maintained by the coordinated successive and rapid contraction of the constrictor muscles. The pharynx, which was dilated for reception of the bolus by the caudal stylopharyngeus muscle, is then shortened and in effect drawn onto and over the bolus by the longitudinal fibers of the constrictor muscles. The caudal end of the pharynx relaxes to receive the food, which is then hastened through the esophagus by a wave of peristalsis that commences just beyond the cricopharyngeal fibers. This last movement is probably coordinated by a local reflex, unlike the preceding events, which are controlled by a deglutition center in the brainstem.

Fluid is swallowed in essentially the same way. It passes mainly through the piriform recesses, and the initial impetus may be sufficient to project it well into the esophagus.

THE ABDOMINAL CAVITY

Some general observations concerning the abdominal cavity are necessary before the description of the digestive system continues.

The abdomen is the portion of the trunk that lies caudal to the diaphragm. It contains the largest of the body cavities, which is continuous at a plane passing through the sacral promontory and the pubic brim with the more caudal and very much smaller pelvic cavity (see Fig. 2.2). The more cranial (intrathoracic) part of the abdominal cavity is protected by the hindmost ribs and costal cartilages and is rather restricted in the variations in its size; the more caudal part is supported by the skeleton only on its dorsal aspect and is therefore more variable. The pelvic cavity has the most extensive bony support and the most constant size, although even here a certain latitude is allowed by changes in the soft tissue components of its walls (see Fig. 29.25A and B).

The structure of the abdominal and pelvic walls has been described with the locomotor apparatus. Comparative features, including conformation and the factors that influence it in different species, are considered in later chapters. The abdominal and pelvic cavities contain the peritoneal sac; the stomach, small and large intestines, and associated liver and pancreas; the spleen; the kidneys, ureters, bladder, and urethra (in part); the ovaries and most of the reproductive system in the female and a smaller part of the reproductive tract in the male; the adrenal glands; and many nerves, blood vessels, and lymph nodes and vessels.

Peritoneal Structures

An incision through the whole thickness of the abdominal wall enters the peritoneal cavity, which is a division of the celom that is bounded by a delicate serous membrane, the peritoneum. The *peritoneal cavity* is completely enclosed in the male, but in the female a potential communication with the exterior exists at the abdominal opening of each uterine tube. The peritoneal cavity contains only a small amount of serous fluid because the abdominal organs are excluded from the space by their peritoneal covering. The organs suspended from the abdominal roof within the peritoneal reflections are termed *intraperitoneal.* The term, though misleading, emphasizes the difference between this and the alternative retroperitoneal arrangement of other organs, such as kidneys, that are directly joined to the abdominal wall. Fig. 3.32 may make the distinction plain and also shows the division of the peritoneum into a parietal part lining the walls (parietes), a visceral part directly enshrouding the organs (viscera), and a series of double folds connecting the parietal to the visceral parts. These folds are often collectively known as *mesenteries,* but properly this term is restricted to the fold suspending the small intestine (and more specifically only the jejunum and ileum); certain similar folds are conveniently named *mesocolon, mesovarium,* and so on, according to the organ

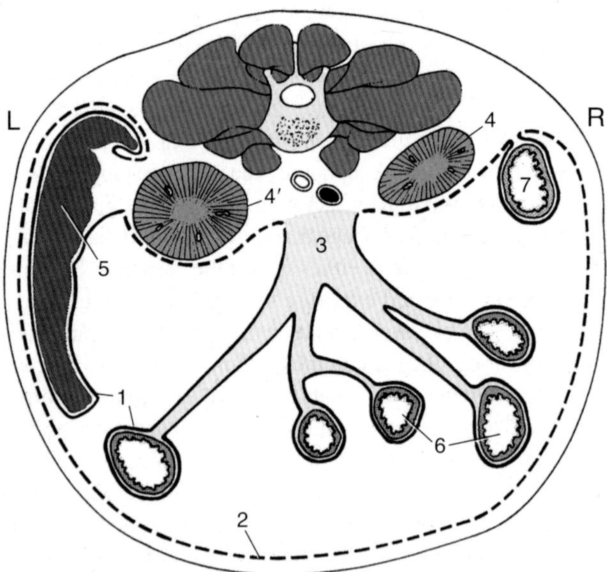

Fig. 3.32 Schematic transverse section through the abdomen of the dog. *1,* Visceral peritoneum *(continuous line)*; *2,* parietal peritoneum *(broken line)*; *3,* root of mesentery; *4* and *4′,* right and left kidneys (retroperitoneal); *5,* spleen; *6,* jejunum; *7,* descending duodenum; *L,* left; *R,* right.

that they support. Others, for example, the greater omentum, have names less immediately revealing.

A small outpouching (infracardiac bursa) of the parietal peritoneum extends a little way into the mediastinum within the thorax along the right face of the esophagus where it penetrates the diaphragm.

The *peritoneum* consists of a single layer of flattened mesothelial cells supported by a fibroelastic tissue that attaches, more or less firmly according to position, to the underlying structures. A considerable amount of fat is often stored below the peritoneum, and some locations are especially favored. In the healthy animal the peritoneal cavity is reduced to a series of clefts between the closely packed abdominal organs. Most clefts are of capillary dimensions, and the total volume of the peritoneal fluid is therefore small—a few milliliters in the dog. The fluid is nonetheless of vital importance, for it lubricates the viscera, allowing them to slip freely over each other or against the abdominal wall in the performance of their own functions or when displaced by other activities. The large surface area (2 m^2 in humans) of the peritoneum aids rapid removal, and drugs are sometimes administered by intraperitoneal injection. Toxins are also readily absorbed, and because the warm and moist peritoneal cavity affords ideal conditions for bacterial growth, inflammation of the peritoneum is never regarded lightly.

Inflamed serous sheets have a tendency to stick together, a feature that may become organized and permanent with time. This is the reason the surgeon often turns in the edges of the wound to bring serosal surfaces together when closing an incision. Adhesion between organs that are normally free to move over each other is a possible and undesirable sequel to infection or trauma of the peritoneum. Clearly, any attachment that limits mobility may interfere with normal function. However, it must also be noted that adhesion of apposed serosal surfaces (with the obliteration of the intervening space) is commonplace in development and explains the definitive position and arrangement of many organs and mesenteries.

In early development the gastrointestinal tract pursues a sagittal course through the body cavity. It is attached along its whole length to the roof of the embryonic trunk by a primitive dorsal "mesentery," but only a portion of the foregut (the part that becomes the stomach and first part of the duodenum) and a short caudal portion of the hindgut have similar ventral attachments. The parts of the dorsal mesentery associated with the differentiating organs are assigned appropriate names and may be listed in succession: (dorsal) *mesogastrium, mesoduodenum, mesojejunum, mesoileum, mesocolon,* and *mesorectum*. The ventral connection to the stomach is known as the ventral mesogastrium. The mesojejunum and mesoileum together constitute the (great) mesentery of adult anatomy. Most portions of the dorsal mesentery persist in more or less unmodified form (at least in the dog), but the mesogastria have a more complicated fate dictated by the later development of the stomach.

The dorsal mesogastrium becomes drawn out and folded on itself during development and is then known as the *greater omentum*. The folding creates a pouch, the omental bursa, enclosing a portion of the peritoneal cavity. However, the pouch is flattened and its walls brought into close contact so that the cavity is potential, not actual. The greater omentum of the dog is turned caudally between the viscera and the abdominal floor, and its walls are described as parietal (ventral) and visceral (dorsal) because of their relationship to the abdominal wall and viscera. It is the first structure to appear when the abdominal floor is opened. The later growth of the liver reduces access to the interior of the bursa to a narrow opening known as the *epiploic* (omental) foramen, through which the cavity of the omental bursa remains in open, if restricted, communication with the major part of the peritoneal cavity. The main features of the arrangement are shown in Figs. 3.33 and 3.61.

The differential growth and the secondary attachments that determine the adult arrangement vary considerably among species, and those details that possess a practical importance are mentioned in context. In most species the greater omentum is lacelike, which is an effect produced by the deposition of fat in strands along the course of the blood vessels; in ruminants so much fat may be present that the omentum appears to consist entirely of this tissue. The omentum has no intrinsic capacity for movement but is liable to be shifted about the abdomen by the movements of other structures. Because it possesses the common tendency of serous membranes to adhere when inflamed, it is often found attached in regions of infection and helps to wall them off. The surgeon may stitch the greater omentum over a closed incision of a viscus as extra insurance against leakage.

The no less complicated arrangement of peritoneal folds that develops, mainly in the pelvic cavity, in association with the urogenital organs is best described with these organs (p. 174).

Visceral Topography

The general disposition of the viscera is determined by the form of the cavity in which they are retained, and their detailed arrangement is influenced by individual features of attachment, motility, and distention. Because the peritoneal cavity is hermetically sealed and most abdominal contents are incompressible, any change in the position or contours of one organ must be followed by adjustment of the abdominal wall or by a reciprocal change in a neighboring organ. The weight of the abdominal contents is considerable, especially in the larger herbivores. They "float" within the serous fluid, and the gravitational forces are opposed actively and passively by the tension developed by the structures of the abdominal wall, by the cranial pull on the diaphragm exerted by the negative

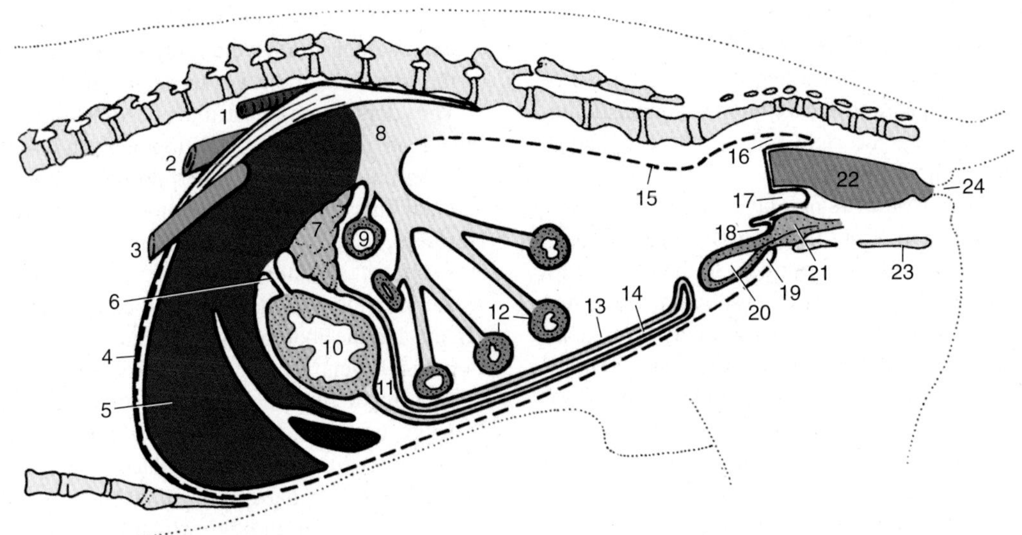

Fig. 3.33 Paramedian section of the abdominal cavity of a dog to show the disposition of the peritoneum (schematic). *1,* Aorta; *2,* esophagus; *3,* caudal vena cava; *4,* diaphragm; *5,* liver; *6,* lesser omentum; *7,* pancreas; *8,* root of mesentery; *9,* transverse colon; *10,* stomach; *11,* omental bursa; *12,* small intestine; *13,* deep wall of greater omentum; *14,* superficial wall of greater omentum; *15,* parietal peritoneum; *16,* pararectal fossa; *17,* rectogenital pouch; *18,* vesicogenital pouch; *19,* pubovesical pouch; *20,* bladder; *21,* prostate; *22,* rectum; *23,* ischium; *24,* anus.

pressure within the thorax, and, to a lesser and uncertain extent, by the mesenteries and vessels that support particular organs.

The essence of the situation can be conveyed schematically (Fig. 3.34). It can be seen that the internal pressure varies at different heights within the abdomen. It is less than the ambient pressure in the most dorsal part, equal to it at one particular level, and increasingly greater toward the abdominal floor. This concept explains the concavity of the upper part of the flank very evident in cattle and also the tendency for air to rush into the rectum when exploration of this part is clumsily performed. Clearly, the local internal pressures also vary with respiratory changes in intrathoracic pressure and with posture.

The mesenteries and other attachments influence visceral topography in a varying manner. The attachments, for example, between the liver and the diaphragm, anchor organs quite firmly. The others are too frail, and the organs to which they attach must be held in place by mutual contact and by the "lift" of the diaphragm. Certainly, they drop as soon as air is introduced into the peritoneal cavity. The potbellied appearance familiar in many older people is alleged to be in part a consequence of the loss of elasticity in the lungs with resulting reduction of the diaphragmatic "pull." The unusually thick intima of some of the arteries that supply abdominal organs may allow them

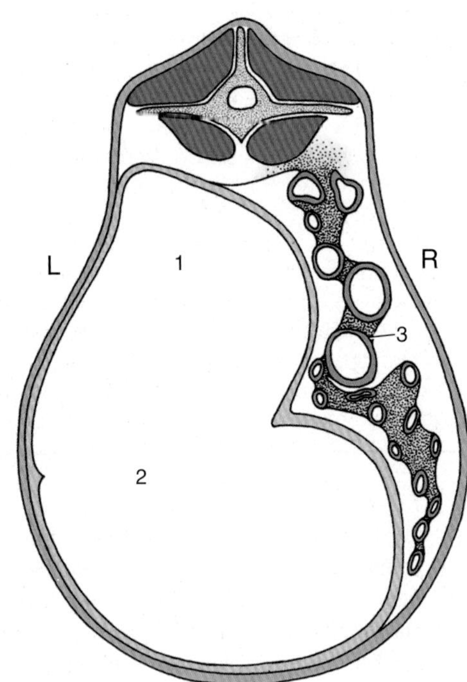

Fig. 3.34 Section through the abdomen of a goat. The greater pressure in the lower part of the abdomen causes the convex form of the lower part of the abdominal wall. The pressure within the upper part of the abdomen is below that of the atmosphere, and the flank is sunken. *1,* Gas in upper part of rumen; *2,* ingesta in the lower part of rumen; *3,* intestines; *L,* left; *R,* right.

to bear some weight when the enclosing mesenteries are fully stretched.

The viscera commonly conform to a fixed pattern in dead animals. However, the assumptions that each hollow organ possessed a fairly constant "normal" form in the live animals have been destroyed by imaging methods. Therefore, it is sufficient to say that detailed assertions of normal form and position have no place in the description of the hollow organs. When the positions of the abdominal organs need to be described, it is generally sufficient to relate them to the abdominal wall by means of everyday expressions.

THE STOMACH

The stomach is the dilated part of the digestive tract where digestion is initiated. It is succeeded by the intestine, which consists of a proximal small intestine (the principal organ of digestion and absorption in most species) and a distal large intestine (generally much shorter and especially concerned with the dehydration of the food residue).

There is considerable diversity, much of it due to dietary habits, among mammals in the form and function of stomach and intestines, which are collectively known as the gastrointestinal tract (Figs. 3.35 and 3.36). The concentrated diet of carnivores is most easily digested, and these animals have a small and simple stomach (Fig. 3.35A) and a relatively short and uncomplicated intestine. The fodder of herbivores has a lower nutritive value and must be consumed in large amounts. Moreover, celluloses and other complex carbohydrates, major parts of the diet, need to be broken down by symbiotic microorganisms for their enzymatic breakdown and utilization. This relatively slow process requires the provision of a large fermentation chamber to create an environment favorable to the multiplication and activity of the microorganisms. Such a chamber is supplied by a greatly enlarged and subdivided stomach (e.g., ruminants) or by a voluminous and complicated large intestine (e.g., horses). Species-specific details are found later in the book, and the following description is largely confined to the dog and cat.

The *stomach* (ventriculus)* receives food from the esophagus and retains it for a time before discharging it into the duodenum, the first part of the small intestine. The stomach of the dog has a relatively modest capacity, ranging from 0.5 to 6.0 L according to breed, and conforms to a pattern that is common to most carnivores and indeed to many other mammals, including humans. It consists of two distinct parts that converge and join at a ventral angle (Fig. 3.37). The larger part, into which the esophagus opens at the cardia, lies mainly to the left of the median plane, well forward under cover of the ribs and in direct contact with the liver and the diaphragm. The cardia is relatively distensible and rapidly expands to accommodate a meal. The second part is narrower, has thicker walls, and is more constant in appearance because it is less affected by the presence of a meal. It passes to the right to continue into the duodenum at the pylorus (Fig. 3.35B). The cranial (parietal) aspects of both parts are mainly in contact with the liver, whereas the more numerous relations of the caudal (visceral) surface include the intestinal mass, left kidney, pancreas, and greater omentum. The left part of the margin is applied to the hilar region of the spleen.

*The alternative term *gaster*, derived from the Greek, is the root of most clinical terms: for example, gastritis and gastrectomy.

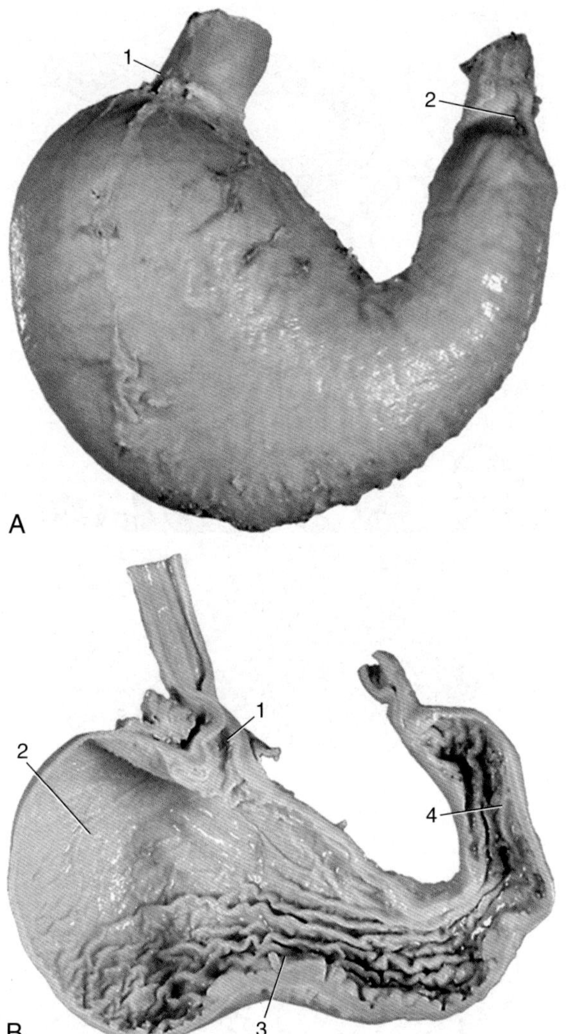

Fig. 3.35 (A) Visceral surface of stomach (dog). *1,* Cardia; *2,* pylorus. (B) Interior of stomach (dog). *1,* Cardiac opening; *2,* fundus; *3,* body; *4,* pyloric antrum.

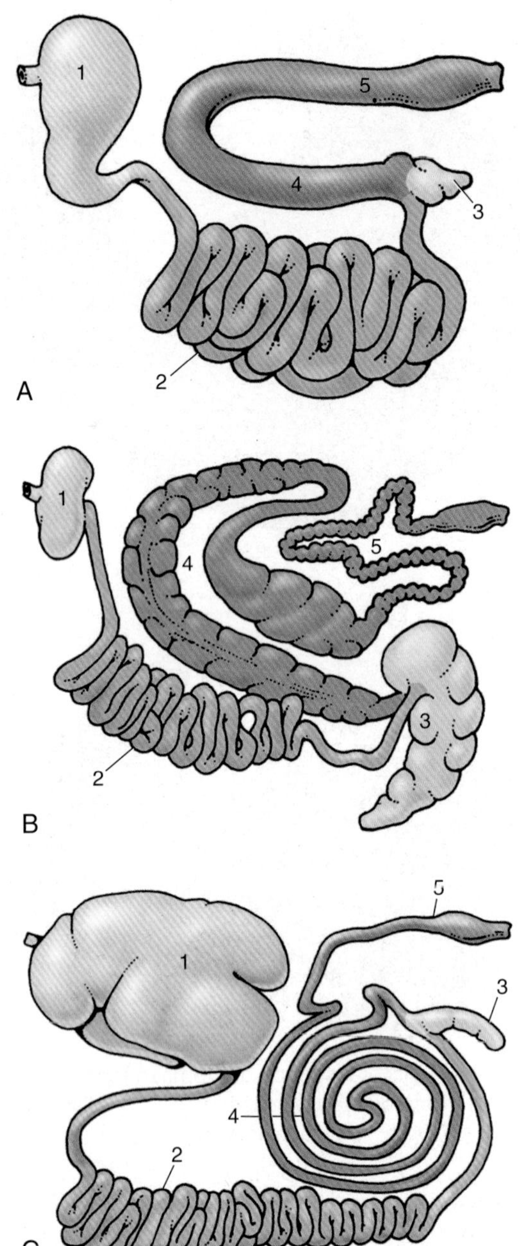

Fig. 3.36 Gastrointestinal tracts of (A) the dog, (B) the horse, and (C) cattle laid out in one plane. *1,* Stomach; *2,* small intestine; *3,* cecum; *4,* ascending colon; *5,* descending colon.

The large left sac is divided between a blind *dome (fundus)* rising above the cardia and a *body (corpus)* extending from the cardia to the ventral angle. On the basis of the terminal muscular thickenings, the more tubular right or pyloric part is divided between a more proximal pyloric antrum and a more distal pyloric canal (Fig. 3.35B). The margin separating the two surfaces is divided between greater and lesser curvatures, each of which runs between the cardiac and pyloric openings. The convex greater curvature attaches to the greater omentum, of which a part (gastrosplenic ligament) connects the spleen with the stomach. The shorter, concave lesser curvature is connected with the liver by the lesser omentum. This curvature is marked by a sharp change in direction known as the *angular notch* (incisura).

The *stomach wall* is composed of layers corresponding to those of the esophagus and intestine. The external peritoneum or *serosa* covers the entire organ, adhering to the underlying muscle, except along the curvatures, where it is reflected to continue into the omenta; its absence from the curvatures makes them the parts most likely to burst when the organ is excessively distended.

The next coat is of *smooth muscle* and is arranged in three overlapping but incomplete layers. The external layer is more or less longitudinal, continues the outer muscle of the esophagus, and is concentrated along the curvatures, although it spreads more widely over the pyloric part. The middle layer is disposed in hoops, and those most proximal form a weak sphincter around the cardia; beyond this the pattern is interrupted by the projection of the fundus, but it is resumed at a lower level. It then continues to the pyloric canal, where the hoops are bunched together on the lesser curvature, forming a muscular knot (that in some species produces an obvious projection into the lumen) and fanning out on the greater curvature to sometimes constitute proximal and distal pyloric sphincters. The innermost layer is very incomplete but compensates for the deficiencies in the circular muscle; particularly stout fascicles arch above the cardia before continuing distally to each side of the lesser curvature, extending toward, but not beyond, the angular notch (Fig. 3.37).

The thin *submucosa* internal to the muscle is separated from the mucosa proper by a plexiform muscularis mucosae. It contains major arterial and venous plexuses and also a wealth of elastic fibers that help the muscularis mucosae throw the mucosa of the empty organ into the folds (rugae) that provide the characteristic surface relief (Fig. 3.37 and Fig. 3.38A). These folds are predominantly longitudinal in orientation, although individually tortuous; they are completely effaced only when the stomach is grossly distended.

The entire gastric mucosa has innumerable gastric pits. The pits, invisible to the naked eye, are depressions but account for the surface folding seen in histologic sections (Fig. 3.38B). The surface epithelium of columnar, mucus-secreting cells continues into the pits and even extends into the uppermost parts of the gastric glands that deliver their products into the depth of the pits. This epithelium is largely responsible for the protective coat that makes gastric mucosa slimy to the touch. The gastric glands are of three varieties, termed *cardiac, proper gastric* (fundic), and *pyloric,* although it must be stressed that in many species, including the dog, their distribution does not exactly coincide with the

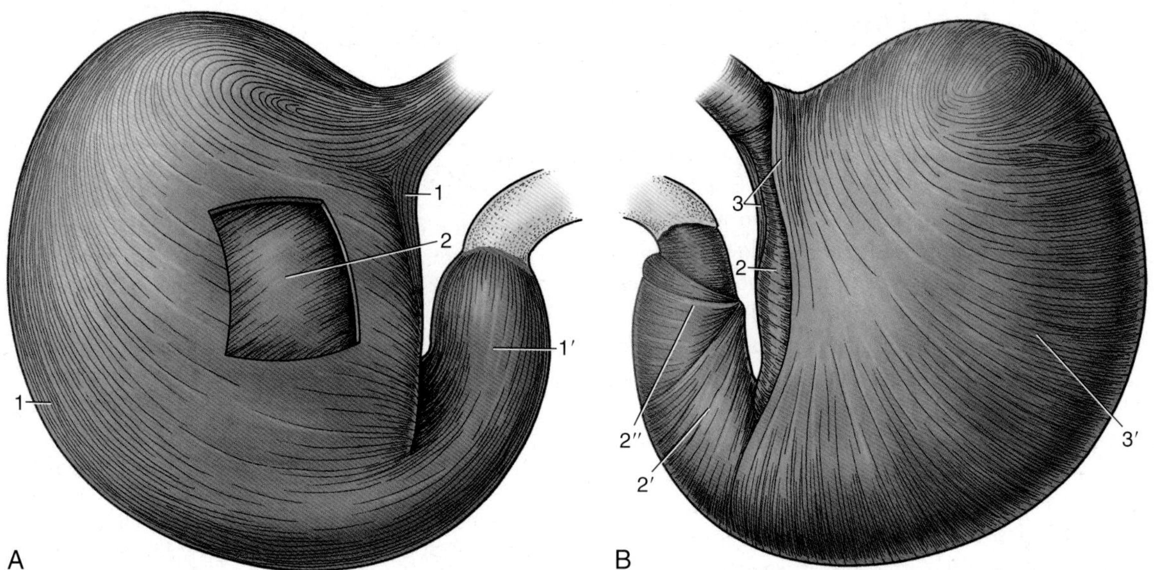

Fig. 3.37 The tunica muscularis of the canine stomach. (A) Parietal surface after removal of the serosa. (B) Stomach turned inside out with the mucosa removed. The tunica muscularis comprises outer longitudinal, middle circular, and inner oblique layers. The longitudinal layer clothes the curvatures *(1)* and the pyloric part *(1′)* but is thin over the body. The circular layer surrounds the body *(2)* and is especially prominent on the pyloric part *(2′)*, where it furnishes the pyloric sphincters *(2″)*. The oblique layer *(3)* is thickest along the lesser curvature, where it forms two lips that fuse over the cardia (cardiac loop); it is thin where it lines the fundus and body *(3′)*.

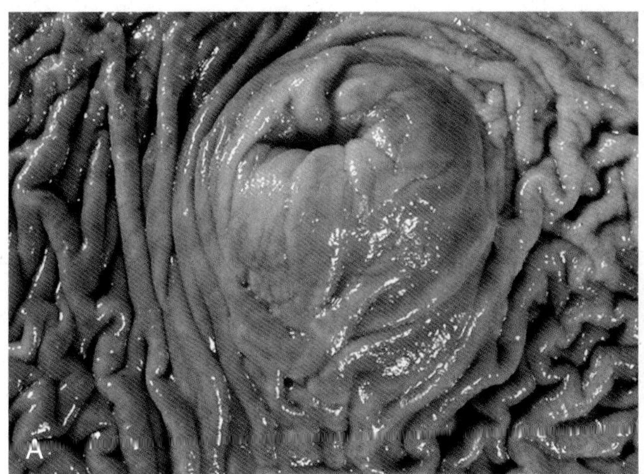

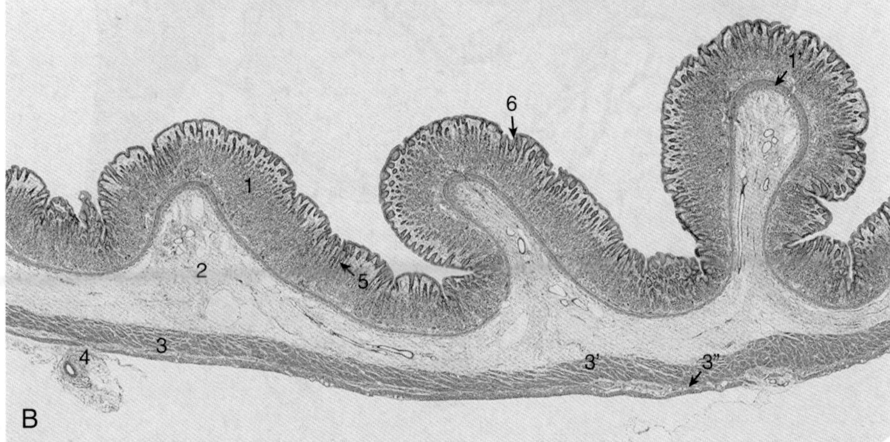

Fig. 3.38 (A) Protruding cardia surrounded by longitudinal folds or rugae. (B) Glandular region of stomach of cat. Glandular region shows 3 rugae or folds. *1*, tunica mucosa; *1′*, lamina muscularis mucosae; *2*, tunica submucosa; *3*, tunica muscularis composed of inner oblique *(3′)* and outer longitudinal *(3″)* layers; *4*, tunica serosa is thin with a blood vessel; *5*, gastric glands located in lamina propria; *6*, gastric pit (hematoxylin and eosin stain).

gross regions bearing the same names. The cardiac and pyloric glands produce additional mucus, whereas the proper gastric glands alone produce pepsin and hydrochloric acid, which are important parts of digestive juice. The enzyme is produced by the more numerous (chief) cells, the acid by the fewer parietal cells. There also are mucus-secreting cells. It is claimed that the proper gastric glandular region has a somewhat darker hue than the remainder of the mucosa.

The *blood supply* to the stomach comes from all three chief branches of the *celiac artery* and is particularly generous along the two curvatures (Fig. 3.39). The arteries anastomose quite freely externally and also within the stomach wall. For the most part, the arteries that penetrate the wall pass to the submucosa before branching to form an elaborate plexus from which both the muscular and the mucosal coats are fed. The mucosal branches supply unusually wide-bored capillaries below the epithelium and about the glands.

The veins are similarly arranged and ultimately combine to form trunks that join the portal vein. Numerous arteriovenous anastomoses provide a means of regulating mucosal blood supply, and much blood is diverted from the capillary bed of the fasting organ.

Lymph vessels are present in profusion, particularly in the submucosa. They lead to several gastric nodes, each charged with the drainage of a particular territory.

The stomach is *innervated* by parasympathetic fibers within the two vagal trunks and by sympathetic fibers that reach the organ with the arteries. The efferent fibers of both sets are accompanied by more numerous afferent fibers. Parasympathetic fibers of the vagus nerve synapse on ganglion cells in intramural plexuses within the submucosa and between the muscle coats and exert a high measure of control over gastric motility. In the proximal stomach, vagal activity suppresses muscular contraction and leads to adaptive relaxation, whereas in the distal stomach, vagal stimulation causes intense peristaltic activity. Vagal stimulation of distal antral motility is mediated by acetylcholine, but the identity of the inhibitory mediator is not well established and it may be vasoactive intestinal peptide. The intramural plexuses are involved in the local reflexes in which the stomach wall reacts to direct stimulation. Sympathetic and parasympathetic fibers also innervate the surface epithelium and glands, but only parasympathetic fibers end on the intragastric endocrine cells.*
Division of the vagal nerves, either the main trunks or selected branches, reduces gastric activity and secretion.

*There are several varieties of these cells, the most important of which is the gastrin-secreting cells scattered singly within the epithelium of gastric glands, especially those of the antral region. The release of gastrin is stimulated by the vagal nerves and also, more directly, by distention of the stomach by a meal. Gastrin is passed into the portal circulation, returning within the arterial blood to promote increased activity, both glandular and muscular, of the stomach wall.

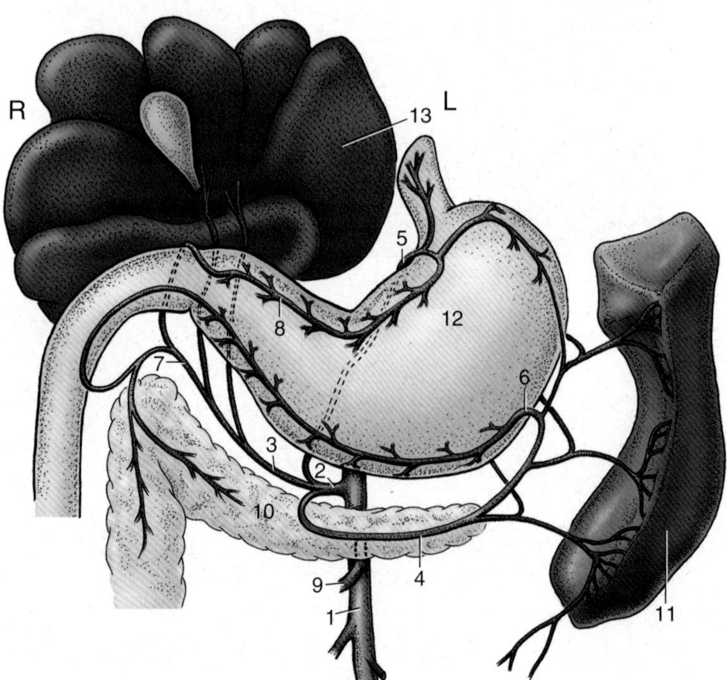

Fig. 3.39 Distribution of the celiac artery of the dog (ventral view). *1,* Aorta; *2,* celiac artery; *3,* hepatic artery; *4,* splenic artery; *5,* left gastric artery; *6,* left gastroepiploic artery; *7,* gastroduodenal artery; *8,* right gastric artery; *9,* cranial mesenteric artery; *10,* pancreas; *11,* spleen; *12,* stomach; *13,* liver; *L,* left; *R,* right.

The empty stomach is small and contracted toward the fixed point of the esophageal entrance such that it is entirely within the rib cage and fails to reach the abdominal floor. The wall is generally inert except for occasional weak peristaltic contractions, and little secretion from the glands occurs. Any residual peristaltic activity ceases as soon as food is offered (or anticipated). Secretion increases as a reflex response to the taste of food or the effort of mastication. When food does arrive, it first collects in layers (because as yet no mixing movements are present) largely in the body, to expand it in all directions but principally ventrally and caudally. A motor response is delayed and slowly builds to a peak. Peristaltic contractions commence near the cardia and course distally, accelerating and becoming more vigorous when they reach the muscular pyloric antrum. The terminal segment contracts en masse to move the ingesta into the duodenum while the peristaltic wave is still some distance from the pylorus. Radiographic studies suggest that the pylorus is open for about one third of the time. It is probable that emptying is dependent more on intermittent increase in the intragastric pressure than on the regular peristaltic activity.

The effects of feeding on topography and relations of stomach with other organs are considerable, especially in animals kept under regimens that allow them to feed seldom but to repletion. The fully distended stomach may extend almost to the umbilicus—or even beyond this in the puppy—pushing the intestinal mass dorsally and caudally. The liver is pushed to the right while the spleen, tethered to the left part of the greater curvature, follows the expansion of that side of the stomach.

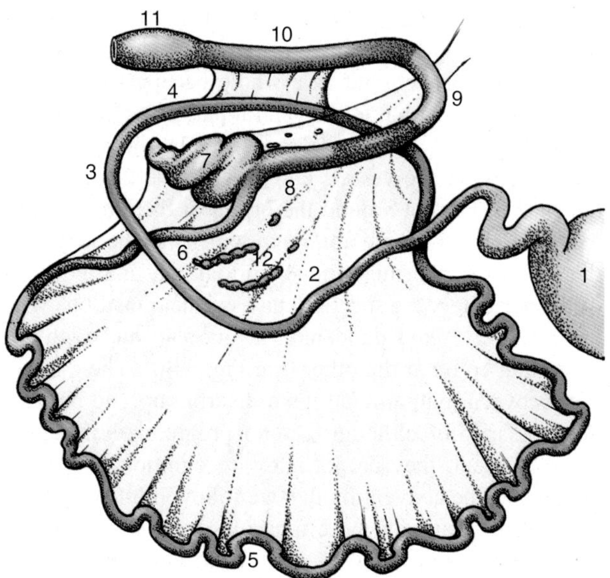

Fig. 3.40 Intestinal tract of the dog (schematic). *1,* Stomach; *2,* descending duodenum; *3,* caudal flexure; *4,* ascending duodenum; *5,* jejunum; *6,* ileum; *7,* cecum; *8,* ascending colon; *9,* transverse colon; *10,* descending colon; *11,* rectal ampulla; *12,* jejunal lymph nodes.

THE INTESTINE

The intestine* commences at the pylorus and continues to the anus. It is divided between the proximal small intestine (intestinum tenue) and the distal large intestine (intestinum crassum), which are parts that do not always differ as much in caliber as their names suggest. However, the boundary is made obvious by the outgrowth of a blind diverticulum, the cecum, at the origin of the large intestine (Fig. 3.40). The small intestine consists of three parts: an initial duodenum, which is short and rather closely fixed in position, and the jejunum and ileum, which are carried by the great mesentery. The large intestine also comprises three parts; recognition of the blind-ending cecum presents no problem, but the separation of colon from rectum is arbitrarily put at the pelvic inlet. The rectum joins the short anal canal that leads to the exterior, but this canal is not part of the intestine in the strict sense.

The length of the intestine may be given in absolute terms or, more usefully, in measures of body length, and neither figure may reflect the reality. The dog, in keeping with its diet, has a relatively short gut, which is perhaps some three or four times its body length in life. Intestinal length in herbivores varies with the nature of the gastrointestinal adaptation but may be as much as 25 times the body length in sheep.

THE SMALL INTESTINE

The *duodenum* is short and is closely attached to the abdominal roof by a short mesoduodenum. The initial portion continues from the pyloric part of the stomach and passes toward the right body wall before being deflected caudally to descend to a point between the right kidney and the pelvic inlet. It then passes medially, behind the root of the mesentery, before ascending a short distance; it ends by bending ventrally to enter the mesentery, where it is continued as the jejunum. The more constant relations of the dog's duodenum are to the liver at its origin, thereafter to the right body wall laterally, to the pancreas and later the right kidney medially, and, overall, to other parts of the intestinal mass. Although the first part of the duodenum is not expanded to form a distinct "duodenal bulb" or "cap" (so commonly the site of ulcers in people), its functional independence is retained.

* The Greek word *enteron* provides the stem for many terms: *enteritis, mesentery,* and so forth.

The *jejunum* and *ileum* are less closely fixed in position, but although the arrangement of individual coils continually adjusts, this gut as a whole occupies a more or less constant position in the ventral part of the abdominal cavity (Fig. 3.41). The coils are carried by the mesentery, which conveys the vessels and nerves. The mesentery is bunched at its root around the origin of the cranial mesenteric artery from the aorta and widens to the length of the gut at its other margin. The initial and final portions of the mesentery are shortest and ease the transitions with the relatively fixed duodenum at one end and with the ascending colon at the other (see Fig. 3.40). The distinction between jejunum and ileum is arbitrary and perhaps unnecessary, for although certain progressive structural changes occur, they do not allow recognition of a sharp boundary. The convention that we follow limits the ileum to a short, relatively more muscular (and hence firmer) final portion with a direct peritoneal connection to the cecum.

The *jejunum* fills those parts of the abdomen that are not preempted by other viscera. In the dog, in which the large intestine is relatively small, the jejunum lies more or less symmetrically about the midline, between the liver and stomach cranially and the urinary bladder caudally. It lies on the abdominal floor, though separated from the parietal peritoneum by the intervention of the greater omentum. The coils are quite mobile and have some pattern to their arrangement despite the haphazard appearance. The mainly sagittal coils of the proximal part lie largely cranial to the more transverse coils of the distal part (see Fig. 3.41). The *ileum* pursues a rather direct cranial, dorsal, and dextral course toward its junction with the large intestine. In life the intestine is not uniformly full, and at any moment most parts are flattened and molded by the pressures of adjacent viscera. The lumen may be locally obliterated, and when a passage is retained, it is more often than not reduced to a narrow channel along one margin: a "keyhole" form is seen when this is viewed in section. This occurrence also explains the narrow streaks that are the common representation of the small intestine in radiographs obtained after the administration of a barium suspension. Segmental and peristaltic movements continually alter the configuration in life.

The intestine is composed of the usual four tunics (Fig. 3.42). The luminal surface has a velvety appearance because of the innumerable tiny but densely packed projections known as the *intestinal villi*. They are finger-like in the dog and horse but broader and leaflike in many species (Fig. 3.43). In addition to the interspecific differences, variations in form and dimension may be present at different locations along the length of the small intestine. The appearance and the detailed morphology may be profoundly influenced by changes in diet (early weaning) or disease (microbial infections). The villi greatly increase

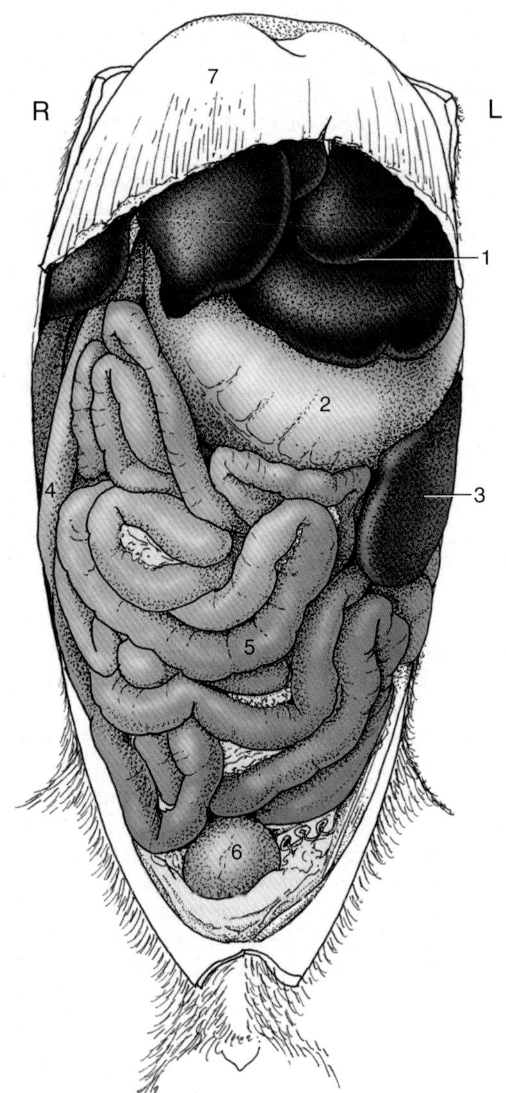

Fig. 3.41 Ventral view of the abdominal organs of the dog after removal of the greater omentum. *1,* Liver; *2,* stomach; *3,* spleen; *4,* descending duodenum; *5,* jejunum; *6,* bladder; *7,* diaphragm; *L,* left; *R,* right.

the area of epithelium available for absorption, and the efficiency of the process is enhanced by very generous subepithelial capillary plexuses (Fig. 3.43B). Microscopic intestinal glands (crypts) open to the surface between the bases of the villi. The crypts produce a mucous secretion, which coats the surface of the bowel, and various enzymes that contribute to the further digestion of carbohydrate and protein breakdown products.

Larger (Brunner's) glands confined to the submucosa of the duodenum, especially its initial part, also secrete a protective mucus. A proportion of the cells lining the crypts, perhaps 1% of the total population, belong to the enteroendocrine (enterochromaffin) system (p. 209). These types of cells include the gastrin-producing cells of the stomach as well as those in the small and the large

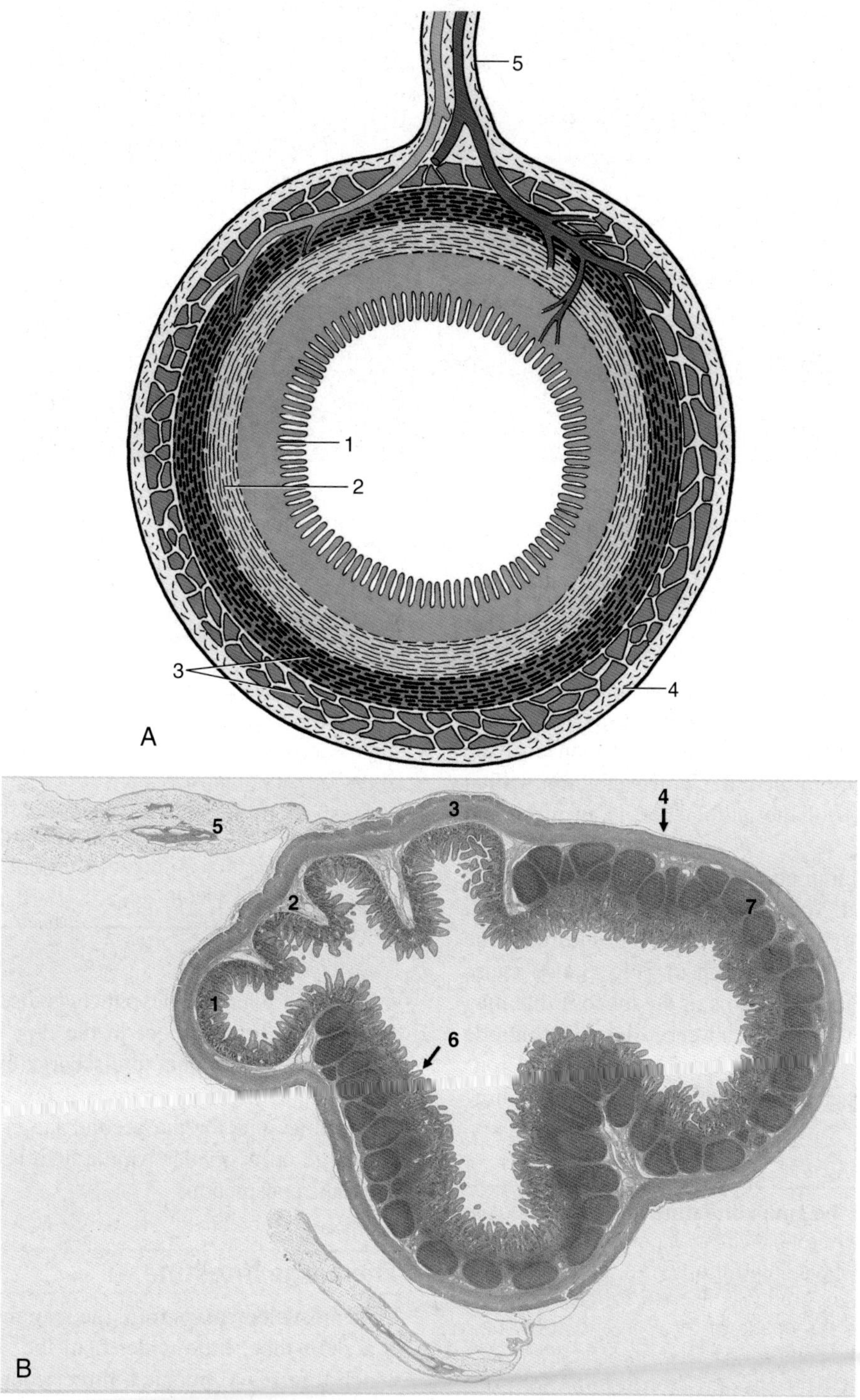

Fig. 3.42 (A) Schematic transverse section through the gut. (B) Transverse section through pig ileum (hematoxylin and period acid–Schiff stain). The artery and vein reach the gut via the mesentery; the larger branches fail to reach the antimesenteric border. *1,* Mucosa; *2,* submucosa; *3,* muscle layer; *4,* serosa; *5,* mesentery; *6,* intestinal villi projecting into the lumen; *7,* Peyer's patches.

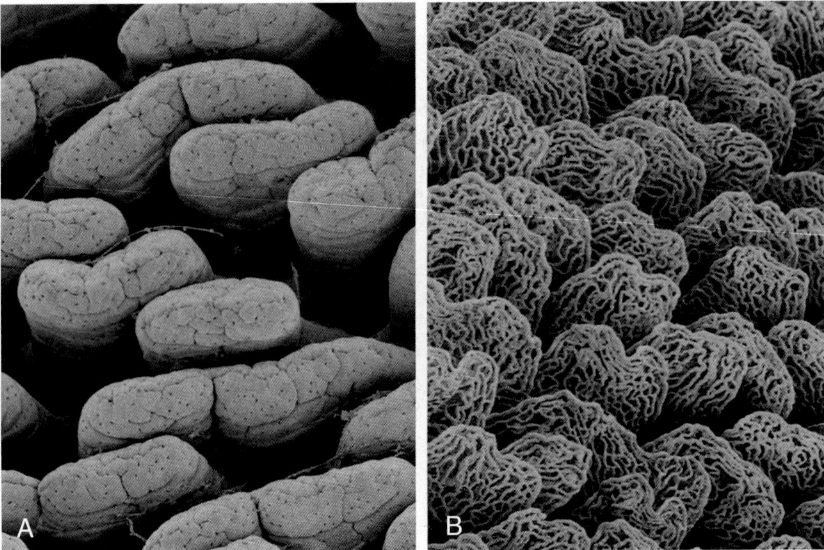

Fig. 3.43 Scanning electron micrographs (A) of rat duodenal villi and (B) of a vascular cast of the same tissue demonstrating subepithelial capillary plexuses.

intestine, and they produce a number of hormones that influence various aspects of gastrointestinal activity. The intestinal components of the series, unlike the components of the stomach, are under regulation by intrinsic nerves of the organ wall and largely outweigh the influence of the extrinsic nerve supply to the gut. Cholecystokinin, which provokes contraction of the gallbladder, is an important member of the set.

The mucosa is rich in nodules of lymphoid tissue, both solitary and clumped. The folding of mucosa and the villi increase the absorptive surface area of the intestine. The larger aggregations (Peyer's patches* [Fig. 3.44]) cause visible depressions and elevations of the mucosa that may become more obvious with the absence of a covering pile of villi. These aggregations tend to be more numerous and individually larger toward the junction with the large intestine.

The epithelium of the small intestine renews throughout life through the mitotic division of cells in the depths of the crypts. The cells lining the crypts, continuously recruited in this way, gradually ascend to the surface, spread to embrace the bases of the villi, and continue up them to the summits where they are finally shed into the gut lumen. The passage from the bottom of a crypt to the summit of a villus takes about 3 days and involves a prodigious wastage—one calculation suggests a loss of about 1 g of epithelial cells for every centimeter stretch of the human small intestine every day. The process has the fortunate consequence of permitting rapid renewal of the integrity of the gut lining after extensive damage, such as the necrosis and loss by sloughing of the surface layer that occurs in certain infections in various domestic species. While repair is in train, the villi are reduced in size, and they remain so until a sufficient number of epithelial cells has become available.

*These patches may be initial sites for the accumulation, after ingestion, of the infective agents responsible for the transmissible spongiform encephalopathies ("new variant" Creutzfeldt Jacob disease, bovine spongiform encephalopathy [BSE], scrapie) that have claimed so much attention in recent years.

Both the liver and the pancreas discharge into the duodenum. The arrangement in the dog is for the bile duct and one pancreatic duct to discharge by separate openings on a (major duodenal) papilla a few centimeters beyond the pylorus and for the second larger pancreatic duct to discharge on a smaller papilla a little farther on. Neither papilla is conspicuous.

The Large Intestine

In its most elementary form the mammalian large intestine is a short tube, little wider than the small intestine from which it arises to pursue a direct course to the anus. The large intestine in the dog is somewhat more complicated, although still simple if compared with that in herbivores (Fig. 3.45). As in most species, it is clearly divided into cecum, colon, and rectum, and the colon is itself differentiated into ascending, transverse, and descending parts (Fig. 3.45/*3–5*). The cecum is a blind-ending piece of gut that arises at the junction of the ileum and colon. The division of the colon follows from the rotation of the embryonic

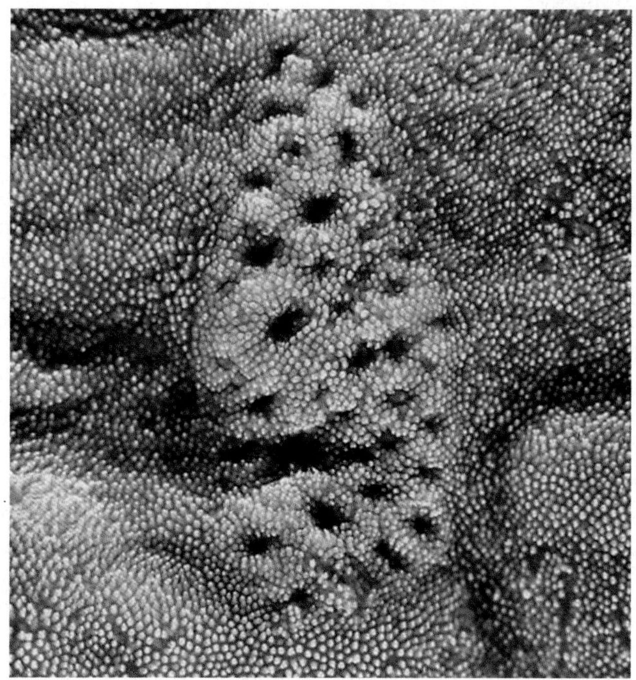

Fig. 3.44 Patch of aggregated lymph nodules in ileum (horse).

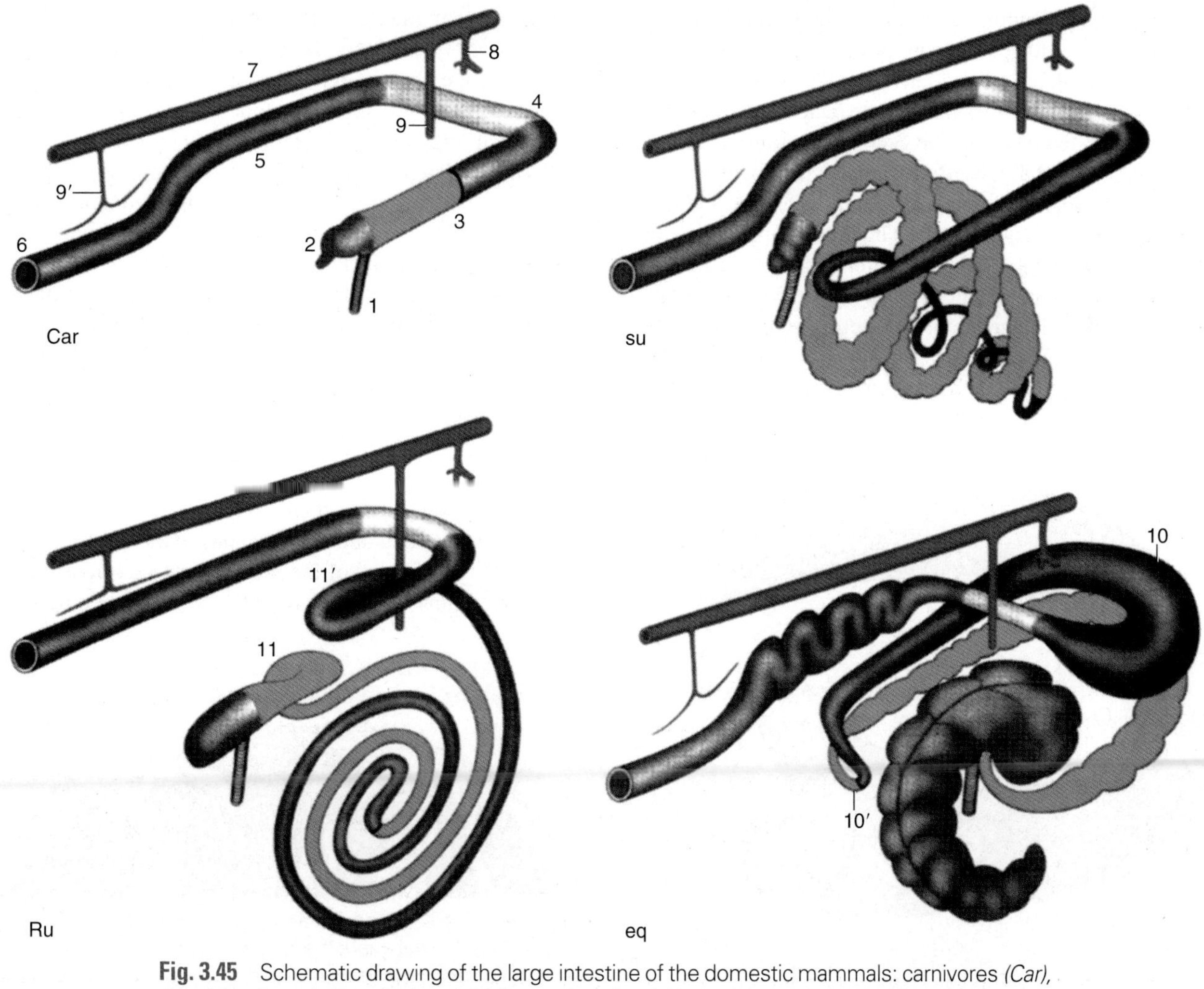

Fig. 3.45 Schematic drawing of the large intestine of the domestic mammals: carnivores *(Car)*, the pig *(su)*, ruminants *(Ru)*, and the horse *(eq)*. Cranial is to the *upper right*. *1*, Ileum; *2*, cecum; *3*, ascending colon; *4*, transverse colon; *5*, descending colon; *6*, rectum and anus; *7*, aorta; *8*, celiac artery; *9* and *9′*, cranial and caudal mesenteric arteries; *10* and *10′*, dorsal diaphragmatic and pelvic flexures of ascending colon; *11* and *11′*, proximal and distal loops of ascending colon.

gut, which imposes a conformation on the adult organ that resembles a question mark (when viewed from below; see Fig. 14.15).

The canine *cecum* is unusual in having no direct connection with the ileum; however, it is conventional to regard the cecum as the first part of the large intestine. The cecum of the dog is short and at first sight appears even shorter because it is drawn into a spiral and held against the ileum by folds of peritoneum. It is only slightly wider than the small intestine and tapers slightly toward its rounded blind extremity. The lumen communicates with the interior of the colon, immediately beyond the ileocolic junction, through an opening that is guarded by an inner, circular, muscular ring (the cecocolic sphincter) (Fig. 3.46).

The caliber of the smooth, externally featureless *colon* is uniformly and significantly, though not remarkably, greater than that of the small intestine. The colon is suspended throughout its length by a moderately long mesocolon, which allows it some mobility, and its position and relations vary within certain limits. The flexures that divide the colon into ascending, transverse, and descending parts are not precisely fixed. The short ascending part continues the axis of the ileum from a junction defined internally by an ileocolic opening of similar appearance and construction to that at the origin of the cecum. The transverse part runs across the abdomen from right to left, between the stomach cranially and the mass of small intestine and cranial mesenteric artery caudally. The descending part is the longest. It follows the left flank before edging medially to enter the pelvic cavity, where it becomes the rectum without any visible demarcation. The term *rectum* implies a straight course, but often this part of the bowel is deflected to one side by pressure from other viscera, most usually a distended bladder. The *rectum* is the most dorsal of the pelvic viscera and lies above the reproductive organs, bladder, and urethra. Its cranial part has the same relationship to the peritoneum as the colon, but this relationship changes as the mesorectum shortens and the serosal covering is reflected laterally to continue into the parietal peritoneum of the pelvic cavity and ventrally to continue over the urogenital organs. The terminal part is wholly retroperitoneal and is directly attached to the vagina in the female, to the urethra in the male, and to the pelvic diaphragm in both sexes.

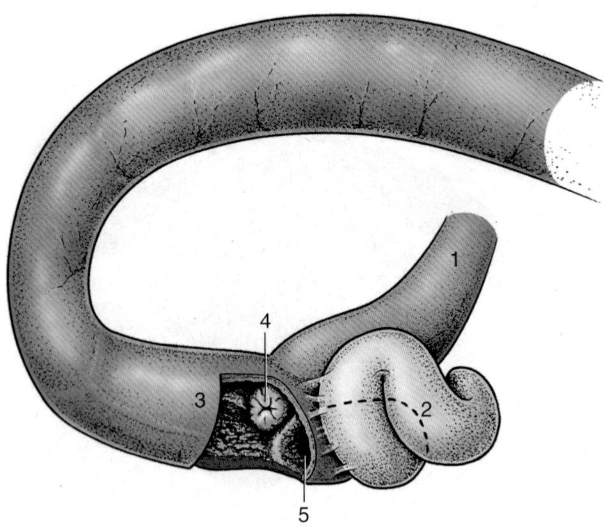

Fig. 3.46 The ileocolic junction and its relation to the cecum in the dog. *1,* Ileum; *2,* cecum; *3,* ascending colon; *4,* ileal orifice surrounded by annular fold; *5,* cecocolic orifice.

The mucosa of the large intestine lacks villi. No permanent mucosal folds are present, but there are numerous scattered lymph nodules, especially in the rectum, where they tend to be conspicuous because of the depressions and pits in the summits of the swellings. In many species, including the horse and pig among domestic animals, the outer muscle coat of the large intestine is concentrated mainly in a number of bands (teniae) that, on shortening, pucker the gut so that a linear series of sacculations (haustra) is produced (see Figs. 21.12 and 21.18). Such bands are not present on the intestine of the dog and cat.

The *anal canal* joins the bowel to the exterior. It is a short passage that is derived from the proctodeum, the invagination of the surface ectoderm. The lumen is constricted at the rectoanal junction where the mucosa is thrown into longitudinal folds, normally pressed together to occlude the orifice (Fig. 3.47). Anal continence, however, depends primarily on the presence of two sphincters; the internal anal sphincter is merely a thickening of the circular smooth muscle of the gut, but the external sphincter is striated, of somatic origin, and under voluntary control (Fig. 3.48).

Many glands are always present in the anal region, both in the mucosa and in the surrounding skin. Most are small, but the dog and cat also possess two so-called anal sacs (sinus paranasales). Each is roughly the size of a hazelnut (in the dog) and is located ventrolateral to the anus between the internal and external sphincters (see Figs. 3.47 and 15.4). The fundus of the sac secretes an evil-smelling fluid that drains through a single duct to an opening near

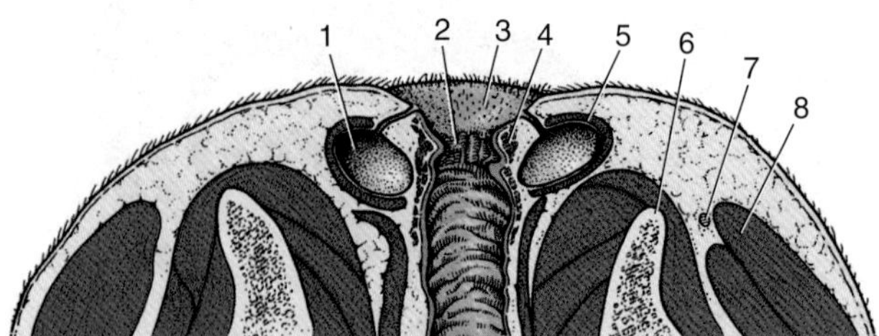

Fig. 3.47 Dorsal (horizontal) section through the canine anal canal. *1,* Anal sac; *2,* columnar zone of the anal canal; *3,* cutaneous zone; *4,* internal anal sphincter; *5,* external anal sphincter; *6,* ischium; *7,* sacrotuberous ligament; *8,* gluteus superficialis.

the anocutaneous junction. The sac is compressed at defecation, expelling the secretion, which probably serves as a territorial marker. Such sacs are found in most carnivores and are most notorious in the skunk.

The blood supply to the intestinal tract is provided mainly by the *cranial and caudal mesenteric arteries*. However, the initial part of the duodenum is supplied by the hepatic branch of the celiac artery, and the caudal part of the rectum by rectal branches of the internal pudendal artery. The cranial mesenteric artery supplies the bulk of the small intestine, the ileocecocolic junctional region, and the midpart of the colon through its three primary divisions; the details of branching vary among species and also, though to a lesser extent, among individuals. The distribution of the smaller caudal mesenteric artery is restricted to the descending colon and cranial part of the rectum. The knowledge of arterial branching and richness of anastomoses is of help in surgical procedures (Figs. 3.42 and 3.49). The arterial anastomoses ensure the survival of the intestine even following the complete obstruction of a major supplying vessel. The chain of anastomoses continues beyond the territories of the mesenteric arteries to connect with those of the celiac and internal pudendal arteries.

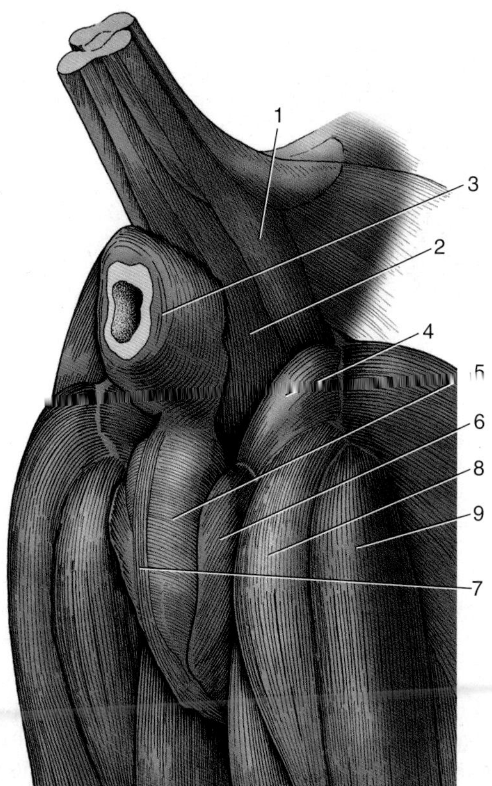

Fig. 3.48 The muscles of the perineal region of the male dog. *1,* Coccygeus; *2,* levator ani; *3,* external anal sphincter; *4,* internal obturator; *5,* bulbospongiosus; *6,* ischiocavernosus; *7,* retractor penis; *8,* semimembranosus; *9,* semitendinosus.

The *veins* are broadly comparable and join to form the cranial and caudal mesenteric veins, two of the main radicles (the splenic vein is the third) of the portal vein (Fig. 3.50). Certain tributary veins connect with systemic veins at the extremities of their territories, which are the thoracic esophagus and anal canal, parts that normally drain by systemic routes. Congestion within the portal circulation (p. 127) may lead to enlargement of submucosal veins in both these (and other) parts but is much more important in human than in veterinary medicine. The gut wall contains a considerable proportion of the lymphocyte population and represents an important component of the body's defense mechanism.

The *lymphatic drainage* of the small intestine, in particular, is copious because some of the products of digestion are absorbed by this route. When these products include fat, the lymph is milky and the intestinal lymphatic vessels ("lacteals") are unusually conspicuous. The flow is directed toward certain nodes through which the lymph percolates before joining the cisterna chyli, the dilated origin of the thoracic duct, the most important lymphatic vessel (p. 245). In the dog these nodes are large but few and are centralized toward the root of the mesentery (see Fig. 3.40), but in other species they may be more numerous and more widely scattered peripherally close to the gut itself.

The intestine receives both *sympathetic and parasympathetic nerves*. The sympathetic pathways lead through the celiac, cranial mesenteric, and caudal mesenteric ganglia, and the postganglionic fibers enmesh the relevant arteries (see Fig. 8.76). The parasympathetic pathways involve both vagal and pelvic nerves. The former supply the intestine to the junction of the transverse and descending parts of the colon; the latter supply the descending colon and rectum. The parasympathetic nerves augment peristalsis, but the effects of intestinal denervation are far less striking than those of gastric denervation.

Under strong vasoconstriction may close the capillary bed of the intestinal wall, leading to abnormal permeability that allows large molecules to overcome the gut barrier; septic shock is then an eventual possibility.

THE LIVER

The liver (hepar) is located in the most cranial part of the abdomen, immediately behind the diaphragm. It is by far the largest gland in the body and performs many functions essential for life. The most obvious is the production of bile, but the parts it plays in protein, carbohydrate, and fat metabolism are even more important and depend on the liver's situation astride the bloodstream draining the gastrointestinal tract. This location ensures that the products of digestion, which are conveyed in the bloodstream after absorption, are presented to the hepatic cells before entering the general circulation.

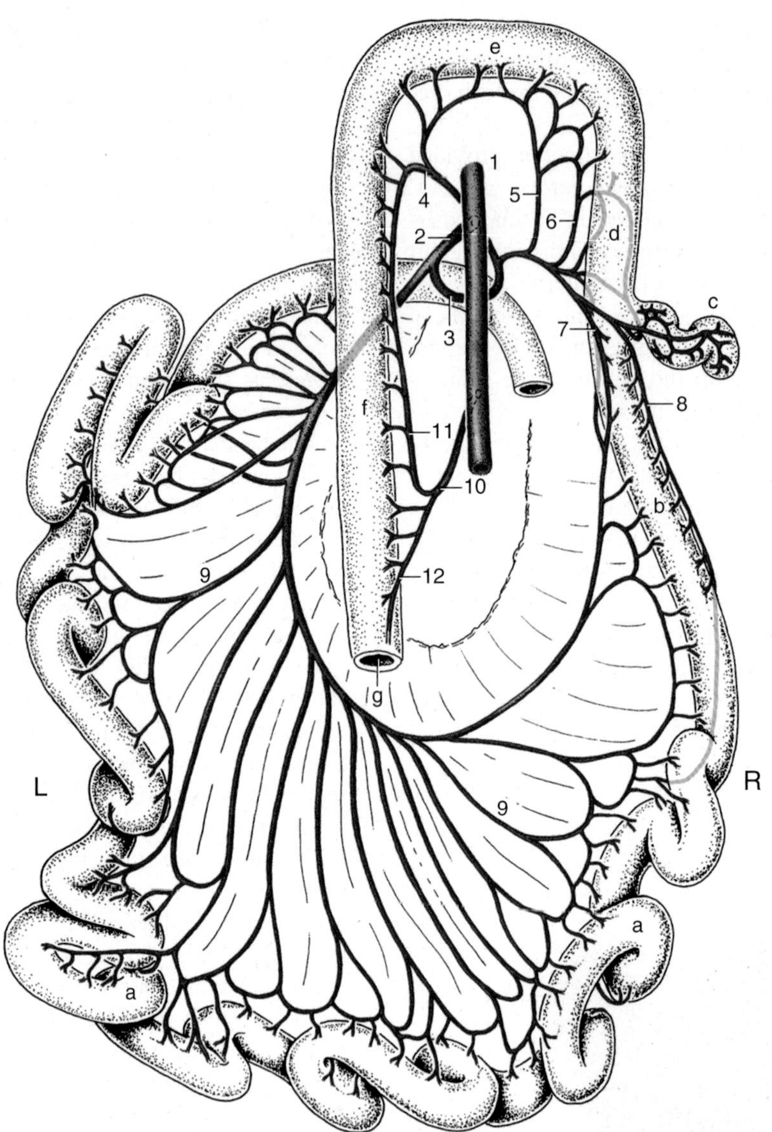

Fig. 3.49 Distribution of the cranial and caudal mesenteric arteries to the intestines of the dog (dorsal view). *a,* Jejunum; *b,* ileum; *c,* cecum; *d,* ascending colon; *e,* transverse colon; *f,* descending colon; *g,* rectum; *L,* left; *R,* right; *1,* aorta; *2,* cranial mesenteric artery; *3,* ileocolic artery; *4,* middle colic artery; *5,* right colic artery; *6,* colic branch of ileocolic artery; *7,* mesenteric ileal branch; *8,* antimesenteric ileal branch; *9,* jejunal arteries; *10,* caudal mesenteric artery; *11,* left colic artery; *12,* cranial rectal artery.

The metabolic functions of the liver explain the wide interspecific variation in size: average values are about 3% to 5% of body weight in carnivores, 2% to 3% in omnivores, and as little as 1% to 1.5% in herbivores. The liver is substantially heavier in the young animal than in the adult and atrophies considerably in old animals. Usually brownish red, the fresh liver is soft and has a characteristic friable consistency.

The adult liver intervenes between the diaphragm cranially and the stomach and intestinal mass caudally. Although this organ is extended across the median plane, the bulk lies to the right in all species (Fig. 3.51). It is not so very asymmetrical in the dog, with the proportions to the right and left of the median plane being about 3:2. In most species, including the dog, the liver is grossly divided into lobes by a series of fissures that extend inward from the ventral margin (Fig. 3.52). Considerable effort has been given to facilitate description of the individual lobes and fissures and their homology among the species. The theoretical pattern, which accords the dog's liver left lateral, left medial, right lateral, right medial, quadrate, and caudate lobes, of which the last is enlarged by papillary and caudate processes, is illustrated here (Fig. 3.53). Modern studies minimize the significance

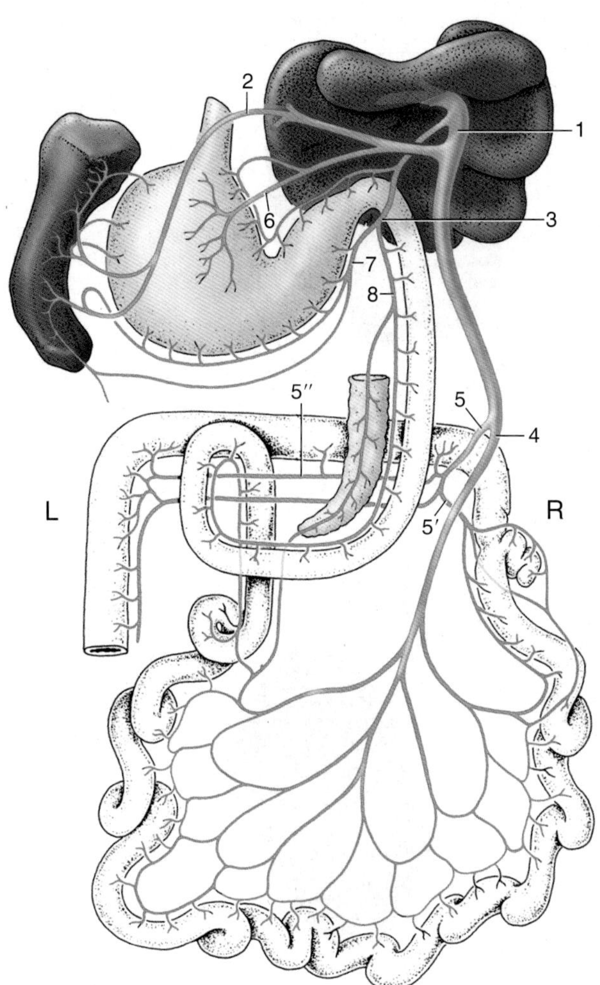

Fig. 3.50 Semischematic dorsal view of the formation of the portal vein (dog). *1,* Portal vein; *2,* splenic vein; *3,* gastroduodenal vein; *4,* cranial mesenteric vein; *5,* caudal mesenteric vein; *5′,* ileocolic vein; *5″,* middle colic vein; *6,* left gastric vein; *7,* right gastroepiploic vein; *8,* cranial pancreaticoduodenal vein.

of the external fissuration and rely more on the internal ramifications of the vessels to establish homologies. Such studies have had the useful by-product of providing the surgeon with the detailed knowledge of the vascular architecture necessary for the safe removal of diseased parts of the human liver.

In life the liver adapts to the forms of neighboring organs, and when fixed in situ, it retains the conformation and impressions they impose. The rather large liver of the dog is therefore bluntly conical, and its cranial surface matches the curvature of the diaphragm against which it is pressed. The concave caudal surface exhibits a large excavation on the left for the stomach, which is then extended over the median plane into a narrow duodenal groove. The dorsal border extends more caudally and reaches farther dorsally on the right side, where it is further extended by the caudate process, which carries a deep impression for the cranial pole of the right kidney. Toward the median plane, this border carries a groove for the passage of the caudal vena cava and, to the left of this, a notch for the esophagus. The gallbladder lies between the quadrate and right medial lobes. It is partly attached, partly free, and in some dogs so deeply embedded that it reaches the parietal surface, thus making contact with the diaphragm (see Fig. 3.53).

The liver is covered in peritoneum except for relatively small areas at the porta (hilus), in the fossa for the gallbladder, and at the origin of certain peritoneal reflections. The right and left triangular, the coronary, and the falciform ligaments that pass to the diaphragm from the parietal surface have fibrous cores and attach the liver firmly. The lesser omentum, which passes from the visceral surface to the stomach and duodenum, is more fragile. A tunica fibrosa encloses the parenchyma beneath the serosa. It enters the substance at the porta and detaches extensions that convey the blood vessels inward, dividing where the vessels divide and thinning at each division. The finer trabeculae pervade the entire organ and divide the liver into innumerable small units, the hepatic lobules of classic description. Although particularly marked in the pig's liver (Fig. 3.54), the lobular pattern is also quite obtrusive in the dog's liver, in which the lobules appear as hexagonal areas (about 1 mm across) on the intact surface and in gross and histologic sections. The histologic section (Fig. 3.54B) shows the relationship of the gallbladder with the liver.

The liver receives a very generous *blood supply* through the *hepatic artery,* a branch of the celiac artery, and the *portal vein.* The relative proportions are not known with certainty for the dog, but it supplies the human liver with only one fifth of the blood but about three fifths of the oxygen. The branches of the hepatic artery that actually enter the liver are effectively end-arteries. However, provision exists for a collateral circulation outside the liver, between the hepatic artery and the other branches of the celiac artery that supply the stomach and duodenum (see Fig. 3.39). The intrahepatic arteries divide in company with branches of the portal vein and tributaries of the hepatic duct. They supply the connective tissue structures en route to the hepatic sinusoids into which both they and the branches of the portal vein eventually discharge.

The *portal vein* is formed by the union of tributaries draining the digestive tract, pancreas, and spleen (see Fig. 3.50). It is connected to systemic veins in the cardioesophageal and rectoanal regions at the extremities of its territory. These connections provide alternative outlets for portal blood when the flow through the liver is obstructed or impaired. The results of obstruction vary among species and reflect the varying effectiveness of the hepatic artery in supplying oxygen. In the dog complete obstruction is rapidly fatal.

All blood delivered to the liver is collected by a single set of veins of which the central veins of the hepatic lobules

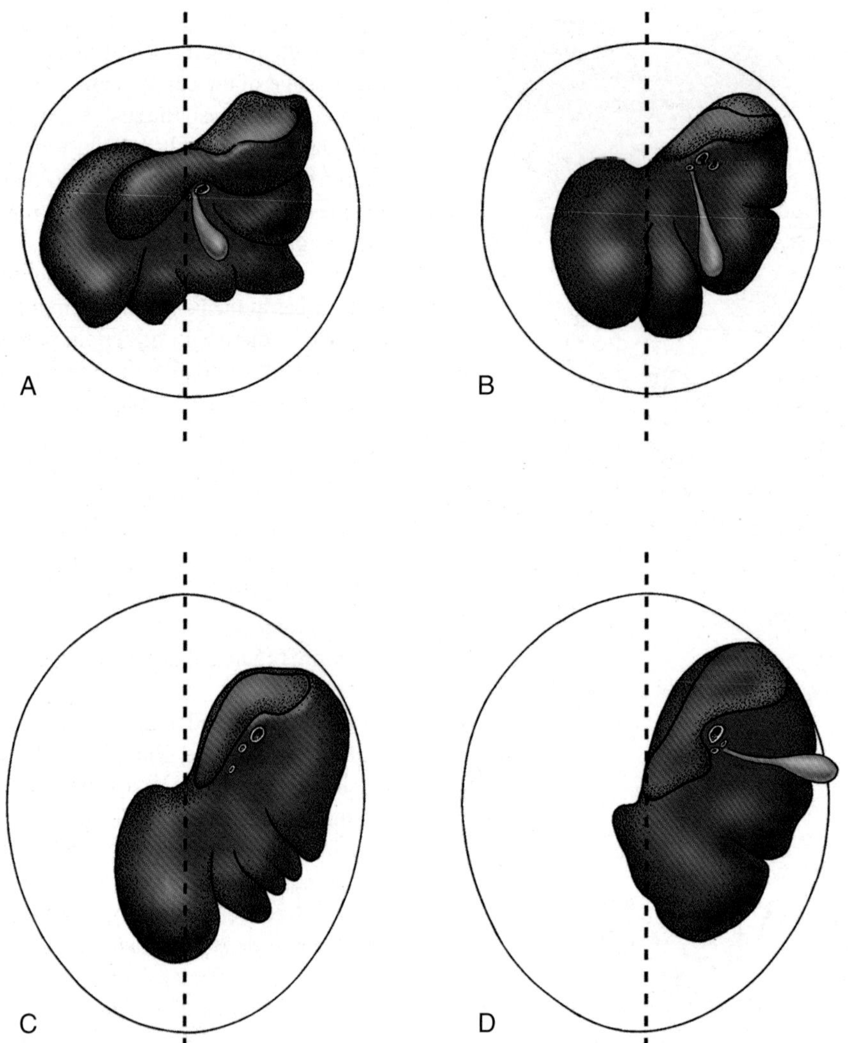

Fig. 3.51 Caudal surface of the liver of the (A) dog, (B) pig, (C) horse, and (D) cattle. The median planes are indicated. The liver is asymmetrical, less so in the dog, more so in the pig and horse, and most in cattle, in which the bulk of the organ is displaced to the right. Note the absence of a gallbladder from the horse liver.

are the smallest radicles. These eventually form the few large *hepatic veins* that open into the caudal vena cava during its passage through the liver. The circulation through the liver is controlled by various sphincters and possesses numerous anastomoses—interarterial, intervenous, and arteriovenous. A relatively rare congenital defect allows portal blood to pass directly to the caudal caval vein.

The liver receives sympathetic and parasympathetic nerves by way of periarterial plexuses and the vagal trunks, respectively.

The *hepatic duct system* begins with microscopic canaliculi within the lobules. These channels open into larger ductules that ultimately form a few large hepatic ducts by successive unions within the connective tissue between the lobules. Before or shortly after leaving the liver at the porta the ducts combine in a single trunk that runs to the duodenum (Fig. 3.55). A tortuous side branch (cystic duct) that arises from the common trunk leads to the pear-shaped gallbladder. The part of the common trunk that is distal to the origin of the cystic duct is known as the *bile duct* (ductus choledochus). Variation in the duct system is common; some hepatic ducts may enter the gallbladder directly, and others may join the main outlet distal to the cystic duct. The gallbladder not only stores the bile but also concentrates it by absorption through the folded mucosa. As is well known, a gallbladder is not essential; it is lacking in the horse, the rat, and certain other species, which compensate by enlargement of the duct system (see Fig. 3.51).

The muscle of the bladder wall and duct, including the sphincter at the entrance to the duodenum, is supplied by parasympathetic nerves. Pain arising from the duct system, common in human patients, is abolished by section of the (sympathetic) splanchnic nerves.

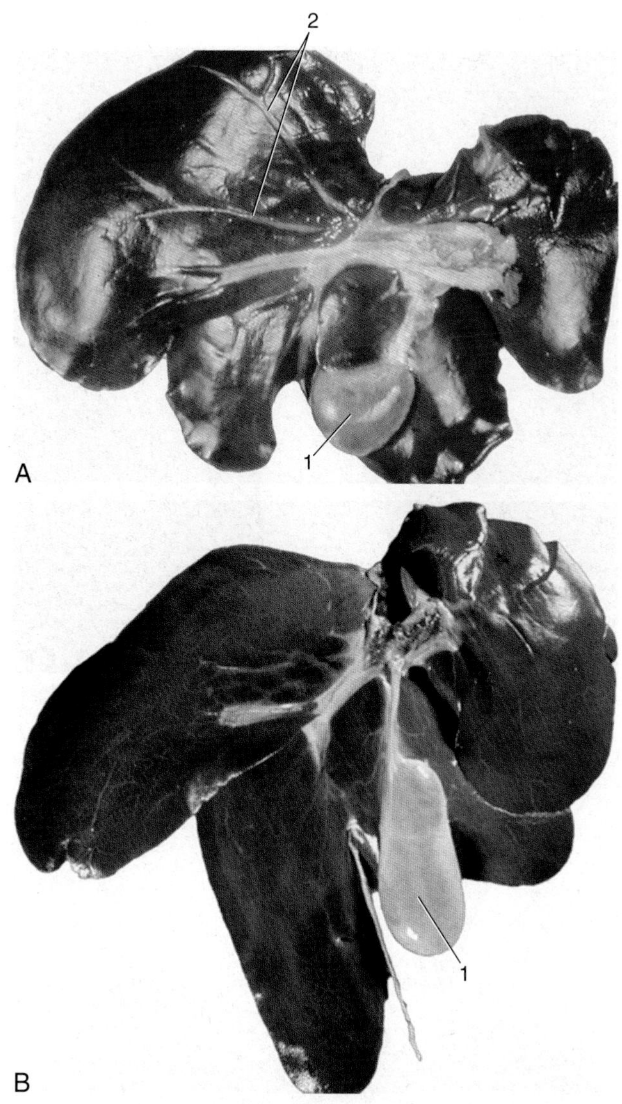

Fig. 3.52 (A) Visceral surface of liver (dog). (B) Visceral surface of liver (pig). *1,* Gallbladder; *2,* hepatic ducts.

THE PANCREAS

The pancreas is a much smaller gland closely related to the duodenum in the dorsal part of the abdominal cavity. It is yellowish and bears some resemblance to the salivary glands, although it is softer and more loosely knit. It combines exocrine and endocrine functions.

The exocrine component, by far the larger, produces a digestive juice that is discharged into the proximal part of the duodenum through one or two ducts. The juice contains enzymes that break down protein, carbohydrates, and fats. The endocrine component comprises the pancreatic islets, which are cell clumps that are scattered between the exocrine acini and are the source of insulin, glucagon, and gastrin. The islets are therefore of prime importance in carbohydrate metabolism (p. 208).

The pancreas is conventionally regarded as consisting of a body and two lobes, a description that suits the canine pancreas but is less apt for those of some other species (Fig. 3.56). When hardened in situ, the canine pancreas is acutely flexed: the apex of the V nestles close to the cranial flexure of the duodenum. The slender right lobe runs within the mesoduodenum. The thicker but shorter left lobe extends over the caudal surface of the stomach toward the spleen, within the greater omentum (see Fig. 3.33/7).

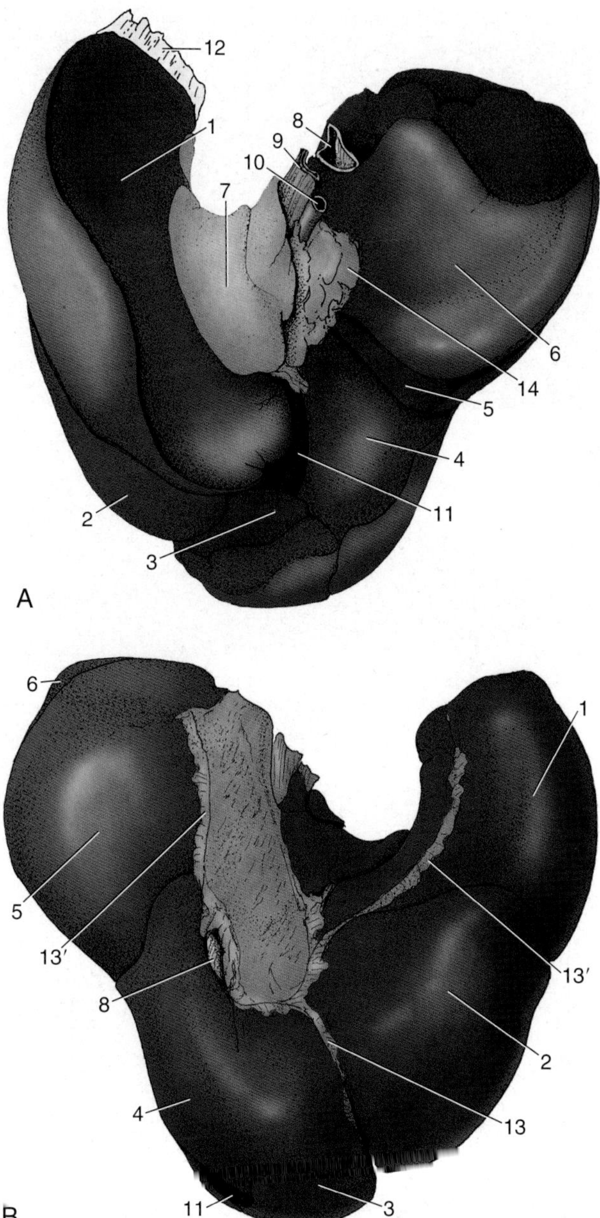

Fig. 3.53 (A) Visceral and (B) diaphragmatic surfaces of the canine liver. *1,* Left lateral lobe; *2,* left medial lobe; *3,* quadrate lobe; *4,* right medial lobe; *5,* right lateral lobe; *6,* caudate process (of caudate lobe); *7,* papillary process (of caudate lobe); *8,* caudal vena cava; *9,* portal vein; *10,* hepatic artery; *11,* gallbladder; *12,* left triangular ligament; *13,* falciform ligament; *13′,* coronary ligaments; *14,* lesser omentum.

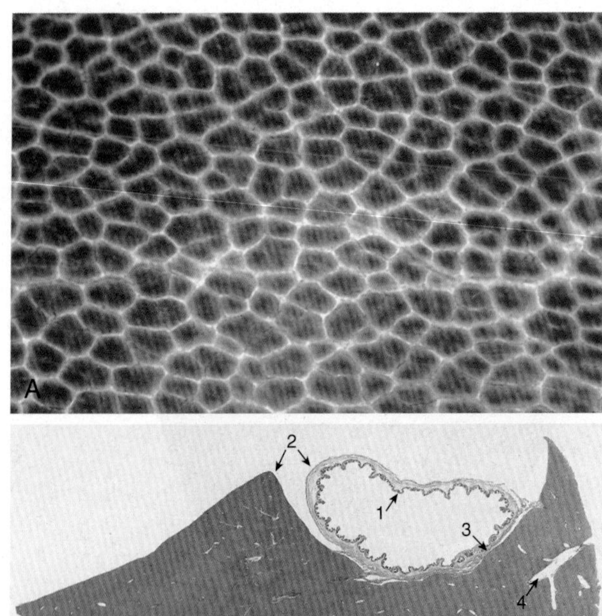

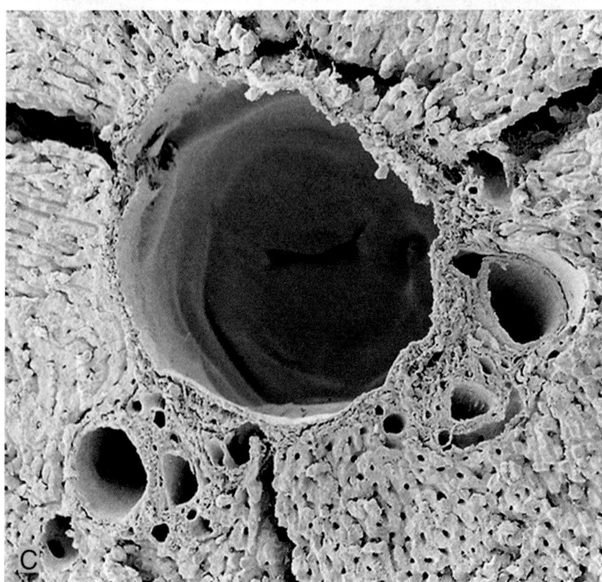

Fig. 3.54 (A) Surface of liver (enlarged) with clearly defined hepatic lobules (pig). (B) Liver and gallbladder (monkey) (hematoxylin and eosin stain). *1,* Tunica mucosa of gallbladder; *2,* visceral peritoneum covering the liver and gall bladder surface; *3,* tunica adventitia of gallbladder; tunica muscularis is very thin; *4,* hepatic portal vessels. (C) Scanning electron microscope image of a corrosion cast of hepatic vessels (rat); note the valve within the central vein.

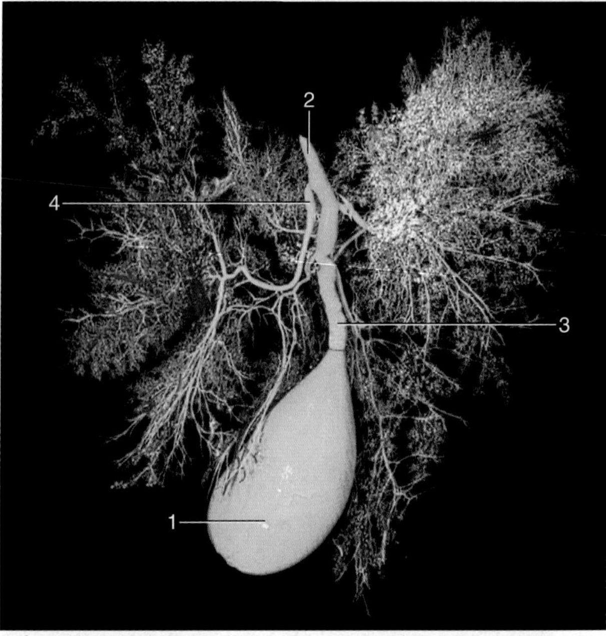

Fig. 3.55 The bile drainage system of the dog. *1,* Gallbladder; *2,* bile duct; *3,* cystic duct; *4,* hepatic ducts.

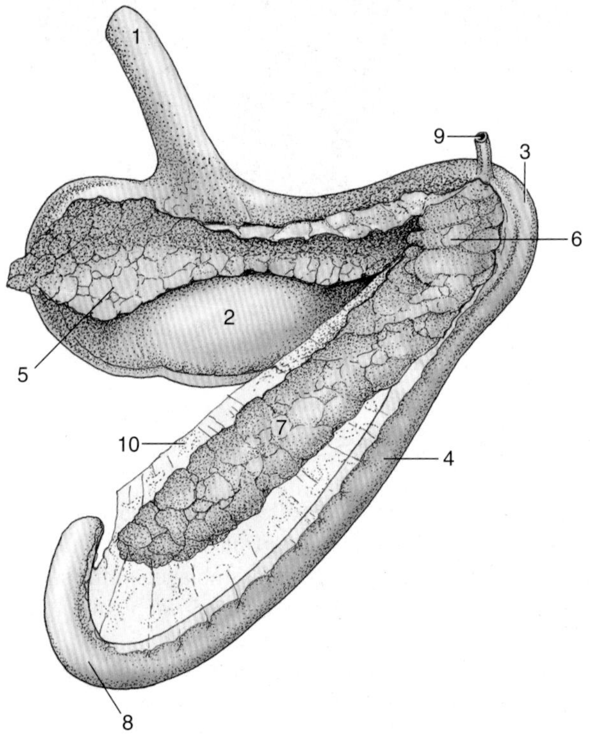

Fig. 3.56 The pancreas of the dog (caudal view). *1,* Esophagus; *2,* stomach; *3,* cranial flexure of duodenum; *4,* descending duodenum; *5,* left lobe of pancreas; *6,* body; *7,* right lobe; *8,* caudal flexure of duodenum; *9,* bile duct; *10,* mesoduodenum.

The pancreas arises from two primordia that bud from the proximal part of the duodenum. The buds later merge, but in many species evidence of the dual origin of the pancreas is provided by its duct system. A greater pancreatic duct commonly drains the part of the pancreas that arises from the ventral primordium and opens into the duodenum together with, or just beside, the bile duct. A lesser (accessory) duct emerges from the part of the pancreas formed by the dorsal primordium and opens on the opposite aspect of the gut. This is the arrangement usually found in the dog, although the terminal part of one duct sometimes regresses. Because the duct systems of the two lobes communicate within the gland, the absence of one or the other outlet is of no significance. In some species only one duct commonly survives.

The generous blood supply is from the *cranial and caudal pancreaticoduodenal arteries,* of which the former branches from the celiac artery and the latter from the cranial mesenteric artery. The veins drain to the portal vein. The gland is supplied by both sympathetic and parasympathetic nerves.

THE DEVELOPMENT OF THE DIGESTIVE APPARATUS

The foregut and hindgut end blindly at the oral and cloacal membranes, circumscribed median areas where the endoderm and ectoderm are in direct contact, with no intervening mesoderm (see Fig. 3.2). These membranes form the floors of surface depressions known as the *stomodeum* and *proctodeum*. The depressions are deepened by the relatively rapid growth of the surrounding tissue; when the membranes break down the depressions become confluent with the gut, extending it at each end by a short passage lined with ectoderm. The cranial extension forms the larger part of the mouth, the caudal extension the anal canal.

The foregut differentiates to form the pharynx, esophagus, stomach, and first part of the duodenum together with the structures formed by outgrowth from these parts. The midgut forms the remainder of the small intestine, the cecum, and the larger part of the colon. The hindgut forms the distal part of the colon, the rectum, and, after partitioning, part of the urogenital tract.

The Mouth

The stomodeum, carried ventrally in the folding process, comes to lie between the swelling of the forebrain dorsally and that over the developing heart ventrally. The oral membrane soon breaks down, and thereafter it is no longer possible to recognize the extent of the ectodermal contribution to the lining of the mouth.

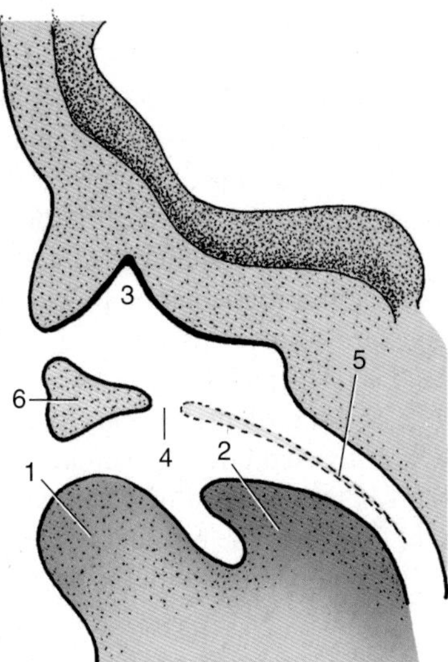

Fig. 3.57 Sagittal section through the nasal and oral cavity of a young embryo. *1,* Lower lip; *2,* tongue; *3,* nasal cavity; *4,* primitive choana (future incisive duct); *5,* position of future secondary palate; *6,* primary palate.

The mouth is built up by the forward growth of certain processes that appear around the margins of the oral plate. Dorsally, a frontal process appears as the result of a spurt in growth of the paraxial mesoderm around the forebrain. Laterally and ventrally, the margin is formed by the mandibular arch, the first of the thickenings (see later) that develop in the mesoderm lateral to the presumptive pharynx.

The frontal process is initially a simple prominence. Soon bilateral thickenings, olfactory placodes, appear in the covering ectoderm immediately bounding the oral depression. These placodes sink below the surface when growth of the surrounding mesoderm throws up a rim around each. The rim has the form of a horseshoe with a ventral interruption, leading to a groove extending to the mouth. The interruption divides the lateral and medial parts of the rim, which are known hereafter as the lateral and medial nasal processes. The mandibular arches also expand and grow toward each other at this time and soon fuse ventral to the oral depression, forming the continuous shelf of the lower jaw and mouth floor. In addition, the upper end of each mandibular arch detaches a maxillary process that extends forward between the frontal and mandibular processes to enclose the mouth laterally. The various swellings gradually merge.

The depressions in which the olfactory placodes are contained originally communicate with the oral cavity, but these connections are lost when the placodes sink more deeply within blind pits, the nasal fossae, that now excavate the upper jaw. The tissue that remains between these pits and the mouth constitutes the primary palate. Communication between nose and mouth is regained when the pits eventually break through into the mouth cavity at two openings known as the *primitive choanae* (Fig. 3.57).

The disruption is considerable, and only the most rostral part of the primary palate survives.

The definitive nasal cavities arise from a fresh subdivision of the temporarily combined nasal and oral spaces. The inner aspect of each maxillary process sends out a flange, the palatine process, which first hangs ventrally to the side of the developing tongue. At a certain stage it undergoes a very rapid reorientation in which it is swung inward and upward to meet its fellow on the other side (Fig. 3.58A and B). The palatine processes fuse with each other, with the residue of the primary palate, and with the lower edge of the septum between the nasal fossae; a horizontal shelf is thus formed between the nasal fossae and the mouth. Fusion of the residual primary palate (the region of the incisive papilla) with the palatine processes is almost complete but leaves open the small passages that become the incisive ducts. The shelf that now divides the nasal and oral cavities constitutes the secondary (definitive) palate, which later differentiates into rostral hard and caudal soft parts. The timing of this process is critical because the stage at which the secondary palate forms is normally soon followed by a marked widening of the head. If reorientation of the palatine processes is delayed, they are too short to bridge the gap and fail to fuse with each other and with the ventral edge of the nasal septum, leaving the secondary palate divided by a median fissure through which the nasal and oral cavities communicate. The consequences of this anomaly (cleft palate) can be severe, not least because of resulting difficulties in feeding from the teat.

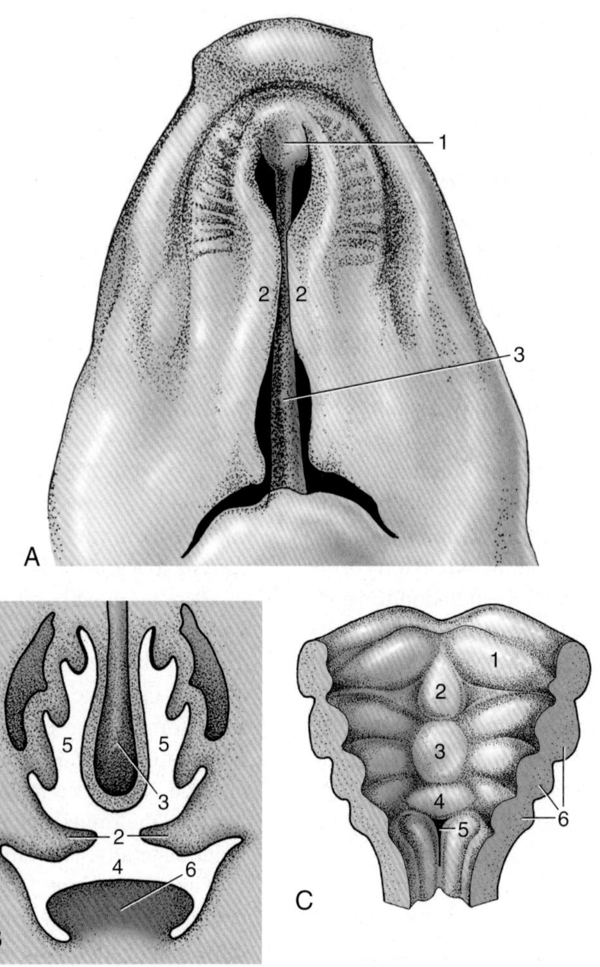

Fig. 3.58 (A) Ventral view of the development of the palate (pig). (B) Transverse section through oral and nasal cavity before closure of the secondary palate. *1,* Primary palate; *2,* palatine processes (secondary palate); *3,* nasal septum; *4,* oral cavity; *5,* nasal cavity; *6,* tongue. (C) Development of the tongue in the floor of the oral cavity. *1,* Distal (lateral) tongue swelling; *2,* median tongue swelling; *3,* proximal tongue swelling; *4,* primordium of epiglottis; *5,* laryngeal entrance; *6,* pharyngeal arches.

The division of the mouth cavity into its vestibular and central parts is foreshadowed by the appearance of ectodermal thickenings that run parallel to the margins of both the maxillary and mandibular processes. These thickenings are soon transformed into grooves, known as labiogingival grooves, as they mark the division of the lips from the outer aspect of the gums. The deepening of the grooves creates and then enlarges the vestibular space. A second, similar formation internal to the labiogingival groove of the mandibular process separates the gum from the tongue now developing in the floor of the mouth.

The salivary glands, both major and minor, are formed from solid outgrowths of epithelium that push into the underlying mesenchyme. These branch repeatedly and become canalized to form both gland acini and ducts. It is tempting to suppose that their sites of origin correspond with the points of entry of the adult ducts; however, some evidence suggests that the openings may be relocated when grooves in the oral epithelium are bridged over, extending the ducts.

The *tongue* develops in the floor of the mouth through a complicated mergence of several swellings (Fig. 3.58C). One, a median (distal) tongue swelling, appears on the pharyngeal floor between the lower ends of the mandibular arches and later fuses with more lateral swellings that appear over the adjacent parts of these arches. A more caudal (proximal) swelling extends from the floor onto the ventral parts of the second, third, and, possibly, fourth pharyngeal arches. The caudal swelling divides as follows: the caudal part becomes the epiglottis, and the rostral part blends with the other contributions to the tongue. The thyroid gland develops from the pharyngeal floor between the median and proximal swellings. The substance of the tongue is supposed to derive mainly from myotomes of occipital somites. It is alleged that material from these myotomes migrates forward under the floor of the mouth, and although the evidence is not wholly convincing, the theory satisfactorily accounts for the innervation of the lingual muscles by the hypoglossal nerve, the nerve specific to the occipital somites. The sensory supply to the lingual epithelium involves the mandibular, fascial, glossopharyngeal, and vagus nerves, which are the nerves associated with the first, second, third, and fourth arches, respectively. The separation of the tongue from the floor is gradual. It is more complete for the part that forms the body than for that that forms the root.

The first indications of the *teeth* are ribbon-like thickenings of epithelium internal to the labiogingival thickenings. The thickenings extend as plates, dental laminae, into the subjacent mesenchyme (Fig. 3.59); soon thereafter a linear series of knoblike swellings buds from the deep margin of each. The swellings represent the enamel organs of the temporary teeth, and their number corresponds to the dental formula of the species. Occasionally disparity occurs when primordia appear (and possibly develop quite far) for teeth that later regress without erupting. The upper incisors of ruminants are examples of teeth whose development is aborted in this way.

The mesenchyme condenses against the free surfaces of each bud. The mesenchyme, now known as the *dental papilla,* fills the depression created by the invagination of the bud. The whole tooth germ, the enamel organ together with the dental papilla, is enclosed by a mesenchymal thickening that merges with the papilla at its base, forming the dental sac or follicle.

The enamel organ consists of an inner epithelium (over the concave surface applied to the dental papilla), an outer epithelium (over the convex surface facing the dental follicle), and an intervening sparsely cellular tissue (enamel reticulum) (see Fig. 3.59). The cells of the inner dental epithelium are known as *ameloblasts* because they produce enamel. Enamel formation begins over the center of the crown but soon spreads outward from this focus. As the

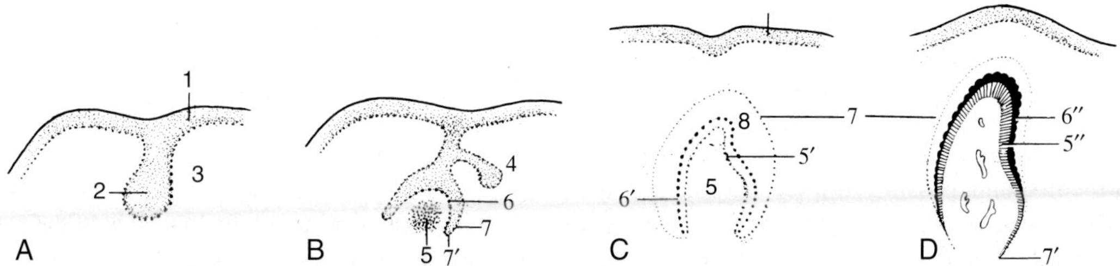

Fig. 3.59 (A) Development of dental plate. (B) Development of an enamel organ. (C) Enamel organ. (D) Deciduous tooth before eruption. *1,* Epithelium of oral cavity; *2,* dental plate; *3,* mesenchyme; *4,* bud of a permanent tooth; *5,* dental papilla; *5′,* odontoblasts (differentiated from the outer cell layer of the papilla); *5″,* dentin; *6,* inner dental epithelium (future ameloblasts); *6′,* ameloblasts; *6″,* enamel; *7,* outer dental epithelium; *7′,* transition of inner and outer dental epithelia (where root formation occurs); *8,* enamel reticulum.

layer thickens, the ameloblasts retreat in a centrifugal direction until finally they meet and fuse with the outer dental epithelium to form an epithelial cuticle over the crown.

Meanwhile, certain cells of the mesodermal papilla have become arranged in a sheet facing the ameloblasts. Because they produce dentin, they are known as *odontoblasts*. The first dentin also appears toward the center of the crown, a little later than the first deposition of enamel. Thereafter dentin deposition also spreads out in all directions. As the layer thickens the odontoblasts withdraw in a centripetal direction, and when dentin production has ceased, they remain as a covering to the pulp, which is the surviving less differentiated portion of the original papilla.

The root of the tooth is initially ensheathed by a prolongation of the enamel organ not producing enamel. The sheath later breaks down when the follicular tissue produces cement to encase the dentin of the root.

After the enamel organs of the temporary teeth have appeared, the dental lamina undergoes extensive destruction. However, its free edge remains to produce a second crop of buds, the enamel organs of the replacement teeth; these buds remain dormant until activated to replicate the sequence that created the temporary teeth.

The Pharynx

Many details of the development of the pharyngeal region are more appropriately considered in Chapters 2 and 6. The pharynx is initially flattened dorsoventrally and widest immediately behind the oral plate, but the initial form is altered by the unequal growth of the mesoderm flanking the endodermal tube (Fig. 3.60). This mesoderm forms serial thickenings, the pharyngeal (branchial) arches, which protrude into the pharyngeal lumen and bulge on the surface of the neck. The internal modeling of the lumen defines a series of pouches with which corresponding grooves coincide externally (see Fig. 3.60). The number of arches (and therefore of pouches) is disputed. It is most commonly assumed that five arches exist, representing the first four and the sixth of the somewhat longer series found in other vertebrates. Each arch develops an internal skeleton and musculature with which a particular cranial nerve is associated; their fates are tabulated elsewhere (p. 52). Each pouch has a specific fate (see Fig. 6.5). The features of immediate interest include the contributions of the first and, possibly, the second pouches to the cavity of the middle ear, which is a fate revealed in the adult by the site of entry of the auditory tube into the nasopharynx. The ventral part of the second pouch forms the tonsillar sinus, a landmark providing some clue to the former position of the oral plate.

The outgrowth of the lower respiratory tract at the caudal limit of the pharynx is considered in the following chapter.

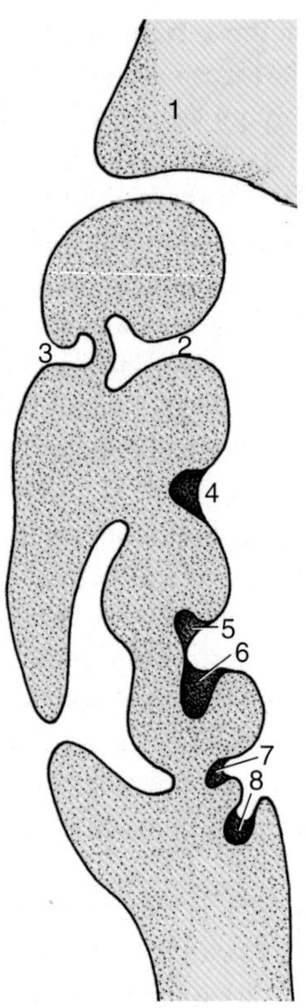

Fig. 3.60 Dorsal section of the left side of the pharynx showing the development of the pharyngeal arches and pouches. *1,* Maxillary process; *2,* pharyngotympanic tube (future auditory tube); *3,* external auditory meatus; *4,* palatine tonsil (in tonsillar sinus); *5,* parathyroid gland III; *6,* thymus; *7,* parathyroid gland IV; *8,* ultimobranchial body.

The Caudal Part of the Foregut

A fusiform enlargement identifies the stomach at an early stage. The foregut between this enlargement and the pharynx becomes the esophagus, which is initially very short but elongates as the heart descends from the neck into the thorax. The esophagus is involved in the origin of the lower respiratory tract (p. 156) but, apart from this, presents little of interest. At one stage, the proliferation of the endodermal lining obstructs the lumen, but the passage is later restored.

The development of the stomach involves displacement, reorientation, and differential enlargement. The displacement carries it to a position ventral to the caudal thoracic segments. Reorientation appears to involve rotations about two axes. Rotation about the long axis of the stomach spindle carries the originally dorsal aspect to the left, where it is later distinguished as the greater curvature. The dorsal mesogastrium, which becomes the greater omentum, shares in the process. Rotation about a vertical axis swings the cranial (cardiac) extremity to the left and the caudal (pyloric) one to the right (Fig. 3.61). In most species the most conspicuous change in shape is an asymmetrical

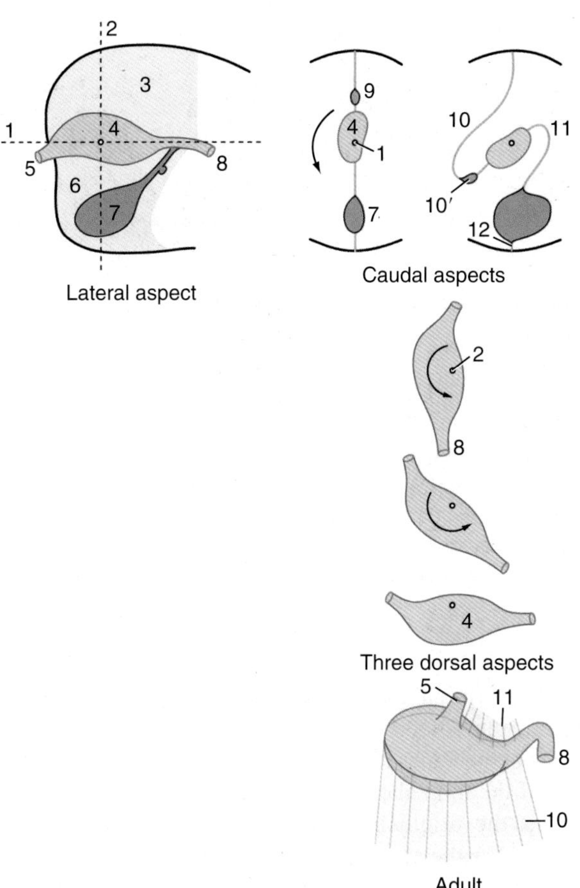

Fig. 3.61 The reorientation of the developing simple stomach. It rotates counterclockwise (as seen from behind) around a longitudinal axis (caudal aspects *[1]*) and continues counterclockwise (as seen from above) around a dorsoventral axis (three dorsal aspects *[2]*). *1,* Longitudinal axis; *2,* dorsoventral (vertical) axis; *3,* dorsal mesogastrium; *4,* stomach primordium; *5,* esophagus; *6,* ventral mesogastrium; *7,* developing liver; *8,* duodenum; *9,* developing spleen; *10,* greater omentum; *10′,* omental bursa; *11,* lesser omentum; *12,* developing ligaments of the liver.

enlargement to the left of the cardia that produces the fundus; a much more radical reshaping is required in ruminants. In the human fetus the gastric glands are capable of secretion by midterm.

The short portion of foregut between the gastric spindle and the midgut forms the initial part of the duodenum, which terminates at the entrance of the bile and pancreatic ducts.

The Liver and Pancreas

The liver appears as an endodermal diverticulum at the junction of the foregut and midgut. It quickly divides into a cranial branch, which forms the gland tissue and hepatic ducts, and a caudal branch, which forms the gallbladder and cystic duct (Fig. 3.62).

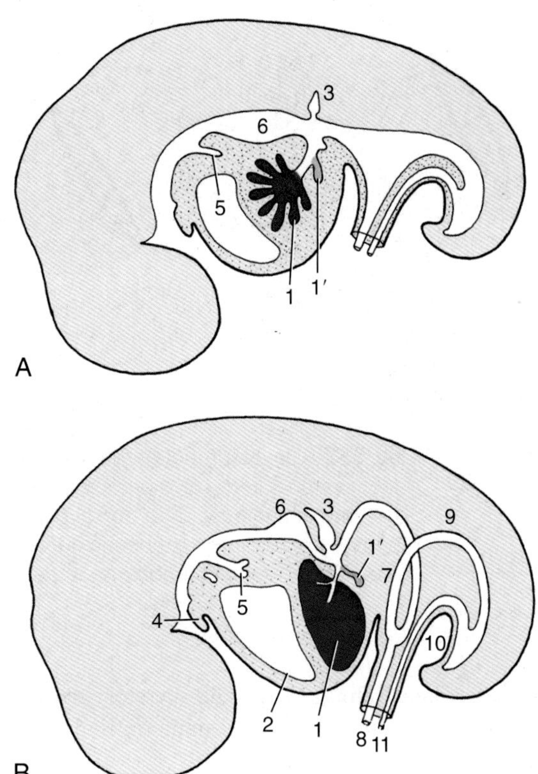

Fig. 3.62 Development of the liver. (A) Early development: a cranial branch *(1)* of the endodermal diverticulum invades the septum transversum; a caudal branch *(1′)* forms the gallbladder and cystic duct. (B) A later stage, in which the developing liver expands caudally into the abdominal cavity. *1,* liver; *1′,* gallbladder; *2,* pericardium and heart; *3,* dorsal primordium of pancreas; *4,* tongue; *5,* tracheobronchial diverticulum; *6,* stomach; *7,* loop of midgut; *8,* vitelline duct; *9,* hindgut; *10,* cloacal membrane; *11,* allantoic stalk.

The cranial branch extends finger-like processes into the splanchnic mesoderm of the adjacent septum transversum, carried here with the formation of the head fold. As the processes penetrate the mesoderm, they engage with the vitelloumbilical system of veins, which arrive here from the extraembryonic membranes. Very soon a three-dimensional spongework of hepatic cell-cords and plates is formed, surrounded on all sides by thin-walled blood vessels, which is a precocious realization of the adult arrangement. Attenuation of the connection between the liver and the gut forms the lesser omentum.

The growth of the liver, extremely rapid in younger embryos, is a major factor in the temporary herniation of the midgut (see later). Although its growth slows later, the liver remains disproportionately large (in comparison with that in the adult) until well after birth. One relevant factor is the exercise of an erythropoietic activity before

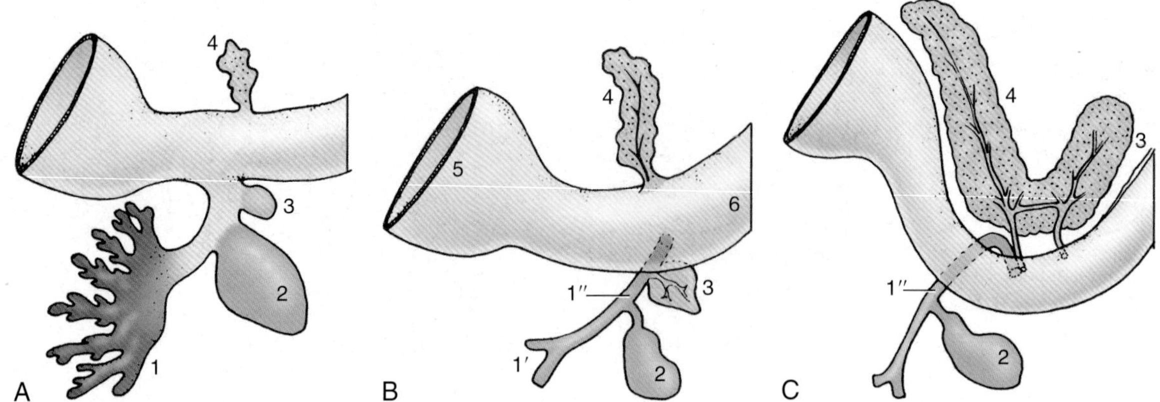

Fig. 3.63 Development of the pancreas. (A) Early stage. (B) A later stage showing separate duct systems in the two primordia. (C) The two primordia have fused after the migration of the ventral pancreas. The dorsal pancreas now drains mainly via the ventral duct system. *1,* Liver primordium; *1′,* hepatic ducts; *1″,* bile duct; *2,* gallbladder; *3,* ventral primordium of pancreas; *4,* dorsal primordium of pancreas; *5,* stomach; *6,* duodenum.

birth that is later relinquished. The secretory and metabolic functions are established by midterm in the human fetus.

The pancreas arises from the same portion of the foregut as the liver. There are initially two primordia: one is dorsal and the second is ventral and associated with the hepatic outgrowth (Fig. 3.63). These later fuse, allowing combination of the two duct systems, following which one or the other may lose its connection with the gut. The islet tissue develops by budding from the ducts. Both endocrine and exocrine components are competent well before birth.

The celiac artery is associated with the postpharyngeal part of the foregut.

THE MIDGUT

The midgut forms the intestine, from the entry of the bile duct to the junction of the transverse and descending parts of the colon. Its initial wide connection with the yolk sac is quickly lost.

The early growth of the midgut is very rapid, causing it to hang in a loop from an elongated mesentery in which the midgut (cranial mesenteric) artery runs. The expanding liver claims so large a part of the abdominal cavity that insufficient room remains for the intestine. The long mesentery then permits the midgut to slip out of the abdominal cavity into the umbilical cord, a process known as *physiologic herniation,* where growth continues. The cranial limb of the herniated loop becomes the small intestine. The appearance of a diverticulum, the future cecum, indicates the division of the caudal limb into the terminal part of the small intestine and the initial part of the colon. The cranial limb grows more rapidly and soon becomes much coiled. The key event is the rotation of the loop about the arterial axis (Fig. 3.64), which carries the originally caudal limb forward on the left, then across the abdomen before it passes caudally on the right side, completing a rotation through approximately 270 degrees. This rotation, clockwise when viewed from above, brings the intestines more or less into their adult disposition when they are returned to the abdomen (Fig. 3.65). The return is possible because the rate of liver increase slows and falls behind the general growth of the embryo. The final arrangement may depend on local shortenings of the mesentery and fusions of apposed peritoneum-clad surfaces.

The Hindgut

The hindgut develops into the descending colon and the rectum, parts supplied by the caudal mesenteric artery in the adult. Initially the gut ends blindly against the cloacal plate. Except in the horse and ruminants, in which the descending colon shows a secondary increase in length, significant changes affect only the terminal part of the hindgut. A bud, the allantois, grows from its ventral aspect toward and through the umbilical opening in the abdominal wall; once outside the embryo it enlarges to form the capacious allantoic sac (see Fig. 5.66). A wedge of tissue (urorectal septum) enlarging in the angle between the gut and this diverticulum thrusts toward the cloacal membrane (Fig. 3.66). When it meets the membrane, the wedge divides the gut into two separate tubes: the dorsal one is continuous with the descending colon, and the

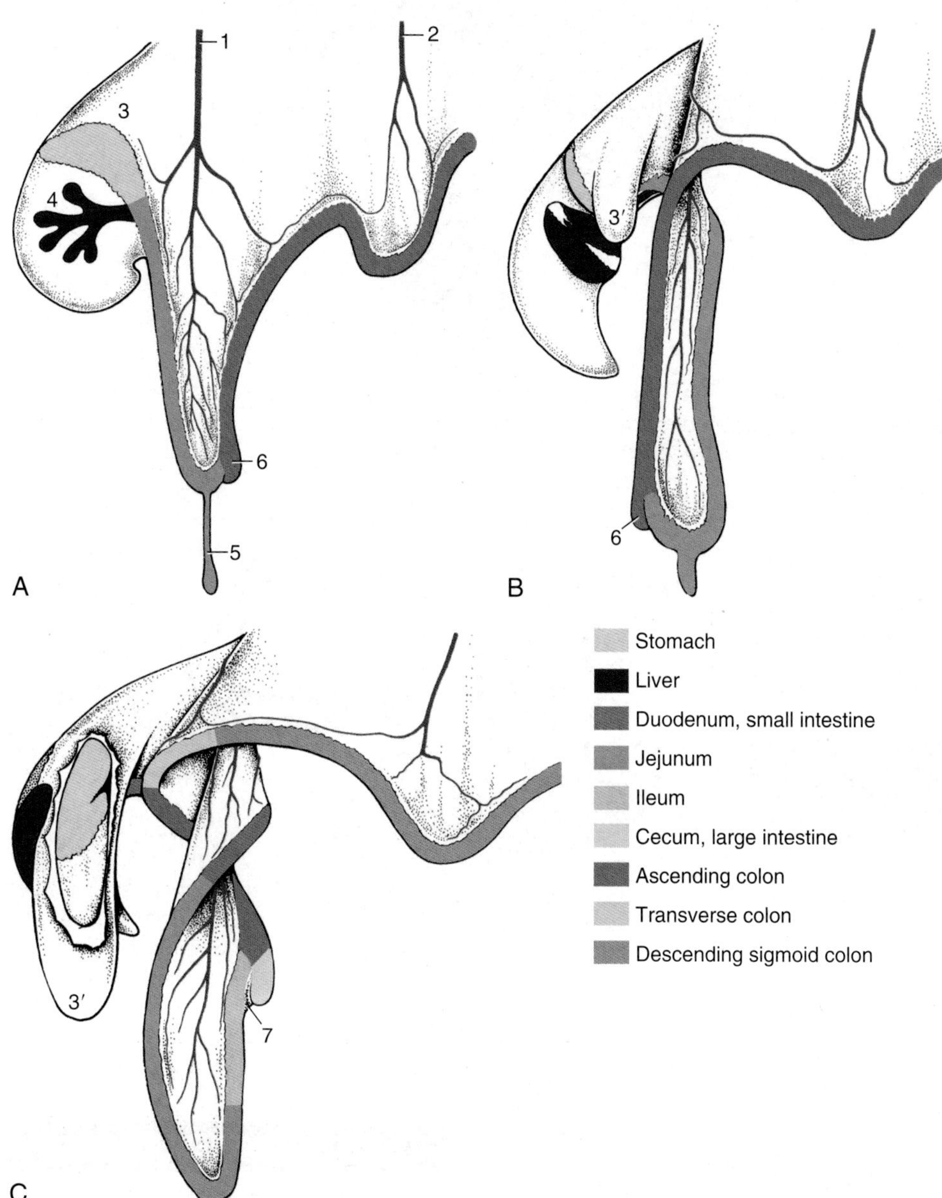

Fig. 3.64 (A to C) Three stages in the growth and rotation of the canine midgut, in left lateral views. *1,* Cranial mesenteric artery; *2,* caudal mesenteric artery; *3,* dorsal mesogastrium; *3′,* greater omentum, fenestrated in (C) to expose stomach; *4,* ventral mesogastrium with developing liver; *5,* vitelline duct; *6,* cecal primordium; *7,* ileocecal fold.

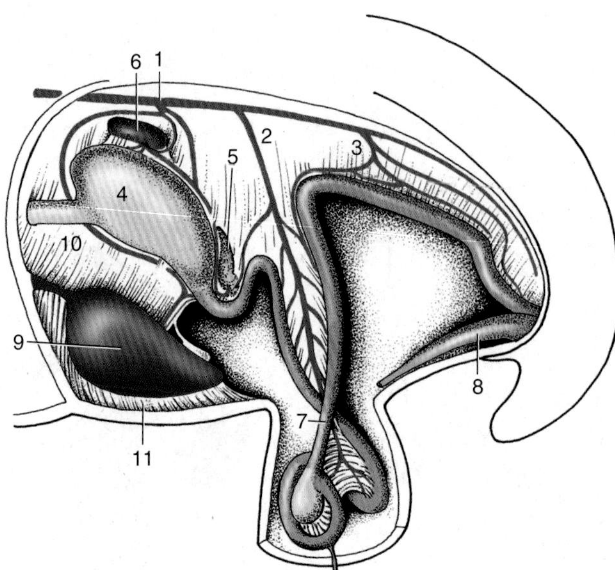

Fig. 3.65 Development of the intestinal tract during the rotation process. The midgut loop is herniated into the extraembryonic celom. *1,* Celiac artery; *2,* cranial mesenteric artery; *3,* caudal mesenteric artery; *4,* stomach; *5,* pancreas; *6,* spleen; *7,* loop of midgut; *8,* bladder expansion of the urogenital sinus; *9,* liver; *10,* lesser omentum; *11,* falciform ligament.

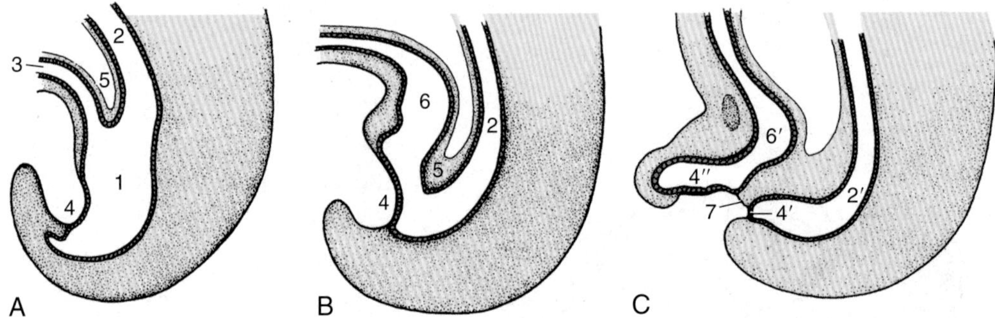

Fig. 3.66 Division of the distal part of the hindgut into the rectum and urogenital sinus. (A) Formation of the allantois and beginning of the caudal extension of the urorectal septum *(5).* (B) The urorectal septum now approaches the cloacal membrane. (C) Complete division of the urogenital sinus and anorectal canal. *1,* Cloaca; *2,* hindgut; *2′,* anorectal canal; *3,* allantois; *4,* cloacal membrane; *4′,* anal membrane; *4″,* urogenital membrane; *5,* urorectal septum; *6,* primitive urogenital sinus; *6′,* urogenital sinus; *7,* tissue bridge ventral to future anus.

ventral one is continuous with the allantois and destined to form the lower urogenital tract. Meanwhile, proliferation of mesoderm beneath the ectoderm around the proctodeum has deepened the pit, which is added to the gut upon breakdown of the dorsal part (anal membrane) of the cloacal membrane. The result is the anal canal leading to the exterior.

COMPREHENSION CHECK

Using an embryologic framework, discuss the in vivo arrangement of the digestive tract. Also, demonstrate an understanding of the projections of various digestive organs on the body surface.

The Respiratory Apparatus

4

The essential organs of respiration are the lungs. The ancillary organs include the airways, which lead air to and from the lungs for gas exchange with bloodstream. The nose is also included, although it may alternatively be considered among the organs of special sense because it evolved as the organ of olfaction. The pharynx, in which the air and food streams cross, is more conveniently considered among the digestive organs, although its upper part (nasopharynx) is purely an airway. A short account of the development follows the description of the adult anatomy.

THE NOSE

The nose* (nasus) in the broad sense comprises the external nose, the paired nasal cavities, and the paranasal sinuses. A case may be argued for also including the nasopharynx.

The true extent of the external nose is not readily apparent because it lies within general features of the muzzle; its margins correspond with the cartilaginous and flexible skeleton of the muzzle (Fig. 4.1). The external nose is divided internally into two cavities, the nasal vestibules, each of which is entered through a nostril and leads through a region of constriction to the much larger nasal cavity placed beyond. The form and size of the nostrils, their orientation, and the nature of the surrounding integument all show considerable species differences. The integument around the nostrils, which is naked and sharply demarcated from the unmodified skin in all domestic species other than the horse, is known as the nasal (carnivores, small ruminants), nasolabial (cattle), or rostral (pigs) plate. The nasal plate may be divided by a median groove or philtrum (Fig. 4.1/*2*). The plate is moist to touch because of the secretions of the underlying glands in cattle and pigs and from secretions of the nasal mucosa, principally the lateral nasal glands, in dogs.

Many cartilages support and shape the external nose. The rostral part of nasal septum creates the right and left vestibules and includes a small bone (os rostrale) in the pig. Other cartilages, such as alar cartilage, attach to the free edges of the septum, support the dorsal and lateral margins, and determine the form of the opening of the nostrils. For example, the large alar cartilage creates the unique comma form of the equine nostril, which is divided into a ventral part, the so-called true nostril leading to the nasal cavity, and a dorsal part, the false nostril leading to a skin-lined diverticulum occupying the nasoincisive notch (see Fig. 18.3). The nostril is round in the pig, but in most other species it is prolonged laterally by a slitlike extension. The form of the nostril may be altered actively by the actions of facial muscles on the lateral "wing" (ala) or passively by the increased airflow in strenuous breathing or sniffing. These changes can be very pronounced in the horse, leading to compression and almost complete obliteration of the diverticulum.

The integument meets with the mucosa in the vestibule at a sharply defined line. Near this line the long ducts of the serous lateral glands open along with the prominent opening of the nasolacrimal (tear) duct on the vestibule floor in the horse; the opening is less easily found in other species, either because the tissues are less pliant (cattle) or because it is placed more deeply (dog). This arrangement aids humidification of the incoming air.

The *nasal cavities* occupy a large part of the face and extend caudally up to the transverse bony septum at the rostral end of the cranial cavity (Fig. 4.2). The use of conformation of the head to estimate the cavities' size is grossly misleading because several features greatly reduce the extent of the cavities to below expectation. First, certain bones bounding the cavity are thickened by air spaces (paranasal sinuses) that communicate with the cavity but do not form part of it. Second, the embedded portions of the upper cheek teeth occupy a surprising amount of space, especially in the horse. Third, the very delicate mucosa-covered turbinate bones (conchae) project into the interior of the cavities from the dorsal and lateral walls. And last, the walls are covered by a mucosa locally thickened by vascular plexuses (Figs. 4.3–4.5).

The right and left cavities are divided by the nasal septum, which is largely cartilaginous but is ossified in its most caudal part (the perpendicular plate of the ethmoid bone). The septum meets the upper surface of the hard palate, which separates the nasal and mouth cavities, but the details vary greatly among species (Fig. 4.5). In the horse the septum meets the whole length of the hard palate so that each nasal cavity communicates with the pharynx through a separate opening (choana) (see Fig. 18.11). In other species (e.g., ox, dog) the caudal part of the septum fails to meet the palate, and a single opening is shared by the two sides (Figs. 4.4/*7* and 25.9).

The *conchae,* which are coiled fragile laminae that intrude on the cavity, have a complicated and variable pattern. Classified by topography (and not by morphology),

*The Greek word for nose, *rhin*, provides the stem for many medical terms, for example, *rhinitis*.

they comprise a caudal system (of ethmoidal conchae) constituting the lateral mass or labyrinth of the ethmoid bone and a rostral (nasal) system in which large dorsal and ventral (and a much smaller middle) conchae predominate (see Figs. 4.2 and 25.9). The numerous ethmoidal conchae are separated by narrow clefts (ethmoidal meatuses) and have a highly complicated pattern in species with a sharp sense of smell (Fig. 4.4/*5* and *6*). The dorsal and ventral nasal conchae create meatuses of the middle and more rostral parts of the cavity. The form of the conchae varies with the species and the location. Rostrally, the lamina does not recurve to meet itself and thus bounds a recess of the nasal cavity; more caudally the coil meets itself or the lateral nasal wall to enclose a space that is part of the paranasal sinus system. The major conchae define dorsal, middle, and ventral meatuses branching from a common meatus against the septum, and the arrangement looks like the letter E in transverse section (Fig. 4.5). The dorsal meatus leads directly to the fundus of the nasal cavity and presents air to the olfactory mucosa. The middle meatus usually gives access to the sinus system. The ventral and common meatuses provide the principal airway leading to the pharynx. The stomach tube is passed through the wide space at the junction of the meatuses.

The nasal mucosa blends with the underlying periosteum. In some parts the mucosa is thin, but elsewhere, and especially ventrally, it is much thickened by the inclusion of cavernous blood spaces that make it a semi-erectile tissue (Fig. 4.5/*8*). The mucosa may become congested and thicker in conditions such as head cold so as to greatly impede the airflow and resulting in stuffiness.

Apart from olfaction, the nasal cavity warms the air passing over the highly vascular mucosa, humidified by the vapors of tears and serous nasal secretions, and cleans by interaction with the mucus. The mucous glands create a carpet of mucus on nasal mucosa that entraps particles in the incoming air. The mucous carpet is moved toward the pharynx by the ciliary action of the lining epithelium and is then swallowed. The human species may swallow as much as half a liter of mucus unconsciously each day.

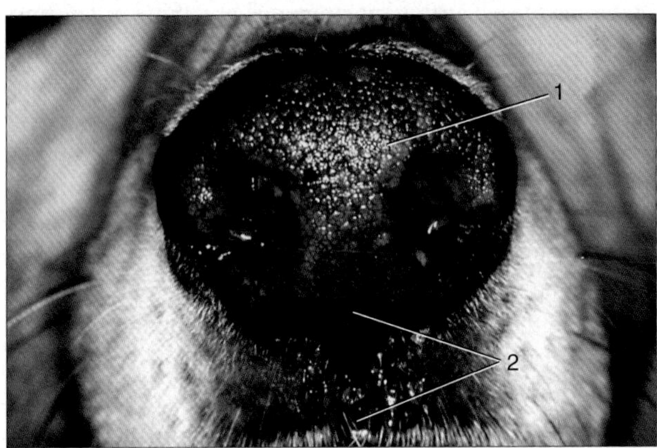

Fig. 4.1 The canine muzzle. *1,* Nasal plate; *2,* philtrum.

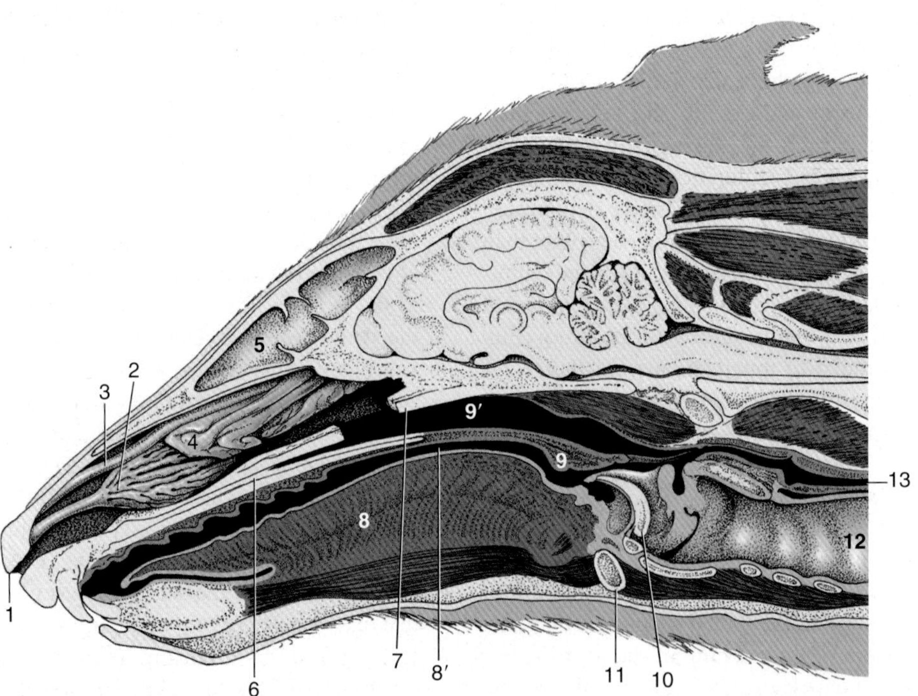

Fig. 4.2 Paramedian section of the canine head; the nasal septum has been removed. *1,* Right nostril; *2,* ventral nasal concha; *3,* dorsal nasal concha; *4,* ethmoidal conchae; *5,* frontal sinus; *6,* hard palate; *7,* vomer, resected; *8,* tongue; *8′,* oropharynx; *9,* soft palate; *9′,* nasopharynx; *10,* epiglottis; *11,* basihyoid; *12,* trachea; *13,* esophagus.

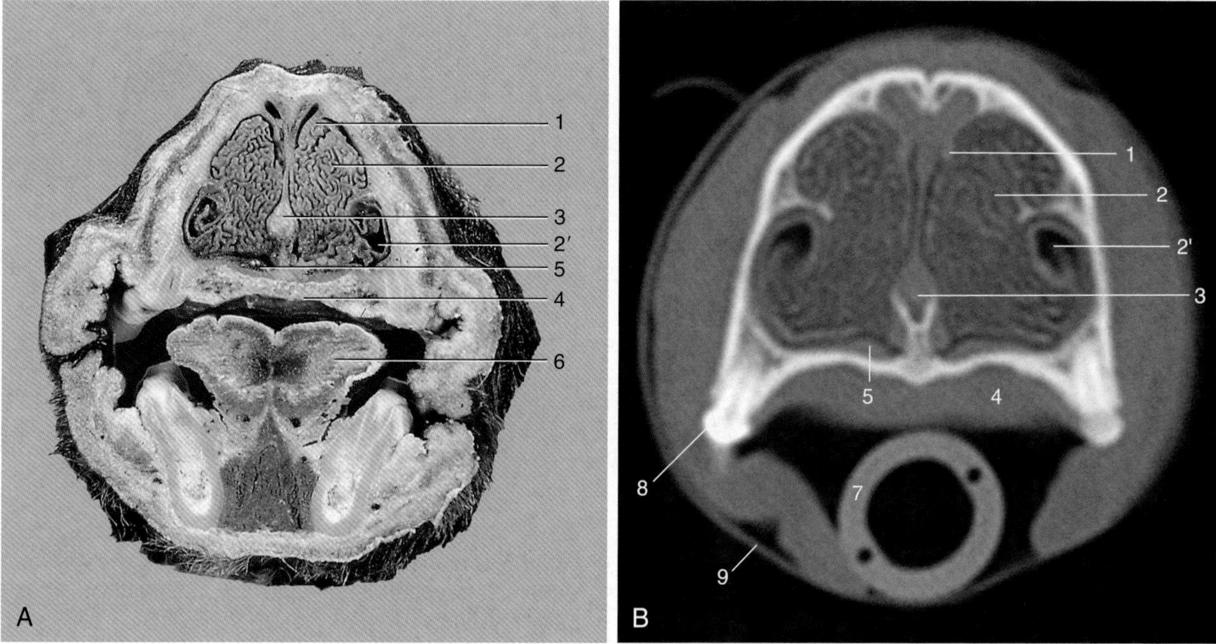

Fig. 4.3 (A) Transverse section of the canine head at the level of P2. (B) Computed tomography (CT) scan taken at the same level but without the tongue and structures of the lower jaw. *1,* Dorsal concha; *2,* ventral concha; *2′,* recess of ventral concha; *3,* nasal septum; *4,* hard palate; *5,* venous plexus in nasal mucosa; *6,* tongue; *7,* endotracheal tube; *8,* P2; *9,* tape to keep endotracheal tube against hard palate during CT procedure.

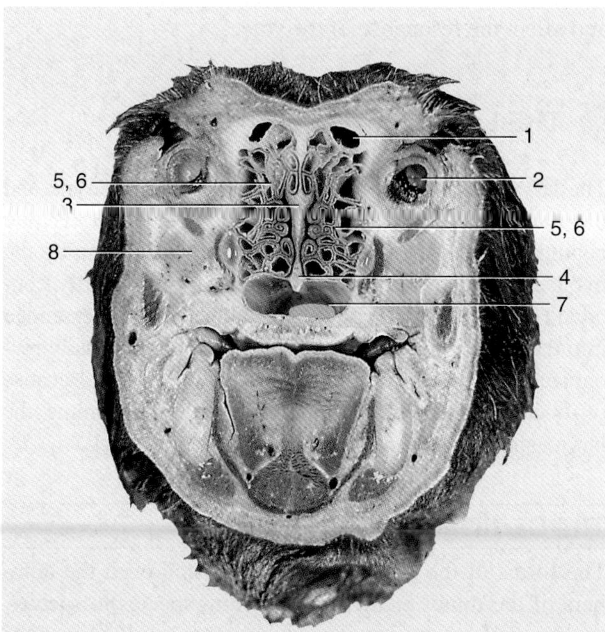

Fig. 4.4 Transverse section of the canine head at the level of the eyeball. *1,* Frontal sinus; *2,* eyeball; *3,* ethmoid bone; *4,* vomer; *5* and *6,* ethmoidal conchae; *7,* choana; *8,* zygomatic gland.

The paranasal sinuses are diverticula of the nasal cavity that develop postnatally through the separation of the inner and outer tables of the skull bones (Fig. 4.6). These processes alter the conformation of the head, which is especially striking in pigs and cattle (Figs. 4.7 and 25.11) because certain sinuses do extend dorsal and even caudal to the cranial cavity. The narrow openings of the sinuses slow the exchange of the air with the nasal cavity and are also prone to blockage by congested mucosa in inflammation. Because no all the sinuses are of equal clinical importance, the surface projections of only those commonly involved in disease are considered in the topographical chapters.

All species have *frontal and maxillary sinus systems,* neither communicating with its contralateral counterpart. The frontal system consists of one or more spaces within the bones at the border between the nasal and cranial cavities. In most species the various frontal compartments open separately into the ethmoidal meatuses in the nasal fundus, but in the horse the frontal sinus communicates with the nasal cavity indirectly via the caudal maxillary sinus.

The *maxillary sinus system* occupies the caudolateral part of the upper jaw, above the caudal cheek teeth. Its

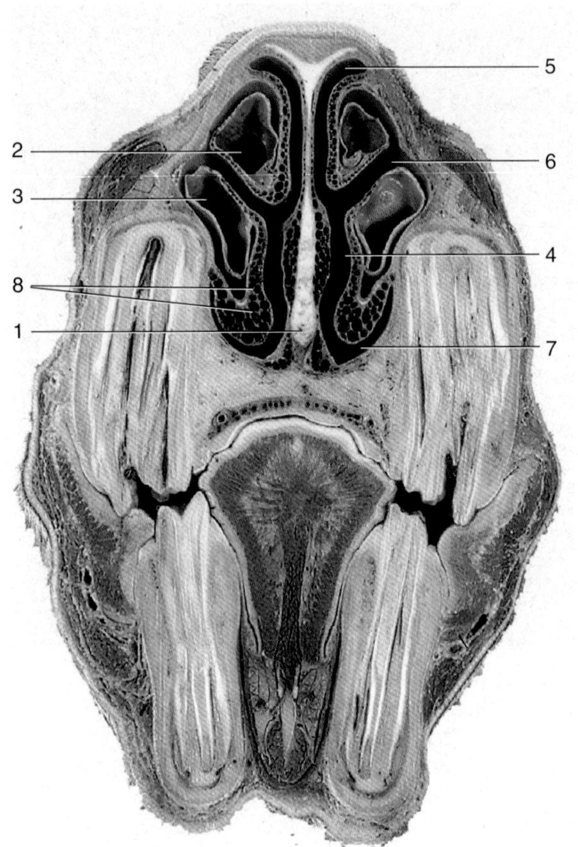

Fig. 4.5 Transverse section of the equine head at the level of P4. *1*, Nasal septum; *2*, dorsal concha; *3*, ventral concha; *4*, common meatus; *5*, dorsal meatus; *6*, middle meatus; *7*, ventral meatus; *8*, venous plexus in nasal mucosa.

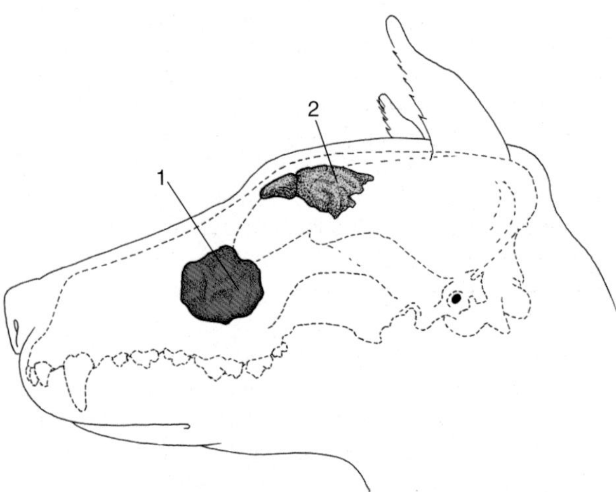

Fig. 4.6 Paranasal sinuses in the dog. *1*, Maxillary recess; *2*, frontal sinus.

extensions into the hard palate, the sphenoid bones, the medial aspect of the orbit, and the ventral concha seen in some species are described as separate sinuses or as diverticula. The horse's maxillary sinus has caudal and rostral parts that are connected to the middle nasal meatus. In the dog the maxillary cavity communicates freely with the cavity of the nose and is known as the *maxillary recess*.

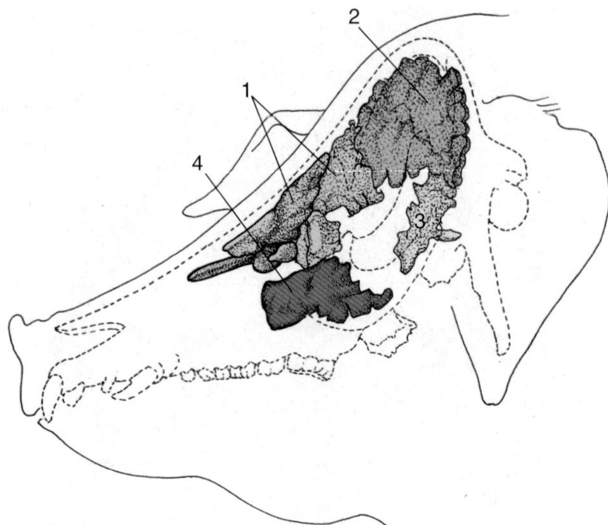

Fig. 4.7 Paranasal sinuses in the pig. *1*, Rostral frontal sinus; *2*, caudal frontal sinus; *3*, sphenoidal sinus; *4*, maxillary sinus.

The function of the sinuses is obscure, but they offer some thermal and mechanical protection to the orbit and nasal and cranial cavities, enlarge the skull areas available for muscular attachment without unduly increasing weight, and affect the resonance of the voice.

THE LARYNX

The larynx forms the connection between the pharynx and the tracheobronchial tree. It lies below the pharynx and behind the mouth, suspended from the cranial base by the hyoid apparatus. In most species the larynx is partly contained between the rami of the mandible and partly extended into the neck, where its cartilaginous skeleton is easily recognized on palpation of the living animal (Fig. 4.8). Because of its connection with the tongue and hyoid apparatus, the larynx shifts its position when the animal swallows.

The Cartilages

The forms of the laryngeal cartilages, and even the numbers of the minor elements, vary from species to species, but few differences are of great practical significance. The major, consistently present cartilages comprise the median epiglottic, thyroid, and cricoid cartilages and the paired arytenoid cartilages (Figs. 4.9 and 4.10).

The *epiglottic cartilage* is most rostral. It consists of a small stalk and a large leaflike blade. The stalk is embedded between the root of the tongue, the basihyoid, and the body

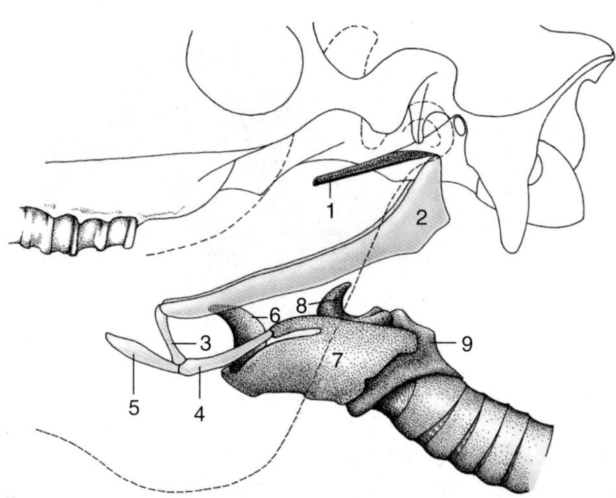

Fig. 4.8 Hyoid apparatus suspending the larynx from the base of the skull (horse). The *broken line* indicates the mandible. *1,* Cartilage of auditory tube; *2,* stylohyoid; *3,* keratohyoid; *4,* thyrohyoid; *5,* lingual process of basihyoid; *6,* epiglottic cartilage; *7,* thyroid cartilage; *8,* arytenoid cartilage; *9,* cricoid cartilage.

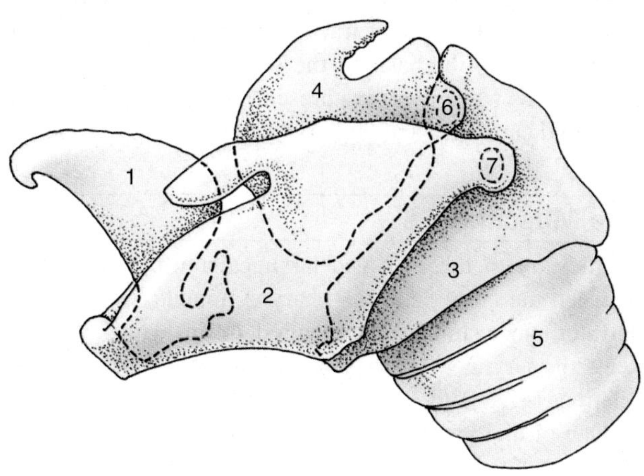

Fig. 4.9 Lateral view of the equine laryngeal skeleton. The outlines of those parts of the cartilages that are covered by others are indicated by broken lines. *1,* Epiglottic cartilage; *2,* thyroid cartilage; *3,* cricoid cartilage; *4,* arytenoid cartilage; *5,* trachea; *6,* cricoarytenoid joint; *7,* cricothyroid joint.

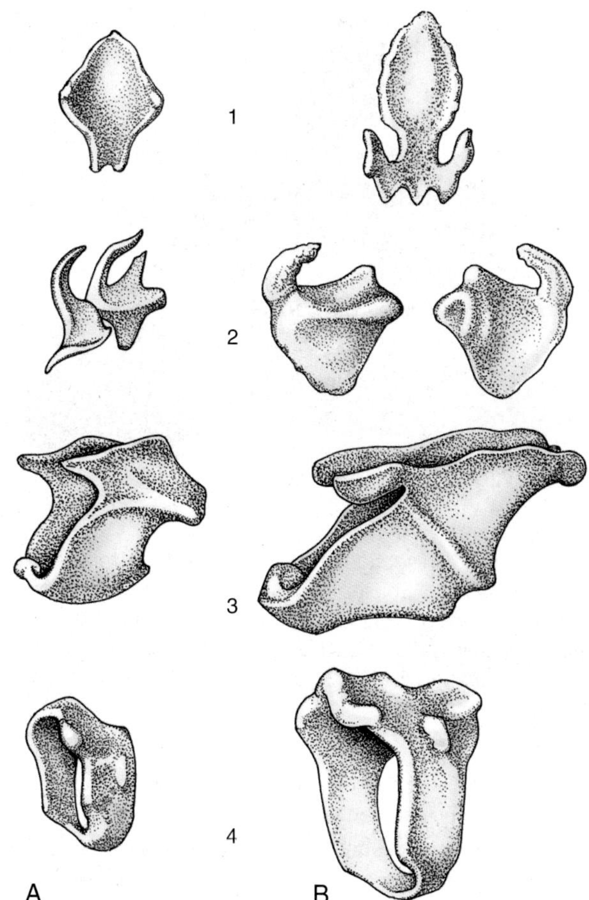

Fig. 4.10 Laryngeal cartilages of (A) the dog and (B) the horse. *1,* Epiglottic cartilage; *2,* arytenoid cartilage; *3,* thyroid cartilage; *4,* cricoid cartilage.

of the thyroid cartilage and is attached to all of these structures. At rest, the blade inclines dorsorostrally behind the soft palate (the retrovelar position), but it may be tilted backward to partially cover the entrance to the larynx when the animal swallows. It is composed of elastic cartilage and is flexible.

The *thyroid cartilage,* the largest of the series, partly encloses the cricoid and arytenoid cartilages. It consists of two lateral plates that fuse to a varying degree ventrally and form a major part of the laryngeal floor (Fig. 4.10/*3*). The body formed by this ventral fusion is least extensive in the horse, in which a large, forward-pointing notch provides a convenient route of entry for laryngeal surgery. The most rostral part of the body is generally thickened and corresponds to the "Adam's apple," which is more salient in the human than in domestic species. The rostral and caudal extremities of the dorsal edge of each lamina articulate with the thyrohyoid cartilage and the arch of the cricoid cartilage, respectively. The thyroid cartilage is hyaline and so may become more brittle with age because of focal calcification and ossification.

The *cricoid cartilage* is fashioned like a signet ring, consisting of an expanded dorsal "seal" (lamina) and a narrower ventral arch (Fig. 4.10/*4*). The dorsal part carries a median crest and, on its rostral rim, two facets for the arytenoid cartilages. The arch carries a facet on each side for articulation with the thyroid cartilage. The cricoid cartilage is also hyaline and subject to the aging process.

The *arytenoid cartilages* have a very irregular form best described as pyramidal (Fig. 4.10/*2*). The details are of little importance, so it is sufficient to recognize only a few features. A caudal facet articulates with the rostral margin of the cricoid lamina, and from it radiate (1) a vocal process that projects ventrally into the laryngeal lumen, and to which the vocal fold attaches; (2) a muscular process that extends laterally; and (3) a corniculate process that extends

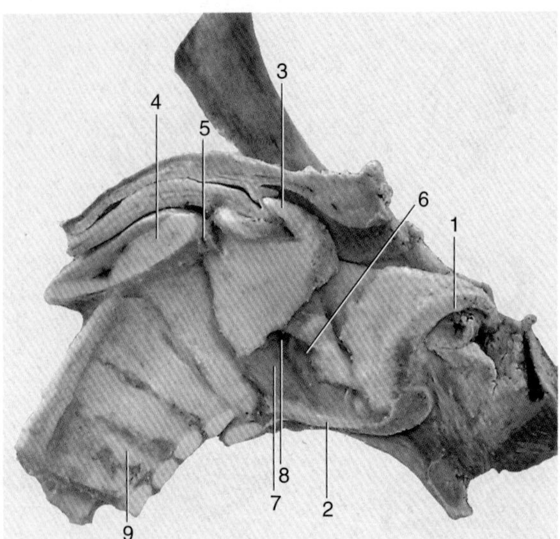

Fig. 4.11 Median section of the equine larynx after removal of the mucosa. *1,* Epiglottic cartilage; *2,* sectioned body of thyroid cartilage; *3,* corniculate process of arytenoid cartilage; *4,* sectioned lamina of cricoid cartilage; *5,* cricoarytenoid joint; *6,* ventricularis; *7,* vocalis; *8,* laryngeal ventricle; *9,* tracheal rings.

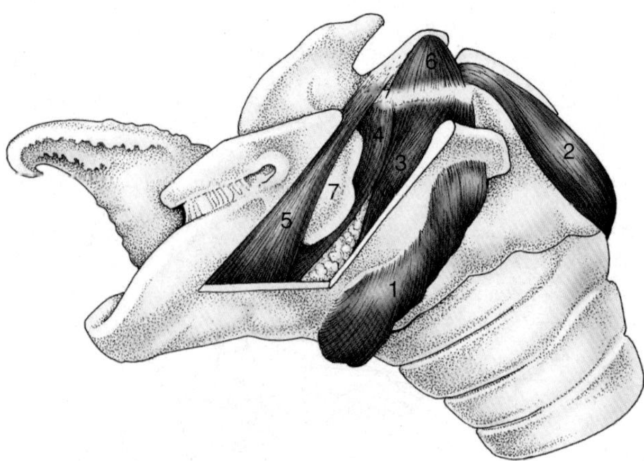

Fig. 4.12 Intrinsic muscles of the equine larynx. *1,* Cricothyroideus; *2,* cricoarytenoideus dorsalis; *3,* cricoarytenoideus lateralis; *4,* vocalis; *5,* ventricularis (*4* and *5* together: thyroarytenoideus); *6,* arytenoideus transversus; *7,* laryngeal ventricle.

dorsomedially, forming the caudal margin of the laryngeal entrance with its fellow of the other side. The arytenoid cartilage is mainly hyaline, but the *corniculate process* is elastic.

Among the smaller and less prominent cartilages are the elastic *cuneiform processes* that support mucosal folds passing from the epiglottis to the arytenoids. These processes do not occur in all species, and when present, they may be free or fused with the epiglottis or with the arytenoid cartilages. A discrete nodule of hyaline cartilage, the *interarytenoid cartilage,* may be found between the arytenoid cartilages dorsally.

The Articulations, Ligaments, and Membranes

In most mammals a synovial articulation is present between the thyrohyoid cartilage and the dorsorostral angle of the thyroid cartilage. Rotation occurs about a transverse axis common to the right and left joints. The joints between the dorsocaudal angles of the thyroid cartilage and the lateral facets of the cricoid cartilage also allow rotation about a common transverse axis. The third pair of synovial joints is formed between the arytenoid and cricoid cartilages (Figs. 4.9 and 4.11). They are more complex and allow rotation about both sagittal and transverse axes as well as sliding movements that bring the two arytenoid cartilages closer together or carry them farther apart. Movement at the cricoarytenoid joints is the most important factor in regulating the size of the glottic opening, the narrow stretch of the lumen of the larynx. All of these joints possess the usual attributes of synovial joints.

The cartilages are additionally joined by various membranes and ligaments that balance the laryngeal musculature and determine the resting posture of the larynx. Elastic membranes join the epiglottis to the thyroid and arytenoid cartilages, the thyroid to the cricoid cartilage, and the cricoid cartilage to the first tracheal ring. Other, less elastic ligaments form the basis of the vocal folds (and the vestibular folds when these are present) that pass between the arytenoid cartilages and the laryngeal floor.

The Musculature

In addition to the extrinsic laryngeal muscles that pass between the larynx and the pharynx, tongue, hyoid bone, and sternum, a suite of small, paired, intrinsic muscles connects the laryngeal cartilages and influences their mutual relations (Fig. 4.12).

One of these muscles, the *cricothyroideus* (Fig. 4.12/*1*), is somewhat set apart from the rest through its superficial position and its innervation by the cranial laryngeal nerve, a branch of the vagus. This muscle runs between the lateral surfaces of the thyroid lamina and cricoid arch ventral to the cricothyroid joint. Its contraction moves the dorsal part of the cricoid (and the attached arytenoid cartilages) caudally, thereby tensing the vocal folds. The rest of the laryngeal muscles are deeper, attach to the arytenoid cartilage, and are innervated by the caudal (recurrent) laryngeal branch of the vagus nerve. The *cricoarytenoideus dorsalis* (Fig. 4.12/*2*) arises from the dorsal surface of the cricoid lamina, and its fibers converge rostrolaterally to insert on the muscular process of the arytenoid cartilage. Its contraction abducts the vocal process and the vocal folds to widen the glottis. The *cricoarytenoideus lateralis* (Fig. 4.12/*3*) takes origin from the rostroventral part of the cricoid arch and passes dorsally to an insertion on the muscular process. It is therefore an adductor of the vocal processes and thus narrows

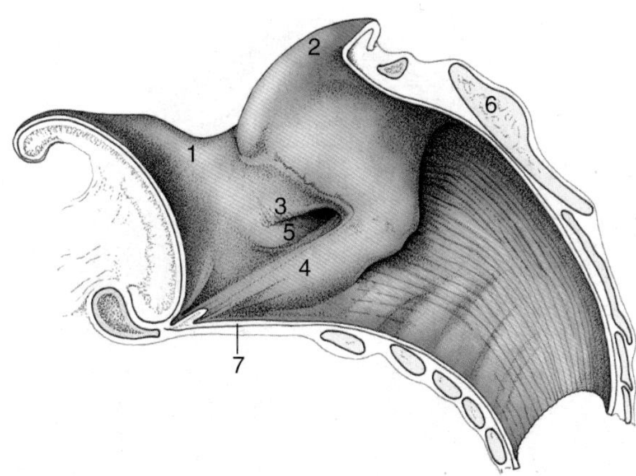

Fig. 4.13 Median section of the equine larynx. *1,* Epiglottis; *2,* corniculate process of arytenoid cartilage; *3,* vestibular fold; *4,* vocal fold; *5,* laryngeal ventricle; *6,* lamina of cricoid cartilage; *7,* cricothyroid ligament.

the glottis. The *thyroarytenoideus* arises from the cranial part of the laryngeal floor (chiefly the thyroid cartilage) and runs dorsocaudally to insert on the muscular process and adjacent part of the arytenoid cartilage. In certain species (horse and dog included) it is divided into two units, a rostral ventricularis (Fig. 4.12/*5*) and a caudal vocalis (Fig. 4.12/*4*), which occupy the vestibular and vocal folds. The *thyroarytenoideus* muscle adjusts the tension of the fold(s) and forms part of the sphincter arrangement. The *arytenoideus transversus* (Fig. 4.12/*6*) runs from the muscular process of the arytenoid cartilage to a median raphe (sometimes containing the interarytenoid nodule); some fibers may cross the midline to reach the arytenoid cartilage of the other side. The muscle approximates the arytenoid cartilages and completes the sphincter.

The Cavity of the Larynx

The cavity of the larynx may be divided into three sections arranged in series (Figs. 4.13 and 18.35). The vestibule extends from the laryngeal entrance to the rostral margin of the arytenoid cartilages and vocal folds. The glottic cleft is bounded by the arytenoid cartilages dorsally and the vocal folds ventrolaterally and can vary in size. The third, infraglottic, cavity is of fixed dimensions and leads smoothly to the lumen of the trachea (Fig. 4.14).

The structures bounding the *entrance to the larynx* (aditus laryngis) project into the lumen of the pharynx. They may protrude through the intrapharyngeal ostium into the nasopharynx, where they may be grasped by the free margin of the soft palate and its continuation by the palatopharyngeal arches. The rostral part of the wall of the entrance is provided by the epiglottis, the lateral parts by the (aryepiglottic) folds extending between the epiglottis and the arytenoid cartilages, and the caudal part by the corniculate processes of the arytenoid cartilages. All of the features on the interior of the *vestibule* are not found

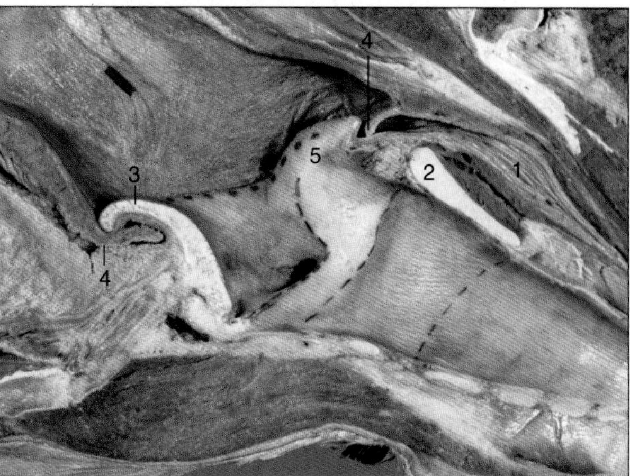

Fig. 4.14 Sagittal section of junction of pharynx with larynx (horse). *1,* Esophagus; *2,* cricoid lamina; *3,* epiglottis; *4,* palatopharyngeal arch; *5,* corniculate process of arytenoid cartilage.

in every species. In some animals a vestibular fold runs roughly parallel to the vocal fold but at a more rostral level (Fig. 4.13/*3*). This fold pairs with an outpouching of the mucosa to form a ventricle or diverticulum that is entered between the vestibular and vocal folds (see Fig. 18.35). These features are especially prominent in the horse and receive more attention later. The mucous membrane bounding the vestibule is tightly adherent to the epiglottic and arytenoid cartilages but is looser in other places where it rests on fat.

The *glottic cleft* (rima glottidis) is narrower than the vestibule. The dorsal part of the glottis cleft is bounded by the vocal processes and adjacent parts of the arytenoid cartilages, and the ventral part is bounded by the vocal folds (the folds and the arytenoid cartilages constitute the glottis). The cleft, laterally compressed and diamond-shaped, varies in dimensions and disappears when the glottis is closed. The vocal folds run caudodorsally from the rostral part of the laryngeal floor to their attachments on the arytenoid cartilages. Each fold contains a ligament in its free margin and, lateral to it, the vocalis muscle, which is surrounded on most sides by fat. The vestibular folds, when present, have a similar construction but form no part of the glottis in the strict sense. The mucosa is tightly adherent to the arytenoid cartilages and along the free margin of the folds; it is much looser elsewhere.

The *infraglottic cavity* has few features of interest: its form reflects that of the cricoid cartilage. It may be slightly smaller where it continues into the trachea. The mucosa is relatively firmly attached.

The *laryngeal mucous membrane* contains numerous mucous glands (especially massed within the ventricles when these are present) and also lymphoid aggregations (especially in the infraglottic region). The nature of the epithelium varies across regions with its use. This epithelium is stratified squamous about the entrance to minimize risks of abrasion from food and also the free edges of the folds, which at times are abruptly brought together. Elsewhere, the epithelium is pseudostratified and ciliated like the epithelium lining most respiratory passages. The sensory innervation is from the cranial and caudal (recurrent) laryngeal nerves; the boundary between the territories coincides with the glottis.

The Mechanism of the Larynx

The larynx protects the lower respiratory passages against entry of food and drink and produces voice (phonation). On swallowing, the larynx is drawn forward, and the epiglottis, tilted somewhat backward by coming against the root of the tongue, forms a partial cover to the laryngeal entrance. The resemblance between the outlines of the epiglottis and the aditus suggests a much closer fit than actually occurs. Solid foods are swiftly carried over the laryngeal entrance by the pharyngeal muscles, whereas fluids are deflected by the epiglottis through the piriform recesses of the pharyngeal floor. It is known that removal of the larger part of the human epiglottis does not interfere with normal swallowing. A second, active protection is provided at a deeper level by the glottis, which is closed by the adduction of the vocal folds. Inhibition of inspiration at this time further reduces the risk that food will be drawn into the larynx. In fact, food comparatively rarely "goes down the wrong way," but when it does, its contact with the vestibular mucosa initiates reflex coughing.

On inspiration, abduction of the vocal folds may widen the rima glottidis, but the effect is pronounced only when breathing is unusually vigorous. Although the dorsal cricoarytenoideus is the abductor and the lateral cricoarytenoideus muscle is the adductor (Fig. 4.15/*5* and *6* and *arrows*), both muscles are supplied by the caudal (recurrent) laryngeal nerve.

Closure of the glottis also occurs when free passage of air to or from the lungs must be prevented. A buildup of expiratory forces against a closed glottis allows for a forceful expulsion when the air is eventually released, as during coughing to clear the lower passages of mucous accumulations or foreign matter. Sustained closure with elevation of the intrathoracic pressure is also used in activities such as defecation, micturition, and parturition. The blockage of the escape route for air helps maintain the intrathoracic pressure and, by so stabilizing the diaphragm, aids the action of the muscles of the abdominal wall. The skeleton of the thorax can also be more effectively fixed to provide a firm base for muscles attaching to the ribs when the glottis is closed. This combination of activities is well illustrated in ourselves when we attempt to lift a heavy weight or to draw the trunk toward a handhold above the head.

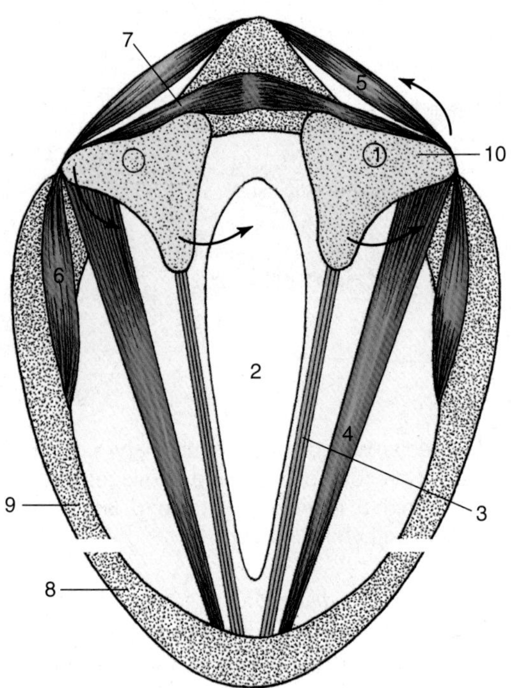

Fig. 4.15 Schematic transverse section of the larynx. *Arrows* on the *left* indicate action of cricoarytenoideus lateralis *(6)* on arytenoid cartilage, and *arrows* on the right, action of cricoarytenoideus dorsalis *(5)* on arytenoid cartilage *(10)*. *1,* Location of the cricoarytenoid joint; *2,* glottic cleft; *3,* vocal ligament in vocal fold; *4,* thyroarytenoideus; *5,* cricoarytenoideus dorsalis; *6,* cricoarytenoideus lateralis; *7,* arytenoideus transverse; *8,* thyroid cartilage; *9,* cricoid cartilage; *10,* arytenoid cartilage.

The *production of voice* is a further important function of the larynx. Humans can produce more complex sounds than other species even though the larynx is no more complex. An animal in which the larynx had to be surgically removed due to malignant disease can produce some sounds through the expulsion of air from the esophagus. Even normally the laryngeal sounds are much modified and "colored" by the resonance chambers provided by other cavities of the head. Some controversy exists over the mechanism of sound production in the larynx. The airstream is made to vibrate as it passes through the glottis. The pitch is controlled by the thickness, the length, and the tension of the vocal folds and is thus to some extent variable and to some extent determined by permanent (or semipermanent, in that a boy's voice breaks with growth) and individual features of laryngeal anatomy. The tension of the folds, or of part of them, is varied by the cricothyroideus muscle, which acts as the coarse adjustment, and the vocalis muscle, as the fine adjustment. Most authorities believe that the folds are made to vibrate passively by the flow of air passing between them. An alternative theory suggests that the muscles contract and relax at the appropriate rate. However, this latter theory is weak because some tones of the human voice exceed 200 cycles per second and

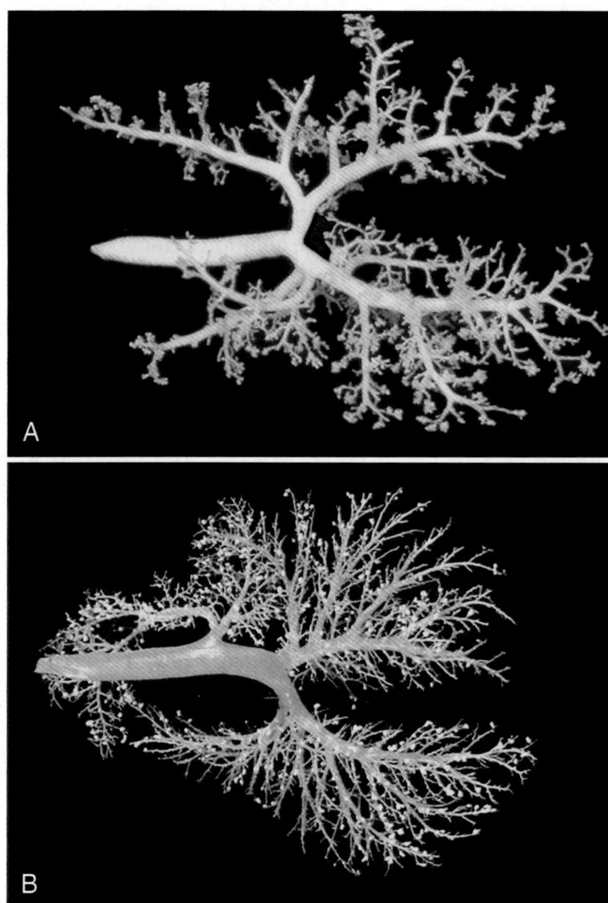

Fig. 4.16 Dorsal views of corrosion casts of the bronchial tree and lungs of (A) the cat and (B) the calf.

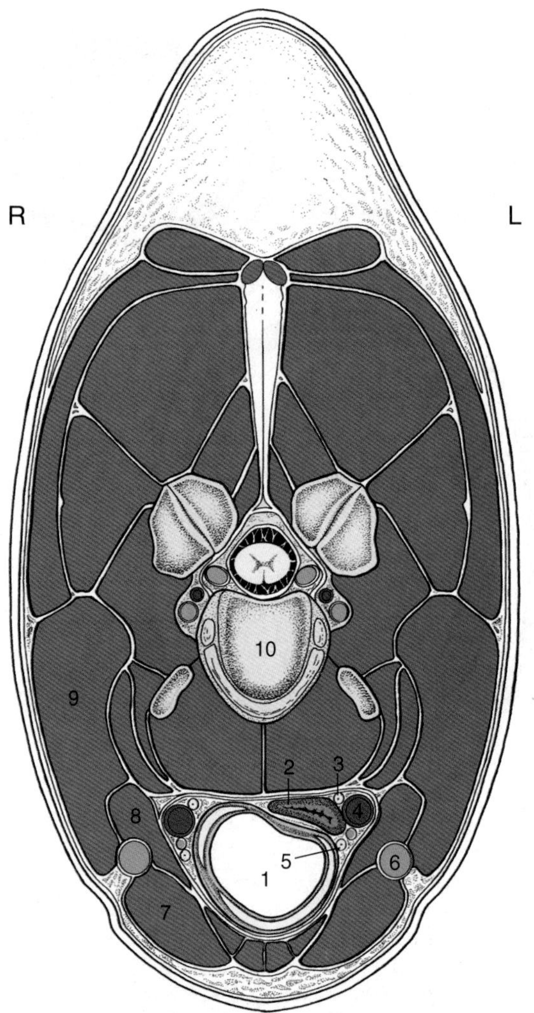

Fig. 4.17 Transverse section of the neck (horse) at the level of the fourth cervical vertebra. *1,* Trachea; *2,* esophagus; *3,* vagosympathetic trunk; *4,* common carotid artery; *5,* caudal (recurrent) laryngeal nerve; *6,* external jugular vein; *7,* sternocephalicus; *8,* omohyoideus; *9,* brachiocephalicus, *10,* body of the fourth cervical vertebra; *L,* left; *R,* right.

tonic contraction of the vocalis muscle occurs with stimuli repeated 67 times per second. Electromyographic studies show that purring in cats is produced by fast twitching of the laryngeal muscles and the diaphragm. The laryngeal muscles rapidly narrow and widen the glottis, causing the respiratory air to vibrate and make the sound.

THE TRACHEA

The trachea and bronchi form a continuous system of tubes conducting air between the larynx and the smaller passages (bronchioli) in the lungs. They have a very similar construction and together are sometimes termed the *tracheobronchial tree*.

The trachea leads from the larynx through the visceral space of the neck, enters the mediastinum at the thoracic inlet, and continues to its terminal bifurcation above the heart. The bifurcation lies in the region of the fourth to sixth intercostal spaces but varies with the species and with the respiratory phase. The two chief bronchi diverge from the line of the trachea to quickly enter the corresponding lungs at their roots (Fig. 4.16) and ramify in patterns described later (p.150). In ruminants and pigs a separate tracheal bronchus arises proximal to the tracheal bifurcation to enter the cranial lobe of the right lung. The cervical part of the trachea maintains a more or less median position, although its relationship to the esophagus alters at different levels and in different postures of the head and neck (see Figs. 3.29 and 4.17/*1*). Other relations in the neck include the ventral strap muscles of the neck and the carotid sheath and its contents. The common carotid artery commences ventrolaterally but gradually climbs to a dorsolateral position where the trachea originates from the larynx.

The thoracic part of the trachea is deflected slightly to the right where it crosses the aortic arch. It is related ventrally to the cranial vena cava, to the arteries arising from the aortic arch, and to various tributaries and branches of

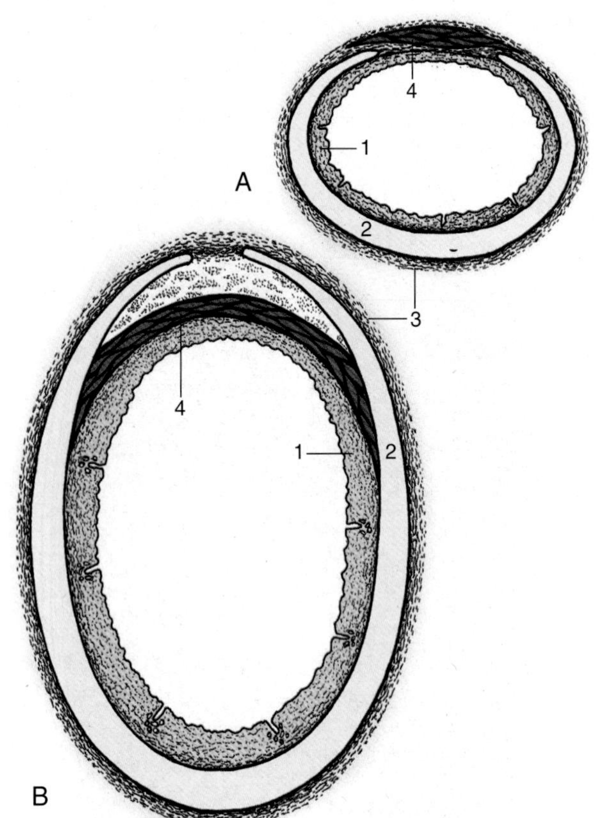

Fig. 4.18 Transverse sections of the (A) canine and (B) bovine tracheas. *1,* Mucous membrane; *2,* tracheal cartilage; *3,* adventitia; *4,* tracheal muscle (external in dogs, internal in cattle).

these vessels. It is related dorsally to the esophagus and related variously to mediastinal lymph nodes. In young subjects it is related to the thymus.

The wall of the trachea is composed of an inner mucosa, a fibrocartilaginous middle layer, which prevents its collapse, and an adventitia (in the neck) or serosa (in the thorax) (Fig. 4.18). The mucosa, which is pseudostratified ciliated epithelium as in the infraglottic part of the larynx, may show slight longitudinal folding when the lumen is narrowed. It contains both unicellular and multicellular mucous glands that produce a protective covering of mucus that is continuously moved toward the larynx by the epithelial cilia. This mucus eventually reaches the pharynx and is swallowed without being noticed. Excessive mucus accumulations may irritate the mucosa, stimulating coughing to clear the airway. The fibrocartilaginous coat is composed of numerous strips of cartilage that are bent to form "rings" that are incomplete dorsally, where the ends may fail to meet or may overlap. The edges of the strips are connected to each other by sheets of rather elastic connective tissue continuous with the perichondrium. The smooth tracheal muscle (Fig. 4.18/*4*) bridges the gap within the "ring" in most species but is placed externally in the dog and the cat.

The trachea is attached to the diaphragm indirectly by the pulmonary ligaments and mediastinal connective tissue and also, more effectively, by the negative intrapleural pressure that couples the lungs to the chest wall, including the diaphragm. These attachments allow the necessary adjustments in length during extension of the neck or contraction of the diaphragm. Variations in diameter are regulated by the tracheal muscle. In addition to these functional changes, there are permanent species and regional variations in the cross-sectional form and area of the trachea.

The structure of the larger bronchi is identical to that of the trachea except that their outer surfaces merge with the peribronchial connective tissue (and through this with the stroma of the lung). With further divisions of the bronchi, the cartilage rings are gradually replaced by irregular plaques, and they finally disappear to mark the transition into bronchioles.

Variations in the diameter of the bronchi and bronchioli are relatively greater and more significant than those of the trachea.

Before proceeding, one may need to reread the section on the shape and function of the thoracic cavity (p. 45-47).

THE PLEURA

Each lung is invested by a serous membrane, the pleura, which also lines the corresponding "half" of the thoracic cavity. Thus, two pleural membranes exist, each arranged as a closed invaginated sac. The space between the right and left sacs forms the mediastinum, a more or less median partition in the thorax within which the heart and other thoracic organs are situated (Fig. 4.19/*7*).

The part of the pleura that clothes the lung directly is known as the visceral or pulmonary pleura (Fig. 4.19/*4*). It is reflected around, and also behind, the root of the lung to become continuous with the mediastinal pleura, which in turn is continuous with the costal and diaphragmatic pleura; these last three parts are together termed the *parietal pleura.*

In the healthy animal the pleural cavity is a potential rather than an actual space, and it contains only a small amount (a few milliliters) of serous fluid, which is thinly spread over the pleural surface and facilitates the smooth movement of the lung against the chest wall and of one lung lobe against another. The pressure within the pleural cavity, which is about −5 cm H_2O in the neutral resting position of the chest, represents the difference between the forces that tend to recoil the lung and those that tend to expand the chest. The pressure is not uniform throughout the pleural cavity, and in addition to the expected dorsoventral gradient, local and partly unexplained differences exist. These variations in intrapleural pressure account for regional differences in the expansion and aeration of the lungs. The prevailing negative pressure explains why a surgical or traumatic opening in the chest wall causes an

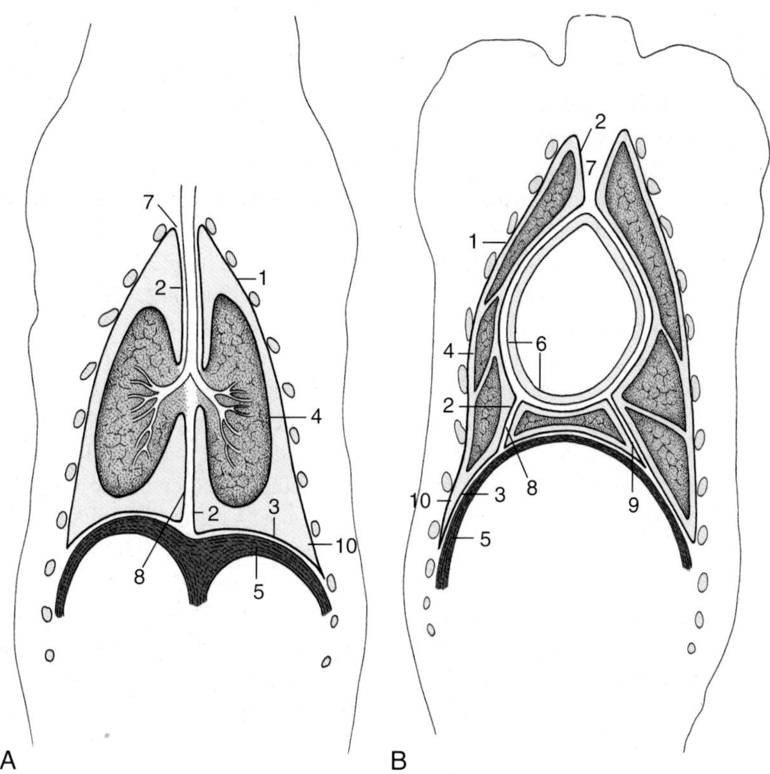

Fig. 4.19 Schematic dorsal sections of the pleural cavities (dog) (A) at the level of the tracheal bifurcation and (B) at the level of the heart. *1* to *3*, Parietal pleura, later subdivided; *1*, costal pleura; *2*, mediastinal pleura; *3*, diaphragmatic pleura; *4*, visceral pleura; *5*, diaphragm; *6*, parietal and visceral pericardium; *7*, cranial mediastinum; *8*, caudal mediastinum; *9*, plica venae cavae; *10*, costodiaphragmatic recess.

inrush of air into the pleural cavity, collapsing the lung and producing the condition known as *pneumothorax*.

The pleural sac is always more extensive than the lung, and in certain regions, facing surfaces of parietal pleura are directly applied to each other. The most important example of such an arrangement is found caudal to the basal border of the lung, where the peripheral part of the diaphragmatic pleura rests against the costal pleura lining the chest wall (the costodiaphragmatic recess; Fig. 4.19/*10*). Although the extent of the recess varies with the phase of respiration, it remains considerable even in full inspiration, and the potential of this portion of the pleural sac is therefore never realized (see Fig. 4.22/*6*). A similar but smaller costomediastinal recess is present ventral to the lung (Fig. 4.20/*12*).

Cranially, the costal and mediastinal portions of the pleura come together to form a dome, the cupula pleurae, which may extend in front of the first rib, where it is obviously vulnerable to injury (Fig. 4.21/*8′*). The mediastinum is not symmetrical but is deflected to the left at certain levels. The important deflection of the caudal mediastinum is produced by the greater size of the base of the right lung.

A special fold (plica venae cavae) of the pleura of the right sac extends between the diaphragm and pericardium and carries the caudal vena cava in its free dorsal border (Fig. 4.20/*3* and *9*). This triangular partition helps define a recess into which the accessory lobe of the right lung fits (see Fig. 4.21).

Considerable practical significance attaches to the strength of the mediastinum, which varies much among species. In some, for example, the ruminants, the mediastinum is thick and able to withstand a considerable pressure difference between the two pleural cavities and potentially tolerate collapse of one lung. In others, for example, the dog, cat, and horse, it is very delicate and ruptures readily. Indeed the horse is among those species in which the mediastinum of the dead specimen always presents numerous small openings that place the right and left pleural cavities in communication.

THE LUNGS

The right and left lungs (pulmones,* [pl]) are enclosed into their respective pleural sacs and are free except at the roots, where they are attached to the mediastinum.

* Both the Latin term, *pulmo,* and its Greek equivalent, *pneumon,* are used as stems in the production of medical terms; *pulmonitis* and *pneumonia* both describe inflammation of the lungs.

Their size is determined by the dimensions of the thorax and the phase of respiration. The lungs are normally kept expanded by the air pressure within the respiratory tree. Their elastic recoil leads to their collapse once the air enters into the pleural cavities following trauma, surgery, or dissection. They have a soft, spongy texture, and the residual air in them, even when collapsed, causes them to crepitate when squeezed and to float when placed in water. In contrast, the unexpanded lungs of the fetus or stillborn animal that has not breathed feel solid and sink when immersed. The healthy lungs are a fresh pink in many slaughterhouse specimens but a much deeper red in lungs obtained from animals that were not bled. The frequently patchy coloration is produced by uneven distribution of blood. The lungs of animals that spent their lives in heavily polluted atmospheres acquire a grayish tinge from deposition of soot or other inhaled particles (Table 4.1).

Anatomic descriptions are generally based on specimens hardened in situ before the thorax was opened; at death such lungs retain their size, which is intermediate between those adopted in full inspiration and full expiration (Fig. 4.22). The two lungs are grossly alike and mirror each other in shape. The right lung is always larger, most obviously in the cattle, partly owing to the skewed position of the heart. Each lung resembles the half of a cone and has following features: an apex toward the thoracic inlet; a wide, concave base facing the diaphragm; a convex costal surface fitted against the lateral chest wall; an irregular medial surface modeled on the contents of the mediastinum; a thick dorsal border occupying the gutter between the vertebrae and ribs; and a thin border that comprises a ventral part bordering the costomediastinal recess and a basal (caudoventral) part bordering the costodiaphragmatic recess (Figs. 4.20 and 4.22). The ventral part is indented over the heart (cardiac notch; incisura cardiaca).

The *mediastinal surface of the lungs* carries many indentations, including the large and deep cardiac impression, which is naturally larger on the left lung. The impression extends to the ventral border, which is deeply notched at this level in most species and which allows the heart (or more accurately, the pericardium) direct contact with the thoracic wall (see Fig. 4.22). The root of the lung, situated dorsal to the cardiac impression, is formed by the bunching together of the chief bronchus and the pulmonary artery, veins, lymphatics, and nerve. The reflection of the mediastinal pleura onto the lung, which covers the root, extends caudal to the root in a tapering fashion that leaves bare an area of lung that is directly joined by mediastinal connective tissue to the corresponding part of its partner. In some species, including the dog and the cat, the empty part of the reflection, which is known as the pulmonary ligament, extends onto the base of the lung, which thus has additional attachment to the diaphragm. In ruminants and pigs the bronchus that arises from the trachea before its bifurcation together with the associated vessels creates a smaller second root of the right lung (Figs. 4.23 and 4.17B).

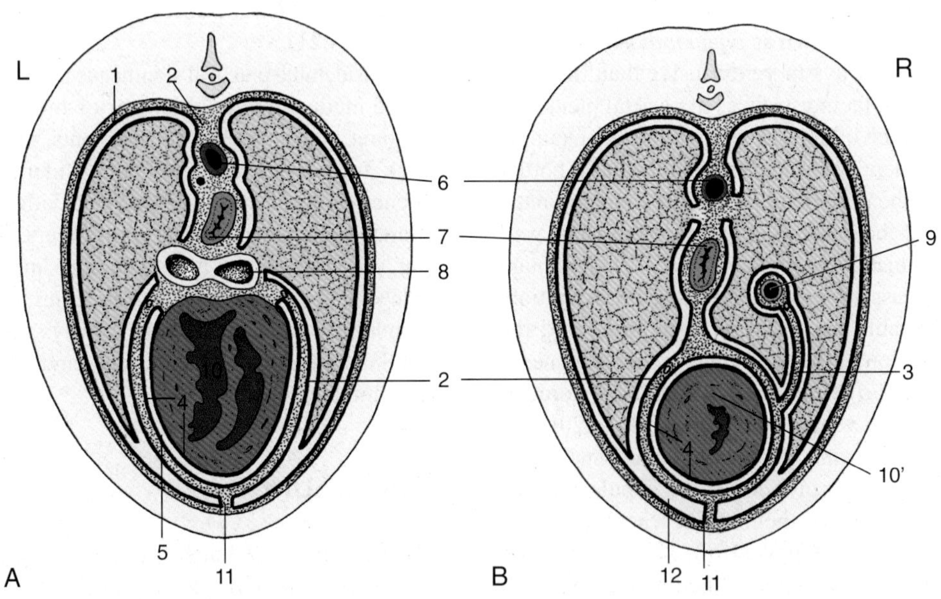

Fig. 4.20 Schematic transverse section of the thorax (A) at the level of the heart and (B) at the transition of heart to caudal mediastinum. *1,* Costal pleura; *2,* mediastinal pleura; *3,* plica venae cavae; *4,* parietal and visceral pericardium; *5,* pericardial space; *6,* aorta; *7,* esophagus; *8,* tracheal bifurcation; *9,* caudal vena cava; *10,* heart; *10′,* apex of heart; *11,* sternopericardial ligament; *12,* costomediastinal recess; *L,* left; *R,* right.

The base of the right lung reveals the small accessory lobe, which is separated from the medial surface of the caudal lobe by a fissure that widens at its dorsal limit to accommodate the caudal vena cava in its passage between the caval foramen of the diaphragm and the right atrium. The accessory lobe sits, as it were, astride the vein.

In most species one or more fissures extend into the substance toward the root, dividing each lung into parts that are commonly equated with lobes. The lobes, however, are properly defined not by the fissures but by the branching of the bronchial tree. The left lung consists of cranial and caudal lobes and the right one of cranial, middle, caudal, and accessory lobes. The cranial lobe is commonly subdivided by an external fissure, whereas the right lung of the horse lacks a middle lobe. The fissures are much deeper in the lungs of the dog and the cat than in those of other species. The deeper fissures may allow the parts to slip over each other more easily, thus facilitating the adaptation of the lungs to the pronounced changes in thoracic form that occur in animals that employ a bounding gallop.

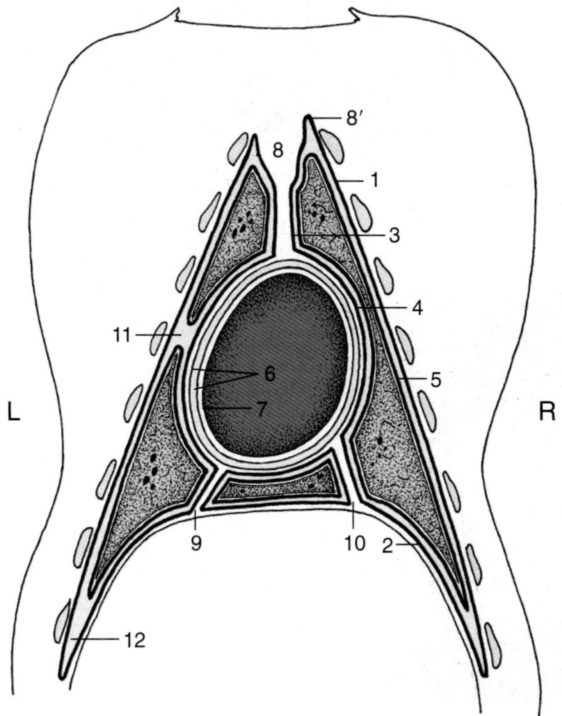

Fig. 4.21 The distribution of the pleura and pericardium, schematic. The *heavy lines* indicate the pleura. *1* to *4*, Parietal pleura, later subdivided; *1*, costal pleura; *2*, diaphragmatic pleura; *3*, mediastinal pleura; *4*, pericardial pleura; *5*, visceral (pulmonary) pleura; *6*, parietal pericardium: its outer fibrous layer tightly adheres to its inner serous layer; *7*, visceral pericardium, adherent to heart (epicardium); *8*, cranial mediastinum; *8′*, cupula pleurae; *9*, caudal mediastinum; *10*, plica venae cavae; *11*, left cardiac notch; *12*, costodiaphragmatic recess; *L*, left; *R*, right.

The bulk of the lung substance is provided by the bronchi, pulmonary vessels, and peribronchial and perivascular connective tissue. Both right and left chief bronchi, upon entering the lung at its root, detach a bronchus to the cranial lobe before continuing caudally (Figs. 4.17 and 4.24). The two generations of subdivisions that follow next have a fairly consistent pattern of origin, but subsequent ramifications are less predictable. The number of bronchial generations before their transition into bronchioles varies among species and also among the parts of a single lung. In mice and other small animals only four or five generations of bronchi are present, whereas more than a dozen may be necessary in large animals. The consistency in the pattern of the first branchings allows the recognition of the so-called bronchopulmonary segments, specific portions of the lung supplied by identifiable bronchi and partly defined by connective tissue septa that extend from the peribronchial and perivascular tissue (and are responsible for the surface marbling where they impinge on the visceral pleura). Although bronchopulmonary segmentation has been studied in domestic species, it has yet to find important application. It is the elasticity of the connective tissue stroma that allows the lungs to expand on inspiration and collapse on subsequent expiration. Loss of this elasticity, which occurs naturally with aging (but also in certain pathologic conditions), reduces respiratory efficiency.

The structure of the major bronchi resembles that of the trachea, but with each successive division the supporting

TABLE 4.1 COMPARATIVE ANATOMY OF THE LUNGS

	Horse & Sheep	Ox & Pig	Dog & Cat
Pleura	Thick	Thick	Thin
Intlobular Connective Tissue			Little
Connective Tissue Around Lobules	Partial	Completely	None
Non-Respiratory Bronchioles	Many generations and last one ending in alveolar duct/short respiratory bronchiole	Many generations and last one ending in alveolar duct/short respiratory bronchiole	Terminal bronchiole ends respiratory bronchiole that divides many times

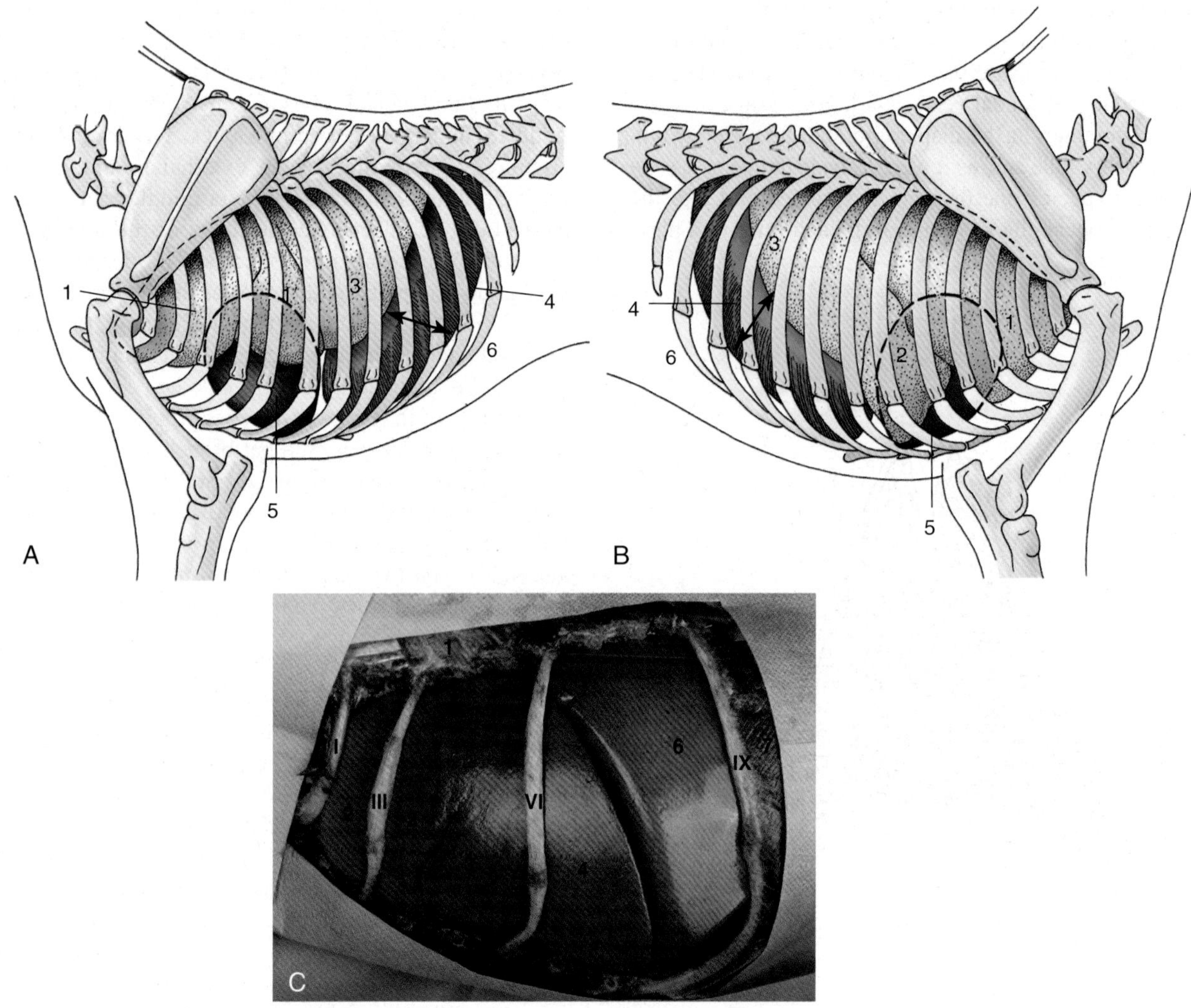

Fig. 4.22 Semischematic drawings of the thoracic organs of the dog on the left (A) and right (B) sides. The outline of the heart is indicated by a *broken line*. *1,* Cranial lobe; *1′,* caudal part of left cranial lobe; *2,* middle lobe; *3,* caudal lobe; *4,* diaphragm; *5,* heart; *6,* costodiaphragmatic recess *(arrow)*. (C) shows left view of the lung. *2,* Cranial part of the cranial lobe; *3,* fissure, *4,* caudal part of the cranial lobe; *6,* caudal lobe; *7,* intercostal muscles I, III, VI, and IX indicate the rib numbers.

cartilages become smaller and more irregular, whereas the muscle expands to enclose the lumen on all sides. The lumen is lined by a pseudostratified epithelium comprising tall ciliated columnar cells interspersed with goblet and serous-secreting cells and with stem cells that proliferate to repair depletions of the other types. Larger glands are included within the submucosa of the major bronchi. The transition from bronchus to bronchiole is defined by the disappearance of the last cartilage plate and by the submucosal glands. Bronchioles are narrow—less than 1 mm in diameter—and also pass through several generations. The last of these is characterized by the loss of goblet cells and their replacement by the nonciliated epithelial cells (Clara cells) thought to secrete a component of lung surfactant and act as germinal cells for the bronchiolar epithelium. The terminal bronchioles have scattered alveolar outpouchings on their walls that are continued by alveolar ducts, thence by alveolar sacs, and ultimately by the saclike alveoli—the spaces where gaseous exchange takes place through a flattened epithelium closely related to the pulmonary capillaries. Patency of the finer passages, which are unsupported by cartilage, is ensured by elastic fibers that anchor them to the pulmonary stroma. At the first breath, the alveoli fill with air and dilate, although for a time they remain significantly smaller than those in the adult (Fig. 4.25).

The identification of the lungs of individual species is most conveniently based on the degrees of lobation and lobulation. The lungs of horses show almost no lobation and very inconspicuous lobulation externally (Fig. 4.26), those of ruminants (Fig. 4.27) and pigs are conspicuously lobated and lobulated (though not uniformly in sheep and

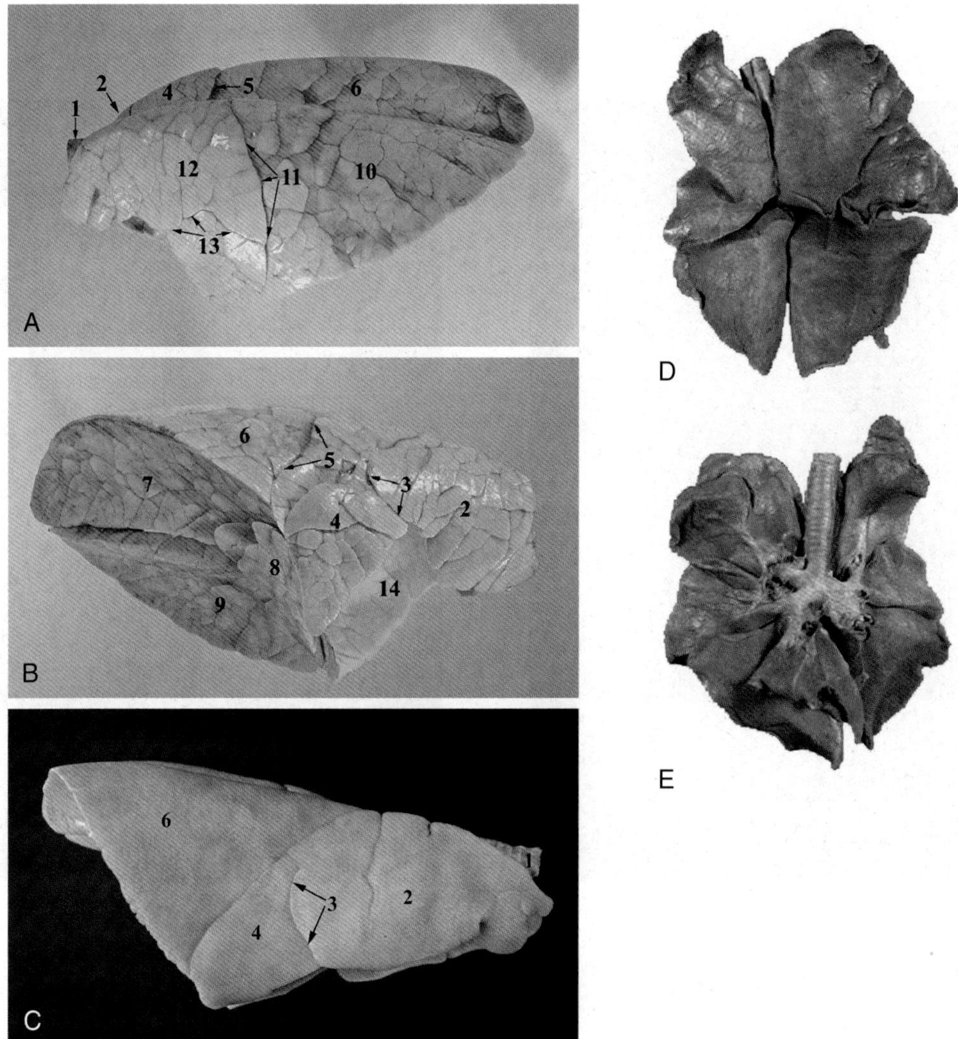

Fig. 4.23 Left dorsolateral view (A) and right ventro-lateral view (B) of lungs of a pig. (C) shows a lateral view of the right lung of a cat. *1*, Trachea; *2*, cranial lobe of the right lung; *3*, cranial interlobar fissure of the right lung; *4*, middle lobe of the right lung; *5*; caudal interlobar fissure of the right lung; *6*; caudal lobe of the right lung (costal surface); *7*, caudal lobe of the right lung (diaphragmatic surface); *8*, accessory lobe of the right lung; *9*; caudal lobe of the left lung (diaphragmatic surface); *10*, caudal lobe of the left lung; *11*, cranial interlobar fissure of the left lung; *12*, cranial lobe of the left lung; 12, cranial lobe of the left lung; *13*, intralobar fissure of cranial lobe of the left lung; *14*, cardiac impression; (D) Dorsal and (E) ventral surfaces of the lung of a dog.

goats), and those of carnivores are very deeply fissured into lobes but show little external evidence of lobulation (see Fig. 4.23).

The *pulmonary arteries* generally follow the bronchi (see Fig. 4.24), but the pulmonary veins sometimes run separately, alternating in position with the bronchoarterial associations. The pattern varies not only with the species but also with location in a single lung, an observation that currently does not have major clinical significance. A set of bronchial arteries arises from the aorta to supply the bronchi and associated connective tissue wholly independently of the pulmonary arteries (Fig. 4.28). A corresponding set of bronchial veins may return this blood to the right atrium via the azygous vein, but often the bronchial flow is returned entirely to the left atrium. Arteriovenous anastomoses appear to be absent, making the lung an effective filter to prevent the further spread of emboli and tumor cells. This feature also accounts for the frequent occurrence of abscesses and tumor metastases in lung tissue secondary to disease of other organs.

Lymph drains to the tracheobronchial and mediastinal lymph nodes, directly or after initial passage through

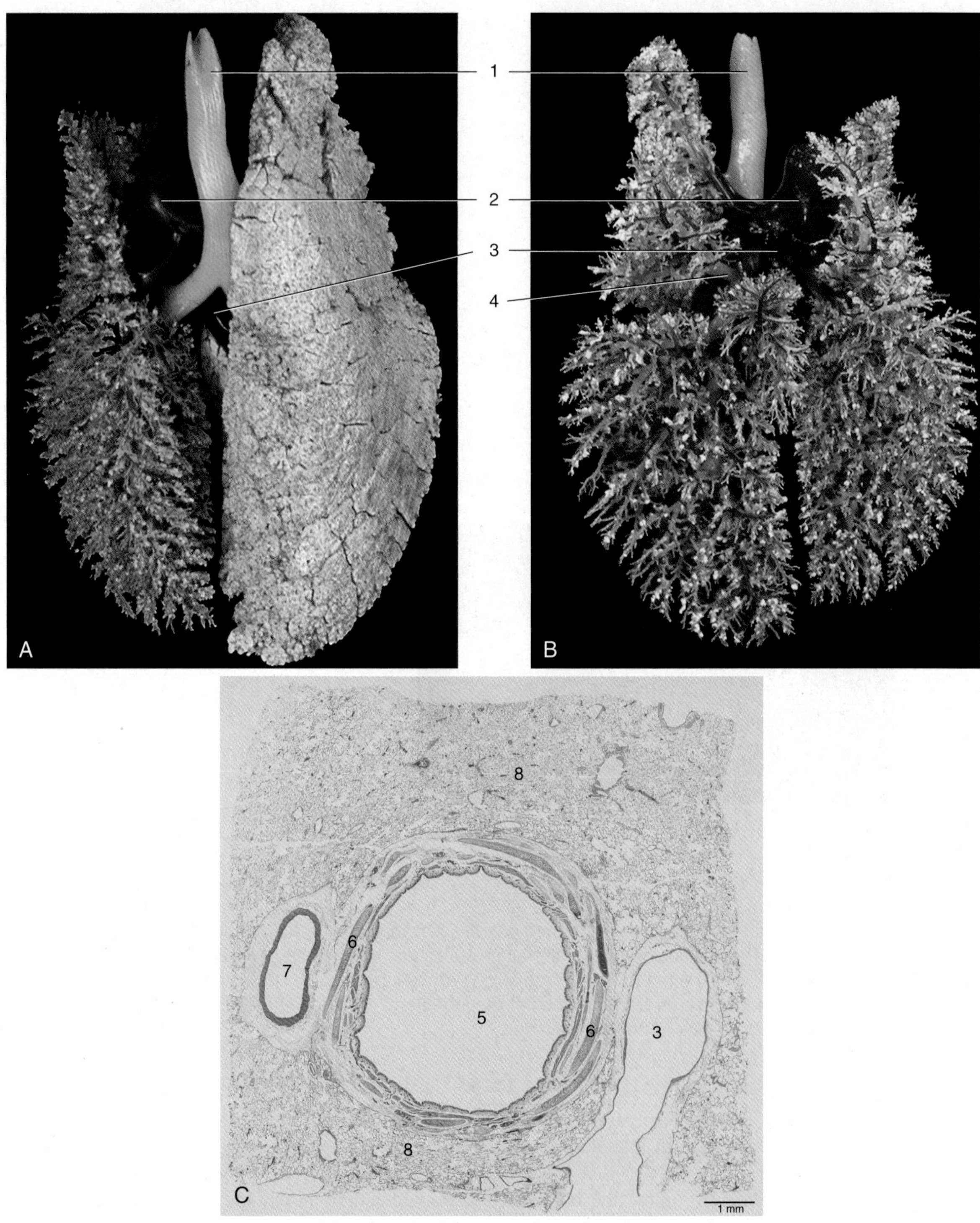

Fig. 4.24 (A) and (B) Dorsal view of the bronchial tree *(yellow)* and accompanying blood vessels and (C) histological section of the pig (corrosion cast). *1,* Trachea; *2,* pulmonary trunk; *3,* pulmonary veins; *4,* tracheal bronchus; *5,* bronchus; *6,* plaques of hyaline cartilages; *7,* pulmonary artery; *8,* gas exchange area.

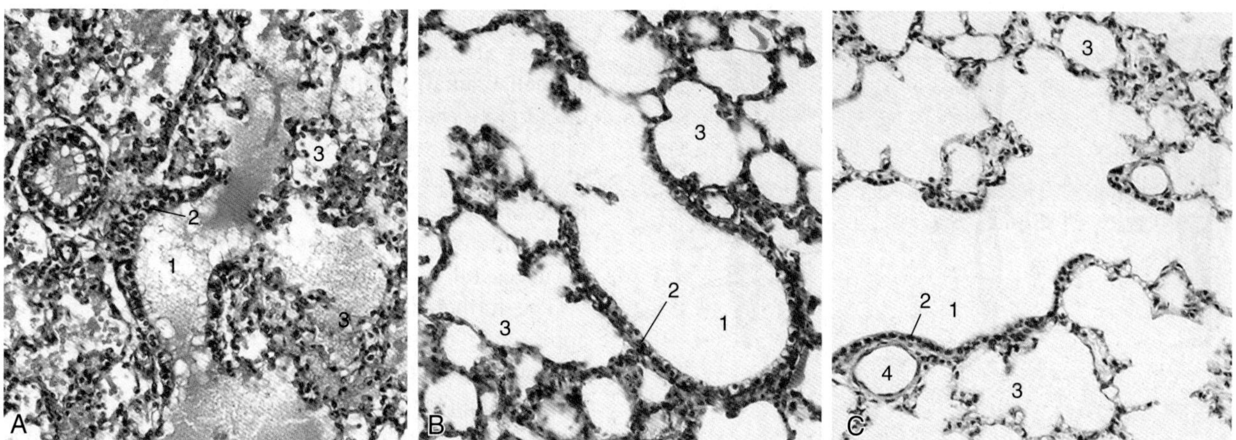

Fig. 4.25 (A) Lung of pig fetus (140×); note presence of fluid in bronchioles and alveoli. (B) Lung of 1-day-old piglet (140×). (C) Lung of an adult pig (140×). *1,* Terminal bronchioles; *2,* bronchiolar exocrinocyte (Clara) cells; *3,* alveolar sac; *4,* bronchiole.

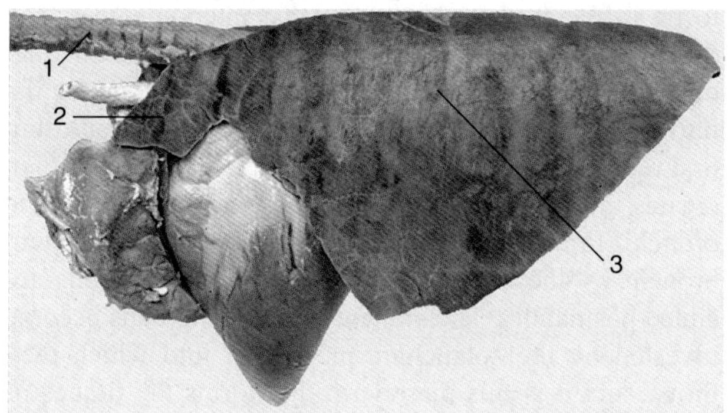

Fig. 4.26 Left lateral view of the equine lungs. Note the poor lobation and lobulation. *1,* Trachea; *2,* cranial lobe; *3,* caudal lobe.

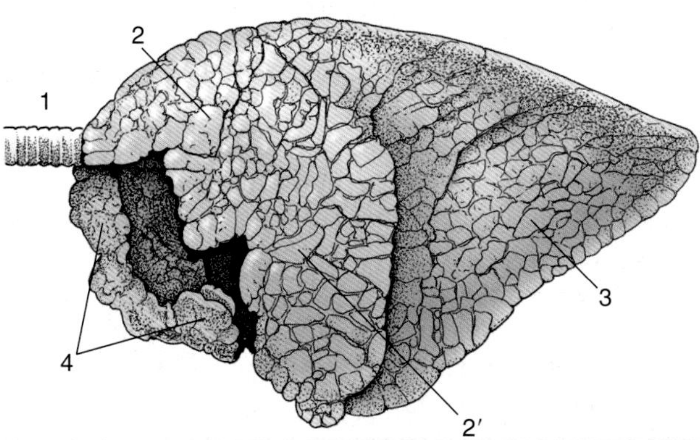

Fig. 4.27 Left lateral view of the bovine lungs. Note the definite lobation and lobulation. *1,* Trachea; *2* and *2′,* cranial and caudal parts of left cranial lobe; *3,* caudal lobe; *4,* right cranial lobe.

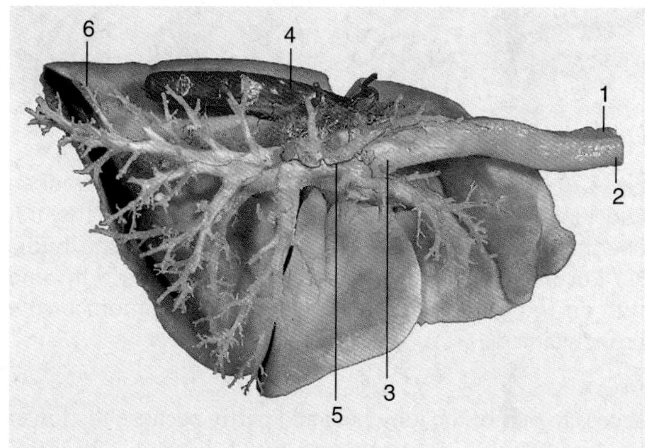

Fig. 4.28 Corrosion specimen of the lungs and part of the aorta of a dog. On the *right* side the resin in the bronchioli and smaller bronchi has been removed to expose the main tracheobronchial tree. *1,* Esophagus; *2,* trachea; *3,* tracheal bifurcation; *4,* aorta; *5,* bronchial artery; *6,* caudal lobe of left lung.

small pulmonary nodes set on the bronchial tree within the lung substance. However, the details are complicated, vary among species, and, when of pathologic relevance receive notice in later chapters.

The nerves to the lungs are delivered through a pulmonary plexus within the mediastinum to which both sympathetic and parasympathetic (vagal) fibers contribute. The efferent fibers pass to the bronchial glands and musculature and to the blood vessels. Afferent fibers come from the bronchial mucosa (cough reflex), from vessels, and from stretch receptors. Vagal section has been found to relieve pain in inoperable bronchial carcinoma in human patients.

The features of the lungs of greatest clinical significance are their projection on the surface of the body and their radiographic appearance. The projections vary among species and with the phase of respiration and are described later. Moreover, the areas that can be usefully auscultated and percussed are more limited than might initially be supposed, partly because the upper part of the forelimb denies

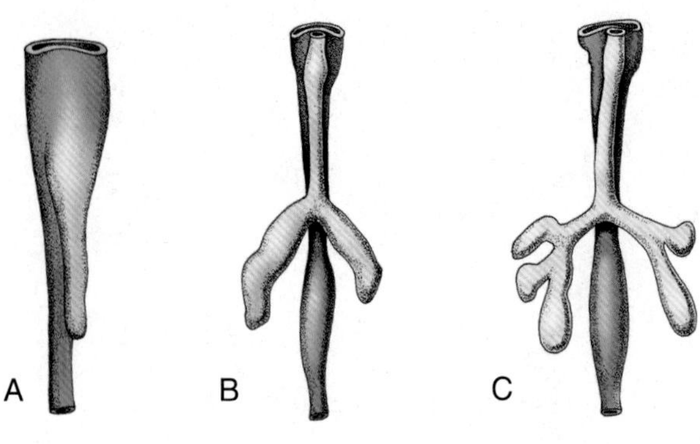

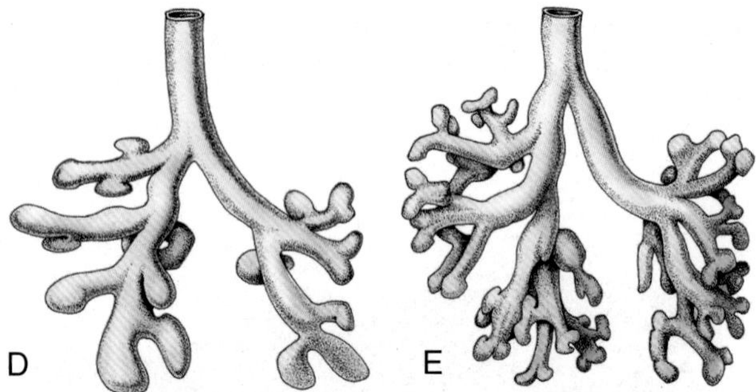

Fig. 4.29 Five stages in the development of the trachea and lungs (ventral view). (A) Caudal growth of the tracheobronchial tube. (B) Its division into two lung buds. (C) Further division into three bronchi on the right and two on the left. (D) and (E) Further development of the bronchial tree.

access to part of the lung field and partly because the lower border of the lung is too thin to provide much useful information. Because radiography of the lungs is performed mainly in small animals (dogs and cats), the relevant observations on their appearance on radiographs and figures can be found in Chapter 13.

THE DEVELOPMENT OF THE RESPIRATORY APPARATUS

The development of the nose was considered in the previous chapter in relation to the development of the mouth and face (p. 131). The larynx, trachea, and lungs find a common origin in a ventral outgrowth from the foregut, directly caudal to the second of the two swellings that form the tongue (Fig. 4.29). The primordium extends caudally as a (tracheobronchial) groove in the pharyngoesophageal floor; the groove is later converted into a tube by infolding and fusion of its lips. Fusion commences caudally and extends forward until the esophagus and pharynx are divided from the respiratory tract, except for a small cranial opening that persists as the entrance to the larynx. The fact that the initial development has the form of a groove rather than a tube is important, because it explains the wide variety of communications between the esophagus and trachea that may occur as congenital anomalies when the process of division has been locally unsuccessful.

The further differentiation of the larynx includes the appearance of the separate cartilages and muscles by condensation and differentiation of the mesoderm of the neighboring pharyngeal arches. The epiglottis has a somewhat different origin, developing as a caudal division of the second of the two median swellings that give rise to the tongue.

After separation from the esophagus, the caudal end of the respiratory tract grows down the neck and comes to lie in the median mesoderm that intervenes between the two forward-pointing extensions of the celom that become the pleural cavities. The apex of the tract splits into two lung buds (Fig. 4.29B), whose further splitting first reproduces the pattern of the bronchial tree and then creates the smaller respiratory passages that succeed the bronchi. In humans about 18 divisions succeed the stem bronchi by the time of birth, and further divisions are added postnatally. The branches of the lung buds become invested by the splanchnic mesoderm into which they thrust, and it is this mesoderm that forms the tissues of the respiratory organs other than the lining epithelium (which is, of course, supplied by the foregut endoderm). The histologic development of the lungs encompasses three phases named after the dominant microscopic characters: the first (*glandular*) phase establishes the bronchial pattern, the second (*canalicular*) phase establishes the respiratory portion of the lung, and the third and final (*alveolar*) phase is concerned with the development of the alveoli.

The production of surfactant, a substance secreted by certain alveolar cells that reduces the surface tension to allow alveolar expansion when breathing commences, is of rather late occurrence. The respiratory distress syndrome of the newborn is associated with immaturity of this feature of development.

COMPREHENSION CHECK

Discuss the clinical significance of differences in the gross and subgross anatomy of the lungs of cattle, horse, dog, and pig.

The Urogenital Apparatus

5

The official name, *apparatus urogenitalis,* brings the urinary and reproductive organs together under one heading. The chief justification for this convention lies in the common origin of certain elements of the two systems in the intermediate mesoderm and adjacent part of the celomic epithelium. Also, the urinary and reproductive systems of the adult share the final portions of the tracts, urethra in the male and the vestibule in the female.

Because of the close developmental associations of the urinary and reproductive systems, we have chosen in this chapter to precede the account of the adult anatomy with a review of the development. However, the general layout of the urogenital apparatus is provided in Figs. 5.1 and 5.2.

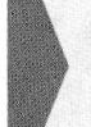

THE DEVELOPMENT OF THE UROGENITAL APPARATUS

Development of the Urinary Organs

The intermediate mesoderm reflects in muted fashion the segmentation that is so evident in the adjoining somites. It soon forms in its caudal domain a continuous solid longitudinal (nephrogenic) thickening from which arise, in craniocaudal and temporal sequence, three attempts at the formation of an excretory organ. The first attempt, which is transient and nonfunctional, constitutes the pronephros and forms in the presumptive neck region. The second attempt, the mesonephros, forms in the thoracic and lumbar regions and is functional through a large part of embryonic life. The third attempt, the metanephros, forms in the lumbar region and becomes the adult kidney (Fig. 5.3).

All three structures have a series of excretory tubules as their essential histologic feature. In the *pronephros* one end of each tubule turns caudally to meet its neighbor to form a continuous pronephric duct (Fig. 5.3/*4*), which grows at its caudal end to open into the cloaca. The duct survives the regression of the pronephric tubules, which are nonfunctional, and becomes the drainage of the mesonephric tubules that now appear.

Each of the many mesonephric tubules resembles a rather simple version of the nephron of the adult kidney (see Fig. 5.27). The blind end is invaginated by a capillary tuft to form a filtration mechanism and the connection of the other end with the pronephric duct, now more appropriately termed the *mesonephric duct,* provides an outlet for the urine. The *mesonephros* may be a very prominent organ at its apogee, when it projects from the roof of the abdomen (Fig. 5.4). Its size varies among species and is in inverse proportion to the permeability (and thus the excretory efficiency) of the placenta. The mesonephros is supplanted by the metanephros when it begins its craniocaudal regression. Parts, however, survive to be given fresh use by the male reproductive system (Fig. 5.5).

The *metanephros* has two primordia. One is provided by an outgrowth, the ureteric bud, from the lower end of the mesonephric duct close to its opening into the cloaca. This bud grows cranially into the metanephric blastema constituted by the caudal part of the nephrogenic cord (Fig. 5.3/*5*). The extremity of the bud undergoes a dozen or so dichotomous divisions. Branches of the later orders become the collecting tubules of the kidney, whereas those of the first few orders are later reabsorbed into the terminal expansion of the duct in a variable fashion that accounts for the specific forms of the renal pelvis and calices. The outer part of the metanephric mass forms the capsule and interstitium of the kidney, and cellular condensation in the inner part creates the cell cords that are transformed into nephrons. One end of each cell cord makes contact with a connecting duct, and once canalization has occurred, a continuous passage is established (Fig. 5.6). The other extremity of the nephron becomes invaginated by a vascular tuft supplied

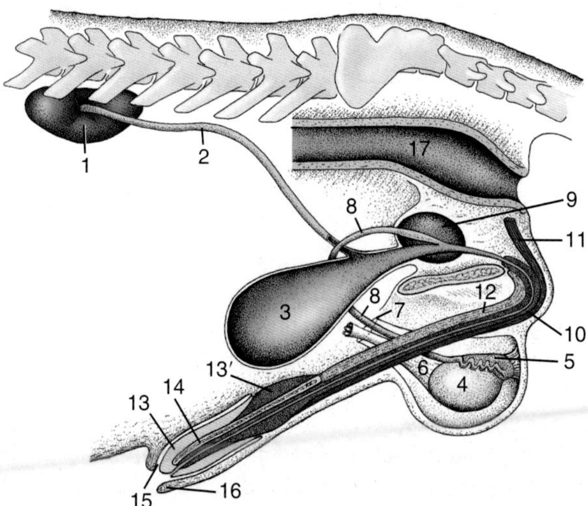

Fig. 5.1 The male urinary and reproductive organs (dog). *1,* Right kidney; *2,* ureter; *3,* bladder; *4,* testis; *5,* epididymis; *6,* spermatic cord; *7,* vaginal ring; *8,* deferent duct; *9,* prostate; *10,* corpus spongiosum (spongy body); *11,* retractor penis; *12,* corpus cavernosum (cavernous body); *13,* glans penis; *13′,* bulb of glans; *14,* os penis; *15,* preputial cavity; *16,* prepuce; *17,* rectum.

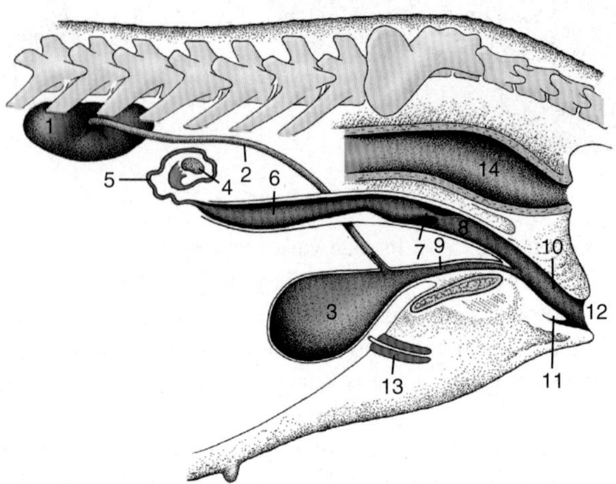

Fig. 5.2 The female urinary and reproductive organs (bitch). *1,* Right kidney; *2,* ureter; *3,* bladder; *4,* ovary; *5,* uterine tube; *6,* uterine horn; *7,* cervix; *8,* vagina; *9,* urethra; *10,* vestibule; *11,* clitoris; *12,* vulva; *13,* vaginal process; *14,* rectum.

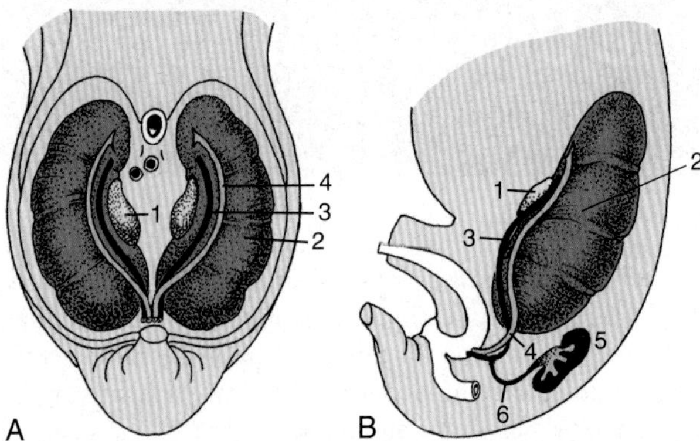

Fig. 5.4 (A) Ventral and (B) lateral views of the abdominal roof in a pig embryo of 2.5 cm. The pronephric duct drains the mesonephros and is now more aptly termed the *mesonephric duct. 1,* Developing gonad; *2,* mesonephros; *3,* mesonephric duct; *4,* paramesonephric duct; *5,* metanephros; *6,* ureter.

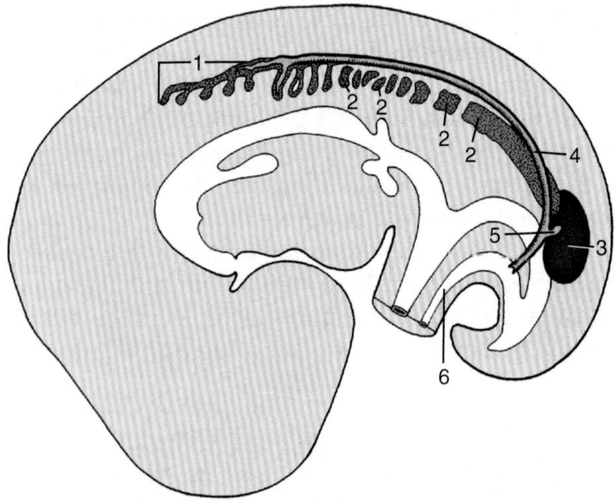

Fig. 5.3 Differentiation of the intermediate mesoderm. *1,* Pronephros; *2,* mesonephros, segmented cranially but continuous caudally; *3,* metanephros; *4,* pronephric (later mesonephric) duct; *5,* ureteric bud; *6,* urachus.

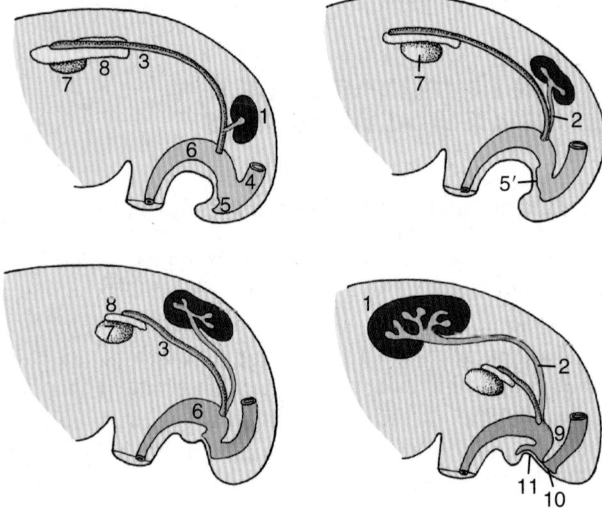

Fig. 5.5 The development of the metanephros from two primordia (metanephric cord and ureteric bud). Note the gradual regression of the mesonephros. *1,* Metanephros; *2,* ureteric bud (future ureter); *3,* mesonephric (deferent) duct; *4,* rectum; *5,* cloaca; *5′,* cloacal membrane; *6,* urogenital sinus; *7,* gonad; *8,* remnant of mesonephros (future epididymis); *9,* urorectal septum; *10,* anal membrane; *11,* urogenital membrane.

from a local branch of the aorta; this structure forms the glomerulus (see also Fig. 5.27).

The horizontal division of the cloacal region of the hindgut forms the lower urinary passages. The division itself is due to the caudal growth of a wedge of mesoderm, the urorectal septum, present within the angle between the hindgut and the allantoic bud. The septum eventually reaches the cloacal membrane, which is thus divided into dorsal (anal) and ventral (urogenital) parts (Fig. 5.5/*9*). The fusion site corresponds to the perineal body. The breakdown of the anal membrane transforms the dorsal passage into a continuous rectoanal canal. A similar process in the urogenital membrane opens the ventral passage to the surface of the body. This urogenital passage differentiates into a cranial part, the future bladder and allantois, and a caudal part, from which the urethra is formed.

The bladder then appears as a widening that is continued cranially by the allantoic duct and caudally by an undilated urethra. The allantoic duct or *urachus* (Fig. 5.3/*6*) can be followed through the umbilical opening to an extraembryonic expansion (the allantois) in which urine accumulates and which is discarded at birth. The part of the duct within the fetus then shrivels and is finally represented only by the cicatrix or scar on the apex of the bladder. The caudal part of the primordium is transformed into the urethra—the entire urethra in the female but only the short pelvic urethra in the male (in which the penile urethra develops with the genital system). The definitive positions of the openings

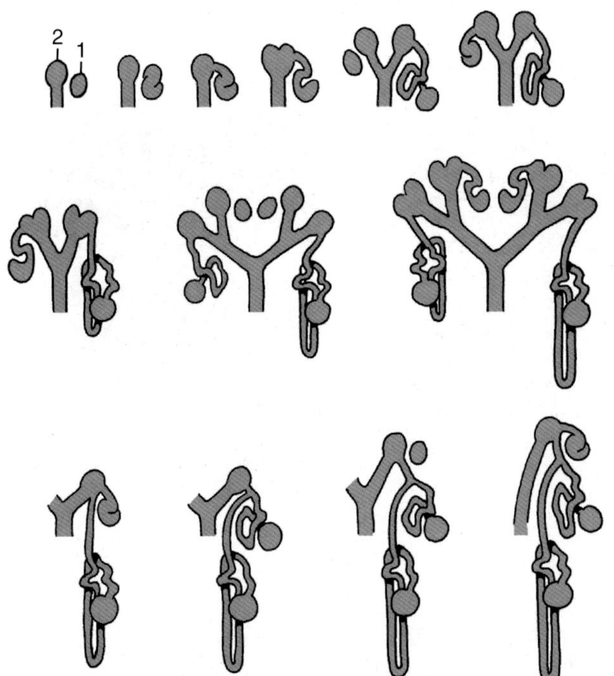

Fig. 5.6 This series of schematic drawings depicts the connections between developing nephrons *(1)* and branches *(2)* of the ureteric bud. Note the dichotomous division of the drainage system (ureteric bud).

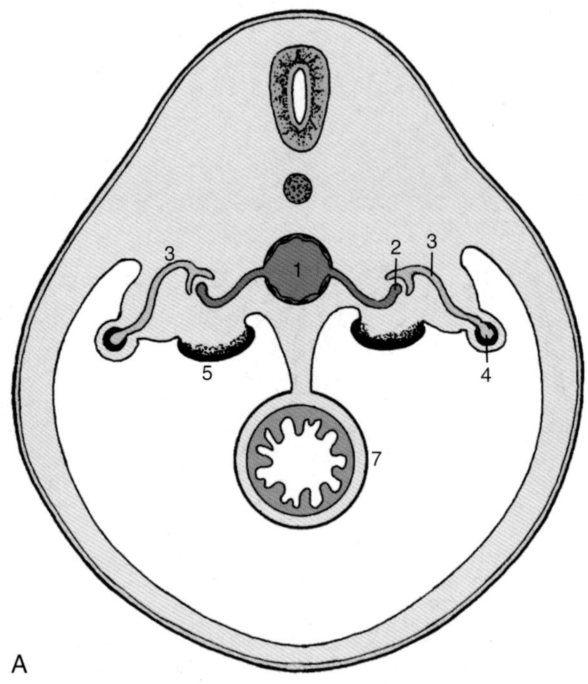

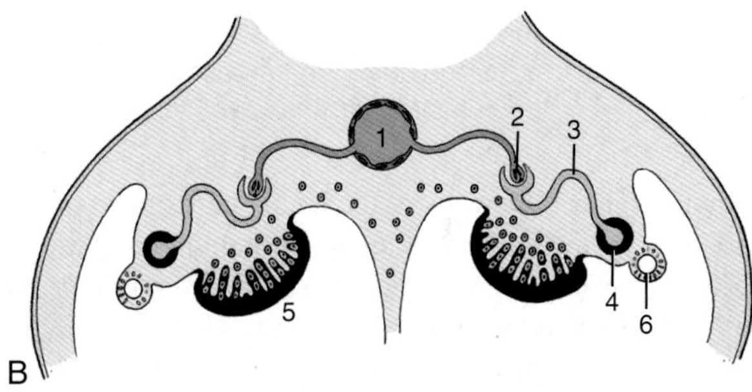

Fig. 5.7 (A) Early development of the indifferent gonad. (B) Invasion of the gonad by epithelial cords, which then incorporate primordial germ cells. *1,* Aorta; *2,* capillary tuft (in nephron); *3,* nephron (tubule); *4,* mesonephric duct; *5,* gonad; *6,* paramesonephric duct; *7,* gut.

of the mesonephric and metanephric ducts result from the incorporation of their lower ends within the larger passage. The rearrangement brings the opening of the metanephric duct (ureter) into the bladder and situates that of the mesonephric duct (deferent duct) more caudally within the urogenital sinus (see Fig. 5.5). In this process the mesoderm of the mesonephric duct provides the epithelium of the dorsal trigonal region of the bladder (p. 172) and the hindgut endoderm that of the remaining part. The outer layers of the bladder wall differentiate from local mesoderm.

Development of the Male Reproductive Organs

The early stages of morphologic differentiation of the reproductive organs follow a pattern common to the two sexes. In both, the gonadal primordium appears as a thickening of the celomic epithelium on the medial aspect of the mesonephros. It projects as a swelling when the underlying mesenchyme proliferates (Fig. 5.7A/*5*). Cords of cells that develop from the covering epithelium penetrate the interior of the swelling (Fig. 5.7B/*5*). These cords shortly incorporate the primordial germ cells, which rather surprisingly have a distant origin in the endoderm of a restricted portion of the yolk sac, where they are identifiable by their large size. They reach the gonad by migration over the gut and its mesentery, but carriage in the bloodstream also seems possible.

An early indication that *the gonad* will become a testis is provided by a marked mesenchymal condensation (tunica albuginea) below the celomic epithelium. Now isolated from the surface epithelium, the cords increase in size and in complexity of arrangement (Fig. 5.8/*3*). They connect to a plexus or network (rete) within the testis. On the other side the plexus makes contact with the blind ends of the few tubules that have survived the general regression of the mesonephros (Fig. 5.8B/*3–5*). Differentiation within the cell cords permits recognition of two cell lineages. One provides the sustentacular (Sertoli) cells of the seminiferous tubules. The second, contributed by the primordial germ cells, provides the germinal epithelium. During fetal development the primordial germ cells differentiate into gonocytes, which after birth give rise to spermatogonia. At puberty, the spermatogonia proliferate and differentiate to supply cells that undergo meiosis and spermiogenesis to form male gametes (see Fig. 5.39). Sections through the adult testis show seminiferous tubules cut in

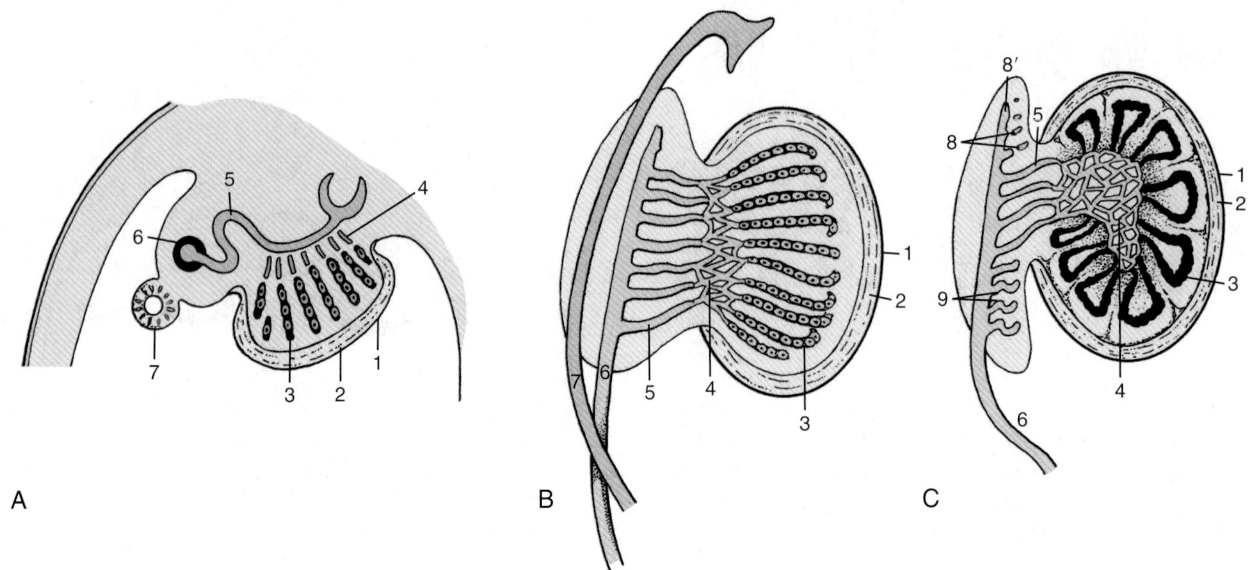

Fig. 5.8 Three stages in the development of the testis. (A) The epithelial cords are isolated from the surface epithelium by the formation of the tunica albuginea. (B) The epithelial cords, rete, and mesonephric tubules have interconnected. (C) The epithelial cords become seminiferous tubules, and the mesonephros is gradually transformed into part of the epididymis. *1,* Celomic epithelium; *2,* tunica albuginea; *3,* epithelial cords, seminiferous tubules; *4,* rete testis; *5,* mesonephric tubules, efferent ductules; *6,* mesonephric (later deferent) duct; *7,* paramesonephric duct; *8,* cranial remnant of mesonephric tubules (aberrant ductules); *8′,* remnant of *6* (appendix of epididymis); *9,* caudal remnant (paradidymis).

various planes. The walls of the highly convoluted tubules are lined by a stratified germinal epithelium consisting of cells in various stages of differentiation. Supporting Sertoli cells nourish the germ cells. The Leydig cells produce the steroid testosterone that is essential if spermatogenesis is to continue. Their progenitors, like those of Sertoli and primordial germ cells, presumably migrate from the mesonephros during fetal development to become embedded in a mesenchymal interstitium, and around puberty, when the process of spermatogenesis is initiated, a second generation of Leydig cells develops.

The initial formation of *the seminiferous cords* is followed in later fetal life by canalization of the cords to create a series of passages leading to the mesonephric duct, which thus becomes the outlet for the gamete products of the testis. The peripheral parts of the cords become seminiferous tubules, the central parts become the rete testis, and the mesonephric tubules become the efferent ductules (Fig. 5.8C). The first part of the mesonephric duct convolutes and forms the duct of the epididymis within the dense connective tissue of that organ; the remaining part retains a straighter course, and as the deferent duct (Fig. 5.5/*3*), it opens into that part of the cloaca that becomes the urogenital sinus (Fig. 5.5/*6*). Glandular proliferation of the lining of the duct toward its termination produces the ampullary thickening, whereas in most species but not in carnivores, a subterminal budding enlarges as the vesicular gland (Fig. 5.9/*5*). In some species a final short passage, the ejaculatory duct, persists, but in others later adjustments cause the deferent and vesicular ducts to open separately. Gonadal enlargement causes the testis to hang within a fold (mesorchium) arising from the regressing mesonephros. The duct is carried within this supporting fold, which in its caudal stretch inclines medially to form with its neighbor the genital fold of peritoneum that helps subdivide the peritoneal cavity of the pelvis. The testis later migrates outside the abdomen (p. 163) before the initiation of spermatogenesis.

The division of the cloaca has been described (p. 136). The caudal part of the sinus constitutes the pelvic part of the urethra. Outgrowths from its lining differentiate into the prostate and bulbourethral glands in a species-characteristic fashion (Fig. 5.9). The greater part of the male urethra lies within the penis and has a different origin. Thickenings appear around the margin of the urogenital membrane in the indifferent stage (Fig. 5.10). One thickening, ventral and median, constitutes the *genital (phallic) tubercle* or swelling (Fig. 5.10/*1*), which gives rise to the greater part of the penis; other thickenings that are more lateral in position contribute the scrotum. A further *urogenital fold* that appears medial to each scrotal swelling makes an additional contribution to the penis. A groove extends along the (initially) dorsal surface of the genital tubercle; it is gradually closed by the approach and merging of these urogenital folds. This process is rather complex because

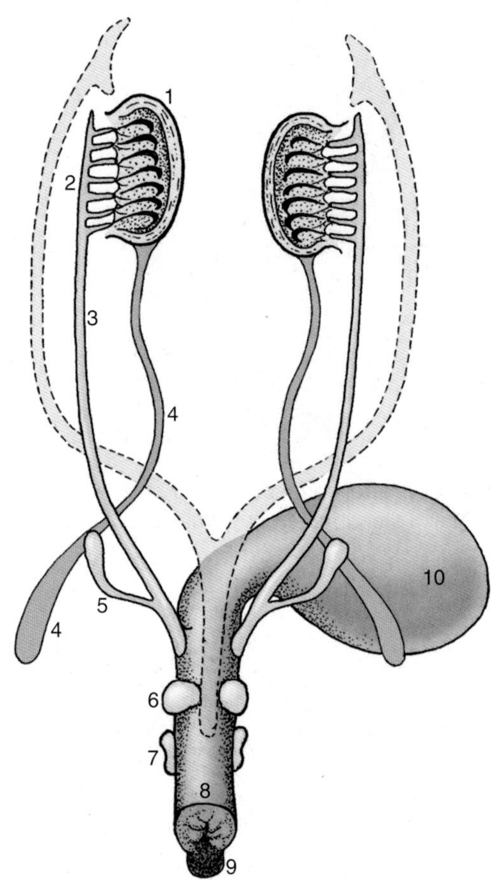

Fig. 5.9 Differentiation of the urogenital sinus. Note the budding of the prostate and bulbourethral glands and the enlargement of the genital tubercle. The regressed paramesonephric ducts are indicated by the *broken lines*. *1*, Testis; *2*, epididymis; *3*, deferent duct; *4*, gubernaculum; *5*, vesicular gland; *6*, prostate; *7*, bulbourethral gland; *8*, urogenital sinus (urethra); *9*, genital tubercle; *10*, bladder.

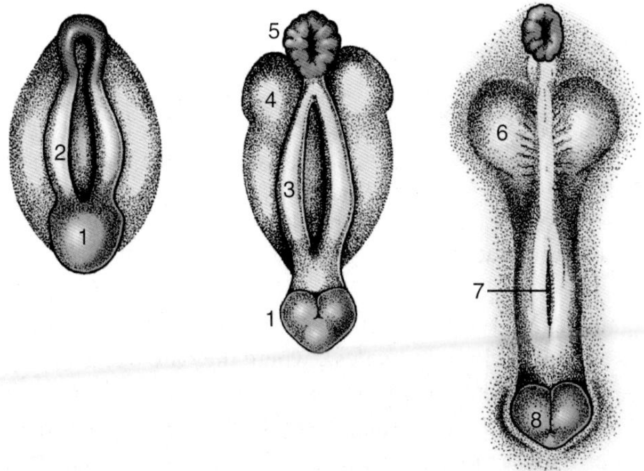

Fig. 5.10 Development of the male external genitalia. *1*, Genital tubercle; *2*, cloacal fold; *3*, urogenital fold; *4*, lateral (scrotal) swelling; *5*, anus; *6*, scrotum; *7*, groove closing to form the penile urethra; *8*, glans penis.

the lining of the penile urethra is provided by an extension of the endoderm of the urogenital sinus, although the initial swellings have ectodermal coverings. The corpus spongiosum (spongy body) of the penile urethra directly continues the bulbar tissue of the pelvic urethra, while the corpus cavernosum penis forms within the genital swelling. The lateral swellings grow and join together to form the scrotum, which retains evidence of its bilateral origin in a median raphe and septum.

Differentiation of the male efferent duct system, accessory glands, and external genitalia depends on the presence of testosterone, the male sex hormone produced by the developing testes. The testes also produce several other hormones—for example, the antimüllerian hormone (AMH) and insulin-like factor 3 (descendine), respectively responsible for the disappearance of the müllerian duct and the outgrowth of the gubernaculum, respectively. Without exposure to these three hormones the genital tract would develop in the female direction. Removal of the pituitary by decapitation in the fetal period does not disturb the production of these hormones by the testis (Fig. 5.11A and B).

Development of the Female Reproductive Organs

The initial stages of gonadal development resemble those described for the male. Later, the cell cords fragment into cell clusters, each enclosing an immigrant germ cell. The cords penetrate less deeply into the interior of the gonad than in the male. The primordial follicles are formed here. Rete formation is less pronounced in the ovary, and because no connection is established with mesonephric tubules, no uninterrupted tubular outlet for the escape of gametes is created (Fig. 5.12).

Consequently, follicular rupture releases the female gametes at the surface of the ovary by tissue breakdown, a process made easier by the absence of a thick tunica albuginea. The same feature allows for the formation of further sex cords and the establishment of additional follicles during a large part of prenatal life; indeed in certain species this process may continue for a time after birth. Even so, it ceases eventually, and the number of female gametes is then at its maximum. It is afterward depleted by loss through atresia and, to a much smaller extent, through ovulation. Ovarian descent is very limited in most species, being greatest in the ruminants, in which the ovaries shift caudally to the abdominopelvic boundary.

The duct system of the female is largely provided by the *paramesonephric ducts* (Fig. 5.12/7), which have only vestigial importance in the male. These ducts develop first by invagination of the celomic epithelium lateral to the mesonephric ducts and second by active growth in the direction of the urogenital sinus within the genital folds. In contrast, the mesonephric ducts regress in craniocaudal sequence (Fig. 5.13), and only remnants survive within the broad

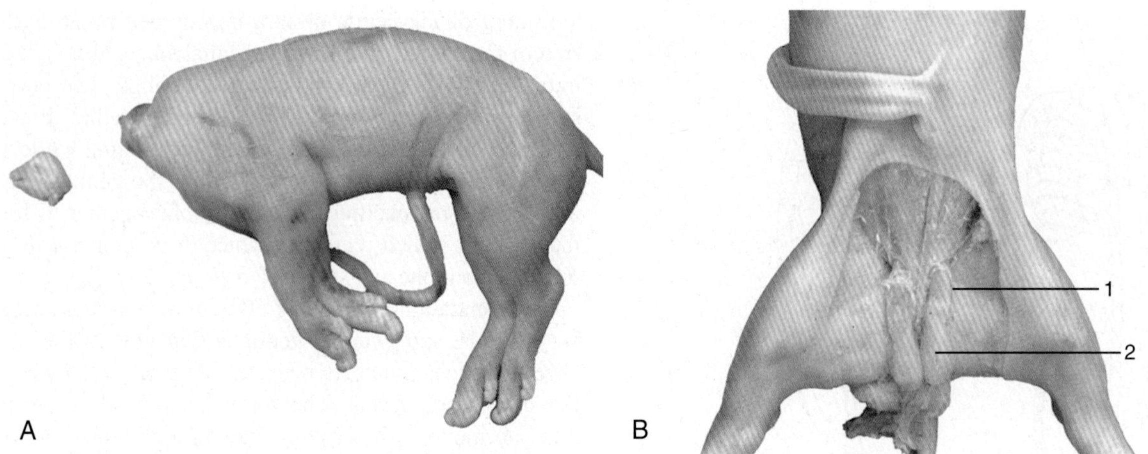

Fig. 5.11 (A) Pig (fetus) (near term), decapitated in utero 42 days after conception. (B) Fetus shown in (A) with inguinal area dissected to show gubernacula unaffected by removal of pituitary gland. *1,* testis; *2,* gubernaculum.

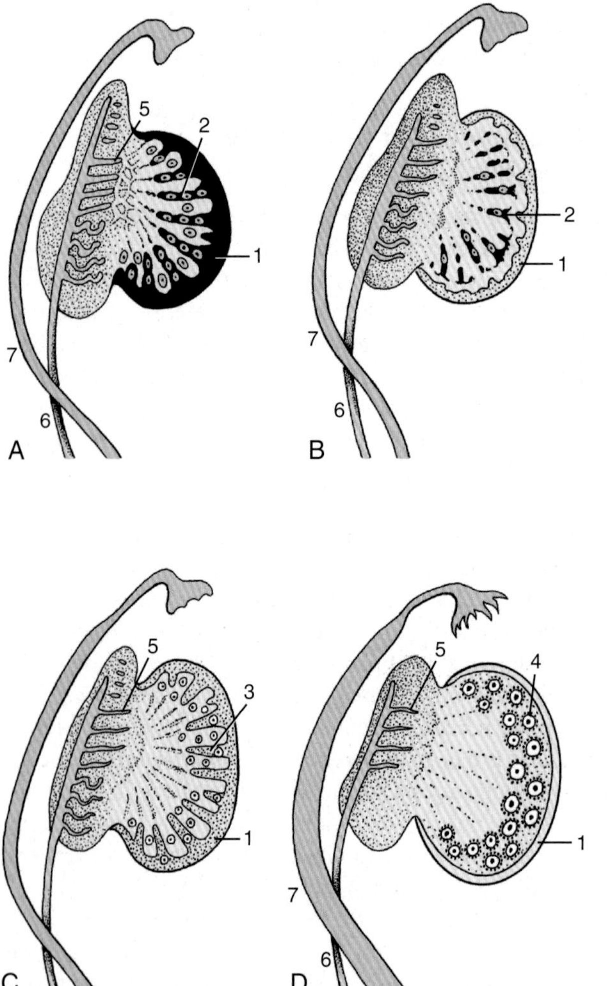

Fig. 5.12 (A) to (D), Successive stages in the development of the ovary. *1,* Celomic epithelium; *2,* epithelial cords, penetrating (A) and regressing (B); *3,* second formation of sex cords (C); *4,* primitive follicles; *5,* remnants of mesonephric tubules; *6,* mesonephric duct; *7,* paramesonephric duct (D).

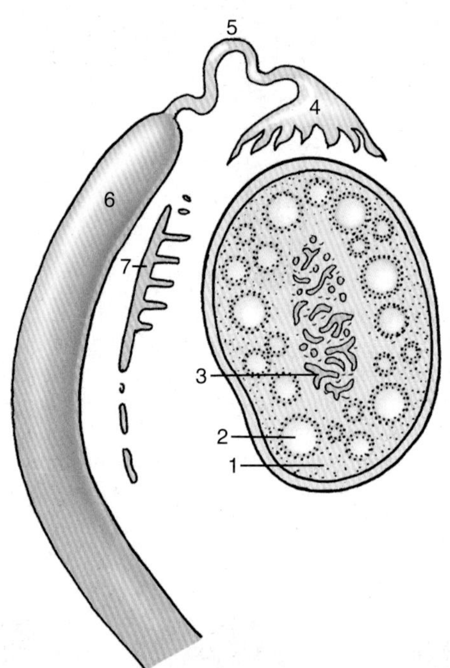

Fig. 5.13 Differentiation of paramesonephric duct and regression of mesonephric duct. *1,* Interstitial tissue of the ovary; *2,* primitive follicles; *3,* ovarian rete; *4,* infundibulum; *5,* uterine tube; *6,* uterine horn *(4, 5,* and *6* differentiate from paramesonephric duct); *7,* remnants of the mesonephric tubules and duct (epoöphoron and paroöphoron).

ligaments and in the vaginal wall (ducts of Gartner, ductus epoöphori longitudinales), where they are occasionally the seat of anomalous processes. The cranial part of each paramesonephric duct runs lateral to the mesonephric duct but crosses it more caudally, where it inclines to meet and fuse with its fellow (Fig. 5.14/*6*). The cranial end of each paramesonephric duct remains open to the peritoneal cavity (abdominal ostium of the uterine tube), but the caudal end of the united duct initially ends blindly against a solid

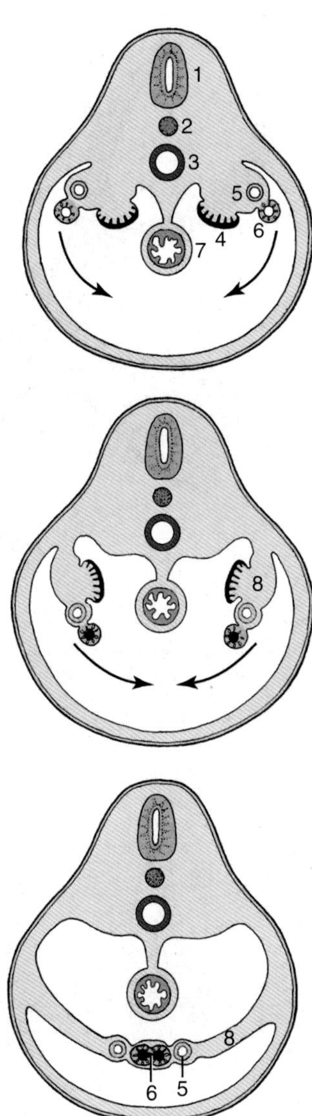

Fig. 5.14 Transverse sections (from cranial to caudal) through the caudal part of the abdomen, illustrating the creation of the genital fold in the female embryo. *1,* Neural tube; *2,* notochord; *3,* aorta; *4,* gonad; *5,* mesonephric duct (regressing); *6,* paramesonephric duct (merged in the caudal section); *7,* gut; *8,* genital fold.

outgrowth from the dorsal wall of the urogenital sinus (Fig. 5.15). The uterine tubes and the horns, body, and cervix of the uterus form from the paramesonephric ducts; their caudal parts fuse to an extent that varies with the species and accounts for the very different form and proportions of the uterus of adult animals (p. 186) (Fig. 5.16). The supporting genital fold becomes the broad ligament with its various parts. The vaginal lumen appears within the solid outgrowth from the sinus, although a tissue partition, the hymen, may persist near the junction with the fused paramesonephric ducts. A hymen is present only in virgin animals and is rarely well formed in domestic species. There is dispute over the contribution of the urogenital and paramesonephric epithelia to the lining of the vagina in the adult, and some writers suggest that the boundary may divide regions with different responses to hormonal influences that are observed in some species.

The urogenital sinus becomes the vestibule with relatively little further change. Epithelial outgrowths form the vestibular glands in species-variable fashion. The external genital parts are formed from the same structures as in the male; the genital tubercle and lateral folds (swellings) appear first (Fig. 5.17). The former produces the clitoris, but the lateral folds, which form the labia majora of human anatomy, regress—with a possible reservation for the bitch. The labia of the vulva in domestic species are provided by the *urogenital folds* (Fig. 5.17/*3*) that appear medial to the lateral swellings and correspond to the labia minora of women.

The Process of Testicular Descent

The descent of the testis into a scrotal position is necessary in most mammals to obtain normal fertility. The process depends on the existence of a mesenchymal condensation, the *gubernaculum testis,* within a detachment from the genital fold that leads from the testis toward and through the inguinal canal (Fig. 5.18). At a certain critical period of development (which varies in timing among different species) the distal part of the gubernaculum, which extends through the inguinal canal to the groin, enlarges very rapidly and considerably (Fig. 5.19A and B). The gubernaculum is invaded by an extension of the peritoneal lining of the abdomen. In this way the vaginal process, which provides the space into which the testis will be drawn, is formed (Fig. 5.18/*3*). The invasion by the vaginal process divides the gubernaculum into three parts: the proximal part (pars propria) is enclosed by the inner (future visceral) peritoneal lining of the process; the second part (pars vaginalis) surrounds the outer (future parietal) peritoneal lining of the process; and the third part (pars infravaginalis) lies distal to the invagination and is thus continuous with the other parts. The swelling of the gubernaculum commences distally, causing it to exert pressure on the body wall about the superficial ring of the inguinal canal. The swelling displaces the testis distally, toward the abdominal entrance of the canal. The swelling then gradually extends proximally, and at its peak the part adjacent to the testis (and within the inguinal canal) is as thick as the testis itself (Fig. 5.19A and B). At this stage any slight increase in intraabdominal pressure may be sufficient to expel the testis from the abdomen into the inguinal canal, although for a time its return to the abdomen is still possible. The descent is complete and irreversible once the core of the gubernaculum has regressed (Fig. 5.20). A well-timed gubernacular regression is therefore as indispensable to normal descent as is the earlier swelling. Because the timing is critical and the process is subject to various disturbances, it is not surprising that abdominal retention and abnormal descent are both relatively frequent. Failure of the

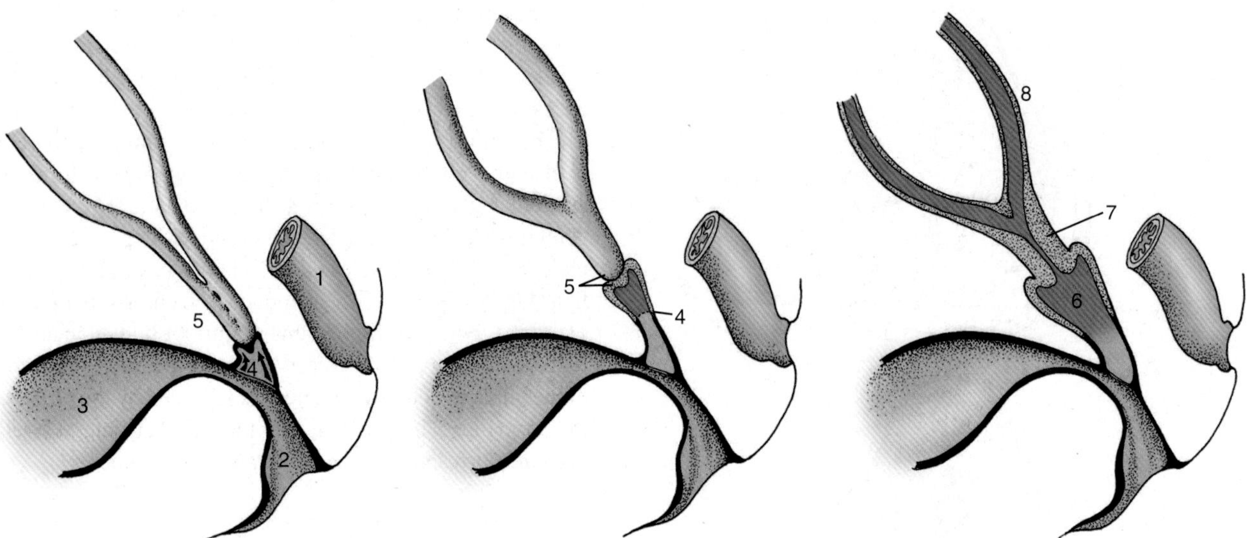

Fig. 5.15 The fusion of the combined paramesonephric ducts with a bud from the urogenital sinus forms the vagina. *1,* Rectum; *2,* caudal part of urogenital sinus (vestibule); *3,* cranial part of urogenital sinus (bladder, urethra); *4,* bud from urogenital sinus; *5,* fused paramesonephric ducts; *6,* vagina; *7,* cervix uteri; *8,* uterine horn.

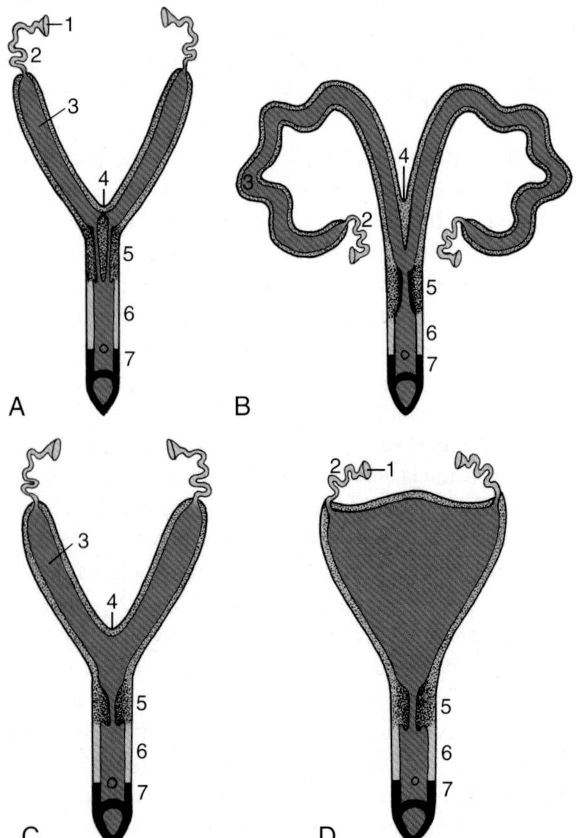

Fig. 5.16 Different degrees of fusion of the paramesonephric ducts. (A) Uterus duplex (rabbit). (B) Uterus bicornis (small body: sow, cow). (C) Uterus bicornis (large body: mare). (D) Uterus simplex (woman). *1,* Infundibulum; *2,* uterine tube; *3,* uterine horn; *4,* fusion site of the two ducts; *5,* cervix; *6,* vagina; *7,* vestibule.

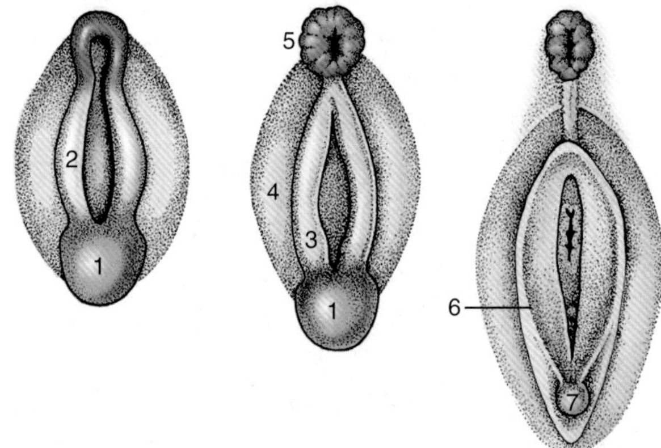

Fig. 5.17 Development of the female external genitalia. *1,* Genital tubercle; *2,* cloacal fold; *3,* urogenital fold; *4,* lateral swelling; *5,* anus; *6,* labia of vulva; *7,* clitoris.

testis to appear in the groin is known as cryptorchidism (hidden testis). It takes various forms: it may be unilateral or bilateral, and the testis may be held within the abdomen or trapped within the inguinal canal. As a result of the higher temperature to which an undescended testis is exposed, spermatogenesis is not initiated at puberty. The condition is clearly undesirable, and although unilaterally cryptorchid animals may be fertile, they should be excluded from breeding because the condition is often hereditary.

Similar structures are formed in the female sex but do not develop significantly, except in the bitch among domestic mammals, in which the existence of the vaginal process is occasionally troublesome (p. 448).

In several species when a twin pregnancy occurs, the circulation of the two fetuses can become interconnected, resulting in the exchange not only of cells but also of hormones (see Fig. 29.18). The hormonal influence of the male fetus can interfere with the development of the female cotwin. In cattle this interference can result in a "freemartin," in which the ovary and the female duct system are severely underdeveloped or absent. It can also result in the outgrowth of the gubernacula in the female twin (see Fig. 35.8A and B). Very seldom, this problem can also occur in a pig fetus that is interconnected with a male fetus in utero.

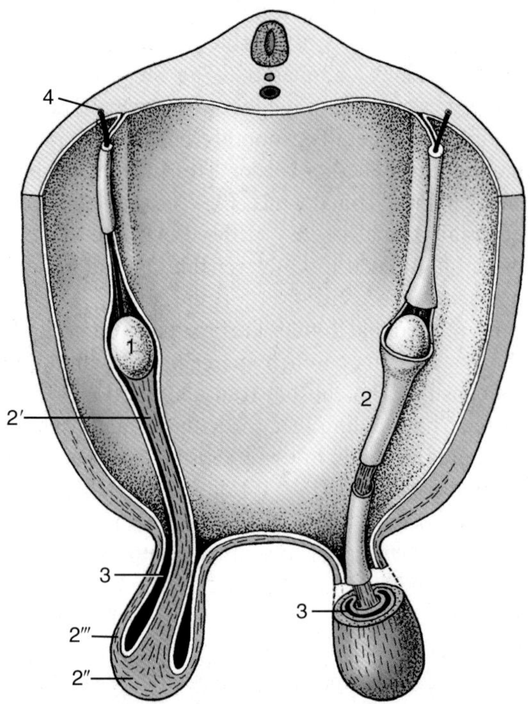

Fig. 5.18 Schematic representation of the testis and gubernaculum within the peritoneal fold in which descent takes place. *1,* Testis; *2,* gubernaculum; *2′,* pars propria; *2″,* pars infravaginalis; *2‴,* pars vaginalis; *3,* vaginal process; *4,* testicular artery.

THE URINARY ORGANS

The urinary system comprises paired kidneys that form the urine from the blood; ureters that convey the urine from the kidneys; the bladder, where urine is stored until it can be discharged conveniently; and the urethra, through which it finally passes to the exterior. As almost the entire male urethra also conveys the reproductive products, it is usually described with the reproductive organs.

The Kidneys

The kidneys have the maintenance of the milieu intérieur as their prime task. They do this by filtering the plasma, initially extracting an enormous volume of fluid before subjecting this ultrafiltrate to further processing in which useful substances are selectively reabsorbed, waste substances are concentrated for elimination, and the volume is adjusted by the conservation of sufficient water to maintain the composition of the plasma within the appropriate range. Some figures may give an impression of the dimensions of this task. In large dogs (and animals of similar size), 1000 to 2000 L of blood perfuse the kidneys daily; the 200 to 300 L of fluid that are filtered from this volume are later reduced by reabsorption until only 1 or 2 L of urine remain to be discharged.

The kidney produces and releases two endocrine hormones: renin, which plays a vital role in the regulation of systemic blood pressure, and erythropoietin, which influences erythropoiesis. Both are produced within the juxtaglomerular complexes, localized regions of intimate association between arterioles formed by the union of

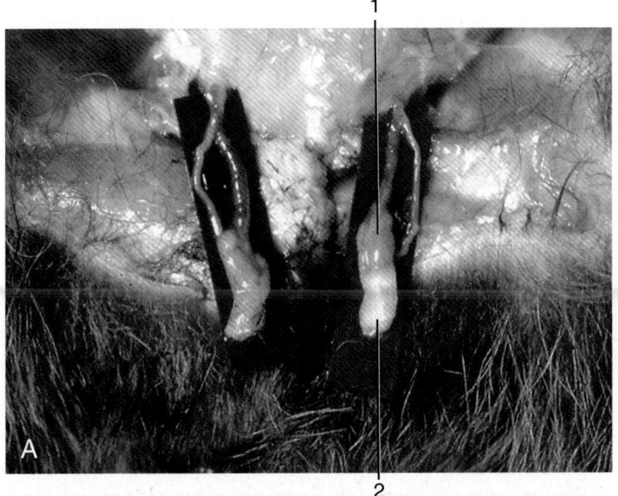

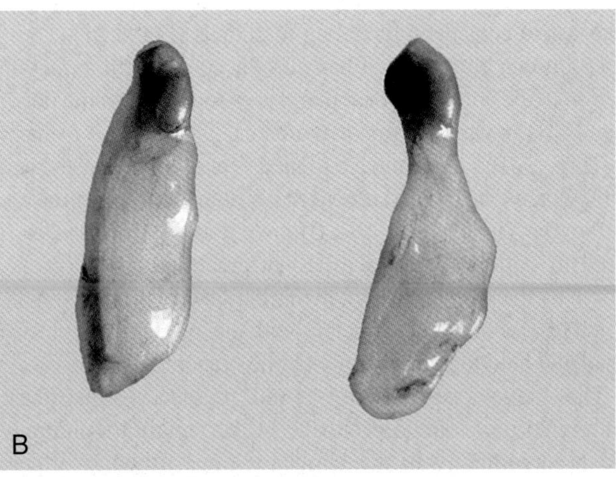

Fig. 5.19 Stages in the process of gubernacular swellings. The testis and gubernaculum have already passed the inguinal canal. Inguinal area of newborn pup. (A) *1,* Testis; *2,* exposed gubernaculum. (B) Testis and gubernaculum of pig fetus (110 days).

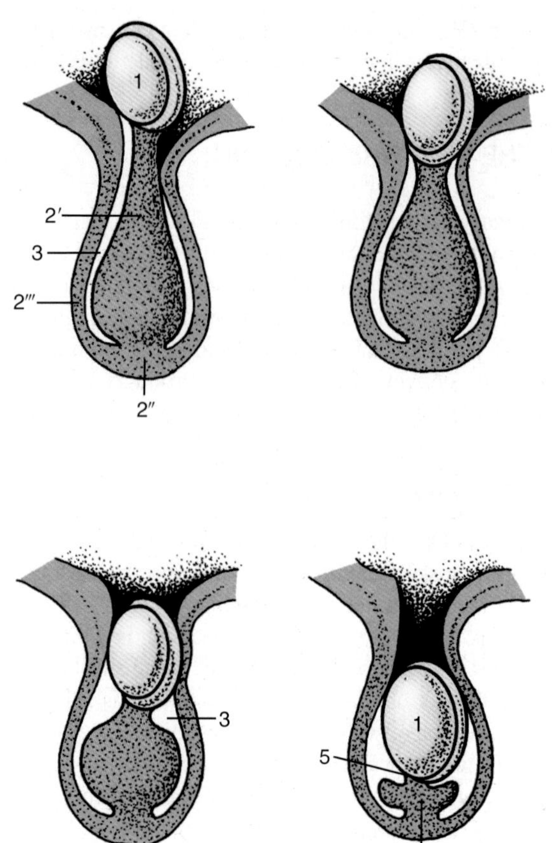

Fig. 5.20 Successive stages in gubernacular regression in the pig fetus. Observe the migration of the testis caused by this regression. *1*, Testis and epididymis; *2*, gubernaculum; *2′*, pars propria; *2″*, pars infravaginalis; *2‴*, pars vaginalis; *3*, vaginal process; *4*, ligament of the tail of the epididymis; *5*, proper ligament of the testis.

afferent glomerular capillaries with adjacent portions of the distal convoluted tubules (p. 209).

The kidneys are firm, reddish brown glands whose appearance varies considerably among mammals (Fig. 5.21). The most familiar form, which has introduced the term *kidney-shaped* to the common vocabulary, is encountered in the dog (Fig. 5.21D), cat, and small ruminants. The kidneys of the pig (Fig. 5.21C) are a much flattened version, whereas those of the horse (Fig. 5.21E) are more heart-shaped. In contrast, the bovine kidneys (Fig. 5.21B) have a surface deeply fissured to outline many lobes. Even greater subdivision is shown by the kidneys of certain marine species (Fig. 5.21A), which resemble trusses of grapes with the lobes only slightly fused and held together mainly by the branching "stalk."

The kidneys are usually found pressed against the abdominal roof, one to each side of the vertebral column, and predominantly in the lumbar region, although often extending forward under the last ribs. Their positions change by half the length of a vertebra with each breath. They are rarely symmetrical; in domestic animals, other than pigs, the right one is about half a kidney length in advance of its fellow. The cranial extremity of the right kidney commonly fits into a fossa of the liver, which helps fix its position. The left one, lacking this lodgment, is more mobile and is more likely to sag within the abdomen. The pendulous left kidney of ruminants is thrust into the right half of the abdomen by the large stomach. In general, kidneys pressed against the abdominal roof are largely retroperitoneal, whereas those suspended at a lower level have a more extensive peritoneal covering (Fig. 5.22).

Each kidney lies within a splitting of the sublumbar fascia, which also holds considerable fat (sometimes enough to hide the kidney completely). The fat protects against distorting pressures from neighboring organs. The surface of a kidney is generally smoothly convex except for an indentation of the medial border. This indentation leads to a concealed space (renal sinus; Fig. 5.23) occupied by the dilated origin (renal pelvis) of the ureter, the vessels and nerves passing to and from the renal hilus, and more fat.

The general organization of the kidney, as shown through a section that divides the organ into dorsal and ventral "halves," has its parenchyma enclosed within a tough fibrous capsule. The capsule restricts the kidney's ability to expand. The swelling that occurs in certain disease conditions therefore tends to compress the tissue and narrow the internal passages. The capsule strips readily from the healthy kidney but adheres in response to inflammation.

The *parenchyma* is visibly divided into an outer cortex and an inner medulla (see Fig. 5.23). The *cortex* is distinguished by its reddish brown color and finely granular appearance. The *medulla* consists of a dark purplish outer zone, from which stripes (medullary rays) extend into the cortex, and a paler, grayish red, and radially striated inner zone that extends toward the renal sinus. The gross arrangement of the medulla shows very marked species differences. In many species the medulla is arranged as several (or even many) roughly pyramidal discrete masses. In kidneys of this type a portion of the cortex is associated with each pyramid and caps its base. The apex of the pyramid points toward the renal sinus and forms a *papilla* that fits into a cuplike expansion (calix) of the renal pelvis. Each medullary pyramid with its associated cortex constitutes a *renal lobe.* Kidneys that retain this organization are said to be *multipyramidal* or multilobar. In some multipyramidal kidneys, such as those of cattle (Fig. 5.23A), the boundaries between the lobes are revealed by the fissures that penetrate from the surface; in others, including those of pigs, no external evidence of lobation is present (Fig. 5.23B).

All mammalian kidneys pass through a multipyramidal phase in their development, although in most species the number of lobes is later dramatically reduced (Fig. 5.24). In some species, including the dog, horse, and sheep, all the pyramids finally fuse to form a single medullary mass that confines the cortex to the periphery, where it forms a continuous shell. Even this *unipyramidal* or unilobar type of kidney retains some evidence of its complex ontogeny; a slight scalloping of the corticomedullary junction, punctuated by the arteries that mark the interlobar boundaries, shows

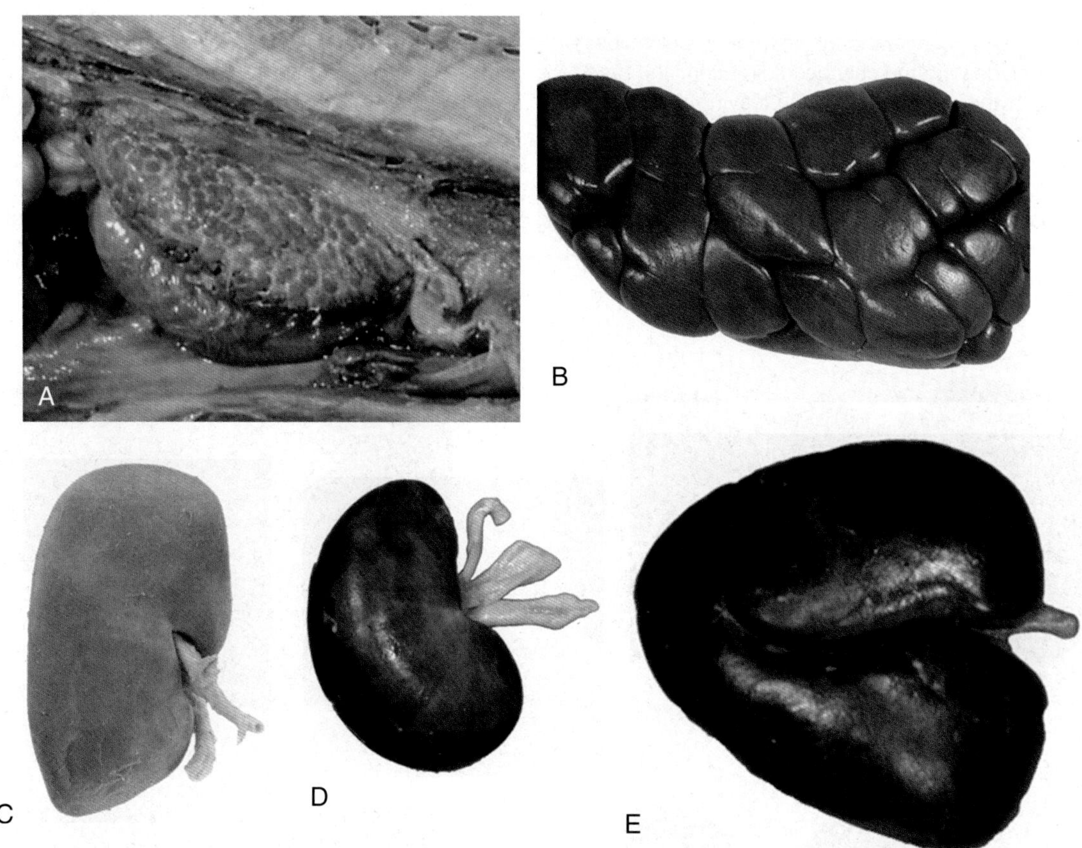

Fig. 5.21 Kidneys of (A) a dolphin, (B) a cow, (C) a pig, (D) a dog, and (E) a horse.

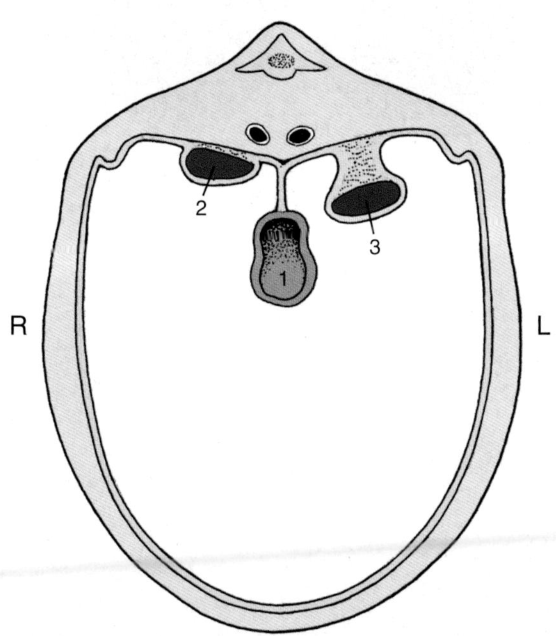

Fig. 5.22 Schematic representation of the position of the kidneys in relation to the peritoneal cavity. *1,* Gut; *2,* right kidney (retroperitoneal); *3,* left kidney (intraperitoneal: pendulous or "floating"); *R,* right; *L,* left.

where the pyramids fused. The fusion joins the papillae in a common crest (Figs. 5.25 and 5.26) that may be modeled to reveal its composite origin; it is so modeled in the dog and goat but not in the horse.

The renal tubules are lined by epithelium are supported by a connective tissue interstitium and are estimated to number several hundred thousand or even a million in canine kidneys.

Each *nephron* begins with a blind expansion that is invaginated by a cluster of capillaries known as a *glomerulus* (Figs. 5.27/*1* and 5.28). The glomerulus and its epithelial covering together constitute a *renal corpuscle* (Fig. 5.27/*1'*), a structure just large enough to be visible to the unaided eye, especially if the capillaries are congested. The corpuscles are scattered throughout the cortex and give it a finely granular appearance.

The remaining part of the nephron forms a long tubule differentiated into several successive segments. The first, the proximal convoluted tubule, is very tortuous and is located close to the corpuscle from which it arises (Fig. 5.27/*2*). This part gradually straightens and enters one of the narrow rays that penetrate the cortex from the medulla. The tubule then forms a long hairpin loop (formerly known as the loop of Henle) within the medulla. The first part of the loop, the descending limb, is relatively narrow and runs through the medulla to approach the papilla before turning back. The ascending limb is generally thicker, although the change in caliber need not coincide with the change in direction, and runs back to regain the medullary ray. On leaving this point, the tubule forms a second or distal convoluted part that is also placed close to the corpuscle of origin (Fig. 5.27/*4*). A short junctional section then runs to join a collecting tubule within the medullary ray. Each *collecting tubule* (Fig. 5.27/*5*), which serves many nephrons, runs through the medulla before opening into a larger vessel, a *papillary duct,* close to the apex (Fig. 5.27/*6*). Several score of papillary ducts drain into the renal pelvis. The papillary ducts can be clearly demonstrated in resin-injection specimens (see Fig. 5.24). The perforated (cribriform) areas where they discharge are confined to the apices of independent papillae or to specific regions of a common crest. Variations in the location of the corpuscles and in the overall length and proportions of the tubules have functional importance.

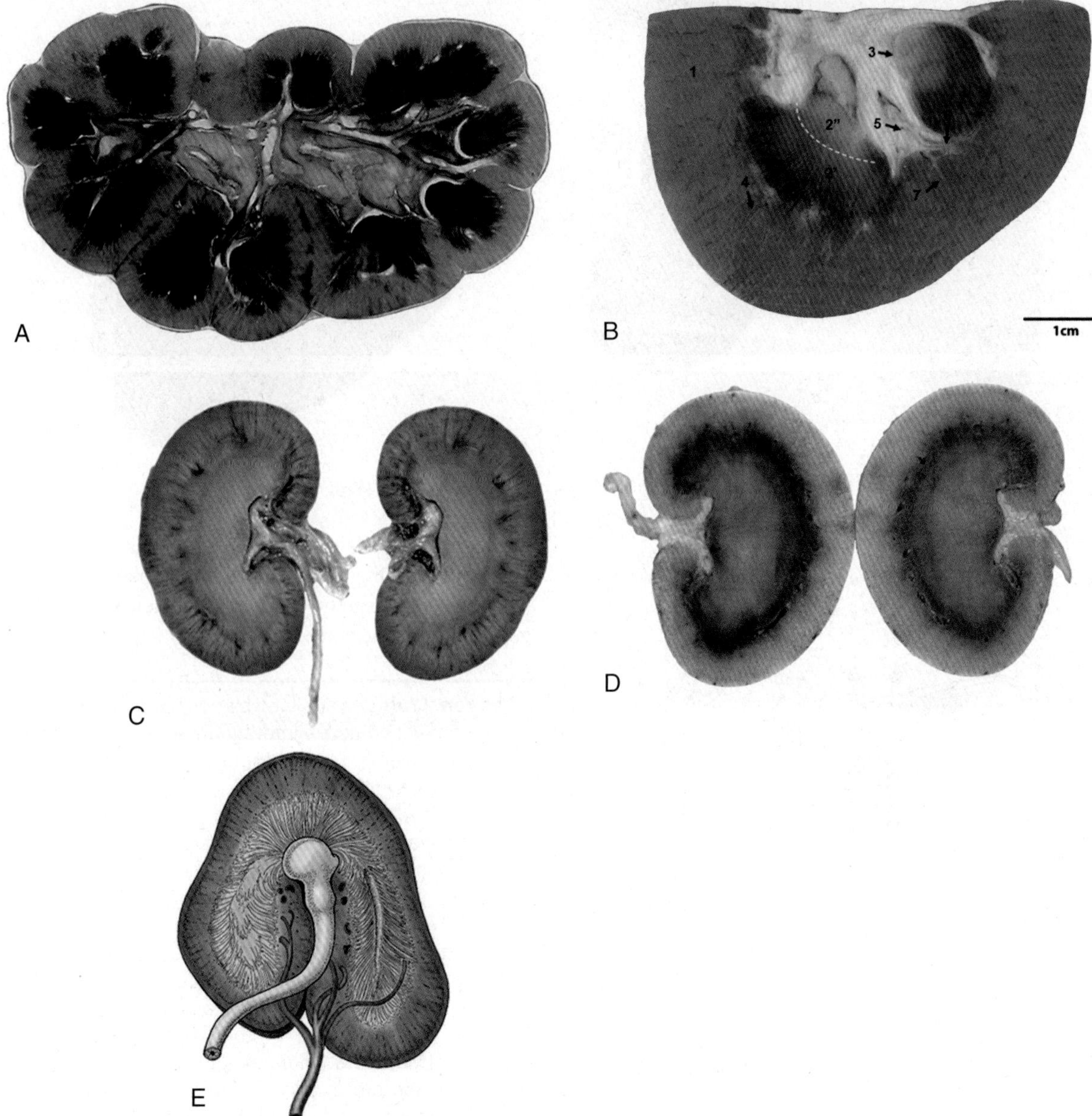

Fig. 5.23 Sectioned kidneys of (A) 1, Cortex; 2, medulla divided into lobes and 3, renal calyces; 4, medullary rays in cortex; inner (2′) and outer (2″) zones medulla (separated by the dotted line), and lobar (5), arcuate (6) and interlobular (7) vessels Notice the complexity of the renal pelvis decreases from cow to horse. F shows section of the pig kidney showing cortex (1), medulla (2) divided into lobes and renal calyces (3). Notice the medullary rays (4) in cortex, inner (2′) and outer (2″) zones medulla (separated by the dotted line), and lobar (5), arcuate (6) and interlobular (7) vessels.

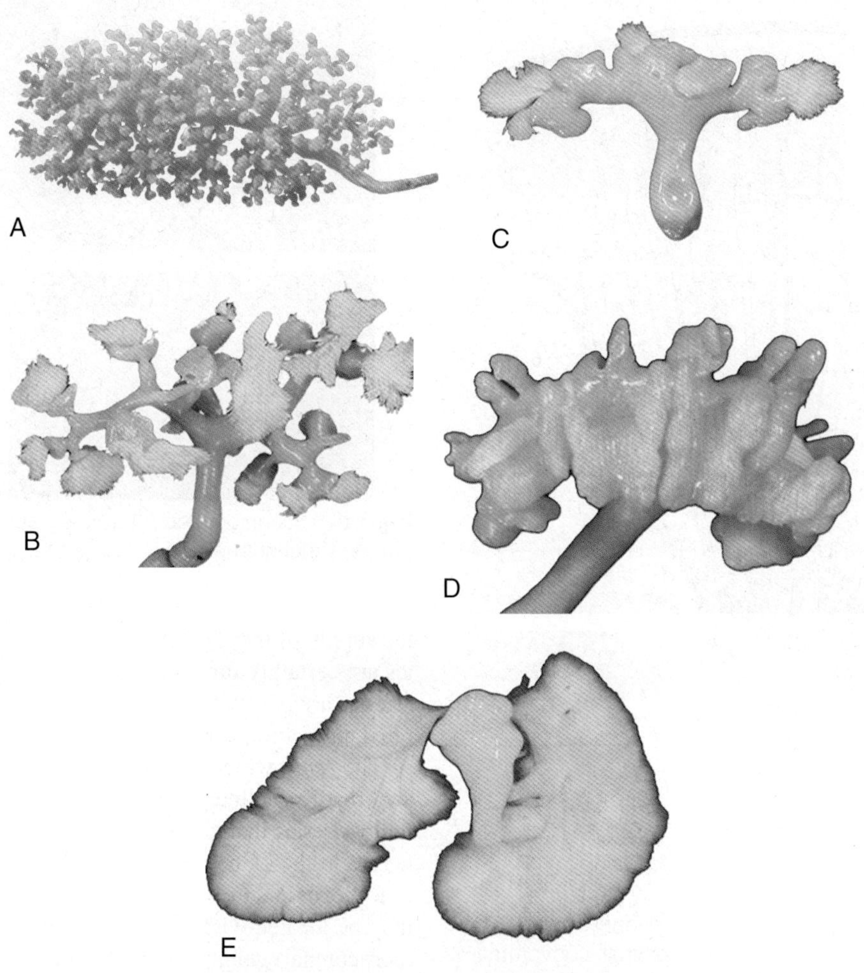

Fig. 5.24 Corrosion casts of the renal pelvis. (A) Dolphin; note the branched renal pelvis with many calices. (B) Cow; note the papillary ducts extending from the calices. (C) Pig; the renal pelvis becomes confluent; again note the papillary ducts. (D) Dog; the renal pelvis is one cavity, but note the ridges between the renal papilla. (E) Horse; one simple renal pelvis and many papillary ducts open into the renal pelvis.

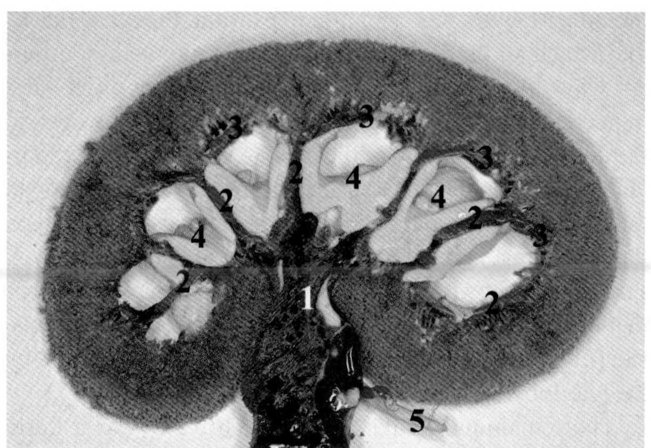

Fig. 5.25 Corrosion cast of canine kidney. *1*, Renal vein and artery; *2*, interlobar arteries and veins; *3*, arcuate arteries and veins; *4*, renal pelvis and the pelvic recesses; *5*, ureter.

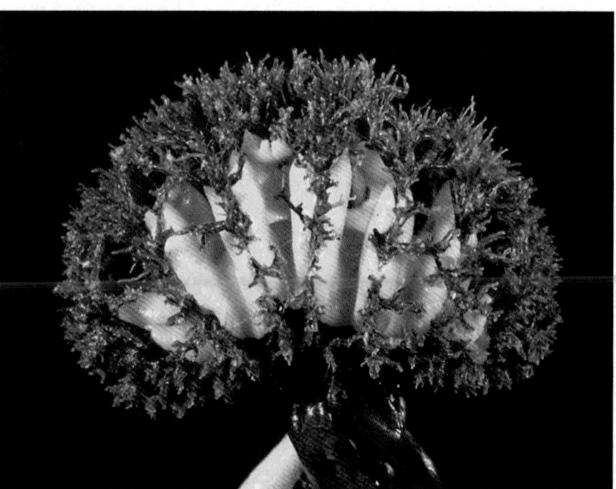

Fig. 5.26 Corrosion cast of renal pelvis, renal artery (red), and renal veins (blue) of a goat. The depressions of the ridges of the renal papillae are clearly visible.

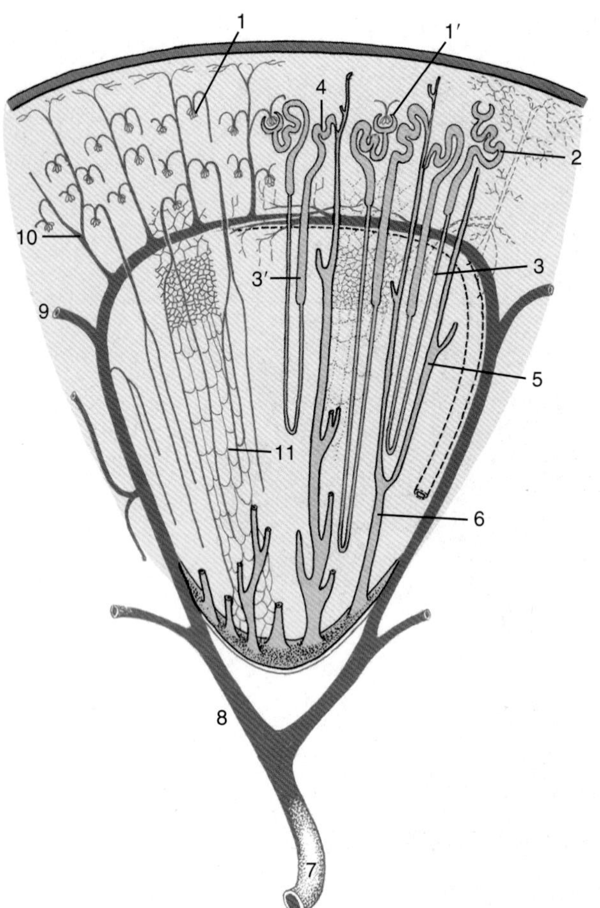

Fig. 5.27 Schematic drawing of a kidney lobe. *1,* Glomerulus; *1′,* renal corpuscle; *2,* proximal convoluted tubule; *3,* descending limb of nephron; *3′,* ascending limb; *4,* distal convoluted tubule; *5,* collecting tubule; *6,* papillary duct; *7,* renal artery; *8,* interlobar artery; *9,* arcuate artery; *10,* interlobular artery; *11,* capillary plexus.

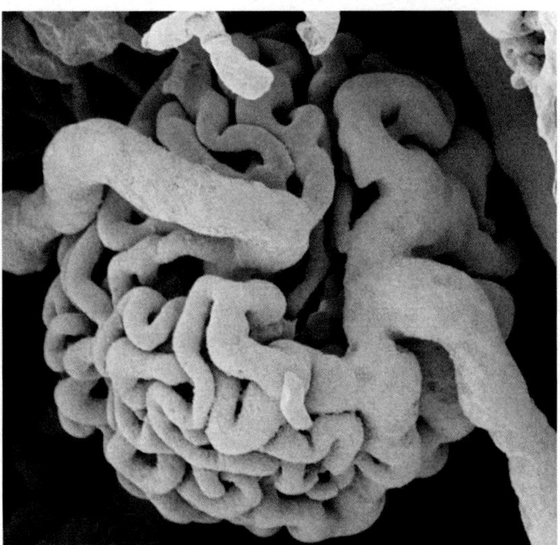

Fig. 5.28 Scanning electron micrograph of a corrosion cast of a rat renal glomerulus.

Each kidney is supplied by a *renal artery,* a branch of the abdominal aorta, which may carry more than a tenth of the total output of the left ventricle! The renal artery divides into several *interlobar arteries* (Fig. 5.27/*8*) that follow the divisions, former or extant, between the renal pyramids at the corticomedullary junction. These vessels are prominent in gross sections of the kidney. They give rise to branches known as *arcuate arteries* that curve over the bases of the pyramids (Fig. 5.27/*9*). These in turn give origin to numerous *interlobular arteries* that supply the units or lobules into which the cortex is divided by the medullary rays (Fig. 5.27/*10*). Each interlobular artery gives rise to many branches that supply individual glomeruli. The glomerular capillaries rejoin in one emissary vessel at the distal pole of the glomerulus, and this vessel then supplies a further capillary plexus around the tubules (Fig. 5.27/*11*). The flow of blood through this second capillary bed is countercurrent to the direction of the urine flow. The vessels that issue from the juxtamedullary corpuscles (those in the innermost layer of the cortex) have a particular importance in the supply of the medulla. However, the interlobular arteries are certainly functional end-arteries, and the interlobar arteries are possibly functional end-arteries. Of course, the renal circulation is more complicated than described here.

The *veins,* which lead ultimately to the caudal vena cava, are broadly satellite. Lymphatic vessels drain to nodes of the lumbar series that accompanies the aorta. The sympathetic nerves to the kidneys are routed through the celiacomesenteric plexus and thence along the renal arteries. The synapses may be located within the major ganglia or within smaller (aorticorenal) ganglia within peripheral parts of the plexus. The vagus nerve contributes the parasympathetic supply.

The Renal Pelvis and Ureter

In cattle the ureter is formed by the coming together of the short passages that lead from the calices that enclose individual renal papillae (Figs. 5.24B). In most domestic species the ureter begins in a common expansion, the *renal pelvis,* into which all the papillary ducts open—although in different ways in different species (Figs. 5.24). Few differences in pelvic anatomy are of practical significance. However, in the dog and cat the form of the renal pelvis obtains an importance lacking in the other species from its ready depiction in radiographs. The renal pelvis of these animals is molded on the renal crest and extends flanges dorsal and ventral to it. Each flange shows a number of local expansions or recesses that are divided from each other by projections of renal tissue (Fig. 5.29). Neighboring recesses are also separated by the interlobar vessels.

The remaining tubular part of each *ureter* has a fairly even caliber. It mostly travels sagittally against the abdominal roof and may exhibit occasional sharp changes in direction. Each ureter bends medially upon entering the pelvic cavity to enter the genital fold in the male or the broad ligament in the female for its journey over the dorsal surface

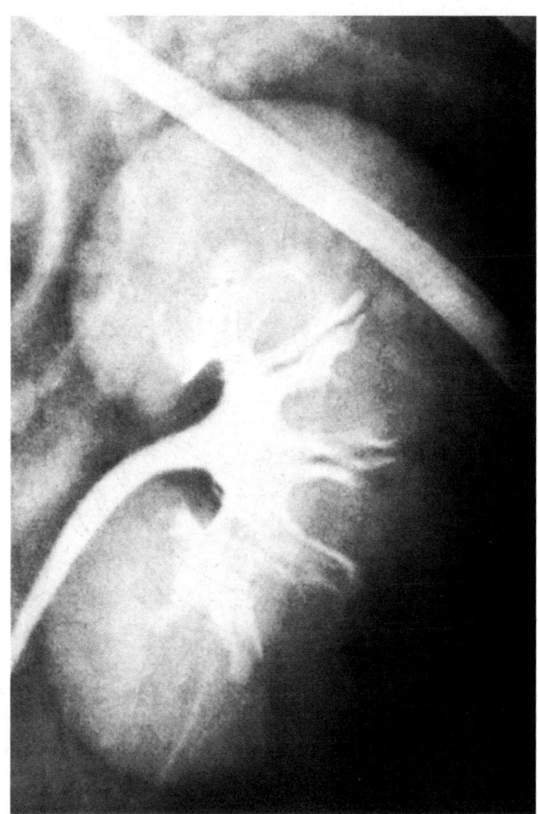

Fig. 5.29 Radiograph of the renal pelvis of a dog. Note the pelvic recesses.

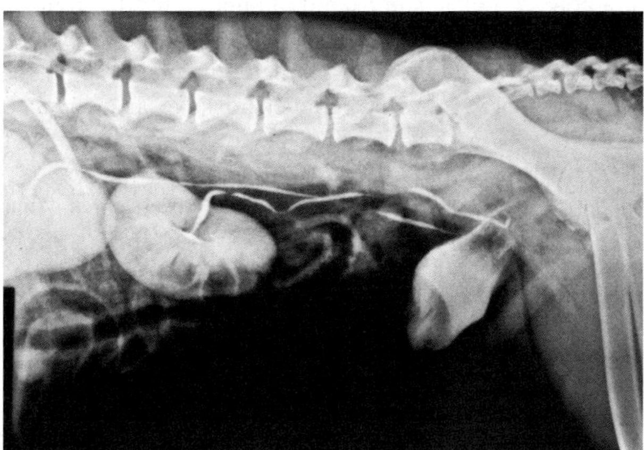

Fig. 5.30 Radiograph of the renal pelves, ureters, and bladder of a dog.

before opening into the bladder near its neck (Fig. 5.30). In the male the ureter passes dorsal to the corresponding deferent duct.

The ureter penetrates the bladder wall very obliquely, thereby guarding against reflux of urine into the ureter when the bladder fills up (Fig. 5.31). However, the angle does not prevent further filling of the bladder because the resistance is overcome by peristaltic contractions of the ureteric wall. The wall of the renal pelvis and ureter possesses an external adventitia, a well-developed middle muscularis, and an internal mucosa.

The Urinary Bladder

The distensible nature of the *bladder* creates variability in size, position, and relationships. When fully contracted, it is small and globular with thick walls and negligible lumen. It is confined to the pelvic cavity in the larger species but extends into the abdomen in carnivores. The enlarged bladder is pear shaped and has a cranial vertex (apex), an intermediate body, and a caudal neck that narrows to the internal urethral orifice at the junction with the urethra. The continuing distention carries an ever-increasing portion of the bladder into the abdomen. But the neck remains fixed within the pelvis through its continuity with the urethra (Fig. 5.32/*11*).

The initial filling of the bladder does not cause an immediate increase in internal pressure. However, considerable filling of the bladder leads to sharp rise in pressure and an urge to urinate followed by actual act of urination by most of the domestic animals. The house-trained dog may resist the urge, leading to discomfort and, later, pain as the bladder continues to fill and distend to an extent at which the apex of the bladder rests cranial to the umbilicus and creates the risk of rupture. Though the outline of the grossly distended bladder is smooth, that of the more modestly distended organ is irregular (see Fig. 5.30).

The contracted bladder in the larger species is largely retroperitoneal. However, it becomes intraperitoneal after even moderate expansion. Three folds continue this serosal covering onto the abdominal and pelvic walls (Fig. 5.33). Paired *lateral vesical folds* convey the round ligaments of the bladder; these vestiges of the umbilical arteries retain narrow lumina to let some blood reach the cranial part of the bladder. The third, *median vesical fold,* is empty in the adult, but in the fetus it supports the urachus, the constricted cranial continuation of the bladder that leaves the abdomen through the umbilical foramen before expanding externally into the allantoic sac. The urachus and umbilical arteries rupture at birth; the urachus remains as a scar on the bladder vertex, but the umbilical arteries become the round ligaments. The folds in the adult bound the ventral pair of the several excavations into which the pelvic peritoneal cavity is divided (see Figs. 22.6 and 22.7).

The constant dorsal relations of the bladder are to the uterus and vagina within the broad ligament in the female and to the deferent duct (and perhaps the vesicular glands) within the genital fold in the male. The bladder may also make indirect contact with the rectum through these folds. The ventral surface touches the pelvic and abdominal floor. Other relations of the intraabdominal part of the bladder are less predictable because of size and shape changes.

The loose attachment of the mucosa and its ability to stretch allow marked change in the appearance of the bladder's interior. The surface, much folded when the

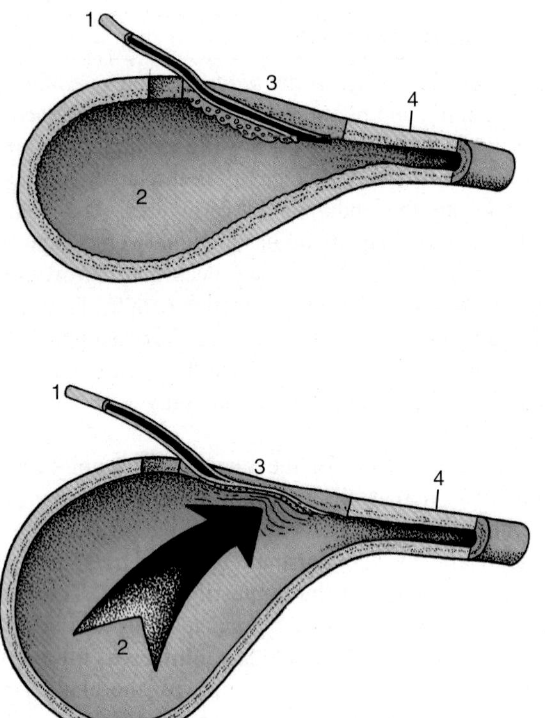

Fig. 5.31 *Top,* The ureterovesical junction. *Bottom,* Because of its oblique passage through the wall, the ureter is compressed *(arrow)* as the intravesical pressure rises. *1,* Ureter; *2,* bladder lumen; *3,* bladder wall; *4,* bladder neck.

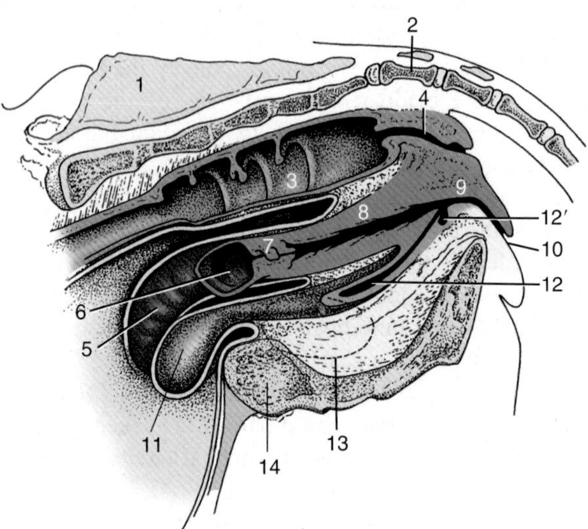

Fig. 5.32 Median section of the bovine pelvis. *1,* Sacrum; *2,* first caudal vertebra; *3,* interior of rectum; *4,* anal canal; *5,* exterior of right uterine horn; *6,* interior of stump of left uterine horn; *7,* cervix; *8,* vagina; *9,* vestibule; *10,* vulva; *11,* exterior of bladder; *12,* urethra; *12′,* suburethral diverticulum; *13,* obturator foramen; *14,* pelvis symphysis.

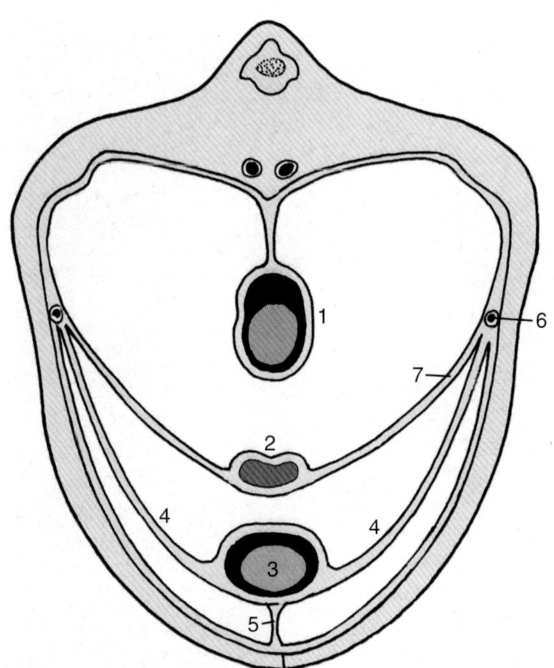

Fig. 5.33 Peritoneal disposition in the caudal part of the abdomen. *1,* Colon; *2,* uterus; *3,* bladder; *4,* lateral vesical ligaments; *5,* median vesical ligament; *6,* ureter; *7,* broad ligament of uterus (mesometrium).

lumen is small, becomes generally smooth when the bladder fills. However, two particular folds resist effacement. They run from the slitlike orifices of the ureters, converge at the exit from the bladder, and fuse to form a median *urethral crest* that continues into the pelvic urethra (Fig. 5.34/*5*). The triangle bounded by the ureteric and urethral openings is termed the *trigone;* it appears to have a different origin from the remainder of the bladder wall (p.159) and is believed to have an enhanced sensitivity (Fig. 5.34/*4*). The bladder epithelium is of the transitional kind.

The *bladder muscle* is arranged in three sheets that exchange fascicles. The muscle is probably entirely detrusor—available to squeeze and empty the bladder—and fails to form an often described internal sphincter. Many writers now believe that, in place of this sphincter, some muscle bundles form a series of arcades whose summits are directed toward the orifice; they therefore dilate rather than occlude the exit when they contract. If this latter belief is accurate, continence depends on the tension passively exerted by the elastic elements within the mucosa and on the action of the external sphincter, the striated urethralis. This interpretation is consistent with the demonstration that in certain species (dog, goat) the proximal part of the urethra forms part of the urine reservoir, expanding as the bladder fills. The functional boundary between bladder and urethra would thus appear to be represented by the cranial limit of the urethralis in these species.

Autonomic fibers reach the bladder through the sympathetic hypogastric and parasympathetic pelvic nerves; the latter innervate the detrusor muscle. Sensory fibers are routed through the pudendal nerve. The main blood supply

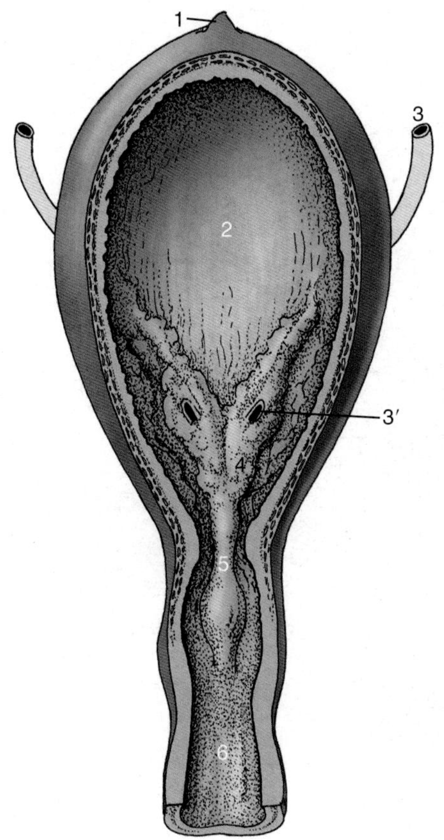

Fig. 5.34 The interior of the urinary bladder. *1,* Scar of urachus; *2,* bladder; *3,* ureter; *3′,* ureteric orifice; *4,* trigone of bladder; *5,* urethral crest; *6,* urethra.

is from the vaginal (or prostatic) artery, but, as has been mentioned, it is supplemented by the reduced umbilical arteries.

The Female Urethra

The female urethra runs caudally on the pelvic floor below the reproductive tract. It passes obliquely through the vaginal wall to open ventrally at the junction of vagina and vestibule (Fig. 5.35). It is conspicuously short and wide in mares. In some animals, such as the cow and sow, it opens together with a suburethral diverticulum (Fig. 5.32/*12′*), and in others, such as the bitch, it opens on a hummock. Both arrangements create difficulties when catheterization of the bladder is attempted.

When a *diverticulum* is present, it is enclosed within the urethralis, which surrounds the urethra along most of its length. The cranial fascicles of the urethralis encircle the urethra, while the caudal ones support it within U-shaped loops that arise and end on the vaginal wall. Contraction of this part of the muscle closes the urethra by pressing the two organs together and also narrows the vagina. The urethralis obtains a somatic innervation through the pudendal nerve, but sympathetic and parasympathetic involvement is also described. The urethral submucosa contains many veins that constitute a form of erectile tissue that may contribute to continence by assisting mucosal apposition. These features apart, the structure of the urethra continues that of the bladder.

THE MALE REPRODUCTIVE ORGANS

The male reproductive organs include paired gonads, the testes, which produce both male gametes (sperm) and hormones; paired gonadal duct systems, each consisting of an epididymis and deferent duct (ductus deferens), which convey the exocrine products of the testes to the urethra; a suite of accessory glands, which contributes the bulk of the semen; the male urethra, which extends from the bladder to the free extremity of the penis and serves for the passage of both urine and semen; the penis, the male copulatory organ, which deposits the semen within the reproductive tract of the female; and skin adaptations, the scrotum and the prepuce, developed in relation to the testes and the penis.

The Testes and Their Adnexa

The Testis

The testis combines endocrine and exocrine components within a common capsule. The endocrine component functions normally at the core temperature of the body, but in most mammals the successful production of the male gametes requires a temperature a few degrees lower than that within the abdomen. However, spermatogenesis does occur normally at the core temperature in a few mammals (described as *testicond,* e.g., elephants, hyraxes) that have intra-abdominal testes. In many small mammals (chiefly found among rodents, insectivores, and bats) the testes descend from the abdomen into the scrotum transiently for the breeding season. This descent is brought about by contraction of the cremaster muscle sac found in these species.

The testes are solid ellipsoidal organs whose bulk bears no fixed proportion to the body size. They are conspicuously small in cats and impressively large in sheep and goats. Their orientation also varies. They are carried with their long axes vertical in ruminants (necessitating a deep and pendulous scrotum), horizontal in horses and dogs, and tilted toward the anus in pigs and cats. These differences are broadly correlated with the position of the scrotum, which is below the caudal part of the abdomen in ruminants, perineal in pigs and cats, and intermediate in position in horses and dogs (Fig. 5.36). Each testis is separately suspended within the scrotum by a spermatic cord, a bundle of structures that includes the deferent duct and the supplying vessels and nerves enclosed within a double covering of peritoneum.

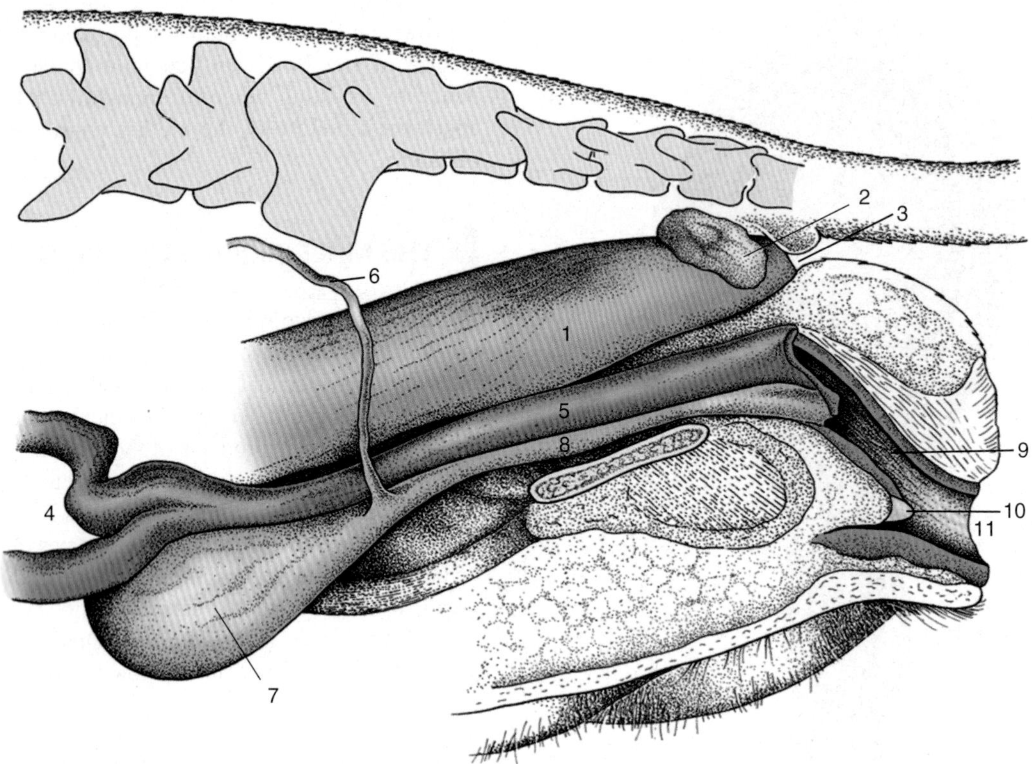

Fig. 5.35 Pelvic organs of the bitch. The lateral pelvic wall and the lateral wall of the vestibule have been removed. *1,* Rectum; *2,* anal sac; *3,* anus; *4,* uterus; *5,* vagina; *6,* ureter; *7,* bladder; *8,* urethra; *9,* vestibule; *10,* clitoris; *11,* vulva.

The outer surface of the testis is made smooth by the direct peritoneal investment, except at the poles and along one margin, where the testis is attached to the *epididymis,* a structure formed by the coiled initial portion of the external duct system. The peritoneum covers a thickish capsule (*tunica albuginea*) composed mainly of dense connective tissue but sometimes including smooth muscle. The larger branches of the testicular artery and vein form a visible pattern within the capsule. The parenchyma is contained under moderate pressure and pouts through any incision of the capsule. Although slight swelling of the parenchyma can be accommodated by the assumption by the testis of a more globular form, any significant expansion raises the intratesticular pressure and produces severe pain, especially in inflamed testes (orchitis).* The capsule detaches septa and trabeculae that divide the parenchyma into lobules. The septa are not always conspicuous, but in those species in which they are well developed, they may be seen to converge on a substantial thickening (mediastinum testis), which may be axial or displaced toward the side bordering the epididymis (Fig. 5.37).

The soft, yellowish or brownish parenchyma consists of intermingled seminiferous tubules and interstitial tissue (Fig. 5.38). The greater part (60% in boars and stallions, 90% in rams and bulls) of the parenchyma is formed by the tubules, where spermatogenesis occurs. Each *seminiferous tubule* (Fig. 5.38) is much contorted and also looped so that both ends open into the rete testis (Fig. 5.38/*5*), a plexus of spaces within the mediastinum. Within the seminiferous tubules two cell types can be discerned: the Sertoli cells, which support and nourish the germ cells by the production of hormones and growth factors, and the seminiferous epithelium (Fig. 5.39). The rete drains by a dozen or so efferent ductules (Fig. 5.38/*6*) that pierce the capsule to join the head of the epididymis. The interstitial tissue consists of massed interstitial (Leydig) cells supported by a delicate connective tissue framework containing small blood and lymphatic vessels (Fig. 5.39).

*Many derivative terms are based on the alternative name, *orchis,* derived from the Greek.

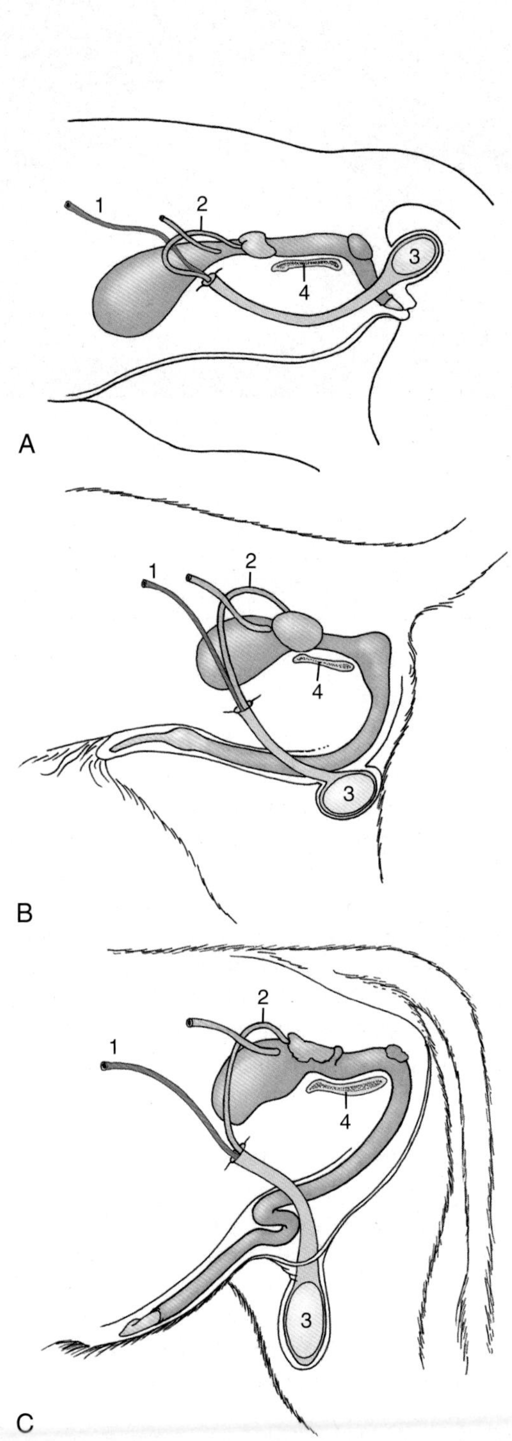

Fig. 5.36 The perineal, intermediate, and inguinal positions of the scrotum exhibited by the (A) tomcat, (B) dog, and (C) bull. *1,* Testicular artery; *2,* deferent duct; *3,* testis; *4,* pelvic symphysis.

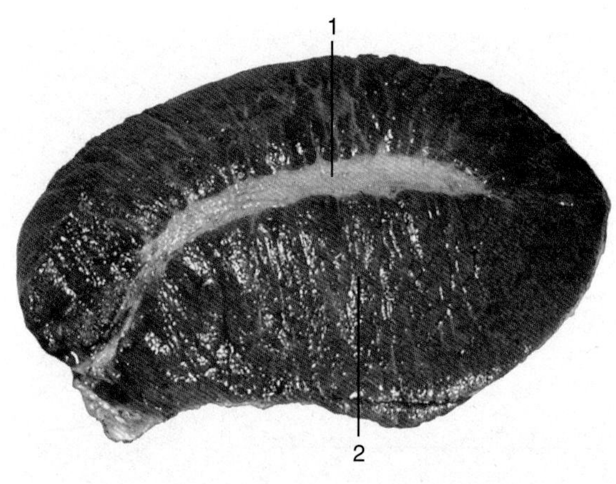

Fig. 5.37 Median section of testis (bull). *1,* Mediastinum testis; *2,* testicular parenchyma.

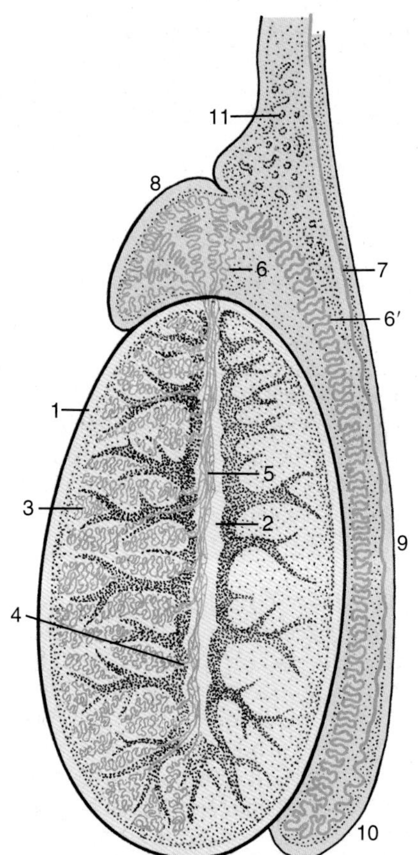

Fig. 5.38 Longitudinal section of a testis and epididymis, schematic. *1,* Tunica albuginea; *2,* mediastinum; *3,* seminiferous tubules; *4,* straight tubules; *5,* rete testis; *6,* efferent ductules; *6′,* epididymal duct; *7,* deferent duct; *8,* head of epididymis; *9,* body of epididymis; *10,* tail of epididymis; *11,* pampiniform plexus.

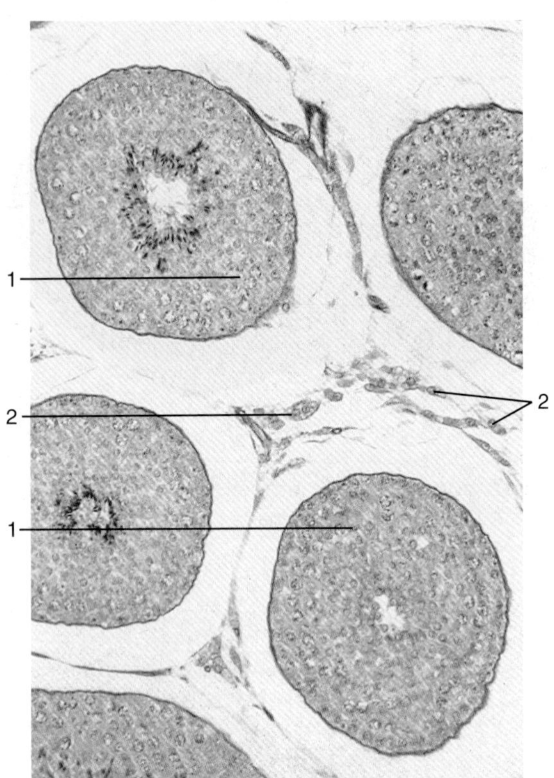

Fig. 5.39 Testis (dog) (140×). *1,* Seminiferous tubules (showing spermatogenesis); *2,* interstitial tissue with androgen-producing (Leydig) cells.

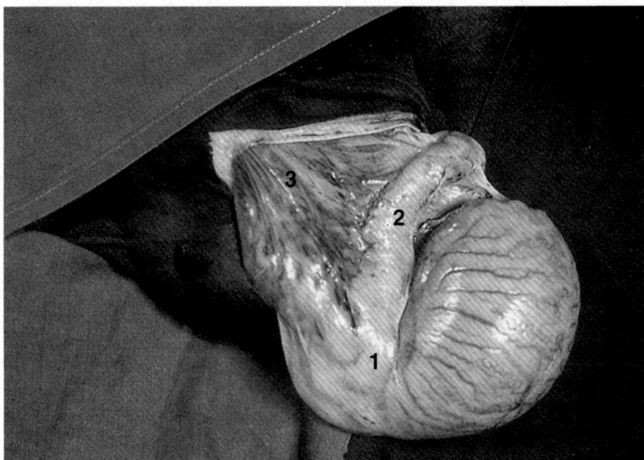

Fig. 5.40 Testis (horse). *1,* Head of epididymis; *2,* body of epididymis; *3,* pampiniform plexus.

Endocrine Component

The endocrine functions of the testis are performed by the interstitial (Leydig) cells, responsible for androgen production, and the sustentacular (Sertoli) cells, responsible for inhibin production. Both types are normally under the pulsatile but more or less tonic control of gonadotropins (luteinizing hormone [LH] and follicle-stimulating hormone [FSH], respectively) produced in the pituitary (p. 204). Among other functions, the sustentacular cells produce activin and inhibin, which regulate the synthesis and release of FSH through mechanisms that may be direct or mediated via the hypothalamus. Androgens clearly have distinct local function but are also responsible for secondary sex characteristics such as the maturation of the accessory sex glands, male skeletomuscular development, skin characteristics, and even the prenatal differentiation of certain brain and spinal cord nuclei. These hormones are also partly responsible for the behavior typical of the male. They also act on hypothalamus to exert a negative feedback on pituitary gonadotropin secretion. In the fetal period, active production of androgens may take place without pituitary control. The interstitial cells in this period are also responsible for the production of insulin-like factor 3, which is associated with gubernacular outgrowth and thus with testicular descent. In the fetal period the sustentacular cells produce *antimüllerian hormone* (AMH), which exerts an inhibitory effect on the paramesonephric ducts (p. 159), causing the disappearance of most of the female duct system.

The Epididymis

A firm organ, the epididymis is largely formed by the numerous convolutions of the single epididymal duct within a connective tissue matrix. It is attached along one of the longer borders—dorsal in the dog, caudomedial in the bull—of the testis and usually spreads some distance over both poles (Fig. 5.40). It is conventionally divided into three rather arbitrary parts—head, body, and tail—that do not always correspond to functions.

The head (Fig. 5.38/*8*) is firmly attached to the testicular capsule. It receives the efferent ductules, which immediately or after some coiling join to form the wider *epididymal duct* (Fig. 5.38/*6′*). The body may be less completely attached to the surface of the testis and creates an intervening space called *testicular bursa* (homologous with the ovarian bursa) (see Fig. 5.41/*3*). The tail is firmly attached to the testis by the proper ligament of the testis and also to the parietal layer of the enveloping peritoneal sac by the ligament of the tail of the epididymis (Fig. 5.41/*7* and *8*). The tail finally tapers, and the duct emerges to continue as the deferent duct (Fig. 5.41/*4*). The epididymis appears spongy in section because the coiled duct is inevitably cut across many times.

The Deferent Duct

The deferent duct is undulating where it emerges but gradually straightens when followed toward the abdomen (Fig. 5.42). It first runs medial to the epididymis as it heads toward the testicular vessels that form the bulkier components of the spermatic cord. The constituents of the cord remain together as they pass through the inguinal canal but disperse at the vaginal ring (see Figs. 5.36). The duct here turns caudomedially to pass under the ureter before gaining the dorsal surface

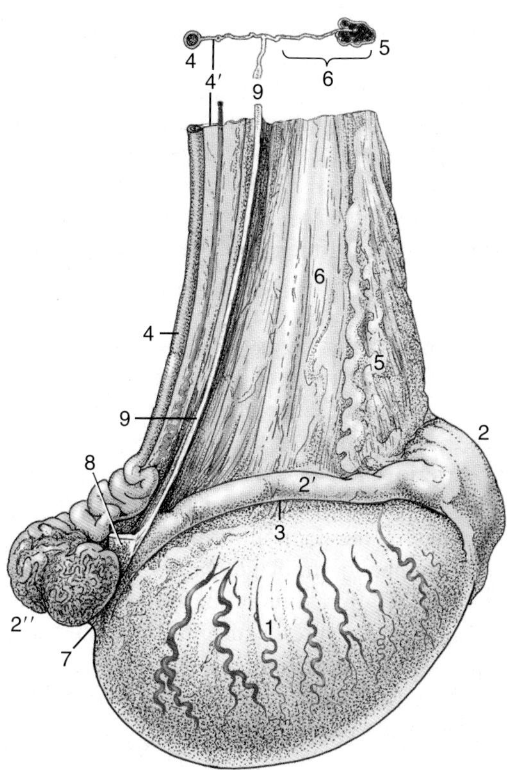

Fig. 5.41 Lateral view of the right testis of a stallion. *1,* Testis; *2,* head of epididymis; *2′,* body of epididymis; *2″,* tail of epididymis; *3,* testicular bursa; *4,* deferent duct; *4′,* mesoductus deferens; *5,* pampiniform plexus; *6,* mesorchium; *7,* proper ligament of testis; *8,* ligament of tail of epididymis; *9,* cut edge of fold connecting visceral and parietal layers of the vaginal tunic.

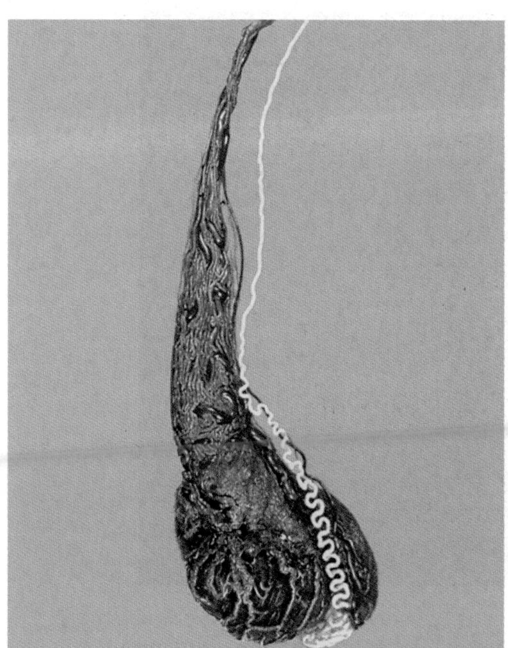

Fig. 5.42 Corrosion cast (dog) of testicular artery *(red),* pampiniform plexus *(blue),* and deferent duct *(yellow).*

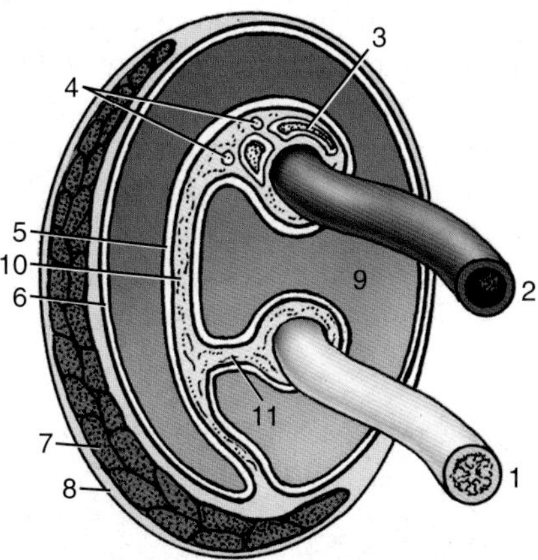

Fig. 5.43 Transverse section of the spermatic cord and its immediate investments, schematic. *1,* Deferent duct; *2,* testicular artery (coiled); *3,* pampiniform plexus; *4,* testicular nerves and lymph vessels; *5,* visceral layer of vaginal tunic; *6,* parietal layer of vaginal tunic; *7,* cremaster muscle; *8,* external spermatic fascia; *9,* vaginal cavity; *10,* mesorchium; *11,* mesoductus.

of the bladder (see Fig. 5.36). It penetrates the prostate before finally entering the urethra a little way beyond the urethra's origin from the bladder. The abdominal part continues to be supported by a peritoneal fold (mesoductus), which joins its contralateral partner to produce a horizontal genital fold above the bladder. The greater part of the duct is of uniform appearance with a rather narrow lumen relative to the thick muscular wall. In most species the subterminal stretch lying on the bladder is enlarged into the *ampulla of the deferent duct* or ampullary gland (see Fig. 5.51/*4*) through the proliferation of the glandular tissue in the mucosa but not with real widening of the lumen. In most domestic mammals a second accessory gland, the vesicular gland, grows from the duct close to its termination (described later). The short, shared passage is known as the *ejaculatory duct.*

The Vaginal Tunic and Spermatic Cord

The peritoneal process (vaginal tunic) that encloses the testis is an evagination of the lining of the abdomen through the inguinal canal. The narrow proximal part surrounding the spermatic cord widens distally to form a flasklike expansion within the scrotum that encloses the testis and epididymis. The parietal and visceral layers of the tunic are connected by a fold that extends from the vaginal ring to the tail of the epididymis (see Fig. 5.41).* The cavity between the parietal and visceral layers (Fig. 5.43/*9*) normally contains only a minute amount of serous fluid.

*The mesorchium is the visceral tunic between the fold (Fig. 5.41) and the epididymal border of the testis but also includes the long peritoneal fold that conveys the testicular vessels and nerves from their origin at the abdominal roof to the testis; it thus forms a considerable portion of the spermatic cord. The narrow fold that attaches the deferent duct to the pelvic and abdominal walls and (more distally) to the mesorchium is the mesoductus deferens.

It communicates with the peritoneal cavity of the abdomen through the vaginal ring, a narrow slitlike opening placed within the internal opening of the inguinal canal. Sometimes a loop of small intestine or another abdominal organ herniates into the peritoneal process through the vaginal ring. It is worth mentioning that in human infants the neck of the peritoneal process usually becomes obliterated shortly after birth, isolating the cavity about the testis.

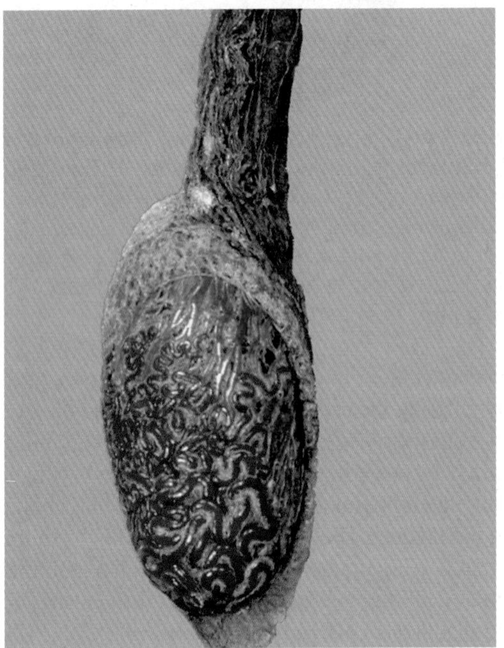

Fig. 5.44 Corrosion cast of vessels, arteries in red and veines in blue, within and on the testis and the pampiniform plexus (bull).

The spermatic cord varies in length and shape according to the position and orientation of the testis. It is shortest and most compact in those species in which the testis hangs vertically. The bulk of the cord is provided by the *testicular artery* and veins, both remarkably modified. The artery branches from the abdominal aorta and first pursues a fairly direct course toward the vaginal ring to join rest of the constituents of the spermatic cord. The more distal part is extraordinarily convoluted—one account describes no less than 7 m of artery packed within a 10-cm stretch of cord (Figs. 5.44 and 5.45A and B). The testicular veins that run to the caudal vena cava constitute a very elaborate close-meshed *pampiniform plexus* in which the contortions of the artery are embedded (Fig. 5.45B). Arteriovenous anastomoses are present between the coiled testicular artery and its epididymal branches and the veins of the pampiniform plexus (Fig. 5.46). A generous lymphatic drainage passes to lymph nodes placed about the bifurcation of the aorta. In some species a small lymph node is present near the inguinal canal. The lymph conveys a substantial fraction of the hormone production of the testis. The inconspicuous testicular nerves are of sympathetic origin.

The Scrotum

The scrotum has an external median groove dividing it into right and left compartments and also betraying a striking asymmetry of the testes. The lower part of the scrotum is molded on the testes and adjusts as their position varies with the ambient temperature (Fig. 5.47).

The relatively thin scrotal skin is well provided with both sweat and sebaceous glands. It is sometimes rather bare but hidden by hair in the cat and densely covered by

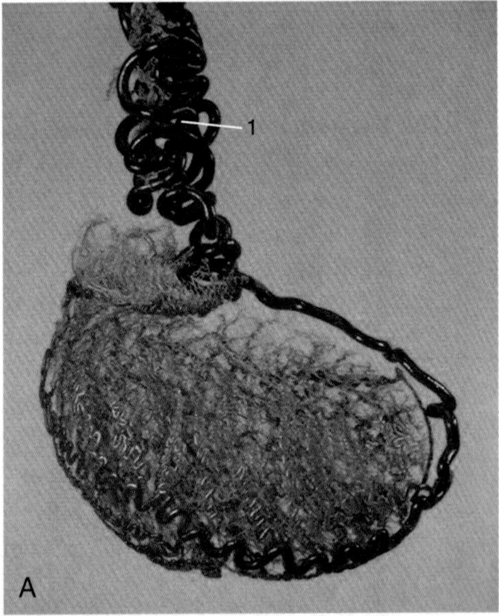

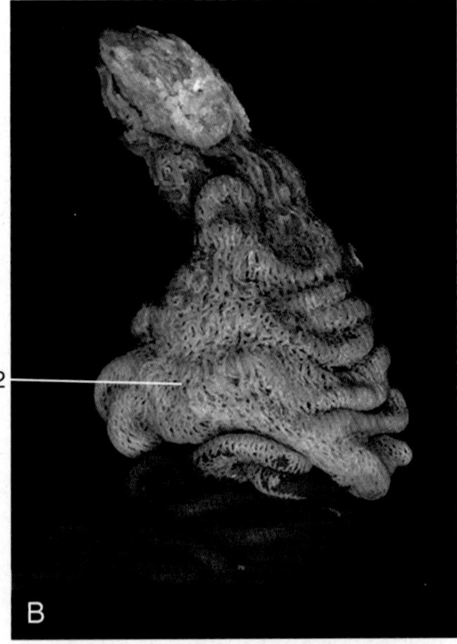

Fig. 5.45 (A) and (B) Vascularization of the equine testis. Observe the course of arterial branches on the testicular surface. *1,* Testicular artery (red, becoming very tortuous as it approaches the testis); *2,* part of the pampiniform plexus.

fleece in sheep of certain breeds. When bare, it is often pigmented. The scrotal skin adheres to a tough fibromuscular layer (*tunica dartos*), which also extends as a septum between the compartments that separately lodge the testes. Internal to the dartos, a (spermatic) fascia is present in several layers, which are believed to correspond to the layers of the abdominal wall. The predominant layer is the *external spermatic fascia,* which can be clearly separated from the dartos (Fig. 5.48). The loose intermediate stratum allows the vaginal tunic independent movement within the scrotal sac; in addition to its functional significance (see later), this arrangement facilitates castration by the closed method (in which the testis is brought to the exterior within the vaginal tunic before the cord is severed proximally). The dense external spermatic fascia that supports the vaginal tunic also invests the *cremaster,* a slip of muscle that passes onto the cord on detachment from the caudal margin of the internal oblique muscle of the abdomen.

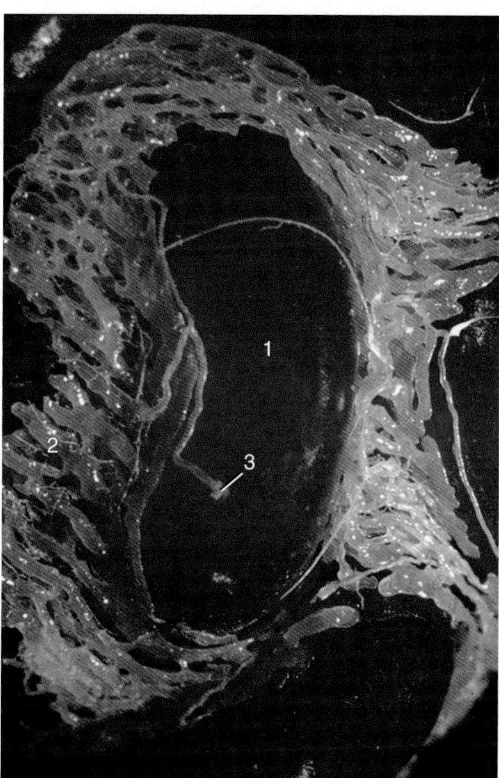

Fig. 5.46 Corrosion cast of the testicular artery. *1,* Coil of artery; *2,* pampiniform plexus; *3,* arteriovenous anastomosis (plexus filled via this anastomosis).

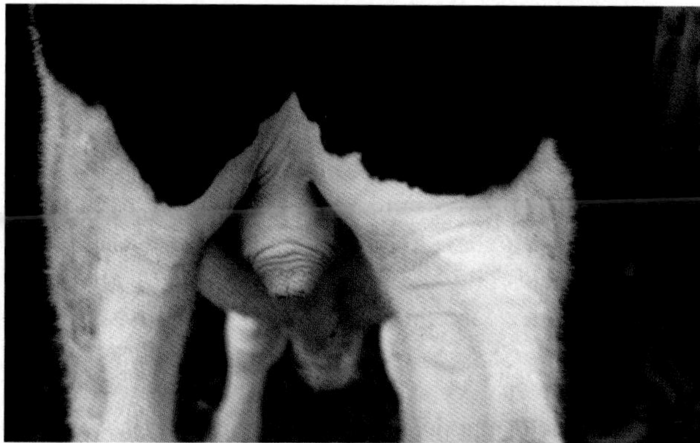

Fig. 5.47 Scrotum of a bull. The musculature in the tunica dartos is contracted, causing elevation of the scrotum.

Testicular Function

Most wild mammals are seasonal breeders, a characteristic that is reflected in changes in the morphology and activity of the reproductive organs of both sexes. In contrast domesticated males have an active seminiferous epithelium throughout the year with at most only slight variation in sperm output. Although the process of spermatogenesis is not described, the reader is reminded that the serial cell divisions and maturation processes that constitute the cycle are not synchronous in every part of the seminiferous epithelium. Instead, adjacent segments show successive stages so that a "lucky" longitudinal section of a tubule displays the different stages of the process occurring as a wave spreading along its length (see Fig. 5.39).

The process of spermatogenesis cannot proceed normally at the core temperature of the body in most

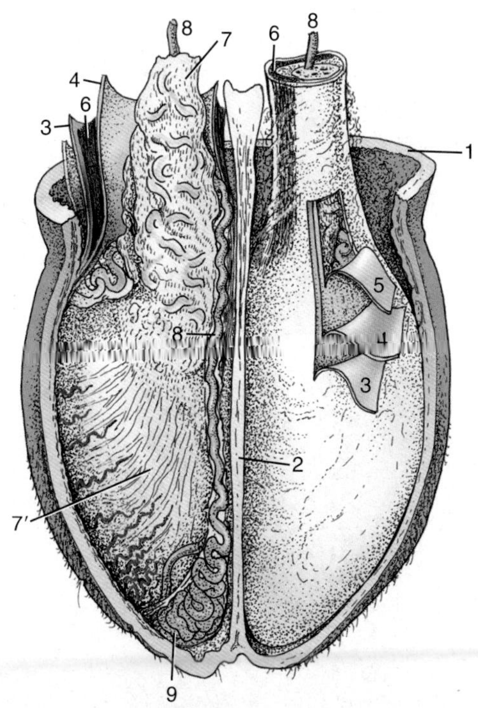

Fig. 5.48 Cranial view of the opened scrotum of a bull; the investments of the testis have been partly dissected. *1,* Scrotal skin and dartos; *2,* scrotal septum; *3,* external spermatic fascia; *4,* parietal layer of vaginal tunic; *5,* visceral layer (dissected from surface of testis); *6,* cremaster muscle; *7,* visceral layer of vaginal tunic covering structures in spermatic cord; *7',* visceral layer on testis; *8,* deferent duct; *9,* tail of epididymis.

mammals. The seminiferous epithelium is damaged in testes that fail to descend into the scrotum (the "cryptorchid condition"), and these do not produce sperm. Similar changes are evident in testes that return to the abdomen after having descended successfully, and in scrotal testes that are overheated by an unusually thick covering of hair or fleece. Because the interstitial tissue is less susceptible to temperature, the libido and potency may be normal in cryptorchid animals that are infertile.

Many factors help maintain the appropriate endotesticular temperature. The exposed position of the scrotum, the absence of fat within the scrotal fascia, and the intracapsular situation of large testicular vessels all favor heat loss by radiation (Fig. 5.49); the generous supply of sweat glands allows additional loss through evaporation from the skin surface. Perhaps more important, the extensive contact between the arterial and venous vessels within the cord precools the arterial blood (see Fig. 5.45). The opportunities for heat loss are such that the testicular temperature could be lowered excessively in colder climates. Countermeasures are available. Contraction of the tunica dartos, which is directly sensitive to temperature change, tightens and bunches the scrotum, thereby reducing the exposed surface and also drawing the testes toward the warmer trunk (see Fig. 5.47). The testes may also be separately raised within the scrotum by contraction of the cremaster muscles, which pull on the vaginal tunics; being striated, these muscles react briskly to pull the testes away from potentially harmful stimuli.

Castration has been used to manage animal populations and to promote particular carcass qualities. The routine castration is now questioned because food are animals are

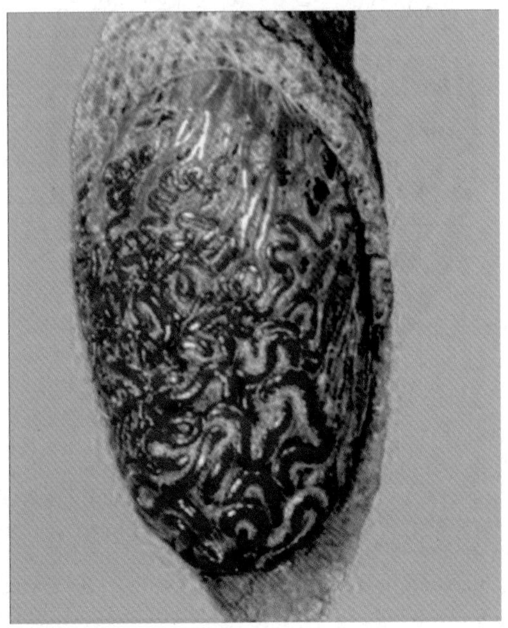

Fig. 5.49 Testicular arteries *(red)* and veins *(blue)* on the surface of the bovine testis and the pampiniform plexus.

slaughtered at earlier ages than before and are selectively bred for particular meat qualities. The direct influence of castration on the reproductive organs is considered in some detail for cattle on Chapter 29.

The Pelvic Reproductive Organs

The Male Urethra

The male urethra extends from an internal orifice at the bladder neck to an external orifice at the free extremity of the penis. It is thus divisible into an internal or pelvic part and an external or spongy part; here, *spongy* refers to the very vascular tissue that surrounds the urethra on its leaving the pelvic cavity. The spongy part is largely incorporated within and is considered a part of the penis. The pelvic part is joined by the deferent and vesicular (or combined ejaculatory) duct(s) a short distance from its origin from the bladder; by far the greater part of the urethra thus serves to discharge both urine and semen.

Although the pelvic urethra shows regional and specific variations, it consists essentially of a mucosal tube successively invested by a vascular submucosa and a muscular tunic. The mucous membrane is thrown into longitudinal folds in the inactive state. The initial part also carries a dorsal crest that continues from the urethral orifice to end in a thickening (*colliculus seminalis*). The colliculus displays on its sides the slitlike orifices of the deferent ducts and the much smaller openings through which the many prostatic ducts discharge (Fig. 5.50/*7*). Similar but more distal openings mark the entry of the ducts of other accessory glands (Fig. 5.50/*8*). The submucosa contains a rather inconspicuous system of connecting blood spaces that is continuous with the vastly more generous spongy investment of the second part of the urethra. The major component of the muscle coat is the striated urethralis that encircles the tube.

The urethra is embedded in fat and other connective tissues where it lies on the pelvic floor. The dorsal surface is related to the rectum and, with species differences, to various accessory reproductive glands; usually only a narrow median strip that faces directly into the rectogenital pouch is covered by peritoneum. The urethra is easily palpated per rectum, a procedure that may stimulate rhythmic activity of its muscle.

The Accessory Reproductive Glands

The full set comprises ampullary, vesicular, prostate, and bulbourethral glands, although not all of these are present in every species (Fig. 5.51). The *ampullary glands* have been sufficiently described.

Paired *vesicular glands* (Fig. 5.51/*5*) are present in all domestic species except the dog and cat. Each buds from the distal part of the deferent duct in the embryo, and this relationship commonly persists. In the pig the later absorption of the ejaculatory duct into the urethra causes the vesicular gland to open separately. These glands vary greatly in appearance; in the horse they are large, externally smooth, and bladder-like, resembling the human organs that were formerly known as seminal *vesicles*. This term is inappropriate because in most species the glands are knobby and thick-walled with rather narrow, branched lumina. The vesicular glands lie wholly or partly within the genital fold, each lateral to the corresponding deferent duct.

A *prostate* (Fig. 5.51/*6*) is present in all domestic species. In some it consists of two parts: one is diffusely spread within the wall of the pelvic urethra, and the other is a compact body placed external to the urethralis. Both parts drain by many small ducts. The small ruminants have only the diffuse or disseminate part and the horse only the compact part. The disseminate part is vestigial in the dog and cat, but the compact part is very large and globular and so well developed that it surrounds the urethra entirely (dog) or almost so (cat).

Paired *bulbourethral glands* (Figs. 5.51/*7* and 5.52), compound tubular glands with a secretory epithelium, lie on the dorsal aspect of the urethra close to the pelvic exit. They are found in all species other than the dog (although they are vestigial in the cat). They are of moderate size in horses and ruminants but are very substantial in the pig, in

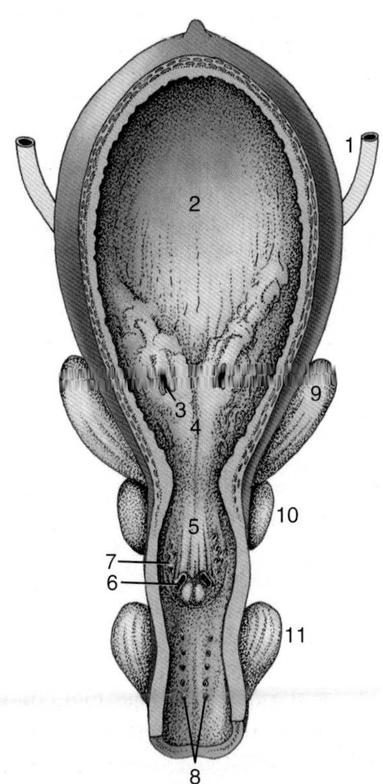

Fig. 5.50 Ventral view of the opened bladder and urethra of a stallion. *1,* Ureter; *2,* bladder; *3,* ureteric orifice; *4,* trigone of bladder; *5,* urethral crest and seminal colliculus; *6,* opening of ejaculatory duct; *7,* multiple openings of prostatic ducts; *8,* multiple openings of bulbourethral ducts; *9,* vesicular gland; *10,* prostate; *11,* bulbourethral gland.

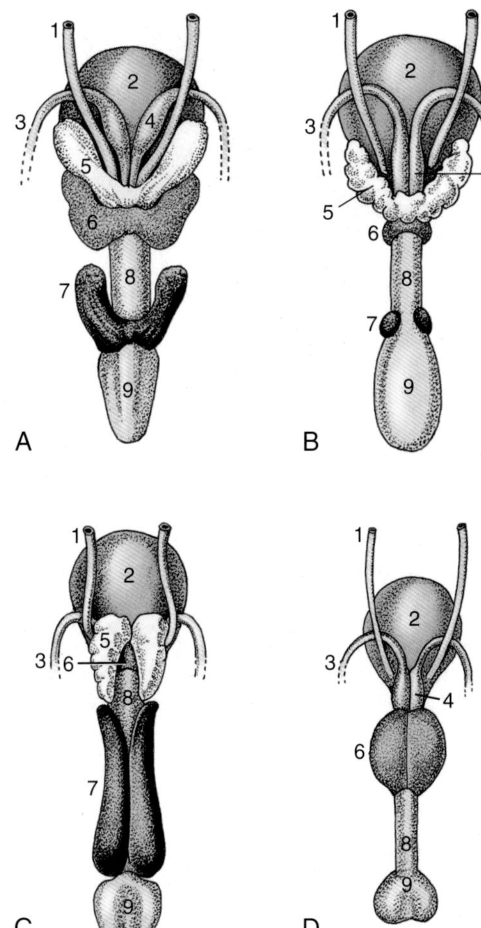

Fig. 5.51 Accessory reproductive glands of the (A) stallion, (B) bull, (C) boar, and (D) dog, dorsal view. *1,* Ureter; *2,* bladder; *3,* deferent duct; *4,* ampullary gland; *5,* vesicular gland; *6,* body of prostate; *7,* bulbourethral gland; *8,* urethra, *9,* bulb of penis.

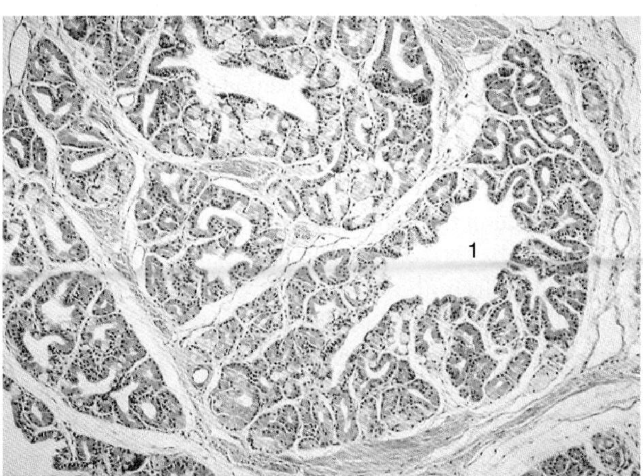

Fig. 5.52 Bulbourethral gland (goat) (hematoxylin and eosin; 70×), a compound tubular gland lined with a columnar secretory epithelium. *1,* Collecting duct.

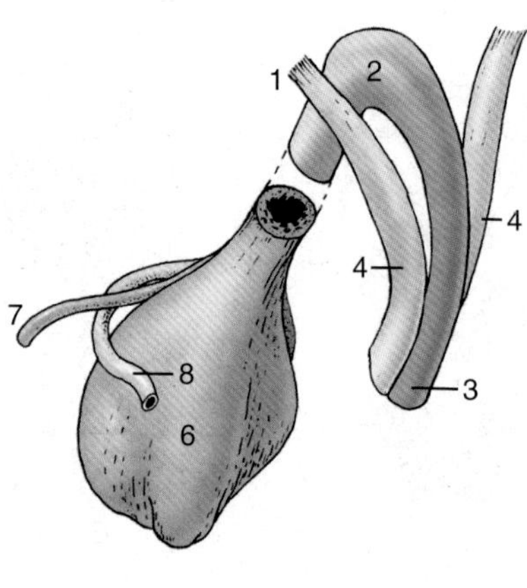

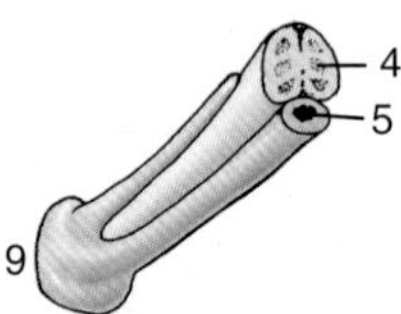

Fig. 5.53 Schematic drawing of the components that constitute the equine penis at its root *(top)* and at its apex *(bottom)*. *1,* Crus penis; *2,* bulb; *3,* corpus spongiosum; *4,* corpus cavernosum; *5,* urethra; *6,* bladder; *7,* ureter; *8,* deferent duct; *9,* glans.

which they appear as rather irregular elongated cylinders placed to each side of the urethra. They may drain by one or by several ducts.

All the larger glands possess well-developed capsules and internal septa in which much smooth muscle is present that expels the secretion at the appropriate time.

The Penis and Prepuce

The penis is suspended below the trunk and is partly contained between the thighs, where it is anchored to the floor of the pelvis by a suspensory ligament in the large species. In the quiescent state, the free extremity is concealed within an invagination of the abdominal skin, the prepuce, which opens at a variable site behind the umbilicus. The organ is mainly constructed of three columns of erectile tissue (Fig. 5.53). These are independent caudally where they constitute the root of the penis, but their major parts are combined in the body of the penis.

The paired *crura of the penis* (Fig. 5.53/*1*), widely separated origins from the ischial arch, converge, bend to run forward under the pelvic floor, and join. Each consists of a core of cavernous tissue enclosed within a thick connective tissue casing (tunica albuginea), and the complex is known as a *corpus cavernosum* (Fig. 5.53/*4*). A septum exists between the two corpora cavernosa in the proximal part of the body, but in most species this structure weakens and ultimately disappears toward the apex of the penis. In carnivores the septum is complete. The combined structure is grooved ventrally to accommodate the third component, the urethra within its enveloping vascular sleeve, the *corpus spongiosum* (Fig. 5.53/*3*). The blood spaces within the crura and corpus cavernosum communicate freely.

The corpus cavernosum does not extend to the apex of the penis, which is formed by an expansion of the corpus spongiosum. The corpus spongiosum commences at the pelvic outlet with the sudden enlargement of the meager spongy tissue of the pelvic urethra. The expansion constitutes the *bulb of the penis* (Fig. 5.53/*2*), a bilobed structure that tapers to continue as a more uniform sleeve. The corpus spongiosum is more delicate than the corpus cavernosum, having larger blood spaces separated by thinner septa. Its cranial expansion over the distal end of the corpus cavernosum, usually known as the *glans* (Fig. 5.53/*9*), forms the apex of the whole organ. Because the corpus spongiosum surrounds the urethra, the urethral orifice is brought to the very extremity of the penis; indeed, in small ruminants a free urethral process prolongs the urethra well beyond this point.

Species Differences in Penis Structure

There are other pronounced species differences in penis structure, such as the transformation of the corpus cavernosum into the os penis in the dog and cat. The glans too differs in its form; it is minimally developed in the pig, insubstantial in the ruminants, and large and mushroom shaped in the horse. It is most specialized in the dog, in which it presents bulbar proximal and long cylindrical distal parts. The penis of the cat is unique (among domestic species) in that it retains its embryonic posture of pointing caudoventrally from the ischial arch, which affects the manner of copulation.

The construction of the corpus cavernosum also exhibits major differences. In some species it contains small blood spaces enclosed within and divided by substantial amounts of tough fibroelastic tissue. This *fibroelastic type* of penis, found in the boar and ruminants, requires relatively little additional blood to become erect (Fig. 5.54A). The penis of the ruminants also has a sigmoid flexure in the part of its body carried between the thighs. The *musculocavernous type* of penis, found in the stallion and, in atypical form, in the dog, has larger blood spaces separated by delicate septa (Fig. 5.54B). This muscular penis requires a greater quantity of the blood to achieve erection, which is accompanied by significant increase in both length and girth.

The prepuce or sheath is a tubular fold consisting of an external layer (lamina externa), continuous with the general integument, and an internal layer (lamina interna) that faces the free end of the penis; the internal layer continues as the covering of the free part of the penis after reflection in the depth of the preputial cavity. Both the internal layer and the penile covering are hairless but often well provided with smegma-secreting glands and lymphoid tissue. In the newborn male the penis and sheath are fused, and separation is

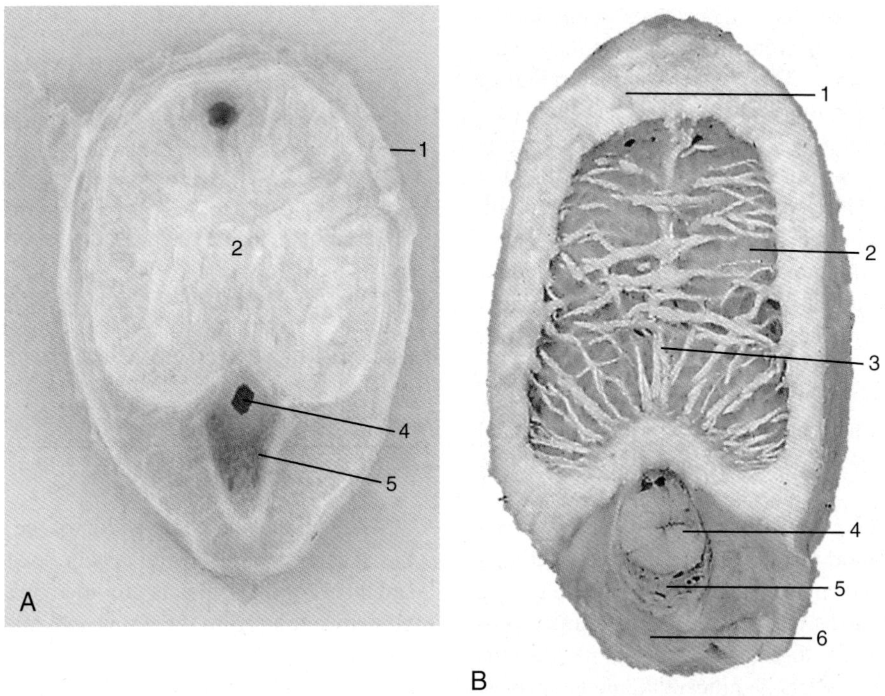

Fig. 5.54 Transverse sections of the fibroelastic penis of a bull (A) and the musculocavernous penis of a stallion (B). *1,* Tunica albuginea; *2,* corpus cavernosum; *3,* septum; *4,* urethra; *5,* corpus spongiosum; *6,* bulbospongiosus.

gradually achieved during the period before puberty (p. 705). The attachments of the adult prepuce are sufficiently loose to allow the internal lamina to be reflected onto the erect penis when it is protruded through the preputial orifice.

Certain muscles are associated with the penis. The *bulbospongiosus* is the thick extrapelvic continuation of the urethralis. It begins abruptly and extends distally to end on the surface of the corpus spongiosum, at a variable distance beyond the point at which this structure is incorporated within the penis. The powerful paired *ischiocavernosi* arise from the ischial arch, almost enclose the crura, and follow them to their fusion. The *retractor penis* is also paired. The two muscles arise from the caudal vertebrae and descend through the perineum, bending laterally to pass around the anal canal, to reach the penis. Unlike the other muscles associated with the penis, the retractors are mainly composed of smooth muscle fibers. Narrow slips of striated muscle (*cranial* and *caudal preputial*) may pass onto the prepuce and attach near its opening. The caudal muscles are less frequently encountered and retract the prepuce, thus uncovering the extremity of the penis. The cranial muscles protract the prepuce. Both caudal and cranial muscles must be regarded as detachments of the cutaneous trunci and are best developed in the bull but lacking in the stallion.

The penis obtains its exclusive (in the horse, principal) *blood supply* from *the artery of the penis,* a terminal branch of the internal pudendal. The artery of the penis has a very short course, and at the ischial arch it quickly divides to form an artery of the bulb, which enters the bulb of the penis and supplies the corpus spongiosum; a deep artery, which pierces the tunica albuginea to supply the corpus cavernosum; and the dorsal artery, which passes apically on the dorsal border of the organ to supply the free end. The dorsal artery may be reinforced by anastomosis with the obturator artery (horse) and generally by anastomosis with the external pudendal artery for the supply of the prepuce. The veins are broadly satellite. Interspecific details are considered in the later chapters if they are significant.

The nerves to the penis accompany the vessels. The motor fibers are predominantly parasympathetic and from the pelvic nerves.

Sperm Transport in the Male Tract: Erection of the Penis

The sperm are immotile when released into the lumen of the seminiferous tubules, where they float in fluid secreted by the sustentacular (Sertoli) cells of the epithelial lining. Their passage through the rete testis into the head of the epididymis is effected by the current generated by the combination of the testicular secretory pressure and the resorption of fluid by the lining of the efferent ductules. Onward progress through the epididymis appears to depend on several factors, among which spontaneous peristalsis of the muscular epididymal duct is probably most important. Hydrostatic pressure may continue to play a part, and in many species the sperm have themselves acquired the capacity for coordinated movement by the time they reach the tail of the epididymis. The physiologic maturation of the sperm—which take some days to complete their passage through the epididymis—may be a result of aging and specific molecules in their environment. Fertilization with epididymal sperm, especially the one from the tail, has been achieved under experimental conditions. Secretory activity of the lining of the epididymal duct is maintained by androgens, and it is possible that these substances also have a direct influence on sperm. The deferent duct also exhibits peristalsis, which gradually moves the sperm toward the ampullary region. In sexually inactive animals, sperm are lost from here by seepage into the urethra and flushed away by urine. A few may be resorbed by the lining of the duct system.

This regular but slow emission of sperm contrasts with the vigorous ejaculation that occurs during coitus through a penis erected by the engorgement of the cavernous and spongy spaces. The penis thus stiffened and enlarged protrudes its free extremity to enter the vagina. The details of the process, which differs significantly among species, largely depend on the structure of the penis. The fibroelastic penis needs little additional blood to fully distend the cavernous spaces, does not increase greatly in size, and uses effacement of the preexisting sigmoid flexure for its protrusion. Moreover, because relatively little additional blood is required, full erection of the fibroelastic penis may be achieved rapidly. The cavernous spaces are much larger and more dilatable in the musculocavernous penis possessed by horses and dogs. In these species a much greater increase in both length and girth occurs. The process requires more time for its completion.

Erection of penis in two distinct phases. In the first stages of sexual excitement, blood flow into the penis increases as the walls of the supplying arteries relax, with simultaneous obstruction of the venous outflow. The pressure within the cavernous spaces rises rapidly and soon equals that within the arteries that deliver blood to the corpus cavernosum via the crura and to the corpus spongiosum via the bulb. The venous outflow is restricted at the proximal extremity of the organ, where the veins are compressed against the ischial arch; this has more effect on the drainage of the crura and corpus cavernosum than on that of the corpus spongiosum, whose more distal outlet is as yet unaffected (see Fig. 15.20).

The process continues and intensifies after intromission. Rhythmic contractions of the ischiocavernosus and bulbospongiosus muscles now begin, impelling blood forward through the corpus cavernosum and corpus spongiosum. The internal pressures fluctuate in time with this activity. The additional blood pumped distally within the corpus cavernosum cannot escape because the emissary veins are compressed; the pressure therefore rises further. In contrast, the contractions of the bulbospongiosus produce only intermittent rises in pressure because some blood continues to escape at the free extremity of the penis; the effect of this flow is to massage the urethra, which supplies a further impulse to the forward movement of semen when ejaculation takes place.

In most species the pressures drop rapidly after ejaculation, first reaching that within the arteries and then dropping to the resting pressure (a mere 15 to 20 mm Hg). As the blood escapes, the penis shrinks, becomes more flaccid, and is returned to the prepuce. The return is brought about by the active involvement of the retractor penis muscles (see Fig. 29.34).

The volume and composition of the ejaculate vary with the species and also with recent sexual activity. Only a small part of the semen is provided by the sperm-rich fraction emanating from the testes and epididymides, the bulk coming from the accessory reproductive glands. Because semen volume depends on the bulk of these glands, it could be anticipated that the ejaculate would be greatest in the boar. The various contributions to the semen are very imperfectly mixed when expelled into the urethra. The semen is moved through the urethra by the activity of striated muscles (urethralis, bulbospongiosus), and its ejaculation into the vagina or cervix (according to the species) is therefore forceful.

THE FEMALE REPRODUCTIVE ORGANS

The female reproductive organs include paired female gonads, or ovaries, which produce both female gametes (ova) and hormones; paired uterine tubes, which capture the ova on their release from the ovaries and convey them to the uterus; the uterus, in which the fertilized ova are retained and nourished until prenatal development is complete; the vagina, which serves both as copulatory organ and as birth canal; and the vestibule, which continues the vagina to open externally at the vulva but which also doubles as a urinary passage (see Fig. 5.2).

Age and functional changes in these organs are particularly obtrusive. Age changes include the rapid growth and maturation associated with puberty and also regression as the capacity for reproduction wanes. Functional changes include those that are relatively transient and recur with each reproductive cycle as well as other, more lasting ones that are associated with pregnancy and giving birth. This initial account concentrates on the description of the organs of the mature nonpregnant animal; the growth and functional changes are left for later comment. Even so, a few general terms are introduced at this point to help the reader.

Female mammals generally accept the male only close to the time of ovulation, a period characterized by various structural changes, general excitability, and specific behavioral features; the period is known as *heat* or *season* in lay language and as *estrus* more technically. Estrus recurs with varying frequency according to a program that is characteristic for each species although subject to environmental modification. In certain wild mammals the breeding season is confined to a certain part of the year, and sexual receptivity, with the concomitant structural and behavioral changes, occurs only once (monestrous species) or perhaps several times (seasonally polyestrous species) within this period. In other (truly polyestrous) species the cycle is repeated throughout the year; the adoption of the polyestrous mode often distinguishes domestic and laboratory species from their wild progenitors. The condition in which female receptivity is continuous and not linked to ovulation occurs only in women and some higher primate species (e.g., bonobo); in most of the latter it appears to be more common among, if not confined to, menagerie specimens.

The estrous cycle is divided into several phases. Estrus, the climax, is prefaced by proestrus, a period of follicular development; it is followed by a period of luteal activity divided between metestrus and diestrus. In monestrous species a lengthy period of sexual inactivity (anestrus) occurs before the cycle is renewed with a preparatory period of proestrus. In polyestrous species, proestrus follows directly after diestrus. Proestrus and estrus together represent the follicular phase, which is dominated by the rising levels of estrogen produced in the batch of ovarian follicles and then rapidly developing to maturity and rupture. Metestrus and diestrus represent the luteal phase, when the dominant hormonal influence is exerted by progesterone produced by the corpora lutea that transiently replaces the ruptured follicles.

Animals that have borne young are said to be *parous*, those that have not are *nulliparous*, and *uniparous* and *multiparous* extend this terminology in obvious fashion. Other terms refer to the number of young habitually carried by the gravid female. A mare with its (generally) single foal is monotocous; a sow with its litter of piglets is polytocous.*

The Ovaries

The ovaries possess both gametogenic and endocrine functions. Each ovary is a solid, basically ellipsoidal body, although it is commonly made irregular by the projection from the surface of large follicles and corpora lutea (Fig. 5.55A–F). The irregularity is naturally greatest in polytocous species, in which follicles ripen in batches. The ovaries are much smaller than the testes of conspecific males but, like these, bear no constant proportion to body size. Those of the mare are relatively large and also peculiar in being kidney shaped. Ovaries are usually found in the dorsal part of the abdomen, close to the tips of the horns of the uterus, because they do not shift far from their place of development. This migration is most considerable in ruminants, in which the ovaries come to lie close by the pelvic inlet. Each ovary is suspended within the cranial part (mesovarium) of the broad ligament, the common suspension of the female reproductive tract.

A section through the ovary of a mature animal shows a central looser and more vascular part contained within a denser shell. The *parenchymatous zone* (cortex) is bounded by a tunica albuginea directly below the peritoneum and is strewn with follicles in various stages of development and regression. Each *follicle* contains a single ovum; the stages through which it passes are shown in schematic fashion in Fig. 5.56. The rapid enlargement of the follicles selected to mature in the current cycle is mainly due to the accumulation of the fluid. The cavity within the ruptured follicle, though it may initially fill with blood, is soon occupied by hypertrophy of the granulosa and theca cells that originally lined the space. This produces a solid body, known as the *corpus luteum* (yellow body) on account of its color (Fig. 5.55E). *Corpora lutea* are transient structures that wax and wane between one estrous period and the next (assuming pregnancy does not ensue) (Fig. 5.57A–C). Degeneration of the corpora lutea is characterized by vacuolization of the cytoplasm of the luteal cells due to lipid accumulation and nuclear shrinkage. Although transient, luteal cells are important as the source of progesterone, just as the ripening follicles are the source of estrogen. Corpora lutea finally regress and are replaced by connective tissue scars, corpora albicantes (white bodies). The alternation in the levels of estrogen and progesterone determines the changes in the behavior pattern and in the morphology and activity of the reproductive tract.

The Uterine Tubes

The uterine tubes* are narrow and generally very flexuous. They capture the ova released from the ovaries and convey them toward the uterus; because the tubes also convey the sperm in their ascent, fertilization normally occurs within the tubes.

*Unfortunately, there is some conflict in the use of these terms: many authors reserve *uniparous* and *multiparous* for the senses in which we employ *monotocous* and *polytocous*.

*The obsolete terms *fallopian tubes* and *oviducts* are still encountered, perhaps most commonly in medical writing. Another term, *salpinx*, receives official recognition; though less frequently encountered, it is the stem of such derivatives as *mesosalpinx* and *salpingitis* (inflammation of the uterine tube).

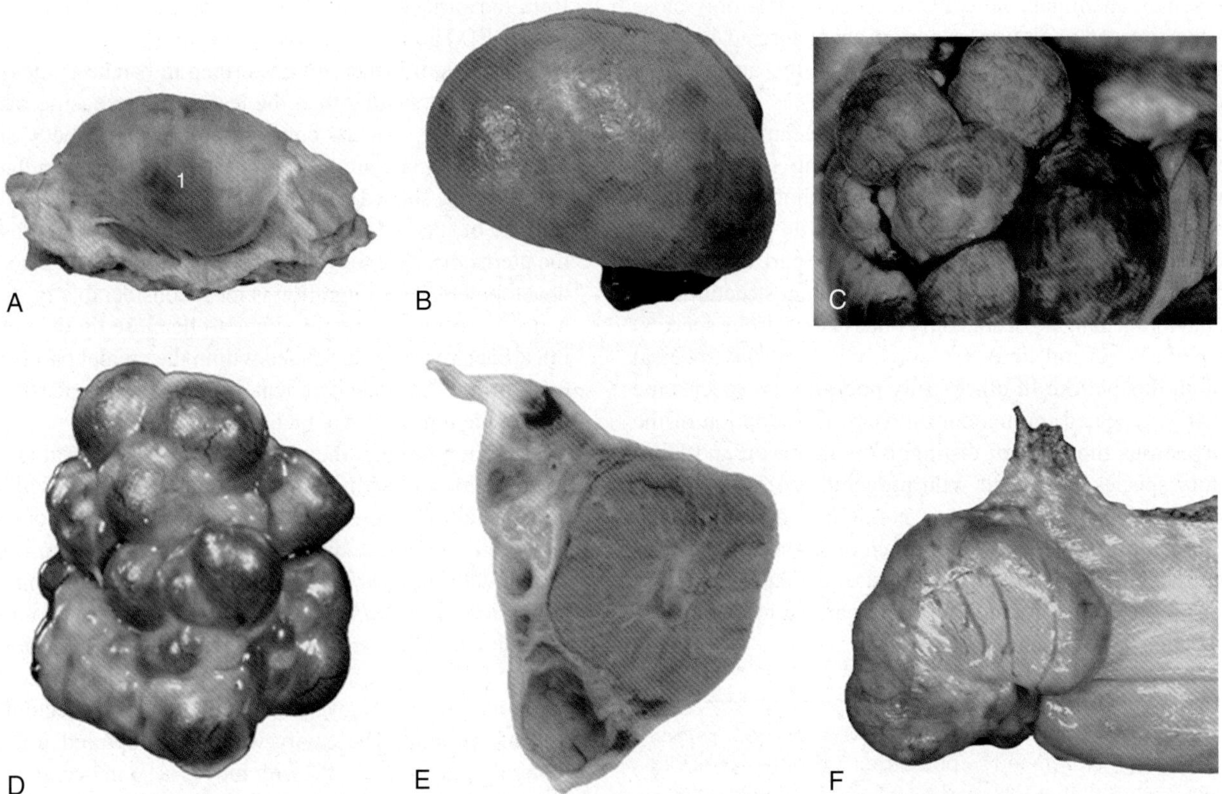

Fig. 5.55 Specific and functional variations in ovarian morphology. (A) Ovary of a cow (monotocous). *1,* Mature follicle. (B) Ovary of a bitch in a quiet stage. (C) Ovary of a bitch exhibiting several mature follicles. (D) Ovary of sow (polytocous) exhibiting mature follicles. (E) Sectioned ovary of a cow containing a large corpus luteum. (F) Ovary of a mare, with ovulation fossa.

The free cranial extremity takes the form of a thin-walled funnel (*infundibulum;* Fig. 5.58/*2*) placed close to the cranial pole of the ovary. The free edge of the funnel is ragged, and the tags (fimbriae) come into contact with and sometimes adhere to the surface of the ovary. A small (abdominal) orifice in the depth of the funnel leads to the longer tubular part that is divided into two more or less equal segments. The proximal segment, known as the *ampulla,* is followed by the more convoluted and narrower *isthmus,* but the distinction between these segments is not equally obvious in all species or at all phases of the cycle (Fig. 5.58/*3* and *4*). The isthmus joins the apex of the horn of the uterus at the uterotubal (salpingouterine) junction, a region of very variable appearance. The junction is gradual in ruminants and pigs and abrupt in horses and carnivores; indeed, in the mare and to a lesser extent also in the bitch and cat, the terminal part of the tube is thrust into the apex of the horn to raise a small papilla perforated by the (uterine) orifice of the tube. Regardless of its appearance, the junction always represents a real barrier, impeding both the ascent of sperm and the descent of ova. The tube wall consists of external serosal, middle muscular, and internal mucosal tunics. The mucosa is folded longitudinally along its whole length from infundibulum to isthmus; secondary and even tertiary folds reduce the lumen of the ampulla to a series of narrow branching clefts. The tube is carried in a side-fold (mesosalpinx) of the part of the broad ligament that supports the ovary.

The Uterus

The uterus,* the womb in popular speech, is the enlarged part of the tract in which embryos arrive to establish a means of physiologic exchange with the mother's bloodstream. It is the part of the tract that displays the most striking specific differences, although the most extreme forms do not occur among domestic species. These differences find a ready explanation in the manner of formation of the reproductive tract (p. 161) from two paramesonephric ducts that grow caudally to meet and fuse with each other and with the median urogenital sinus, the ventral division

*Compound terms are generally derived from the alternative name, *metrium:* for example, *mesometrium* and *metritis;* surgical removal of the uterus, however, is termed *hysterectomy* (Greek, *hystera,* uterus).

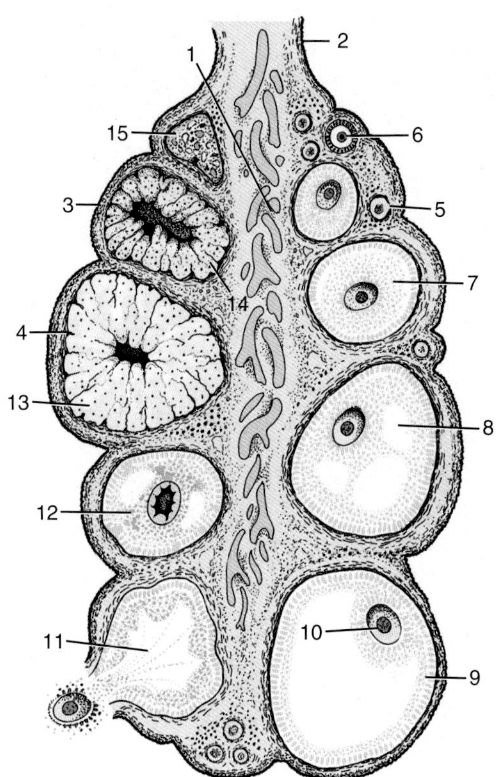

Fig. 5.56 Schematic representation of the different functional stages in ovarian activity. *1,* Medulla; *2,* mesovarium; *3,* surface epithelium; *4,* tunica albuginea (poorly developed); *5,* primordial follicle; *6,* primary follicle; *7,* secondary follicle; *8,* early tertiary follicle; *9,* mature follicle; *10,* oocyte; *11,* ruptured follicle; *12,* atretic follicle; *13,* corpus luteum; *14,* atretic corpus luteum; *15,* corpus albicans.

of the cloaca (Figs. 5.15 and 5.16). In some species, including many rodents, fusion of the ducts is limited to the most caudal portions, which contribute to the vagina. Because of the distinct cranial parts, the uterus consists of paired tubes that open separately into the vagina (double uterus—uterus duplex). In contrast, in women and most other primates, fusion is much more extensive and only the uterine tubes remain paired; a median uterus with a simple undivided lumen is present. In the intermediate variety (bicornuate uterus) found in all major domestic species, the uterus contains a caudal median part from which paired horns diverge cranially to continue as the uterine tubes.

In all domestic mammals the median part of the uterus has two segments. The caudal, very thick-walled segment, the *cervix* (Fig. 5.59/*8*), provides a sphincter controlling access to and from the vagina. A part of the cervix (Fig. 5.59/*9*) (portio vaginalis) usually projects into the vaginal lumen with which it communicates at the external ostium. The lumen of the cervix (cervical canal) is constricted and often almost occluded by mucosal folds. It opens into the *body of the uterus* (Fig. 5.59/*6*) at the internal ostium. The body is generally a rather small segment in domestic species, although the proportions vary see (Fig. 5.16); it is largest in the mare. The division of the interior is not always obvious externally because an internal septum may partially divide an apparently single space. The extent of the cervix, not apparent visually, is easily discovered on rectal palpation, on the basis of its firmness in comparison with the adjacent parts.

The *horns* (cornua) vary greatly in length and are longest in polytocous species. Their disposition also varies from characteristically round in ruminants, to straight and divergent in mares and bitches, to cast into intestine-like loops in sows. The cervix generally lies within the pelvic cavity, interposed between the rectum and the bladder (Fig. 5.32/7), but the body and horns of the uterus typically lie within the abdomen above the mass of intestines.

The uterus possesses serosal, muscular, and mucosal coats that are known as the *perimetrium, myometrium,* and *endometrium,* respectively. The serosal covering reaches the uterus by extension from the supporting broad ligament (mesometrium; Fig. 5.33/7). The muscle is arranged as weak external longitudinal and thicker internal circular layers that are separated by a very vascular stratum of connective tissue. The tissues, especially the external muscle layer, extend (as parametrium) into the supporting broad ligaments. Dense connective tissue intermingles with the muscle of the cervix, making it a very indistensible part of the tract at most times (Fig. 5.60).

The endometrium is thick. Its surface relief varies among species and is most remarkable in ruminants, in which numerous permanent elevations (caruncles) mark the sites where the embryonic membranes firmly attach during pregnancy (Fig. 5.59/7). Numerous tubular glands open on the surface, which is generally lined by a simple columnar epithelium. The mucosa within the cervix is prominently modeled by both longitudinal and circular folds whose interdigitation helps close the passage (Fig. 5.59/*8*). Mucus secreted by cervical glands plugs the canal at most times and so helps seal the uterus from the vagina. The passage is open only at estrus and immediately before, during, and, for a short time, after parturition.

The Vagina

The remainder of the female tract, although sometimes loosely termed the *vagina*, consists of two parts. The cranial part, the vagina in the strict sense (Fig. 5.59/*10*), is a purely reproductive passage that runs from the cervix to the entrance of the urethra. The caudal part, the vestibule, extends from the urethral orifice to the external vulva and combines reproductive and urinary functions. The two

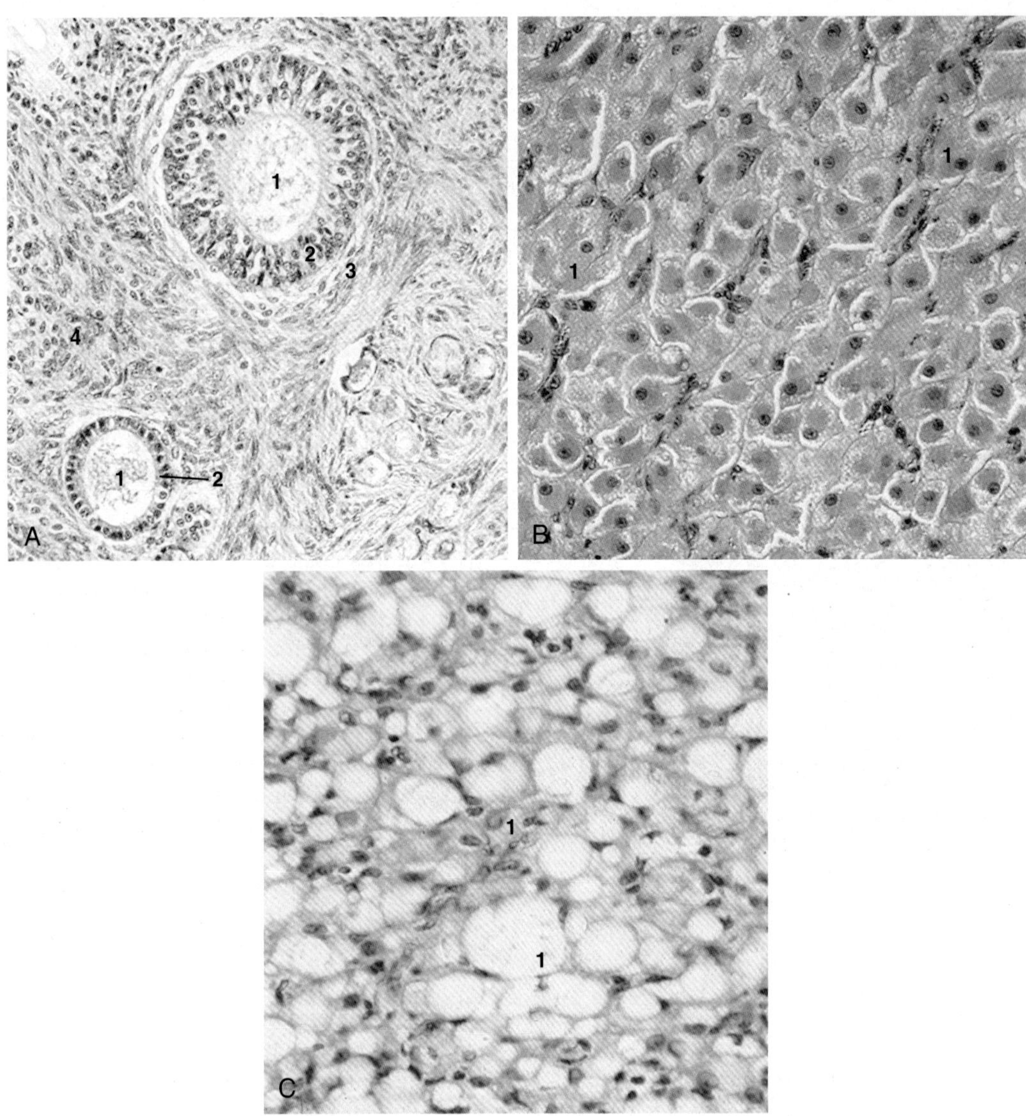

Fig. 5.57 Histologic preparations. (A) Ovary (bitch) in anestrus with preantral follicles (140×). *1,* Oocyte; *2,* granulosa cells; *3,* theca cells; *4,* stroma. (B) Active corpus luteum (queen) (140×). (C) Inactive corpus luteum (queen) (140×). *1,* Degenerating luteal cells.

parts together constitute the female copulatory organ and birth canal.

The *vagina* is a relatively long, thin-walled tube that is distensible in length and width. It occupies a median position within the pelvic cavity, related to the rectum dorsally and the bladder and urethra ventrally (Fig. 5.32/*8*). It is mostly retroperitoneal, although peritoneum does cover the cranial parts of both the dorsal and the ventral surfaces to a variable extent. Incision of this part of the dorsal wall, a relatively easy procedure to perform from within the vagina in larger species, provides a convenient access to the peritoneal cavity (see Fig. 22.6/2 and 8). The corresponding ventral approach is prohibited by the presence of a plexus of veins draining the uterus and vagina.

The vaginal muscle, although weaker, has a similar disposition to that of the uterus. The mucosa is lined by a stratified squamous epithelium that reacts, more emphatically in some species than in others, to changes in hormone levels throughout the estrous cycle. Glands are confined to the cranial part of the vagina, although the moisture may diffuse more widely. The surface is smooth but circular, and longitudinal folds may form when the walls of the inactive organ collapse inward. The intrusion of the cervix into the cranial part of the vagina reduces the lumen of this part to a (generally) ringlike space known as the *fornix* (Fig. 5.59/*10′*).

The junction of vagina and vestibule is supposedly marked in virgin animals by a transverse mucosal fold (hymen). This is best developed in the filly and the gilt, but even in these it is rarely very prominent. It does not survive coitus. The junctional region is less distensible than the parts of the tract cranial and caudal to it.

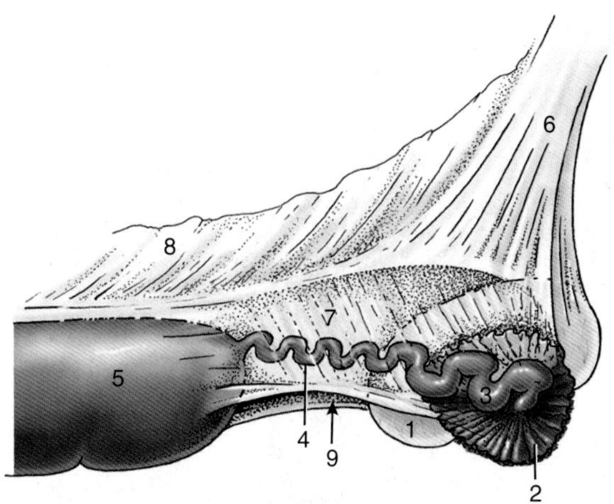

Fig. 5.58 Lateral view of the suspension of the right ovary, uterine tube, and uterine horn of a mare. *1,* Ovary; *2,* infundibulum of tube; *3,* ampulla of tube; *4,* isthmus of tube; *5,* uterine horn; *6,* mesovarium; *7,* mesosalpinx; *8,* mesometrium; *9, arrow* indicates entrance to ovarian bursa.

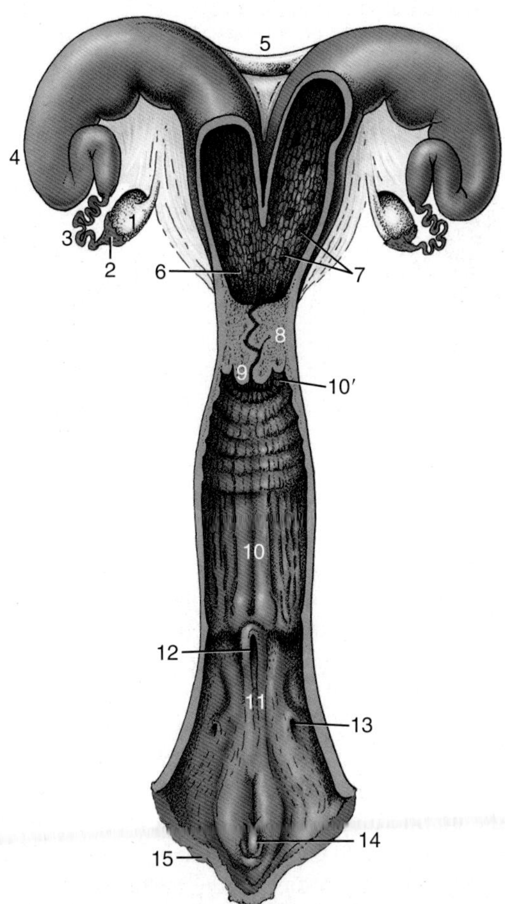

Fig. 5.59 The reproductive tract of a cow, opened dorsally. *1,* Ovary; *2,* infundibulum; *3,* uterine tube; *4,* horn of uterus; *5,* intercornual ligaments; *6,* body of uterus; *7,* caruncles; *8,* cervix; *9,* vaginal part of cervix; *10,* vagina; *10′,* fornix; *11,* vestibule; *12,* external urethral opening; *13,* opening of major vestibular gland; *14,* clitoris; *15,* vulva.

The Vestibule and Vulva

The vestibule, much shorter than the vagina, lies mainly if not entirely caudal to the ischial arch, a circumstance that permits the vagina to slope ventral to its opening at the vulva. The amount of "drop" is variable, among both species and individuals (Fig. 5.61). The resulting inflection of the axis of the genital passage must be borne in mind when introducing a vaginal speculum or other instrument.

The walls of the vestibule are less elastic than those of the vagina and come together at rest, reducing the lumen to a vertical cleft. The urethra opens on the floor, directly caudal to whatever indication of a hymen (Fig. 5.62/*4*) may exist. In some animals such as the bitch, the urethral opening is raised above the general level of the vestibular floor (Fig. 5.35). In others, such as the cow, it is associated with a *suburethral diverticulum* (Fig. 5.32/*12′*). More caudally, the vestibular walls are marked by the entrances of the ducts of *vestibular glands.* In certain species (e.g., bitch) the glands are small but numerous, and the duct orifices form linear series, whereas in others (e.g., cow) a large glandular mass to each side drains by a single duct (Fig. 5.59/*13*). In a few species (e.g., ewe) both minor and major vestibular glands are present. These glands produce a mucous secretion that lubricates the passage at coitus and at parturition. At estrus the odor of the secretion has a sexually stimulating effect on the male. The vestibular wall is exceptionally well vascularized, with a concentration of veins forming a lateral patch of erectile tissue known as the *vestibular bulb* and regarded as the homologue of the bulb of the penis.

The vestibule opens to the exterior at the vulva. The vertical vulvar opening is bounded by labia that meet at dorsal and ventral commissures. Except in the mare, the dorsal commissure is rounded, the ventral one pointed and raised above the level of the surrounding skin. The labia correspond to the (inner) labia minora of human anatomy; the (outer) labia majora are suppressed in domestic species.

The *clitoris,* the female homologue of the penis, lies just within the ventral commissure (Fig. 5.59/*14*). It is formed of two crura, a body and a glans, in the same fashion as its much larger male homologue. Without dissection, only the glans is visible where it projects within a fossa on the vestibular floor, partly enveloped by a mucosal fold constituting a prepuce.

The Adnexa

The *broad ligaments,* the principal attachments of the female reproductive tract, are bilateral sheets that take extended origin from the abdominal roof and pelvic walls. The cranial part of each hangs vertically and suspends the ovary, uterine tube, and horn of the uterus. The caudal part passes more horizontally to attach to the side of the body of the uterus, cervix, and cranial part of the vagina.

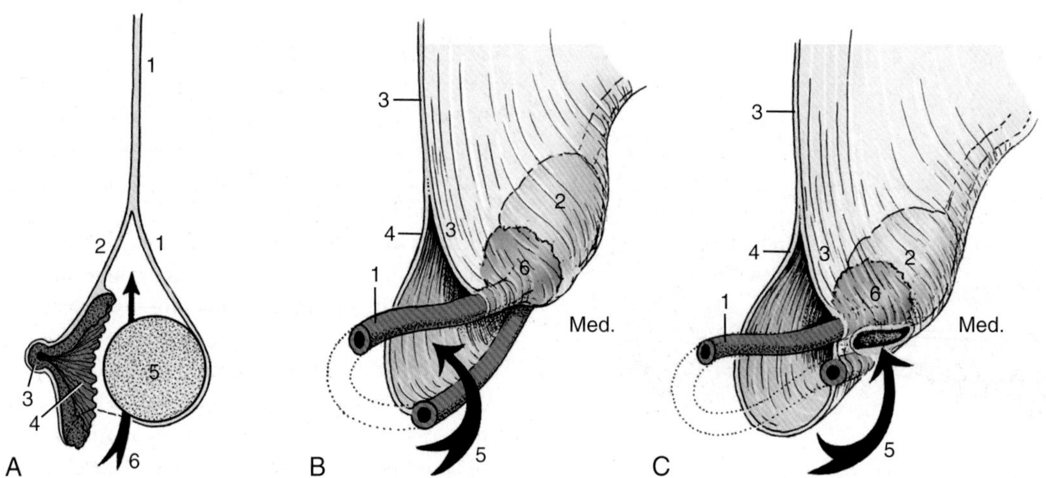

Fig. 5.60 (A) Schematic representations of the ovary and the suspensory system of the ovary and uterine tube and of the varying forms of the ovarian bursa. *1,* Mesovarium; *2,* mesosalpinx; *3,* abdominal opening of uterine tube; *4,* infundibulum; *5,* ovary; *6, arrow* is in the ovarian bursa. (B) Spacious bursa with large entrance (cow, mare). (C) Bursa with constricted entrance and entrapped ovary (bitch). *1,* Uterine tube; *2,* ovary; *3,* mesovarium; *4,* mesosalpinx; *5, arrow* entering the ovarian bursa; *6,* infundibulum; *Med.,* medial.

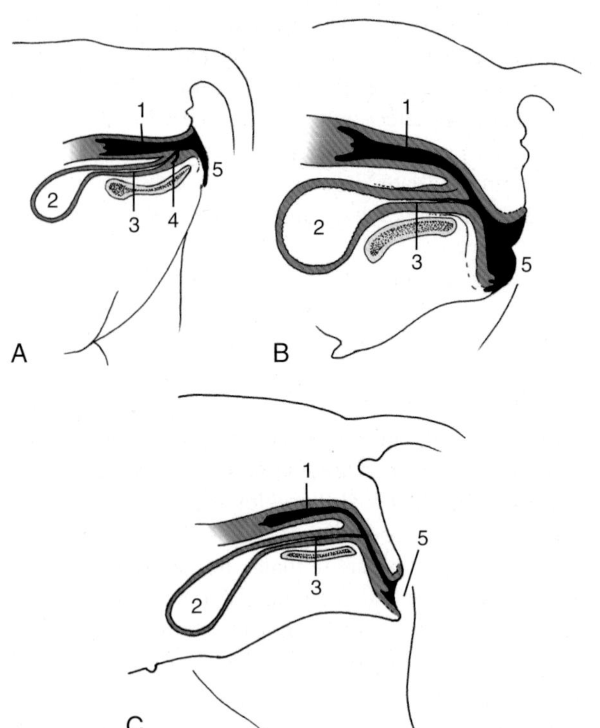

Fig. 5.61 Variation in the position of the vestibule in relation to the ischial arch in the (A) cow, (B) mare, and (C) bitch. *1,* Vagina; *2,* bladder; *3,* urethra; *4,* suburethral diverticulum; *5,* vulva.

The right and left caudal parts with their visceral inclusion divide the pelvic cavity into dorsal and ventral spaces (Figs. 5.33/7). Different parts of the broad ligaments obtain the specific designations already mentioned (e.g., mesovarium). These ligaments are unlike most peritoneal

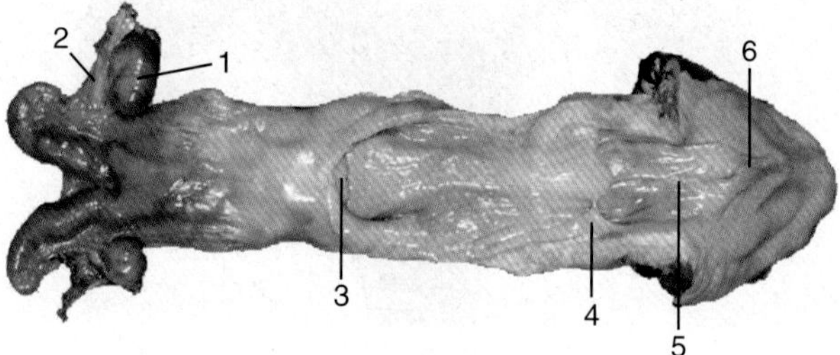

Fig. 5.62 Uterus and opened vagina of the cow. *1,* Ovary; *2,* uterine tube; *3,* cervix; *4,* hymen; *5,* vestibule; *6,* glans of clitoris.

folds because the serosal membranes are held apart by considerable amounts of tissue, mainly smooth muscle; this sometimes makes it difficult to point to the exact boundary between the uterus and its adnexa. The muscle enables the ligaments to take an active part in the support and disposition of the reproductive organs in addition to conveying vessels and nerves.

When followed distally from its attachment to the abdominal roof, the *mesovarium,* which supports the ovary, releases a lateral fold (mesosalpinx) that passes onto the uterine tube (Figs. 5.58/7 and 5.60A). Mesosalpinx and mesovarium enclose a pouch, the *ovarian bursa,* into which the ovary projects. The bursa may be shallow and unable to hold the ovary (mare; Fig. 5.58/9) or deep and so enclosed by the fusion of apposed serosal surfaces that the ovary is permanently trapped (bitch; Fig. 5.60C). In certain nondomestic species (e.g., mouse) fusion is so complete that the space within the bursa no longer communicates with the peritoneal cavity. The walls of the bursa may contain so much fat that the ovary is quite hidden. The mesovarium also supports a fibromuscular band, the proper ligament of the ovary, which extends from the caudal pole of the ovary to the adjacent tip of the horn of the uterus.

The large part of the broad ligament that passes onto the horn and body of the uterus helps to give the organ the shape characteristic of the species. The two serosal membranes are very widely separated by fat where they attach to the cervix and especially to the vagina and make the lateral part of the vagina retroperitoneal. A cord of fibrous tissue and smooth muscle, the *round ligament of the uterus,* passes from the tip of the horn of the uterus toward (and in the bitch, through) the inguinal canal, supported by a special fold of peritoneum detached from the lateral surface of the broad ligament.

The muscles and fasciae associated with the female reproductive organs are best considered in topographical contexts for those animals such as ruminants in which they have special importance (p. 692). It will be recalled that the pelvic outlet is closed by a musculofascial partition of complicated form and structure. The dorsal part, the pelvic diaphragm, closes the outlet about the anus. The ventral part, the *urogenital diaphragm* (membrana perinei), closes the outlet about the vestibule. Muscle forms the principal component of the pelvic diaphragm, whereas the fasciae predominate in the urogenital diaphragm.

The blood supply to the female reproductive organs is obtained from several sources. The *ovarian artery,* a direct branch of the aorta, supplies the ovary and branches in varying patterns to the uterine tube and cranial part of the horn of the uterus. The ovarian artery assumes an extraordinarily convoluted course and, depending on species, is more or less closely related to the ovarian vein. The uterine branch anastomoses with the uterine artery within the broad ligament (Fig. 5.63/*1′* and *2*).

The *uterine artery* arises as an indirect branch of the internal iliac artery (except in the mare) and runs forward within the broad ligament. It detaches a series of anastomosing branches to the body and horn of the uterus; the most cranial anastomoses with the ovarian artery, the most caudal with the vaginal artery. Thus, an arterial arcade is established, running the length of the uterus and supplied from both ends (Fig. 5.64). It is thought that more blood supply may occur to areas such as implantation sites in the uterus, and a reduced supply to certain parts may result in runts, which are so common in pigs. The more caudal parts of the tract are variously supplied by branches of the *internal pudendal* and *vaginal arteries;* some more important species differences are mentioned elsewhere.

The veins, broadly satellite to the arteries. The plexiform *ovarian vein* is relatively much larger, the *uterine vein* relatively much smaller, than the accompanying artery (Fig. 5.63). A prominent and elaborate venous plexus present on the ventral aspect of the uterus and vagina drains both organs via any of the paired ovarian,

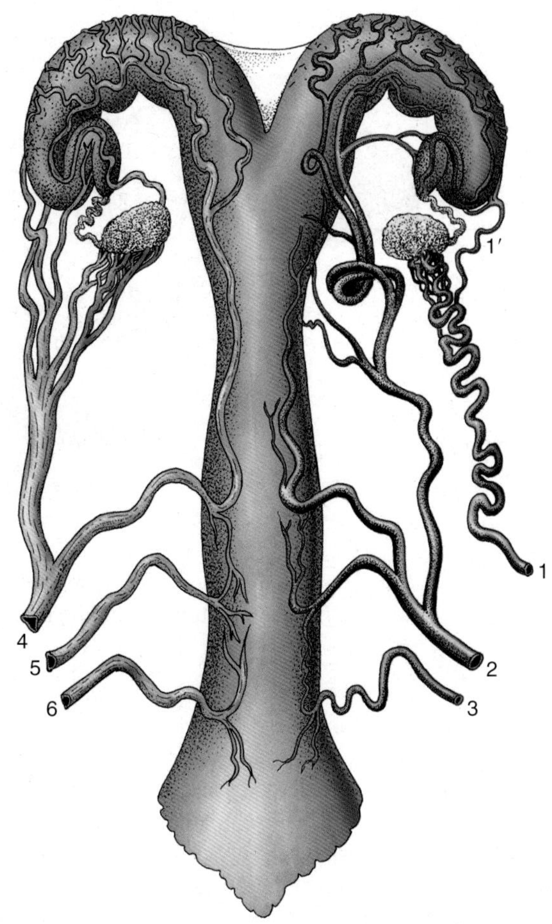

Fig. 5.63 Semischematic ventral view of the blood supply to the reproductive tract of the cow. The arteries are depicted on the right side, the veins on the left. *1,* Ovarian artery; *1′,* uterine branch; *2,* uterine artery; *3,* vaginal artery; *4,* ovarian vein; *5,* accessory vaginal vein; *6,* vaginal vein.

uterine, and vaginal veins. The close relation between the artery and ovarian vein, best seen in ruminants and sows, provides a means for the countercurrent transfer of the luteolytic hormone (prostaglandin) from venous to arterial blood (p. 198).

The lymphatics from the ovaries and more cranial parts of the tract pass to the aortic and medial iliac nodes, and those from more caudal parts to the medial iliac and other nodes within the pelvis.

Innervation of the female reproductive organs is provided by both sympathetic and parasympathetic fibers, by routes that have yet to be fully clarified. Although sympathetic fibers run to the ovary including the ripening follicles together with the ovarian artery, their denervation hardly disturbs ovarian function. The fibers to the uterine tube, uterus, and vagina mainly follow the other arteries to form plexuses within the broad ligaments and the genital organs themselves. In the caudal part of the broad ligaments these fibers are augmented by other sympathetic fibers that travel by way of the plexus located in the retroperitoneal pelvic tissue.

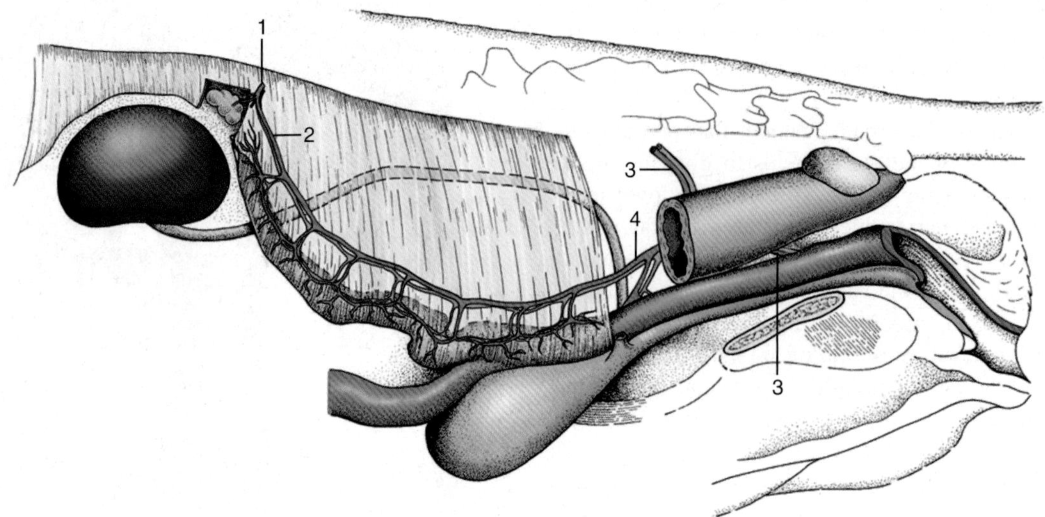

Fig. 5.64 Semischematic drawing of the blood supply of the female reproductive tract (bitch). *1,* Ovarian artery; *2,* uterine branch of the ovarian artery; *3,* vaginal artery; *4,* uterine artery.

The parasympathetic fibers branch from the pelvic nerves and reach the genital organs via the pelvic plexus. A large proportion goes to erectile tissue.

Both sympathetic and parasympathetic fibers seem to be concerned with uterine activity, although their precise roles in stimulation and inhibition are still controversial. The uterus is able to coordinate contractions and accomplish a normal birth even after denervation.

Age and Functional Changes to the Female Tract

Only a general account of the important age and functional changes is presented in this chapter, which glosses over the many species differences that affect all aspects but particularly the timing and duration of events.

Age and Cyclic Changes

The *juvenile* reproductive organs are disproportionately small. At birth the ovaries provide no evidence of their future endocrine role, which is not established until shortly before puberty, when ripening follicles and the corpora lutea that replace them produce the hormones that stimulate the growth, tissue differentiation, and activity of the reproductive tract as well as the manifestation of female behavior. In contrast, the gametogenic or exocrine function was established in the young fetus with the migration of primordial germ cells into the ovary. These immigrant cells proliferate rapidly to produce a population of perhaps 3 million at its maximum, but this number soon begins to be progressively reduced in a process that continues to puberty and beyond. Only a few hundred thousand generally survive at birth and, because no later accession to their number is possible, the later release of female gametes is much more stingy than that of male gametes. Each surviving oocyte is initially surrounded by a single layer of flattened epithelial (granulosa) cells to form the structure known as the *primordial follicle*. Most primordial follicles remain in arrested development or undergo atresia, but some transform into primary follicles that are distinguished by the enlargement of the oocyte and its enclosure within a covering of granulosa cells that have assumed a cuboidal conformation.

Growth of reproductive organs is initially isometric, keeping pace with general somatic growth. After puberty the actions of ovarian hormones, cumulative over the first few cycles, bring about a rapid enlargement and a better differentiation of the component tissues. Follicles in all stages of development may now be found within the ovaries together with corpora lutea and replacement scars (Fig. 5.56).

There is a continuous slow growth of many follicles within the adult ovaries. In the ovary of anestrous animals, the follicles grow to the early antral stage (Fig. 5.57A) but then degenerate. The onset of the breeding season is heralded by a more rapid development of a few, which are chosen from this larger population through a yet poorly understood mechanism. These favored follicles enlarge at an exponential rate under the influence of FSH of the pituitary. Their growth is explained by the proliferation of granulosa and theca cells and the accumulation of follicular fluid. This fluid increasingly distends a central vesicle (antrum) into which the ovum projects, raised on a mound of cells (cumulus oophorus) and enclosed within a cellular covering (corona radiata). The follicle is bounded by a two-layered capsule (theca interna and externa) differentiated

TABLE 5.1 SOME SPECIFIC PARAMETERS IN REPRODUCTION

Species	Puberty (mo)	Cycle Length (days; range)	Duration of Estrus	Ovulation	Pregnancy Duration (days)
Dog	6–9	≥90	9 days	3 days after the beginning of estrus	62
Cat	6–9	Variable	7–10 days	24 h after coitus	63–65
Horse	20	21 (19–22)	5–6 days	1–2 days before the end of estrus	330
Cattle	6–18	21 (18–24)	18 h	10–12 h after the end of estrus	280
Sheep	6–12	17 (16–18)	24–36 h	30–36 h after the beginning of estrus	150
Goat	4–8	21	24–36 h	30–36 h after the beginning of estrus	150
Pig	5–10	21 (19–21)	48–72 h	35–45 h after the beginning of estrus	114

from the surrounding stroma (Fig. 5.56). As each follicle grows it shifts toward the surface of the ovary, where it forms an increasingly salient projection. The granulosa cells of the ripening follicle produce estrogen, and it is the peak level of production of this hormone that induces both the behavioral pattern and the structural changes that characterize the animal in heat.

Estrogen has an epitheliotropic effect most evident in promoting proliferation of the vaginal epithelium and simple lengthening of the uterine glands. It also causes edema and hyperemia of the tissues of the reproductive tract; edema may produce a visible swelling of the vulva, but congestion of the endometrium may lead in some species (notably the bitch) to the appearance of blood in the external discharge. It also enhances the irritability of the myometrium that is detectable through the uterus, including the cervix, which becomes more responsive to manipulation.

Ovulation occurs late in estrus or shortly after its termination and is stimulated by LH, also of pituitary origin. Ovulation is spontaneous in most species, but in some, including the cat, the mechanical stimulus of coitus is necessary to set in train the events that culminate in follicular rupture (Table 5.1). Once shed into the peritoneal cavity, an ovum is soon gathered into the expanded end of the uterine tube. Because the ovum is nonmotile, the most likely mechanisms are the production of a current in the suspending fluid by the ciliary beat of the tubal epithelium and grasping movements of the muscular fimbriae, which are closely applied to the surface of the ovary at this time. Both mechanisms would be assisted by the surface irregularity provided by adherent corona cells.

The space within the vacated follicle fills with blood when rupture has been attended by considerable hemorrhage, but any clot is soon replaced by proliferation of the surviving granulosa and internal theca cells to form a solid body, the *corpus luteum* (Fig. 5.57B). This structure grows rapidly and may soon equal in size the follicle that it replaces. It produces progesterone, the hormone that continues the preparation of the uterus for the reception of the embryo and for the maintenance of pregnancy. In animals that become pregnant the corpus luteum survives well into or throughout pregnancy (according to species), but it regresses quite rapidly in cycles that are infertile (Fig. 5.57C). Responsibility for its regression rests with a luteolytic hormone (prostaglandin) produced by the "empty" uterus. The effects of progesterone reinforce those produced by previous exposure to estrogen and stimulate further growth of the uterine glands, which now become branched, tortuous, and more active, secreting the so-called uterine milk that nourishes the embryo before implantation. Progesterone also dampens the activity of the myometrium.

The transport of ova within the tube is achieved by the combination of ciliary and muscular activity. If mating has occurred the ova rendezvous with the sperm within the ampulla. Although sperm may reach this site within a few minutes of coitus, a longer sojourn within the female tract is required before they become capable of fertilization. According to species, semen is initially deposited within the vagina or the cervix, where it forms a coagulum from which some sperm soon emerge. Even when the semen is deposited in the vagina, churning movements soon bring some sperm into contact with the cervical mucus, which protects and guides the sperm on their upward path. Even so, the movement of sperm would be slow if they depended on their own puny efforts; transport is mainly effected by muscular contractions, evoked by prostaglandin within the semen, and by oxytocin reflexly released into the bloodstream at coitus. Only 1% or 2% of the many millions within an ejaculate deposited within the vagina succeed in passing the cervical barrier. The uterotubal junction, the next major impediment, is successively negotiated by even fewer sperm (and these necessarily of normal motility). In species in which intrauterine deposition of sperm takes place, the uterotubal junction is the first barrier. Movement within the tube is more erratic because the muscular contractions are ill coordinated. In most species sperm remain fertile for a day or two after coitus, and many apparently find temporary refuge in cervical glands and other niches.

Fertilization activates the ovum, and cleavage begins within a short time. Its later fate is considered in the following section.

The Course of Pregnancy

The evolution of the gravid uterus affects its size, position, form, and relations that become increasingly evident with advancing pregnancy. The principles effecting change in size are more or less the same in all animals, but the other aspects vary among species and are best considered separately for each (see the appropriate later chapters). The increase in size may ultimately be as much as 100-fold (as in the cow), but the greater part of this change is represented by the contents of the uterus, which comprise the fetal membranes and fluids in addition to the conceptus(es). The more modest growth of the organ involves all its components. The endometrium remains hyperemic and edematous, and the myometrium enlarges owing to a vast increase in the size of individual muscle cells. Despite this hypertrophy, the uterine wall is unable to keep pace with the growth of the contents, and it stretches markedly—so much so that in rats and other species of similar size it becomes transparent. The broad ligaments share in the increase and come to contain large amounts of muscle. The arteries enlarge greatly as it becomes necessary to satisfy an ever-increasing demand for blood. Activity of the cervical glands continually renews the mucous plug that seals the cervical canal.

Implantation involves reaction from the apposed epithelial layers of the blastocyst and endometrium, and in some species considerable erosion of maternal tissue occurs during attachment (see later). This erosion occurs mainly in species in which the blastocyst remains small before implantation and either seeks out a nidus (nest) in a cleft of the endometrium or burrows into its substance. The blastocysts of domestic species grow considerably before implantation and remain centrally within the lumen of uterus. In domestic ungulates the implantation is probably delayed significantly longer than the 2 weeks after coitus suggested for many other mammals.

Implantation and the initial development of the fetal membranes concludes the *preembryonic period,* the first of the three periods into which development is conventionally divided. Its principal features may be summarized as follows: the intrauterine migration and eventual settlement of the blastocyst, and its rapid transformation from a spherical to a threadlike form in many species (which include the ruminants and pig but not the horse).

The second or *embryonic period* includes the establishment of a fully functional placenta, the differentiation of the various tissues and organ systems, and the initiation of various functions, most notably an embryonic circulation. By the end of this period the external conformation is sufficiently developed to identify the major taxon—order and, perhaps, family—to which the embryo belongs, though not yet the particular species.

The remaining part of the intrauterine development is somewhat arbitrarily and imprecisely assigned to a third, or *fetal, period.** Organogenesis continues throughout the fetal period and, for many organs, well into postnatal life, but the changes that now bring the different systems into the levels of structural and functional competence necessary for survival after birth are less dramatic than those that took place earlier. The rapid growth, which is the foremost characteristic of the fetal period, continues into postnatal life without significant interruption around the time of birth (Fig. 5.65).

The early transformations and the complexities of organogenesis provide ample opportunity for death or malformation in the first two periods. This is probably true for all mammals, although data are most reliably available for the human and the pig. Some losses and abnormalities are due to intrinsic defects of the conceptus, some to an unreceptive state of the uterus, and some to exposure of the mother to any of a variety of environmental insults. It is known, for example, that chromosomal abnormality of structure or number is demonstrable in about 10% of clinically detectable human pregnancies, including spontaneous early abortions, and it is believed to be even more common in conceptuses lost at earlier stages, before there was awareness of pregnancy. In contrast, chromosomal abnormality is identified in a much smaller proportion, perhaps 0.5%, of human infants delivered at term. Although the fertilization rate in pigs is high, possibly exceeding 95% in some herds, it has been estimated that only 60% or so of conceptuses come to term. Most deaths occur within the first 40 days (of a gestation period of 114 days), but because conceptuses lost at an early stage are generally resorbed and leave no trace, the figure must be interpreted with caution. The rates of fertilization and delivery at term for other species vary too much from herd to herd and stud to stud to be conveniently summarized.

The environmental insults that may affect development include ionizing radiation, viral infections, inorganic and organic chemicals, including some that are constituents of plants (e.g., clover, soya and certain other legumes, *Veratrum californicum*) potentially present in pasture or other feedstuffs. Many of these agents are better known from their effects in the laboratory than in the field, and although some are lethal, others are more likely to produce abnormalities that are survivable, if only for a time. Such agents (teratogens) are most likely to produce abnormality when exposure occurs during the embryonic period, when

*Because many processes continue uninterrupted from one period to the next, there is unavoidable overlap and inconsistency in the use of the terms *embryo* and *fetus*.

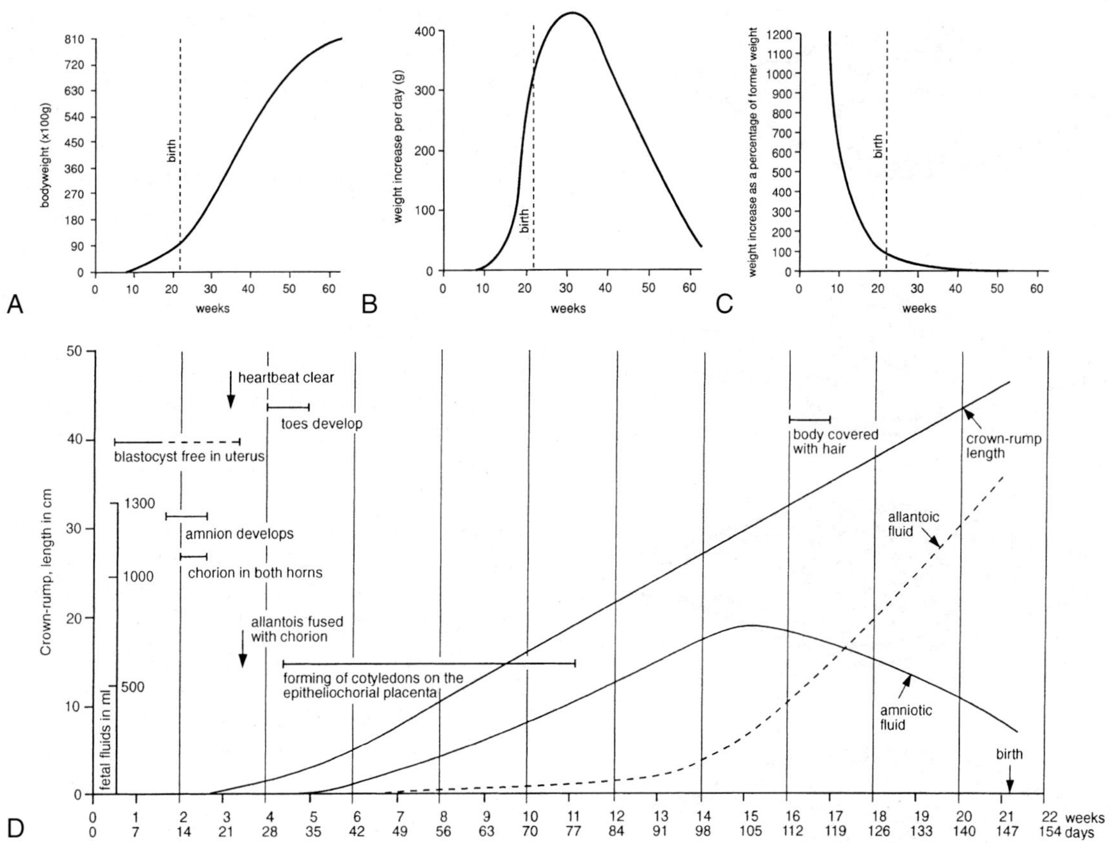

Fig. 5.65 The growth of lambs. (A), (B), and (C) record the growth in weight of lambs during fetal and early postnatal life. (D) Schematic summary of metrical and other features of the development of the fetal lamb and its adnexa.

so many complicated and critically timed procedures are under way.

Infectious agents such as bovine viral diarrhea (BVD), hog cholera (swine fever) (HCV), border disease virus (BDV), and human rubella and cytomegalovirus can cause fetal death, resulting in abortion or stillbirth and producing defects of brain and eye especially or growth retardation in young born to mothers infected in early pregnancy. Fetuses infected at a later stage with BVD or HCV become immunotolerant to these viruses and may be born apparently healthy. Because they are persistently infected, they represent a real danger to other livestock on the farm.

Fetal Membranes and Placentation

We have insufficient space to describe the formation of the embryonic or fetal membranes but include diagrams (Fig. 5.66) as reminders of the principal points. The definitive gross arrangement is shown for the dog (Fig. 5.67A), horse (Fig. 5.67B), and ruminant (Fig. 5.67D and E) conceptuses. The fetal membranes and the endometrium participate in the formation of the placenta, an organ that facilitates physiologic exchange and hormone production. A provisional placenta, furnished by a vascularized yolk sac, may provide a useful organ of exchange in early pregnancy. This omphaloplacenta is important in the first third or so of equine pregnancy (Fig. 5.68), but in most species the chorioallantoic placenta, the definitive placenta of eutherian mammals, becomes competent at a relatively earlier stage. In the definitive arrangement, the chorion, intimately associated with the endometrium, is vascularized by vessels that reach it by following the allantoic outgrowth from the hindgut. The stalk of the allantois (urachus), the accompanying vessels that become the umbilical arteries and veins, and the ensheathing connective tissue (the fetal variety known as *Wharton's jelly*) constitute the umbilical cord, which persists as the communication between fetus and placenta until ruptured in the course of birth or shortly thereafter.

The *chorioallantoic placenta* takes many forms that may be classified in several complementary ways. The first system refers to the gross distribution of the chorionic villi, minute outgrowths of the chorionic surface that engage with depressions of the endometrial surface to provide the areas of exchange. The horse and the pig have a *diffuse* placenta in that the villi are spread in small clumps (microcotyledons) over virtually the entire surface of the

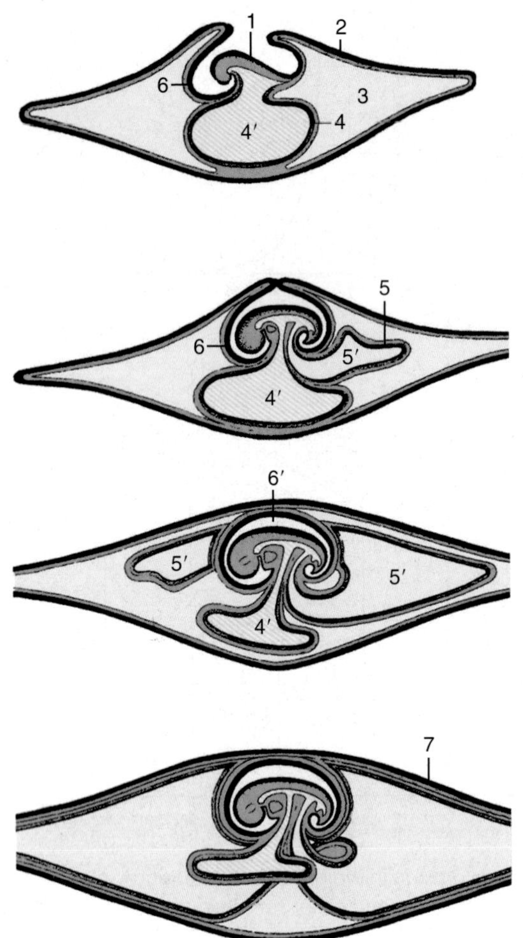

Fig. 5.66 Schematic representations of the formation of extraembryonic membranes. *1,* Embryo; *2,* chorion; *3,* extraembryonic celom; *4,* yolk sac; *4′,* yolk sac cavity; *5,* allantois; *5′,* allantoic cavity; *6,* amnion; *6′,* amniotic cavity; *7,* chorioallantois.

chorion (Fig. 5.67B and C). In ruminants the villi develop in scattered patches or cotyledons opposite the endometrial caruncles; each cotyledon and associated caruncle forms a separate unit or placentome, which collectively constitute a *cotyledonary placenta* (Fig. 5.67D and E). In the dog and the cat the villi develop in a band of chorion that encircles the trunk of the embryo, forming a zonary placenta* (Fig. 5.67A). In the fourth and last type, *discoidal placenta,* which commonly occurs in primates and rodents but not in domestic species, the villi are concentrated in one large patch (Fig. 5.69).

The second system refers to the tissue layers that separate the fetal and maternal bloodstreams. Initially, six layers are present: chorionic capillary endothelium, connective tissue, epithelium, endometrial epithelium, connective tissue, and capillary endothelium. The tissue barrier at the areas of exchange is always later reduced, sometimes only by the closer approach of the two sets of capillaries but often by tissue loss. In theory, the six layers persist in the *epitheliochorial placenta* seen in the mare and sow. They are reduced to four, by the loss of the endometrial epithelium and connective tissue, in the *endotheliochorial placenta* seen in dogs and cats (Fig. 5.70), and they suffer the ultimate reduction to one layer, embryonic endothelium, in the *hemoendothelial placenta* of bats. Ruminants were long described as having a *syndesmochorial placenta,* in which only the uterine epithelium had been lost; modern studies discount this loss, and it is now believed that these animals also have *epitheliochorial placentas*.

The third system refers to the loss of maternal tissue that occurs at birth. In some species the fetal and maternal layers part cleanly, no maternal tissue is shed, and the description *nondeciduate* is appropriate. When implantation is interstitial, considerable maternal loss may be expected; the human placenta is of this *deciduate* type. Minor loss of uterine tissue occurs in an intermediate semideciduate type found in ruminants (Table 5.2).

The histologic system appears to define different degrees but offers incomplete explanations of variations of placental permeability. The barrier may not be exactly as implied by the description. Moreover, the placenta evolves and changes in structure during pregnancy, and significant regional differences may exist side by side. Freely diffusible molecules cross from one circulation to the other, and in this respect the human hemochorial placenta certainly allows more rapid passage than the "thicker" epitheliochorial placenta of the larger domestic species. The transport of larger molecules depends on other factors, including specialized unidirectional mechanisms.

Differences in the barrier to the passage of immunoglobulin G (IgG) are of particular veterinary significance. In some species a mechanism exists for the transfer of maternal antibodies to the fetus to confer some immediate protection on the newborn. This prenatally acquired immunity is denied to offspring of species (including horses and farm animals) with epitheliochorial placentas, and their neonates rely on colostrum, the milk first produced, as the source of antibodies for temporary protection.

Fetal antigens, present in plasma or borne by blood cells, may leak into the maternal bloodstream with potentially damaging consequences. The classic illustration is furnished by the hemolytic disease of human infants (erythroblastosis fetalis). This condition develops in a second or later child confronted by antibody produced by a Rhesus-negative mother in reaction to a previous Rhesus-positive child. Antibody production by the mother develops so slowly that the child (usually the first) provoking the response generally escapes serious harm. Similar

*In the dog a permanent zone of leaking blood creates marginal hematomas (Fig. 5.67A). In the cat this zone is diffuse and temporary and therefore not as striking as that of the dog.

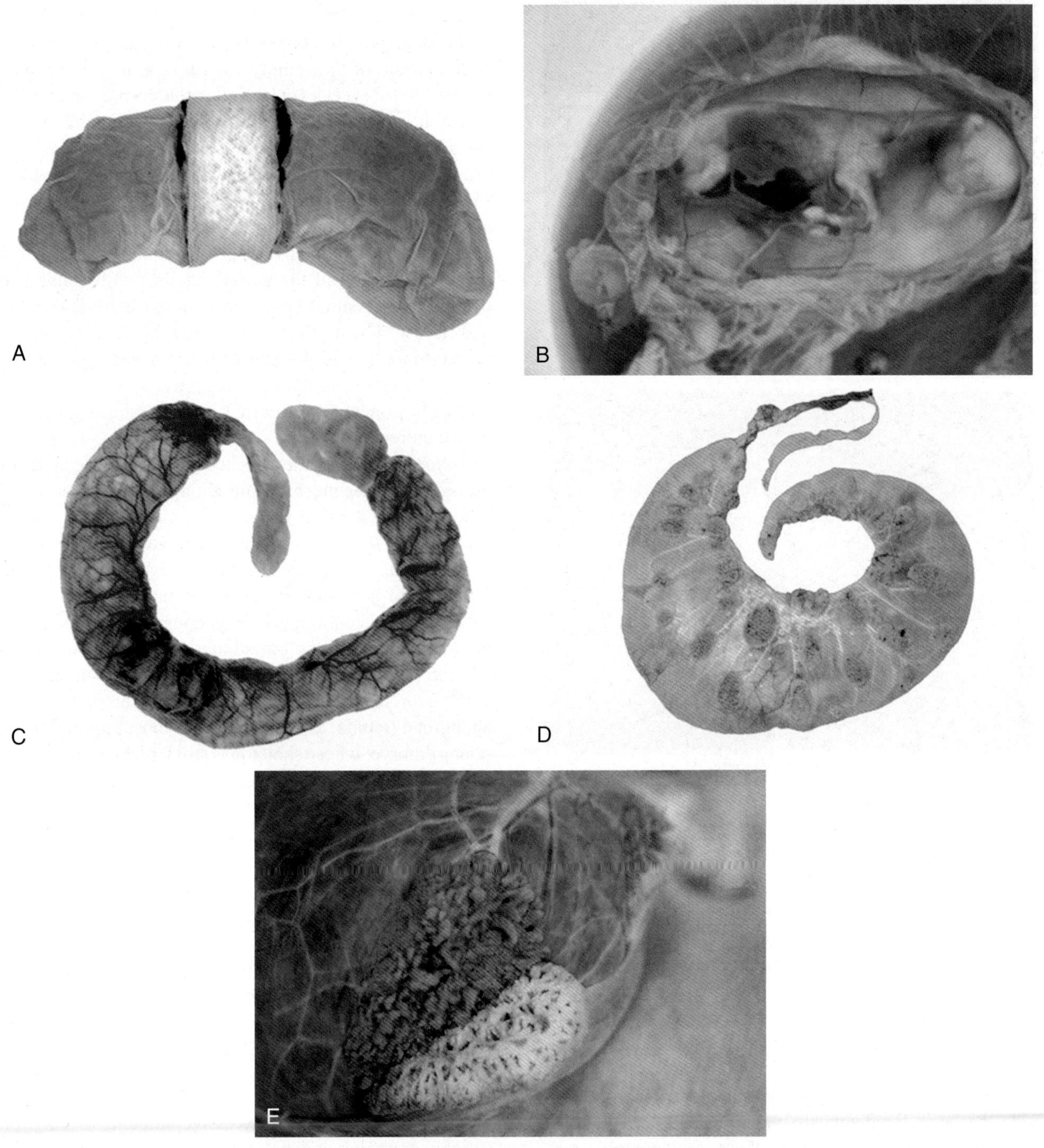

Fig. 5.67 Placentation in a number of species. (A) The most intense interaction between the fetal membranes and the endometrium in domesticated species is found in carnivores with the zonary placenta. (B) The placenta of the horse fetus is not very complex. The villi do not penetrate deep into the endometrium. (C) A similar situation exists in the pig. (D) The placenta of ruminants is a cotyledonary placenta with many placentomes (cow). (E) The partial separation of the maternal and fetal part of the placentome is demonstrated.

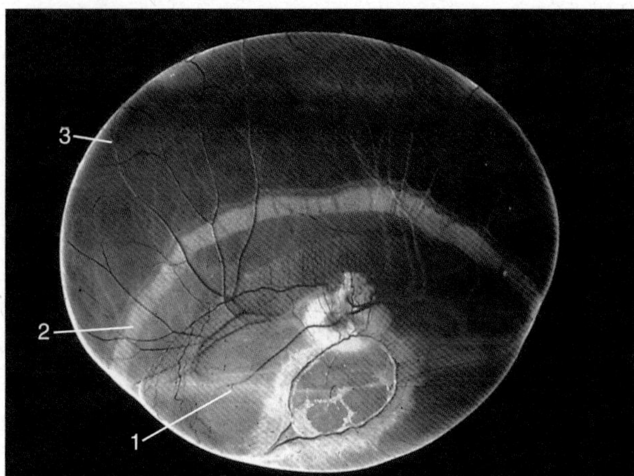

Fig. 5.68 Young conceptus (horse). *1,* Yolk sac; *2,* chorionic girdle; *3,* allantochorion.

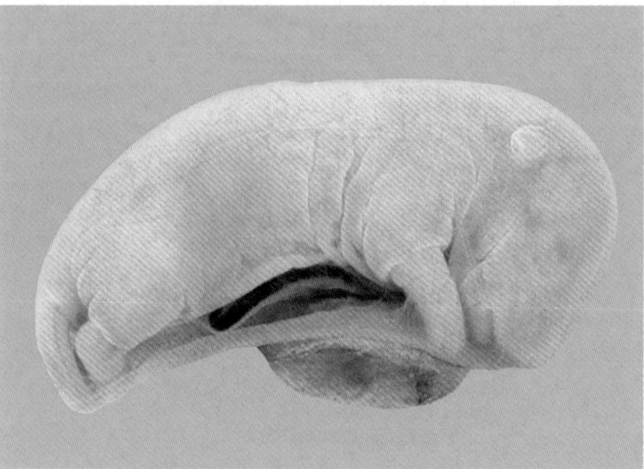

Fig. 5.69 Discoidal placenta of a rat.

conditions occur in other species, including horses and pigs, but damage to their offspring can be prevented by denying them access to colostrum, which contains the relevant antibody.

The endocrine functions of the placenta are both complex and lacking in uniformity among species, even between those that are closely related. The horse is of unusual interest in this context because equine chorionic gonadotropin is produced from structures unique to Equidae: the endometrial cups (Fig. 5.71 and p. 564). Elevated concentrations of steroid hormones in blood and urine provide the basis for diagnosis, including the do-it-yourself tests for pregnancy in women. Tests of comparable reliability, simplicity, and economy are not yet available for domestic species, for which reliance is still largely placed on clinical procedures, including ultrasonography.

The placenta is one (though not the only) source of other hormones relevant to pregnancy. Lactogen, a hormone related to growth hormone, acts with other hormones to develop the mammary glands for the approaching lactation, while relaxin, which is also secreted by the corpus luteum, helps prepare the reproductive tract and pelvic parietes for parturition (p. 564); later, acting in synergy with oxytocin, the latter stimulates the expulsive activity of the myometrium.

Prostaglandin is a product not of the placenta but of the endometrium of the "empty" uterus, and its production is delayed for 2 weeks (or so) after the corpus luteum first forms. It leaves the uterus in the uterine vein, and in some species, including ruminants, it reaches the ipsilateral ovary after countercurrent transfer to the ovarian artery. In others, for example, the horse, in which contact between artery and vein is less close, it reaches the ovaries via the general circulation. Within the ovary, prostaglandin promotes luteolysis (regression of the corpus luteum) with consequent decline and eventual cessation of progesterone secretion and release. The production of prostaglandin is stimulated by oxytocin, but in pregnancy the conceptus produces a factor that blocks endometrial receptivity to oxytocin, thus indirectly protecting the corpus luteum, whose integrity is now required.

Before we conclude the account of the fetal membranes and placenta, brief attention may be given to the fluids contained within the amniotic and allantoic cavities. These fluids, dramatically released at the time of birth—the "breaking of the waters"—actually have rather important functions to perform throughout gestation, and at certain stages they account for a very considerable fraction of the total content of the gravid uterus. The fluid within the amniotic cavity immediately surrounds and supports the embryo or fetus, cushioning it against compression and abdominal trauma. This protection is most required by the young embryo, whose skeleton is still largely unformed and whose external covering—hardly yet to be called skin—is delicate and vulnerable to trauma. Later, when these structures are better developed, the amniotic fluid tends to be reduced in amount (see Fig. 5.65). At its maximum, it measures about 3 to 5 L in cattle and perhaps a little more in horses; in pigs it varies around 100 mL, and it is about 10 to 30 mL in dogs and cats. The amniotic fluid has a brisk turnover with roughly matched production and resorption in the short term. In early stages, the fluid is a dialysate from vessels of the embryonic skin and amnion; later, once rupture of the urogenital membrane has opened a passage from the bladder, it consists largely of urine, and as more is added, the fluid already present is reduced by being swallowed. Deficient and excessive amounts of this fluid (oligohydramnios and polyhydramnios, respectively) are possible complications of pregnancy, the former often indicating anomalous development of the kidneys, the latter potentially open to correction by the addition of a "sweetener" to encourage deglutition. This fluid is not normally a significant contributor to that present in the respiratory passages of the fetus and newborn, contrary to some suggestions. Being slightly mucoid, amniotic fluid has additional value as a lubricant of the birth canal at parturition.

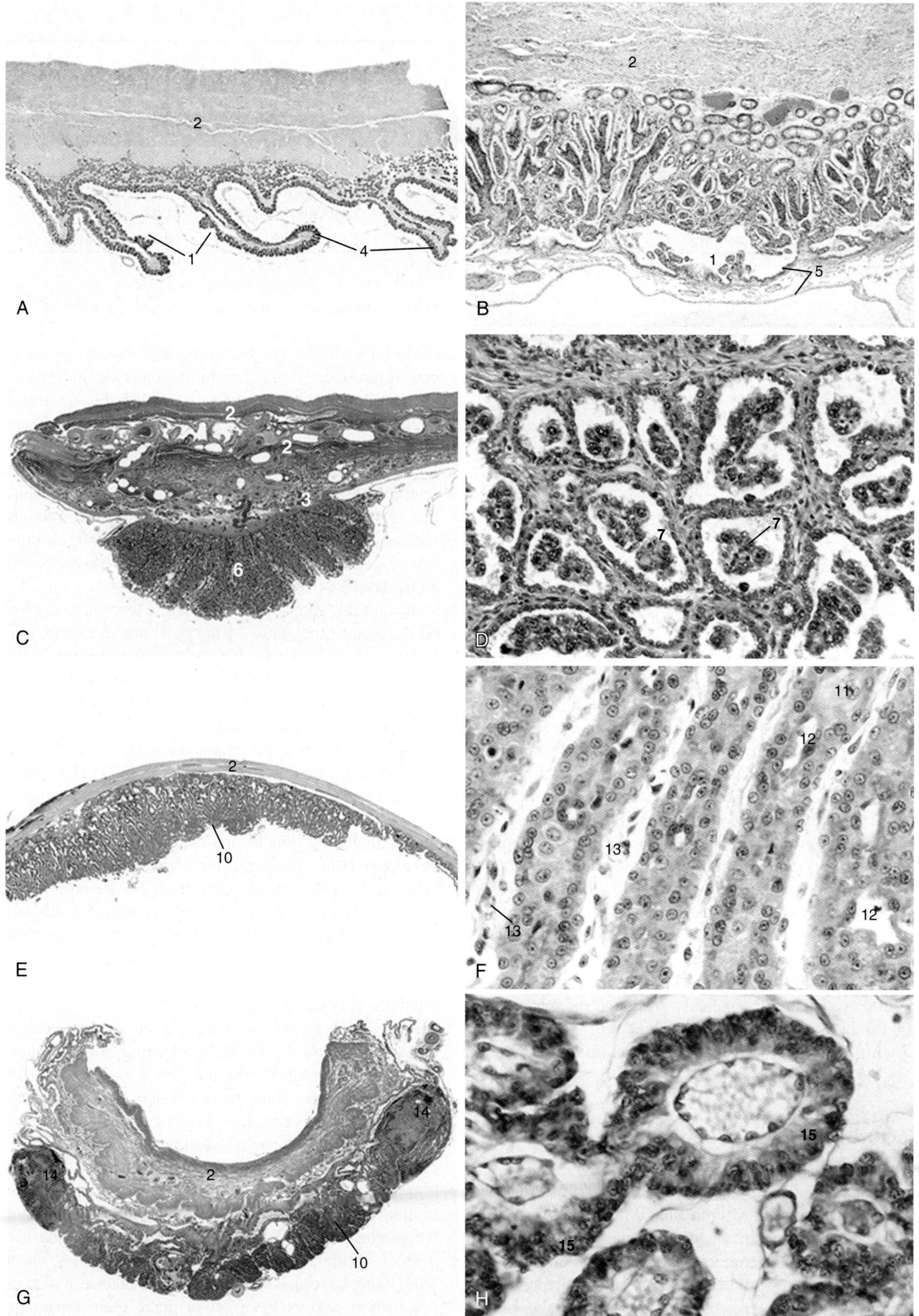

Fig. 5.70 (A) to (H) Placental histology; (H) for label descriptions. (A) Diffuse folded villous placenta (pig) (4×). (B) Diffuse villous placenta (horse) (28×). (C) and (D) Cotyledonary villous placenta (cow) (4×; 140×). (E) and (F) Zonary labyrinthine placenta (cat) (4× and 279×). (G) and (H) Zonary labyrinthine placenta (dog) (4× and 279×). *1,* areola; *2,* myometrium; *3,* endometrial glands; *4,* primary fold; *5,* allantochorion; *6,* placentome; *7,* trophoblastic giant cells; *8,* uterine septum; *9,* chorionic villi; *10,* placental labyrinth; *11,* decidual cell; *12,* maternal capillaries; *13,* fetal capillaries; *14,* marginal hematomas; *15,* trophoblast cells.

TABLE 5.2 **PLACENTAL CLASSIFICATION**

	Carnivores	Horse	Ruminants	Pig
Gross form	Zonary and labyrinthine	Diffuse	Cotyledonary	Diffuse and folded
Histologic type	Endotheliochorial	Epitheliochorial	Epitheliochorial	Epitheliochorial
Separation	Semideciduate	Nondeciduate	Semideciduate	Nondeciduate

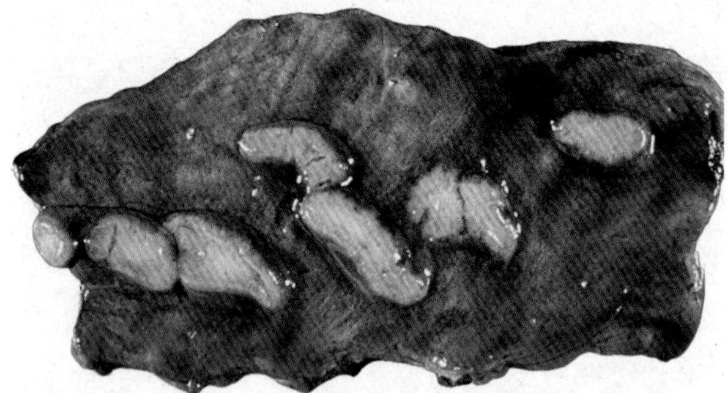

Fig. 5.71 Endometrial cups (mare) during early pregnancy. These cups are responsible for the production of the pregnant mare's serum gonadotropin (PMSG).

The allantoic cavity is large in all domestic species, but the human allantois fails to expand and is soon reduced to a negligible vestige. It is possibly the consequent lack of medical interest that explains the relative paucity of information concerning the formation, turnover, and role of allantoic fluid. The allantoic cavity does, of course, receive urine through the urachus before the urethral route is established, and this process helps maintain the osmotic pressure of the fetal plasma at a level that prevents fluid loss to the maternal bloodstream. A second function may be to maintain sufficient radial pressure to hold the chorion tight against the endometrium in those species in which the placental attachment is less firm. There is rather more allantoic than amniotic fluid in the large species, and amounts are about the same in dogs and cats. Although there is about 100 mL in the pig at midterm, the quantity is reduced to very little at full term. However, the quantities are rather variable in all species.

Parturition and the Puerperal Period: The Neonate

Parturition is initiated mainly by the fetus, although the mother is not without all influence. Mares, for example, tend to give birth when conditions in the stable are quiet and settled. The endocrine control of birth is complicated and beyond the scope of this book, but certain preparatory changes in the tissues may be mentioned. These take some time to develop, affect many structures, and largely comprise an increase in their water content and loosening of the larger collagen accumulations. The most familiar effect is the in-sinking of the tailhead of cows to the side as parturition impends. Similar but concealed changes soften the caudal reproductive tract, including most significantly the cervix. In some species there is considerable weakening of the pelvic symphysis, but articular changes in domestic animals are limited to some loosening of the sacroiliac joints. After parturition the reproductive organs tend to return toward their former condition, although the restoration after the first pregnancy is never complete. The uterine muscle contracts directly after delivery, and this organ loses much of the weight it gained during pregnancy within a few days.

Before this chapter is concluded, a few sentences may be devoted to the status of the newborn, which exhibits interspecific differences that are both striking and important. Neonates of so-called precocial species possess a remarkable ability to fend for themselves more or less at once (Fig. 5.72), whereas those of altricial species are initially much more reliant on maternal care and the warmth and protection of a nest (Fig. 5.73). The young of the ungulate orders, both perissodactyls and artiodactyls, are generally precocial; those of carnivores and primates, including human infants, are predominantly less developed. Young rodents are divided between the two categories; those like rats (myomorphs) are born naked, unable to maintain body temperature independently, and barely capable of struggling to reach the dam's teats, and their eyelids are joined and external ear canals closed by epithelial fusion. In contrast, guinea pigs and their close relatives (caviomorphs) are born fully haired, mobile, equipped with vision and hearing, and able to seek and ingest solid food within hours of being born (although they may take milk during the first 2 or 3 weeks). The differences among domestic species are significant if less extreme. Foals, like most newborn ungulates, are able to stand and attend their mothers almost at once; their skeletons are well developed, and most secondary ossification centers are not only present but also well advanced in modeling toward their adult form. Relatively efficient locomotor coordination allows them to follow the herd or flock within a short time. Kittens and puppies, on the other hand, have skeletons that are less mature, and many ossification centers have yet to make their appearance (Fig. 5.74); the forelimb musculature is sufficiently developed and controlled to enable them to scramble toward

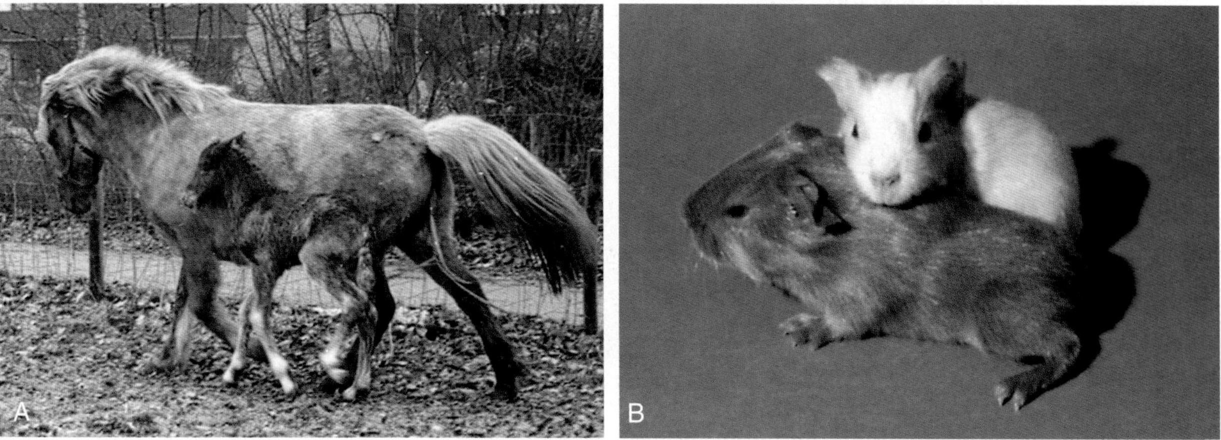

Fig. 5.72 Developmental status shortly after birth. (A) Neonatal foal with mother (the mare has yet to discharge the fetal membranes [afterbirth]). (B) Newborn guinea pigs, which are born in a more developed state.

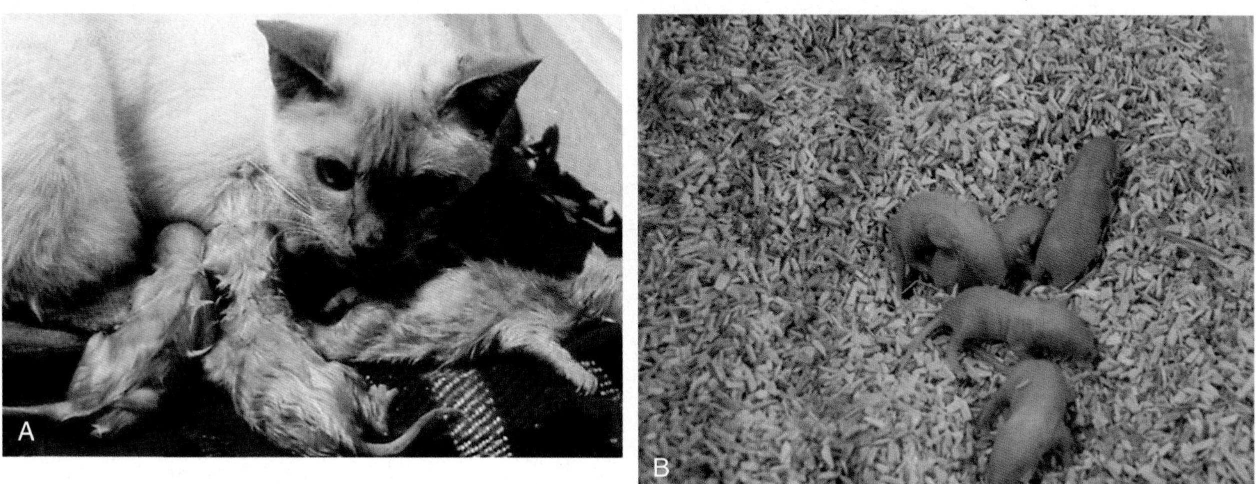

Fig. 5.73 Developmental status shortly after birth in altricial species. (A) Newborn kittens. (B) Three-day-old mouse pups.

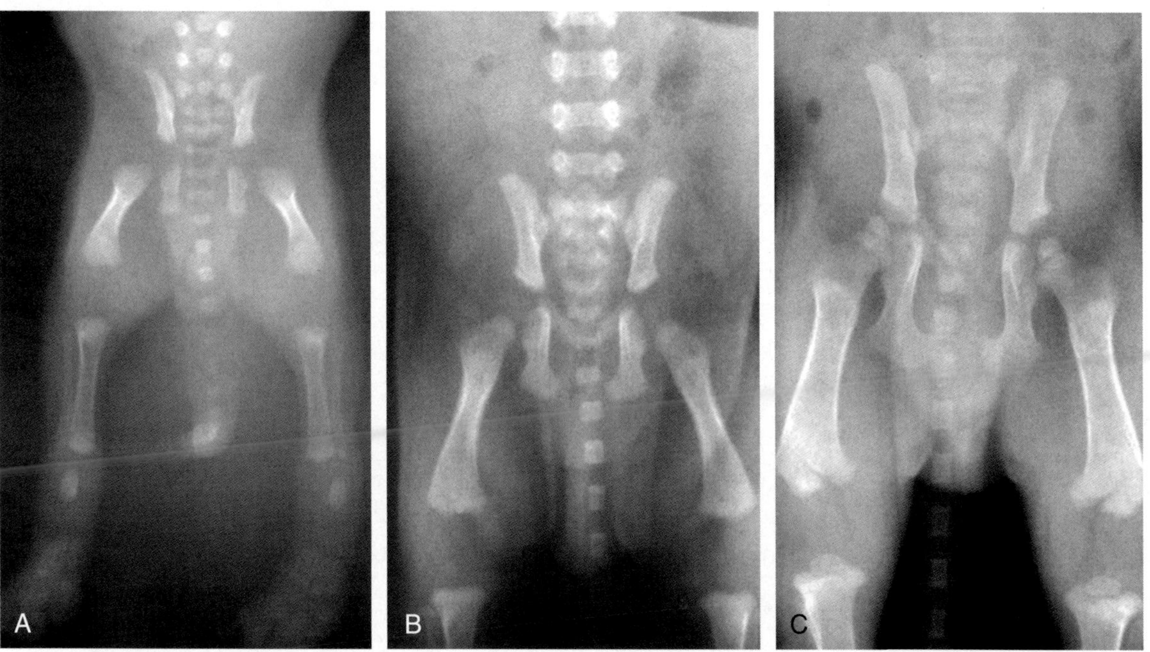

Fig. 5.74 Progress of skeletal ossification in the puppy (A) 1, (B) 14, and (C) 28 days after birth.

the teats, but that of the hindlimbs is less competent and contributes little to this progress. The development of the sense organs is somewhat retarded, and the eyelids do not part until the tenth day or shortly thereafter. These differences in neonatal status are gradually "ironed out" and most mammals—ourselves excluded—show comparable maturity by the end of the usual lactation period.

COMPREHENSION CHECK

Demonstrate how embryologic development leads to the gross anatomic arrangement of the male reproductive system and facilitate normal sperm development.

Using a dog or a cat cadaver, understand the surgical approach to remove the ovaries and the uterus.

The Endocrine Glands

6

The endocrine or ductless glands are those that deliver their secretory products (hormones) into the blood, lymph, or tissue fluid, which transports them to the target organs. Although each gland has its particular and distinctive function, they collaborate with the nervous system to maintain the internal environment and the appropriate general and specific responses to external and internal stimuli. In comparison with the effects of the nervous system, the hormones' effects are slow to start but last longer.

The study of the anatomy of the glands, the production and the chemistry of the hormones, the responses of the target organs, and the complicated interplay of the various endocrine tissues with one another and with the nervous system is entitled *endocrinology*. Because of its clinical implications, the endocrinology is one of the most important and most active branches of biology. This chapter is mainly concerned with the gross anatomy of the glands.

The endocrine organs are collectively termed an *endocrine system*. However, it must be understood that the individual organs are scattered, achieve no physical continuity, and have very diverse embryologic origins, targets, and functions. They are united only by their general subservience to the central nervous system (hypothalamus), the similar patterns of their target organ effects, and some common structural features; these last comprise the epithelioid character of the secretory cells, the absence of drainage ducts, the sparse supporting frameworks, the generous vascularity, and the intimate association with blood vascular or other transport media (Fig. 6.1).

Three types of endocrine organs may be recognized pragmatically. The first group includes the few discrete primary endocrine organs: the hypophysis (pituitary gland), the epiphysis (pineal gland), and the thyroid, parathyroid, and adrenal glands. The second comprises those organs that combine major endocrine functions with other important related functions: the pancreas, testes, ovaries, and placenta. The last group are the unobtrusive endocrine components of organs with quite different primary functions; the brain, kidneys, liver, thymus, heart, and gastrointestinal tract are the best examples. There are notable species differences.

THE HYPOPHYSIS

The hypophysis or pituitary gland, sometimes called the master gland, produces certain hormones that directly influence the activities of other endocrine glands. It acts as the relay between the nervous and humoral mechanisms that jointly control certain functions.

The hypophysis is a dark ellipsoidal body measuring about 1 × 0.75 × 0.5 cm in the medium-sized dog. It is suspended below the hypothalamus by a narrow, fragile stalk and is received into a depression (hypophyseal fossa or sella turcica) of the cranial floor that is defined by rostral and caudal crests of bone. A covering of dura directly invests the gland and also roofs the depression, extending from its margins to embrace and confine the hypophyseal stalk from all sides; this arrangement (diaphragma sellae) makes it exceedingly difficult to remove the brain at autopsy with the hypophysis attached.

Features of Clinical or Experimental Interest A large venous channel (cavernous sinus) to each side of the hypophysis provides a longitudinal connection between the ophthalmic plexus (and thus the veins of the face) rostrally and the external jugular vein and vertebral venous plexus caudally (p. 300); transverse (intercavernous) sinuses rostral and caudal to the gland complete an encircling venous ring. The internal carotid artery (or the emissary vessel from the rete mirabile that replaces this in the cat, ruminants, and pig [p. 298]) runs through the cavernous sinus to join the arterial circle below the brain. The optic chiasm is directly rostral to the hypophysis (see Fig. 8.22/*21* and *24*), and laterally, flanking the cavernous sinus, are the cranial nerves that supply the adnexa of the eye (the oculomotor, trochlear, ophthalmic, and abducent nerves).

Pathologic growth or a physiologic increase in the size of the hypophysis, which occurs in pregnancy, may exert pressure on these structures, especially on the optic nerves. Specific features in topography affect both the manner of expansion and the most convenient surgical approach. This approach is made via the nose and the sphenoidal sinus (within the cranial base, rostroventral to the hypophyseal fossa) in human patients but more directly from below, via mouth, pharynx, and sphenoid, in the dog. A temporal approach has been used in the pig.

Although the hypophysis appears to be a solid unitary organ, its parts have very different origins and functions, and it includes certain spaces. One part, the *neurohypophysis* (posterior lobe), is formed by a downgrowth of the hypothalamus; the stalk that persists as the connection with the brain includes an extension of the third ventricle. The other

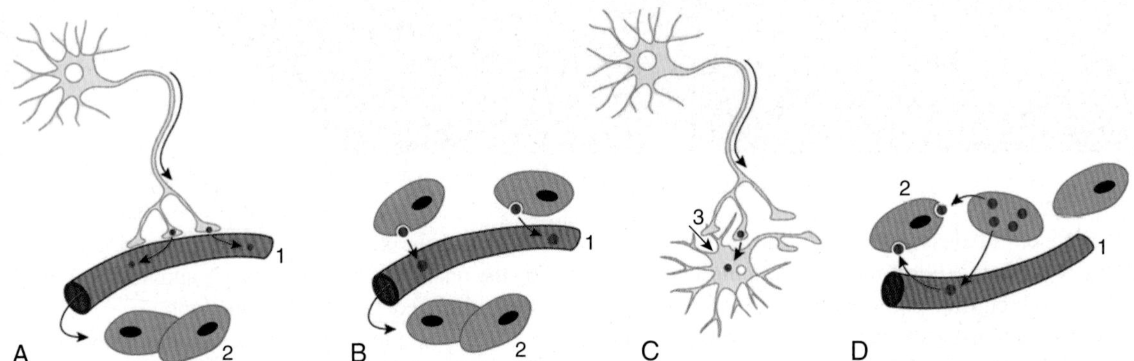

Fig. 6.1 The various ways in which peptides reach their targets: (A) neuroendocrine, (B) endocrine, (C) neurotransmitter, neuromodulator (action on postsynaptic membrane), and (D) paracrine (localized hormone action). *1,* Bloodstream; *2,* target cell; *3,* synapse.

part, the *adenohypophysis* (anterior lobe), is formed by an epithelial outgrowth of the roof of the developing mouth. It contains a flattened vestigial space, the hypophyseal cleft. The tissue caudal to the cleft is directly applied to the neurohypophysis and is distinguished as the pars intermedia (intermediate lobe). The topographical relationships of the three "lobes" show some interspecific differences (Fig. 6.2).

The adenohypophysis produces several hormones commonly designated by acronyms: growth (somatotropic) hormone (STH); gonadotropic hormones—follicle-stimulating (FSH) and luteinizing (LH); adrenocorticotropic hormone (ACTH); thyroid-stimulating hormone (TSH); and prolactin. The intermediate part produces α-melanocyte-stimulating hormone (MSH). The production of all these hormones is controlled by regulating hypophysiotropic hormones and releasing or inhibitory factors such as gonadotropin-releasing hormone (GnRH), somatostatin (SS), growth hormone–releasing hormone (GRH), and corticotropin-releasing hormone (CRH), to name the most important. They are produced by neurosecretory cells in several hypothalamic nuclei, particularly the paraventricular nucleus, preoptic area, arcuate nucleus, and periventricular nucleus. These hormones are secreted from their axon terminals and are discharged into fenestrated capillaries within the median eminence (see Fig. 8.67/6); these releasing and inhibitory hormones are conveyed to a sinusoidal network within the adenohypophysis (Fig. 6.3).

The hormones stored and later released into the circulation by the neurohypophysis include oxytocin and vasopressin. Oxytocin stimulates contraction of the smooth muscle of the uterus and the myoepithelial cells of the udder. Vasopressin stimulates vasoconstriction and promotes fluid reabsorption by the kidneys. These substances are produced by magnocellular neurosecretory neurons within the supraoptic and paraventricular nuclei of the hypothalamus and are conveyed along the axons for direct release via the neurohypophyseal capillary bed into the main circulation.

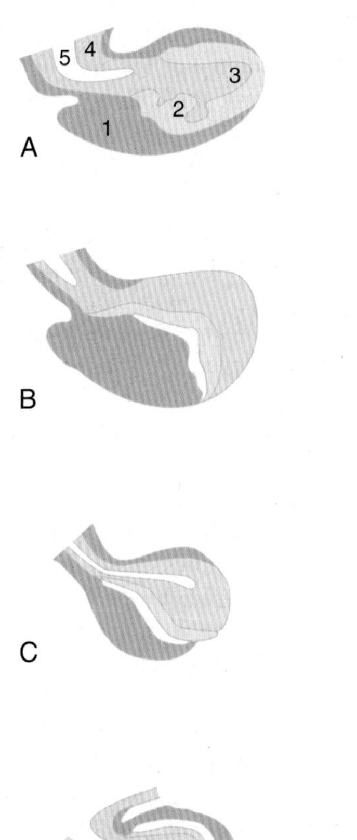

Fig. 6.2 Median sections of the hypophysis of the (A) horse, (B) ox, (C) pig, and (D) dog. The rostral extremity of the gland is to the *left.* *1,* Adenohypophysis; *2,* intermediate part; *3,* neurohypophysis; *4,* hypophyseal stalk; *5,* recess of third ventricle.

The neurohypophysis is supplied by small branches from the internal carotid artery (or substitute vessel) and the arterial circle (of Willis) of the brain. The adenohypophysis is supplied indirectly; rostral hypophyseal arteries, also from the internal carotid, expend themselves within the

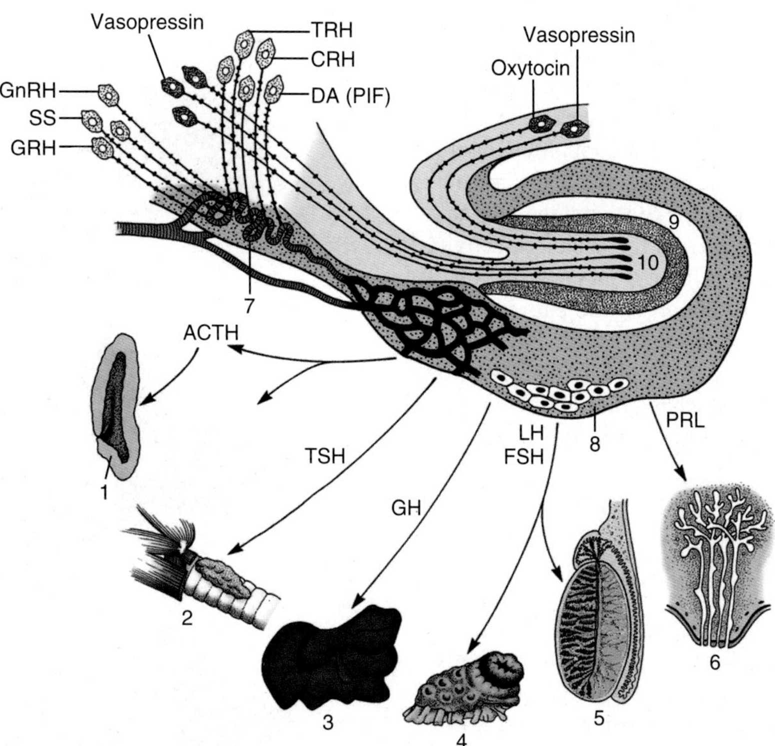

Fig. 6.3 Organization of the brain–pituitary–peripheral organ axis. *ACTH,* adrenocorticotropic hormone; *CRH,* corticotropin-releasing hormone; *DA,* dopamine; *FSH,* follicle-stimulating hormone; *GH,* growth hormone; *GnRH,* gonadotropin-releasing hormone; *GRH,* growth hormone–releasing hormone; *LH,* luteinizing hormone; *PIF,* prolactin-inhibiting factor; *PRL,* prolactin; *SS,* somatostatin; *TRH,* thyrotropin-releasing hormone; *TSH,* thyroid-stimulating hormone. *1,* Adrenal cortex; *2,* thyroid; *3,* liver; *4,* ovary; *5,* testis; *6,* mammary gland; *7,* median eminence; *8,* anterior lobe of pituitary; *9,* intermediate lobe of pituitary; *10,* neural lobe of pituitary.

floor of the hypothalamus, whence the blood is conveyed through the stalk by a portal system of veins. The capillary network of the adenohypophysis subsequently drains into the cavernous sinus.

Certain regions of the brain, collectively known as the *circumventricular organs* (CVOs), directly receive chemosensory stimulation from bloodborne substances. This occurs as a result of the fenestration of perfusing capillaries, unlike the tight blood-brain barrier elsewhere, which allow exchange of large molecules between the plasma and the extracellular milieu of the CVOs. The proximity of CVOs to the system of ventricles within the brain also suggests a role for the cerebrospinal fluid in the diffusion of the chemical messengers. The neurons within the different regions are of course able to communicate through synaptic connections in the usual way but also allow CVOs to use neurohormonal mechanisms to influence peripheral function. The CVOs comprise the subfornical organ, the pineal gland, the subcommissural organ, the area postrema, the posterior lobe of the pituitary, the median eminence, and the vascular organ of the lamina terminalis (see Fig. 8.67). These organs are broadly concerned with homeostatic and autonomic function (feedback regulation) and induce peripheral effects through secretion of chemicals that are carried into the general circulation by the fenestrated capillaries.

THE EPIPHYSIS

The epiphysis or pineal gland is a small, darkly pigmented outgrowth from the dorsal aspect of the brain at the caudal end of the roof of the third ventricle and directly before the rostral colliculi (see Fig. 8.22/11). In certain species the epiphysis is related to a large outpouching (epiphyseal recess) of the pia-ependyma that roofs the ventricle. It is concealed between the cerebral hemispheres and cerebellum in the intact brain.

The epiphysis is solid but is not always homogeneous because foci of calcification ("brain sand") often develop with advancing age. It produces melatonin, an indolamine derived from serotonin, which has an antigonadotropic circadian effect. Tumors that destroy the secretory tissue have been noted to be frequently associated with precocious puberty.

The melatonin secretion by the pineal gland is controlled through a polysynaptic pathway by the endogenous circadian clock located in the hypothalamic suprachiasmatic nucleus (SCN). The autonomic innervation of the pineal gland runs via the superior cervical ganglion. Melatonin is secreted as a sleeping hormone during the night and acts on many brain areas, including the SCN and the pituitary. The brain knows that it is day from the enhanced activity of the SCN and knows that it is night from the secretion of melatonin. The action of melatonin on the pars tuberalis is important for seasonal hormonal fluctuations. Fine-tuning of the biological clock in the SCN can be achieved by gradual changes in daylight, which regulate both long-term (seasonal) and short-term (diurnal) variation in gonadal activity.

THE THYROID GLAND

The thyroid gland lies on the trachea directly behind, and sometimes overlapping, the larynx. Its form varies greatly: in the dog and the cat the gland consists of separate masses that are occasionally connected by an isthmus (Fig. 6.4A); in the horse paired lobes are widely dissociated but connected by an insubstantial isthmus (Fig. 6.4B); in cattle the lobes are connected by a wide isthmus of parenchymal tissue (Fig. 6.4C); in small ruminants the isthmus is inconstant and when present is a mere connective tissue strand. In pigs and humans the thyroid has a more compact form and exhibits a relatively large median (pyramidal) lobe in addition to the lateral lobes to provide a cover on the trachea that extends toward the thoracic inlet (Fig. 6.4D).

The gland develops as a median outgrowth from the part of the pharyngeal floor that contributes to the tongue (p. 133). The primordium extends caudally on the ventral surface of the trachea before dividing at its apex into divergent processes that extend dorsolaterally to reach the boundary between the trachea and the esophagus (Fig. 6.5/2). In most mammals the connection with the developing tongue (thyroglossal duct) is never patent, and it later regresses in its entirety.

The mature gland is enclosed within a connective tissue capsule that is loosely attached to neighboring organs. The gland has many follicles that gives it substance, generally brick-red, and a rather granular texture. The surface of the intact organ is irregular in some species (e.g., cattle) but smooth in others (e.g., dog). The tissue is relatively firm, and this consistency, allied to the form, size, and location, enables the lobes to be identified in larger species by palpation caudal to the larynx although not in healthy dogs.

The size of the thyroid gland varies greatly, depending to a large extent on the iodine content of the diet. Because iodine deficiency leads to enlargement (goiter), iodine is added to table salt in many parts of the world. In dogs

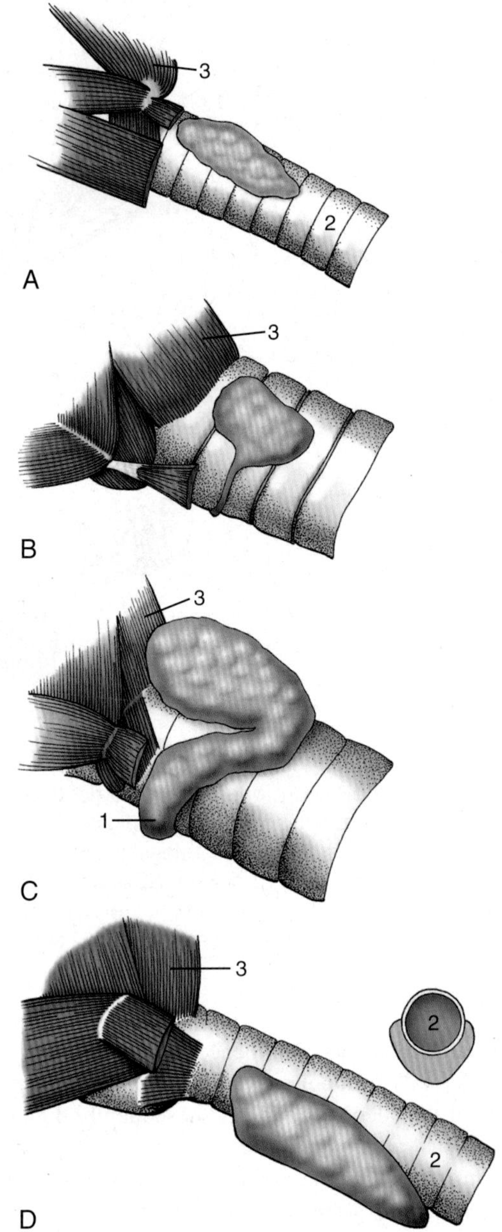

Fig. 6.4 The thyroid gland of the (A) dog, (B) horse, (C) cattle, and (D) pig. The *inset* to (D) illustrates the subtracheal connection in transverse section in the pig. *1,* Isthmus; *2,* trachea; *3,* cricopharyngeus.

the relative weight of the thyroid may vary by a factor of as much as 6, although the increasing use of commercial foods (of uniform composition) now tends to reduce this variation. Average dimensions in medium-sized dogs are of the order of 6 × 1.5 × 0.5 cm. Accessory masses of thyroid tissue are sometimes located along the cervical trachea and are occasionally carried into the thorax by the descending heart.

The gland is mainly supplied by the *cranial thyroid artery,* which arises from the common carotid artery and arches around the cranial pole. A subsidiary supply is

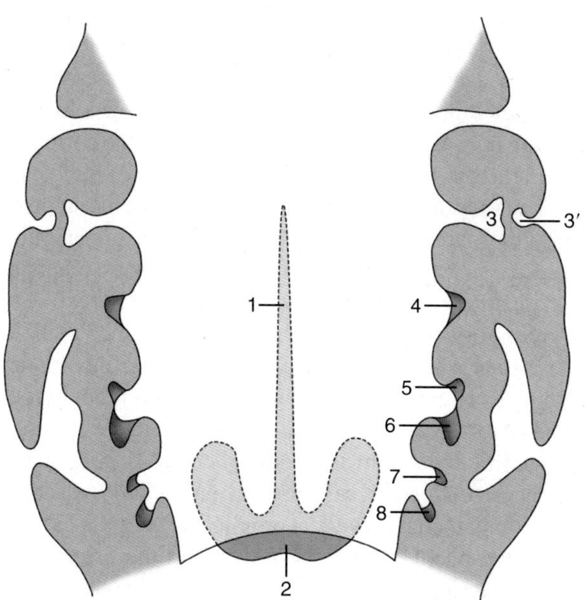

Fig. 6.5 The pharyngeal primordia of certain endocrine structures; dorsal view, schematic. *1*, Thyroglossal duct; *2*, thyroid gland; *3*, first pharyngeal pouch; *3′*, external acoustic meatus; *4*, palatine tonsil (second pouch); *5*, parathyroid III; *6*, thymus; *7*, parathyroid IV; *8*, ultimobranchial body.

occasionally provided by a caudal thyroid artery, which takes a more proximal origin. In the dog the two vessels are connected by a substantial anastomosis along the dorsal margin. The venous drainage is to the internal jugular vein. The glandular tissue receives both *sympathetic and parasympathetic fibers* routed through the cranial cervical ganglia and the laryngeal branches of the vagus nerves, respectively. The fibers are predominantly vasomotor, and denervation has little effect on secretory activity. The main lymph drainage of the thyroid in the dog proceeds to the cranial deep cervical nodes.

A small portion of the parenchyma is provided by parafollicular (or C) cells. These appear to have their origin in the ultimobranchial bodies that derive from epithelial clusters of the fourth pharyngeal pouches that are invaded by neural crest cells (Fig. 6.5/*8*). C cells produce calcitonin, a hormone antagonistic to parathormone in some species. This hormone also seems to play a role in fetal bone growth, and it protects the maternal skeleton against excessive demineralization.

The thyroid hormones, which regulate metabolism and growth, are produced by the follicular cells that compose the bulk of the parenchyma. They are stored in the follicular fluid and later broken down to yield the final products, which are released into the bloodstream.

THE PARATHYROID GLANDS

The parathyroid glands, usually four, also develop from the pharyngeal lining; one pair (parathyroids III or external parathyroid glands) comes from the third pharyngeal pouches, the other (parathyroids IV or internal parathyroid glands) from the fourth pouches (Fig. 6.5/*5* and *7*). In the dog, cat, and small ruminants the parathyroid glands generally become recessed or embedded within the substance of the thyroid gland and frequently escape notice in routine dissections. Once exposed, they can be identified by their pale color, which contrasts with the brick-red thyroid tissue. In cattle and the horse they are usually located close to the thyroid gland.

The parathyroids III are carried down the neck by the developing thymus and come to rest at various levels, generally near the carotid bifurcations but much farther caudally in the horse (in which they may approach the thoracic inlet). They are distinguished from lymph nodes on the basis of their paleness and lack of the smooth and glistening exterior. These glands are usually located at the rostral end of the thyroid gland in the dog and at the caudal end in the cat. The close relationship of the parathyroid glands to the thyroid points to the need for caution in thyroid surgery.

The parathyroid hormone (parathormone) plays a vital role in regulating the absorption of calcium from the gut, its mobilization from the skeleton, and its excretion in the urine. The production of parathormone is largely regulated by the calcium plasma concentration.

THE ADRENAL GLANDS

The retroperitoneal and paired adrenal glands lie against the roof of the abdomen near the thoracolumbar junction. They are usually located craniomedial to the corresponding kidney (more directly medial in the horse). The glands are closely connected with the aorta on the left and the caudal vena cava on the right. They adhere to the blood vessels when the kidneys shift from their accustomed positions (e.g., the left kidney of the ruminant; see p. 685).

Although generally elongated, the glands are often asymmetrical and quite irregular, being molded on neighboring vessels (Fig. 6.6/*1*). It is difficult to specify their size. They are relatively larger in wild than in related domestic forms, in juvenile than in adult individuals, and in pregnant and lactating females than in those reproductively inactive. The adrenal glands of a medium-sized dog commonly measure about 2.5 × 1 × 0.5 cm.

Adrenal glands are firm, solid bodies that fracture readily when flexed. The fractured (or sectioned) surface exposes the division of the interior into an outer cortex and an inner medulla. The cortex, covered by a fibrous capsule, is yellowish and radially striated; the much darker medulla has

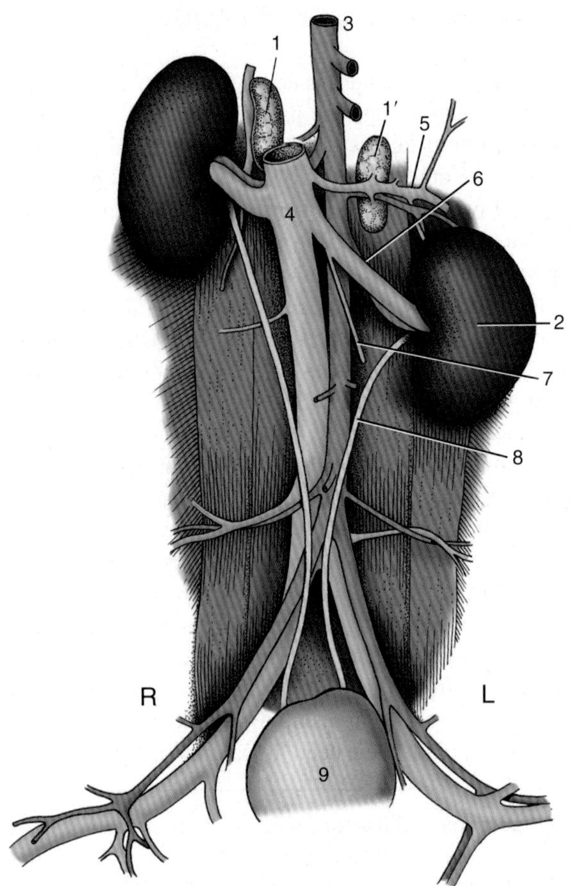

Fig. 6.6 The topography of the canine adrenal glands. *1, 1′,* Right and left adrenal glands; *2,* left kidney; *3,* aorta; *4,* caudal vena cava; *5,* phrenicoabdominal vessels; *6,* renal vessels; *7,* ovarian vein; *8,* ureter; *9,* bladder.

a more uniform appearance. The two parts also contrast in origin, in microscopic structure, and in function (Fig. 6.6B).

The cortex is mesodermal and derived from a patch of celomic epithelium close to the gonadal fold. On gross inspection, certain color changes vaguely suggest a subdivision into several concentric shells (zones), but these distinctions become clear only in microscopic preparations. The outer zone produces the mineralocorticoid hormone. The subjacent zones produce glucocorticoids and certain sex steroids.

The medulla is of ectodermal origin, being contributed by a parcel of the cells that migrates from the neural crest to provide the neurons of the peripheral sympathetic ganglia. The medullary cells produce the transmitter substances norepinephrine and epinephrine and thus share with the sympathetic nervous system in the control of the body's response ("flight or fight") to acute stress situations. These cells obtain the additional designation *chromaffin* from their marked affinity for the salts of chromium and other heavy metals.

The adrenal glands are variously but always generously vascularized by small branches from the aorta as well as the renal, lumbar, phrenicoabdominal, and cranial mesenteric arteries. After perfusing the gland, the blood pools within a central vein from which emissary vessels lead through a hilus to join the caudal vena cava or a tributary. Though not easily found, fine nerves within the cortex subject the tissue to hypothalamic control. Nerve bundles are more readily demonstrated within the medulla; appropriately, they are predominantly sympathetic preganglionic fibers passing to the medullary cells, which are equivalent to sympathetic postganglionic neurons elsewhere.

Accessory masses of both cortical and medullary tissues occur. Those of cortical tissue may be incorporated within any of several organs but are most commonly found attached to the capsule of the adrenal gland itself. Accessory chromaffin cells form the bodies known as *paraganglia,* which are endocrine cell clusters particularly associated with sympathetic nerves; a prominent example is found within the plexus on the aorta, close to the origin of the cranial mesenteric artery. Similar clumps of nonchromaffin cells, usually assigned to the parasympathetic system, are best known from the carotid and aortic bodies (described in Chapter 7, p. 227).

OTHER ENDOCRINE TISSUES

The other endocrine tissues are incorporated within organs of composite function. The most familiar example is provided by the endocrine component of the pancreas, the pancreatic islets, also known as the *islets of Langerhans.* The general anatomy of the pancreas has already been described (p. 129). The endocrine component comprises many hundred (or thousand) islets of varying size unevenly distributed among the predominant exocrine tissue. The islets are not normally visible to the naked eye, but the larger ones—of pinhead size—can be made apparent by the use of intravital dyes. The islet tissue has the same origin as the exocrine pancreas and buds from the epithelial cords at an early stage; it remains solid when the remainder of the "tree" canalizes.

The islet cells are of several types, the two most numerous being the alpha and beta types, which produce glucagon and insulin, respectively. These hormones affect carbohydrate metabolism, and their role is best known from the diabetes that develops when insufficient insulin is produced by the islet tissue. The pancreas is also the source of certain other hormones, including somatostatin and pancreatic polypeptide. Other less numerous cells manufacture gastrin; the distinction and functions of yet other types are in dispute. The relative frequencies of the different types are not the same in all parts of the pancreas, and some evidence exists that different ratios occur in the parts that originate from the dorsal and ventral primordia.

The endocrine components and functions of the testes (p. 176), ovaries (p. 192), and placenta (p. 198) were sufficiently mentioned in Chapter 5.

The endocrine components of other organs are even more discrete and thus are not described because they make no gross representation. The most important examples are the renin-producing juxtaglomerular complexes within the kidney and the variety of enteroendocrine cells scattered within the gastric and intestinal epithelia (p. 120). The numbers, distinctions, and functions of the enteroendocrine cell types are inadequately known. Although mainly scattered singly, these cells are so numerous that they would constitute a considerable gland if massed together. They are considered to belong to the so-called APUD* cell system (now shown to be of endodermal not neuroectodermal origin, as formerly supposed) and are believed to produce gastrin, secretin, glucagon, vasoactive intestinal peptide, gastric inhibitory peptide, and several other hormones.

COMPREHENSION CHECK

Explain how embryologic development influences the gross anatomic location of the endocrine organs.

Develop a figure to demonstrate the role of endocrine organs in the development of skeleton.

* An acronym for *a*mine *p*recursor *u*ptake and *d*ecarboxylation.

7 The Cardiovascular System

The study of blood vascular and lymphatic systems officially is termed *angiologia. Angiology* strictly means the study of vessels, but its scope is conveniently enlarged to include the heart, spleen, and various lymphatic organs.

A circulatory system is essential to any organism that exceeds that relatively trivial size at which diffusion can deliver the metabolic fuel and take away the waste. That critical size is quickly realized in the rapidly growing embryo. Although the circulatory system is not the first to be laid down, it is the first body system to reach a "working state."

The circulatory organs and the blood cells have a common origin in clusters of mesenchymal cells that first appear in the wall of the yolk sac. The outermost cells of these "blood islets" are arranged as an endothelium whereas the remaining cells, hemocytoblasts or stem blood cells, float within a fluid plasma. The islets first formed are soon supplemented by others that appear in the mesoderm of the chorioallantois and within the body of the embryo; as the various patches spread and link up they form a diffuse system of connecting vessels that is then extended further by branching from existing channels. The principal vessels thus form independently of one another and in relation to the appearance and growth of the regions and organs of the embryo.

The heart also appears early because pumping is required for proper circulation. It is formed by differentiation of channels within a part of the mesoderm appropriately known as the *cardiogenic area*. This area lies in front of the oral membrane of the discoidal embryo, and the heart rudiments are related from the outset to the most rostral of the tissue spaces that later coalesce to form the celomic cavity, which divides the somatopleure from the splanchnopleure. The cardiogenic area, including both heart and pericardial rudiments, becomes folded ventrally and carried caudally in the process that converts the embryonic disk into a cylindrical body (p. 91). At this stage the heart consists of paired endothelial (endocardial) tubes placed ventral to the foregut, but these tubes shortly fuse to form a single median organ that gradually shifts caudally to the level of the thoracic somites (Fig. 7.1/*5* and *7*).

At the outset, the heart is connected at one end with vessels that become the aorta and at the other with vessels that form the vitelline (omphalomesenteric) veins, the umbilical veins, and the cardinal veins, which drain the yolk sac, the chorioallantoic placement, and the body, respectively. The ventral aorta, continuous with the heart, is soon joined to an independently formed dorsal aorta by a system of aortic loops contained within the pharyngeal (branchial) arches lateral to the pharynx (Fig. 7.2). It is possible to trace the origin of certain arteries of adult anatomy from the six pairs of aortic arches that develop (although not all persist). The developing circulatory system responds to changing functional requirements by refashioning the pattern of vessels, always retaining obsolescent parts until their replacements have become operative.

Descriptions of the development of the heart itself and of the particularly dramatic changes that occur in the circulation at birth are found later in this chapter.

THE HEART

The heart (cor) is the central organ that pumps blood continuously through the blood vessels by rhythmic contraction. The adult heart has right atrium, left atrium, right ventricle, and left ventricle (Fig. 7.3). The two atria and the two ventricles are separated by an internal septum, but the atrium and ventricle of each side communicate through a large opening. The heart consists of two pumps that are combined within a single organ. The deoxygenated (venous) blood enters the right atrium and

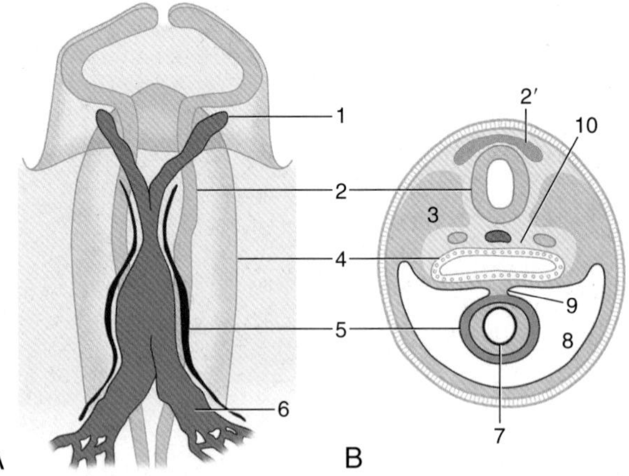

Fig. 7.1 (A) Ventral view of the cranial part of a 15-day-old pig embryo after fusion of the endocardial tube. (B) Transverse section of a seven- to eight-somite embryo taken at the level of 5. *1*, First aortic arch; *2*, neural tube; *2′*, neural crest; *3*, somite; *4*, foregut; *5*, epimyocardial wall of the fused endocardial tubes; *6*, vitelline vein; *7*, endocardial tube; *8*, pericardial cavity; *9*, dorsal mesocardium; *10*, notochord and dorsal aortae.

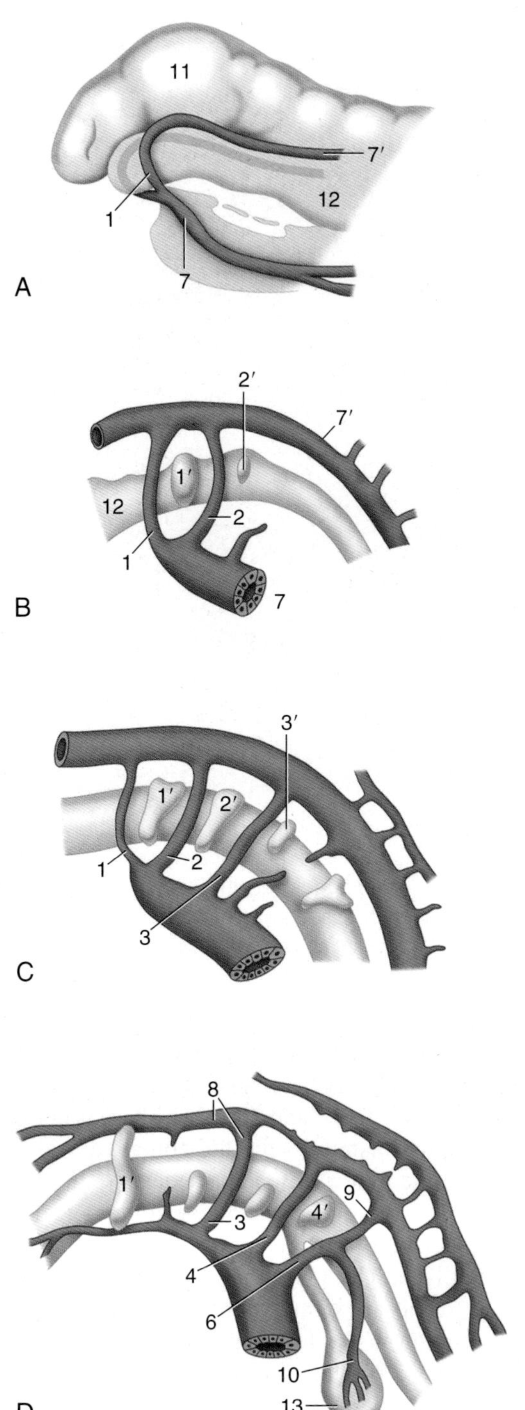

Fig. 7.2 (A) to (D) Left lateral views of the aortic arches and their transformation. (A) Dorsal and ventral aortae are connected by the first aortic arches. (B) First and second aortic arches are present. (C) The first arch begins to disappear, the third is complete, and the fourth and sixth develop. (D) The third arch and the cranial part of the dorsal aorta are now transformed into the internal carotid artery, and the sixth gives rise to the pulmonary trunk and ductus arteriosus. *1–4* and *6,* Aortic arches; *1′–4′,* pharyngeal pouches; *7* and *7′,* ventral and dorsal aortae; *8,* internal carotid artery; *9,* ductus arteriosus; *10,* left pulmonary artery; *11,* brain vesicle; *12,* foregut; *13,* lung bud.

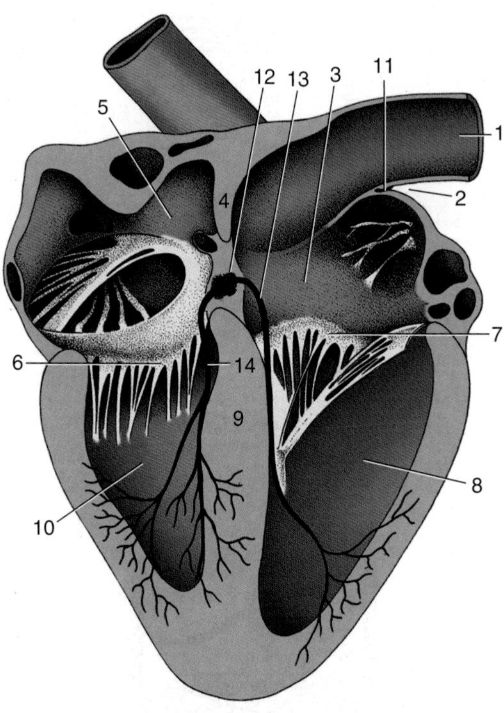

Fig. 7.3 Section of the heart exposing the four chambers. *1,* Cranial vena cava; *2,* terminal sulcus; *3,* right atrium; *4,* interatrial septum; *5,* left atrium; *6,* left atrioventricular valve; *7,* right atrioventricular valve; *8,* right ventricle; *9,* interventricular septum; *10,* left ventricle; *11,* sinoatrial node; *12,* atrioventricular node; *13* and *14,* right and left limbs of atrioventricular bundle.

is ejected to the lungs via the pulmonary trunk. The left pump receives the oxygenated blood from the lungs via the pulmonary veins and ejects it into the aorta for distribution to the body (Fig. 7.4).

The size of the heart varies considerably among species and also among individuals but generally forms 0.75% of the body weight. The heart is typically and relatively larger in smaller species and animals of smaller size but larger in athletic animals such as the Thoroughbred horse and Greyhound. The heart becomes larger (hypertrophied) with exercise. However, the construction, the form, and the general position of the heart are similar among mammals. The differences in topography are mentioned in later chapters because of their significance in clinical examination.

THE PERICARDIUM AND THE TOPOGRAPHY OF THE HEART

The heart is almost completely invested by and fits snugly in the *pericardium* (Fig. 7.5). The pericardium makes a serous sac, but its very tight fit around the heart reduces the lumen to a mere capillary space that contains a small amount of serous fluid to facilitate the easy movement of the heart wall in the pericardial sac (Fig. 7.5/4). The visceral and

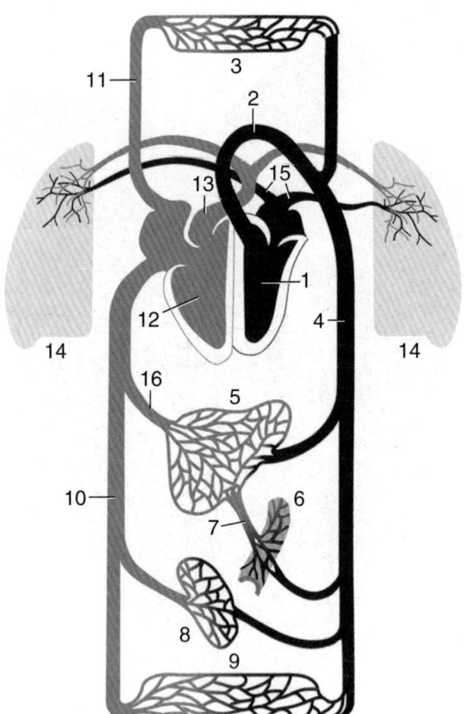

Fig. 7.4 Schematic drawing of the systemic and pulmonary circulation. *1,* Left ventricle; *2,* aorta; *3,* capillary bed of head, neck, and forelimb; *4,* abdominal aorta; *5,* liver; *6,* capillary bed of intestines; *7,* portal vein; *8,* capillary bed of kidneys; *9,* capillary bed of caudal part of the body; *10,* caudal vena cava; *11,* cranial vena cava; *12,* right ventricle; *13,* pulmonary trunk; *14,* capillary bed of lungs; *15,* pulmonary vein; *16,* hepatic veins.

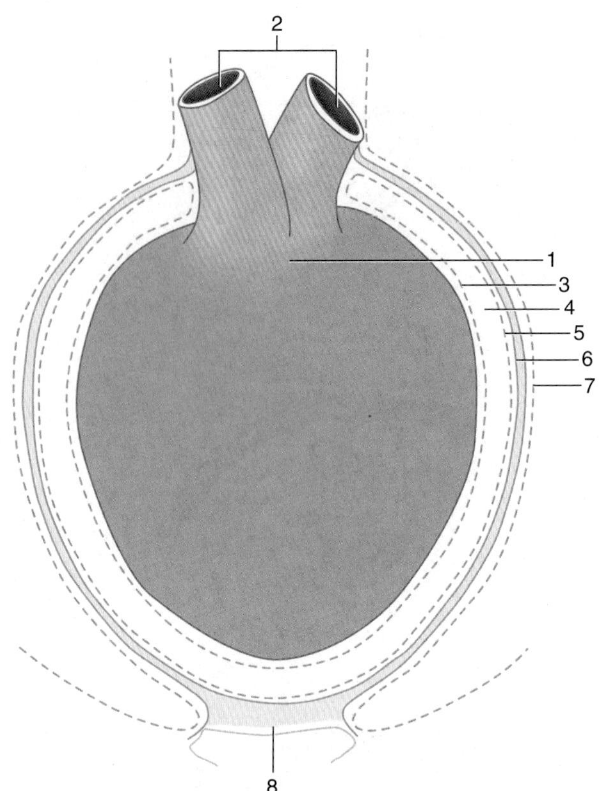

Fig. 7.5 Schematic illustration of the pericardium. *1,* Heart; *2,* great vessels; *3,* visceral pericardium (epicardium); *4,* pericardial cavity (exaggerated in size); *5,* parietal pericardium; *6,* connective tissue layer of the parietal pericardium; *7,* mediastinal pleura; *8,* sternopericardial ligament.

parietal layers of the pericardium continue into each other at a complicated reflection that runs over the atria and the roots of the great vessels. The visceral layer is so closely adherent to the epicardium that it may be described as an epicardial component. The parietal layer has a thick external fibrous covering (Fig. 7.5/*6*) that blends with the adventitia of the great vessels dorsally and forms a ligament at the ventral apex of the sac to attach to the sternum (*sternopericardial ligament;* Fig. 7.5/*8*) or to the diaphragm (*phrenicopericardial ligament*). These attachments place a severe restraint on the mobility of the heart, although slight movement does occur with each respiratory excursion.

Although the pericardium distorts to accommodate the changing form of the heart during the cardiac cycle, its fibrous component prevents any significant distention in the short term. It may stretch over longer periods if the heart becomes enlarged by exercise or disease or if an effusion or accumulation of inflammatory fluid occurs within the pericardial cavity.

The heart (within the pericardium)* is included within the mediastinum, the partition that separates the right and left pleural cavities (see Fig. 4.20A). It is conical and is placed asymmetrically within the thorax, and the larger part (about 60%) lies to the left of the median plane (see Figs. 13.13B and 20.8). The base is dorsal and reaches approximately to the horizontal (dorsal) plane that bisects the first rib; in some species (e.g., the dog) it is tilted in varying degrees to face craniodorsally. The apex is placed close to the sternum, opposite the sixth costal cartilage. The long axis that joins the center of the base to the apex thus slopes caudoventrally, with some deviation to the left imposed by the skewed orientation (Fig. 7.6). The projection of the heart on the chest wall extends between the third and sixth ribs (or thereabouts). Thus, much of the heart is covered by the forelimb, which makes clinical examination a challenge, especially in larger animals (See Chapters 20 and 27).

The heart displays some lateral compression to conform to the shape of the thorax of most quadrupeds. This shape of the heart better defines right and left surfaces (which are also crossed by the corresponding phrenic nerves) make a better fit with the corresponding lungs. The cardiac notch in the ventral border of each lung allows the heart a restricted contact with the chest wall, which is normally greater on the left side because of

*This qualification, necessary for strict accuracy, may be assumed in later references to the relations of the heart.

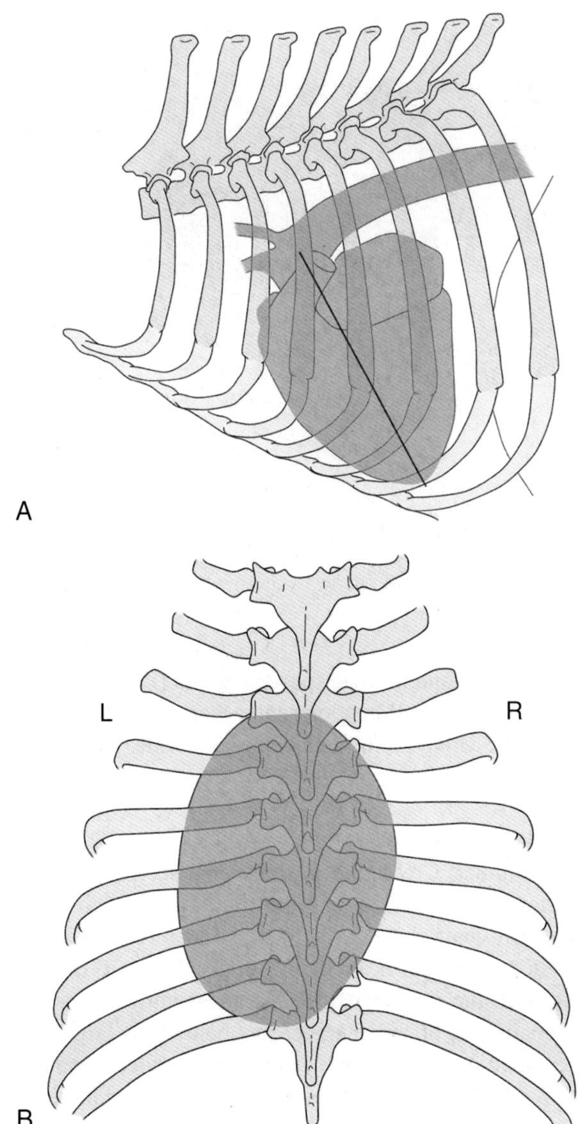

Fig. 7.6 Schematic drawings to show the position of the canine heart, based on radiographs. (A) Left lateral view; the caudoventrally sloping long axis *(red line)* of the heart is indicated. (B) Dorsoventral view showing the asymmetrical position of the heart. *L*, left; *R*, right.

the asymmetrical position (see Fig. 13.5). The cranial aspect is extensively related to the thymus (in the young animal), but the caudal surface faces toward the diaphragm and may be indirectly related through it to cranial abdominal organs a point of importance in certain species such as cattle (see Chapter 28).

General Anatomy of the Heart

The base of the heart is formed by the thin-walled *atria*, which are clearly separated from the ventricles by an encircling *coronary groove* that contains the main trunks of the coronary vessels within a concealment of fat. The right and left atria combine in a continuous U-shaped formation that embraces the origin of the aorta; the formation is interrupted craniosinistrally where each atrium ends in a free blind appendage, the auricle (Fig. 7.7A/*1*), which overlaps the origin of the pulmonary trunk. The margins of the atria are often crenated.

The thick walled *ventricles* provide a much larger and much firmer part of the heart. Although the ventricles merge externally, their separate extents are defined by shallow grooves that descend toward the apex. The *paraconal (left) groove* runs close to the cranial aspect of the heart (Fig. 7.7A); the *subsinuosal (right) groove* runs close to the caudal aspect (Fig. 7.7B). Both grooves convey substantial vessels that follow the edges of the interventricular septum, and together they reveal the asymmetrical disposition of the ventricles. The right chamber lies as much cranially as to the right of the left one (see Fig. 7.10). Additional branches of the coronary vessels extend some distance over the ventricular surface in a less constant pattern, but these apart, the external surface is smooth and featureless. Although it is not apparent externally, a fibrous skeleton separates the atrial from the ventricular muscle mass.

The Right Atrium

The right atrium lies mainly on the right, although the auricular cul-de-sac extends to the cranial face of the pulmonary trunk to appear on the left side. The greater part forms a chamber (sinus venarum) into which the principal systemic veins discharge (Fig. 7.8/*1*). The caudal vena cava enters the caudodorsal part of this chamber, above the opening of the much smaller vein (*coronary sinus*) that drains the heart itself. The cranial vena cava opens craniodorsally at the *terminal crest* (Fig. 7.8/*7*). An azygos vein enters variously. When a *right azygos* is present (as in the horse, dog, and ruminants), it enters dorsally, either by joining the cranial vena cava (Fig. 7.8/*6*) or by discharging between the caval openings; when a *left azygos* is present (as in ruminants and the pig), it joins the coronary sinus close to its termination after winding around the caudal aspect of the base from the left side (Fig. 7.9A/*12*).

The interior of the atrium is smooth between the vein entrances, which are unobstructed by valves. Its roof dips between the caval openings, being indented by the passage of pulmonary veins returning across the right atrium to enter the left atrium. The ridge produced by the indentation (*intervenous tubercle;* Fig. 7.8/*5*) prevents confrontation between the caval streams by deflecting both ventrally, toward the atrioventricular ostium (Fig. 7.8/*3*) that occupies much of the floor. A depressed membranous area (*fossa ovalis;* Fig. 7.8/*8*) of the septal wall is present caudal to the tubercle; it corresponds to the foramen ovale of fetal life. In sharp contrast, the interior of the auricle (Fig. 7.8/*1′*) is made irregular by a series of ridges (musculi

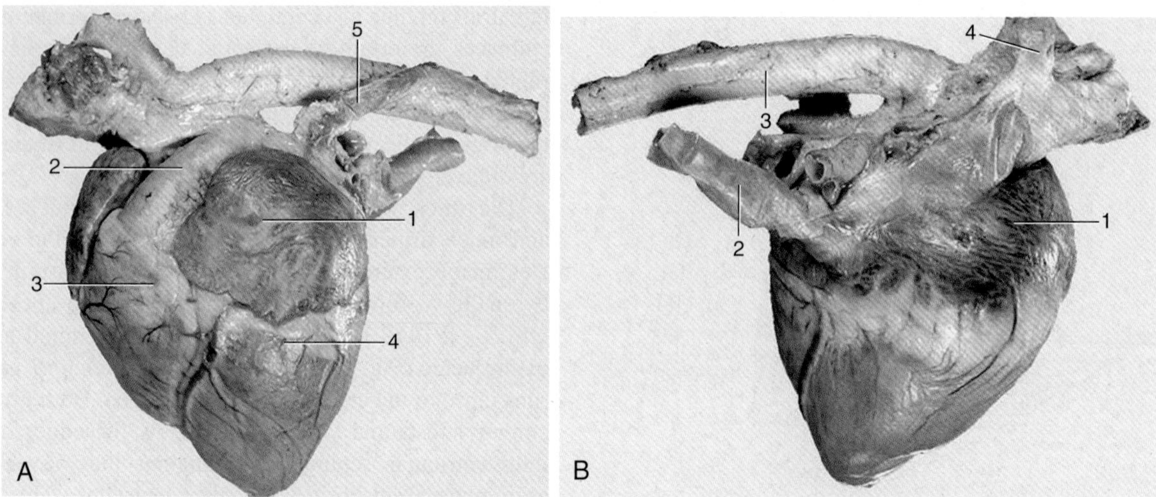

Fig. 7.7 (A) Left view of the heart. *1,* Left auricle; *2,* pulmonary trunk; *3,* right ventricle; *4,* left ventricle; *5,* left azygous vein. (B) Right view of the heart. *1,* Right atrium; *2,* caudal vena cava; *3,* aorta; *4,* right azygos vein (opening into the cranial vena cava).

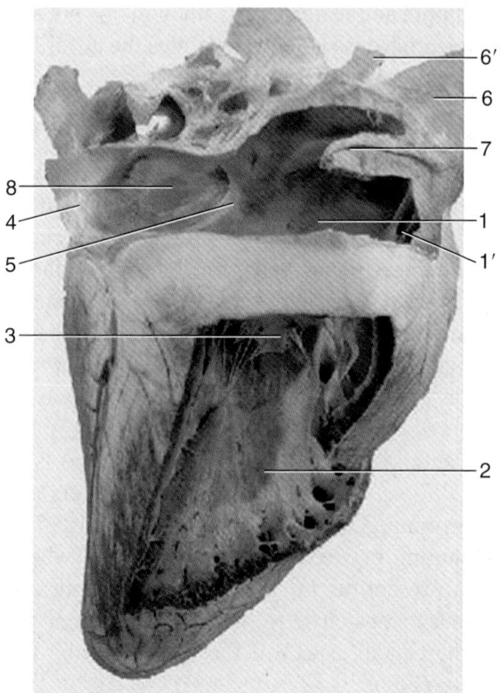

Fig. 7.8 Overview of the interior of the right atrium and right ventricle of the equine heart. *1,* Right atrium; *1′,* right auricle; *2,* right ventricle; *3,* right atrioventricular valve; *4,* caudal vena cava; *5,* intervenous tubercle; *6,* cranial vena cava; *6′,* right azygos vein; *7,* terminal crest; *8,* fossa ovalis.

pectinati) that branch from the terminal crest that marks the boundary between the auricle and the main compartment.

The Left Atrium

The form of the left atrium is generally similar to that of the right atrium. It receives the pulmonary veins, which enter separately or in groups at two or three sites: craniosinistral, craniodextral, and in some species, caudal (Fig. 7.9/*11*i and *11′*). The septal wall may present a scar marking the position of the valve of the fetal foramen ovale. The auricle resembles that on the right side.

The Right Ventricle

This chamber, Crescentic in transverse section, the right ventricle is wrapped around the right and cranial aspects of the left ventricle (Fig. 7.10). It is incompletely divided by a stout muscular beam (supraventricular crest) that projects from the roof cranial to the atrioventricular ostium. The main part of the chamber lies below this large elongated opening, whereas the extension to the left, the *conus arteriosus* (Fig. 7.11), leads directly to the much smaller circular exit into the pulmonary trunk.

The *right atrioventricular (tricuspid) valve* is composed of three flaps or cusps that attach to a fibrous ring that encircles the opening. The cusps are fused at their attachment but part toward the center of the opening, where their free margins are thick and irregular, especially in later life. Each cusp is joined by fibrous strands (chordae tendineae) that descend into the ventricular cavity to insert on projections from the walls (*papillary muscles*). Generally, three papillary muscles are present, and the chordae tendineae are so arranged that they connect each cusp to two muscles and each muscle to two cusps (Fig. 7.11/*2* and *3*). The arrangement prevents eversion of the cusps into the atrium during ventricular contraction (systole). The lumen of the ventricle is crossed by a thin band of muscle (*trabecula septomarginalis*) that passes from the septal wall to the outer wall (see Fig. 7.17B/*2*). It provides a shortcut for a bundle of the conducting tissue, thus ensuring a more nearly simultaneous contraction of all parts of the ventricle (see Fig. 7.3). The muscle is further modified by the many

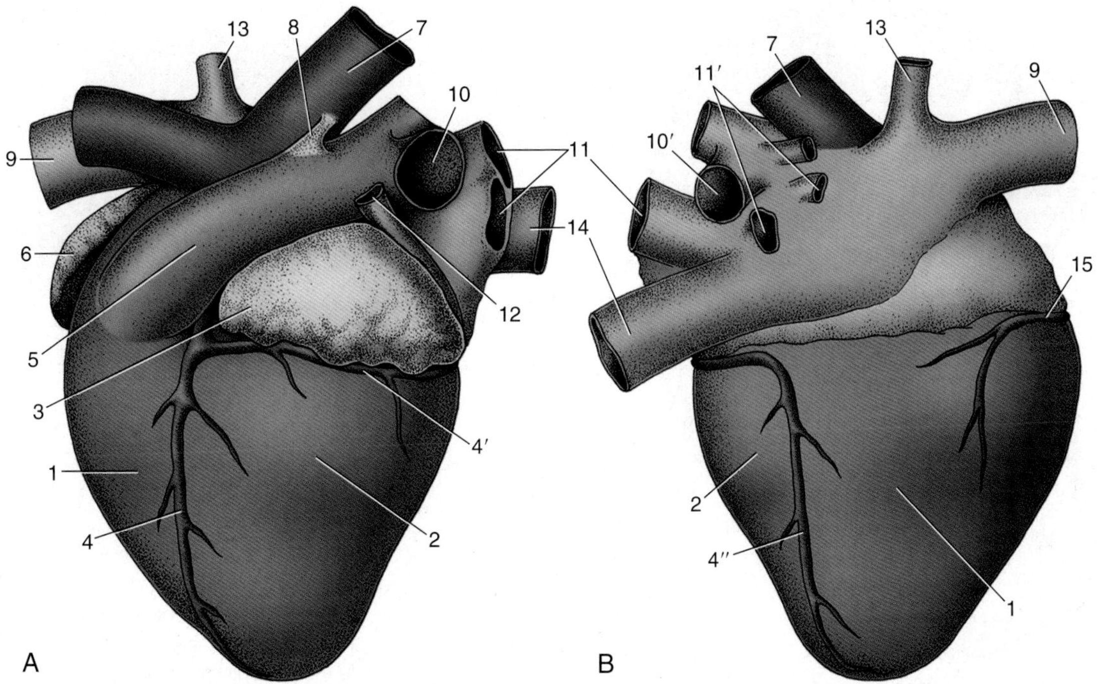

Fig. 7.9 (A) Left and (B) right views of the bovine heart. *1,* Right ventricle; *2,* left ventricle; *3,* left auricle; *4,* paraconal interventricular branch of left coronary artery (a.); *4′,* circumflex branch of left coronary a.; *4″,* subsinuosal interventricular branch of left coronary a.; *5,* pulmonary trunk; *6,* right auricle; *7,* aorta; *8,* ligamentum arteriosum; *9,* cranial vena cava; *10* and *10′,* left and right pulmonary arteries; *11* and *11′,* left and right pulmonary veins; *12,* left azygos vein (v.); *13,* right azygos v.; *14,* caudal vena cava; *15,* right coronary a.

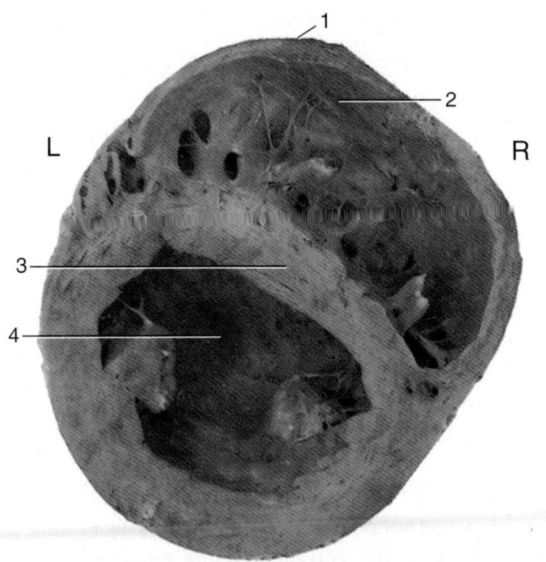

Fig. 7.10 Transverse section through the ventricles. Note the different thicknesses of the walls of the right and left ventricles. *1,* Most cranial point; *2,* right ventricle; *3,* interventricular septum; *4,* left ventricle; *L,* left; *R,* right.

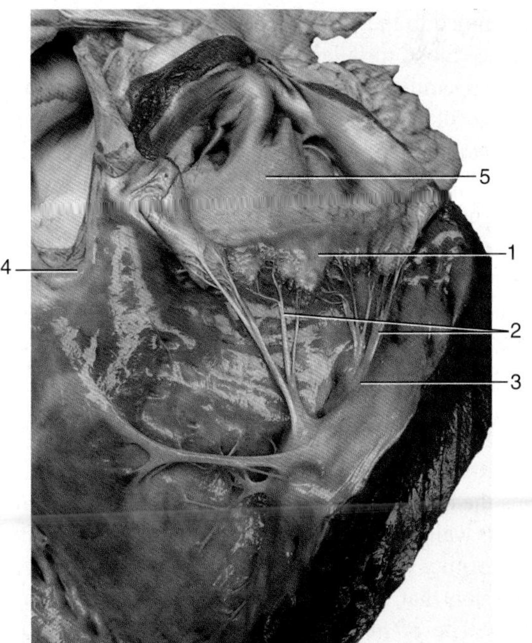

Fig. 7.11 Cranioventral view of the interior of the right ventricle. *1,* Cusp of right atrioventricular valve; *2,* chordae tendineae; *3,* papillary muscles; *4,* pulmonary valve; *5,* right auricle.

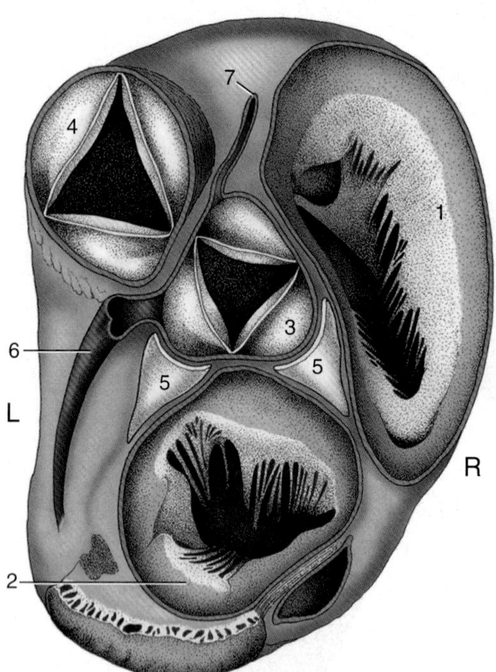

Fig. 7.12 Dorsal view of the base of the bovine heart after removal of the atria. The ossa cordis on both sides of the aortic valve have been exposed. *1,* Right atrioventricular valve; *2,* left atrioventricular valve; *3,* aortic valve; *4,* pulmonary valve; *5,* ossa cordis; *6,* left coronary artery; *7,* right coronary artery; *L,* left; *R,* right.

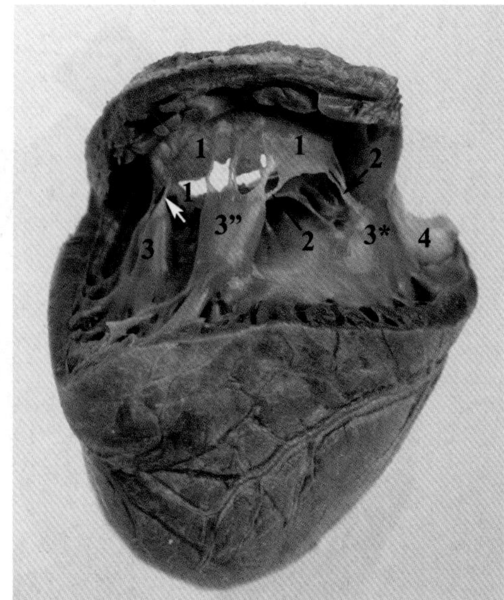

Fig. 7.13 Tricuspid valve and the right ventricle of the dog. *1,* Cusps of the tricuspid valve, magenta: parietal cusp, blue: angular cusp, green: septal cusp; *2,* chordae tendineae; *3,* papillary muscle (Mm. papillares parvi); *3",* papillary muscle (M. papillaris magnus); *3*,* papillary muscle (M. papillaris subarteriosus); *4,* pulmonary valve.

irregular ridges (trabeculae carneae) that give the lower part of the wall a spongy appearance. These ridges, which are confined to the "inflow" part of the cavity, are thought to reduce blood turbulence.

The opening into the pulmonary trunk lies at a more dorsal level than the atrioventricular ostium and is craniosinistral to the origin of the aorta. It is closed during ventricular relaxation (diastole) by the backflow of blood forcing together the three cusps that arise around its margin and constitute the *pulmonary valve* (Fig. 7.12). The cusps are semilunar and deeply hollowed on the arterial side, fitting together tightly when the valve is closed; thickenings of the contact areas, sometimes pronounced in older animals, improve the seal (Fig. 7.13).

The Left Ventricle

The left ventricle is circular in section (see Fig. 7.10) and forms the apex of the heart as a whole. Except toward the apex, its wall is much thicker than that of the right ventricle, in conformity with the greater work demands; however, the impression that the left chamber is also much smaller is illusory. The *left atrioventricular (bicuspid or mitral) valve* that closes the atrioventricular ostium generally has only two major cusps but is otherwise comparable to that of the right side. It lies largely to the left of the median plane (Figs. 7.12/*2* and 7.14/*3*). The exit to the aorta takes a more central position within the heart.

The *aortic valve,* generally resembling the pulmonary valve, shows a different orientation of its cusps (Fig. 7.12/*3*). The nodular thickenings in the free margins of the aortic cusps are conspicuous.

The Structure of the Heart

The thick middle layer of the wall (*myocardium*) is composed of cardiac muscle, which is a variety of striated muscle peculiar to this organ. It is covered externally by the visceral pericardium (*epicardium*) and internally by the *endocardium,* a thin smooth-surfaced layer continuous with the lining of the blood vessels.

The atrial and ventricular parts of the muscle are separated by a fibrous skeleton that is formed mainly by the conjunction of the rings that encircle the four heart orifices. The skeleton contains islands of fibrocartilage in which nodules of bone (*ossa cordis*) may develop (Fig. 7.12/*5*). Although these bones appear precociously in the hearts of cattle, they are not confined to this species, as is sometimes suggested. Near the entrance of the coronary sinus, the fibrous skeleton allows passage to the *atrioventricular bundle,* which conducts the impulse to contract and constitutes the only direct connection between the atrial and ventricular muscles. Delicate extensions of the fibrous tissue also provide the cores of the cusps of the various valves.

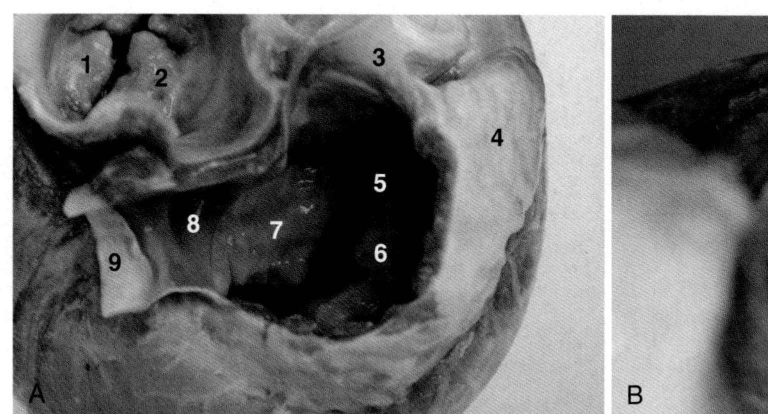

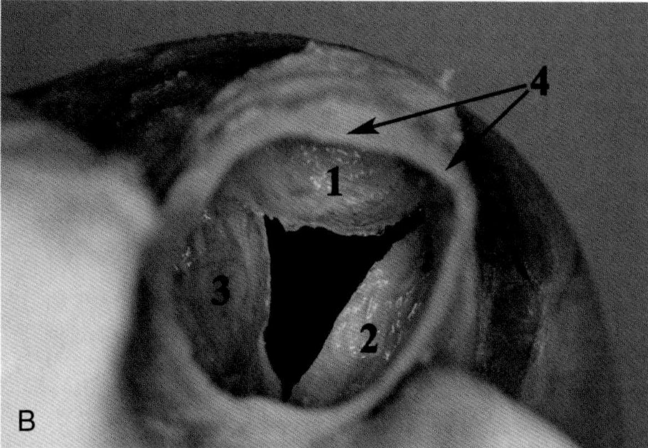

Fig. 7.14 (A) Atrioventricular openings of the dog (dorsal view): *1,* Parietal cusp of the left atrioventricular valve; *2,* septal cusp of the left atrioventricular valve; *3,* cranial vena cava; *4,* right auricle; *5,* angular cusp of the right atrioventricular valve; *6,* parietal cusp of the right atrioventricular valve; *7,* septal cusp of the right atrioventricular valve; *8,* opening of the coronary sinus; *9,* caudal vena cava. (B) Semilunar valves of the pulmonary trunk: *1,* Intermediate semilunar valve; *2,* right semilunar valve; *3,* left semilunar valve; *4,* pulmonary trunk.

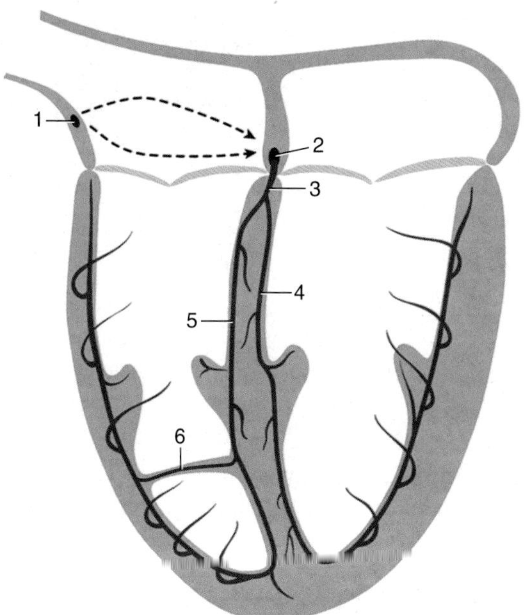

Fig. 7.15 Schematic drawing of the conducting system of the heart. The *broken lines* and *arrows* suggest the passage of the excitation wave through the atrial wall. *1,* Sinoatrial node; *2,* atrioventricular node; *3,* atrioventricular bundle; *4,* left limb; *5,* right limb; *6,* branch of right limb traversing the septomarginal band.

The atrial muscle is thin—indeed, the auricular wall may be translucent between the pectinate ridges. It is arranged in superficial and deep bundles; some of the former are common to both atria, but the remainder, and all of the deep bundles, are confined to one. It has been postulated that the fascicles that surround the various systemic and pulmonary venous inlets act as throttles to oppose reflux of blood into the veins during atrial systole.

The much thicker ventricular muscle is also arranged in superficial and deep bundles. Some superficial bundles coil around both chambers, utilizing the septum to complete a figure-of-eight course. Others, like the deeper bundles, encircle only the one chamber. The arrangement of the muscles and their contraction mechanisms are actually very complicated.

The inherent rhythm of the heart is controlled by a pacemaker, a small, richly innervated *sinoatrial node* of modified cardiac fibers (nodal myofibers) (Fig. 7.16A). This node, which is not apparent to the naked eye, lies below the epicardium of the right atrial wall ventral to the cranial caval opening (see Fig. 7.3/*11*). With each heart cycle a wave of excitation arises in the sinoatrial node and spreads throughout the atrial muscle to reach the atrioventricular node (Figs. 7.15 and 7.16B and C). In ungulates, specialized conductive tissue is present subendocardially in the atrium, mainly on the pectinate muscle. From the *atrioventricular node* an excitatory stimulus passes rapidly throughout the whole ventricular myocardium via the *atrioventricular bundle,* which is largely composed of Purkinje fibers, modified cardiac muscle fibers that conduct impulses much more rapidly than those of the common sort (see Fig. 7.15). The atrioventricular node consists of modified nodal and Purkinje fibers and is found within the interatrial septum, cranial to the opening of the coronary sinus; it is richly innervated. This node gives origin to the *atrioventricular bundle,* which penetrates the fibrous skeleton before dividing into right and left limbs (crura) that straddle the interventricular septum (Fig. 7.17A and B). Each limb continues ventrally close to the endocardium and branches to reach all parts of the heart muscle; part of the right bundle travels to the outer

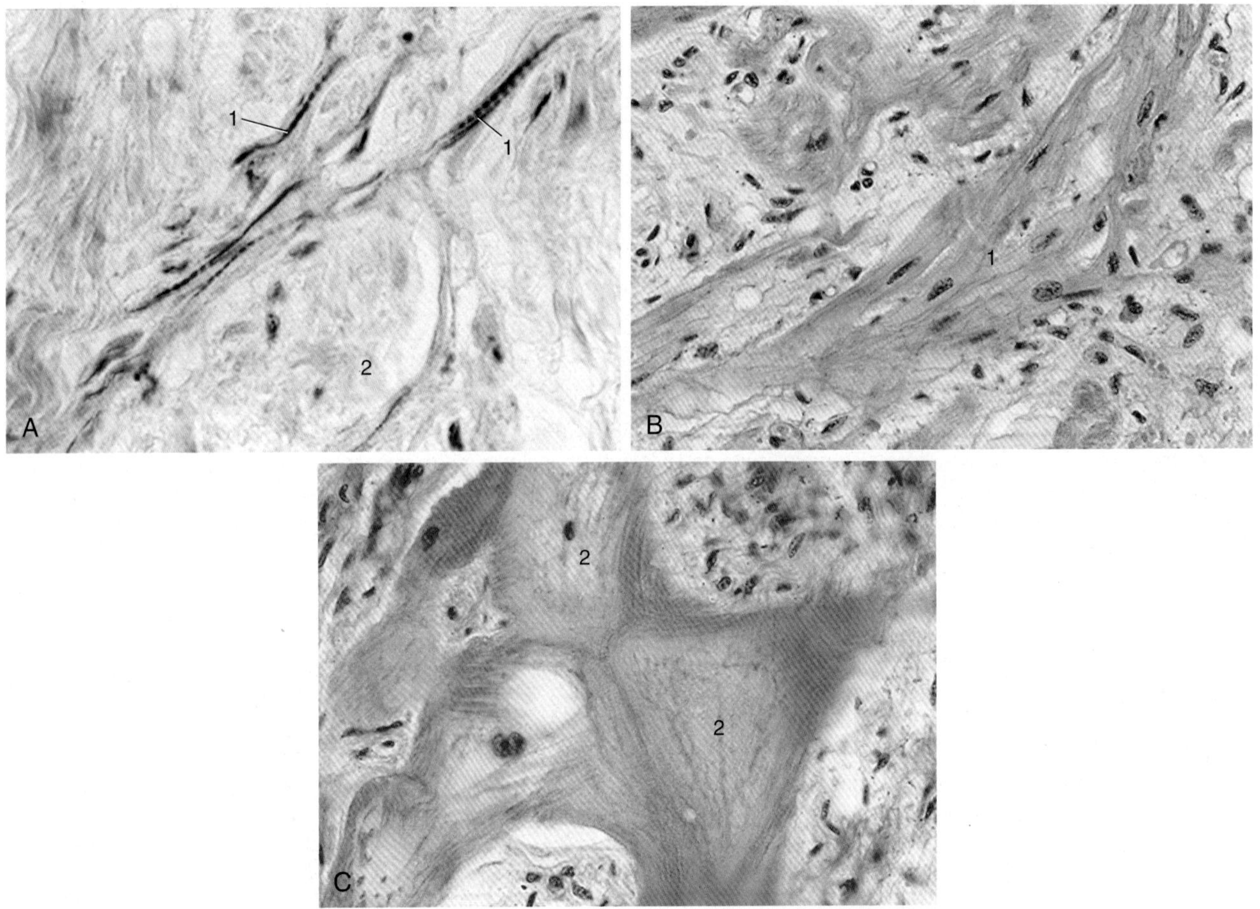

Fig. 7.16 (A) Sinoatrial node of the equine heart. *1,* Nodal myofibers; *2,* bundle of nerve fibers (hematoxylin and eosin [HE]; magnification ×279). (B) and (C) Atrioventricular node of equine heart (HE; magnification ×279). *1,* Nodal myofibers; *2,* Purkinje cells with abundant glycogen.

wall by way of the septomarginal band. The main conducting structures are not difficult to display by dissection of the beef heart.

Cardiac Vessels and Nerves

The heart is lavishly supplied with blood, receiving about 15% of the output of the left ventricle. The supply is led through the coronary arteries that spring from two of the three sinuses above the semilunar cusps at the beginning of the aorta (Fig. 7.18).

The *left coronary artery* is usually the larger. It arises above the caudosinistral cusp and reaches the coronary groove by passing between the left auricle and the pulmonary trunk; it divides almost at once. The left (paraconal) interventricular branch follows the like-named groove toward the apex of the heart (Fig. 7.19/*2′*). The trunk continues as a circumflex branch (Fig. 7.19/*2″*) that follows the coronary groove toward the caudal aspect of the heart, where it may terminate close to the origin of the right (subsinuosal) interventricular groove (horse and pig) or continue into it (carnivores and ruminants) (Figs. 7.20A and B and 7.21).

The *right coronary artery* arises above the cranial cusp (Fig. 7.18/*6*) and reaches the coronary groove after passage between the right auricle and pulmonary trunk. It pursues a circumflex course that either fades toward the origin of the subsinuosal groove or turns into it in those species in which the left artery has the restricted distribution. Both coronary arteries send other branches, of varying size and constancy of position, to neighboring parts of the atrial and ventricular walls. Very small twigs extend some distance into the cores of the valve cusps (Fig. 7.22).

Anastomoses are not formed between the main branches of the coronary arteries but are numerous between the lesser branches. Even so, sudden closure of one of these small vessels leads to local infarction of the cardiac muscle.

Blood is returned to the heart principally through the *great cardiac vein* that opens separately into the right atrium via the coronary sinus (Fig. 7.20/*3* and *4*). Rather surprisingly, many very small (thebesian) veins open directly into all four heart chambers.

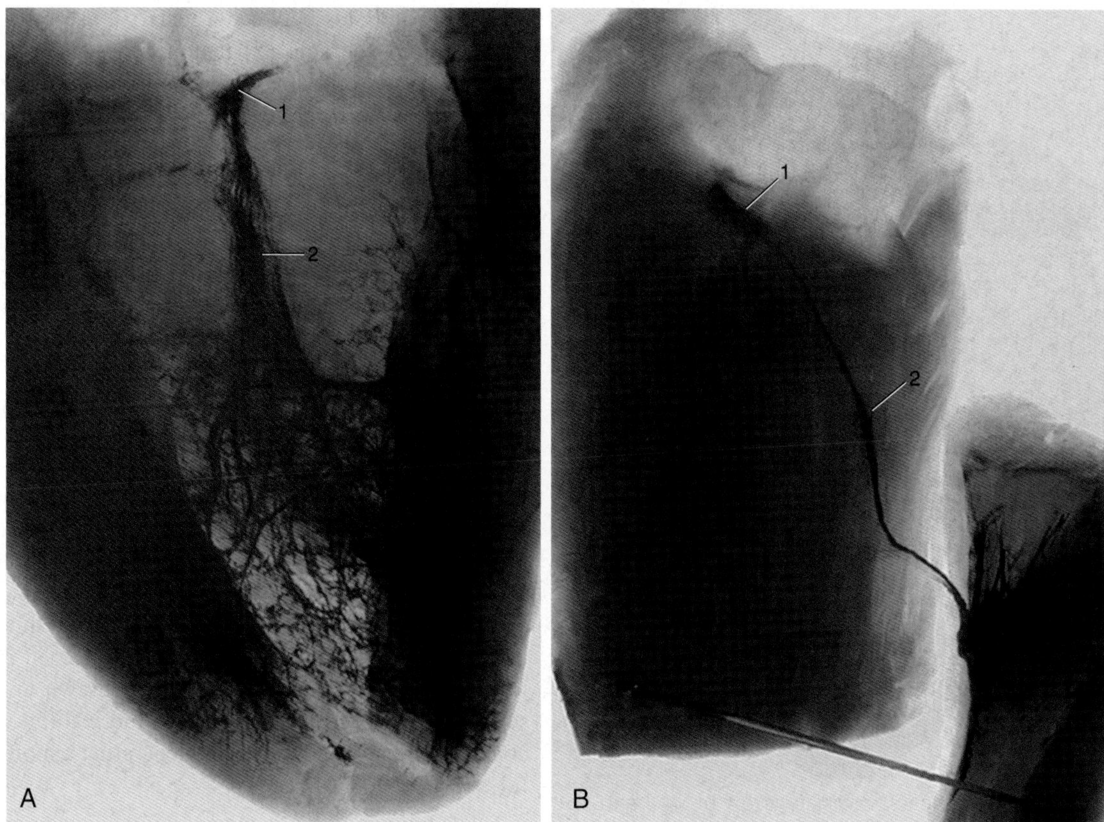

Fig. 7.17 (A) Cleared specimen of left ventricle. *1,* Atrioventricular node; *2,* left crus of atrioventricular trunk (injected blue). (B) Cleared specimen of right ventricle. *1,* Atrioventricular node; *2,* right crus of the atrioventricular trunk, continuing into the moderator band.

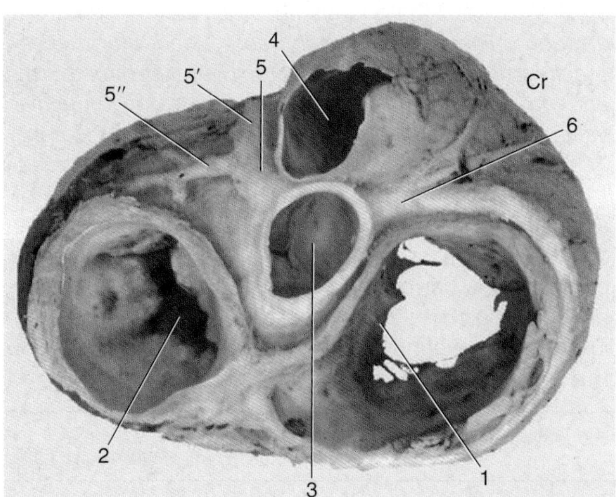

Fig. 7.18 Dorsal view of the base of the heart after removal of the atria. The coronary arteries are exposed. *1,* Right atrioventricular valve; *2,* left atrioventricular valve; *3,* aortic valve; *4,* pulmonary valve; *5,* left coronary artery; *5′,* paraconal interventricular branch; *5″,* circumflex branch; *6,* right coronary artery; *Cr,* cranial.

The innervation of the heart is topographically complicated. A sympathetic contribution is routed through the caudal cervical and first few thoracic ganglia of the sympathetic trunk. The postganglionic fibers form cardiac plexuses within the cranial mediastinum before extending to the heart wall (Fig. 7.23). Parasympathetic fibers branch from the vagus nerves, either directly or after short passage within the recurrent laryngeal nerves. They end on nerve cells in the heart wall, especially within and about the sinoatrial and atrioventricular nodes. Many of the postganglionic fibers pass to the nodes, but others reach the periphery of the heart by following the atrioventricular bundle and its branches.

Functional Anatomy

The heart has an exacting task because 60%, 80%, and 100% of the total volume of blood in humans, dogs, and horses, respectively, passes through the heart each minute. This efficient pumping requires coordinated contraction because asynchronous contraction (fibrillation) of heart muscle, especially of the ventricles, is ineffectual and is rapidly fatal. The sinoatrial node, the pacemaker, generates

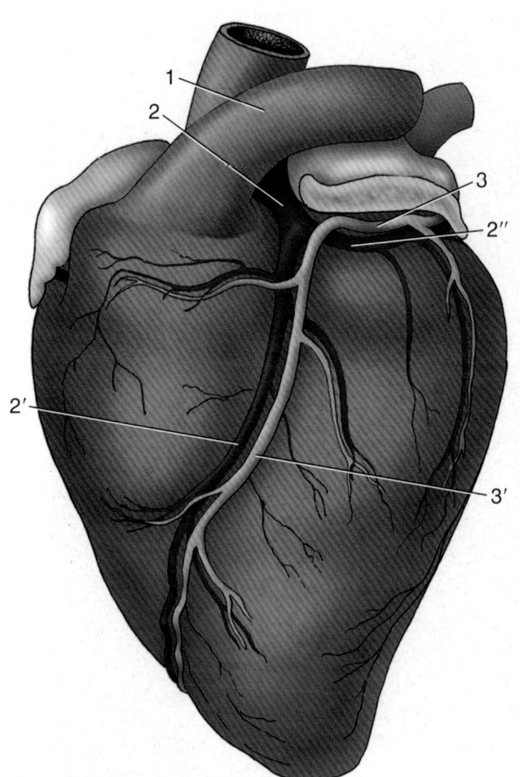

Fig. 7.19 Branching of the left coronary artery of the heart, viewed from the left. The left auricle has been shortened. *1,* Pulmonary trunk; *2,* left coronary artery; *2′,* paraconal interventricular branch; *2″,* circumflex branch; *3,* great cardiac vein (continued by the coronary sinus on the right side of the heart); *3′,* paraconal interventricular tributary of *3.*

a wave of excitation that normally spreads to the atrial muscle to reach the atrioventricular node (Figs. 7.15/*2* and 7.17A and B). It has the highest rate of spontaneous activity when relieved of external stimuli but is regulated by the fine balance of accelerating sympathetic and retarding vagal inputs. Following a short delay at the atrioventricular node to permit completion of atrial contraction, the impulse then spreads to the ventricular muscle through the atrioventricular conducting tissue. Although ventricular contraction is almost synchronous, the subendocardial layer, which includes the papillary muscles, gains a slight lead.

Blood enters the atria for as long as the pressure within the veins exceeds that within the heart. Several factors of uncertain and varying magnitude contribute to the venous pressure. The force exerted upstream (*vis a tergo*) is the summation of the following: *the residual pressure imparted to the blood by ventricular contraction; the forces exerted by muscles, visceral activity, and arterial pulsation; and the contraction of the diaphragm (the so-called abdominal pump) expelling blood from the caudal vena cava and its large tributaries within the abdomen.* The downstream force (*vis a fronte*) oscillates between a negative aspirating effect (provided by thoracic expansion and atrial relaxation) and a positive pressure developed on atrial systole. A lateral pressure may be exerted by contraction of the muscular coat of the great veins. Gravity also plays a part, sometimes assisting and sometimes impeding flow according to posture. Much blood flows directly into the ventricles through open atrioventricular ostia, and only a "topping-up" effect is exerted by the atrial contraction, which coincides with the last stage of ventricular relaxation. When the atria do contract, some blood may reflux into veins (despite the conjectured throttle mechanism already mentioned) as evidenced by a jugular pulse mostly seen in cattle.

The pulmonary and aortic (arterial) valves are closed during ventricular relaxation. Ventricular contraction closes the atrioventricular valves while papillary muscles prevent eversion of the cusps into the atria. As the contraction develops, blood forces the arterial valves open, and the conducting arteries are expanded by this sudden input. The right ventricular lumen is squeezed in a bellows action in which the outer wall is drawn toward the septum (Fig. 7.24), and the more cylindrical left ventricle contracts radially and in length, generating a more powerful effect.

Auscultation Closure of the heart valves produces distinctive sounds that are audible on auscultation, and these sounds provide valuable information about the condition of the valves. Because of intervening tissues of varying densities, the projections of the heart valves on the chest wall are not necessarily the spots (puncta maxima) where the sounds are most clearly heard. *As a rough guide, the pulmonary, aortic, and left atrioventricular valves are best auscultated over the third, fourth, and fifth ribs of the left side, and the right atrioventricular valve is best auscultated over the fourth rib on the right. The arterial valves are somewhat dorsal to the atrioventricular valves.* Percussion is also used as a means of evaluating the size of the heart. The quality of cardiac dullness contrasts with the high pitch obtained when percussion is performed over the lungs. The boundary of the cardiac area is not sharply defined because the lung tissue covering the heart varies in thickness about the cardiac notch.

The Development of the Heart

The primitive heart, the single median structure formed by the fusion of paired rudiments, is carried ventral to the foregut by the reversal process reshaping the head end of the embryo (p. 91). Though initially consisting of a simple endothelial tube, the heart soon acquires an investment of mesoderm that forms the myocardial and epicardial components of its wall. The cranial part of the tube, which will

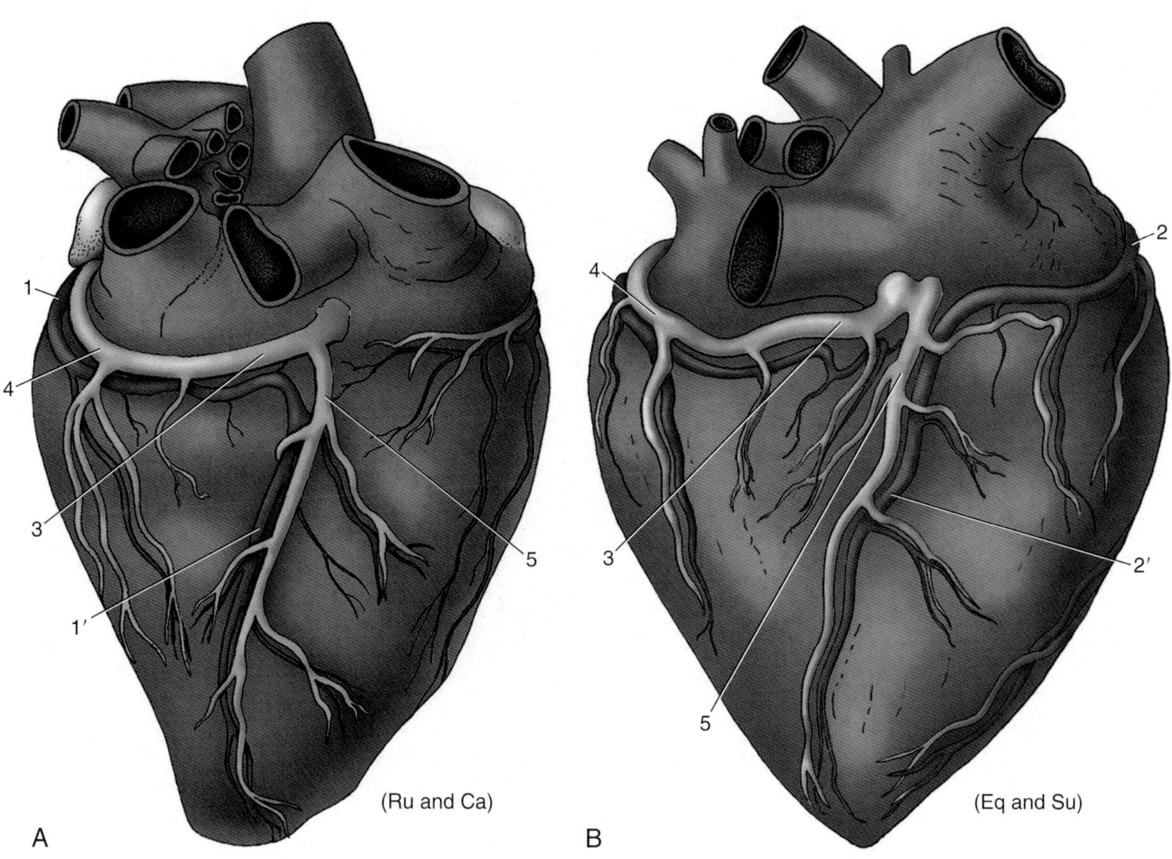

Fig. 7.20 Patterns of coronary circulation of the heart viewed from the right. (A) Situation in ruminants *(Ru)* and carnivores *(Ca);* the right (subsinuosal) interventricular branch *(1′)* is a continuation of the left coronary artery. (B) Situation in the horse *(Eq)* and pig *(Su);* the right (subsinuosal) interventricular branch *(2′)* is a continuation of the right coronary artery. *1,* Circumflex branch of left coronary artery; *2,* right coronary artery; *3,* coronary sinus; *4,* great cardiac vein; *5,* middle cardiac vein.

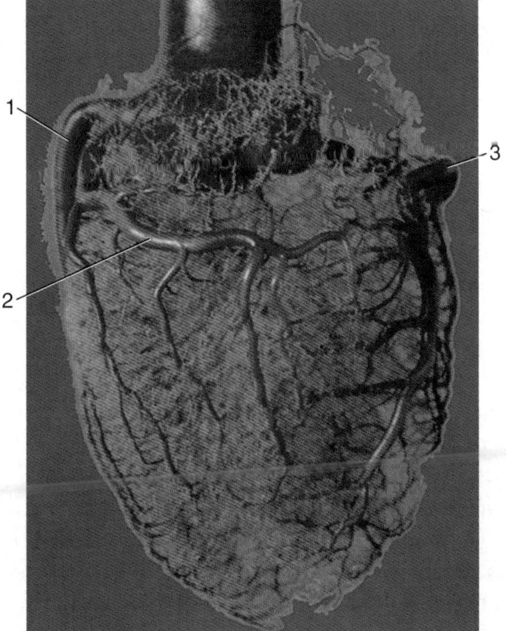

Fig. 7.21 Corrosion cast of aorta and coronary circulation (pig). *1,* Left coronary artery; *2,* ramus circumflexus; *3,* right coronary artery.

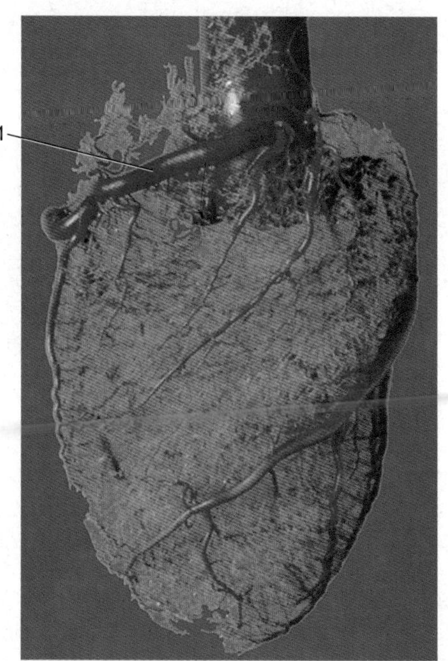

Fig. 7.22 Corrosion cast of aorta and coronary circulation (pig). *1,* Right coronary artery.

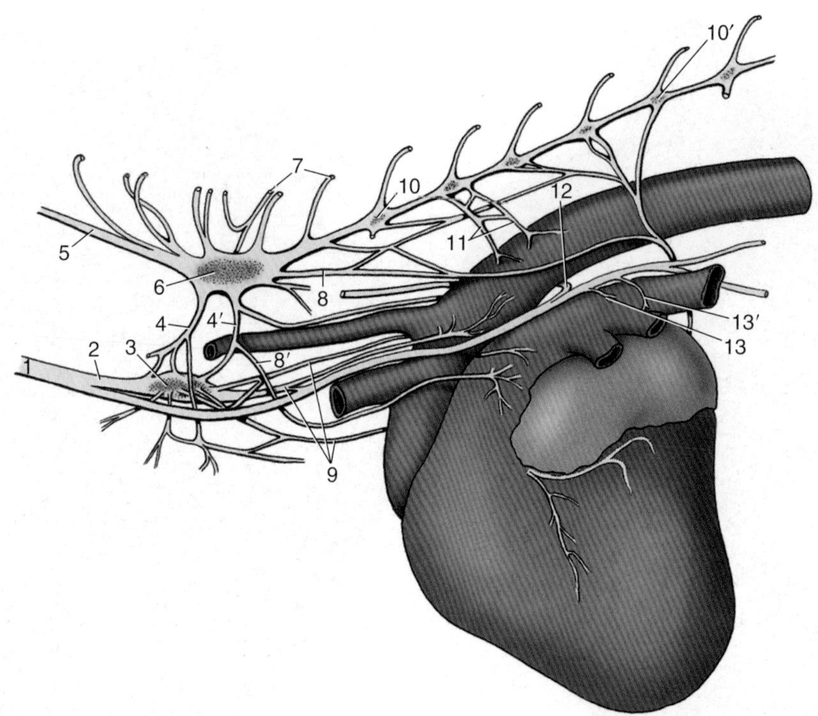

Fig. 7.23 Cardiac nerves and related ganglia of the dog; left lateral view. *1,* Vagosympathetic trunk; *2,* sympathetic trunk; *3,* middle cervical ganglion; *4* and *4′,* cranial and caudal limbs of ansa subclavia; *5,* vertebral node; *6,* cervicothoracic ganglion; *7,* communicating branches; *8* and *8′,* caudodorsal and caudoventral cervicothoracic cardiac nodes; *9,* vertebral cardiac nodes; *10* and *10′,* third and seventh thoracic ganglia; *11,* thoracic cardiac nodes; *12,* left recurrent laryngeal node; *13* and *13′,* cranial and caudal vagal cardiac nodes.

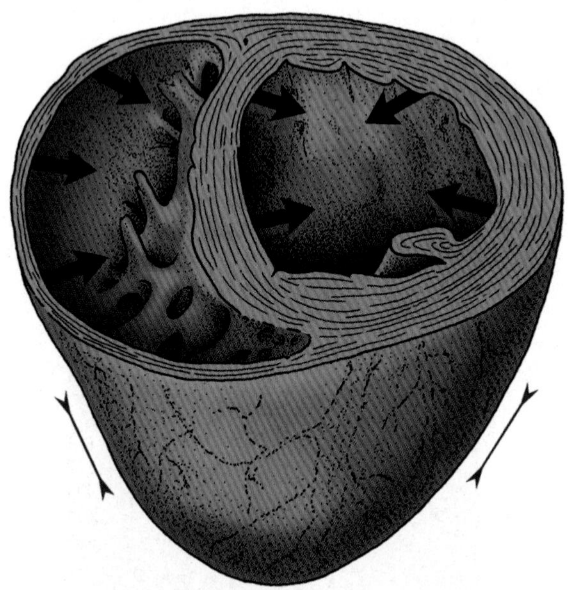

Fig. 7.24 Schematic drawing of the mode of contraction of the left and right ventricles. The wall of the left ventricle contracts radially, whereas the right ventricular lumen is squeezed in a bellows action. *Arrows* indicate direction of contraction.

later form the truncus arteriosus and ventricles, is at this stage contained within the pericardial cavity and suspended by a fold (dorsal mesocardium) extending between the myoepicardium and the pericardial wall (Fig. 7.1B/*9*). The caudal part, which forms the atria and sinus venosus, first lies caudal to the pericardial cavity embedded within the septum transversum. The enclosed (truncoventricular) part of the heart grows more rapidly than the pericardial space and is forced into a flexure whose apex is directed ventrocaudally and somewhat to the right. The atrial expansions of the initially paired endothelial tubes have now fused in a single common atrium continuous with the sinus venosus; this presents an unpaired transverse part that receives the paired horns created by the entry of the veins (Fig. 7.25).

The four heart chambers at this stage, in caudocranial sequence, are *sinus venosus, atrium, ventricle,* and *truncus arteriosus*. The atrium and ventricle are separated by a constriction called the *atrioventricular canal,* whereas the transition from ventricle to truncus forms the *arterial conus* (bulb of the heart). The truncus continues rostrally into the aortic arches, which now appear in the mesoderm to each side of the pharynx (see Fig. 7.2B). The sinus venosus receives the cardinal, vitelline, and umbilical systems of veins that extend from the body of the embryo,

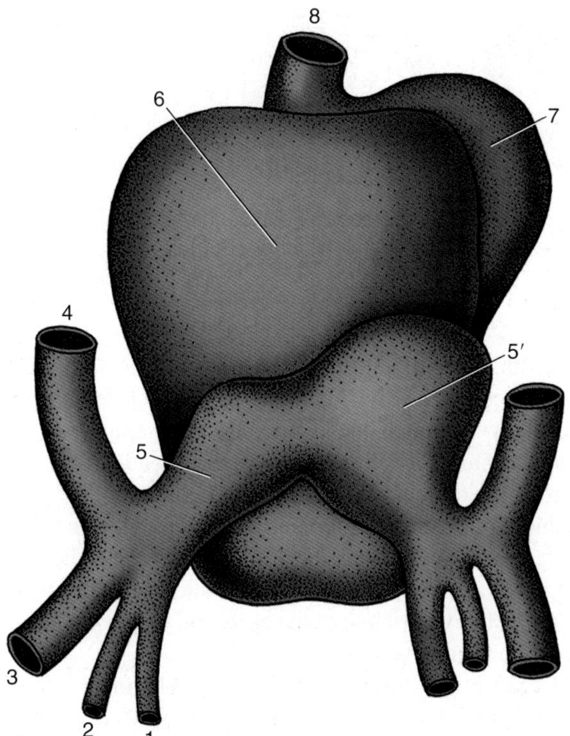

Fig. 7.25 Dorsal view of the developing heart. *1,* Vitelline vein (v.); *2,* umbilical v.; *3,* caudal cardinal v.; *4,* cranial cardinal v.; *5* and *5′,* left and right horns of sinus venosus; *6,* atrium, *7,* ventricle; *8,* truncus arteriosus.

the yolk sac, and the chorioallantois, respectively (see Fig. 7.25). The bifid character of the sinus venosus persists for a time, but its wide communication with the atrium gradually shifts toward the right as the amount of blood entering the left horn is diminished after the obliteration of the left umbilical and left vitelline veins. When the sinus is eventually incorporated within the atrium, the undivided part and the right horn contribute the sinus venarum of the adult right atrium, but the left horn is reduced to the coronary sinus. By this stage the sinus venosus and common atrium have also become included within the pericardial cavity, where they lie dorsal to the ventricle.

The appearance and subsequent growth of a crescentic ridge, known as the *septum primum*, initiates the division of the common atrium into right and left chambers (Fig. 7.26/*2*). This ridge projects ventrally into the lumen and at its ends grows toward thickenings of the wall of the atrioventricular canal known as the *endocardial cushions* (Fig. 7.26/*6*). The opening between its free margin and the cushions is known as the *ostium primum* (Fig. 7.26/*4*). The ostium primum is gradually occluded by the further enlargement of the cushions, but before closure is complete, a number of perforations appear within the septum and coalesce to form a fresh communication, the *ostium secundum* (Fig. 7.26/*5*), between the two atria. The definitive division of the atria is achieved by a second crest (Fig. 7.26/*3*) that now appears to the right of the primary partition. The concave free ventral margin of this second

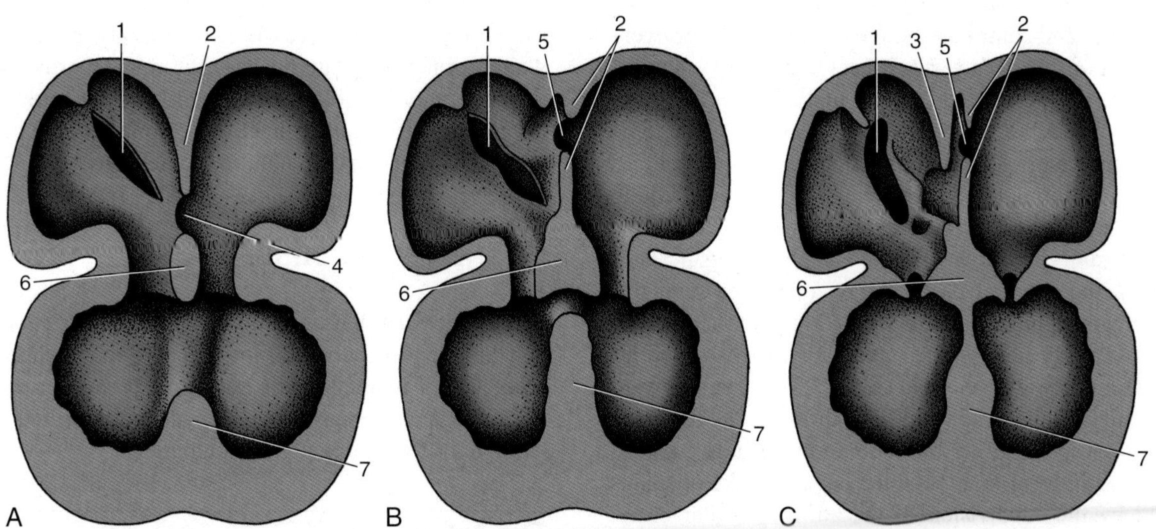

Fig. 7.26 (A) to (C) The partitioning of the atrium and ventricle, schematic. (A) The primary atrial septum has formed, and development of the interventricular septum has begun. (B) The primary atrial septum has fused with the endocardial cushions, and a secondary foramen *(5)* has been formed. (C) The secondary atrial septum has formed, and a passage (foramen ovale) between primary and secondary septa connects the right and left atria. Note the fusion of the interventricular septum with the endocardial cushions. *1,* Sinoatrial opening; *2,* primary atrial septum; *3,* secondary atrial septum; *4,* ostium primum; *5,* ostium secundum; *6,* fused endocardial cushions; *7,* interventricular septum.

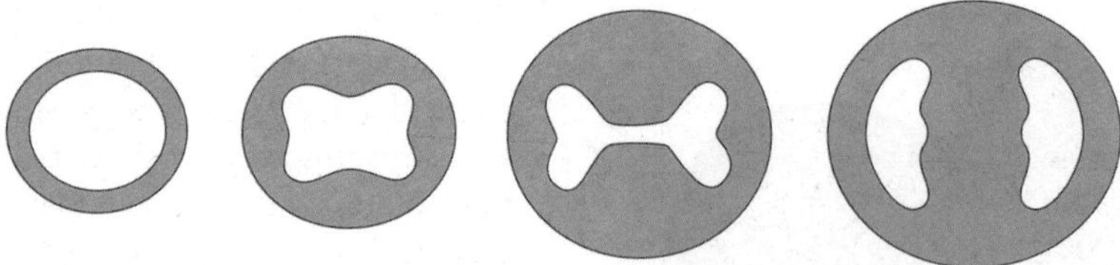

Fig. 7.27 *Left to right,* Partitioning of the atrioventricular canal by the endocardial cushions. The single atrioventricular canal is gradually divided into right and left atrioventricular openings.

crest overlaps the ostium secundum, reducing the passage between the atria to a narrow space, the foramen ovale, between the two septa (Fig. 7.26C). The remnant of the septum primum forms the valve of the foramen ovale. The final closure of the opening is accomplished after birth by the apposition and subsequent fusion of the valve to the septum secundum (p. 241).

Further growth and eventual mergence of the endocardial cushions divide the canal into the two openings that become the right and left atrioventricular ostia (Figs. 7.27 and 7.28B).

The septation of the truncus arteriosus and bulbus is achieved by the appearance, growth, and fusion of two endocardial ridges that run along the length of the truncus. The left one is known as the *septal ridge*, the right one as the *parietal* or *dorsal ridge*. Fusion of the ridges commences at the distal extremity of the truncus and gradually extends proximally, producing a partition that ends in a free edge arched over the common ventricle (Fig. 7.28B/*2* and *3*). The lower end of the parietal ridge expands within the ventricle and contributes to the closure of the atrioventricular ostium. The septal ridge fuses with the most cranial part of the interventricular septum that has been developing in the meantime.

This interventricular septum first appears as a falciform crest formed through local thickening of the myocardium at the apex of the ventricle; as it extends it divides the common cavity into right and left chambers (Fig. 7.26/*7*). Although the external conformation of the heart at this stage already approximates its final form, the truncus arteriosus (although now divided internally) appears to arise solely from the right ventricle (Fig. 7.28A). The two ventricles still communicate with each other over the free edge of the interventricular septum but are in separate communication with the atria through the paired slitlike openings created by the subdivision of the atrioventricular canal. The right atrioventricular opening is substantially bounded by the right part of the caudal endocardial cushion, less extensively by the cranial cushion, and partly, as already mentioned, by the parietal ridge of the truncus. These three contributions each form a separate cusp of the valve, and the truncus ridge contributes the parietal cusp.

The left atrioventricular valve has a similar origin, mainly from the cranial and caudal endocardial cushions but with a small additional (lateral) cushion forming the parietal cusp. The division of the ventricles is largely completed by fusion of the interventricular septum with the caudal cushion; it is finally achieved by fusion of the lower edge of the truncus septum with the right part of the caudal cushion and with the interventricular septum. Because the same process completes the aortic part of the truncus, the output of the heart is now divided into two streams: one from the left ventricle into the aorta and one from the right ventricle into the pulmonary trunk.

Because the process of heart development requires highly precise meeting and fusion of various elements, heart malformations are among the most common congenital abnormalities, affecting up to 1% of all human births. Heart malformations are also frequent in domestic animals. The more common malformations are defects of the cardiac septa, atresia or stenosis of the pulmonary or aortic trunks, or some combination of these anomalies (e.g., the tetralogy of Fallot: pulmonary stenosis, enlarged overriding aorta, ventricular septal defect, and hypertrophy of the right ventricle). Failure of closure of the oval foramen is generally without functional significance, but most other malformations are incompatible with normal life after birth. Surgical correction is neither practicable nor advisable in those affected animals that do not die spontaneously.

THE BLOOD VESSELS

The arteries, capillaries, and veins form a continuous system lined by an unbroken low-friction endothelium. The other layers of their walls vary greatly in construction, thickness, and even presence, in evident or presumed adaptation to different functional requirements.

The Arteries

The arterial wall is composed of three concentric tunics (Fig. 7.29A and B). The endothelium of the inner one (*tunica interna*) is supported by a thin layer of specialized connective tissue that is bounded externally by a well-developed, fenestrated elastic sheet, the inner elastic membrane (Fig. 7.29/*2*). The subendothelial connective tissue is frequently affected by arteriosclerotic changes

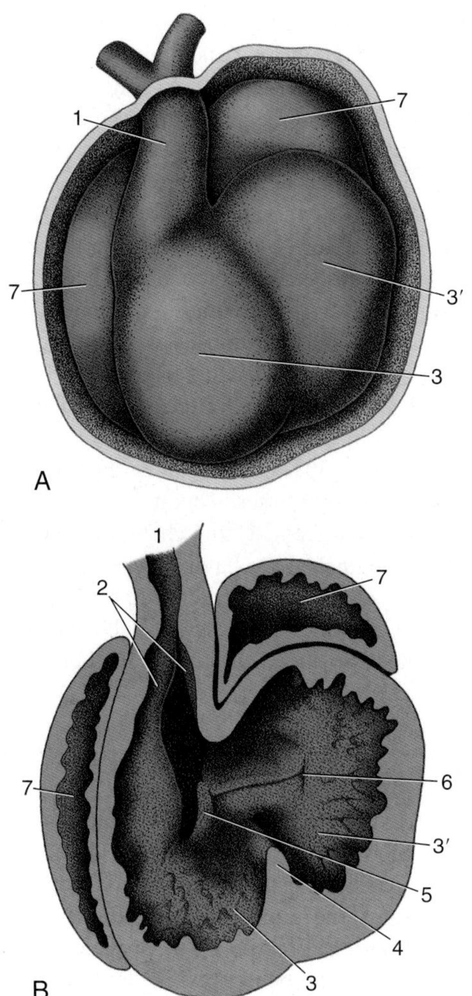

Fig. 7.28 The partitioning of the truncus arteriosus. (A) Ventral view of the developing heart. (B) The ventral part of the heart has been removed to expose the developing ridges *(2)* in the truncus arteriosus. *1,* Truncus arteriosus; *2,* ridges in truncus; *3,* right ventricle; *3′,* left ventricle; *4,* interventricular septum; *5,* right atrioventricular canal; *6,* left atrioventricular canal; *7,* atrium.

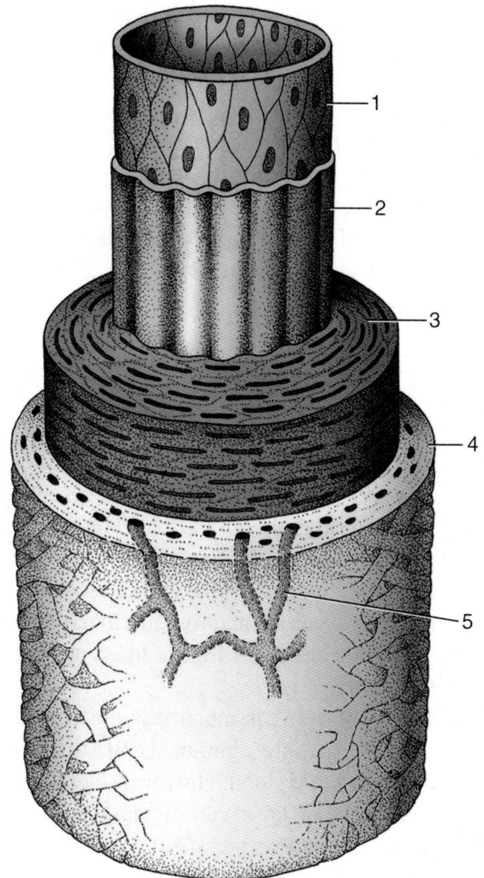

Fig. 7.29 The components of the arterial wall. *1* and *2,* Tunica interna (*1,* endothelium; *2,* inner elastic membrane); *3,* tunica media; *4,* tunica adventitia; *5,* vasa vasorum.

(hardening of the arteries), particularly though not exclusively in humans. The middle tunic (*tunica media*) is the thickest and most variable layer. It is composed of an elaborately organized admixture of elastic tissue and smooth muscle in varying proportions (Fig. 7.29/*3*). The outer tunic (*tunica adventitia*) is predominantly fibrous and grades into the fibroareolar tissue that limits expansion of the artery (Fig. 7.29/*4*).

The differences in the structure of the media results in three major classes of arteries. A few very large arteries that stretch upon receiving the systolic output of the ventricles have a media composed predominantly of concentric, fenestrated elastic membranes with relatively little muscle interspersed. The elastic tissue stretches to absorb and store the energy followed by its release upon recoil to aid the flow of blood toward the periphery. These elastic or conducting arteries are the first part of the aorta, certain of its major branches, and the pulmonary trunk.

The media of most named arteries and others of smaller size is composed largely of many closely spiraled layers of smooth muscles. The caliber of these muscular or distributing arteries is closely controlled by an autonomic innervation.

The smallest arteries, known as *arterioles,* principally regulate the resistance to the flow of blood and hence the peripheral blood pressure. The muscle, reduced to a few layers, is progressively shed. The openings of arterioles into capillaries are guarded by sphincters that regulate the vascular perfusion of capillary bed (Fig. 7.30).

The Capillaries and Sinusoids

The capillaries are reduced to narrow endothelial tubes supported by a very delicate connective tissue investment. They allow escape of fluid from the blood into the tissue interstitium at the arterial end followed by the resorption of some fluid toward the venous end (see Fig. 7.30). They permeate almost every tissue with varying densities. The capillaries have complete endothelium that allows transcellular transport of the fluid. However, some capillaries (fenestrated) present in intestinal villi and renal glomeruli have minute pores.

Sinusoids constitute a special type of capillary found in certain organs, including the liver, spleen, and bone marrow. They are wider, less regular, and more commonly fenestrated than ordinary capillaries, and their endothelial cells are able to extract colloidal substances from the blood.

The Veins

Although thinner walled, the larger veins have a construction similar to that of arteries. The smallest ones, the venules, may pass through several successive confluences before acquiring smooth muscle. The tunica interna of veins is always thin, lacks an elastic membrane, and is involved in the formation of the valves (see p. 25). The media is relatively weak, is mainly muscular, and has little admixture of elastic elements. Elastic fibers are more plentiful in the adventitia.

The structure of veins is much less uniform than that of arteries, but the specific significance of structural adaptations is not well understood. However, clear indications exist that the muscular layer can increase in thickness in response to elevated venous pressure (e.g., the digital veins of horses).

Arteriovenous Anastomoses

Direct connections between small arteries and veins exist in many parts of the body where they are used to short circuit the capillary bed (Fig. 7.31). One purpose of such connections is to shunt blood away from tissues of intermittent activity when they are resting; good examples are supplied by the thyroid gland and the gastric mucosa. Arteriovenous anastomoses are also concerned with temperature regulation and are plentiful in the digits, external ears, and nose. Paradoxically, they appear to be used in two ways. They open in a cold environment to prevent local overchilling of the appendages. The anastomoses also promote heat loss by increasing the throughput of blood close to the body's surface in overheated animals. The panting dog uses the circulation of blood through the many arteriovenous anastomoses within the tongue to promote the evaporation of saliva from the surface, which compensates to some degree for the restricted distribution of sweat glands in canine skin.

In the pig, up to 30% of the total cardiac output sometimes passes through arteriovenous anastomoses. The structure of these interconnecting channels is not uniform. Some are distinguished by having very muscular walls, and in others the muscle cells take on a peculiar epithelioid character; these epithelioid cells are believed to swell in response to specific chemical stimuli, thereby closing the channel.

Erectile Tissue

Erectile or cavernous tissue is a vascular specialization consisting of many close-packed, endothelium-lined spaces. The spaces are usually closed, but they are directly fed by arterioles and rapidly engorge under appropriate nervous stimulation. Erectile tissue provides a large part of the structure of the penis (p. 184) and the clitoris. In modified form it is also found in the teat wall, the nasal

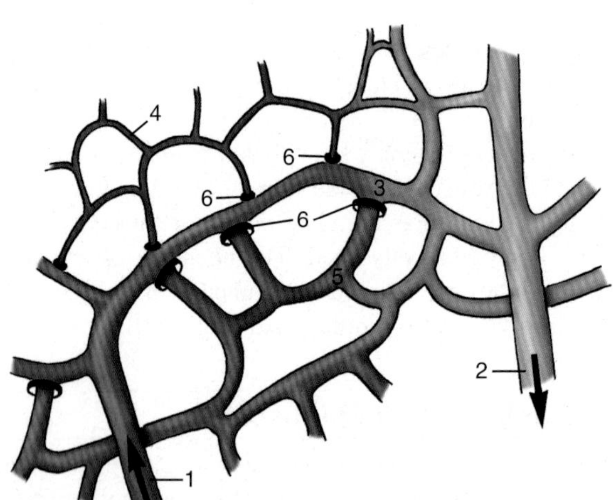

Fig. 7.30 Schematic drawing of a capillary plexus. *1,* Arteriole; *2,* venule; *3,* communicating (low-resistance) channel; *4,* closed capillaries; *5,* open capillaries; *6,* precapillary sphincters. *Arrows* indicate direction of blood flow.

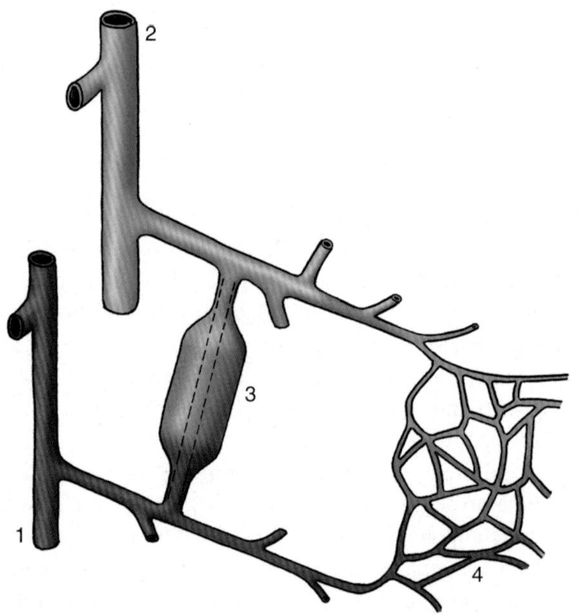

Fig. 7.31 Precapillary arteriovenous anastomosis. *1,* Artery; *2,* vein; *3,* arteriovenous anastomosis; *4,* capillary plexus.

mucosa, the vomeronasal organ, and a few other sites. A simultaneous response of the genital and nasal erectile tissue is common and may occur because perception of odors plays a significant part in the sexual behavior of many animals.

"Blood cushions" formed by a concentration of veins are associated with the gastrointestinal tract. One of veterinary interest is provided by the ileal papilla of the horse (Chapter 21), which has a considerable capacity for engorgement. In the human anal mucosa pads formed by the underlying veins are believed to contribute to closure of the orifice.

Vascularization and Innervation of the Vessel Wall

Like other tissues, blood vessel walls require nutrition. Diffusion from the lumen is sufficient to supply the needs of smaller vessels but requires supplementation by an intramural circulation for those of larger size. The supplying arteries (vasa vasorum) most often arise at some distance from the stretch of wall they feed, frequently coming from collateral branches. They penetrate the adventitia from outside and ramify within this layer and the adjoining part of the media (Fig. 7.32/*1*). They do not penetrate beyond the middle of the media in arteries. The tunica intima is never vascularized unless diseased.

Arteries and veins receive both a motor innervation and a sensory innervation. The vasomotor nerves control the diameters of the lumina of the arteries and hence the peripheral resistance. Most are vasoconstrictor fibers of sympathetic origin. Some pass directly to the great arteries from sympathetic plexuses within the mediastinum, but most first travel within local nerve trunks from which they later emerge to enmesh the peripheral arteries. The afferent supply is concerned in local and general vascular reflexes; some fibers mediate the sensation of pain perceived from arterial lesions.

In addition, certain specific sites are much more richly supplied with nerves whose endings respond to pressure or chemical stimuli. These baroreceptor and chemoreceptor concentrations, of great importance in the regulation of the circulation, are confined to arteries originating in the pharyngeal (branchial) arches: the internal carotid arteries, the aortic arch, the right subclavian artery, and the pulmonary trunk. The best known examples of each type, the carotid sinus and carotid body (glomus caroticum), are found in close association at the origin of the internal carotid artery (Fig. 7.33).

The carotid sinus may be recognized in the cadaver as a slightly expanded and especially distensible stretch at the origin of the internal carotid. Its baroreceptors respond to pressure changes that alter the mechanical tension in its wall. The carotid body is a neighboring nodule (sometimes palpable) composed of a richly vascularized mass of epithelioid cells. The chemoreceptors respond to changes in oxygen and carbon dioxide tension and hydrogen ion concentration in the perfusing blood. The afferent fibers from both receptor types travel in the carotid sinus branch (known to physiologists as the nerve of Hering) of the glossopharyngeal nerve to project on centers within the brainstem.

The less familiar receptor areas in the other arteries named are similar but less important. Specific differences exist, and in some animals they appear to decline in importance with the attainment of maturity.

Patterns of Arterial Distribution

We have already mentioned certain more obvious features of arterial distribution: the increase in total cross-sectional area at each branching, the variation in the angle

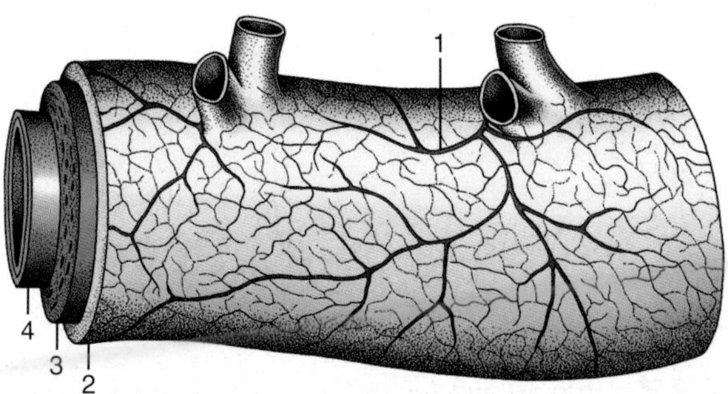

Fig. 7.32 Vasa vasorum in the wall of a large artery. *1,* Vasa vasorum; *2,* tunica adventitia; *3,* tunica media; *4,* tunica interna.

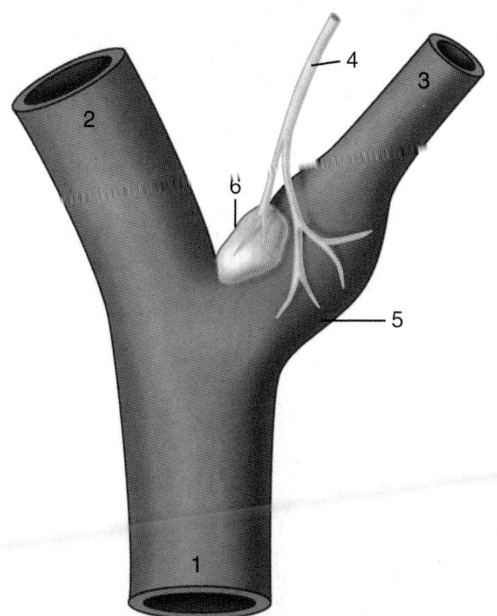

Fig. 7.33 Baroreceptors and chemoreceptors at the origin of the internal carotid artery (a.). *1,* Common carotid a.; *2,* external carotid a.; *3,* internal carotid a.; *4,* carotid sinus branch of the glossopharyngeal nerve; *5,* carotid sinus (baroreceptor); *6,* carotid body (chemoreceptor).

of branching, the preference for protected courses within the limbs, and the generosity of interarterial anastomoses (p. 25). Amplification of the description of certain features is required.

Collateral Circulation

Few arteries of any size terminate in capillary beds without first detaching side or collateral branches. Most collateral branches, whether large or small, anastomose with their neighbors, connections that may not be apparent on dissection because so many are concealed within muscles and other organs (Fig. 7.34). The anastomoses enlarge when the bloodstream is diverted from its normal route by occlusion of a principal trunk; the widening initially is due to relaxation and stretching of the wall but later is due to reconstruction of the anastomotic links. Thus, provided that sufficient blood can pass in the meantime, tissues deprived of their usual sources of supply generally survive, though possible temporary loss of function of the ischemic parts may occur. Experiments have shown that healthy dogs have a fair chance of survival even if the aorta is ligated (caudal to the origin of the renal arteries). The ability to develop an adequate collateral circulation is increased when the obstruction develops slowly but is markedly lessened by sudden onset of obstruction, aging, or pathologic changes in the vessel wall.

The blockage of end-arteries produces a cone-shaped infraction. By strict definition, the end-artery is a rarity, but "functional" end-arteries, in which the collateral connections are of insufficient caliber, are more common (Fig. 7.35). The adequacy of collateral circulation cannot be assessed from purely morphologic evidence. For example, intramuscular arteries appear to anastomose freely, but the occlusion of one frequently leads to local necrosis. The consequences of obstruction of the central artery of the retina and many small vessels within the brain that lack adequate anastomoses are immediate and catastrophic. This situation may be contrasted with the liberal anastomoses between the major arteries that join to form the arterial circle on the ventral surface of the brain. Although anastomoses between finer branches of the coronary arteries are also poor and usually incapable of maintaining an adequate collateral circulation, not all coronary emboli are fatal. Much of the outcome may depend on the size and specific site of the infarct and on immediate medical care.

Anastomoses between small arteries within the limbs are especially numerous in the regions of the joints and sometimes form visible networks or retia; a prominent

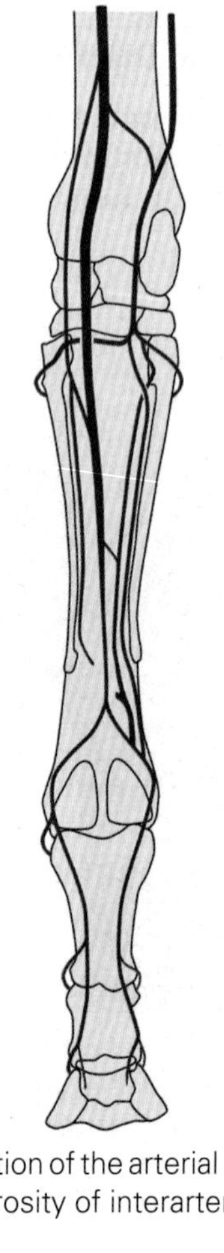

Fig. 7.34 This illustration of the arterial pattern of the equine limb shows the generosity of interarterial anastomoses.

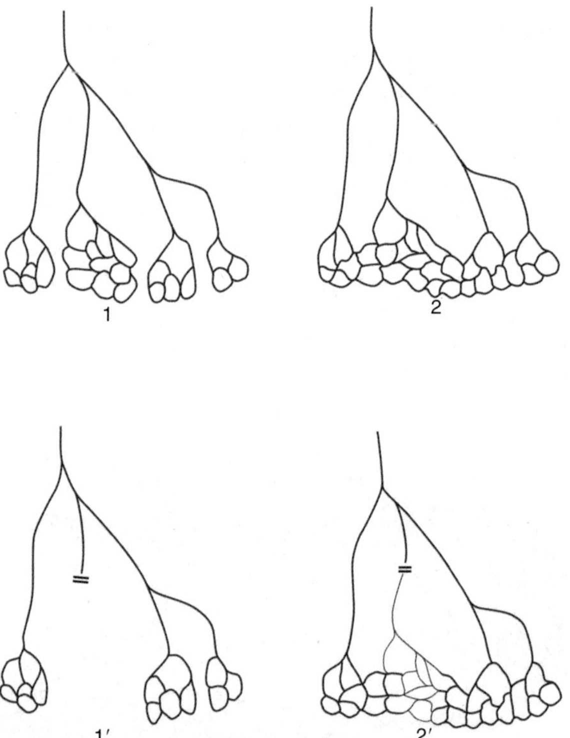

Fig. 7.35 True *(1)* and functional *(2)* end-arteries. Closure *(double black lines)* of an end-artery leads to necrosis of the tissue it supplies *(1′)*. In the case of a functional end-artery *(2)*, a potential but inadequate alternative route exists *(2′)*.

example exists over the dorsal aspect of the carpus of the horse (rete carpi dorsale).

The retia just described are not to be confused with the so-called retia mirabilia of more restricted occurrence. Retia mirabilia are found where a main trunk splits more or less at once into a leash of parallel vessels. The "bipolar" arrangement has parallel trunks reuniting later, as in the arteries to the brain in some species (Fig. 7.36/*7*) and, on a diminished scale, in the renal glomeruli (see Fig. 5.28). In the "unipolar" arrangement, the branches remain separate as found within the limbs of slow-moving arboreal creatures (sloths, lemurs) and in the thoracic cavity of whales and other diving mammals. No convincing explanations exist of the adaptive value of most of these arrangements; the renal glomeruli, however, are the obvious exception (p. 170).

SYSTEMATIC ANGIOLOGY

This section provides an outline of the arterial and venous trees derived from dog as a model. Only a few most salient comparative features are discussed here; the vascularization of particular organs and regions of special functional or clinical importance are included in other chapters.

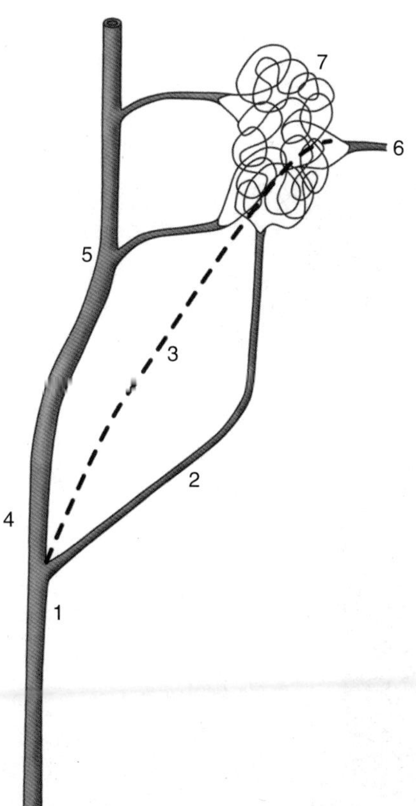

Fig. 7.36 A rete mirabile interposed on the blood supply to the bovine brain. *1,* Common carotid artery (a.); *2,* occipital a.; *3,* internal carotid a. (regresses after birth); *4,* external carotid a.; *5,* maxillary a.; *6,* branch from rete to arterial circle of the brain; *7,* rostral epidural rete mirabile.

The Pulmonary Circulation

The Pulmonary Arteries

The *pulmonary trunk* arises from the pulmonary orifice of the right ventricle on the craniosinistral aspect of the heart. It is slightly expanded at its origin, where it presents a small sinus above each cusp of the pulmonary valve. The trunk (Fig. 7.9A/*5*) passes between the two auricles and then bends caudally over the base of the heart, where it is joined on its right face by the ligamentum arteriosum, the fibrosed remnant of the ductus arteriosus (p. 241). After penetrating the pericardium, it divides into right and left *pulmonary arteries,* each directed to the hilus of the corresponding lung in company with the principal bronchus and pulmonary veins (Fig. 7.9/*10* and *10'*). The course of the right artery carries it ventral to the trachea.

The pulmonary arteries make their initial branching before entering the lung (see Fig. 4.23); their further ramifications have already been briefly noted (p. 153).

The Pulmonary Veins

The pulmonary veins open variously into the roof of the left atrium. They form two clusters in the dog: one for the veins draining each lung. In some other species the veins draining the caudal lobes of both lungs form a separate third cluster. Valves are absent from these veins.

The Systemic Circulation

The Systemic Arteries

The Aortic Arch. The origin of the aorta is similar to that of the pulmonary trunk but is from the left ventricle. The initial portion, the aortic bulb, is concealed between the atria and forms sinuses above the three cusps of the aortic valve; the right coronary artery arises from the cranial sinus, the left artery from the caudosinistral sinus (Fig. 7.18/*5* and *6*). Beyond this, the aorta arches cranially, dorsally, and caudally, penetrating the pericardium to ascend within the mediastinum to reach the sinistroventral aspect of the vertebral column about the level of the seventh thoracic vertebra (Fig. 7.37). In addition to the *coronary arteries* (p. 218) the first part of the aorta gives origin to the *paired subclavian* and paired *common carotid arteries*. These vessels amalgamate at their origins to form a short, cranially directed *brachiocephalic trunk* in the larger species (Fig. 7.38). In the dog and pig the left subclavian artery remains distinct and takes a separate, more distal origin (Fig. 7.37/*4*). The common carotid arteries supply structures of the head.

The *subclavian artery* (Fig. 7.37/*4*) supplies blood to the forelimb and to structures of the neck and cervicothoracic junction. It winds around the cranial border of the first rib to enter the limb through the axilla to become the axillary artery. The subclavian detaches four branches in its intrathoracic course. The first, the *vertebral artery* (Fig. 7.37/*6*), runs craniodorsally, dives between the scalenus and longus colli muscles, and then passes through the successive

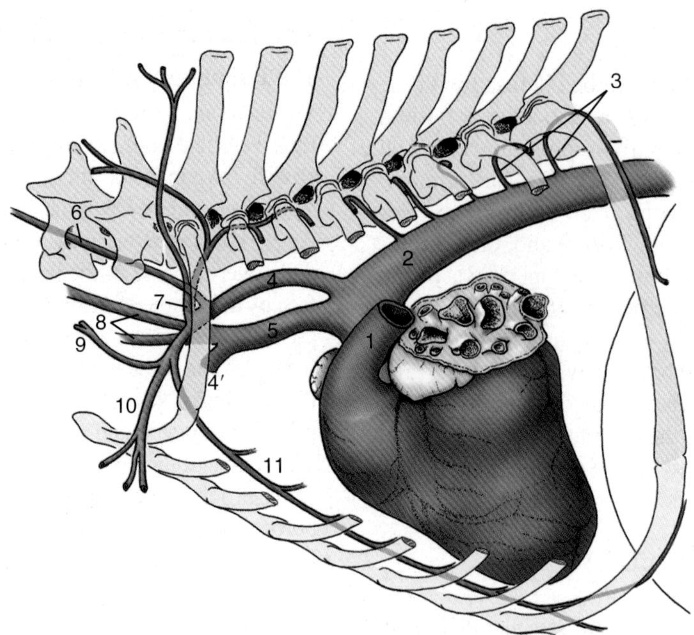

Fig. 7.37 Branching of the aortic arch in the dog. (In this series of figures, not all arteries depicted are named.) *1,* Pulmonary trunk; *2,* aorta; *3,* intercostal aa.; *4,* left subclavian a.; *4′,* right subclavian a.; *5,* brachiocephalic trunk; *6,* vertebral a.; *7,* costocervical trunk; *8,* left and right common carotid aa.; *9,* superficial cervical a.; *10,* axillary a.; *11,* internal thoracic a.

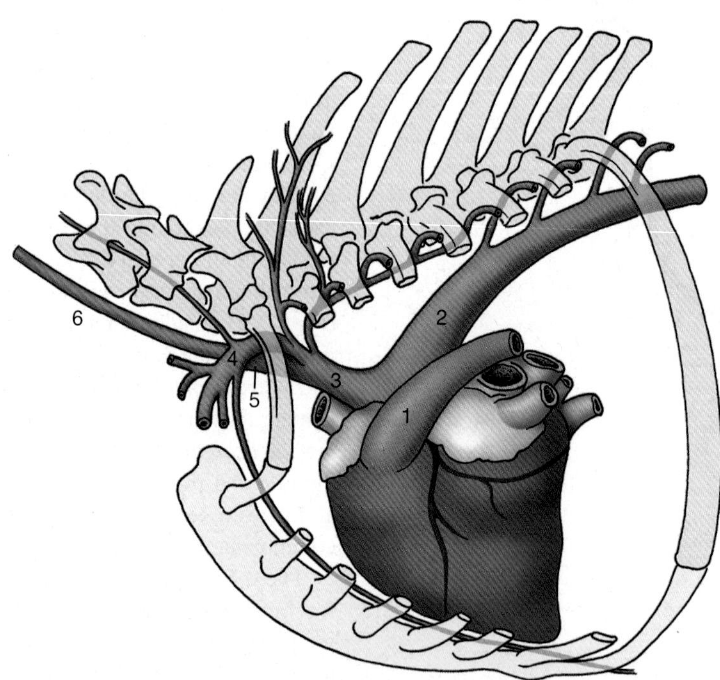

Fig. 7.38 Branching of the aortic arch in the horse. The arteries to the head and neck and to the forelimbs originate from a short brachiocephalic trunk *(3)*. *1,* Pulmonary trunk; *2,* aortic arch; *3,* brachiocephalic trunk; *4,* left subclavian artery; *5,* bicarotid trunk; *6,* left common carotid artery.

transverse foramina of the sixth to first cervical vertebrae. After receiving the termination of the occipital artery, it enters the vertebral canal within the atlas and there divides into a basilar artery to the brain and the ventral artery of the spinal cord (p. 299). Twigs are detached en route to the vertebral column, covering muscles, and contents of the vertebral canal.

The larger second branch, the *costocervical trunk* (Fig. 7.37/*7*), provides the first few dorsal intercostal arteries and the *deep cervical artery,* which ascends the neck within the dorsal cervical musculature that it supplies.

The *internal thoracic artery* (Fig. 7.37/*11*), the third branch, curves ventrally within the mediastinum to pass between the transversus thoracic and the sternum. It follows the sternum and tunnels below the diaphragm to continue as the cranial epigastric artery of the abdominal floor. Collateral branches include twigs to the pleura, thymus, and pericardium, perforating branches to the pectoral muscles and thoracic mammary glands, and ventral intercostal arteries. The more caudal ventral intercostal branches arise from a common trunk, the musculophrenic artery, which follows the lateral attachment of the diaphragm. The *cranial epigastric artery* divides into superficial and deep branches; the latter follows the deep face of the rectus abdominis to an anastomosis with the caudal epigastric artery within the substance of this muscle. The superficial branch passes to the superficial fascia, where it assists in the supply of the abdominal mammary glands.

The *superficial cervical artery* (Fig. 7.37/*9*), the fourth branch, arises from the subclavian opposite the origin of the internal thoracic. It supplies muscles of the ventral part of the neck, the cranial part of the shoulder, and the upper arm.

Aortic arch

- Coronary aa. *(supply heart musculature)*
- Brachiocephalic trunk
  - Right subclavian a. *(supplies forelimb, neck structures, and cervicothoracic junction)*
    - Vertebral a. *(supplies vertebral column, covering muscles, and vertebral canal content)*
    - Costocervical trunk
      - Deep cervical a. *(supplies dorsal cervical muscles)*
    - Internal thoracic a.
      - Ventral intercostal aa. *(supply intercostal muscles)*
      - Cranial epigastric a. *(rectus abdominis muscles and abdominal mammary glands)*
      - Musculophrenic a. *(supplies structures of diaphragm)*
    - Superficial cervical a. *(supplies muscles at base of neck, cranial part of shoulder, and upper arm)*
  - Common carotid aa. *(supply structures of head)*
- Left subclavian a. *(its branches correspond to those of the right subclavian artery)*

a. stands for artery and aa. stands for arteries

The Axillary Artery. The *axillary artery* (Fig. 7.39/*1*), the magistral trunk of the forelimb, crosses the axilla to continue distally over the medial surface of the arm. It becomes the brachial artery when level with the teres major tuberosity (Fig. 7.39/*6*). The axillary gives

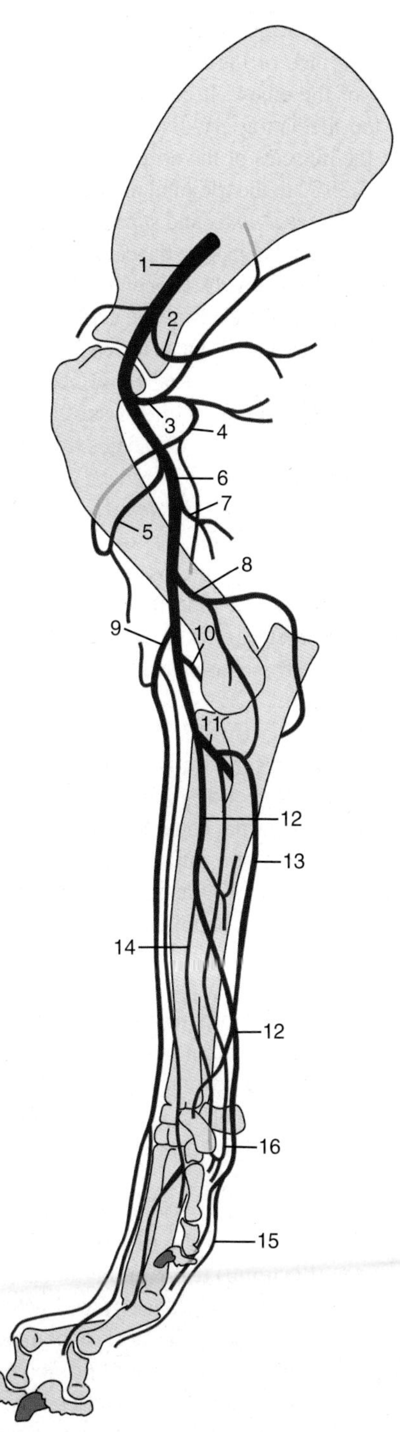

Fig. 7.39 Arteries of the canine forelimb. *1,* Axillary artery (a.); *2,* lateral thoracic a.; *3,* subscapular a.; *4,* caudal circumflex humeral a.; *5,* cranial circumflex humeral a.; *6,* brachial a.; *7,* deep brachial a.; *8,* collateral ulnar a.; *9,* superficial brachial a.; *10,* transverse cubital a.; *11,* common interosseous a.; *12,* median a.; *13,* ulnar a.; *14,* radial a.; *15,* superficial palmar arch; *16,* deep palmar arch.

external and *lateral thoracic arteries* to the chest wall and one important collateral branch to the limb, the *subscapular artery* (Fig. 7.39/*3*), which runs dorsally along the caudal border of the scapula between the subscapularis and teres major to supply branches to the muscles of the shoulder.

The *brachial artery* (Fig. 7.39/*6*) passes obliquely over the medial surface of the humerus to reach the craniomedial aspect of the elbow. It continues into the forearm and becomes the median artery. Its collateral branches include several to the muscles of the arm, principally the *deep brachial* (Fig. 7.39/*7*) to the tricipital muscles; toward the elbow it detaches *collateral ulnar* and *superficial brachial arteries* (Fig. 7.39/*8* and *9*) that pass to the caudal and cranial aspects of the forearm, respectively. Branches of the superficial brachial run subcutaneously beside the cephalic vein and superficial branch of the radial nerve to reach the dorsum of the paw. The *transverse cubital artery* (Fig. 7.39/*10*) is detached just proximal to the elbow joint. A substantial branch, the *common interosseous artery,* originates from the main artery distal to the elbow.

The *common interosseous artery* (Fig. 7.39/*11*) detaches the *ulnar artery* (Fig. 7.39/*13*) for the digital and carpal flexors and the caudal interosseous artery, which runs between the radius and ulna to reach the palmar arches of the proximal metacarpus. A cranial interosseous artery penetrates the interosseous space to supply the dorsal muscles of the forearm.

The *median artery* (Fig. 7.39/*12*) runs down the caudomedial aspect of the forearm in company with the median nerve and under protection of the flexor carpi radialis. It passes through the carpal canal to end by concurring with branches of the common interosseous in forming palmar arterial arches (Fig. 7.39/*15* and *16*) from which the palmar aspect of the forepaw is supplied.

The paw receives its principal blood supply on its palmar aspect where (deep) palmar metacarpal and (more superficial) palmar common digital arteries run at the boundaries of the metacarpal bones before dividing at their distal ends into proper palmar digital arteries that follow the axial borders of the digits. The corresponding but narrower dorsal common and proper digital arteries follow a similar pattern.

The Common Carotid Artery. The common carotid arteries arise separately in the dog (Fig. 7.37/*8*) and by a short common (bicarotid) trunk in ungulates (Fig. 7.38/*5*). Each crosses the ventrolateral face of the trachea (or esophagus on the left) to ascend the neck accompanied by the vagosympathetic trunk before dividing above the larynx into external and internal carotid arteries. The *caudal* and *cranial thyroid arteries* are the only significant collateral branches of the common carotid artery, and the cranial thyroid artery gives off the laryngeal and pharyngeal branches.

The *external carotid artery,* the larger of the terminal branches, appears as the direct continuation of the parent trunk (Fig. 7.40/*1* and *2*). In the dog it shortly detaches the

Axillary a. *(supplies forelimb)*
- External thoracic a. *(supplies superficial pectoral muscle)*
- Lateral thoracic a. *(supplies muscles of chest wall such as latissimus dorsi)*
- Subscapular a. *(supplies muscles of shoulder and scapula)*

Brachial a.
- Deep brachial a. *(supplies tricipital muscles)*
- Collateral ulnar a. *(supplies triceps)*
- Superficial brachial a. *(supplies dorsal surface of paw)*
    - Cranial superficial antebrachial a.
        - Dorsal common digital aa.
- Transverse cubital a.
- Common interosseous a.
    - Ulnar a. *(supplies digital and carpal flexors ulnar and humeral heads of deep digital flexor and flexor carpi ulnaris)*
    - Cranial interosseous a. *(supplies dorsal muscles of forearm)*
    - Caudal interosseous a. *(supplies metacarpal and digital areas)*
        - Superficial palmar arch
            - Palmar common digital aa.
        - Deep palmar arch
            - Palmar metacarpal aa.

Median a. *(supplies palmar aspect of paw)*
- **Radial a.**

(The small arteries of the forepaw arise from anastomoses not listed.)

occipital artery, which branches from the internal carotid in some other species, and is continued as the maxillary artery (Fig. 7.40/*11*).

The external carotid in this narrow sense forms a short dorsally convex arch resting on the pharynx and covered by the mandibular gland and digastricus muscle. It has the following branches:

- The *occipital artery* (Fig. 7.40/*4*) runs to the condyloid fossa, where it divides into several branches that supply, among other structures, the middle and internal ear and the caudal meninges. The largest branch, effectively the continuation of the stem, passes to the atlantal fossa to an anastomosis with the vertebral artery and participates in the supply to the brain (p. 299).
- The *cranial laryngeal* and *ascending pharyngeal arteries* (Fig. 7.40/*5* and *6*) are the principal supplies to the larynx and pharynx, respectively. The large *lingual artery* (Fig. 7.40/*7*) pursues a rostroventral course over the pharynx to enter the tongue between the genioglossus and hyoglossus muscles. It principally supplies the tongue, but one of the collateral branches detached is to the palatine tonsil, which is of potential importance to the surgeon (p. 376).
- The *facial artery* (Fig. 7.40/*8*) arises near the angle of the jaw and runs within the intermandibular space

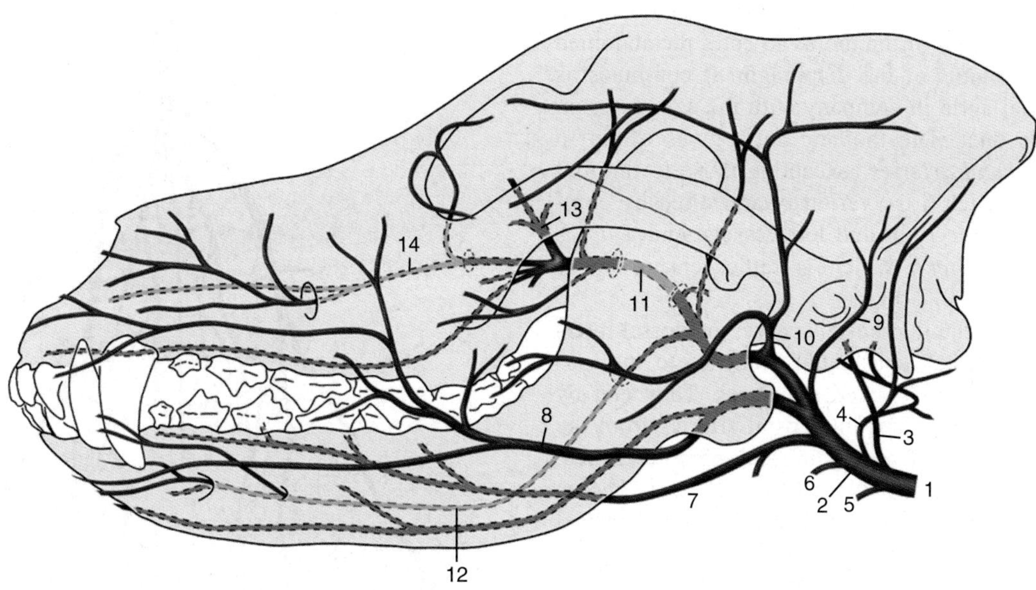

Fig. 7.40 Arteries of the canine head. *1,* Common carotid artery (a.); *2,* external carotid a.; *3,* internal carotid a.; *4,* occipital a.; *5,* cranial laryngeal a.; *6,* ascending pharyngeal a.; *7,* lingual a.; *8,* facial a.; *9,* caudal auricular a.; *10,* superficial temporal a.; *11,* maxillary a.; *12,* inferior alveolar a.; *13,* external ophthalmic a.; *14,* infraorbital a.

before winding around the ventral border of the mandible, where it is conveniently located for pulse taking in larger species. It then divides into various branches for the lips, lateral nose, and angle of the mouth. The relatively large *caudal auricular artery* (Fig. 7.40/*9*) generously supplies the external ear and associated muscles. The *parotid artery* supplies the parotid gland.

- The *superficial temporal artery* (Fig. 7.40/*10*) winds onto the face and runs forward to supply the masseter. In the dog it branches to the upper and lower eyelids and dorsum of the nose. The position and firm support of one of the branches (transverse facial artery) suit it to pulse taking in larger species.
- The *maxillary artery* (Fig. 7.40/*11*) passes through the alar canal to enter the pterygopalatine fossa. Before reaching the canal, its main branch is the *inferior alveolar artery* (Fig. 7.40/*12*), which enters the mandible to supply the alveoli and teeth and, through mental branches that emerge from the bone, the lower lip and the chin region. Other maxillary branches pass to the tympanic cavity, muscles of mastication, and cranial meninges (the last passing through the oval foramen). No branches are detached from the stretch of artery within the canal, but a sheaf of diverging vessels comes off directly as it reaches the pterygopalatine fossa. The most important is the *external ophthalmic artery* (Fig. 7.40/*13*) going to the contents of the orbit (p. 329). Others include the *ethmoidal artery* to the nasal cavity, the *major* and *minor palatine arteries* to the hard and soft palates, respectively, and the continuation (*infraorbital artery*) of the main trunk into the superior alveolar canal (Fig. 7.40/*14*).
- The *internal carotid artery* (Fig. 7.40/*3*) enters the cranial cavity through the jugular foramen and carotid canal, taking a rather indirect course in the dog (p. 384). It divides within the cavity into divergent caudal and rostral branches that concur with their contralateral counterparts and forms an arterial circle with the basilar artery to supply the brain (p. 299).

Common carotid a.

- Caudal thyroid a.
- Cranial thyroid a.
- External carotid a.
  - Occipital a. *(supplies middle and internal ear, and meninges)*
  - Cranial laryngeal a. *(supplies larynx)*
  - Ascending pharyngeal a. *(supplies pharynx)*
  - Lingual a. *(supplies tongue and palatine tonsil)*
  - Facial a. *(supplies lips, lateral nose, and angle of the mouth)*
  - Caudal auricular a. *(supplies external ear and associated muscles)*
  - Parotid a. *(supplies parotid gland)*
  - Superficial temporal a. *(supplies masseter and upper and lower eyelids)*
  - Maxillary a.
    - Inferior alveolar a. *(supplies alveoli and teeth)*
    - External ophthalmic a. *(supplies the orbital contents)*
    - Ethmoidal a. *(supplies nasal cavity)*
    - Palatine aa. *(supply hard and soft palate)*
    - Infraorbital a. *(supply alveolar canal)*
- Internal carotid a. *(supplies brain along with basilar artery)*

The Thoracic Aorta. The thoracic aorta runs caudally below the roof of the thorax to enter the abdomen by the aortic hiatus of the diaphragm. It continues as the abdominal aorta in company with the azygous vein and thoracic duct. The thoracic aorta gives origin to *dorsal intercostal arteries* (excepting those to the first few spaces), which arise variously and often by common trunks for the right and left vessels, and a *bronchoesophageal artery,* which is rather erratic in its origin.

In addition to the intercostal spaces, the dorsal intercostal arteries detach substantial branches to the vertebral column and associated structures. They end by anastomosing with ventral intercostal arteries from the internal thoracic artery and its musculophrenic branch. The corresponding artery behind the last rib is known as the *dorsal costoabdominal.* The bronchoesophageal artery gives rise to bronchial branches for the tissues of the lungs and esophageal branches for much of the thoracic esophagus.

Thoracic aorta
- Dorsal intercostal aa. *(supply intercostal muscles and vertebral column)*
- Bronchoesophageal a.
  - Bronchial branches *(supply lung tissue)*
  - Esophageal branches *(supply thoracic esophagus)*
- Dorsal costoabdominal a. *(supply area behind last rib)*

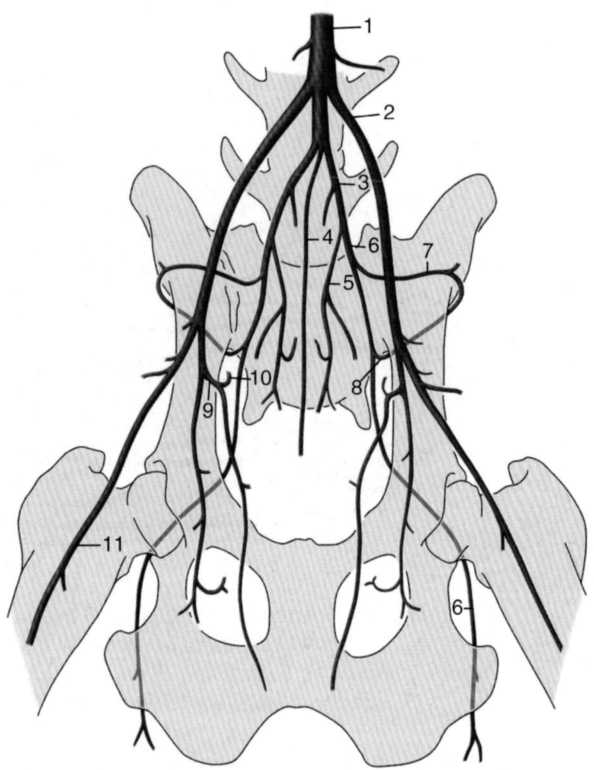

Fig. 7.41 Termination of the canine abdominal aorta (ventral view). *1,* Aorta; *2,* external iliac artery (a.); *3,* internal iliac a.; *4,* median sacral a.; *5,* internal pudendal a.; *6,* caudal gluteal a.; *7,* iliolumbar a.; *8,* cranial gluteal a.; *9,* deep femoral a.; *10,* pudendoepigastric trunk; *11,* femoral a.

The Abdominal Aorta. The abdominal aorta follows the roof of the abdomen, related to the caudal vena cava on its right and the psoas muscles on its left. Shortly after releasing the paired external iliac arteries, the abdominal aorta terminates in the dog below the last lumbar vertebra by branching off the internal iliac arteries and then continues as the much smaller *median sacral artery* that extends into the tail (Fig. 7.41/*2–4*). Along its course the abdominal aorta detaches both visceral and parietal branches.

The visceral arteries have been considered with the organs they supply. They comprise the unpaired celiac (p. 118), cranial mesenteric (p. 125), and caudal mesenteric (p. 125) arteries and the paired renal (p. 170) and testicular (p. 178 or ovarian [p. 191]) arteries. The unpaired vessels represent the arteries of the caudal foregut, midgut, and hindgut of the embryo (see Fig. 3.65).

The collateral parietal branches begin with the caudal phrenic and cranial abdominal arteries, which share a common *phrenicoabdominal* origin in the dog. They also include the paired *lumbar arteries* to the tissues and structures of the back, the *deep circumflex iliac* to the flank, the *external iliac artery* to the hindlimb, and the *internal iliac artery,* which serves both pelvic viscera and pelvic walls.

It is worth drawing attention at this point to the existence of several pathways, established by anastomosis, that mitigate the effects of constriction or blockage of the aorta (e.g., by thrombosis, especially common in the cat). The collateral pathways include those formed along the spinal cord by anastomoses between successive lumbar arteries, those along the gut formed by connections between the principal visceral arteries, and those within the abdominal floor formed by the cranial and caudal epigastric arteries.

The External Iliac Artery. The principal artery of the hindlimb, the external iliac artery arises close to the termination of the aorta and runs obliquely over the abdominal roof to leave the abdomen by the vascular lacuna above the caudodorsal corner of the flank (Fig. 7.42/*3*). It detaches one branch within the abdomen, the *deep femoral artery* (Fig. 7.42/*12*), which is the common origin of the pudendoepigastric trunk and an important branch to the adductor muscles of the thigh. The short *pudendoepigastric trunk* (Fig. 7.42/*13*) ends by giving rise to the *caudal epigastric* and *external pudendal arteries.* The former

Abdominal aorta

- Phrenicoabdominal aa. *(supply the diaphragmatic structures and the abdominal wall)*
- Lumbar aa. *(supply the tissue and structures of the back)*
- Celiac a. *(supplies the liver, spleen, and stomach with the named arteries)*
  - Left gastric a.
  - Hepatic a.
    - Hepatic branches
    - Right gastric a.
    - Gastroduodenal a.
    - Cranial pancreaticoduodenal a.
    - Right gastroepiploic a.
  - Splenic a.
    - Pancreatic branches
    - Short gastric aa.
    - Left gastroepiploic a.
- Cranial mesenteric a. *(supplies intestinal tract)*
  - Caudal pancreaticoduodenal a.
  - Jejunal aa.
  - Ileal aa.
  - Ileocolic a.
    - Middle colic a.
    - R. colic a.
    - Cecal aa.
- Renal aa. *(supply the kidneys)*
- Testicular *(ovarian)* aa. *(supply testes or ovaries)*
- Caudal mesenteric a. *(supplies intestinal tract)*
  - Left colic a.
  - Cranial rectal a.
- Deep circumflex iliac aa. *(supply flank region)*
- External iliac aa. *(supply hindlimb)*
- Internal iliac aa. *(supply pelvic wall and pelvic viscera)*
- Median sacral a. *(supplies tail)*
  - Lumbar a. VI
- Median caudal a.

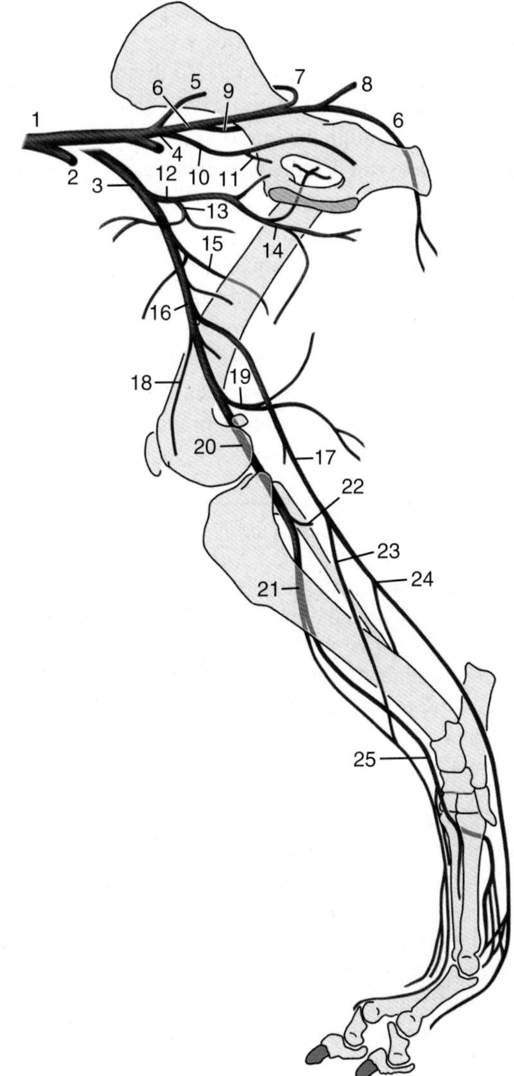

Fig. 7.42 Arteries of the canine hindlimb. *1,* Abdominal aorta; *2,* left external iliac artery (a.); *3,* right external iliac a.; *4,* left and right internal iliac arteries; *5,* median sacral a.; *6,* caudal gluteal a.; *7,* cranial gluteal a.; *8,* lateral caudal a.; *9,* iliolumbar a.; *10,* internal pudendal a.; *11,* vaginal (prostatic) a.; *12,* deep femoral a.; *13,* pudendoepigastric trunk; *14,* medial circumflex femoral a.; *15,* lateral circumflex femoral a.; *16,* femoral a.; *17,* saphenous a.; *18,* descending genicular a.; *19,* distal caudal femoral a.; *20,* popliteal a.; *21,* cranial tibial a.; *22,* caudal tibial a.; *23,* cranial branch of the saphenous a.; *24,* caudal branch of the saphenous a.; *25,* dorsal pedal a.

divides in similar fashion to the cranial epigastric; the latter passes through the inguinal canal to supply structures in the groin, including the prepuce in the male and the caudal mammary glands (via the caudal superficial epigastric artery) in the bitch.

On leaving the abdomen, the external iliac continues as the *femoral artery* (Fig. 7.42/*16*). Its first part has a superficial position in the femoral triangle—between the sartorius and pectineus—where it raises a visible ridge and is ideally located for pulse taking. It then burrows more deeply among the muscles to cross the medial surface of the femur to gain the caudal aspect of the thigh; it continues directly over the capsule of the stifle joint as the *popliteal artery*. The femoral artery has many branches, named and unnamed, to the muscles of the thigh, but most do not require individual notice. The *saphenous artery* (Fig. 7.42/*17*), which is detached in midthigh, is a more important vessel in carnivores than in the larger species, and it descends over the medial aspect of the limb before dividing into cranial and caudal branches. The cranial branch (Fig. 7.42/*23*) supplies the dorsal crural muscles before crossing the dorsal aspect of the hock to continue as the *dorsal common digital arteries*. The caudal branch (Fig. 7.42/*24*) takes a deep course between the muscles of the caudal aspect of the leg (crus), which it supplies, crosses the caudal face of the hock, and terminates as the plantar common digital arteries, which are comparable to the corresponding forelimb arteries.

The *popliteal artery* (Fig. 7.42/*20*) divides into cranial and caudal tibial arteries. The *cranial tibial artery* (Fig. 7.42/*21*) passes through the interosseous space between the tibia and fibula to run distally with the deep peroneal nerve. It crosses the dorsal aspect of the hock (as the dorsal pedal artery; Fig. 7.42/*25*) and gives rise to the dorsal metatarsal arteries among other branches. One of these metatarsal arteries reinforces the caudal branch of the saphenous on the plantar aspect of the limb after passing between the second and third metatarsal bones. The *caudal tibial artery* (Fig. 7.42/*22*) is of little account in carnivores. The following list includes various muscular branches not mentioned in the text.

External iliac a. *(principal supply of hindlimb)*
- Deep femoral a. *(supplies adductor muscles)*
  - Pudendoepigastric trunk
    - Caudal epigastric a. *(supplies rectus abdominis muscle)*
    - External pudendal a. *(supplies groin structures, prepuce, and caudal mammary glands)*

Femoral a. *(used for pulse taking in femoral triangle area)*
- Lateral circumflex femoral a.
- Proximal, middle, and distal caudal femoral aa.
- Saphenous a.
  - Cranial branch *(supplies dorsal caudal muscles)*
    - Dorsal common digital aa. *(supply digits)*
- Caudal branch *(supplies caudal muscles of leg/crus)*
  - Plantar common digital aa. *(supply digits)*

Popliteal a. *(supplies stifle region, gastrocnemius, and popliteal muscles)*
- Cranial tibial a. *(supplies cranial tibial muscles)*
  - Dorsal pedal a. *(supplies metatarsal region)*
    - Dorsal metatarsal aa.
    - Plantar metatarsal aa.
- Caudal tibial a.

The Internal Iliac Artery. The internal iliac artery supplies the pelvic viscera and walls, including the overlying muscles of the gluteal region and those of the proximocaudal part of the thigh. The artery continues caudoventrally from its origin, and in the dog it has a single branch, the *umbilical artery* (Fig. 7.43/*5*), a rather unimportant vestige of the placental supply of the fetus (p. 239). The proximal part of the umbilical artery carries a little blood to the cranial part of the bladder; the distal part is transformed into the round ligament of the bladder within the lateral vesical fold.

The internal iliac artery terminates by dividing into the caudal gluteal and internal pudendal arteries. The parietal branch, the *caudal gluteal artery* (Fig. 7.43/*6*), turns out of the pelvis with the sciatic nerve. This trunk, with its *iliolumbar* and *cranial gluteal* (Fig. 7.43/*7*) branches, supplies the muscles about the lumbosacral junction and those of the gluteal and proximocaudal femoral regions; the structures of the last-named region include the proximal parts of the hamstring muscles in which the caudal gluteal terminates.

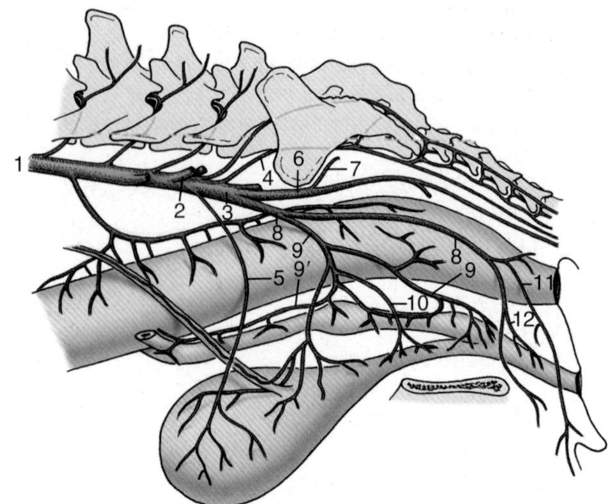

Fig. 7.43 Arteries of the female pelvis, left lateral view (bitch). *1,* Abdominal aorta; *2,* external iliac artery (a.); *3,* internal iliac a.; *4,* median sacral a.; *5,* umbilical a.; *6,* caudal gluteal a.; *7,* cranial gluteal a.; *8,* internal pudendal a.; *9,* vaginal a.; *9′,* uterine a.; *10,* urethral a. (frequently a branch of the vaginal a.); *11,* ventral perineal a.; *12,* a. of the clitoris.

The second terminal branch, the *internal pudendal artery* (Fig. 7.43/*8*), supplies the pelvic viscera (see also pp. 553 and 687). Its branches are differently named and disposed in the two sexes. The first branch is the prostatic artery in the male dog and the vaginal artery (Fig. 7.43/*9*) in the female. The *prostatic artery* supplies the middle rectal artery to the penultimate part of the rectum and various branches to the caudal parts of the ureter and bladder, the prostate, and the first part of the urethra. The *vaginal artery* also supplies the rectum and urinary organs in addition to the uterus and vagina. Its cranial branch, the uterine artery, forms the caudal part of the arterial arcade within the broad ligament (p. 463).

The next artery, the *urethral artery* (Fig. 7.43/*10*), is the same in both sexes. It supplies the caudal part of the pelvic urethra. The terminal branches of the internal pudendal are the ventral perineal artery and the artery of the penis or clitoris. The *ventral perineal artery* (Fig. 7.43/*11*) supplies a caudal rectal artery to the last part of the rectum and branches to the scrotum (or labia of the vulva). The *artery of the penis* runs the length of the upper border of this organ to the region of the bulbus glandis; it becomes known as the *dorsal artery of the penis* after detachment of a branch to the penis bulb, which also supplies the corpus spongiosum and pars longa glandis, and a deep branch to the corpus cavernosum (p. 456 and Fig. 15.20). The *artery of the clitoris* (Fig. 7.43/*12*) is similar but on a less substantial scale.

Internal iliac a.

- Umbilical a. *(unimportant vestige)*
- Caudal gluteal a. *(through its branches supplies muscles about lumbosacral junction and gluteal and proximocaudal femoral area)*
  - Iliolumbar a.
  - Cranial gluteal a.
- Internal pudendal a. *(supplies pelvic viscera)*
  - Prostatic *(vaginal)* a. *(supplies parts of rectum, urethra, ureter, bladder and prostate (vagina and uterus in female))*
    - A. of deferent duct
    - Caudal vesicle a.
    - Middle rectal a.
  - Urethral artery *(supplies caudal part of urethra)*
  - Ventral perineal a.
    - Caudal rectal a. *(supplies last part of rectum and to scrotum)*
  - Artery of penis *(clitoris) (supplies bulbus glandis)*
    - Artery of bulb *(supplies bulb of penis)*
    - Deep artery *(supplies corpus cavernosum)*
    - Dorsal artery *(supplies corpus spongiosum and pars longa glandis)*

The Systemic Veins

The systemic veins return blood to the heart through the cranial vena cava, caudal vena cava, and coronary sinus. The *coronary sinus* returns the bulk of the blood from the heart wall in ruminants and pigs it is joined by the left azygos vein. In the horse and the dog, the equivalent (azygos) territory is drained by the right azygos.

The Cranial Vena Cava. The cranial vena cava is formed close to the entrance to the chest by the union of the external jugular and subclavian veins, which drain the head and neck and the forelimb, respectively. In the dog the subclavian and jugular veins of each side join in a common trunk, which then combines with its fellow; another arrangement is the union of the two jugulars in a single bijugular trunk, which is then joined by the subclavian veins. The cranial vena cava runs through the cranial mediastinum, ventral and to the right of the trachea, and is related to the brachiocephalic trunk (dorsally at its origin, later at its left face). It is joined by various tributaries broadly corresponding to branches of the subclavian artery and by the larger right azygos vein toward its termination (Fig. 7.44/*3*)—unless the latter makes separate entry to the right atrium as in the horse.

The *azygos vein* (Fig. 7.44/*3*) is formed by the union of the first lumbar veins and passes through the aortic hiatus into the chest, where it receives intercostal veins from the caudal and middle intercostal spaces. Right and left veins are present in the embryo, but the main trunk is the right azygos vein in horses and dogs and the left one in ruminants and pigs—unless, as is usual in ruminants, both remain of some size. The right azygos vein arches ventrally, passing in front of the root of the right lung to reach the terminal part of the cranial vena cava or the adjacent part of the right atrium (horse). The left vein arches in front of the root of the left lung and must then run caudally, over the left atrium, to reach its confluence with the coronary sinus (Fig. 7.9A/*12*). The cranial intercostal veins that do not drain into this system join various tributaries of the subclavian or go directly to the cranial vena cava. The special importance of the azygos system in draining the plexus within the vertebral canal is considered elsewhere (p. 300).

The *subclavian vein* generally corresponds to the subclavian artery, and most tributaries in the upper part of the limb are satellite to arterial branches. However, in the distal part of the limb are important unaccompanied superficial veins connected with the deeper veins at various levels. These veins also drain into the *cephalic vein* (Fig. 7.44/*13*), which runs between the pectoral and brachiocephalic muscles in the arm to join the external jugular vein in the lower part of the neck.

Two pairs of jugular veins exist within the neck. The deep *internal jugular* (Fig. 7.44/*5*) runs with the common carotid artery within the visceral space of the neck; however, except in the dog and cat, it is very much reduced in size or even absent in postnatal animals. Even in the dog and cat it is of minor importance. The *external jugular vein* (Fig. 7.44/*6*) is formed near the angle of the jaw by the union of linguofacial and maxillary veins. Its course through the neck occupies a (jugular) groove between the brachiocephalicus dorsally and the sternocephalicus ventrally in the larger species; in the dog it lies on the sternocephalicus. It is easily raised for intravenous injection and blood sampling, and in the larger species it is the first choice for these procedures. The linguofacial vein is in general the principal drainage of the more superficial and more rostral structures of the head, whereas maxillary vein drains deeper and more caudal territory including the contents of the cranial cavity (see Fig. 11.44).

The Caudal Vena Cava. The caudal vena cava is formed on the roof of the abdomen, near the pelvic inlet, by the union of the right and left common iliac veins, each formed in its turn by the union of an *internal iliac vein,* which drains the pelvic walls and much of the contents of the pelvic cavity, and an *external iliac vein,* which drains the hindlimb (Fig. 7.44/*25* and *31*). The external iliac vein and the bulk of its tributaries are satellite to arteries. The independent medial and lateral saphenous veins of the leg (Fig. 7.44/*35* and *37*) drain the superficial veins of the foot.

Within the abdomen, the caudal vena cava is joined by additional tributaries draining the abdominal roof and large *renal veins,* before it dips ventrally to tunnel through the liver and subsequently the diaphragm at the caval foramen. It enters the thoracic cavity at a relatively ventral level and pursues a course within the free edge of the plica venae cavae between the caudal and accessory lobes of the right lung (see Fig. 4.21B/*9*). It joins the right atrium dorsal to the inlet of the coronary sinus.

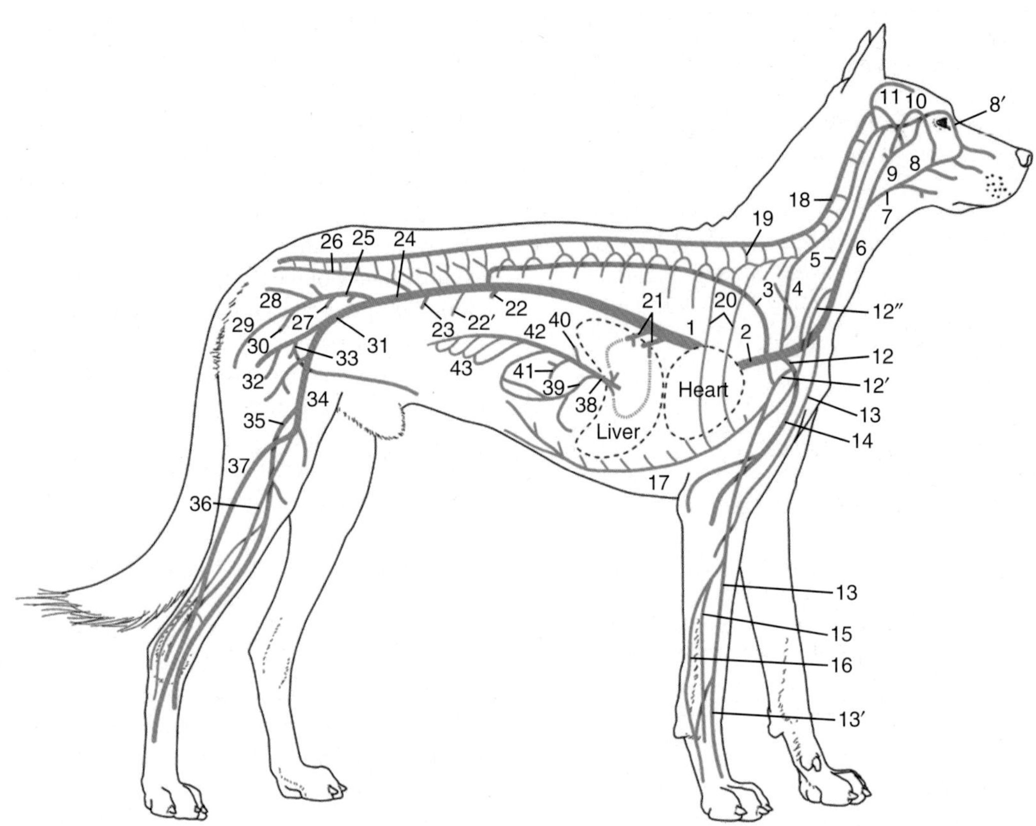

Fig. 7.44 Schematic representation of the venous system (dog). *1,* Caudal vena cava; *2,* cranial vena cava; *3,* azygous vein (v.); *4,* vertebral v.; *5,* internal jugular v.; *6,* external jugular v.; *7,* linguofacial v.; *8,* facial v.; *8′,* angularis oculi v.; *9,* maxillary v.; *10,* superficial temporal v.; *11,* dorsal sagittal sinus; *12,* subclavian v.; *12′,* axillobrachial v.; *12″,* omobrachial v.; *13,* cephalic v.; *13′,* accessory cephalic v.; *14,* brachial v.; *15,* radial v.; *16,* ulnar v.; *17,* internal thoracic v.; *18,* vertebral venous plexus; *19,* intervertebral v.; *20,* intercostal veins (vv.); *21,* hepatic vv.; *22,* renal v.; *22′,* testicular or ovarian v.; *23,* deep circumflex iliac v.; *24,* common iliac v.; *25,* right internal iliac v.; *26,* median sacral v.; *27,* prostatic or vaginal v.; *28,* lateral caudal v.; *29,* caudal gluteal v.; *30,* internal pudendal v; *31,* right external iliac v.; *32,* deep femoral v.; *33,* pudendoepigastric trunk; *34,* femoral v.; *35,* medial saphenous v.; *36,* cranial tibial v.; *37,* lateral saphenous v.; *38,* portal v.; *39,* gastroduodenal v.; *40,* splenic v.; *41,* caudal mesenteric v.; *42,* cranial mesenteric v.; *43,* jejunal vv.

In its intrahepatic course the caudal vena cava receives the *hepatic veins,* which drain the liver (Fig. 7.44/*21*).

The *portal vein* drains the spleen, the intra-abdominal digestive organs, the caudal part of the thoracic esophagus, and the bulk of the rectum (Figs. 7.44/*38* and 7.45). It is formed variously from three main tributaries (see Fig. 3.50/*2, 4,* and *5*). The splenic tributary corresponds to the celiac artery (excluding its hepatic branches) and therefore drains the last part of the esophagus, the stomach, parts of the duodenum and pancreas, and the spleen. The cranial and caudal mesenteric veins drain the territories of the like-named arteries and usually join in a common trunk before combining with the splenic vein.

The last part of the rectum and the anal region differ from the remainder of the gut in draining toward the internal iliac vein. The veins of this part form one of the portosystemic

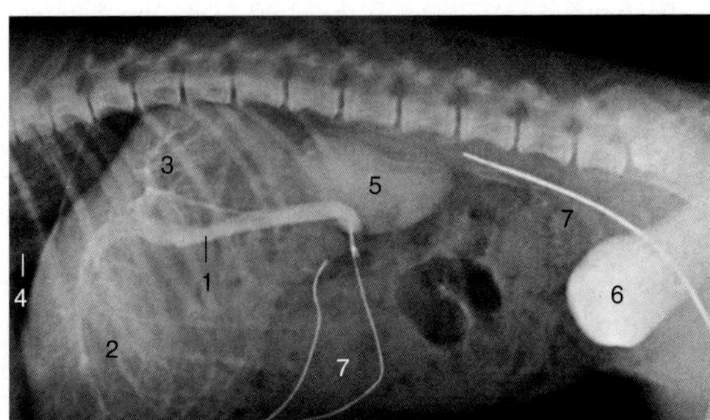

Fig. 7.45 Cannulation of the portal vein of a dog. *1,* Portal vein; *2,* branches to the quadrate, left medial and lateral liver lobes; *3,* branches to the remaining liver lobes; *4,* caudal vena cava; *5,* kidney; *6,* bladder, filled with opaque medium; *7,* catheters.

connections that provide alternative (although not very capacious) outlets from the portal drainage territory that are used when the intrahepatic circulation is impaired, as, for example, by cirrhosis (hepatic fibrosis).

THE CIRCULATION IN THE FETUS AND THE CHANGES AFTER BIRTH

During fetal life the placenta combines the roles that are later performed by the lungs, the digestive tract, and the kidneys. The blood is therefore replenished with oxygen, provided with nutrients, and cleansed of waste in its circulation through the placenta. It is returned to the fetus by two large umbilical veins that wind within the umbilical cord and join as one where they enter the body at the navel (Fig. 7.46/*11*). The single intra-abdominal umbilical vein runs forward to penetrate the liver at the umbilical fissure before it divides. It detaches collateral branches that vascularize the left portions (umbilical moiety) of the liver, and a further branch bends toward the right to make a wide connection with the portal vein (Fig. 7.46/*12*), which vascularizes the right portions (portal moiety). A direct continuation of the umbilical trunk, the ductus venosus (Fig. 7.46/*9*), tunnels through the substance of the liver, bypassing the hepatic circulation, to join the caudal vena cava. The ductus venosus, present in all young embryos, soon becomes vestigial in those of the horse and pig. It persists in other species but varies in caliber and importance and tends to become reduced toward term. The division of the liver into umbilical and portal moieties has obvious functional and possibly also clinical importance. The portal moiety is less generously supplied with oxygen, thus stimulating more active hemopoiesis; the umbilical moiety is more likely to suffer from infections acquired in utero.

The caudal vena cava (Fig. 7.46/*8*) receives the umbilical blood after its passage through the liver and adds it to the deoxygenated blood returned from the hindpart of the body. The oxygen content of the caudal caval stream is therefore already lower than that of the placental return before it reaches the heart, where the stream impinges on the cranial margin of the foramen ovale (Fig. 7.47/*2* and *4*). This structure divides the stream into two: one part continues into the right atrium (Fig. 7.47/*3*), and the other passes through the foramen ovale into the left atrium (Fig. 7.47/*8*). The relative sizes of the two streams change as gestation advances: a continuing shift of the margin of the foramen to the left increases the flow into the right atrium. The right stream mixes with the return from other systemic veins (Fig. 7.47/*1*), and the oxygen content of the blood passed to the right ventricle is thus further diminished. This blood is ejected into the pulmonary trunk (Fig. 7.47/*6*), which in the fetus communicates with the aorta through a wide channel, the ductus arteriosus (Fig. 7.47/*7′*). The ductus enters the aorta beyond the origin of the brachiocephalic trunk and is as wide as the pulmonary trunk (it is in fact its direct continuation—the right and

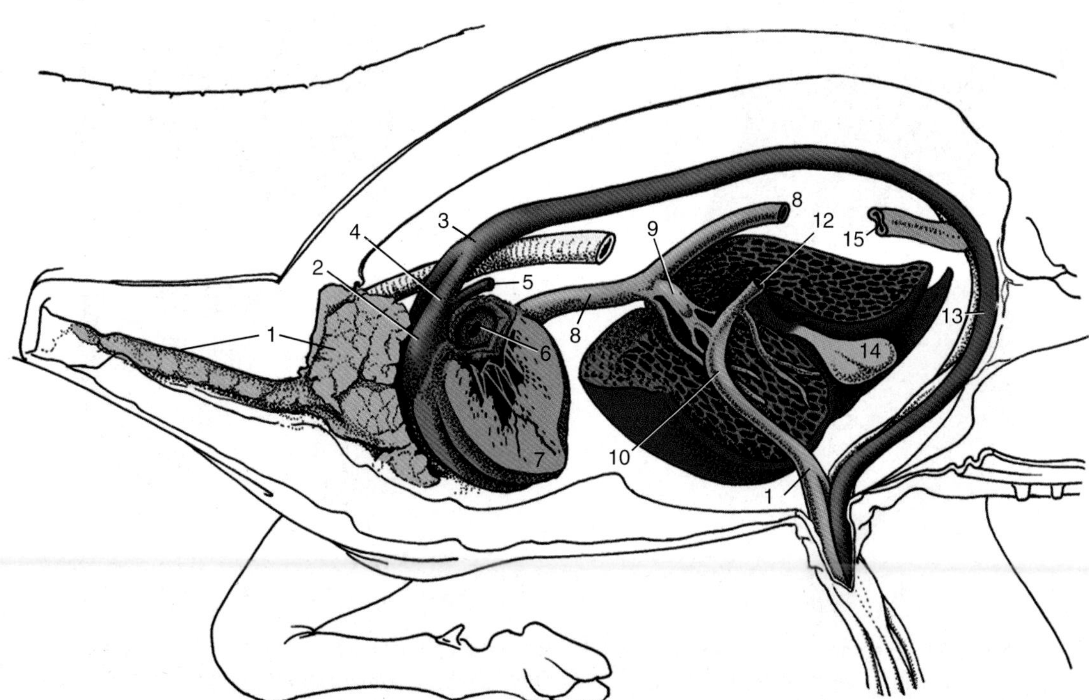

Fig. 7.46 Semischematic drawing of fetal circulation (calf). *1,* Thymus; *2,* pulmonary trunk; *3,* aortic arch; *4,* ductus arteriosus; *5,* pulmonary artery; *6,* foramen ovale; *7,* wall of left ventricle; *8,* caudal vena cava; *9,* ductus venosus; *10,* junction of umbilical and portal branches within the liver; *11,* umbilical vein; *12,* stump of portal vein; *13,* left umbilical artery; *14,* gallbladder; *15,* descending colon.

left pulmonary arteries [Fig. 7.47/*7*] are the side branches). The ductus arteriosus receives most of the output of the right ventricle because the vascular bed of the unexpanded lungs offers considerable resistance to blood flow.

The small flow that is returned to the left atrium from the lungs mixes there with the greater volume of blood that passed through the foramen ovale. The blood that enters the aorta (Fig. 7.47/*10*) is therefore relatively well oxygenated; part of this stream enters the coronary and carotid arteries. The head and brain are therefore favored by receiving a richer supply of oxygen than is given to organs supplied from those branches of the aorta that arise distal to the entry of the ductus arteriosus; these later branches receive the mixed output of both ventricles. The placenta receives the greater share of the flow through the descending aorta (Fig. 7.47/*10′*) by way of the umbilical arteries (Fig. 7.47/*11*); these vessels branch from the internal iliac arteries and leave the fetus at the umbilicus, together with the allantoic duct (Fig. 7.46/*13*). The fetal bloodstream is brought into close apposition to the maternal bloodstream within the placenta, although the intervening tissue barrier varies in thickness and permeability among species (p. 196).

Postnatal changes in the circulation may occur over many hours or even days to result in a pattern of adult circulation. The permanent closure of the redundant fetal channels requires a much longer time. The arrest of the placental circulation may precede or follow the initiation of pulmonary ventilation according to the circumstances of parturition. The umbilical vessels are either bitten across by the mother (e.g., puppy) or are ruptured, being unable to support the weight of the offspring (e.g., calf). In both circumstances little hemorrhaging occurs because the rough treatment stimulates contraction of the muscle in the vessel wall. The arterial stumps are slowly transformed into the round ligaments of the bladder. The stump of the umbilical vein outside the abdomen shrivels, and the intra-abdominal part is in time transformed into the round ligament of the liver. The raw umbilical surfaces provide potential entry to infection ("navel ill"), and the allantoic duct and thrombosed vein are convenient routes for its spread.

The ductus venosus closes within a few hours or days after birth, with the result that the portal vein perfuses all parts of the liver.

The loss of the umbilical return reduces both the volume and the pressure of the caudal caval stream. This change,

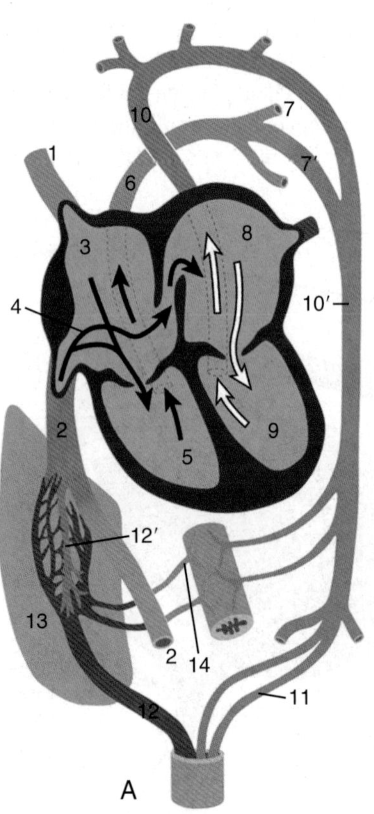

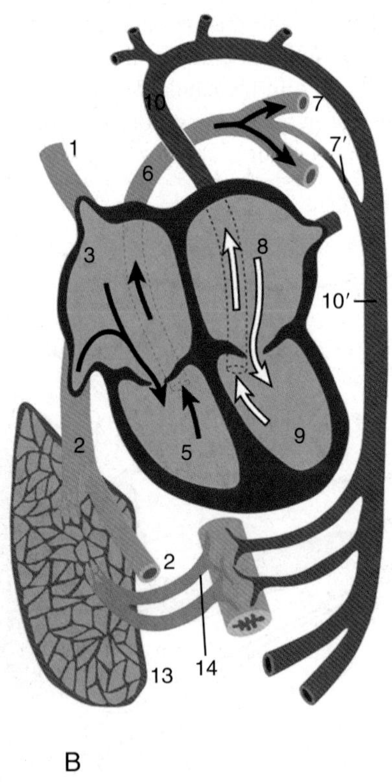

Fig. 7.47 Diagrams of the (A) fetal and (B) postnatal circulatory systems. *1,* Cranial vena cava; *2,* caudal vena cava; *3,* right atrium; *4,* arrow entering oval foramen; *5,* right ventricle; *6,* pulmonary trunk; *7,* pulmonary artery; *7′,* ductus arteriosus (in [B], vestige); *8,* left atrium; *9,* left ventricle; *10,* aortic arch; *10′,* descending aorta; *11,* umbilical artery; *12,* umbilical vein; *12′,* ductus venosus; *13,* liver; *14,* portal vein. *Black arrows* indicate blood entering and exiting the right chambers of the heart while the *white arrows* indicate the blood movement in the left chambers of the heart. coming into the right side of the heart and *white arrows* indicated.

combined with the concurrent increase in left atrial pressure, halts the shunt through the foramen ovale. Contraction of the muscular wall of the ductus arteriosus is stimulated by the raised oxygen tension of the perfusing blood; it is not effected at once, and for some hours or days blood may shunt in either direction according to the relative pressures in the aorta and pulmonary artery. Expansion of the lungs reduces the resistance of their vascular bed, and the drop in pulmonary arterial pressure results in the flow through the ductus normally comes from the aorta. The passage of blood through the constricted tube causes vibration of its wall, which may be detected on auscultation as a *continuous murmur* during the first day or two of postnatal life in calves and foals. Permanent structural changes eventually obliterate the lumen, converting the duct into a fibrous structure (ligamentum arteriosum); however, for some time after birth the ductus dilates in circumstances that produce hypoxia, and it is often found widely open in the neonatal postmortem specimen.

The increased venous return from the lungs raises the pressure within the left atrium, forcing the valve of the foramen ovale against the atrial septum, which closes the foramen (see Figs. 7.26 and 7.47). The valve is a simple flap in carnivores but more elaborate and tubular in ungulates, in which muscle causes it to crumple, improving closure. Although fibrosis eventually seals the valve in place, this process takes some time, and it is not uncommon for the opening to be patent to a probe for months or even years; such patency is rarely of significance. The increased workload now placed on the left ventricle leads to its muscular hypertrophy and thickening of the walls.

THE ORGANIZATION OF THE LYMPHATIC SYSTEM

The lymphatic system is integral to the body's defense from a variety of pathogens and from abnormal endogenous molecules. It includes all the lymphatic organs: thymus, tonsils, spleen, lymph nodes and hemal nodes, and the diffuse lymphatic tissue and lymphatic nodules present in many mucous membranes. The circulating lymphocytes, as well as the lymphocytes and plasma cells spread across the body, also participate in this protective system.

Two types of functionally distinct lymphocytes are recognized: T lymphocytes and B lymphocytes. Both result from antigen-independent proliferation and differentiation of stem cells in the primary lymphatic organs: T cells come from the thymus, and B cells come from the bursa of Fabricius in birds and the bone marrow in mammals. From the primary organs, both types of lymphocytes seed the secondary lymphatic organs, within which B and T lymphocytes undergo antigen-dependent proliferation and differentiation into effector cells that either attend to the disposal of particular antigens or provide the memory cells, which become temporarily inactive. There is, in addition, a reserve population of undifferentiated lymphocytes.

The brief introduction to the system presented in Chapter 1 emphasizes the role of the lymphatic capillaries and larger vessels in returning an important fraction of the tissue fluid to the circulating blood. This role justifies the inclusion of these vessels, and of the nodes through which the lymph is passed, within the broad concept of a circulatory system (see Fig. 1.34). The framework that supports the lymphatic nodules (germinal centers) contains phagocytic cells that remove particulate matter, including microorganisms on occasion, from the lymph; this element must be included within the widely diffused macrophage or mononuclear phagocytic system that also encompasses the tissue macrophages and the endothelium of the hepatic, splenic, and bone marrow sinusoids.

There also are lymphoepithelial structures comprising aggregations of unencapsulated lymph nodules within various mucosae. These are conveniently genetically termed *tonsils,* although the name is most often used specifically for those in the pharyngeal region (Fig. 7.48/*2*). Pharyngeal and palatine tonsils, which are mentioned on page 108, and others are found in the mucosae of the larynx, intestine, prepuce, and vagina and other parts of the female tract. The common features that distinguish tonsils from lymph nodes are the absence of a capsule, the close relationship to

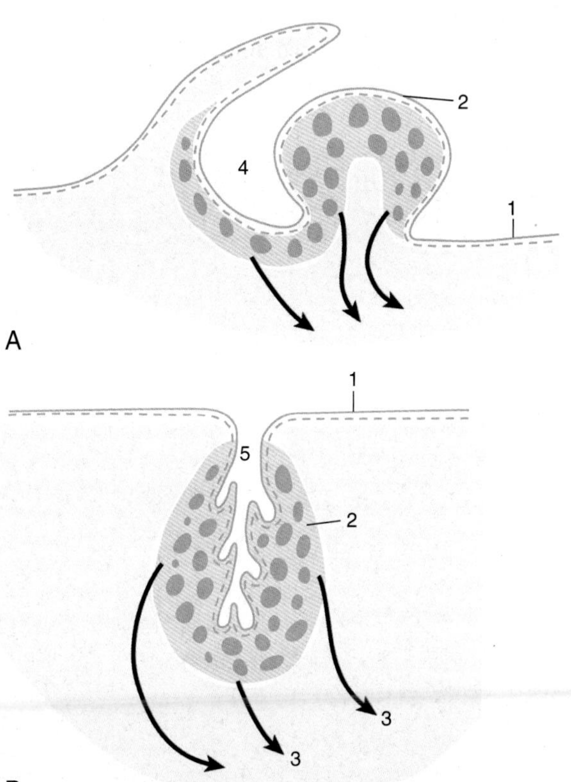

Fig. 7.48 Schematic drawing of the palatine tonsils of (A) the dog and (B) cattle. The tonsils of the dog develop around a fossa but protrude into the oropharynx. Those of cattle surround the tonsillar sinus within the oropharyngeal wall. *1,* Epithelium; *2,* palatine tonsil; *3,* efferent vessels *(arrows)*; *4,* tonsillar fossa; *5,* tonsillar sinus.

a moist epithelial surface, and the position at the origin of a lymphatic drainage pathway.

In addition to the ordinary lymph node, a second variety of similar structure, called *hemal nodes*, is positioned across the bloodstream (Fig. 7.49). These nodes are not found in all species and are most familiar in sheep, in which their dark color (due to the contained blood) contrasts them with the white fat in which they are commonly embedded. They are found mainly below the roof of the abdomen and thorax. A so-called third variety, the hemolymph node, is probably only a lymph node that contains red blood cells in its sinuses as a result of hemorrhage in its tributary field.

It is uncertain whether lymph vessels develop independently and later make secondary entry to veins, bud from existing veins, or arise by a combination of these methods. Both methods account for the existence of the lymphaticovenous connections between the major lymphatic trunks and the great veins at the entrance to the chest. In some (nondomestic) mammals additional connections are described, often with renal veins, which develop in response to obstruction of normal flow.

Lymph nodes initially form as mesenchymal condensations placed along the lymphatic capillary plexus. They are later populated by lymphocytes that emigrate from the central lymphoid organ, the thymus. All lymphoid structures are especially well developed in juveniles.

As already mentioned (p. 27) there are important species differences in the disposition of the components of the lymph nodes. In most animals, the lymph nodules are located in the peripheral cortex close to where the afferent lymph vessels penetrate the capsule (Figs. 7.50 and 7.51). The central medulla consists of loose lymphoreticular tissue where the efferent vessels take origin to leave the node in the indented hilar region. In contrast, in porcine nodes, the "cortical" tissue is central, and most nodules lie alongside the trabecular sinuses. The afferent vessels penetrate the capsule at one or more sites and follow the trabeculae to reach the centrally located nodules. The periphery of the node is largely occupied by loose lymphoreticular tissue (Fig. 7.52), and it is from here that the efferent lymph vessels emerge.

THE TOPOGRAPHY OF LYMPHATIC DRAINAGE

The applied importance of the lymphatic drainage has been stressed, and accounts of its organization in different species are presented later. Because these accounts are necessarily fragmented by the regional character of the later chapters, it may be useful to give a short general account here. We begin with Figs. 7.53 and 7.54, which show the palpable lymph nodes of the dog and the cat.

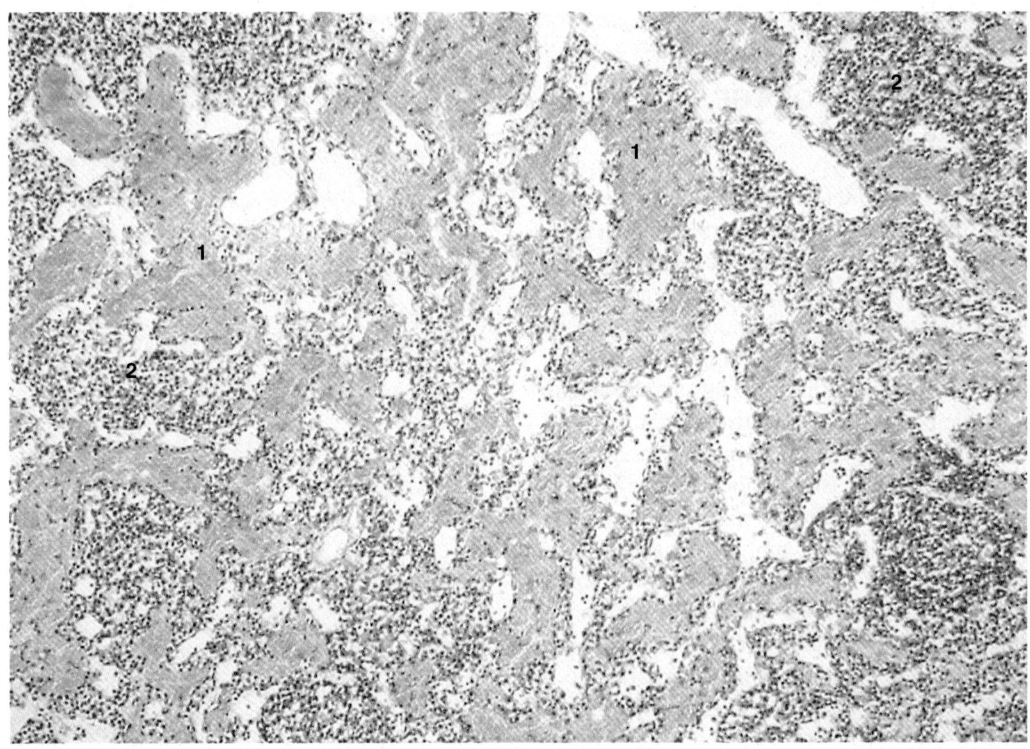

Fig. 7.49 Hemal node of sheep (hematoxylin and eosin; magnification ×70). *1*, Erythrocytes; *2*, lymphocytes.

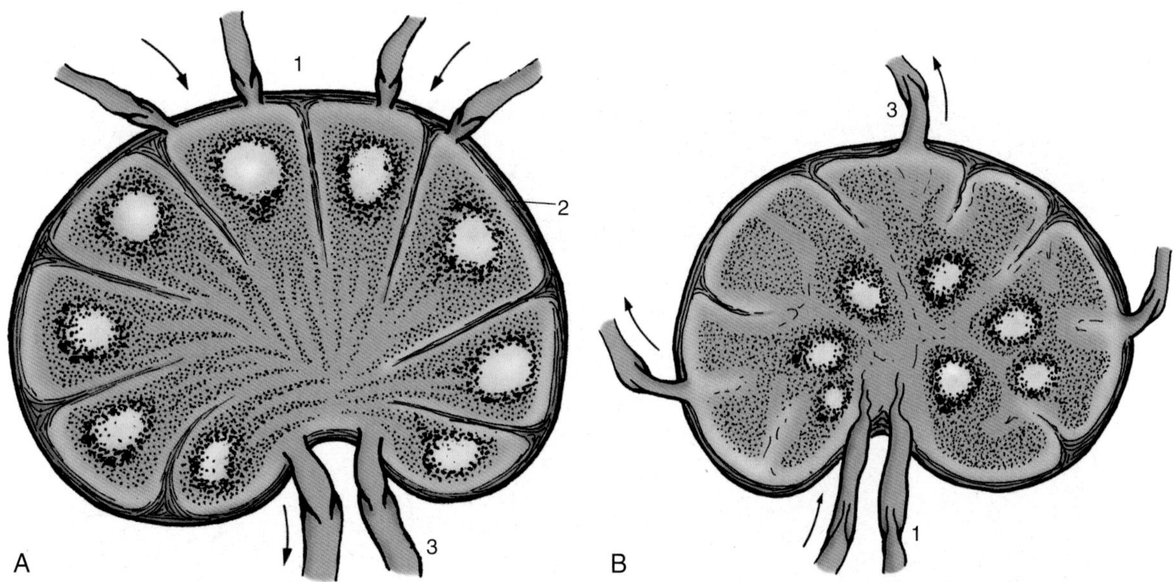

Fig. 7.50 (A) Structure of a lymph node in which the germinal centers (lymph nodules) occupy the cortical region. (B) In the pig the germinal centers lie centrally. *Arrows* indicate the direction of lymph flow. *1,* Afferent lymphatics; *2,* subcapsular sinus; *3,* efferent lymphatics.

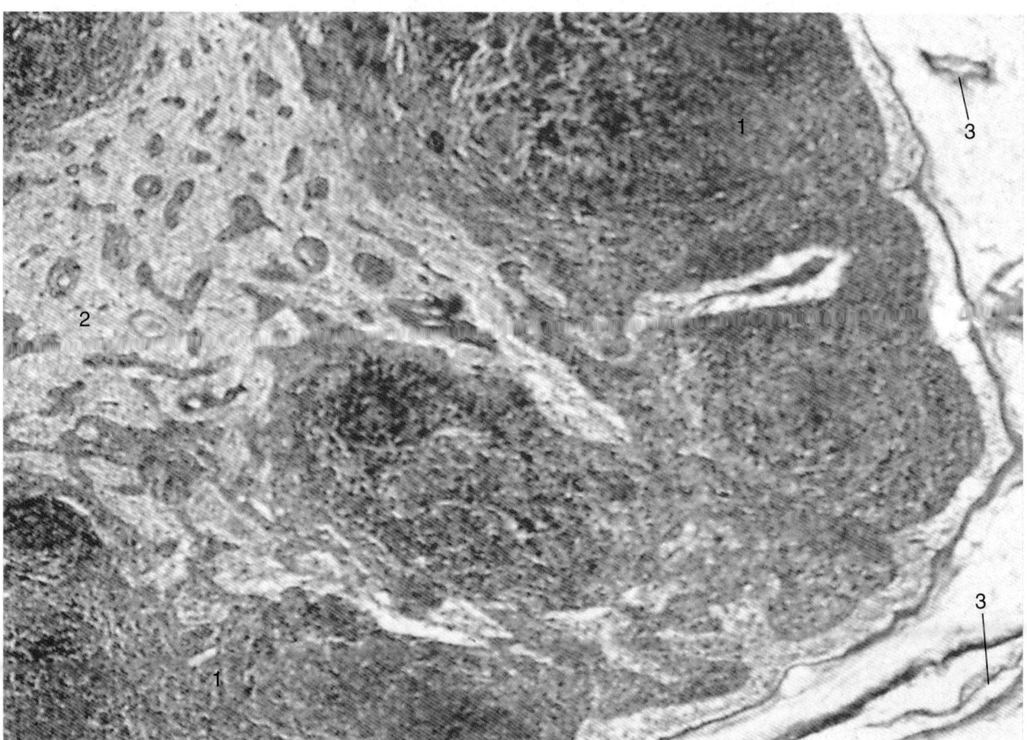

Fig. 7.51 Lymph node (dog) (magnification ×28). *1,* Cortex with lymph nodules; *2,* medulla; *3,* afferent lymph vessels.

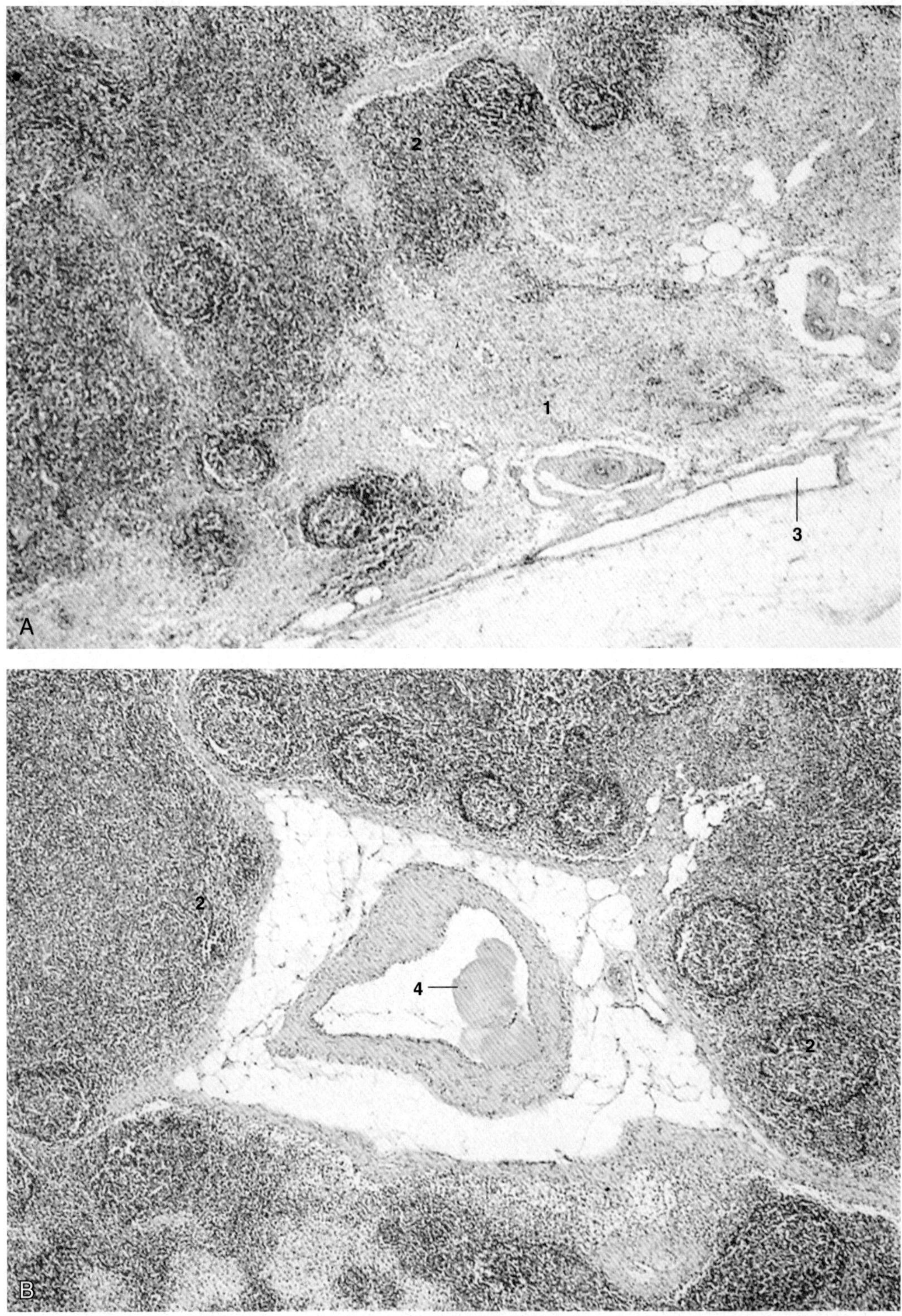

Fig. 7.52 (A) and (B) Lymph node (pig) (magnification ×28). *1,* Loose lymphoreticular tissue; *2,* lymph nodules in centrally located "cortex"; *3,* efferent lymph vessels; *4,* centrally located afferent lymph vessel, with valve.

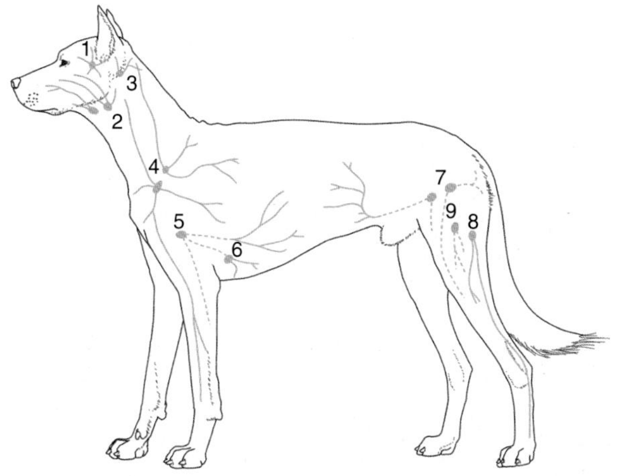

Fig. 7.53 Palpable lymph nodes of the dog. *1,* Parotid; *2,* mandibular; *3,* lateral retropharyngeal (inconstant); *4,* superficial cervical; *5,* axillary; *6,* accessory axillary (inconstant); *7,* superficial inguinal; *8,* popliteal; *9,* femoral (inconstant).

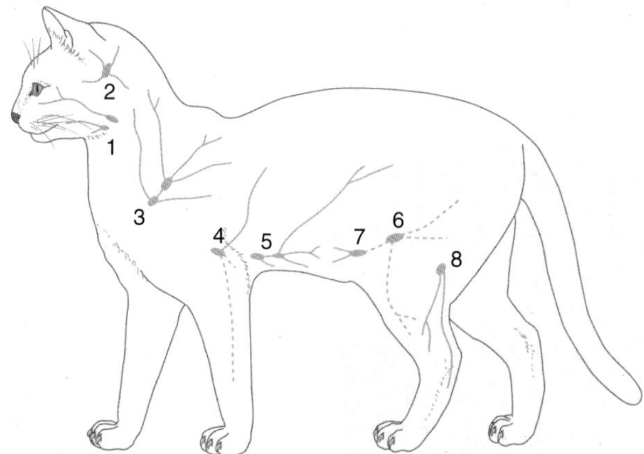

Fig. 7.54 Palpable lymph nodes of the cat. *1,* Mandibular; *2,* lateral retropharyngeal; *3,* dorsal superficial cervical; *4,* axillary; *5,* accessory axillary; *6,* superficial inguinal; *7,* caudal epigastric; *8,* popliteal.

The Lymph Nodes of the Head

Three lymphocenters are present in the head. The *parotid center* consists of one or more nodes placed on the masseter close to the temporomandibular joint and commonly covered by the parotid gland (Fig. 7.55/*2*). These nodes receive lymph from dorsal structures of the head, including skin, the dorsal bones of the skull, the contents of the orbit, and the masticatory muscles (in part).

The *mandibular center* (Fig. 7.55/*1*) comprises a group of nodes placed within the intermandibular space or more caudally by the angle of the jaw. They drain structures of the muzzle, the salivary glands, the intermandibular space (including the tongue), and a further part of the masticatory muscles.

The *retropharyngeal center* consists of two groups of nodes, medial and lateral; the former (Fig. 7.55/*4*) lie against the roof of the pharynx, and the latter (Fig. 7.55/*3*) are contained within the atlantal fossa. Together, they drain deeper structures of the head and adjacent parts of the neck, including the pharynx and larynx; one or the other also receives lymph that has already passed through the more peripheral centers. In most species the medial group receives the output from the lateral retropharyngeal, parotid, and mandibular nodes; in cattle this role is taken by the lateral group (see in Chapter 25).

The Lymph Nodes of the Neck

The *superficial cervical center* (Fig. 7.55/*6*) lies in front of the shoulder, under cover of the lateral superficial muscles of the neck. It consists of one or more nodes that drain a very wide but predominantly superficial territory. It extends from the nape to the middle of the trunk and includes the proximal part of the forelimb. The outflow is usually to the lymphatics at the thoracic inlet (Fig. 7.55/*12*).

The *deep cervical center* (Fig. 7.55/*5*) comprises a chain of nodes usually arranged in cranial, middle, and caudal groups but often irregular in disposition. The nodes are placed along the trachea within the visceral space of the neck and mainly drain deeper and more ventral structures. Much of this lymph percolates through successive nodes of the chain before entering one of the major lymphatic channels at the entrance to the chest.

The Tracheal Duct

In most species the tracheal duct (Fig. 7.55/*12*) is a large paired vessel that follows the course of the trachea within the neck. Except in the horse, it takes origin in the retropharyngeal nodes that serve as the collecting center of the head. It may be augmented by tributaries from deep cervical nodes before it joins the thoracic (on the left side) or right lymphatic duct. Alternatively, one or both tracheal ducts may enter the corresponding jugular or other vein at the venous confluence at the entrance to the thorax (see Fig. 1.34). In the horse the flow may be interrupted by serial passage through deep cervical nodes (see in Chapter 18).

The Lymph Nodes of the Forelimb

One *axillary center* exists. The principal nodes are contained within the axilla where they lie on the medial muscles of the shoulder. Additional nodes may be found in relation to the first rib or more caudally on the chest wall. In the horse alone, a more distal group of cubital nodes is placed over the medial aspect of the elbow. The center drains the deeper structures of the entire limb and the more superficial structures of the distal segments, and the collection goes to one of the major lymphatic or venous channels at the entrance to the chest.

The Lymph Nodes of the Thorax

Four lymphocenters attend to the drainage of the thoracic walls and contents. The nodes within certain groups are

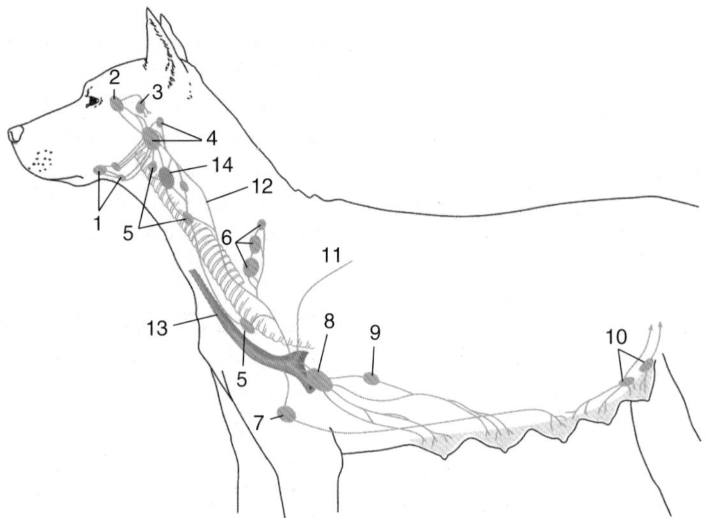

Fig. 7.55 Lymph drainage of the head, neck, and mammary glands of the dog. *1,* Mandibular nodes; *2,* parotid node; *3,* lateral retropharyngeal node; *4,* medial retropharyngeal nodes; *5,* cranial and caudal deep cervical nodes; *6,* superficial cervical nodes; *7,* sternal node; *8,* axillary node; *9,* accessory axillary node; *10,* superficial inguinal nodes; *11,* thoracic duct; *12,* tracheal duct; *13,* external jugular vein; *14,* thyroid gland.

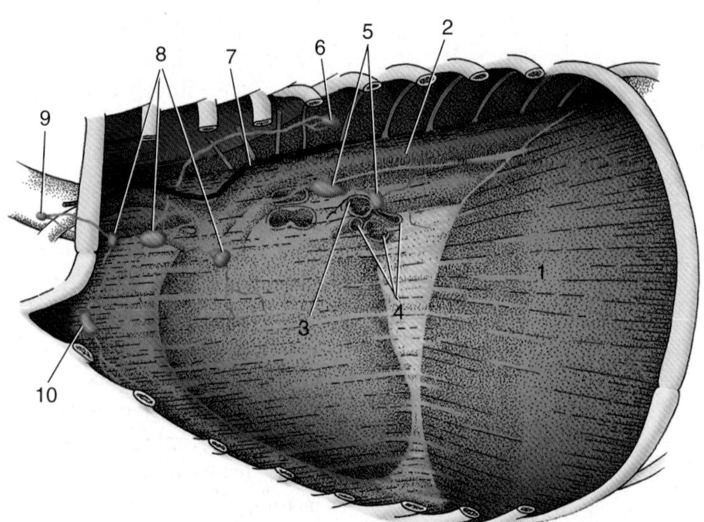

Fig. 7.56 Thoracic lymph nodes in the dog. Left lung removed; the outline of the heart is visible within the mediastinum. *1,* Diaphragm; *2,* thoracic aorta; *3,* left bronchus; *4,* pulmonary vessels; *5,* tracheobronchial nodes; *6,* intercostal node; *7,* thoracic duct; *8,* cranial mediastinal nodes; *9,* caudal deep cervical node; *10,* sternal node.

rather diffusely spread, and it is not always easy to decide their correct designation.

The *dorsal thoracic center* comprises two groups of small, inconstant nodes. The intercostal set (Fig. 7.56/*6*) is found within the upper parts of a few intercostal spaces. The thoracic aortic set is dispersed along the course of the vessel. The center drains the back and the deeper tissues of the thoracic wall and sends its outflow, possibly after serial passage through several nodes, to the thoracic duct or the mediastinal nodes (Fig. 7.56/*8*).

The *ventral thoracic center* consists of cranial sternal nodes (Fig. 7.56/*10*) by the manubrium of the sternum and, only in ruminants, caudal sternal nodes placed against both surfaces of the transversus thoracic muscle. The center drains the deeper structures of the ventral part of the thoracic wall and sends its efferent flow either to mediastinal nodes or to one of the larger collecting vessels.

The *mediastinal center* is divided into a group of nodes within the cranial mediastinum (Fig. 7.56/*8*), a middle

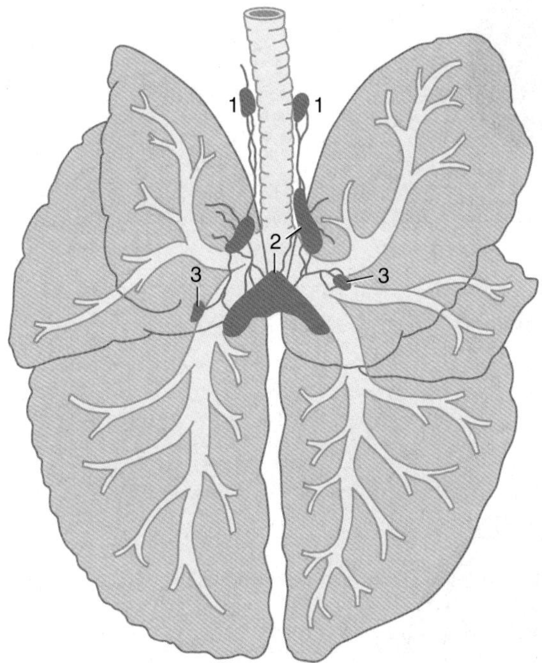

Fig. 7.57 Lymph nodes associated with trachea and lungs of the dog. *1,* Cranial mediastinal nodes; *2,* tracheobronchial nodes; *3,* pulmonary nodes.

group about the base of the heart, and a caudal group (absent in carnivores) near the esophagus as it approaches the diaphragm (see in Chapter 27). The various nodes drain structures of the thoracic wall, mainly after first passage of the lymph through other primary nodes, and thoracic viscera. They provide a secondary station for lymph from the lungs that has already passed through tracheobronchial nodes. The outflow goes to the large collecting vessels at the entrance to the chest, in part after serial passage through several nodes.

The *bronchial center* consists of groups of tracheobronchial nodes placed about the tracheal bifurcation and, in many animals, small pulmonary nodes embedded within the substance of the lung (Figs. 7.56/*5* and 7.57). The former groups are individually named (left, middle, right, and [in ruminants and pigs] cranial tracheobronchial nodes) according to their relationships to the major bronchi. They collect lymph from the lungs and send it in inconstant fashion to middle and caudal mediastinal nodes and sometimes directly to the thoracic duct.

The Thoracic Duct

The thoracic duct is the major lymph-collecting channel. It arises from the cisterna chyli, which receives lymph from the abdomen, pelvis, and hindlimbs (see Fig. 1.34/*5* and *7*). The cisterna has a very irregular, even plexiform, shape, and although it is mainly contained between the aorta and the vertebrae at the thoracolumbar junction, it may also extend ventrally around the vena cava and the origin of the celiac artery. The thoracic duct

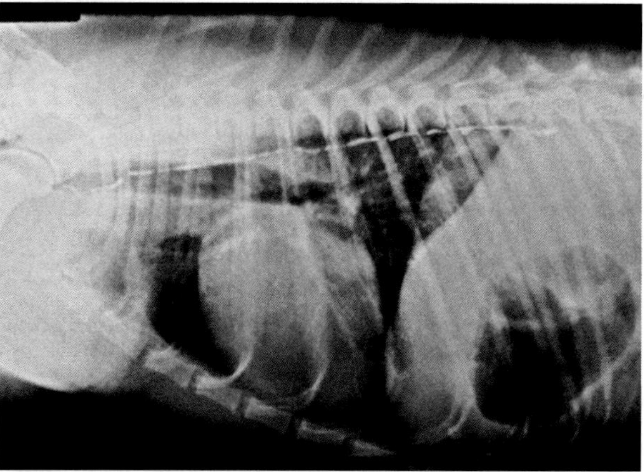

Fig. 7.58 Lymphangiogram of the canine thoracic duct.

passes through the aortic hiatus into the mediastinum. Its further course takes it cranially and ventrally, over the left face of the trachea, to a termination within one of the veins, most often the left jugular vein, that form the cranial vena cava or the vena cava itself (Fig. 7.58). The duct receives additional lymph from the structures and nodes of the left side of the chest. A separate right lymphatic duct provides similar drainage for cranial thoracic structures of the right side and proceeds to a similar termination. One or both commonly receive the corresponding tracheal duct(s).

The Lymph Nodes of the Abdominal Viscera and Loins

The roof of the abdomen is drained by a *lumbar center* containing various nodes spread along the abdominal aorta and possibly also within the spaces between the lumbar transverse processes (Fig. 7.59). Usually those (renal) nodes (Fig. 7.59/*7*) that are associated with the kidneys are larger than others in the series. In addition to draining the structures of the loins, kidneys, and adrenal glands, these nodes may receive some lymph from reproductive organs. The flow is to the cisterna chyli (Fig. 7.59/*5*) directly or after serial passage.

Three centers associated with the drainage of the abdominal viscera have territories broadly corresponding to those of the celiac, cranial mesenteric, and caudal mesenteric arteries. They show very considerable interspecific distinctions and include the following (Fig. 7.60). The *celiac center* comprises splenic, gastric (subdivided in ruminants), hepatic, and pancreaticoduodenal nodes (Fig. 7.60/*1–4*). The *cranial mesenteric center* consists of cranial mesenteric nodes toward the root of the mesentery and more peripheral jejunal, cecal, and colic nodes (Fig. 7.60/*5–7*). The *caudal mesenteric center* comprises caudal mesenteric nodes associated with the descending colon (Fig. 7.60/*8*). The three centers give rise to various visceral trunks that converge on the cisterna chyli.

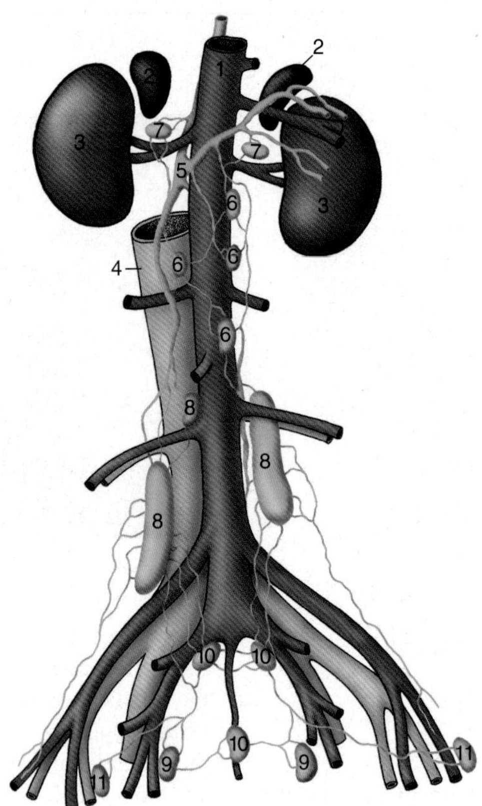

Fig. 7.59 Lymph drainage of the canine lumbosacral area, ventral view. *1,* Aorta; *2,* adrenals; *3,* kidneys; *4,* caudal vena cava; *5,* cisterna chyli; *6,* lumbar aortic nodes; *7,* renal nodes; *8,* medial iliac nodes; *9,* hypogastric nodes; *10,* sacral nodes; *11,* deep inguinal (iliofemoral) nodes.

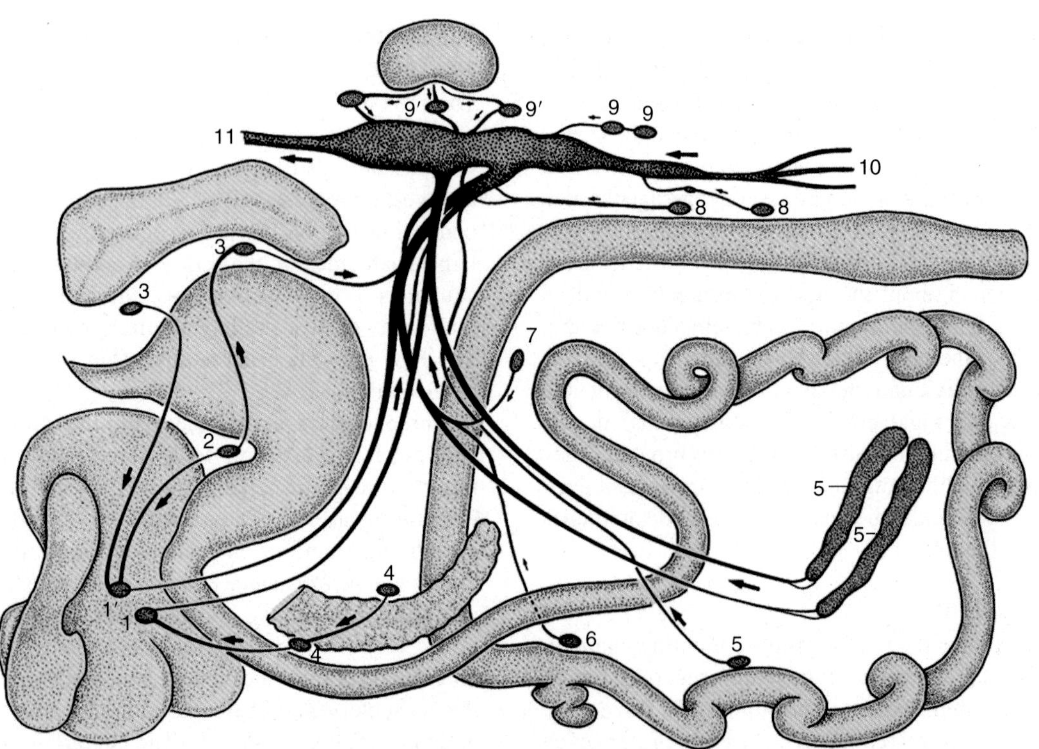

Fig. 7.60 Lymph drainage from the organs in the canine abdominal and pelvic cavities (schematized). *1* and *1′,* Right and left hepatic nodes; *2,* gastric node; *3,* splenic nodes; *4,* pancreaticoduodenal nodes; *5,* jejunal nodes; *6,* right colic node; *7,* middle colic node; *8,* caudal mesenteric nodes; *9,* lumbar aortic nodes; *9′,* renal nodes; *10,* efferents from the iliosacral region; *11,* continuation of cisterna chyli as thoracic duct.

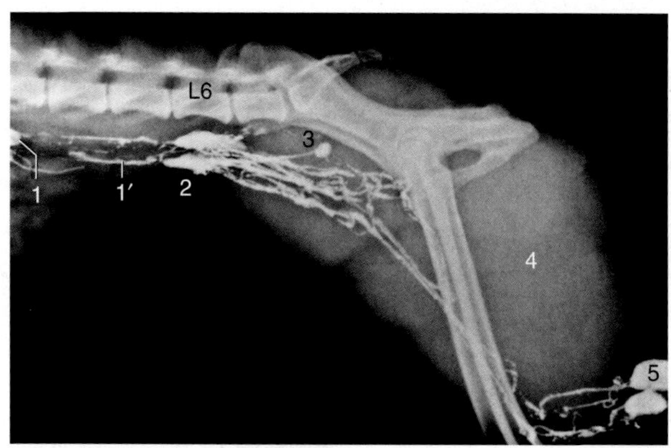

Fig. 7.61 Lymphangiogram of the canine lumbar area, pelvis, and thigh. *1,* Lumbar aortic lymph node; *1′,* lumbar trunks; *2,* medial iliac nodes; *3,* hypogastric node; *4,* thigh muscles; *5,* popliteal nodes; *L6,* sixth lumbar vertebra.

The Lymph Nodes of the Hindlimb, Pelvis, and Abdominal Wall

Although an inconveniently large territory to consider together, the hindlimb, pelvis, and abdominal wall cannot be subdivided because the responsibilities of certain nodes do not coincide with the usual division of the body. The most peripheral *popliteal center,* which consists of a node (or nodes) placed within the popliteal fossa caudal to the stifle (Figs. 7.53/*8* and 7.61/*5*), drains the distal part of the limb. The efferent flow is directed to the medial iliac center (except in the horse, in which it passes to deep inguinal nodes).

The *ischial center* contains the ischial node placed on the lateral aspect of the sacrosciatic ligament (of ungulates [see in Chapter 31]—no comparable node exists in carnivores). It collects from the muscles and skin of the rump and proximal thigh and sends its outflow to various nodes of the iliosacral center.

The nodes of the *deep inguinal* (iliofemoral) *center* are placed along the course of the external iliac artery or its femoral continuation (Fig. 7.59/*11*). They primarily drain part of the thigh but also accept lymph from the popliteal nodes for onward passage to the iliosacral center.

The more peripheral *superficial inguinal center* includes the superficial inguinal nodes of the groin, the subiliac nodes of the flank fold (except in the dog), the coxal node, and the nodes of the paralumbar fossa of cattle (Figs. 7.55/*10* and Chapter 31). The superficial inguinal nodes are also named *scrotal* or *mammary* because they drain the external male reproductive organs or the udder (in dogs, caudal mammary glands) in addition to the groin region. The subiliac node drains skin and deeper structures extending from the midflank to the thigh. The efferent lymph passes to the iliosacral center, directly or after passage through the deep inguinal nodes.

The *iliosacral center* is a very large, widely spread collection of nodes placed against the roof of the caudal part of the abdomen and within the pelvic cavity (see Fig. 7.59). The main components are the medial iliac nodes (Fig. 7.59/*8*), near the origin of the external and internal iliac arteries and, though not in the dog, the lateral iliac about the branching of the deep circumflex iliac vessels. There are other nodes on the walls (sacral nodes) and about the viscera (hypogastric and anorectal nodes) in the pelvic cavity. These various small nodes are the primary filtration centers for adjacent structures and secondary stages in the drainage of the hindlimb and reproductive and other pelvic organs. The lymph from these nodes flows to the medial iliac nodes that give origin to the lumbar trunks.

The Lumbar Trunks

The lumbar trunks are formed mainly by efferent vessels from the medial iliac nodes. They form a plexus on the roof of the abdomen, where they are augmented by part of the lumbar outflow before they expand as the cisterna chyli (Figs. 7.59/*5* and 7.61/*1′*). This structure also receives visceral trunks from the digestive organs.

THE SPLEEN

The spleen* is contained within the left cranial part of the abdomen, where it is joined to the greater curvature of the stomach by inclusion within the greater omentum. The spleen's precise position depends on the degree of filling of the stomach and on its own blood content. The basic form is very dissimilar in the various domestic species, being dumbbell-shaped in the dog and cat, straplike in the pig, a broader oblong shape in cattle, and falciform in the horse (Fig. 7.62). Its capsule extends trabeculae into the interior. In some species (carnivores) the capsule and trabeculae are very muscular, in others (ruminants) much less so, and these differences determine the extent of the physiologic variation in size. When relaxed, the spleen of the dog and cat increases many times from its contracted state.

The soft tissue contained within the supporting framework is divided between red and white pulp. Red pulp consists of spaces in series with the blood vessels and is occupied by a concentrated cellular elements of the blood. The white pulp, which is divided into foci that are usually just visible to the naked eye, is formed of lymph nodules within a supporting reticuloendothelial framework. This tissue has the usual lymphogenic and phagocytic properties.

The functions of the spleen are blood storage, the removal of particulate matter from the circulation, the destruction of worn-out erythrocytes, and the production of lymphocytes. The blood storage function is familiar to all who have experienced a "stitch in the side," the pain that sometimes accompanies physical stress and is associated with contraction of the splenic capsule.

The spleen is supplied by the generously sized splenic artery, a branch of the celiac artery (see Fig. 3.39/*4*). The

*The official name, *lien,* is the stem for many descriptive terms—for example, a. lienalis, the splenic artery.

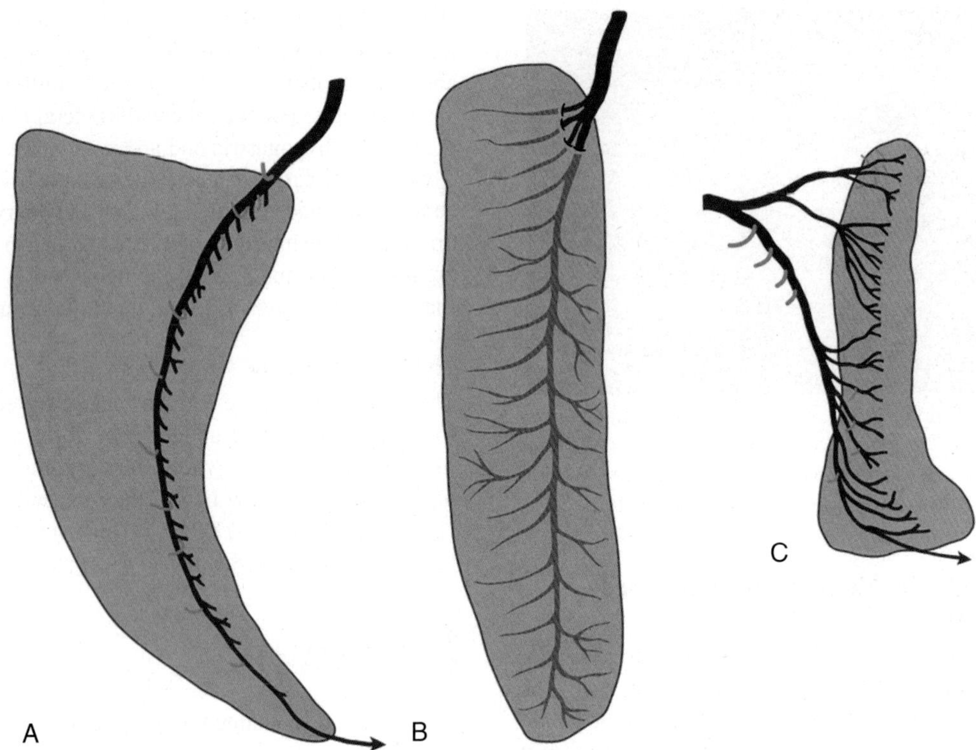

Fig. 7.62 Visceral surfaces of the spleens of (A) horse, (B) cattle, and (C) dog to show the distribution of the splenic arteries. Branches to other structures are shown in *blue*.

venous drainage through the splenic vein leads to the portal vein (see Fig. 3.50/*1* and *2*). Important specific features in the arrangement of these vessels exist. The artery and vein may pass undivided through a confined hilus (ruminants; Fig. 7.62B); may run the length of the organ, detaching branches at intervals (horse, pig; Fig. 7.62A); or may divide as they approach the spleen into branches that vascularize splenic compartments that are normally independent, although they do communicate (dog, cat; Fig. 7.62C). The lymph vessels found in the capsule and trabeculae do not extend into the pulp. The sympathetic and parasympathetic nerves approach with the artery.

The spleen develops from a mesodermal condensation within the dorsal mesogastrium (which becomes the greater omentum) (see Fig. 3.65/*6*). The part of the sheet intervening between the stomach and the spleen may be specifically distinguished as the gastrosplenic ligament.

THE THYMUS

The thymus is of greatest importance in the young animal. It begins to regress about the time of puberty and may eventually almost disappear. Even when a more sizable vestige persists, it will be found to consist largely of fat and fibrous elements.

The thymus has a paired origin from the third pharyngeal pouch (see Fig. 6.5/*6*). Although some uncertainty exists about the precise contributions made by the endoderm and subjacent mesoderm to thymus development, an ectodermal contribution is even conjectured in some species. The buds grow down the neck beside the trachea and invade the mediastinum, in which they extend to the pericardium. The cervical part regresses prematurely in many species (including the dog), and the thymus then appears as a single, median organ. At its peak the thymus is a lobulated structure that fills the ventral part of the cranial mediastinum, fitting about the other contents of this space.

The thymus tissue is divided into a cortex and medulla. The cortex produces the immunocompetent T lymphocytes, which enter the bloodstream for distribution to and multiplication in the peripheral lymphoid organs (nodes and scattered lymph nodules). The medulla is formed of epithelioid cells of more speculative significance (Fig. 7.63). Because of its relevance to the postnatal development and maintenance of immunologic competence, the thymus is of vital importance.

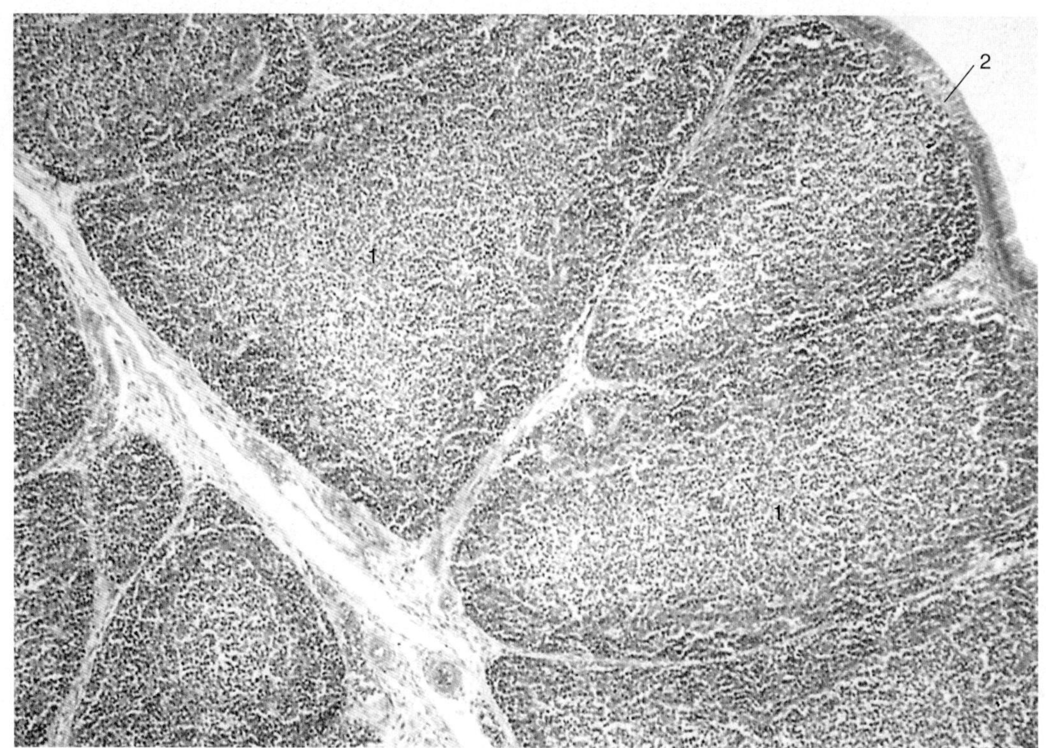

Fig. 7.63 Thymus of calf (hematoxylin and eosin; magnification ×70). *1,* Thymic lobules; *2,* capsule.

COMPREHENSION CHECK

Create a list of the organs that have backup arterial blood supply.

Using embryologic foundation, compare the structure of the fetal and postnatal heart, and detail the transition of the heart from fetal to postnatal life.

Practice auscultation on species of your choice. Imagine you hear a "murmur." Work through different types of murmurs and their structural origins.

8 The Nervous System

INTRODUCTORY CONCEPTS

Every living organism must be able to react appropriately to changes in its environment if it is to survive. The detection of these environmental changes, their subsequent integration and interpretation, and finally, the production of a behavioral response are the function of the nervous system, incomparably the most complicated of the body systems.

The immense complexity of the nervous system occurs at the microscopic level and, as such, cannot be appreciated by a review of its gross structure. Ongoing advances in research methods, including the development of genetic, molecular, and optical tools, has allowed us to examine and manipulate the activity of individual cells and circuitry, but sufficient detailed knowledge of the complex and diverse connections making up the neural circuits of the nervous system still eludes us. Nevertheless, there is much to be learned from a description of the organization of the nervous system and the general functional regions, of the brain in particular, keeping in mind that there is much we still do not understand.

The approach in this chapter is the presentation of an initial description of the basic organization, cells, and circuitry of the nervous system followed by a more detailed region-by-region description of neural development, morphology, and function. We use it knowing that more complete functional analyses will be provided by concurrent or later courses of physiology and neurology.

THE SUBDIVISIONS OF THE NERVOUS SYSTEM

Although the nervous system forms a single, integrated whole, it is useful to discuss several anatomic and functional divisions (Fig. 8.1). The most fundamental division can be made on an anatomic basis, distinguishing the *central nervous system*—consisting of the brain (Fig. 8.1/*1*) and spinal cord (Fig. 8.1/*2*)—from the *peripheral nervous system* (Fig. 8.1/*3*), which includes the spinal nerves, which travel throughout the body and limbs, and the cranial nerves, which travel in the head. Although these two parts of the nervous system function closely together, they have distinct embryologic origins, as we discuss later in the chapter, and also respond differently to injury—that is, the peripheral nervous system has some capacity for regeneration of damaged fibers, but the central nervous system does not regenerate.

The peripheral nervous system is further divided functionally into *afferent* and *efferent* divisions. The afferent component of the peripheral nervous system, also termed the *sensory* component, conducts impulses *toward* the spinal cord and brain (Fig. 8.1/*4*); the efferent, or *motor* component of the peripheral nervous system conveys impulses *away from* the brain and spinal cord (Fig. 8.1/*5*). Each of the afferent and efferent components of the peripheral nervous system is further subdivided into the *somatic* and *visceral* systems. The *somatic system* is concerned with both sensory and motor functions that determine the relationship of the organism to the outside world. They include detection of stimuli in the skin and tissues of the limbs and torso as well as behavioral actions such as locomotion. The somatic system is sometimes referred to as the *voluntary system,* because there is a greater conscious awareness and greater voluntary control of somatic functions than of the visceral functions. The *visceral system* is concerned with sensory and motor functions that relate to the internal viscera: the regulation of the blood pressure and heart rate, the control of glandular activity and digestive processes, and so forth. The motor component of the visceral peripheral nervous system is also referred to as the autonomic nervous system, discussed in more detail here and later in the chapter.

There are several significant subdivisions of the sensory or afferent system that warrant further description. The *general* classification refers to that part of the sensory system that senses pressure, stretch, temperature, and noxious stimuli from tissues throughout the body and head. The *special* classification refers to those senses in the head for vision, audition, taste, smell, and balance.

General somatic afferent pathways originate in receptors within the skin and deeper somatic tissues of the body wall and limbs. The pathways that arise from skin receptors are concerned with the *exteroceptive* sensations, such as touch, temperature, and pain, that respond to stimuli delivered from outside the organism. Receptors within the deeper tissues, the *proprioceptive* category, include stretch and tension receptors in muscle and joint capsules. These receptors provide information about the position and movements of the muscles and body segments relative to one another. General somatic afferent fibers are present in all spinal nerves and in cranial nerve V, the trigeminal nerve (see Table 8.2).

General visceral afferent pathways originate in the receptors of vessels and glands and the viscera of the head

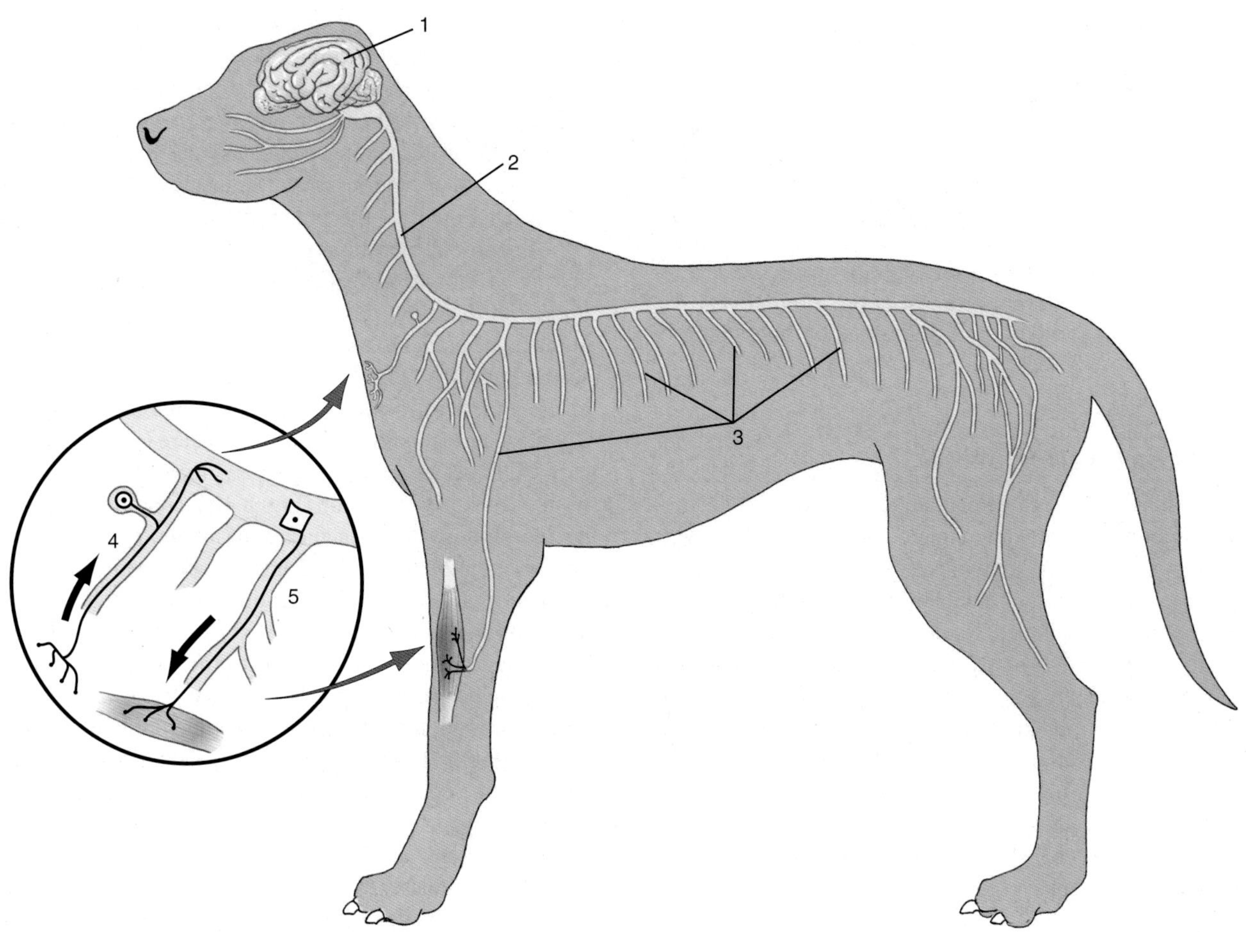

Fig. 8.1 The nervous system can be divided into the central nervous system, comprised of the *(1)* brain plus *(2)* spinal cord, and the peripheral nervous system, comprised of the peripheral nerves *(3)* and associated ganglia. The peripheral nervous system is further divided into the sensory, or afferent system *(4)* and the motor or efferent system *(5)*. See text for details.

and trunk that respond largely to stretch and chemical stimuli. The fibers of this division are found in the cranial nerves III, V, VII, IX, and X and all spinal nerves

Special somatic afferent pathways have a more restricted origin within certain special sense organs of the head: the retina of the eye and the cochlear and vestibular components of the inner ear, which are concerned with vision, hearing, and balance, respectively. Special somatic afferent fibers are thus found only within two cranial nerves, the optic (II) and vestibulocochlear (VIII) nerves.

Special visceral afferent pathways arise from the special sense organs of smell and taste. Fibers conveying olfactory information are confined to the olfactory nerve (I); those conveying gustatory (taste) information are confined to a small group of cranial nerves, VII and IX.

Efferent or motor systems are divided more simply:

- *Somatic efferent* pathways innervate striated muscles. In the body and limbs, these are the muscles that arise from somites. In the head, striated muscles arise from the pharyngeal, or branchial, arches. Somatic efferent fibers are found in all spinal nerves and in all cranial nerves except those that are exclusively sensory nerves (I, II, VIII).
- *Visceral efferent* pathways—that is, the autonomic nervous system, innervate the smooth muscle of blood vessels, viscera, heart muscle, and glands. The autonomic system has two major divisions—the sympathetic and parasympathetic components. Most organs receive innervation from both components (p. 313). The sympathetic and parasympathetic components are often described as having antagonistic actions on each organ, although "balancing" might better describe their cooperative role. Visceral efferent fibers of the *sympathetic division* leave the central nervous system via the spinal nerves in the thoracolumbar regions of the spinal cord; those of the *parasympathetic division* are found in a small group of cranial nerves (III, VII, IX, X) and in spinal nerves in the sacral region of the spinal cord. Many visceral efferent fibers travel to their target organ by joining with other nerves so that they obtain a very widespread peripheral distribution.

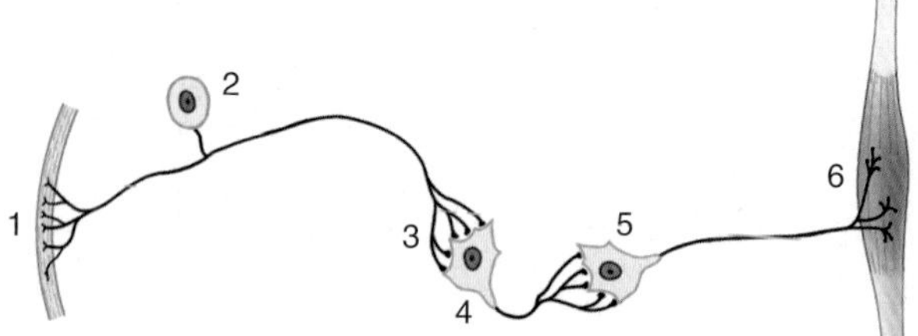

Fig. 8.2 A simplified receptor:effector neural circuit. *1*, Skin receptor; *2*, afferent or sensory neuron; *3*, synapses on interneuron; *4*, interneuron; *5*, efferent or motor neuron; *6*, striated muscle (effector). See text for details.

The Structural Elements

The cellular basis for the remarkable functioning of the nervous system is the network of interconnected cells known as *neurons*. Neurons are highly specialized cells in which the membrane properties of excitability and conductivity are extremely well developed. Rapid, transient changes in electrical potentials travel along neuronal membranes and then are transmitted between neurons within the same circuit through connections known as *synapses*. A brief description of a highly simplified circuit will serve to explain the manner in which neurons subserve an organism's behavioral reaction to an environmental stimulus (Fig. 8.2). A stimulus, such as change in pressure or temperature, is first detected by a receptor organ (*1*) Regardless of the type of stimulus, the neuron associated with the receptor (*2*), normally a *sensory neuron* in the peripheral nervous system, translates this change into an electrical potential, and the impulse, or *action potential,* travels the length of the neuron before transmission, via one or more synapses (*3*), to the next neuron in the circuit. This second neuron (*4*), located in the central nervous system, receives and in turn transmits the electrical signal to a third neuron within the central nervous system (*5*). This neuron, the motor neuron, transmits the signal out of the central nervous system to an effector organ in the periphery, normally a muscle (*6*), resulting in muscle contraction and ultimately movement. Although this description is an oversimplification of any particular neuronal circuitry, it illustrates that the properties of neurons and their organization into anatomic circuits form the underlying basis for nervous system function.

The typical *neuron* consists of the perikaryon, or cell body, containing the nucleus from which extend numerous elongated processes (Fig. 8.3). The processes, which vary considerably in number, length, and form, are of two varieties, the dendrites and the axon. Dendrites are multiple and highly branched, and they transmit impulses toward the cell body; the axon is always single at its origin at the cell body and conveys impulses away from the cell body. This general morphology underlies four functional regions of the neuron: *inputs* from other neurons or receptors are received as synapses on dendrites (Fig. 8.3/*1*); the membrane of the cell body is positioned to support *integration* of the signals from each dendrite (Fig. 8.3/*2*); generation of a new electrical signal occurs at the junction of the cell body with the axon; and then *transmission* of the impulse along the axon occurs, toward synaptic connections with other neurons or with muscle cells (Fig. 8.3/*3*). The arrangement of the processes results in a wide variety of neuronal morphology (Fig. 8.3D), but superficially permits a simple classification. Most neurons are *multipolar* in that they possess a number (often a very large number) of branching dendrites that join the perikaryon at scattered points (Fig. 8.3A). Some neurons, predominant in the peripheral nervous system, are bipolar or unipolar. *Bipolar* neurons possess dendrites that are joined in a common trunk before reaching the perikaryon at a site remote from the origin of the axon (Fig. 8.3B). Neurons with bipolar morphology exist in the retina of the eye and in the olfactory epithelium. The dendrites and axon of a *unipolar* neuron are directly contiguous along a single process (conventionally known as the axon), and the perikaryon is attached to the axon by a short process (Fig. 8.3C). All sensory neurons in the peripheral nervous system are unipolar in morphology. In both bipolar and unipolar neurons, the integration and generation of the new electrical signal occurs at the confluence of the dendrites rather than at the cell body (Fig. 8.3B and C).

The different varieties of neurons have specific distributions that are related to their particular functions. Clearly, a much branched dendritic tree enables a neuron to receive impulses from many sources. Similarly, a much branched axon makes connection with and stimulates many cells. The first arrangement allows a convergence of impulses from various origins; the second provides for a divergence or diffusion of a message. An axon may establish synaptic connections with the bodies, dendrites, or axons of other neurons, or in the case of the axon of a motor neuron, with the cell membrane of muscle cells. Most neurons establish many synapses: some have many thousands of synaptic sites. Synapses have a variable morphology, but only an elementary description is required here. The synapse is a specialization of both the membrane of the transmitting, or presynaptic, cell, and of the receiving, or postsynaptic, cell. The cell membranes of each are separated by a very narrow gap. An action potential, arriving at the presynaptic terminal membrane, does not jump from cell to cell; instead, it causes the release of a specific chemical transmitter substance that diffuses across the gap. This chemical transmitter is normally stored in vesicles in the presynaptic terminal, awaiting the arrival of the action potential. The arrival of the action potential initiates fusion of the presynaptic vesicle membrane with the cell membrane of the presynaptic terminal, causing release of the chemical transmitter into the synaptic gap. When this substance arrives at the cell membrane of the postsynaptic cell, it binds to receptors embedded in the postsynaptic membrane. These

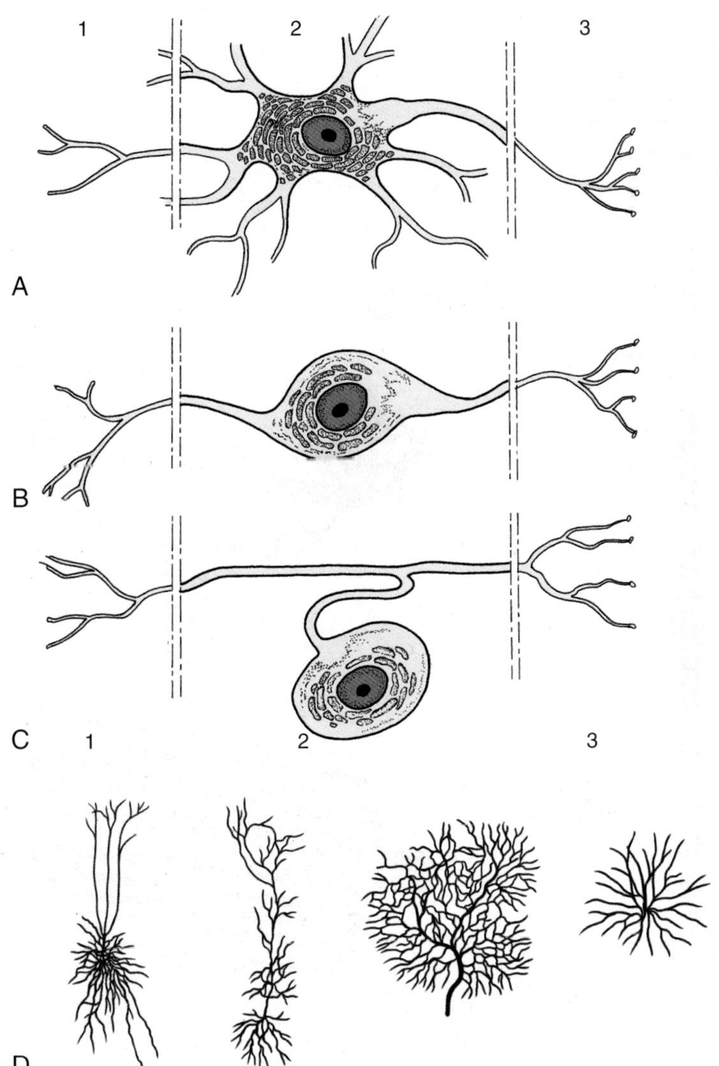

Fig. 8.3 (A–C) Schematic diagrams of (A) multipolar, (B) bipolar, and (C) unipolar neurons. *1,* Receptor side (dendrites); *2,* cell body (perikaryon); *3,* effector side (axon). (D) Drawings of actual neurons.

receptors, once bound with the transmitter, produce one of two effects: they can either depolarize or excite the postsynaptic membrane, thus contributing to a new action potential, or they can hyperpolarize the membrane, producing an inhibitory effect by making the generation of an action potential less likely. The existence of both excitatory and inhibitory synapses, sometimes on the same cell, provides a means for a great diversity of response. Many transmitter substances are known; the most common are acetylcholine, glutamate, GABA (gamma-aminobutyric acid), noradrenaline, serotonin, and many neuropeptides. This description of synaptic activity as being excitatory or inhibitory is, for brevity's sake, an oversimplification of the complexities of synaptic transmission in the nervous system. Many postsynaptic receptors neither directly contribute to nor inhibit the generation of an action potential but instead make the postsynaptic cell more or less responsive to other transmitters at nearby synapses. This response, termed *neuromodulation,* permits the fine-tuning of a neuron's response to particular inputs, thus contributing to the subtle nuances of chemical neurotransmission.

Neurons are supported by other specialized cells. The supporting cells of the brain and spinal cord, which are much more numerous than neurons, are known as *neuroglia* and consist of two main types: *astrocytes* and *oligodendrocytes.* In brief, astrocytes assist in nutrition of neurons, maintenance of the extracellular environment, and neurotransmission; oligodendrocytes provide axons within the brain and spinal cord with cell membrane sheaths that insulate the axons from their surroundings and speed action potential conductance. The cell membrane sheaths, termed *myelin,* are formed by

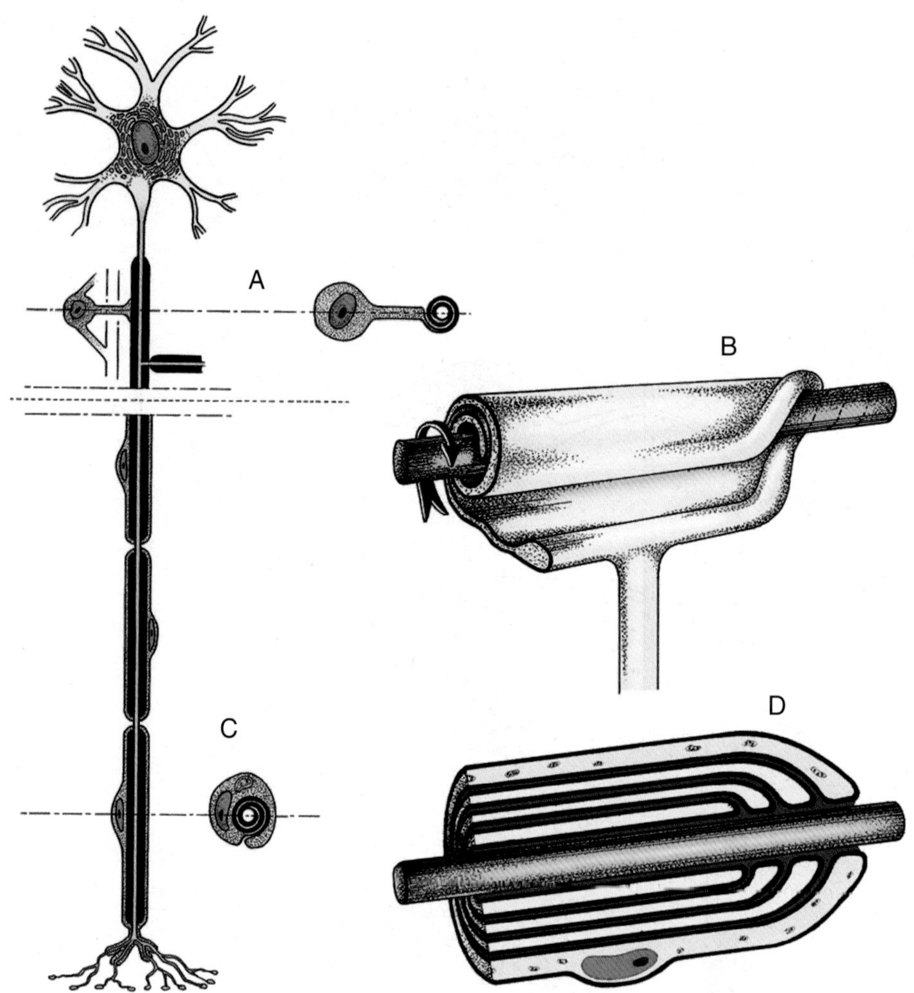

Fig. 8.4 (A) and (B) Neuron with its axon enwrapped within a myelin sheath supplied by oligodendrocytes within the central nervous system. (C) and (D) Once the axon leaves the central nervous system, myelin is provided by Schwann cells in the peripheral nervous system. In both cases, the myelin consists of concentric plasmalemma layers forming an insulating sheath.

the concentric wrapping of oligodendrocyte membrane around the axon (Fig. 8.4).

Myelin imparts a white color to nerve fibers seen *en masse,* and groups of myelinated axons in the brain and spinal cord are termed *white matter.* Within white matter of the brain and spinal cord, axons of common origin, destination, and function tend to be aggregated together into *fasciculi* or *tracts.* Most tracts are named by the combination of their origin employed as prefix with their destination employed as suffix. Thus, the spinocerebellar tracts originate in the spinal cord and terminate in the cerebellum; the converse is true for the cerebellospinal tracts. Groups of perikarya, or neuronal cell bodies, in the brain and spinal cord are termed *nuclei* and, when set off by the whiteness of adjacent fiber bundles, take on a gray or beige color; this effect permits the distinction of *gray matter* from white matter of the brain and spinal cord.

Within the peripheral nervous system (outside the brain and spinal cord), axons receive insulation similar to that of axons in the brain and cord, but from another type of supporting cell, the *Schwann cell* (also termed *neurolemmocyte;* Fig. 8.4). Peripheral axons are grouped together and are protected, supported, and subdivided by connective tissue sheaths and septa, forming the *peripheral nerves.* The presence of neuronal perikarya in the peripheral nervous system is limited to those of sensory afferent and visceral efferent or autonomic neurons, and they are found in aggregations known as *ganglia.* Autonomic ganglia on peripheral nerves and sensory ganglia on peripheral nerve roots may form visible swellings; they may also be distinguished by their color and texture, which are darker and firmer than the related nerves or nerve roots.

Stimulus-Response Function of the Nervous System

Having established these fundamental points, we may now return to consider the stimulus-response apparatus in more detail (see Fig. 8.2). Each neuron in the nervous system is part of one or multiple circuits that have specific behavioral functions. Although not all behavior can be seen as a direct response to a sensory stimulus, we can consider that behavior is produced ultimately as a result of processing of sensory stimuli. This processing can occur either immediately when stimuli are detected—that is, as simple reflex movement—or as a result of longer term processing of previously received and integrated sensory stimuli—stored as memory, for example—which can contribute to self-initiated, more complex behavior. Nevertheless, it is valuable to consider reflexive behavior first, because the underlying neural circuitry contains many of the basic elements of more complex behavior and is itself useful in a clinical context.

The *monosynaptic reflex arc* is often described as the most simple reflex, in that only two neurons, and the synaptic connection between them, are involved in the reflex circuit. This is actually an uncommon arrangement, in that all other known reflexes involve multiple neurons. The monosynaptic reflex, generally termed the *stretch* or *myotatic reflex,* is associated with most muscles, the most familiar example of which is the patellar or knee-jerk reflex (Fig. 8.5). This reflex is the rapid, brief contraction of the quadriceps femoris muscle elicited by an appropriate tap on the patellar ligament, the functional continuation of the quadriceps femoris (*1*). The tap stretches the muscle and stimulates receptors termed *muscle spindles* within the muscle belly (*2*), which detect changes in length; activation of the muscle spindle generates action potentials in the sensory afferent neurons (*3*), innervating the spindle, and these impulses are transmitted along sensory axons within the femoral nerve to reach the spinal cord. Within the spinal cord gray matter, the sensory neurons form excitatory synapses onto those motoneurons that innervate the quadriceps muscle (*4*). The axons of these motoneurons in turn exit the spinal cord and travel in efferent direction within the femoral nerve, (*5*) to innervate the muscle fibers of the quadriceps muscle (*6*). Motoneuron excitation results in muscle fiber excitation and contraction to produce the brief extension of the stifle joint. This reflex is useful clinically and is elicited when the animal is not weight bearing, in order to produce detectable joint extension. Its essential function for the animal, however, is to maintain extensor muscle activation when the animal is weight-bearing, such that the limbs remain extended against gravity (see Fig. 8.48).

In all reflexes other than the stretch reflex, neurons are interposed in the circuitry between the afferent and efferent neurons (Fig. 8.6/*3*). These neurons are conventionally

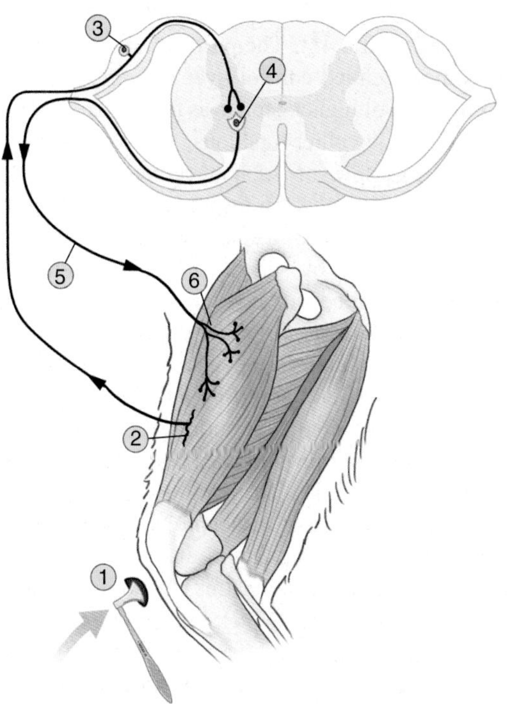

Fig. 8.5 The monosynaptic patellar reflex. The stretch on the tendon *(1)* stimulates muscle spindles *(2)*, generating action potentials that travel via the afferent neuron *(3)* to the spinal cord. The impulse is then transmitted to the efferent neuron *(4)*, whose axon *(5)* innervates the quadriceps muscle *(6)*.

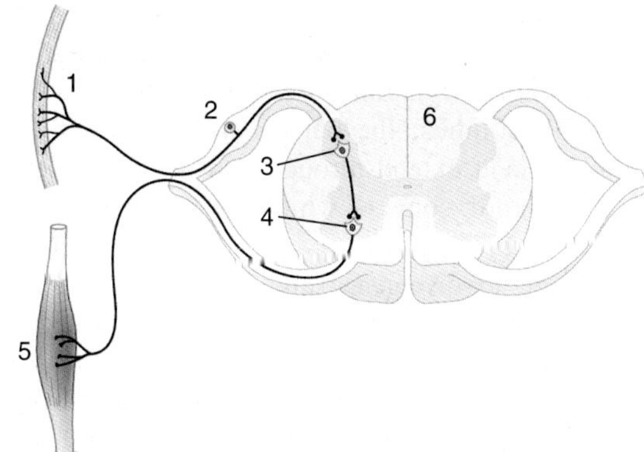

Fig. 8.6 Schematic representation of a reflex chain in which an interneuron is interposed. *1*, Skin receptor; *2*, afferent neuron; *3*, synapse on interneuron; *4*, synapse at efferent neuron; *5*, muscle; *6*, spinal cord.

known as *interneurons,* although several synonyms exist. Furthermore, all reflexes, including the stretch reflex, involve complex collateral circuitry in which additional neurons not directly interposed between the afferent and efferent neurons are stimulated or inhibited. This arrangement is enabled by the presence of collateral branches of sensory afferent axons within the central nervous system such that the initial sensory signal is divergently distributed within this system and is used by multiple neural circuits (see Figs. 8.7 and 8.48). The purpose of such divergence includes more refined control over the reflex movements and notification of higher centers as to the state of the afferent activity, among other functions.

A good example of such a refined and integrated response is provided by the response to a noxious stimulus applied to the limb of a standing animal. The noxious stimulus is detected by sensory neurons specialized for this modality, termed *nociceptors*. The reflex response, termed the *withdrawal* or *flexor reflex*, is the flexion of all joints of the stimulated limb, such that the limb is withdrawn from the offending stimulus. This action occurs through the coordinated contraction of many flexor muscles across several joints of the limb. The signal from nociceptor activation is distributed within the spinal cord by collateral branching of nociceptor afferent axons, each branch of which synapses upon an individual interneuron, which in turn transmits this excitation to multiple flexor motoneurons (Fig. 8.7/*2*). Furthermore, the smooth flexion of the limb joints is facilitated by the relaxation of antagonistic extensor muscles that would normally be active in the standing animal. This process necessitates, again through divergence of the same afferent signal, excitation of a different set of interneurons that are capable of inhibiting extensor motoneurons of the same limb. The pathways involved in producing this coordinated activation and inhibition of appropriate muscles extend through several segments of the cord to reach and excite or inhibit the efferent neurons that supply the flexor and extensor muscles of the stimulated limb (Fig. 8.7/*3*). At the same time, the animal has to adjust to the removal of support from one of its limbs by redistributing its weight over the other limbs; the pathways necessary for this wider adjustment extend through considerable stretches of the spinal cord, some of which cross to the contralateral side (Fig. 8.7).

In addition to divergence and integration of afferent information within the spinal cord to coordinate these movements, some information travels cranially to reach brain regions specialized for equilibrium, so that the animal can maintain its balance while standing on three legs. To this complexity of the reflex response is added the inevitable relay of initial nociceptor activation to those regions of the brain involved in decision making, such that the animal can assess the situation and consider whether a more general response, such as flight from or retaliation against the aggressor, would be appropriate. This considered response involves integrative circuitry of various degrees of complexity, extending through the cord and brain, and drawing on those higher centers that are concerned with memory and judgment. Thus, the relationship between reflexive movements and more complex cognitively driven behavior is a continuum, a function of the integration and processing of multiple afferent inputs by increasingly sophisticated neural circuitry.

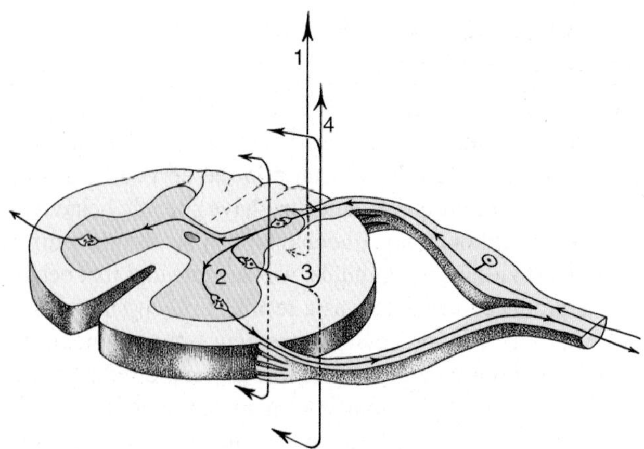

Fig. 8.7 The course of fibers within the spinal cord. Some afferent fibers in the dorsal funiculus travel directly toward the brain *(1)*; others end on interneurons in the dorsal horn. From here impulses can be transmitted directly to efferent neurons *(2)* or to other interneurons that transmit impulses caudally or cranially within the spinal cord *(3)*, some extending to the brain *(4)*.

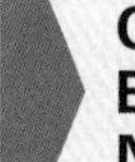

GENERAL MORPHOLOGY AND EMBRYOLOGY OF THE CENTRAL NERVOUS SYSTEM

Introductory Survey

The brain* and spinal cord† are continuous without any clear demarcation. The brain is a very irregular organ whose shape conforms very approximately to the cranial cavity in which it is lodged, whereas the slender elongated cord has a more regular and uniform appearance.

The size of the brain does not bear a linear relationship to that of the animal from which it came but is relatively smaller in large species and is proportionately larger in more advanced mammals. The ratio of brain mass to body mass is of the order of 1:50, 1:200, and 1:800 in the human, dog, and horse, respectively. As a general rule, domestication of a species leads to a smaller brain to body mass ratio than in nondomesticated species of the same kind; the process is not reversed by putting domesticated animals back into the wild. Perhaps more important is the relative development of particular parts of the brain; mammals possess a relative preponderance of phylogenetically newer parts, particularly in the cerebrum generally and in "higher" mammals specifically, in comparison with other forms.

* The official term, *encephalon*, is rarely encountered but provides a much used stem—*encephalitis* and *electroencephalography*.

† The official term is *medulla spinalis*. Unfortunately, medulla (marrow) is used in several contexts. The term *medulla tout court* generally signifies medulla oblongata, the hindmost part of the brainstem.

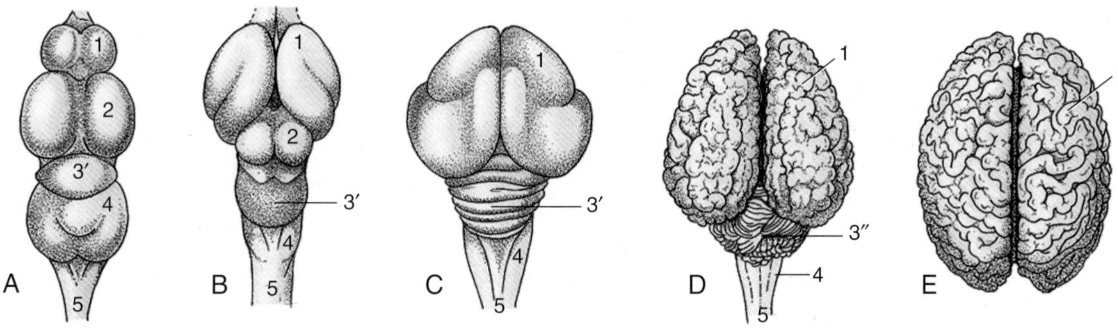

Fig. 8.8 Vertebrate brains illustrating the phylogenetic development. The increase in volume and complexity of the telencephalon and cerebellum is most striking. (A) Fish (carp); (B) reptile (python); (C) bird (duck); (D) mammal (cattle); (E) mammal (human). *1*, Telencephalon; *2*, mesencephalon; *3′ and 3″*, metencephalon *(3′* archicerebellum in *A-C; 3″* neocerebellum in D*)*; myelencephalon; *5*, spinal cord.

The great size and complexity of the human cerebral hemispheres provide the extreme example of this evolutionary trend (Fig. 8.8).

An initial survey of the brain as a whole is given here, followed by an account of its development. Detailed descriptions of the parts of the central nervous system follow in this chapter. Repeated consultation should be made to the figures indicated so that the structures named can be located and identified.

Dorsal views show the cerebral hemispheres and cerebellum as the dominant features of the mammalian and avian brain; only a small part of the medulla oblongata is visible in continuity with the spinal cord (Fig. 8.8 C, D). The semiovoid cerebral hemispheres are divided from each other by a deep longitudinal fissure and from the cerebellum by a transverse fissure; when the brain is in situ, both fissures are occupied by folds of the tough dural membrane that lines the cranial cavity. In many domestic mammals, each hemisphere is molded to display ridges (gyri) and grooves (sulci) in patterns that differ significantly among the various species. The cerebellum has an even more pronounced surface folding, the purpose of which is to increase the area available for neural processing.

The ventral aspect of the brain is flatter overall and reveals the subdivisions of the brain more clearly (see Fig. 8.19). The caudalmost part is the medulla oblongata, which widens cranially until it terminates at a prominent transverse ridge. This ridge represents the ventral surface of the next part of the brain, the pons. The ridge is formed by the transverse fibers of the pons, which can be followed dorsally over the lateral aspect to join the cerebellum (Fig. 8.19). The midbrain is located cranial to the pons and is represented on the ventral aspect of the brain by two divergent columns, the crura cerebri or cerebral peduncles (Fig. 8.19/*12*). They continue rostrally to disappear into the depths of the hemispheres. They are separated by the interpeduncular fossa, a shallow depression on the ventral midline of the midbrain (Fig. 8.19/*13*). The forebrain lies rostral to this depression; its most prominent ventral median features of the forebrain are the hypothalamus (to which the hypophysis [pituitary gland] is attached by a stalk) and the crossing or chiasm formed by the optic nerves. The larger part of the forebrain is provided by the paired cerebral hemispheres, which have as their most prominent ventral features the rounded piriform lobes (Fig. 8.19/*3*), flanking the crura cerebri, and the rostrally located olfactory tracts (Fig. 8.19/*2*), which originate in the olfactory bulbs that project at the rostral extremity. The superficial origins of the cranial nerves, all except the trochlear (IV) pair, are also visible on the ventral surface.

The cerebral hemispheres and cerebellum dominate the dorsal aspect of the brain, and when they are removed, all that remains is referred to as the *brainstem,* which is directly continuous with the spinal cord (see Fig. 8.22).

Development

The anatomy of the brain is most easily understood by reference to its development. As such, a general account is provided here; additional details are mentioned as appropriate during descriptions of regional neuroanatomy.

The nervous system makes a very early appearance, becoming evident at the embryonic disk stage as an elongated thickening (neural plate) of the ectoderm that overlies the notochord and paraxial mesoderm. The lateral parts of the neural plate are soon raised above the surrounding surface by growth of the underlying mesoderm and form bilateral neural folds that slope toward an axial crease, the neural groove. As the process continues, the edges of the folds become increasingly prominent and then bend inward toward each other; eventually they meet and fuse, converting the neural groove into a neural tube (Fig. 8.9). The tube, which is the primordium of the brain and spinal cord, then sinks ventral to, and is separated from, the overlying nonneural ectoderm, which fuses dorsal to the neural tube to produce a continuous ectodermal layer. At the same time, cells at the crest of the neural folds, at the junction with

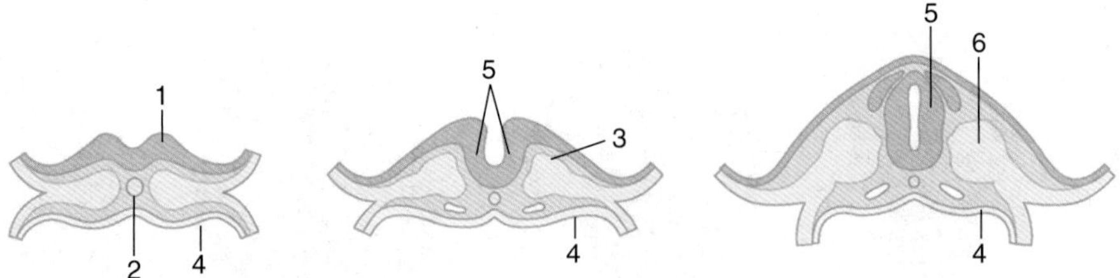

Fig. 8.9 *Left to right,* Three stages in the closure of the neural plate. *1,* Neural plate; *2,* notochord; *3,* paraxial mesoderm; *4,* endoderm; *5,* neural tube; *6,* somite.

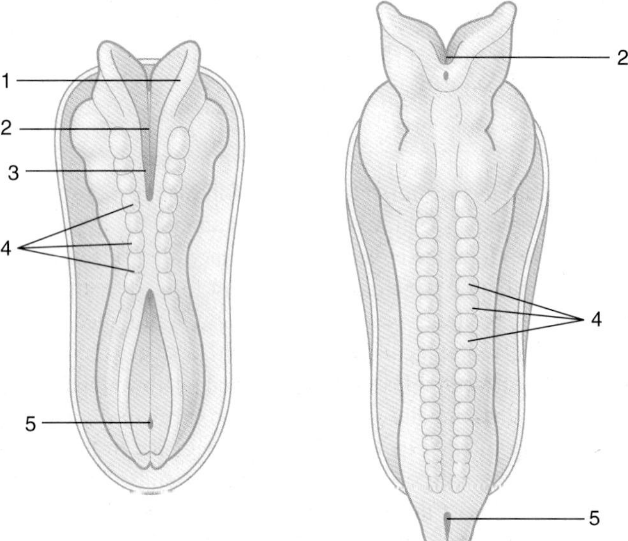

Fig. 8.10 Dorsal views of developing embryos. Two stages in the formation and fusion of the neural folds are illustrated. *1,* Neural fold; *2,* neural groove; *3,* rostral neuropore; *4,* somites; *5,* caudal neuropore.

the nonneural ectoderm, separate from the folds to form continuous cords, the neural crests, that run almost the whole length of the tube at its dorsolateral aspects. Neural crest cells that remain adjacent to the neural tube eventually develop into neurons, which populate peripheral ganglia (i.e., peripheral sensory neurons and neurons of the visceral motor system), and those neural crest cells that migrate away from the neural tube produce neurons of the enteric nervous system, the medullary parts of the adrenal glands, glia, skin melanocytes, and a variety of craniofacial connective tissues.

Closure of the neural tube initially occurs in the presumptive occipital region, which will become the junction of the spinal cord and brain, but fusion soon spreads rostrally and caudally until only two small openings (neuropores; Fig. 8.10/*3* and *5*) remain to provide communication at the surface of the embryo between the lumen of the tube and the amniotic cavity. These openings do not persist long: the rostral neuropore closes first, and the caudal one remains open for another day or two while the tube continues to lengthen at its caudal extremity by extension and subsequent infolding of the neural plate. The abnormal persistence of these openings produces relatively common defects of the brain and spinal cord in which nerve tissue may be exposed on the surface of the body. Failure at the rostral extremity leads to malformation of the forebrain and midbrain with accompanying anomalies of the skull; it is known as *anencephaly,* and although the term implies complete failure of brain development, it can show considerable variation in severity. Most forms are incompatible with life after birth. Failure at the caudal extremity is more common and is known as *spina bifida.* It is associated with defective closure of the vertebral arches. Children and young animals with this malformation may live after birth, though with severe functional disturbance; affected animals are not usually permitted to survive.

The part of the neural tube that forms the brain is wider from the outset and shows localized expansions even before the tube is completely closed. These define three primary brain vesicles: prosencephalon (forebrain), mesencephalon (midbrain), and rhombencephalon (hindbrain). The remaining, more uniform part of the tube becomes the spinal cord. The differentiation of the wall of the neural tube is initially similar along the length of the tube but becomes greatly modified later in the part that becomes the brain, increasingly so toward its rostral extremity. The spinal cord develops more uniformly, and its differentiation is considered first.

A transverse section of the tube at its formation reveals three concentric layers in its structure (Fig. 8.11A). These are unequally developed around the circumference, which is divisible into thick lateral parts connected by thinner dorsal and ventral regions known as the *roof plate* and the *floor plate.* The innermost layer (Fig. 8.11A/*1*) bounding the lumen of the tube is a continuous layer of neuroepithelial cells—these cells are similar to those that remain as the ependyma lining the adult derivatives of the lumen, the central canal, and the ventricular system of the adult spinal cord and brain. During early development, these neuroepithelial cells proliferate rapidly, and although some daughter cells remain in place adjacent to the lumen, most cells migrate outward into the middle (mantle) layer of the wall of the neural tube (Fig. 8.11A/*3*). These migrating cells are neural stem cells, precursors of neurons and glia. The mantle layer itself becomes the gray matter of the brain and spinal cord, containing neuronal cell

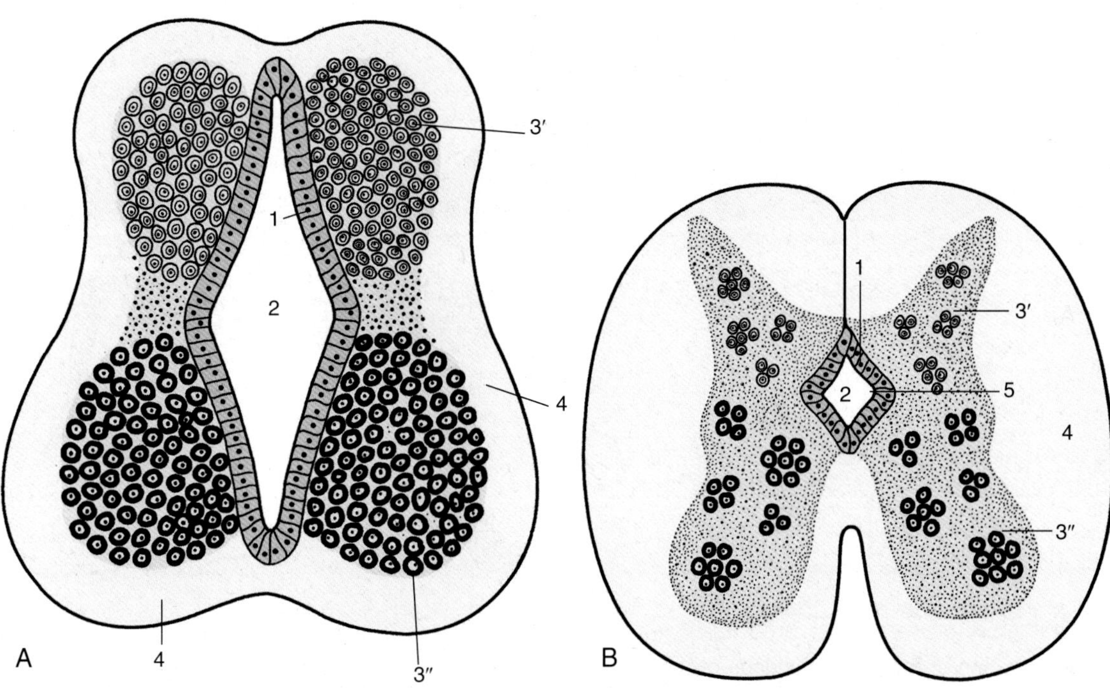

Fig. 8.11 (A) Differentiation of the neural tube. *1*, Neuroepithelial (ependymal) layer; *2*, central canal; *3′* and *3″*, mantle layer (*3′*, dorsal column, alar lamina; *3″*, ventral column, basal lamina); *4*, marginal layer. (B) Further differentiation of the neural tube (spinal cord). *1*, Neuroepithelial layer; *2*, central canal; *3′*, dorsal column of mantle layer; *3″*, ventral column of mantle layer; *4*, marginal layer; *5*, longitudinal limiting groove, or sulcus limitans.

bodies and innumerable neuronal processes. Some of these processes—namely, the axons of developing neurons—grow laterally in the tube, extending outward to form the outer (marginal) layer of the neural tube. The marginal layer (Fig. 8.11A/*4*) eventually becomes the white matter of the spinal cord, in which fibers descend or ascend along the length of the spinal cord for various distances.

As the number of cells of the mantle layer expands through cell division and migration, the mantle layer becomes arranged in dorsal and ventral columns that bulge into the lumen of the tube, columns that are separated by a longitudinal limiting groove (Fig. 8.11B/*5*). The dorsal bulge (alar plate) provides the dorsal horn or dorsal column of the gray matter of the cord; its constituent neurons are those receiving synaptic input from sensory or afferent neurons, among other inputs. The ventral bulge (basal plate) becomes the ventral horn or ventral column of spinal gray matter, which is the location of cell bodies of motor or efferent neurons; both dorsal and ventral horns also contain many interneurons. Neurons with somatic functions segregate from those with visceral functions, and four groups of neurons are then arranged in dorsoventral sequence: somatic afferent, visceral afferent, visceral efferent, and somatic efferent (Fig. 8.12). The roof and floor plates provide passages for nerve fibers that pass from one side of the cord to the other, known as *commissures*.

Further growth of the alar and basal plates causes the lateral parts of the tube wall to expand outward in all directions, submerging the roof and floor plates and creating the dorsal median sulcus and the ventral median fissure that divide the adult cord into its right and left halves. A serial segmentation along the rostrocaudal length of the spinal cord is created by the appearance of the dorsal and ventral roots associated with the spinal nerves. The dorsal roots develop as newly forming axons of developing sensory neurons, differentiating from local condensations of neural crest cells located just lateral to the cord. The axon processes of these sensory neurons extend medially into the cord to reach and penetrate the outer marginal layer. Branches of these axons can extend over several segments before entering the mantle layer to terminate on neurons in the developing dorsal columns; some branches do not synapse within the spinal cord but turn cranially and extend within the marginal layer to reach the developing brain (see Fig. 8.7). The ventral roots are formed by axons of developing motor neurons within the ventral columns. These axons extend laterally through the marginal layer to emerge on the surface of the cord. The appearance of the dorsal roots on the dorsolateral surface of the spinal cord and of the ventral roots on the ventrolateral surface of the cord divides the white matter into dorsal, lateral, and ventral funiculi (Fig. 8.13/*7–9*).

Although the cellular development of the nervous system is not described, two points must be made. In most parts of the brain and spinal cord, the full complement of neurons

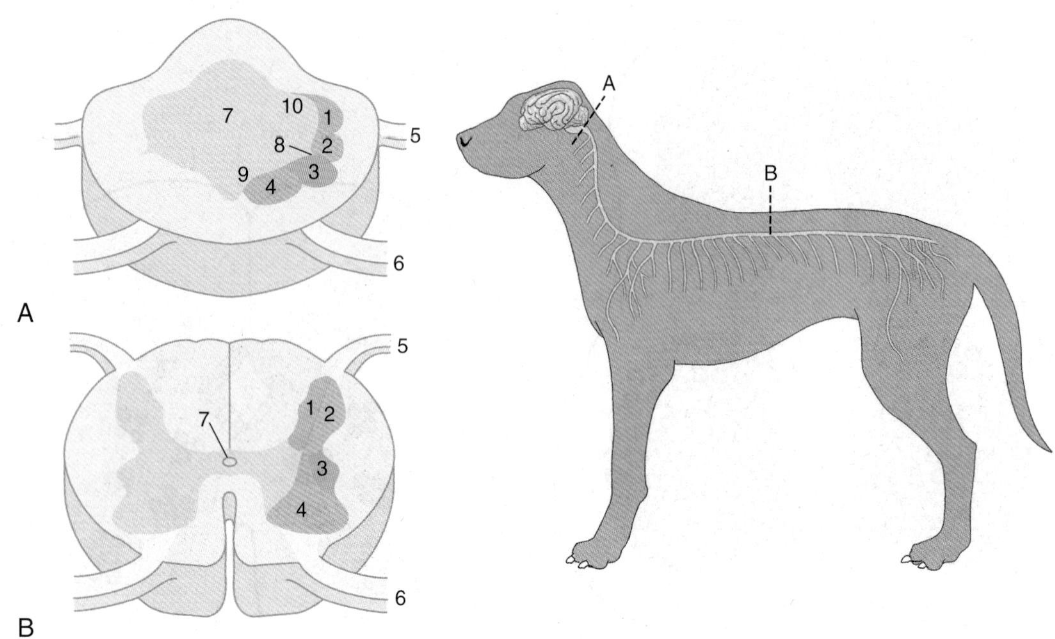

Fig. 8.12 Organization of the gray substance of the (A) medulla oblongata and (B) spinal cord. *1*, Somatic afferent column; *2*, visceral afferent column; *3*, visceral efferent column; *4*, somatic efferent column (lower motor neurons); *5*, dorsal root; *6*, ventral root; *7*, central canal or fourth ventricle; *8*, sulcus limitans; *9*, basal lamina; *10*, alar lamina.

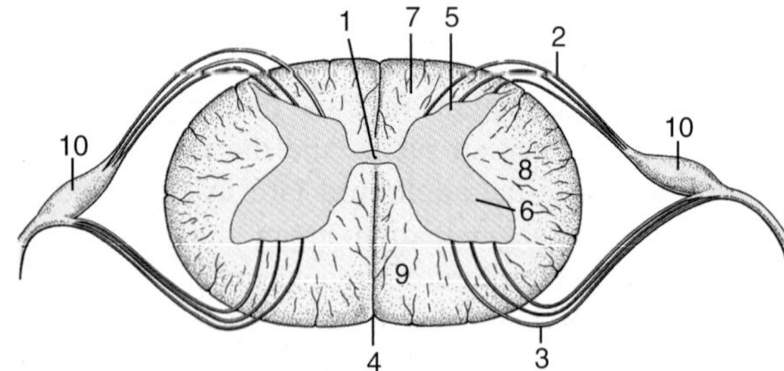

Fig. 8.13 Transverse section of spinal cord showing the subdivision of the white substance by the dorsal and ventral roots of the spinal nerves. *1*, Central canal; *2*, fibers of dorsal root; *3*, fibers of ventral root; *4*, ventral median fissure; *5*, dorsal horn; *6*, ventral horn; *7*, dorsal funiculus; *8*, lateral funiculus; *9*, ventral funiculus; *10*, dorsal root ganglion.

is established shortly after, if not before, birth. However, contrary to former beliefs, in some regions there is a significant, more protracted postnatal recruitment of neural stem cells in areas such as the cerebellum and hippocampus that continues into later life. There is strong evidence that neural stem cells persist, albeit in small numbers, in the adult stages and can be recruited to produce new neurons under certain conditions. The second point relates to the process of myelination of axons within the central nervous system. Different tracts within the brain and cord acquire adequate insulation (essential to their function) at different stages of development, including well after birth. There are important species differences in this process.

During the early development of the brain, three primary brain vesicles, the prosencephalon (forebrain), mesencephalon (midbrain), and rhombencephalon (hindbrain), are evident before closure of the neural tube. At this time, the prosencephalon or forebrain has already extended the evaginations that become the optic cups and eventually form the retina of the eyes. The brain grows more rapidly than the nonneural tissues that surround and enclose it in the embryo, and these constraints enforce a remodeling of its form such that three flexures appear. The most caudal flexure bends the brain ventrally at its junction with the cord. A second flexure at midbrain level occurs almost simultaneously and is sufficiently pronounced to bring the ventral surfaces of the forebrains and hindbrains close together; this relationship is later reversed by the third, or dorsal, flexure, which folds the hindbrain dorsally on itself (Fig. 8.14). The formation of the major divisions of the brain is completed by the appearance of paired lateral evaginations from the alar region of the prosencephalon. These outgrowths, the future cerebral hemispheres, constitute the telencephalon; the unpaired median portion of the prosencephalon, hereafter known as the diencephalon, differentiates into the adult thalamus and related structures. The telencephalon expands in all directions but chiefly in a curve that extends dorsally and caudally to overlap the diencephalon (see Fig. 8.32).

Directly caudal to the developing telencephalon and diencephalon, the midbrain, or mesencephalon, remains undivided. The alar region at this level becomes the tectum of the midbrain, and the basal region the tegmentum of the midbrain. The hindbrain develops cranially into the

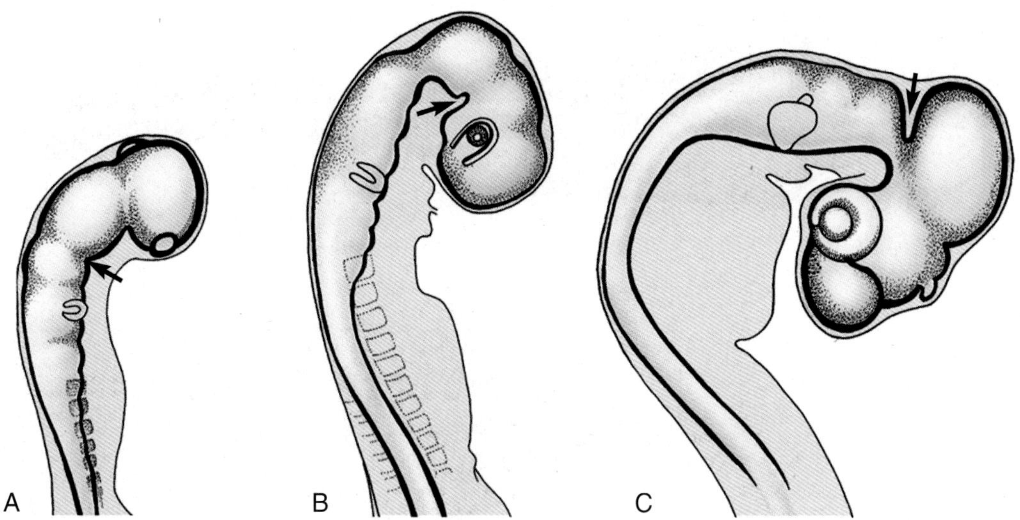

Fig. 8.14 Formation of the (A) caudal ventral, (B) rostral ventral, and (C) dorsal flexures *(arrows)*.

TABLE 8.1 DERIVATIVES OF THE NEURAL TUBE

Primary Division	Subdivisions	Major Derivatives	Lumen
Prosencephalon	Telencephalon	Cerebral cortex	Lateral ventricles (paired)
		Basal nuclei	
		Limbic system	
	Diencephalon	Epithalamus	Third ventricle
		Thalamus	
		Hypothalamus	
Mesencephalon		Tectum (corpora quadrigemina)	Mesencephalic aqueduct
		Tegmentum	
Rhombencephalon	Metencephalon	Cerebellum	Rostral part of fourth ventricle
		Pons	
	Myelencephalon	Medulla oblongata	Caudal part of fourth ventricle
Remainder of neural tube		Spinal cord	Central canal

metencephalon and caudally into the myelencephalon. The basal plate of the metencephalon develops into the structures of the pons in the adult, whereas the alar plate undergoes a bilateral expansion dorsally, becoming the cerebellum. The myelencephalon develops into the medulla oblongata of the adult, continuous caudally with the spinal cord.

Throughout neural development, the lumen of the original neural tube persists and undergoes modification in shape and size along with the flexures and expansions of the neural tube, eventually becoming the canal and ventricular system of the adult central nervous system. The origin of the major components and ventricles of the brain may be conveniently summarized in tabular form (Table 8.1).

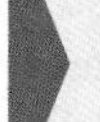

DESCRIPTIVE ANATOMY OF THE CENTRAL NERVOUS SYSTEM

The Spinal Cord

The spinal cord (medulla spinalis) is an elongated structure that is more or less cylindrical but with some dorsoventral flattening and certain regional variations in form and

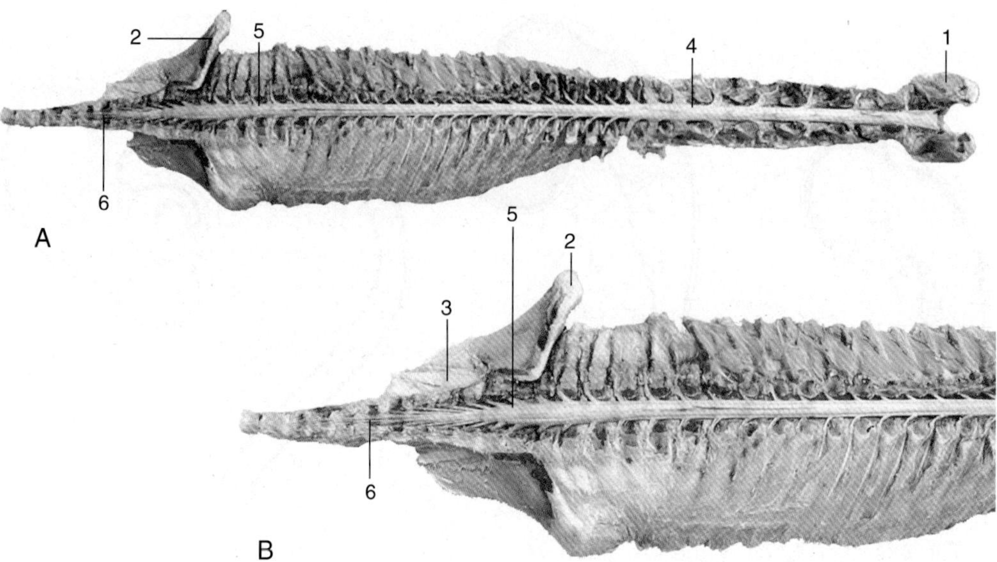

Fig. 8.15 (A) Dorsal view of the spinal cord and the vertebral pedicles of the horse. The spinal cord is shorter than the vertebral canal (ascensus medullae spinalis). (B) Enlargement of the caudal part. *1,* Atlas; *2,* ilium; *3,* sacrum; *4,* cervical intumescence; *5,* lumbar intumescence; *6,* cauda equina.

dimensions. The most important of these are the thickenings (*intumescentiae;* Fig. 8.15) of the regions that give origin to the nerves supplying the forelimbs and hindlimbs and the final caudal tapering (*conus medullaris*). The spinal cord lies within the vertebral canal, formed by the alignment of the series of vertebrae, and is divided into segments along its craniocaudal length. Each spinal segment is defined by its association with a pair of spinal nerves, formed by the union of a dorsal root arising from dorsolateral margin of the spinal cord, containing sensory afferent fibers, and a ventral root, containing motor efferent fibers, arising ventrolaterally as described (p. 27). The segments, and corresponding spinal nerves, are grouped and named according to the region of the body: from cranial to caudal, these are cervical, thoracic, lumbar, sacral, and caudal. The number of segments in each group varies among species and is identical to the corresponding number of vertebrae for each species except in the cervical region, where there is always one less cervical vertebra than cervical spinal segment. The position of the spinal segments relative to the corresponding vertebrae varies along the length of the cord. Species-specific details are discussed in later chapters, but the most consistent and notable disparity is in the lumbar region, where the short craniocaudal length of each of the caudalmost lumbar segments and of the sacral and caudal spinal segments results in the cranial displacement of these segments to lie within the lumbar vertebrae. The relationship between the spinal nerves and corresponding vertebrae remains consistent along the length of the spinal column, however, with the result that the last lumbar, and the sacral and caudal spinal nerves necessarily must travel caudally within the vertebral canal before exiting at their corresponding vertebrae. This group of nerves, thought to resemble the tail of a horse, is termed the *cauda equina* and represents the innervation of much of the perineum, tail, and pelvic viscera (Fig. 8.15/*6* and Fig. 12.9/*9*). The location of the cauda equina serves as a convenient access for anesthesia of these structures, particularly in obstetric cases.

A simple transverse section shows a central mass of gray matter perforated in the midline by a small central canal, which is the derivative of the lumen of the embryonic neural tube (Figs. 8.13/*1* and 8.11A and B/*2*). The gray matter, which has a crude resemblance to a butterfly or an *H,* is commonly described as exhibiting dorsal and ventral horns or columns; the former is a rather misleading term because the *horns* extend the length of the cord (Fig. 8.16). The dorsal horn corresponds to the embryonic alar plate. It contains neurons receiving afferent input from sensory axons entering the cord through the dorsal root as well as innumerable interneurons. Somatic sensory input synapses on dorsomedially located interneurons and visceral afferent neurons synapse on dorsolaterally located interneurons (Fig. 8.17). The ventral horn is derived from the basal plate; it is composed in part of the cell bodies of somatic efferent, or motor neurons, which are located ventrally, and visceral efferent neurons, which form an additional lateral horn confined to the thoracolumbar and sacral regions of the cord.

The neurons within each column are more specifically grouped according to their functional and topical associations, but this grouping is not grossly discernible.

The white matter that surrounds the gray matter is divided into three funiculi on each side (Fig. 8.18/*I–III*). The dorsal

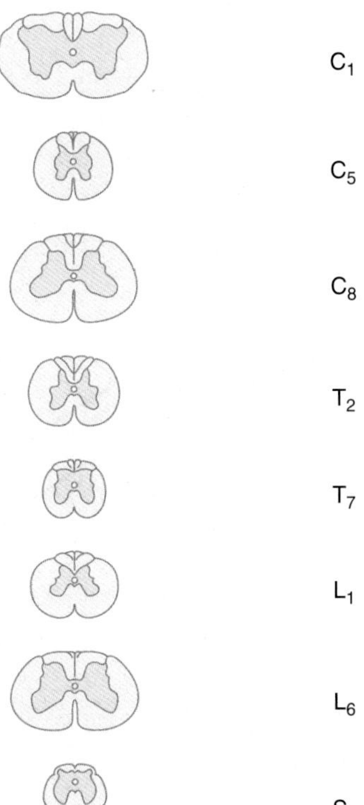

Fig. 8.16 Transverse sections of the canine spinal cord (the vertebral levels are indicated: *C*, cervical; *T*, thoracic; *L*, lumbar; *S*, sacral). Note the changes in diameter of the cord and in the relative proportions of gray *(darker)* and white *(lighter)* substance.

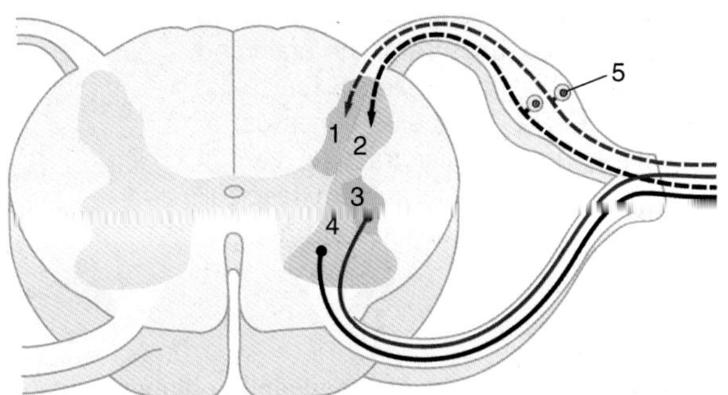

Fig. 8.17 Schematized subdivision of the gray substances in the spinal cord. *1*, Input from somatic afferent neurons; *2*, input from visceral afferent neurons *(1* and *2* form the dorsal horn); *3*, visceral efferent neurons; *4*, somatic efferent neurons *(3* and *4* form the ventral horn); *5*, dorsal root ganglion.

funiculus is contained between a shallow dorsal sulcus, extended deeply by a median glial septum, and the line of origin of the dorsal roots of the spinal nerves (see Fig. 8.13). The lateral funiculus is contained between the lines of the dorsal and ventral roots, and the ventral funiculus between the line of the ventral roots and a ventral fissure that penetrates far into the white matter, although it leaves a considerable commissure connecting the right and left halves. This ventral fissure is occupied by a mass of pia that appears as a glistening streak on the ventral surface of the cord.

The funiculi are composed of ascending and descending nerve fibers, of which many are grouped within bundles (fasciculi or tracts) of common origin, destination, and function (see Fig. 8.18). Although the details vary among species, the dorsal funiculus is almost entirely composed of ascending tracts (Fig. 8.18/*1* and *2*), as are the most lateral regions of the lateral funiculi (Fig. 8.18/*5* and *6*). Most of the lateral funiculi and the ventral funiculi contain both ascending and descending tracts.

The Hindbrain

The hindbrain (rhombencephalon) comprises the medulla oblongata, pons, and cerebellum. These parts differentiate from the caudal brain vesicle shortly after closure of the neural tube. Thinning of the roof plate in this region weakens the structure and causes the vesicle to flatten as the pontine flexure develops. The flattening splays the lateral wall of the neural tube outward so that the luminal surfaces come to face dorsomedially; the alar plates are now lying lateral to the basal plates (Fig 8.24). The part of the hindbrain caudal to the pontine flexure (the myelencephalon) becomes the medulla oblongata of adult anatomy. The rostral part is the metencephalon, which becomes the pons and cerebellum in the adult. The parts of the roof plate caudal and rostral to the cerebellum remain thin and form the rostral and caudal medullary vela (velum, singular) that form the roof of the lumen, known as the *fourth ventricle* in the adult (see Fig. 8.24).

The Medulla Oblongata and Pons

The medulla oblongata and pons together form the caudal regions of the brainstem, and internally there is no distinct division between them. Externally, the pons corresponds in extent to the large transverse group of axons that [illegible] its ventral and lateral aspects and continues into the cerebellum as the *middle cerebellar peduncles* (see Fig. 8.22/*9*).

Although the medulla oblongata continues the spinal cord caudally, it widens toward its rostral end as the result of the developmental flattening of the myelencephalon. The medulla oblongata's ventral surface is marked by a median fissure continuous with that of the cord and flanked by longitudinal ridges, the *pyramids* (Fig. 8.19/*17*). Many of the constituent fibers of the pyramids decussate (cross to the opposite side) at the transition of spinal cord and medulla, forming interlacing bundles within the fissure. More cranially, a lesser transverse ridge, the *trapezoid body,* crosses the ventral surface of the medulla oblongata directly caudal to the transverse fibers of the pons. The other noteworthy features on the ventral surface of the pons and medulla are the superficial origins of many of the cranial nerves. The trigeminal nerve (V) appears at the lateral aspect of the transverse pontine fibers; the abducent nerve (VI) emerges caudal to this and more medially, through the trapezoid body lateral to the pyramid; the facial (VII) and

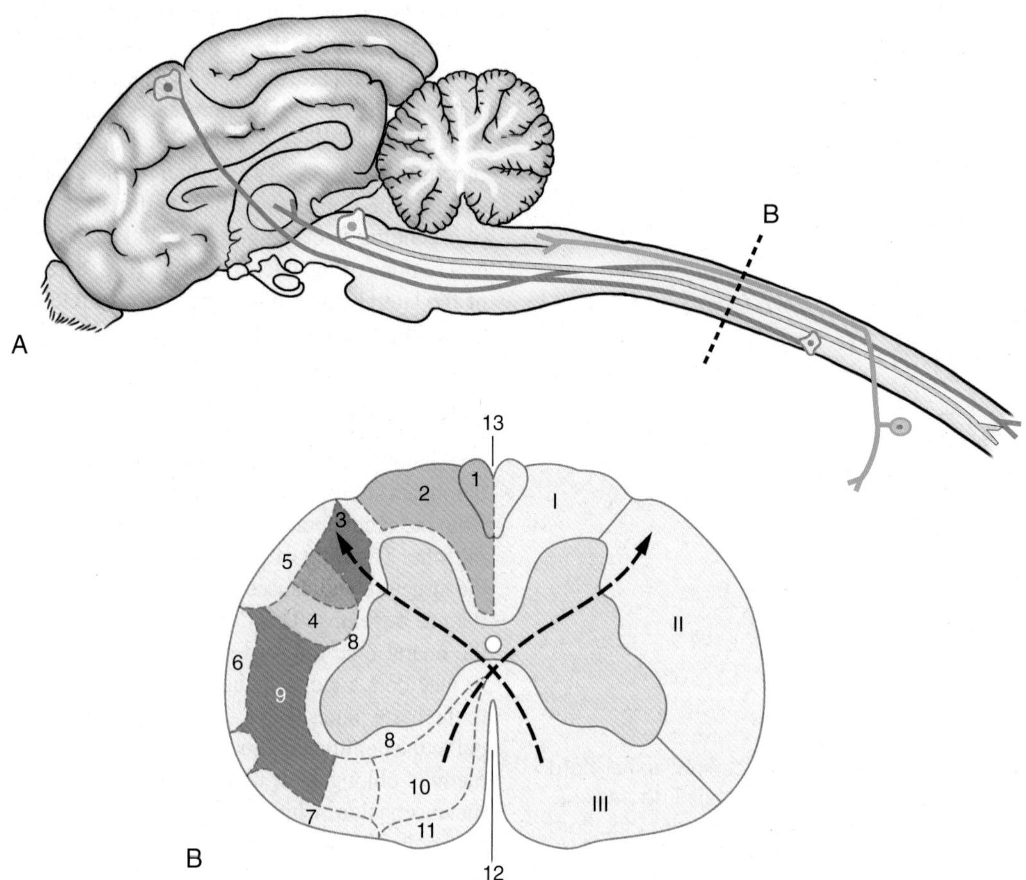

Fig. 8.18 (A) Principal ascending and descending tracts of the spinal cord, showing the locations of the cell bodies and axon pathways. (B) Hypothetical transverse section at the level indicated shows the the relative location of principal tracts. The *curved dotted arrows* indicate the crossing of the pyramidal tracts, which occurs at the juncture of the brain and spinal cord. (The drawing has been simplified for the sake of clarity.) *I*, Dorsal funiculus; *II*, lateral funiculus; *III*, ventral funiculus; *1*, fasciculus gracilis; *2*, fasciculus cuneatus; *3*, lateral corticospinal tract; *4*, rubrospinal tract; *5*, dorsal spinocerebellar tract; *6*, ventral spinocerebellar tract; *7*, spino-olivary and olivospinal tracts; *8*, propriospinal system (fasciculi proprii); *9*, spinothalamic tract; *10*, ventral corticospinal tract; *11*, vestibulospinal tract; *12*, ventral median fissure; *13*, dorsal median sulcus.

vestibulocochlear (VIII) nerves appear to continue the trapezoid body laterally; the glossopharyngeal (IX), vagus (X), and accessory (XI) nerves arise from the lateral aspect of the medulla oblongata in close succession; and the hypoglossal nerve (XII) takes a more ventral origin in line with that of the abducent nerve and the ventral roots of the spinal nerves (Figs. 8.19 and 8.20).

It is helpful to study a median section of the brain (Fig. 8.21) before examining the dorsal aspect of the medulla oblongata and pons. This section shows that the fourth ventricle is located close to the dorsal surface of the brainstem. The ventricle is covered by a tented roof formed in part by the ventral surface of the cerebellum and in part by the *rostral* and *caudal medullary vela* (Fig. 8.21/*15* and *15'*), which extend from the cerebellum to the midbrain and from the cerebellum to the closed caudal part of the medulla oblongata, respectively. Exposure of the dorsal surface of the medulla and pons requires the removal of the cerebellum by transection of its peduncles attaching it to the pons, an operation that almost inevitably destroys the fragile vela (Fig. 8.22).

The *fourth ventricle* is diamond shaped from a dorsal view (see Fig. 8.22) and is aptly named the *rhomboidal fossa;* its widest part is at the pontine-medullary junction. The margins of the fossa are provided by the three pairs of cerebellar peduncles. The floor is irregular and is marked by a *median sulcus* on the midline and paired *lateral (limiting) sulci.* The most rostral part of the rostral velum, a part that occasionally survives removal of the cerebellum, contains the superficial origins of the trochlear nerves (IV), the only nerves to emerge from the dorsal aspect of the brain.

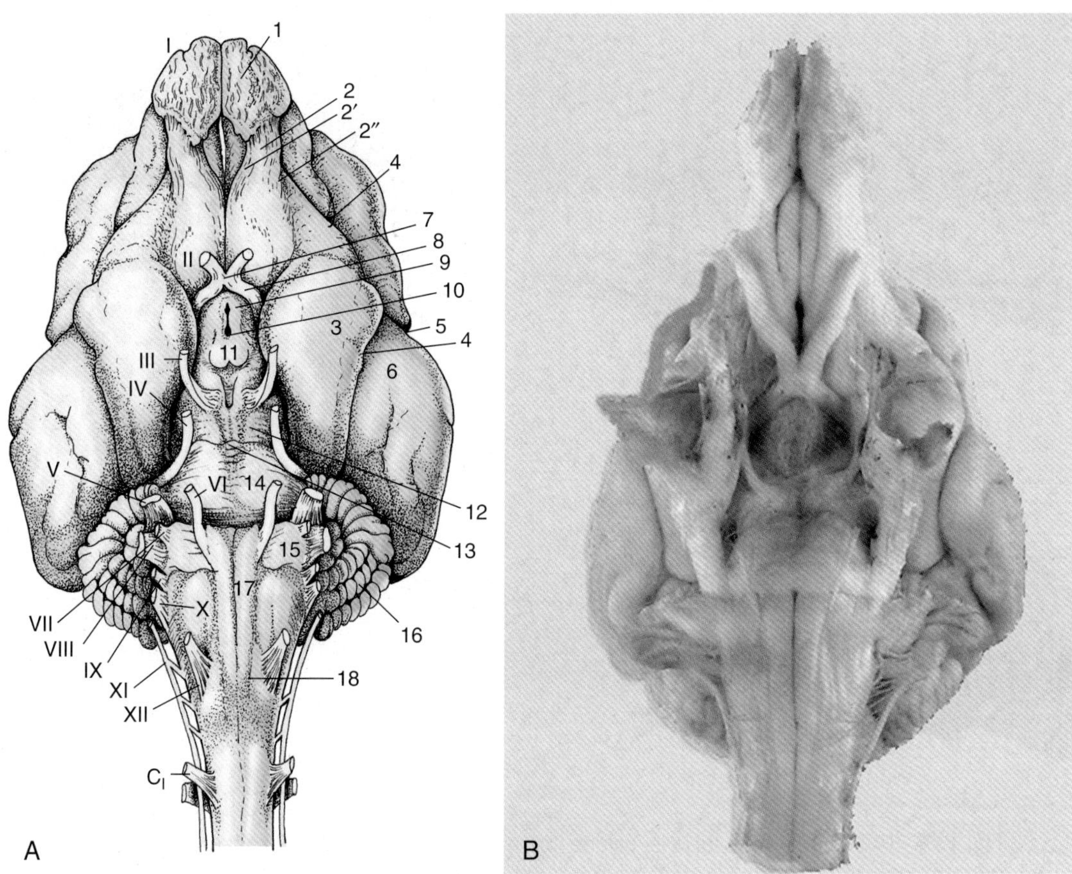

Fig. 8.19 (A) Ventral view of the canine brain. *1*, Olfactory bulb; *2*, olfactory tract; *2′*, medial olfactory tract; *2″*, lateral olfactory tract; *3*, piriform lobe; *4*, rhinal sulcus; *5*, sylvian sulcus; *6*, ectosylvian gyrus; *7*, optic chiasm; *8*, optic tract; *9*, tuber cinereum; *10*, infundibulum (the hypophysis has been detached and the third ventricle is opened); *11*, mammillary body; *12*, crus cerebri; *13*, interpeduncular fossa; *14*, pons; *15*, trapezoid body; *16*, cerebellar hemisphere; *17*, pyramidal tract; *18*, crossing of pyramidal tracts. *I–XII* designate the appropriate cranial nerves; C_1, Cervical nerve 1. (B) The real specimen of the dog.

On either side of the caudal part of the fourth ventricle, the dorsal surface of the medulla oblongata is represented by inconspicuous eminences, the *gracile* and *cuneate nuclei* (Fig. 8.23/5 and 7), which are the cranial terminations of the similarly named *gracile* and *cuneate fasciculi* of the dorsal funiculus of the spinal cord. These nuclei transmit somatosensory information from the body and limbs, as discussed later in the chapter.

The principal features of the *internal anatomy* of the medulla oblongata and pons are as follows: the nuclei of the cranial nerves, the olivary and pontine nuclei, the reticular formation, and certain ascending and descending fiber tracts that connect the spinal cord with higher regions of the brain. These structures are described here but without excessive attention to establishing their topographic relationships.

The Nuclei of the Cranial Nerves

The nuclei of the cranial nerves represent the continuation of the four functional components, somatic afferent, visceral afferent, visceral efferent, and somatic efferent, that compose the gray matter of the spinal cord (see Fig. 8.12). These components are supplemented by two additional components, special somatic afferent and special visceral afferent, that are carried by cranial nerves in connection with the innervation of receptors for special senses, which have no counterparts in the trunk or limbs (i.e., hearing, balance, taste).

Recall that in the spinal cord, the regions receiving somatic and visceral afferent input are located together in the dorsal gray column whereas the somatic and visceral motor neurons are located in the ventral column. In the medulla, the widening of the roof of the fourth ventricle and flattening of the brainstem cause these components to be arranged medial to lateral (see Fig. 8.12). These components now exhibit a lateromedial rather than dorsoventral sequence, with a lateral somatic afferent column and a medial somatic efferent column. Certain of the columns also fragment into discrete parts (nuclei), and at some levels

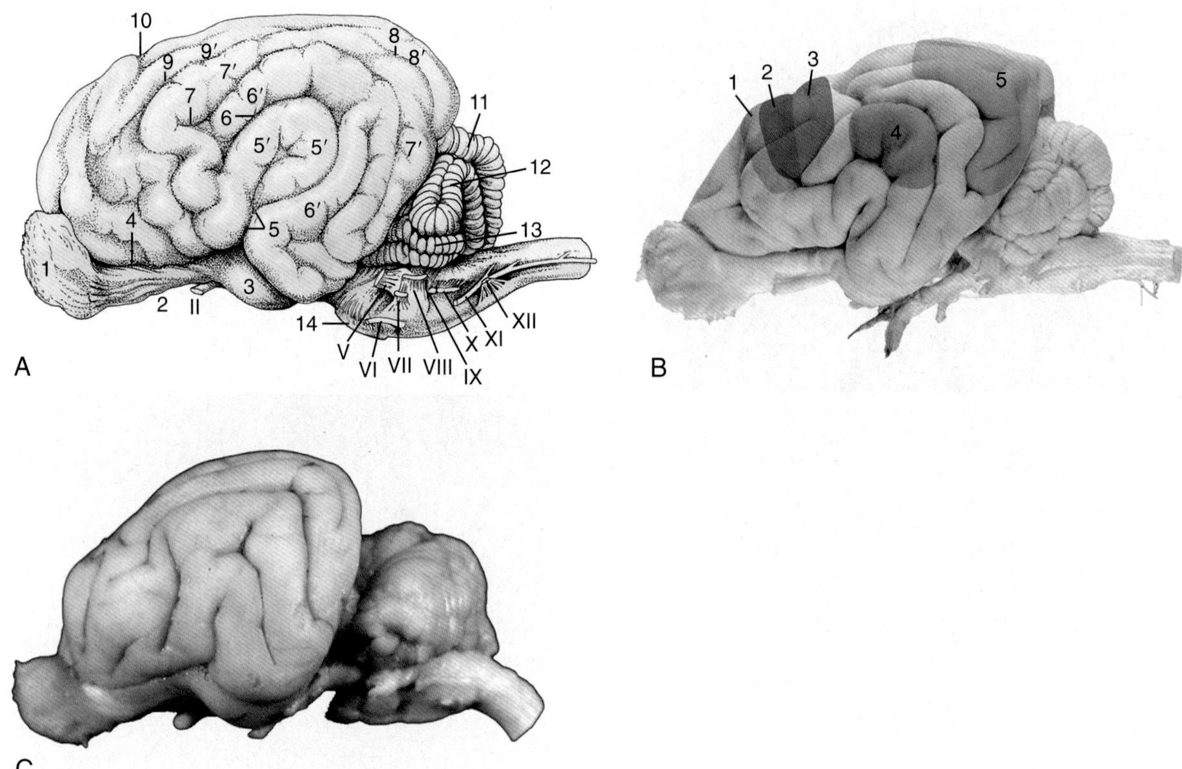

Fig. 8.20 (A) Lateral view of the canine brain. *1,* Olfactory bulb; *2,* olfactory tract; *3,* piriform lobe; *4,* rhinal sulcus; *5,* sylvian sulcus; *5′,* sylvian gyrus; *6,* ectosylvian sulcus; *6′,* ectosylvian gyrus; *7,* suprasylvian sulcus; *7′,* suprasylvian gyrus; *8,* ectomarginal sulcus; *8′,* ectomarginal gyrus; *9,* coronal sulcus; *9′,* coronal gyrus; *10,* cruciate sulcus; *11,* cerebellar vermis; *12,* cerebellar hemisphere; *13,* paraflocculus; *14,* pons; *II* and *V–XII* designate the appropriate cranial nerves. (B) Lateral view of the canine brain. *1,* motor cortex; *2,* overlap of motor and somatosensory cortex; *3,* somatosensory cortex; *4,* auditory cortex; *5,* visual cortex (C) Lateral view of the feline brain.

the relationships are further adjusted to allow the intrusion of the additional components. The consequences are that those cranial nerves that contain more than one functional component arise from more than one nucleus and that certain nuclei give rise to similar components of more than one nerve. The general arrangement of the six components is illustrated in Fig. 8.25 in a schematic fashion.

The *somatic efferent column* serves muscles that have originated from somites and branchiomeres of the head. Its medial part is fragmented into a long *hypoglossal nucleus* and a smaller *abducent nucleus* within the floor of the fourth ventricle (and *trochlear* and *oculomotor nuclei* within the tegmentum of the midbrain). The fibers from the oculomotor, abducent, and hypoglossal nuclei take the expected courses to emerge on the ventral aspect of the brain, close to the midline and in line with one another and the ventral roots of the spinal nerves (see Fig. 8.19). Those that compose the trochlear nerve emerge from the dorsal aspect of the brain after decussation within the rostral medullary velum (Fig. 8.22/*IV*); this is an aberrant course for a cranial nerve, for which there is no satisfactory explanation.

The lateral (branchiomeric) portion of the somatic efferent column (see Fig. 8.25) supplies the striated masticatory, facial, laryngeal, and pharyngeal muscles through the trigeminal, facial, glossopharyngeal, vagus, and accessory nerves. This portion is divided into the motor *nuclei* of the *trigeminal* and *facial nerves* (Fig. 8.25/*16* and *17*) and the nucleus ambiguus (Fig. 8.25/*14*) shared by the glossopharyngeal and vagus nerves. The fibers emerge from the ventrolateral surface of the brainstem but do not always take the most direct internal course to do so.

The *visceral efferent column* supplies the autonomic (parasympathetic) motor component of certain cranial nerves. The lateral of the efferent columns (Fig. 8.24/*4*), it is divided into the *parasympathetic nucleus of the vagus* nerve (Fig. 8.25/*13*), the *caudal salivatory nucleus* of the glossopharyngeal nerve, and the *rostral salivatory nucleus* of the facial nerve (Fig. 8.25/*15*) (and, in the midbrain, the parasympathetic nucleus of the oculomotor nerve [Fig. 8.25/*18*]). The vagal parasympathetic fibers are distributed to the cervical, thoracic, and abdominal (but not pelvic) viscera, whereas parasympathetic fibers in the glossopharyngeal and facial nerves are distributed

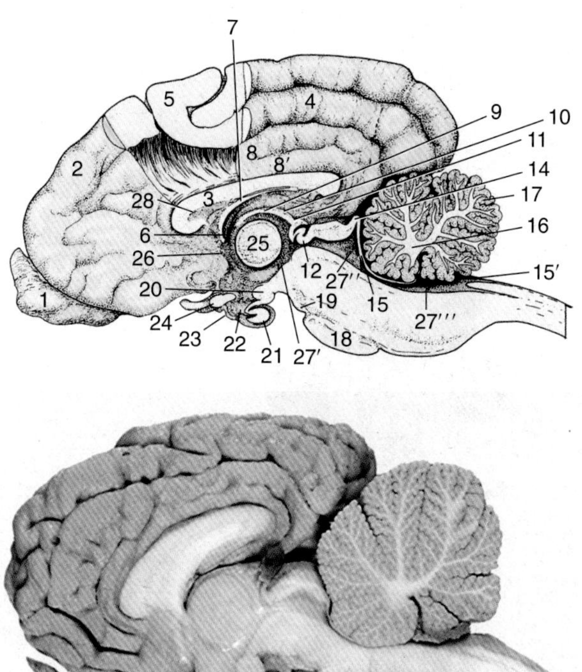

Fig. 8.21 Median section of the canine brain. Part of the medial wall of the hemisphere has been removed. *1*, Olfactory bulb; *2*, hemisphere; *3*, corpus callosum; *4*, splenial sulcus; *5*, cerebral cortex; *6*, interventricular foramen; *7*, fornix; *8*, cingulate gyrus; *8′*, supracallosal gyrus; *9*, thalamus; *10*, epithalamus; *11*, epiphysis; *12*, posterior commissure; *13* and *14*, commissures of rostral and caudal colliculi; *15*, rostral medullary velum; *15′*, caudal medullary velum; *16*, corpus medullare; *17*, cerebellar cortex; *18*, pons; *19*, crus cerebri; *20*, mammillary body; *21*, hypophysis; *22*, infundibulum; *23*, tuber cinereum; *24*, optic chiasm; *25*, interthalamic adhesion; *26*, anterior commissure; *27*, third ventricle; *27″*, mesencephalic aqueduct; *27‴*, fourth ventricle; *28*, septum telencephali (pellucidum).

to glands of the head. Further rostrally, parasympathetic fibers within the oculomotor nerve innervate the smooth intrinsic muscles of the eyeball.

The *visceral afferent column* (Fig. 8.24/*2* and *3*) is in fact double and is made up of neurons receiving either visceral or special visceral afferent inputs. It forms a single very long nucleus (*nucleus of the solitary tract* [Fig. 8.25/*10*]) that is subdivided in relation to the associated facial, glossopharyngeal, and vagus nerves. Many neurons receive visceral input from the caudal part of the mouth and the cervical, thoracic, and abdominal viscera; the special component, which is concerned with taste, is distributed among the facial, glossopharyngeal, and vagus nerves.

The *somatic afferent column* (Fig. 8.24/*1*) extends from the cervical part of the spinal cord through the medulla and pons into the mesencephalon. It is broken into several nuclei. The rostralmost extent, the *mesencephalic nucleus of the trigeminal nerve* (Fig. 8.25/*7*), is concerned with proprioception; it presents a unique feature, the inclusion of the primary afferent neuron cell bodies within the central nervous system (the one exception to an otherwise inviolable rule that the cell bodies of primary afferent neurons are located within peripheral ganglia). The two exteroceptive nuclei (Fig. 8.25/*7*) are the *principal sensory nucleus of the trigeminal nerve* within the pons and *the nucleus of the descending (spinal) tract of the trigeminal nerve,* which extends from the level of the pons into the cervical part of the spinal cord.

The *special somatic afferent column* is associated with the optic and vestibulocochlear nerves and therefore with the special somatic senses of vision (II), balance (vestibular division of VIII), and hearing (cochlear division of VIII) (Fig. 8.25/*6*, *8*, and *9*). The afferent pathways of these important senses are considered elsewhere; our present purpose is to locate the relevant nuclei within the brainstem. The four closely related *vestibular nuclei* are spread through part of the medulla oblongata and pons, medial to the caudal cerebellar peduncle. The two (dorsal and ventral) *cochlear nuclei* are located within the most rostral part of the medulla oblongata close to the entry of the eighth nerve.

The fiber composition of the nerves is summarized conveniently in Table 8.2.

Other Internal Features

The *olivary nuclear complex* occupies a position in the caudal part of the medulla oblongata, dorsolateral to the pyramidal tract, where it sometimes raises a gentle surface swelling (Fig. 8.26/*10*). It is composed of several parts and varies considerably in form among species, generally taking the form of a nuclear lamina folded onto itself to form a bag. It has an important function in the regulation of motor feedback (pp. 288–289). Several other nuclei within the pons (Fig. 8.27) are also concerned with motor control.

The *reticular formation* is a diffuse system of nuclei and fiber tracts (Figs. 8.26/*8* and 8.28/*13*) that extends from the spinal cord to the forebrain and occupies a large part of the core of the medulla oblongata and pons. It is discussed on p. 284.

The principal fiber tracts that pass through the pons and medulla are summarized here but are discussed later in this chapter along with their functional morphology. The large descending corticospinal tract that forms the *pyramid* on the ventral surface of the medulla (Fig. 8.26/*11*) and the ascending tract known as the *medial lemniscus* (Fig. 8.28/*9*) are prominent in transverse sections. The medial lemniscus consists of axons arising from neurons in the gracile and cuneate nuclei, axons that initially travel ventrally from the nuclei (as the deep [internal] arcuate fibers), then cross the midline in the ventral part of the caudal medulla before turning rostrally as the prominent medial lemniscal bundle. Also traversing the pons and medulla are axons of the trigeminothalamic and cervicothalamic tracts, which arise from the principal sensory nucleus of the trigeminal nerve

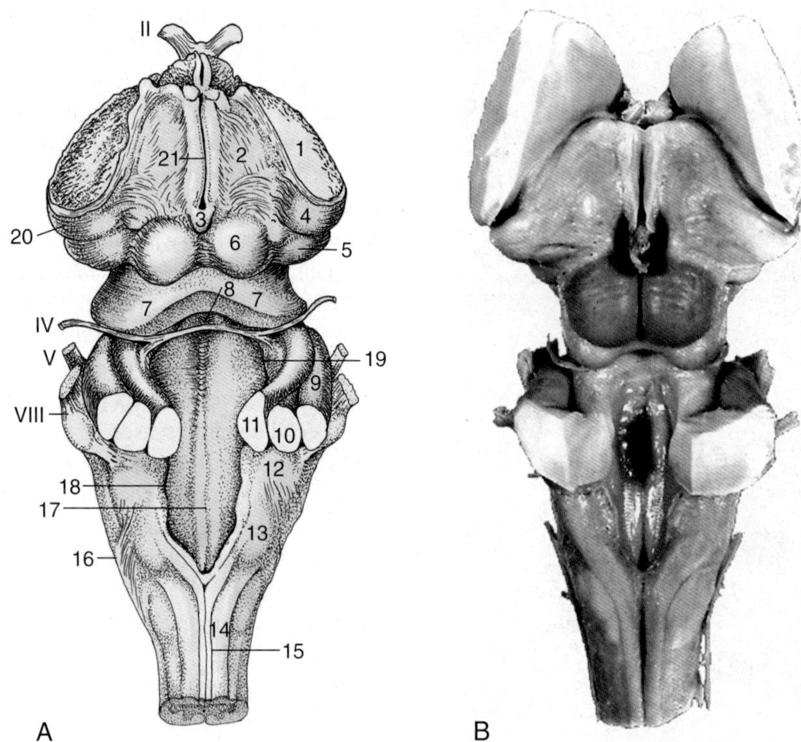

Fig. 8.22 (A) Dorsal view of the canine brainstem with the cerebellum removed and the fourth ventricle opened. *1*, Cut fibers of internal capsule; *2*, dorsal part of thalamus; *3*, epiphysis; *4*, lateral geniculate body; *5*, medial geniculate body; *6*, rostral colliculus; *7*, caudal colliculus; *8*, decussating fibers of trochlear nerves in the rostral velum; *9*, middle cerebellar peduncle; *10*, caudal cerebellar peduncle; *11*, rostral cerebellar peduncle; *12*, dorsal cochlear nucleus; *13*, cuneate tubercle; *14*, fasciculus cuneatus; *15*, fasciculus gracilis; *16*, superficial arcuate fibers; *17*, median sulcus; *18*, medial eminence; *19*, sulcus limitans; *20*, optic tract; *21*, margin of roof of third ventricle; *IV*, *V*, and *VIII* designate the appropriate cranial nerves. (B) Dorsal view of equine brainstem.

and the lateral cervical nucleus in the spinal cord, respectively. The three cerebellar peduncles are also prominent here, the composition, origin, and destination of which are described later.

The Cerebellum

The cerebellum is a roughly globular, multiply and deeply fissured mass that is located above the pons and medulla oblongata and is connected to the brainstem by three peduncles on each side (Fig. 8.22/*9–11*). It is separated from the cerebral hemispheres cranially by the transverse fissure occupied by the membranous tentorium cerebelli (p. 295) when the brain is in situ in the skull.

The cerebellum consists of two large *lateral hemispheres* and a narrower median region named the *vermis* owing to its supposed resemblance to an earthworm. Deep to both of these regions, a small *flocculonodular lobe* is separated by deep fissures from the larger mass (see Fig. 8.20). Smaller fissures divide each region into lobules and these into yet smaller units known as *folia.* The lobules are individually named, but neither their names nor their exact forms are important.

The arrangement of the gray matter and white matter sharply contrasts that found in the spinal cord and medulla oblongata. In the cerebellum the bulk of the gray matter is arranged as an external cortex that encloses the white matter, or "medulla" (see Fig. 8.21). The cortex is highly folded to accommodate the large amount of gray matter required for neural processing. The medulla, consisting of myelinated axon tracts arising from the peduncle and radiating through the various lobes, lobules, and folia, form a branching structure with some resemblance to a tree. Because of this appearance and because of an ancient belief that it is the seat of the soul, it is sometimes known as the *arbor vitae*—tree of life. A series of paired nuclei are embedded among the white matter of the medulla; the most important of these are the *fastigial nuclei* (Fig. 8.27/*13*) close to the midline, the *lateral cerebellar (or dentate) nucleus* (Fig. 8.27/*15*) laterally, and the *nuclei interpositi* (Fig. 8.27/*14*) between the former two.

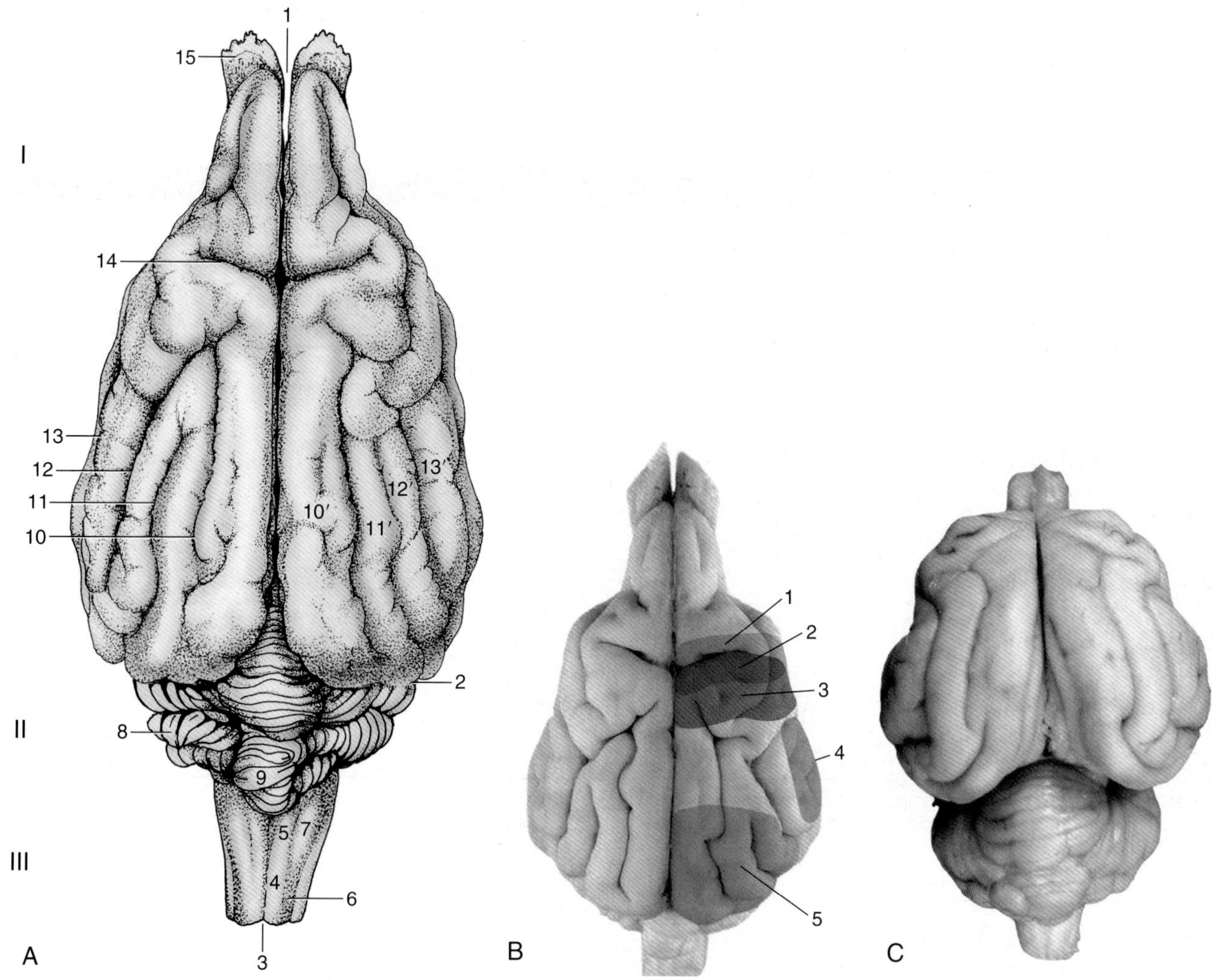

Fig. 8.23 (A) Dorsal view of the canine brain. *I*, Cerebral hemispheres; *II*, cerebellum; *III*, medulla oblongata. *1*, Longitudinal fissure; *2*, transverse fissure; *3*, dorsal median sulcus; *4*, tractus gracilis; *5*, nucleus gracilis; *6*, tractus cuneatus; *7*, nucleus cuneatus; *8*, cerebellar hemisphere; *9*, cerebellar vermis; *10*, marginal sulcus; *10′*, marginal gyrus; *11*, ectomarginal sulcus; *11′*, ectomarginal gyrus; *12*, suprasylvian sulcus; *12′*, suprasylvian gyrus; *13*, ectosylvian sulcus; *13′*, ectosylvian gyrus; *14*, cruciate sulcus; *15*, olfactory bulb. (B) The real specimen of the dog. *1*, motor cortex; *2*, overlap of motor and somatosensory cortex; *3*, somatosensory cortex; *4*, auditory cortex; *5*, visual cortex. (C) The real specimen of the cat.

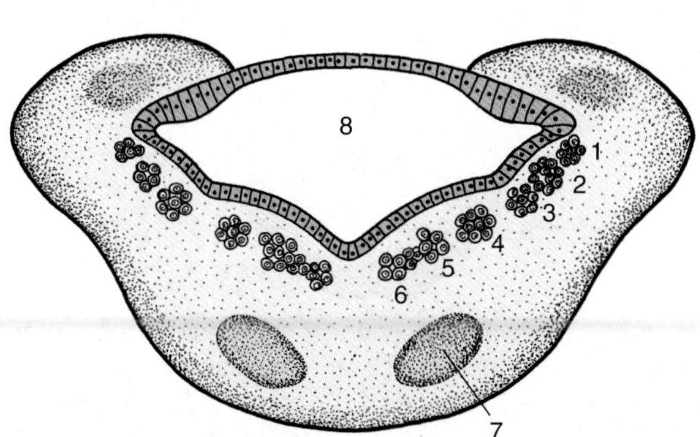

Fig. 8.24 Schematic transverse section of the metencephalon. The special somatic afferent nuclei are not shown. *1*, Somatic afferent column; *2*, visceral afferent column; *3*, special visceral afferent column; *4*, visceral efferent column; *5* and *6*, somatic efferent column; *7*, nuclei of pons; *8*, fourth ventricle.

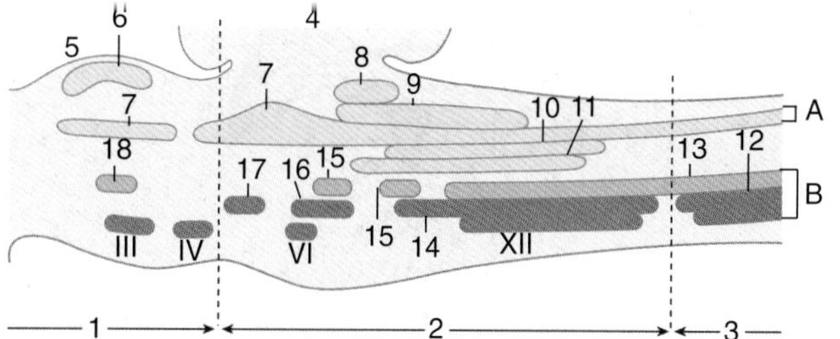

Fig. 8.25 Schematic representations of the brainstem showing the nuclei in an adult mammal. *Roman numerals* are used for nuclei of some cranial nerves. (A) Afferent nuclei; (B) efferent nuclei. *1*, Mesencephalon; *2*, rhombencephalon; *3*, spinal cord; *4*, cerebellum; *5*, tectum mesencephali; *6*, rostral colliculus (special somatic efferent [SSA]); *7*, trigeminal nuclei (somatic efferent [SA]); *8*, cochlear nuclei (SSA); *9*, vestibular nuclei (SSA); *10*, solitary nucleus of VII, IX, X (visceral afferent [VA]); *11*, *11′*, gustatory nuclei of VII, IX (special visceral afferent [SVA]), respectively; *12*, motor nucleus of XI (somatic efferent [SE]); *13*, motor nucleus of X (visceral efferent [VE]); *14*, nucleus ambiguus of IX, X (SE); *15*, salivatory nuclei of VII, IX (VE); *16*, motor nucleus of VII (SE); *17*, motor nucleus of V (SE); *18*, parasympathetic nucleus of III (VE).

TABLE 8.2 CRANIAL NERVE COMPONENTS[a]

		Components					
Number	Name	Somatic Efferent	Visceral Efferent	Somatic Afferent	Special Somatic Afferent	Visceral Afferent	Special Visceral Afferent
I	Olfactory		–	–	+		
II	Optic	–	–	–	+	–	–
III	Oculomotor	+	+	–	–	–	–
IV	Trochlear	+	–	–	–	–	–
V	Trigeminal	+	–	+	–	–	–
VI	Abducent	+	–	–	–	–	
VII	Facial	+	+	–	+	+	
VIII	Vestibuloco-chlear	–	–	–	+	–	–
IX	Glossopharyn-geal	+	+	–	–	+	+
X	Vagus	+	+	–	–	+	+
XI	Accessory	+	+			+	–
XII	Hypoglossal	+	–	–	–	–	–

[a]Certain points are controversial: notably, the nerve trunks followed by fibers conveying proprioceptive information from various muscles of the head and the precise distribution of the medullary component of the accessory nerve.

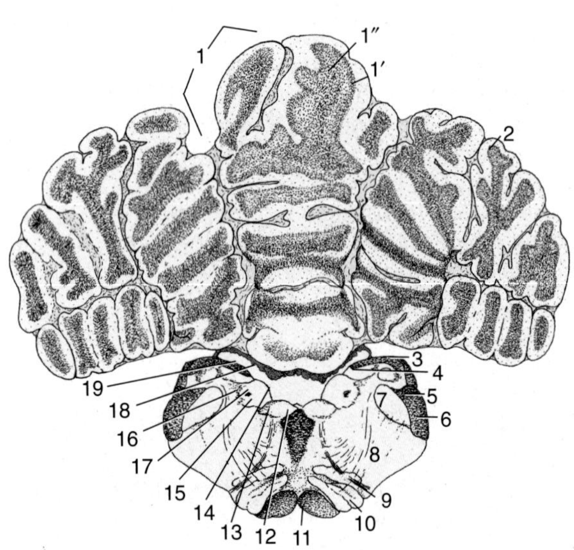

Fig. 8.26 Transverse section of the canine brain at the level of the hypoglossal nerve (XII). *1*, Cerebellar vermis; *1′*, cortex; *1″*, medulla; *2*, cerebellar hemisphere; *3*, fasciculi gracilis and cuneatus; *4*, gracile and cuneate nuclei; *5*, caudal cerebellar peduncle; *6*, spinal tract of the trigeminal nerve; *7*, nucleus of the spinal tract of the trigeminal nerve; *8*, reticular formation; *9*, root of hypoglossal nerve; *10*, caudal olivary nucleus; *11*, pyramidal tract; *12*, medial longitudinal tract; *13*, motor nucleus of XII; *14*, sulcus limitans; *15*, motor nucleus of X; *16*, solitary tract (special visceral afferents of VII, IX, and X); *17*, solitary nucleus; *18*, choroid plexus; *19*, fourth ventricle.

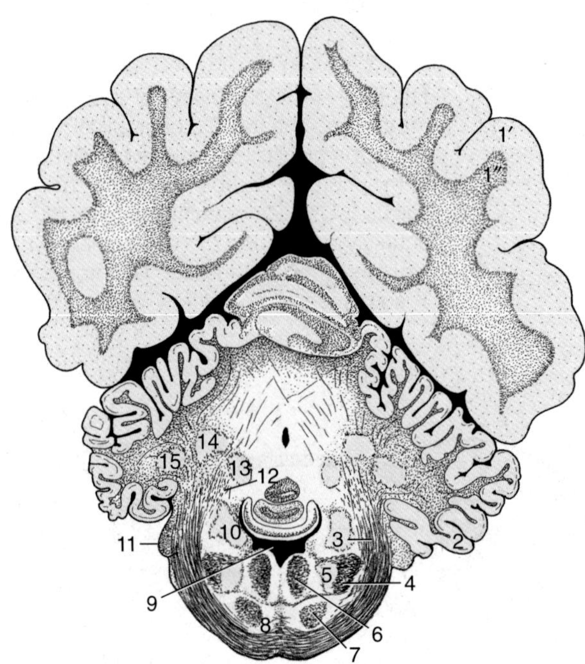

Fig. 8.27 Transverse section of the canine brain at the level of the middle cerebellar peduncle. *1′*, *1″*, cerebral hemisphere: *1′*, neocortex; *1″*, fibers; *2*, paraflocculus lateralis; *3*, middle cerebellar peduncle; *4*, spinal tract of the trigeminal nerve; *5*, nucleus of the spinal tract of the trigeminal nerve; *6*, medial longitudinal fasciculus; *7*, pyramidal tract; *8*, pontine nuclei; *9*, fourth ventricle; *10*, nuclei of the vestibulocochlear nerve (VIII); *11*, root of VIII; *12*, rostral cerebellar peduncle; *13*, fastigial nucleus; *14*, nucleus interpositus; *15*, lateral cerebellar nucleus.

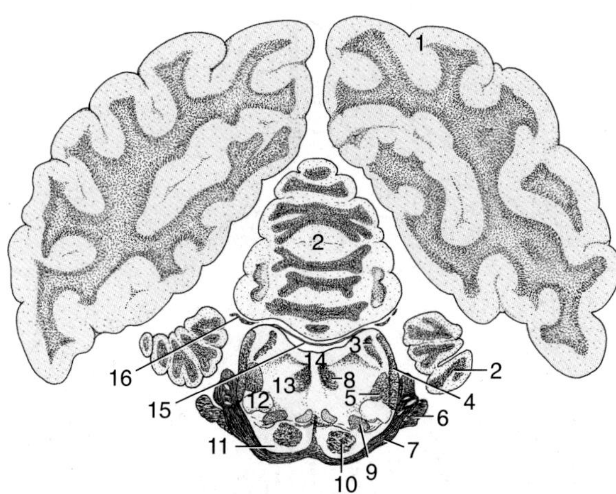

Fig. 8.28 Transverse section of the canine brain at the level of the trigeminal nerve. *1*, Cerebral hemisphere; *2*, cerebellum; *3*, rostral cerebellar peduncle; *4*, lateral lemniscus; *5*, rubrospinal tract; *6*, root of V; *7*, middle cerebellar peduncle; *8*, medial longitudinal fasciculus; *9*, medial lemniscus; *10*, pyramidal tract; *11*, pontine nuclei; *12*, nucleus of lateral lemniscus; *13*, reticular formation; *14*, fourth ventricle; *15*, rostral medullary velum; *16*, root of IV.

Axons traveling in the three *cerebellar peduncles* form the attachments of the cerebellum on each side. The cerebellum is also attached to the brainstem by the caudal and rostral medullary vela (Fig. 8.21/*15,15'*). The caudal peduncle (Fig. 8.22/*10*) connects the cerebellum with the medulla oblongata and is largely composed of afferent fibers entering the cerebellum, of which some run from origins within the spinal cord and others run from the vestibular nuclei, the olivary nucleus, and the reticular formation. The middle peduncle (brachium pontis; Fig. 8.22/*9*) is also composed of afferent fibers; these arise from pontine nuclei. The rostral peduncle (brachium conjunctivum; Fig. 8.22/*11*) is attached to the midbrain; it is largely composed of efferent fibers leaving the cerebellum to synapse in the red nucleus, reticular formation, and thalamus. The rostral peduncle also includes a considerable afferent component that continues the ventral spinocerebellar tract. The three peduncles are compressed closely together at their attachments to the cerebellum.

The functions of the cerebellum are concerned with the control of balance, the coordination of postural and locomotor activities, and motor planning. Balance, including head and eye movements, is largely controlled within the flocculonodular node. The vermis and medialmost portions of the hemispheres are concerned with the feedback regulation of motor function of axial and limb muscles. The lateral hemispheres are involved in planning motor movements. There is somatotopic representation in the cerebellar cortex, in that adjacent regions of the body are represented by corresponding adjacent areas in the cortex.

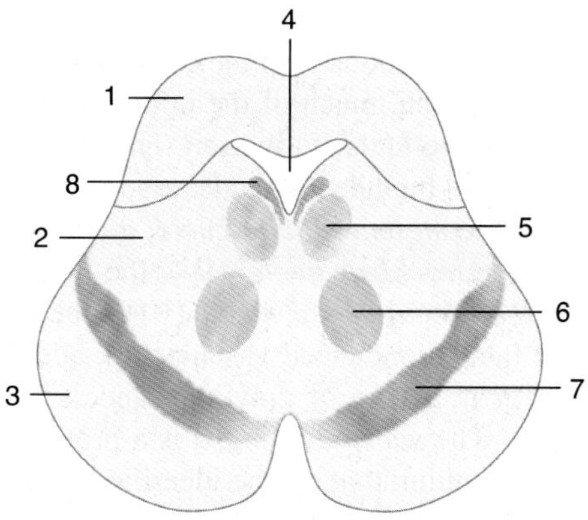

Fig. 8.29 Schematic transverse section of the mesencephalon. *1*, Tectum; *2*, tegmentum; *3*, crus cerebri; *4*, mesencephalic aqueduct; *5*, oculomotor nucleus (III); *6*, red nucleus; *7*, substantia nigra; *8*, locus coeruleus.

The cerebellum does not project directly to lower motor neurons and so does not initiate movement. Instead, the cerebellum coordinates movements by continually adjusting the output of upper motor neurons. Thus, damage to the cerebellum produces incoordination but not paralysis.

THE MIDBRAIN

The midbrain, or mesencephalon, is a fairly short portion of the brainstem that better preserves the basic organization of the neural tube than do other parts of the brainstem.

The midbrain is represented on the ventral surface of the intact brain by the *crus cerebri* (cerebral peduncles Fig. 8.19/*12*), the interpeduncular fossa, and the superficial origin of the oculomotor nerves (III). The midbrain is concealed dorsally by the overhanging cerebral hemispheres and cerebellum. Its lumen, the mesencephalic aqueduct, is a simple canal joining the much larger cavities of the third and fourth ventricles. The mesencephalon has a stratified structure, comprising from dorsal to ventral: tectum, tegmentum, and cerebral peduncle (Fig. 8.29).

The *tectum* lies dorsal to the aqueduct. Its major features are four rounded surface swellings (see Fig. 8.22). The paired caudal swellings, the *caudal colliculi,* are widely spaced and are joined by a substantial commissure. They serve as important integration centers for auditory pathways (p. 287). The brachium, an axonal tract from of the caudal colliculus to the ipsilateral medial geniculate body in the thalamus, is visible as a distinct ridge. The *rostral colliculi* are closer together and are joined to the lateral geniculate bodies of the thalamus by similar but less obtrusive brachia. The rostral colliculi, an important integration center for visual pathways, are involved in somatic reflexes initiated by visual input, such as head movements and startle responses.

The *tegmentum* constitutes the core of the midbrain and is directly continuous with the corresponding region of the pons. As such, much of the midbrain tegmentum is formed by the reticular formation. The principal mesencephalic nuclei include the nuclei associated with cranial nerves—the *mesencephalic nuclei of the trigeminal nerves* (V), the *trochlear nuclei* (IV), the *principal and parasympathetic oculomotor nuclei* (III)—the *red nuclei* (named for their pronounced vascularity), and the *periaqueductal gray,* a core of gray substance surrounding the aqueduct. The *substantia nigra* is a prominent lamina in the tegmentum that can be identified in transverse sections by its darker color, which is due to the gradual accumulation of melanin pigment within the constituent neurons. Like the red nucleus, it is associated with the basal nuclei (p. 277) in the control of voluntary movement.

The *crura cerebri* are visible on the ventral surface of the brain. They comprise fiber tracts that travel from the telencephalon to the caudal brainstem. These fibers converge as they emerge from the telencephalon, although they are separated by the interpeduncular fossa (see Fig. 8.19/*13*). The oculomotor nerves (III) also emerge in this region, directly rostral to the pons.

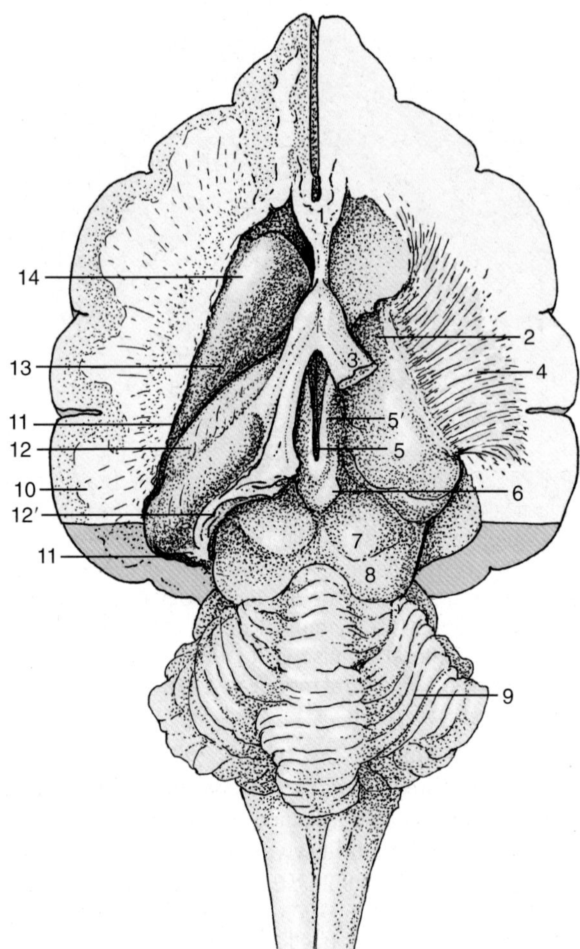

Fig. 8.30 Dorsal view of the canine brain. Part of the left hemisphere has been removed, opening the lateral ventricle. On the right, the hippocampus and basal nuclei have also been removed, exposing the thalamus and the internal capsule. *1,* Septal nuclei; *2,* dorsal surface of thalamus; *3,* fornix (cut); *4,* internal capsule; *5,* dorsal part of third ventricle; *5′,* habenular nuclei (in roof of third ventricle); *6,* epiphysis; *7,* rostral colliculus; *8,* caudal colliculus; *9,* cerebellum; *10,* cut lateral wall of hemisphere; *11,* lumen of lateral ventricle; *12,* hippocampus; *12′,* cut-edge of denticulate gyrus; *13,* tail of caudate nucleus; *14,* head of caudate nucleus.

The Forebrain

The forebrain comprises the diencephalon and the paired cerebral hemispheres (telencephalon). The hemispheres overlap the dorsolateral aspects of the diencephalon, to which they are connected by extensive fiber tracts.

The Diencephalon

The diencephalon (there is no convenient alternative name) forms the most rostral part of the brainstem. Only its most ventral part, the hypothalamus, is visible on the external surface of the intact brain (see Fig. 8.19), but it is more extensively revealed in median section (see Fig. 8.21). The diencephalon has three parts: epithalamus, thalamus (including subthalamus), and hypothalamus, which develop in relation to the roof, walls, and floor of the third ventricle, respectively.

The *epithalamus,* the most dorsal part, comprises the pineal gland (*epiphysis cerebri*), habenular striae, habenulae, and habenular commissure (Fig. 8.30). The *pineal gland* (Fig. 8.30/*6*) is a small, median body projecting dorsally from the brainstem behind an evagination of the roof of the third ventricle that is composed only of pia and ependyma. The pineal gland plays an important role in sexual development and behavior; it is believed to be particularly concerned in the seasonal regulation of ovarian activity in response to changing day length. The pineal gland produces melatonin, which is important in circadian and seasonal rhythms (p. 206). The *habenulae* are nuclear complexes that develop within the most dorsal parts of wall of the third ventricle. They have important functions relating to emotion, motivation, and reward. The nuclei receive fibers (*habenular stria*) from the hippocampus and other parts of the telencephalon and send fibers to mesencephalic nuclei. The left and right habenular nuclei are interconnected via the *habenular commissure* (Fig. 8.30/*5′*).

The *thalamus* is the largest component of the diencephalon. It develops within the lateral walls of the third ventricle, but in many species, including domestic species, the wall of each side of the thalamus expands medially into the ventricle to connect right and left sides. This, the intermediate mass or *interthalamic adhesion,* reduces the ventricle to an encircling annular space (Fig. 8.31/*3*). The relations of the thalamus are difficult to envisage because of its deep position and lack of separation from neighboring structures. It

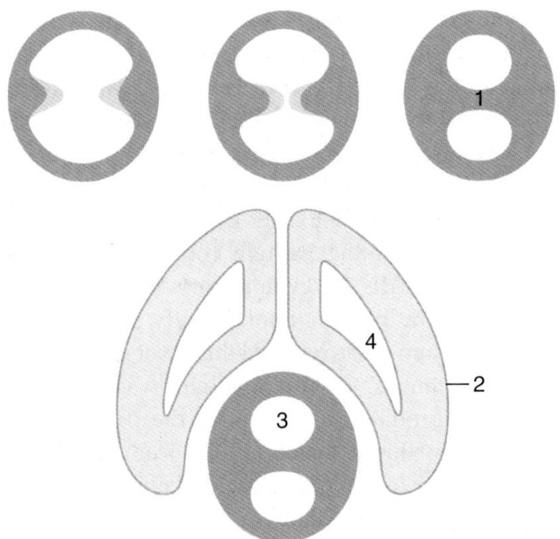

Fig. 8.31 *Top left to right,* The formation of the interthalamic adhesion *(1)* by median fusion of outgrowths of the lateral walls of the diencephalon. *2,* Telencephalon; *3,* third ventricle; *4,* lateral ventricle.

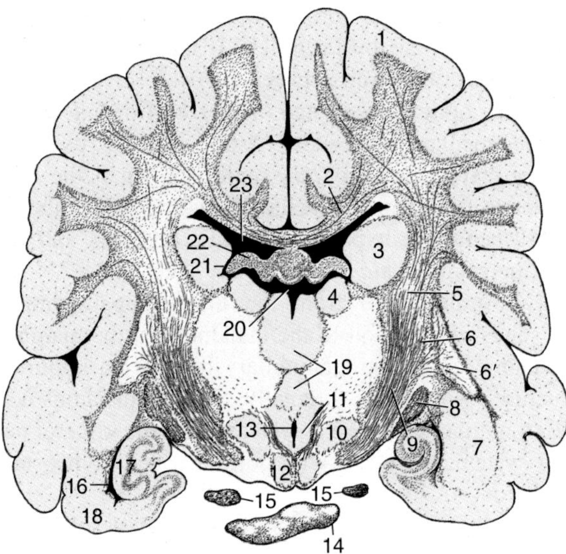

Fig. 8.32 Transverse section of the canine brain at the transition between the crus cerebri and internal capsule. *1,* Cerebral hemisphere; *2,* corpus callosum; *3,* caudate nucleus; *4,* thalamic nuclei; *5,* internal capsule; *6* and *6′,* lentiform nucleus: *6,* globus pallidus; *6′,* putamen; *7,* amygdala; *8,* optic tract; *9,* crus cerebri; *10,* hypothalamic nuclei; *11,* mammillothalamic tract; *12,* mammillary body; *13,* ventral part of third ventricle; *14,* hypophysis; *15,* oculomotor nerve; *16,* ventral part of lateral ventricle; *17,* hippocampus; *18,* piriform lobe; *19,* interthalamic adhesion; *20,* dorsal part of third ventricle; *21,* interventricular foramen; *22,* fornix; *23,* lateral ventricle.

extends rostrally to the *lamina terminalis grisea* and to the midbrain caudally. Its dorsal surface contacts the fornix, a telencephalic structure, and the floor of the lateral ventricle; its ventral surface is continuous with the hypothalamus; and its lateral face is enclosed by an internal capsule of white matter containing axons ascending to and descending from the cerebral cortex (see Fig. 8.30).

The thalamus is composed of a very large number of nuclei named according to their topographic relationships to one another. These nuclei have various specific functions and collectively form one of the most important relay and integration centers of the brainstem. Nuclei in the ventral thalamus receive information from most afferent systems (excluding the pathways concerned with olfaction) and also provide relays on feedback control systems of motor pathways (Fig. 8.32).

The *subthalamus* contains the subthalamic and endopeduncular nuclei and the zona incerta. The subthalamic nucleus acts as a relay station for the extrapyramidal motor pathway, whereas the other nuclei serve as links between the limbic system and the somatic and visceral motor systems.

The *metathalamus,* the caudolateral part of the thalamus, comprises the *lateral* and *medial geniculate bodies* (Fig. 8.33/*3* and *5*), whose presence and position were noted in the description of the midbrain. The lateral geniculate body, although not conspicuous in itself, is joined by the optic tract, which sweeps caudodorsally over the surface of the thalamus. The medial geniculate body lies ventromedial to the lateral geniculate body and receives acoustic fibers, the brachium, via the caudal colliculus (p. 287). The nuclei within the lateral and medial geniculate bodies relay visual and acoustic information, respectively, to the cerebral cortex.

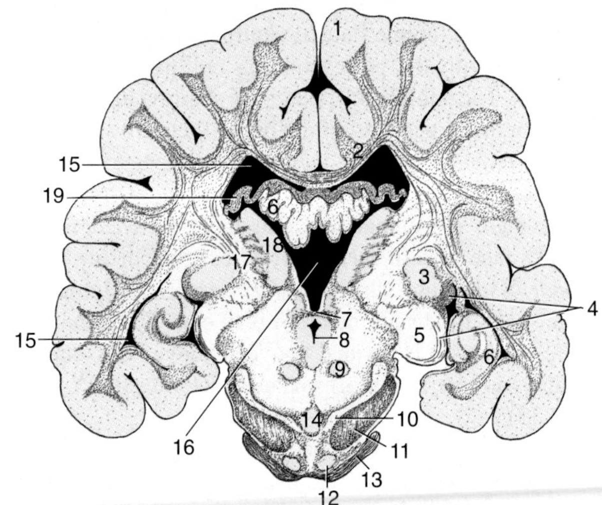

Fig. 8.33 Transverse section of the canine brain at the boundary between the mesencephalon and diencephalon. *1,* Cerebral hemisphere; *2,* corpus callosum; *3,* lateral geniculate nucleus; *4,* optic tract; *5,* medial geniculate nucleus; *6,* hippocampus; *7,* caudal commissure; *8,* mesencephalic aqueduct; *9,* red nucleus; *10,* substantia nigra; *11,* crus cerebri; *12,* rostral extension of pontine nuclei; *13,* middle cerebellar peduncle; *14,* interpeduncular nucleus; *15,* lateral ventricle; *16,* third ventricle; *17,* internal capsule; *18,* thalamic nuclei; *19,* fornix.

The *hypothalamus* forms the ventralmost parts of the lateral walls of the third ventricle. It appears on the external surface of the brain between the *preoptic region* (rostral to the optic chiasm) and the cerebral peduncles and interpeduncular fossa caudally (see Fig. 8.19). Its salient surface features are, first, the region known as the *tuber cinereum,* from which extends the stalk or infundibulum that suspends the hypophysis below the brain, and second, the rounded *mammillary body* (see Fig. 8.21) that receives information from the hippocampal complex and sends information to the thalamus via the mammillothalamic tract. The mammillary body is an important structure for memory. Internally, the hypothalamus contains a number of nuclei associated with the visceral nervous system as well as with hormonal and homeostatic regulation.

The *hypophysis,* or pituitary gland, is a dark solid body. It is located within a recess of the floor of the cranial cavity and is usually left behind when the brain is removed because the infundibulum, hollowed by a recess of the third ventricle, is easily torn across. The hypophysis is also held in place by a fold of dura mater (p. 295). The functions of the hypophysis are described elsewhere (p. 203).

The Telencephalon (Cerebrum)

The telencephalon consists of the paired hemispheres and the *lamina terminalis grisea,* the thin plate forming the rostral wall of the third ventricle with the vascular organ of the lamina terminalis (see Fig. 8.67/*7*). Because the hemispheres develop as outgrowths of the diencephalon, their walls and lumina (lateral ventricles) remain in direct continuity with the corresponding regions of the diencephalon. The adult hemispheres are semiovoid structures that form the largest part of the brain; their growth causes them to extend caudally over the brainstem to reach to within a short distance of the cerebellum. This growth brings them close together, and their flattened medial surfaces face toward each other across the narrow *longitudinal fissure* into which the *falx cerebri,* a connective tissue sheet, fits when the brain is in situ. The remainder of the outer wall is divided between convex dorsolateral and flattish ventral (basal) surfaces (see Figs. 8.23, 8.32, and 8.33).

The walls of the hemispheres thicken unequally. Much of the medial wall of each hemisphere remains particularly thin, and in fetal life a part rolls inward, invaginating the pia mater and blood vessels covered by the ependymal lining into the ventricle, where it develops into the *choroid plexus* (p. 296) associated with this cavity. This structure produces the cerebrospinal fluid. The ventrolateral (striatal) part of the wall becomes much thickened when a number of large nuclei, the basal nuclei, develop within it. The alternation of these nuclei with the fiber tracts in which they are embedded lends this region a striated appearance when exposed by section (see Fig. 8.32); it is therefore appropriately known as the *corpus striatum.* The remainder of the wall is initially known as the *pallium,* but when it acquires an external covering of gray substance, by migration of cells from the ependyma during development, it is more frequently termed the *cortex,* although this term strictly designates only the outer gray substance.

Three regions of the pallium (or cortex) are distinguished on the basis of evolutionary history, structure, and function. The paleopallium initially served a purely olfactory function; it has retained this association in highly developed mammals. The archipallium was also initially concerned with olfaction, but unlike the paleopallium, it has largely lost this association. The youngest part, the neopallium, made a very modest initial appearance in vertebrate history but has undergone a spectacular enlargement in mammals, in which it is both the largest and the functionally dominant part of the mammalian telencephalon. These parts are now described separately but in a different order for convenience. First, it may be helpful to dispose of the concept of a *rhinencephalon* ("smell-brain") of primary olfactory function. Although it is true that the telencephalon of lower vertebrates developed specifically in relation to this sense, many parts have since discarded their original function and acquired new roles. The term *rhinencephalon* therefore no longer describes the functions of these parts at all adequately, and because it is now used in many conflicting ways, there is little in favor of its retention.

The Paleopallium

The paleopallium is confined to the basal part of the brain; it is separated from the neopallium by the *rhinal sulcus* (Fig. 8.34/*4*) on the lateral surface and, although less clearly, from the archipallium medially. Its rostral extremity is provided by an appendage, the olfactory bulb (Fig. 8.34/*1*), that fits into a recess of the ethmoid bone. The surface apposed to the bone is made shaggy by the entrance of the numerous filaments that together form the olfactory nerve (I); these arise from receptors within the nasal mucosa and pass through the many perforations in the cribriform plate of the ethmoid bone. In the olfactory bulb, the olfactory stimuli are conveyed to second-stage neurons. The bulb is continued caudally by the *common olfactory tract* (see Fig. 8.19/*2*), which soon divides into medial and lateral divisions separated by a triangular area. The *medial tract* runs toward the medial aspect of the hemisphere (precommissural area), where the information is conveyed to third-stage neurons. Some of the continuing fibers terminate within certain cortical gyri; others pass through the narrow *anterior commissure* in the rostral wall of the third ventricle to reach the corresponding region of the opposite hemisphere. The *lateral tract* continues caudally to join the large *piriform lobe* (see Fig. 8.19/*3*), the most salient feature of the basal surface of the hemisphere;

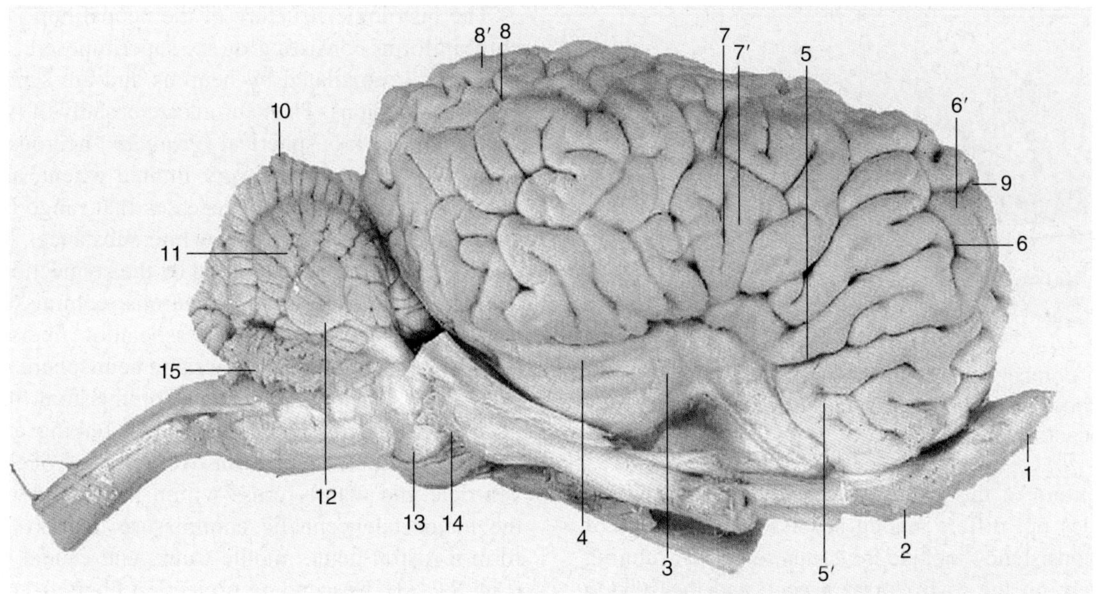

Fig. 8.34 Lateral view of the equine brain. *1,* Olfactory bulb; *2,* olfactory tract; *3,* piriform lobe; *4,* rhinal sulcus; *5,* sylvian sulcus; *5′,* sylvian gyrus; *6,* ectosylvian sulcus; *6′,* ectosylvian gyrus; *7,* suprasylvian sulcus; *7′,* suprasylvian gyrus; *8,* ectomarginal sulcus; *8′,* ectomarginal gyrus; *9,* cruciate sulcus; *10,* cerebellar vermis; *11,* cerebellar hemisphere; *12,* paraflocculus; *13,* pons; *14,* crus cerebri; *15,* caudal medullary velum.

not all the fibers in this tract reach the piriform lobe; some synapse on deeper structures such as the amygdala.

The Basal Nuclei

The basal nuclei are a group of large nuclei positioned dorsal to the paleopallium; they consist of the *caudate nucleus* and the *putamen* (which together are referred to as the *striatum,* or *neostriatum*) and the *globus pallidus,* or *paleostriatum.* The basal nuclei coordinate activity between the cerebral cortex and thalamus and play an important role in the initiation and regulation of movement. The *caudate nucleus* (Fig. 8.32/*3*) has the general form of a comma with a large head bulging into the floor of the main part of the lateral ventricle, a body following the caudal bend of the ventricle, and a tail close to the roof of ventral extension of the ventricle (Fig. 8.30/*13* and *14*). The caudate nucleus and the more laterally located *putamen* are functionally one structure, although anatomically they appear as two nuclei separated by a band of white matter that is composed of the axons of the internal capsule passing to and from the cerebral cortex. The *globus pallidus,* the other component of the basal nuclei, is also located laterally and, when combined with the putamen, is referred to as the *lentiform nucleus* (Fig. 8.32/*6* and *6′*). The lentiform nucleus is separated from the thalamus by the caudal portion of the internal capsule. The nucleus accumbens, the reward center, is located in the ventral part of the neostriatum.

The other components of the basal nuclei complex are the smaller *amygdala* (Fig. 8.32/*7*), located near the tail of the caudate nucleus, and the *claustrum,* which is interposed between the lentiform nucleus and neopallium. It is separated from these structures by other white matter tracts; the one on the lateral face of the claustrum is known as the *external capsule.*

The Neopallium

The neopallium makes up the majority of the telencephalon: all of the telencephalon that is visible in dorsal view and the bulk of that visible in lateral and medial views is neopallium. It is commonly referred to as the *cerebral cortex.* It is divided from the ventrally located paleopallium by the rhinal sulcus on the lateral side of the hemisphere (Fig. 8.20/*4*) and from the archipallium, described later, by the splenial sulcus medially (Fig. 8.21/*4*). In mammals of smaller size, rats and mice for example, the outer surface of the neopallium is smooth; however, in larger mammals, including domestic species, it displays a complicated arrangement of alternating ridges (*gyri*) and grooves (*sulci*) (see Fig. 8.23). Though it is tempting to regard the presence of more intricate gyri and deeper sulci as evidence of greater intelligence and increased capacity for complex responses, the immediate underlying cause appears to be physical. The ridges, which are mainly longitudinal, are produced by restraints imposed on the expanding telencephalic vesicle by the rigid corpus striatum and corpus callosum, and additional folding is necessary to maintain the relationship between volume (which increases by the cube) and cortical area (which increases by the square) in large brains.

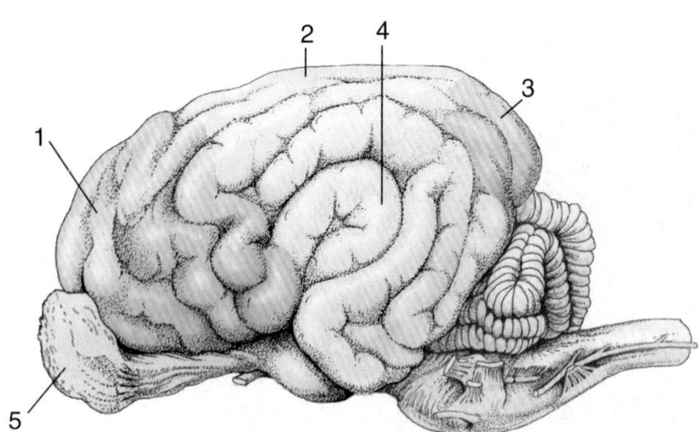

Fig. 8.35 Cortical lobes of the canine brain, lateral view. *1*, Frontal lobe; *2*, parietal lobe; *3*, occipital lobe; *4*, temporal lobe; *5*, olfactory lobe.

The pattern of the gyri is reasonably constant within one species but differs among species. The features of greatest consistency include the *cruciate sulcus,* running transversely on the rostrodorsal aspect, and the *sylvian sulcus* on the lateral side. Although other features provide useful landmarks for the investigator seeking to establish the functional significance of particular cortical areas, the names of most are of little consequence to the student. A simpler, rather arbitrary division of more general utility distinguishes four regions or lobes named for their proximity to overlying bones; this division recognizes *frontal, parietal,* and *occipital lobes* in rostrocaudal sequence and a *temporal lobe* lying lateral to the last two. Only the frontal lobe is clearly demarcated because it is bounded caudally by the cruciate sulcus (see Figs. 8.23/*14* and 8.35). Functional regions of the cerebral cortex have also been identified through experimentation. Thus we can locate the motor cortex, the sensory cortex, the auditory cortex and the visual cortex (Figs. 8.20B and 8.23B).

The concept of somatotopy is a characteristic of many structures in the brain and spinal cord but is expressed most highly in the cerebral cortex and to a lesser extent in the cerebellar cortex and so is discussed here. The fibers and cell bodies within many tracts and relaying nuclei and within areas of the cerebral and cerebellar cortices preserve very orderly point-to-point arrangements that reflect the topography of the parts of the body from which afferent impulses arise or to which efferent impulses are delivered. These do not always, or even usually, reproduce the true physical proportions but represent the parts of the body in relation to the densities of their innervation. The representations take the form of grotesque caricatures, sometimes known as *homunculi*—although *animalcula* would better fit veterinary anatomy—in which very sensitive, densely innervated body regions such as the lips and muzzle of the horse, or regions capable of very refined and accurate movements, such as the fingers of a human or the prehensile tail of a monkey, are of exaggerated size. The concept of somatotopy is of great importance in the consideration of the significance of pathologic lesions, in the conduct of neurosurgery, and in experimental stimulation.

The histologic structure of the neopallium is remarkably uniform, consisting of six superimposed strata that are densely populated by neurons and are separated by cell-free divisions. The neurons are broadly of two types: some more or less spherical (*granular*) neurons are provided with processes of very limited extent, and other, pyramidal, neurons have processes that range more distantly within the underlying white substance. The pyramidal neurons can be classified by the connection of their axon fibers into association neurons, commissural neurons, or projection neurons. Association fibers connect parts of the neopallium of the same hemisphere after passage directly below the cortex. Commissural fibers connect the two hemispheres, generally linking equivalent contralateral parts. They run over the roof of the lateral ventricle and mainly cross within the corpus callosum, the major telencephalic commissure that is shaped to form a rostral genu, middle trunk, and caudal splenium (Fig. 8.21/*3*). Descending projection fibers from the cortex connect with lower parts of the central nervous system; most converge on the internal capsule squeezed between the basal nuclei and thalamus (Figs. 8.36/*7* and 8.37/*1*). In their courses to, from, and within the capsule the projection fibers are ordered according to their functional associations and somatotopic relationships.

The Archipallium

The part of the cortex known as the *archipallium* is concerned with the correlation of olfactory with other sensory information but has acquired additional functions in modern mammals. It forms part of the limbic system, which comprises the cingulate, supracallosal, and geniculate gyri; the hippocampal formation; and the dentate gyrus.

The archipallium is not a conspicuous feature of the telencephalon in domestic mammals. The enormous development of the neopallium has caused the archipallium to be displaced to the medial wall of the cerebral hemisphere; it is further reduced in prominence because a large part is rolled inward to lie on the floor of the lateral ventricle. The archipallium is topographically divided by the corpus callosum into a dorsal part that remains on the medial surface of the hemisphere named the *cingulate* and *supracallosal gyri* between the splenial sulcus and the corpus callosum (Fig. 8.21/*8* and *8'*) and a ventral part composed of the inflected portion, usually known as the *hippocampus* (Fig. 8.38/*2*), located deep in the hemisphere. The archipallium is curved in conformity with the shape assumed by the expanding telencephalon and fits around the dorsal, caudal, and ventral aspects of the thalamus. This arrangement is difficult to envisage, and it is helpful to remember that the archipallium is interposed between the olfactory bulb and the hypothalamus. The pathway is thus bent into a hairpin loop by the expansion of the hemisphere (Fig. 8.39); the proximal limb extends, with a ventral

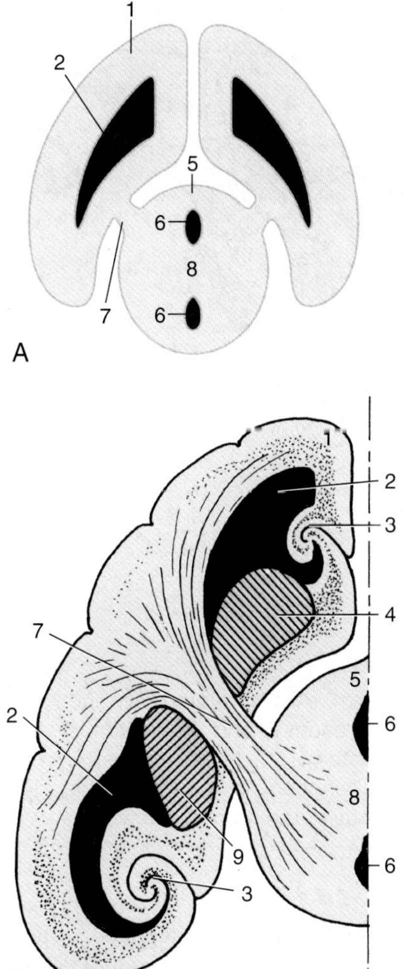

Fig. 8.36 (A) The connection between the cerebral hemisphere and diencephalon via the internal capsule *(7)*. (B) The lateral ventricle, basal nuclei, and hippocampus form concentric arches over the internal capsule. *1*, Cerebral hemisphere; *2*, lateral ventricle; *3*, hippocampus; *4*, caudate nucleus; *5*, diencephalon; *6*, third ventricle; *7*, internal capsule; *8*, interthalamic adhesion; *9*, globus pallidus and putamen.

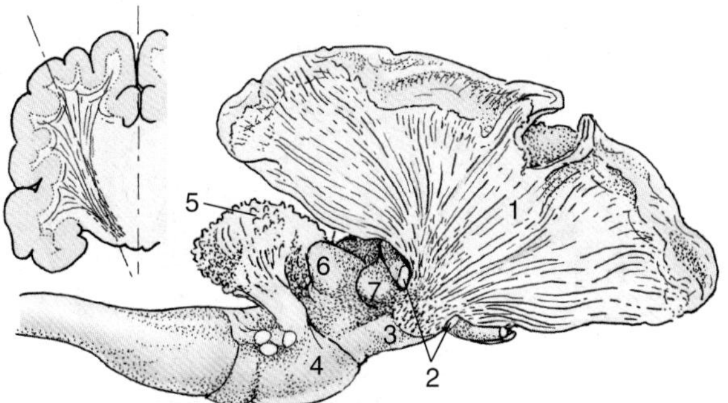

Fig. 8.37 The internal capsule in the canine brain. A part of the cerebral cortex and the cortex of the cerebellum have been removed. The resected part of the telencephalon is indicated in the inset. *1*, Fibers of the internal capsule; *2*, optic tract, partly removed; *3*, crus cerebri; *4*, pons; *5*, corpus medullare of cerebellum; *6*, caudal colliculus; *7*, medial geniculate body.

concavity, caudally toward the apex of the loop, where a spiral twist sets the distal limb on a parallel returning course.

The proximal limb is formed by the medial surface gyri; ventral to this run the longitudinal association fibers (*cingulum*) that originate in the septal area. The fibers of this multisynaptic pathway enter the caudal extremity of the hippocampus and form a covering for it. The fibers leaving the hippocampus run rostrally over its surface, gradually consolidating into a thick bundle, the fornix. The *fornix* lies directly below the corpus callosum at its start but then deviates ventrally as it passes rostrally; it curves around the rostral extremity of the thalamus to enter the hypothalamus, where it terminates within the mammillary body (Figs. 8.38 and 8.40). The right and left hippocampi are joined by the *commissure of the fornix*. There are thus three telencephalic commissures: the large corpus callosum of the neopallium, the anterior commissure of the paleopallium, and the commissure of the fornix (also known as the archipallial fornical commissure).

When the fornix parts company with the corpus callosum, it remains connected to it by a thin vertically oriented septum that increases in depth toward its rostral end. This *septum telencephali (pellucidum)* forms part of the medial wall of the lateral ventricle (see Fig. 8.21/*28*). It is a bilateral structure, each sheet of which is separated from its neighbor by a narrow, completely enclosed cleft, and its ventrorostral part contains *septal nuclei* in which fibers from the medial olfactory tract terminate.

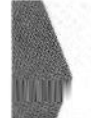

THE FUNCTIONAL MORPHOLOGY OF THE CENTRAL NERVOUS SYSTEM

Despite the pretensions of the heading, this section deals only with certain rather fundamental topics involving, for the most part, relatively discrete structured pathways.

Processing of Somatic Afferent Information

The term *somatic afferent* is applied to those sensory pathways that receive and convey information from the wide array of peripheral receptors scattered throughout the skin and the deeper somatic tissues. The term does not apply to the afferent pathways from the retina of the eye or the inner ear (referred to as *special afferent pathways*) or those from receptors in the viscera (*visceral afferent pathways*).

The somatic afferent system transmits a variety of sensory modalities: touch, pressure, vibratory sensation, thermal sensation, pain, as well as kinesthetic or *proprioceptive* sensations such as muscle length, muscle

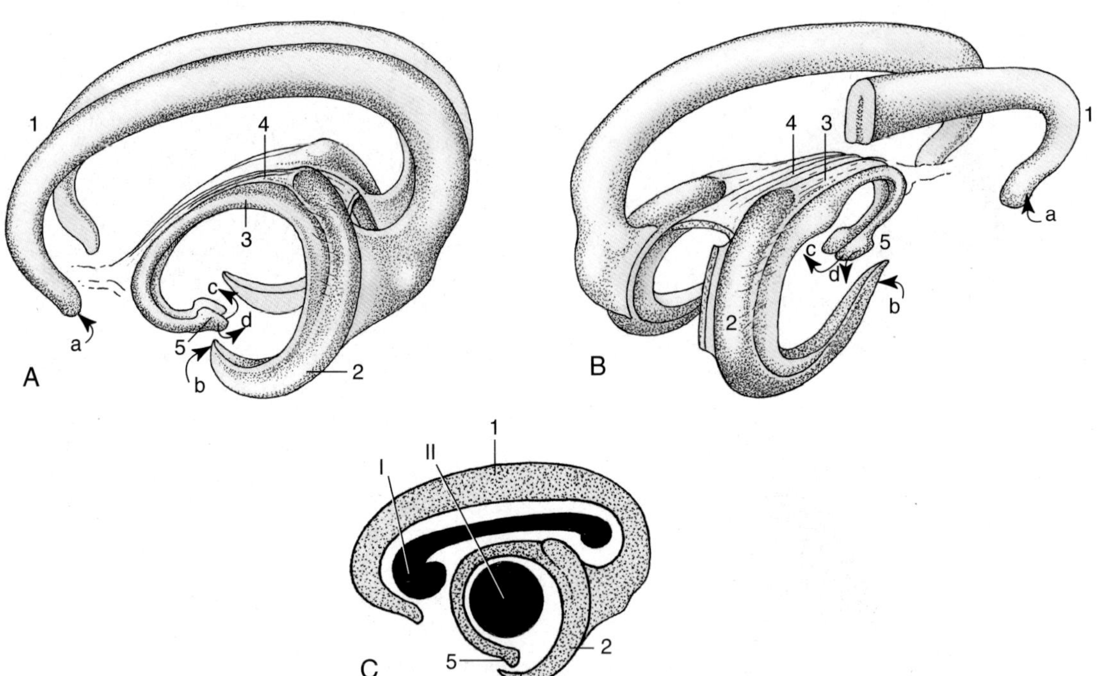

Fig. 8.38 Three-dimensional representations of the archipallium. (A) Left lateral view and (B) right caudolateral view. (C) The positions of the corpus callosum *(I)* and the thalamus *(II)* are shown in lateral projection. *1*, Supracallosal and cingulate gyri; *2*, hippocampus; *3*, fornix; *4*, commissure of fornix; *5*, hypothalamus with mammillary body. *a*, Input from the medial olfactory tract; *b*, input from the piriform lobe; *c*, output to the mammillothalamic tract; *d*, output to the brainstem.

tension, and joint angulation. The cell bodies of the primary sensory neurons, which transmit all these sensations to the central nervous system, are located within the dorsal root ganglia of the spinal nerves (and, for these same senses in the head, in the sensory ganglion of the trigeminal nerve). The axons of these sensory neurons enter the central nervous system by the dorsal roots of the spinal nerves (and the afferent root of the trigeminal nerve). The axons branch upon entering the central nervous system. Some of these branches synapse onto interneurons within the adjacent gray matter; a subset of these interneurons in turn project onto motor neurons in the ventral gray matter of the same or neighboring segments. The axons of motor neurons leave the central nervous system and travel as a component of peripheral nerves to reach and synapse upon skeletal muscle in the periphery. The complete route just described—from peripheral somatic receptors to somatic afferent pathway to interneuron to motor neuron to peripheral motor neuron axon to muscle—forms the neural circuit that provides the anatomic basis for local reflex responses. (For only the *myotatic reflex,* also termed the *tendon jerk,* the interneuron is not present in this circuit; see Fig. 8.5.)

Other branches of the primary sensory axons connect directly, or through interneurons, with higher centers in the brain or spinal cord, thus providing pathways that initiate more complex integrated responses. These ascending pathways, described in more detail later, form some of the white matter tracts of the spinal cord. Once in the brain, these pathways ultimately reach the somatosensory area of the cerebral cortex, providing the mechanism for conscious perception of these various somatic sensations. Additionally, as these pathways ascend to and through the brain, they produce collateral branches at different levels to connect to numerous brain regions.

The Lemniscal System

There are two main ascending pathways that reach the somatosensory region of the cerebral cortex. The first, termed here the *lemniscal system* though other names are used, transmits information that provides a high degree of spatial discrimination of touch, an accurate assessment of the intensity of pressure, repetitive vibratory sensation, and muscle and joint proprioception. Spinal interneurons are not involved in this pathway. Instead, some of the axonal branches of the primary sensory neurons, after entering the spinal cord, pass at once to the dorsal funiculus of the cord, that component of the spinal white matter located dorsally (see Fig. 8.7). These primary sensory axons adopt a very orderly arrangement within the dorsal funiculus (see Fig. 8.18); those that enter through sacral nerves—that is, most caudally—occupy the most medial

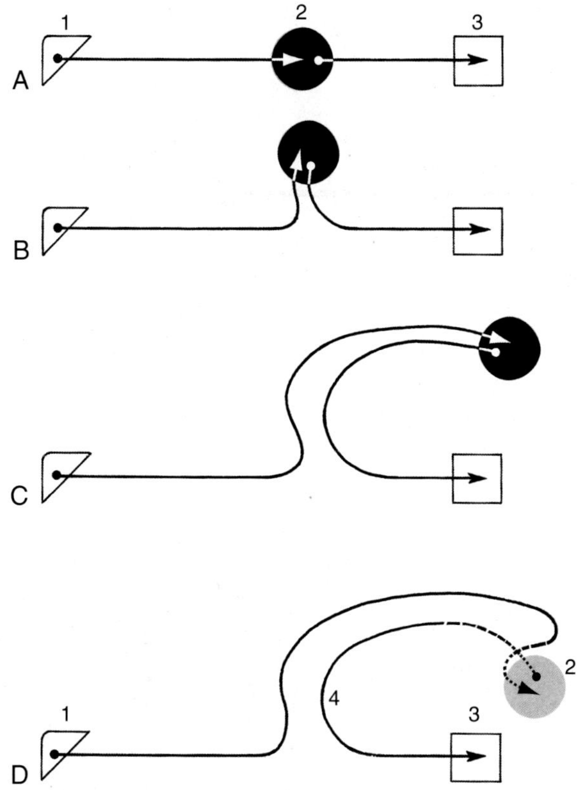

Fig. 8.39 (A) Diagram illustrating conjectured course of fibers running to and from the hippocampus. Because of differential growth of various parts of the brain, the hippocampus extends first (B) dorsally, then (C) caudally, and finally (D) laterally. *1*, Olfactory bulb; *2*, hippocampus; *3*, hypothalamus; *4*, fornix.

positions, whereas those that enter at more cranial levels assume progressively more lateral positions. A glial septum that appears within the dorsal funiculus at midthoracic level divides it into two parts: the medial division, which constitutes the *gracile fasciculus,* contains axons from the hindlimb and caudal trunk; the lateral division, the *cuneate fasciculus,* contains axons from the forelimb, the cranial part of the trunk, and the neck. Both tracts end within corresponding nuclei, *gracile and cuneate nuclei,* within the dorsal part of the medulla oblongata, where they raise slight surface elevations, the gracile and cuneate tubercles (Fig. 8.22/*13* and *14*). The axons of the second-stage neurons—that is, neurons located within the gracile and cuneate nuclei—leave the ventral aspects of the nuclei and at once decussate, or cross, to the opposite side and turn rostrally as the large axon tract known as the medial lemniscus. The *medial lemniscus* runs cranially within the ventral part of the medulla, dorsal to the pyramid and close to the midline, to reach a specific part of the *caudoventral nuclear complex of the thalamus* (MCV) (Fig. 8.41). After synapses within the thalamus, axons of third-stage neurons travel within the white matter projection termed the *thalamic radiation* to the somatosensory area of the cerebral cortex (neopallium) (see Figs. 8.20B/*2,3* and 8.23B/*2,3*). This is a cortical area directly caudal to the cruciate sulcus. In addition to information transmitted via spinal somatic sensory pathways, the lemniscal pathway receives somatic sensation from the head and neck at the level of the brainstem, where the medial lemniscus is joined by axons transmitting somatic sensory information from the lateral cervical nucleus, the nucleus of the descending tract of the trigeminal nerve,

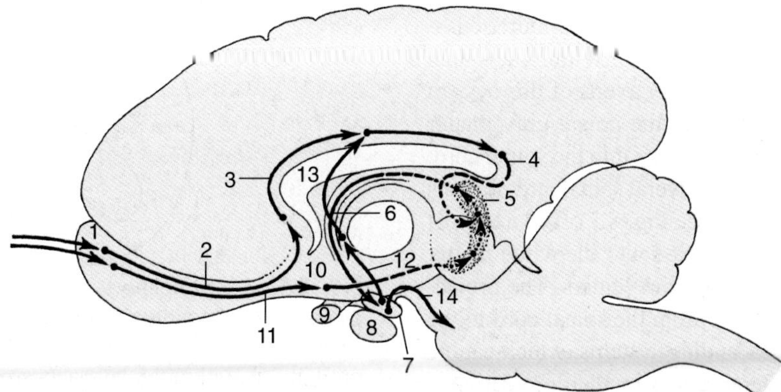

Fig. 8.40 A simplified conjectured diagram of the relay scheme of the limbic system. The *solid arrows* indicate the relay of information from the olfactory bulbs through the structures of the limbic system. The fiber tracts indicated by *dotted lines* are bent laterally out of the plane of the drawing. *1*, Olfactory bulb; *2*, medial olfactory tract; *3*, cingulum (in gyri supracallosus and cinguli); *4*, gyrus dentatus; *5*, hippocampus; *6*, fornix; *7*, mammillary body; *8*, hypophysis; *9*, optic chiasm; *10*, piriform lobe; *11*, lateral olfactory tract; *12*, mammillothalamic tract; *13*, projection fibers entering the cingulum; *14*, projection fibers to reticular formation.

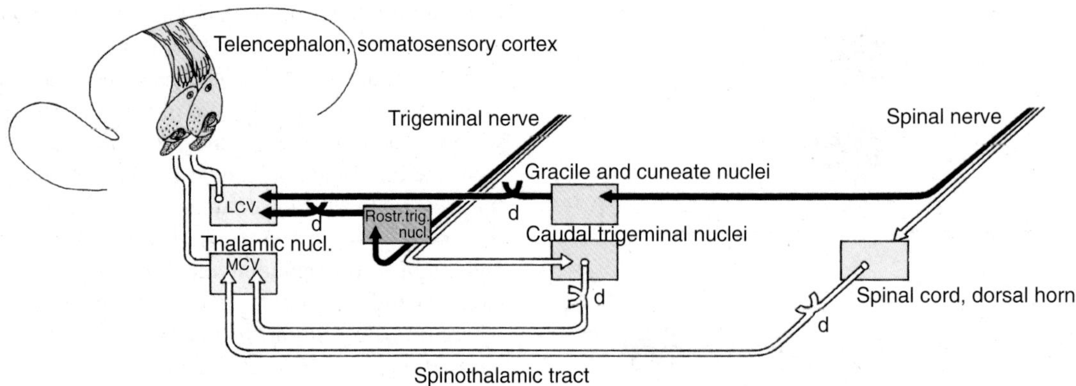

Fig. 8.41 The lemniscal *(black)* and extralemniscal *(white)* projections from the trunk and head to the telencephalon. *d*, Decussation; *LCV*, lateral part; MCV, medial part of the caudoventral thalamic nucleus.

and the rostral (principal) sensory nucleus of the trigeminal nerve after a decussation within the metencephalon (Figs. 8.41 and 8.42).

The somatotopic organization of the lemniscal pathway is preserved throughout its length, including the thalamic nucleus and the cortex. The somatotopic representation of the body within the cortex is of contralateral parts of the body and reflects the density of the sensory innervation of each body region rather than its absolute size. There is also some segregation within the cortex by sensory modality.

The Extralemniscal System

The extralemniscal system transmits a second subset of somatic afferent modalities, characterized by slower propagation and less precise localization of the originating stimuli. The information conveyed is composed of cruder varieties of touch and pressure sensation, temperature sensation, and, most important, pain sensation. Within the spinal cord, branches of the primary sensory axons of this system synapse on interneurons located in the dorsal gray matter within a segment or two of axonal entry into the spinal cord. The information is processed via several spinal interneurons before leaving the dorsal horn (see Fig. 8.7). The axons of these second-stage neurons then pass into the white matter of the cord and ascend to higher brain centers. The projection of pain signals in particular from the spinal cord to the brain occurs via multiple ascending systems, which can be divided into medial and lateral groups by their projections.

The tracts of the medial group tend to project and synapse upon regions throughout the brainstem up to the level of the diencephalon. This group is made up of the spinothalamic tract (see Fig. 8.42) that projects to the medial and intralaminar thalamic nuclei; the spinoreticular tract, composed of axon bundles located bilaterally within the ventral and ventrolateral regions of the spinal white matter that synapse within the reticular formation of the brainstem

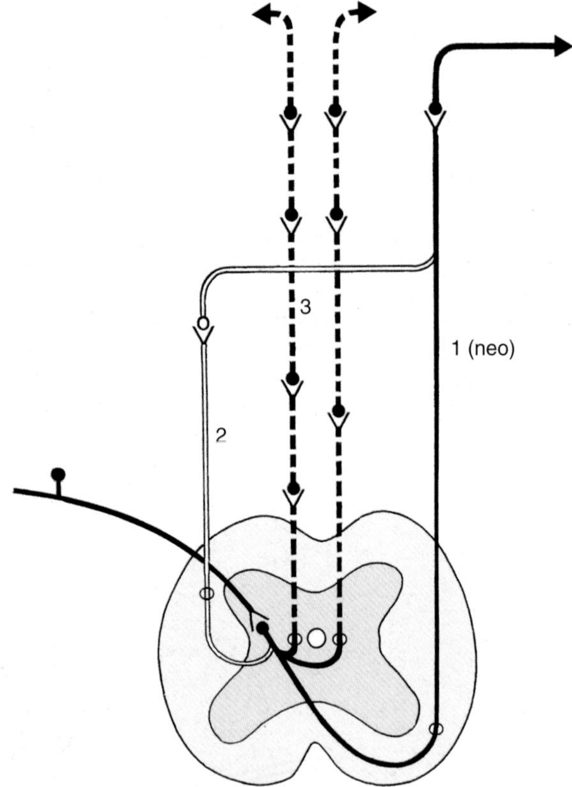

Fig. 8.42 A simplified scheme of the extralemniscal projections ascending from the spinal cord to the telencephalon. The *solid black* and *white* lines represent the projections within the lateral system; the *interrupted black lines* represent the bilateral and multisynaptic projections within the medial system. The (paleo) spinothalamic tract is not represented in this scheme. *1*, Spinothalamic tract; *2*, spinocervicothalamic tract; *3*, spinoreticulothalamic tract.

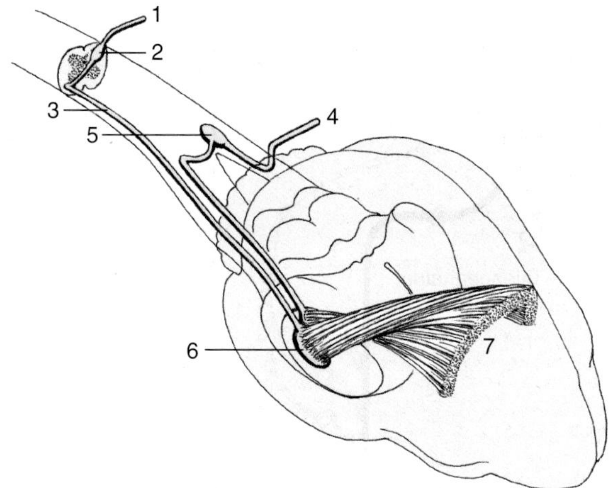

Fig. 8.43 Three-dimensional representation of the extralemniscal projection in the dog. *1,* Spinal nerve; *2,* dorsal horn of spinal cord; *3,* spinothalamic tract; *4,* trigeminal nerve; *5,* nucleus of the spinal tract of the trigeminal nerve; *6,* medial part of the caudoventral thalamic nucleus; *7,* somatosensory cortex.

as far rostrally as the thalamus; and a loosely organized group of ascending propriospinal axons that originate and end repeatedly in the spinal gray matter, forming a multisynaptic relay system for information to ascend to the brain. These three main components of the medial group show little variation among vertebrates, in contrast to the lateral group described next.

The lateral group is made up of tracts projecting onto the medial caudoventral nuclear complex of the thalamus, similar to the lemniscal pathways. The tracts making up the lateral group include the (neo)spinothalamic tract, the spinocervicothalamic system, and the second-order dorsal column pathway (Figs. 8.42 and 8.43).

The (neo)spinothalamic tract constitutes the classic pain tract of primates, including humans. It is entirely crossed and ascends within the spinal cord white matter on the ventrolateral aspect of the spinal cord and then through the brainstem toward the MCV.

The spinocervicothalamic system is well developed in subprimate mammals, particularly carnivores. Second-order axons arising from spinal interneurons ascend ipsilaterally as the spinocervical tract, located in the dorsolateral region of the spinal white matter, and synapse in the lateral cervical nucleus, located at the junction of the spinal cord and brainstem. The third-order axons that arise from this nucleus cross the midline and follow the medial lemniscus to end in the MCV, where they overlap the projection site of the (neo)spinothalamic tract.

The third system has been found in cats. It is composed of second-order axons from spinal interneurons that, surprisingly, ascend as a component of the spinal dorsal columns alongside the axons of primary afferent neurons of the lemniscal system. The postsynaptic, pain-conveying axons of this third system synapse in ipsilateral dorsal column nuclei. From neurons in the dorsal column nuclei, third-order axons cross the midline and also run to the MCV.

For sensory information from the head and neck traveling in the extralemniscal system, second-order axons arise from the caudal part of the descending trigeminal nucleus. These axons either join the lateral system and ascend to synapse in the MCV or join the medial system and ascend to the reticular formation of the thalamus. The third-order axons arising in the thalamus project to an area of the somatosensory cortex rostral to the area allocated to the lemniscal system.

Models have been proposed to explain the respective roles of the lateral and medial pain-signaling systems in the generation of pain sensation and behavior. It has been proposed that the lateral and medial systems contribute differentially to the psychological dimensions of pain experience: one suggestion is that the lateral system conveys information regarding the sensory-discriminative dimensions of pain, whereas the medial is mainly involved in the motivational-affective dimension via the reticular formation, medial thalamus, and limbic system. Another model suggests that the lateral system is tuned preferentially to the sudden onset of noxious stimuli and thus may be related to the threat modality of pain. In contrast, the medial system is tuned to persistent components of pain and is thus better suited to mediate signals relating to existing tissue damage.

Subconscious Proprioceptive Pathways

The pathways transmitting information about the position and movement of the limbs—that is, proprioceptive information—to the somatosensory cortex have already been described as a component of the lemniscal system. An entirely different set of pathways transmits the same proprioceptive information to the brain but only as far as the cerebellum. These pathways are considered subconscious proprioceptive pathways as they do not terminate in the cerebral cortex. The pathways commence in the usual way with primary sensory axons arising from muscle and joint receptors that terminate on interneurons in spinal gray matter within the initial and adjacent spinal segments. The axons of the second-stage neurons travel cranially as the *dorsal* and *ventral spinocerebellar tracts* constituting the lateralmost regions of spinal white matter (Fig. 8.18/*5* and *6*). The dorsal tract takes a direct ipsilateral pathway that enters the cerebellum through the caudal cerebellar peduncle; the information it conveys is obtained from stimulation of muscle spindles. In contrast, the ventral spinocerebellar tract is concerned mainly with transmitting information arising from tendon receptors. The axons of the ventral tract decussate within the cord close to their origins; they then ascend to midbrain level before they turn caudally to enter the cerebellum through the rostral cerebellar peduncle. A second decussation within the cerebellar medulla restores the axons of the ventral tract to the side of the origin of the stimulus before they terminate within the cerebellar cortex. These two tracts transmit information only from the trunk and hindlimbs; the equivalent representation of the forelimb follows a different pathway that is not described here.

A further diffuse ascending pathway is provided within the reticular formation, the subject of the following section. It provides a means for integrating information conveyed by the pathways previously described with information from other afferent systems, somatic and visceral, general and special.

The Reticular Formation

The reticular formation extends throughout the brainstem as a diffuse arrangement of neurons interspersed with axon tracts. In the evolutionary sense, it is an old system. Despite the lack of obvious organization, closer analysis permits the recognition of numerous nuclei of varying size and architecture; some are sufficiently distinctive for their homologues to be recognizable in different species.

The reticular formation is connected to all projection systems within the central nervous system, whether afferent or efferent, and has reciprocal connections with the major integration centers within the brain. Thus, among its many ascending, descending, and transverse connections, there are such tracts as reticulocerebellar and cerebelloreticular and reticulothalamocortical and corticoreticular. The inescapable inference is that the reticular formation plays an important role in modulating the activities of these integration centers.

The reticular formation occupies a large part of the brainstem; it forms the main substance of the medulla, pons and midbrain, and when it reaches the thalamus, it contributes some of the nuclear groups of this complex structure. It also extends into the cervical part of the spinal cord.

The reticular formation may be divided into parts distinguished by morphology and location. The medial part, the *periventricular gray,* is located adjacent to the ventricular system of the brain. It has proved impossible to analyze in detail but appears to provide multisynaptic pathways composed of an indeterminable number of neurons with short and much branched processes. The *second component* exhibits a more obvious organization with more readily identifiable nuclei and ascending and descending tracts. For example, the reticular nuclei of the thalamus receive an input from lower parts of the reticular formation as the *spinoreticulothalamic tract* and project diffusely on the entire neopallium. This tract is an important component of the reticular system and may be a route, complementary to the spinothalamic tract, for somatic sensory information to reach the cortex. It contains axons that project for long distances and conduct more rapidly than those found in the spinothalamic tract.

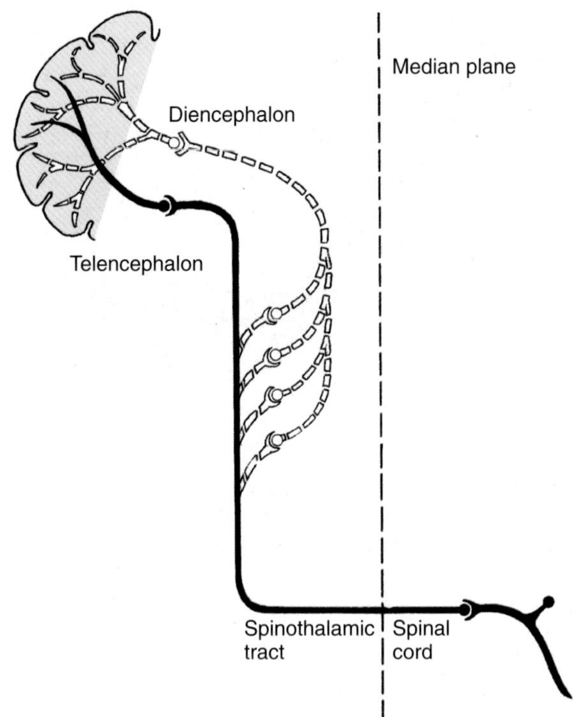

Fig. 8.44 A multisynaptic ascending tract *(white dotted line)* to the telencephalon via the reticular formation. The collateral tract in this example represents the extralemniscal projection *(solid black line).*

One extensive reticular ascending pathway that ultimately projects beyond the thalamus to the cortex is known as the *ascending reticular activating system (ARAS).* The ARAS receives inputs through collateral branches from all sensory systems, whether somatic or visceral (Fig. 8.44). Its activation arouses the animal, making it more conscious of its circumstances and surroundings; diminution of ARAS activity induces lethargy or sleep. The ARAS has been regarded as an important component of the seat of consciousness, although most neurologists would assert that "there is no single place where consciousness dwells."

The reticular system also plays an essential role in motor control by means of descending pathways from the telencephalon that synapse on reticular nuclei. In turn, these nuclei project axons to synapse on lower motor neurons of the brainstem and cord.

Special Somatic Afferent Pathways

The Visual Pathways

Visual information is conveyed from the retina by the optic nerve. After entering the cranial cavity through the optic foramen, the nerve converges to meet its fellow in the optic chiasm on the ventral surface of the brain. At the chiasm, there is a partial decussation of axons from each retina. The proportion of axons crossing to the opposite side is inversely correlated with the degree of binocular vision in a particular species. In ungulates, the binocular field of vision is small, and a very large percentage (85% to 90%) of fibers cross. Carnivores have a more binocular vision and a corresponding smaller proportion (75%) of axons cross in those species. Approximately 50% cross in primates, in which binocular vision is best developed. In birds, all axons were thought to cross, and it was considered that birds had no binocular vision—that is, that each eye was thought to see completely separate parts of the visual field. However, newer information indicates that some birds have an even larger field of binocular vision than humans.

After reassortment of axons at the chiasm, these axons then continue on as the optic tracts, which arch over the lateral surface of the thalamus (Fig. 8.22/*20*). Most axons terminate within the lateral geniculate nucleus of the thalamus, which forms a swelling on dorsolateral surface of the thalamus. The axons of the second-order neurons then project, via the optic radiation within the internal capsule, to the visual cortex, which is located within the occipital lobe of the cerebrum. The visual cortex is the cortical region responsible for conscious visual perception (Fig. 8.45/*6*).

Those optic tract fibers that do not synapse in the lateral geniculate nuclei project onto various mesencephalic nuclei. A proportion of these optic tract axons synapse in the pretectal region, an area near the border between the thalamus and the midbrain. Second-order neurons in the pretectal region then project to and synapse on neurons of the oculomotor nerve located in the midbrain that are responsible for reducing pupillary diameter in response to light. Optic tract fibers also synapse in the rostral colliculi, an important visual integration center in the midbrain responsible for controlling direction of gaze. Axons arising from the rostral colliculi also end on lower motor neurons in the cervical spinal cord and constitute the tectospinal tract, part of the so-called extrapyramidal motor system.

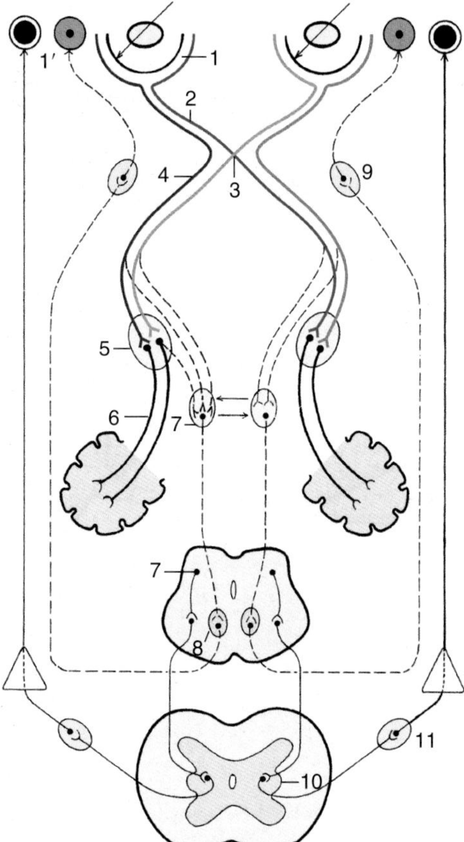

Fig. 8.45 A simplified schema of the visual and pupillary reflex pathways. *Thick solid lines* indicate special somatic visual fibers; *thin solid lines*, sympathetic fibers; and *interrupted lines*, parasympathetic fibers. *1*, Retina; *1′*, dilated and constricted pupils; *2*, optic nerve; *3*, optic chiasm; *4*, optic tract; *5*, lateral geniculate nucleus; *6*, optic radiation; *7*, rostral colliculus and pretectal nuclei; *8*, oculomotor nucleus (parasympathetic part); *9*, ciliary ganglion; *10*, lateral visceral efferent column; *11*, cranial cervical ganglion.

Vestibular Pathways

The vestibular axons arising from the vestibular sensory apparatus in the inner ear travel within the common vestibulocochlear nerve (CN VIII) that enters the brain at the level of the trapezoid body. These axons then terminate on, or detach collateral branches to, neurons of the vestibular nuclei (Fig. 8.46/*2*). Some vestibular axons enter the caudal cerebellar peduncle to synapse within the vestibular portion of the cerebellum. The second-order axons that arise from neurons in the vestibular nuclei are divided between those that also pass to the cerebellum and the remainder, which travel to the spinal cord via the vestibulospinal tract and to the brainstem via the medial longitudinal fasciculus. Within the spinal cord, vestibulospinal axons project via a series of interneurons onto lower motor neurons of the ipsilateral ventral gray matter. The vestibulospinal tracts are part of the extrapyramidal system. Those second-order fibers that follow the medial longitudinal fasciculus (Fig. 8.46/*4*) and the reticular formation proceed to synapse on the nuclei of the cranial nerves supplying the external ocular muscles.

Finally, the axons that lead to conscious perception of vestibular stimuli travel from the vestibular nuclei via the lateral lemniscus and thalamic nuclei to a particular region of the cerebral cortex of the temporal lobe.

Auditory Pathways

The axons of the cochlear component of the vestibulo cochlear nerve synapse within the dorsal and ventral cochlear nuclei located on the dorsal surface of the brainstem

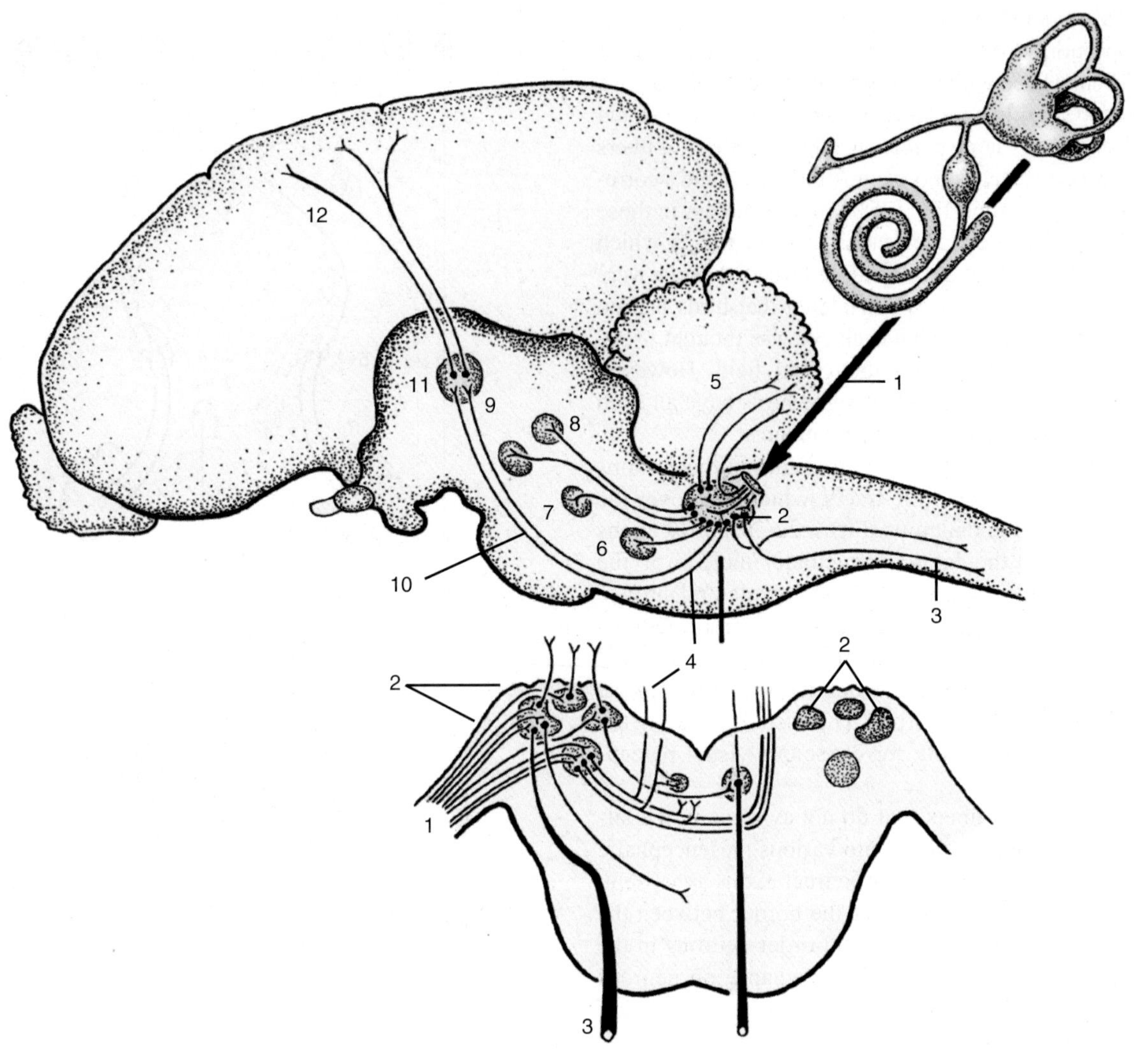

Fig. 8.46 A simplified scheme of the vestibular pathways. *1,* Vestibular fibers in vestibulocochlear nerve; *2,* vestibular nuclei; *3,* vestibulospinal tract; *4,* medial longitudinal fasciculus; *5,* vestibulocerebellar tract; *6,* abducent nucleus; *7,* trochlear nucleus; *8,* oculomotor nucleus; *9,* red nucleus; *10,* vestibulothalamic tract (in lateral lemniscus); *11,* thalamic nuclei; *12,* thalamocortical projection fibers.

(Fig. 8.47/*1* and *2*). The second-order axons from the ventral cochlear nucleus then proceed to synapse within either an ipsilateral or a contralateral nucleus of the trapezoid body (Fig. 8.47/*3*). The pathway is then continued by axons of third-stage neurons carried within the lateral lemniscus. A proportion of these axons synapse within the nucleus of the lateral lemniscus (Fig. 8.47/*5*), a second group of axons travels to and synapses within the caudal colliculus (Fig. 8.47/*6*), and a third set of axons, concerned with the conscious perception of sound, travels farther rostrally to synapse in the medial geniculate nucleus of the thalamus, which in turn sends axons to the auditory cortex, located within the temporal lobe.

The second-order axons that emerge from the dorsal cochlear nuclei join the ipsilateral or contralateral lateral lemniscus and thereafter follow the same courses as those that proceed from the ventral cochlear nuclei.

Somatic Motor Pathways

Somatic motor activity is regulated hierarchically within the central nervous system by separate groups of neurons termed the *lower motor neurons* and *upper motor neurons.*

Lower motor neurons are neurons that have cell bodies located within the central nervous system and axons that leave the central nervous system to synapse upon muscle fibers in the periphery—these are the neurons that have been named motor neurons up to this point. The axons of lower motor neurons form the motor component of peripheral nerves. The cell bodies of those lower motor neurons,

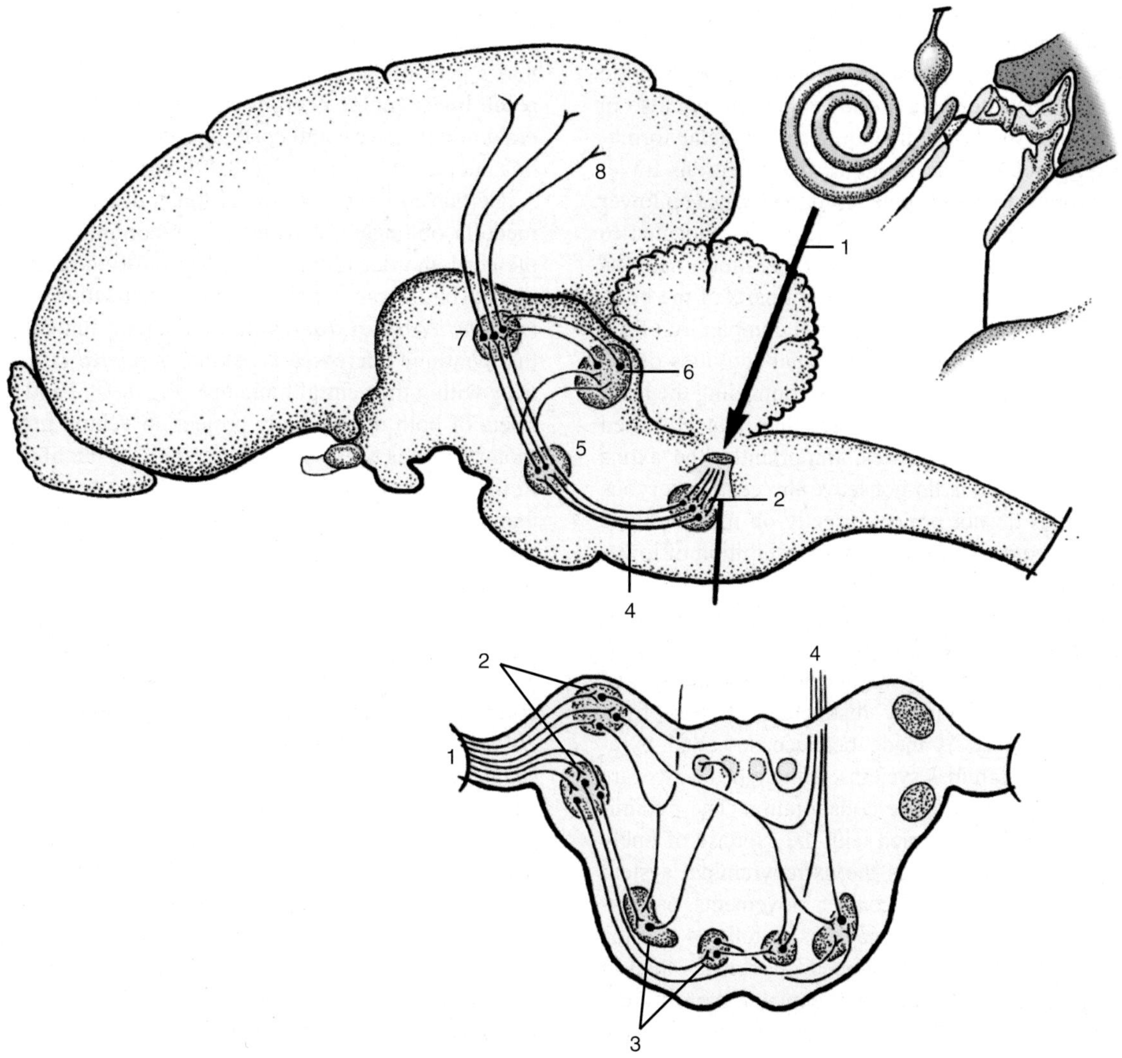

Fig. 8.47 A simplified scheme of the auditory pathways. *1*, Cochlear fibers in the vestibulocochlear nerve; *2*, cochlear nuclei (dorsal and ventral); *3*, nuclei in trapezoid body; *4*, lateral lemniscus; *5*, nucleus in lateral lemniscus; *6*, caudal colliculus; *7*, medial geniculate nucleus; *8*, projection fibers for conscious perception.

which innervate the skeletal muscle of the neck, trunk, and limbs, are located within the ventral portion of the gray matter of the spinal cord (Figs. 8.12/*4* and 8.13/*6*) and their axons travel in the peripheral nerves of the neck, trunk, and limbs (Fig. 8.48). The cell bodies of those lower motoneurons that innervate the skeletal muscle of the head are located within somatic motor nuclei in the brainstem, and their axons travel in the cranial nerves that contain somatic efferent components. The number of lower motor neurons innervating a particular muscle varies with the precision of performance required of that muscle (p. 23). Lower motor neurons are the efferent component of local reflex responses that involve the muscles in question (Fig. 8.48) but are also importantly controlled by the activity of upper motor neurons.

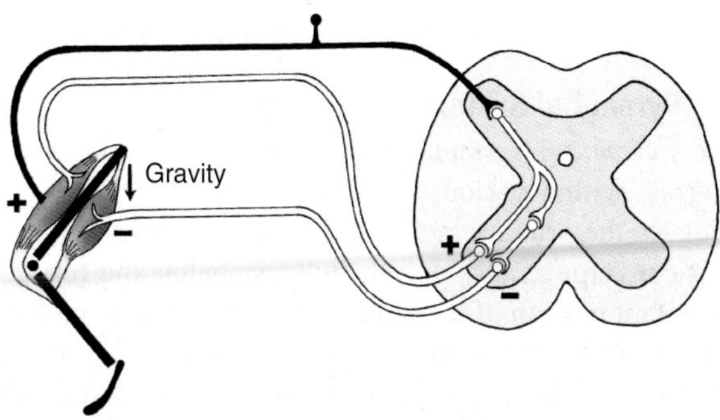

Fig. 8.48 A myotactic reflex arc. Gravity *(arrow)* stretches the extensor muscle, stimulating its contraction via the reflex arc. To allow shortening of the extensor muscle, the flexor muscle is inhibited at the same time by a collateral fiber and an inhibiting interneuron.

The *upper motor neurons* are involved in more complicated reflexes and also initiate voluntary movements. The cell bodies of upper motor neurons are located in the brain, within the motor area of the neopallium but also in other regions of the brain, including the reticular formation and red nucleus. The axons of these neurons travel through the brainstem and spinal cord to synapse on lower motor neurons. The amount of cortical area allocated to upper motor neurons controlling the lower motor neurons and, ultimately, the muscles of different parts of the body vary in extent with the importance and complexity of the movements of these parts in the habitual activities of the species. Thus the region of the cortex controlling the hand in humans is relatively much larger than that allocated to the whole limb in ungulates. Importantly, the axons of upper motor neurons do not leave the central nervous system and thus do not project directly on muscle fibers but exert their control by excitation or inhibition of lower motor neurons.

The axonal connections between the upper and lower motor neurons follow pathways that vary considerably among species in their relative development and details of organization. The primary distinction, derived from human neuroanatomy, is made between so-called pyramidal and extrapyramidal systems, although the two are coordinated and work in close collaboration. The pyramidal system is mostly concerned with the exercise of finely adjusted movements, whereas the extrapyramidal system is employed in the control of coarser movements, particularly in stereotyped locomotor patterns. It follows that the pyramidal system is better developed in primates than in domestic species, a distinction that explains the different consequences of lesions to the pyramidal pathway. Severe damage to the pyramidal pathway produces a complete and permanent paralysis of the contralateral voluntary musculature in primates, but the effects in domestic species are mainly confined to disturbance of contralateral postural reactions from which partial recovery occurs after a few days. Both pyramidal and extrapyramidal systems are provided with elaborate feedback mechanisms that allow for the continuous monitoring and adjustment of motor activity.

The Pyramidal System

The *pyramidal system* takes origin from upper motor neurons within various regions of the neopallium, particularly the primary motor area. The axons of these neurons converge as they exit the telencephalon and form an important portion of the internal capsule; in their passage they preserve the orderly point-to-point arrangement of the cortical motor representation. They then continue over the lateral aspect of the thalamus to enter the crus cerebri on the ventral surface of the brain (Fig. 8.32/*9*); after traversing the ventral portion of the pons, they reappear on the surface as the pyramids of the medulla oblongata (Fig. 8.19/*17*). Three fiber groups may be distinguished within the system: *corticospinal fibers* continue through the medulla oblongata into the spinal cord; *corticobulbar fibers* peel off at appropriate levels of the brainstem to reach lower motor neurons in motor nuclei of contralateral cranial nerves; and *corticopontine fibers* pass to various nuclei in the pons (Fig. 8.49/*a–c*).

Certain of the corticospinal fibers decussate within the medulla oblongata, and the others continue directly into the cord and decussate only when close to their terminations. The fibers with a medullary decussation form a *lateral corticospinal tract* within the lateral funiculus; those that continue uncrossed constitute a *ventral corticospinal tract* within the ventral funiculus (Fig. 8.18/*3* and *10*). The fibers of both tracts finally project on ventral gray matter motor neurons of the side contralateral to the fibers' origin in the cortex. In domestic species, as in the generality of mammals, a short interneuron is often interposed between the upper and lower motor neuron; in primates, corticospinal fibers synapse directly with lower motor neurons in the spinal cord.

There are other differences among species. In primates and carnivores, pyramidal fibers reach all levels of the cord; in the dog about 50% terminate in cervical segments, 20% in thoracic segments, and 30% in lumbosacrocaudal segments. In contrast, the pyramidal system of ungulates appears to have terminated completely by the level of origin of the brachial plexus (Fig. 8.50), although some corticospinal axons appear to travel the length of the spinal cord within the dorsal funiculus—the route, incidentally, that represents most of the corticospinal system in rodents. The proportion of fibers that decussate within the medulla oblongata also varies: about 50% do so in ungulates, 75% in primates, and all, or almost all, in the dog and cat.

The corticopontine fibers synapse on neurons in the nuclei of the ventral pons (Fig. 8.51/*1*); the axons of these second-order neurons then decussate and pass within the transverse fibers of the pons to enter the cerebellum through the middle cerebellar peduncle. Further successive synapses occur within the cerebellar cortex and then within the deep nuclei of the cerebellum (Fig. 8.51/*8*). From these cerebellar nuclei, axons travel back to the cerebral cortex via a relay through ventral thalamic nuclei (Fig. 8.51/*11*). This arrangement constitutes a pyramidal feedback system.

The Extrapyramidal System

The extrapyramidal motor system encompasses all brain areas involved in regulating motor functions that are not included within the pyramidal system. It is more complicated and involves various multisynaptic pathways that relay within a series of nuclei dispersed through the brain, from the telencephalon to the medulla oblongata. Some of these nuclei are large, grossly visible structures; others are small or diffuse, constituting a descending reticular system within the reticular formation of the brainstem. Tracts originating in the tectum of the midbrain and in the lateral

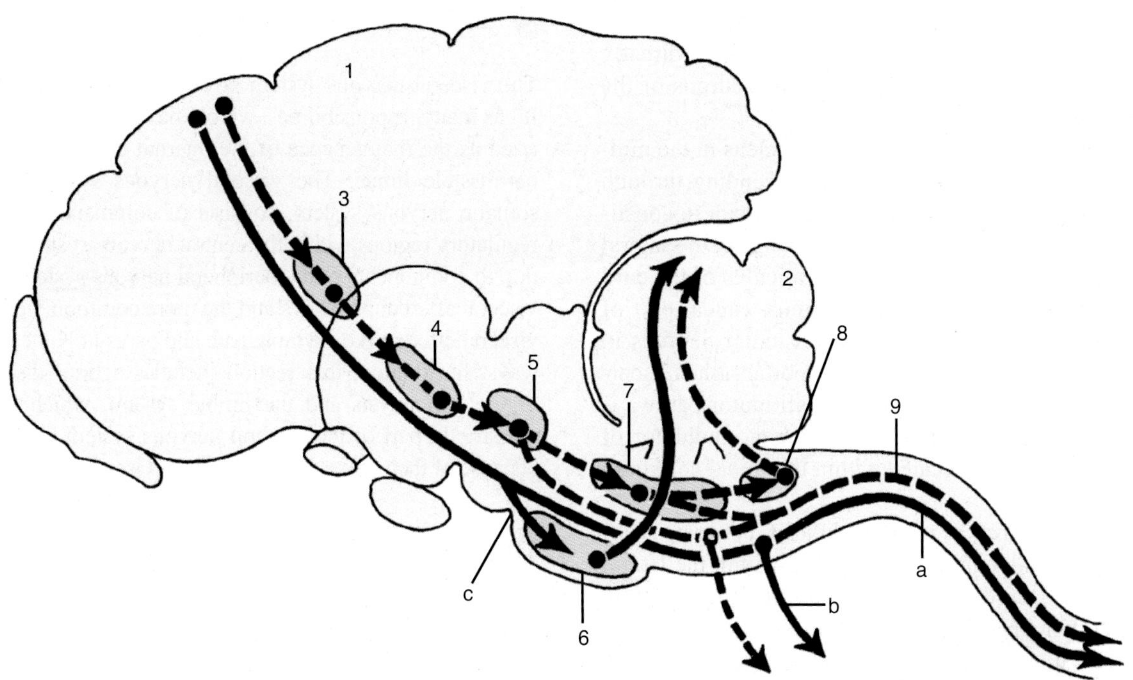

Fig. 8.49 Relay diagram of the pyramidal *(solid lines and arrows)* and the extrapyramidal *(interrupted lines and arrows)* systems. *1*, Motor cortex; *2*, cerebellum; *3*, basal nuclei; *4*, substantia nigra (mesencephalon); *5*, red nucleus (mesencephalon); *6*, pontine nuclei (metencephalon); *7*, reticular formation; *8*, olivary nucleus; *9*, rubrospinal tract; *a*, corticospinal fibers; *b*, corticobulbar fibers; *c*, corticopontine fibers.

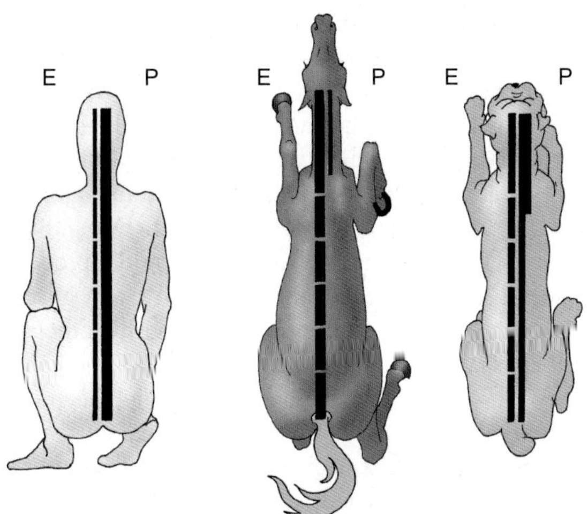

Fig. 8.50 Comparison of the pyramidal *(P)* and extrapyramidal *(E)* systems of the human, horse, and dog. The multisynaptic composition of the extrapyramidal system is indicated by the interruptions in this column; the width of a column is an indication of its relative importance.

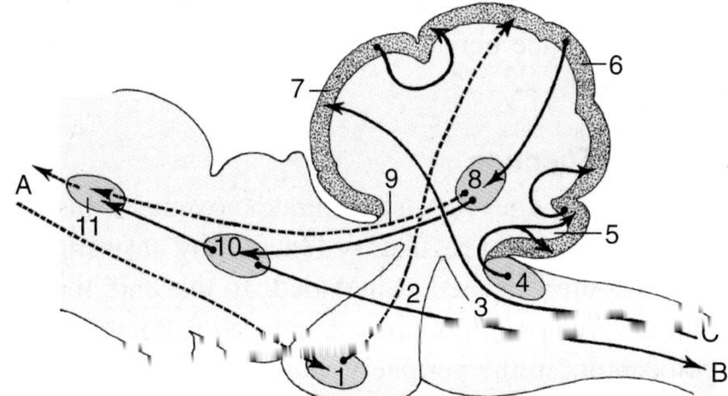

Fig. 8.51 Some important fiber connections of the cerebellum. The connections with the neocortex are represented by *broken lines*. *A*, Tracts to and from the neocortex; *B*, tracts to the motor column of the spinal cord (extrapyramidal); *C*, proprioceptive tracts; *1*, pontine nuclei; *2*, middle cerebellar peduncle; *3*, caudal cerebellar peduncle; *4*, cochlear nuclei; *5*, flocculonodular lobe of the cerebellum; *6*, neocerebellum; *7*, rostral cerebellar lobe; *8*, cerebellar nuclei; *9*, rostral cerebellar peduncle; *10*, red nucleus; *11*, thalamic nuclei.

vestibular nucleus in the medulla are dealt with in the discussion of visual and vestibular pathways (p. 284).

The extrapyramidal system in part originates from regions of the cerebral cortex, including the primary motor area. Activity from these regions is relayed through a series of brain structures referred to collectively as the basal nuclei, which include the caudate nucleus, subthalamic nuclei, and substantia nigra, before returning via the thalamus to the cortex, thus forming a subcortical feedback loop. Other extrapyramidal output from the cortex reaches the red nucleus of the mesencephalon, the reticular formation, and the olive in the medulla oblongata (see Fig. 8.49). Only the red nucleus and the reticular formation contain neurons that project directly (or via interneurons) on the lower motor neurons of the brainstem and spinal cord.

The axons from neurons in the red nucleus in the midbrain decussate immediately before descending through the ventrolateral part of the medulla oblongata to constitute a discrete *rubrospinal tract* bordering on the lateral corticospinal tract within the lateral funiculus of the cord (Fig. 8.18/*4*). This tract reaches the most caudal part of the cord, projecting en route on lower motor neurons in the ventral gray matter. This is an important tract in carnivores and is the best developed of all motor pathways in ungulates (see Fig. 8.50). It serves as a modulator of neural circuits that are located within the spinal cord gray matter.

The reticulospinal system is divided between well-defined dorsal and ventral tracts located within the lateral funiculus and a third (pontine reticulospinal) tract within the ventral funiculus (Fig. 8.18/*II* and *III*).

The activities of the various nuclei and connecting tracts of the extrapyramidal system are closely coordinated and so finely balanced that damage to any part may seriously impair the animal's ability to maintain posture or to execute intended movements. Different parts of the system play different roles: some are facilitatory, others inhibitory, and yet others facilitatory through removal of inhibitory influences. The numerous feedback circuits associated with the extrapyramidal system maintain the necessary balance between these facilitatory and inhibitory influences.

Cerebellar Function

The cerebellum does not itself initiate movement. Instead, it serves an essential regulatory function by ensuring that movements are executed as intended. To this end, the cerebellum receives a continuous stream of information from proprioceptors in the periphery via the subconscious proprioceptive pathways, from the vestibular apparatus via the vestibular nuclei, and from the pyramidal and extrapyramidal motor pathways via relays within the olivary nuclear complex (see Fig. 8.51). Thus, the cerebellum receives information about the current position and movements of the limb segments and of the head (proprioception and vestibular input) as well as information about the motor commands that have been sent to lower motor neurons controlling the limbs and head (pyramidal and extrapyramidal input). The cerebellum compares both inputs and sends any necessary corrective actions back to pyramidal and extrapyramidal circuits. The most important output from the cerebellum runs from the cerebellum to the thalamic nuclei and thence to the motor cortex and basal nuclei; other pathways travel to the contralateral red nuclei, the reticular formation, and the vestibular nuclei (for the coordination of vestibular reflexes).

THE VISCERAL NERVOUS SYSTEM

The visceral nervous system governs the visceral functions. It has many responsibilities, which may be generally summarized as the maintenance of the internal environment within permissible limits. The visceral nervous system, like the somatic nervous system, consists of command centers and regulatory regions within the central nervous system, in addition to components of the peripheral nervous system, such as visceral afferent pathways and the more commonly discussed visceral efferent (i.e., sympathetic and parasympathetic) pathways. In addition, this section includes a brief discussions of the hypophysis and the limbic system, which although not strictly part of the visceral nervous system are included because of their close association with visceral function.

The Hypothalamus

The hypothalamus is an important integration center for many visceral, endocrine, and behavioral functions, all of which work to keep the animal alive. These functions include the control of biologic rhythms, appetite, water balance, body temperature, cardiovascular performance, sexual behavior and activity, sleep, and emotion. The hypothalamus must receive and coordinate information from most other parts of the nervous system, including visceral information as well as ostensibly somatic information. Information on the somatic activities is relayed via the thalamic nuclei to which the somatic afferent pathways lead. Information concerning visceral function is received from mesencephalic nuclei and the medullary reticular formation. For example, the nucleus of the solitary tract in the medulla is the principal visceral sensory nucleus that receives topographically organized input from major organ systems by way of the glossopharyngeus (IX) and vagus (X) nerves. This nucleus is the region of initial processing of visceral, cardiovascular and respiratory, and gustatory information, which it then projects to the hypothalamus. A further very important contribution to the hypothalamus comes from the telencephalon, specifically the prefrontal cortex, and especially from the hippocampus, via the fornix. This arrangement enables emotional inputs to be related to and coordinated with the visceral and somatic information. Hypothalamic input from peripheral organ systems is also possible by way of blood-borne signals.

The hypothalamus regulates activity through both neural and endocrine mechanisms, sometimes in combination. Axonal pathways from the hypothalamus extend to the brainstem and spinal cord by direct routes or by multisynaptic pathways within the reticular formation, in which final integration takes place. Hypothalamic regions that exert control over visceral efferent neurons—namely, preganglionic sympathetic and parasympathetic neurons (see later)—are anatomically distinct, in that caudal hypothalamic regions control sympathetic functions whereas more cranial regions exert control over parasympathetic functions. Other hypothalamic projections provide a feedback to the forebrain routed through rostral thalamic nuclei.

The endocrine pathways operate through neurosecretory cells whose products either may enter the bloodstream directly for general distribution or may be conveyed specifically to the hypophysis by means of a system of portal vessels (see Fig. 6.3).

Anatomically, the hypothalamus is largely concealed, and only the caudal parts—namely, the tuber cinereum and mammillary bodies—are exposed on the ventral surface of the brain (Figs. 8.19/*9* and *11* and 8.21/*20* and *23*).

The Hypophysis

The hypophysis (pituitary gland; Figs. 8.21 and 8.52), which is attached to the hypothalamus by the infundibulum, has two parts. One, the neurohypophysis (or posterior lobe), is an outgrowth of the brain itself; the other, the adenohypophysis, develops from oral ectoderm (p. 203) and consists of anterior and intermediate lobes. Interspecific differences in the topographic interrelationship of the lobes are not of present concern (see Fig. 6.2).

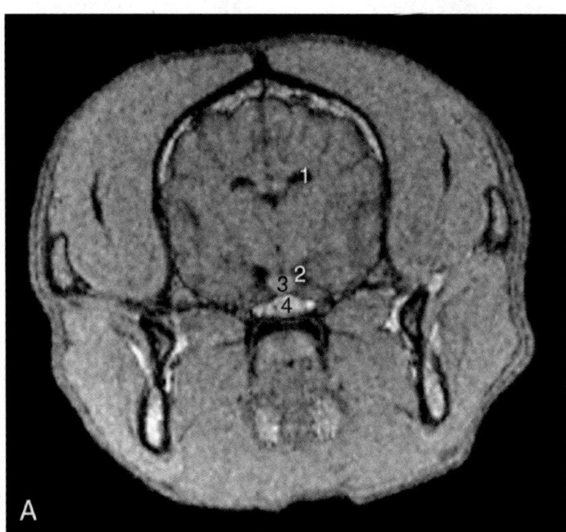

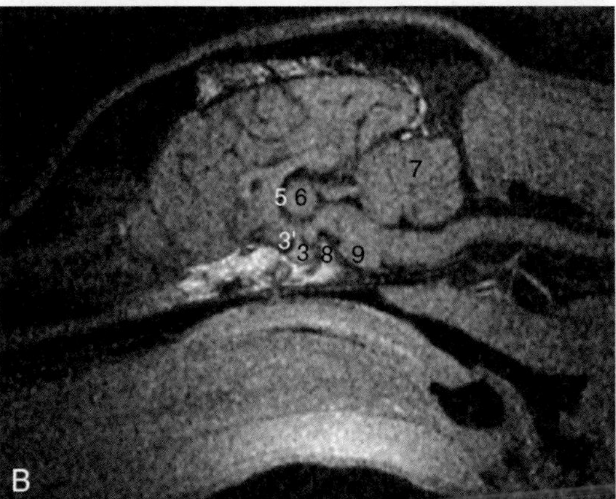

Fig. 8.52 (A) Transverse image at the level of the pituitary fossa and (B) median image of 1-mm-thick T1-weighted gradient-echo magnetic resonance slices of the canine head. *1*, Lateral ventricle; *2*, basal cistern; *3*, pituitary gland; *3′*, infundibulum; *4*, fat in sphenoid bone; *5*, third ventricle; *6*, interthalamic adhesion; *7*, cerebellum; *8*, dorsum sellae; *9*, pons.

The three lobes produce or store several hormones (p. 204). The posterior lobe hormones (vasopressin and oxytocin) are produced by neurosecretory cells within the supraoptic and paraventricular nuclei of the hypothalamus and are conveyed along the axons for direct release into the neurohypophysial capillary bed (see Fig. 6.3).

Visceral Afferent Pathways

There are both general and special visceral afferent pathways. Special visceral afferent pathways are concerned with taste and smell and are discussed later. The receptors of the general visceral afferent pathway are located within viscera and blood vessels; most of these receptors are mechanoreceptors responsive to pressure, stretch, and, less commonly, flow, although a minority are chemoreceptors responsive to the carbon dioxide content of the blood. The axons that convey impulses from these receptors travel within peripheral nerves and may travel alongside other axons of visceral or somatic origin. The cell bodies of primary sensory neurons carrying visceral afferent information are located within the dorsal root ganglia of all spinal nerves (and the equivalent ganglia of certain cranial nerves) alongside those transmitting somatic afferent information; the axons from these cell bodies project on interneurons and projection neurons within the visceral afferent column of the spinal cord and brainstem (Fig. 8.12/*2*).

Within the central nervous system, short chains of interneurons provide for simple local visceral reflexes that utilize visceral efferent pathways, discussed in the next section, and thus have their last two relays within the visceral efferent column and the peripheral autonomic ganglia. Visceral afferent information also reaches the brain via projection neurons that form ascending pathways that follow somatic systems, both lemniscal and extralemniscal, to end, like the somatic afferent system, within nuclei of the ventrocaudal thalamus. A final projection to the cortex may give rise to conscious perception of visceral sensation, although most visceral activity goes unnoticed. (The sense of fullness arising from digestive organs or the bladder is among the visceral activities of which awareness is most common.) Pronounced contraction and serious overdistention of visceral organs may be perceived as pain. Pain of visceral origin may be "referred" to the surface of the body, presumably as a consequence of the convergence of the cutaneous somatic and visceral afferent pathways on the same neurons at some point along their course.

The special visceral afferent pathway concerned with taste follows a similar route to that taken by the general visceral sensory modalities. The axons course from the taste buds in the oral cavity within the facial, glossopharyngeal, and vagus nerves and terminate in the nucleus of the solitary tract. The more complicated olfactory pathways are described elsewhere (see Fig. 8.40).

Visceral Efferent Pathways

Unlike the afferent component, the efferent component of the visceral nervous system, sometime referred to as the *autonomic nervous system,* is arranged in two divisions, sympathetic and parasympathetic, distinguished by morphology, pharmacology, and physiology. The final conducting pathway of both divisions, unlike that of the somatic system, consists of two motor neurons in succession: the first has its cell body, or perikaryon, within the central nervous system, and the second is located within a peripheral ganglion (Fig. 8.53). The two successive motor neurons are most frequently distinguished as the preganglionic and the postganglionic neurons and together are equivalent to the lower motor neuron of the somatic system.

The parasympathetic and the sympathetic divisions of the autonomic nervous system are distinguished anatomically by the nonoverlapping distribution of the preganglionic neurons within the central nervous system. The cell bodies of the preganglionic neurons of the sympathetic division are located within the lateral (visceral efferent) column of the spinal cord gray matter, between the first thoracic and middle lumbar segments (with some interspecific variation) (see Fig. 8.75). The cell bodies of the sympathetic postganglionic neurons are found in paravertebral ganglia of the sympathetic chain or in the subvertebral ganglia on the aorta; both groups are relatively close to the spinal cord.

The cell bodies of the parasympathetic preganglionic neurons are restricted to the brainstem; to the nuclei of the oculomotor, facial, glossopharyngeal, and vagus nerves; or to the lateral gray matter columns of the sacral segments of the cord (see Fig. 8.74). The cell bodies of parasympathetic postganglionic neurons are located within small ganglia in close proximity to or actually incorporated within the walls of the organs they supply.

The neurotransmitter released onto visceral smooth muscle by postganglionic sympathetic neurons is norepinephrine and that by postganglionic parasympathetic neurons is acetylcholine; both are released with a host of neuropeptides. The two divisions therefore react differently to autonomic agonist and antagonist drugs.

In spite of the nonoverlapping arrangement of sympathetic and parasympathetic preganglionic neurons, the two systems have broadly similar distributions with respect to visceral organ innervation and are frequently described as antagonist: one inhibits while the other stimulates a particular activity. This rule is less absolute than was once supposed, and their roles are better regarded as collaborative. The more diffuse anatomy of the peripheral sympathetic nerves (which are described later) and the use of norepinephrine as a transmitter indicate the more general effects produced by sympathetic activity, in contrast to those of parasympathetic activity, which are often local, affecting single specific functions.

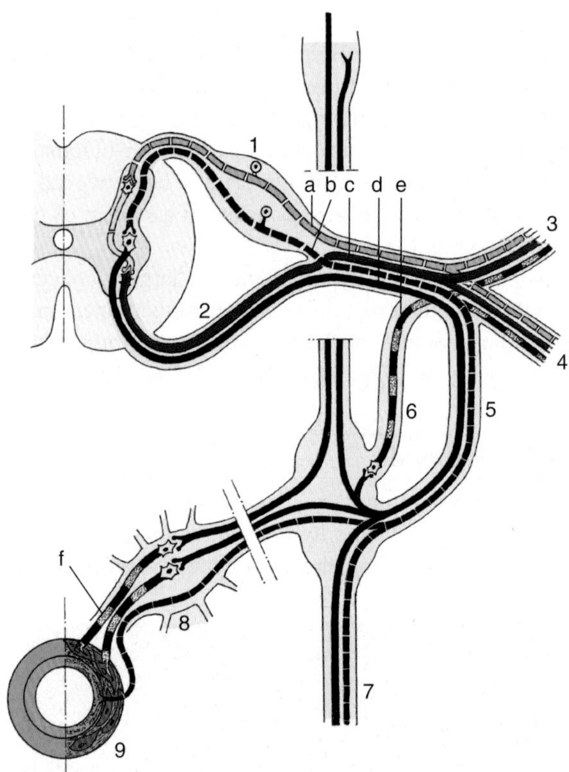

Fig. 8.53 Comparison of the organization of the visceral *(black)* and the somatic *(red)* nervous systems at the thoracolumbar level of the spinal cord. Afferent fibers are indicated by *interrupted lines*, efferent fibers by *solid lines*. The postganglionic sympathetic fibers are indicated by *alternating black and stippled lines*. *1*, Dorsal root ganglion; *2*, ventral root; *3*, dorsal branch of spinal nerve; *4*, ventral branch of spinal nerve; *5 and 6*, white (preganglionic) and gray (postganglionic) communicating branches, often fused; *7*, sympathetic trunk with ganglia; *8*, prevertebral ganglion; *9*, gut; *a*, somatic afferent fibers; *b*, visceral afferent fibers; *c*, somatic efferent fibers; *d*, visceral efferent fibers (preganglionic sympathetic); *e*, postganglionic sympathetic (to peripheral structures); *f*, postganglionic sympathetic (to abdominal organs).

The Limbic System

The limbic system is a series of forebrain structures that control somatic and visceral behavior associated with strong emotions, such as rage and fear. Anatomically, the limbic system has a complex organization and is composed of the limbic cortex and many subcortical nuclei. The cortical part of the limbic system forms a ring at the medial surface of the cerebral hemisphere, including, among other structures, the cingulate and supracallosal gyri, the piriform lobe, and the hippocampus. The subcortical part is composed of the hypothalamus, septal area, amygdala, habenular nuclei, and dorsal part of the mesencephalic tegmentum. There are numerous associations between these structures and other regions of the brain. The limbic system is often considered to be primarily a "visceral brain" because many of its major functions are expressed through visceral motor activity. The types of behaviors most influenced by the limbic system are those essential for the preservation of the individual or the species.

Olfactory inputs that relay through the piriform lobes may influence many structures of the system. Of all the sensory inputs, olfaction exhibits the most profound effects on visceral motor activities that are associated with emotional behavior such as eating, rage, sexual activity, fear, and drinking. The limbic system also receives optic, auditory, exteroceptive, and enteroceptive stimuli.

The efferent pathways from the cortical limbic regions involve nearly all the subcortical nuclei of the system. A major portion of the influences of the limbic cortex is mediated through the efferent systems of the amygdaloid nuclei. Electrical stimulation of the amygdala produces a wide variety of visceral and somatic reactions and many behavioral reactions, such as aggression and anxiety.

The hippocampus is concerned with memory functions, such as the processing of recently acquired memory and its more permanent consolidation. The hypothalamus also plays an essential part in the limbic system's control of emotional expression and behavior through its integration of autonomic, endocrine, and somatic functions.

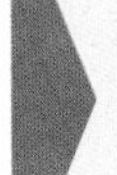

THE TOPOGRAPHY, ENVIRONMENT, AND VASCULARIZATION OF THE BRAIN AND SPINAL CORD

Topography

The brain and spinal cord are contained within a continuous space provided by the cranial cavity of the skull and the vertebral canal, which is formed by successive bony rings and connecting ligaments and disks of the vertebral column.

The *cranial cavity* lies directly behind the nasal cavities. It is smaller than is commonly supposed, the form and extent of the cranial cavity not easily being predicted from the external appearance of the head and skull because the paranasal sinuses, horns, muscular ridges, and other projections of the skull, as well as the temporal muscles, all contribute significantly to the conformation of this part of the head. The closest agreement between the external contours and the cavity within the cranium is found in the newborn of all species; among adults, this agreement is best retained in cats and in dogs of brachycephalic breeds. Fortunately, the exact location of the brain is rarely of practical significance except in humane slaughter techniques mentioned in later chapters. It is probably sufficient to know that the caudal limit of the cavity extends to the caudal wall of the skull—thickened by the frontal sinus in cattle—but that the rostral limit shows considerable variation; in dogs and cats, the rostral limit of the cranial cavity is associated with the caudal margin of the zygomatic processes of the frontal bones and in horses and cattle with the rostral level of these processes. In pigs and small ruminants, the rostral limit of the cranial cavity extends to the middle of the orbit.

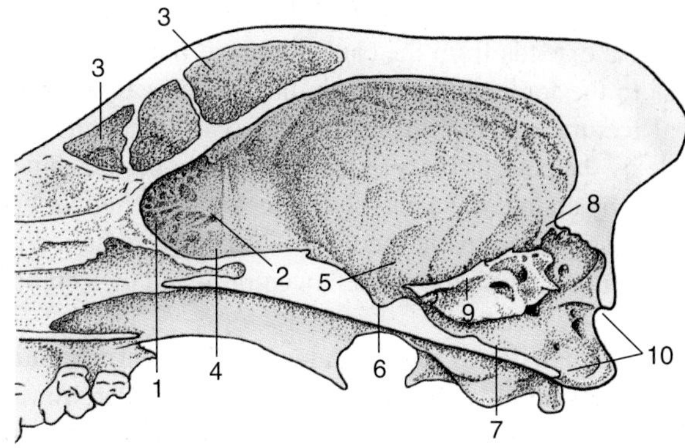

Fig. 8.54 Sagittal section of the cranium of the dog. *1*, Cribriform plate; *2*, ethmoid foramen; *3*, frontal sinus; *4*, rostral fossa; *5*, middle fossa; *6*, hypophysial fossa; *7*, caudal fossa; *8*, tentorium cerebelli osseum; *9*, petrosal crest; *10*, foramen magnum.

The interior of the cranial cavity shows a fairly close correspondence with the contours of the brain, although significant intracranial space is required for the meninges and intermeningeal spaces that surround the brain and for the capacious intracranial venous sinuses. Although the roof (calvaria) of the cavity remains largely undivided, the base is divided into three fossae; these need not be described in detail because the main features are depicted in Fig. 8.54. The rostral fossa is formed by the sphenoid and ethmoid bones and extends to the level of the optic canals, the passages of exit of the optic nerves. The rostral fossa contains the olfactory bulbs embedded within recesses of the cribriform plate (Fig. 8.54/*1*) and the rostral parts of the cerebral hemispheres. The middle fossa extends from the optic canals to the sharp petrosal crests (Fig. 8.54/*9*) that project inward from the petrous temporal bones of the lateral walls. The floor of the middle fossa is formed by the sphenoid bone, which carries the median hypophysial fossa (sella turcica) into which the hypophysis fits; it also contains various foramina—the orbital fissure and the round and oval foramina—that were encountered in the previous description of the skull (p. 54). This middle fossa, the widest part of the cranial cavity, contains the temporal and parietal lobes of the cerebral hemispheres. The caudal fossa extends from the caudal limit of the hypophysial fossa to the foramen magnum in the caudal wall. Its principal features are the invaginations from the lateral walls made by the petrous parts of the temporal bones (each perforated by an internal acoustic meatus) and the jugular and hypoglossal foramina in the floor. The caudal fossa lodges the midbrain, pons, and medulla ventrally and the cerebellum dorsally.

The caudal, dorsal, and lateral walls of the entire cranial cavity are smoothly joined together. The most prominent internal feature of the cranial cavity is the tentorium cerebelli osseum (Fig. 8.54/*8*), a large projection at the junction of the dorsal and caudal walls forming the middle portion of the tentorium cerebelli within the transverse fissure of the brain. The tentorium contains passages for branches of the dorsal intracranial venous sinuses.

The *vertebral canal* is widest within the atlas cranially and tapers rapidly within the sacrum caudally; between the two extremes, it is most expanded where it contains the cervical and lumbar enlargements of the spinal cord, from which arise the nerves that form the forelimb and hindlimb plexuses, respectively (see Fig. 8.15). The topography of the spinal cord is of considerable importance in veterinary practice because injections into the canal are frequently made, particularly injections of local anesthetic, with the intention of blocking specific spinal nerves; in addition, there is sometimes a need to locate central nervous lesions to specific vertebral levels, a procedure made possible by the association of specific sensory and motor deficits with particular spinal segments.

Even with the inclusion of its meningeal wrappings, the spinal cord is considerably smaller than the vertebral canal (Fig. 8.55). It is also considerably shorter in craniocaudal length. This discrepancy is due to the unequal growth between the spinal cord and vertebral column, which begins well before birth and continues after. The relative shift in position (ascensus medullae) results in the more cranial location of spinal cord segments in comparison with their original corresponding vertebrae. This shift is most pronounced in more caudally located segments and explains the position of the tapered end of the spinal cord (*conus medullaris*) in the lumbar or sacral region of the vertebral column. The level at which the cord ends varies among species (and, in early life, with age); it is within L5 or L6 in the pig, L6 in ruminants, L6 or L7 in the dog, S2 in the horse, and rather variably between L6 and S3 in the cat (Fig. 8.56).

The cranial shift in position of the more caudally located segments also explains the peculiar arrangement of the associated spinal nerves. The spinal nerves associated

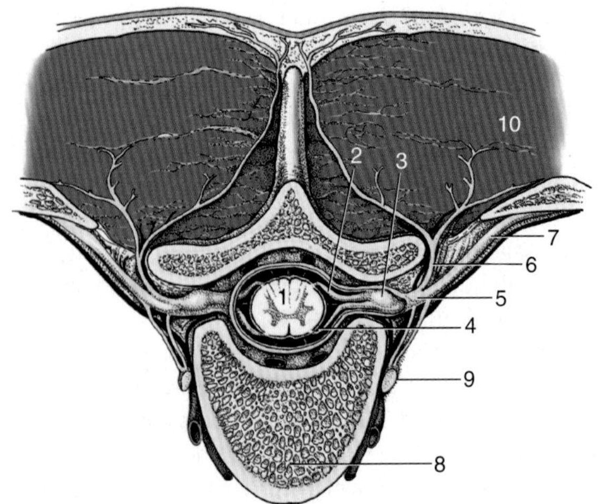

Fig. 8.55 Transection of the vertebral column to show the formation of a spinal nerve. *1*, Spinal cord; *2*, dorsal root; *3*, spinal ganglion; *4*, ventral root; *5*, spinal nerve; *6*, dorsal branch of spinal nerve; *7*, ventral branch of spinal nerve; *8*, body of vertebra; *9*, sympathetic trunk; *10*, epaxial muscles.

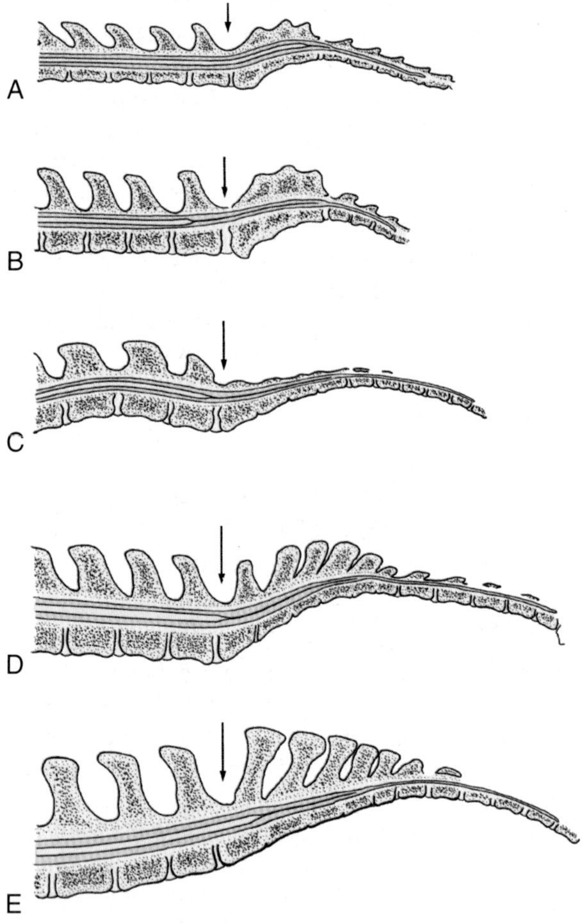

Fig. 8.56 Median section of the vertebral canal and spinal cord of (A) cat, (B) dog, (C) pig, (D) cattle, and (E) horse. The lumbosacral interarcuate space is indicated by an *arrow*. Notice the difference in caudal extent of the spinal cord in the different species. The thin extension of the spinal cord is the filum terminale that ends on the caudal vertebrae (not shown).

with the lumbar and sacral spinal segments travel caudally within the vertebral canal to reach their corresponding vertebrae to exit the canal. This collection of caudally directed spinal nerves on each side of the conus medullaris is known as the cauda equina because of its superficial resemblance to a horse's tail (see Fig. 12.9/*9*).

The Meninges and Fluid Environment

The brain and spinal cord are surrounded by three continuous membranes or meninges composed of connective tissue that exhibit important topographic differences in their cranial and vertebral parts.

The tough outermost membrane, the *dura mater,* is fused with the inner periosteum of the skull bones; it splits from this within the margin of the foramen magnum to form a free tube of connective tissue separated from the wall of the vertebral canal by a distinct epidural space. The *epidural space* is occupied by fat, more fluid in life than in the postmortem specimen, and by the internal vertebral venous plexus; the fat and vessels together cushion the spinal cord and allow it to adjust to the movements of the neck and back (see Fig. 8.55). The dural tube is attached at its caudal end, where the several meninges finally combine in a fibrous strand (filum terminale) that fuses with the upper surface of the caudal vertebrae.

The fusion of the cranial dura with the periosteum obliterates the epidural space within the skull, and the cranial venous sinuses thus come to be enclosed within the thickness of the combined periosteum and dura. In addition to lining the cavity, the cranial dura forms certain folds that project inward and limit movements of the brain; these are a considerable hindrance to the removal of the intact brain at autopsy. One, the *falx cerebri,* extends ventrally from the dorsal and rostral cranial walls and serves to separate the two cerebral hemispheres; caudally the falx cerebri joins a second, transverse fold, the *membranous tentorium cerebelli,* which separates the cerebellum from the cerebrum (Fig. 8.57/*7*). The tentorium is ossified in its median part. A third specialization of the dura surrounds the dorsal aspect of the hypophysial fossa in which the hypophysis is seated, forming a diaphragm around the infundibular stalk.

A capillary space, the *subdural space,* divides the dura from the *arachnoid,* the first of the two more delicate inner meningeal membranes. This subdural space normally contains only a minute amount of a clear lymphlike fluid but may be enlarged by effusion of blood after an injury. The subdural space of the spinal cord is crossed by a bilateral series of triangular (*denticulate*) ligaments, each of which alternates with the origins of the spinal nerves; they attach the inner meninges to the dural tube and thus indirectly suspend the spinal cord within the dura along its craniocaudal length (Fig. 8.58/*4*). The outer part of the arachnoid forms a continuous membrane molded against the dural tube. The inner part of the arachnoid is composed of numerous fine trabeculae and filaments (imaginatively compared to a spider's web, hence the name *arachnoid*), which join the innermost meningeal membrane, the *pia mater.*

The *pia mater* covers the surface of the brain and spinal cord and follows every change in their contours. The pia mater is firmly attached to the outer surface of the brain and cord, and branches from arteries traveling within the pia penetrate the brain and spinal cord substance. These vessels are initially enclosed by pial sleeves, but as the vessels continue into the brain and spinal cord substance, the connective tissue of the pia soon merges with the vascular walls. In the spinal cord, a thickening of the pia fills the ventral fissure of the cord, where it appears as a glittering silver line.

All three meninges form cuffs around the roots of origin of the cranial and spinal nerves.

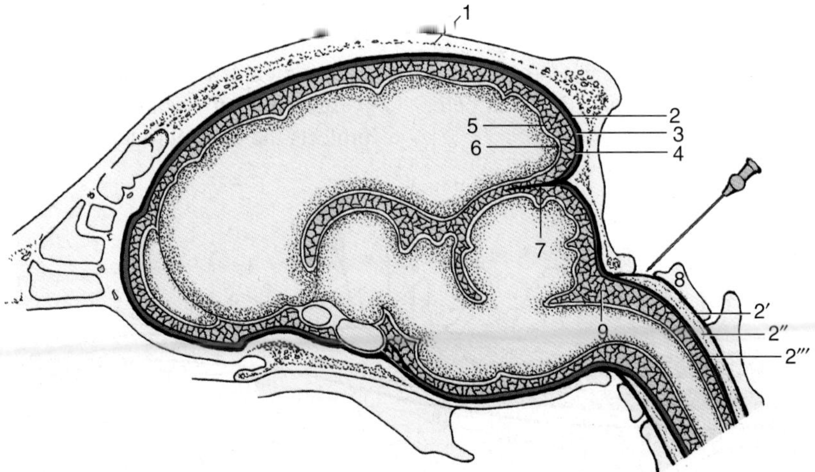

Fig. 8.57 Schematic representation of the meninges of the brain. The needle points to the atlanto-occipital space and the cerebellomedullary cistern. *1,* Calvaria; *2,* dura mater (also connected to the bone as periosteum); *2′,* periosteum of vertebral canal; *2″,* epidural space (with fat); *2‴,* dura mater of spinal cord; *3,* subdural space; *4,* arachnoid; *5,* arachnoid space; *6,* pia mater; *7,* membranous tentorium cerebelli; *8,* atlas; *9,* cerebellomedullary cistern.

The *subarachnoid space* exists as the space between the pia and outer part of the arachnoid, traversed by the arachnoid trabeculae. The space containing the clear, watery cerebrospinal fluid is much wider than the subdural space but less uniform, particularly in its cranial part (see Fig. 8.57).

The widest parts ("cisterns") of the cranial *subarachnoid space* are located ventrally between the more prominent parts of the ventral surface of the brain and dorsally in the angle between the cerebellum and the dorsal aspect of the medulla. The dorsal widening, the *cerebellomedullary cistern,* is especially large and may be accessed in the living animal by a needle passed between the atlas and the skull through the foramen magnum (see Fig. 8.57). Cisternal puncture is employed in both clinical and experimental work for obtaining samples of cerebrospinal fluid. The spinal subarachnoid space is fairly uniform but widens around the conus medullaris, a fortunate circumstance because the subarachnoid space in the vertebral canal is accessed most easily by a dorsal route through the lumbosacral intervertebral space (Fig. 8.59).

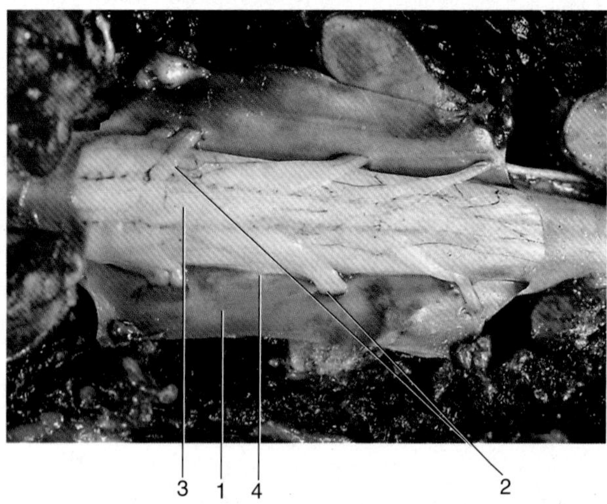

Fig. 8.58 Dorsal view of the opened vertebral canal. The dura mater has been dissected and is reflected. *1,* Dura mater; *2,* dorsal rootlets of a spinal nerve; *3,* spinal cord (covered by pia mater); *4,* denticulate ligament.

The cerebrospinal fluid within the subarachnoid space forms a water jacket that buoys up and protects the soft brain and cord. It is largely a product of the ependymal lining of the ventricular system within the brain, and most of the cerebrospinal fluid is produced at the *choroid plexuses.* The choroid plexuses are tufts of capillaries covered with ependyma that invaginate into the ventricles at specific locations throughout the brain (Fig. 8.60/*6* and *9*). An additional contribution to cerebrospinal fluid is made by the pial vessels.

The ventricles are the adult derivative of the lumen of the embryonic neural tube; the ventricles have complicated shapes, but because they are illustrated (Fig. 8.61) and the details have little veterinary significance, they need not be described. It is more important to understand their relationship to the choroid plexuses. The plexuses of each of the two lateral ventricles and of the third ventricle, which merge within the interventricular foramen, develop within a fold of pia that becomes entrapped between the expanding telencephalic vesicles and the roof of the diencephalon (Fig. 8.62). The plexuses of the fourth ventricle develop separately within the pia over the caudal medullary velum. In the course of development, these plexuses invaginate into the lumen of the fourth ventricle; parts later reemerge into the arachnoid space by herniating through paired lateral openings in the roof (Fig. 8.63).

The clear colorless *cerebrospinal fluid* is formed from the blood plasma by ultrafiltration through the "blood–cerebrospinal fluid barrier" at the choroid plexuses. Ependymal cells of the choroid plexuses are joined together with tight junctions, thus forcing any substances other than water or small lipophilic molecules to be transported through the cells to reach the ventricles. The fluid has a higher concentration of potassium and calcium ions and a lower concentration of sodium, magnesium, and chloride ions than the plasma; it is also rather deficient in glucose and, most important, contains little protein because the barrier is impermeable to larger molecules, which of course include those of many antibiotics and other drugs.

In addition to its mechanical role, the cerebrospinal fluid protects the brain through its chemical buffering capacity,

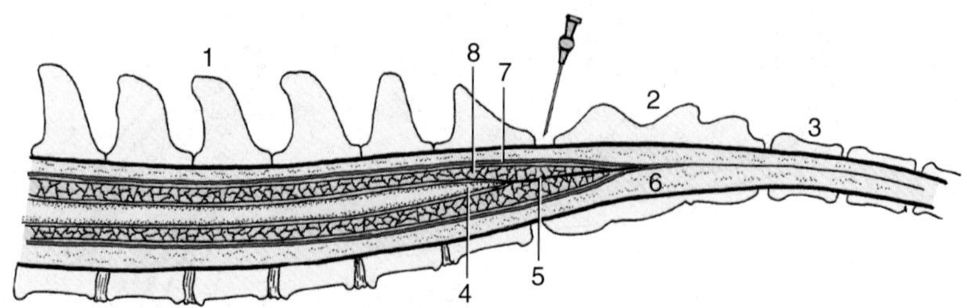

Fig. 8.59 Schematic median section of the vertebral canal and its contents. The needle points to the lumbosacral interarcuate space. *1,* Lumbar vertebra; *2,* sacrum; *3,* caudal vertebra; *4,* conus medullaris; *5,* filum terminale; *6,* epidural space; *7,* dura mater; *8,* arachnoid space with cerebrospinal fluid.

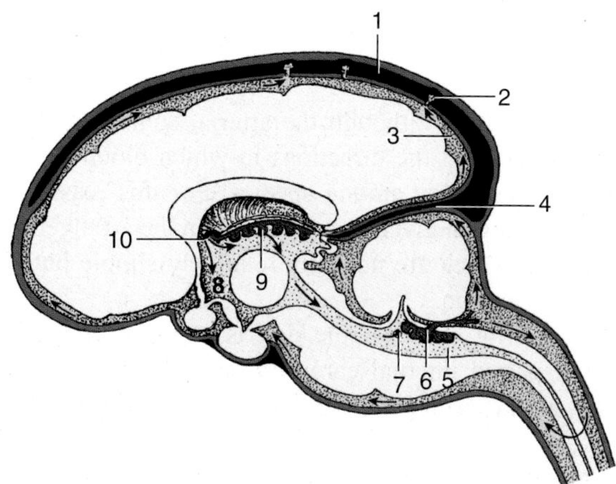

Fig. 8.60 The production and circulation of cerebrospinal fluid (sagittal section). The blood vessels are shown in *black*, the choroid plexuses are red, the subarachnoid spaces are *stippled blue*, the ventricles are *stippled yellow*, and the nervous tissue is *solid yellow*. The direction of the flow of the cerebrospinal fluid is indicated by *arrows*. The cerebrospinal fluid is secreted by the choroid plexuses *(6, 9)* of the lateral, third, and fourth ventricles. It escapes into the subarachnoid space via the aperture of the fourth ventricle *(7)*. The cerebrospinal fluid is transferred to the systemic circulation *(1)* at the arachnoid villi *(2)*. *1*, Dorsal sagittal sinus; *2*, subarachnoid space; *3*, membranous tentorium cerebelli; *4*, fourth ventricle; *5*, choroid plexus of fourth ventricle; *6*, aperture of fourth ventricle; *7*, third ventricle; *8*, choroid plexus of third ventricle; *9*, interventricular foramen, connecting the lateral and third ventricles.

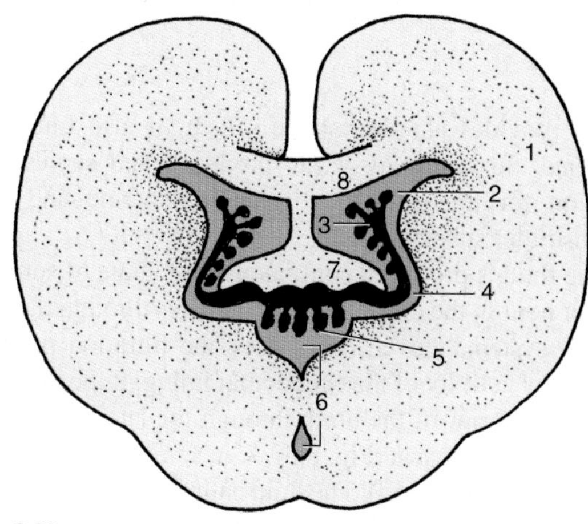

Fig. 8.62 Schematic section of the brain illustrating the interrelations of the third and lateral ventricles and their choroid plexuses. *1*, Cerebral hemisphere; *2*, lateral ventricle; *3*, choroid plexus of lateral ventricle; *4*,interventricular foramen; *5*, choroid plexus of third ventricle; *6*, third ventricle; *7*, fornix; *8*, corpus callosum.

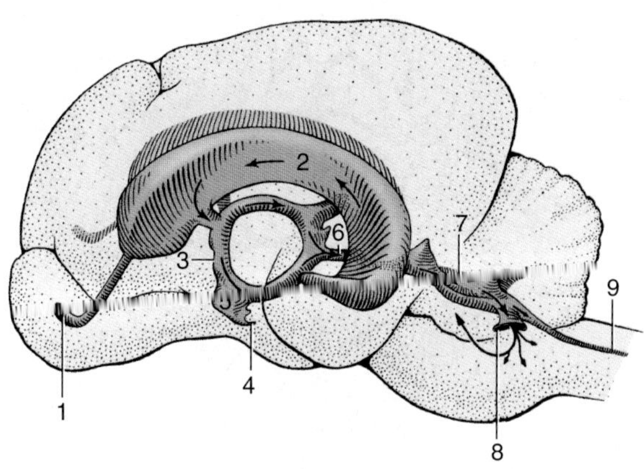

Fig. 8.61 Lateral view of a cast of the ventricles of the brain of the dog. *1*, Cavity of olfactory bulb; *2*, lateral ventricle; *3*, third ventricle; *4*, infundibular recess; *5*, optic recess; *6*, mesencephalic aqueduct; *7*, fourth ventricle; *8*, lateral recess; *9*, central canal.

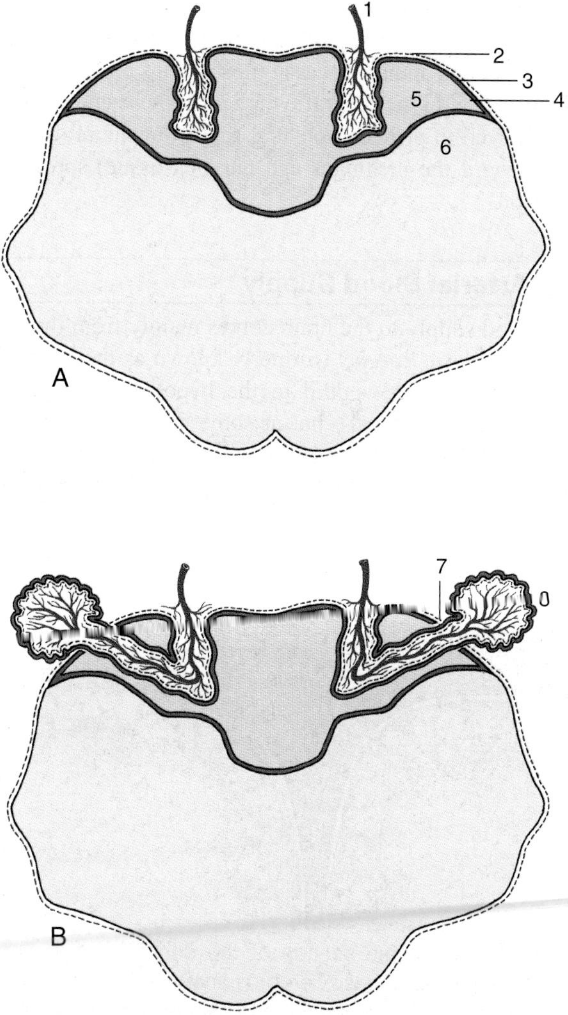

Fig. 8.63 (A) The formation of the choroid plexus in the roof of the fourth ventricle and (B) its later extension into the subarachnoid space. *1*, Blood vessel invagination; *2*, pia mater; *3*, caudal medullary velum; *4*, ependyma; *5*, fourth ventricle; *6*, myelencephalon; *7*, aperture of fourth ventricle; *8*, choroid plexus extending into subarachnoid space.

which provides a rather stable milieu. It also transports nutrients, flushes away waste products, and serves as a medium for the diffusion of neuroendocrine and neurotransmitter substances.

The fluid is produced continuously, at a rate of some 30 mL per hour in the dog, and first circulates through the ventricular system, moved onward by the filtration pressure and ciliary activity of the ependymal lining. It then escapes from the interior of the brain through the lateral apertures of the fourth ventricle (Fig. 8.60/*7;* in some species there is a third median opening). The fluid bathes the brain and cord before returning to the blood, mostly through the arachnoid villi (Fig. 8.64/*10*), which are projections of the arachnoid and subarachnoid space that pierce the dura to enter the dorsal sagittal venous sinus of the brain; these formations become increasingly prominent with age. (Obliteration of the villi results in hydrocephalus because drainage of the fluid is hampered while its production continues and is not influenced by a feedback mechanism.) A smaller part of the fluid percolates along the meningeal cuffs that surround the cranial and spinal nerves at their origins and is eventually absorbed by perineural lymphatics; these connections are believed to provide potential routes for the retrograde (i.e., toward the meninges and nervous tissue) spread of infection.

The Arterial Blood Supply

The blood supply to the brain comes mainly from the *circulus arteriosus cerebri* (formerly known as the circle of Willis), which lies ventral to the hypothalamus, where it forms a ring around—but at some distance from—the infundibular stalk. The appearance of the circle and the pattern of its major branches are remarkably constant among mammals, although the arterial sources that supply the circle and the directions in which blood flows in certain vessels vary among species. For this reason, the initial description given here is based on the arrangements in the dog, which are not only relatively simple but also the most common.

The arterial circle of the dog is supplied from three sources: paired internal carotid arteries laterally and the basilar artery caudally (Fig. 8.65). The *internal carotid artery* (Fig. 8.65/*5*) arises as a terminal branch of the common carotid at the level of the pharynx. The internal carotid then travels toward the base of the skull. In many species the artery makes immediate entry to the cranial cavity through a carotid foramen in the cranial floor, but in the dog it must first traverse a tunnel (*carotid canal*) in the bone medial to the tympanic bulla. The artery leaves the rostral end of the tunnel and forms a loop that first carries

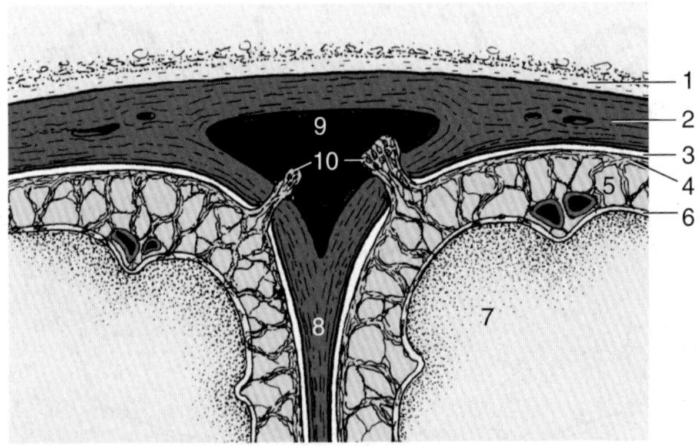

Fig. 8.64 Transverse section of the dorsal sagittal sinus and adjacent meninges. Cerebrospinal fluid is transferred from the subarachnoid space to the sinus via the arachnoid granulations (villi). *1,* Roof of cranial cavity; *2,* fused dura mater and periosteum; *3,* subdural space; *4,* arachnoid; *5,* subarachnoid space; *6,* pia mater; *7,* cerebral hemisphere; *8,* falx cerebri; *9,* dorsal sagittal sinus; *10,* arachnoid granulations (villi).

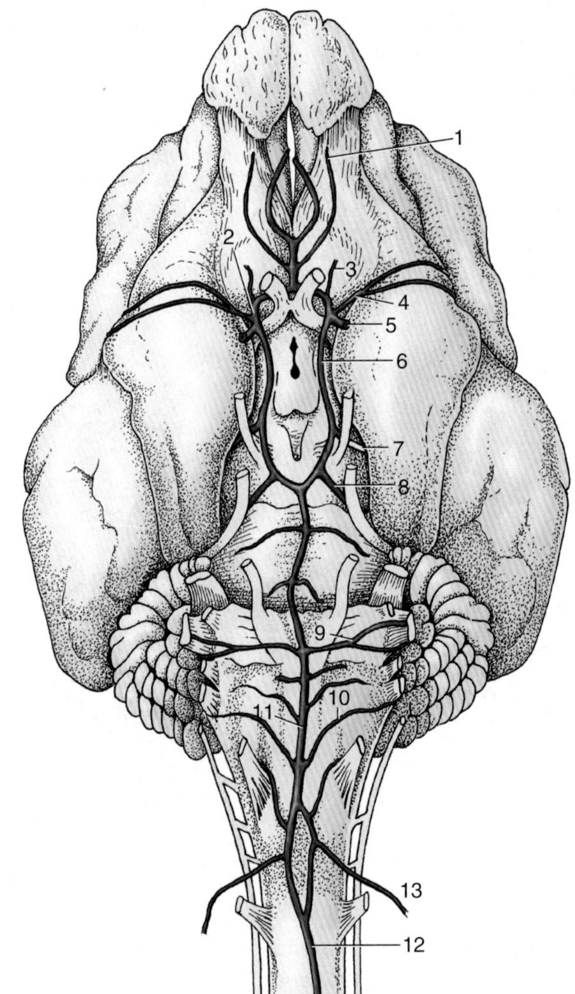

Fig. 8.65 Arteries on the ventral surface of the canine brain. *1,* Internal ethmoidal artery (a.); *2,* rostral cerebral a.; *3,* internal ophthalmic a., *4,* middle cerebral a.; *5,* internal carotid a.; *6,* caudal communicating a.; *7,* caudal cerebral a.; *8,* rostral cerebellar a.; *9,* labyrinthine a.; *10,* caudal cerebellar a; *11,* basilar a.; *12,* ventral spinal a.; *13,* vertebral a.

it ventrally, then dorsally, before it finally enters the cranial cavity. It then penetrates the outer meninges, a process that involves passage through the cavernous venous sinus enclosed within the dura, before dividing into rostral and caudal branches. The rostral branch of right and left internal carotid arteries unite across the midline to complete the rostral half of the circle. From this rostral portion, both the rostral and middle cerebral arteries arise. The caudal branch of each internal carotid artery anastomoses with the *caudal communicating artery,* a branch of the *basilar artery* (Fig. 8.65/*6*). The basilar artery originates farther caudally as single artery (Fig. 8.65/*11* and see later) but divides into right and left branches at the level of the midbrain before each branch joins the internal carotid arteries to complete the circle. The caudal cerebral and rostral cerebellar arteries leave the caudal half of the circle; the fifth major artery to the brain, the caudal cerebellar, leaves the single basilar artery directly (Fig. 8.65/*10*).

The blood within the basilar artery has a composite origin. The artery appears to be the direct continuation of the small ventral spinal artery but is greatly reinforced by anastomosis with the vertebral artery (Fig. 8.65/*13*), which passes into the vertebral canal through the atlas. The *vertebral artery* itself receives anastomotic branches (dog and horse) from the occipital artery (another branch of the common carotid) before entering the canal, and it would thus appear that the occipital artery also contributes to the supply of the brain. However, the vertebral artery is the main if not sole supply to the occipital lobes of the cerebral hemispheres and other caudal parts of the brain.

The arrangement is more complicated in many other species (Fig. 8.66). In these, the internal carotid connects with other arteries of the head, especially the maxillary, before joining the arterial circle. The internal carotid at this level may be a small vessel initially, but in many species it enlarges closer to the brain and detaches many tortuous branches, which then rejoin to form the original single channel before meeting up with the arterial circle. This arrangement, which may present a rather tangled appearance, is known as a *rete mirabile* and has a rather enigmatic significance; the arrangement enhances the efficiency of the blood-cooling mechanism that is discussed shortly. In some species, the lumen of the part of the internal carotid artery proximal to the rete becomes obliterated, sometimes only a considerable time after birth; when this happens, the distal artery from the rete that delivers blood to the brain is wholly of external carotid origin (see Fig. 7.36). This arrangement is found in both sheep and cattle, although these species differ in other features of the arterial supply to the brain (p. 648).

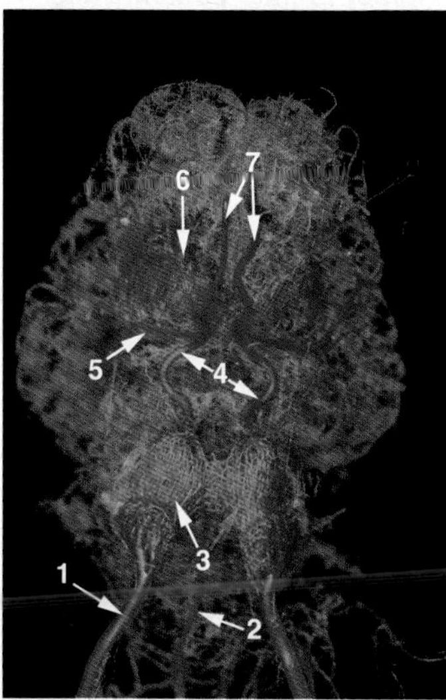

Fig. 8.66 Corrosion cast of the pig's brain (ventral view). *1,* Internal carotid artery; *2,* Basilar artery; *3,* Rete mirabile; *4,* cerebral arterial circle; *5,* middle cerebral artery; *6,* rostral cerebral artery; *7,* internal ethmoidal artery.

The brain, particularly its gray substance, has very high metabolic requirements, and the arterial supply is commensurate with them, amounting to 15% or 20% of the cardiac output. Nevertheless, the vessels that actually penetrate the brain are uniformly small, a feature that may be related to the need to avoid large, pulsating arteries within the delicate brain tissue. Moreover, in sharp contrast to the wide anastomoses between the large vessels supplying the brain, any intracerebral anastomoses are narrow and mostly connect functional end-arteries. This fact, coupled with the very limited regeneration capacity of brain tissue, explains why occlusion or rupture of a small sole vessel, being the only effective blood supply to some vital nucleus or tract, can have serious functional consequences. Notorious examples are provided by the small arteries within the human corpus striatum, where an infarct is often the cause of a stroke.

The permeability of the blood capillaries of the nervous tissue is greatly reduced in comparison with that in other tissues, forming the blood–brain barrier. The main structural component of this barrier is composed of tight junctions between endothelial cells of brain capillaries, such that all substances to enter the brain tissue, other than small lipid-soluble molecules, must be transported through capillary endothelium. The blood–brain barrier is maintained through close cellular communication between brain endothelial cells and the pericytes and astrocytes surrounding these capillaries. There are several regions in the brain where the blood–brain barrier as described is not present; these regions, termed the circumventricular organs are described in detail elsewhere ((Fig. 8.67) (p. 204).

The spinal cord is supplied by three arteries that run its craniocaudal length. The largest, the *ventral spinal artery,* follows the surface of the ventral fissure of the cord; paired *dorsolateral spinal arteries* run close to the furrow fissure from which the dorsal roots of the spinal nerves arise. All three vessels are periodically reinforced

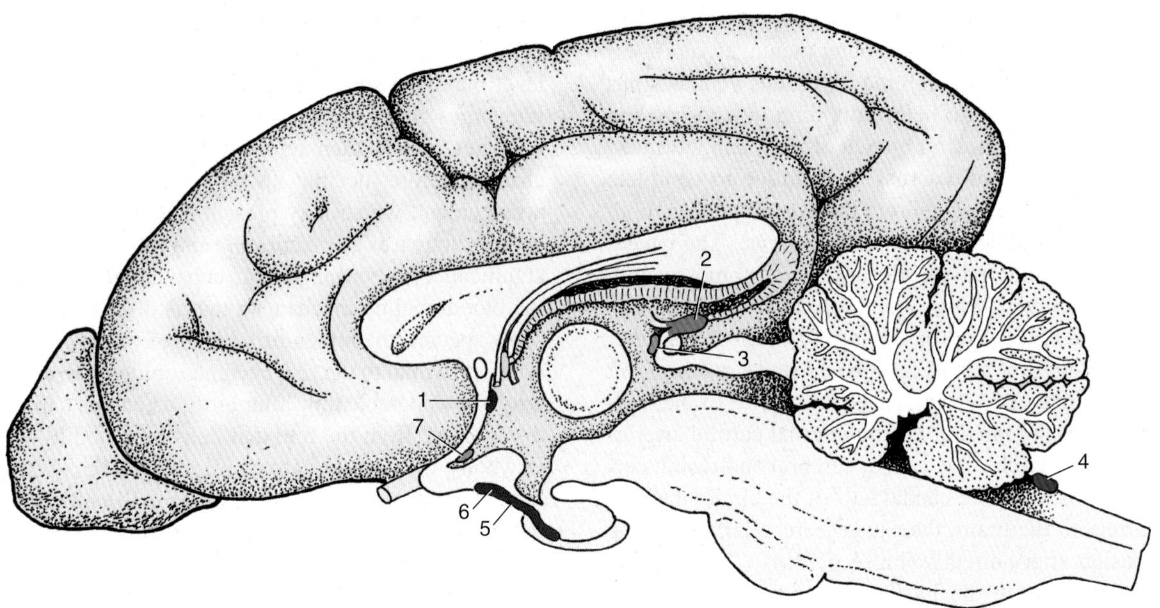

Fig. 8.67 Schematic median section of the canine brain with an indication of the locations of the circumventricular organs. *1*, Subfornical organ; *2*, pineal body; *3*, subcommissural organ; *4*, area postrema; *5*, posterior and intermediate lobes of pituitary; *6*, median eminence; *7*, vascular organ of lamina terminalis.

by branches from regional arteries: vertebral arteries in the neck and intercostal, lumbar, and sacral arteries in the trunk. These vessels enter at the intervertebral foramina, often in the form of narrow vessels that accompany the roots of the spinal nerves; they form plexuses on the surface of the cord with which the major longitudinal arteries connect. This theoretically regular pattern is subject to much variation, both specific and individual, in which many expected reinforcing arteries are lacking, the plexus is unevenly developed, and stretches of the longitudinal trunks are attenuated.

Branches of the ventral spinal artery supply the "core" of the cord, the gray substance, and the adjacent layer of white matter by an approach through the ventral fissure (see Fig. 19.5). The greater part of the white substance is supplied by radial branches from the dorsolateral arteries and surface plexus. Internal anastomoses between the two sets of vessels, although common, are of questionable efficiency.

The Venous Drainage

A complicated system of venous sinuses within the cranial cavity and vertebral canal is connected at intervals to the exposed regional veins. The cranial sinuses enclosed within the dura mater are divided into dorsal and ventral systems, between which there is only limited communication. The dorsal system collects blood from the dorsal parts of the brain and the diploë of the bones of the cranial vault. It includes a dorsal sagittal sinus within the falx cerebri (Fig. 8.64/9). The *dorsal sagittal sinus* receives numerous tributary veins directly from the cerebral hemispheres, and it is joined toward its caudal end by the *straight sinus,* which runs within the ventral part of the falx and collects blood from a major vein draining deeper parts of the brain. The dorsal sinus splits (in a variable manner) into bilateral *transverse sinuses* within the tentorium cerebelli; each later divides—one branch leaving the skull through a foramen, the other connecting with the ventral system.

The ventral or *basilar system* drains the ventral part of the brain (and other cranial contents and walls) and also receives a major inflow from a vein that enters the cranial cavity from the orbit after draining much of the face, including the nasal cavity. The rostral part of the longitudinal trunk of the ventral system, the *cavernous sinus* (Fig. 8.68/6), is connected with its fellow both rostral and caudal to the hypophysis. It divides caudally into the *basilar sinus,* which continues through the foramen magnum as the main component of the internal vertebral plexus, and a branch that receives a connection from the dorsal system before emerging through a ventral foramen to contribute to the maxillary vein.

The flow of blood into the cranial cavity from the face is noteworthy for two reasons. First, it provides a potential pathway for the spread of infection from the face to the cranial contents. Second, it provides for cooling of the arterial supply particularly to the hypothalamus, the part of the brain responsive to and concerned with the regulation of body temperature. The cooling is due to the passage of the internal carotid artery (or rete mirabile) through the cavernous sinus, where the arterial vessel is surrounded by cooler

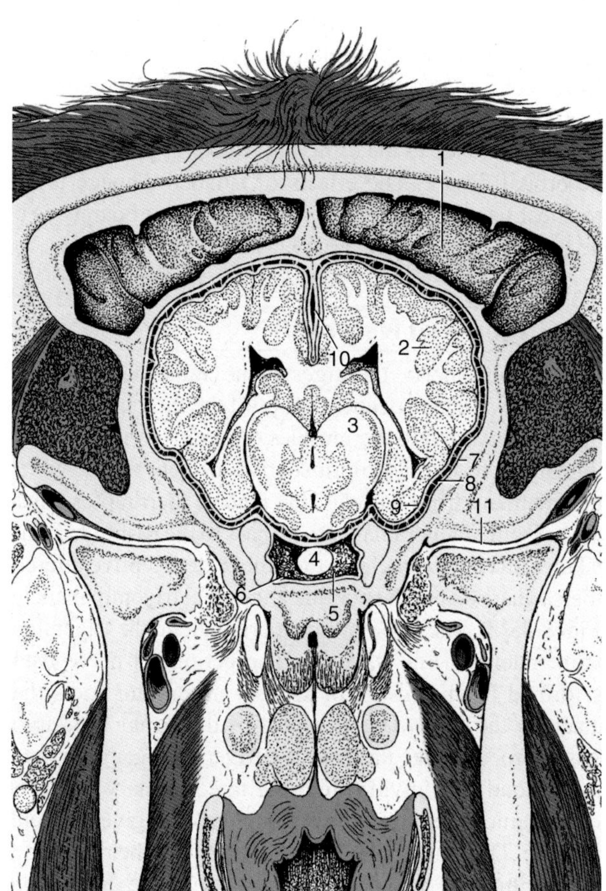

Fig. 8.68 Position of the brain in relation to the roof of the bovine skull. Some features of the meninges are also shown. *1*, Frontal sinus; *2*, cerebral cortex; *3*, diencephalon; *4*, hypophysis; *5*, sella turcica; *6*, cavernous sinus; *7*, dura mater; *8*, arachnoid; *9*, pia mater; *10*, falx cerebri with dorsal sagittal sinus; *11*, temporomandibular joint.

venous blood drained from the nose and superficial structures of the head. An additional mechanism for protecting the brain from damaging hyperthermia is provided by the course of the common carotid artery, which is located close to the trachea at no great depth below the skin. These relationships promote heat loss, especially because any physical exertion that tends to raise body temperature also increases the flow of air within the upper respiratory tract.

The *vertebral venous plexus* is probably more important clinically. It runs the whole length of the vertebral column and drains blood from the vertebrae, the adjacent musculature, and the structures within the vertebral canal. It gives rise to segmental veins that leave the canal through the intervertebral foramina to join the principal venous channels of the neck and trunk: the vertebral, cranial caval, azygous, and caudal caval veins (see Fig. 7.43/*18*). The major part of the plexus consists of paired longitudinal channels within the epidural space ventral to the cord. They are composed of paired crescent-shaped segments that extend between successive intervertebral foramina (see Fig. 26.5). The enlarged midpart of each segment swings toward and is generally joined to its neighbor over the middle of the vertebra, producing a ladder-like pattern of vessels. The connections with segmental veins through the intervertebral foramina form a plexus around the emerging spinal nerves, protecting them from injury.

The veins composing the plexus are thin walled and, being without valves, may pass blood in either direction. They are capacious and adjust in size to compensate for variations in venous return to the heart induced by the intrathoracic pressure changes that accompany respiration. Because the system provides alternative channels to the major systemic veins, and its location within the bony vertebral canal protects the vessels from external compression, its presence may mitigate the effects of jugular obstruction (when the neck is compressed) or caudal caval obstruction (when pressure within the abdomen is raised). The intermittency of flow caused by these several factors facilitates the spread of septic or neoplastic disease to the vertebral column; blood diverted into the vertebral plexus when the flow through other channels is impeded may be temporarily held stagnant, allowing tumor seeds or microorganisms to settle within the tributaries that issue from the bones.

A further point of clinical importance lies in the risk of hemorrhage when epidural or subarachnoid puncture is performed. The risk is greatest at the atlanto-occipital space, where tributaries of the plexus most often encircle the dural tube.

There are no lymphatics in the central nervous tissue.

THE CRANIAL NERVES

The names and sequence of the cranial nerves should now be familiar. Although these nerves lack the relative uniformity of makeup and distribution pattern that is found with the spinal nerves, it is possible to arrange them in three groupings: those exclusively concerned with special senses (the olfactory, optic, and vestibulocochlear nerves); those that supply head muscles of somitic origin (the oculomotor, trochlear, abducent, and hypoglossal nerves); and those primarily concerned with structures of pharyngeal arch origin (the trigeminal, facial, glossopharyngeal, vagus, and accessory nerves). However, it is probably more convenient to deal with them in numerical—that is, in rostrocaudal—sequence.

THE OLFACTORY NERVE (I)

The fibers that compose the olfactory nerve arise as the central processes of the olfactory cells of the nasal mucosa. They are collected into a number of filaments that separately traverse the cribriform plate to join the adjacent surface of the olfactory bulb (see Fig. 8.19/*1*). The further course of the olfactory pathways has been described (p. 276).

The short course and deep location protect these nerves against casual injury, and though they may be involved in infectious or neoplastic disease, interference with the sense of smell is more often due to blockage of the air passages leading to the olfactory mucosa. The filaments are surrounded by meningeal sheaths enclosing extensions of the subarachnoid space, which provide potential routes for the spread of infection from the nose to the cranial cavity.

The vomeronasal organ is also part of the olfactory system (see p. 337).

The Optic Nerve (II)

The optic nerve mediates the visual sense and is in fact a brain tract connecting the retina with the diencephalon (from which it originated). The intracranial part of the nerve extends from the optic chiasm (Fig. 8.19/*7*), where varying proportions of the fibers decussate (p. 284), to the optic foramen at the apex of the orbital cone; the intraorbital course is described elsewhere (p. 331) (see Fig. 9.17/*9*). The optic nerve is also enclosed within extensions of the meninges, and the dura blends with the sclera where the nerve joins the eyeball. Section of the nerve obviously results in blindness of that eye.

The Oculomotor Nerve (III)

The oculomotor nerve consists of somatic efferent fibers from the principal (motor) nucleus and visceral efferent fibers from the parasympathetic nucleus (of Edinger-Westphal), both of which are within the tegmentum of the midbrain (see Fig. 8.25/*III* and *18*). Fibers of both nuclei emerge together as the oculomotor nerve from the ventral aspect of the midbrain, close to the midline (see Fig. 8.19). In its intracranial course, the oculomotor nerve travels close to the trochlear, abducent, and ophthalmic nerves and to the cavernous sinus and then passes through the orbital fissure alongside these structures. The nerve divides within the orbit to supply the dorsal, medial, and ventral recti, the ventral oblique, and the levator muscle of the upper eyelid (some writers also include part of the retractor bulbi). The preganglionic parasympathetic fibers synapse within the small ciliary ganglion placed on one of the branches (Figs. 8.45/*9* and 8.71/*1* and *6*). From here, postganglionic fibers pass within the short ciliary nerves to supply the intraocular ciliary and constrictor pupillae muscles. Isolated injury of the oculomotor nerve and its involvement in disease are not common; the effects can be deduced from consideration of the actions of the muscles it supplies (p. 331).

The Trochlear Nerve (IV)

The trochlear nerve, which is small, provides somatic efferent innervation to the dorsal oblique muscle. The nucleus of origin within the tegmentum of the midbrain gives rise to a fiber bundle that decussates internally before emerging from the rostral medullary velum (Fig. 8.22/*8*). The nerve then follows the edge of the tentorium cerebelli to the floor of the cranial cavity. In some species it makes a separate entrance to the orbit, but usually it passes through the orbital fissure. The effects of isolated damage to the trochlear nerve, rare as for others, are those of paralysis of the dorsal oblique muscle (p. 327).

The Trigeminal Nerve (V)

The trigeminal nerve, the largest of the cranial nerves, is sensory to the skin and deeper tissues of the face and provides motor innervation to the muscles of first pharyngeal (mandibular) arch origin. Proprioceptive afferent fibers, which include many from muscles that receive their motor innervation from other cranial nerves, pass to the rostral trigeminal mesencephalic nucleus; the other exteroceptive afferent fibers synapse onto the pontine and spinal trigeminal nuclei (Fig. 8.25/*7*). The efferent fibers originate in the trigeminal motor nucleus (Fig. 8.25/*17*). The peripheral nerve itself is formed by the fusion of sensory and motor roots that attach to the ventrolateral aspect of the pons. The larger sensory root carries the massive trigeminal ganglion and, just beyond this, divides into the three primary branches (ophthalmic, maxillary, and mandibular) that give the trunk its name. The mandibular branch unites with the motor root to constitute the mixed mandibular nerve; the ophthalmic and maxillary divisions remain purely sensory at this level, although peripheral connections with other cranial nerves introduce somatic and visceral efferent fibers into certain branches. The mandibular nerve emerges through the oval foramen in the floor of the cranial cavity. The ophthalmic and maxillary nerves run rostrally to emerge through the orbital fissure and round foramen, respectively (in ruminants the two openings are combined).

The three primary divisions are initially each restricted to a different process of the embryonic face, a fact that explains the crisply defined adult territories (cf. the dermatomes of the trunk). The ophthalmic nerve supplies the frontonasal process, the primordium of the forehead and nose regions; the maxillary nerve supplies the maxillary process, the primordium of the upper jaw, and associated parts; and the mandibular nerve supplies the mandibular process, the primordium of the lower jaw, and associated parts, which include the masticatory and other first pharyngeal arch muscles (Fig. 8.69).

The *ophthalmic nerve* (Fig. 8.69/*1*), for which the convenient notation is V-1, divides into three divergent branches (lacrimal, frontal, nasociliary) soon after entering the orbit. The *lacrimal nerve* (Fig. 8.69/*3*) passes to the lateral part of the orbital perimeter and, after detaching branches to the lacrimal gland and other deeper structures, emerges to supply the skin about the lateral angle of the eye. The more considerable territory of the *frontal nerve*

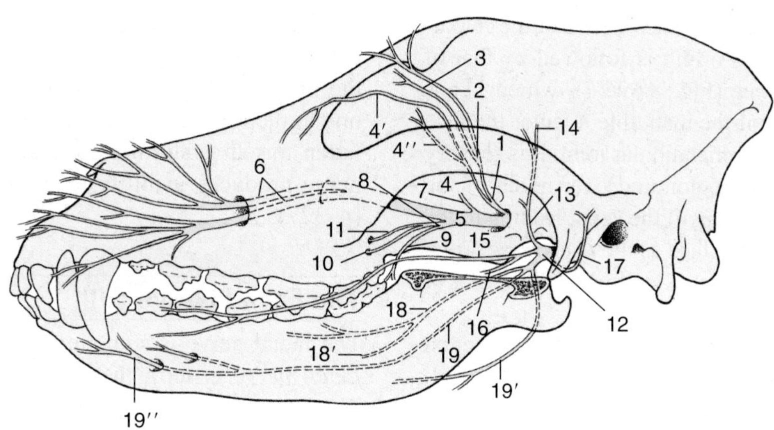

Fig. 8.69 Distribution pattern of the trigeminal nerve (n.) of the dog. *1,* Ophthalmic n.; *2,* frontal n.; *3,* lacrimal n.; *4,* nasociliary n.; *4′,* infratrochlear n.; *4″,* long ciliary n.; *5,* maxillary n; *6,* infraorbital n.; *7,* zygomatic n.; *8,* pterygopalatine n.; *9,* lesser palatine n.; *10,* greater palatine n.; *11,* caudal nasal n.; *12,* mandibular n.; *13,* masticatory n.; *14,* deep temporal n.; *15,* buccal n.; *16,* pterygoid n.; *17,* auriculotemporal n.; *18,* lingual n.; *18′,* sublingual n.; *19,* inferior alveolar n.; *19′,* mylohyoid n.; *19″,* mental n.

(Fig. 8.69/*2*) includes much of the upper eyelid, the forehead, and, through branches that penetrate the bone, the mucosa of the frontal sinus.

The *nasociliary nerve* (Fig. 8.69/*4*) runs toward the medial wall of the orbit. One branch, the *infratrochlear nerve* (Fig. 8.69/*4′*), emerges on the face after supplying structures at the medial angle; it supplies another portion of the mucosa of the frontal sinus and in small ruminants detaches the principal nerve to the horn. Other branches of the nasociliary nerve include long ciliary and ethmoidal nerves. The *long ciliary nerves* (Fig. 8.69/*4″*) penetrate the posterior aspect of the eyeball to supply sensitive tissues, including the cornea; the *ethmoidal nerve* first reenters the cranial cavity through the ethmoidal foramen and subsequently passes to the nasal cavity via the cribriform plate before dividing into medial and lateral branches to the mucosa.

The *maxillary nerve* (V-2) runs across the wall of the pterygopalatine fossa ventral to the orbit (Fig. 8.69/*5*). It bears, or lies close to, the pterygopalatine ganglion, but the relationship is purely topographic. It then enters the infraorbital canal at the maxillary foramen, where it becomes known as the *infraorbital nerve* (Fig. 8.69/*6*) in anticipation of its reappearance on the face at the infraorbital foramen.

Collateral branches of the maxillary nerve detach within the pterygopalatine fossa. They include the *zygomatic nerve* (Fig. 8.69/*7*), which supplies the lower eyelid and adjacent skin and is the origin of the principal nerve of the horn in cattle.

The second branch of the maxillary nerve, the *pterygopalatine nerve* (Fig. 8.69/*8*), detaches the *lesser palatine nerve* (Fig. 8.69/9) to the soft palate; the *greater palatine nerve* (Fig. 8.69/*10*), which reaches the hard palate after traversing the palatine canal and supplies both the palatine mucosa and the floor of the nasal vestibule; and the *caudal nasal nerve* (Fig. 8.69/*11*), which passes through the pterygopalatine foramen to supply mucosa of the ventral part of the nasal cavity, maxillary sinus, and palate.

Within the infraorbital canal, the *infraorbital nerve* (Fig. 8.69/*6*), being the continuation of the maxillary nerve, detaches short twigs to the alveoli of the cheek teeth and nasal mucosa and longer rostral alveolar branches that continue within the bone, beyond the infraorbital foramen, to the alveoli of the canine and incisor teeth. After emerging at the infraorbital foramen, the infraorbital nerve supplies various labial and nasal branches to the structures of the muzzle, including some branches that run back over the nose to the edge of the infratrochlear territory. Although covered by muscle at its emergence from the infraorbital foramen, the infraorbital nerve can usually be palpated, stimulated by pressure, or blocked by injection of local anesthetic solution.

On leaving the cranium, the *mandibular nerve* (V-3) detaches several branches in close succession that pass to the masseter, temporalis, medial and lateral pterygoid, tensor veli palatini, and tensor tympani muscles (Fig. 8.69/*12*). There are minor variations in their pattern, and the nerves to the masseter and temporalis are often initially joined as a short masticatory nerve (Fig. 8.69/*13*). The *masseteric nerve* passes to the masseter muscle between the coronoid and condylar processes of the mandible. The *deep temporal nerves* (Fig. 8.69/*14*) run dorsomedially to the temporalis muscle. The otic ganglion lies close to the origin of the pterygoid nerves (Fig. 8.69/*16*).

The next branch from the mandibular nerve, the *buccal nerve* (Fig. 8.69/*15*), is sensory to the tissues of the cheek, which it reaches after first passing between the pterygoideus and temporalis and then between the maxillary tuber and mandible. Its origin is followed by that of the *auriculotemporal nerve* (Fig. 8.69/*17*), which bends around the caudal border of the mandible to enter the face a little ventral to the temporomandibular joint. It is sensory to the skin of the temporal region and over much of the external ear, including the lining of the canal leading to the eardrum. It continues onto the face as the *transverse facial branch,* supplying a strip of skin extending to the corner of the mouth.

The mandibular nerve continues between the medial and lateral pterygoid muscles before dividing into its end-branches, the lingual and inferior alveolar nerves.

The *lingual nerve* (Fig. 8.69/*18*) detaches twigs to the oropharyngeal mucosa before dividing into a deep branch that enters the tongue, and a superficial branch, the *sublingual nerve* (Fig. 8.69/*18'*), that runs medial to the mylohyoideus below the mucosa of the oral floor that it supplies. The branch of the lingual nerve to the tongue is joined by the *chorda tympani,* a branch of the facial, which contains axons of preganglionic visceral efferent fibers to salivary glands that synapse in the adjacent mandibular ganglion as well as gustatory (special visceral afferent) fibers innervating the taste buds of the rostral two-thirds of the tongue. Other sensory fibers in the lingual nerve supply general sensation (general somatic afferent) in the same rostral two-thirds of the lingual mucosa.

The *inferior alveolar nerve* (Fig. 8.69/*19*) detaches the *mylohyoid nerve* (Fig. 8.69/*19'*) to supply motor innervation to the mylohyoideus and rostral belly of the digastricus before entering the mandibular canal at the mandibular foramen. The inferior alveolar nerve supplies sensory innervation to the lower cheek teeth before a large part reappears at the mental foramen as the *mental nerve* (Fig. 8.69/*19"*, which supplies tissues of the lower lip and chin. In some species several mental branches exit through as many foramina. Although also covered by muscle, the mental nerve(s) can be palpated, compressed, and blocked at their emergence from the foramina.

Injuries to, or disease of, the branches of the trigeminal nerve produce sensory deficiencies in their territories and sometimes manifest as chronic facial irritation; some branches are frequently blocked for minor surgery of the head. Destructive lesions of the mandibular nerve produce paralysis of the muscles that close the jaw; when the lesion is unilateral, the resulting atrophy may be more obvious than any motor disability. A temporary idiopathic bilateral paralysis of the trigeminal musculature, characterized by a dropped jaw, has been reported in dogs.

The Abducent Nerve (VI)

The fibers of the abducent nerve originate within the caudal brainstem and emerge from the brain close to the midline, as is typical for general somatic efferent fibers (see Fig. 8.19). The fibers travel intracranially to the orbital fissure (or the foramen orbitorotundum); within the orbit, the nerve divides into a branch to the lateral rectus and one to the retractor, although the exact innervation of the latter muscle is still controversial. Injury to the abducent nerve produces inability to deviate the eyeball laterally (p. 327).

The Facial Nerve (VII)

The facial nerve is sometimes known as the *intermediofacial nerve,* a term that indicates its composite nature. The intermediate component is a visceral one with sensory (including gustatory) and motor (parasympathetic) functions; the facial component is the nerve of the second pharyngeal arch whose main distribution is to the muscles of the face (mimetic musculature).

The facial nerve arises close to the vestibulocochlear nerve at the lateral extremity of the trapezoid body (Fig. 8.20/*VII* and *VIII*), and the two nerves run within common meningeal covering to the internal acoustic meatus of the petrous temporal bone. The facial nerve enters the facial canal within the bone that leads, via a sharp caudal convexity ("genu"), to the stylomastoid foramen, where the nerve appears at the surface of the skull. The facial nerve contains the appropriately named *geniculate ganglion* at the corner of the convexity within the facial canal. With the exception of a small branch to the stapedius muscle, the branches of the facial nerve detached within the facial canal represent the intermediate (visceral) component and those detached after leaving the bone the motor component (Fig. 8.70/*1*).

Within the facial canal, the *greater petrosal nerve* branches from the main nerve at the level of the ganglion and emerges through an independent foramen. It initially contains only parasympathetic axons but is shortly joined by sympathetic fibers to form a composite autonomic nerve, the *nerve of the pterygoid canal.* This nerve runs through the pterygoid canal to reach the pterygopalatine ganglion within the pterygopalatine fossa (Fig. 8.71/*7* and *11*). The nerve of the pterygoid canal is discussed more fully later (p. 313). The stapedial nerve, which arises next within the canal, is motor to the stapedius muscle of the middle ear. The next branch, the chorda tympani (Fig. 8.71/*13*), crosses the tympanic cavity to emerge at the petrotympanic fissure, after which it converges on and becomes incorporated within the lingual branch of the mandibular nerve (p. 338).

After the facial nerve emerges from the stylomastoid foramen, its first branches are the *internal* and *caudal auricular nerves,* which supply muscles of the external ear and several branches to hyoid muscles, including the caudal belly of the digastricus. The main trunk enters the face by turning around the mandible, where it is first contained between the masseter and the parotid gland. It divides at

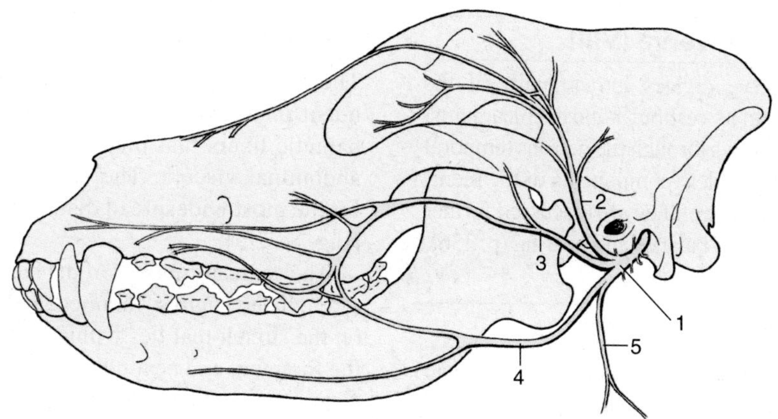

Fig. 8.70 Distribution pattern of the facial nerve (n.) of the dog. *1,* Facial n.; *2,* auriculopalpebral n.; *3,* dorsal buccal branch; *4,* ventral buccal branch; *5,* cervical branch.

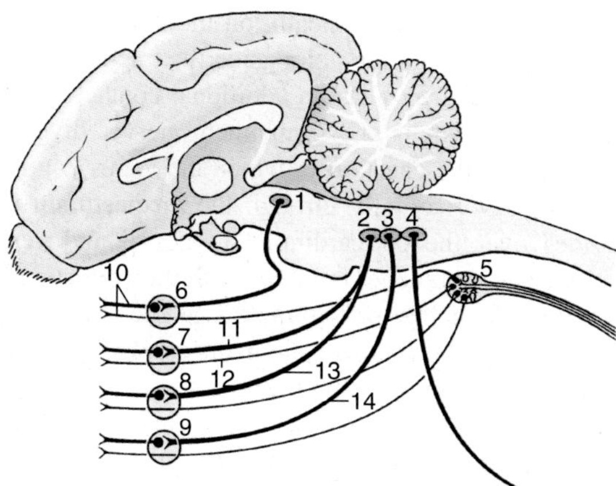

Fig. 8.71 Schematic representation of the autonomic innervation of structures of the head. *1,* Parasympathetic oculomotor nucleus (III); *2,* parasympathetic facial nucleus (VII); *3,* parasympathetic glossopharyngeal nucleus; *4,* parasympathetic vagus nucleus; *5,* cranial cervical ganglion; *6,* ciliary ganglion; *7,* pterygopalatine ganglion; *8,* mandibular ganglion; *9,* otic ganglion; *10,* short ciliary nerves; *11,* greater petrosal nerve; *12,* deep petrosal nerve; *13,* chorda tympani; *14,* tympanic plexus, short petrosal nerve.

about this level (although there are species differences) into three terminal branches, the auriculopalpebral nerve and the dorsal and ventral buccal nerves.

In some species the *auriculopalpebral nerve* (Fig. 8.70/*2*) is detached before the main trunk reaches the face, and it is then less vulnerable to injury from superficial trauma to the side of the head. It crosses the zygomatic arch, traveling toward the space between the upper eyelid and external ear, before dividing into branches that supply the muscles of the eyelids (excluding the levator palpebrae superioris) and the auricular muscles in front of the external ear.

The *dorsal buccal branch* (Fig. 8.70/*3*), which may take the form of a group of divergent branches, crosses the masseter en route to the muzzle.

In some species the *ventral buccal branch* (Fig. 8.70/*4*) may take a path similar to that of the dorsal branch at a slightly more ventral level, but in others it takes a divergent course, first running within the intermandibular space before entering the face with the parotid duct and facial vessels, where they cross the mandible in front of the masseter. Together, the buccal branches supply the muscles of the cheek, lips, and nostrils. Their peripheral branches join with those of the trigeminal nerve at various levels, and many of the smaller trunks combine motor (facial) and sensory (trigeminal) fibers.

The effects of injury or disease clearly depend on the site of the lesion. Lesions that are situated more centrally, which tend to have more serious origins, affect the whole facial field and lead to loss of secretory activity by the lacrimal and salivary (except the parotid) glands in addition to muscular paralysis. Lesions involving the main trunk near its exit from the bone paralyze the entire facial musculature, whereas more peripheral lesions may spare some function, depending on their site and the specific and individual variations in the branching pattern. Lesions confined to the auriculopalpebral nerve produce drooping of the external ear and narrowing of the palpebral fissure with inability to close the eye. Damage to the buccal branches may paralyze the muscles of the lips and cheeks, allowing food to collect in the oral vestibule. It may also lead to deformation of the muzzle, which is made asymmetrical by the unopposed activity of the muscles on the sound side. The alteration in appearance is not always very striking, and the uninjured side, toward which the muzzle is pulled, may sometimes appear to have the more distorted aspect. The distortion tends to be more pronounced in the horse and sheep than in other domestic species. It is important to be aware that in unilateral facial spasm, seen occasionally in the dog, the nose may be drawn toward the affected side.

The auriculopalpebral nerve is sometimes blocked to facilitate examination of the eye.

The Vestibulocochlear Nerve (VIII)

The vestibulocochlear nerve divides intracranially at the internal acoustic meatus into its vestibular and cochlear parts, which make their separate ways through the petrous temporal bone to the vestibular and cochlear components of the membranous labyrinth of the inner ear. They are discussed further with the special sense organs of balance and hearing (p. 336).

The Glossopharyngeal Nerve (IX)

The glossopharyngeal nerve combines fibers that innervate structures of third pharyngeal arch origin with important visceral efferent (parasympathetic) and afferent components. It is motor to part of the palatopharyngeal musculature and to certain salivary glands and sensory to mucosa of the root of the tongue, palate, and pharynx. In addition, there is an important branch to the carotid sinus and body.

The glossopharyngeal nerve arises from the ventrolateral aspect of the medulla oblongata, from the most rostral rootlets of the linear series of rootlets that also give origin to the vagus and the medullary part of the accessory nerve (Figs. 8.19 and 8.20). It runs with these nerves to the jugular foramen and at about this level bears two small and rather indistinct ganglia. The first branch, the *tympanic nerve,* enters the tympanic cavity, where it participates with branches of the facial and internal carotid (sympathetic) nerves in forming a plexus from which a nerve leads to the otic ganglion for the supply of the parotid gland (Fig. 8.71/*3* and *14*).

The main trunk travels closely with the vagus and accessory nerves and at this level detaches the *carotid sinus branch,* which proceeds to the carotid sinus, where it terminates in baroreceptors within the sinus wall and chemoreceptors of the carotid body. The glossopharyngeal nerve then turns rostroventrally, parallel to the stylohyoid, before dividing into pharyngeal and lingual branches. The *pharyngeal branches* include one to the stylopharyngeus caudalis; the others become dispersed within the pharyngeal plexus to which the vagus also contributes. Although most fibers are sensory to the mucosa, it is likely that some fibers provide motor innervation to pharyngeal musculature.

The larger *lingual branch* enters the tongue parallel to the lingual artery, the lingual branch of the mandibular nerve, and the hypoglossal nerve. It is sensory to the mucosa of the root of the tongue (including the taste buds in this area) and motor to the levator palatini muscle and the glands of the soft palate.

Damage to the glossopharyngeal nerve, which is most common in horses as the result of inflammation of the guttural pouch, may lead to difficulties in swallowing. Because the vagus may also be affected, it is difficult to know the extent to which the paresis of palate and pharynx is due to glossopharyngeal involvement. Experimental studies suggest that the role of the glossopharyngeal nerve is more important than many writers have claimed.

The Vagus Nerve (X)

The vagus nerve is the nerve of the fourth and subsequent pharyngeal arches. It also contains the parasympathetic fibers that innervate the cervical, thoracic, and abdominal viscera. The second component gives it by far the most widespread distribution of any cranial nerve (Fig. 8.72/*5*).

The vagus forms part of the bundle of nerves that passes through the jugular foramen. It bears two small ganglia on the stretch that lies within and immediately external to the foramen, and beyond this the vagus runs in close association with the glossopharyngeal and accessory nerves. After the glossopharyngeal nerve turns rostrally, the vagus continues caudally, running close to the cranial cervical ganglion. It then continues down the neck in close contact with the sympathetic trunk, with which it is bound within a common fascial sheath, on the dorsal margin of the common carotid artery, alongside the trachea. The left vagosympathetic trunk has an additional contact with the esophagus. The vagus and sympathetic nerves diverge at the entrance to the chest, after which the vagus continues more or less horizontally through the mediastinum until it divides over the pericardium into dorsal and ventral branches. These branches combine with the corresponding contralateral branches to form the dorsal and ventral vagal trunks that enter the abdomen along the corresponding borders of the esophagus. Within the abdomen, the two nerves branch freely, participating with the sympathetic fibers in forming the plexuses from which the abdominal viscera are supplied (p. 315).

The first significant branch from the main trunk after the vagus nerve leaves the skull is an *auricular branch* that takes part in the innervation of the skin of the external ear. This is followed by *pharyngeal branches* that combine with those of the glossopharyngeal, cranial laryngeal, and sympathetic nerves in forming the pharyngeal plexus. An extension of the plexus supplies the cervical esophagus. The *cranial laryngeal nerve* goes to the larynx, where it divides into an external branch for the cricothyroid muscle and an internal branch for the laryngeal mucosa from the aditus to the glottis. This internal branch makes connections with the recurrent laryngeal nerve (described later). The *depressor nerve* to the heart is formed partly of fibers from the cranial laryngeal nerve and partly of fibers from the main vagal nerve; it is difficult to follow because in most animals it rejoins the main trunk for its further progress through the neck and thorax to the heart.

The thoracic portion of the vagus detaches *cardiac branches* that form a mediastinal plexus with sympathetic fibers also innervating cardiac muscle. A large *caudal (recurrent) laryngeal nerve* is also detached within the thorax. The recurrent laryngeal nerve of the right side changes direction by winding around a branch of the

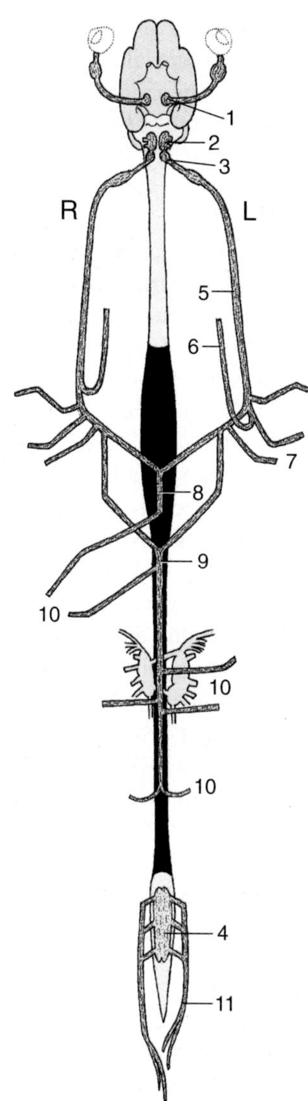

Fig. 8.72 Origin and distribution of the parasympathetic nervous system. Ventral view, schematic. *1*, Parasympathetic oculomotor nucleus; *2*, rostral and middle parasympathetic nuclei of the medulla oblongata; *3*, dorsal vagal nucleus; *4*, sacral outflow; *5*, vagus nerve; *6*, recurrent laryngeal nerve; *7*, parasympathetic fibers to heart and lungs; *8*, ventral vagal trunk; *9*, dorsal vagal trunk; *10*, parasympathetic fibers to the abdominal organs; *11*, pelvic nerves; *L*, left; *R*, right.

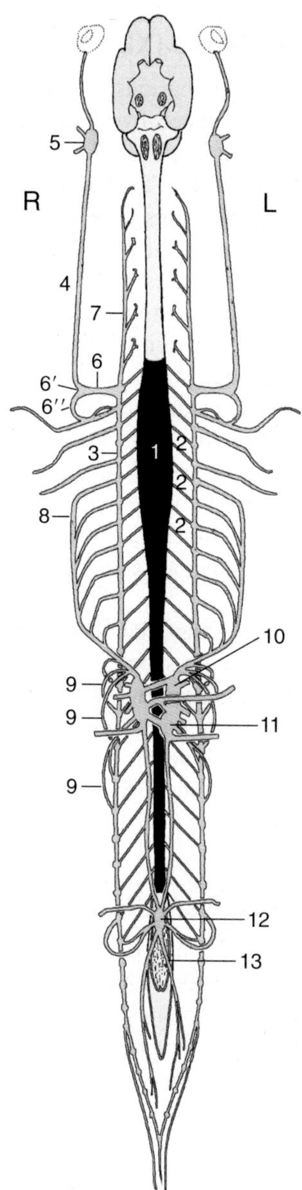

Fig. 8.73 Origin and distribution of the sympathetic nervous system. Ventral view, schematic. The parasympathetic nuclei in brain and spinal cord are indicated in gray. *1*, Sympathetic outflow from T1 to L3; *2*, communicating branches; *3*, and *4*, sympathetic trunk; *5*, cranial cervical ganglion; *6*, cervicothoracic ganglion; *6¢*, middle cervical ganglion; *6^2*, ansa subclavia; *7*, vertebral n.; *8*, greater splanchnic n.; *9*, lesser splanchnic nn.; *10*, celiac ganglion; *11*, cranial mesenteric ganglion; *12*, caudal mesenteric ganglion; *13*, hypogastric n.

subclavian artery, and the left one winds around the aorta. The recurrent laryngeal nerve reascends the neck ventral to the common carotid artery in a course that leads it back to the larynx, where it supplies the bulk of the intrinsic laryngeal musculature (all but the cricothyroideus) and the mucosa caudal to the glottis. Small twigs from the recurrent laryngeal nerve detached en route pass to the cardiac plexus and to the trachea and esophagus. The distribution of the main trunk is completed by pulmonary branches that combine in a common plexus with sympathetic nerves.

Damage to the vagus nerve and its branches may be manifested in a variety of ways, including difficulties in swallowing and altered functioning of the heart and the other viscera. Degeneration of the recurrent laryngeal nerve is especially common in horses, producing the condition known as roaring (p. 515); it also occurs in dogs.

The Accessory Nerve (XI)

The accessory nerve is curiously formed of two roots. The spinal root is provided by axons that emerge midway between the dorsal and ventral roots of the first five (or so) spinal nerves (Figs. 8.19 and 8.20). These roots combine in a trunk that runs cranially within the spinal subarachnoid space to enter the skull through the foramen magnum; it then approaches the cranial root, which is formed by the most caudal rootlets of the glossopharyngeal–vagus series. There is only brief contact between the two roots, and although some fibers may be exchanged, the cranial root then amalgamates with the vagus to which it probably furnishes the fibers that reach the laryngeal musculature via the recurrent laryngeal nerve. It is the spinal root that forms the accessory nerve of descriptive anatomy. This nerve passes through the jugular foramen to divide within the atlantal fossa into dorsal and ventral branches.

The *dorsal branch* runs caudally over the splenius and serratus ventralis before it supplies the brachiocephalicus, omotransversarius, and trapezius. The *ventral branch* supplies only one muscle, the sternocephalicus, which it enters close to its cranial attachment.

There is no convincing explanation for the curious detour made by the spinal fibers of this nerve.

The Hypoglossal Nerve (XII)

The hypoglossal nerve is motor to the intrinsic and extrinsic muscles of the tongue, which are derived from the myotomes of occipital somites. After leaving the ventral aspect of the medulla oblongata (see Fig. 8.19), the nerve passes through the hypoglossal canal before crossing the nerves of the vagus group to continue toward the tongue, which it enters ventral to the glossopharyngeal nerve. It ramifies within the tongue substance to reach the various muscles.

A destructive lesion of this nerve paralyzes the ipsilateral muscles, allowing a deviation of the tongue toward the normal side. A marked atrophy of the denervated side eventually develops.

THE SPINAL NERVES

A general account of the formation and distribution of the spinal nerves has been given (see p. 27). That account described the formation of each nerve by the union of dorsal and ventral roots and its later division into dorsal and ventral primary branches or rami, which diverge from each other on passing through the intervertebral foramen (Fig. 8.55). The term *rami* rather than the general term *branch* is used here to refer to the most proximal dorsal and ventral branch of each spinal nerve, to avoid confusion with further divisions of these nerves. The rather consistent pattern of distribution of the dorsal rami may be represented by a single description; important regional features of the ventral rami require separate attention.

The Dorsal Rami

As a rule, the dorsal rami are considerably smaller than the ventral and have simpler distributions. Each dorsal ramus divides into a medial branch that supplies the local part of the epaxial musculature of the neck, trunk, or tail and a lateral branch that is distributed to the dorsal part of the skin segment (dermatome) served by the particular spinal nerve. These areas extend from the dorsal midline for a variable distance over the animal's side. The territories served by the dorsal rami of the first few cervical nerves extend rostrally onto the poll region of the head in addition to supplying skin over the neck; the dorsal rami of the spinal nerves at the cervicothoracic junction supply skin over the upper part of the shoulder; those of the middle and caudal thoracic and lumbar regions serve increasingly larger areas of the skin of the chest wall and flank. The dorsal rami of the sacral spinal nerves serve more restricted areas. Inconspicuous connections between neighboring nerves form a continuous plexus through which exchange of fibers blurs the boundaries between the dermatomes supplied by individual nerves; indeed, it is probable that every part of the skin receives sensory fibers from two, if not three, spinal nerves.

The Ventral Rami

The larger ventral rami supply the hypaxial muscles, including those of the limbs (excepting the thoracic girdle muscles supplied by the eleventh cranial nerve and the rhomboideus supplied in some species by dorsal rami) and the remaining skin of the neck, trunk, and limbs. Except in the thoracic region, where a more precise segmental distribution is retained, the ventral rami are also joined with their cranial and caudal neighbors by connecting branches. These connections are greatly exaggerated at the levels of origin of the nerves to the forelimb and hindlimb, where they constitute the brachial and lumbosacral plexuses, respectively.

The Cervical Ventral Rami

The cutaneous distribution of the first two cervical ventral rami extends rostrally to the external ear and the masseteric and throat regions. The more caudal cervical ventral rami, in addition to providing sensory innervation to dermatomes of the neck region, also provide motor axons to the phrenic nerve and to the brachial plexus, discussed later.

In domestic species the *phrenic nerve,* the nerve supplying the diaphragm, is generally formed by the fifth, sixth, and seventh cervical nerves. Axons that contribute to the phrenic nerve leave the large ventral rami to run ventrally over the scalenus muscle to join in a trunk (see Fig. 1.38) that winds below the muscle to enter the mediastinum between the two first ribs. The phrenic nerve runs caudally within the mediastinum, crossing the lateral surface of the pericardium, to reach the diaphragm; the right nerve utilizes the plica venae cavae in the last part of its course (see Fig. 13.14/*12* and Fig 13.15/*6*). The phrenic nerves ramify within the diaphragm to which they are the sole motor innervation; their sensory fibers are supplemented by others channeled through intercostal nerves. It is worth emphasizing that the diaphragmatic muscle is skeletal muscle and phrenic nerves contain somatic efferent fibers; it must not be inferred from the normally involuntary nature of breathing that phrenic nerves contain visceral efferent—in other words, autonomic—fibers. Experiments in some species have shown that bilateral section of the phrenic nerves has little effect, although respiratory distress may become evident when the animal is severely stressed.

The Brachial Plexus

The brachial plexus is a network of nerves that supplies sensory and motor innervation to almost all structures of the forelimb—except for the trapezius, omotransversarius, brachiocephalicus, and rhomboideus—and the skin over the upper shoulder region.

The plexus is usually formed by contributions from the last three cervical and first two thoracic nerves; the fifth cervical nerve sometimes participates, and the contribution of the second thoracic nerve is then reduced or lacking. The plexus reaches the axilla by passing between the parts of the scalenus and quickly splits into peripheral nerves that diverge toward their separate destinations (Fig. 8.74). Several of these nerves have very restricted local distributions, and bare mention of their names and destinations is all that is required; they include the *long thoracic nerve* (Fig. 8.74/*9*) to the serratus ventralis, the thoracodorsal nerve (Fig. 8.74/*9′*) to the latissimus dorsi, the *cranial and caudal pectoral nerves* (Fig. 8.74/*3* and *9″*) to the pectoral muscles (including the subclavius), the *subscapular nerve* (Fig. 8.74/*2*) to the subscapularis, and the *lateral thoracic nerve* (Fig. 8.74/*9″*) to the cutaneous trunci and to skin over the ventral part of the thorax and abdomen. The other nerves, described here, require fuller description. There are some interspecies differences, but these are rarely of importance except in the manus.

The *suprascapular nerve* (Fig. 8.74/*1*) leaves the cranial part of the brachial plexus (C6–C7). It passes between the supraspinatus and subscapularis to reach the cranial margin of the neck of the scapula, around which it winds to the lateral aspect of the bone, where it is distributed to supply the supraspinatus and infraspinatus muscles. Like other nerves directly apposed to bone, it is vulnerable to injury;

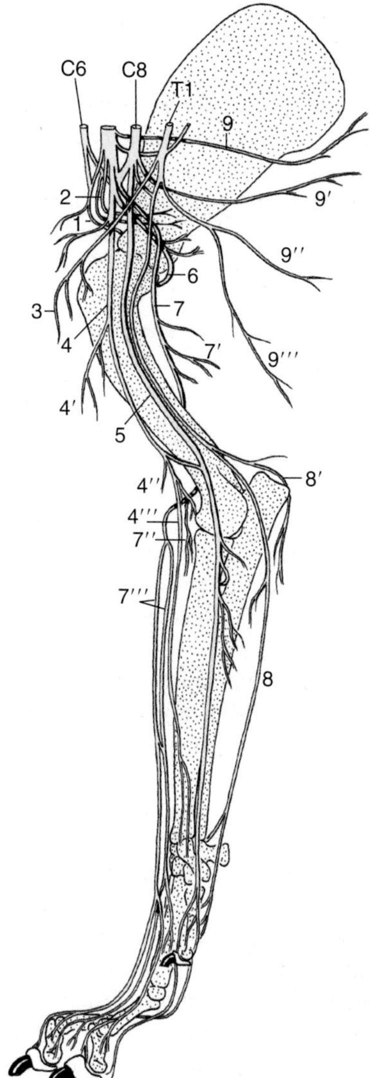

Fig. 8.74 The nerves of the right forelimb of the dog; medial view. *1*, Suprascapular nerve (n.); *2*, subscapular nerves (nn.); *3*, cranial pectoral nn.; *4*, musculocutaneous n.; *4′*, proximal muscular branch; *4″*, distal muscular branch; *4‴*, medial cutaneous antebrachial n.; *5*, median n.; *6*, axillary n.; *7*, radial n.; *7′*, muscular branches to triceps; *7″*, muscular branches to extensors; *7‴*, cranial cutaneous antebrachial n.; *8*, ulnar n.; *8′*, caudal cutaneous antebrachial n.; *9*, long thoracic n.; *9′*, thoracodorsal n.; *9″*, lateral thoracic n.; *9‴*, caudal pectoral n.; *C6* and *C8*, sixth and eighth cervical nn.; *T1*, first thoracic n.

in this case it is usually stretched against the scapula when the limb is overabducted or violently retracted. The resulting paralysis of the lateral shoulder muscles does not affect the standing posture but may result in an obvious lateral movement of the shoulder joint ("shoulder slip") during the stride. The condition occurs most frequently in horses, in which it is also known as "sweeny"; it manifests itself after a time by obvious wasting of the muscles beside the scapular spine.

The *musculocutaneous nerve* (Fig. 8.74/*4*) is also of cervical origin (C7–C8). After a short course within the axilla, the nerve provides a proximal branch (Fig. 8.74/*4′*), which supplies and terminates in the coracobrachialis and biceps in the upper part of the arm. In the dog, the main part of the nerve continues into the distal third of the arm, where a communicating branch passes distocaudally to the median nerve. The remaining trunk of the musculocutaneous nerve passes under the terminal part of the biceps brachii, where it forms a distal branch (Fig. 8.74/*4′*), which supplies the brachialis, and the medial cutaneous nerve of the forearm (Fig. 8.74/*4″*), which crosses the flexor aspect of the elbow before ramifying in skin.

In ungulates, the musculocutaneous nerve loops around the axillary artery to join the median nerve; further distally, the musculocutaneous fibers again separate from the median nerve in the upper and lower parts of the arm, where they form the proximal and distal muscular branches of the musculocutaneous nerve. In the horse alone, the cutaneous branch extends beyond the carpus to the fetlock.

Damage to the main musculocutaneous trunk is an unlikely injury; it would paralyze the main flexors of the elbow, although compensation would probably be found from activity of the carpal and digital extensors.

The *axillary nerve* (C8) (Fig. 8.74/*6*) passes behind the shoulder joint to reach the lateral aspect of the limb. En route it supplies the teres major, teres minor, capsularis, and deltoideus—the true flexors of the shoulder joint. It also supplies small branches to the distal part of the brachiocephalicus, which, it will be recalled, is of deltoid origin. A cutaneous branch supplies skin over the cranial aspect of the arm and forearm.

The three remaining branches of the plexus have the most complicated courses and the most extensive distributions. The *radial nerve* (Fig. 8.74/*7*) arises from the last two cervical and first thoracic nerves (C7–T1). It first runs distally within the arm, caudal to the brachial artery, before diving between the long and medial heads of the triceps to follow the spiral groove of the humerus, which leads it to the craniolateral aspect of the limb. The nerve supplies branches to the various heads of this muscle (Fig. 8.74/*7′*) and to tensor fasciae antebrachii and anconeus. In the lower part of the arm, the radial nerve supplies a further set of branches (Fig. 8.74/*7″*) to all carpal and digital extensor muscles, including the anomalous ulnaris lateralis. A cutaneous branch or branches (Fig. 8.74/*7*) descends over the craniolateral aspect of the forearm and carpus to reach the dorsal surface of the digits. In the horse, this cutaneous contribution ends at the level of the carpus, and more distal innervation is assumed by the musculocutaneous nerve.

Damage to the radial nerve can have three obvious consequences: paralysis of the elbow extensors, paralysis of the carpal and digital extensors, and anesthesia of the denervated skin regions. The combination of all three disabilities points to injury proximal to the middle of the arm, the combination of the second and third points to injury in the distal part of the arm, and a purely sensory deficit suggests injury beyond the origin of the distal motor branches. Injury in the arm is quite common because in places only a thin layer of muscle separates the radial nerve from the humerus, and the nerve may be involved in fracture or tumor of this bone. Extensive damage to the radial nerve proximal to the origin of the branches to the triceps is serious because it prevents fixation of the elbow, prohibiting the limb from bearing weight; the foot is dragged with its dorsal surface on the ground. More distal lesions are less serious because the elbow can be fixed, and most animals learn to compensate for paralysis of the forearm muscles by flicking the limb forward and planting the foot quickly to prevent toe drag.

The *median nerve* (Fig. 8.74/*5*) comes mainly from the last cervical and first thoracic nerves (C8–T1). It runs down the medial surface of the arm caudal to the main artery and enters the forearm muscle over the medial collateral ligament of the elbow joint, where it provides motor innervation to many of the carpal flexors. It inclines caudally, passes under the flexor carpi radialis, and maintains this protected situation until it reaches the carpus. It divides in the distal part of the forearm, or within the carpal canal, into two or more divisions that descend through the carpal canal to supply most structures of the palmar part of the foot. The median nerve supplies most of the flexor muscles of the carpus and digit in a pattern that overlaps (but does not quite coincide) with the distribution of the ulnar. Therefore, damage confined to the median nerve is not usually manifested through any abnormality of posture or gait.

The *ulnar nerve* (Fig. 8.74/*8*) leaves the caudal part of the plexus (C8–T2). It runs down the arm adjacent to and possibly conjoined with the median nerve before deviating in the direction of the olecranon to cross the caudal aspect of the elbow joint. Within the arm it detaches the caudal cutaneous antebrachial nerve. The main trunk is severely depleted by detachment of the branches to the carpal and digital flexor muscles in the upper part of the forearm, and the narrow continuation runs down the caudal aspect of the forearm. It finally divides a short distance above the accessory carpal bone. The dorsal branch of this division emerges between the tendons of the ulnar carpal flexor and ulnaris lateralis and descends over the lateral face of the accessory bone to supply the skin on the lateral aspect of the forefoot. The palmar branch continues through the carpal canal and later supplies the interosseous and other small muscles of the foot. It also supplies sensory branches to skin and deeper structures. The distribution within the foot is in close collaboration with the median nerve, partly through combined trunks. The innervation of the forefoot, a topic of considerable practical importance in horses, is later considered separately.

Damage confined to the ulnar nerve is unlikely to impair locomotion; the sensory deficits show considerable interspecies variation.

The Thoracic Ventral Rami

The thoracic ventral rami show a more strictly segmental distribution than is found in other regions. The first two thoracic rami contribute to the brachial plexus, but generally the thoracic ventral rami provide the intercostal nerves that run ventrally within the intercostal spaces, either directly below the pleura or between the two intercostal muscle layers; the relation varies according to location and species. Apart from supplying the intercostal muscles, the intercostal nerves detach lateral cutaneous branches that supply a band of skin over the lateral aspect of the chest wall and ventral cutaneous branches that supply the skin of the ventral chest wall; the more caudal thoracic rami also supply sensory innervation to the abdominal floor. In the sow, bitch, and cat, the lateral cutaneous branches detach branches to supply sensory innervation to the thoracic mammary glands.

The last thoracic ventral branch (costoabdominal nerve) is slightly different in its course and distribution because it runs behind the last rib. It joins with the lumbar ventral branches to supply the flank.

The Lumbar Ventral Rami

The lumbar and sacral ventral rami form a continuous plexus, best developed where the last three or four lumbar and first two sacral nerves form the lumbosacral plexus that supplies the hindlimb. The more cranial lumbar ventral rami have a considerable importance in cattle because they are frequently blocked for abdominal surgery. They are given individual names; in species (including cattle) in which there are six lumbar nerves, the first ventral ramus is known as the *iliohypogastric,* the second is known as the *ilioinguinal,* and the third and fourth combine to form the *genitofemoral nerve.* In species with seven lumbar nerves the first two ventral rami are distinguished as the *cranial and caudal iliohypogastric;* the third supplies the ilioinguinal and also makes a contribution to the genitofemoral nerve. The genitofemoral nerve divides into a femoral branch that supplies the skin over the medial aspect of the thigh and a genital branch that supplies the spermatic fasciae, the scrotum, and the prepuce.

It is important to note that the ventral rami travel in a caudoventral direction rather than strictly ventral—this feature is most obvious in the lumbar rami but is apparent with the caudalmost thoracic rami, the intercostal nerves. Thus, the locations of their corresponding dermatomes and the locations where these nerves can most easily be accessed for injection of local anesthetic solution are both considerably more caudal than would naturally be supposed (see Fig. 28.2). The lumbar nerves pass through the transversus close to the tip of the transverse processes and then run deep to the internal oblique toward the abdominal floor (see Fig. 1.37). In addition to supplying the flank and rectus muscles, the lumbar nerves detach lateral and ventral cutaneous branches; the former appear subcutaneously at increasingly dorsal levels as the series is followed caudally.

The Lumbosacral Plexus

The lumbosacral plexus that gives origin to the nerves of the hindlimb (with the minor exceptions of those to certain proximal skin areas) is an enhancement of the continuous plexus described previously. It usually begins at the ventral ramus of the fourth lumbar nerve and ends with that of the second sacral nerve (L4–S2); it thus has an additional root in species possessing seven lumbar nerves (Fig. 8.75).

The *femoral nerve* (Fig. 8.75/*1*) arises from the cranial part (L4–L6) of the plexus and pursues a course through the psoas muscles to reach the gap between the dorsocaudal corner of the flank and the iliopsoas muscle. It is accompanied by the external iliac artery and vein, and on entering the thigh it runs in a protected position between the sartorius and pectineus. It soon detaches the saphenous nerve, and after a very short further course it dives between the rectus femoris and vastus medialis to branch within and innervate the quadriceps mass (Fig. 8.75/*1′*). Severe damage to this nerve, though relatively infrequent, has serious consequences because paralysis of the quadriceps prevents fixation of the stifle joint, rendering the whole limb incapable of supporting weight. No compensation for this defect is possible.

The *saphenous nerve* (Fig. 8.75/*1″*) innervates the sartorius before continuing to supply skin over the medial aspect of the limb from the stifle to the metatarsus.

The *obturator nerve* (Fig. 8.75/2) has broadly the same origin (L4–L6) as the femoral nerve. It follows the medial aspect of the shaft of the ilium to reach the obturator foramen, through which it passes to the adductor muscles of the thigh; this group of muscles comprises the gracilis, pectineus, adductor, and obturator externus—and obturator internus in ruminants and the pig.* The close relationship of the obturator nerve to the pelvis is potentially dangerous, because it exposes the nerve to the risk of laceration in fractures and

*The variation may be more apparent than real; it has been suggested that the internal obturator of Artiodactyla is actually an intrapelvic part of the external obturator.

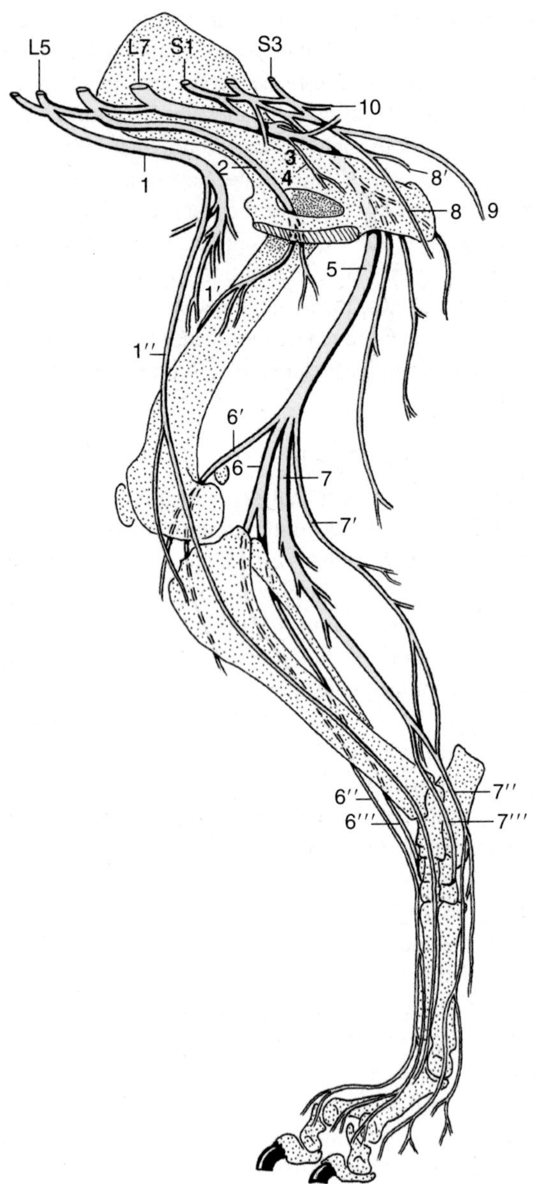

Fig. 8.75 The lumbar and sacral nerves of the dog; medial view. *1*, Femoral n.; *1′*, branches to quadriceps; *1″*, saphenous n.; *2*, obturator n.; *3*, pelvic n.; *4*, branch to obturator internus, gemelli, and quadratus femoris; *5*, sciatic n.; *6*, peroneal n.; *6′*, lateral cutaneous sural n.; *6″*, superficial peroneal n.; *6‴*, deep peroneal n.; *7*, tibial n.; *7′*, caudal cutaneous sural n.; *7″*, medial plantar n.; *7‴*, lateral plantar n.; *8*, pudendal n.; *8′*, deep perineal n.; *9*, caudal cutaneous femoral n.; *10*, caudal rectal n.; *L5* and *L7*, fifth and seventh lumbar nn; *S1* and *S3*, first and third sacral nn.

to the risk of compression during calving and foaling. The risk is less in species in which the young are small relative to the pelvic cavity. The effects of injury vary depending on the location of the damage along the extent of the nerve, but consequences of injury are greater in heavier animals and are exaggerated by a requirement to walk on smooth ground, when the limb tends to slip sideways.

The remaining branches of the lumbosacral plexus arise from a common *lumbosacral trunk* that is largely formed by the last lumbar and first two sacral nerves, along with a smaller contribution from the penultimate lumbar nerve. The trunk leaves the pelvis through the greater sciatic foramen and almost at once detaches three branches before continuing on as the sciatic nerve.

The *short cranial gluteal nerve* supplies the tensor fasciae latae, the middle and deep gluteal, and in some species part of the superficial gluteal muscles, a group that—contrary to the usual expectation—includes both flexor and extensor muscles of the hip.

The *caudal gluteal nerve* supplies the superficial gluteal muscle and the vertebral heads of origin of the hamstring muscles (biceps femoris, semitendinosus, and semimembranosus). These parts of the hamstrings are thought to represent an assimilation of elements of the superficial gluteal. It thus supplies extensor muscles of the hip.

The *caudal cutaneous femoral nerve* (Fig. 8.75/*9*) supplies skin over the caudal aspect of the thigh.

The *sciatic nerve* (Fig. 8.75/*5*) continues the lumbosacral trunk distally, passing between the middle and deep gluteal muscles before turning into the thigh caudal to the hip joint, where it is protected by the greater trochanter of the femur. It then runs between the biceps femoris laterally and the semitendinosus medially before dividing into its terminal branches, the common peroneal (fibular) and tibial nerves, at a level that varies among species. In the proximal part of its course, the sciatic detaches twigs to the internal obturator (unimportant except in ruminants and pigs), gemelli, and quadratus femoris (Fig. 8.75/4); other muscular branches that may appear to arise directly from the sciatic nerve are usually associated with its common peroneal and tibial divisions.

The *common peroneal nerve* (Fig. 8.75/*6*), the lesser of the terminal branches, arises from the lumbar roots of the lumbosacral trunk. It runs first with the tibial nerve but separates from this nerve to pass over the lateral head of the gastrocnemius to enter the leg. It detaches a branch, the lateral sural nerve (Fig. 8.75/*6′*), to the skin over the lateral aspect of the leg before dividing into superficial and deep branches when close to the head of the fibula. The *superficial peroneal nerve* (Fig. 8.75/*6″*) supplies skin over the dorsal aspect of the leg and entire foot, except in the horse, in which it fades about the level of the fetlock joint. The *deep peroneal nerve* (Fig. 8.75/*6‴*) supplies the dorsolateral muscles of the leg (flexors of the hock and extensors of the digits) and is also sensory to the structures of the foot. Because the sensory innervation of pedal structures varies considerably, the details are deferred to the accounts of individual species.

Paralysis of the common peroneal nerve produces overextension of the hock and flexion of the digits, which may be rested on their dorsal surfaces. The foot may be passively placed to support weight, and in time compensation may be possible (cf. radial paralysis, p. 310). There is also a considerable sensory deficit.

The *tibial nerve* (Fig. 8.75/*7*) arises from the sacral roots of the lumbosacral trunk. It detaches important proximal muscular branches to the pelvic heads of the hamstring muscles before freeing itself from the sciatic trunk to enter the leg by passing between the two heads of the gastrocnemius. About this level it first detaches a caudal sural nerve (Fig. 8.75/*7′*) to the skin of this aspect of the leg and later detaches distal muscular branches to the gastrocnemius, soleus, popliteus, and caudal crural muscles. The nerve continues as an almost exclusively sensory trunk (although it will supply short digital muscles) within the fascial plate between the common calcanean tendon and the caudal crural muscles; it ends by dividing into medial and lateral plantar nerves when level with the point of the hock. The *plantar nerves* (Fig. 8.75/*7″* and *7‴*) continue into the plantar aspect of the foot to supply sensation to plantar structures chiefly but with some dorsal penetration that varies among species.

Section of or severe damage to the tibial nerve is manifest as overflexion of the hock and overextension of the digits. Similar damage to the sciatic trunk combines the effects of common peroneal and tibial nerve injuries, rendering the limb largely incapable, although fixation of the stifle joint by the unaffected quadriceps, supplied by the femoral nerve, may allow it to support some weight.

The Sacral and Caudal Ventral Rami

The sacral ventral rami caudal to and overlapping the roots of the lumbosacral plexus give rise to other important individual nerves. The *pelvic nerves* (Fig. 8.75/*3*), composed primarily of parasympathetic axons, are considered in the following section.

The *pudendal nerve* (Fig. 8.75/*8*) arises from various sacral nerves (S1–S3 in the dog, S2–S4 in ruminants, S[2]3–S4 in the horse). It is sensory to the rectum, perineal skin, and internal and external reproductive organs and motor to much of the striated perineal musculature. The nerve has both physiologic and applied importance, but because of species variation, it suffices here to say that the pudendal nerve takes an oblique course through the pelvis toward the ventral part of the pelvic outlet (see Fig. 29.5/*7*). The nerve provides deep and superficial perineal nerves in addition to various cutaneous branches and finally continues as the dorsal nerve of the penis (or clitoris). The *superficial perineal branch* supplies the skin of the anus, vulva, and ventral perineal region.

The *deep perineal nerve* supplies the ventral part of the striated musculature of the perineum, particularly that of the reproductive organs. The main trunk also supplies branches to the skin of the prepuce and scrotum in the male and of the caudal part of the udder in ungulates.

The *caudal rectal nerves* (Fig. 8.75/*10*) arise from the most caudal sacral nerves, sometimes overlapping the origin of the pudendal nerve. They supply sensory fibers to the rectum, anus, and perianal skin and motor fibers to the dorsal perineal striated musculature, including the levator ani. The division of territory between these nerves and the pudendal nerve is rather variable.

The ventral rami of the caudal nerves supply the ventral or depressor muscles of the tail.

In the standing animal, extensor muscles of the limbs must be continually active to support the body against gravity. Thus, damage to those nerves innervating the major extensor muscles of the limbs—that is, the radial, femoral, and sciatic nerves—produce obvious clinical signs and severe consequences for the animal.

THE PERIPHERAL AUTONOMIC NERVOUS SYSTEM

The appropriate regulation of visceral activities involves both afferent and efferent functions. Visceral afferent pathways, however, are in general indistinguishable in structure and arrangement from their somatic afferent counterparts. In contrast, the visceral efferent pathways are clearly distinguished from their somatic efferent pathways. These distinctions include the existence of two neurons in series (the preganglionic, myelinated fiber and a postganglionic thinly myelinated fiber), the location of the last neuron in the chain within a peripheral ganglion, and the restriction of the location of the preganglionic cell bodies to specific nuclei of the brainstem and particular regions of the cord (Figs. 8.72 8.73, and 8.76). Thus the term *autonomic nervous system* was originally, and is still best, defined as wholly efferent. Moreover, certain anatomic, physiologic, and pharmacologic features distinguish the two contrasting divisions of the autonomic system—sympathetic and parasympathetic—whereas no similar distinction exists for visceral afferent pathways. Visceral afferent fibers are, nonetheless presumed to be included in all cranial and spinal nerves, if only because of the ubiquitous distribution of blood vessels.

Before we move to more detailed descriptions of the specifics of the parasympathetic and sympathetic systems in the next section, one general distinction relates to the nature of the actions of the two systems—namely, that the activities of the parasympathetic system tend to be more discrete than those of the sympathetic system. Acetylcholine is used at the synapse between the postganglionic parasympathetic neuron and the target organ, and because acetylcholine is liberated and destroyed locally, its effects tend to be very specific. The narrower localization of parasympathetic responses is further assisted by the location of parasympathetic ganglia close by or even within the target organ. In contrast,

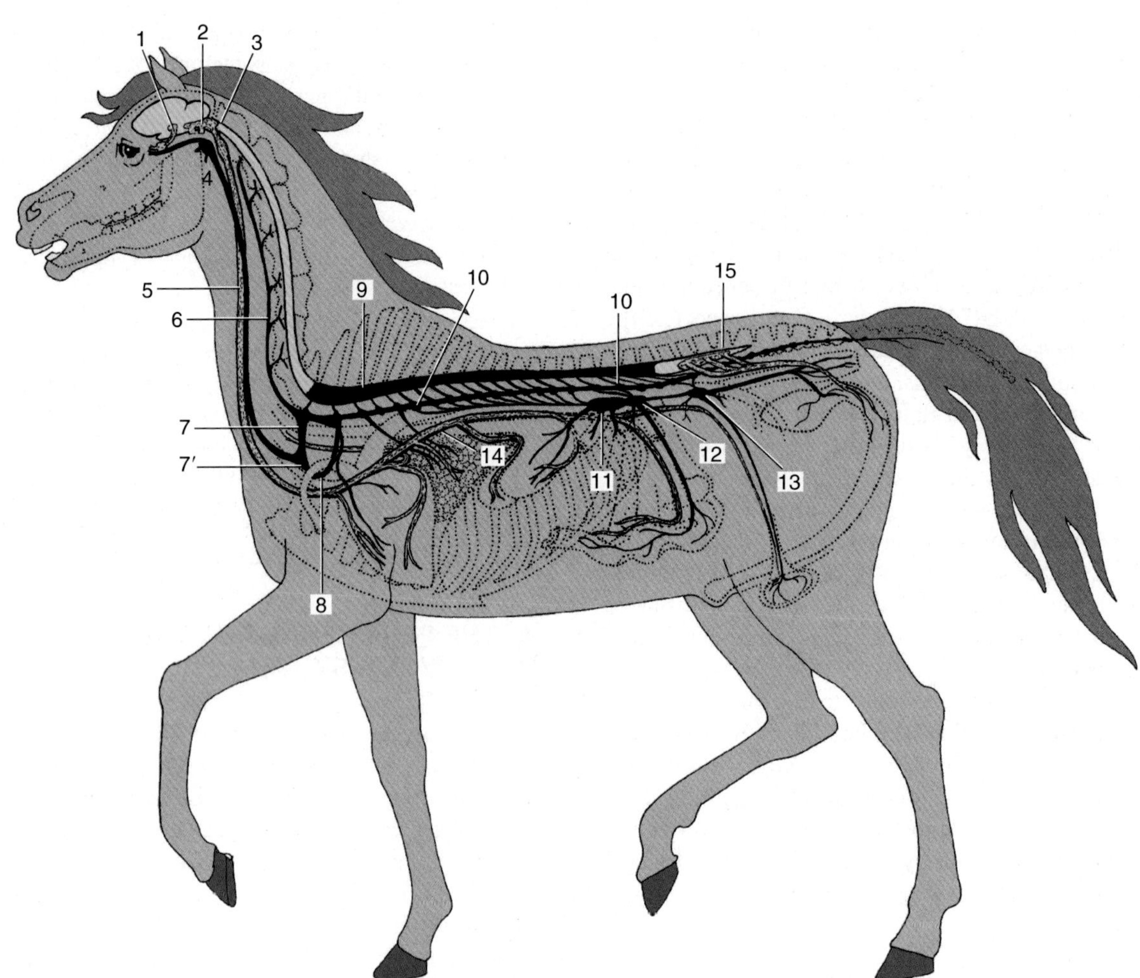

Fig. 8.76 Distribution of sympathetic (black) and parasympathetic (dotted yellow) nervous systems, semischematic. *1,* Parasympathetic oculomotor nucleus; *2,* salivatory nuclei (rostral and middle parasympathetic nuclei); *3,* dorsal vagal nucleus; *4,* cranial cervical ganglion; *5,* vagosympathetic trunk; *6,* vertebral nerve; *7,* cervicothoracic ganglion; *7′,* middle cervical ganglion; *8,* ansa subclavia; *9,* sympathetic outflow from spinal cord; *10,* sympathetic trunk with paravertebral ganglia; *11,* celiac ganglion; *12,* cranial mesenteric ganglion; *13,* caudal mesenteric ganglion; *14,* vagus nerve with distribution to thoracic and abdominal organs; *15,* sacral outflow of parasympathetic nervous system.

norepinephrine is used as the neurotransmitter at the last synapse of the sympathetic pathway except where epinephrine is produced by the adrenal medulla, from which it is released into the bloodstream, evoking a mass sympathetic response. Additionally the sympathetic ganglia are located closer to the central nervous system, such that sympathetic postganglionic fibers radiate more widely before reaching their target organ, resulting in more general and less discrete sympathetic responses.

The Parasympathetic System

The preganglionic cells of the parasympathetic system are restricted to a number of discrete nuclei within the brainstem and to the lateral gray column of a short stretch of the second, third, and possibly fourth sacral spinal cord segments (see Fig. 8.72). The aptly designated craniosacral outflow is thus confined to the oculomotor, facial, glossopharyngeal, vagus, and pelvic nerves, in that only these nerves contain parasympathetic fibers.

The cranial parasympathetic pathways generally travel in cranial nerves alongside somatic axons, and exclusively parasympathetic bundles of axons are found only close to the target organs. The grossly visible features of these cranial nerves have previously been described, so the following account focuses specifically on cranial parasympathetic outflow.

The most rostral parasympathetic nucleus, the parasympathetic oculomotor nucleus, lies within the midbrain in association with the motor nucleus of the third cranial nerve. The parasympathetic preganglionic fibers emerge from the main trunk of the nerve within the orbit to constitute the oculomotor (short) root of the ciliary ganglion. Beyond the ganglion, the postganglionic fibers proceed as the short ciliary nerves, which also incorporate sympathetic and sensory fibers; these nerves penetrate the sclera to form the ciliary plexus from which the parasympathetic fibers extend to the ciliary and pupillary sphincter muscles (Fig. 8.71/*6* and *10*).

The parasympathetic component of the facial nerve originates in the rostral parasympathetic (salivatory) nucleus of the medulla oblongata (Fig. 8.71/*2*). The preganglionic fibers are incorporated within the main facial trunk, run through the somatic geniculate ganglion without interruption, and later leave in the chorda tympani and the greater petrosal nerve (Fig. 8.71/*11* and *13*). The chorda tympani joins with the lingual nerve from which the parasympathetic fibers later emerge to synapse within the mandibular ganglion; the postganglionic fibers supply the mandibular and sublingual salivary glands.

The greater petrosal nerve is joined by the deep petrosal (sympathetic) nerve (Fig. 8.71/*12*) to constitute the nerve of the pterygoid canal, which leads to the pterygopalatine ganglion (Fig. 8.71/*7*). The postganglionic parasympathetic fibers join the lacrimal nerve (after passage through the zygomatic nerve) en route to the lacrimal gland and various other branches of the maxillary nerve and then to glands within the nasal and palatine mucosae.

The parasympathetic component of the glossopharyngeal nerve originates from the middle parasympathetic nucleus in the medulla oblongata (Fig. 8.71/*3*). The preganglionic fibers pass through the somatic ganglion of this nerve before joining the tympanic plexus; from this they proceed to and synapse in the otic ganglion (Fig. 8.71/*9*). The postganglionic fibers are carried via the pterygoid nerve and a communicating branch of the auriculotemporal nerve to the parotid gland.

The parasympathetic component of the vagus nerve constitutes the bulk of the nerve; indeed, the vagus is composed completely of parasympathetic fibers distal to the origin of the recurrent laryngeal nerve (Fig. 8.72/*5* and *6*). The preganglionic parasympathetic fibers synapse in numerous small ganglia scattered along the nerve plexuses that supply and are often located within the tissues of the target organs. The plexuses include the cardiac and pulmonary plexuses within the chest (Fig. 8.72/*7*) and the gastric, hepatic, mesenteric, gonadal, and renal plexuses within the abdomen formed by the convergence of branches of the vagal trunks with sympathetic nerves (Fig. 8.72/*10*). Broadly, the dorsal vagal trunk supplies hepatic and gastric plexuses, and the larger ventral vagal trunk supplies celiac, mesenteric, renal, and gonadal plexuses.

The fibers of the sacral parasympathetic outflow are initially incorporated in certain sacral ventral rami, from which they emerge to constitute the pelvic nerves (Fig. 8.72/*11*). These nerves form a retroperitoneal plexus, being joined by sympathetic fibers delivered by the hypogastric nerves that descend from the caudal mesenteric ganglion. Numerous small ganglia are found scattered in the plexus, whereas other (terminal) ganglia are embedded within the walls of predominantly pelvic viscera: the descending colon, rectum, bladder, uterus, and vagina (in the female); accessory reproductive glands (in the male); and the genital erectile tissue. The parasympathetic pathways synapse exclusively in the terminal ganglia, whereas some sympathetic peripheral synapses are divided among the plexus and terminal ganglia.

The Sympathetic System

The preganglionic axons of the sympathetic system originate from sympathetic preganglionic neurons located in the lateral gray column of the thoracolumbar part of the spinal cord (Fig. 8.73/*1*) and pass into the ventral roots of the thoracic and first several lumbar nerves. They continue into the spinal nerves and then leave the ventral rami, becoming the myelinated communicating branches (Fig. 8.73/*2*), which join the ganglia of the sympathetic trunk (Figs. 8.53/*5* and *7* and 8.73/*3*). These bilateral trunks run the length of the neck and back, and each has a segmental arrangement, although strict correspondence of the ganglia with spinal nerves is evident only in the thoracic and cranial lumbar regions.

The cervical part of the trunk begins at the large, spindle-shaped, cranial cervical ganglion placed close to the base of the skull (Fig. 8.73/*5*). The cervical trunk is associated with the vagus within the carotid sheath and forms the vagosympathetic trunk that proceeds down the neck. Whereas the vagus contains parasympathetic axons travelling caudally to innervate thoracic and abdominal viscera, the sympathetic trunk in the neck contains sympathetic axons travelling cranially to innervate structures of the head. The two components part company at the entrance to the chest, where the sympathetic trunk often bears a middle cervical ganglion by the first rib (Fig. 8.76/*7'*). The thoracic part of the sympathetic trunk then continues subpleurally, over the line of the costovertebral articulations, before passing dorsal to the diaphragm to enter the abdomen. Its thoracic part contains regularly spaced ganglia, although the first one or two are fused with caudal cervical ganglia to form the large cervicothoracic ganglion deep to the head of the first rib (Fig. 8.76/*7*). The lumbar part of the trunk, which lies between the psoas musculature and vertebral bodies, at first also carries a regular arrangement of ganglia, but the arrangement later becomes more erratic in that some caudal lumbar ganglia split into two or, less commonly, fuse with their neighbors. The sacral part is even less regular, and right and left trunks may fuse, temporarily or finally, before extending into the tail, where it rapidly fades (Fig. 8.73/*3*).

The locations of preganglionic sympathetic neurons are restricted to the thoracic and lumbar spinal segments, so it follows that only the thoracic and cranial lumbar ganglia are connected by myelinated communicating branches. However, all spinal and many cranial nerves are joined by unmyelinated communicating branches of postganglionic fibers destined for vessels, skin glands, and so forth. It should be stressed that the body wall and limbs are innervated only by these postganglionic sympathetic fibers. Sympathetic fibers contributing to most cervical nerves join within a single trunk, the vertebral nerve, which runs from the cervicothoracic ganglion through the foramina of successive cervical transverse processes (Fig. 8.73/*7*). The postganglionic sympathetic fibers traveling along with the first two cervical nerves and alongside cranial nerves extend from the cranial cervical ganglion; many form the internal carotid nerve that follows the internal carotid artery.

Several alternative fates are possibly with the preganglionic sympathetic fibers that enter the sympathetic chain, each to project on many ganglion cells. Some fibers synapse immediately within the local ganglion, others run cranially or caudally within the trunk to synapse within ganglia that are more cranial or caudal in the series, and yet others pass uninterruptedly through the trunk to proceed to a second set of (prevertebral) ganglia placed about the origin of the visceral branches of the abdominal aorta (Figs. 8.73/*10* and *11* and 8.76/*11* and *12*). This last group constitutes the splanchnic nerves, which are rather variable in arrangement; usually one *greater splanchnic nerve* is formed by preganglionic fibers that leave the trunk from about the sixth to the penultimate thoracic ganglia, with *lesser thoracic and lumbar splanchnic nerves* arising at more caudal levels (Fig. 8.73/*8* and *9*).

The viscera and vessels of the head receive their sympathetic innervation via the cranial cervical ganglion (Fig. 8.71/*5*). The postganglionic fibers that emerge from this ganglion radiate in a number of directions that carry them into the territories of the cranial nerves and the first two cervical nerves. Though many fibers pass through parasympathetic ganglia, they of course do so without interruption. The details are of rather limited clinical importance (although relevant to experimental work), and only a few points are presented here (see Fig. 8.71).

One large group of fibers follows the internal carotid artery into the cranial cavity and there provides twigs to the intracranial vessels and fiber bundles that join various nerves, especially the trigeminal and those to the extraocular muscles. Another group of fibers passes through the ciliary ganglion to the eyeball for ultimate distribution to the dilator pupillae. At a more proximal level, the *internal carotid nerve* gives off the deep petrosal nerve, which combines with the greater petrosal nerve (Fig. 8.71/*11*) in its passage through the pterygoid canal to the pterygopalatine ganglion (Fig. 8.71/*7*). These fibers are ultimately dispersed with the various nerves that supply structures within the orbit, nasal cavity, sinuses, and palate.

Other branches participate with parasympathetic fibers in forming a plexus within the tympanic cavity from which the parotid gland is supplied after passage beyond the otic ganglion. Yet other bundles of fibers entwine the external carotid artery and its branches.

The thoracic organs—heart, trachea, and lungs—are supplied by postganglionic fibers that form cardiac and pulmonary plexuses within the mediastinum after leaving the thoracic portion of the sympathetic trunk. These

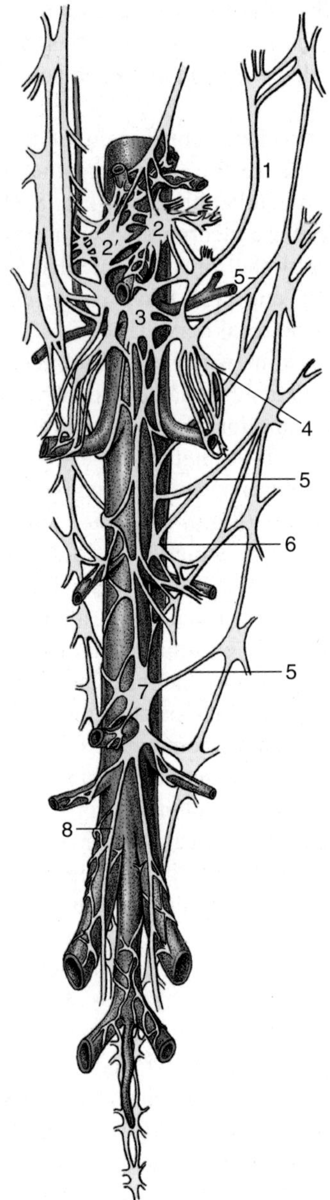

Fig. 8.77 Ganglia and plexuses of the abdominal cavity. Ventral view. *1*, Greater splanchnic nerve ; *2*, left celiac ganglion; *2'*, right celiac ganglion; *3*, cranial mesenteric ganglion; *4*, renal ganglion; *5*, lumbar splanchnic nerves; *6*, gonadal ganglion; *7*, caudal mesenteric ganglion; *8*, right hypogastric nerve.

plexuses combine with the corresponding parasympathetic component (see Fig. 8.76).

The abdominal and pelvic organs receive their sympathetic innervation through the various splanchnic nerves that lead to the celiac, cranial mesenteric, renal, aorticorenal, gonadal, and caudal mesenteric ganglia placed on the ventral face of the aorta by the origins of the visceral arteries. The preganglionic fibers synapse in these ganglia, and the postganglionic fibers that emerge from intricate plexuses (combining vagal contributions) enmesh, and run parallel to, the visceral arteries from which they obtain their names (Fig. 8.77).

TABLE 8.3 ACTIONS CONTROLLED BY THE AUTONOMIC NERVOUS SYSTEM

Sympathetic Innervation			Parasympathetic Innervation	
Source	**Effect**	**Target Organ**	**Effect**	**Source**
Cranial thoracic segment via cranial cervical ganglion	Dilation of pupil	Iris	Contraction of pupil	Oculomotor n. via ciliary ganglion
Cranial thoracic segment via cranial cervical ganglion	Relaxation: Accommodation for distant vision	Ciliary muscle	Contraction: Accommodation for near vision	Oculomotor n. via ciliary ganglion
Cranial thoracic segment via cranial cervical ganglion	Vasoconstriction and contraction of myoepithelial cells	Salivary glands	Vasodilation and secretion	Facial n. via mandibular ganglion Glossopharyngeal n. via otic ganglion
Cranial thoracic segment via cranial cervical ganglion	Vasoconstriction	Lacrimal gland	Secretion	Facial n. via pterygopalatine ganglion
Cranial thoracic segments	Increased activity	Heart	Reduced activity	Vagus n. via cardiac ganglia
Thoracic and lumbar segments	Vasoconstriction in some tissues, e.g., skin; vasodilation in others, e.g., skeletal muscle	Blood vessels	Vasodilation, and possibly vasoconstriction in some vessels	
Cranial thoracic segments	Relaxation	Bronchi	Constriction	Vagus n.
Caudal thoracic segments	Secretion	Adrenal medulla		
Caudal thoracic and lumbar segments via abdominal ganglia	Decreased activity	Gastrointestinal tract	Increased motility and secretion	Vagus n. and pelvic nn.
Lumbar segments via abdominal ganglia	Relaxation	Bladder wall	Contraction	Pelvic nn.
		Erectile tissue	Vasodilation	Pelvic nn.

n., nerve; nn., nerves.

The pelvic organs are supplied with postganglionic fibers that leave the caudal mesenteric ganglion within the paired hypogastric nerves (Fig. 8.77/*8*). These fibres enter the pelvic cavity below the peritoneum to form a common pelvic plexus with the parasympathetic pelvic nerves (Fig. 8.76). As already mentioned, the sympathetic contribution to the pelvic plexus includes preganglionic sympathetic fibers that synapse in peripheral locations within the pelvis.

Summary of Autonomic Innervation

Certain effects of the autonomic nervous system are tabulated (Table 8.3) by way of illustration, but for more controversial points, such as the innervation of the bladder and urethra, or those requiring more detailed description, the reader is referred to modern works of physiology.

COMPREHENSION CHECK

Knowledge of the cellular components, the neural pathways, and the gross structure of the nervous system has not yet provided us with a thorough picture of how the nervous system works. What more must be understood to inform our understanding of how the nervous system functions and produces behavior?

9 The Sense Organs

In order to detect changes in the environment, animals must necessarily have mechanisms to sense these changes. The sense organs are receptive structures, located in the head and throughout the skin, muscles, and internal organs, that are each able to detect changes in specific sensory modalities, including pressure, light, sound, and stretch. Some sensory receptors are part of the nervous system proper—the receptors in the skin and throughout the body that detect noxious stimuli, for example—but most receptors are composed of both neural and nonneural tissue. Stretch receptors located in muscle, known as *muscle spindles,* are composed largely of specialized muscle cells. The eye is a highly complex structure of which only the retina is of neural origin. Regardless of its composition, each receptor is connected with a sensory neuron that transmits information about the activity of the receptor, in the form of a series of action potentials, to the central nervous system.

Many of the senses are conscious, meaning that the animal is aware of what it has registered. However, there are sensory systems associated with muscle and viscera of which the animal is less aware and through which it is in touch with the "internal environment" of its own body.

The sense organs are generally classified into those of special sense—eye, ear, smell, taste—and the more general senses of touch, pressure, and pain. The organs of special sense are described first.

THE EYE

The eye, the organ of vision, consists of the eyeball and various adnexa—accessory structures such as the ocular muscles that move the eyeball, the lids that protect it, and the lacrimal apparatus that keeps its exposed parts moist. Most of the adnexa are housed in the orbit, where the eyeball is embedded in generous quantities of fat. The eyelids arise from the bony margins of the orbit and, like curtains, are intermittently drawn over the exposed part of the eye (blinking) to distribute the tears or lacrimal fluid for protection; they are kept across the eye during sleep, when vision is not required.

The eyes of the domestic mammals protrude more from the surface of the face than those of primates, ourselves included. Their position in the head is related to the animal's environment, habits, and method of feeding. In general, predatory species (cat, dog) have eyes set well forward, to provide a large field of binocular vision that allows for focus on near objects and for the perception of depth (Fig. 9.1). Prey species (herbivores: horses, ruminants, rabbits) carry their eyes more laterally so that the right and left fields of vision hardly overlap; consequently, these animals have a large field of vision but little capacity for binocular vision.

When an animal is emaciated, the orbital fat is reduced and the eyes sink within the orbits, giving the face a gaunt appearance.

THE EYEBALL

The eyeball (bulbus oculi) of the domestic mammals is nearly spherical but with some anteroposterior* compression in horses and cattle. In addition, the cornea, the transparent part of the eyeball, bulges from the anterior surface by virtue of its smaller radius of curvature (Fig. 9.2).

The optic axis is the straight line passing through the highest point on the cornea, the *anterior pole,* and the highest point on the posterior surface, the *posterior pole* of the eyeball. The *equator* is an imaginary line about the eyeball that, like that of the Earth, is equidistant from the poles. A *meridian* is one of the many lines passing from pole to pole that intersect the equator at right angles. The optic nerve (Fig. 9.2/*6*) leaves the eyeball slightly ventral to the posterior pole.

The eyeball has three thin tunics that, being in close apposition, form a laminated sheet that surrounds the partly liquid, partly gelatinous center. The three tunics are (1) an external fibrous tunic, the only complete tunic, that provides form and protection to the eyeball; (2) a middle vascular tunic, rich in blood vessels and smooth muscle, that supplies nutrients to the eyeball and contributes to the regulation of the shape of the lens and size of the pupil; and (3) an internal nervous tunic, consisting largely of nervous tissue, that is the layer most directly concerned with vision—the translation of visual stimuli into nerve impulses for interpretation by the brain.

The Fibrous Tunic

The fibrous tunic of the eyeball is made up of very dense collagenous tissue that, by resisting the internal pressure, gives the eye shape and stiffness. It consists of the sclera and cornea, which meet at the *limbus* (Fig. 9.2/*7*).

* *Anterior* and *posterior,* in front of and behind, respectively, are used instead of *rostral* and *caudal* to refer to the eye.

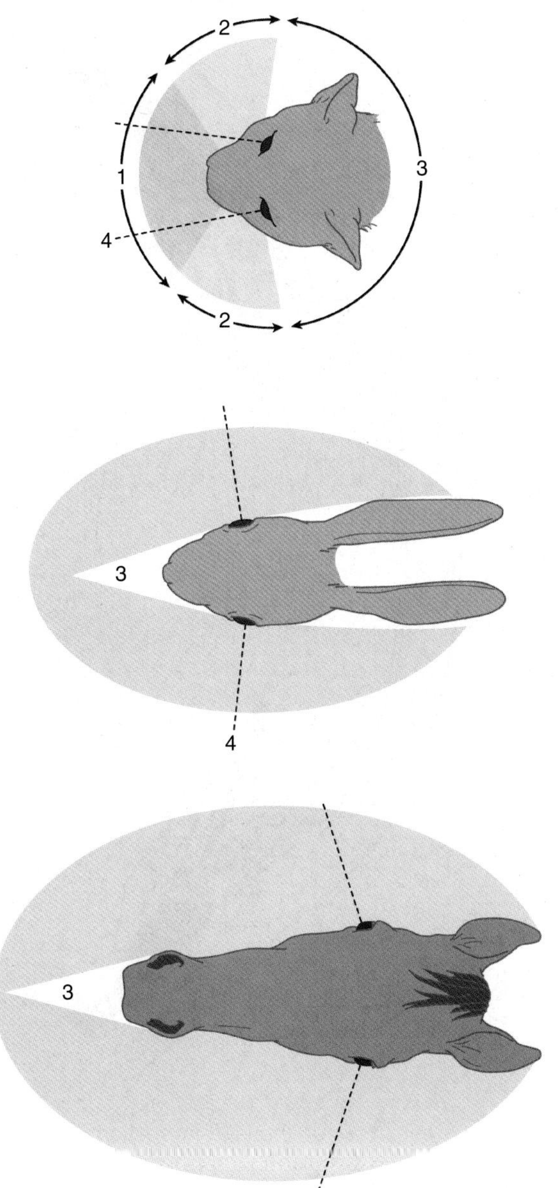

Fig. 9.1 Visual fields of *(top to bottom)* cat, rabbit, and horse. *1,* Binocular vision; *2,* monocular vision; *3,* blind area; *4,* visual axis of eye in central position.

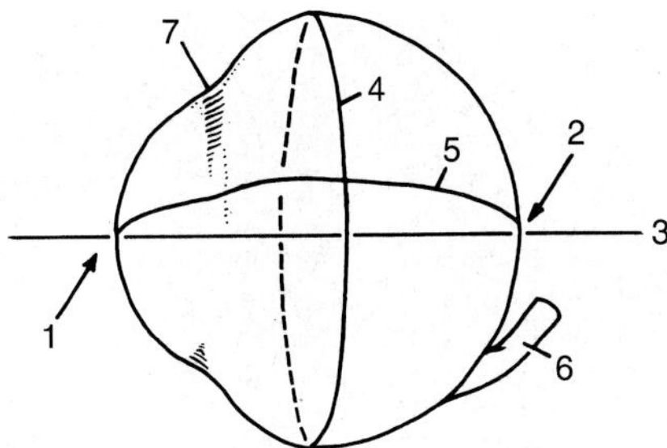

Fig. 9.2 Medial view of right eyeball. *1,* Anterior pole; *2,* posterior pole; *3,* optic axis; *4,* equator; *5,* a meridian; *6,* optic nerve; *7,* limbus.

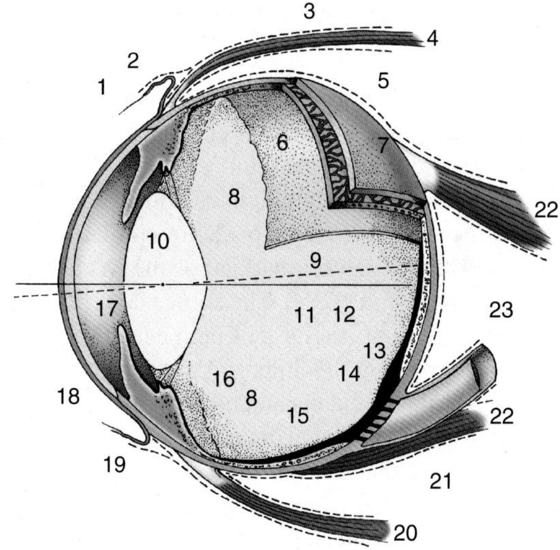

Fig. 9.3 Eye opened to show the three tunics, which have been drawn thicker than they actually are. *1,* Limbus; *2,* upper fornix; *3,* deep muscular fascia; *4,* dorsal rectus muscle; *5,* vagina bulbi; *6,* choroid; *7,* sclera; *8,* ora serrata; *9,* retina; *10,* lens; *11,* optic axis; *12,* visual axis; *13,* area cribrosa; *14,* optic disk; *15,* retina; *16,* ciliary body; *17,* iris; *18,* cornea; *19,* conjunctiva; *20,* ventral rectus muscle; *21,* optic nerve; *22,* retractor bulbi; *23,* sheath of optic nerve.

The *sclera* is the opaque posterior part of the fibrous tunic. It consists of a dense feltwork of collagenous and elastic fibers and is generally white ("the white of the eye"), though with a bluish tinge; in some species it contains pigmented cells that render it gray. Ventral to the posterior pole, the sclera consists of a small cribriform area (Fig. 9.3/*13*) through which the fibers of the optic nerve pass. The nerve is surrounded by a connective tissue sheath that continues the dura mater to the sclera. The sclera is also pierced by several small ciliary arteries and nerves and by larger veins known as *vorticose veins*. The sclera provides attachment to the tendons of the ocular muscles anterior to the equator. Posteriorly, except for the areas taken up by the retractor bulbi muscle, the sclera is covered by a thin membrane (vagina bulbi; Fig. 9.3/*5*) that separates it from the retrobulbar fat, which forms a socket in which the eyeball can rotate. Near the limbus, the sclera is covered by conjunctiva (see later), which provides a connection to the inside of the lids (Fig. 9.3/*19*).

The *cornea,* which forms about one quarter of the fibrous tunic and bulges forward (Fig. 9.4), is composed of a special kind of dense connective tissue arranged in lamellar form. It is generally recognized that, in addition to the careful arrangement of its fibers, transparency is not only a structural but also a physiologic phenomenon and depends on the continuous pumping out of interstitial fluids, a process that occurs in the posterior epithelium. The main bulk

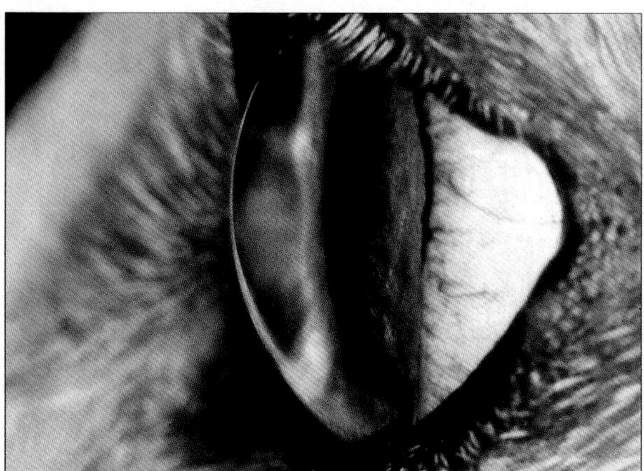

Fig. 9.4 Curvature of canine cornea.

of the cornea, the *substantia propria,* is continuous with the sclera (Fig. 9.5/*6* and *9*) and is encased by anterior and posterior limiting membranes and epithelial layers. The anterior epithelial layer is continuous with the epithelium of the conjunctiva, whereas the posterior epithelial layer is continuous with the anterior surface of the iris across the iridocorneal angle (Fig. 9.5/*4*). The cornea does not contain blood vessels; nutrients for its cells permeate the substantia propria from vessels in the limbus or are carried to its surfaces in the lacrimal fluid and aqueous humor. The surface of the cornea is very sensitive owing to the presence of free nerve endings near the anterior epithelium. They arise from the long ciliary nerves, which are branches of the ophthalmic nerve (described later).

The Vascular Tunic

The vascular tunic of the eye (also known as the *uvea*) lies deep to the sclera to which it is apposed. It consists of three zones: choroid, ciliary body, and iris, in posteroanterior sequence (see Fig. 9.3). The choroid, the most posterior zone, lines the sclera from the optic nerve almost to the limbus; the ciliary body is a thickened zone opposite the limbus; the iris projects into the cavity of the eyeball posterior to the cornea. The iris is the only internal structure readily seen through the cornea without the use of an instrument such as an ophthalmoscope. The principal function of the vascular tunic is to provide a blood supply to structures of the eye, but it also serves to suspend the lens, regulate the lens curvature, and adjust the size of the pupil by means of the smooth muscle in the ciliary body and iris (see Fig. 9.5).

The *choroid* contains a dense network of blood vessels embedded in heavily pigmented connective tissue. The network is supplied by the posterior ciliary arteries and is drained by the vorticose veins. A flat sheet of capillaries on the internal surface is responsible for the nutrition of the external layers of the nervous tunic (retina), which lies deep (internal) to the choroid. The blood in these capillaries produces the redness of the fundus (interior

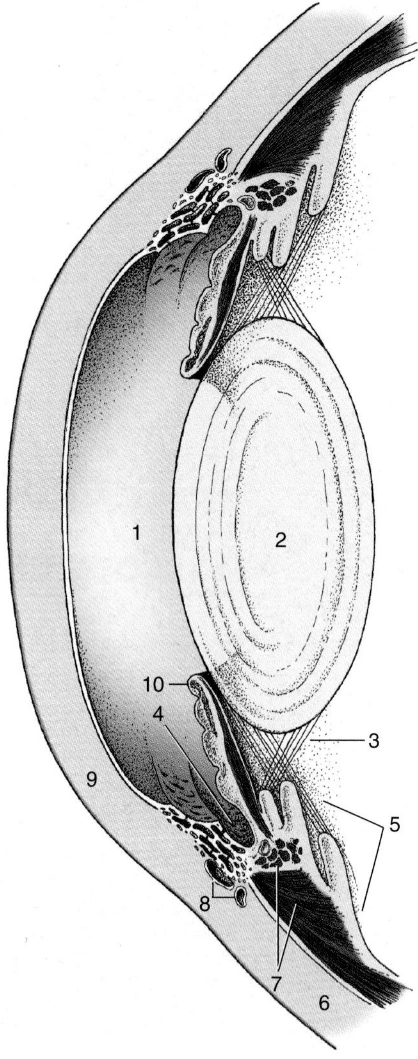

Fig. 9.5 Anterior part of the eye in section. *1,* Anterior chamber; *2,* lens; *3,* zonular fibers; *4,* iridocorneal angle; *5,* ciliary body; *6,* sclera; *7,* ciliary muscles; *8,* venous plexus of sclera; *9,* cornea; *10,* iris with the sphincter and dilator muscles shown.

surface of the posterior hemisphere) seen when the eye is examined with an ophthalmoscope. In the dorsal part of the fundus, the choroid forms a variously colored, light-reflecting area known as the *tapetum lucidum* (Fig. 9.6). This is an avascular layer (cellular in carnivores, fibrous in ruminants and horses) between the capillaries and the network of larger vessels. The tapetal cells contain crystalline rods arranged in such a way that light striking them is split into its components, which results in the characteristic iridescence. In the fibrous tapetum, the packaging of the collagen has the same effect. The tapetum makes the eyes of animals "shine" when they look toward a light, such as the headlights of an oncoming car. The eyes of the human and the pig do not have a tapetum and therefore do

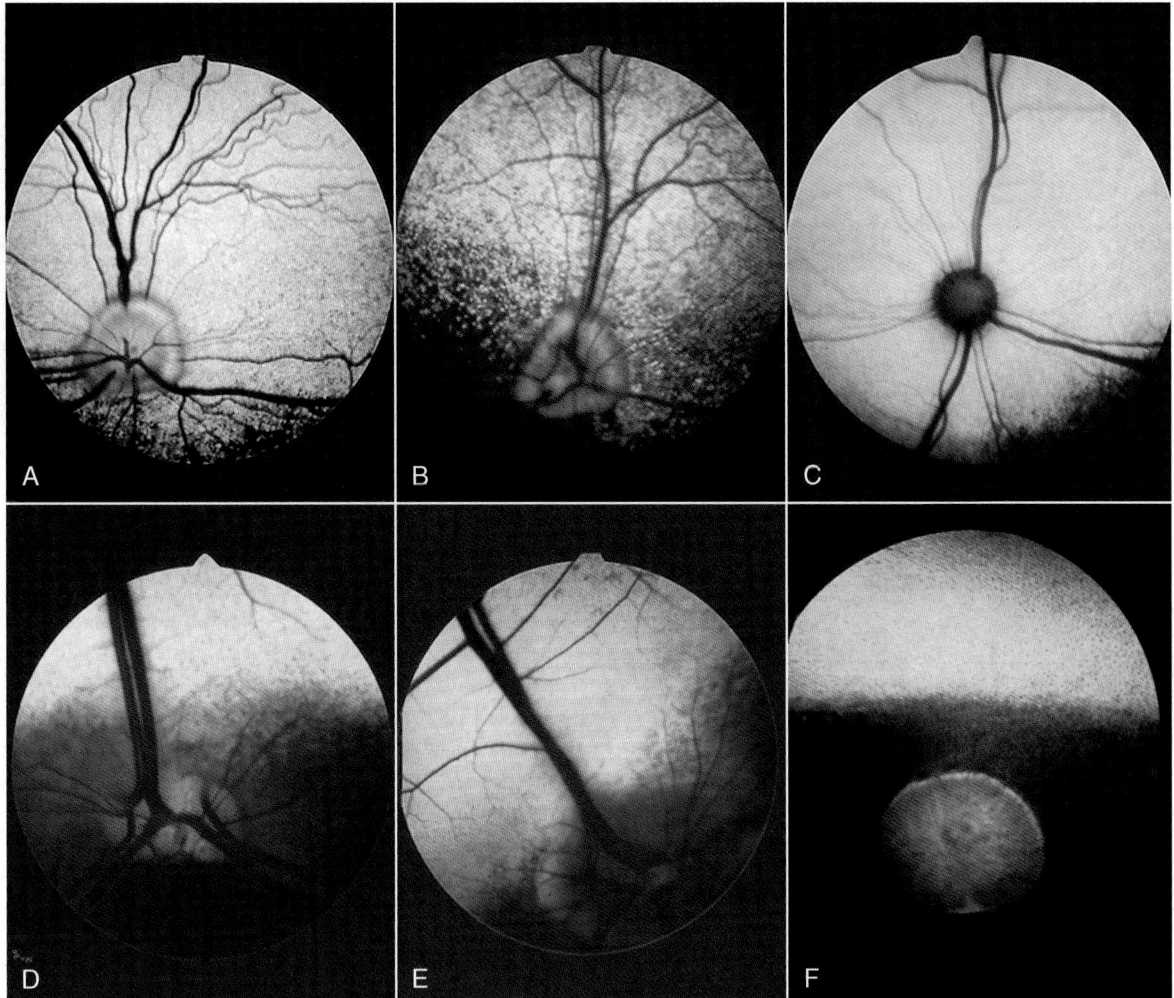

Fig. 9.6 Fundus of the eye of (A) Dutch Sheepdog, (B) Old English Sheepdog, (C) cat, (D) cow, (E) goat, and (F) horse.

not give this effect. It is believed that the tapetum is a nocturnal adaptation: by reflecting incident light, it increases the stimulation of the light-sensitive receptor cells in the overlying retina and thus aids vision in dark places. The choroid adheres closely to the pigmented external layer of the retina, so that the pigmented layer remains attached to the choroid when the bulk of the retina is removed during dissection. The retina is without pigment where it overlies the tapetum lucidum.

Toward the limbus, the choroid thickens to form the *ciliary body* (Fig. 9.5/*5*). This structure is a raised ring with ridges converging toward the lens in the center; anteriorly the ring is continued by the iris. One can best understand the ciliary body when seeing it in its entirety by looking into the anterior part of the eye from behind (Figs. 9.7/*2* and 9.8). The radial ridges, known as the *ciliary processes,* extend *zonular fibers* (Fig. 9.5/*3*) to the equator of the lens, suspending it around its periphery. Between the ciliary body and the sclera is the smooth *ciliary muscle* (Fig. 9.5/*7*), which functions in accommodation, the ability of the eye to focus on near or distant objects by changing the shape of the lens (described later).

The third and smallest part of the vascular tunic is the iris (Fig. 9.5/*10*), which is suspended between the cornea and lens. It is a flat ring of tissue attached at its periphery to the sclera (by the pectinate ligament; Fig. 9.12/*7*) and to the ciliary body. The opening in the center is the *pupil* (Fig. 9.9) through which light enters the posterior part of the eye. The size of the pupil and therefore the amount of light reaching the retina are regulated by two smooth muscles in the iris: the sphincter (constrictor) muscle and the dilator muscle. The sphincter lies near the pupillary margin, but the fibers of the dilator are arranged radially and, on contraction, enlarge the pupil. Irregular outgrowths (iridic granules; Fig. 9.9) containing coils of capillaries are often seen on the upper and lower pupillary margins of ungulates; their significance is not known, although there are suggestions that they act as "shades."

The iris divides the space between the lens and cornea into anterior and posterior chambers that communicate

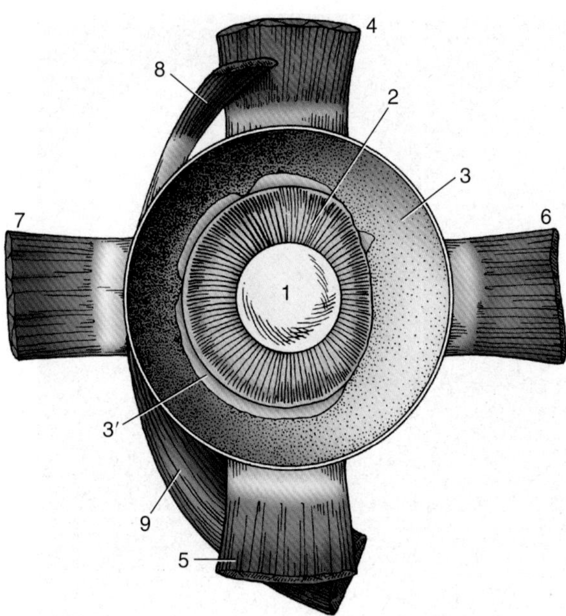

Fig. 9.7 Anterior half of the left equine eye, viewed from behind. *1*, Lens; *2*, ciliary body; *3*, choroid covered by pigmented outer layer of retina; *3′*, remnants of inner nervous layer of retina, which has been removed; *4*, *5*, *6*, and *7*, dorsal, ventral, medial, and lateral rectus muscles; *8* and *9*, dorsal and ventral oblique muscles.

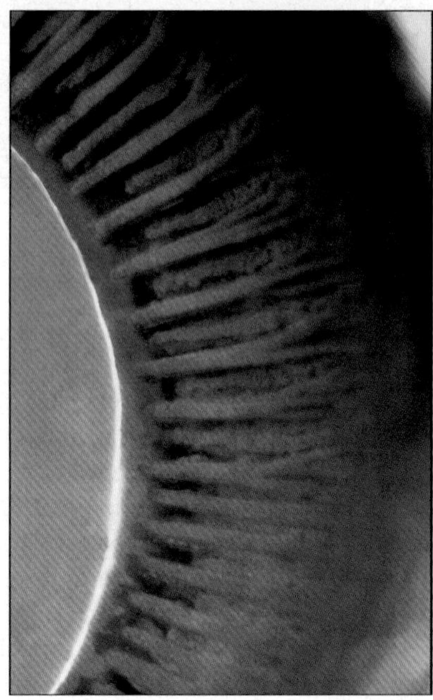

Fig. 9.8 Posterior view of ciliary body with ciliary processes (horse).

through the pupil (see Fig. 9.9). Both are filled with *aqueous humor*, a clear watery fluid (described later).

The iris consists of three layers: an anterior epithelial layer that is continuous across the iridocorneal angle and blends with the posterior epithelium of the cornea; a middle layer of connective tissue stroma that contains the two smooth muscles; and a posterior layer of pigmented epithelium that is the forward extension of the pigmented layer of the retina mentioned earlier. The posterior layer is known as the iridic part of the retina and is adjacent to the dilator muscle (Fig. 9.5/*10*).

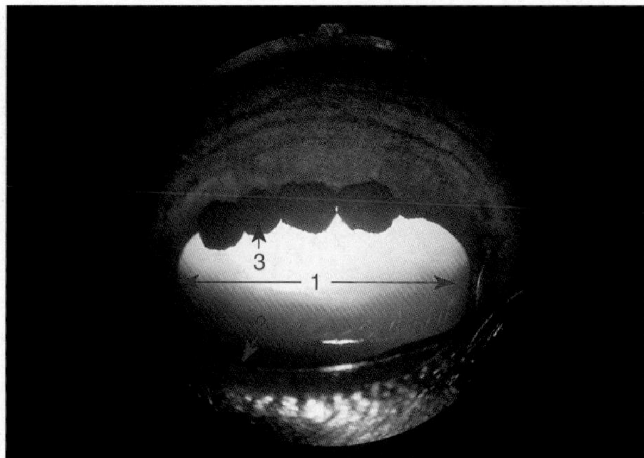

Fig. 9.9 Anterior surface of the equine iris with characteristic iridic granules. *1*, Pupil; *2*, pupillary margin; *3*, iridic granule.

The color of the iris determines the "color of the eye" and depends both on the number of pigmented cells present in the stroma and on the type of pigment present in the cells. If the pigmented cells (melanocytes) are tightly packed, the iris is dark brown (Fig. 9.10); with fewer cells the iris is lighter and yellowish; a minimum of pigmented cells results in a bluish appearance. In albino animals, pigment is absent from the iridic part of the retina, such that the iris is totally devoid of pigment; albino eyes appear red because the blood in the capillaries is not obscured by pigment.

The Internal Tunic

The internal or nervous tunic of the eyeball contains the light-sensitive receptor cells and is known as the *retina* (Fig. 9.3/*9* and *15*). The retina develops as an extension of the brain to which it remains connected by the optic nerve. The retina begins where the nerve penetrates the choroid; shaped like a hollow cup, it lines the inner surface of the eye and ends at the pupillary margin. Only the posterior two thirds or so of the retina can be reached by light entering the pupil. Consequently, only that portion (*pars optica retinae*) is provided with photoreceptor cells and is relatively thick. The remaining anterior third is without photoreceptors and is therefore "blind" (*pars ceca retinae*) and constitutes the pigmented layer that continues on to the ciliary body and the back of the iris. The edge caused by the abrupt decrease in retinal thickness at the junction of optic and blind parts is the *ora serrata* (Fig. 9.3/*8*); it also demarcates the choroid from the ciliary body. The two layers of the retina develop from the inner and outer layers of the optic cup with which the eye makes its appearance in

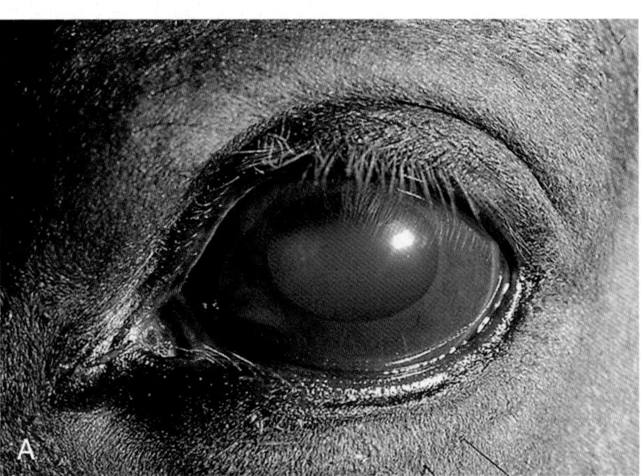

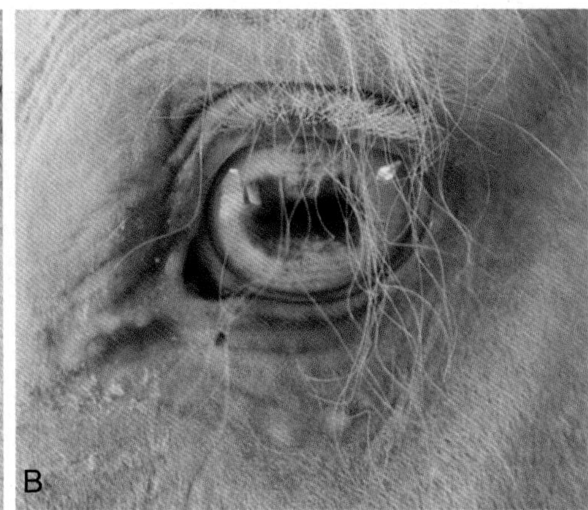

Fig. 9.10 (A) Left equine eye. Note the brown pigmentation of the iris. (B) Left equine eye of an albino animal. Note the absence of pigment.

the embryo. The gap between the layers of the optic cup, though obliterated postnatally, remains a weakness where delamination produces "detachment" of the retina.

The presence of large amounts of retinal and choroidal pigment makes the interior of the posterior part of the eye dark like the inside of a camera so that the pupil appears black. The black walls absorb scattered and reflected light and prevent it from striking the retina a second time, which would contribute to blurred vision.

The layers in the pars optica retinae are as follows, beginning at the choroid and moving inward: a single layer of pigmented cells; a neuroepithelial layer containing the photoreceptor cells—that is, the rods and cones (the rods, so far as we know, are concerned with black and white [night] and the cones with color [day] vision) (Fig. 9.11/*2*); a layer of bipolar ganglion cells (Fig. 9.11/*3*); and a layer of multipolar ganglion cells whose nonmyelinated axons, lying internal (deep) to the cells, pass to the optic disk, where they aggregate to form the optic nerve (Fig. 9.11/*4*). It is clear from this arrangement that light passes through all layers except the first before reaching and stimulating the rods and cones.

The area where the axons of the fourth layer converge to leave the eye, the *optic disk,* can easily be seen when the fundus is examined with an ophthalmoscope (see Fig. 9.6). Because the axons here turn in toward the cribriform area of the sclera, there is no room for receptor cells; the optic disk, therefore, is a blind spot. In contrast, an area of maximum optical resolution (macula) is located a short distance dorsolateral to the optic disk. It is believed that when we examine objects intently, we focus them on the macula. It is not known whether animals do the same. In some species the macula is faintly visible with the ophthalmoscope. The *visual axis* is the line connecting the macula, the center of the lens, and the object viewed. It does not quite coincide with the optic axis because the macula is slightly dorsal to the posterior pole of the eyeball (see Fig. 9.3).

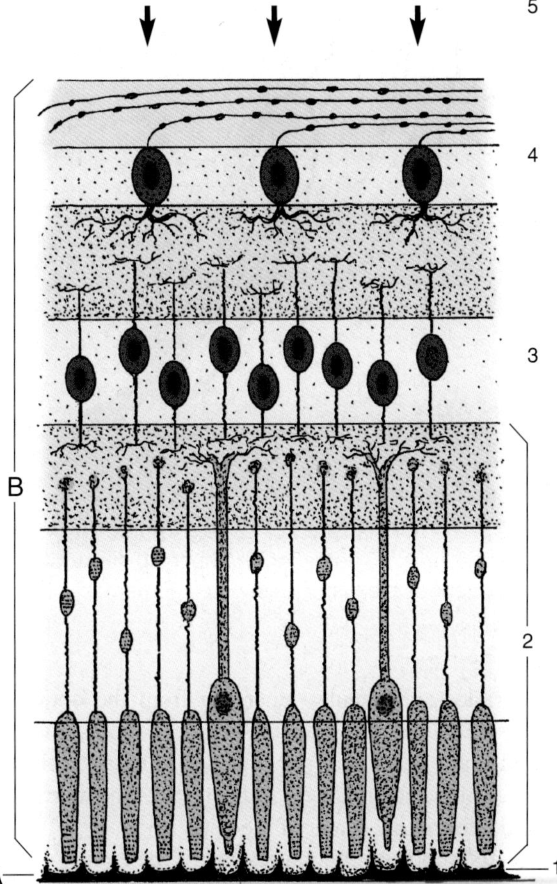

Fig. 9.11 (A) Outer pigmented layer and (B) inner neuroepithelial layer of retina. *1,* Pigmented cells; *2,* receptor cells (rods and cones); *3,* bipolar ganglion cells; *4,* multipolar ganglion cells; *5,* incoming light *(arrows).*

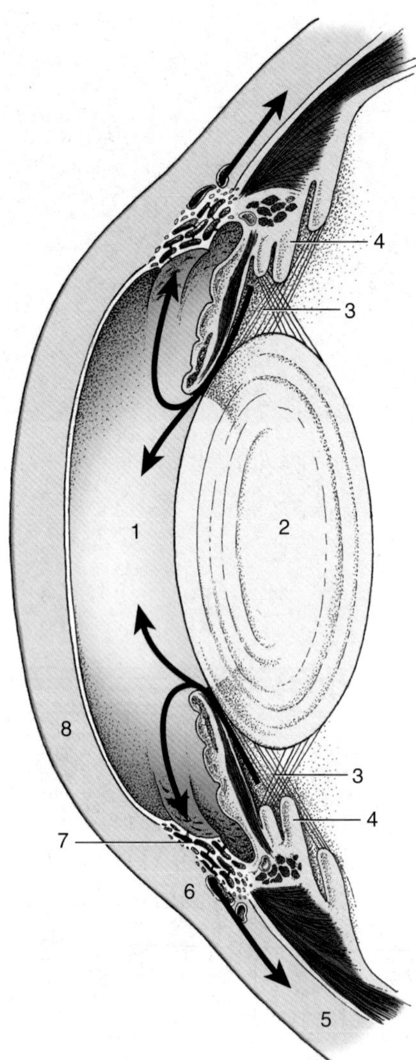

Fig. 9.12 The flow *(arrows)* of aqueous humor. *1,* Anterior chamber; *2,* lens; *3,* posterior chamber; *4,* ciliary body; *5,* sclera; *6,* venous plexus; *7,* pectinate ligament; *8,* cornea.

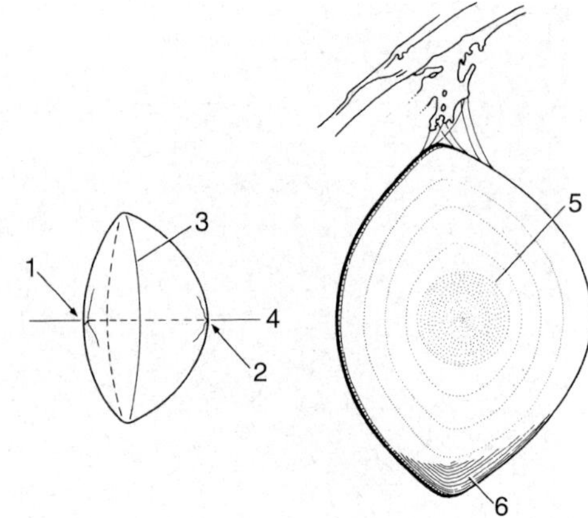

Fig. 9.13 Bovine lens; on the *right,* a meridional section. *1,* Anterior pole with lens star; *2,* posterior pole with lens star; *3,* equator; *4,* optic axis; *5,* nucleus; *6,* layers of lens fibers, shown only in part.

Arterioles and venules emerging from the optic disk spread out in various species-specific patterns to nourish and drain the retina (see Fig. 9.6). The arterioles are branches of the central artery of the retina, which arrives at the optic disk in the center of the optic nerve.

The anteroposterior compression of the equine eyeball has led to the assumption that the horse has a ramp retina. A ramp retina is one in which all parts of the retina are not equidistant from the posterior pole of the lens; the distance from the lens becomes progressively greater as the retina is followed dorsally. Presumably, as increasingly closer objects are viewed, they are focused on the more dorsal parts of the retina; focal length is automatically increased, and little accommodation of the lens is required (p. 516).

The Refractive Media of the Eyeball

Now that the layers of the wall of the eyeball have been explained, the interior of the eyeball is described by following the path taken by light entering the eye.

Light first enters the *cornea,* an integral part of the supporting fibrous tunic. Although dense and tough, it has the quality of being transparent and thus enables light to enter the eye. The cornea plays a major role in refraction; that is, it is capable, as is the lens, of bending light so that what is seen by the animal is miniaturized sufficiently to be focused on the retina.

The rays next encounter the *aqueous humor* filling the space between cornea and lens. The aqueous humor is a clear watery fluid that, apart from its refractive properties, plays an important role in the maintenance of intraocular pressure. It is continuously produced by cells of the ciliary processes and enters the system in the posterior chamber, caudal to the iris. From here it passes through the pupil into the anterior chamber and thence through the spaces in the trabecular tissue (pectinate ligament) at the iridocorneal angle. These spaces carry the fluid to venous sinuses in the sclera and thus into the bloodstream (Fig. 9.12). In the healthy eye, the rate of production balances the rate of drainage, maintaining a constant pressure. Interference with drainage allows excess fluid to accumulate, causing the intraocular pressure to rise (glaucoma). This serious condition is less common in domestic animals than it is in humans.

The *lens* (Fig. 9.13), in contrast to its liquid neighbors, is a solid structure, though sufficiently elastic to be able to change in shape. It is biconvex and has anterior and posterior poles, an equator, and a central axis that coincides with the optic axis of the eye. The posterior surface is usually more convex than the anterior. The lens has an outer capsule that is thicker anteriorly and thickest at the equator, where the zonular fibers of the ciliary body

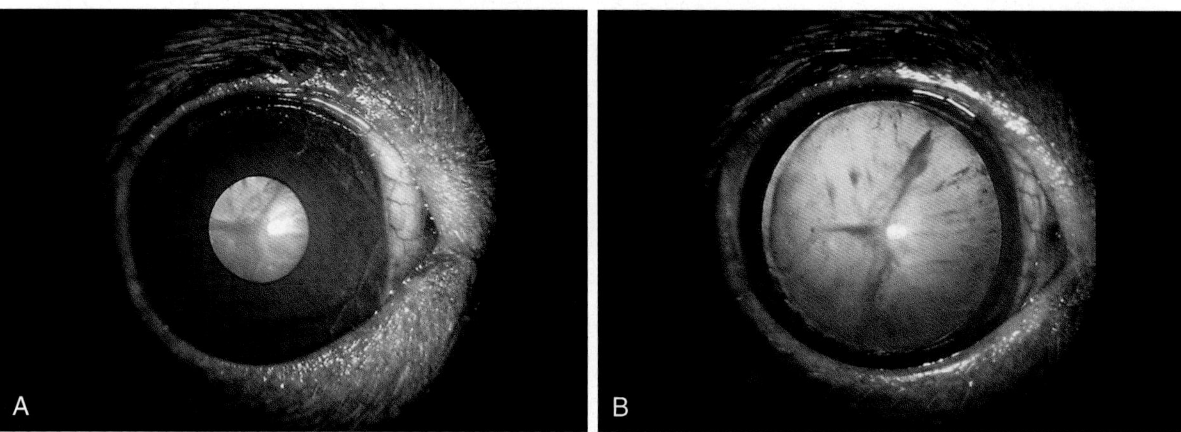

Fig. 9.14 (A) Slightly constricted canine pupil. Cataract of lens visible. (B) Canine pupil in mydriasis (enlarged pupil). Lens is now totally visible; opacity is seen to affect the entire lens.

are attached. The capsule of the lens is elastic and is permanently under tension, which, if unopposed by the pull exerted at the periphery, would cause the lens to assume a more spherical shape. The substance of the lens consists of very regularly arranged fibers. They form concentric sheets that can be peeled off like the layers of an onion. Within each sheet, the fibers are arranged so that they loop from a point on the anterior surface to one on the posterior surface. Their ends are cemented to the ends of other fibers, forming visible sutures shaped like little three-pointed stars (radii lentis; Fig. 9.13/*1* and *2*). In the peripheral, or cortical, part of the lens the fibers are relatively soft; they are firmer and thinner toward the center of the lens where they form a harder nucleus. Owing to its elastic properties the cortex can be molded so that the lens changes shape during accommodation. In many older animals the lens becomes cloudy, impairing vision; the condition is known as cataract (Fig. 9.14).

Accommodation. As previously mentioned, the elastic capsule of the lens would squeeze the relatively soft cortex of the lens into a rounder shape unless opposed by the zonular fibers that arise from the ciliary processes, which exert a constant radial pull on the equator. This pull flattens the lens into the resting shape adapted for far vision and present during sleep. When the animal wants to focus on a near object, the muscle on the surface of the ciliary body contracts, thickening the ciliary body. This change displaces the processes toward the lens and thus relaxes the zonular fibers. The lens, released from the tension at its equator, rounds out and brings the object into focus. In comparison with the muscle in humans, the ciliary muscle, and therefore, the ability to accommodate, is poorly developed in domestic animals.

After passing through the lens the light rays enter the *vitreous body.* A gel-like mass consisting mainly of water (vitreous humor), the vitreous body has a stroma of fine transparent fibers that condenses into a membrane at the surface. The body occupies the space between lens and retina and holds the latter against the choroid. In the embryo, the lens is nourished by the hyaloid artery, a branch of the central retinal artery that passes through the vitreous body. The artery usually degenerates after birth, and the lens is then nourished by diffusion (Fig. 9.15). Unlike the aqueous humor, the vitreous humor is not continuously replaced; it is therefore constant in volume.

The Adnexa of the Eye

The structures that protect and move the eyeball include the orbital fasciae, the ocular muscles, the eyelids and tunica conjunctiva, and the lacrimal apparatus; most are contained within the *orbit.* This structure is a cone-shaped cavity on the lateral surface of the skull that is delimited externally by a bony margin (base of cone). In the carnivores and pig the bone is deficient laterally, but the ring is completed by the *orbital ligament* (see Fig. 2.31/*1*). The wall of the human orbit is entirely osseous, but in the domestic mammals the lateral and ventral parts are formed by the fibrous periorbita, one of the orbital fasciae (described later).

The Orbital Fascia

The eyeball is surrounded by three roughly conical fascial layers. The most external of these is the periorbita, which has just been mentioned; internal to the periorbita are superficial and deep muscular fasciae (Fig. 9.16).

The *periorbita* is attached near the optic foramen at the apex of the cone. It blends with the periosteum at the orbital margin and on the medial and dorsal walls of the orbit. Elsewhere (mainly laterally and ventrally) it is free and forms a substantial fibrous partition between orbital and extraorbital structures (Fig. 9.17/*11*). The periorbita splits at the orbital margin. One part is continued as the periosteum of the facial bones; the other, the *orbital septum* (Fig. 9.17/*2*), forms two semilunar folds with thickened free margins (tarsi) that stiffen the edges of the upper and lower eyelids. The *trochlea* (Fig. 9.17/*6*), a flat piece

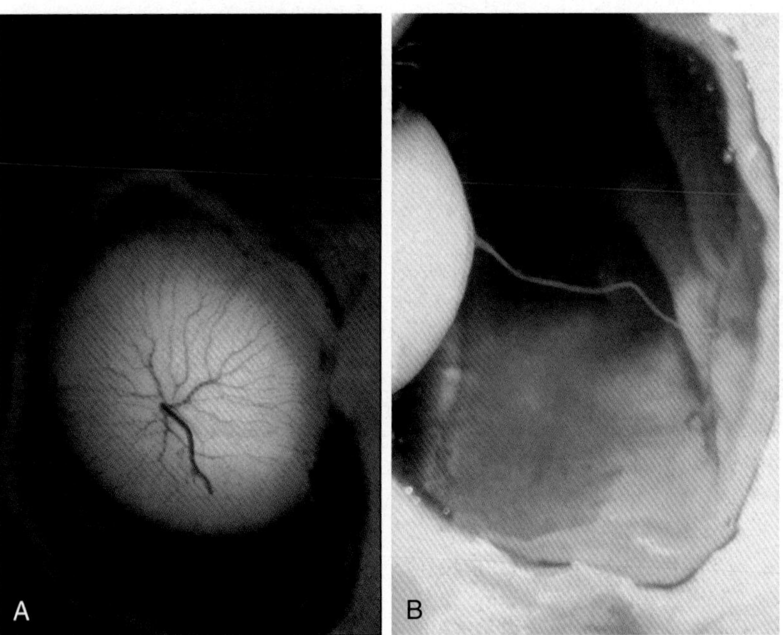

Fig. 9.15 (A) Posterior surface of lens (newborn puppy) showing remnant of hyaloid artery. (B) Persistent hyaloid artery (dog).

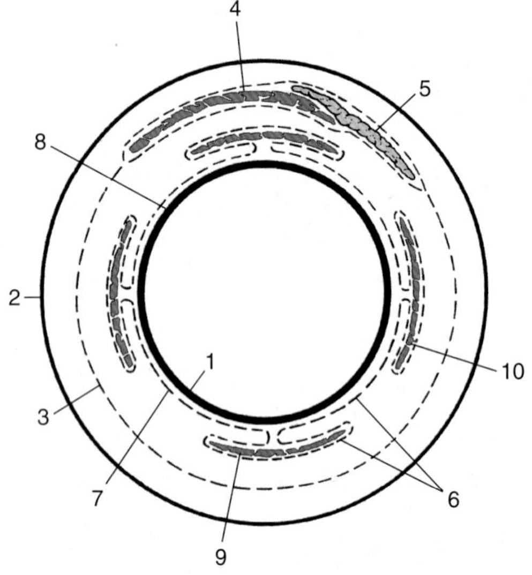

Fig. 9.16 Schematic representation of the orbital fasciae: transection of orbital structures at the level of the eyeball. Part of the deep muscular fascia *(6)* forms the vagina bulbi *(7)*. *1,* Eyeball; *2,* periorbita; *3,* superficial muscular fascia; *4,* levator palpebrae; *5,* lacrimal gland; *8,* episcleral space; *9,* ventral rectus muscle; *10,* lateral rectus muscle.

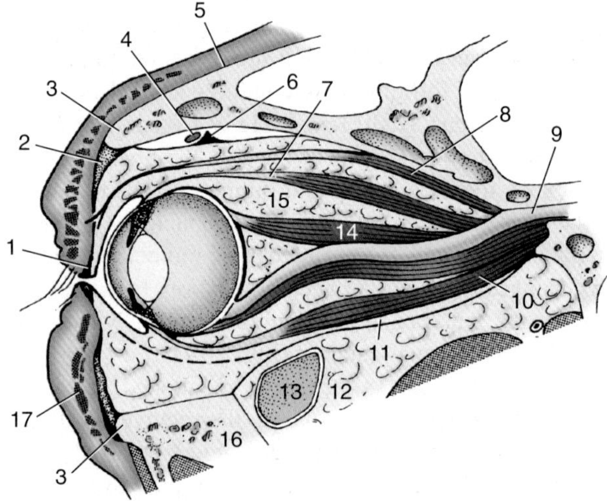

Fig. 9.17 Right bovine eye cut along orbital axis, rostromedial surface. *1,* Tarsus; *2,* orbital septum; *3,* orbital margin; *4,* dorsal oblique muscle; *5,* periosteum of face; *6,* trochlea; *7,* dorsal rectus muscle; *8,* levator palpebrae superioris; *9,* optic nerve in optic foramen; *10,* ventral rectus muscle; *11,* periorbita; *12,* extraperiorbital fat; *13,* lacrimal bulla, a caudal recess of the maxillary sinus; *14,* retractor bulbi; *15,* intraperiorbital fat; *16,* zygomatic arch; *17,* orbicularis.

of cartilage embedded in the dorsomedial wall close to the orbital margin, provides a pulley around which the dorsal oblique muscle winds to change direction by nearly 90 degrees.

The loose and fatty *superficial muscular fascia* lies within the periorbita and envelops the levator palpebrae superioris and the lacrimal gland (Fig. 9.16/*3*). The *deep muscular fascia* is more fibrous; it arises from the eyelids and from the limbus of the eyeball, which it closely invests. It is reflected around the muscles attaching to the eyeball and then around the optic nerve, providing each with a fascial envelope. Where the deep muscular fascia is applied to the eyeball, it is known as the *vagina bulbi* (Fig. 9.16/*7*), although it is separated by a narrow episcleral space. The

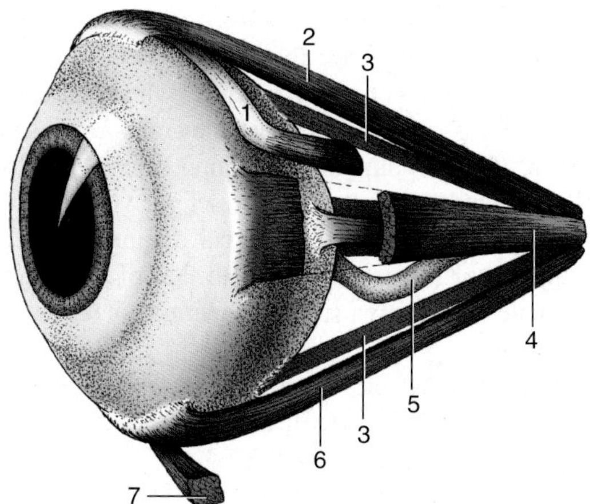

Fig. 9.18 Ocular muscles. *1,* Dorsal oblique muscle (m.); *2,* dorsal rectus m.; *3,* retractor bulbi; *4,* medial rectus m.; *5,* optic nerve; *6,* ventral rectus m.; *7,* ventral oblique m.

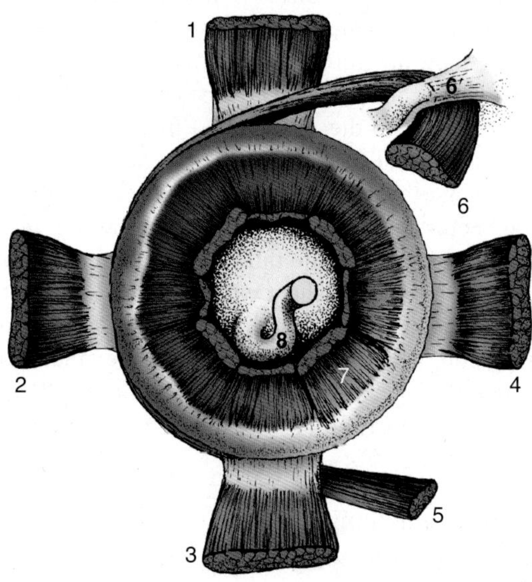

Fig. 9.19 Stumps of ocular muscles viewed from behind the left eyeball. *1,* Dorsal rectus muscle (m.); *2,* lateral rectus m.; *3,* ventral rectus m.; *4,* medial rectus m.; *5,* ventral oblique m.; *6,* dorsal oblique m.; *6',* trochlea; *7,* retractor bulbi; *8,* optic nerve.

presence of this space facilitates the movement of the eyeball against the retrobulbar fat, which is advantageous during enucleation to free the eyeball while leaving the vagina bulbi and the retrobulbar structures in place.

The Muscles of the Eyeball

The muscles that move the eye are located behind the eyeball. All except one originate in the vicinity of the optic foramen at the apex of the orbital cone. There are four rectus muscles, two oblique muscles, and a retractor.

The four *rectus muscles*—dorsal, ventral, medial, and lateral—insert anterior to the equator of the eyeball by wide but very thin tendons (see Fig. 9.7). The *dorsal* and *ventral oblique muscles* attach to the eyeball near the equator and act to rotate the eyeball around the visual axis (Fig. 9.18/*1* and *7*). The dorsal oblique muscle arises close to the optic foramen and passes forward on the dorsomedial wall of the orbit before it is deflected around the trochlea to end on the dorsolateral surface of the eyeball beneath the tendon of the dorsal rectus muscle. A small synovial sheath protects the muscle as it passes around the trochlea, which in fact is its functional origin. If this muscle were to contract by itself, it would pull the dorsal part of the eyeball medially.

The *ventral oblique muscle,* uniquely, does not arise from the vicinity of the optic foramen. Instead, it takes its origin from a depression in the ventromedial wall of the orbit, passing laterally below the eyeball and the tendon of the ventral rectus muscle before inserting on the ventrolateral part of the eyeball. Its contraction, if isolated from the action of the other muscles, would rotate the eyeball around the visual axis so that the dorsal portion of the eyeball would move laterally. The *retractor bulbi* (Fig. 9.17/*14*) arises from the vicinity of the optic foramen but is inserted on the eyeball posterior to the equator. It forms a nearly complete muscular cone about the optic nerve (Fig. 9.19/*7*). The reasons for the absence of the retractor in the humans are not understood.

The movements of the eyes are much more complex than the origins and insertions of the individual muscles suggest. The activity of muscles of the eyeball are closely coordinated, such that tension is increased or decreased appropriately in opposing muscles for smooth transition from one eye position to another. The most difficult actions to explain are those of the oblique muscles because there is no significant rotation around the visual axis in any usual movement. Their participation is required for the following reason. The rectus muscles arise slightly medioventral to the point where the visual axis, if extended caudally, would strike the skull. That is, the visual axis does not coincide with the axis of the orbital cone. As a result, the dorsal rectus muscle, as one example, would not simply elevate the cranial pole of the eyeball but would also rotate the eyeball so that its dorsal part moved slightly medially. This slight intorsion is reflexively resisted by the ventral oblique, and the result is a smooth elevation of the anterior pole. The reverse happens in depression of the eyeball, in which the ventral rectus and the dorsal oblique muscles are involved.

An additional striated muscle within the orbit is considered here for convenience. The *levator palpebrae superioris* (Fig. 9.17/*8*) does not attach to the eyeball but passes over it to enter and elevate the upper eyelid.

In addition to these striated muscles, there are three sheets of smooth muscle associated with the eyeball, although they are rarely observed during routine dissection. The orbital muscle consists of a sheet of circular (with regard to the visual axis) fibers applied to the internal surface of the periorbita. A ventral longitudinal sheet of smooth muscle extends from the sheath of the ventral rectus muscle into the lower lid as the inferior tarsal muscle and into the third eyelid (described later). A medial longitudinal sheet extends from the sheath of the medial rectus muscle and from the trochlea into the upper eyelid, as the superior tarsal muscle, and into the third eyelid. Tension in these sheets maintains the normal protruded position of the eye and retracted position of the eyelids.

The Eyelids and Conjunctiva

The eyelids (palpebrae) are two musculofibrous folds of which the upper is the more extensive and more mobile. The free margins of the lids meet at the medial and lateral *angles of the eye* and bound an opening known as the *palpebral fissure.* The eyelids consist of three layers: skin, a middle musculofibrous layer, and a mucous membrane, known as the *palpebral conjunctiva,* facing the eye (Fig. 9.20). The skin of the lids is thin and delicate and is covered with short hairs; it may also carry a few prominent tactile hairs.

The *musculofibrous layer* is formed by the orbicularis oculi, the orbital septum, the aponeurosis of the levator muscle, and the smooth tarsal muscle. The orbicularis oculi closes the eyelids. It lies directly under the skin and can be dissected away from the remaining layers, which are closely intermingled. The orbital septum arises from the margin of the orbit; the aponeurosis of the levator and the tarsal muscle originate in the orbit. Toward the free margin of the eyelid, these components are succeeded by the *tarsus* (Fig. 9.20/*2′*), a platelike fibrous condensation that stabilizes the edge of the lid. The ends of the two tarsi are anchored to the orbital margin by medial and lateral *palpebral ligaments* that ensure an elongated palpebral fissure when the eye is closed. Deep to the tarsus and opening onto the edge of the lid by a row of tiny openings is a series of *tarsal glands* (Fig. 9.20/*6*) that secrete a fatty material. Just in front of these glandular openings are the cilia (eyelashes), which are usually more prominent and numerous on the upper than on the lower lid; conspicuous cilia are absent from the lower lid of carnivores. Small ciliary and sebaceous glands are associated with the roots of the cilia; inflammation of one of these glands is known as a *stye* (hordeolum).

The *palpebral conjunctiva* is a thin, transparent mucous membrane that forms the posterior surface of the lid. It is reflected at the base of the lids to continue on the sclera as the *bulbar conjunctiva,* which ends at the limbus, although the epithelium continues as the anterior epithelium of the cornea. The potential space between the lids and the eyeball is known as the *conjunctival sac,* and their dorsal and ventral extremities are the *fornices* (Fig. 9.3/*2*). The transparency of the conjunctiva renders the smaller blood vessels visible, especially when they are congested in infections. Those in the bulbar conjunctiva move with this loosely attached layer; the deeper scleral vessels do not. This arrangement allows the clinical distinction between inflammation of the conjunctiva and that of deeper structures. A pale conjunctiva suggests anemia, shock, or internal hemorrhage.

A slight mucosal elevation, the *lacrimal caruncle,* is present in the medial angle of the eye; it bears a few fine hairs in the large species (Fig. 9.21/*2*).

Between the lacrimal caruncle and the eyeball is a dorsoventrally oriented conjunctival fold known as the *third eyelid* (Fig. 9.21/*6*). Unlike a true lid, it is covered with conjunctiva on both sides and is invisible when the eye is closed. The third eyelid is supported by a T-shaped piece of

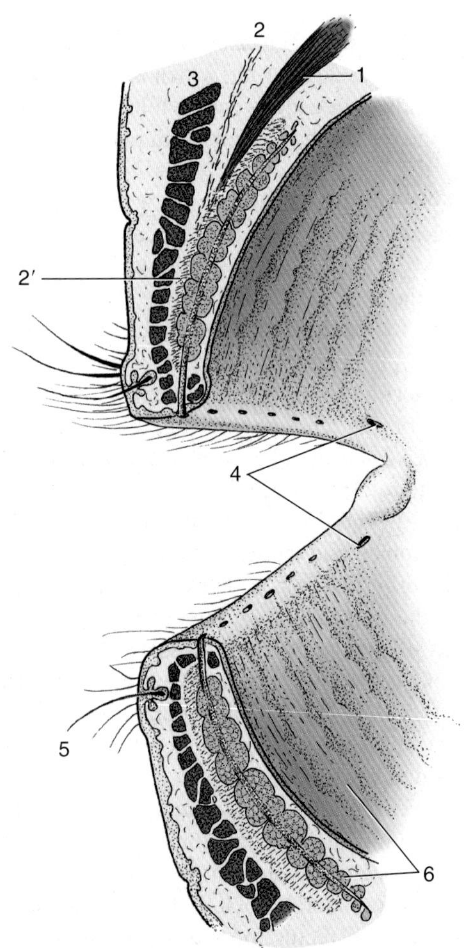

Fig. 9.20 Eyelids, sectioned and viewed obliquely from behind. *1,* Levator palpebrae superioris; *2,* orbital septum; *2′,* tarsus; *3,* orbicularis oculi; *4,* puncta lacrimalia; *5,* cilium with associated ciliary and sebaceous glands; *6,* tarsal glands.

cartilage (Fig. 9.21/*6'*) whose bar lies in the free edge of the fold and whose stem points backward into the orbit medial to the eyeball. The stem of the cartilage is surrounded by an additional lacrimal gland, the *gland of the third eyelid;* pigs and cattle also have a second, deeper gland. The secretion of these glands enters the conjunctival sac on the bulbar, or inner, surface of the third eyelid. The third eyelid is kept retracted by a smooth muscle (m. [muscle] orbitalis, previously described) and innervated by sympathetic fibers. The third eyelid slides passively over the eyeball when the eyeball is actively retracted or pushed into the orbit. The lid, in conjunction with the retractor bulbi muscle, is thought to provide added protection to the protruding eyes of animals.

The Lacrimal Apparatus

The lacrimal apparatus consists of the lacrimal gland proper, the gland(s) associated with the third eyelid, several small accessory glands, and a duct system that conveys the lacrimal fluid (tears), into the nasal cavity for evaporation. The *lacrimal gland* is flat and lies between the eyeball and the dorsolateral wall of the orbit (Fig. 9.21/*9*). Its secretion is drained by many minute ducts into the dorsal fornix of the conjunctival sac, where it mixes with the secretions of the accessory glands. Blinking movements distribute the lacrimal fluid over the exposed part of the eye, which is thus kept moist; the tears carry away foreign material and supply the cornea with nutrients. The fluid is repelled by the fatty secretion of the tarsal glands along the edge of the lids and normally pools at the medial angle of the eye in the so-called lacrimal lake, a shallow depression surrounding the lacrimal caruncle. The lacrimal fluid is then drawn by capillary action into the duct system through the puncta lacrimalia, described later (Fig. 9.20/*4*). Lacrimal fluid escapes over the edge of the lower eyelid onto the face only when produced in excessive amounts or when normal drainage is impaired.

The *puncta lacrimalia* are minute slits, one on the edge of each lid next to the caruncle. Each punctum leads to a short, narrow *canaliculus* through which the fluid flows to the much longer *nasolacrimal duct* (Fig. 9.21/*3*). The beginning of the nasolacrimal duct is slightly enlarged, forming the *lacrimal sac,* which occupies a funnel-shaped fossa near the bony margin of the orbit. The nasolacrimal duct runs rostrally, at first within the thickness of the maxilla, and then on its internal surface, where it is covered by nasal mucosa. In some species, the duct ends deep in the nasal cavity, and in others it extends to the nostril.

The tear film washing the eye consists of three layers. The outermost lipid layer is derived from the secretion of the tarsal glands; it helps spread the tears evenly and retards the breakup of the film. The thick middle aqueous layer is derived from the lacrimal glands; it moistens and nourishes the cornea. The innermost mucinous layer is produced by goblet cells in the conjunctiva and holds the tear film intimately apposed to the cornea. Tear flow can be increased by drugs or reflexively after stimulation of the conjunctiva, cornea, or nasal mucosa. Weeping as an expression of emotion does not occur in domestic animals.

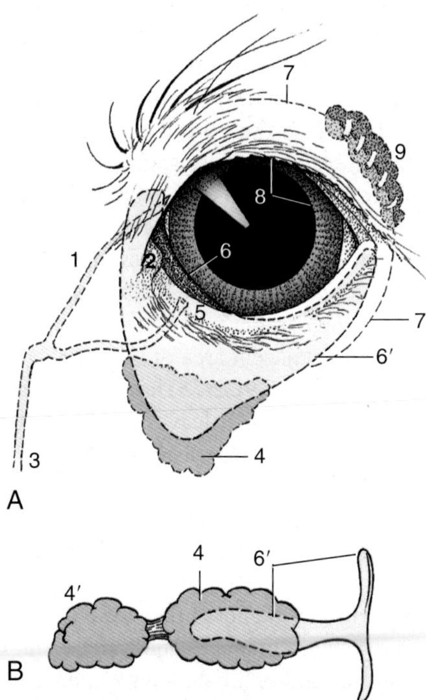

Fig. 9.21 (A) Left eye of dog showing third eyelid and lacrimal apparatus. (B) Isolated cartilage of the third eyelid and associated glands of a pig. *1,* Upper canaliculus; *2,* lacrimal caruncle; *3,* nasolacrimal duct; *4,* gland of third eyelid; *4',* deep gland of third eyelid; *5,* punctum lacrimale; *6,* third eyelid; *6',* cartilage of third eyelid; *7,* position of conjunctival fornix; *8,* pupil; *9,* lacrimal gland.

The Blood Supply of the Eye

The blood supply to the eyeball and its adnexa is complex (Fig. 9.22 and 9.23). The blood supply to the human eye enters the orbit with the optic nerve, but in domestic mammals this route is represented by a rudimentary internal ophthalmic artery (Fig. 9.22/*2*). The principal blood supply is instead carried by the *external ophthalmic artery* (Fig. 9.22/*3*), a branch of the maxillary artery as it passes ventral to the orbit to supply more rostral structures of the face. The arteries arising from the external ophthalmic and malar arteries (a further, smaller branch of the maxillary) can be divided into three groups: (1) those supplying the eyeball, (2) those supplying ocular muscles, and (3) those leaving the orbit to supply adjacent structures, regardless of whether these are associated with the eye:

1. The branches of the external ophthalmic artery for the eyeball penetrate the sclera to reach the vascular tunic and the retina. *Short posterior ciliary arteries*

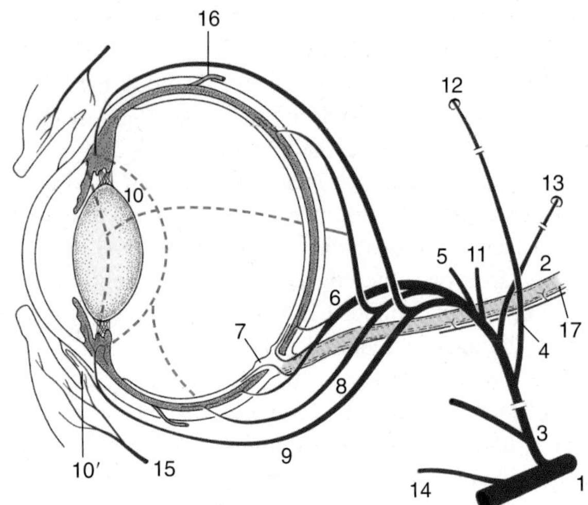

Fig. 9.22 The principal arteries (aa.) supplying the eye. *1,* Maxillary artery (a.); *2,* rudimentary internal ophthalmic a.; *3,* external ophthalmic a.; *4,* anastomosis between external and internal ophthalmic aa.; *5,* lacrimal a. to lacrimal gland and upper lid; *6,* short posterior ciliary aa.; *7,* retinal aa.; *8,* long posterior ciliary aa.; *9,* anterior ciliary aa., substantial branches to *10* in horse, lesser branches in the other domestic species; *10,* greater arterial circle of the iris; *10′,* annular pericorneal network; *11,* muscular branches; *12,* supraorbital a. and foramen; *13,* external ethmoidal a. and foramen; *14,* malar a.; *15,* palpebral branches; *16,* vorticose veins; *17,* optic nerve.

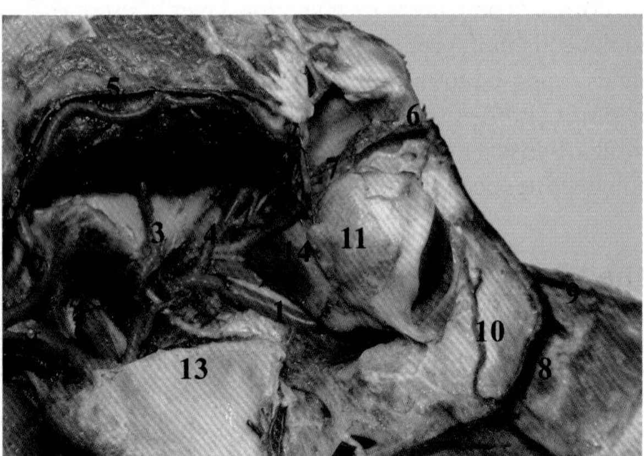

Fig. 9.23 Blood supply of the orbital fossa *1,* Maxillary artery; *2,* Superficial temporal artery; *3,* Caudal deep temporal artery; *4,* Rostral deep temporal artery; *5,* Superficial temporal vein; *6,* Angular ocular vein; *7,* Ophthalmic plexus; *8,* Facial vein; *9,* Dorsal nasal vein; *10,* Inferior palpebral vein; *11,* Lacrimal gland; *12,* Temporomandibular joint (mandibular fossa); *13,* Ramus mandibulae (cut); *14,* Infraorbital nerve.

(Fig. 9.22/*6*) penetrate near the optic nerve and supply the adjacent choroid in addition to supplying the nerve. The short posterior ciliary arteries then form the *central artery of the retina,* the parent vessel for the retinal arteries (Figs. 9.22/*7* and Fig. 9.6). *Long posterior ciliary arteries* (Fig. 9.22/*8*) pass through the sclera somewhat closer to the equator. The *anterior ciliary arteries* (Fig. 9.22/*9*) penetrate near the limbus and supply the anterior portion of the choroid, the ciliary body, and the iris. These arteries anastomose to form the *greater arterial circle of the iris* (Fig. 9.22/*10*), from which numerous fine branches pass toward the pupil and into the ciliary body. Capillaries near the limbus nourish the cornea by diffusion. The anterior ciliary arteries also send branches to the conjunctiva. The principal venous return is through several *vorticose veins* (Fig. 9.22/*16*) that emerge from the sclera near the equator. The extraocular veins of carnivores and ruminants form substantial venous plexuses within the periorbita. Venous blood returning from the retina leaves at the optic disk through small veins associated with the short posterior ciliary arteries.

2. The arteries supplying the ocular muscles enter the muscles proximally. The absence of larger vessels in the distal ends accounts for the reduced bleeding when the muscles are transected at these ends during enucleation.
3. Only four of the arteries that leave the orbit will be described. The *lacrimal artery* (Fig. 9.22/*5*) passes forward in the lateral part of the orbital cone and, after supplying the lacrimal gland en route, crosses the dorsolateral part of the orbital margin to supply lateral parts of the eyelids and conjunctiva. The *supraorbital artery* (Fig. 9.22/*12*) passes dorsally and leaves the orbit by the supraorbital foramen. It ramifies subcutaneously medial to the orbit and may send branches into the upper eyelid. Because carnivores lack the supraorbital foramen and artery, their cyelids are supplied by long branches of the superficial temporal artery. The *malar artery* (Fig. 9.22/*14*) arises directly from the maxillary and passes over the ventral wall of the orbit to the medial angle of the eye, where it supplies the eyelids and also the adjacent area of the face. The *external ethmoidal artery* (Fig. 9.22/*13*) has the shortest intraorbital course of the four. It leaves the orbit through the ethmoidal foramen and supplies the ethmoid labyrinth of the nasal cavity.

Most of the arteries described also take part in supplying the fat, fascia, and nerves within the orbit. There are interspecies variations, but they are rarely of practical concern. However, it may be noted that the external ophthalmic artery in ruminants branches and forms a small arterial network (rete mirabile ophthalmicum) upon entering the orbit. The various arteries, except the malar, arise from this network.

The Nerve Supply of the Eye

The nerve supply to the eye and its accessory structures is derived from no fewer than six cranial nerves (denoted here by roman numerals). Most of them enter the orbital cone, but some reach accessory structures directly.

The *optic nerve* (II) enters the orbit through the optic foramen and contains axons arising from the innermost layer of the retina. It is rather slack in order to allow for the movements of the eye and is covered by meninges that it acquired during development as the stalk of the optic cup.

Though the name of the *oculomotor nerve* (III) implies that it controls movement of the eyeball, it does not innervate all the ocular muscles. It enters the orbit through the orbital foramen (fissure; foramen orbitorotundum in ruminants and the pig) and sends branches to the levator palpebrae; the dorsal, medial, and ventral recti; the ventral oblique; and part of the retractor bulbi muscles.

The *trochlear nerve* (IV) accompanies the third nerve and innervates the dorsal oblique muscle.

The ophthalmic and maxillary divisions of the *trigeminal nerve* (V) send branches to the eye. The *ophthalmic nerve* passes through the orbital foramen and supplies the following sensory branches: long ciliary nerves to the eyeball, especially the cornea; a lacrimal nerve to the eyelids and conjunctiva of the lateral angle; a supraorbital nerve that accompanies the supraorbital artery through the supraorbital foramen to supply the upper eyelid and skin medial to the orbit; an infratrochlear nerve (not present in all species) sensory to structures near the medial angle of the eye; and an ethmoidal nerve that follows the ethmoidal artery to innervate the caudal part of the nasal cavity. The *maxillary nerve* has only one relevant branch, the zygomatic nerve, which supplies the lateroventral segment of the eyelids and conjunctiva via a zygomaticofacial branch and the skin caudal to the orbit via a zygomaticotemporal branch. In horned cattle, the zygomaticotemporal branch furnishes the clinically important cornual nerve to the horn. These sensory nerves to the orbit provide the afferent limbs of the palpebral and corneal reflexes that stimulate the orbicularis oculi to close the eyelids when the lids or cornea are touched.

The *abducent nerve* (VI) enters through the orbital foramen. It innervates most of the retractor bulbi and the lateral rectus muscles.

The auriculopalpebral branch of the *facial nerve* (VII) passes between the eye and ear and thus approaches the eyelids from a caudal aspect. It innervates the orbicularis oculi. It may be blocked to immobilize the lids or to relieve the "pressure" that tension in the muscle may exert on a painful globe. The levator palpebrae is not immobilized by this block.

Sympathetic postganglionic nerve fibers arise from the cranial cervical ganglion and follow arteries or the ophthalmic nerve to the orbit, where they innervate the orbital muscle and the dilator of the pupil. Tension in the orbital muscle keeps the eyeball protruded, the third eyelid retracted, and the palpebral fissure open. Active dilation of the pupil (mydriasis) is initiated by fear, excitement, or pain.

Parasympathetic preganglionic nerve fibers enter the orbit within the oculomotor nerve. They synapse in the ciliary ganglion, and the postsynaptic fibers, forming the short ciliary nerves, innervate the ciliary muscle and the constrictor of the pupil. They control both the accommodation of the lens and the constriction of the pupil (miosis) in response to light.

The axons of the long ciliary nerve, a branch of the ophthalmic nerve, form the afferent limb of the **corneal reflex**, which is the closure of the lids when the cornea is touched. The efferent limb of this reflex is the auriculopalpebral branch of the facial nerve. This reflex is used clinically when monitoring deep anesthesia.

Both the orbital muscle and the dilator muscle of the pupil receive sympathetic input. Loss of sympathetic innervation results in a sunken eye, protrusion of the third eyelid, and constriction of the pupil (miosis), a collection of clinical signs known as **Horner's syndrome**.

THE EAR

The ear as a whole is sometimes called the *vestibulocochlear organ* because it not only enables the animal to hear but also gives it a sense of balance. The mechanical stimuli produced by sound waves are transformed into nerve impulses in the *cochlea*, and the movement of fluid and the action of gravity on receptors within the *vestibular apparatus* provide the animal with a sense of the position and movement of the head. Both functions are performed in the *internal ear,* the most medial of the three subdivisions of the ear as a whole, the other subdivisions being the middle ear and the external ear. Only the external ear is visible in the intact animal; the other two are hidden within the temporal bone (Fig. 9.24/*24*).

The External Ear

The external ear consists of two parts, the auricle and the external acoustic meatus (Fig. 9.24/*1* and *2*). The auricle, or pinna, is the "ear" as it is understood by the layperson, the part that sticks out from the head. The external acoustic meatus is the canal that leads from the base of the auricle to the eardrum (tympanic membrane) stretched across an opening in the temporal bone.

The auricle is shaped like a funnel; distally it is wide open to receive the sound, and more proximally it is rolled up to form a tube that bends medially for connection with the external acoustic meatus. The particular shape of the auricle is determined by the supporting *auricular cartilage* (Fig. 9.25). In most domestic mammals, the cartilage is sufficiently stiff to keep the auricle erect at all times. In many breeds of dogs and in certain other animals, the cartilage is relatively soft, allowing the auricle to collapse; even so, most dogs can prick their ears.

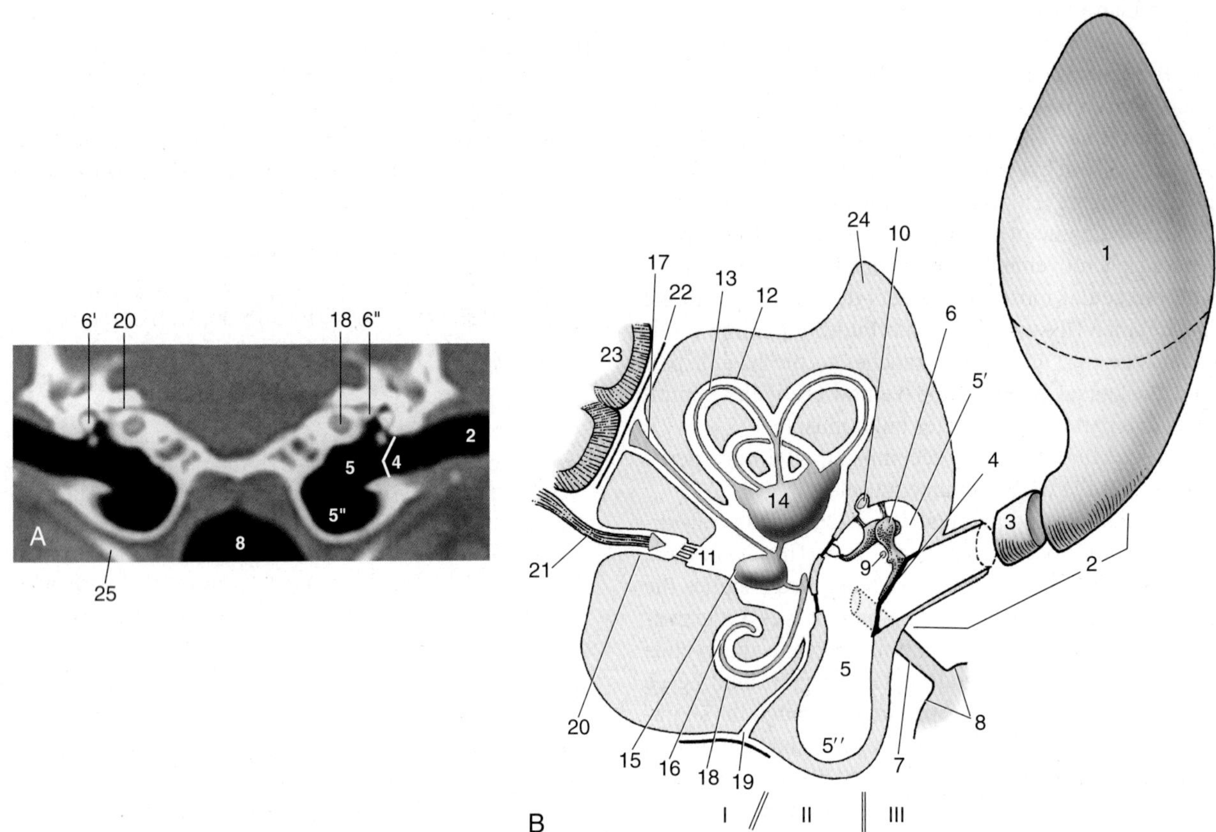

Fig. 9.24 (A) Transverse image of a 2-mm-thick computed tomography slice of the canine tympanic bullae and petrous temporal bones. (Bone settings were used.) (B) Schema of the right ear, caudal view. Note that the sizes of the structures shown are out of proportion to one another. *I,* Internal ear; *II,* middle ear; *III,* external ear. *1,* Auricle; *2,* external acoustic meatus; *3,* annular cartilage; *4,* tympanic membrane; *5,* tympanic cavity; *5′,* epitympanic recess; *5″,* tympanic bulla; *6,* auditory ossicles; *6′,* malleus; *6″,* base of stapes in vestibular window; *7,* auditory tube; *8,* nasopharynx; *9,* chorda tympani; *10,* facial nerve; *11,* vestibule; *12,* semicircular canals; *13,* semicircular ducts; *14,* utriculus; *15,* sacculus; *16,* cochlear duct; *17,* endolymphatic duct; *18,* cochlea; *19,* perilymphatic duct; *20,* internal acoustic meatus; *21,* vestibulocochlear nerve in internal acoustic meatus; *22,* meninges; *23,* brain; *24,* petrous temporal bone; *25,* stylohyoid bone.

In domestic animals, the auricle can be turned toward the source of sound; right and left auricles can move independently so that each can focus on separate sounds. A complex set of *auricular muscles,* all voluntary, is responsible for the movement of the ear. These muscles arise from various points on the skull and adjacent fasciae and attach to the base of the auricle. A flat, palpable (scutiform) cartilage rostral to the ear redirects the pull of some muscles. The auricular muscles are innervated by branches of the facial nerve.

The *external acoustic meatus* begins where the rolled-up part of the auricular cartilage narrows and ends at the eardrum (Fig. 9.24/*2*). The meatus therefore has a distal cartilaginous and a more proximal osseous part. It is lined with skin that contains sebaceous and tubular ceruminous glands. The latter secrete the earwax (cerumen), which is thought to prevent dust from reaching the delicate tympanic membrane. The ear of the dog is of the most clinical interest. Unfortunately, its external acoustic meatus is curved, making passage of the straight otoscope for the examination of the proximal part of the meatus and eardrum difficult.

The Middle Ear

The middle ear is housed in the temporal bone and is essentially the small air-filled space known as the *tympanic cavity* (Fig. 9.24/*5*). It is lined with a thin mucous membrane and communicates with the nasopharynx by the auditory tube (Fig. 9.24/*7*). The lateral wall of the cavity incorporates the tympanic membrane (Fig. 9.24/*4*). The medial wall is formed by the petrous part of the temporal bone, which houses the internal ear. It contains two windows

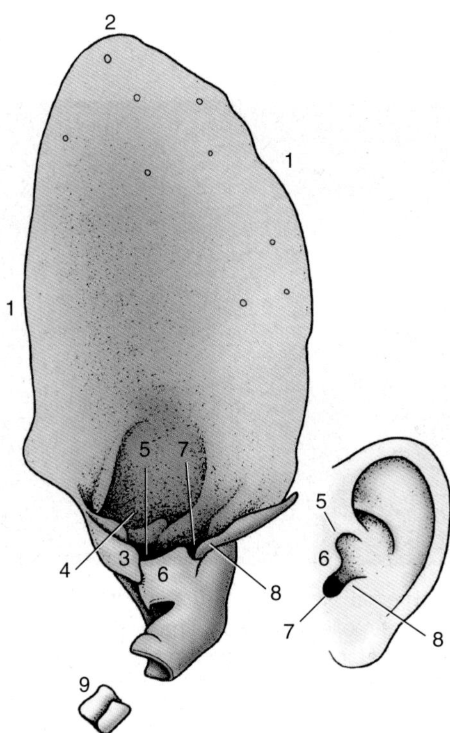

Fig. 9.25 Left auricular cartilage of dog *(left)* compared with human ear *(right)*. *1,* Helix; *2,* apex; *3,* medial crus of helix; *4,* lateral crus of helix; *5,* pretragic notch; *6,* tragus; *7,* intertragic notch; *8,* antitragus; *9,* annular cartilage.

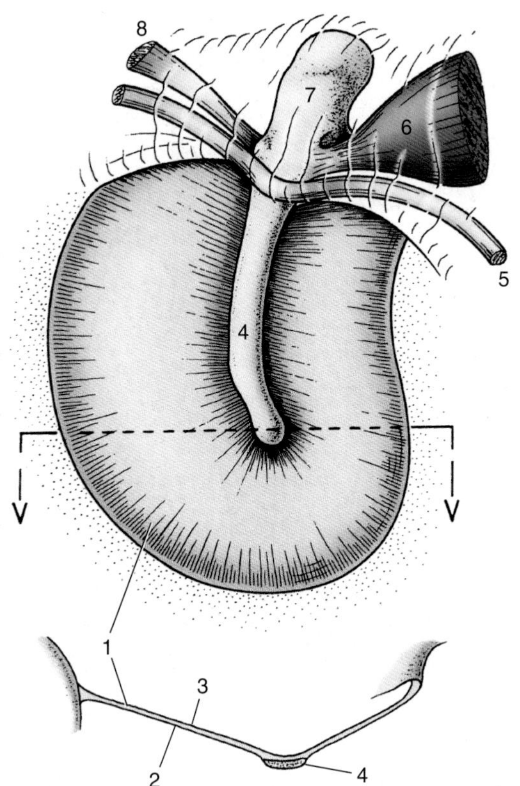

Fig. 9.26 Medial surface *(top)* and transverse section *(bottom;* location of section indicated by *dotted lines and arrows)* of canine tympanic membrane. *1,* Tense part of tympanic membrane; *2,* medial surface; *3,* lateral surface; *4,* handle of malleus; *5,* chorda tympani; *6,* tensor tympani muscle; *7,* head of malleus; *8,* one of the ligaments associated with the malleus.

(fenestrae), closed in the natural state, through which the mechanical stimuli produced by sound waves enter the internal ear for translation into nerve impulses. The more dorsal *vestibular window* connects the tympanic cavity with the vestibule of the internal ear. In the live animal, the vestibular window is in contact with the stapes, the most medial of the auditory ossicles in the middle ear (Fig. 9.24/*6*). The other window, the *cochlear window,* leads to the cavity of the cochlea (Fig. 9.24/*18*). It is closed by the thin secondary tympanic membrane. Ventral to the two windows, the medial wall of the tympanic cavity bulges over the cochlea, forming the promontory.

The tympanic cavity may be divided into dorsal, middle, and ventral parts. The dorsal part of the tympanic cavity, the epitympanic recess, is situated dorsal to the level of the tympanic membrane and is compressed from side to side and slanted laterally. It contains the chain of three auditory ossicles and the two associated muscles. The middle part includes the tympanic membrane in its lateral wall and opens rostrally into the nasopharynx via the auditory tube. The ventral part is an enlarged bulbous extension of the temporal bone known as the *tympanic bulla* (Fig. 9.24/*5″*). The bulla varies in prominence among species; in some it is subdivided into numerous bony cells. The function is not known with certainty but may be to improve the perception of sounds of very low and very high frequencies.

The *tympanic membrane* (Fig. 9.26) is a thin partition separating the lumen of the external acoustic meatus from that of the tympanic cavity. Like the tympanic cavity, it is slanted so that its dorsal part is more lateral than its ventral part, and its surface area is thus considerably larger than that of the transected external acoustic meatus. The dog's eardrum on average measures 10 × 15 mm; its long axis is oriented rostrocaudally. Its outer, laterally facing surface is covered with an epidermis continuous with that of the meatus, whereas its medial surface is continuous with the mucosa lining the tympanic cavity. A layer of fibrous tissue between the epidermis and mucosa firmly attaches the edges of the membrane to the osseous tympanic ring of the temporal bone. The tympanic ring is interrupted dorsally by a notch that extends onto the roof of the external acoustic meatus. The part of the tympanic membrane attached to the tympanic ring is tense; the part that closes the notch is flaccid.

The handle of the malleus (Fig. 9.26/*4*), the most lateral of the ear ossicles, is embedded in the medial surface of the tympanic membrane. Tension in the chain of ossicles pulls the tympanic membrane medially, hollowing its

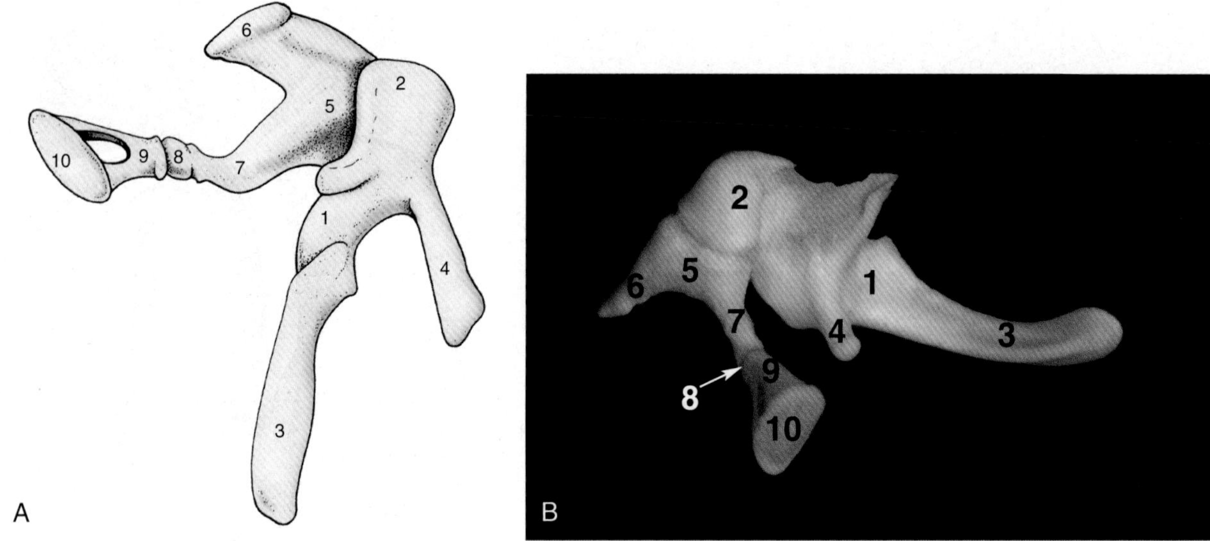

Fig. 9.27 (A) Left auditory ossicles of the horse, craniomedial view. (B) Left auditory ossicles of the dog. *1,* Malleus; *2,* head of malleus; *3,* handle of malleus; *4,* rostral process; *5,* incus; *6,* short crus; *7,* long crus; *8,* os lenticulare; *9,* head of stapes; *10,* base (footplate) of stapes.

lateral surface. The handle shines through the thin membrane and is visible as a light band (stria mallearis) when the eardrum is examined with an otoscope (see Fig.11.43 A and B).

Auditory Ossicles

The transmission of sound waves across the tympanic cavity is mediated by the three auditory ossicles (Fig. 9.24/*6*) known, in lateromedial sequence, as *malleus, incus*, and *stapes* (Latin names for hammer, anvil, and stirrup, from their rather fanciful resemblance to these objects).

The handle (manubrium) of the *malleus* (Fig. 9.27A/*3* and B) is embedded in the tympanic membrane, as previously mentioned, so that the head of the malleus protrudes above the membrane by a few millimeters. The head articulates with the body of the *incus,* and the latter articulates with the head of the stapes by means of its long crus. The base (footplate) of the *stapes* sits in the vestibular window in the medial wall of the tympanic cavity.

The oscillations of the tympanic membrane transmitted by the handle of the malleus are magnified and transmitted to the vestibular window by lever action through the chain of ossicles. The base of the stapes is set in motion, causing the fluid in the internal ear to vibrate. The vibration stimulates the receptor cells in the cochlea, and sound is perceived.

The mechanism of sound transmission from the outside to the internal ear may not in fact be quite so simple. There is evidence that some sound waves are also transmitted to the fluid through the walls of the tympanic cavity and directly through the cochlear window.

The auditory ossicles are attached to the wall of the epitympanic recess by several ligaments, and their relationships can be altered by two small muscles (tensor tympani and stapedius). These muscles tense the tympanic membrane and the chain of ossicles to decrease the amplitude of their vibrations during lower frequencies and protect the system from damage caused by sudden overload (see p. 304 for their innervation).

Auditory Tube

This structure, often called the *eustachian tube*, connects the tympanic cavity with the nasopharynx (Fig. 9.24/*8*). It is short with a narrow lumen that is laterally compressed and usually collapsed. The tube is confined by an inverted cartilaginous trough except along its ventral border. The membranous wall of the horse's auditory tube evaginates through this ventral defect in the cartilaginous support to form the large, thin-walled *guttural pouch* dorsolateral to the nasopharynx (see p. 511).

The *pharyngeal openings of the auditory tubes* are located in the lateral walls of the nasopharynx and are marked by accumulations of lymphoid tissue (tubal tonsils) (see Fig. 18.11/*8*). The cartilage of the auditory tube extends into the medial wall of the pharyngeal opening and stiffens it. The auditory tubes allow equalization of the pressures on the two sides of the delicate eardrums. The pressure sometimes becomes unbalanced, for example, during rapid elevation changes, and its sudden restoration causes a popping sensation. The auditory tubes temporarily open each time we swallow or yawn. This opening permits

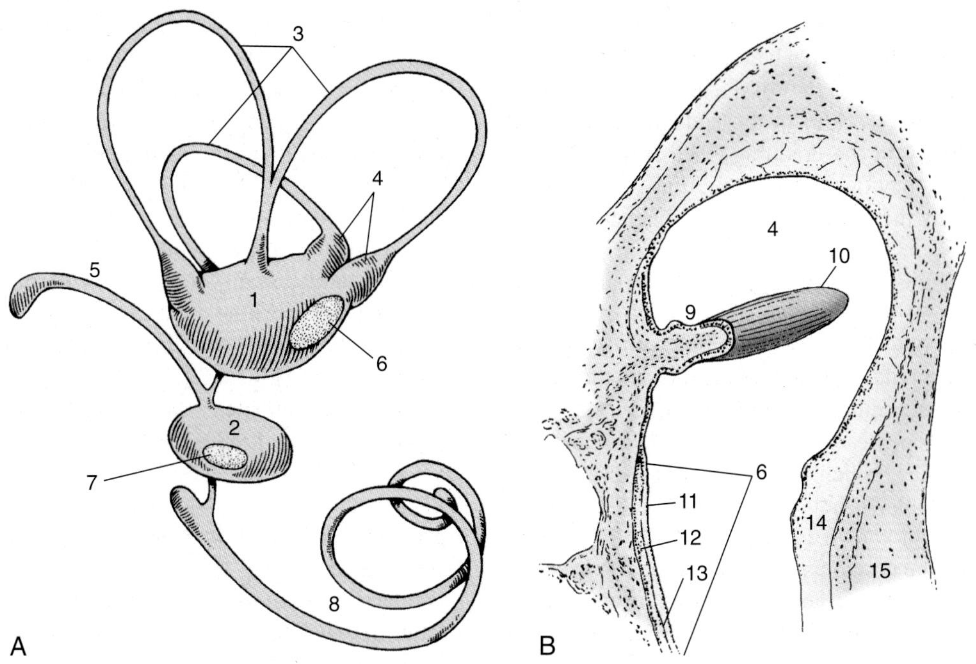

Fig. 9.28 (A) Membranous labyrinth. (B) Section of ampulla. *1,* Utriculus; *2,* sacculus; *3,* semicircular ducts; *4,* ampullae containing ampullary crests; *5,* endolymphatic duct; *6 and 7,* maculae; *8,* cochlear duct; *9,* ampullary crest; *10,* cupula containing sensory hairs; *11,* layer of neuroepithelial hair cells; *12,* statoconia; *13,* gelatinous layer of macula; *14,* perilymphatic space; *15,* wall of osseous labyrinth.

the slight secretion from the goblet cells and the glands in the lining of the tympanic cavity to escape.

The Internal Ear

The mechanical stimuli produced by sound and by the positional changes of the head are transformed into nerve impulses in the internal ear. This is a delicate mechanism, no larger than about 12 mm across in the dog, and is completely enclosed in the very hard petrous temporal bone for protection and proper functioning (see Fig. 9.24A). It is exposed to sound vibrations on the lateral surface, and the electrical impulses into which these vibrations are converted leave the internal ear in nerve fibres of the vestibulocochlear nerve, which passes through the internal acoustic meatus on the medial surface.

The internal ear consists of a closed system of tiny membranous ducts and cavities known, because of its complexity, as the *membranous labyrinth* (Fig. 9.28A). It contains endolymph whose movement inside the system stimulates sensory cells in the membranous wall. Two enlargements in the center of the membranous labyrinth are known as the *utriculus* and *sacculus*. From the *utriculus* arise three semicircular ducts, and the sacculus is attached to the spiral cochlear duct. Although these structures are all closely related to each other developmentally and anatomically, their functions are distinct. The utriculus, sacculus, and semicircular ducts are concerned with detection of head position and movement, whereas the cochlear duct is concerned with hearing.

The *semicircular ducts* stand roughly at right angles to one another and are designated anterior, posterior, and lateral; one end of each duct is widened, or ampullated, close to the utriculus. The endolymph within the ducts is set in motion by movements of the head, applying force on receptive structures known as *ampullary crests* in each ampulla (Fig. 9.28/*9* and *10*). An important component of the ampullary crests are hair cells, so-called because of their cilia, which project into the ampulla. Forces exerted by the motion of the endolymph cause the cilia to bend, stimulating the hair cells to release neurotransmitter onto closely associated sensory neurons of the vestibular portion of the vestibulocochlear nerve, which in turn send impulses to the central nervous system.

Two further receptor areas called *maculae* (Fig. 9.28/*6* and *7*) are present in the walls of the utriculus and sacculus. They monitor the position of the head with respect to gravity. Like the ampullary crests, the maculae are bathed in endolymph and also contain hair cells. Instead of reacting to movement of the endolymph, however, the cilia of the macular hair cells are embedded in a gelatinous substance in which a layer of crystals (statoconia) is adhered. When the gelatinous layer of the maculae faces toward the ground, the cells are maximally stimulated by the gravitational pull on the statoconia. The maculae detect the *position and linear movements* of the head, whereas the ampullary crests detect the *rotational movements* of the head.

The sacculus gives origin to the endolymphatic duct, which ends blindly in the epidural space (Fig. 9.24/*17*). It is thought to function in the resorption of the endolymph secreted by the epithelial lining of the membranous labyrinth.

The membranous labyrinth is housed in a similar but slightly larger *osseous labyrinth,* a complex excavation in the temporal bone. The central chamber of the osseous labyrinth, the vestibule, houses the utriculus and the sacculus. The semicircular ducts lie within the osseous semicircular canals. The cochlear duct lies within the bony spiral canal of the cochlea, which is an excavation very similar to the inside of a snail's shell. The center of the cochlea is an osseous pyramid known as the *modiolus* (Fig. 9.29/*2*). Running around the modiolus is the spiral canal, the actual lumen of the cochlea, which ends blindly at the apex of the modiolus. Projecting into the spiral canal from the modiolus is an osseous shelf, the spiral lamina (Fig. 9.29/*5*), which terminates in the blind end of the spiral canal of the cochlea. The spiral lamina itself is hollow, forming the spiral canal of the modiolus.

Because the osseous labyrinth is slightly larger than the membranous labyrinth it encloses, there is a minute space between the two that contains perilymph. The perilymphatic space is only of significance in the area associated with the cochlea, where it forms two chambers, the scala tympani and the scala vestibuli, described below.

The bony spiral canal of the cochlea is divided into three channels (Fig. 9.29/A*6–8*), by a split longitudinal membrane, all running around the modiolus to the apex of the cochlea. The membrane arises centrally from the spiral lamina and, after splitting, attaches to the outside wall of the spiral canal. The uppermost channel is the scala vestibuli (Fig. 9.29/*6*), the middle one is the cochlear duct (Fig. 9.29/*7*), and the lowest is the scala tympani (Fig. 9.29/*8*). The two scalae communicate at the apex of the cochlea around the blind end of the cochlear duct. At the base of the cochlea, the scala vestibuli communicates with the perilymphatic space in the vestibule, and the scala tympani ends at the secondary tympanic membrane of the cochlear window (described previously; see Fig. 9.24).

An enlarged transverse section of the spiral canal of the cochlea shows the composition of the split membrane, particularly the part that forms the walls of the triangular cochlear duct (Fig. 9.29/*7*). The simplest of these walls separates the cochlear duct from the scala vestibuli; it consists of a single layer of cells and is known as the *spiral membrane* (Fig. 9.29A/*12*). The wall of the cochlear duct facing the scala tympani is complex by virtue of an arrangement of multiple rows of hair cells and other cells found in it, termed the *spiral organ* (Fig. 9.29A/*13*). Its connective tissue base is the basilar lamina, the characteristics of which play an important role in the transduction of different sound frequencies.

The functioning of the cochlea is described here briefly. In the middle ear, the mechanical movements of the base of the stapes vibrate the vestibular window, as described previously. Movement of the vestibular window in turn compresses the perilymph in the closed system of perilymphatic spaces in the inner ear. Because fluids are incompressible, pressure exerted on the fluid in the scala tympani results in a pressure wave traveling up to the apex of the bony cochlea. As the pressure wave passes, the force serves to move the pliable basilar lamina of the cochlear duct. This movement bends the cilia of the hair cells in the basal lamina, causing release of neurotransmitter onto closely associated sensory neurons associated with the cochlear portion of the vestibulocochlear nerve. The details of how

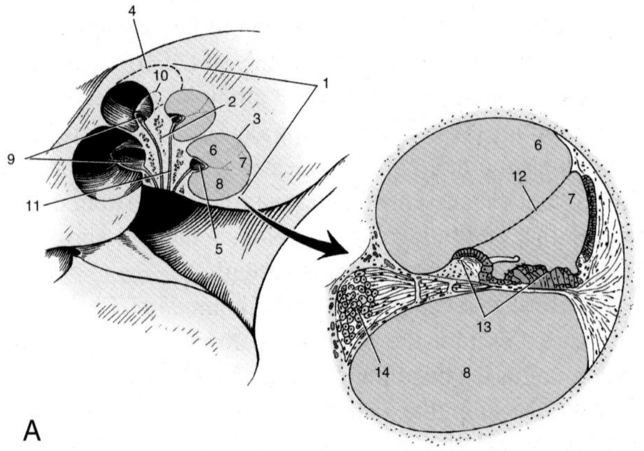

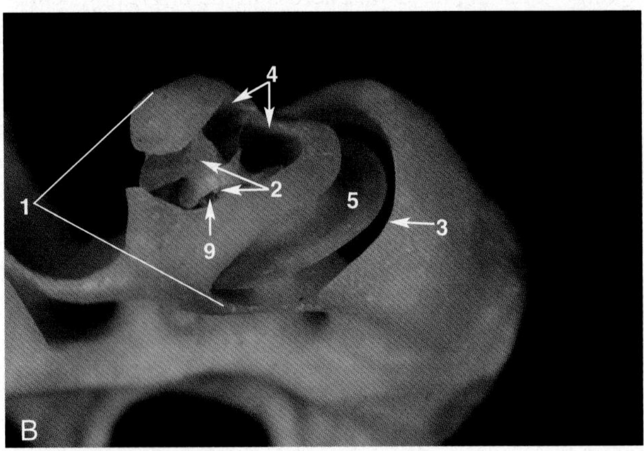

Fig. 9.29 Cochlea and enlarged cochlear duct. Schematic (A) and of the dog (B). *1,* Cochlea; *2,* modiolus; *3* and *4,* spiral canal of cochlea; *5,* osseous spiral lamina; *6,* scala vestibuli; *7,* cochlear duct; *8,* scala tympani; *9* and *10,* spiral canal of modiolus; *11,* longitudinal canals; *12,* spiral membrane; *13,* spiral organ; *14,* spiral ganglion.

the movements of the basilar membrane act on the hair cells is complex and beyond the scope of this book. Suffice it to say that the width and compliance of the basilar lamina results in transduction of lower frequency waves by the spiral organ located near the apex of the cochlea and that of higher frequency sounds by more proximal regions of the basilar membrane and spiral organ.

The impulses generated in cochlear fibers travel toward the modiolus to ganglion cells housed in the spiral canal. The aggregate of these cells forms the *spiral ganglion* (Fig. 9.29A/*14*), which also winds around the modiolus. From the spiral ganglion, the impulses travel along nerve fibers within canals to the base of the modiolus, where the fibers join to form the cochlear part of the vestibulocochlear nerve.

The vestibulocochlear nerve (cranial nerve VIII) is composed of vestibular and cochlear parts as it enters the internal acoustic meatus. As previously mentioned, the branches of the vestibular portion arise from the maculae in the utriculus and sacculus and the ampullae in the semicircular canals, conveying impulses concerned with balance; the cochlear portion arises from the base of the cochlea to mediate the impulses concerned with hearing.

The anatomy of the internal and middle ear is complicated by the passage of the facial nerve through this area (Fig. 9.24/*10*). The facial nerve enters the internal acoustic meatus together with the vestibulocochlear nerve and, within an osseous facial canal, traverses the temporal bone to emerge at the stylomastoid foramen. The facial canal makes a sharp kneelike bend within the temporal bone, and at this point the nerve is enlarged by the geniculate ganglion. From this ganglion arises the major petrosal nerve, which regulates secretion of the lacrimal and nasal glands. The chorda tympani, regulating the sublingual and mandibular glands but also relaying taste from the rostral two thirds of the tongue, leaves the facial nerve a little more distally. The chorda tympani is so named because, for a short segment of its course, it lies on the upper part of the tympanic membrane (Fig. 9.26/*5*). Both major petrosal and chorda tympani nerves leave the temporal bone through foramina on the rostroventral aspect of the bone. The facial nerve also supplies the stapedius muscle. (The tensor tympani is activated through the mandibular division of the trigeminal nerve [V3].)

THE OLFACTORY ORGAN

The sense of smell is overwhelmingly better developed in domestic mammals than in humans; this is particularly true of the dog, which can detect airborne substances in incredibly low concentrations. Much of an animals' contact with the environment and with other animals is made through olfaction, underscoring the importance of this sense in animals' sensory experience. This capability is exploited when dogs are used to "point" at game, to follow a scent in tracking fugitives, or to detect drugs and explosives, and when dogs and pigs are trained to find buried truffles. Dams recognize their offspring largely by the sense of smell, wild animals identify the extent of their territory by odorants on the ground, and wild herbivores test the air for the scent of predators.

The olfactory organ is of course situated in the nose. In animals with a well-developed sense of smell, it consists of a relatively large area of *olfactory mucosa* covering the lateral wall and the ethmoidal conchae in the caudal part of the nasal cavity. Although claimed to be a little more yellowish than the respiratory mucosa rostral to it, the olfactory mucosa cannot convincingly be identified by gross inspection. Histologic sections show the presence of olfactory cells that, like the photoreceptors in the retina, are bipolar neurons. Their dendrites reach the surface of the epithelium, presenting several minute olfactory hairs (cilia) to the air in the nasal cavity. The axons of the cells combine to form the fascicles of the olfactory nerve (cranial nerve I) that pass through the cribriform plate to the nearby olfactory bulb situated at the rostralmost part of the brain. Serous *olfactory glands* below the olfactory epithelium moisten the surface of the epithelium, presumably to wash away previously perceived odorants no longer present in the air.

The *vomeronasal organ** found in the nasal cavity is also concerned with olfaction. It consists of two narrow, parallel ducts that are embedded in the hard palate, one to each side of its junction with the nasal septum. The ducts, which are supported laterally, ventrally, and medially by thin cartilages, are lined in part with olfactory mucosa (Fig. 9.30A and B). Caudally they end blindly, but rostrally they open into the incisive ducts, which in most mammals connect the nasal and oral cavities through openings in the hard palate. The communication with the oral cavity is lacking in horses and donkeys. This organ has received considerable attention from animal behaviorists and reproductive physiologists because of its involvement in sexual activity, particularly in the lip-curl (flehmen) reaction demonstrated by male animals aroused by the odor of vaginal secretion or urine from estrous females (Fig. 9.31A and B). Whether the flehmen reaction as well as the accompanying extension of the head helps the odorants reach the vomeronasal organ is still a matter of speculation. Experimental

*A vomeronasal organ is not found in human adults; it makes an appearance during development but later regresses, although vestiges occasionally survive within the nasal septum. Because stimulation of the vomeronasal organ is known to affect the activity of gonadotropin-releasing hormone (GnRH) neurons, it is interesting to learn that these neurons have an unusual origin in the olfactory placodes. Their definitive locations are diffusely and variously spread (according to species) within the hypothalamic region of the brain.

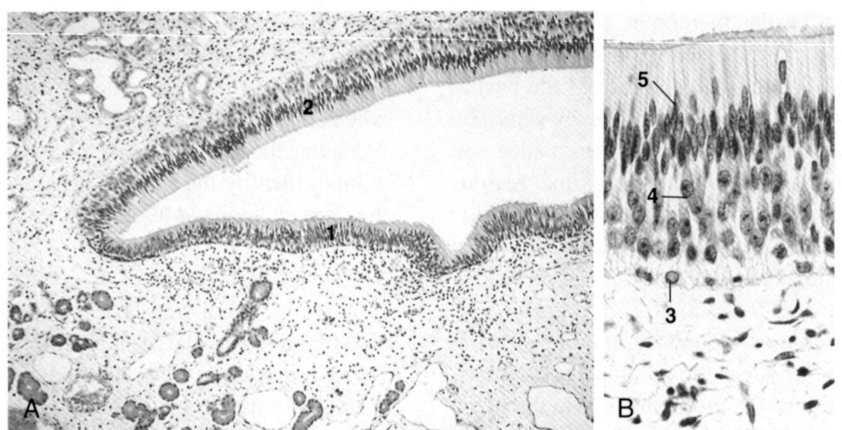

Fig. 9.30 (A) Vomeronasal organ (pig) (hematoxylin and eosin [HE]; magnification ×70). (B) Vomeronasal organ (pig) (HE; magnification ×279). *1,* Ciliated pseudostratified columnar respiratory epithelium; *2,* pseudostratifed columnar epithelium, enlarged in (B), consisting of *3,* basal cells; *4,* sustentacular cells; and *5,* neurosensitive cells.

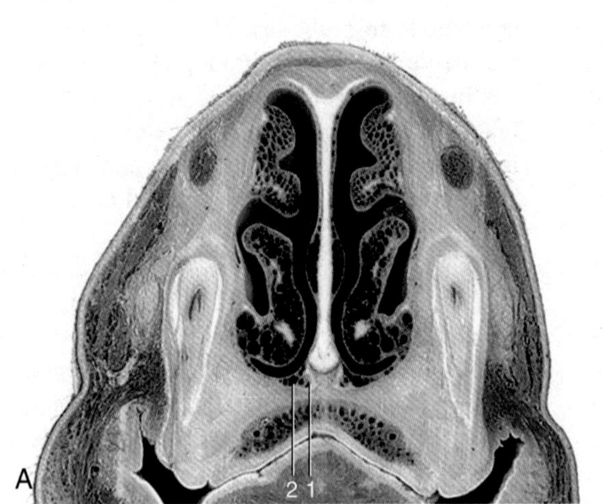

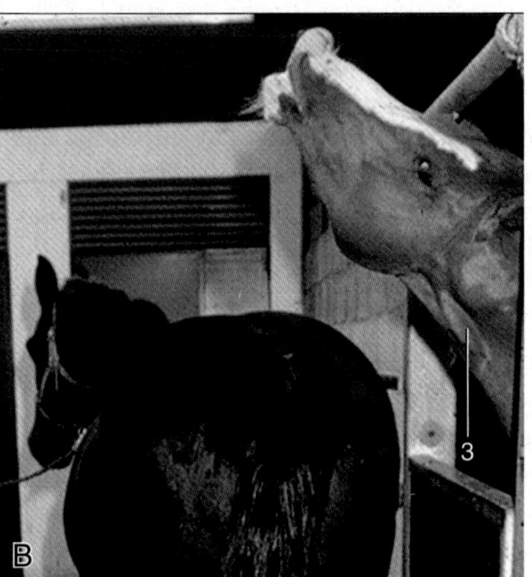

Fig. 9.31 (A) Transverse section of vomeronasal organ of horse. (B) During the flehmen reaction the head is fully extended, accentuating several features of the neck. *1,* Vomeronasal cartilage; *2,* vomeronasal duct; *3,* jugular groove.

blockage of the incisive ducts modifies but does not eliminate the flehmen reaction and other responses of bulls exposed to the pheromones contained within the vaginal secretion of cows in heat.

THE GUSTATORY ORGAN

The receptors for the sense of taste are the *taste buds* (Fig. 9.32), microscopic nests of cells mainly associated with the papillae of the tongue, although small numbers are also found in the soft palate and in the vicinity of the epiglottis. Taste buds are about as tall as the epithelium in which they lie and communicate with the oral cavity by taste pores through which solutions enter to stimulate the receptor cells. Taste pores cannot be seen with the naked eye.

The taste buds consist of sustentacular or supporting cells in addition to the receptor or *gustatory cells.* The gustatory cells have elongated nuclei and at their free tips bear microvilli (taste hairs) that project into the taste pore. Glands deep to the lingual papillae discharge a serous secretion on the surface of the epithelium. It is believed that the secretion cleanses the taste pores and enhances perception by the gustatory cells.

To be discerned, food substances have to be in solution. One of the reasons food is insalivated is to dissolve parts for sampling by the taste buds. The principal taste sensations are sweetness, sourness, and saltiness. In the dog sweetness and saltiness appear to be perceived in the rostral two thirds of the tongue, where taste buds are present on the fungiform papillae. Sour substances are perceived over the entire tongue. The caudal third of the tongue,

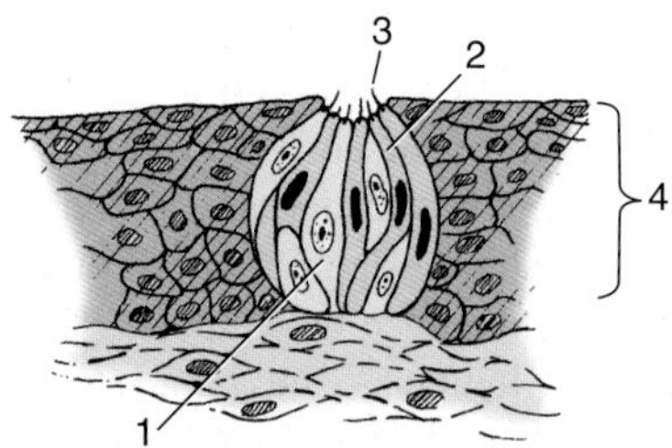

Fig. 9.32 Histologic section of a taste bud. *1*, Sustentacular cell; *2*, gustatory cells; *3*, taste pore; *4*, epithelium.

which incorporates the vallate and foliate papillae, therefore seems to respond only to what tastes sour.

The afferent pathways transmitting these sensations to the brain are similarly divided. In the rostral two thirds of the tongue, the sensory fibers travel first in the lingual nerve and then pass into the chorda tympani, which we encountered in the description of the ear. Neuronal cell bodies associated with these fibers are located in the geniculate ganglion of the seventh cranial nerve, and the centrally directed axons of these sensory neurons then enter the medulla oblongata. The afferent fibers innervating taste buds in the caudal third of the tongue travel in the glossopharyngeal nerve (and to a small extent in the vagus) to the medulla oblongata.

THE CUTANEOUS SENSE

As mentioned at the beginning of the chapter, much of the more immediate environment is experienced by the animal through its skin. This sense, referred to as *exteroception,* includes sensations such as touch, pressure, pain, heat, and cold; touch is a light stimulus such as is produced by a fly on the haircoat, and pressure is a stronger and deeper stimulus such as a horse feels from a saddle or girth. The receptors responsible for the detection of these stimuli vary considerably in structure. Unfortunately, because many intermediate forms exist, it is difficult to classify them and assign clear-cut functions to each kind. The simple classification given here is probably adequate for the purpose of this book.

The sensory receptors of the skin can be divided according to strictly anatomic criteria into free nerve endings and nerve endings that bear terminal corpuscles. The *free nerve endings* are tufts formed by the branches of nerve fibers that terminate either in fine points or in button-like swellings; they are found principally in the epidermis, and their purpose is to detect noxious, or painful, stimuli (Fig. 9.33/*1*). The *corpuscular endings* fall into three kinds: bulbous, lamellar, and meniscoid. The bulbous corpuscles, which are encapsulated terminal tufts of nerve fibers found in the dermis, are thought to respond to heat or cold (Fig. 9.33/*2*). The lamellar corpuscles are large (2–3 mm) and each consists of many concentric lamellae (flattened cells) surrounding the distal end of an afferent nerve fiber; they

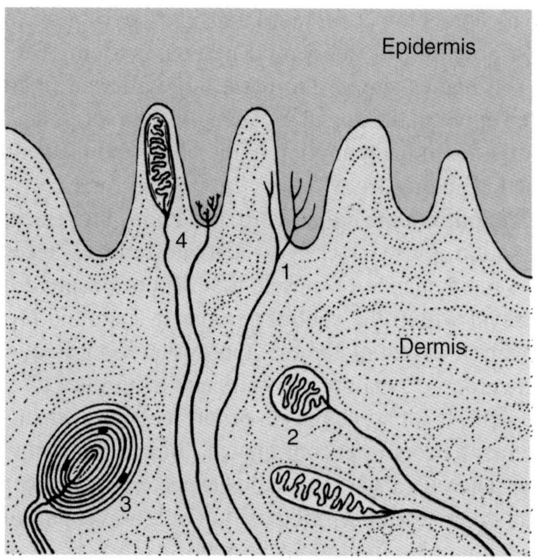

Fig. 9.33 Sensory nerve endings of the skin, schematic. *1*, Free nerve endings (pain); *2*, bulbous corpuscles (heat or cold); *3*, lamellar corpuscles (vibration); *4*, meniscoid nerve endings (touch).

are found in the subcutis and are thought to be pressure receptors (Fig. 9.33/*3*). Meniscoid corpuscles are small cup-shaped disks (menisci) at the ends of nerve fibers with which they contact "tactile" cells; they are found, usually encapsulated, both in the papillary layer of the dermis and free in the adjacent epidermis and are thought to be touch receptors (Fig. 9.33/*4*).

A special cutaneous sense is mediated by the *tactile hairs.* They are long hairs that protrude from the head and are substantially thicker than the hairs forming the haircoat. The cat's whiskers are good examples, but all domestic mammals have them, principally in association with the muzzle and eyes. The roots of tactile hairs are surrounded by blood sinuses, the walls of which are densely populated with afferent nerve endings (see Fig. 10.12). When the tips of the tactile hairs are touched, the movement is amplified by fluid movement in the sinuses, exciting the sensory nerve fibers, which transmit this message to the central nervous system (see also p. 346).

PROPRIOCEPTION

Proprioception, or kinesthesia, is the sense of the position and movement of body segments, and it relies upon the presence of receptors embedded in skeletal muscle, tendons, joint capsules, and ligaments. These specialized receptors respond to stretch or force and provide information on muscle length, muscle tension, and the amount of joint flexion in addition to the rate at which these changes occur. The immediate detection of this information is of utmost importance for control of movement, and the largest, fastest conducting afferent fibers in the body innervate these receptors to permit rapid transmission of proprioceptive information to the central nervous system. The sensory cell bodies supporting these large afferent fibers are located either in the dorsal root ganglia near the spinal cord or in the trigeminal ganglion in the head, and the centrally projecting axons from these sensory neurons carry this information into the spinal cord and brain. Proprioceptive information is used locally to activate reflexes necessary for the maintenance of muscle tone. Proprioceptive fibers also travel within the central nervous system and provide information essential for the appropriate coordination of muscle groups to maintain posture and to produce effective movement. If for some reason proprioception is disturbed, movements become uncoordinated, a condition known as *ataxia*. There is also a conscious aspect to proprioception in that we are aware of the position and movement of our limbs without having to look at them.

ENTEROCEPTION

Enteroception is the sense of stretch or pain arising from the viscera. Sensory receptors present in the viscera are activated in response to dilation, to contraction or spasm (colic), and to chemical irritation. These sensations are usually perceived as unpleasant or painful, and when the affected organ is in the abdominal cavity, they are often accompanied by reflex contraction of the abdominal muscles and cessation of abdominal breathing. A rigid abdomen is an important accompanying diagnostic sign.

Referred pain, although important in human medicine, is of unknown significance in animals. The most widely known example in humans is the pain referred to the presternal region, neck, shoulders, and inner aspect of the left arm in humans with angina pectoris, a lack of oxygen to the heart tissue due to an inadequate blood supply. Afferent fibers arising from receptors in the viscera travel in the same spinal cord pathways as somatic sensory fibers innervating those cutaneous regions, which develop at the same embryologic level. It is thought that the predominance of somatic fibers in these spinal pathways is in part responsible for the incorrect perception that activity in visceral receptors is pain is arising instead in nearby somatic tissues.

COMPREHENSION CHECK

Olfaction and audition are much better developed in domestic animals than in humans, whereas vision is less important. How do these differences inform us about the total sensory experience of domestic animals in comparison with ours?

The Common Integument

10

The term *common integument* encompasses ordinary skin with its covering of hair and variety of skin glands as well as more specialized parts such as claws, hoofs, and horns. The skin completely encloses the body and blends with the mucous membranes at the various natural openings. The integument offers protection against wear and tear as well as entry of pathogens and other environmental toxicants. It is critical for thermoregulation (p. 343) and impermeable to water while preventing the body from drying out. Conversely, the integument prevents excessive water uptake in aquatic mammals. Certain lipid substances can penetrate skin and are used (in the form of ointments) as vehicles for administration of medication.

The pigment granules in certain cells impart color to the skin, protect it against ultraviolet radiation, and reflect solar heat to protect in increases in body temperature. It is known that skin and coat color affect the adaptability of animals to life in sunny climates. The color of naked and nonpigmented areas is also affected by the perfusion of blood vessels in deeper layers, examples of which are blushing in humans, the pallor of anemia or shock, the blue tint (cyanosis) of lack of oxygen, and the yellow (icterus) of jaundice. Very spectacular color changes, such as that for which the chameleon is famous, do not occur in mammals, although mention may be made of the garish coloration of the skin of the mask and perineum of male mandrills and related monkeys.

THE STRUCTURE OF SKIN

Some recapitulation and amplification of the earlier account (p. 7) of basic skin structure is now required. Skin is composed of two parts: a superficial epithelium (epidermis) and a tough fibrous layer (dermis) that rests on a stratum of loose connective tissue (subcutis) (see Fig. 1.7).

The *epidermis* is continuously renewed. The surface cells are sloughed in flakes (e.g., dandruff) or as smaller particles (those of human skin accounting for much household dust) and are replaced by cell division in the deepest layer followed by migration of daughter cells toward the surface. As the epidermal cells migrate superficially, they undergo a series of molecular changes leading to their deaths, thus rendering them incapable of reacting to the various influences once they reach the surface. The sequence of changes, shown in Fig. 10.1, imposes an obvious stratification. The deepest layer (*stratum basale*) is closely molded on the irregularities of the underlying dermis and has a considerably greater area than the surface of the body (Fig. 10.1/*1*). As the cells move into the *stratum spinosum,* they shrink and draw apart, though remaining connected by intercellular bridges (desmosomes). The process of keratinization (cornification) now begins, and in the next layer (*stratum granulosum*) the cells contain scattered keratohyalin granules (Fig. 10.1/*4*). In some regions this layer is followed by a narrow *stratum lucidum* composed of flattened cells that have already lost their nuclei and distinct outlines but obtain a homogeneous appearance from the even dispersal of the granules. Finally, the outermost squamous layer (*stratum corneum*; Fig. 10.1/*6*) is densely packed with the fibrous protein keratin, the true horny substance, which is transformed keratohyalin. It is keratin that gives epidermal specializations (e.g., hair, hoof, and horn) their hardness and their strength.

The epidermal layers are thickest and most clearly differentiated where the skin is exposed to hard usage, as on the footpads of a dog (Fig. 10.2). Where abrasion is less severe, as in haired regions, the epidermis is much thinner, and neither the stratum granulosum nor the stratum lucidum may be clearly represented. The thickness of the epidermis depends on the mitotic rate within the stratum basale, which is adjusted by a substance (epidermal chalone) that inhibits cell division. Although cell production and loss normally match to maintain an even epidermal thickness, this balance may be disturbed in certain circumstances.

There are no blood or lymphatic vessels in the epidermis, which is nourished by diffusion from the subjacent dermis.

The *dermis* is largely composed of collagen bundles, thickly felted together, as can be demonstrated by teasing leather (tanned dermis). Elastic fibers, which are also present, make the skin pliable and are able to restore its shape after being wrinkled or deformed. These fibers also draw apart the edges of a wound, making it gape (Fig. 10.3). Chronic tension damages the structure of the dermis, rupturing the connective tissue bundles; subsequent repair is usually by lighter scar tissue. The white lines (striae) of abdominal skin that appear after the completion of a pregnancy, especially in women, is an example.

The dermis is generously vascularized and innervated. It is also invaded by hair follicles and sweat, sebaceous, and other glands growing from the epidermis (see Fig. 1.7).

The interface for diffusion between the epidermis and the dermis is enlarged by the complicated molding of these components. The finger-like and ridgelike projections

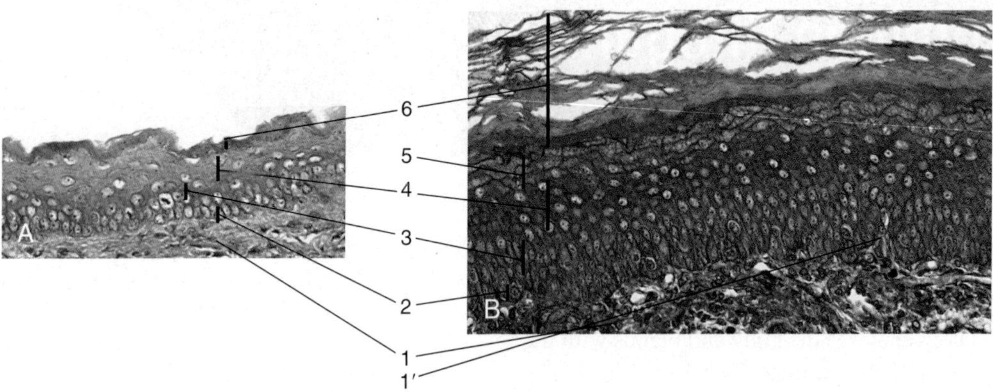

Fig. 10.1 Structure of the adult skin (Crossmon). (A) Skin from the canine flank. (B) Skin from a worn feline footpad; note the increased keratinization and the presence of a stratum lucidum and dermal papillae. *1,* Dermis; *1′,* dermal papilla; *2,* stratum basale; *3,* stratum spinosum; *4,* stratum granulosum; *5,* stratum lucidum; *6,* stratum corneum.

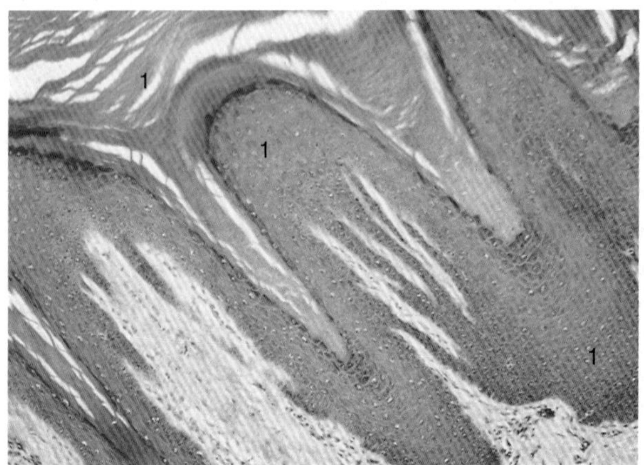

Fig. 10.2 Stratified squamous epithelium of a footpad of a dog (hematoxylin and eosin; magnification ×70). *1,* Very thick stratum corneum.

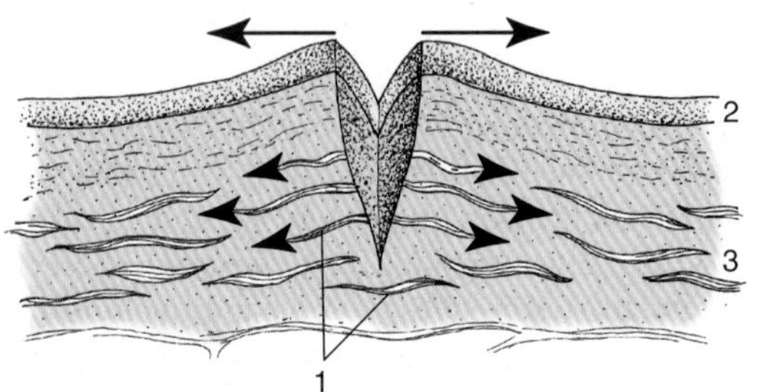

Fig. 10.3 Skin incision; elastic fibers in the dermis cause the wound to gape *(arrows)*. *1,* Elastic fibers; *2,* epidermis; *3,* dermis.

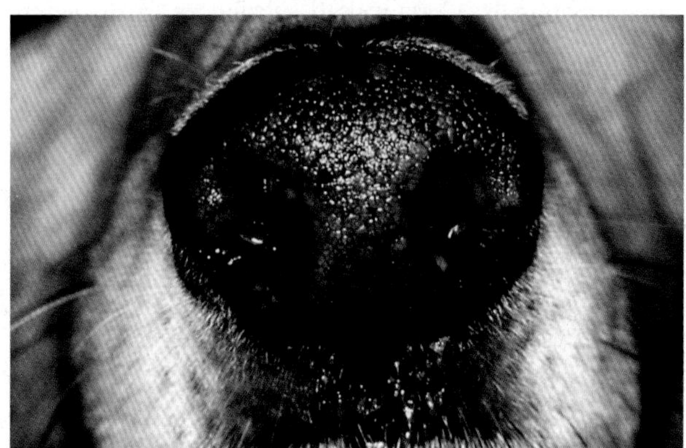

Fig. 10.4 The nose print in the dog can be used for identification of an individual.

(papillae; Fig. 10.1/*1′*) of the dermis fit closely into reciprocal depressions of the epidermis, and under normal conditions adhesion between the two structures is not easily disturbed. Trauma, such as that caused by the rubbing of an ill-fitting boot or shoe, sometimes separates them forcibly, and interstitial fluid then collects in a blister. The raw surface of the dermis exposed following the rupture of the blister normally is rapidly covered by the growth of the epithelium from the margins.

The larger dermal ridges and papillae, generally developed where the covering epithelium is thickest, are reflected by corresponding epidermal contours. These contours are permanent and individually distinct and provide a means of identification, widely used in ourselves (fingerprinting) and less commonly used in other species (nose printing of dogs and cattle; Fig. 10.4).

The *subcutis* consists of loose connective tissue interspersed with fat. It varies in amount according to situation and is thin or even absent where movement is undesirable (e.g., over the lips, eyelids, and teats). It is particularly ample in dogs and cats, whose easily shifted skin can be grasped in large folds over much of the body (Fig. 10.5). In the pig and the human, the subcutis contains more substantial accumulations of fat, even in relatively ill-nourished individuals; this part constitutes the panniculus adiposus familiar in sliced bacon.

The clinical significance of the effects of dehydration or edema of the subcutis has been mentioned (p. 7).

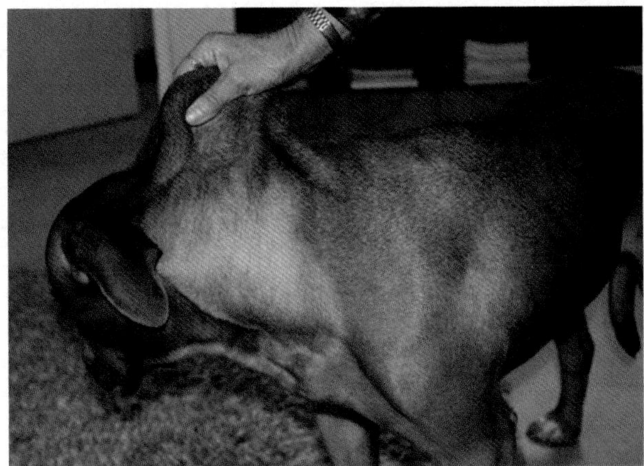

Fig. 10.5 Loose skin on the neck of a dog. Ample subcutis permits shifting of the skin.

The *cutaneous blood vessels* come from the vessels that supply the fasciae and superficial muscles. The arteries form a series of networks within the dermis. The most superficial network lies at the bases of the papillae and provides end-arteries that enter the papillae to release numerous capillaries that nourish the basal epidermal cells. Other capillary plexuses surround the hair follicles and associated glands (see Fig. 1.7). When the body temperature is raised, vasodilation of superficial vessels promotes heat loss—directly by surface radiation and indirectly by favoring the activity of the glands that produce sweat, which then evaporates. Conversely, the surface vessels constrict in cold environments or when the internal temperature drops. The blood flow is partly regulated by opening or closing of numerous anastomoses connecting the cutaneous arteries with veins. The skin vessels normally contain a considerable volume of blood, but much can be recalled to the musculature and internal organs after hemorrhage or shock.

Skin has a rich *sensory innervation*. The nerves accompany the vessels through the fasciae and form networks within the dermis. From these, fibers disperse to a variety of sensory receptors; some even penetrate a little way into the epidermis (see Fig. 9.33). Other (autonomic) fibers regulate the caliber of the smaller vessels, control the activity of skin glands, and excite the arrector pili muscles that attach to the hair follicles.

The epidermis develops from the embryonic ectoderm. This structure is initially a single layer of cells lying on a bed of mesenchyme that in time gives rise to the dermis (Fig. 10.6A). Long before birth the ectodermal cells begin to proliferate, pushing new cells toward the surface to produce a multilayered epithelium, while local condensations grow into the mesenchyme as the epithelial buds from which hair and glands differentiate. By the time of birth the skin of domestic mammals has a basically adult character, unlike that of many rodents and other small mammals that are born naked.

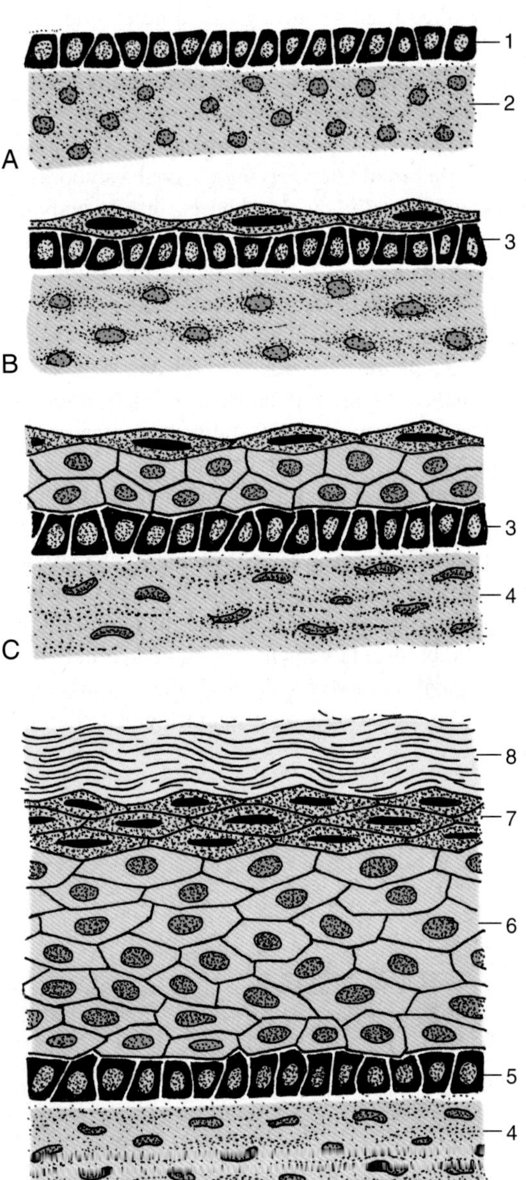

Fig. 10.6 Development of skin, schematic. (A) Skin of an early embryo. (B) Differentiation of epidermis and dermis. (C) Further differentiation of the epidermis. (D) Complete differentiation of the epidermis and dermis. *1*, Ectoderm; *2*, mesoderm (mesenchyme); *3*, primitive stratum basale; *4*, dermis; *5*, stratum basale; *6*, stratum spinosum; *7*, stratum granulosum; *8*, stratum corneum.

HAIR

Hair is a mammalian feature, diagnostic of the class. In most species a thick haircoat is spread over the body, except about the mouth and other openings and on the surfaces of the feet; in a few, including the domestic pig (though not its ancestors), the covering is sparse (see Fig. 10.10E). The individual hairs take a variety of intergrading forms, but only three need be distinguished here: straight, rather stiff guard hairs provide a "topcoat"; fine, wavy wool hairs provide an "undercoat"; and stout tactile hairs of restricted distribution are associated with touch receptors.

Guard hairs mostly lie close against the skin and sweep uniformly in broad tracts, giving the coat a smooth appearance disturbed only by the whorls, crests, and partings formed where different streams converge and combine or diverge from one another. The regularity of the arrangement is significant because it promotes the runoff of rain, preventing the chilling that would occur if water were allowed to penetrate the pile to reach the skin. Occasionally, animals are born with a disturbed coat pattern, which may seriously impair their ability to withstand severe weather.

Each hair grows from a tiny pit or follicle to protrude above the surface of the skin. The follicle develops from an ectodermal bud that grows into the underlying mesenchyme during the embryonic stage of life. The bud branches give rise to skin glands (Fig. 10.7). The distal end of the bud forms a bulbous enlargement, which is then indented by a mesenchymal (dermal) papilla to form a primitive hair follicle. The epithelial cells lying against the papilla multiply, forming a hair matrix; the cells produced here keratinize and combine to form a primitive hair that grows through the center of the bud until it rises above the epidermis on the surface of the skin. Its passage takes it past the sebaceous glands that develop to the side of the follicle, and this arrangement allows the hair to obtain the oily coating so important for its health. Although the ectoderm differentiates in this way, the mesoderm also condenses so that the tiny sheath around the embedded part of the hair acquires an outer mesodermal component.

Fig. 10.8 shows only the essential features of a hair. It must suffice here to say that, in essence, a hair consists of a flexible column of closely consolidated and heavily keratinized, and hence dead, epithelial cells. Their arrangement permits the distinction of a medulla or core, a cortex, and an outer "scaly" cuticle. The variation in proportions and the arrangement of the parts permit the microscopic determination of the origin of a hair sample. In general, hairs with a thick medulla are straight and rather brittle, whereas those in which the cortex predominates are stronger and more pliable.

The proximal end of the follicle is joined by a tiny arrector pili muscle passing from an attachment near the dermal

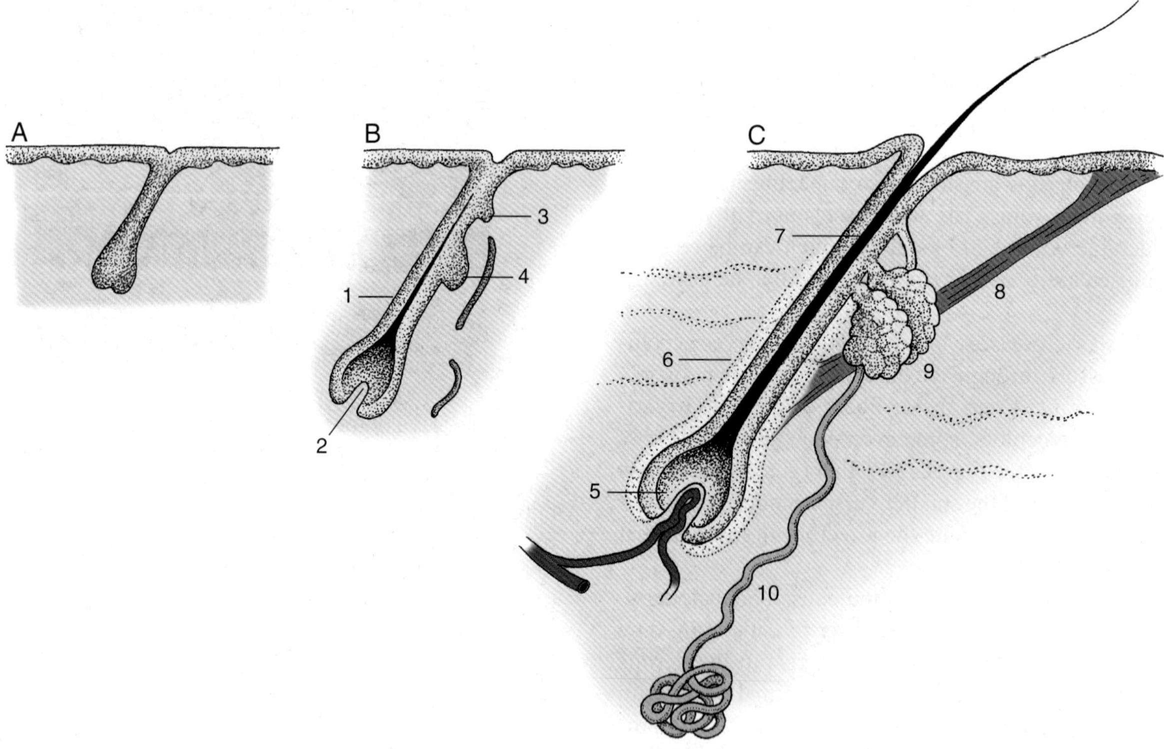

Fig. 10.7 Development of hair and associated sebaceous and sweat glands, schematic. (A) Ectodermal bud growing into mesenchyme. (B) Differentiation of the bud; indications of glands appear. (C) Hair follicle with accessory structures. *1,* Primitive hair follicle; *2,* dermal papilla; *3,* bud of sweat gland; *4,* bud of sebaceous gland; *5,* bulb (hair matrix) of hair; *6,* hair follicle; *7,* root of hair; *8,* arrector pili muscle; *9,* sebaceous gland; *10,* sweat gland. In the adult, many glands open independently, not into hair follicles.

papillae (Fig. 10.7/*8*). The involuntary contraction of this muscle, which may be stimulated by a low ambient temperature, causes erection of the hair; the en masse erection of hairs traps more air and improves the insulation of the body. Although functionally unimportant in the human species, the effect is very obvious in our relatively naked skin when little mounds (goose pimples) appear over the courses of the arrector muscles. The fight-or-flight reaction mediated by the sympathetic nervous system raises the hackles that give an animal a threatening appearance.

There are many local variations in the form and development of guard hairs. Familiar examples are the stiff, sparsely scattered bristles of pigs (see Fig. 10.10E), the coarse hair of the mane and tail of horses, the long tail hairs of cattle, the fetlock tufts of horses, and the feathering of the tail and limbs of certain breeds of dogs. The hormone-dependent local variations particularly evident in the human species include the male beard and the sexually dimorphic distribution of body hair. Baldness as an accompaniment of advancing age is especially a problem of the human male. Testosterone, which is responsible for the growth of the beard and coarse body hair, paradoxically seems to trigger early baldness in genetically predisposed individuals; a reduced blood level of thyroxine, which initiates and controls hair growth, also plays some part.

Hairs have restricted lives and are discarded sooner or later. Although hair shedding in humans is a continuous process involving only a few hairs at a time, most other species, especially wild species, shed many hairs at a time in a seasonal fashion. Even domesticated animals protected from the more extreme climatic changes show a recurrent pattern with peaks in the spring and fall; spring shedding lasts about 5 weeks in dogs. Shedding is more obvious in animals not regularly groomed to remove dead hair. Cats also molt most heavily in spring, with less substantial

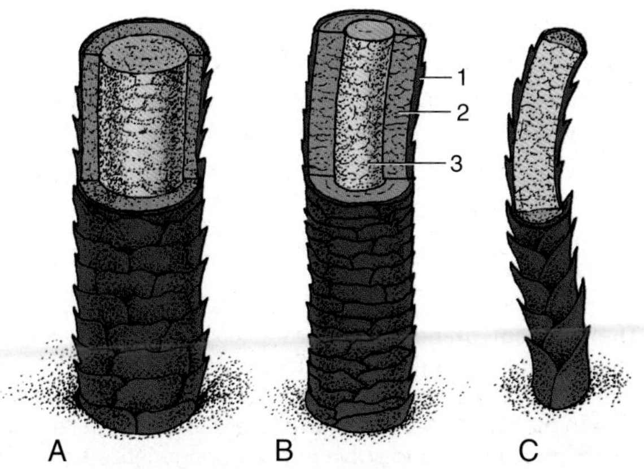

Fig. 10.8 Schematic representation of three kinds of hair. (A) Guard hair with thick medulla. (B) Guard hair with thick cortex and thin medulla. (C) Wool hair; the cortex is absent. *1*, Cuticle; *2*, cortex; *3*, medulla.

loss through the summer and fall followed by attaining of prime condition in winter. For the same reason, the pelts of furbearing species are harvested in winter, although the number of harvested pelts has fallen with changing social attitudes.

The seasonal replacement begins with a slowing of the growth of existing hair mainly owing to a rise in seasonal temperature. As growth slows (in the so-called catagen phase) the hair matrix and covering papilla both atrophy (Fig. 10.9B). No growth occurs in the ensuing (*telogen*) phase when the follicle, including the papilla, shortens, causing a larger part of the hair to project above the skin in simulation of growth (Fig. 10.9D). When growth resumes, the follicle, with its matrix now reactivated, lengthens, and as it again extends away from the surface, it loses its grip on the old hair, which falls out. A replacement hair then forms in the active growth (*anagen*) phase that follows to emerge on the surface of the skin.

Wool hairs provide the soft undercoat. They are thin, wavy, and in most species, shorter and more numerous than the guard hairs by which they are concealed. The distinction between hair fiber types is not always clear-cut, and intermediate forms exist to complicate description, especially in the sheep.* Wool is not, of course, confined to sheep among domestic animals. Cashmere and Angora goats, Angora rabbits, and alpacas all produce wools of distinctive quality that are utilized in the production of luxury yarns and textiles.

In many species, including mature dogs and cats, several hairs share a single follicle opening (Fig. 10.10B–D). The

*The coat of wild sheep and of extant primitive breeds exhibits an outer coat of very coarse, hollow-cored guard hairs, known as *kemp*, which conceals and protects, by facilitating the runoff of rain, a short undercoat of much finer wool fibers. The growth of both fiber types is seasonally restricted and is succeeded by a spring molt when the shed wool forms tangled mats that are eventually cast. The wool is harvested by being gathered from the pasture and plucked directly from the animals. Evolution of the fleece under domestication has been characterized by loss of pigmentation and by reduction in the amount of kemp, partly by depletion of the number of kemp hairs and partly by the transformation of a proportion of these into finer and more typical forms of hair. The wool now grows continuously and at a more rapid rate, though showing seasonal variation, and elimination of the spring molt introduces the necessity for shearing. The more rapid growth results in increased fiber length in the annual wool clip; other changes affect fiber waviness (crimp) and introduce greater diversity in the relative incidences of fibers of different diameters. The variations in these acquired features account for the characters, and therefore the values, of the fleeces of different breeds. The coarse, hairy fleece of some is most appropriate for the less valuable carpet trade, whereas the improved fleece of others is suited to the production of finer yarns and fabrics. The weight of wool produced annually also varies widely with breed, ranging from as little as 3 to as much as 20 pounds (1.4 to 9 kg).

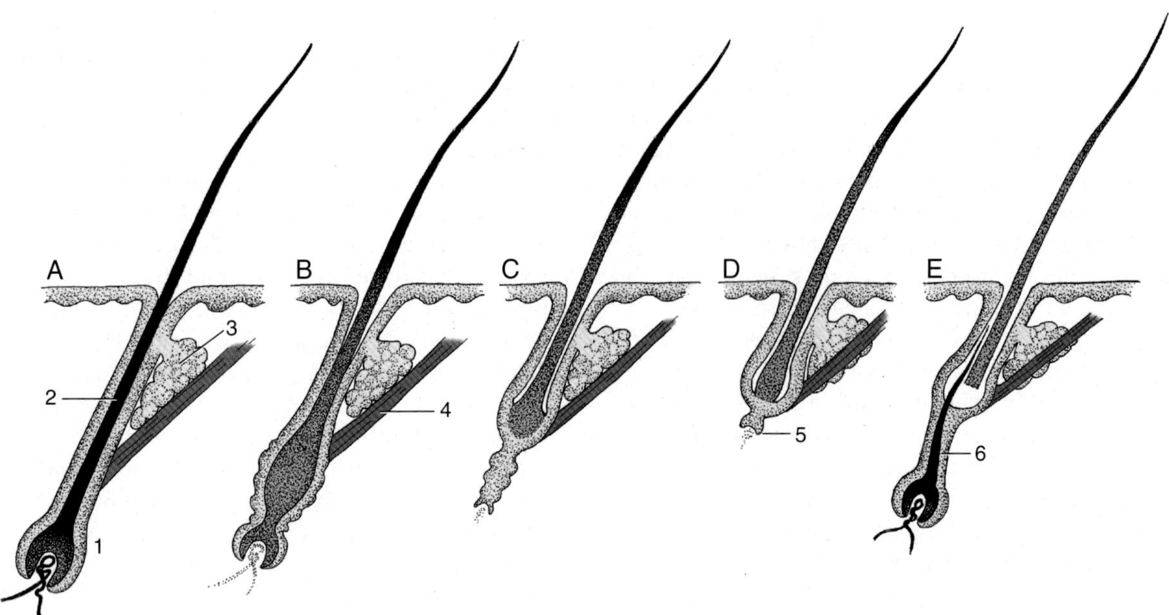

Fig. 10.9 Phases of the hair cycle. (A) Fully functional hair follicle; anagen phase. (B) Follicle begins to atrophy; early catagen phase. (C) Further atrophy of follicle; late catagen phase. (D) Atrophied follicle; hair is displaced distally and new hair matrix begins to form; telogen phase. (E) New hair matrix established and new hair begins to grow; early anagen phase. *1,* Hair follicle; *2,* root of hair; *3,* sebaceous gland; *4,* arrector pili muscle; *5,* new hair matrix; *6,* new hair.

central (primary) hair is longest and of the guard type, but the surrounding (secondary) hairs are shorter and softer; they provide the undercoat and may be designated wool hairs because they have little medulla.

Tactile hairs are substantially thicker and generally protrude beyond the neighboring guard hairs. Most are found on the face, principally on the upper lip and about the eyes, although others are scattered (in species-variable fashion) on the lower lip, the chin, and elsewhere on the head. The cat, whose whiskers are particularly good examples (Fig. 10.11), also possesses a cluster of similar hairs at the carpus. Tactile hair follicles reach deep into the subcutis or even the superficial muscles. They are characterized by the presence of a venous sinus filled with blood and located between inner and outer layers of the dermal sheath (Fig. 10.12). The nerve endings responsive to mechanical stimulation are also contained within the dermal sheath (Fig. 10.12A). The stimulus provided by disturbance of the hair is amplified by wave motion in the blood. The follicles of tactile hairs appear early in development, before those of the coat hairs, and their staged appearances provide useful criteria for aging embryos.

The skin of dogs and cats presents minute scattered tactile elevations (toruli tactiles) usually associated with special (tylotrich) guard hairs; the roots of these are surrounded by venous sinuses similar to, though smaller than, those of true tactile hairs. These elevations are also sensitive to touch (Fig. 10.13).

The restricted distribution of various pigments creates a distinct pattern of coats as seen in breeds such as Holstein cattle and Dalmatian dogs. The pigments, polymers of melanin ranging from black, through brown and red, to lighter shades are present in granule form* within cells of the epidermis, hair follicles, and hair. The pigments protect the skin from potentially harmful ultraviolet radiation and are unnecessary within those epidermal regions that are covered by a dense coat of hair. In most mammals, unlike in humankind, skin pigmentation is therefore restricted to a few exposed parts that include the modified area associated with the external nose. It may be lacking here in white-coated individuals that obtain equivalent protection from a thickened stratum corneum.

*The pigment granules are produced within melanocytes, specialized cells of neural crest origin that are confined to the basal layer of the epidermis and hair follicles. The granules move to the tips of the dendritic processes of the melanocytes and are pinched off and subsequently phagocytized by neighboring cells (keratinocytes) in a process that continues until widespread. Melanin production is influenced by many factors including sufficiency of copper and, by the melanocyte-stimulating hormone. Melanin production may be affected by season (white fur in lagomorphs and mustelids in winter) and age.

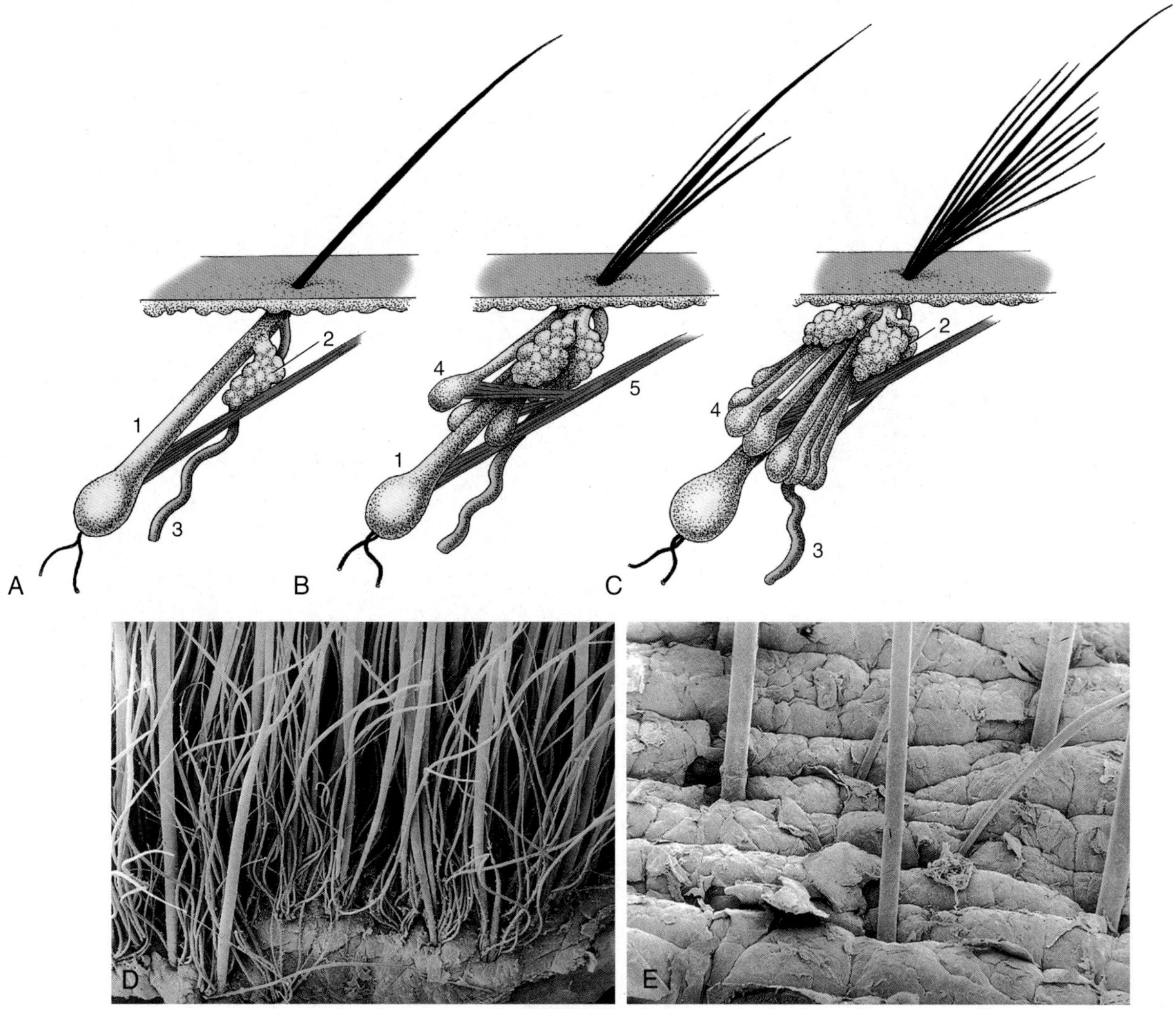

Fig. 10.10 Hair follicles of the dog: (A) simple follicle present shortly after birth; (B) follicle present during the first few months after birth; (C) complex adult follicle; the primary hair is surrounded by several secondary hairs. (D) Scanning electron micrograph of adult canine skin; note one or two follicles without primary (guard) hairs. (E) "Naked" skin of a pig with sparse primary hairs (bristles) and surface debris. *1*, Primary hair follicle; *2*, sebaceous gland; *3*, duct of sweat gland; *4*, secondary hair follicle; *5*, arrector pili muscle.

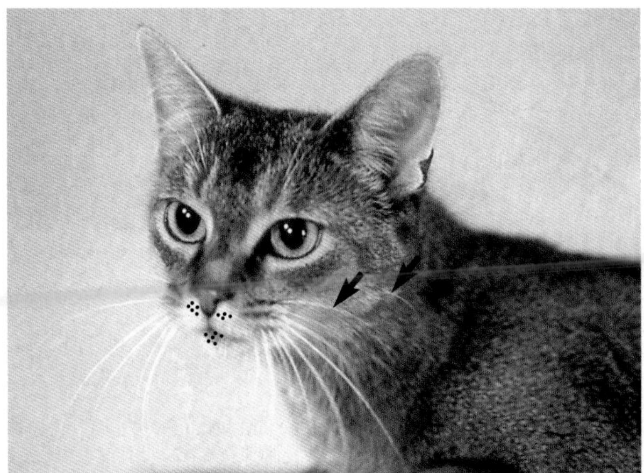

Fig. 10.11 Tactile hairs on the head of the cat. The *dots* on the lips show the position of the circumoral glands. The *arrows* point to the buccal (tactile) hairs.

FOOTPADS

The footpads (tori) are the cushions on which animals walk. They are covered by a naked, densely cornified epidermis (see Fig. 10.2). The dermis is unremarkable, and the bulk of their substance is provided by a thick, resilient subcutis, an admixture of collagenous and elastic fibers interspersed with adipose tissue.

Footpads are best developed in plantigrade mammals (e.g., bears), in which digital, metacarpal (metatarsal), and carpal (tarsal) pads are all present (Fig. 10.14). In the digitigrade dog and cat, only digital and metacarpal (metatarsal) pads make ground contact; there is a carpal pad of no obvious use but no corresponding tarsal pad (Fig. 10.15).

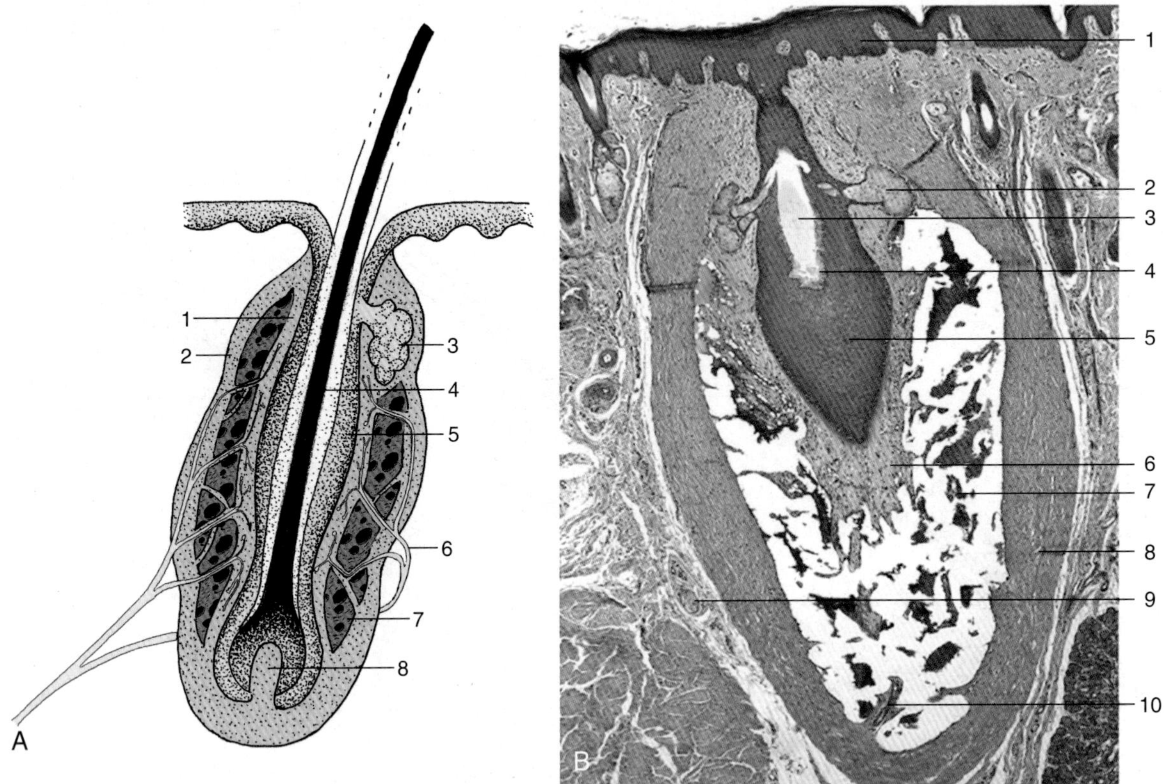

Fig. 10.12 (A) Schematic longitudinal section of a tactile hair follicle. *1* and *2,* Internal and external walls of blood sinus; *3,* sebaceous gland; *4,* root of hair; *5,* epidermal wall of hair follicle; *6,* nerve ending in wall of blood sinus; *7,* blood sinus; *8,* dermal papilla. (B) Tactile hair follicle of calf (Crossmon). *1,* Epidermis; *2,* sebaceous gland; *3,* hair; *4* and *5,* inner and outer hair root sheath; *6* and *7,* trabeculated blood sinus; *8,* inner and outer layer dermal sheath; *9,* nerve ending; *10,* trabecula.

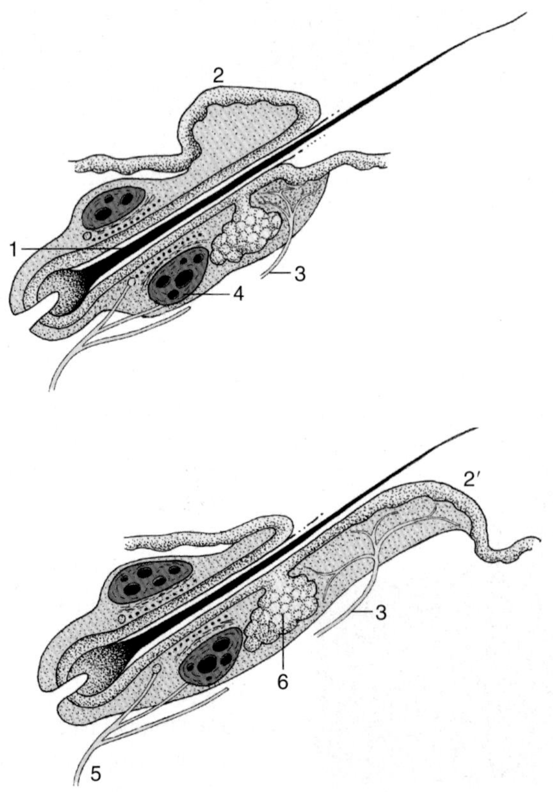

Fig. 10.13 Tylotrich hairs below *(top)* and above *(bottom)* tactile elevations (*2* and *2′*). *1,* Root of hair; *3,* nerve endings associated with tactile elevations; *4,* blood sinus; *5,* nerve endings associated with blood sinus; *6,* sebaceous gland.

Only digital pads, called *bulb* in ruminants and pigs and *frog* in horses, located in the hoof are functional and in contact with the ground in ungulates. The bulbs of the pig are softer than those of ruminants and well set off from the sole (see later) (Fig. 10.16/*1*).

The digital cushion (pulvinus digitalis) deep to the frog of the horse consists of an apex and a base. The apex lies deep to the horny frog on the ground surface of the hoof (Fig. 10.17/*4*), whereas the base helps shape the palmar (plantar) surface, forming the swellings at the heels. These, the bulbs of the heels (Fig. 10.17/*3*), do not make contact with the ground and are covered by periople, the softer horn produced at the junction of the skin with the wall of the hoof. The horse, unlike the other domestic ungulates, also has rudimentary metacarpal (metatarsal) pads ("ergots"; Fig. 10.17/*2*) embedded in a tuft of hair behind the fetlock joint and vestigial carpal (tarsal) pads (chestnuts; Fig. 10.17/*1* and *1′*).

The subcutis of the canine footpads, porcine bulbs, and equine frog contains sweat glands whose ducts channel through the thick, cornified epidermis. The secretions function as territorial or trail markers.

NAILS, CLAWS, AND HOOFS

The basically similar structures enclosing the distal phalanx appear strikingly different. Their origins as local modifications of skin are reflected in their retention of epidermal, dermal, and subcutis layers (though perhaps in

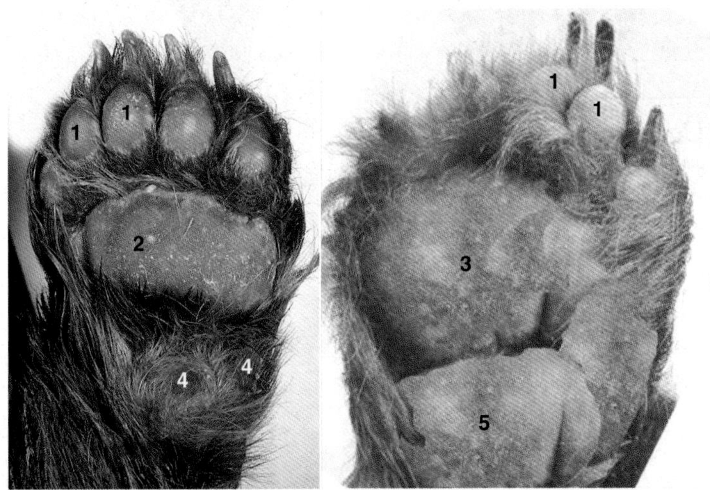

Fig. 10.14 Footpads of a bear, forelimb *(left)* and hindlimb *(right)*. *1,* Digital pads; *2,* metacarpal pad; *3,* metatarsal pad; *4,* carpal pads; *5,* tarsal pad, fused with the metatarsal pad.

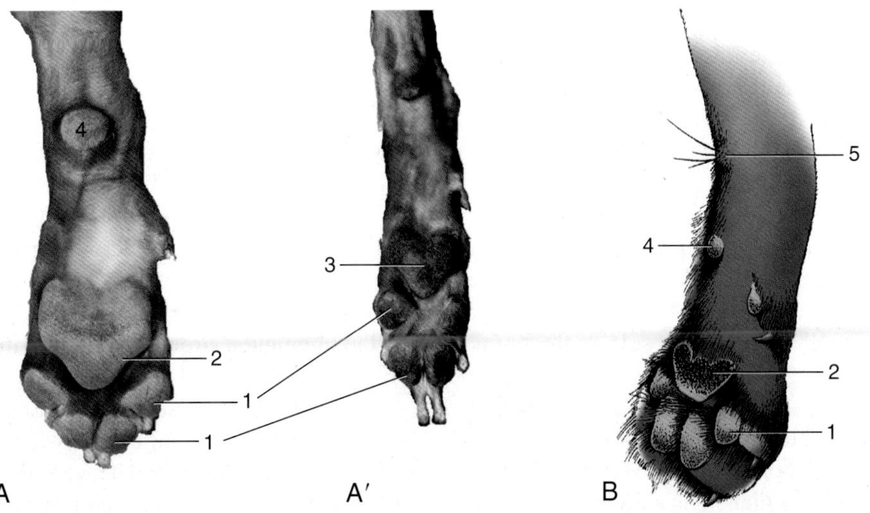

Fig. 10.15 Footpads of canine (A) forelimbs and (A′) hindlimbs and of (B) feline forelimb. *1,* Digital pads; *2,* metacarpal pad; *3,* metatarsal pad; *4,* carpal pad; *5,* carpal gland and associated tactile hairs.

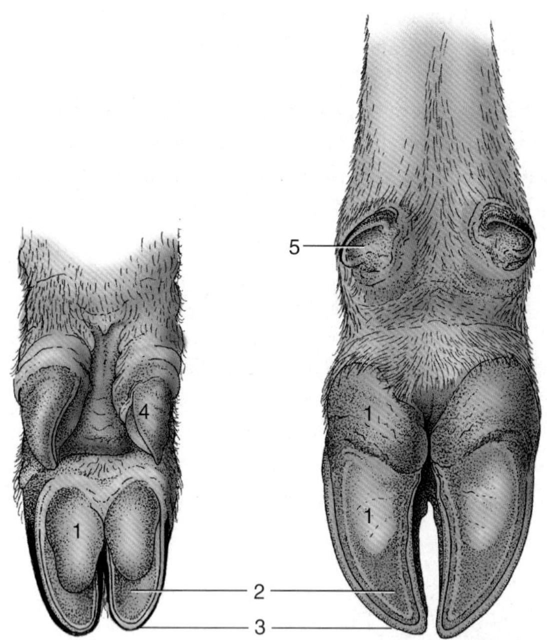

Fig. 10.16 Palmar surface of foot of the pig *(left)* and of a cow *(right)*. *1,* Bulb (digital pad) of hoof; *2,* sole of hoof; *3,* wall of hoof; *4,* hoof of accessory digit; *5,* rudimentary hoof of dewclaw.

greatly altered form). Nails, claws, and hoofs serve primarily to protect the underlying tissues, but each is also used for other purposes, such as scratching and digging or as a weapon. The equine hoof, the most complex, reduces concussion on foot impact. Fig. 10.18 shows the correspondences among these appendages, each of which presents three parts: wall, sole, and associated pad. It is only in ungulates that the last forms part of the horny structure; it corresponds with the digital bulb of primates and the digital pad of carnivores.

The *nail* (wall) of primates grows from the epidermis covering a curved fold of dermis at its base. The epidermis under most of the nail produces a little horn that helps maintain adhesion as the nail gradually slides distally. The dermis under this rather unproductive portion of the epidermis is gathered into a few low, longitudinal folds (laminae) that interdigitate with corresponding epidermal laminae; increased dermoepidermal contact strengthens the bond between the nail and the deeper tissues. The epidermis underlying the free border of the nail produces small amounts of soft "sole horn" (Fig. 10.18/*2*).

The wall of the *claw* of carnivores can be likened to a nail that has been laterally compressed and so has obtained a sharp dorsal border. Its proximal part and the germinal layer from which it is derived are similarly shaped and are lodged with the associated dermis within the unguicular crest of the distinctively shaped distal phalanx (Fig. 10.18D). The epidermis deep to the

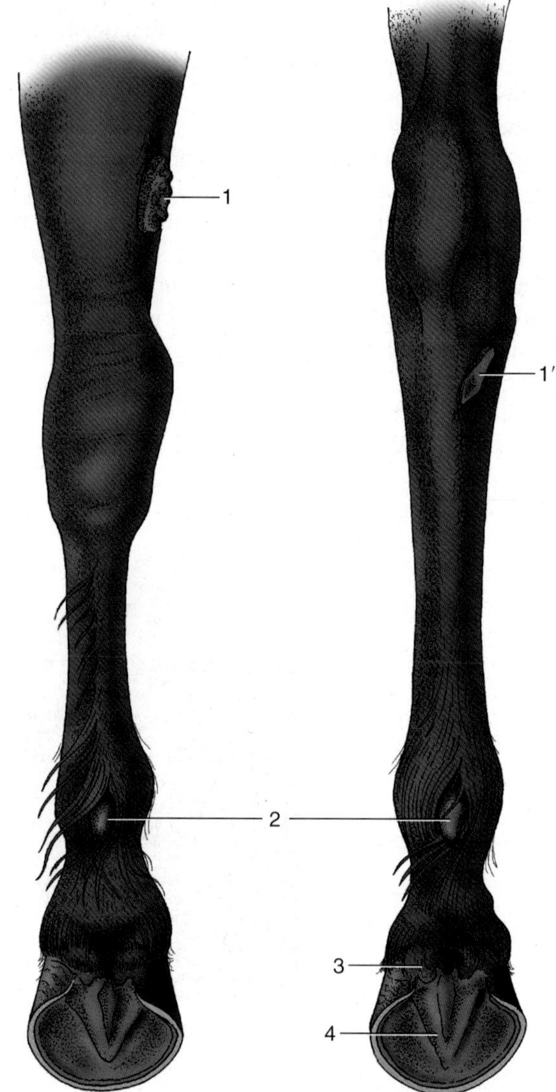

Fig. 10.17 Left forelimb *(left)* and left hindlimb *(right)* of the horse, caudal view. *1* and *1′,* Chestnuts above carpus and below hock, respectively; *2,* ergots; *3,* bulbs of the heels; *4,* frog.

wall is minimally productive. The dermis that covers the unguicular process fuses with the periosteum, and as with the primate nail, longitudinal interdigitations between dermal and epidermal laminae strongly bond the claw to the dorsal border of the bone. The space between the free margins of the wall on the undersurface of the unguicular process is filled with flaky "sole horn" (Fig. 10.18/*5*).

The wall of the *horse's hoof* is also strongly curved, and the sides are sharply inflected to form the so-called bars (Fig. 10.19E/*2″*). The space between the bars is occupied by the frog, the part of the footpad that makes contact with the ground. The sole horn that fills the ground surface between wall and frog meets the wall at a junction known as the white line (zona alba; Fig. 10.19/*5*). The wall grows distally from

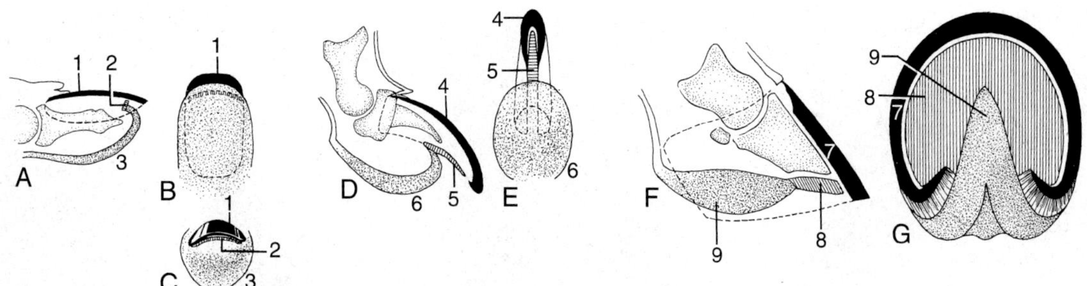

Fig. 10.18 Schematic representations of (A)–(C) nail, (D) and (E) claw, and (F) and (G) hoof. (A) Longitudinal section, (B) palmar surface, and (C) head-on view of human fingertip. (D) Longitudinal section and (E) palmar surface of canine claw. (F) Longitudinal section and (G) ground surface of equine hoof. *1,* Nail (wall); *2,* "sole horn" of nail; *3,* bulb of finger; *4,* wall of claw; *5,* "sole" of claw; *6,* digital pad; *7,* wall of hoof; *8,* sole of hoof; *9,* frog.

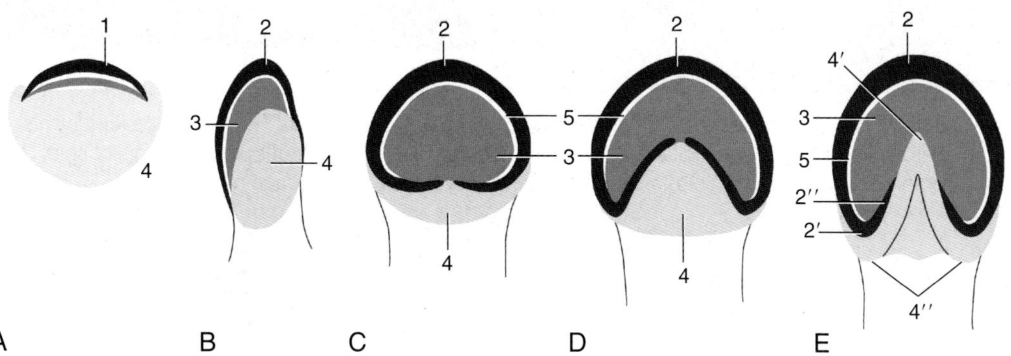

Fig. 10.19 An interpretation of the phylogenetic "development" of the horn structures associated with the distal phalanx. (A) Human fingertip. (B) Pig hoof. (C) Rhinoceros hoof. (D) Tapir hoof. (E) Horse hoof. *1,* Nail; *2,* wall of hoof; *2′* and *2″,* heel and bar (of horse); *3,* sole; *4,* footpad (bulb in human finger and pig); *4′* and *4″,* frog and bulbs of the heels (of horse); *5,* white line.

the epidermis over a bulging (coronary) dermis* studded with numerous papillae directed toward the ground. The epidermis covering these papillae produces horn tubules that run distally, toward the weight-bearing margin of the wall. The tubules are embedded in less structured intertubular horn formed by the epidermis over the interpapillary regions of the dermis; the combination of horn types gives the tissue a finely striated appearance. The (laminar) epidermis deep to the wall is again only minimally productive. It is arranged as several hundred well-formed laminae that tightly interdigitate with an equal number of dermal laminae (see Chapter 23, p. 600), bonding the wall to the underlying distal phalanx. One should remember that this is a living bond that allows the wall to slide gradually toward the ground, where its distal border is worn away. A band of soft horn (periople) lies over the external surface of the wall near its junction with the skin (Fig. 10.20/*1*). It descends with the wall and dries to a protective glossy layer. The band widens at the back of the hoof, where it covers the bulbs of the heels and part of the frog.

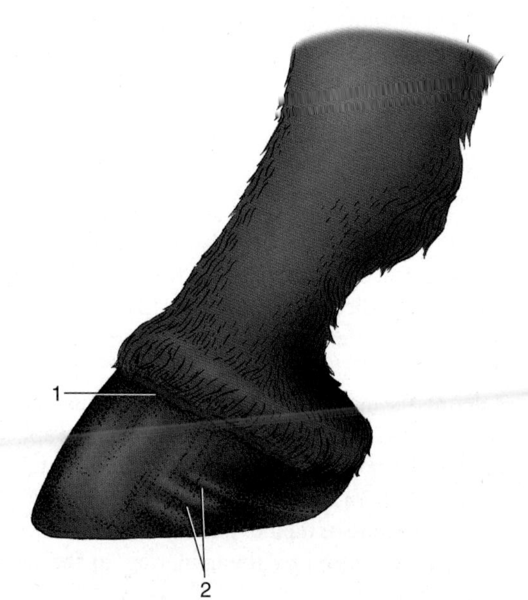

Fig. 10.20 Equine hoof. *1,* Periople; *2,* rings indicating uneven horn growth.

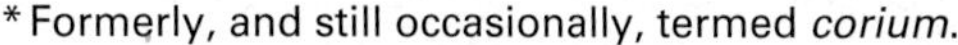

* Formerly, and still occasionally, termed *corium.*

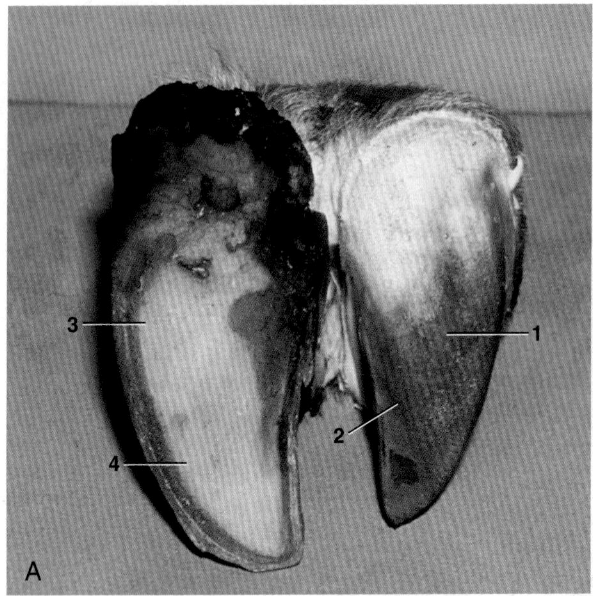

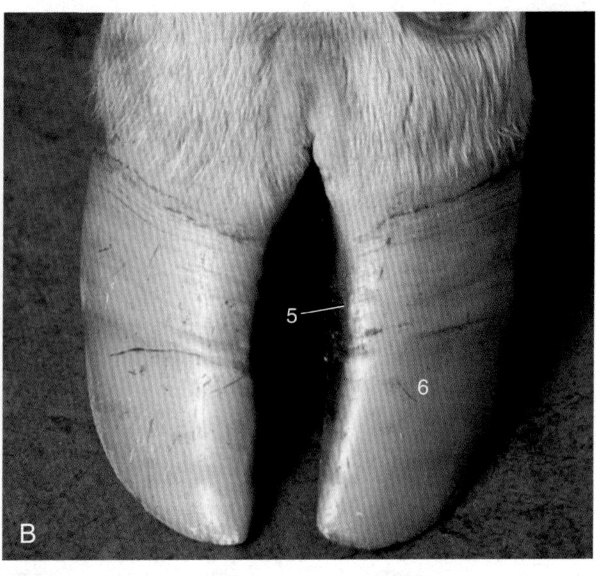

Fig. 10.21 (A) Bovine foot, palmar view. (B) Bovine foot, dorsal view. The horn shoe (epidermis) has been pulled off one digit in (A), exposing the dermis. *1,* Dermis of bulb; *2,* dermis of sole; *3,* horn of bulb; *4,* horn of sole; *5,* dorsal border of hoof; *6,* abaxial surface of hoof.

The hoofs of *ruminants and the pig,* although resembling those of the horse in principle, differ in several respects: the wall is sharply bent to form a dorsal border (like that of the claw); the footpad (bulb) is relatively large and furnishes the entire caudal part of the hoof (Fig. 10.19B/*4*); the sole between the bulb and wall is small; and the interdigitating laminae are less developed (Fig. 10.21/*2*).

In all species, periods of disturbed or lessened horn production create ridges on the wall parallel to the formative region at the junction with the skin (Fig. 10.20/*2*).

Fuller accounts of these specializations are found in the appropriate later chapters.

HORNS

The horns of domestic ruminants have osseous bases provided by the cornual processes of the frontal bones. Unlike antlers, which are shed and replaced yearly, horns are permanent* and grow continuously after their first appearance soon after birth.

The dermis is tightly adherent to the cornual process and bears numerous short papillae that are slanted apically, ensuring that the horn elongates and thickens as it grows (Fig. 10.22). The horn substance resembles that of the hoof in being an admixture of tubules and intertubular horn. The horn (epiceras) produced by the epidermis at the base is

*Uniquely, the horns of the American Pronghorn are shed annually.

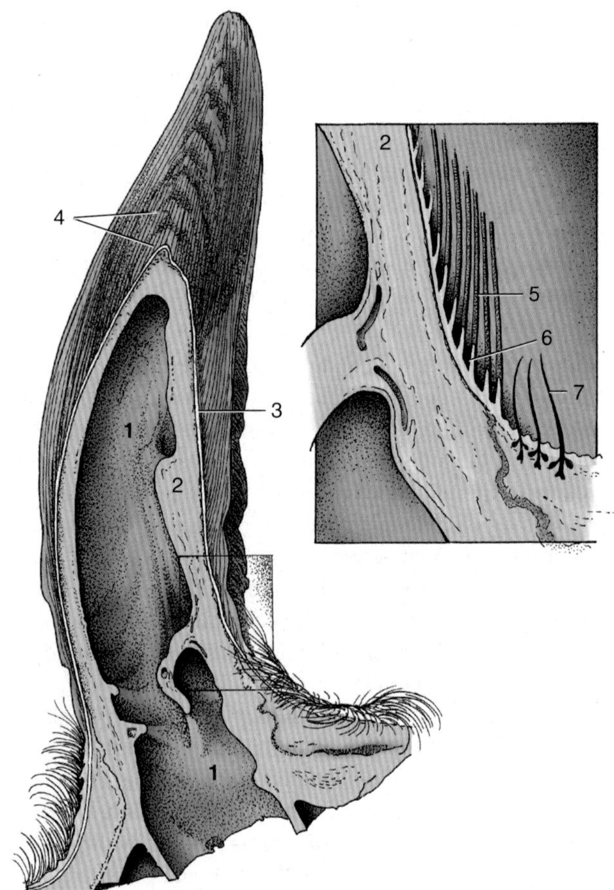

Fig. 10.22 Longitudinal section of bovine horn. *1,* Caudal frontal sinus extending into horn; *2,* cornual process of frontal bone; *3,* combined periosteum, dermis, and noncornified stratum of epidermis; *4,* horn tubules separated by intertubular horn; *5,* horn tubules *(inset)*; *6,* dermal papilla; *7,* hair.

soft and somewhat transparent, resembling the periople of the hoof. It gives the horn its glossy sheen.

Except the naturally polled breeds, the horns are found in both males, who have larger horns, and females. Their shape is strongly characteristic of the breed and reflects the shape and size of the cornual process. In cattle, these processes are invaded by the frontal sinuses (Fig. 10.22/*1*), a feature that may have implications for the dehorning of an adult animal.

The horny shell separates from the bony core on maceration, explaining the (obsolete) zoologic designation Cavicornia (hollow-horned animals) sometimes given to ruminants with permanent horns. Ruminants of the deer family (Cervidae) have antlers and are specifically excluded from this grouping. Antlers are sturdy outgrowths of the skull that are initially covered with skin but become exposed when the skin dies. The dead skin, or velvet, is removed by being rubbed against trees and other objects. The osseous processes lose their blood supply when exposed, die, and are shed, and the animal is left relatively defenseless until a new set of antlers grows next season.

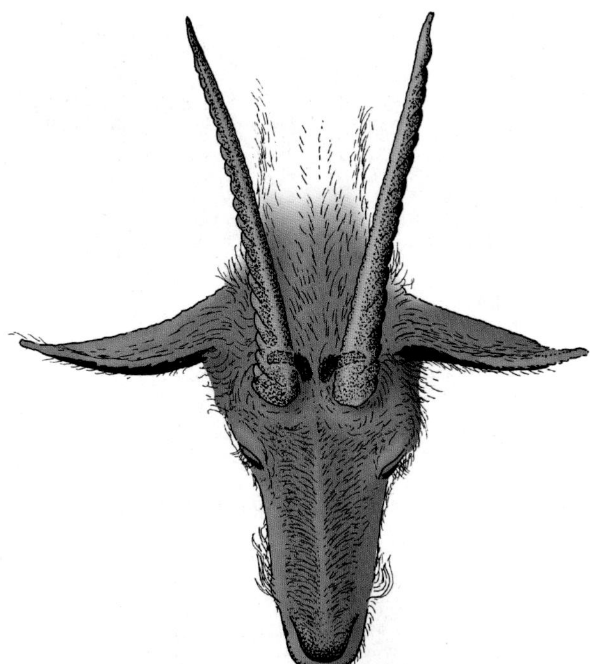

Fig. 10.23 Horn glands caudomedial to the base of the horns in the goat.

SKIN GLANDS

The glands of the skin develop as epidermal sprouts that invade the underlying mesoderm. They generally develop from primitive hair follicles and retain these connections; the ducts deliver the secretion into the adult follicles from which it oozes onto the skin surface beside the projecting hairs. Two basic types, sweat and sebaceous glands (Fig. 10.7/*9* and *10*), are distinguished, but each occurs in various subvarieties and in more definitely specialized forms.

THE SEBACEOUS GLANDS

Sebaceous glands produce a fatty secretion (sebum) that lubricates and waterproofs the skin and coat. It also promotes the spread of sweat, retards bacterial growth, and, in certain instances, serves as a territorial marker that is recognized by other members of the species. The odor of the wet dog is due to these glands. Certain substances (pheromones) present in sebum are known to be sexually attractive. Their rate of production is controlled by steroid hormones (androgens generally promote secretion, and estrogens retard secretion). A good illustration of a selective effect of androgens is found in the reaction of the so-called acne region of the human adolescent. The sebum of the fleece of sheep, known as *lanolin* commercially, is used as a base for ointments, in cosmetics, and as a cleansing agent in soaps. The secretions of certain specialized glands (e.g., the preputial glands of musk deer and the anal glands of the civet) have long been collected for use by the perfume industry.

The major localized accumulations of sebaceous glands found in domestic animals and large enough to be visible to the naked eye are listed; several are associated with skin pouches.

Circumoral Glands (Fig. 10.11)

Circumoral glands are large glands found in the lips of cats, which use them to mark their territories. The secretion is deposited directly by the animal's rubbing its head against an object or ingratiatingly against its owner and indirectly after transference to the body during grooming.

Horn Glands (Fig. 10.23)

Horn glands are musk or scent glands present in goats of both sexes, caudomedial to the horn base (or at the corresponding site in polled animals). They are larger and more productive in the breeding season; stimulated by testosterone, those of males produce a secretion with an odor so pungent that some owners insist on their surgical removal.

Glands of the Infraorbital Pouch (Fig. 10.24)

Some glands in sheep are contained in a cutaneous pouch, called the *infraorbital pouch,* rostral to the eye and opening ventrolaterally on the face. The pouch wall contains both sebaceous and tubular serous glands whose mixed secretion stains the skin when it escapes from the pouch. The glands, which serve as territorial markers, are larger in rams.

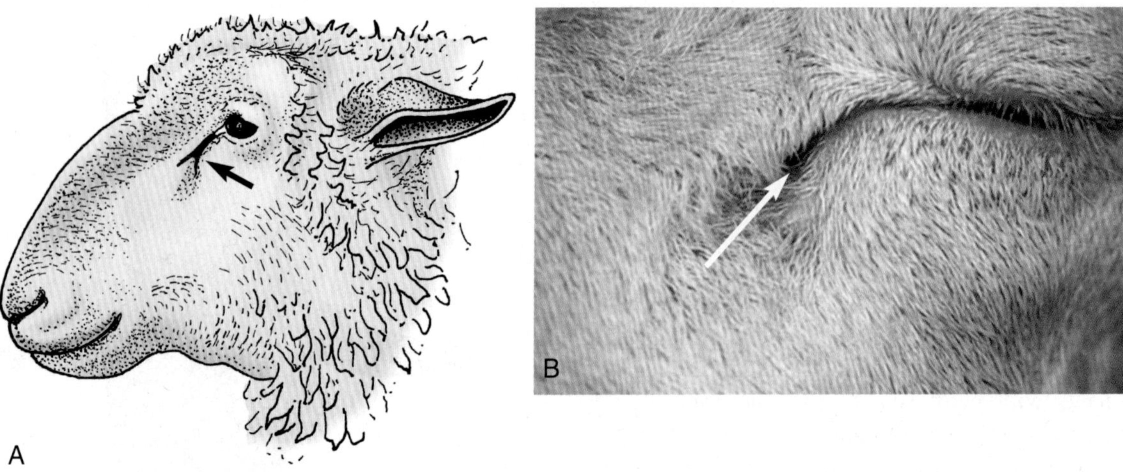

Fig. 10.24 (A) and (B) Infraorbital pouch *(arrow)* of the sheep.

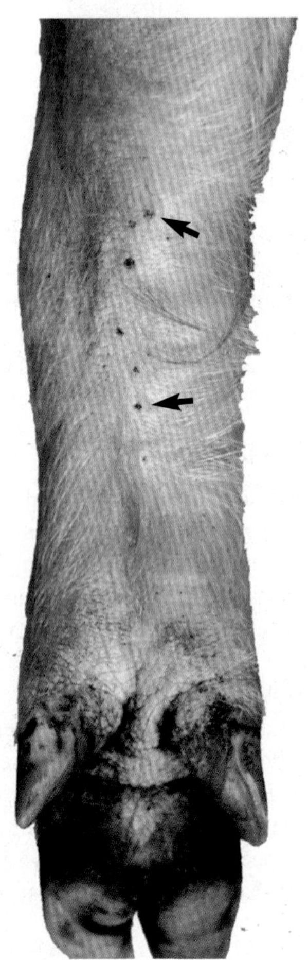

Fig. 10.25 Carpal glands *(arrows)* of the pig, palmar view.

Carpal Glands (Fig. 10.25)

Pigs and cats have carpal glands. In pigs they surround several cutaneous invaginations on the mediopalmar aspect of the carpus. They are found in both sexes and serve to indicate territorial claims; boars are said to make particular use of them when "marking" sows during copulation.

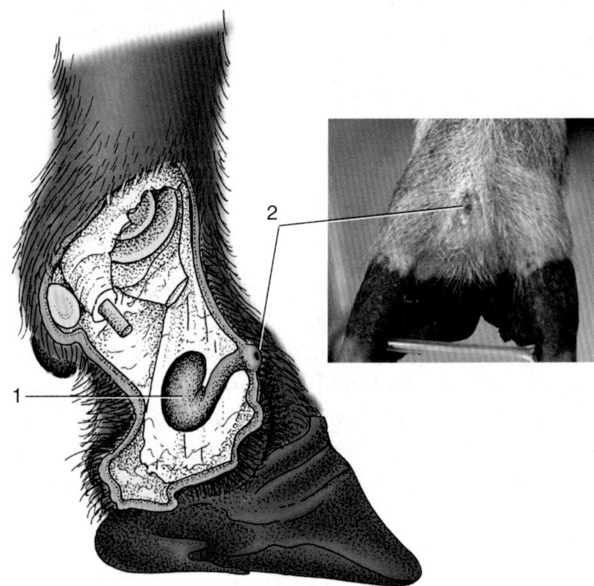

Fig. 10.26 Interdigital pouch *(1)* of the sheep and its opening *(2)*.

The location of the glands in the cat is marked by a tuft of a few tactile hairs proximal to the carpal pad. The site is betrayed by a palpable thickening of the skin (Fig. 10.15B/*5*).

Glands of the Interdigital Pouch (Fig. 10.26)

Interdigital pouches are found on the forelimbs and hindlimbs of sheep of both sexes. The pouches are tubular invaginations of the skin whose walls contain branched sebaceous and serous glands. The waxy secretion is discharged through a single opening above the hoofs and serves as a "trail marker." Many gregarious wild species have similar glands.

Glands of the Inguinal Pouch (Fig. 10.27)

Inguinal pouches, found near the base of the udder or scrotum of sheep, contain both sebaceous and sweat glands.

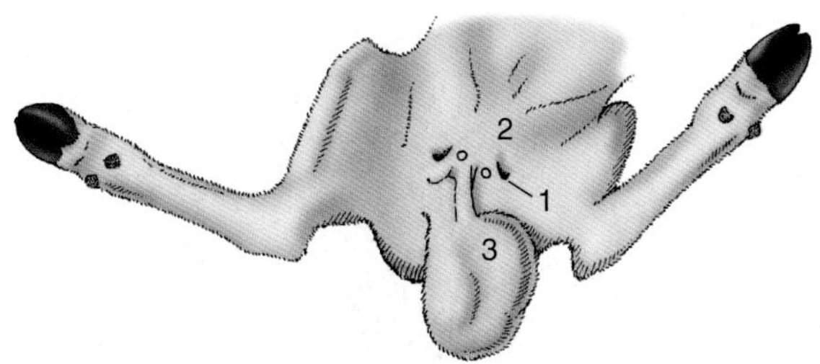

Fig. 10.27 Inguinal region of the ram. *1,* Inguinal pouch; *2,* rudimentary teat; *3,* scrotum.

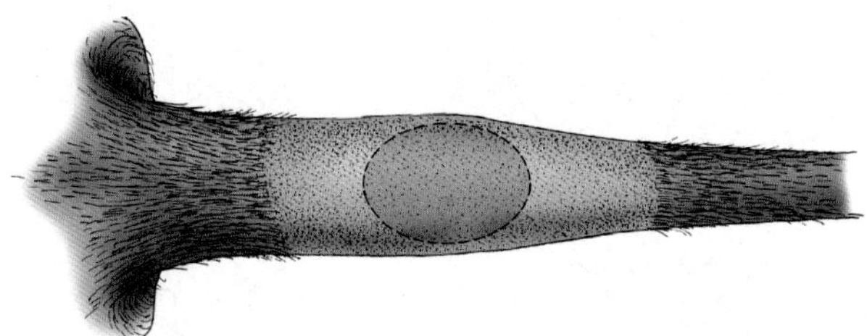

Fig. 10.28 Location of the tail glands of the dog *(dark pink area with dotted outline).*

The secretion escapes as a brown waxy substance whose odor may assist the lamb to find the udder.

Preputial Glands (Fig. 35.11)

Sebaceous and apocrine sweat glands within the prepuce produce secretions that combine with desquamated cells to form the crumbly substance known as *smegma.* They are best developed in the boar, in which they are massed within a dorsal diverticulum of the preputial cavity (see Chapter 35). Their secretion gives the boar its characteristic odor. They are present but less offensive in other species (which lack the diverticulum).

Tail Glands (Fig. 10.28)

Collections of large sebaceous and serous glands are found in an oval patch on the dorsal surface of the tail of certain carnivores. The skin over these glands is often defined by its sparser hair and yellowish color. Activity is greatest during the breeding season. The patch is situated more proximally in cats, toward the root of the tail, than in dogs (Fig. 10.28).

Circumanal Glands (Fig. 10.29)

Some sebaceous glands are restricted to the perianal skin of certain carnivores (circumanal glands), including dogs, where they drain into (and are believed to influence) special sweat glands. It is probably their secretion that excites the particular attention paid to the anal region when dogs confer.

Glands of the Anal Sacs (Fig. 10.30)

Sebaceous and serous glands are found in the walls of the anal sacs, cutaneous pouches that open beside the anus

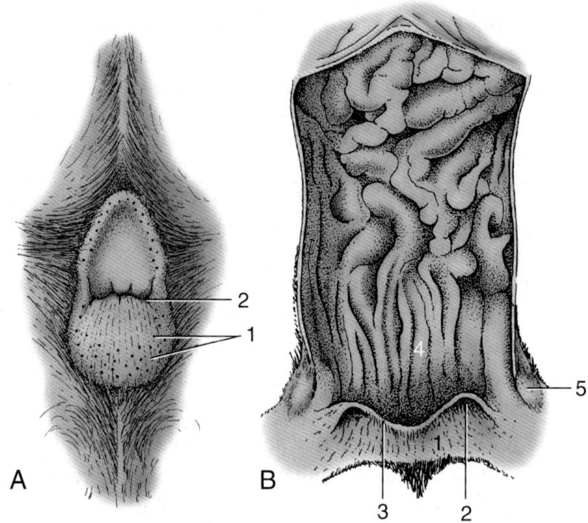

Fig. 10.29 (A) Cutaneous zone of the canine anal canal. (B) Feline anal canal opened dorsally. *1,* Cutaneous zone with circumanal glands forming a ring around the anus of the dog; *2,* opening of the right anal sac; *3,* anocutaneous line; *4,* columnar zone; *5,* right anal sac.

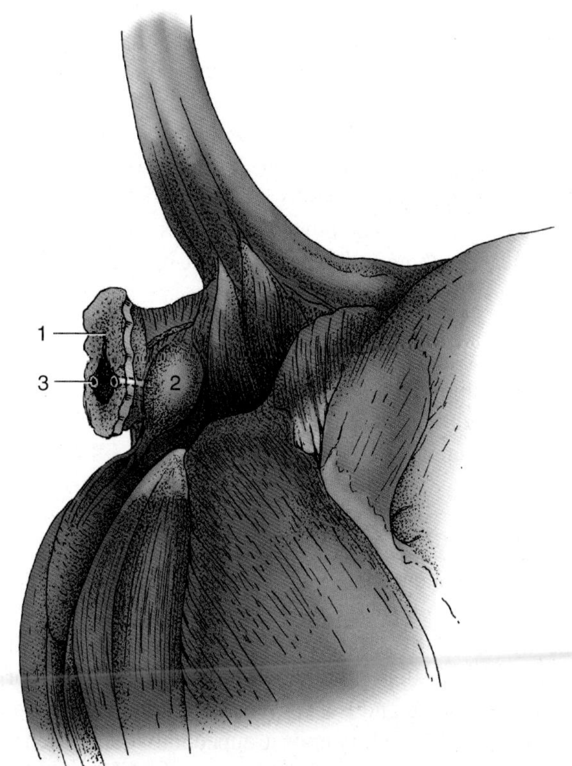

Fig. 10.30 Exposed right anal sac of a dog. *1,* Anus; *2,* anal sac; *3,* opening of excretory duct of anal sac (emphasized; see Fig. 10.29A/*2*).

of carnivores (Fig. 10.29/*2*). The secretion, which is particularly foul smelling, is expressed during defecation and apparently serves as a marker. It is well known that skunks can forcefully expel the contents of the sacs to fend off aggressors.

The Sweat Glands

Sweat glands are scattered over the entire body but are somewhat sparse in carnivores and pigs. Two types are distinguished by (a probably erroneous interpretation of) the histology of the secretory process. Apocrine sweat glands discharge an albuminous sweat into hair follicles over most of the body.* Eccrine glands secrete a more watery sweat directly onto certain naked, or nearly naked, regions of the skin (e.g., the nasolabial plate of cattle and the footpads of dogs). The apocrine variety predominates, and its secretion and subsequent evaporation are important in salt metabolism and temperature regulation. The secretion is degraded by bacteria, which form substances that provide the characteristic body odor. The product of the eccrine variety is thought to play a lesser role in temperature regulation.

Most mammals possess fewer glands and sweat less profusely than humans. However, impressions can be misleading because the sweating that does occur tends to be masked by the more generous coat. The horse sweats abundantly and also produces an especially albuminous sweat that froths when worked by movement of the skin and coat ("lathering up"). Certain breeds of cattle, mostly tropical, also sweat visibly along the neck and over the flanks. Surprisingly, the Asiatic buffalo has fewer sweat glands than cattle and resorts to wallowing in water in compensation. Among domestic species, dogs and cats sweat least, although the skin of short-haired individuals sometimes feels moist. Sweat glands are present in the footpads of dogs and cats. In dogs, excessive activity of these glands may, in cold climates, lead to snow- or ice-balling on digital hair, making it painful to walk. This issue may be important in breeding of sled dogs. Arctic wolves lack these glands.

The Mammary Glands

Mammary glands (mammae) are greatly modified, much enlarged sweat glands whose secretion nourishes the young. The modified milk (colostrum) produced immediately after parturition transfers immunoglobulins to the newborn. Each mammary gland is a compound tubuloalveolar gland that consists of secretory units grouped into lobules defined by intervening connective tissue septa (see Chapter 29). The mammary glands develop as epithelial buds that grow

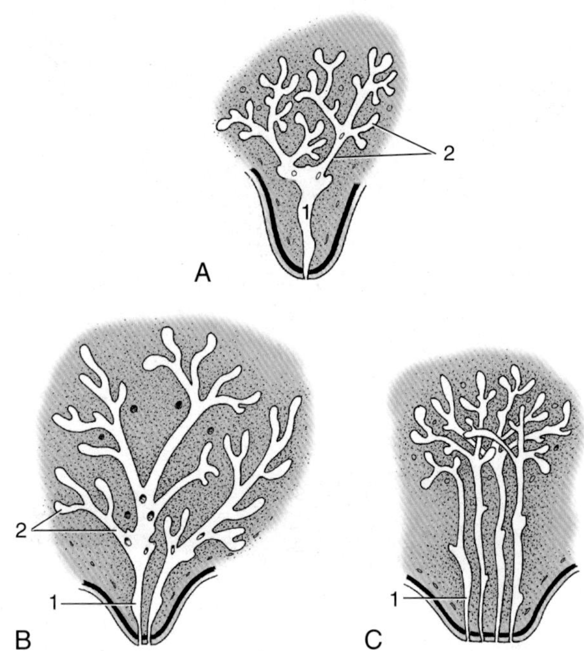

Fig. 10.31 Developing duct systems growing proximally from the tip of the fetal teat. (A) Cow, ewe, and goat. (B) Mare and sow. (C) Bitch and cat (only four primary sprouts are shown). *1,* Primary sprout, which gives rise to the lactiferous sinus; *2,* secondary and tertiary sprouts, which give rise to the lactiferous ducts.

into the underlying mesenchyme from linear ectodermal thickenings (mammary ridges). These ridges may extend from the axilla to the groin (as in carnivores and pigs) or may be of more limited extent, restricted to the axilla (as in elephants), the thorax (as in women), or the groin (as in ruminants and horses). Usually more buds appear than survive in the adult, and although most extra buds soon regress, some persist to give rise to *supernumerary teats.* These teats may be independent or may be attached to other, better developed glands (see Fig. 10.33A/*7*). They are unsightly, and because they may interfere with milking, they are often removed from the udders of cows and goats.

Proliferation of the mesenchyme surrounding the bud raises a teat (papilla) on the surface of the body. One or more epidermal sprouts grow from the mammary bud into the connective tissue of the teat and begin to canalize at about the time of birth. Each sprout is destined to form a separate duct system with associated glandular tissue. The mammary gland arising from only one sprout has a single duct system leading to a single orifice on the tip of the teat (Fig. 10.31A).

The number of sprouts results in a corresponding number of separate duct systems, each with an associated glandular mass and separate orifice. The growth of the ducts and gland tissue is continued after puberty and especially during the first pregnancy, forming the swelling that pushes the teat away from the body wall. The process is controlled

*There are important species differences. The distribution and other features of human (and other primate) sweat glands differ significantly.

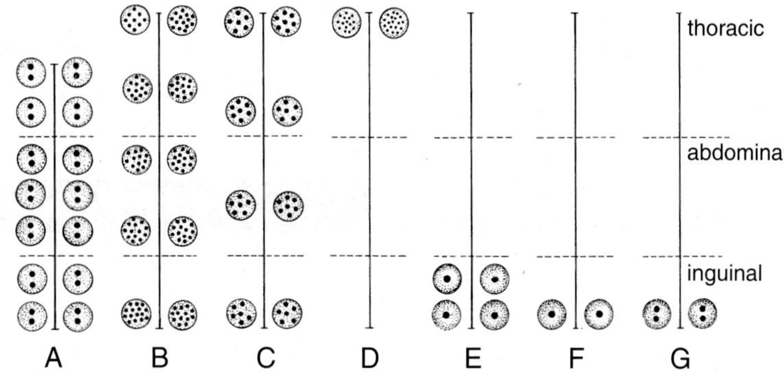

Fig. 10.32 Distribution of mammary glands in certain mammals. *Dots* indicate the number of orifices on the teat. (A) Sow. (B) Bitch. (C) Cat. (D) Woman. (E) Cow. (F) Ewe and she-goat. G, Mare.

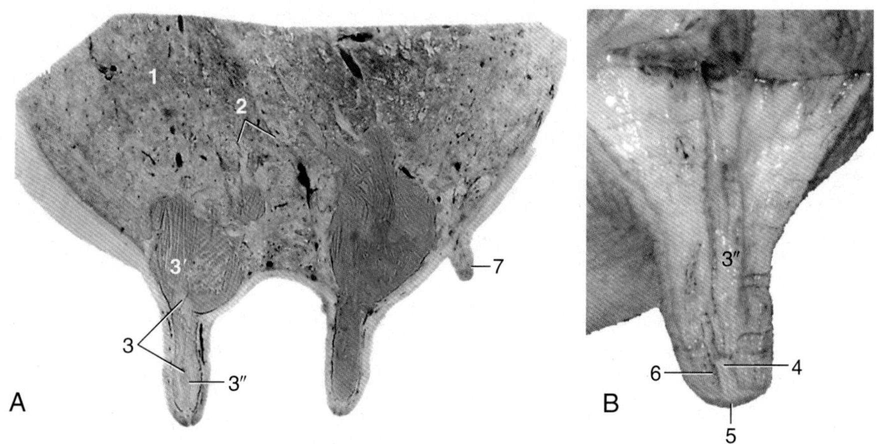

Fig. 10.33 (A) Sagittal section of udder, showing teat and gland sinuses and lactiferous ducts filled with latex (cranial quarter, *green*; caudal quarter, *blue*). (B) Section of teat. *1*, Parenchyma of gland; *2*, lactiferous ducts of various diameters; *3*, lactiferous sinus; *3′*, gland sinus; *3″*, teat sinus; *4*, papillary duct; *5*, teat orifice; *6*, teat sphincter; *7*, supernumerary teat.

by the intricate interplay of several hormones from the hypophysis, ovaries, and other endocrine glands.

Each of the units formed along the trunk of a lactating sow (see Fig. 10.31B) is composed of glandular tissue supported and enclosed by a fibrous tissue framework in which the mammary vessels and nerves run. The whole formation is pervaded with fat and covered by skin. The mammary glands in species such as ruminants and horses may appear to merge in a single consolidated complex called the udder. This term is also applied to the even more distinctly separated mammary glands in the sow. The numbers of mammary glands (as well as their duct systems) in the domestic species is shown schematically in Fig. 10.32.

The more detailed organization is illustrated by reference to the cow. The glandular tissue is arranged in lobules, each 1 mm or perhaps a little more in diameter and consisting of about 200 alveoli. The milk drains to an intralobular duct that joins others to form a larger interlobular duct (Fig. 10.33/*2*). Interlobular ducts lead in their turn to a system of lactiferous (milk-carrying) ducts that ultimately convey the milk to the relatively large cavity known as the *lactiferous sinus* (Fig. 10.33/*3*). The lactiferous ducts of successive orders increase in diameter but diminish in number so that only 10 or so enter the sinus. Unlike most ducts, they have alternating narrow and dilated portions where contraction of the muscular wall of the narrow portions holds the milk in the expansions before it is "let down" when the cow suckles or is milked. The lactiferous sinus extends into the teat and is incompletely divided into gland and teat sinuses (Fig. 10.33/*3′* and *3″*) by a constriction. The teat sinus is continued by the papillary duct (Fig. 10.33/*4*), which opens at the tip of the teat, where the orifice is surrounded by a smooth muscle sphincter (Fig. 10.33/*6*).

Corresponding parts can be identified in other species, including those in which each gland contains several small lactiferous sinuses, each served by a separate duct system and each opening independently.

It must be stressed that mammary glands are fully developed and fully functional only at the height of lactation. They are then large and show a predominance of yellow glandular tissue over the paler fibrous stroma. When the dam weans her young, involution sets in, the parenchyma regresses (see Chapter 29), and the connective tissues now form the bulk of the organ. However, the gland never quite reverts to its prelactation size, and it grows a little more with each pregnancy.

Mammary buds also form in male embryos and persist to give rise to the rudimentary teats found on the ventral surface of the trunk (carnivores and pig) or on the cranial surface of the scrotum (ruminants). They are less common in horses but occasionally appear beside the prepuce. In certain species such as rats, however, the male glands regress completely.

COMPREHENSION CHECK

Demonstrate your understanding of the structure of the skin, its functions, and comparative anatomy of its modifications in the foot of the dog, cattle, and the horse.

Part II

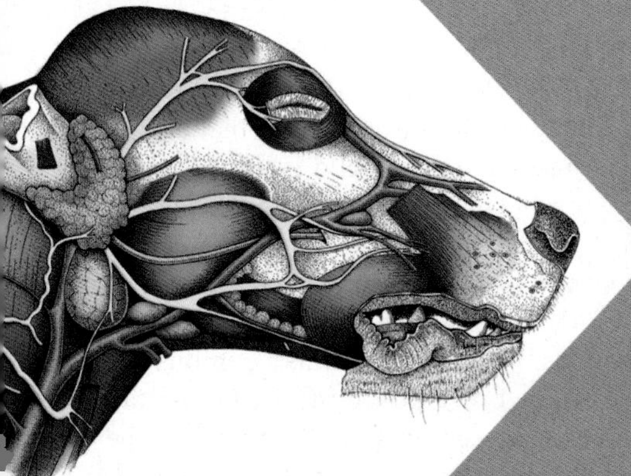

Dogs and Cats

The Head and Ventral Neck of the Dog and Cat

11

This chapter is the first of a series that covers the regional anatomy of the two companion animals, the dog and cat. Although the dog and cat are included in different suborders of Carnivora (Canoidea and Feloidea, respectively), the general anatomies are sufficiently alike to consider them together. Although cats rival and in many countries now surpass dogs in popularity, it is both conventional and convenient (because of the greater wealth of literature) to base the initial accounts on the dog and follow them with mention of the clinically significant differences in the cat. Dogs, of course, differ considerably among themselves. The description here refers to animals of moderate size and generalized conformation, such as are represented by the Beagle. The reader is also reminded that the systemic chapters are largely based on the anatomy of the dog, which supplies the bulk of their illustrations.

CONFORMATION AND EXTERNAL FEATURES

Conformation varies much more considerably in dogs than in other domesticated species. The preferences of fanciers have produced a variety of breeds that are strikingly different from one another and from their common wolf ancestor. The current popularity of purebred cats has increased awareness of the variation among breeds, even if the differences are much less considerable than among dogs. In both species this variation is nowhere better expressed than in the head.

The appearance of the dog's head is largely determined by the shape of the skull, the position and size of the eyes, and the form and carriage of the ears. The ears may be held erect, hang from the side, or have an intermediate carriage that is erect at the base and pendulous toward the tip. Certain differences are permanent attributes of a breed, but others are no more than temporary expressions of mood.

The skull of the adult dog is characterized by a well-developed facial part, large orbits and temporal fossae, incomplete postorbital bars, prominent tympanic bullae, and the absence of supraorbital foramina. It is widest behind the eyes, where the zygomatic arches are widely spread. Breed differences in the skull largely relate to the relative length of the facial part. Dolichocephalic, brachycephalic, and mesaticephalic or mesocephalic (long, short, and intermediate head length, respectively) breeds are recognized (Fig. 11.1). In dolichocephalic breeds like the Greyhound, the head is long and narrow. The dorsal surfaces of nose and cranium form two nearly parallel planes that are divided at the level of the eyes by a break (nasofrontal angle or stop) where the cranium descends to the level of the nose. The long facial part is often accompanied by an underbite jaw (brachygnathism). The external sagittal crest is well developed for attachment of the temporal muscles, and the zygomatic arches project less than in the other groups. In brachycephalic breeds, like the English Bulldog and the Pekingese, the facial part is short and the cranium wide and globular. The stop is pronounced, and the dorsal surface of the cranium is convex and has a much reduced external sagittal crest. In some breeds the fontanelles remain open throughout life. Numerous skin folds mark the face, and the eyes are widely spaced. Brachycephalic breeds are most often prognathic—the term indicating that the lower jaw protrudes in front of the upper jaw (Fig. 11.1C). Most breeds belong to the mesaticephalic type, in which the length of the skull is more harmoniously proportional to its width.

The face of the dog is more expressive of emotion than that of other species, able to indicate aggressive intent (Fig. 11.2), submission, and pain, even if unable to particularize them. Age is also clearly revealed in dogs of pigmented coat by a "graying" that begins at the upper lip and later spreads, reaching the area around the eyes by about the eighth year or a little later (Fig. 11.3).

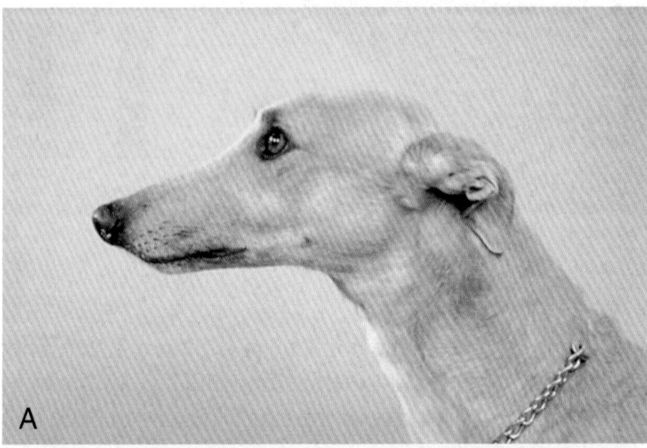

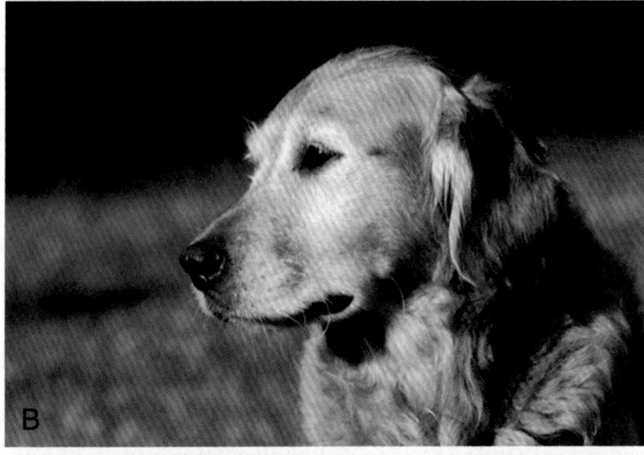

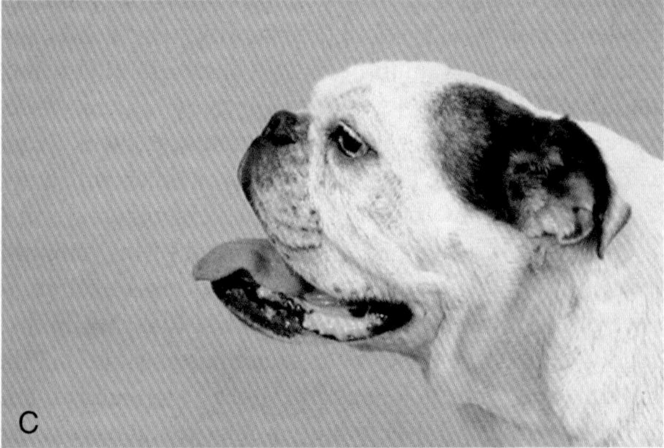

Fig. 11.1 Representatives of (A) dolichocephalic, (B) mesaticephalic, and (C) brachycephalic breeds.

Redundancy of facial skin is a feature of several breeds such as the Bulldog, Shar-Pei (Fig. 11.4), and Bloodhound. In extreme form it may result in frontal folds that obscure the vision, and because the upper eyelid is turned inward (entropion), it may irritate the cornea through contact with hairy skin.

In cats, in contrast to the breeds of dogs just mentioned, the skin on the scalp is tight and barely sufficient to close large wounds. The cat's head also exhibits features distinctive of breed or type. In most cats the face is relatively short, but in certain Oriental breeds, especially the Siamese, it is proportionally longer and the whole head is more wedge-shaped with a less pronounced stop. In contrast, Persian cats have very short "pushed-in" faces; when exaggerated, this trait may be associated with blockage of tear ducts, leading to persistent weeping (Fig. 11.5). The eyes and orbits are relatively large and face more directly forward than those of dogs, providing a wider field of binocular vision (see Fig. 9.1). The ears are wide at the base and are carried erect, except in

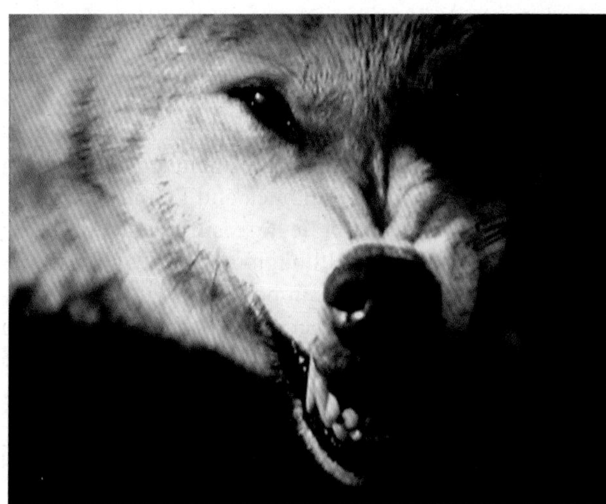

Fig. 11.2 Clear sign of aggressive intent of a dog.

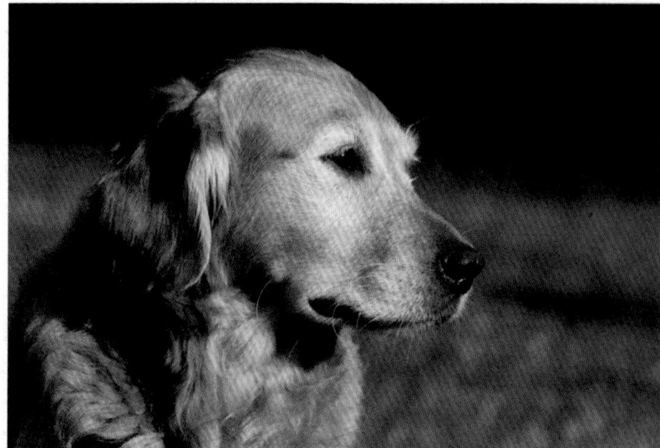

Fig. 11.3 Graying beginning at the upper lip and around the eye.

the Scottish Fold, in which the distal part of the pinna flops. The contrast between the rather short, rounded ears of most European breeds and the larger pointed ears of the Oriental has little practical importance but contributes much to breed "character." Tactile hairs (whiskers) are prominent (see Fig. 10.11).

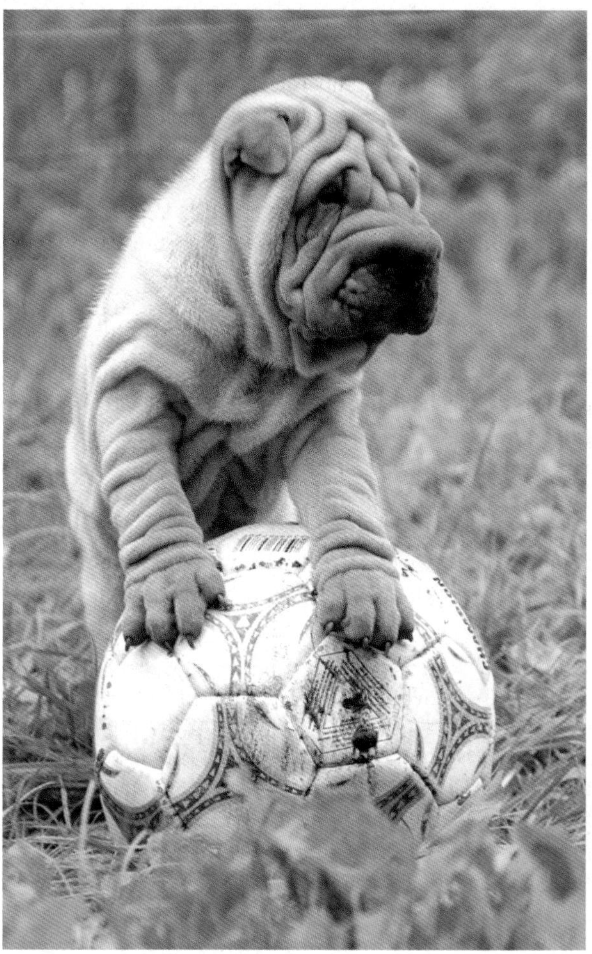

Fig. 11.4 Redundancy of skin in a Shar Pei.

SUPERFICIAL STRUCTURES

Much of the surface of the skull can be palpated because it is either directly subcutaneous or covered only by a thin layer of muscle. Palpable features of the face include the infraorbital and mental foramina and the ridge over the long root of the upper canine tooth. In the cat the infraorbital foramen is small and not easily found on palpation; it lies very close to the orbit.

Masticatory Muscles

The masticatory muscles are massive. The temporalis and masseter prevent direct access to the lateral plate of the frontal and parietal bones and the ramus of the mandible. The boundary between these muscles is provided by the zygomatic arch, which is relatively vulnerable to traumatic separation at the oblique suture between the zygomatic and temporal bones (see Fig. 2.34).

Skull

The brain case is surmounted by the sagittal crest and by the nuchal crest, which connects the caudal end of the sagittal crest with the base of the ear, providing the dorsal boundary of the triangular caudal (nuchal) surface of the skull. Both crests are palpable, although little of the nuchal surface can be appreciated. In the puppy's skull the cranial exceeds the facial part in size, being relatively much wider than it is in the adult (see Fig. 1.18); the sagittal crest has yet to form, and the nuchal crest, although visible on

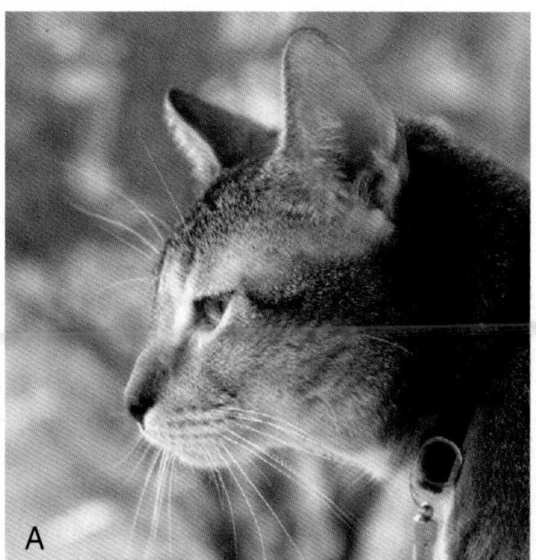

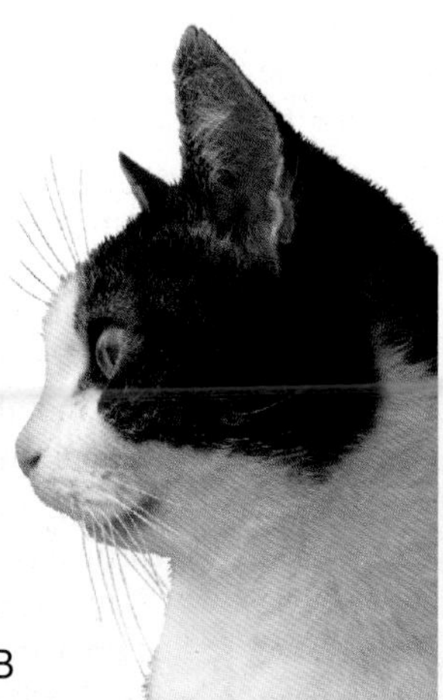

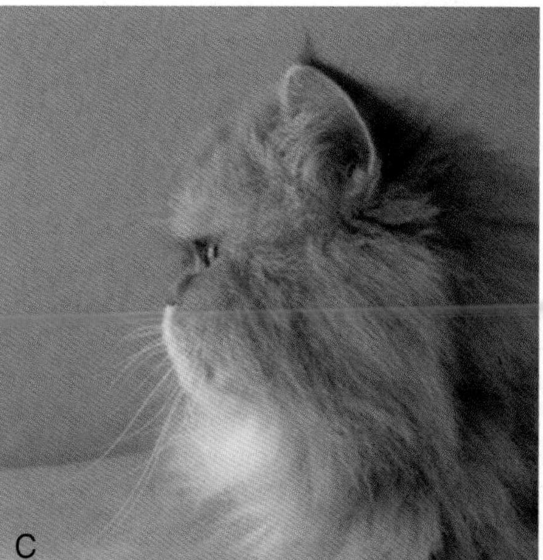

Fig. 11.5 Representatives of cats with (A) long heads (Abyssinian), (B) medium-sized heads (European short hair), and (C) short heads (Persian).

the skull, is not palpable. The fontanelle, characteristic of the neonatal skull, may persist into adult life in certain toy breeds, in which it remains a palpable feature. The ventral border of the mandible and the prominent angular process at its caudal end are easily palpated. The halves of the mandible meet in a cartilaginous joint that persists throughout life.

Salivary Glands and Lymph Nodes

The parotid and mandibular glands and the mandibular lymph nodes can be palpated caudal to the mandible. The mandibular gland is embraced by the maxillary and linguofacial veins, which join to form the external jugular vein. The parotid duct (Fig. 11.6/*8*) crosses the masseter, midway between two branches of the facial nerve. The duct can sometimes be palpated before it passes deep to the communicating nerves and the facial vessels to open into the cheek cavity. Accessory lobes of the parotid gland may accompany the duct. The end of this duct is occasionally transplanted into the conjunctival sac when the flow of tears is insufficient to keep the conjunctiva moist.

Superficial Vessels

The linguofacial vein is short (Fig. 11.6/*11*). In the dog, the left and right lingual veins unite and form the superficially situated hyoid arch. In the cat, this arch is formed by the left and right linguofacial veins. The facial vein, when followed rostrally, passes first over the mandibular lymph nodes and then along the ventral border of the masseter before crossing the face obliquely. It arises from the fusion of prominent dorsal nasal and angularis oculi veins rostral to the eye. These vessels run the risk of injury when surgical access is made to the nasal cavity and frontal sinuses. The angularis oculi vein, which emerges from the orbit, is also vulnerable during enucleation (removal) of the eye. The facial artery and accompanying vein serve the lips, cheek, and muzzle. The side of the nose is supplied by an artery that emerges from the infraorbital foramen.

Superficial Nerves

The distribution of the cutaneous nerves follows the general pattern (see Figs. 8.69 and 8.70). The dorsal branch (Fig. 11.6A/*7*) of the facial nerve runs across the dorsal half of the masseter. The ventral branch takes the more protected course along the ventral edge. They are joined by communicating branches at the rostral border of the muscle. The auriculopalpebral branch of the facial nerve (Fig. 11.6/*6*) passes across the zygomatic arch, where it can be blocked to eliminate blinking (orbicularis oculi muscle) during examination of the eye.

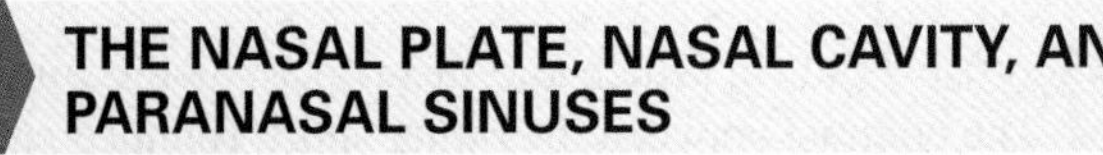

THE NASAL PLATE, NASAL CAVITY, AND PARANASAL SINUSES

The External Nose

The moist bare skin around the nostrils, the nasal plate, is divided by a median philtrum that continues ventrally to groove the upper lip (see Fig. 4.1). The nasal plate is covered with a thick keratinized epidermis. In cats its surface is made up of fine tubercles, but in dogs it is made of irregularly formed plaques and sulci that create a pattern that is believed to be individual and therefore available as a means of identification (nose printing). The nasal plate of dogs has no glands of its own and is kept moist by an overflow of the secretion of glands of the nasal cavity (pp. 139 and 140).

A curved alar cartilage supports the roof and the wing of the nose. The floor is strengthened by a small accessory nasal cartilage. The wing, the thickened dorsolateral portion of the nostril, is the most mobile part. The nostrils of dogs are comma-shaped, with the tail curving laterally beneath the wing. It is suggested that this separation of the wing from the floor of the nostril allows directional scenting (see Fig. 4.1). The alar fold is an extension of the ventral nasal concha, which terminates within the nasal vestibule at a bulbous enlargement fused with the wing of the nostril.

Congenital malformation of the nasal plane is a common finding in brachycephalic dogs and Persian cats. In this condition the cartilage supporting the nostrils is too weak; the resulting collapse of the wings narrows the nostrils, especially during inspiration. This condition can be relieved by surgery, in which parts of the alar folds are removed. The tissue is highly vascular and bleeds profusely when cut.

The Nasal Cavity

The nasal cavity extends from the nostrils to the level of the eyes. Its rostral part, the nasal vestibule, is roughly tubular; caudal to the level of the infraorbital foramen, it widens and gains in height (Fig. 11.7). The nasal vestibule is occupied by the alar fold.

The nasal cavity is divided into two halves by the nasal septum. In dogs, only the caudal and dorsal parts of the septum ossify; the rostral extremity projecting beyond the skull remains cartilaginous, accounting for the passive mobility of the tip of the nose. The middle section of the septum is membranous. A cat's nose is not actively mobile, and its cartilages resemble shortened canine nasal cartilages.

In dogs, the cavity is more tightly filled with nasal and ethmoidal conchae than in other species, and the intervening meatuses are narrow. The rostral half lodges the dorsal and ventral conchae. The dorsal one (Fig. 11.7/*3*) is a simple plate where it arises from the nasal bone, and it widens

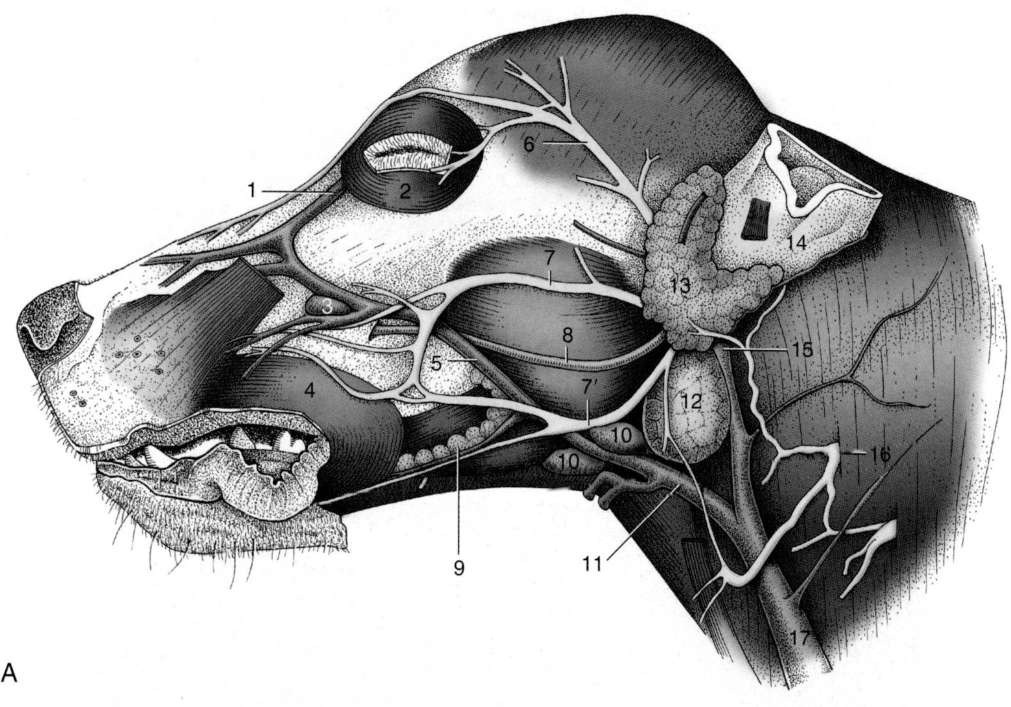

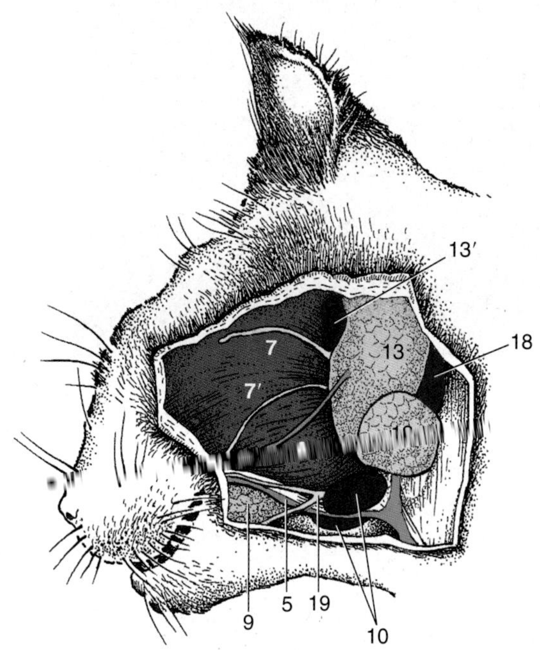

Fig. 11.6 Superficial dissection of (A) canine and (B) feline heads. *1,* Angularis oculi vein; *2,* orbicularis oculi; *3,* facial lymph node; *4,* orbicularis oris; *5,* facial vein; *6,* auriculopalpebral nerve; *7* and *7′,* dorsal and ventral buccal branches of facial nerve; *8,* parotid duct; *9,* buccal salivary glands; *10,* mandibular lymph nodes; *11,* linguofacial vein; *12,* mandibular gland; *13,* parotid gland; *13′,* parotid lymph node; *14,* base of ear; *15,* maxillary vein; *16,* second cervical nerve; *17,* external jugular vein; *18,* lateral retropharyngeal lymph node; *19,* facial nerve, ventral branch.

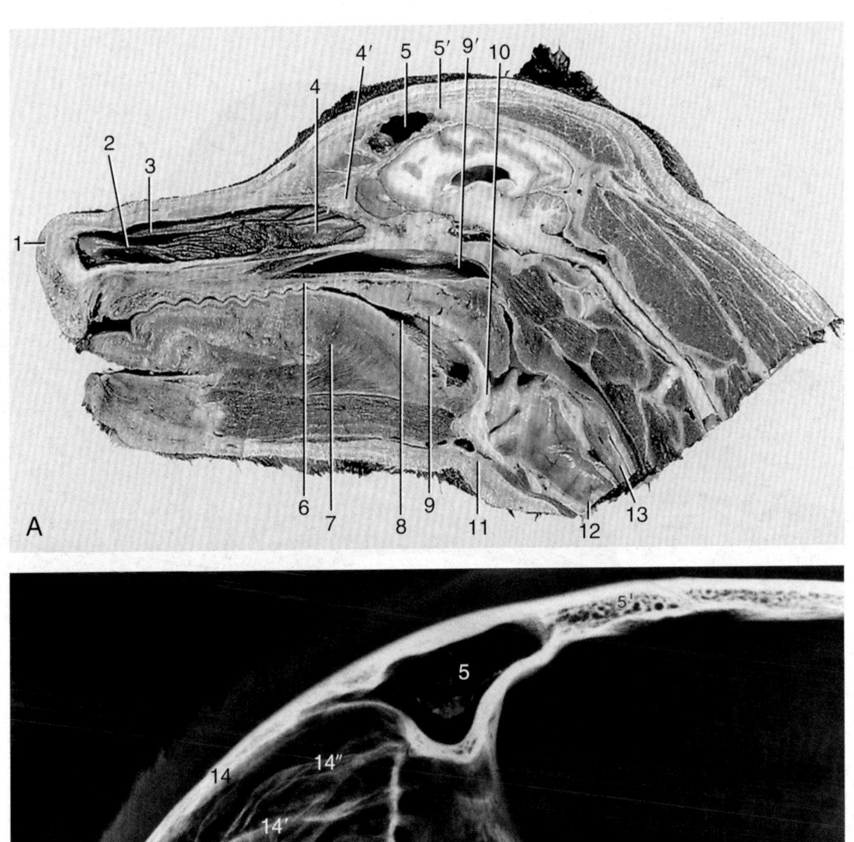

Fig. 11.7 (A) Paramedian section of the canine head. (B) Tomogram of the feline nasal cavity. *1,* Right nostril; *2,* ventral nasal concha; *3,* dorsal nasal concha; *4,* ethmoidal conchae; *4′,* cribriform plate; *5,* frontal sinus; *5′,* frontal bone; *6,* hard palate; *7,* tongue; *7′,* vomer; *8,* oropharynx; *9,* soft palate; *9′,* nasopharynx; *10,* epiglottis; *11,* basihyoid; *12,* trachea; *13,* esophagus; *14,* nasal bone; *14′,* horizontal crest of nasal bone; *14″,* dorsal part of nasal cavity invaded by ethmoidal conchae; *15,* optic canal; *15′,* hypophyseal fossa.

caudally to attach to the ethmoid. The ventral concha is thick but short, arises from the maxilla, and breaks into many scrolls that greatly enlarge the area that is covered by a richly vascularized mucosa (Fig. 11.7/*2*). The concha extends from the level of the first to the third premolar teeth and is attached to the conchal crest on the medial surface of the maxilla. This crest creates a linear shadow that is a very distinctive radiographic feature (Fig. 11.7B/*14′*). The ventral concha is continued rostrally by the alar fold. The caudal half of the nasal cavity is almost filled by ethmoidal conchae covered with olfactory mucosa. These conchae also invade the lower part of the frontal sinus. The olfactory mucosa in the German Shepherd reportedly covers an area of 150 cm^2 and possesses more than 20 million receptors. The olfactory membrane differs little from the remainder of the mucous membrane, although it may be slightly thicker and grayer. Collectively, the ethmoidal conchae are larger than the nasal conchae, a difference indicating the dog's keen sense of smell (see Fig. 11.10/*11*).

The nasal cavity of cats resembles the one of brachycephalic dogs. However, the ventral nasal concha is smaller, compensated for by enlargement and development of the

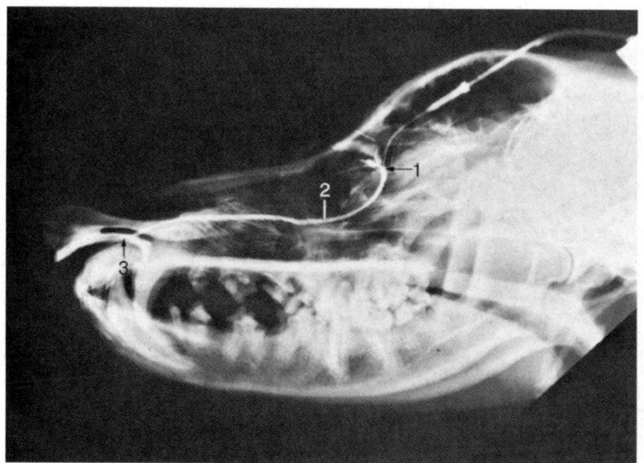

Fig. 11.8 Contrast medium outlining the canine nasolacrimal duct in a radiograph. *1*, Position of ventral punctum; *2*, nasolacrimal duct; *3*, opening of duct at the nostril.

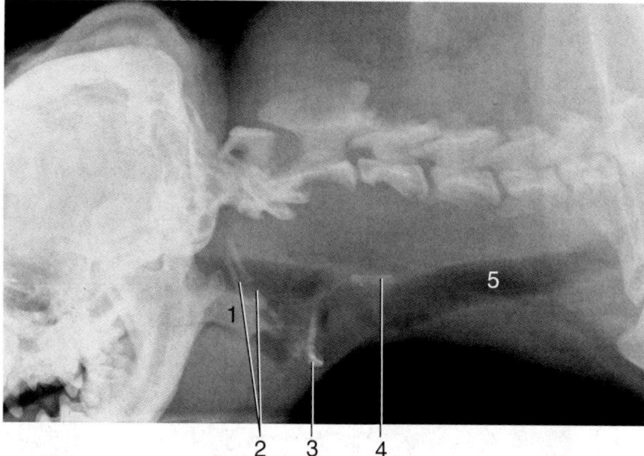

Fig. 11.9 Radiograph of the cramped pharyngeal region of the brachiocephalic dog. (The space available is rather cramped.) *1*, Soft palate; *2*, hyoid apparatus; *3*, basihyoid; *4*, cricoid cartilage; *5*, trachea.

middle concha and its lamellae. The middle concha reaches to the level of the entrance of the maxillary recess that it covers.

In both species, the nasolacrimal duct (Fig. 11.8) opens where the floor of the vestibule meets the alar fold and is visible when the nostril is spread. As often as not, there is a second, more caudal opening level with the canine tooth. The duct is described more extensively later. The duct of the lateral nasal gland opens at the rostral end of the dorsal nasal concha, but because it is only about 0.5 mm in diameter, it can be difficult to identify, even at dissection. The gland lies in the lateral nasal wall close to the entrance of the maxillary recess. Its secretion may have a social significance that accounts for the nose-to-nose sniffing common when dogs meet. In cats, the lateral nasal gland and its duct are not visible macroscopically; the secretion is mucous instead of serous.

A few much smaller nasal glands found on the rostral part of the septum open at the caudal limit of the vestibule and contribute marginally to the wetness of the nose. The watery secretions of the lacrimal, lateral nasal, and scattered minor nasal glands moisten the nasal plate.

The nasal cavity has an extremely good blood supply from both the external and internal carotid arteries; anastomoses occur between the internal carotid artery and the maxillary arteries (the main branch of the external carotid artery) of both sides. The maxillary artery is the major supply to the nasal cavity. Ligation of the external carotid artery in dogs (in cases of persistent nose bleeding) gives rise to collateral connections between corresponding vessels of both sides.

The Paranasal Sinuses

The sinus system of the dog is poorly developed. The sinuses may even be absent in brachycephalic dogs, but the absence may not cause any clinical symptoms. The frontal sinus is the largest, occupies much of the frontal bone including its zygomatic process, and is separated from its fellow by a median septum. It may extend to the level of the temporomandibular joints in larger animals (especially if long-headed) (Fig. 11.11). The three cavities (lateral, medial, and rostral) of each of the frontal sinus communicate separately with the nasal cavity via nasofrontal openings (ethmoidal meatuses). The lateral compartment is the largest, has ethnoturbinates in its rostral part, and may be subdivided by incomplete septa. The medial and rostral compartments are also filled with ethmoturbinates, which hamper identification of these compartments on radiographs. The ethmoturbinates are covered with olfactory mucosa, in contrast to the sinus walls, which are lined with nonolfactory mucoperiosteum.

The sinus system of the cat comprises frontal, sphenoidal, and maxillary compartments, of which the frontal is the most important (Figs. 11.7B and 11.12/*1*). Its position generally corresponds to that in the dog, but the compartment is undivided and extends rather far ventrally within the medial wall of the orbit. The communication with the nasal cavity is in its rostral part and may provide ineffective drainage in the bacterial sinusitis that is corrected with surgical drainage. In mature cats, the sinus can be surgically approached just lateral to the midline, on the line connecting the rostral margins of the supraorbital processes. In 3- to 4-month-old kittens the approach is made midway between the line connecting the rostral margins of the supraorbital processes and that connecting the medial angles of the eyes.

In both dogs and cats, the maxillary sinus (Fig. 11.10/*13*) communicates so freely with the nasal cavity that the term *nasal recess* is preferred. It is not a true sinus because it is not formed between two plates of maxillary bone, being bounded by the maxilla laterally and the ethmoid medially. The recess occupies the face immediately rostral to the orbit, above the roots of the last three cheek teeth, and communicates with the middle meatus by a wide nasomaxillary

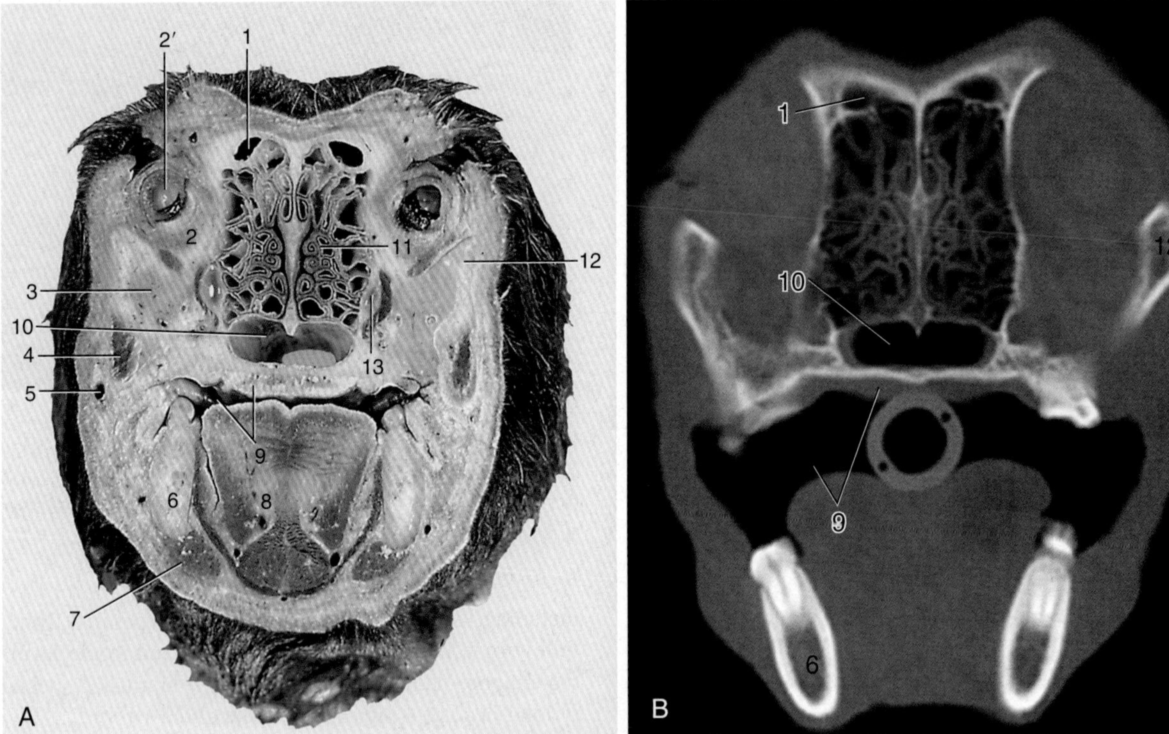

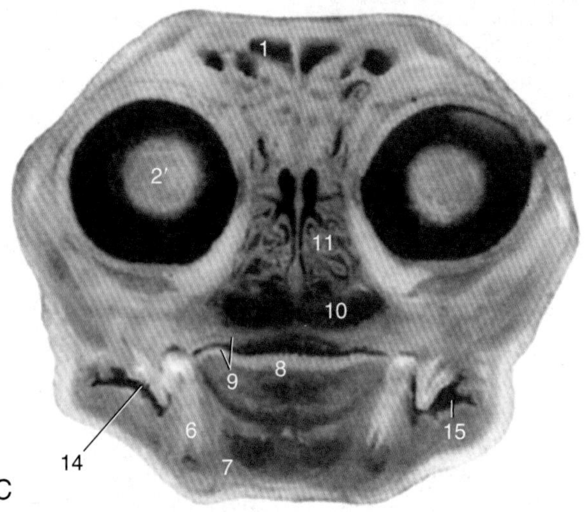

Fig. 11.10 Transverse sections of (A) canine and (C) feline heads through the rostral part of the orbit, rostral surface. (B) Computed tomography scan (bone window) of canine head at the level of (A). *1,* Frontal sinus; *2,* orbital structures; *2′,* eye; *3,* zygomatic gland; *4,* masseter; *5,* facial vein; *6,* mandible; *7,* digastricus; *8,* tongue; *9,* oral cavity and hard palate; *10,* choana; *11,* ethmoidal conchae; *12,* zygomatic arch; *13,* maxillary recess; *14,* sectorial teeth, P^4 engaging M_1; *15,* oral vestibule.

opening flanked by the nasal conchae. The recess houses on its lateral wall the broad, flat, lateral nasal gland, which appears as a thickening of the mucosa. Root abscesses of the sectorial tooth P^4 may break into the recess and later onto the surface of the skull. Surgical drainage is most conveniently achieved by the extraction of the sectorial tooth to open a passage to the mouth; the presence of the infraorbital canal makes the direct lateral approach unwise.

In cats, a small sphenoidal sinus is present; the similar cavity found in dogs is filled with ethmoturbinates.

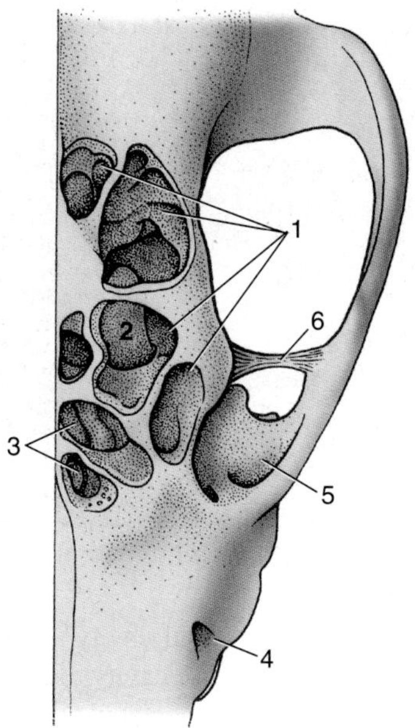

Fig. 11.11 The canine frontal sinuses, dorsal view. *1*, Lateral frontal sinus; *2*, ethmoidal concha invading the sinus; *3*, medial and rostral frontal sinuses; *4*, infraorbital foramen; *5*, orbit; *6*, orbital ligament.

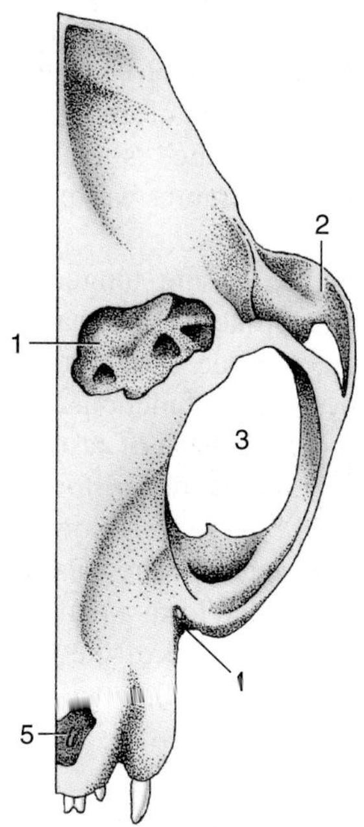

Fig. 11.12 The feline frontal sinus, dorsal view. *1*, Frontal sinus, opened; *2*, zygomatic arch; *3*, orbit; *4*, position of infraorbital foramen; *5*, nasal aperture.

THE MOUTH

The wide gape of carnivores is due to the caudal situation of the angles of the mouth and the correspondingly short cheeks. The interior of the mouth, including the oropharynx,

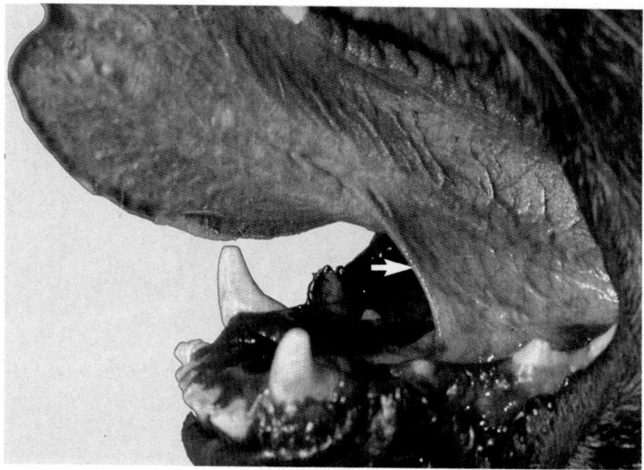

Fig. 11.13 Tongue with frenulum *(arrow)*.

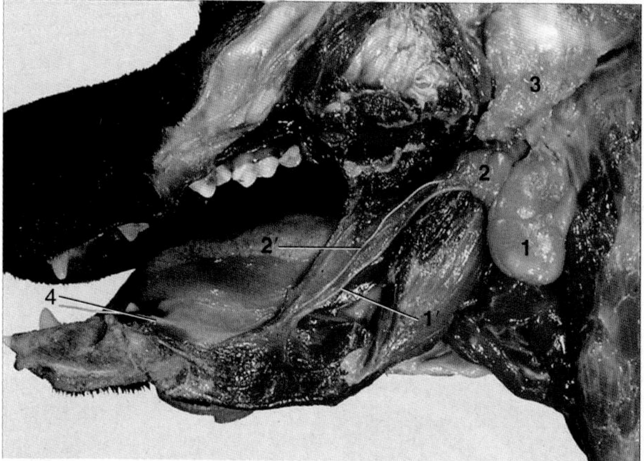

Fig. 11.14 Salivary glands. *1*, Mandibular gland; *1′*, mandibular duct; *2*, sublingual gland, monostomatic part; *2′*, its duct; *3*, parotid gland; *4*, sublingual caruncle.

is therefore easily examined. The edge of the lower lip carries blunt papillae. The upper lip is pendulous and presses on the lower one, which is everted near the commissure in certain breeds with ample head skin, such as the Spaniel (Figs. 11.6A and 11.13). The resulting folds predispose to infection. The general looseness of the lips creates a large vestibule—an advantage for the administration of liquid medicines, which then escape behind the cheek teeth into the central cavity.

The ducts of the parotid (Figs. 11.6 /*13* and 11.14/*3*) and zygomatic (see Figs. 11.10/*3* and 11.27/*8*) salivary glands open into the vestibule: the former by a single orifice in a small papilla opposite the upper fourth premolar P^4 and the latter by a row of four or five orifices on a mucosal ridge a little farther caudally. The ducts of the mandibular and compact (monostomatic) sublingual glands open to the floor of the mouth at the sublingual caruncle. They run below the mucous membrane that connects the side of the tongue with the gums; when a duct is damaged, saliva may escape to form a large mucosal swelling (ranula) lateral to the tongue. The larger salivary ducts are occasionally cannulated to remove obstructions or to inject a contrast

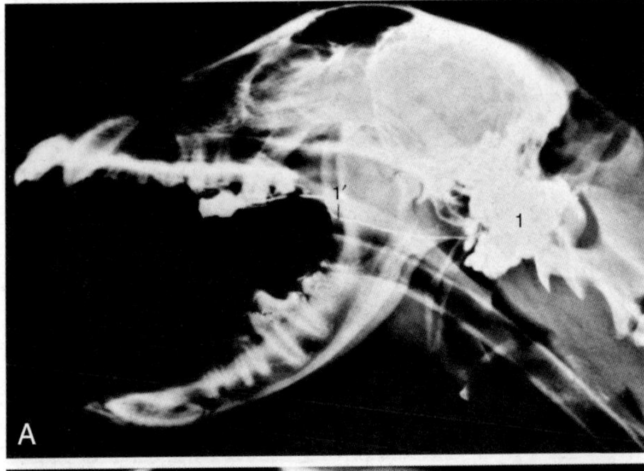

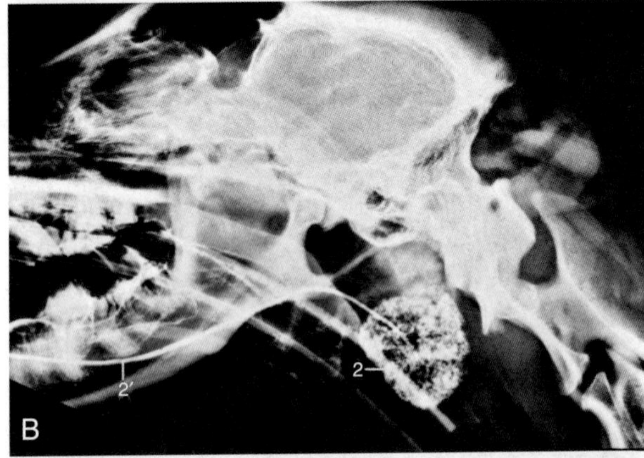

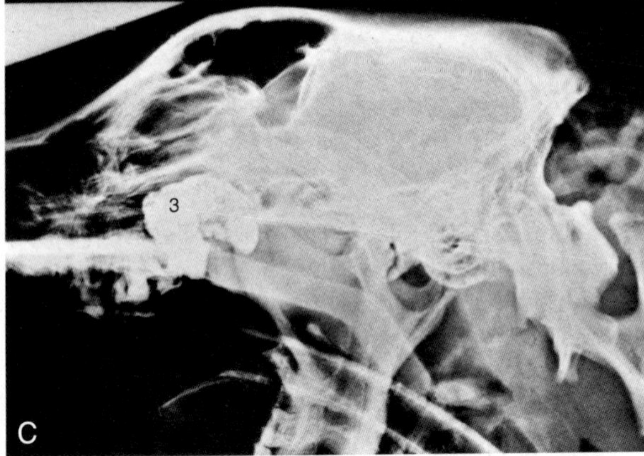

Fig. 11.15 Contrast medium outlining canine (A) parotid, (B) mandibular, and (C) zygomatic glands. *1,* Parotid gland; *1′,* duct; *2,* mandibular gland; *2′,* duct; *3,* zygomatic gland.

medium for radiographic examination (sialography; Fig. 11.15).

The oral cavity proper, like the nasal cavity above it, widens from front to back before contracting at the level of the palatoglossal arches, beyond which it is continued by the oropharynx.

The hard palate presents transverse ridges and a prominent incisive papilla (see Fig. 3.5). The slit to each side of the incisive papilla opens into an incisive duct that extends caudodorsally for 1 or 2 cm through the palatine fissure to open onto the floor of the nasal cavity. Before doing so, the duct communicates with the cavity of the vomeronasal organ. The flehmen reaction associated with the perception of pheromones is exhibited in both dogs and cats but is less clearly demonstrated than in animals such as the horse (Fig. 11.16).

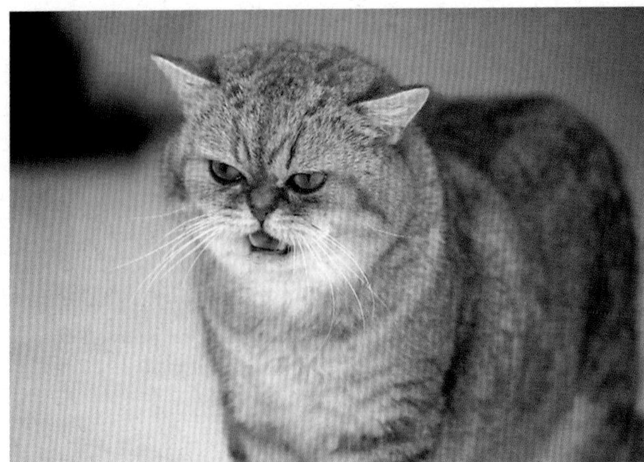

Fig. 11.16 Tomcat demonstrating flehmen.

The oral mucosa, generally pink, may be pigmented locally. The wide and flat apex of the tongue is depressed centrally (like a spoon) when liquids are lapped. A short median rod (lyssa) of connective, muscular, and cartilaginous tissue is embedded close to the ventral surface of the tongue. Its significance is not known, although a fanciful connection with rabies was postulated in former times.

The dorsal surface of the tongue is roughened by papillae. Filiform papillae predominate but are replaced by stouter conical papillae toward the root; both have protective and mechanical functions. Other papillae are concerned with the perception of taste; round fungiform papillae are dotted among the filiform papillae; foliate papillae, represented by a few shallow grooves, are present on the lateral border, near the palatoglossal arch; and four to six vallate papillae form a rostrally open V on the root (Fig. 11.17). The tongue of the newborn is fringed with lacelike (marginal) papillae that persist for the first 2 weeks and are thought to assist in fitting the tongue to the dam's teat.

The oral cavity of the cat is short and wide and is easily examined in cooperative subjects (Fig. 11.18). The abrasive nature of the cat's tongue is due to the strong keratinization of the epithelium of the large conical papillae that replace the delicate filiform papillae of most species. The caudally directed and hook-shaped papillae on the dorsum of the tongue assist with grooming but also trap hair and other fine objects (Figs. 11.19 and 11.20). Hairs removed from the coat during grooming therefore accumulate in the stomach (hairballs), and may be expelled with the feces or ejected through the mouth.

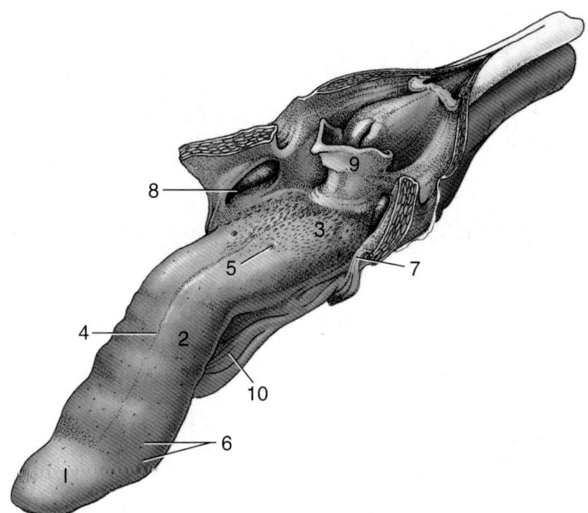

Fig. 11.17 The tongue of the dog. The soft palate and the esophagus are sectioned in the median plane. *1,* Apex; *2,* body; *3,* root, forming floor of oropharynx; *4,* median groove; *5,* vallate papilla; *6,* fungiform papillae; *7,* palatoglossal arch; *8,* palatine tonsil in tonsillar fossa; *9,* epiglottis; *10,* frenulum.

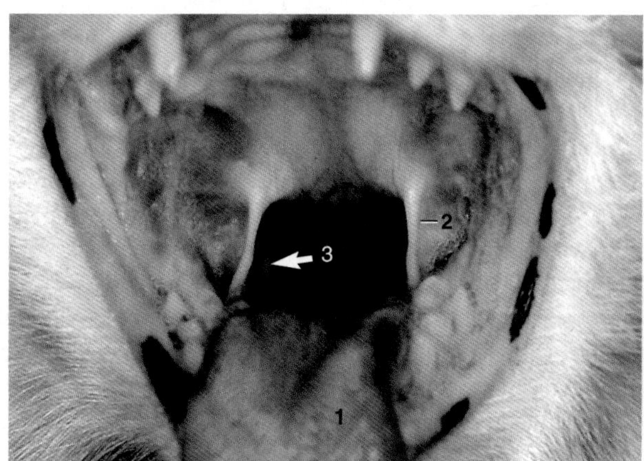

Fig. 11.18 Oropharynx (cat). *1,* Tongue; *2,* palatoglossal arch; *3,* position of right palatine tonsil *(arrow).*

In addition to diffuse labial salivary glands, the lips of cats contain large sebaceous and apocrine glands. The secretion of these circumoral glands is used in grooming and may be frequently rubbed off on objects, apparently as a scent marker substance (see Fig. 10.11).

Congenital clefts of the primary (harelip) or secondary palate have been reported in cats, especially Siamese. In dogs, the incidence of cleft palate is higher in brachycephalic breeds, although other breeds (Labrador, Cocker Spaniel) may be affected. The primary palate forms the lips and premaxilla, and the secondary palate forms the hard and soft palates. The incomplete closure of these structures is attributed to inherited recessive or irregular dominant traits and to exposure to toxic agents or intrauterine viral infections, especially those occurring at a very specific time in fetal development (25th to 28th day in dogs).

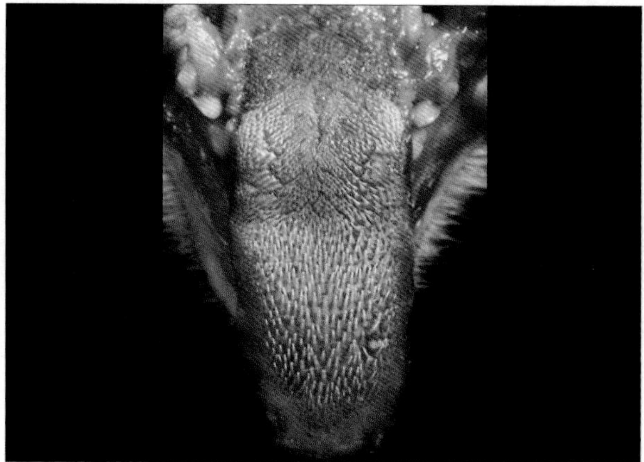

Fig. 11.19 Tongue (cat) with papillae.

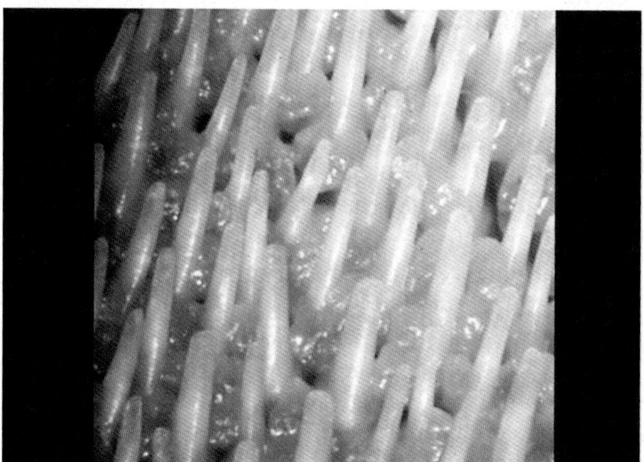

Fig. 11.20 Enlargement showing caudally directed keratinized filiform papillae on the tongue (cat).

Fractures of the mandible and separation at the symphysis, often as the result of traffic accidents, are fairly common in both species. Concurrent involvement of the maxilla, nasal structures, teeth, and soft tissues of the face is more frequent in cats that have fallen from heights.

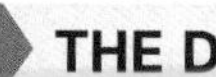

THE DENTITION

Much of the general description of the teeth was based on the dentition of the dog, in which the most remarkable features are the prominence of the canine teeth and the marked regional specialization of the others (see Fig. 3.16). The upper dental arch, despite having fewer teeth, is slightly longer than the lower one; the upper teeth

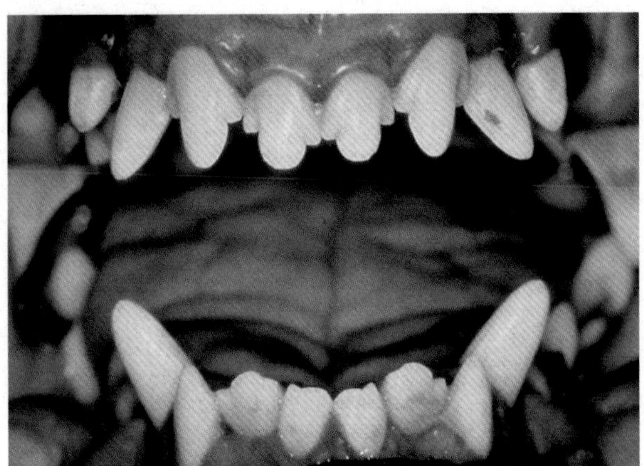

Fig. 11.21 Trilobular form of upper incisors.

therefore bite on the buccal side of the lower ones in a shearing action. This feature precludes lateral movement of the lower jaw, making grinding impossible. There is little occlusal contact between upper and lower teeth except caudally, where some crushing of food is possible. The first few premolars do not touch at all, which creates the so-called carrying space. Dogs and cats bolt rather than chew their food.

The formula for temporary dentition in dogs is

$$\frac{3-1-3}{3-1-3}=28$$

and for the permanent set is

$$\frac{3-1-4-2}{3-1-4-3}=42$$

The Triadan system is also available for reference to specific teeth. In this system, each tooth is assigned a three-digit number. The first digit (in the hundreds place) indicates the quadrant of the mouth: 1(00) indicates the right upper, 2(00) the left upper, 3(00) the left lower, and 4(00) the right lower quadrant. The other two digits indicate the place of the tooth in the dental arcade, 01 being the most mesial. Thus 102 specifies the upper right second incisor, 409 the lower right first molar.

The incisor teeth are rather loosely embedded in the incisive bones and mandible. On eruption the upper incisor crowns present a central cusp flanked by two smaller ones; the mesial cusp is lacking on the lower incisors (Fig. 11.21). These features are lost as wear reduces the incisors to simple prismatic pegs. The wear gives some indication of a dog's age but is not very reliable because of differences in skull size, frequency of malocclusion, and individual variation in the diet and habits (Fig. 11.22). All incisors have a single root. They are mainly for nibbling, both in grooming and when detaching small morsels.

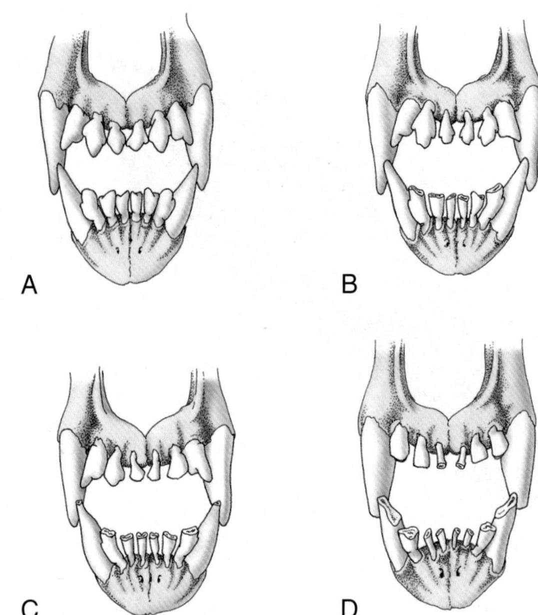

Fig. 11.22 Changes in the canine incisors with increasing age. (A) Six months; (B) about 2½ years; (C) about 6 years; (D) about 10 years.

The root of the canine is especially massive—larger indeed than the crown—and curves caudally to lie dorsal (or ventral) to the first premolar (Fig. 11.23). These teeth are occasionally removed in aggressive dogs. Simple extraction is made impossible by the size and firm implantation of the root; the attempt to draw one free risks fracture of the jaw. It is necessary to resect the bone over the lateral surface of the root before it can be elevated from its socket. Abscesses of the upper canine teeth may fistulate into the nasal cavity.

In adult dogs, there are four premolar teeth, the first of which may have either one or two roots, whereas the others have two. The one exception is the upper fourth premolar or sectorial tooth, which has three roots (Fig. 11.24). The four premolars increase in size and complexity from the first to last in both jaws. The laterally compressed crowns are triangular in profile, presenting small mesial and distal cusps to each side of the principal one. The last upper premolar, P^4, is massive and has a small medial part, with its own root, which encroaches on the hard palate. The molars decrease in size from first to last. The two upper molars, though still tuberculate, have flatter crowns than the premolars and are orientated transversely rather than rostrocaudally (see Fig. 11.24). They have three diverging roots. The first of the lower molars, M_1, the sectorial tooth, is the largest in the lower series. It is flattened from side to side and has two thick divergent roots that occupy most of the width of the jaw. Extraction must be performed carefully to avoid fracture of the mandible. M_2 and M_3 are much smaller; they engage the

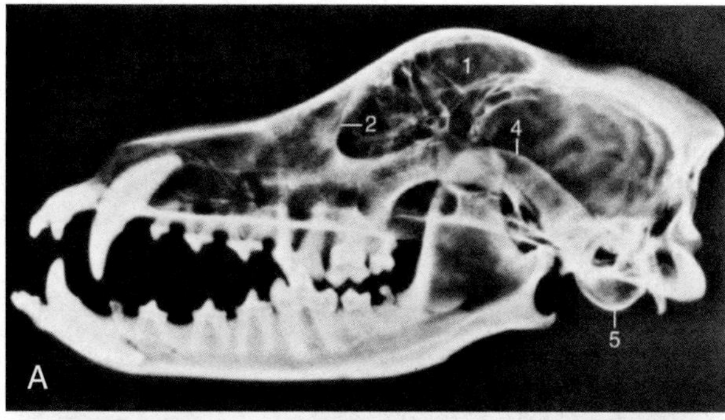

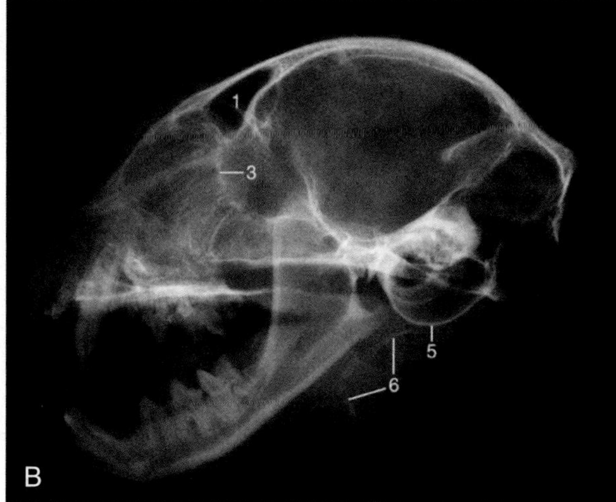

Fig. 11.23 (A) Radiograph of half of a canine skull showing the permanent teeth and their roots. (B) Radiograph of half of a feline head. *1,* Frontal sinus; *2,* orbital rim; *3,* cribriform plate; *4,* zygomatic arch; *5,* tympanic bulla; *6,* hyoid apparatus.

last upper molar and, like it, have flat tuberculate crowns. They also have two roots each.

It is important to know the pattern of the sockets to ensure that no part is left behind after extraction of a tooth (see Fig. 11.24). Multiple roots always diverge, and it is frequently necessary to split a tooth before it can be extracted to avoid causing excessive trauma.

Brachygnathic breeds often have less than the full complement of teeth: upper and lower P1 and M3 are those most often missing. The cheek teeth of these breeds may be more obliquely placed than normal to fit in the foreshortened jaws.

At birth, a puppy is toothless. The first teeth appear within a few weeks, and the deciduous set is complete and functional by the end of the second month. The first replacement tooth erupts after a further month, or little more, and the permanent set is complete by the sixth or seventh month, a remarkably early age (Table 11.1). Permanent teeth erupt earlier in larger breeds of dogs. The temporary teeth in general resemble those of the definitive set but are smaller and sharper. They have long slender roots. A temporary canine is sometimes retained after the replacement tooth has erupted because the latter appears

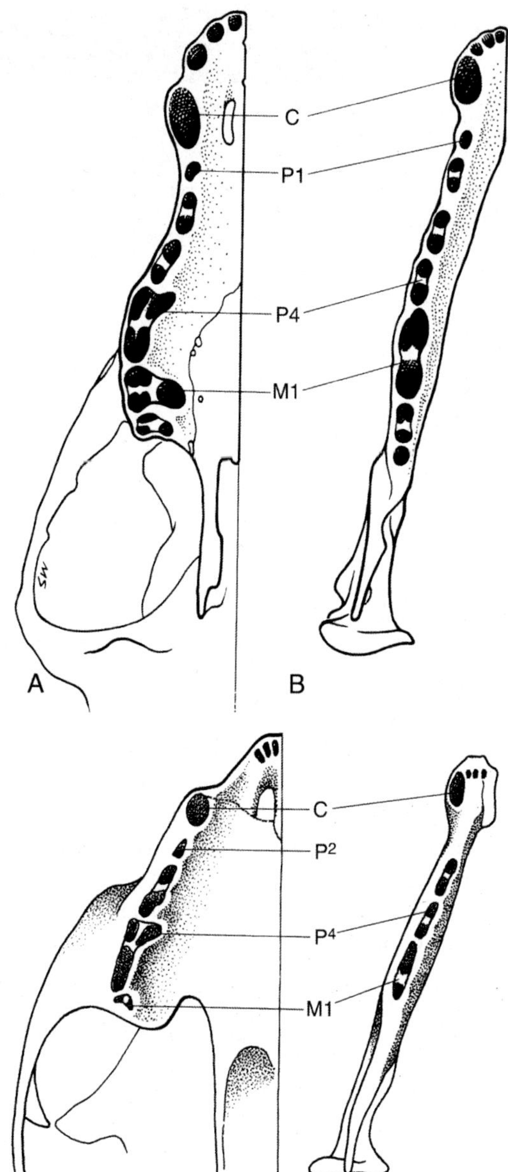

Fig. 11.24 The tooth sockets in *(top)* canine and *(bottom)* feline (A) upper and (B) lower jaws to show the number and disposition of the roots. *C,* canine; *M,* molar; *P,* premolar; *numbers* indicate tooth positions.

beside its predecessor and produces asymmetrical and sometimes insufficient resorption pressure. In such cases the temporary canine is found caudal to its replacement in the upper jaw and lateral to it in the lower jaw. Retained teeth should be removed to allow their replacements to attain their normal positions. The three temporary premolars are properly designated p2, p3, and p4; the tooth known as the *first premolar* erupts several weeks later than these and is part of the permanent dentition (Table 11.1).

The upper teeth are innervated by the infraorbital nerve, and the rostral members of the series can be desensitized by blocking of the nerve within the infraorbital foramen.

TABLE 11.1 ERUPTION DATES OF THE DOG'S TEETH

	Eruption of Temporary Tooth (wk)	Eruption of Permanent Tooth (mo)*
Incisor 1	4–6	3–5
Incisor 2	4–6	3–5
Incisor 3	4–6	4–5
Canine	3–5	5–7
Premolar 1		4–5
Premolar 2	5–6	5–6
Premolar 3	5–6	5–6
Premolar 4	5–6	4–5
Molar 1		5–6
Molar 2		5–6
Molar 3		6–7

*Permanent teeth erupt slightly earlier in large breeds.
Modified from Schummer A, Nickel R, Sack WO: *The viscera of the domestic mammals,* ed 2, New York, 1979, Springer-Verlag; and Evans HE: *Miller's anatomy of the dog,* ed 3, Philadelphia, 1993, Saunders.

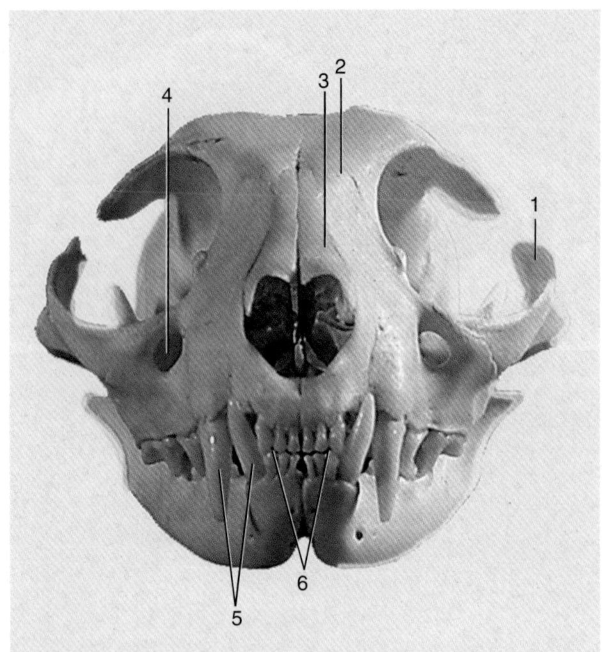

Fig. 11.25 Feline skull, rostral view. *1,* Zygomatic arch; *2,* frontal bone; *3,* nasal bones; *4,* infraorbital foramen; *5,* upper and lower canine teeth; *6,* upper and lower incisors. Upper teeth are in incisive bones and lower teeth in the mandible.

The lower teeth are supplied by the inferior alveolar nerve, which can be blocked at a site a centimeter or so caudal to the last tooth, before it enters the mandible. The rostral members of this series can also be desensitized by blocking of the nerve within the mental foramen.

The cat has sharp and pointed teeth. The formula for the temporary dentition reads

$$\frac{3-1-3}{3-1-2}$$

and for the permanent dentition reads

$$\frac{3-1-3-1}{3-1-2-1}$$

The smaller number of cheek teeth is due to the absence of P^1 and M^2 and of P1, P_2, M_2, and M_3 (see Fig. 3.17). The molar loss deprives the cat of flat-crowned crushing teeth, leaving an exclusively shearing bite (Fig. 11.25). P^4, the upper sectorial, is the only tooth to have three roots, which are implanted only a few millimeters from the ventral wall of the orbit. Its lower counterpart is M_1. It is not uncommon to find that one or more of the smaller incisor teeth have been shed by the time cats settle into middle age, without obvious cause.

In kittens, eruption of deciduous teeth typically begins during the third postnatal week. The permanent teeth are all in place by about 6 months of age. However, there is so much individual and breed variation that the average eruption and replacement dates given in Table 11.2 are unreliable guides to age.

Plaque deposition and consequent periodontal disease are common in both companion species. In cats, such disease is often accompanied by resorptive lesions at the necks of the teeth.

TABLE 11.2 ERUPTION DATES OF THE CAT'S TEETH

	Eruption of Temporary Tooth (wk)	Eruption of Permanent Tooth (mo)
Incisor 1	3–4	3½–5½
Incisor 2	3–4	3½–5½
Incisor 3	3–4	3½–5½
Canine	3–4	5½–6½
Premolar 2	5–6	4–5
Premolar 3	5–6	4–5
Premolar 4	5–6	4–5
Molar 1		5–6

From Schummer A, Nickel R, Sack WO: *The viscera of the domestic mammals,* ed 2, New York, 1979, Springer-Verlag.

THE TEMPOROMANDIBULAR JOINT

The articular surfaces of the temporomandibular joint are nearly congruent. The transverse cylinder provided by the mandible fits within a trough on the undersurface of the zygomatic process of the temporal bone (Figs. 11.23, 11.26, 11.28, and 11.29). The trough is enlarged caudally

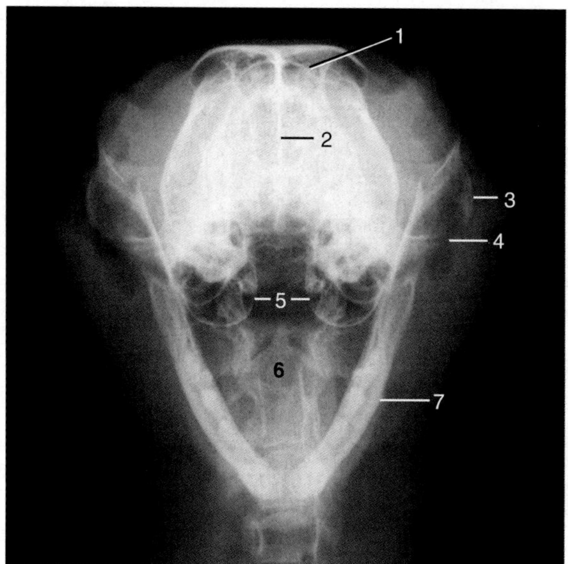

Fig. 11.26 Rostrocaudal open-mouth radiograph of a feline head. *1,* Frontal sinus; *2,* nasal septum; *3,* zygomatic arch; *4,* temporomandibular joint; *5,* tympanic bullae; *6,* axis with dens; *7,* mandible.

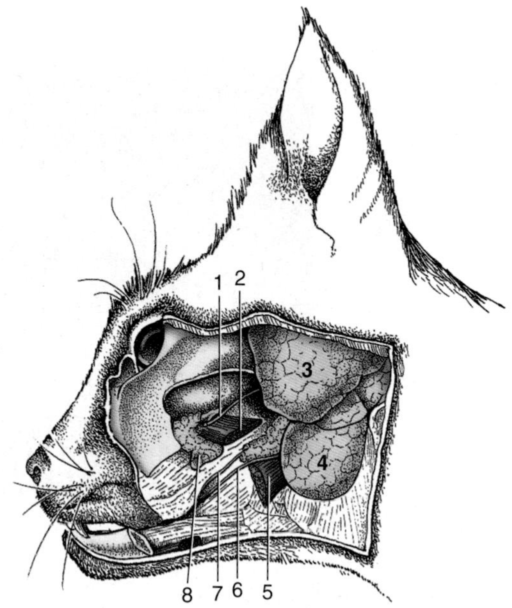

Fig. 11.27 Deep dissection of the feline head to expose the zygomatic salivary gland *(8)*. *1,* Parotid duct, cut; *2,* medial pterygoid muscle; *3,* parotid gland; *4,* mandibular gland; *5,* digastricus muscle; *6,* mandibular duct; *7,* sublingual duct emerging from the rostral end of the monostomatic sublingual salivary gland.

by a prominent retroarticular process that securely cups the cylinder and prevents its luxation in a caudal direction. In keeping with the congruence of the joint, the articular disk is thin. The joint capsule is strengthened by a lateral ligament.

Movement of the mandible is almost exclusively of a hinge nature, but slight protrusion is possible when the mouth is fully open. Lateral movement may be produced by trauma and occasionally is so severe that the coronoid process engages the zygomatic arch, locking the jaws in the depressed position.

The joint lies under cover of the caudal part of the masseter, where the dorsal buccal branch of the facial nerve crosses the border of the muscle. It is rostral to the parotid gland.

The masticatory muscles have been sufficiently described (p. 105-106)

THE SALIVARY GLANDS

Parotid Gland

The parotid gland (see Fig. 11.6) is roughly triangular, relatively thin, and molded around the proximal portion of the auricular cartilage, against which it can be rolled on palpation. It occupies a depression formed by the masseter muscle, the wing of the atlas, and the auricular cartilage. Ventral to the cartilage, it is related medially to the facial nerve and maxillary vein and more rostrally to the parotid lymph node and temporomandibular joint. The parotid duct leaves the cranial aspect of the gland and continues over the lateral aspect of the masseter muscle between the buccal branches of the facial nerve. The duct opens into the vestibule at a small parotid papilla opposite the caudal part of the upper fourth premolar tooth, approximately 5 mm from the margin of the gum. The duct makes a right-angle bend just before opening at the papilla; one can make cannulation of the duct easier by grasping the mucosa just caudal to the opening and pulling it rostrally to straighten the bend.

Zygomatic Gland

The ventral buccal glands comprise a few small, solitary units located in the submucosa, rostral to the masseter muscle, medial to the ventral part of the buccinator, and lateral to the mandible.

The dorsal buccal glands are consolidated in a mass generally known as the *zygomatic gland* (see Figs. 11.10A, 11.27/*28,* and 11.36/*2*). This structure is a large mixed gland located in the ventral part of the orbit, covered by the zygomatic arch, and related medially to the maxillary artery and nerve and medial pterygoid muscle and dorsally to the periorbita. Its swelling, when diseased, may cause protrusion of the eyeball (exophthalmos) or bulging of the oral mucosa near the last upper cheek tooth, where the duct opens into the vestibule. Facial trauma may cause leakage of saliva, and the resulting zygomatic mucocele may produce exophthalmos.

The main duct of the zygomatic gland (Fig. 11.15C) opens on a small papilla lateral to the caudal part of the

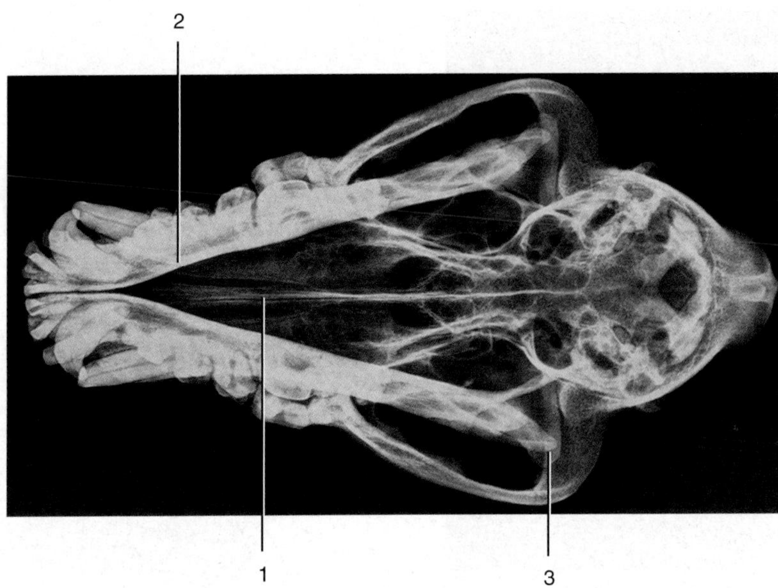

Fig. 11.28 Ventrodorsal radiograph of the canine head. Note the position and size of the brain case. *1,* Nasal septum; *2,* mandible; *3,* temporomandibular joint.

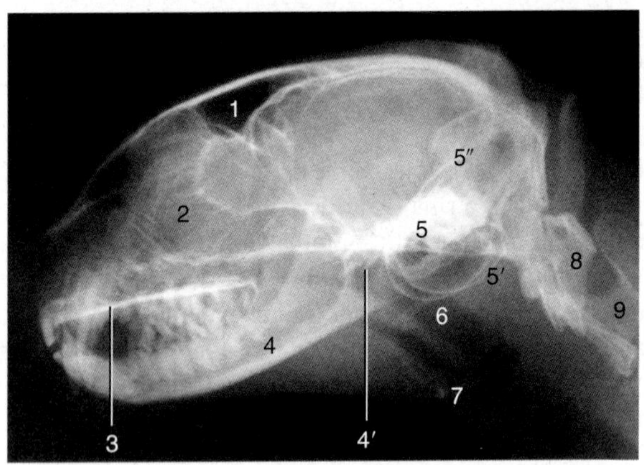

Fig. 11.29 Radiograph of the feline head. *1,* Frontal sinus; *2,* cribriform plate and ethmoidal conchae; *3,* hard palate; *4,* mandible; *4′,* temporomandibular joint; *5,* petrous temporal bone; *5′,* tympanic bullae; *5″,* tentorium cerebelli; *6,* nasopharynx; *7,* basihyoid; *8,* atlas; *9,* axis.

upper first molar tooth. A small ridge connects the main zygomatic and parotid gland duct openings. Usually there are one to four small accessory ducts opening caudal to the main one. These openings are usually obvious and easily cannulated.

Mandibular Gland

The large ovoid mandibular gland is contained within a strong fibrous capsule that gives it form. This capsule, with its firm attachment, makes the gland easily palpable, in contrast to the adjacent mandibular lymph nodes, which "float" under exploring fingers. The gland has these relations: rostrally, the mandibular lymph nodes, sublingual gland, and masseter and digastric muscles; medially, the digastric muscle, external carotid artery, and medial retropharyngeal lymph node; and caudally, the muscles of the neck. Its capsule continues rostrally onto the compact part of the sublingual gland, to which it is firmly fused (see Fig. 11.14). The course of the mandibular duct is described with the sublingual gland.

Sublingual Gland

The narrow compact sublingual gland continues forward from the mandibular gland. It follows the mandibular duct between the digastricus ventrally and the medial pterygoid dorsally and soon gains a position lateral to the root of the tongue, before ending variously at the level of the cheek teeth. Its duct accompanies that of the mandibular gland to the sublingual caruncle; together they raise the sublingual fold, near the body of the mandible. A variable number of lobules of the polystomatic portion of the sublingual gland are present in the sublingual fold, located rostral to the lingual branch of the trigeminal nerve; they open on the floor of the mouth next to the tongue through several ducts. The lingual nerve crosses the lateral surfaces of the mandibular and sublingual ducts just caudal to the level of the orbits.

The slitlike openings of the mandibular and sublingual ducts are recognizable on the lateroventral surface of the lingual caruncles, at the end of the frenulum of the tongue (see Fig. 11.14/*4*). The mandibular duct (Fig. 11.15B), the larger and more rostral of the two, is easily cannulated. The sublingual duct is more difficult to cannulate. In 20% to 40% of dogs the sublingual duct joins the mandibular duct along its course.

The most common clinical condition of the salivary glands in both dogs and cats is the salivary mucocele, which is the accumulation of mucoid saliva leaked from a damaged gland or duct. The sublingual gland is most frequently affected. Extravasated saliva most commonly collects in the subcutaneous tissues of the intermandibular, sublingual tissues (ranula) or cranial cervical area. A less common site is the wall of the pharynx. Treatment requires the removal of the mandibular–sublingual gland complex. Removal of both of these glands does not affect the animal adversely, even if bilateral, but care must be taken to avoid the lingual nerve.

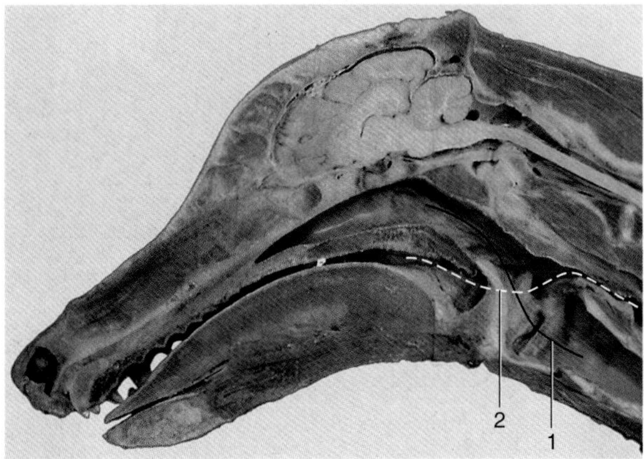

Fig. 11.30 Median section of head and neck. *1,* Route from nasopharynx to trachea *(solid line)*; *2,* route of food from mouth to esophagus *(broken line)*.

The cat's salivary glands are shown in Figs. 11.6B and 11.27.

THE PHARYNX

The auditory tubes open high on the lateral walls of the nasopharynx, immediately rostral to small mucosal cushions measuring about 10 mm long in dogs and 4 mm in cats. Nasopharyngeal polyps, common in cats, originate in the middle ear as focal hypertrophies of the mucosa, develop stalks, and extend through the auditory tube to reach the nasopharynx. There is a flat pharyngeal tonsil in the roof of the nasopharynx. Digital pressure in this area may stimulate respiration.

The dorsoventrally flattened oropharynx extends from the palatoglossal arches, which stand out when the tongue is pulled forward. During normal breathing the soft palate lies on the tongue with its free edge rostral to the epiglottis (Figs. 11.29 and 11.33). In many brachycephalic dogs the soft palate is disproportionally long and rests over the entrance to the larynx, causing respiratory difficulties. The overlong soft palate can be shortened with the use of the palatine vessels laterally and the palatine muscle toward the midline as landmarks. Additional guidance is provided by the wrinkling of the palatine mucosa where it does not lie over muscle. For different reasons, the epihyoid provides a useful landmark where it crosses the lateral wall of the oropharynx. Contact with the oropharyngeal wall during examination of the mouth normally causes dogs to retch; the absence of this (gag) reflex suggests damage to the glossopharyngeal and vagal nerves.

Oral breathing is possible with the palate in the normal position (Fig. 11.30), and the panting dog is a familiar sight. Cats may also breathe through the mouth but more discretely, sitting quietly and letting the air slip in and out through lips slightly parted toward the commissure. Occasionally the mouth is opened more widely, allowing a brief glimpse of the tongue.

The fusiform palatine tonsils occupy fossae in the lateral walls of the oropharynx caudal to the palatoglossal arch and ventral to the soft palate and are covered medially by semilunar folds, which arise from the ventrolateral part of the soft palate (Figs. 11.17/*8* and 11.31). In cats the palatine tonsil is very small and is covered by a mucosal fold.

The tonsils are relatively large in young dogs and often protrude from the fossae; similar protrusion in the adult usually indicates pathologic swelling. In the performance of tonsillectomy the reddish lymphoid tissue that lines the fossa dorsal to the tonsil must also be removed; it is exposed when the main part is retracted from the fossa. The tonsil is related laterally to the lingual nerve and the mandibular and sublingual ducts, all of which are at some risk in this operation. The tonsil is supplied by tonsillar and hyoid branches of the lingual artery, which courses ventrolateral to the tonsil. Sensory innervation to the tonsil is from the glossopharyngeal nerve. The efferent lymph vessels drain to the medial retropharyngeal and mandibular lymph nodes. There are of course no afferents.

On each side the caudal border of the soft palate is continued to the dorsolateral wall of the palatopharyngeal arch. The palatopharyngeal muscle and the mucosa that covers it form this arch.

DEGLUTITION

During the act of swallowing, the regurgitation of food into the nasopharynx and its aspiration into the larynx are both prevented by the coordinated activity of the pharyngeal muscles. These muscles arch over the roof of the pharynx to meet their contralateral fellows at a median raphe, and their contractions occur in sequence but overlap, ensuring that in cooperation they effect the movement of food toward and into the esophagus. The more rostral constrictor muscles also draw the pharynx forward and upward for the better reception of the food bolus as it is passed from the mouth. An essential feature of the process is the sphincter-like closure of the intrapharyngeal ostium that

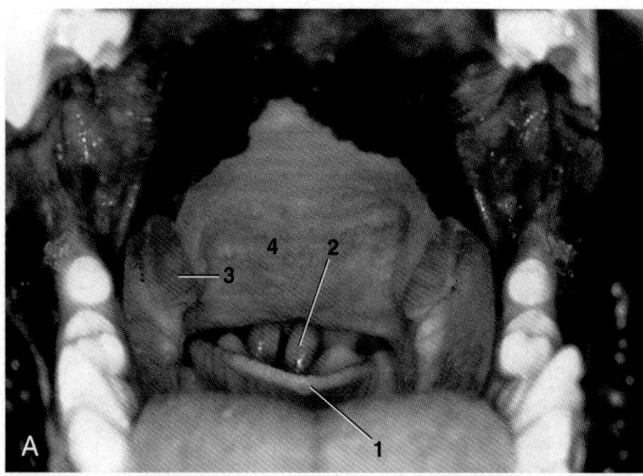

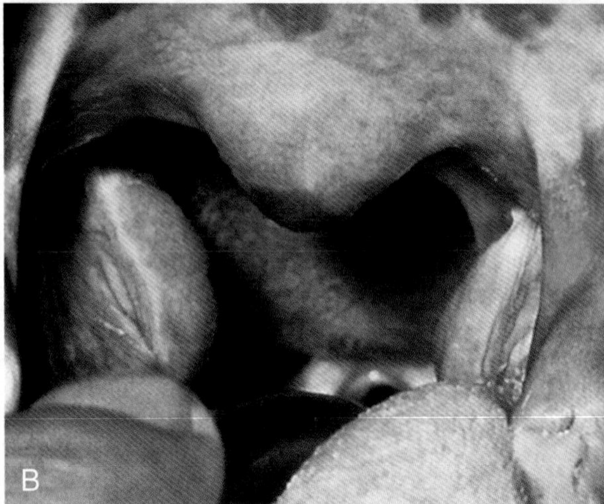

Fig. 11.31 (A) Oropharynx. *1,* Epiglottis; *2,* cuneiform processes of arytenoid cartilages; *3,* palatine tonsils; *4,* soft palate. (B) Palatine tonsils; the caudal part of the soft palate is missing.

involves elevation of the soft palate, in part effected by the small muscles (tensor and levator) that pull the palate taut between the pterygoid bones. The timely relaxation of the cricopharyngeus muscle allows food to escape into the esophagus. During the process, the larynx is raised while its entrance is partially blocked and the glottis closed.

Inappropriate closure of the intrapharyngeal ostium provokes sneezing.

THE LARYNX

The larynx is located caudal to the intermandibular space and ventral to the first two or three cervical vertebrae. Its cranial parts can be examined through the mouth in the sedated dog when the soft palate is raised with a spatula (Fig. 11.31A). Palpation through the skin reveals, in caudorostral succession, the cricoid cartilage (especially its arch), the rounded ventral surface of the thyroid cartilage, and the prominent thyrohyoids that connect the rostral horns of the thyroid cartilage with the basihyoid. The remaining bones of the hyoid apparatus, other than the stylohyoid, are also palpable (Figs. 2.34, 11.9, and 11.32).

The epiglottis resembles a pointed spade that is connected to the body of the hyoid bone and the cranioventral part of the thyroid cartilage. The aryepiglottic folds link the sides of the epiglottis to the dorsal parts of the arytenoid cartilages and their corniculate processes (Figs. 11.31 and 11.33). The channel lateral to the aryepiglottic folds is called the *piriform recess,* through which fluids leave the laryngopharynx for the esophagus during swallowing (Fig. 11.33).

The laryngeal vestibule extends caudally from the entrance to the vocal folds. The vestibular folds are short, but wide plicae of mucosa run from the expanded ventral margins of the arytenoid cartilage to the dorsal surface of the thyroid cartilage. The vocal folds visible through the entrance are formed by the vocal ligaments, straps of elastic fibers continuous caudally with the vocalis muscles. The vocal folds are separated from the more rostral vestibular folds by the large laryngeal ventricles, lateral evaginations of the mucosa that extend to the thyroid cartilage. The opening to the ventricles is about 1.5 mm wide and extends the length of the vocal fold that bounds it. Each ventricle has two parts. One part extends cranially lateral to the vestibule and a separate part caudally lateral to the vocal cord. The secretion of glands within the saccule prevents desiccation of the vestibular and vocal folds. Solitary lymph nodules are present in the walls of the ventricles. The saccules may provide room for the vocal folds to vibrate during barking, a theory supported by the reduction, even absence, of ventricles in the Basenji, a breed of dog that never barks.

The parts of the larynx surrounding the entrance project into the pharynx, and except when the dog swallows or breathes through the mouth, the free border of the soft palate is lodged below the epiglottis, which aligns the laryngeal lumen with that of the nasopharynx (see Fig. 11.33).

The larynx is covered ventrally by the subcutaneous sternohyoid muscles (see Fig. 11.45). It is related laterally to the medial retropharyngeal lymph node, common carotid artery and vagosympathetic trunk, linguofacial vein, and mandibular lymph nodes. It is related dorsally to the caudal part of the laryngopharynx leading to the esophagus.

The sensory nerve supply to the laryngeal mucosa is from the cranial laryngeal nerve, entering the laryngeal cavity through the rostral thyroid notch. The recurrent laryngeal nerves that supply the remainder of the intrinsic laryngeal musculature, except for the cricothyroids (supplied by a branch of the cranial laryngeal nerve), leave the parent vagal trunks within the chest. The right nerve arises level with the middle cervical ganglion and winds dorsally around the subclavian artery to proceed cranially in the angle between the longus colli muscle and the trachea. The left one leaves the vagus level of the aortic arch, which it loops around, distal

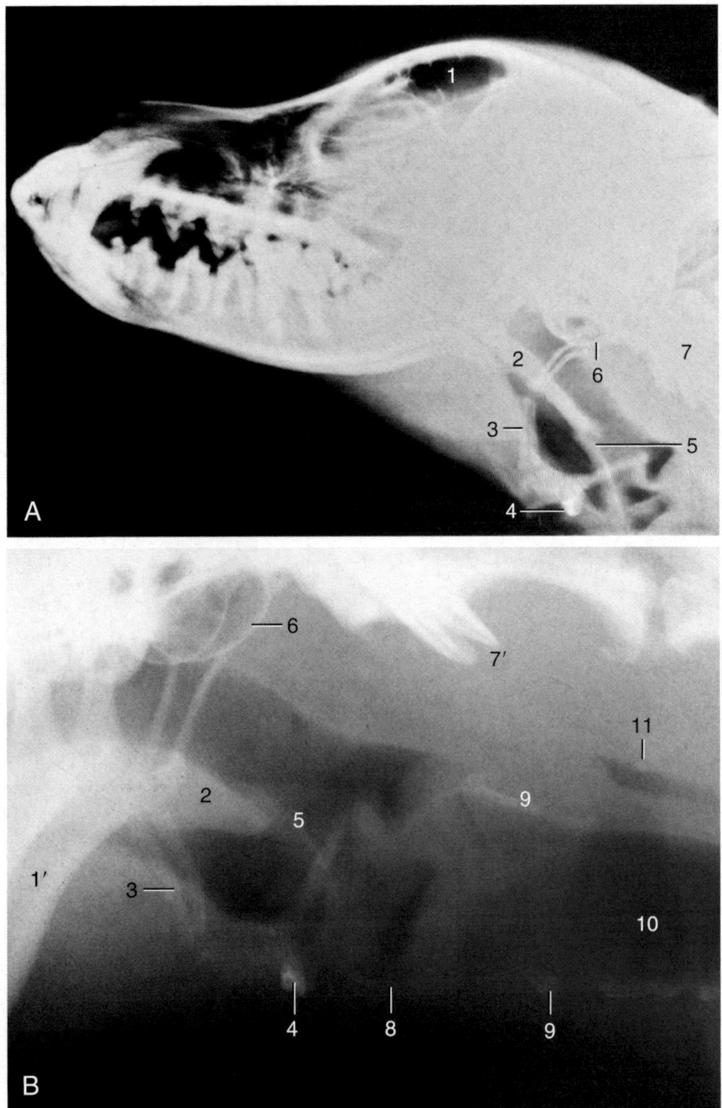

Fig. 11.32 (A) Radiograph of the canine head to show the relation of the hyoid apparatus to the skull and atlas. (B) Enlargement of the laryngeal region of another dog. *1,* Frontal sinus, *1′,* mandible; *2,* soft palate; *3,* hyoid apparatus (epihyoid); *4,* basihyoid; *5,* epiglottis; *6,* tympanic bulla; *7,* atlas; *7′,* wings of atlas; *8,* thyroid cartilage; *9,* cricoid cartilage; *10,* trachea; *11,* air in esophagus.

to the ligamentum arteriosum. It ascends the neck ventromedial to the esophagus. Both nerves supply the trachea and esophagus before terminating at the larynx.

Laryngeal paralysis as a genetic disorder occurs in certain breeds, notably the Bouvier and Leonberger, but it has also been encountered as an occasional disorder of older dogs of other large breeds.

The cranial laryngeal arteries provide the principal blood supply. They originate from the external carotid arteries and, with the cranial laryngeal nerves, pass through the rostral thyroid notches. Satellite veins drain into the external maxillary veins. Lymphatics drain into the medial retropharyngeal lymph nodes.

The cat's larynx is depicted in radiographs (see Fig. 11.29) and in a median section (see Fig. 11.35). The arytenoid cartilages have a simpler shape than those in the dog. The aryepiglottic folds bypass the arytenoid cartilages and connect the sides of the epiglottis directly to the cricoid cartilage. The vocal cords are thick and round; in contrast, the vestibular folds are thin and sharp edged. There is no genuine ventricle, but small pouches of the vestibular mucosa extend lateral to the fold. Solitary lymph nodules are present on the laryngeal surface of the epiglottis, and aggregated nodules (paraepiglottic tonsils) thicken the aryepiglottic folds.

Electromyographic studies show that purring in cats is produced by fast twitching of muscles in the larynx and

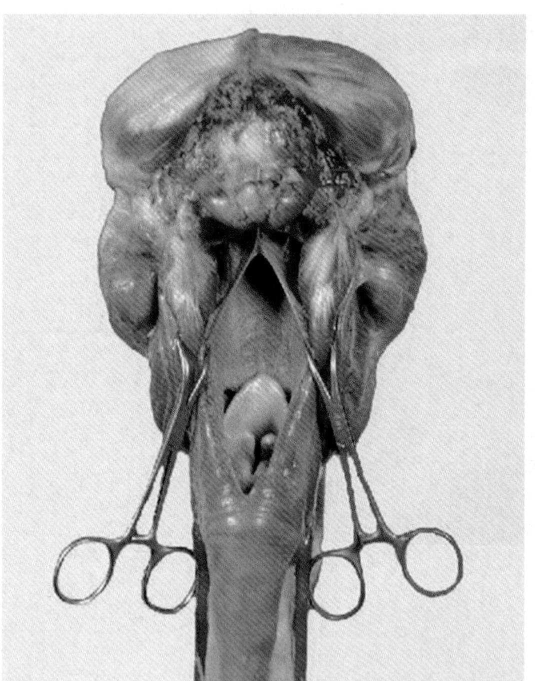

Fig. 11.33 The nasopharyngeal cavity exposed by median incision of the roof. Note the postvelar position of the tip of the epiglottis.

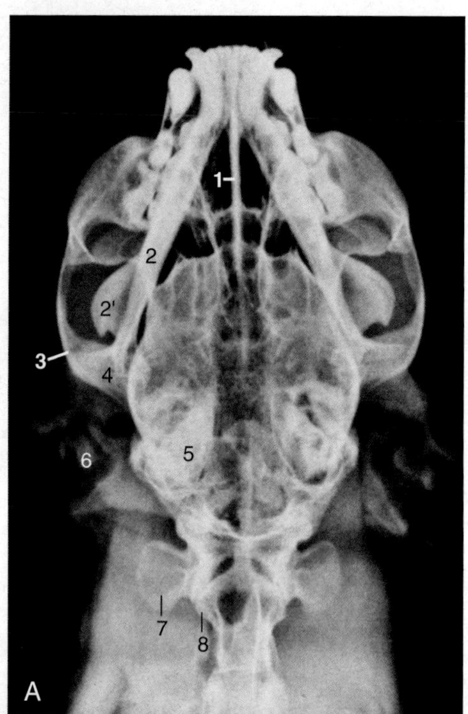

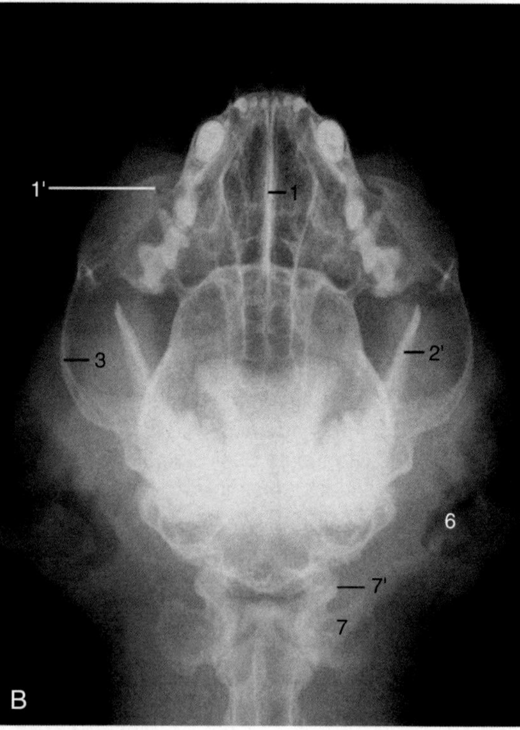

Fig. 11.34 Radiographs of the feline head. (A) Ventrodorsal view. (B) Ventrodorsal view with mouth fully opened. *1,* Nasal septum; *1′,* infraorbital foramen; *2,* mandible; *2′,* coronoid process; *3,* zygomatic arch; *4,* temporomandibular joint; *5,* petrous temporal bone; *6,* external ear; *7,* wing of atlas; *7′,* atlanto-occipital joint; *8,* axis.

diaphragm. The laryngeal muscles rapidly narrow and widen the glottis, causing respiratory air to vibrate and make the sound.

There are differences between the upper airways of brachycephalic and mesaticephalic breeds. In the brachycephalic obstruction syndrome, the nostrils can be stenotic, the pharynx short and narrow with thickened redundant mucosa, the root of the tongue massive, and the soft palate overlong. The progressive dyspnea is caused by increasing body weight, relatively insufficient growth of the laryngeal structures, increasing mass of the pharyngeal mucosa, and insufficient opening of the glottis. In addition, there is progressive collapse of the laryngeal structures and eversion of the laryngeal ventricles because of the increased traction caused by the greater velocity of exhaled air passing the relatively small laryngeal opening.

THE EYE AND ORBIT

The easily palpable margins of the orbit are formed by the frontal, lacrimal, and zygomatic bones, with the gap in the dorsolateral segment closed by the orbital ligament (Fig. 11.11/*6*). Only the medial third of the orbital wall is osseous; the remainder is provided by the periorbita. The orbital axis takes a dorsal, lateral, and anterior direction

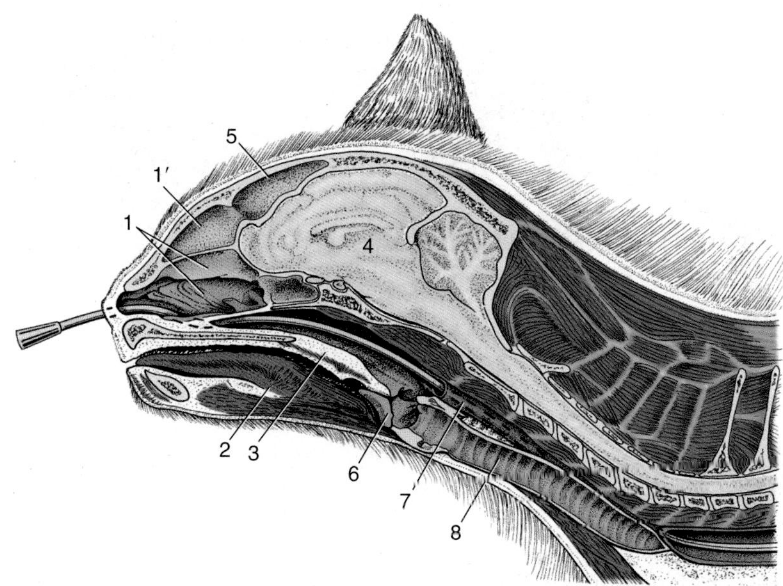

Fig. 11.35 Paramedian section of the feline head and neck. A nasogastric tube is in place. *1,* Nasal cavity; *1′,* dorsal part of nasal cavity; *2,* tongue; *3,* soft palate; *4,* brain; *5,* frontal sinus; *6,* epiglottis; *7,* esophagus; *8,* trachea.

from the apex of the cone. In brachycephalic dogs, particularly those with wide skulls, the axes point more laterally, restricting binocular vision.

The openings into the orbit comprise the optic canal, orbital fissure, duplicated ethmoidal foramina, and fossa of the lacrimal sac. The optic canal transmits the optic nerve and internal ophthalmic artery; the orbital fissure transmits the oculomotor, trochlear, abducent, and ophthalmic nerves; the ethmoidal foramina transmit divisions of the like-named nerve and artery; and the fossa contains the slight enlargement at the origin of the nasolacrimal duct.

The osseous wall of the orbit is related dorsomedially to the frontal sinus and rostromedially to the maxillary recess, creating potential for the spread of infection from these cavities to the orbital structures. The periorbita is related as follows: medioventrally to the medial pterygoid muscle; ventrally to a pad of fat caudal to the orbital margin, the zygomatic gland, and the large deep facial vein; laterally to the zygomatic arch; and caudodorsally to the orbital ligament and temporalis muscle. The dorsolateral aspect of the orbit is accessible to surgery without resection of bone.

The *important maxillary artery and nerve* and their branches to the face and palate course ventral to the orbit between the medial pterygoid and the zygomatic gland (Fig. 11.36). The maxillary artery gives off the external ophthalmic artery, which pierces the periorbita near its apex to supply structures within the cone. The temporalis, which surrounds the coronoid process of the mandible, impinges on the periorbita when the mouth is opened. This impingement may cause pain in conditions such as retrobulbar abscess, which may also drain behind the last cheek tooth in the mouth.

The dimensions of the orbital rim in large and small dogs differ less than might be expected. Because the diameter of the eyeball varies even less, the surgical working "space" is generally narrower in larger dogs. However, the position of the eyeball within the orbit differs markedly. In dolichocephalic dogs the eyeball is deeply placed and the palpebral fissure is small. The eyes of brachycephalic dogs protrude and are more susceptible to injury to the cornea.

The lacrimal gland (Fig. 11.36/*7*) is flat, lobulated, and about 12 to 15 mm in width. It lies between the eyeball and the orbital ligament, dorsal to the lateral angle of the eye. The gland must be identified and removed in enucleation (removal of the eye). The thin edge of the third eyelid is visible in the medial angle of the eye in the resting state. More is seen when the upper and lower lids are retracted with the fingers, whereas full protrusion is obtained by gentle pressure on the eyeball through the upper lid (see Fig. 9.21/*6*). Although the superficial gland that surrounds the cartilage of the third lid is not normally visible, it appears when the eyelid is retracted because the increased retrobulbar pressure pushes it to the fore. Active protrusion of the third eyelid, effected by a specific muscular arrangement, is common in cats and may have an emotional or physical origin. Abnormal retrobulbar pressure may cause the gland of the third eyelid to be everted into the medial angle of the eye, where it appears as a round swelling below a covering of conjunctiva. Subepithelial lymph nodules on the bulbar surface of the third eyelid may become inflamed.

In cross section the eyelids display the external skin, the orbicular muscle of the eye, the tarsal plate, the meibomian glands, and the palpebral conjunctiva. The openings of the tarsal glands (20 to 40 in each lid) can

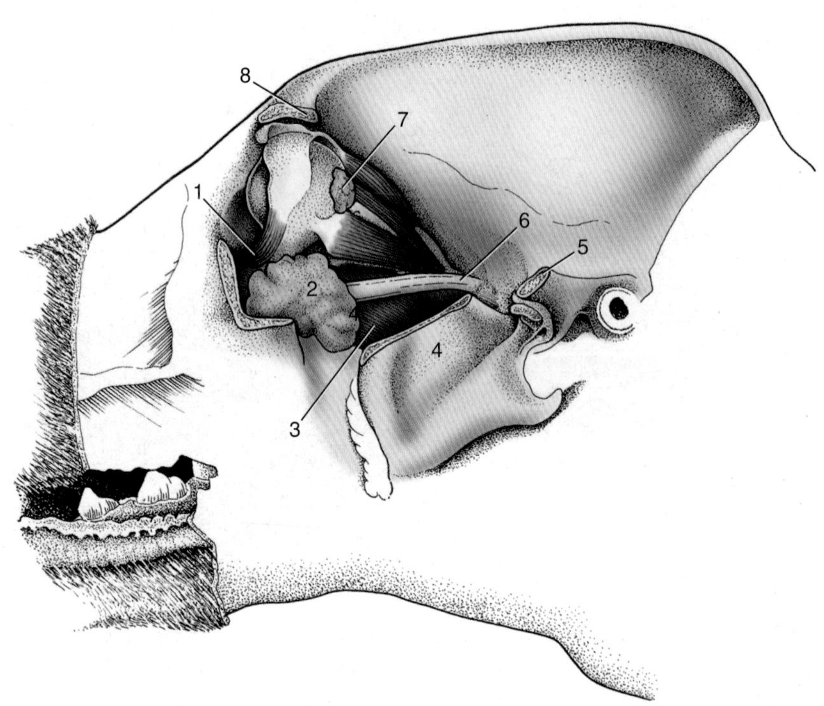

Fig. 11.36 Dissection of the canine orbit and pterygopalatine fossa, lateral view. *1,* Ventral oblique muscle; *2,* zygomatic gland; *3,* medial pterygoid muscle; *4,* coronoid process of mandible, cut; *5,* caudal stump of zygomatic arch; *6,* maxillary nerve; *7,* lacrimal gland; *8,* zygomatic process of frontal bone.

be seen at the lid margins. When the lids are everted, these glands appear as white cords extending 5 to 7 mm from the lid margin under the conjunctiva. Occasionally, aberrant hairs protrude from the openings of the tarsal glands and may irritate the cornea. The eyelashes in dogs are found on the outer surface of the upper lid margin; there are none on the lower lid. Both lids of cats are without lashes.

The orbicular muscle of the eye, rostral to the tarsal plate, is anchored to the orbit by fascia medially and by the retractor muscle of the lateral angle laterally. These attachments preserve the elliptical shape of the palpebral fissure.

The puncta lacrimalia, 2 to 4 mm from the medial angle of the eye, are usually located at the junction of pigmented and nonpigmented epithelia. Although they may be difficult to find or the lower one may in fact be absent or displaced to the bulbar surface of the lid, they can be cannulated. The puncta are the openings to the upper and lower canaliculi, which join to form the lacrimal sac, from which the nasolacrimal duct takes origin (see Fig. 9.21). The duct continues rostrally in the medial wall of the maxilla, deep to the nasal mucosa. An accessory, or more rarely the sole, opening of the nasolacrimal duct may enter the nose at the level of the canine tooth in a significant proportion of dogs. The duct makes an abrupt 90-degree turn about 2 mm before opening onto the floor of the nasal cavity (see Fig. 11.8).

The feline lacrimal system is similar; however, an opening with the oral cavity, located on a small papilla just behind the upper incisor teeth, has been recorded.

One or both puncta may be absent in several dog breeds, as well as Persian cats. If both are absent, a slight depression in the conjunctiva may indicate where the opening would normally have been located.

The eyeball is nearly spherical and relatively large. The cornea is slightly oval, its larger diameter being mediolateral in keeping with the shape of the globe itself. It is slightly thicker at the pole than at the periphery. The canine iris is brown, golden yellow, or bluish, and whether dilated or contracted the pupil remains round. It is said to be smaller in older dogs under standard light conditions. Remnants of the papillary membrane may be seen on its upper margin in puppies up to the age of 5 weeks.

The fundus is illustrated in Fig. 11.37. The triangular tapetum lucidum, which nearly fills the dorsal half, includes the optic disk in large dogs. The retinal vessels radiate from the disk; prominent venules form a partial circle from which tributaries usually spread dorsally, medioventrally, and lateroventrally. Thinner arterioles extend in all directions, many accompanying the venules.

In the cat there is little surgical working space between the eye and the orbital margin. The third eyelid is large, and in certain circumstances it may be drawn completely over the cornea. As in the dog, it responds to retraction of the eyeball. The cornea is relatively

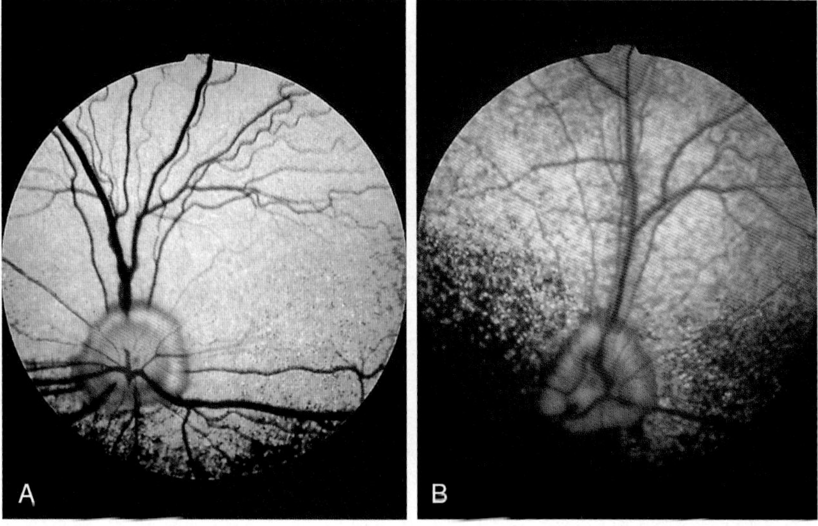

Fig. 11.37 Fundus of eye. (A) Dutch Sheepdog and (B) Old English Sheepdog.

large and permits a wide visual field. The color of the iris ranges from blue through green to golden. In certain breeds iris color is strictly prescribed to meet show standards. Kittens are usually born with blue eyes that later change color.

The pupils of domestic cats are round when dilated but are vertical slits when constricted (those of some wild felids remain round at all times) (Fig. 11.38). The vertical form is due to the dorsoventral orientation of muscle fibers that extend to the periphery of the iris and decussate at the extremities of the pupil. The fundus is dominated by a large tapetum lucidum that surrounds the optic disk. The tapetum of the cat is yellowish green or bluish green and because of its brilliance is thought to be more effective in reflecting light than that of the dog, an advantage that may be a convenience in nocturnal wandering (Fig. 11.39).

THE EAR (SEE P. 331)

External Ear

The external ear consists of the external auditory canal and its cartilaginous extension, the auricle (pinna). The auricle, sometimes known as the *ear leather* to dog fanciers, is shaped like a lopsided funnel, with a small cutaneous pouch on the caudal border a short distance above the ear opening (Figs. 11.40 and 11.41). There is a wide diversity in the shape, size, and posture (erect or folded) of dog ears. Most cats have erect auricles, but an exception is the Scottish Fold cat, in which the most distal portion of the auricle bends rostroventrally beginning at 3 to 4 weeks of age.

The basis of the auricle is a plate of fibroelastic cartilage that is covered by subcutaneous tissue and skin. The skin on the inner (concave) surface adheres more firmly to the cartilage than that on the outer part.

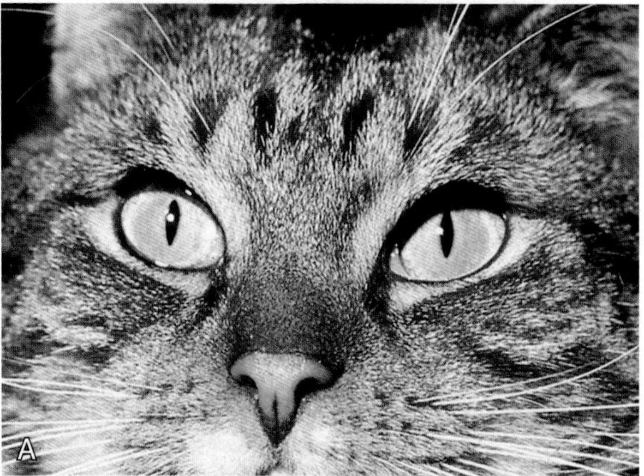

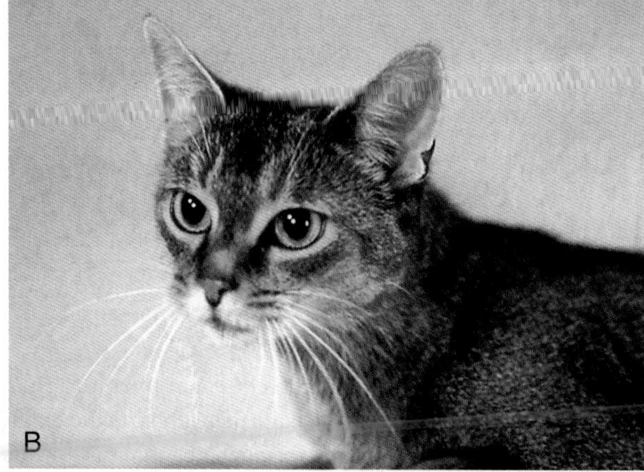

Fig. 11.38 (A) Slit form of constricted feline pupil. (B) Round form of dilated feline pupil.

The features of the auricular cartilage provide important surgical landmarks known as the *helix, antihelix, tragus, antitragus,* and *scapha* (see Fig. 11.41). The tragus, separated from the more caudal antitragus by the intertragic

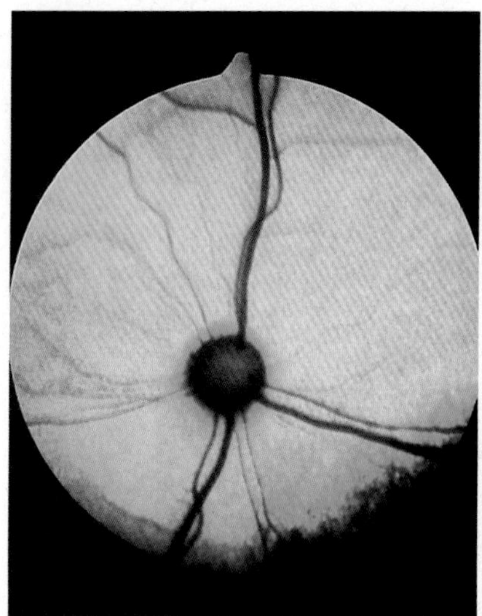

Fig. 11.39 Fundus of eye in a cat.

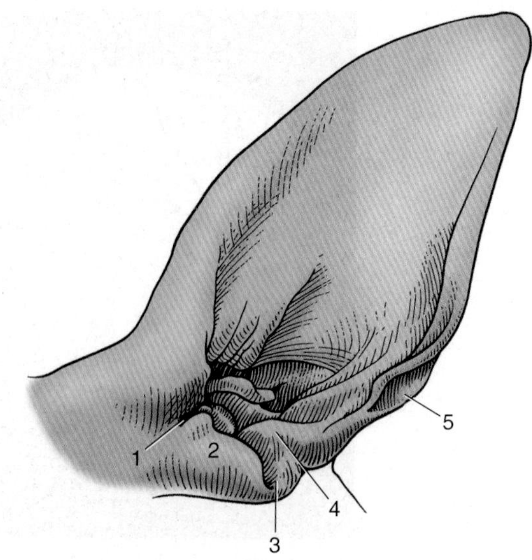

Fig. 11.41 Left canine ear, shaved. *1,* Pretragic notch; *2,* tragus; *3,* intertragic notch; *4,* antitragus; *5,* cutaneous pouch.

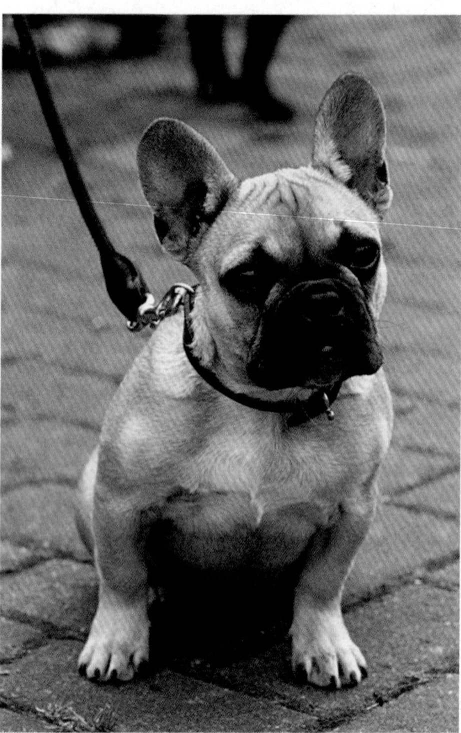

Fig. 11.40 Erect posture of the external ears.

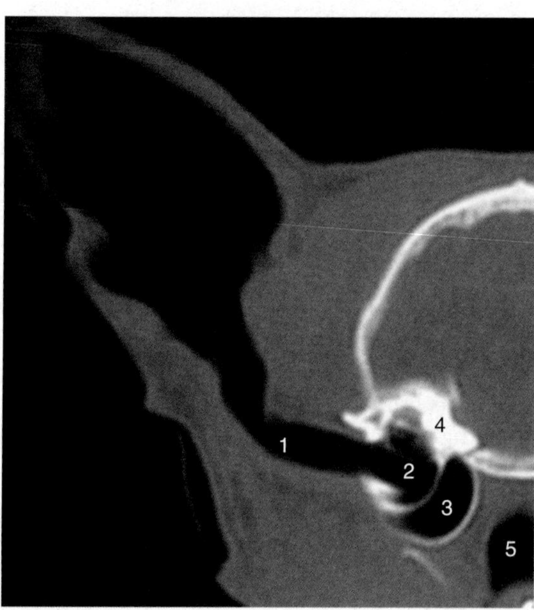

Fig. 11.42 Transverse computed tomography scan (bone window) of half of a feline head showing ear canal and middle ear. *1,* Ear canal; *2,* tympanic cavity; *3,* tympanic bulla; *4,* petrous temporal bone; *5,* nasopharynx.

notch, forms the lateral rim of the ear canal opening. Both consist of rolled-up articular cartilage that supports the external ear opening. The antitragus forms the caudal part of the ear opening and ascends toward the end of the lateral side.

The proximal part of the auricular cartilage is rolled to form a partial tube called the *concha,* which serves as the enlarged entry of the auditory canal. This first part of the canal connects to the short anular cartilage, which terminates in a short osseous external canal. The ear canal is first directed ventrally (auricular cartilage) before turning medially to form the horizontal canal (portion of the auricular and anular cartilages), which is surrounded and supported by the temporal bone. This course hampers passage of the straight otoscope for examination of the proximal part of the canal and the eardrum. The examiner must straighten the canal by pulling the ear first caudally and then ventrally as the otoscope is advanced (Fig. 11.42). The canal is about 7 cm long.

The horizontal ear canal ends at the eardrum. The tympanic membrane consists of an outer epithelial layer, which is a continuation of the skin of the external auditory canal,

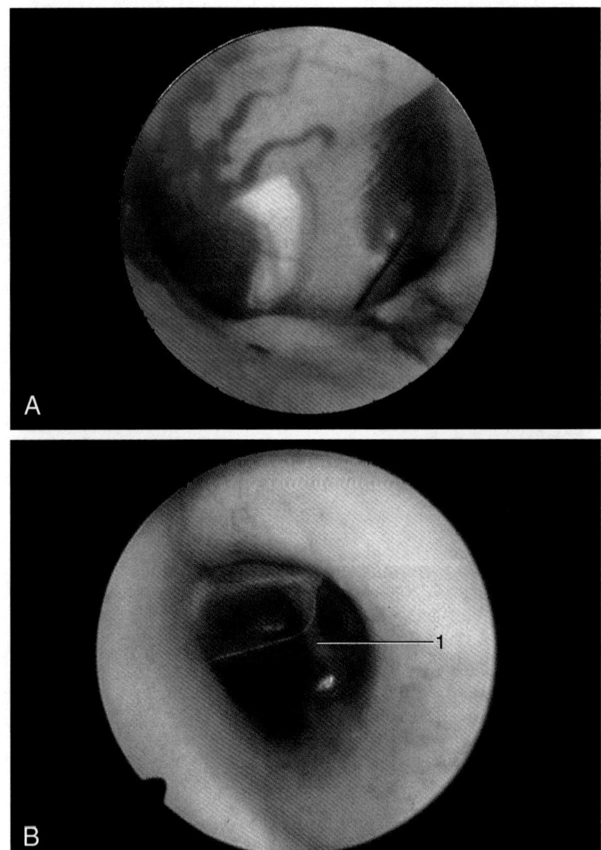

Fig. 11.43 (A) Otoscopic view of eardrum showing handle of malleus. (B) Otoscopic view of the eardrum (cat). *1*, Malleus.

an inner mucosal layer, and a fibrous layer in between. The tympanic membrane is thin, slightly oval, semitransparent, and concave owing to traction on its medial side by the tensor tympani muscle (Fig. 11.43). The tympanic membrane consists of a small upper portion, the pars flaccida, and a large lower portion, the pars tensa (thin, tough, and glistening). The outline of the manubrium of the malleus is clearly visible.

The auricular skin continues as the lining of the auditory canal. This skin is thin, and its lateral part possesses both ceruminous and sebaceous glands. It generally contains only a few hairs, but in some breeds (Poodles) hair is abundant. The skin of the bony part of the ear canal, which is much thinner than that of the cartilaginous portion, is continuous with the epithelial layer of the tympanic membrane. There are no glands or hair follicles here, where because of its thinness, the skin is more sensitive to trauma.

The base of the auricle and the ear canal are related laterally and ventrally to the parotid gland. The facial nerve crosses the ventral surface of the canal deep to the gland before breaking into the auriculopalpebral nerve and the two buccal branches. The former passes dorsally in front of the ear with the superficial temporal vessels. This stretch of the facial nerve also detaches a caudal auricular nerve and a branch to the middle ear. The sensory innervation is provided by the trigeminal, glossopharyngeal, vagus, and second cervical nerves. The innervation of the muscles of the external ear is by the facial nerve.

The veins of the area join the maxillary vein, which descends toward the mandibular gland from its formation by substantial caudal and cranial auricular and superficial temporal veins that may pass through the parotid gland (Fig. 11.44).

The arteries lie more deeply. The external carotid, having detached the caudal auricular artery to the convex surface of the auricle, ends rostroventral to the ear canal by dividing into maxillary and superficial temporal arteries. The latter, with the like-named vein, lies deep to the parotid gland close to the rostral surface of the ear canal.

The caudal auricular artery branches in the convex outer surface of the auricle and sends finer branches to the skin over the concave surface through small holes in the cartilage. Vigorous and repeated head shaking or scratching, in most instances elicited by parasites or infection of the ear canal, may injure the vessels and cause hematomas by rupture of the penetrating small branches. Because such a hematoma is lined by cartilage on both sides, splitting of the auricular cartilage also takes place. Once begun, the bleeding between the cartilages continues until the internal pressure equals the pressure in the feeder arteries.

Middle and Inner Ear

The middle and inner ears show few special features of importance. The auditory tubes are narrow and open on the dorsolateral wall of the nasopharynx, level with the landmark provided by the hamulus of the pterygoid bone, which is palpable through the mouth caudomedial to the last cheek tooth in the dog. The tympanic bullae are large, hemispherical, and, except for a serrated septum in their rostral halves, undivided (see Fig. 11.23).

In the cat, an incomplete bony septum bullae subdivides the middle ear into a small dorsolateral and a large ventromedial compartment. The two compartments communicate with each other through an opening at the caudodorsal margin of the septum near the cochlear window.

The middle ear infections (otitis media) may be drained into the nasopharynx through the bulla, which can be palpated through the oropharynx and soft palate, caudal to the hamulus. The inflated tympanic bulla of the cat is also easily found on palpation through the skin, between the wing of the atlas and the zygomatic arch.

The bulla can be approached surgically from the ventral side, with the use of the medial border of the rostral digastric muscle, the mylohyoid muscle, and the stylohyoid and tympanohyoid cartilages of the hyoid apparatus as landmarks; care should be taken to avoid damage to the nerves of the pharyngeal plexus (Fig. 11.44/*12*) and the vascular supply of the mandibular lymph node.

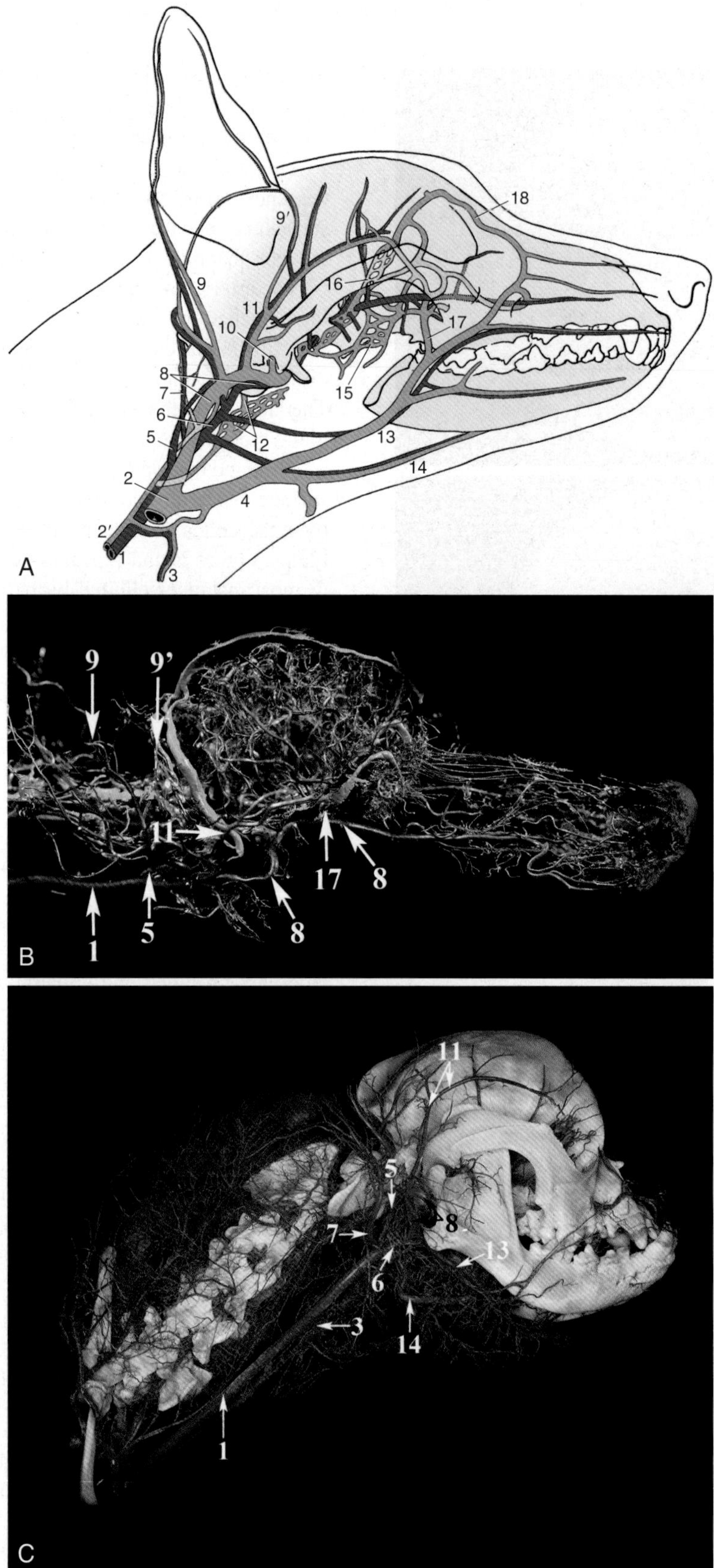

Fig. 11.44 The major arteries *(red)* and veins *(blue)* of the canine head. Schematic (A), corrosion cast without head (B) and with head (C). The ramus of the mandible has been removed. *1,* Common carotid; *2,* external jugular; *2′,* internal jugular; *3,* cranial thyroid; *4,* linguofacial; *5,* internal carotid; *6,* external carotid; *7,* occipital; *8,* maxillary; *9* and *9′,* caudal and rostral auricular; *10,* dorsal emissary; *11,* superficial temporal; *12,* ventral emissary and pharyngeal plexus; *13,* facial; *14,* lingual; *15,* pterygoid plexus; *16,* ophthalmic plexus; *17,* deep facial; *18,* angularis oculi.

Several nerves pass through the middle ear, but only two are of clinical significance. The facial nerve travels in the facial canal of the petrous temporal bone and detaches a branch, the chorda tympani, that enters the cavity of the middle ear.

Postganglionic fibers of the cranial cervical ganglion, located just behind the tympanic bulla, participate in a plexus within the middle ear. The resulting dysfunction is Horner syndrome, a complication of otitis media. The signs are miosis and retraction of the globe, which causes protrusion of the third eyelid, and narrowing of the palpebral fissure. The syndrome usually disappears spontaneously in about 3 months.

THE VENTRAL PART OF THE NECK

It is convenient to describe with the head the part of the neck that lies ventral to the vertebrae. The dorsal part of the neck is dealt with in the next chapter. The skin on the ventral surface of the neck is loose and in some breeds forms longitudinal folds. Subcutaneous fat tends to be concentrated caudally, especially in the depression dorsolateral to the manubrium.

The external jugular vein sinks into this depression after following a course along the lateral surface of the sternocephalic muscle (see Fig. 2.42). It does not lie in a distinct jugular groove as in the larger species. Although it is the principal vein draining the head, it is assisted by small vessels associated with the vertebrae (vertebral vein, internal vertebral plexus) and accompanying the common carotid artery (internal jugular vein) (see Figs. 11.44 and 11.46) that drain mainly the deeper structures. The external jugular vein is formed by tributaries embracing the mandibular gland; these vessels are easily raised by pressure on the jugular and provide an additional means of positively distinguishing the gland from the mandibular lymph nodes (see Fig. 11.6). The large diameter of the jugular vein makes it a convenient alternative to the cephalic when considerable amounts of bloods have to be collected. It is especially useful in the cat, in which the limb veins are naturally small.

Parts of the hyoid and larynx can be palpated immediately caudal to the angle of the mandible. The transverse basihyoid, the most rostral component, is flanked by the ceratohyoid bones, which project forward, and the thyrohyoids, which pass obliquely caudally. Two further prominences, easily identifiable in the midline, are the thyroid prominence and the cricoid cartilage.

THE CONTENTS OF THE VISCERAL SPACE

The visceral space of the neck is enclosed by four superficial and two deep muscles. The sternohyoid muscle ventral to the trachea extends from the manubrium to the basihyoid; it is loosely connected with its fellow in the midline. The sternothyroideus, also thin and straplike, lies lateral to the trachea, ending on the lateral surface of the thyroid cartilage. These are the only structures that intervene between the larynx and trachea and the skin in the cranial half of the neck (Fig. 11.45). They are covered by the sternocephalicus in the caudal half. This muscle consists of two parts, the sternomastoideus and the sterno-occipitalis, which diverge toward the head (Fig. 11.46). The dorsal sterno-occipitalis muscle ends on the back of the skull.

The brachiocephalicus also has two parts in the neck, the cleidomastoideus and the cleidocervicalis. The former passes deep to the sterno-occipitalis to a common insertion with the sternomastoideus on the mastoid process of the temporal bone. The latter sweeps over the lateral surface of the neck to meet its fellow in the dorsal midline (see Fig. 2.55/*2*). The sternocephalicus and brachiocephalicus are fused except caudally, where the separation allows the external jugular vein to become more superficial (see Fig. 11.46).

The deep muscles comprise the longus capitis, ventrolateral to the cervical vertebrae, and the longus colli, which is more medial (Fig. 11.45/*4* and 5). The fascia that covers these muscles ventrally detaches a superficial leaf that encloses the many structures in the visceral space: the esophagus, trachea, thyroid and parathyroid glands, common carotid arteries, vagosympathetic trunks, internal jugular veins, recurrent nerves, and tracheal lymph nodes (see Figs. 11.44 and 11.46). There is no cervical component of the thymus.

The *esophagus* first travels dorsally to the trachea and then takes a position to the left of the trachea from the middle of the neck to the thoracic inlet. This arrangement puts both the trachea and the esophagus in contact with the longus colli in the caudal half of the neck. The esophagus may be felt with the fingertips as a pliable tube sinistrodorsal to the trachea. Because the esophagus has limited ability to expand at the thoracic inlet, large pieces of meat, gristle, or bone may lodge at this location.

The *trachea* continues from the larynx, and its firmness makes it easy to palpate, including the flat dorsal surface between the incomplete tracheal rings. The cervical trachea, especially its caudal part, narrows slightly during inspiration only to recover during expiration. The changes in the thoracic trachea are reciprocal. The tracheal cartilages keep the trachea patent. The trachea may undergo severe narrowing with congenital or acquired degeneration of tracheal cartilages, which is most often observed at the cervicothoracic part. The brachycephalic breeds have relatively narrow tracheas, whereas Dachshunds and Basset Hounds have wide ones. Estimates of the normality of the tracheal diameter may be made by comparing it with the height of the thoracic inlet; in some breeds the ratio may be as high as 0.5, whereas in Bulldogs with very narrow trachea it may be as low as 0.05.

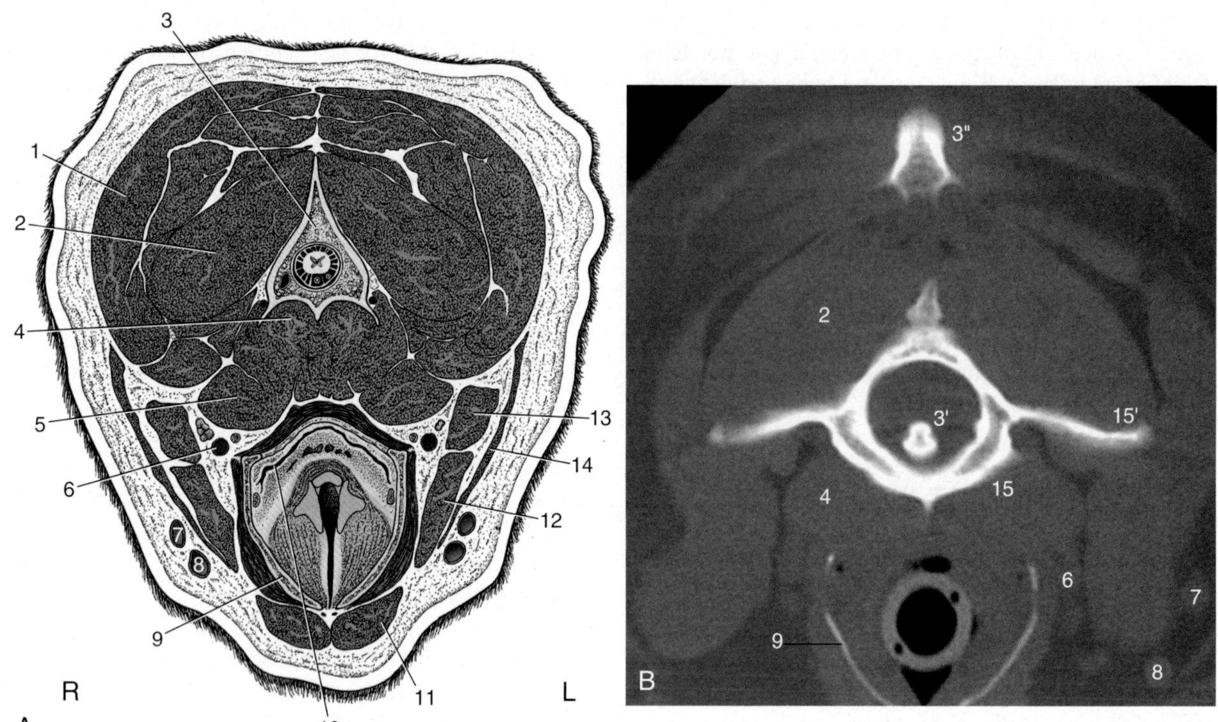

Fig. 11.45 (A) Transverse section of the canine neck at the level of the axis. (B) Corresponding computed tomography scan (bone window) slightly more cranial than (A). *1,* Splenius muscle (m.); *2,* obliquus capitis caudalis m.; *3,* axis; *3′,* dens of axis; 3″, cranial tip of spine of axis; *4,* longus colli m.; *5,* longus capitis m.; *6,* common carotid artery, vagosympathetic trunk, and medial retropharyngeal lymph node; *7,* maxillary vein; *8,* linguofacial vein; *9,* thyroid cartilage (calcified); *10,* laryngopharynx, leading into esophagus; *11,* sternohyoideus m.; *12,* sternomastoideus m.; *13,* cleidomastoideus m.; *14,* sterno-occipitalis m.; *15,* atlas; 15′, wing of atlas; *L,* left; *R,* right.

The trachea is loosely enclosed in a sleeve of fascia. A deeper leaf forms part of the prevertebral fascia that separates the trachea from the longus colli muscle. It also contributes to the carotid sheath, which encloses the vagus and sympathetic nerves, carotid artery, internal jugular vein, and sometimes the tracheal lymph trunk. The carotid sheath is found dorsolateral to the trachea. The recurrent laryngeal nerve follows a similar but independent course.

Each tracheal ring is thickest ventrally and thins along the curves to end dorsally as flexible, potentially overlapping blades. Only the first ring is completely closed in dogs, and it is partially covered by the cricoid cartilage. The dorsal part of the trachea is composed of connective tissue and muscle. In carnivores, this smooth muscle inserts on the external surface of the cartilages some distance from their tips.

The *thyroid gland* consists of two elongated rather flattened lobes placed against and loosely attached to the lateral aspects of the first few tracheal cartilages under cover of the sternothyroid muscle (see Fig. 6.4A). Their caudal poles are sometimes connected across the ventral surface of the trachea by a vestigial isthmus. The two glands are embedded in the deep cervical fascia. The sternocephalicus and sternohyoideus muscles pass immediately lateral to the convex surface of each gland. The recurrent laryngeal nerve passes dorsally. In medium-sized dogs the lobes are about 5 cm long (spanning the first five to eight tracheal rings) and 1.5 cm wide. In immature dogs and brachycephalic breeds, they are larger. In cats each thyroid gland lobe is about 2 cm long and 0.3 cm wide. During development islets of the rapidly proliferating cells of the thyroid primordium separate from the main mass and become incorporated in the developing structures of the branchial arch region and thorax—the reason that some accessory thyroid tissue can be found along the trachea at the thoracic inlet, thoracic portion of the aorta, and within the mediastinum.

The major blood supply to each lobe is provided by a cranial thyroid artery (branching from the common carotid artery). Its thyroid branches include one that follows the dorsal margin caudally to an anastomosis with the much smaller and inconsistent caudal thyroid artery (branching from the brachiocephalic artery), one that follows the ventral margin, and others that pass directly to the cranial pole (and to the external parotid gland). Twigs from all these

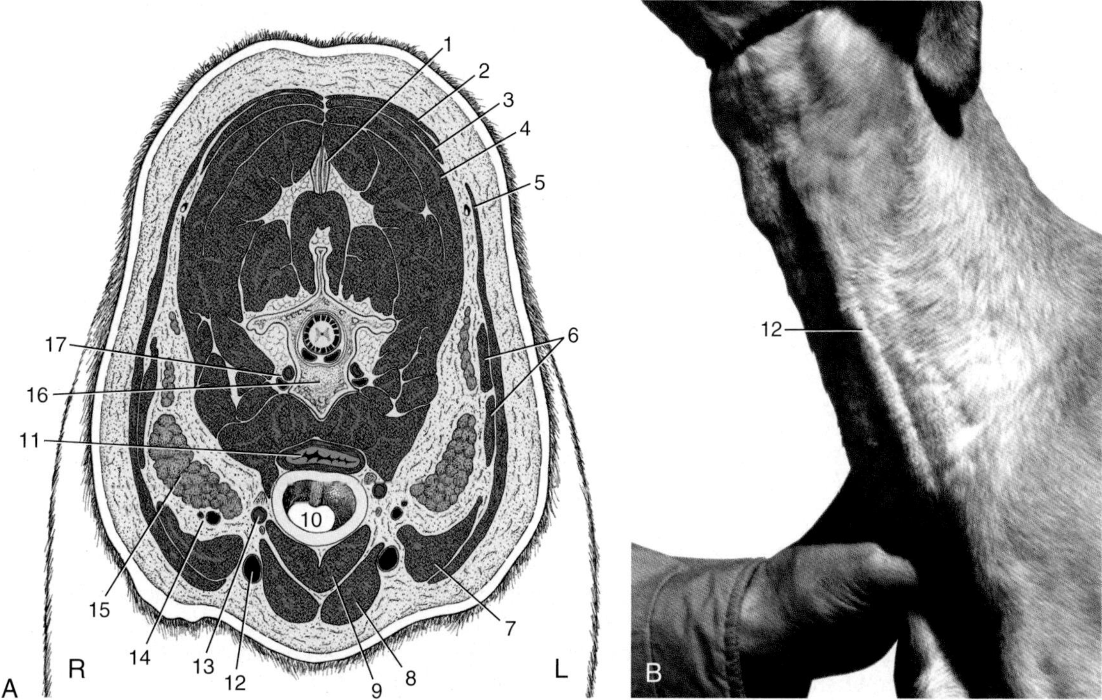

Fig. 11.46 (A) Transverse section of the canine neck at the level of the fifth cervical vertebra. (B) Left external jugular vein raised by thumb pressure at the base of the neck. *1,* Nuchal ligament; *2,* trapezius muscle (m.); *3,* rhomboideus m.; *4,* splenius m.; *5,* cleidocervicalis m.; *6,* omotransversarius m.; *7,* cleidomastoideus m.; *8,* sternocephalicus m.; *9,* sternothyrohyoideus m.; *10,* trachea; *11,* esophagus; *12,* external jugular vein; *13,* common carotid artery, vagosympathetic trunk, and recurrent laryngeal nerve; *14,* superficial cervical vessels; *15,* superficial cervical lymph nodes; *16,* fifth cervical vertebra; *17,* vertebral vessels.

vessels enable the thyroid to be supplied at scattered points around most of its periphery. Blood leaving the gland enters the nearby internal jugular vein, whereas some is conveyed to the large veins at the thoracic inlet by an unpaired (caudal thyroid) vein lying on the ventral surface of the trachea.

Each lobe is closely associated with two *parathyroid glands* (discounting the possible existence of accessory parathyroid tissue) in a relationship of obvious relevance to the performance of thyroid surgery. The external parathyroid gland is generally found close to or against the cranial pole of the thyroid to which it is loosely joined; in cats more often than in dogs, this gland descends unusually far from its site of origin (p. 211) and comes to rest near the caudal pole. The internal parathyroid is located within the connective tissue capsule of the thyroid and may be difficult to discover, especially when completely submerged within thyroid glandular tissue. Recognition is assisted by its pale color, which contrasts with the brownish red thyroid tissue, and can be identified by ultrasound imaging. Although variable, the parathyroid glands on average are about 3 mm in dogs. Partial or complete thyroidectomy may be performed in the treatment of thyroid hyperplasia or neoplasia, the former condition now recognized as occurring with great frequency in cats. The more or less inevitable loss of part of parathyroid tissue during intracapsular thyroidectomy is generally tolerated provided that blood supply to the remaining part is preserved.

The common carotid artery runs dorsolateral to the trachea (though the left one is commonly displaced to the side of the esophagus in the caudal half of the neck). Following its origin from the brachiocephalic trunk about 1 cm apart (sometimes a bicarotid trunk is formed) within the chest, it crosses the lateral surface of the trachea (esophagus on the left) obliquely to gain a dorsolateral position in the neck. After giving off the cranial thyroid artery, the only cervical branch of consequence, the common artery ends at the level of the atlanto-occipital joint by dividing into internal and external carotid arteries. The former enters the skull through the carotid foramen after pursuing a rather unusual course (p. 298).

The internal carotid artery (much smaller than the external one) leaves the medial side of the parent vessel and almost at once displays the bulbous enlargement known as the *carotid sinus* (see Fig. 7.33). It makes its way between deep structures of the head, crossing the lateral surface of the pharynx without detaching any branches, and enters

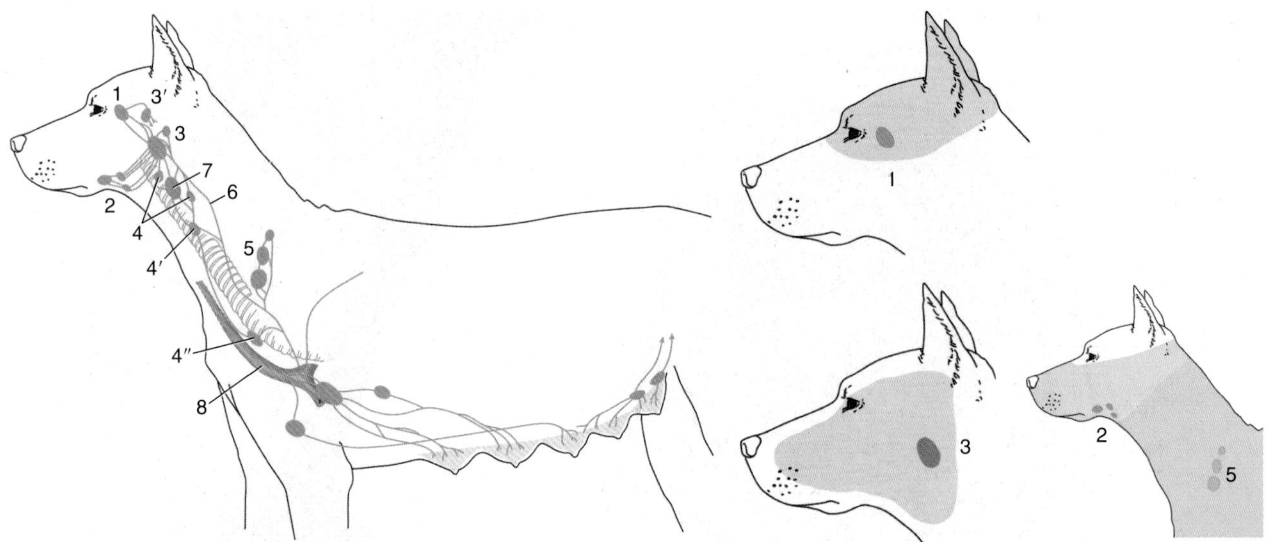

Fig. 11.47 Lymphatic structures of the canine head and neck. The inset shows the approximate areas of drainage of the principal nodes. *1,* Parotid lymph node; *2,* mandibular lymph nodes; *3* and *3′,* medial and lateral retropharyngeal lymph nodes; *4, 4′,* and *4″,* cranial, middle, and caudal deep cervical lymph nodes; *5,* superficial cervical lymph nodes; *6,* tracheal lymph trunk; *7,* thyroid gland; *8,* external jugular vein.

rostral to the tympanic bulla in the skull to supply the brain. Because the internal carotid artery is regressed in the adult cat, the branches of the maxillary artery are main suppliers to the brain.

The external carotid artery forms a sigmoid flexure as it winds its way under the hypoglossal nerve, submandibular salivary gland, and digastric muscle. Its many branches include the occipital, cranial laryngeal, ascending pharyngeal, lingual, facial, caudal auricular, parotid, superficial temporal, and maxillary arteries (see Fig. 7.40). The occipital artery sometimes arises independently from the common carotid.

The internal jugular vein is formed by the confluence of the vertebral vein, the sigmoid sinus, and, occasionally, the vein of the hypoglossal canal. The internal jugular is first associated with the internal carotid artery in the sheath of the common carotid. This vein usually terminates in the caudal part of the external jugular vein, which is the main channel for venous return from the head. It arises from the union of the linguofacial and maxillary veins. In the adult it contains a few ineffective, irregularly spaced valves.

THE LYMPHATIC STRUCTURES OF THE HEAD AND NECK

Except for the unimportant facial node, the lymph nodes of the head are concentrated caudal to the mandible; those of the neck are found at shoulder level and, inconstantly, scattered along the trachea (Fig. 11.47).

Parotid Lymph Node

The parotid lymph node lies on the caudal border of the masseter cranial to the base of the ear, under the rostrodorsal border of the parotid gland. It drains superficial structures such as, broadly, those dorsal to the palate and the ear, including the eyelids and associated glands and the temporomandibular joint. Its efferents drain to the medial retropharyngeal lymph node. The parotid lymph node is not always palpable.

Mandibular Lymph Node

Two or three mandibular lymph nodes are grouped around the facial vein near the angle of the mandible. They drain superficial structures of the face and also the intermandibular space. There is overlap with the region drained by the parotid and the mandibular nodes. Their efferents drain to the medial retropharyngeal lymph node. They are always palpable (Fig. 11.6/*10*).

Medial Retropharyngeal Lymph Node

The large medial retropharyngeal lymph node lies medial to the mandibular gland and sternomastoideus muscle, between the wing of the atlas and the larynx. Coursing along its medial surface is the terminal portion of the common carotid artery, as well as the hypoglossal, vagus, and sympathetic nerves and the internal jugular vein. This node drains deep structures of the head, including the tongue, palatine tonsil, salivary glands, and deep parts of the external ear, and also receives lymph from the other nodes in the head. It also receives afferents from the larynx and esophagus in the upper part of the neck. Its efferents form the tracheal lymph trunk. It cannot be palpated (Fig. 11.47/*3*).

Lateral Retropharyngeal Lymph Node

The lateral retropharyngeal lymph node is located at the caudal border of the parotid and mandibular glands, when present. It drains deep structures dorsal to it and may be palpated.

Tracheal Trunk

The tracheal trunk arises from the caudal pole of the ipsilateral medial retropharyngeal lymph node and runs in or adjacent to the lateral wall of the carotid sheath. The left trunk usually terminates in the thoracic duct, and the right one terminates in the angle formed by the mergence of the right external jugular and the right axillary veins to form the brachiocephalic vein.

Deep Cervical Lymph Nodes

Small, deep cervical lymph nodes are occasionally found in the vicinity of the thyroid gland and the cervical portion of the trachea. They receive afferents from the larynx, thyroid glands, trachea, esophagus, and the cervical vertebrae. They send their efferents in the caudal direction to others in the chain and thence the thoracic duct, tracheal trunk, or cranial mediastinal lymph node. The cranial node of the group is located between the caudal end of the medial retropharyngeal lymph node and the thyroid gland, either dorsomedially to the gland along the carotid sheath or on the pharynx cranial to the thyroid. The middle node is positioned along the carotid sheath or ventral to the trachea, in the middle third of the neck. The caudal node lies on the ventral surface of the caudal third of the cervical trachea.

COMPREHENSION CHECK

Using cadavers and imaging modalities, develop a comprehensive understanding of the relationships of the structures in the ventral part of neck.

Develop a list of the structures that open in the oral cavity, and demonstrate an understanding of their anatomic location.

While enumerating the structures that form the orbit, describe the arrangement of the eye in the orbit along with its musculature, blood supply, and nerve supply.

12 The Neck, Back, and Vertebral Column of the Dog and Cat

The neck and back regions are of increasing clinical importance in the companion animals. This change is due to the better recognition of veterinary physiotherapy as a profession and to mounting evidence that lameness in dogs is frequently referable to back problems.

CONFORMATION AND SURFACE ANATOMY

The length and proportions of the neck vary with the breed; its transverse section, generally circular in smaller dogs, is somewhat compressed from side to side in larger breeds but widens toward the trunk, with which it blends smoothly. Only a few breeds show a significant elevation at the withers. In most the back slopes slightly downward toward the tail. German Shepherd dogs show a much larger slope and walk with strongly flexed stifles and hocks. In some breeds the back is level, and in a few (including the Greyhound) it rises toward the loins after dipping over the thorax. The carriage of the tail is variable. Some conformations are characteristic of certain breeds (e.g., the tightly coiled tail of the Spitz breeds). Dogs may stiffen the tail and hold it level or upright to denote aggressive intent or depress it to cover the anus in the cringing submissive attitude. The back of a sitting dog is almost straight.

Surprisingly little of the vertebral column is palpable, even in moderately lean subjects. The external occipital protuberance is a distinct landmark at the cranial end of the neck, and behind it the wings of the atlas and the spinous process of the axis are easily distinguished, confirming the position of these two vertebrae close to the dorsal surface. The remaining cervical vertebrae are more deeply placed, and it is sometimes only with difficulty—if at all—that their transverse and spinous processes can be appreciated. Only the tips of the spinous processes can be palpated with certainty in the remainder of the column until the tail is reached. The dorsal parts of the scapulae and the iliac crests provide certain landmarks in the regions of the withers and hindquarters.

In cats the dorsal borders of the scapulae are very prominent and bound a hollow over the adjacent part of the vertebral column. Cats in stalking portion lower the trunk between the forelimbs and show pronounced scapular ridges. Cats also vary in the conformation of the neck, trunk, and tail. Many shorthair cats can be described as *cobby,* an adjective suggesting a short, thick neck and a thick, deep, and fairly short trunk that is carried rather close to the ground. Cats of Oriental breeds are more slender and have a longer and narrower trunk raised from the ground on limbs that are proportionally longer, especially behind. The slinky, svelte appearance is accentuated by the longer tail and smooth flat coat. When a cat sits, its back is arched. The neutral carriage of the tail is slightly drooping, but changes from this posture are frequent and revealing to observers of cat behavior. Domestic cats, uniquely and as a behavioral trait acquired in domestication, often carry the tail upright when they are apparently content and at ease. The tucked-under position of the tail of the fearful cat crouching in submission and the side-to-side lashing of the cat in a pugnacious mood or merely irritated by unwanted attention are universally familiar.

THE VERTEBRAL COLUMN (SEE ALSO PP. 31–36)

The dog has 7 cervical, 13 thoracic, 7 lumbar, 3 sacral, and about 20 caudal vertebrae as a rule (Fig. 12.1); the most common variation is the reduction to 6 lumbar vertebrae. The precaudal vertebrae formula is the same in cats, in which the individual bones are generally more slender and differ from those of the dog in subtle ways that are easy to recognize but difficult to define (Fig. 12.2).

The *intervertebral disks* of both dog and cat are relatively thicker than in most species and contribute some 15% and 17% to 20%, respectively, of the total length of the column. Longitudinal growth of the column continues until approximately 12 months of age, when the epiphyses fuse with the bodies of the vertebrae—except in the sacral region, where there is some delay. Table 12.1 records the ages at which the secondary ossification centers of the vertebrae appear and those at which they later fuse.

The contours of the vertebral column do not reproduce the dorsal profile of the standing animal. The convex nape is followed by a relatively straight cervical section. A pronounced but concealed change in direction at the cervicothoracic junction redirects the column on an ascending course in relation to the contour of the back. The caudal thoracic and lumbar segments are fairly straight (depending on the breed), but over the pelvis the column curves ventrally into the tail.

The caudal end of the cervical segment is the most flexible part, and this flexibility enables the dog to reach almost every part of its trunk and limbs with its mouth. Ventral flexion to lower the head to the ground is mainly

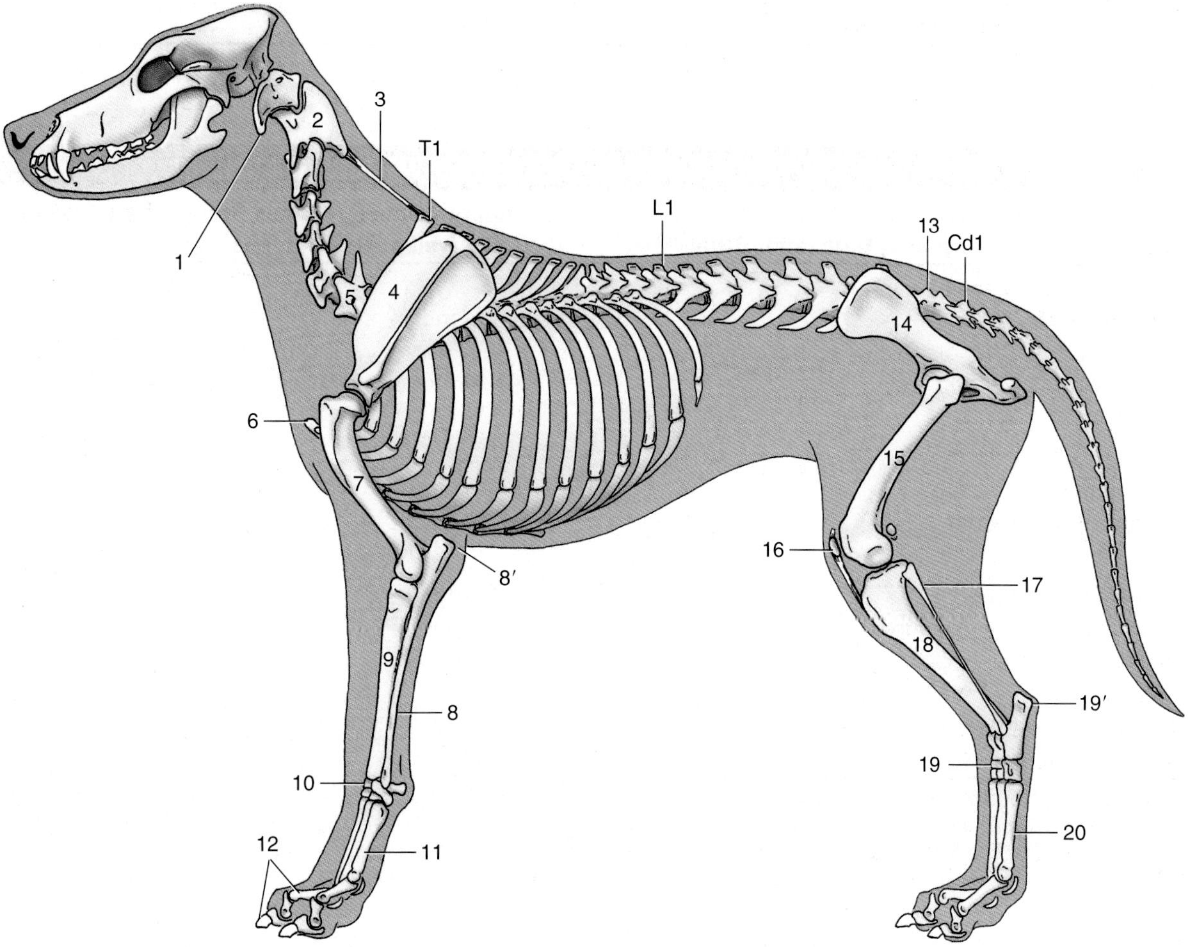

Fig. 12.1 The skeleton of the dog. *1,* Wing of atlas, first cervical vertebra (C1); *2,* spine of axis (C2); *3,* ligamentum nuchae; *4,* scapula; *5,* last cervical vertebra (C7); *6,* cranial end (manubrium) of sternum; *7,* humerus; *8,* ulna; *8′,* olecranon; *9,* radius; *10,* carpal bones; *11,* metacarpal bones; *12,* proximal, middle, and distal phalanges; *13,* sacrum; *14,* hip bone (os coxae); *15,* femur; *16,* patella; *17,* fibula; *18,* tibia; *19,* tarsal bones; *19′,* calcanean tuber; *20,* metatarsal bones; *T1, L1,* and *Cd1,* first thoracic, lumbar, and caudal (tail) vertebrae.

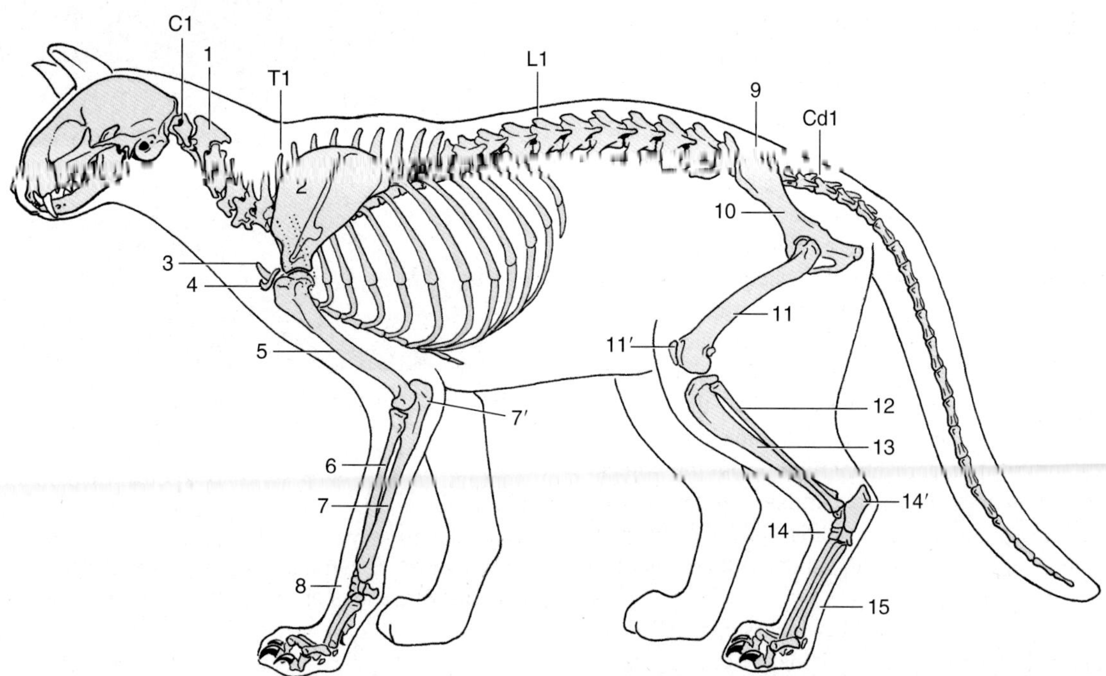

Fig. 12.2 The feline skeleton. *1,* Axis (C2); *2,* scapula; *3,* manubrium of sternum; *4,* clavicle; *5,* humerus; *6,* radius; *7,* ulna; *7′,* olecranon; *8,* carpal bones; *9,* sacrum; *10,* hip bone (os coxae); *11,* femur; *11′,* patella; *12,* fibula; *13,* tibia; *14,* tarsal bones; *14′,* calcaneus; *15,* metatarsal bones; *C1, T1, L1,* and *Cd1,* first cervical, thoracic, lumbar, and caudal (tail) vertebrae.

TABLE 12.1 DEVELOPMENT AND MATURATION OF THE CANINE[a] VERTEBRAL COLUMN

Ossification Centers Present at Birth (after Birth)	Approximate Age When Growth Plate Closure Observed on Radiographs
Vertebrae, except C1 and C2	
Cranial epiphysis (2–8 wk)	7–14 mo[b]
Body	
Caudal epiphysis (2–8 wk)	7–14 mo[b]
Two sides of arch	
Atlas	
Ventral arch	
Two sides of dorsal arch	4 mo[c]
Axis	
Apex of dens (3–4 mo)	3–4 mo[c]
Dens and cranial articular surface	7–9 mo[c]
Intercentrum (3 wk)	4 mo[c]
Body	
Caudal epiphysis (3 wk)	7–9 mo[c]
Two sides of arch	3 mo[c]

[a]Similar information for the cat appears to be lacking.
[b]Based on Hare WCD: Zur Ossifikation und Vereinigung der Wirbelepiphysen beim Hund, *Wien Tierärztl Monatsschr* 48:210–215, 1961.
[c]Based on Hare WCD: *Radiographic anatomy of the cervical region of the canine vertebral column,* JAVMA 139:209–220, 1961.
From de Lahunta, A and Habel RE: *Applied veterinary anatomy,* Philadelphia, 1986, Saunders.

the result of movement in the cranial thoracic joints, and the cervical vertebrae are merely brought into line. Considerable mobility of the caudal thoracic and lumbar joints is necessary for the alternating sagittal flexion and extension of the back in the bounding gallop used by both cats and dogs when moving at speed. The hindlimbs can be placed alongside (if not ahead of) the forelimbs, after which the hindlimb joints and the joints of the column extend to hurl the body forward. Lateral flexion of the joints of the thoracic and lumbar segments is surprisingly free and enables dogs to curl up when sleeping. The spine of the cat is even more supple.

At three locations in the vertebral column the dorsal parts of the vertebral arches are less closely connected and leave relatively wide interarcuate spaces: the atlanto-occipital space between the occipital bone and the first vertebra, the atlantoaxial space between the first and second vertebrae, and the lumbosacral space between the last lumbar vertebra and the sacrum. These interarcuate spaces are of clinical importance because they can be used to allow entry to the vertebral canal for injections or to obtain samples of cerebrospinal fluid. From the clinical point of view it is important to be familiar with the appearance of the vertebral column in radiographs of both juvenile and mature animals, especially at these three junctions (Figs. 12.3, 12.4, and 12.5).

Because of the frequency with which spinal problems are encountered in clinical practice, it may be useful to recapitulate and amplify the descriptions given in Chapter 2.

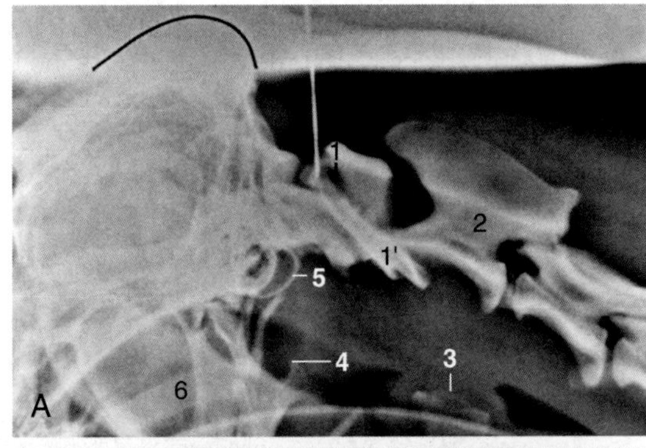

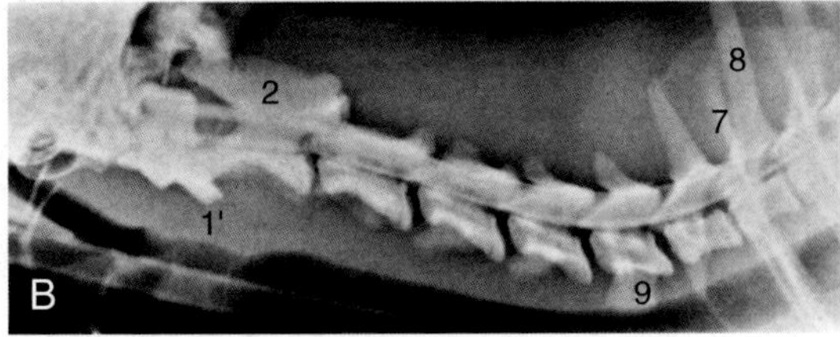

Fig. 12.3 (A) Lateral radiograph of the head–neck junction of an intubated dog. Note the needle placed in the atlanto-occipital space for a cerebrospinal fluid tap. The dorsal contour of the skull is marked. (B) Myelogram of an intubated dog. *1,* Lateral vertebral foramen of atlas; *1′,* wing of atlas; *2,* axis; *3,* cricoid cartilage; *4,* angular process of mandible; *5,* tympanic bulla; *6,* soft palate; *7,* spine of scapula; *8,* spinous process of T1; *9,* ventral tubercle of C6.

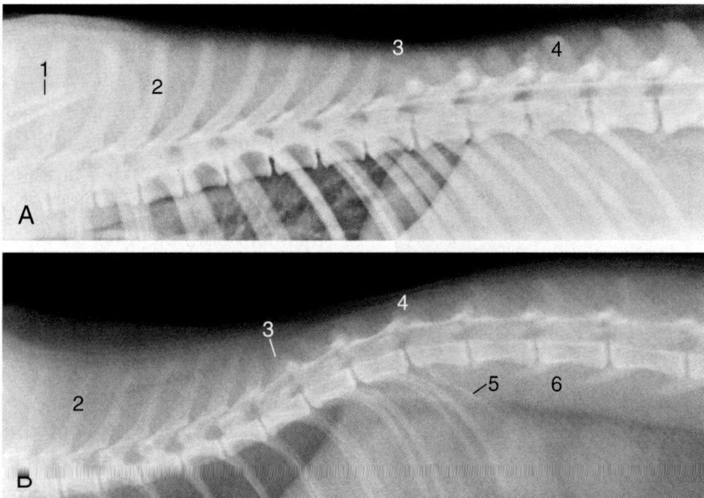

Fig. 12.4 Lateral radiographs of (A) canine and (B) feline thoracic and lumbar vertebrae. Radiograph (A) was obtained after the injection of a contrast agent into the subarachnoid space. *1,* Scapular spines; *2,* spinous process of T5; *3,* anticlinal vertebra (T11); *4,* spinous process of L1; *5,* rudimentary rib; *6,* sublumbar muscles.

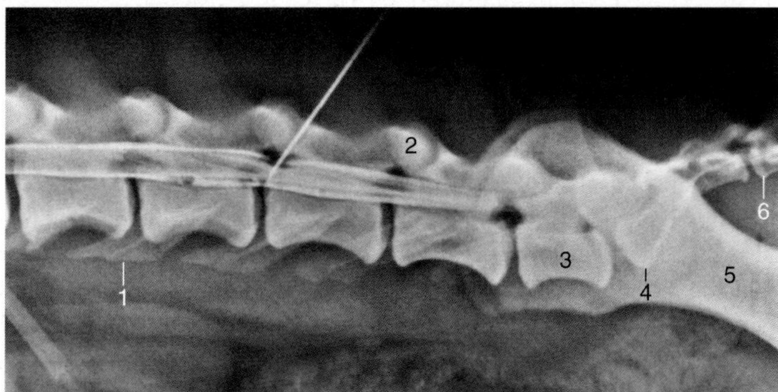

Fig. 12.5 Lateral radiograph of the lumbar area of a dog undergoing a myelogram. A needle is in the interarcuate space between L4 and L5. *1,* Transverse processes of L4; *2,* articular processes; *3,* last lumbar vertebra (L7); *4,* promontory (of sacrum); *5,* shaft of ilium; *6,* first tail vertebra (Cd1).

Atlas

The ventral arch of the atlas is considerably narrower (craniocaudally) than the dorsal arch. The lateral vertebral foramen for the first cervical nerve is close to the cranial border of the dorsal arch; a notch in the cranial border of the wing replaces the alar foramen of other species and transmits the ventral branch of the same nerve. The wings, extended transverse processes, slope caudally and overlap the atlantoaxial junction. The base of the wing is perforated by the transverse foramen (see Fig. 2.7A).

The dorsal and ventral arches of the atlas participate in the deep cranial articular foveae, which receive the occipital condyles. The single joint cavity has a U shape with its dorsal parts widely spaced and only narrowly joined ventrally. The atlanto-occipital membrane extends from the dorsal border of the foramen magnum to the dorsal arch of the atlas, and by attaching laterally to the joint capsules, it closes the atlanto-occipital aperture. This membrane is punctured in the collection of cerebrospinal fluid and in the injection of radiopaque contrast agent into the subarachnoid space (Figs. 12.3 and 12.6).

Axis

The axis is characterized by its length and its enormous spinous process, which overhangs both the dorsal arch of the atlas and the laminae of the third vertebra and carries the caudal articular processes. The cranial extent of the spinous process matches that of the dens, which rests on the dorsal surface of the ventral arch of the atlas (see Figs. 2.7 and 2.8). The dens, the displaced body of the atlas, is the pivot around which the atlas and thus the head rotates. The atlantoaxial

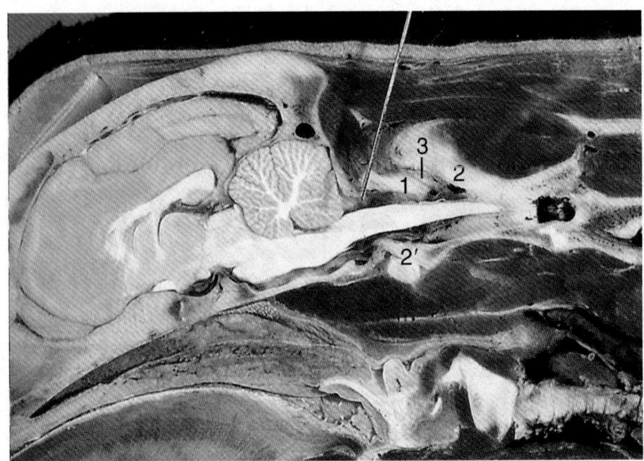

Fig. 12.6 Median section of head and neck (dog); the needle penetrates the atlanto-occipital membrane to enter the subarachnoid cerebellomedullary cistern. *1,* Dorsal arch of atlas; *2,* spinous process of axis; *2′,* dens; *3,* dorsal atlantoaxial ligament.

joint is enclosed by a single joint capsule. The two bones are held in apposition by a thin median ligament (ligamentum apicis dentis), which connects the tip of the dens with the ventral border of the foramen magnum (see Fig. 2.13), and paired (alar) ligaments, which pass obliquely from the dens to the ventrolateral borders of the foramen. The dens is further secured by a transverse ligament connecting the inner walls of the ventral arch of the atlas across its dorsal surface. This transverse ligament allows rotations but prevents impingement of the dens on the spinal cord. The dens plays an important role in stability of the atlantoaxial joint, and aberrant development of the growth plate (early fusion, partial fusion, or nonfusion), seen in miniature breeds (Chihuahua, Toy Pomeranian, Pekingese, and Toy Poodle), leads to instability.

The atlantoaxial membrane closes the interarcuate space; its median part is thickened by elastic fibers that connect the cranial tip of the spine of the axis with the tubercle on the dorsal arch of the atlas (dorsal atlantoaxial ligament) (Fig. 12.6/*3*).

Third to Seventh Cervical Vertebrae

The spinous processes of the remaining cervical vertebrae increase in height and in cranial inclination. The ventral crests are most prominent at the caudal ends of the bodies, marking the positions of the intervertebral disks directly caudal to them. The transverse processes have distinct cranial and caudal extensions (ventral and dorsal tubercles). The ventral tubercle of the sixth vertebra is a nearly sagittal plate that projects considerably below the contour of the body (Fig. 12.3/*9*). The transverse process of the seventh is a rodlike lateral projection that does not overlap the body ventrally. The caudal extremity of that body bears an articular fovea for the head of the first rib. The flat articular surfaces of the synovial joints are nearly horizontal. The cranial articular processes, which provide the ventral component of these joints, narrow the large intervertebral foramina from above.

The wide joint spaces of the atlanto-occipital and the atlantoaxial joints support relatively free vertical and rotational movements. The nuchal ligament extends from the spinous process of the axis to the tip of the first thoracic spinous process; it is then continued by the supraspinous ligament until the third sacral vertebra. The nuchal ligament plays an important role in the support of the head of the dog and must be spared during surgery (see Fig 2.8/*3*). The ligament is not present in cats, but they do possess a supraspinous ligament.

Disorders of the cervical vertebral column, producing compression of the spinal cord, occur in large dogs, especially the Great Dane and the Doberman Pinscher. These disorders may involve deformation of the vertebral arch, malformation of articular facets, vertebral instability of C5–C6 or C6–C7, and dorsal displacement of the vertebral body.

Thoracic Vertebrae

The bodies of the thoracic vertebrae are relatively short but increase in length from the tenth caudally (see Fig. 12.4). The long spinous processes of the first half of the thoracic region are of about equal length. Those of the second half gradually decrease in height; their caudal inclination changes at the eleventh thoracic, the anticlinal vertebra. A more noteworthy change occurs in the orientation of the articular surfaces. On the first 10 (or so) thoracic vertebrae these surfaces lie roughly in a dorsal plane (like those of the cervical vertebrae); caudal to this they are nearly sagittal, and the cranial articular processes enclose the caudal ones (see Fig. 2.10). The articular spaces of the former joints are best depicted in lateral radiographs (Fig. 12.5), and those of the latter, in ventrodorsal radiographs. The more cranial thoracic vertebrae favor lateral movement of the column, whereas the more caudal bones favor sagittal flexion and extension. Other features of the canine and feline vertebrae are the presence of the mammillary and accessory processes. The mammillary processes are short dorsal projections of the transverse processes that first appear at the third thoracic vertebra and, from the eleventh, migrate dorsally to surmount the cranial articular processes. The accessory processes arise from the caudal border of the pedicle and are present from the midthoracic to the midlumbar region; they are confined to the last three thoracic vertebrae in cats (see Fig. 2.11/*1* and *2*).

Lumbar Vertebrae

The lumbar vertebrae continue several features of the thoracic vertebrae. Their bodies are about twice as long as those of the first thoracic vertebrae and are characterized by long transverse processes that sweep cranioventrally, overlapping the preceding vertebra (Fig. 12.7/*1*). The ventral deflection of these processes is even more pronounced in the cat. In comparison with the smaller interarcuate spaces of both lumbar

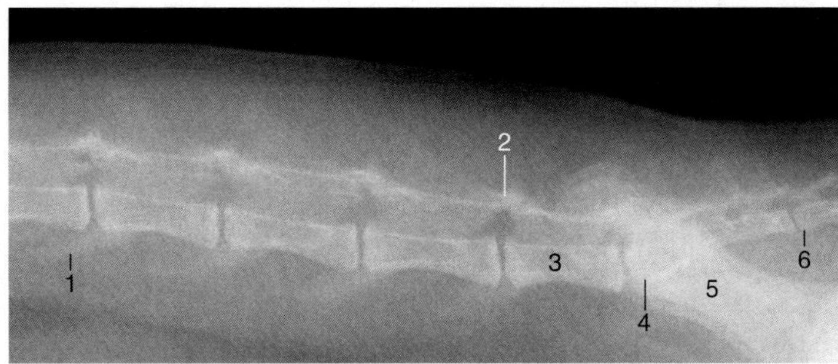

Fig. 12.7 Lateral radiograph of the lumbar region of a cat. *1,* Transverse processes of L4; *2,* articular processes; *3,* last lumbar vertebra (L7); *4,* promontory (of sacrum); *5,* shaft of ilium; *6,* first tail vertebra (CdI).

and thoracic segments, the space at the lumbosacral junction is much better suited to insertion of a needle to access the vertebral canal. It is about 1 cm in diameter (in medium-sized dogs) and lies in the transverse plane of the highest palpable points on the wings of the ilia but about 2 cm deeper. In the cat, the interarcuate space between the last two lumbar vertebrae is also wide enough to allow injection into the vertebral canal.

The mammillary processes are also fused with the cranial articular processes in the lumbar regions.

Sacral Vertebrae

Fusion of the three segments that constitute the sacrum may not be completed until 18 months after birth; fusion involves both the vertebrae and the ossified intervertebral disks. The sacrum is deeply embedded between the wings of the ilia so that only the spinous processes (sacral crest) are palpable through the skin; however, its caudoventral part and the first few (or more) caudal vertebrae can be palpated digitally per rectum. The first sacral vertebra forms a rigid joint with the wing of the ilium.

Caudal Vertebrae

Features of certain caudal vertebrae (usually the fourth to sixth) are the hemal arches, small V-shaped bones attached to the caudal ends of the ventral surfaces (see Fig. 2.12/9). Short hemal processes are found in similar positions on several more segments. They offer protection to the vessels on the ventral surface of the vertebra. Congenital anomalies of the cat tail include the distinctive Manx "bob" and the kinking formerly common in Siamese, which has been largely bred out of the modern breed.

Intervertebral Disks

Intervertebral disks are present in every intervertebral space except that between the first and second cervical vertebrae (p. 36). These disks are functionally important because of their contribution to the flexibility of the spine and to the distribution of pressure over the extremities of the vertebrae. Some degenerative changes occur normally with age, including the metaplastic changes of fibrous tissue, the calcification of the gelatinous nucleus, and, frequently, the separation of the fibrous lamellae of the anulus, the narrow dorsal part of the anulus being most vulnerable. When degeneration is severe, as occurs in particular dog breeds (see later), stretching or total rupture of the dorsal part of the annulus allows disk material to protrude into the vertebral canal, where it may put pressure (through the meninges) onto the spinal cord and nerves, resulting in various and often severe neurologic dysfunctions.

The dorsal longitudinal ligament is well developed in the cervical region, preventing dorsal herniation of disk material into the vertebral canal. In this region, the degenerating disk material protrudes dorsolaterally toward the roots of the spinal nerves, resulting in their compression. Approximately 15% of disk problems in dogs occur in the cervical region; the clinical signs are neck pain, spasms of shoulder muscles, and lameness due to pain referred to a forelimb. The presence of the intercapital ligaments (between the heads of a rib pair passing beneath the dorsal ligament) at the joints T1–T2 to T9–T10 offers almost complete protection against herniation to the greater part of the thoracic cord (see Fig. 2.18). Thoracolumbar lesions account for the remaining 85% of intervertebral disk problems (T11/12 to L1–L2). In the caudal thoracic and lumbar regions of the spine, where the dorsal longitudinal ligament is thinner, dorsal protrusions and consequent spinal cord compressions are more frequent.

Common radiographic findings in cases of disk herniation are narrowing or collapse of the intervertebral disk space, collapse of the synovial joints, narrowing of the intervertebral foramen, and calcified material within the vertebral canal. Misinterpretation of apparent narrowing of intervertebral disk spaces is easy if insufficient attention is paid to the geometry of image formation (p. 5). Furthermore, it should be emphasized that nuclear calcifications are often evident in radiographs of dogs that cause no signs of dysfunction or pain. The intervertebral disks of cats are not immune to degeneration, but for reasons that are obscure, affected animals very often fail to manifest any clinical signs.

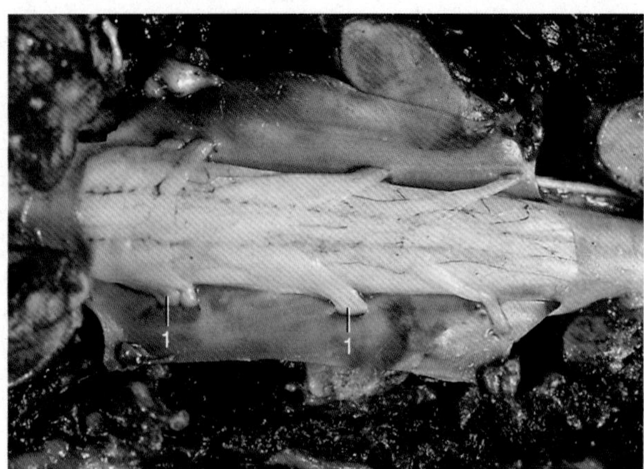

Fig. 12.8 Dorsal view of opened vertebral canal (cat). *1,* Spinal nerves penetrating arachnoid and dura mater.

There are both breed and regional differences in the incidence of disk pathology. Chondrodystrophic breeds, such as the Dachshund and Pekingese, in which the degenerative process is both precocious and accentuated, are particularly prone to protrusions at a relatively early age. In normal dogs, disk disease is characterized by slow fibroid degeneration, most evident between 8 and 10 years of age; mineralization of the disk is unusual. As a result of chronic degenerative disk disease (without clinical signs), spondylosis may develop. The sites most frequently involved are those undergoing the greatest mechanical stress. As a result of the stress, bony spurs are formed ventral and lateral to the intervertebral disk space, leading ultimately to complete fusion of vertebrae. On survey radiographs the presence of spondylosis is often regarded as an incidental finding.

The Vertebral Canal (see also pp. 295–298)

The diameter of the vertebral canal is greatest at the level of the first and second cervical vertebrae. It is reduced in width throughout the cervical spine, increases again in the cranial thoracic region, and becomes narrower in the caudal thoracic region. The diameter widens again in the lumbar region to accommodate the lumbar enlargement of the cord, before gradually narrowing into the tail.

Meninges: The spinal cord and nerve roots are surrounded by three meningeal layers: the tough outer fibrous dura mater, the thin arachnoid membrane lining the inner surface of the dura, and the pia mater, which is attached to the spinal cord. The dura mater adheres to the periosteum of the first two cervical vertebrae but separates thereafter (Fig. 12.8), leaving a relatively narrow epidural space that contains fat. The cerebrospinal fluid in the subarachnoid space and the epidural fat cushion the cord and allow displacement during normal movements of the spine.

The cord is the thickest in the atlas, where it measures about 1 cm. Elsewhere, except for the cervical and lumbar enlargements, it is approximately half that diameter. The cervical enlargement involves cord segments C6–T1, which contain motor neurons innervating muscles of the forelimbs and from which necessarily the nerves forming the brachial plexus arise. For the same reason, the lumbar enlargement, involving cord segments L5–S1, gives rise to the lumbosacral plexus. The craniocaudal positioning of the cord (p. 295) within the vertebral column explains the topography of its segments (Fig. 12.9). Most cervical spinal cord segments are positioned about half a vertebra, and most thoracic segments a whole vertebra, cranial to the vertebra of the same numerical designation. The caudal thoracic and cranial lumbar segments occupy vertebrae of the same designation. From the midlumbar region onward, the cord segments are markedly shorter, generally with the result that the end of the cord is positioned over the last interlumbar joint (Figs. 12.9 and 8.56B). The cervical and lumbosacral enlargements lie in the sixth and seventh cervical vertebrae and the fourth and fifth lumbar vertebrae, respectively. The relative cranial position of the lumbar spinal cord segments is less marked in small dogs, in which the cord may reach the sacrum; in large dogs it may end at L4. The sacral canal contains only spinal nerves and the dural sheath, which extends about 2 cm beyond the caudal termination of the spinal cord. The termination of the cord is said to be variable in cats: all levels from the caudal border of L7 to the caudal border of S3 have been given by different writers. Some of this uncertainty may be due to individual and breed variation, but probably the more cranial limit is likely to be nearer the mark in adults, the more caudal one in young kittens.

The *cauda equina* is the bundle of spinal nerves remaining in the vertebral canal after the termination of the spinal cord. It consists of the spinal nerves L6–Cd5 and includes those that form the sciatic (L6–S1) and pudendal (S2–S3) nerves. Each nerve exits the vertebral canal from its respective intervertebral foramen. Clinically, it may be trapped at the foramen by herniation of the adjacent disk. In the sacrum, the ventral branches of the first two sacral nerves emerge through foramina in the floor of the sacral canal. The "cauda equina syndrome," an important cause of neurologic dysfunction and pain, is a result of entrapment of one or more of the nerves of the cauda equina. The symptoms may include lower back pain, atrophy of muscles innervated by the sciatic nerve, paresis, tail weakness, incontinence of bladder and bowel, and paresthesias (abnormal sensation, possibly provoking self-mutilation). Entrapment may also be caused by bone pathology (e.g., osteochondrosis of the first sacral vertebra) or by secondary hypertrophy of the ligaments.

Puncture of the subarachnoid space is performed for the collection of cerebrospinal fluid and for the injection of contrast media for myelography. Myelograms are performed less often with the availability of more sophisticated imaging

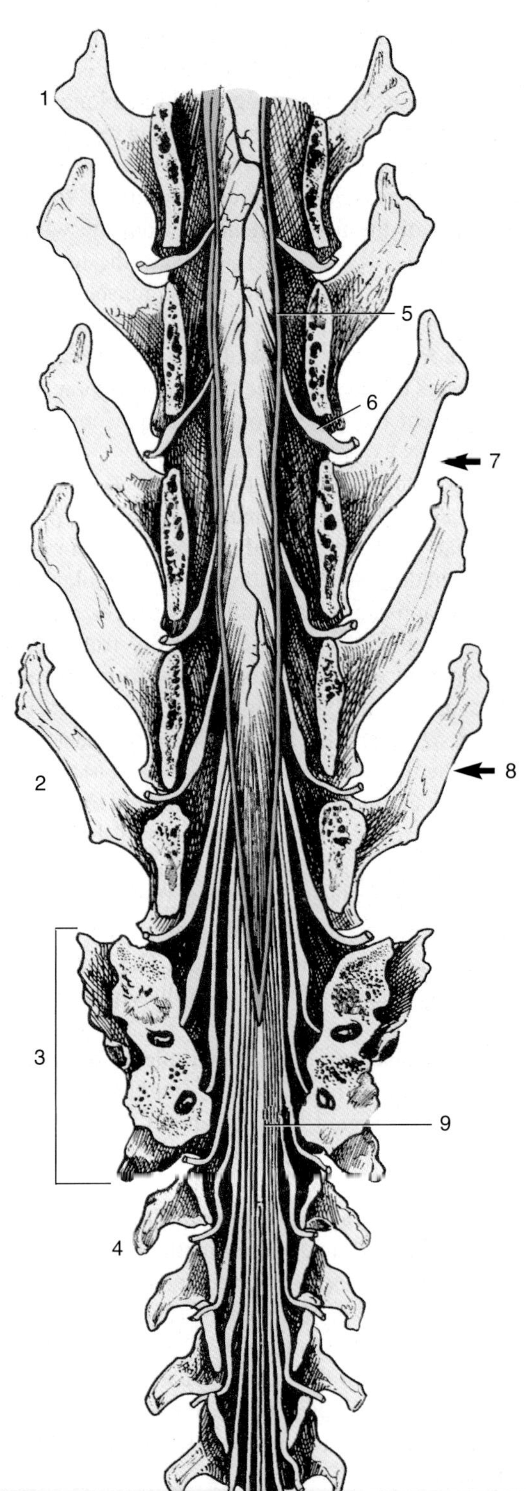

Fig. 12.9 Caudal end of the canine spinal cord in situ, dorsal view. *1,* Third lumbar vertebra; *2,* last lumbar vertebra (L7); *3,* sacrum; *4,* first caudal vertebra; *5,* dura mater; *6,* dorsal root ganglion; *7,* approximate level of L7 cord segment; *8,* end of spinal cord; *9,* cauda equina.

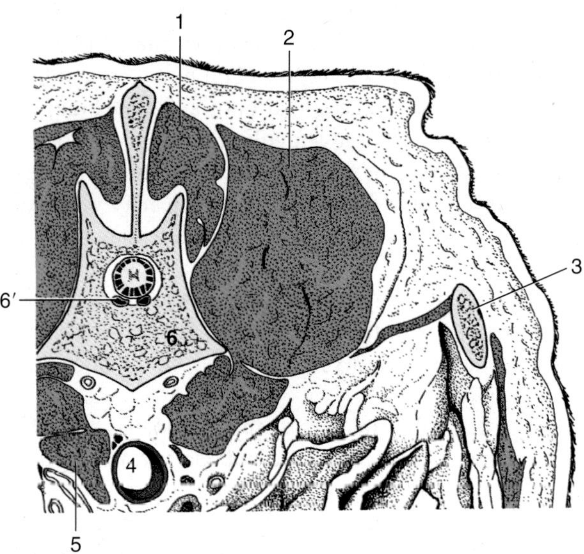

Fig. 12.10 Transverse section of the back of a dog at the level of the first lumbar vertebra. *1,* Multifidus and spinalis muscles (mm.); *2,* longissimus and iliocostalis mm.; *3,* last rib; *4,* aorta; *5,* right crus of diaphragm; *6,* first lumbar vertebra; *6′,* internal vertebral venous plexus.

modalities such as computed tomography and magnetic resonance imaging, but the principle is explained here. Contrast material outlines the subarachnoid space and may thus reveal cord lesions that are not apparent in survey radiographs; a myelogram is especially useful in revealing multiple lesions or when survey radiographs do not match the clinical signs. Recommended sites for puncture are the atlanto-occipital space and the lumbar spine at levels L4–L5 and L5–L6. Atlanto-occipital punctures enter the cerebromedullary cistern of the subarachnoid space (see Fig. 12.6). In this procedure, the neck is strongly ventro-flexed, and an entry is made midway between the external occipital protuberance and the cranial tip of the spinous process of the axis. These landmarks are more easily identified before flexion (Fig. 12.3A). The lumbar puncture (see Fig. 12.7) is also used. Surprisingly, accidental penetration of the spinal cord has minimal clinical effect although it provokes a histologic reaction.

Epidural anesthetics are administered at the lumbosacral or the sacrocaudal intervertebral space. The lumbosacral space is located a little in front of the cranial dorsal iliac spines (see Fig. 12.7). A misleading impression of its size may be obtained by failure to appreciate that a last lumbar spinous process is relatively short and does not approach as closely to the skin as that of the preceding vertebra. The sacrocaudal space is smaller, and the defining features of the vertebrae less obvious, but the space is much closer to the skin.

As in other species, the internal vertebral venous plexus consists of two longitudinal valveless veins on the floor of the vertebral canal, where they are embedded in epidural fat (Fig. 12.10/*6′*; p. 295). The left and right veins often anastomose at different levels; some connections pass below the dorsal longitudinal ligament, and others pass through the vertebral bodies. The plexus receives blood from the spinal cord and vertebrae; it is linked to extensive but less regular external networks and to adjacent great veins (caudal vena cava, azygos vein) by intervertebral veins. These veins, which may be double and triple, cushion the spinal nerves where they leave the vertebral canal.

At the foramen magnum the veins of the internal plexus are continuous with the right and left basilar sinuses that lead from the system of venous sinuses on the floor of the cranial cavity.

Like many other mammals, the dog makes use of its tail to maintain balance when executing various energetic maneuvers, but the tail is also used as a means of communication. Sometimes it is necessary to amputate part of the tail after an injury. A feature relevant to the operation includes the presence of the median caudal artery running below the vertebral bodies. The artery is partly shielded by processes of bone that take the form of separate V-shaped hemal bones located below the fourth to sixth tail vertebrae and hemal processes projecting from the ventral aspect of the more distal vertebral bodies. Obviously, amputation is simplest at the level of an intervertebral disk. It may be mentioned that these disks are not immune from the degenerative processes described earlier.

THE MUSCLES ASSOCIATED WITH THE VERTEBRAL COLUMN (SEE ALSO PP. 42–44)

The muscles directly associated with the neck and back mainly extend between points on the vertebrae (and ribs) (Fig. 12.11), but some also attach to the skull, the ilium, and, for the psoas group, the femur.

Only a superficial acquaintance with these muscles is required in order to appreciate their functional importance and the suitability of the expaxial division for receiving intramuscular injections. A much more detailed knowledge of the locations, construction, and attachments of the individual units is required for those who may contemplate surgery the vertebral column.

The descriptions that follow supply the basic information, which is most conveniently arranged under the following heads: the expaxial division; the hypaxial division, consisting of distinct cervical and lumbar groupings; and those muscles whose actions are confined to the movements of the head.

Epaxial Muscles

The *epaxial muscles* (see Fig. 2.22B) are used for intramuscular injections. Less commonly, they must be separated and detached when access to the vertebral column is necessary. The epaxial muscles comprise three longitudinal systems: iliocostalis, longissimus, and transversospinalis. The hypaxial muscles consist of the longus colli and longus capitis muscles in the cervical and cranial thoracic regions and the psoas muscle in the lumbar region.

The *splenius muscle* is a strong muscle on the dorsolateral aspect of the neck, extending from the withers to the occiput (see Fig. 2.23A/*4*). It covers the longissimus capitis muscle, the semispinalis capitis muscle, and parts of the spinalis et semispinalis cervicis et thoracis muscle. It originates from the spinocostotransverse fascia, the spinous processes of the first three thoracic vertebrae, and the nuchal ligament and inserts on the nuchal crest and the mastoid process.

The iliocostalis muscle is relatively thin (see Fig. 2.23B/*17*) and has only lumbar and thoracic parts. Its bundles span several vertebral segments and, in general, run from caudomedial and dorsal to craniolateral and ventral. The muscle is easily identified over the ribs by the glistening tendons. It arises caudally from the wing of the ilium and also by lumbar fascia from the spinous processes of the lumbar vertebrae. The *lumbar portion* reduces in size cranially and inserts on the last three to four ribs. The thoracic portion arises lateral to the lumbar part but without any sharp demarcation and extends from the twelfth rib to the transverse process of the last cervical vertebrae.

The iliocostalis is lateral to the longissimus system and is covered by the dorsal serratus and the origins of the latissimus and abdominal oblique muscles. The lumbar part of the iliocostalis muscle of the cat is hardly separate from the longissimus.

The *longissimus muscle* is much thicker than the preceding muscle (see Fig. 2.23B). Its bundles are similarly oriented but are largely fused, giving a uniform appearance to the lumbar and thoracic regions. The thoracolumbar part (longissimus dorsi) is credited with the powerful extension of the vertebral column during the propulsive phase of the gallop. It is related medially to the multifidus, and over the thoracic vertebrae, it is covered dorsally by the spinalis et semispinalis (Fig. 12.10/*1* and *2*), although it is separated from both by a fibrous septum that serves as the origin of the last-named muscle. The ventral edge of this septum ends near the transverse processes of the vertebrae and is a landmark in the surgical approach to the intervertebral disks.

The *lumbar part* of the longissimus muscle arises from the wing of the ilium and the lumbar spinous processes, against which it lies. Along its length it detaches several bundles, arranged in a lateral and a medial row, which cover the bases of the lumbar transverse processes before ending on accessory processes of the cranial six lumbar vertebrae. The caudal narrow part, not covered by the middle gluteus, inserts dorsally mainly on the arch of the last lumbar vertebra and the last intervertebral disk, with more limited insertion on the sixth

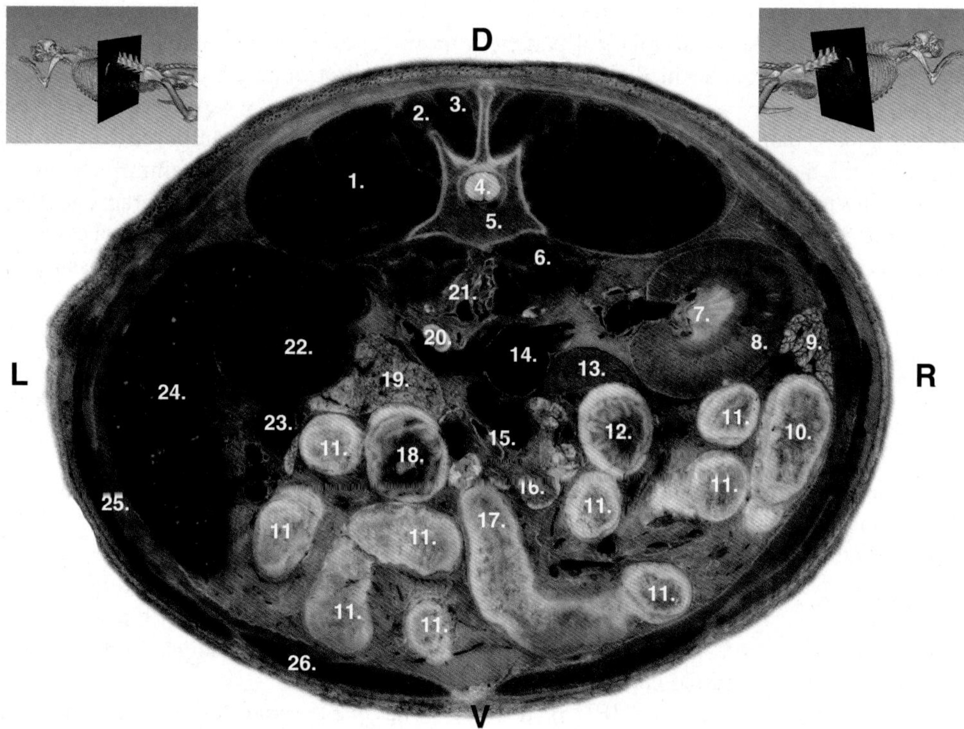

Fig. 12.11 Transverse section of the dog at the level of the 2nd lumbar vertebra. *1,* Iliocostalis and longissimus muscles; *2,* Spinalis and semispinalis muscle; *3,* Multifidi muscles; *4,* Spinal cord; *5,* 2nd lumbar vertebra; *6,* Psoas muscles; *7,* Renal medulla (renal papilla); *8,* Renal cortex; *9,* Pancreas, right lobe; *10,* Descending duodenum; *11,* Jejunum; *12,* Ascending colon; *13,* Liver (caudate process of the caudal lobe); *14,* Caudal vena cava; *15,* Cranial mesenteric artery and vein; *16,* Mesenteric lymph nodes; *17,* Duodenojejunal flexure (terminal part of the ascending duodenum); *18,* Descending colon; *19,* Pancreas, left lobe; *20,* Left adrenal gland; *21,* Abdominal aorta; *22,* Left kidney (cranial pole); *23,* Vessels of the spleen; *24,* Spleen; *25,* Internal, external obliquus and transversus abdominalis muscles; *26,* Rectus abdominis muscle.

and fifth lumbar vertebrae. The longissimus lumborum is covered by a dense aponeurosis separated from the thoracolumbar fascia by fat.

The *thoracic part* (see Fig. 2.23B/*16″*) inserts by medial tendons on the transverse or accessory processes of the thoracic vertebrae and by lateral tendons on the necks of the last seven ribs. The dorsal branches of the thoracic nerves pass between the medial and lateral tendon.

The *cervical part* (see Fig. 2.23B/*16′*) of the longissimus muscle has a triangular form, filling up the angle between the cervical and thoracic vertebrae, and comprises four incompletely separable bundles, which arise from the transverse and articular processes of the first thoracic vertebrae and insert on the transverse processes of the sixth to third cervical vertebrae.

The *longissimus capitis muscle*, strong and flat, lies medial to the longissimus cervicis and splenius muscles (see Fig. 2.23/*16′*). It originates from the transverse processes of the first three thoracic vertebrae and from the caudal articular processes of the last three or four cervical vertebrae. It runs over the dorsal surface of the atlas and inserts on the mastoid process, fused at the level of the atlas with the splenius muscle.

The *longissimus atlantis muscle,* present in only 20% of dogs, arises from the articular processes of the last three cervical vertebrae and ends on the wing of the atlas.

In the cat there is a longissimus *capitis* but not a longissimus *atlantis*. Furthermore, it is not possible to separate the cervical and thoracic longissimus muscles; a shallow longitudinal groove appears to separate the lumbar portion into lateral and medial parts.

The more complex *transversospinalis system* is more intimately related to the vertebrae. Some fascicles connect one vertebra to the next, whereas others span several vertebrae; most are oriented from caudoventral and lateral to craniodorsal and medial, in contrast to the direction taken by the preceding muscles. The transversospinalis system comprises the *spinalis et semispinalis thoracis et cervicis, semispinalis capitis,* and several less important, more obviously segmental muscles (*multifidi, intertransversarii, interspinales,* and *rotatores*) that lie directly on the vertebrae (see Fig. 2.23B/*15*).

The *spinalis et semispinalis thoracis et cervicis* muscles extend from the midlumbar region to the spine of the axis and lie against the lateral surface of the spinous processes (see Fig. 2.24A/*2″* and *2‴*) dorsomedial to the longissimus thoracis. Their fascicles connect spinous and mammillary processes with more cranial spinous processes. They are a powerful muscle incompletely divided into a lateral part, the *spinalis et semispinalis thoracis,* and a medial part, the *spinalis cervicis.*

The *spinalis et semispinalis thoracis* (lateral part) arises from the aponeurosis of the thoracic part of the longissimus muscle and from the midlumbar spinous processes. It inserts on the spinous processes of the sixth thoracic forward to the sixth cervical vertebrae. The tendons that are attached to the last two cervical spines are particularly powerful and form a plate that is fused with the tendon of the medial part of the muscle. In the cat, the *spinalis et semispinalis thoracis* arises from only the tenth or eleventh thoracic spinous process forward.

The *spinalis cervicis* (medial part) lies dorsomedial to the lateral part. It arises from the spinous processes of the sixth to first thoracic vertebrae and continues as a flat muscle with four tendinous inscriptions in its belly on the spinous processes of the fifth to second cervical vertebrae.

The *semispinalis capitis* is a more independent neck muscle lying between the splenius and the cervical components of the preceding muscle (see Fig. 2.23B/*15*). It is clearly divided into the *biventer cervicis* and the *complexus,* which both contact their fellows and the ligamentum nuchae in the median plane. The biventer is the more dorsal and more caudal of the two. It arises from and around the transverse processes of the first few thoracic vertebrae, medial to the longissimus cervicis and capitis, and ends on the occipital bone ventral to the external occipital protuberance. It can be identified by several tendinous inscriptions. The complexus arises from the articular processes of the caudal four cervical vertebrae and first thoracic vertebra and ends on the nuchal crest; it is not segmented.

In the cat, the *biventer* is relatively poorly developed, and it has only two to three tendinous inscriptions. The *complexus,* even less developed, is divided by a distinct strip of tendon that runs horizontally through its middle.

The *multifidus* is more distinctly segmented in the dog than in the cat, especially in the cervical region. The *lumbar* part in the dog consists of 10 to 11 bundles that arise from the mammillary process of the first caudal vertebra, the rudimentary articular processes of the sacrum, and the mammillary processes of the lumbar vertebrae and last two thoracic vertebrae (see Fig. 2.24B/*2'*). As a rule, two segments are passed by each bundle: thus the insertions are to the spinous processes of the sixth lumbar to the tenth thoracic vertebrae. The *thoracic* part comprises nine distinct bundles that arise from the mammillary and transverse processes of most thoracic vertebrae and, after passing two segments, insert on the spinous processes of the first eight thoracic and last cervical vertebrae.

The *cervical* part, which is completely covered by the semispinalis capitis, consists of six individual parts that divide into large lateral and smaller medial bundles.

The *intertransversarii muscles,* divisible into *lumbar, thoracic,* and *cervical* units, are sometimes regarded as being split from the longissimus system. The *lumbar* units are especially well developed in cats, whereas in dogs the muscle is composed of thin bundles. In both species they unite the mammillary and accessory processes of the lumbar vertebrae and last four thoracic vertebrae with the transverse processes of the twelfth to sixth thoracic vertebrae, never passing more than three segments.

The *cervical* intertransversarii are much stronger and are arranged in dorsal, middle, and ventral layers. The dorsal layer is located between the insertions of the longissimus cervicis and capitis muscles and comprises five bundles only partly separable. The middle layer consists of five to six thin, separate parts, of which the deeper fibers run from segment to segment and the superficial ones always pass over one segment. The ventral layer lies dorsal to the longus capitis. It arises from the ventral border, the transverse process of the sixth cervical vertebra, and runs forward, as three digitations, to processes of the fourth to second vertebrae.

The *interspinales* muscles connect the spinous processes of the vertebrae in the lumbar, thoracic, and cervical regions; the lumbar portions are completely covered by the multifidus. The thoracic parts are broader.

Deep *rotator muscles* lie medial to the multifidi in the cranial thoracic region. The eight long rotators extend between the transverse and spinous, spanning two joints; the nine short ones pass between adjacent vertebrae. It is not possible to separate the rotator muscles from the multifidus in the cat.

Cervical Hypaxial Muscles

The *longus colli* is located on the ventral aspect of the cervical and first few thoracic vertebrae. The thoracic part originates from the ventral surface of the first six thoracic vertebrae and inserts on the platelike process of the sixth cervical vertebra. The cervical part originates by separate cervical vertebrae and inserts on the ventral parts of the bodies of more cranial cervical vertebrae near the midline (see Fig. 2.24B/*9*).

The *longus capitis* is a long flat muscle that lies on the lateral and ventral sides of the cervical vertebrae lateral to the longus colli. It arises from the transverse processes of the middle five cervical vertebrae and inserts on the occipital bone between the tympanic bullae.

Lumbar Hypaxial Muscles

The *psoas minor muscle* can be found between the iliac fascia and peritoneum ventrally and the iliopsoas and quadratus lumborum muscles dorsally. It originates from the bodies of the last thoracic and the first four to five lumbar vertebrae. The strong flat tendon has a shiny appearance and inserts on the iliopubic eminence at the pelvic inlet. It stabilizes and flexes the lumbar part of the vertebral column.

The *iliopsoas muscle* consists of the *psoas major* and the *iliacus*. It lies ventral to the quadratus lumborum and dorsal to the psoas minor. The psoas major arises from the bodies of the lumbar vertebrae and passes caudally, medial to the wings of the ilium, where it fuses with the iliacus to form the iliopsoas (see Fig. 2.24B/*11*). The iliacus arises from the wing and shaft of the ilium. The two muscles have a common insertion on the lesser trochanter of the femur. The combined muscle flexes the lumbar vertebral column and plays a role in protraction of the hindlimb.

The *quadratus lumborum* lies directly ventral to the bodies of the last three thoracic vertebrae and the bodies and transverse processes of all the lumbar vertebrae and ends on the medial surface of the wing of the ilium (see Fig. 2.24B/*3*).

Muscles Controlling Movements of the Head

The four straight and two oblique muscles associated with the atlanto-occipital and atlantoaxial joints form a group of their own.

The *rectus capitis dorsalis major* (Fig. 12.12/*2*) arises from the spine of the axis, just cranial to the attachment of the nuchal ligament, and inserts on the nuchal surface of the skull, ventral to the insertion of the semispinalis capitis, by which it is covered.

The *rectus capitis dorsalis minor* (Fig. 12.12/*8*), deep to the preceding muscle, is a short flat muscle; it arises from the dorsal arch of the atlas and inserts on the skull above the foramen magnum.

The *rectus capitis ventralis* comes from the ventral arch of the atlas and goes to the ventral surface of the occipital bone. It lies dorsal to the much larger longus capitis, which inserts close by.

The *rectus capitis lateralis* passes between the ventral arch of the atlas and the paracondylar process of the occipital bone. The recti muscles move the head both up and down and sideways.

The *obliquus capitis cranialis* arises from the cranial surface of the wing of the atlas and inserts on the nuchal surface of the skull.

The larger *obliquus capitis caudalis* arises from the lateral surface of the spine of the axis and inserts on the caudal surface of the wing of the atlas. The obliquus muscles are responsible for rotation of the head at the atlantoaxial joint.

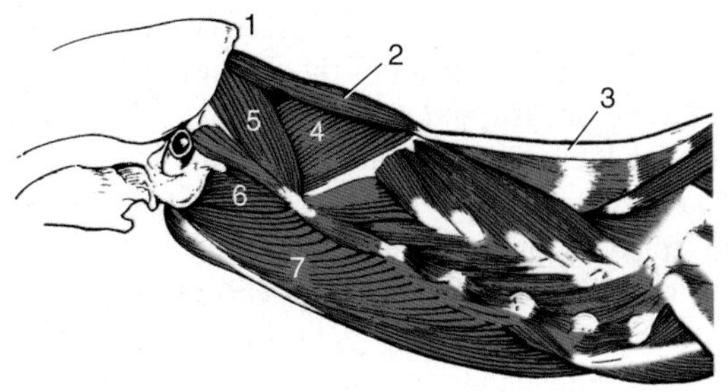

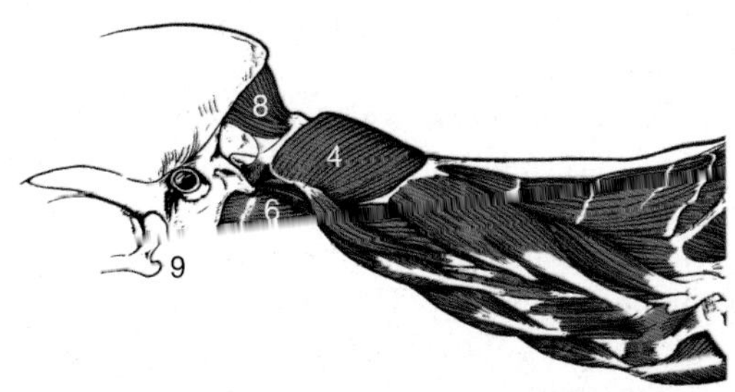

Fig. 12.12 Muscles associated with the canine atlanto-occipital and atlantoaxial joints, lateral view. *1,* External occipital protuberance; *2,* rectus capitis dorsalis major muscle (m.); *3,* nuchal ligament; *4,* obliquus capitis caudalis m.; *5,* obliquus capitis cranialis m.; *6,* rectus capitis ventralis m.; *7,* longus capitis m.; *8,* rectus capitis dorsalis minor m.; *9,* angular process of mandible.

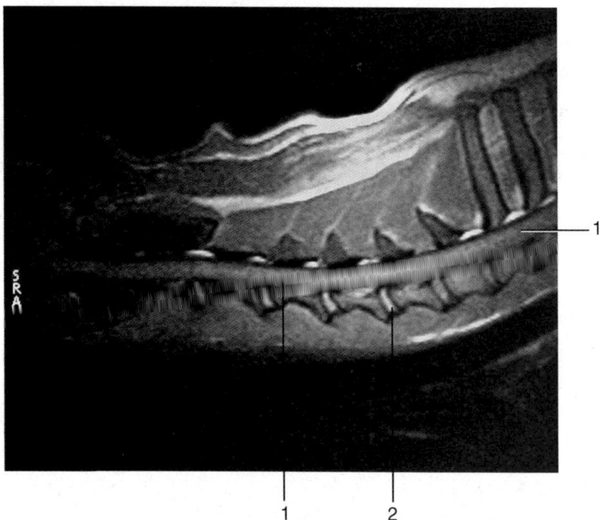

Fig. 12.13 Midsagittal section of cervical region of dog, T2-weighted magnetic resonance image. *1,* Spinal cord; *2,* nucleus pulposus.

CLINICAL CONSIDERATIONS

Muscles of the epaxial and hypaxial divisions must often be separated and detached when access to the vertebral column is necessary. In the neck the ventral approach is most often chosen, although a dorsal approach is also possible. In the lumbar region the dorsal approach is preferred.

The *ventral approach to the cervical vertebrae* (Fig. 12.13) is indicated for disk fenestration in cases of herniation or for the treatment of atlantoaxial instability. The trachea is exposed through a ventral midline incision, midway between the sternomastoid and sternohyoid muscles. Reflection of the trachea to the left protects the esophagus and exposes the paired longus colli muscles, which can be separated longitudinally.

The *dorsal approach to the cervical vertebrae* is indicated for vertebral fractures. This approach includes exposure of the biventer cervicis and the rectus capitis dorsalis major cranially, and the nuchal ligament, the spinalis et semispinalis cervicis, and multifidus cervicis muscles more caudally. The vertebral artery lies in the rectus capitis dorsalis major, ventrolateral to the synovial joint C1/C2 and must be avoided as the dissection is continued laterally.

The *dorsal approach to the caudal cervical and cranial thoracic vertebrae* for dorsal laminectomy (removal of part of the vertebral arch) and fracture repair first exposes the aponeuroses of the trapezius cranially and the rhomboid caudally. Then the subscapulares, splenius, and serratus dorsalis are exposed by lateral retraction of the trapezius and rhomboid muscles and the scapula. Finally, the semispinalis capitis and longissimus cervicis, the nuchal ligament, and the dorsal spines of the vertebrae are exposed by lateral retraction of the splenius and serratus dorsalis. The deep cervical artery passes through the semispinalis capitis.

A *dorsal approach to the thoracolumbar vertebrae* is indicated for dorsal laminectomy and thoracolumbar fractures. Lateral retraction of the lumbar fascia exposes the longissimus lumborum and multifidi caudally and the spinalis et semispinalis thoracis cranially. The multifidus, interspinalis, and rotatores longi are elevated from the spinous processes and vertebral arches. The dorsal branch of each spinal nerve emerges just cranial and ventral to the insertions of the longissimus on the accessory processes.

COMPREHENSION CHECK

Use a cadaver to practice ventral and dorsal approaches to the cervical vertebrae of the dog.

The Thorax of the Dog and Cat

13

CONFORMATION AND SURFACE ANATOMY

The shape of the thorax differs considerably among different breeds, as is well illustrated by the deep, laterally compressed thorax of the Greyhound (Fig. 13.1) and the broad, barrel-shaped one of the Pug (Fig. 13.2). These differences are reflected in the form of the ribs, which are long and relatively straight in the Greyhound, and shorter and strongly curved in the Pug. In cats, corresponding but less pronounced variation distinguishes the Oriental breeds from the Persian.

The small size of the cranial part of the bony thorax and thus of the thoracic inlet is masked by the enclosure of the upper parts of the forelimbs within the skin of the trunk (Fig. 13.3) and by the height of the first few thoracic spinous processes (Fig. 13.4). The dorsal contours of the neck and thorax generally meet without a noticeable elevation at the withers. The skin is loosely attached here, making it a suitable site for the subcutaneous infusion of large volumes of fluid when necessary. The tips of the thoracic spinous processes are individually palpable, together with the spine and the cranial and caudal angles of the scapula to each side. In the standing dog, the cranial and caudal angles are opposite the spinous processes of the first thoracic vertebra and the bodies of the fourth and fifth thoracic vertebrae, respectively. The shoulder joint is located opposite the ventral end of the first rib, and the point of the shoulder is slightly behind the level of the manubrium of the sternum. The gently curved sternum rises between the forelimbs to the thoracic inlet, bringing the easily palpated manubrium a few centimeters cranial to the first pair of ribs. The olecranon projects on the thoracic wall immediately below the ventral end of the fifth intercostal space. However, breed and individual variations in the preceding features are common (Figs. 13.4 and 13.5).

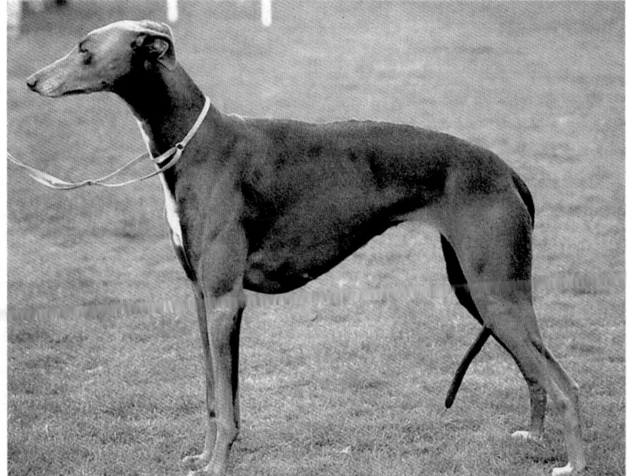

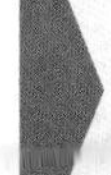

Fig. 13.1 Deep and laterally compressed thorax of the Greyhound.

The epaxial muscles provide a thick covering to the thoracic vertebrae and the dorsal parts of the ribs. The triceps muscles occupy the angle between the scapula and humerus, making it difficult to distinguish the caudal border of the scapula. Medial to the triceps and behind the limb, the lateral parts of the ribs are more thinly covered by the serratus ventralis, latissimus dorsi, scalenus, and obliquus abdominis externus muscles; one can feel the ribs through them (Fig. 13.6). The ventral surface of the thorax is covered by pectoral muscles. The axilla is deep and permits palpation of the first five ribs and the axillary and accessory axillary lymph nodes, especially when they are enlarged. The most extensive exposure of the chest is obtained when the limb is drawn forward.

The thorax of young dogs and cats yields considerably to external pressure, a feature that protects against major damage during traffic accidents. The costochondral joints of certain rib pairs can be brought together by manual compression cranial to the heart. The forelimbs of the cat may be shifted against the trunk (exemplified by the position of the scapulae in the posture adopted by a cat stalking prey) in a free manner (Fig. 13.5).

Pectus excavatum is an uncommon congenital anomaly in both dogs and cats. It is characterized by a concave inward deformation of the caudal sternum and costal cartilages that may cause severe respiratory and circulatory abnormalities.

THE THORACIC WALL AND PLEURA (SEE ALSO PP. 38-39, 45-47, AND 148-149)

The dog generally has 13 rib pairs of which 9 are sternal. Asymmetry of number and the presence of 12 or 14 pairs are both occasionally found. Although the first three to four ribs are almost vertical, the remaining slope increasingly caudoventrally (see Fig. 2.1). The ribs are relatively narrow, resulting in wide intercostal spaces, an advantage in thoracic surgery. The costal cartilages at first continue the

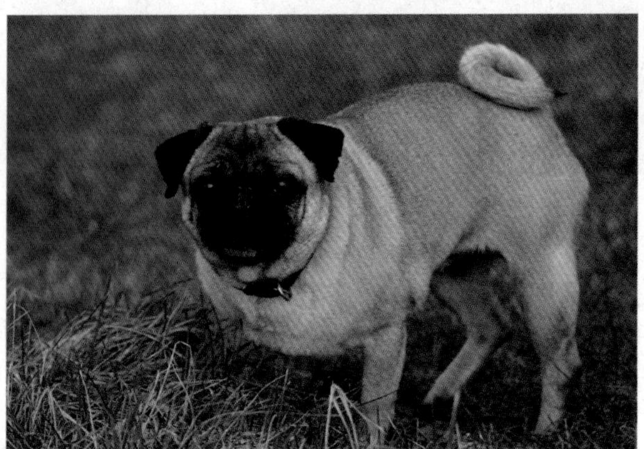

Fig. 13.2 Broad, barrel-shaped thorax of the Pug.

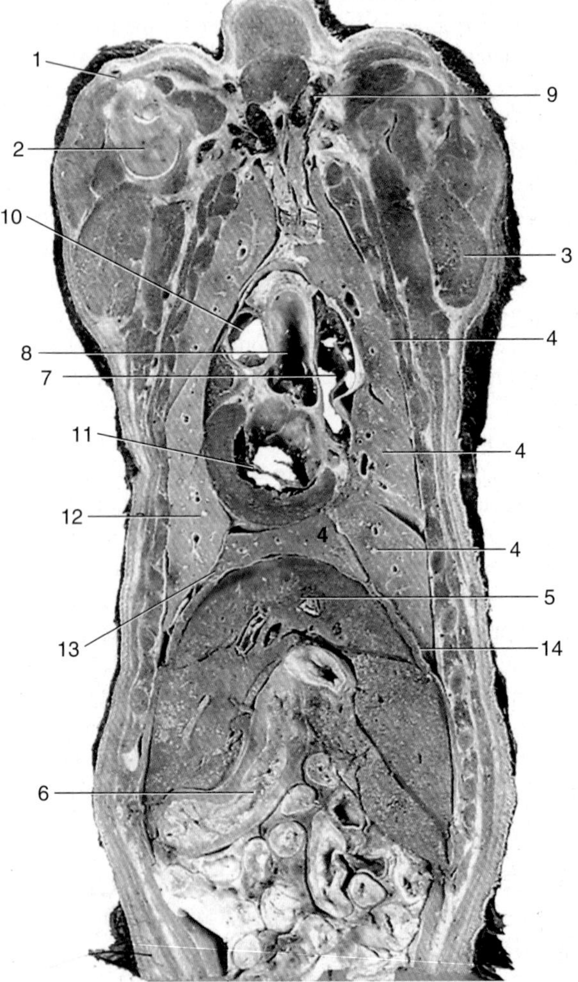

Fig. 13.3 Dorsal section of the canine trunk level with the base of the heart, dorsal view. *1,* Cephalic vein; *2,* proximal end of humerus; *3,* triceps; *4,* cranial, middle, caudal, and accessory lobes of the right lung; *5,* liver; *6,* stomach; *7,* right atrium; *8,* aortic arch; *9,* cranial vena cava; *10,* pulmonary valve; *11,* left atrioventricular valve; *12,* divided cranial and caudal lobes of the left lung; *13,* caudal mediastinum; *14,* diaphragm.

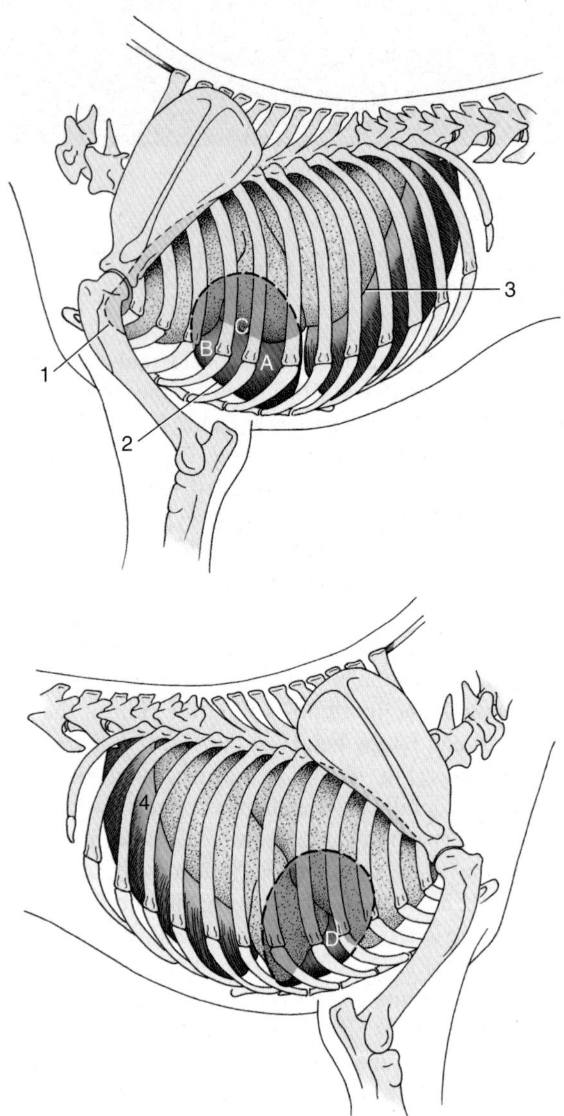

Fig. 13.4 Left and right surface projections of the canine heart and lungs. *Circled letters* on the heart: puncta maxima of left atrioventricular valve *(A),* pulmonary valve *(B),* aortic valve *(C),* and right atrioventricular valve *(D). 1,* Apex of left lung *(broken line)* in cupula pleurae; *2,* heart; *3,* basal border of lung; *4,* diaphragm.

direction of the bony ribs but then bend forward, almost at right angles (see Fig. 13.5), to form the rib "knees." The cartilages of the sternal ribs form synovial articulations with the sternum, which allow expansion of the thorax when the ribs are carried cranially in the "bucket-handle" movement. The cartilages of the four asternal ribs join to form the costal arch, which is easily palpated and may be followed to the vicinity of the xyphoid cartilage (Fig. 13.7/*5*). The slender, cylindrical sternebrae are slightly thickened at their extremities where the costal cartilages attach. Only a thin layer of compact bone encloses the

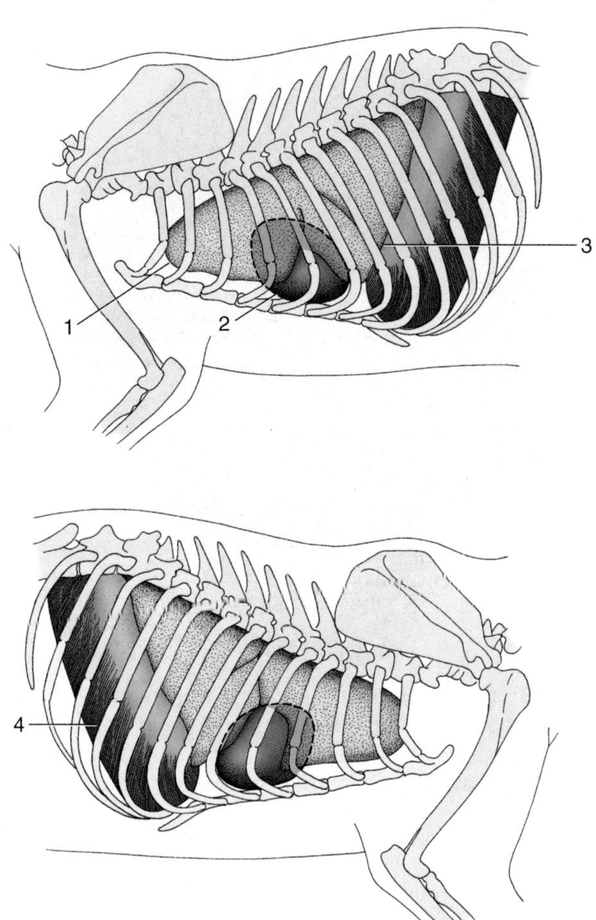

Fig. 13.5 Left *(top)* and right *(bottom)* surface projections of the feline heart and lungs. *1,* Apex of left lung; *2,* heart; *3,* basal border of lung; *4,* diaphragm.

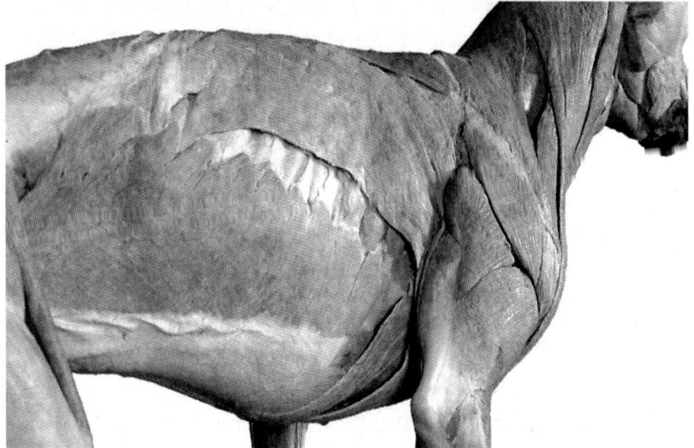

Fig. 13.6 Notice the attachment of the external abdominal oblique muscle on the ribs.

spongy interior of sternebrae; this characteristic, combined with their superficial position, makes them ideal for bone marrow biopsy.

The principal intercostal vessels and nerves run caudomedially to the ribs, under the endothoracic fascia.

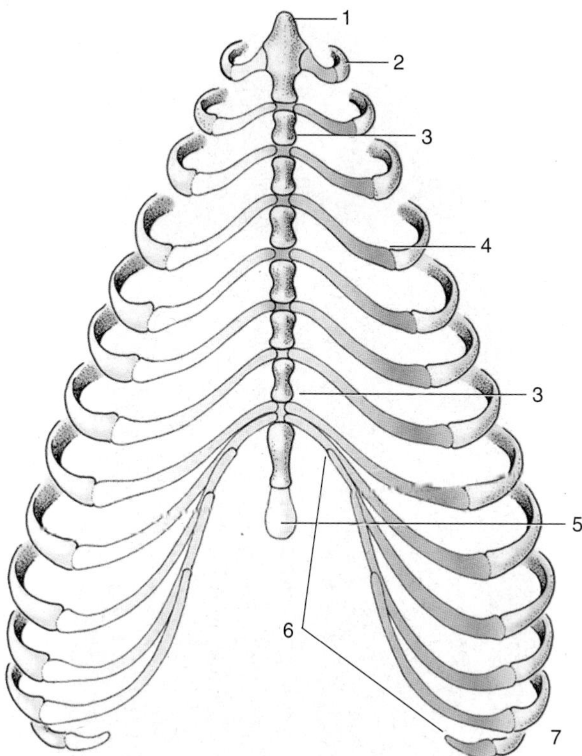

Fig. 13.7 Canine sternum and costal cartilages, ventral view. *1,* Manubrium; *2,* first rib; *3,* sternebra; *4,* costochondral junction; *5,* xiphoid cartilage; *6,* costal arch; *7,* floating rib.

Additional vessels from the internal thoracic trunks follow the cranial borders of the ribs in the ventral parts of the spaces (Fig. 13.8). These locations must be borne in mind when incision or puncture is contemplated. It is helpful to know that the boundary between the scalenus and external abdominal oblique muscles is the fifth intercostal space. The ribs are so much more easily displaced cranially than caudally that a more favorable exposure of the "target" region for clinical procedure may be gained by opening the space immediately caudal to the one that initially seemed most appropriate.

The *diaphragm* arises by right and left crura from the first few lumbar vertebrae and attaches to the medial surfaces of the ribs close to the costal arches and to the sternum. Its strong curvature brings its most cranial point to the level of the 6th or 7th rib. The small, triangular tendinous center transmits the caudal vena cava a little to the right of the median plane. The openings for the esophagus and aorta lie in the fleshy lumbar part, and the former is opposite the upper palpable part of the 10th rib (Fig. 13.9). In lateral radiographs the strongly convex ventral part of the diaphragm presents a simple border that is continued dorsally by the paired outlines of the cupulae (Fig. 13.10A/*4*); the more cranial outline of this double image is provided by the cupula on the "lower" side of a laterally recumbent animal, which is the side subjected to greater forward pressure from the

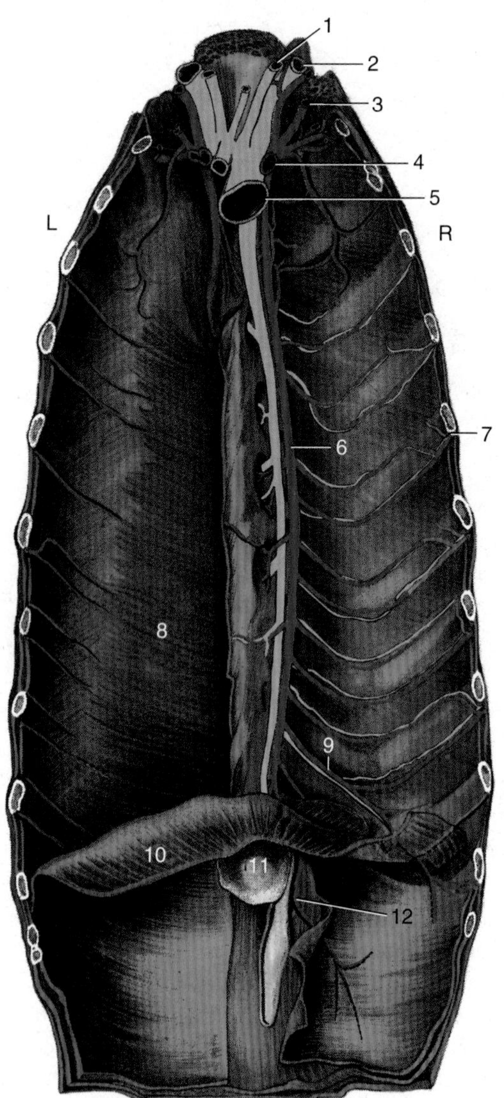

Fig. 13.8 The vessels on the floor of the canine thorax; the transversus thoracis muscle has been removed on the right. *1,* Internal jugular vein; *2,* external jugular vein; *3,* vertebral artery; *4,* right subclavian artery; *5,* cranial vena cava; *6,* internal thoracic artery; *7,* intercostal artery; *8,* transversus thoracis muscle; *9,* musculophrenic artery; *10,* diaphragm; *11,* xiphoid cartilage; *12,* cranial epigastric artery; *L,* left; *R,* right.

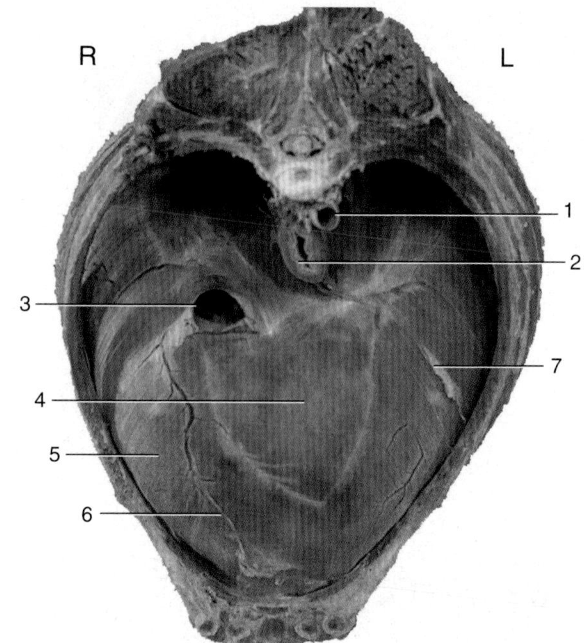

Fig. 13.9 Cranial view of the canine diaphragm. *1,* Aorta; *2,* esophagus; *3,* caudal vena cava; *4,* tendinous center; *5,* sternal and costal parts of diaphragm; *6,* attachment of plica venae cavae; *7,* attachment of caudal mediastinum; *L,* left; *R,* right.

abdominal viscera. The correct identification of the twin elevations is further provided by the gas bubble usually found in the gastric fundus, which is of course located on the left side. The doubling of the outline is less distinct in cats, in which the lighter abdominal organs exert possibly less pressure. Diaphragmatic hernia is the entry of abdominal viscera into the thoracic cavity. It occurs when the diaphragm is torn by a sudden increase in abdominal pressure, which is commonly produced by compression in traffic accidents.

At rest, ventilation depends principally on the diaphragm. However, increased respiratory demand engages other muscles as well. Although some or all of the external intercostal, sternocephalic, ventral serratus, and scalenus may be used to assist at inspiration, the internal intercostal and abdominal muscles may help at expiration.

The most important clinical features of pleural cavities are the cupulae cranially, the caudal reflection of the costal pleura onto the diaphragm, and the presence and extents of the costomediastinal and costodiaphragmatic recesses. Although the cupulae (see Fig. 13.5) project only slightly in front of the first ribs in the dog, they are still susceptible to puncture wounds that appear to be confined to the base of the neck; the resulting entry of air into the pleural cavity (pneumothorax) causes uncoupling of the lung from the thoracic wall and its collapse.

The line of pleural reflection is at the junction between costal and diaphragmatic pleura, and it defines the caudal extent of the pleural cavity. The line runs from the sternum along the 8th costal cartilage, crosses the middle of the 9th cartilage, and then proceeds in a curve that intersects the 11th costochondral junction to reach the dorsal end of the last rib. The two recesses are of course never fully exploited by the lungs. Fluid may be collected through the ventral third of any of the 4th to 7th intercostal spaces of a dog standing or restrained in sternal recumbency. In cases of pneumothorax, air may be aspirated at the dorsal part of

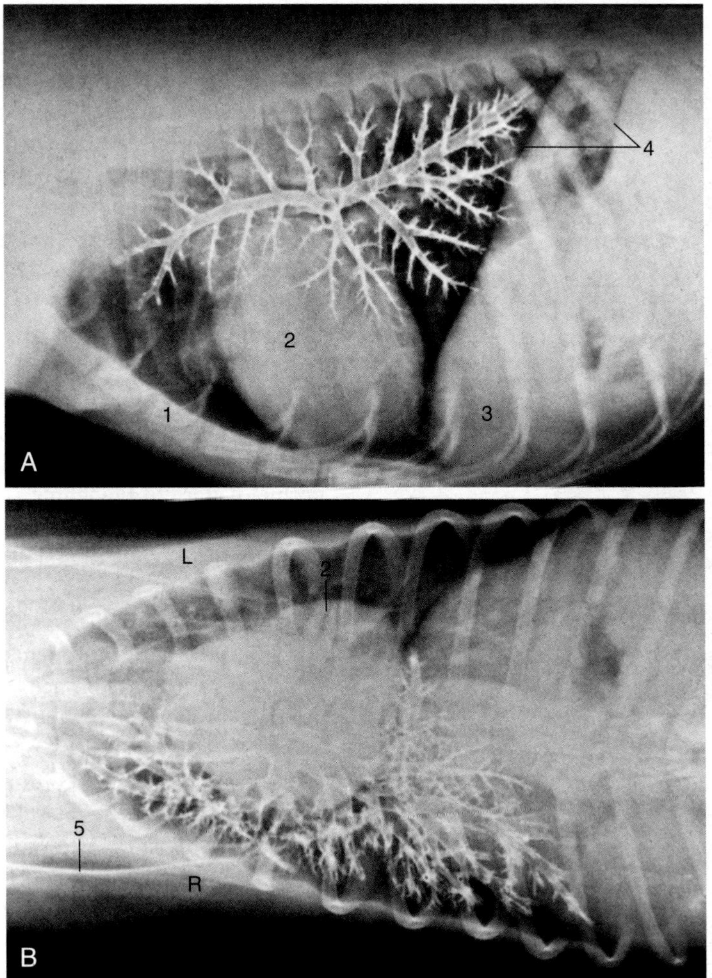

Fig. 13.10 (A) Lateral and (B) ventrodorsal bronchograms of the right canine lung. *1,* Sternum; *2,* heart; *3,* liver behind diaphragm; *4,* paired shadows of the cranial extent of the diaphragm; *5,* scapula; *L,* left; *R,* right.

the 7th or 8th space of dogs similarly placed. The 8th space is optimal for this purpose in the cat.

THE LUNGS (SEE ALSO PP. 149-156)

The lungs of the dog obtain their distinctive appearance from the deep fissures that divide the lobes, sometimes so completely that they remain connected by little more than the branches of the bronchial tree and pulmonary vessels. In consequence, torsion of a lobe is a possible complication of thoracic trauma, perhaps most frequently seen after

traffic accidents. In contrast, lobulation is not evident to the naked eye through the covering pleura. The right lung, always somewhat the larger, possesses cranial, middle, caudal, and accessory lobes (Fig. 13.11); the left one has only a divided cranial lobe and a caudal lobe. The cardiac impression on the medial surface of the left lung is shallower than that on the right. Despite the existence of a small notch between the two parts of the cranial lobe, the left lung practically covers the lateral face of the pericardium. The notch between the cranial and middle lobes of the right lung is larger and restricted to the ventral part of the fourth intercostal space. It is recommended for heart (right ventricular) puncture and for ultrasonic cardiac imaging.

Pulmonary ligaments connect the hilar region of the left lung to the aorta and that of the right lung to the esophagus, which it follows to the hiatus in the diaphragm.

Lung Auscultation The fields for auscultation and percussion of the lungs are triangular: the cranial border is provided by the 5th rib (actually the caudal border of the triceps), the dorsal border is provided by the lateral margin of the back muscles from the 5th rib to the 11th space, and the basal border is provided by the line joining the 6th costochondral junction, the middle of the 8th rib, and the dorsal end of the 11th space. The forelimb may be drawn forward to increase the accessible area by the space of a couple of ribs.

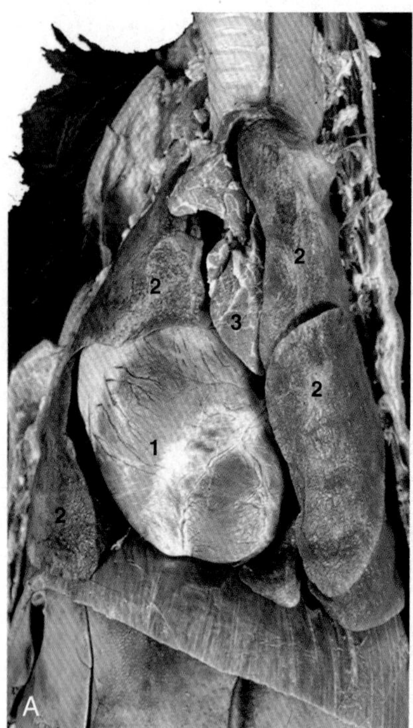

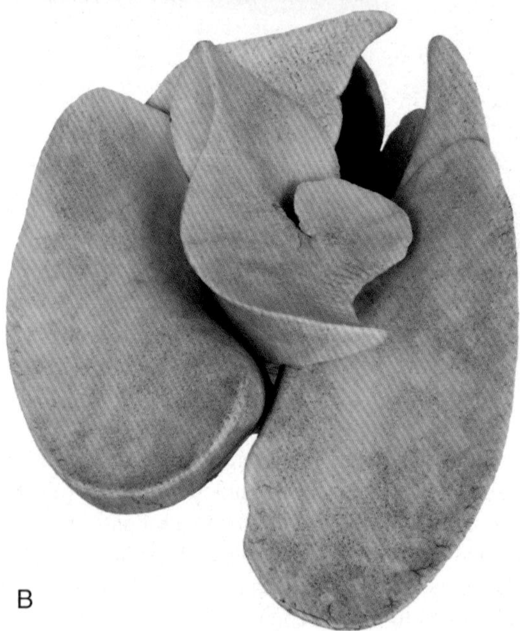

Fig. 13.11 (A) Thoracic viscera of the dog. *1*, Heart; *2*, pulmonary lobes; *3*, thymus. In (B), an inflated specimen, the deep fissures between the lobes of the lung are clearly visible.

In plain radiographs, the principal features of the lungs are made by the vessels and bronchi. The blood within the arteries and veins, which cannot be immediately differentiated, produces a pattern of light streaks radiating from the hilar region toward the periphery, branching and tapering as they go. The bronchi, being filled with air, provide dark streaks that contrast less definitely with the lung parenchyma. Bronchial walls may be invisible or may appear as narrow, whitish lines, especially in older animals, in which the cartilage tends to have calcified. The relationships within the bronchial–vascular triads vary in different regions and in different radiographic views. The components are most clearly depicted when portrayed end on; the dark circles of the bronchial lumina are then flanked by white circles representing the companion vessels. The subpleural connective tissue bordering the interlobar fissures may appear as fine lines when penetrated tangentially on a radiograph view.

Both the bronchial tree and the pulmonary vasculature may be made more evident by the use of an appropriate contrast technique (contrast bronchography: Fig. 13.10; angiocardiography: see Fig. 13.23). The larger divisions of the bronchial tree are then very clearly depicted, and if the normal pattern of branching is known, any deviation may reveal the existence of pathology. A more exact picture of the nature and extent of that pathology may be obtained by the use of bronchoscopy, which also requires familiarity with the branching pattern. The principal bronchi produced at the bifurcation of the trachea are separated by a sharp ridge, the carina. The bronchi that initially branch from the principal bronchi supply the different lobes and are named accordingly. The divisions of the next order, the segmental bronchi, also arise according to a consistent pattern and are each associated with well-defined parts of the lobes. Subsequent divisions into smaller bronchi are less regular and less predictable. The parts of lung associated with the segmental bronchi (the bronchopulmonary segments) constitute the divisions of the lungs on which surgery is based. Various systems of nomenclature such as those based on topography have been devised for the identification.

The branching progressively produces a greater cross-sectional area and reduces resistance to the air as it flows into deeper parts of the lung. This process is similar to that in the upper respiratory system, in which the nostrils, the nasal cavity, the pharynx, the larynx, and the trachea each offers successively less obstruction than the preceding segment. It is estimated that the resistance to the inspiratory airflow in dogs is 79% due to the nasal, 6% to the laryngeal, and 15% to the bronchopulmonary parts of the tract; the corresponding figures at expiration are given as 74%, 3%, and 23%, respectively. The resistance to inspiratory and expiratory air in the nasal cavity is further increased in the brachycephalic breeds of dogs, resulting in breathing difficulty even under resting conditions. Except for their shallowness, the lungs of the cat are not significantly different from those of the dog.

THE MEDIASTINUM (SEE ALSO PP. 150-151)

The fibrous tissue associated with the thoracic organs and between the pleural sacs (fascia endothoracica) is so thin that the mediastinum is reduced in several places to a very

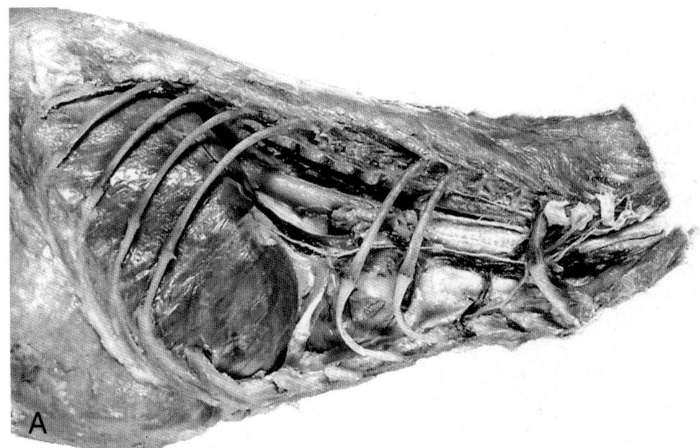

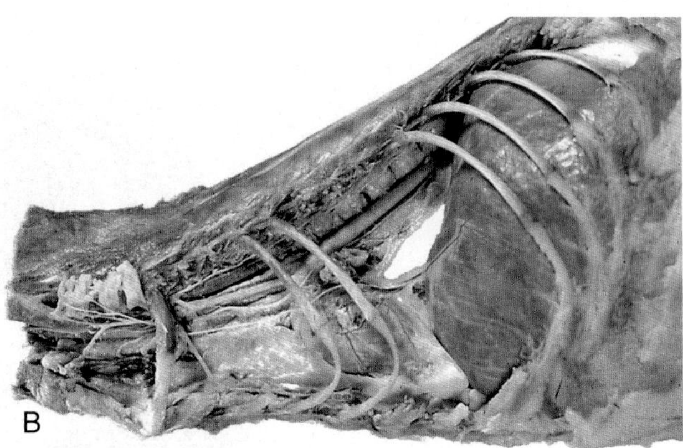

Fig. 13.12 (A) Mediastinum of a cat, right view. In the middle part the heart is the main component. The cranial and caudal mediastinum is thin and, in some places, fragile. (B) Mediastinum, left view. A large opening in the caudal part, probably caused by dissection, indicates the fragility of the structure.

delicate and transparent membrane (Fig. 13.12B) consisting only of apposed right and left pleural sheets. It ruptures easily, and although the two pleural sacs may be regarded as normally independent, most dogs in which pneumothorax has been induced unilaterally show bilateral pneumothorax in radiographs.

The *cranial mediastinum* is wide dorsally where it contains the trachea and esophagus, lying side by side as they pass through the thoracic inlet, and the cranial vena cava and brachiocephalic trunk, with their tributaries and branches, embedded in generous quantities of fat. Ventrally the cranial mediastinum contains lymph nodes, the internal thoracic vessels, fat, and, in the young animal, the thymus. This part narrows with the regression of the thymus, providing more space for the apices of the lungs.

The *dorsal part of the middle mediastinum* is slightly narrower than the heart (Fig. 13.13). It contains the termination of the trachea, the esophagus, the aortic arch, the structures comprising the roots of the lungs, and lymph nodes. Its right surface is flat, but the aorta (Fig. 13.13/4) bulges on the other side to indent the left lung. The middle part at this level contains the heart (within the pericardium), but the ventral part, between the pericardium and sternum, is folded and contains only the phrenicopericardiac ligament, which attaches the pericardium to the sternum and diaphragm more loosely than the corresponding sternopericardiac ligament in larger species.

The triangular *dorsal part of the caudal mediastinum* contains the aorta and the right azygos vein and, more ventrally, the esophagus (Figs. 13.12A and 13.13; also, Figs. 13.14–13.16). The delicate ventral part runs between the pericardium and the diaphragm, which it approaches along a line that is displaced so far to the left that it reaches the thoracic wall near the ninth costochondral junction. There is the usual recess between the mediastinum and the fold enclosing the caudal vena cava that is occupied by the accessory lobe of the right lung.

The infracardiac bursa is a diverticulum of peritoneum that intrudes through the esophageal hiatus of the diaphragm to lie against the right face of the esophagus, extending from the diaphragm to the root of the lung. It is the occasional recipient of a herniated part of an abdominal organ, either as a congenital anomaly or as the result of trauma.

THE HEART (SEE ALSO PP. 219-220)

The canine heart is ovoid. It forms an angle of about 45 degrees with the sternum, with the base facing craniodorsally and the blunt apex resting near the junction of the sternum and the diaphragm, a little to the left of midline (Fig. 13.17 and 13.18). However, the aforementioned angle and the space between the apex and the diaphragm vary more considerably than suggested. The angle is greater and the shape of the heart more conical in deep-chested breeds. Because of the biased position of the heart and the intervention of only a thinner layer of lung tissue between the heart and the left thoracic wall, the heart sounds are more pronounced on the left side (see Figs. 13.10, 13.17, 13.19, and 13.23).

The heart contributes about 0.7% of the body weight on average, but its weight, both absolute and relative, varies considerably. In dogs trained for hunting or racing the heart is two or three times heavier than in fat and less athletic individuals of comparable size.

The left surface presents the auricles (atria) embracing the pulmonary trunk, and below the coronary groove the ventricles are divided by the paraconal interventricular groove (see Fig. 13.14). The right surface presents the atria and the subsinuosal interventricular groove. In reality, the left surface is rotated a little more toward the sternum and the right a little more toward the vertebrae. When one reads counterclockwise from the base, the periphery of the heart

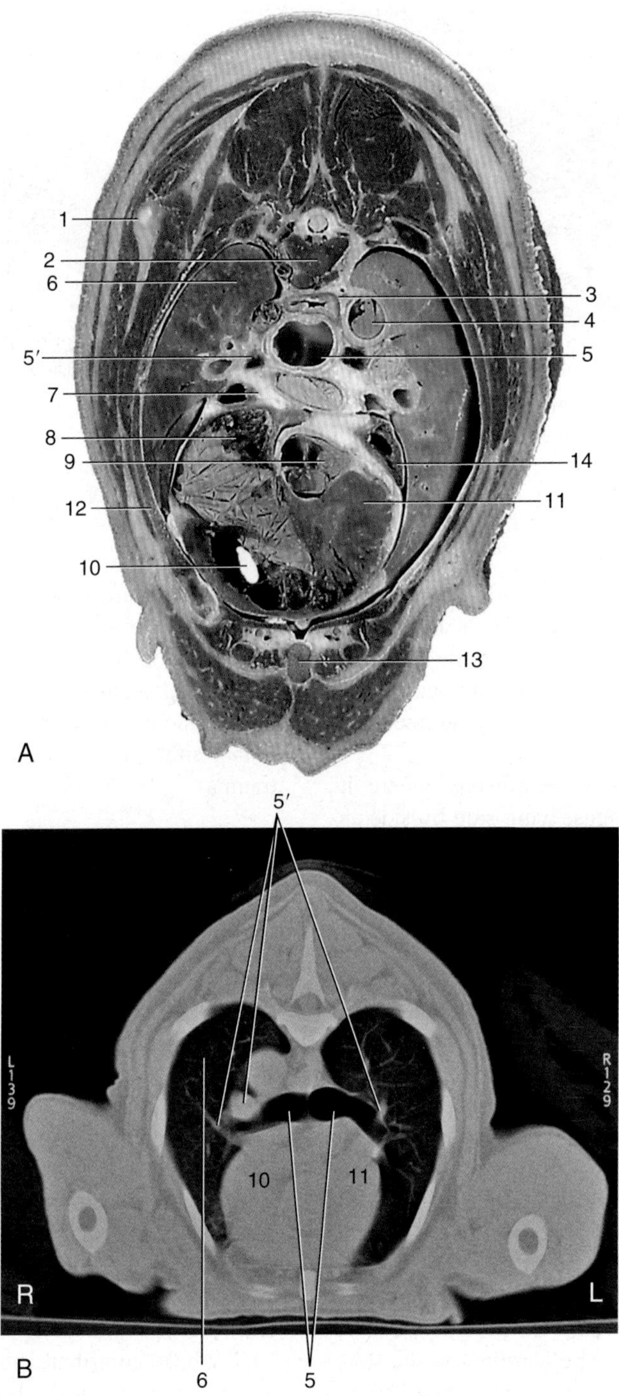

Fig. 13.13 (A) Transverse section of the canine trunk at the level of the sixth thoracic vertebra. (B) Corresponding computed tomography image at a slightly more caudal level. *1,* Caudal angle of scapula; *2,* sixth thoracic vertebra; *3,* esophagus; *4,* aorta; *5,* tracheal bifurcation; *5′,* large blood vessels accompanying principal bronchi are likely right and left pulmonary arteries; *6,* right lung; *7,* tracheobronchial lymph nodes and pulmonary artery; *8,* right atrium; *9,* origin of aorta; *10,* right ventricle; *11,* interventricular septum; *12,* fifth rib; *13,* sternum; *14,* left auricle.

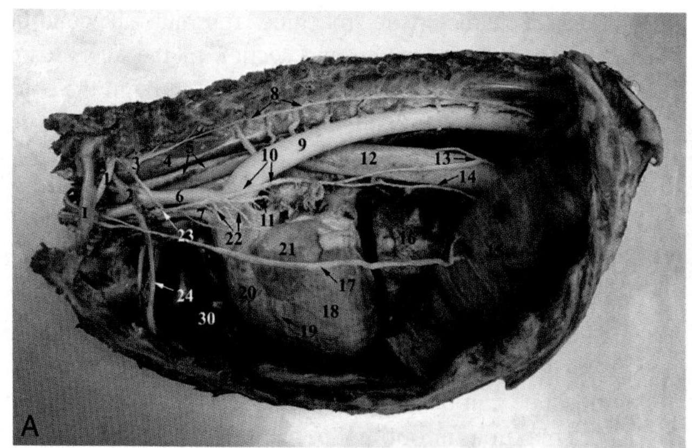

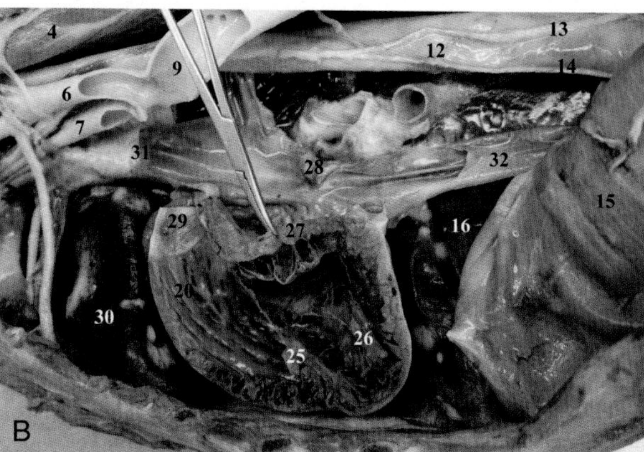

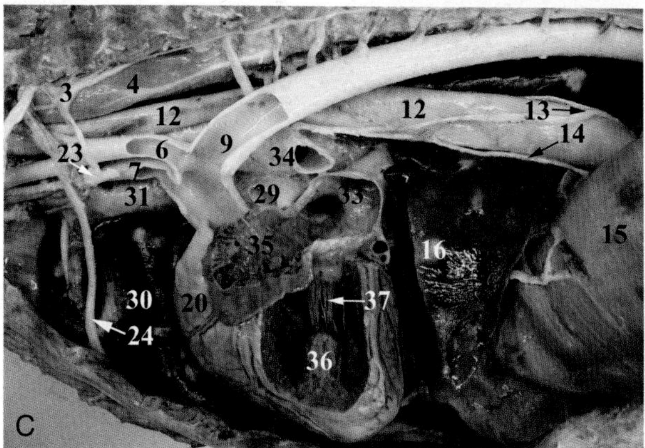

Fig. 13.14 Thoracal cavity of the dog, left side with left lung and mediastinal pleura removed (A) and left side of the heart opened (B) and left of the side of the heart removed (C). *1,* T2 nerve to brachial plexus; *2,* costocervical vein; *3,* left cervicothoracic ganglion; *4,* longus colli muscle; *5,* thoracic duct; *6,* left subclavian artery; *7,* brachiocephalic trunk; *8,* sympathetic trunk; *9,* descending aorta (thoracic part); *10,* vagus nerve; *11,* left recurrent laryngeal nerve; *12,* esophagus; *13,* dorsal branch of vagus nerve; *14,* ventral branch of vagus nerve; *15,* diaphragm; *16,* accessory lobe the right lung; *17,* left phrenic nerve; *18,* left ventricle of the heart; *19,* paraconal interventricular artery, vein, and groove; *20,* conus arteriosus of the right ventricle; *21,* left auricle; *22,* cardiac autonomic nerve; *23,* middle cervical ganglion; *24,* internal thoracic artery and vein; *25,* musculus papillaris magnus; *26,* musculi papillares parvi; *27,* interventricular septum with the septal part of the tricuspidal valve; *28,* intervenosus tubercle; *29,* pulmonary trunk; *30,* cranial lobe of the right lung; *31,* cranial vena cava; *32,* caudal vena cava; *33,* pulmonary veins; *34,* left primary bronchus; *35,* left auricle with the pectinate muscles; *36,* subauricular papillary muscle; *37,* chordae tendineae.

shadow in a left lateral radiograph shows the right auricle, the right ventricle, the left ventricle, and the left auricle (Fig. 13.17/*1–4*); in a ventrodorsal radiograph the sequence is right auricle, right ventricle, left ventricle, and pulmonary trunk (Fig. 13.17/*2, 3, 5,* and *6*). The apex is formed only by the wall of the left ventricle.

It is clearly important to know the relationships of the parts of the heart to external landmarks for auscultation and radiography. The heart extends from the third rib to the sixth intercostal space, and the latter limit roughly coincides with the most cranial extent of the diaphragm (Fig. 13.17A). The projection of the base intersects the middle of the fourth rib; the most dorsal part of the heart reaches approximately to the line connecting the acromion with the ventral end of the last rib. The apex lies just to the left of the second last sternebra. In the standing dog the apex beat is palpable on both sides, low in the fifth or sixth intercostal space. The main contractions are said to be strongest in the lower third of the fourth or fifth space and to be a little more pronounced on the left.

The ductus arteriosus or its replacement, the ligamentum arteriosum (p. 240), is located where the pulmonary trunk is intersected by the left vagus nerve, opposite the fourth rib (see Fig. 13.14). These details are relevant to the diagnosis and surgical treatment of persistent ductus arteriosus, the most common congenital anomaly of the canine cardiovascular system. Among other signs, a persistent ductus

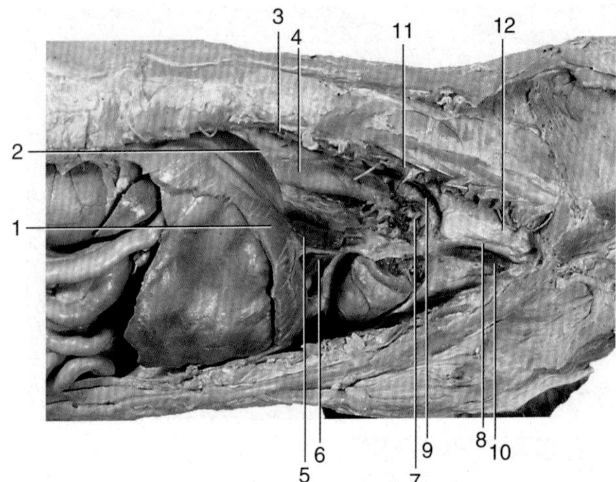

Fig. 13.15 Right lateral view of the canine thoracic cavity; the lung and much of the pericardium have been removed. *1,* Diaphragm; *2,* infracardiac bursa; *3,* sympathetic trunk; *4,* esophagus; *5,* caudal vena cava; *6,* plica venae cavae; *7,* root of lung and phrenic nerve; *8,* right vagus; *9,* right azygous vein; *10,* cranial vena cava; *11,* longus colli; *12,* trachea.

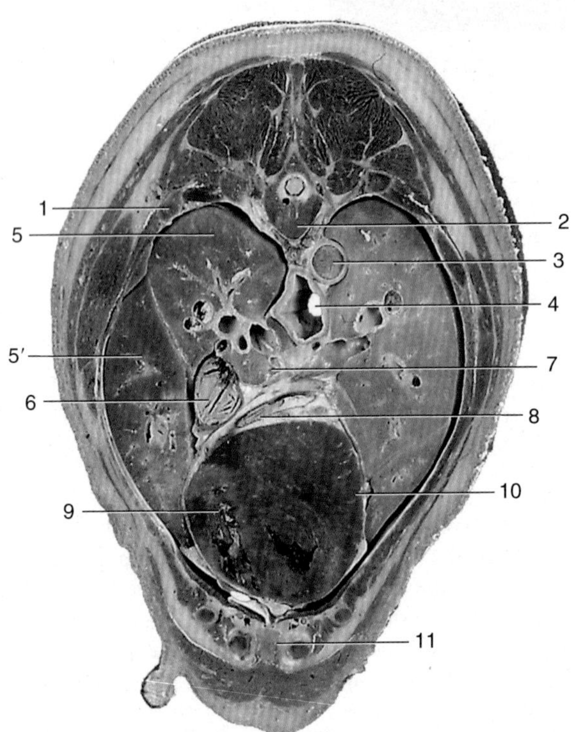

Fig. 13.16 Transverse section of the canine trunk at the level of the seventh thoracic vertebra. *1,* Sixth rib; *2,* seventh thoracic vertebra; *3,* aorta; *4,* esophagus; *5,* cranial lobe; *5′,* middle lobe of right lung; *6,* caudal vena cava; *7,* pulmonary veins passing to left atrium; *8,* great cardiac vein; *9,* right ventricle; *10,* left ventricle; *11,* sternum.

produces a characteristic "machine" murmur. The condition can be treated by ligation and section of the duct. It may be reached by a left lateral thoracotomy through the fourth intercostal space. The same approach provides access to the right ventricle, left auricle, pulmonary trunk, and descending aorta. (The fourth space on the right side may be used to gain access to the main part of the right ventricle, both auricles, the ascending aorta, and both the caval and the azygos veins.)

The heart is more easily auscultated than in the larger species because it is less covered by the forelimbs and a stethoscope can be introduced deeply into the axilla. The puncta maxima for optimal perception of the valve sounds (Fig. 13.4A–D) in the dog may be summarized as shown in Table 13.1. These findings correspond surprisingly closely with those determined at postmortem examinations of dogs diagnosed in life as having valvular lesions, despite the distorting influence of tissues on the conduction of sound.

There are no significant structural peculiarities of the canine heart, although it may be noted that the right atrioventricular valve possesses only two major cusps in many (perhaps most) dogs. No clinical significance attaches to the variation.

In North America many dogs are infested with large heartworms *(Dirofilaria immitis),* which occupy the pulmonary trunk and, in severe cases, the right ventricle, atrium, and caudal vena cava.

The heart of the cat extends from the third (or fourth) to the sixth (or seventh) rib. Little is covered by the forelimb in the standing animal because the triceps reaches no farther than the fourth rib. The long axis of the heart forms a more acute angle with the sternum, which results in a greater area of sternal contact than in most dogs. The contractions are strongest near the ventral ends of the fourth to sixth ribs on the left and the fifth rib on the right (Fig. 13.20). The corresponding puncta maxima are as follows: the left atrioventricular valve—in the fifth and sixth intercostal spaces, level with the shoulder joint; the pulmonary and aortic valves—low in the left second and third intercostal spaces; and the right atrioventricular valve—level with the shoulder joint in the fourth and fifth intercostal spaces. Puncture is difficult because the organ is so small; a needle inserted on either side of the right fifth costochondral junction should enter a ventricle.

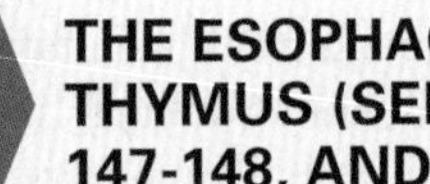

THE ESOPHAGUS, TRACHEA, AND THYMUS (SEE ALSO PP. 110-111, 147-148, AND 250-251)

The *esophagus* enters the thoracic cavity to the left of the trachea but gradually assumes a median position above the trachea within the cranial mediastinum, where it is related

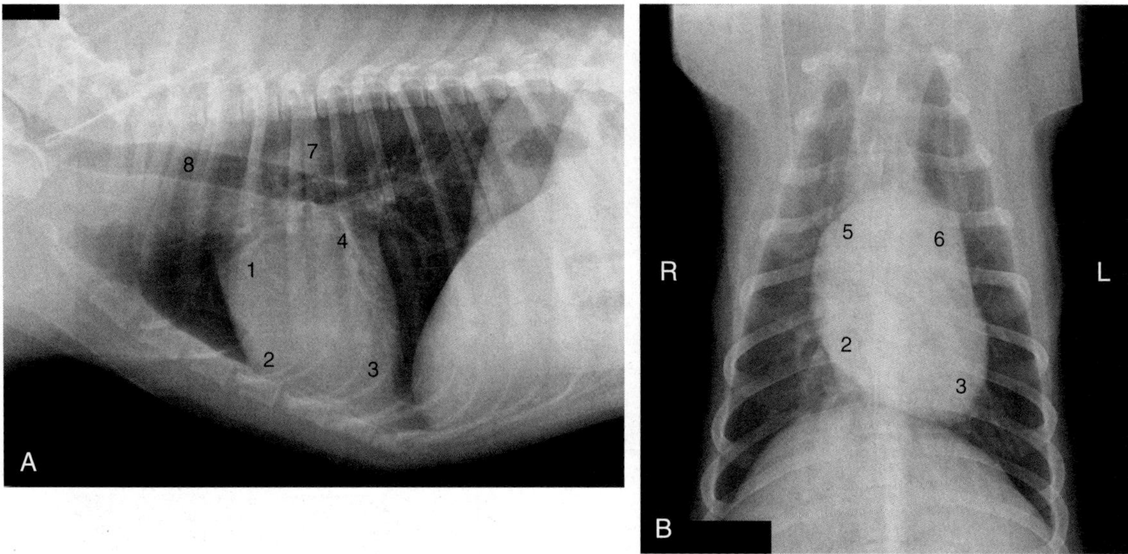

Fig. 13.17 (A) Lateral and (B) ventrodorsal views of the position of the canine heart. *1,* Right auricle; *2,* right ventricle; *3,* left ventricle; *4,* left atrium; *5,* right atrium; *6,* pulmonary trunk; *7,* aorta; *8,* trachea; *L,* left; *R,* right.

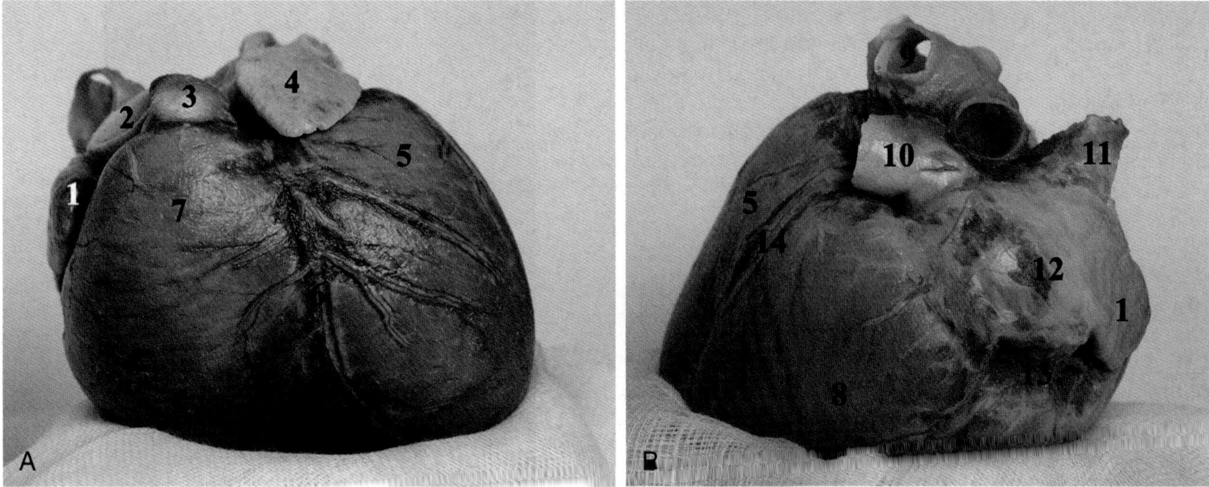

Fig. 13.18 Heart of the dog, (A) auricular surface and (B) right side. *1,* Right auricle; *2,* aorta; *3,* pulmonary trunk; *4,* left auricle; *5,* left ventricle; *6,* interventricular paraconal groove and paraconal interventricular branch of the left coronary artery; *7,* conus arteriosus of the right ventricle; *8,* right ventricle; *9,* pulmonary veins; *10,* caudal vena cava; *11,* cranial vena cava; *12,* sinus venarum cavarum.

to the left subclavian artery, which intervenes between it and the left lung (see Fig. 13.14). It continues dorsal to the trachea and subsequently to the left principal bronchus, where it crosses the heart before passing between the aorta and the azygos vein. Inclusion between these vessels and perhaps also the slight rise over the tracheal bifurcation predispose this part of the esophagus to obstruction by foreign bodies. A potentially more serious interference may be provided by the anomaly in which the right aortic arch persists as part of a constricting ring composed of the aorta to the right, the ligamentum arteriosum dorsally, and the pulmonary trunk and right pulmonary artery to the left (see Fig. 7.2D). More caudally, the esophagus rests on the left atrium and then on the accessory lobe of the right lung before reaching the hiatus in the diaphragm below the 10th thoracic vertebra. A slight narrowing here provides another site for obstruction. The chief blood supply from the bronchoesophageal artery is supplemented by direct branches from the aorta; the most caudal stretch is supplied by branches of the left gastric artery.

Cranial to the heart, a surgical approach to the esophagus is easier from the left. The right approach is favored

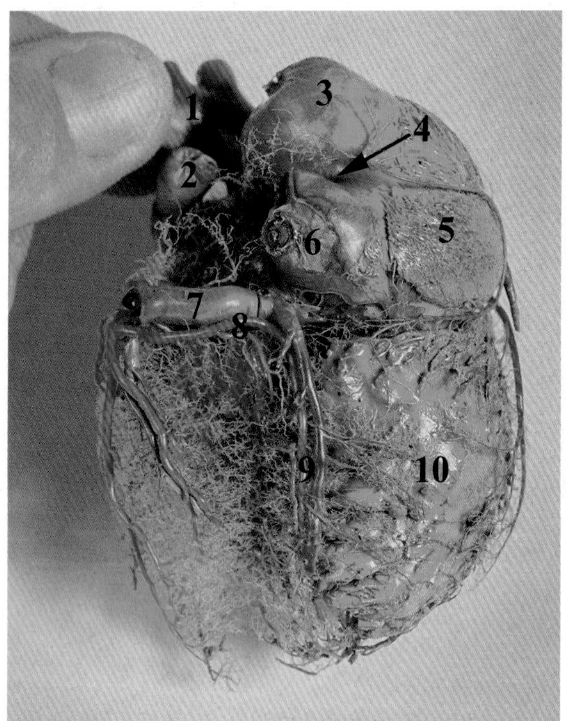

Fig. 13.19 Corrosion cast of the dog's heart (caudal, atrial surface). *1,* Aortic arch; *2,* pulmonary trunk; *3,* cranial vena cava; *4,* impression for the intervenosus tubercle; *5,* right atrium; *6,* caudal vena cava; *7,* vena cordis magna; *8,* circumflex branch of the left coronary artery; *9,* ramus interventricularis subsinosus artery and vena cordis media; *10,* right atrium.

TABLE 13.1 AUSCULTATION OF HEART VALVES

Valve	Intercostal Space
Left atrioventricular valve	Low in fifth on the left at costochondral junction
Pulmonary valve	Low in third on the left
Aortic valve	High in fourth on the left just below the horizontal plane of shoulder joint
Right atrioventricular valve	High in the fourth on the right and just little lower than the location of aorta

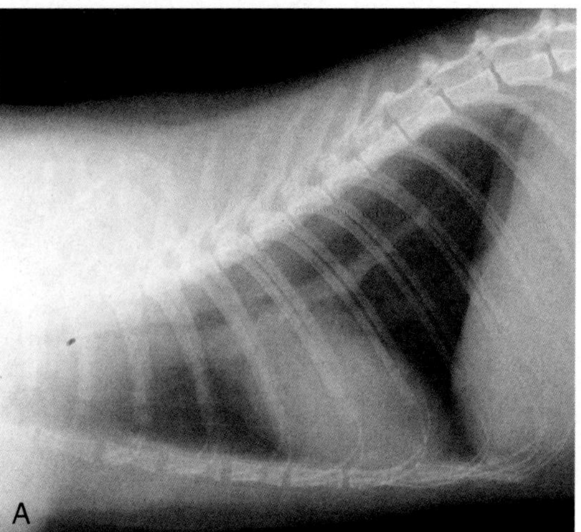

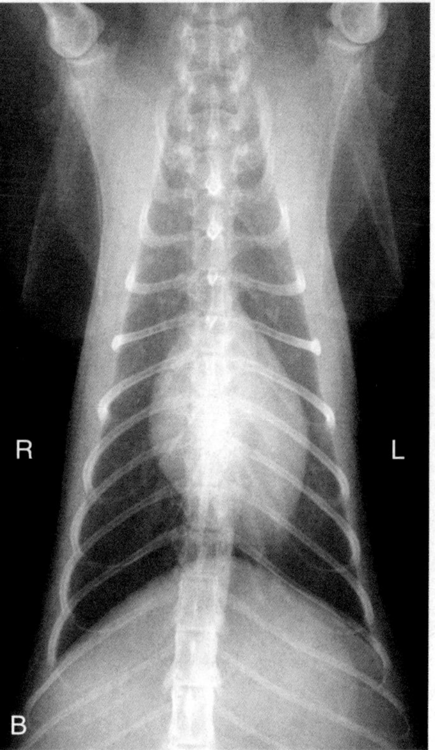

Fig. 13.20 (A) Lateral and (B) ventrodorsal radiographic views showing the position of the feline heart. The ventral ends of ribs 5, 6, and 7 lie on the heart shadow in (A).

at the level of the heart because the azygos vein may be ligated with impunity, unlike the aorta to the left. The caudal section is equally approachable from either side.

The muscle is striated throughout the length of the esophagus in both dog and cat. Only the caudal section is extensively covered by serosa. Glands are present in the submucosa only in the dog. The mucosa is thrown into ridges that are predominantly longitudinal throughout the length of the esophagus of the dog but become oblique in the caudal part of the esophagus of the cat. On barium contrast radiography these oblique folds of the esophagus portray a herringbone pattern caudal to the heart in cats (Fig. 13.21B).

The relationship of the *trachea* to the esophagus has been mentioned. The shift to a position ventral to the esophagus at the level of the aortic arch produces a caudally open angle that is a very prominent feature of lateral radiographs (Figs. 13.17/*8* and 13.20). Changes in this angle may reveal abnormalities of various cranial mediastinal structures. The relations of the trachea in this region are with the brachiocephalic trunk, common carotid arteries, and cranial vena cava. The trachea bifurcates below the fifth or sixth thoracic vertebra, where it lies above the base of the heart. It

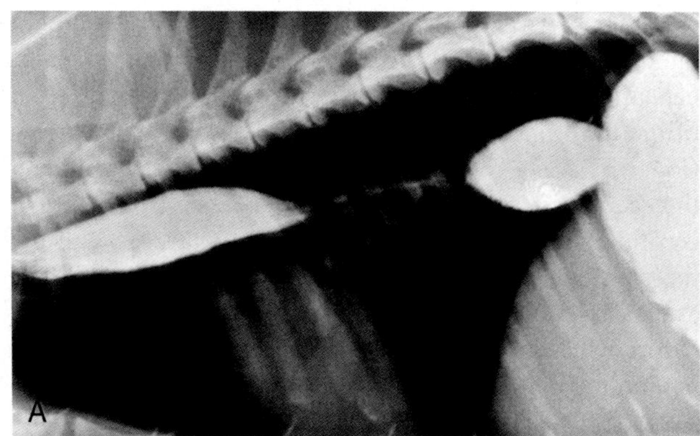

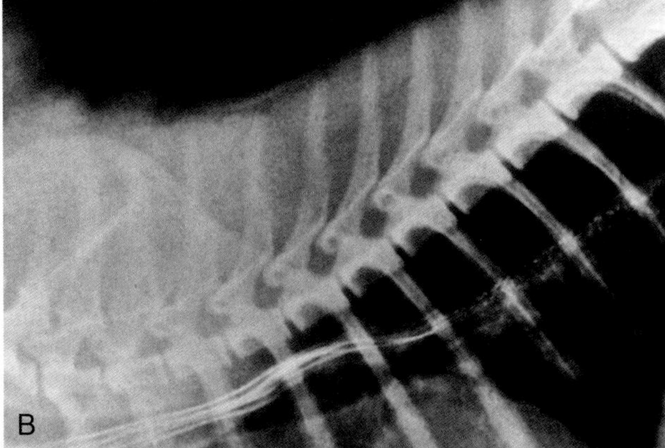

Fig. 13.21 Contrast medium in the esophagus of the (A) dog and (B) cat. Note the herringbone pattern caused by the oblique folds in the caudal part of the feline esophagus.

is continued by the divergent principal bronchi, of which the left is at a slightly more dorsal level despite having the esophagus resting on it.

There are two proposed measures for the evaluation of the tracheal diameter in lateral radiographs. According to one, the tracheal diameter at the level of the third rib should be about three times the width of that rib. The other asserts that the height of the trachea should be about half that of the thoracic inlet. When the latter criterion is used, dogs with severe tracheal hypoplasia can exhibit a ratio that is only a small fraction of the value described. In this condition the deformed tracheal rings are small and thickened and have ends that meet dorsally, displacing the tracheal muscle inward, toward the lumen. It may be part of a wider "brachycephalic syndrome." Stretches of trachea reduced in size but otherwise normal have been recorded in dogs of certain large breeds. Collapse of the trachea along with abnormality of its cartilages, and sometimes also of those of the bronchi, occurs in dogs of miniature breeds.

In the dog, the *thymus* is confined to the thorax, where it occupies the ventral part of the cranial mediastinum, stretching from the thoracic inlet to the pericardium on which it is molded (Figs. 13.11, 13.14, and 13.22). A larger part of the thymus extends onto the left surface of the pericardium than onto the right, producing a characteristic shadow (sail sign) in dorsoventral radiographs of young dogs (those less than a year old). The thymus

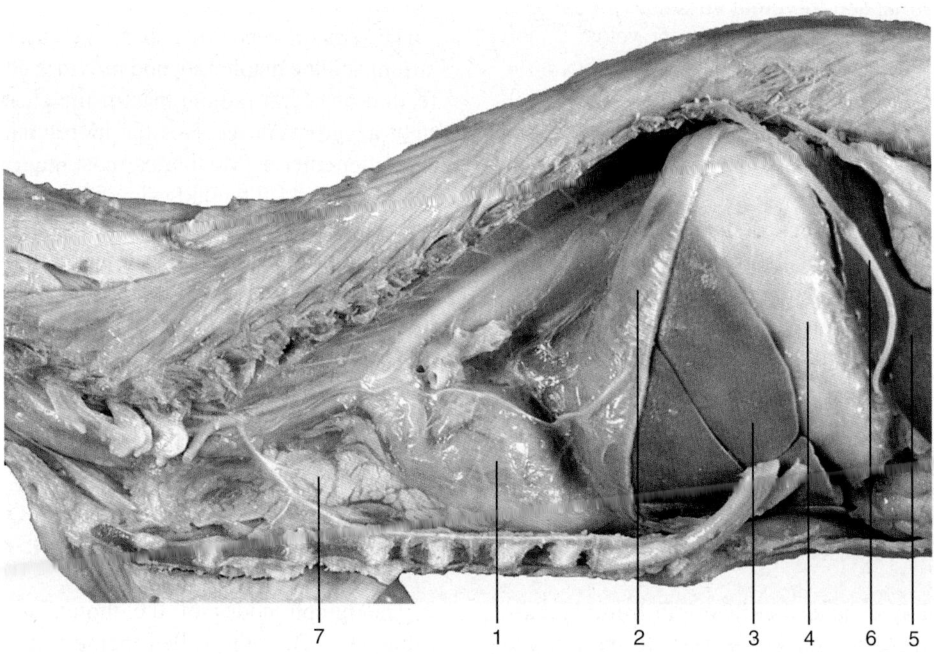

Fig. 13.22 Overview of the feline thorax, demonstrating the thymus. *1,* Heart; *2,* diaphragm; *3,* distended stomach (with attachment of greater omentum); *4,* spleen; *5,* duodenum; *6,* twelfth rib; *7,* thymus.

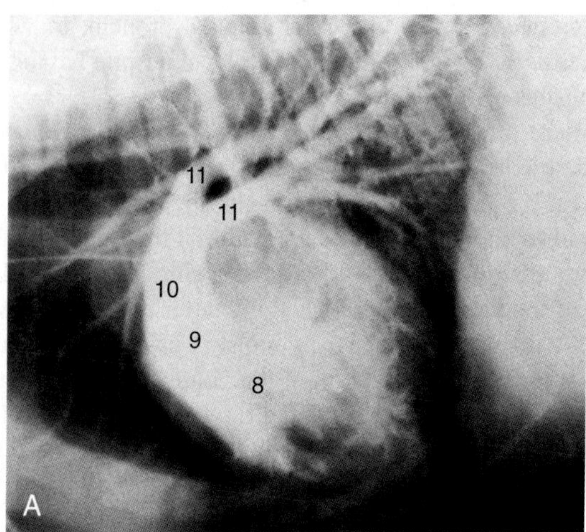

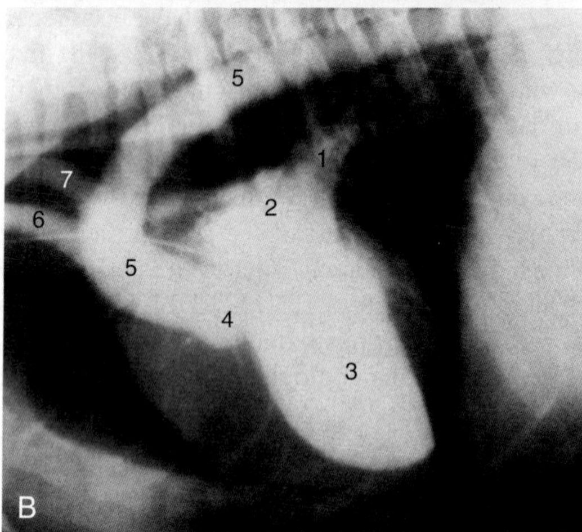

Fig. 13.23 Contrast medium in the canine (A) right and (B) left ventricles marking the great vessels. The catheter is in the cranial vena cava. *1,* Pulmonary veins; *2,* left atrium; *3,* left ventricle; *4,* position of aortic valve; *5,* aorta; *6,* brachiocephalic trunk; *7,* left subclavian artery; *8,* right ventricle; *9,* position of pulmonary valve; *10,* pulmonary trunk; *11,* pulmonary arteries.

consists of right and left lobes, is distinctly lobulated, is pink when fresh, and attains its greatest development at about 6 to 8 weeks. Regression begins about the fourth month but is never complete. Thymic neoplasms may compress the cranial vena cava and esophagus at the thoracic inlet.

THE GREAT VESSELS AND NERVES WITHIN THE THORAX (SEE ALSO PP. 229-230, 232, AND 314-315)

The *aorta* is slightly expanded at its origin from the base of the heart between the pulmonary trunk to the left and the right atrium to the right, providing room for the aortic valve (Fig. 13.23/*4*). It first passes craniodorsally before turning back to follow the vertebrae toward the diaphragm (see Fig. 13.14). Its arch, which is a prominent feature on lateral radiographs (Fig. 13.17/*7*), gives rise to the brachiocephalic trunk and, a short distance farther on at the level of the third intercostal space, to the left subclavian artery (Fig. 13.14/*2*). The brachiocephalic trunk lies ventral to the esophagus and trachea and detaches the two common carotid arteries that accompany these organs through the thoracic inlet before it continues as the right subclavian artery. The subclavian artery gradually shifts to the right before winding around the first rib to enter the forelimb. It is reported that the loss of a subclavian artery is compensated by the enlargement of collateral connections with the vertebral and other arteries.

The *pulmonary trunk* arises from the craniosinistral aspect of the base of the heart to the left of the aorta. It passes dorsocaudally before dividing into divergent left and right pulmonary arteries (Fig. 13.23A/*10* and *11*). Shortly before its division, it is connected to the aorta by the ligamentum arteriosum. The right pulmonary artery, slightly larger than the left, passes across the base of the heart between the venae cavae. Each artery detaches a branch to the cranial lobe before entering the lung for further ramification.

The *cranial vena cava* passes ventral to the trachea, to the right of the brachiocephalic trunk, and in contact with the esophagus on the left side (see Fig. 13.15). It is the most ventral of the major structures that pass through the thoracic inlet and is formed cranial to the inlet by the union of the two brachiocephalic veins, each with tributaries corresponding to the branches of a subclavian artery (see Fig. 7.36), and is augmented by the addition of an external jugular vein.

The *caudal vena cava* spans the gap between the right atrium and the diaphragm and provides a very conspicuous feature of lateral radiographs of the chest. In the dog the right azygos vein receives the more cranial lumbar veins and, after entering the thorax, most intercostal veins; these vessels provide potentially significant connections with the internal vertebral venous plexus. The azygos vein ends by descending in front of the root of the right lung to join the cranial vena cava shortly before the latter opens into the right atrium opposite the third intercostal space.

There are no specific features of interest in the formation, course, or distribution of the phrenic, vagus, and sympathetic nerves.

LYMPHATIC STRUCTURES OF THE THORAX (SEE ALSO PP. 245-247)

The lymph nodes of the thorax are summarized in Table 13.2. The thin-walled thoracic duct begins between the crura of the diaphragm as the continuation of the cisterna chyli. It accompanies the aorta and azygos vein forward and, level with the heart, passes obliquely to the left,

TABLE 13.2 **THORACIC LYMPH NODES**

Lymph Node	Location	Area(s) Drained	Efferent Flow
Intercostal lymph node (see Fig. 7.55/*6*)	Under the pleura at dorsal end of fifth or sixth intercostal space	Dorsal thoracic wall	To cranial mediastinal nodes
Sternal lymph nodes (see Fig. 7.55/*10*)	Beside the sternum at level of second rib	Ventral thoracic wall, diaphragm, mediastinum, and perhaps along with axillary from first three pairs of mammary glands	Directly into veins at thoracic inlet
Cranial mediastinal lymph nodes (see Fig. 7.55/*8*)	With large blood vessels in front of the heart	Mediastinal structures, tracheobronchial nodes, and deep muscles at the base of the neck	Directly into veins at thoracic inlet
Tracheobronchial lymph nodes (Fig. 13.13A)	At tracheobronchial junctions	Lungs, mediastinal structures, and the diaphragm	To cranial mediastinal lymph nodes

crossing the esophagus, to gain a position within the left side of the cranial mediastinum. It follows the esophagus to the thoracic inlet, where it opens into one or other of the larger veins. However, occasionally it ends more caudally by joining the azygos vein or even opening into one of the mediastinal lymph nodes. The duct, which has a diameter of 2 to 3 mm in a medium-sized dog, may be plexiform (see Fig. 7.57). Within the chest it receives additional lymph from various thoracic structures and nodes of the left side; a separate right lymphatic duct provides similar drainage for structures of the right side. One or both commonly receive the corresponding tracheal duct(s). In cats the thoracic duct courses from the left dorsal aspect of the aorta to terminate in the left jugular vein. In both species the thoracic duct may have multiple collaterals.

COMPREHENSION CHECK

Develop an understanding of projections of the lungs and the heart on the chest wall, and use that information for cardiac and pulmonary auscultation.

14 The Abdomen of the Dog and Cat

CONFORMATION AND SURFACE ANATOMY

The cranial boundary of the accessible abdominal wall is easily determined by palpation of the last rib and costal arch. The caudal boundary is discovered from palpation of the ventral part (pecten ossis pubis) of the pelvic inlet between the thighs. Although the wings of the ilia are prominent landmarks, they pertain to the back. The covering of thick muscles does not allow palpation of the lumbar transverse processes themselves, but the tips of the spinous processes provide a guide to the identification of individual vertebrae.

The abdominal cavity is of course larger than these landmarks appear to indicate because the diaphragm bulges far into the rib cage at its cranial end. The organs in this intrathoracic part of the abdomen are protected by the ribs and are in part overlain by the caudal lobes of the lungs. The abdominal cavity is relatively less voluminous than in the large domestic species and has, by and large, the shape of a cone with a bulbous cranial base (Fig. 14.1). Its longitudinal axis, which is steepest in deep-chested breeds, inclines cranioventrally at an angle that varies considerably. Except in fat subjects and heavily pregnant or lactating bitches, the ventral abdominal wall rises from the sternum to the pecten in a straight or even slightly concave line. Dog fanciers use the expression "tucked-up" to describe animals with an especially shallow body depth at the loin. The skin fold that connects the flank with the stifle tends to obscure the shallowness of this part. Advancing pregnancy enlarges the abdomen in both depth and breadth and gives it a more cylindrical or even a barrel shape.

Superficial inguinal lymph nodes may be palpated in the groin, lateral to the bulbus glandis of the penis or in a comparable site in the bitch (Fig. 14.2B/*6*).

MAMMARY GLANDS

The *mammary glands* contribute to the contours during pregnancy and lactation. Dogs generally have five pairs of mammary glands and the cat has four pairs, spread along the ventral aspect of the trunk (see Figs. 10.31C and 10.32B and C). The two cranial pairs are thoracic, the next two abdominal, and the caudalmost pair inguinal in position. A distinct midline separation is noted between the left and right mammary chains. The often staggered pattern makes all teats equally accessible to the pups when the bitch suckles lying on her side. The glands are very small in the virgin (with the teats hidden by hair) but become very swollen, pendulous, and confluent with their ipsilateral neighbors toward parturition and during lactation. The size increase is nearly 10-fold in the cat. They regress greatly in the parous but nonpregnant and nonlactating bitch. The teats, which

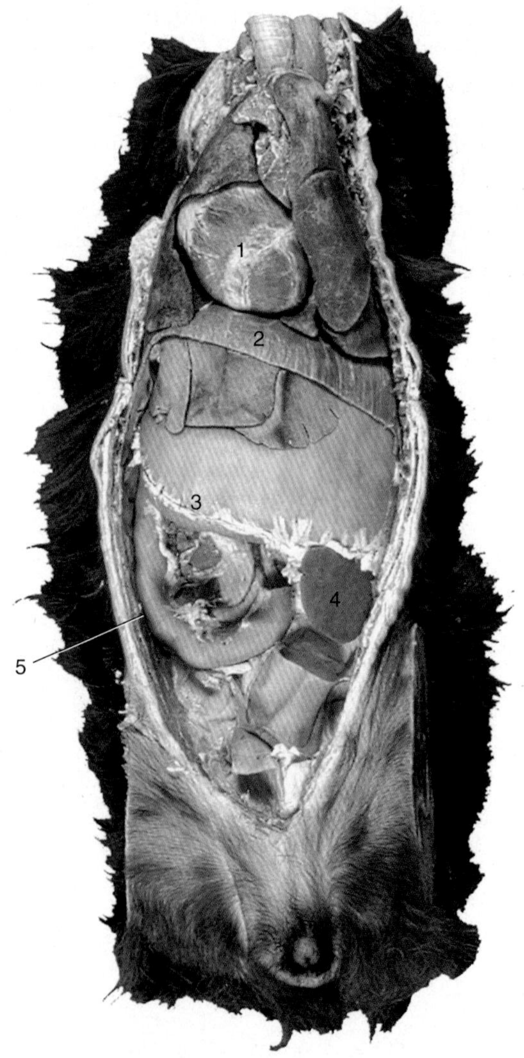

Fig. 14.1 Ventral view of a canine trunk, demonstrating the so-called intrathoracic part of the abdomen. *1,* Heart; *2,* diaphragm; *3,* distended stomach (with attachment of greater omentum); *4,* spleen; *5,* duodenum.

occur in rudimentary form in males, are bare and perforated at their tips by 10 or 12 fine openings in the dog and 4 to 8 openings in the cat.

In dogs and cats, the lateral and internal thoracic and external pudendal arteries are the major sources of blood supply to the mammary glands. The veins are satellite. Both arteries and veins anastomose freely, forming arterial and venous plexuses (Fig. 14.2A), which may cross the midline.

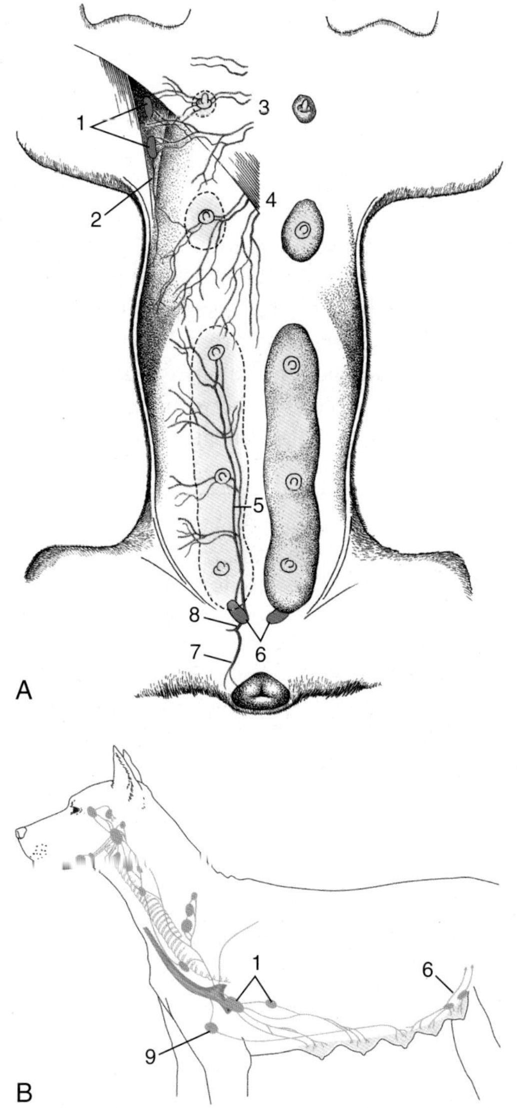

Fig. 14.2 Blood vessels (red) and lymphatics (green) of the canine mammary glands. (A) Ventral view of the mammary glands, blood vessels, and certain lymph nodes. (B) Lateral view of regional lymph nodes. *1,* Axillary and accessory axillary lymph nodes; *2,* branch of lateral thoracic artery; *3,* perforating branches of internal thoracic vessels; *4,* branches of the cranial superficial epigastric vessels; *5,* caudal superficial epigastric artery; *6,* superficial inguinal lymph nodes; *7,* ventral labial branch to vulva; *8,* external pudendal artery; *9,* sternal lymph node.

The lymph drainage pathways are erratic, and some lymph may cross the midline. It is said that in the cat the lymph vessels do not cross the midline nor penetrate the thoracic wall (Table 14.1). The superficial inguinal nodes and caudal glands are related to the vaginal process, which is vulnerable during surgical removal of a diseased gland; injury to the process may cause inadvertent opening of the peritoneal cavity. In both species the superficial inguinal nodes drain the adjacent part of the abdominal wall in addition to the caudal mammary glands. These details of lymph drainage are important because of the high prevalence of mammary tumors in both dogs and cats. In bitches they are the commonest of all tumors and show a disturbingly high (ca. 50%) incidence of malignancy. Although somewhat less common in cats, mammary tumors are even more likely to be malignant in this species.

THE ABDOMINAL WALL (SEE ALSO pp. 47-49)

Abdominal surgery is frequently performed in dogs and cats. Therefore, it is necessary to be familiar with the details even though the ventrolateral abdominal wall is constructed in a common pattern with only a few distinct features mainly concerning the linea alba and rectus sheath; these along with the inguinal canal are more fully described here.

The *linea alba* is the fibrous seam in which the aponeuroses of the right and left oblique and transverse abdominal muscles come together. It extends from the xiphoid process to the pubis and includes the umbilicus at about the level of the third lumbar vertebra. The linea alba is about 1 cm* wide cranial to the umbilicus but gradually narrows behind this point and is reduced to a barely visible line in its caudal third (see Fig. 2.26). Incisions through the linea alba spare the muscles, vessels, and nerves and avoids retraction of the parietal peritoneum from incision edges, which occurs with a median incision. The falciform ligament (see later) and the median ligament of the bladder attach to the dorsal surface of the linea alba, cranial and caudal to the umbilicus, respectively. Umbilical hernias, often associated with an over-wide linea alba and hypoplastic rectus muscles, are common.

The *rectus sheath* is formed by the aponeuroses of the oblique and transverse abdominal muscles. In the dog and cat the aponeuroses of the external and internal oblique muscles pass ventrally (externally) to the rectus muscle over the length of the linea alba. However, the most cranial portion of the internal oblique muscle also detaches an additional lamina that passes dorsally (internally) to the rectus (see Fig. 2.26A). The aponeurosis of the transverse abdominal muscle passes dorsally (internally) to the rectus

*Where we give an indication of weight or measure, we have in mind a subject of the size of a beagle, an animal weighing about 15 to 20 kg. Cats or course vary less if we exclude such atypical breeds as the Maine Coon.

TABLE 14.1 BLOOD SUPPLY AND LYMPH DRAINAGE OF MAMMARY GLANDS

Mammary Glands	Blood supply	Lymph Drainage
Cranial three in dogs and two in cats	Craniolaterally by lateral thoracic artery (from the axillary) and deeply by cranial superficial epigastric artery and perforating branches of the intercostal arteries from the internal thoracic	Axillary, accessory axillary, and sternal nodes; the 3rd pair may also drain caudally;
Two caudal pairs	Caudal superficial epigastric artery from the external pudendal and deeply from the cranial abdominal and deep circumflex iliac arteries	Superficial inguinal (mammary) node in the dog and the caudal epigastric nodes in the cat

muscle in the cranial half of the abdomen, but it changes position to the ventral surface in the caudal portion, leaving the dorsal surface of the rectus covered only by fascia and peritoneum (see Fig. 2.23B). The rectus muscle is adherent to its sheath only at the tendinous inscriptions.

The *inguinal canal* is a potential space between the external and internal abdominal oblique muscles that extends between deep and superficial openings (rings). The deep ring leads from the canal into the abdominal cavity, and the superficial ring leads from the canal to the subcutaneous tissues of the groin. The canal conveys the external pudendal vessels and the genitofemoral nerve in both the sexes, the spermatic cord in the dog and tom, and the vaginal process in the bitch and queen. These all emerge at the superficial inguinal ring, a nearly sagittal slit in the external abdominal oblique aponeurosis about 3 cm lateral to the linea alba, close to where it attaches on the pubis (see Fig. 2.27A/*4'*). Only the caudal end of the ring is palpable. The narrow strip of aponeurosis (see Fig. 2.27A between *4'* and *6*) lateral to the ring forms the only barrier between the structures emerging from the canal and the large femoral vessels and saphenous nerve as they enter the thigh through the vascular lacuna (see Fig. 2.27/*6*).

The deep inguinal ring is visible only from within the abdomen. It is bounded caudolaterally by the caudal border of the external abdominal oblique aponeurosis (*inguinal ligament*), cranially by the unattached border (caudal edge) of the internal abdominal oblique muscle, and medially by the rectus muscle (see Fig. 2.27B). None of these boundaries is palpable in the intact animal. The parietal peritoneum that covers the ring evaginates through the inguinal canal and, then named the vaginal tunic, accompanies the spermatic cord into the scrotum. In the bitch and queen it envelops the round ligament of the uterus and is known as the vaginal process, which is not present in females of other domestic species and is the occasional recipient of herniated abdominal organs (see Chapter 15).

Blood Supply

The ventral abdominal wall is supplied by four paired arteries that come from the sternal and pelvic region. The *cranial superficial epigastric artery* branches off the internal thoracic artery and runs between the abdominal muscles and the skin (Table 14.1). It supplies the region cranial to the level of the umbilicus (it is enlarged in the lactating bitch). The *cranial epigastric artery* runs deep to the rectus, between it and its sheath. The *caudal superficial epigastric artery*, a branch of the external pudendal, is distributed subcutaneously and also supplies the prepuce. The *caudal epigastric artery* arises from the pudendoepigastric trunk and passes forward, first along the lateral border and then on the deep surface of the rectus muscle (see Figs. 14.3 and 2.26). Cranial and caudal sets of vessels anastomose (Fig. 14.2).

Paracentesis of the abdominal wall is most safely performed a short distance caudolateral to the umbilicus to avoid both the fat-filled falciform ligament and risk of injury to a full bladder. The *falciform ligament,* which carries the round ligament of the liver in its free border, is the remnant of the ventral mesogastrium that conveyed the umbilical vein from the umbilicus to the liver in the fetus. The part adjacent to the liver survives, if at all, as a simple peritoneal fold. The blood supply of the falciform ligament arises from along the length of the linea alba. The ligament commonly serves as a major fat storage depot and may become so thickened and enlarged that it complicates the opening and closure of a midline abdominal incision (Fig. 14.13), especially in dogs. Part or all of this obstruction may be excised; care must be taken to place a ligature at the cranial end, before the ligament is totally removed.

GENERAL ASPECTS OF VISCERAL TOPOGRAPHY

The *greater omentum* is extremely well developed and is folded on itself to form a flat sac with superficial and deep leaves that intervene between the intestinal mass and the abdominal floor (see Fig. 3.33). This is the reason that the small intestines are not immediately visible when the abdominal floor is removed (Fig. 14.4). However, the ventral part of the spleen projecting beyond the left

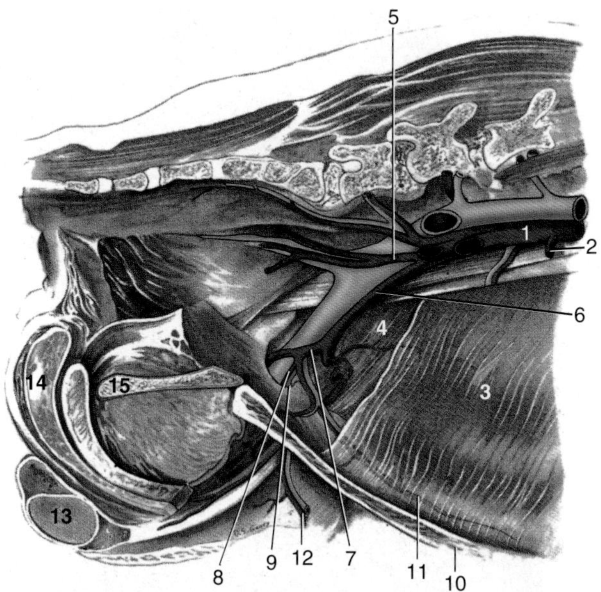

Fig. 14.3 Abdominal wall and pelvic canal of the male dog, showing the breakup of the aorta; medial view. *1,* Aorta; *2,* caudal mesenteric artery (a.); *3,* transversus abdominis; *4,* internal abdominal oblique muscle (m.); *5,* internal iliac a.; *6,* external iliac a.; *7,* deep femoral a.; *8,* pudendoepigastric trunk; *9,* deep inguinal ring; *10,* rectus abdominis m.; *11,* caudal epigastric a.; *12,* external pudendal a.; *13,* left testis; *14,* bulb of the penis; *15,* pelvic symphysis.

costal arch, a part of liver behind the xiphoid process, and the bladder directly before the pubis are visible when the abdominal wall or the floor is removed (Figs. 14.5, 14.6, 14.7, 14.8, and 14.9). The omental bursa exists as a potential space between the leaves. The opening to the omental bursa, the epiploic foramen, is a narrow passage that lies medial to the caudate process of the liver and is bounded dorsally by the caudal vena cava and ventrally by the portal vein.

Being the dorsal mesogastrium, the greater omentum attaches to the greater curvature of the embryonic stomach, as in other species. It arises from the roof of the abdominal cavity, near the caudal part of the liver and the celiac artery. Close to this attachment the left lobe of the pancreas is enclosed in the omentum. The dorsal attachment of the omentum runs between the esophageal hiatus and the epiploic foramen. At this point the greater omentum continues as mesoduodenum, in which the right lobe of the pancreas is situated. The omental bursa is connected to a hilus of the spleen by the gastrosplenic ligament. The omentum is connected to the descending colon caudally by the omental veil.

The superficial leaf of greater omentum (see Fig. 3.33/*14*) passes caudally from its attachment, in direct contact with the ventral abdominal wall to reach the bladder, where it is reflected dorsally to become the deep leaf (see Fig. 3.33/*13*). This structure runs forward between the superficial leaf and coils of the jejunum; at the cranial

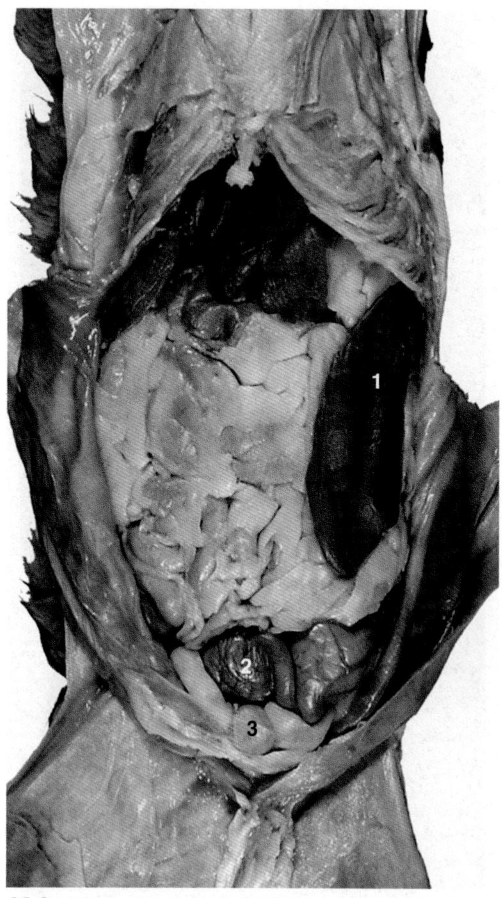

Fig. 14.4 Ventral view of feline abdominal viscera; intestinal loops are concealed by fat-filled greater omentum. *1,* Spleen; *2,* part of gravid uterus with two ampullae; *3,* bladder.

end of the jejunum it passes dorsally, against the caudal (visceral) surface of the stomach, to reach the left lobe of the pancreas, which it encloses and by means of which it gains the roof of the abdominal cavity. The right border of the omental sac is ventral to the descending duodenum. The left extends more dorsally to the level of the kidney and sublumbar muscles and is complicated by an attachment to a hilus of the spleen. The part of the omentum extending between the left crus of the diaphragm and the splenic hilus may be known as the phrenicosplenic ligament. The more generous part between the stomach and hilus forms the gastrosplenic ligament. As a further complication, a sagittal fold (omental veil) with a caudal free border connects the deep leaf with the left surface of the descending mesocolon. The greater omentum always contains fat. , which is first deposited along the small omental vessels, giving the structure a lacy appearance; however, in obese dogs (less so in cats) it forms a more or less continuous layer.

The *lesser omentum* is considerably wider than the short space it has to bridge between the lesser curvature of the stomach and the liver. It blends on the right with

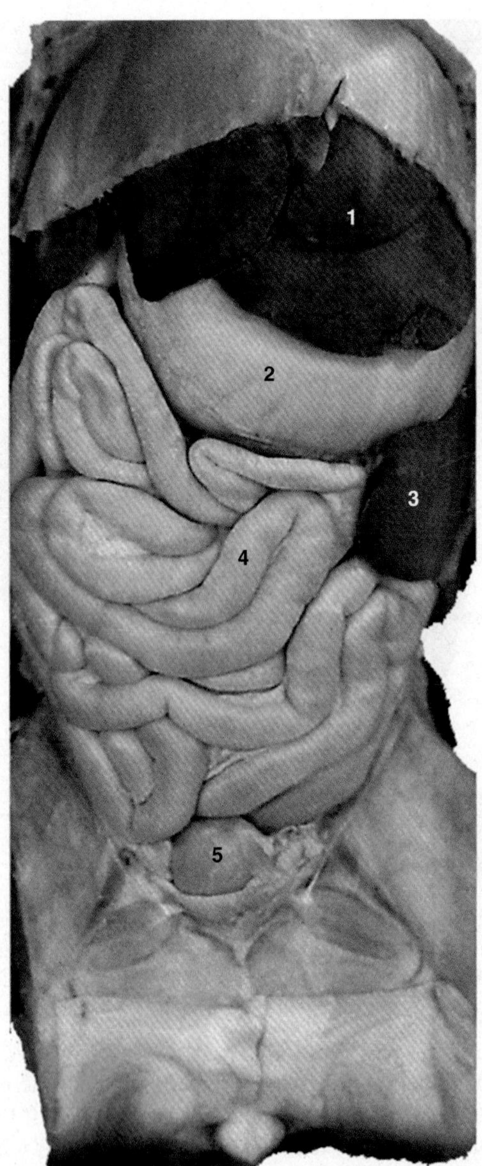

Fig. 14.5 Abdominal viscera of the dog after removal of the greater omentum. *1*, Liver; *2*, stomach; *3*, spleen; *4*, small intestine; *5*, bladder.

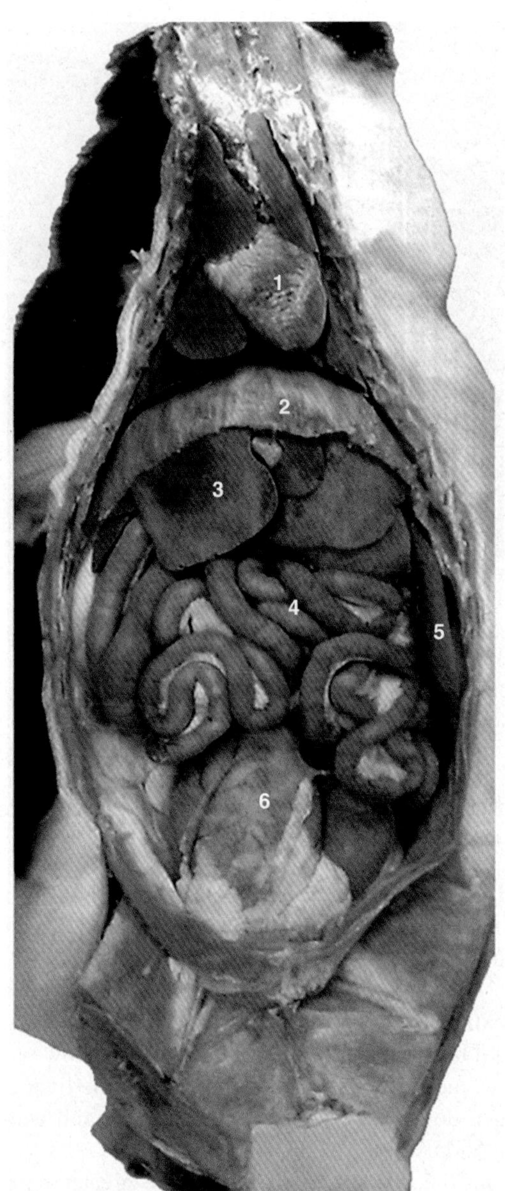

Fig. 14.6 Ventral view of feline viscera after removal of omentum. *1*, Heart; *2*, diaphragm; *3*, liver; *4*, intestine; *5*, spleen; *6*, bladder.

the mesoduodenum, the bile duct marking the boundary between the two. The papillary process of the liver is loosely enveloped by the lesser omentum. The portion of the lesser omentum between the liver and the duodenum is also called the *hepatoduodenal ligament,* and the portion between the liver and the stomach is called the *hepatogastric ligament.*

THE SPLEEN

The spleen (see also p. 249) in dogs and cats is an elongated, roughly dumbbell-shaped organ that lies more or less vertically against the left abdominal wall (Fig. 14.10A/*4*). Its position is much influenced by the distention of the stomach (and by its own capacity to become engorged). The dorsal end reaches the left crus of the diaphragm, passing between the gastric fundus and the cranial pole of the left kidney under cover of (usually) the last two ribs. The larger ventral end may cross the ventral midline, to reach under the costal cartilages of the right side. It then provides a dense triangular shadow on the abdominal floor in lateral radiographs (Fig. 1 4.11A/*3*). A similar shadow between the stomach and left kidney may reveal the position of the organ in ventrodorsal radiographs. In the cat, the ventral part of the spleen is always located outside the rib cage. The parietal surface makes contact (in dorsoventral sequence) with the diaphragm, costal arch, and abdominal muscles. The visceral surface is divided by a hilar ridge

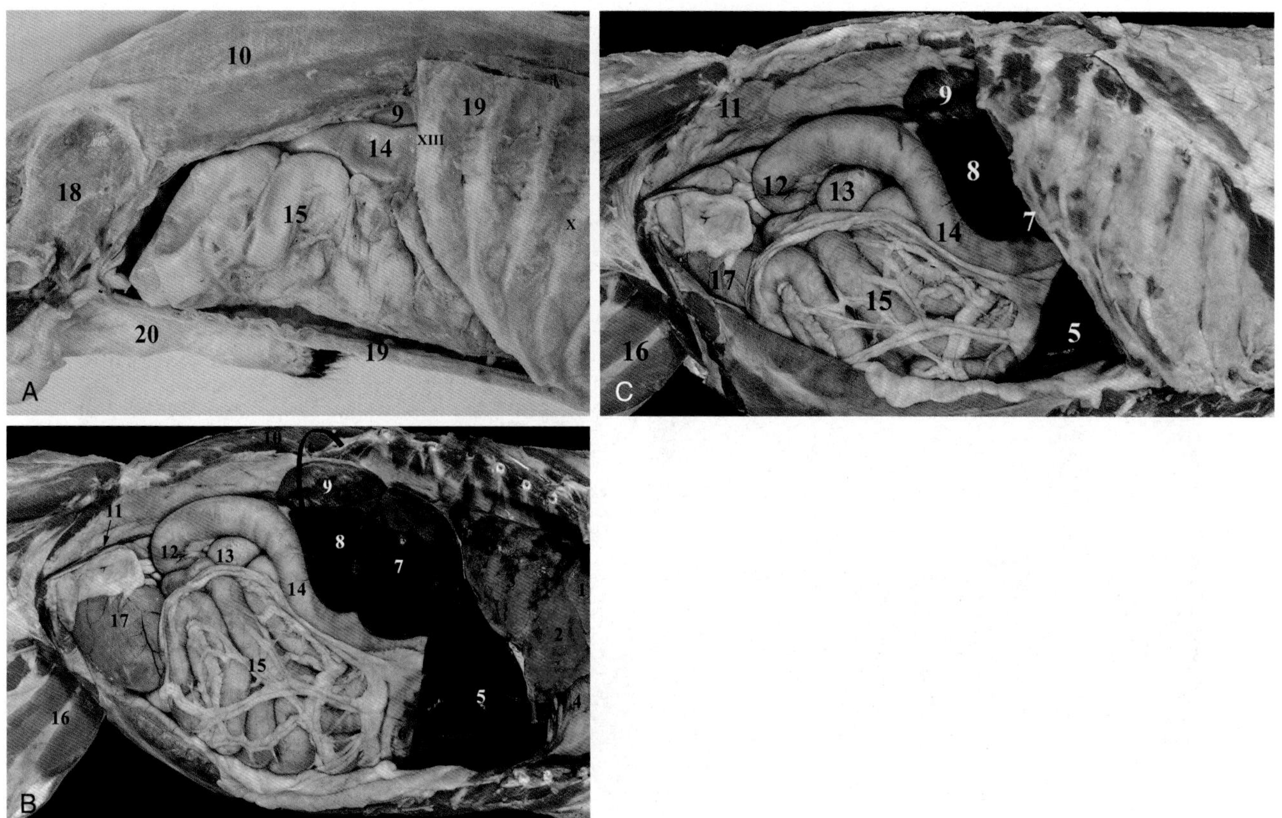

Fig. 14.7 Abdominal cavity of the dog with right abdominal wall removed (A and B) and the ribs removed (B). The black line in B indicates the position of the last rib. *1.* Cranial lobe of the right lung; *2.* Middle lobe of the right lung; *3.* Caudal lobe of the right lung; 4. Heart; 5. Right medial lobe of the liver; *6.* Stomach, greater curvature; *7.* Right lateral lobe of the liver; *8.* Caudate process of the caudate lobe of the liver; *9.* Right kidney; *10.* Longissimus lumborum muscle; *11.* Testicular artery and vein in the genital fold; *12.* Caudal duodenal flexure; *13.* Cecum; *14.* Descending duodenum; *15.* Jejunal loops, covered by the greater omentum; *16.* Sartorius muscle (cranial and caudal part); *17.* Urinary blader; *18.* Ilium (pelvis); *19.* Abdominal muscles (cut); *20.* Bulbus glandis X, XIII: ribs

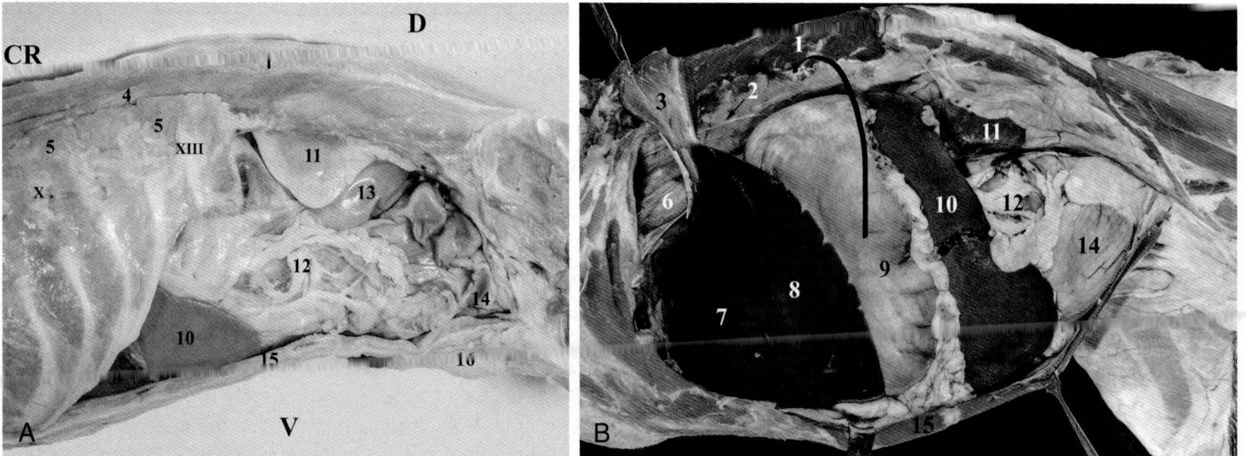

Fig. 14.8 Abdominal cavity of the dog viewed from left side (A) and with ribs removed (B): *1.* Longissimus lumborum muscle; *2.* Sympathetic trunk; *3.* Diaphragm (reflected); *4.* Iliocostalis thoracis muscle; *5.* Serratus dorsalis muscle (caudal part); *6.* Esophagus and the dorsal trunk of the vagus nerve; 7. Left medial lobe of the liver; *8.* Left lateral lobe of the liver; *9.* Stomach; *10.* Spleen; *11.* Left kidney; *12.* Jejunal loops, covered by the greater omentum; *13.* Descending colon *14.* Urinary blader; *15.* Abdominal muscles (cut); black line represents the last (XIII.) rib

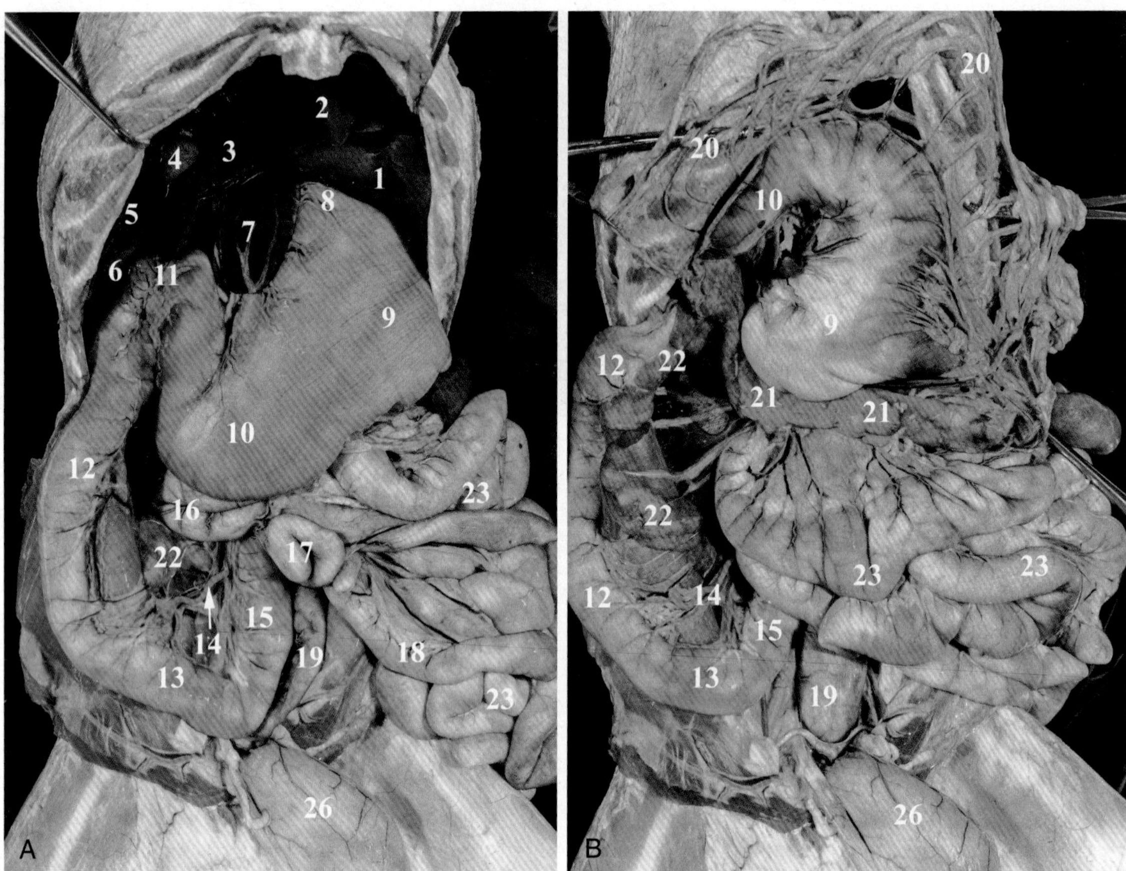

Fig. 14.9 Abdominal cavity of the dog, jejunum flipped to the left (A), stomach and the greater omentum flipped cranially (B), and small intestine removed, colon flipped to the right (fresh specimens): *1.* Left lateral lobe of the liver; *2.* Left medial lobe of the liver; *3.* Quadrate lobe of the liver; *4.* Gallblader; *5.* Right medial lobe of the liver; *6.* Right lateral lobe of the liver *7.* Papillary process of the caudal lobe of the liver (covered by the lesser omentum); *8.* Stomach, cardia; *9.* Stomach, fundus *10.* Stomach, pyloric part; *11.* Cranial duodenal flexure; *12.* Descending duodenum; *13.* Caudal duodenal flexure; *14.* Caudal pancreaticoduodenal artery and vein; *15.* Ascending duodenum ; *16.* Ascending colon; *17.* Cecum; *18.* Ileum; *19.* Descending colon; *22.* Pancreas, right lobe; *23.* Jejunal loops, flipped to the left side; *26.* Urinary blader.

into a cranial strip related to the stomach and a caudal strip related to the left kidney and intestine.

The wide gastrosplenic ligament attaches the spleen to the greater curvature of the stomach, affecting the latter's mobility and location. When the stomach enlarges, the spleen is displaced caudally and ventrally, reaching the pelvic inlet. It may then be palpated through the abdominal wall.

The blood vessels also exert another restraining influence on the spleen. The splenic artery and vein pass (as several divergent branches) to the dorsal end of the spleen. The splenic artery arises as a branch of the celiac artery, and before reaching the spleen, it gives off branches to the left limb of the pancreas. The left gastroepiploic vessels are detached about the middle of the hilus and cross to the greater curvature of the stomach within the gastrosplenic ligament (Fig. 14.12/*3* and *11*). The splenic lymph nodes lie near the splenic vessels, a few centimeters distant from the organ. The spleen has efferent lymphatic vessels (which follow large arteries) but no afferent vessels.

Spleen Function: The spleen serves as an important blood reservoir in the dog and cat, and its size and weight therefore vary widely (Fig. 14.6). The spleen in a resting dog or cat contracts and relaxes rhythmically because of the presence of many smooth muscle fibers throughout the organ. These fibers relax when anesthetics are used, resulting in marked splenic enlargement, and contract because of stress or injection of catecholamines, expelling free blood cells and plasma from the red pulp. The spleen has no parasympathetic nerve supply.

Rupture of the spleen is not uncommon after traffic accidents, but fortunately the organ may be removed without risk to life. The relatively loose attachment of the spleen to the stomach facilitates access to the vascular supply at surgery (splenectomy). During splenectomy, it is important to spare branches of the splenic artery that contribute to the left gastroepiploic artery, which is essential to the integrity of the greater curvature of the stomach (see Figs. 3.39 and 14.12).

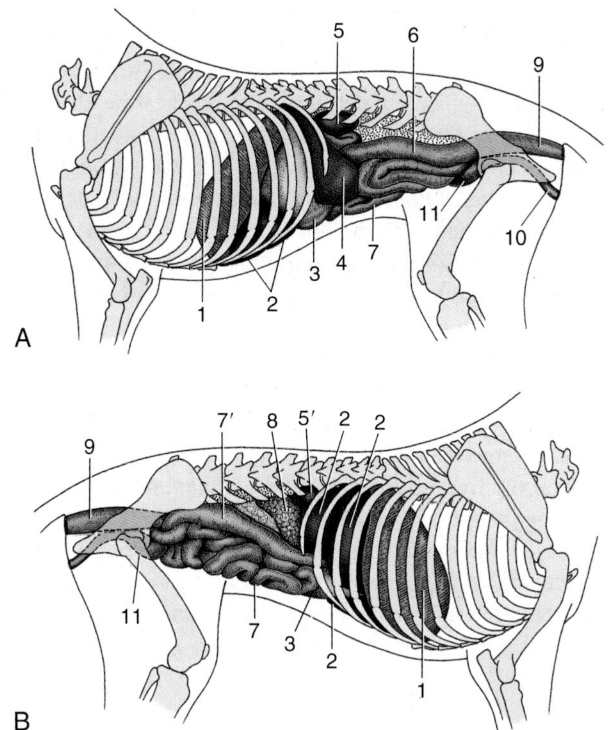

Fig. 14.10 Visceral projections on the (A) left and (B) right canine abdominal walls. *1,* Diaphragm; *2,* liver; *3,* stomach; *4,* spleen; *5* and *5′,* left and right kidneys; *6,* descending colon; *7,* small intestine; *7′,* descending duodenum; *8,* pancreas; *9,* rectum; *10,* female urogenital tract; *11,* bladder.

THE STOMACH

The dog has a simple stomach (see also pp. 115-119) that exhibits the idealized form described on page 125 only when moderately full. The fundus and body merge smoothly and are capable of great expansion, but the cylindrical and thicker-walled pyloric part is less able to enlarge. The fundus projects dorsally to the left of the cardia, against the liver. The cardia is generally wide, a feature that may be related to the ease with which dogs vomit. The pylorus, on the other hand, is narrow, and pyloric stenosis is not uncommon in the young. When the organ is quite empty, the body also becomes more or less cylindrical, and the fundus then forms a bulbous dorsal enlargement. When the organ is greatly distended, all parts except the pyloric canal merge in a common sac. The capacity of the stomach ranges from 0.5 to 6.0 L with the average about 2.5 L, making it relatively large in relation to body size.

The position and relations obviously depend on the degree of fullness but the cardia provides a fixed point opposite the ninth intercostal space. The fundus and body lie mainly to the left of the median plane, in contact with the diaphragm and liver, respectively, but the ventral part of the body crosses to the right before being continued by the pyloric part, which also lies against the liver (Fig. 14.11, 14.13 and 14.14). Indeed, the lesser curvature of the stomach is bound to the porta of the liver by the lesser

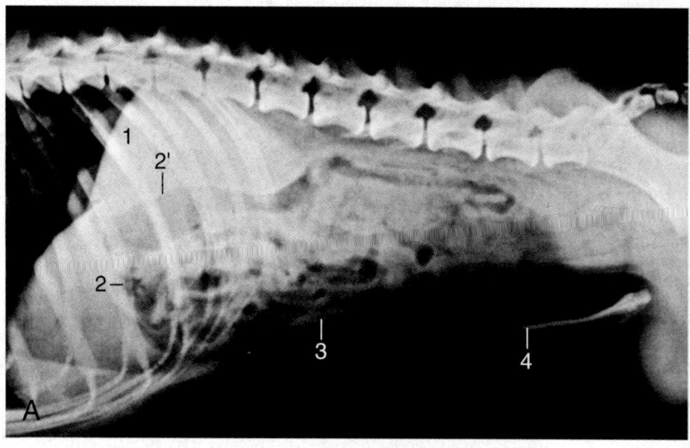

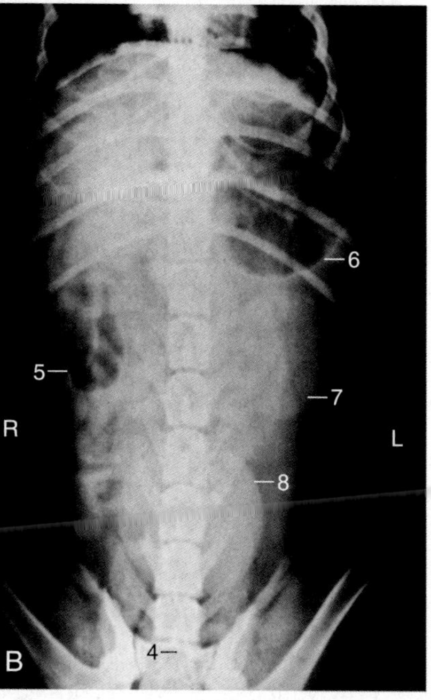

Fig. 14.11 (A) Lateral and(B) Ventrodorsal radiographic view of the canine abdomen. *1,* Liver; *2,* pyloric part of stomach; *2′,* descending duodenum; *3,* spleen; *4,* os penis; *5,* cecum; *6,* fundus of stomach; *7,* left kidney; *8,* bladder; *L,* left; *R,* right.

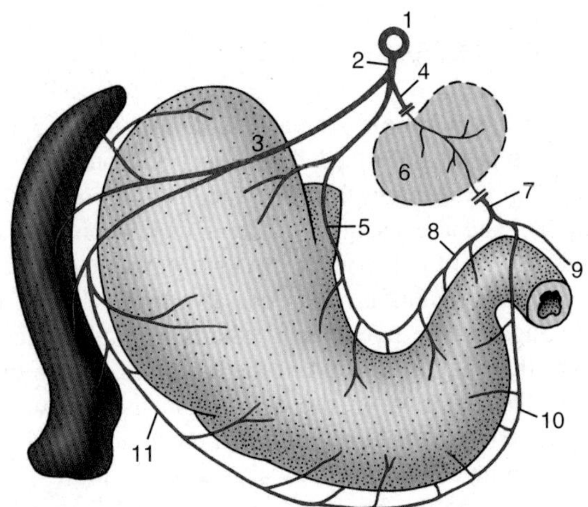

Fig. 14.12 The blood supply of the stomach and spleen, caudal view; schematic. *1,* Aorta; *2,* celiac artery (a.); *3,* splenic a.; *4,* hepatic a.; *5,* left gastric a.; *6,* indication of the liver; *7,* gastroduodenal a.; *8,* right gastric a.; *9,* cranial pancreaticoduodenal a.; *10,* right gastroepiploic a.; *11,* left gastroepiploic a.

omentum. The greater curvature faces mainly to the left, toward the spleen, and ventrally, where it usually lies on the ventral fringe of the liver and on the falciform ligament (Fig. 14.13/*6*). The greater curvature reaches the abdominal floor only when the stomach is greatly distended, and in these circumstances it may be palpated through the abdominal wall. Otherwise, the stomach is out of reach and generally aligned with the 9th to 12th ribs of the left side (Fig. 14.15A). As the stomach expands, its ventral parts (mainly the body) move caudoventrally into broad contact with the abdominal floor and left costal arch, displacing the jejunum from contact with the liver in the process. Excessive distention, not uncommon in this greedy species, may carry the stomach to a level behind the umbilicus. Such gross enlargement also alters its cranial relationships, pushing the liver to the right and the diaphragm forward, reducing the thoracic cavity.

Survey radiographs of the abdomen generally reveal few details of the stomach beyond the gas that naturally collects in the uppermost part of the organ—the fundus in

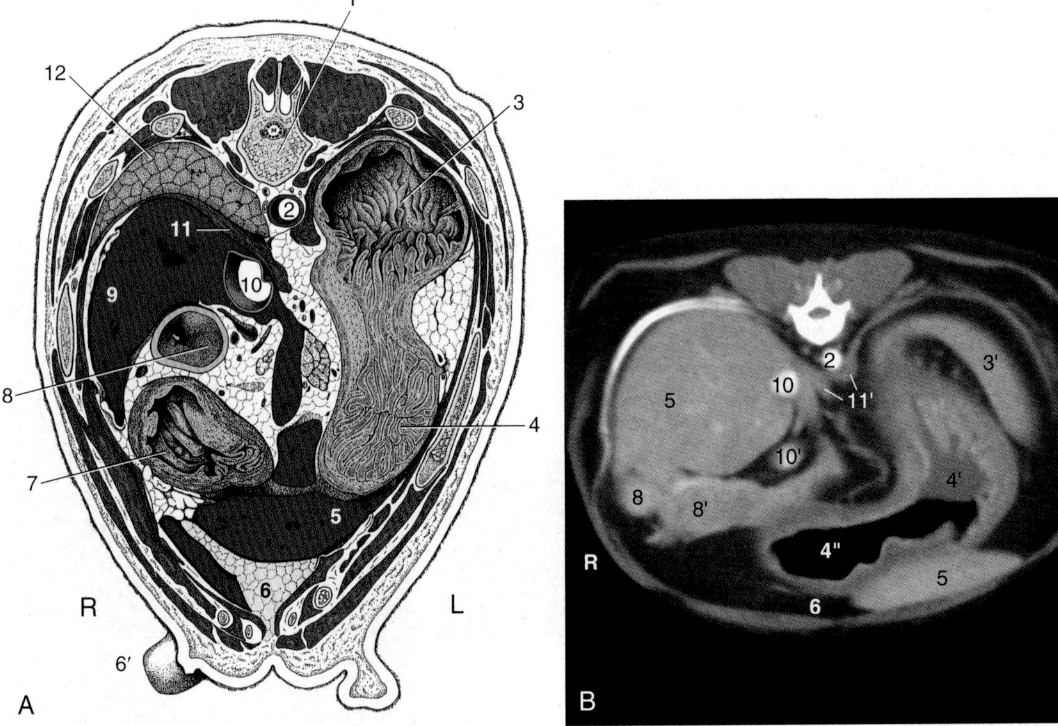

Fig. 14.13 (A) Transverse section of the canine trunk at the level of the 12th thoracic vertebra. (B) Corresponding computed tomography (CT) image slightly more caudal than (A); the dog was lying on its back during the CT procedure. *1,* 12th thoracic vertebra; *2,* aorta; *3,* fundus of stomach; *3′,* spleen; *4,* body of stomach; *4′,* with fluid; *4″,* with gas; *5,* liver; *6,* fat-filled falciform ligament; *6′,* teat; *7,* pyloric part of stomach; *8,* descending duodenum; *8′,* right lobe of pancreas; *9,* caudate process of liver; *10,* caudal vena cava; 10′, portal vein; *11,* diaphragm; *11′,* crura of diaphragm; *12,* right lung; *L,* left; *R,* right.

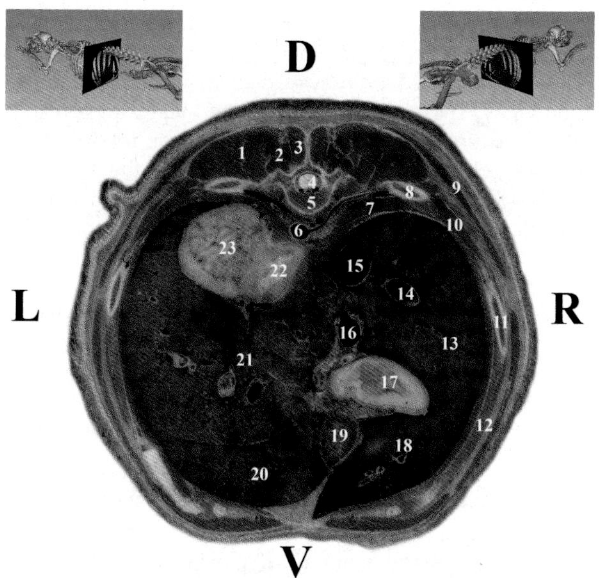

Fig. 14.14 Transverse section of the abdomen of the dog at the level of the 11th thoracic vertebra: *1,* Longissimus muscle; *2,* Semispinalis muscle; *3,* Multifidi muscles; *4,* Spinal cord; *5,* 11th thoracic vertebra; *6,* Descending aorta; *7,* Caudal lobe of the right lung; *8,* 10th rib; *9,* Latissimus dorsi muscle; *10,* Intercostalis muscles; *11,* 9th rib; *12,* Abdominal muscles; *13,* Liver (right lateral lobe); *14,* Right hepatic vein; *15,* Caudal vena cava; *16,* Portal vein; *17,* Pylorus; *18,* Liver (right medial lobe); *19,* Gallbladder; *20,* Liver (left medial lobe); *21,* Liver (left lateral lobe); *22,* Cardia (oesophagus); *23,* Stomach.

the animal standing or in right lateral recumbency. This useful orientation feature is lost when the animal is placed in other positions. A more complete demonstration of the topography is obtained with the administration of a barium meal (Fig. 14.15). The existence of the rugae may be revealed by defects in the outline of the contrast mass; the most satisfactory depiction is obtained after the evacuation of the bulk of the meal, when the residual agent clings to the mucosa and fills the spaces between adjacent rugae.

A number of structures join the stomach to neighboring parts. The fundus is directly bound to the left crus of the diaphragm (gastrophrenic ligament), and there are looser attachments between the cardia and the diaphragm, the lesser curvature and liver (lesser omentum), and the greater curvature and spleen (greater omentum). Except at these reflections, the stomach is completely covered with serosa.

The stomach receives blood from all *three branches of the celiac artery.* The branches to the stomach approach from the right of the fundus and dorsal to the cardia (Fig. 14.12). The *splenic artery* supplies short branches as it crosses the caudal surface of the fundus before reaching the spleen. A more substantial branch (*left gastroepiploic artery*; Fig. 14.12/*11*) follows the greater curvature to an anastomosis with the right gastroepiploic artery (a branch of the hepatic artery). The *left gastric artery* (Fig. 14.12/*5*) supplies the fundus, cardiac region, and a branch to the esophagus before following the lesser curvature to an anastomosis with the right gastric artery (Fig. 14.12/*8*), a further

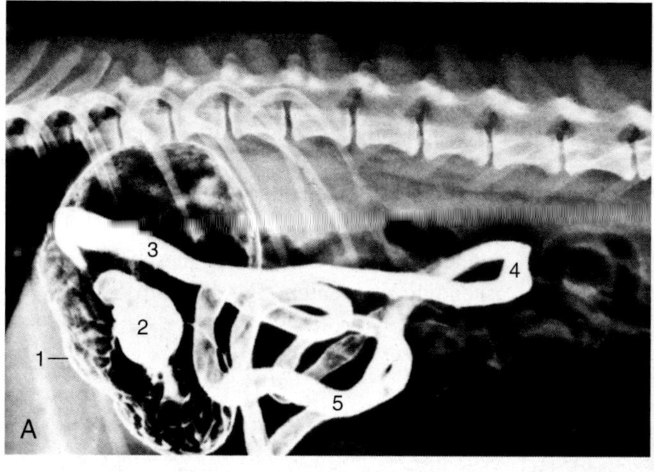

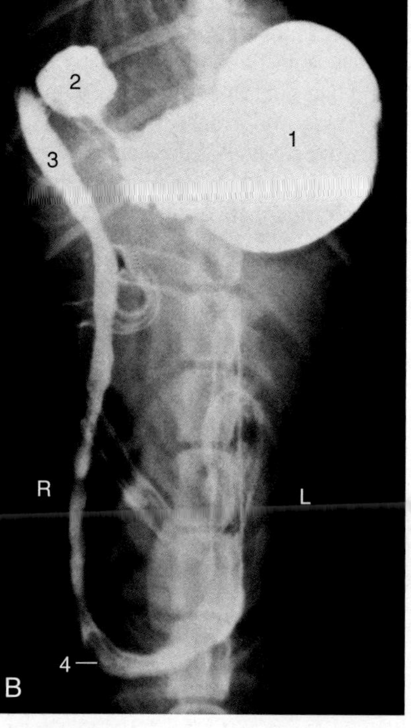

Fig. 14.15 (A) Lateral and (B) ventrodorsal radiographic views of the canine abdomen after administration of a barium suspension. *1,* Stomach; *2,* pyloric part; *3,* descending duodenum; *4,* caudal flexure of duodenum; *5,* jejunum; *L,* left; *R,* right.

branch of the hepatic artery. The arterial arcades that follow the curvatures supply fair-sized branches to adjacent parts of both surfaces. The arteries are mostly accompanied by satellite veins, which contribute as gastrosplenic and gastroduodenal veins to the portal vein. Gastric lymphatics drain into hepatic lymph nodes but may have passed the splenic and gastric nodes first. Large vessels are absent from the strips midway between the curvatures, which are therefore the preferred locations for incision. The parietal surface can be exposed and opened through a midline or paracostal incision (a common procedure for the recovery of foreign bodies), but the visceral surface is inaccessible unless the omental bursa is opened first (see p. 112).

The stomach of the *cat* is more sharply flexed on itself, and the pyloric part reaches little, if at all, into the right half of the abdomen. Gross distention is also less common in cats, which tend to moderate their appetites better than dogs. The cat's stomach is generally similar to that of the dog; its topography and that of the intestines are shown in the radiographs in Figs. 14.15, 14.17 and 14.19) The rugae in the stomach as seen in contrast radiographs are conspicuously fewer and proportionately smaller in cats than in dogs. Pyloric stenosis caused by hypertrophy of the pyloric circular smooth muscle can be encountered in Siamese cats.

Gastric volvulus is relatively common, especially in large deep-chested breeds such as the Great Dane and St. Bernard. In this mishap the distended stomach rotates about the esophagus (usually in a clockwise direction as seen from behind, between 270° and 360°), and this action closes the esophagus at the cardia. The pyloric end of the stomach, less firmly held in place by the lesser omentum and bile duct, moves ventrally and to the left, thereby stretching the cranial part of the duodenum across the ventral surface of the cardia. The ventral leaf of the greater omentum, still attached to the greater curvature of the stomach, covers the ventral aspect of the displaced stomach and is visible at surgical entry of the abdominal cavity. The rotation compresses the veins, causing congestion of the stomach, compression of caudal vena cava and portal vein, and engorgement of the spleen. The correction may also cause ischemia-reperfusion injury. The position of the spleen varies depending on the extent of volvulus, and it may even rotate on its own pedicle. Counterclockwise rotation of the stomach is possible to a maximum of 90°; the pylorus and antrum move dorsally along the right abdominal wall, and in this case, there is no displacement of the omentum over the ventral surface of the stomach.

Removal of foreign objects from the stomach may require *gastrotomy*. In this procedure an incision is made in the hypovascular area between the greater and lesser curvatures and away from the pylorus.

INTESTINES (SEE ALSO PP. 119–125)

Because the general features of the intestinal tract have been described, it is now appropriate to concentrate on its relationships to other organs and to external landmarks and on its attachments and blood supply.

The small intestine is relatively short, perhaps three or four times the body length. Of this length, the *duodenum* contributes, on average, only 25 cm. The short cranial part of the duodenum passes dorsally and to the right, against the visceral surface of the liver, roughly opposite the ninth intercostal space. It is continued caudally beyond the porta as the descending duodenum, which follows the right abdominal wall to reach a point somewhere between the fourth and sixth lumbar vertebrae (Fig. 14.10B/*7'*). In its passage it is related dorsally to the right lobe of the pancreas, ventrally to the jejunal mass, and medially to the ascending colon and cecum (Fig. 14.18/*5*). The mesentery of the descending duodenum begins by being relatively long but shortens toward the caudal flexure, where the gut is closely anchored to the abdominal roof. An additional (duodenocolic) fold with a free caudal border attaches the duodenum to the descending mesocolon at this level. The ascending duodenum (Fig. 14.18/*6*), which begins at the

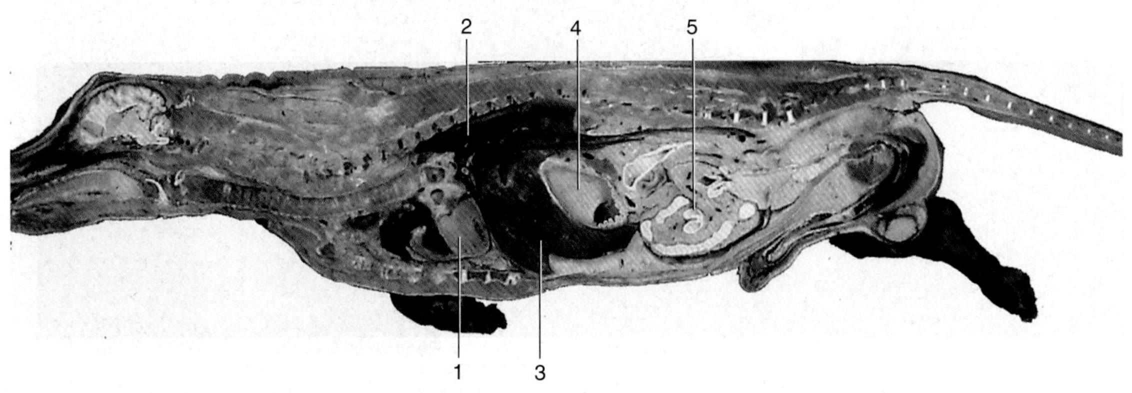

Fig. 14.16 Median section of canine trunk, providing overview of viscera. *1,* Heart; *2,* lung; *3,* liver; *4,* stomach; *5,* intestine.

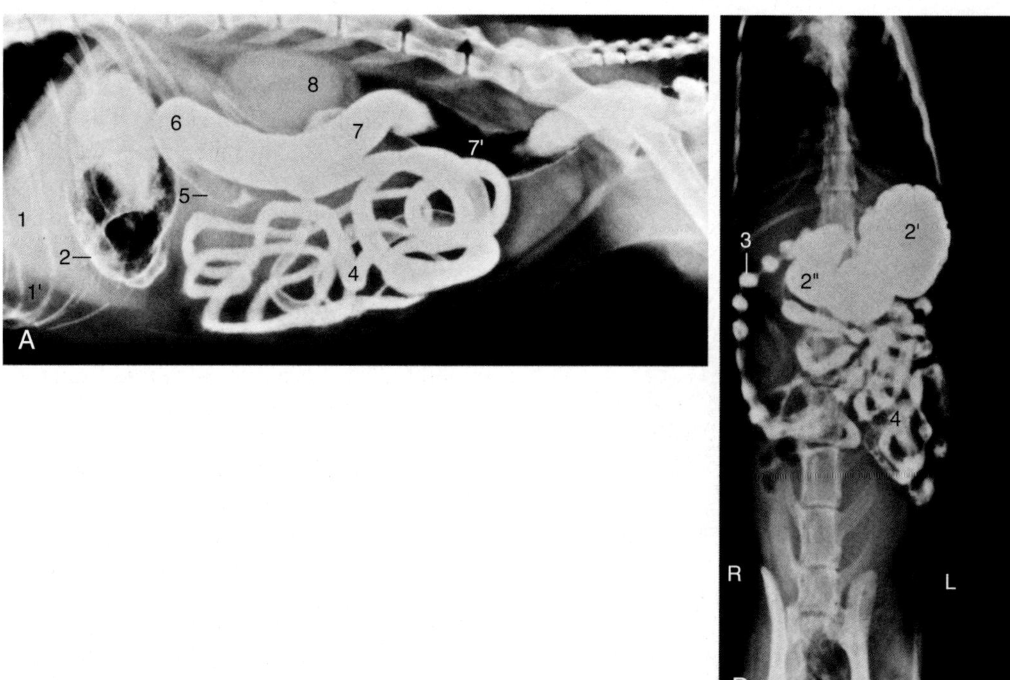

Fig. 14.17 (A) Lateral and (B) ventrodorsal radiographic views of the feline abdomen after administration of a barium suspension. *1*, Liver; *1′*, fat-filled falciform ligament elevating the liver; *2*, gas and barium in stomach; *2′*, fundus; *2″*, pyloric part of stomach; *3*, descending duodenum—the striking "string-of-pearls" appearance (characteristic of cats) is due to segmental peristalsis; *4*, jejunum; *5*, ascending colon; *6*, transverse colon; *7*, descending colon; *7′*, gas in descending colon; *8*, kidneys (superimposed); *L*, left; *R*, right.

caudal flexure, is more tightly tethered than the preceding segment and runs forward, close to the midline, between the descending colon on the left and the root of the mesentery. It turns ventrally at the cranial limit of the root to be continued by the jejunum. Other relations of this part are the medial border of the left kidney dorsally and the jejunal mass ventrally (Figs. 14.11A and 14.15B).

The *jejunum* and short *ileum* form a mass occupying the ventral part of the abdomen between the stomach and the bladder (Figs. 14.5, 14.6, 14.9). The coils of the jejunum are quite mobile, and at first sight their disposition appears to be haphazard; closer inspection shows that there is some pattern to the arrangement. The mainly sagittal coils of the proximal part lie largely cranial to the more transverse coils of the distal part (Fig. 14.11A). The suspending mesentery is relatively long and imposes little restraint, allowing the gut to slip freely over the floor in response to respiratory and other movements. This feature enables the surgeon to exteriorize much of the jejunum to improve the exposure of more dorsal organs. Dorsally, the jejunal mass extends to the descending duodenum on the right and the kidney and sublumbar muscles on the left. The jejunal coils are generally entirely related to the folded greater omentum ventrally; cranially only the deep leaf intervenes between them and the stomach. The *ileum* arises at the caudal end of the mass and passes forward and to the right to open into the ascending colon below the first or second lumbar vertebra.

Small patches of aggregate lymph nodules of varying sizes are present throughout the small intestine; the largest are said to be in the ileum.

In life the intestine is not uniformly full, and at any moment most parts are flattened and molded by the pressures of adjacent viscera. The lumen may be locally obliterated, and when a passage is retained, it is more often than not reduced to a narrow channel along one margin—a "keyhole" section. This fact explains the narrow streaks that are the common representation of the small intestine on radiographs obtained after the administration of a barium meal. Segmental and peristaltic movements continually alter the configuration in life. After the administration of a contrast medium, the duodenum of the cat often displays segmental contractions that are sufficiently pronounced to divide the gut content into a linear series of globular expansions separated by (more or less) empty regions to create a striking "string-of-pearls" effect (Fig. 14.17B). A similar appearance in other regions of the cat's bowel, or in the duodenum of the dog, is probably evidence of abnormality.

The ileocecocolic junction is peculiar in that the ileum and colon are in line and form a continuous tube that is

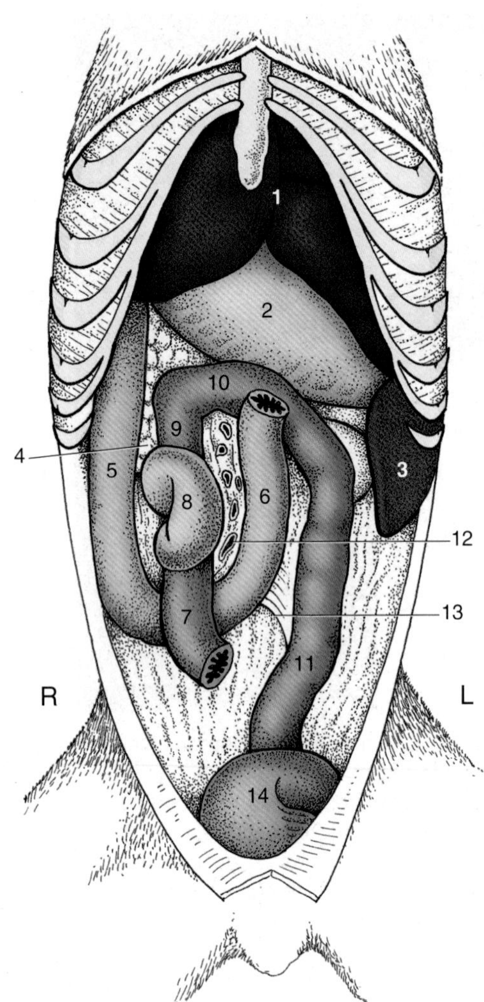

Fig. 14.18 The canine duodenum, cecum, and colon in situ; ventral view. *1,* Liver; *2,* stomach; *3,* spleen; *4,* pancreas; *5,* descending duodenum; *6,* ascending duodenum; *7,* ileum; *8,* cecum; *9, 10, 11,* ascending, transverse and descending colon; *12,* vessels in root of mesentery; *13,* duodenocolic fold; *14,* bladder; *L,* left; *R,* right.

joined by the cecum to one side. (In the other species it is the cecum and colon that meet end to end.) The *cecum* is short, although it varies in length, and twisted (Fig. 14.18/*8* and 14.19/*4*). It is joined to the ileum by a short (ileocecal) fold and is oriented craniocaudally, although its rounded blind end may finally point in any direction. The cecum communicates with the ascending colon through the cecocolic orifice adjacent to the ileal orifice. The cecum lies to the right of the root of the mesentery and is related to the right kidney dorsally, the descending duodenum and pancreas laterally, and the jejunum ventrally. It lies below the second lumbar joint and thus is broadly level with the most caudal part of the costal arch. The cecum of the cat is small and comma shaped. Surprisingly, it can be located on palpation by reference to the firm ileocecocolic junction at the level of the fourth lumbar vertebra. The firmness can be mistaken for a tumor or intussusception (Fig. 14.20/*4*).

The *colon,* 65 cm long on average, is only slightly wider than the small intestine. It is easily recognized by its course cranial to the root of the mesentery and its nearly straight descent on the left toward the pelvis, which it enters dorsal to the bladder (and uterus) (see Figs. 3.45 and 14.19). The short ascending part lies to the right, between the descending duodenum and the root of the mesentery, and generally makes contact with the pyloric part of the stomach. Its narrow mesocolon permits it little mobility. The transverse colon runs from right to left, cranial to the root of the mesentery and ventral to the left lobe of the pancreas (see Fig. 14.18). It is more loosely attached and sinks within the abdomen; usually it is the lowest part of the colon when depicted in lateral radiographs. The free attachment sometimes allows it to fold on itself to appear as no more than a flexure connecting the ascending with the descending colon. The descending colon is by far the longest segment. It passes caudally, to the left of the mesenteric root, to reach the pelvic cavity, where it continues as the rectum (Fig. 14.10A/*6*). It is related dorsally to the left kidney and sublumbar muscles and ventrally to the jejunal mass, and it may lie against the left abdominal wall (Figs. 14.16/*4* and 14.21/*4*). The descending colon is the only segment of the large intestine of the dog that may easily be palpated. No part of the colon lies retroperitoneally.

The prominence of the cecum and colon in plain radiographs of the canine abdomen is determined by the amount of gas and the nature and volume of the digestive residues present (see Fig. 14.19). The cecum almost always contains sufficient gas to provide a reminder of the twisted course of its lumen. This convenient identifying feature is not found in cats, in which the simpler conformation rarely allows gas to be retained (see Fig. 14.20).

The *blood supply* of the intestines comes mainly from the *cranial and caudal mesenteric arteries* with a part of the duodenum supplied by the *cranial pancreaticoduodenal branch of the gastroduodenal artery* (from the celiac artery). The details are shown in Fig. 14.22 and 14.23. The descending colon and rectum receive blood from the caudal mesenteric artery that, in both cats and dogs, branches off the aorta near the fifth lumbar vertebrae. The veins form the portal vein, with the exception of those from the caudal rectum, which are directed toward the caudal vena cava.

Enterotomy is an incision into the intestine, and it may be needed for biopsy, removal of foreign objects, or resection of ischemic parts of the intestines. The resection will require anastomosis to restore the intestinal tract.

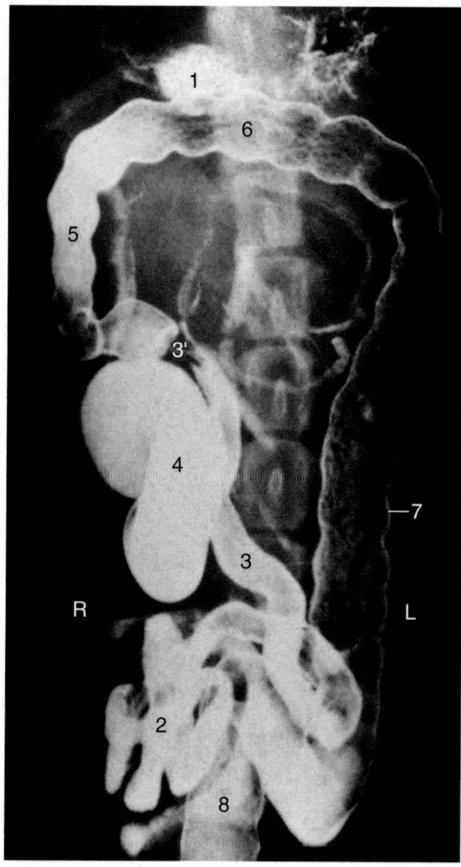

Fig. 14.19 Ventrodorsal radiographic view of the canine abdomen after administration of a barium suspension. *1,* Residue of barium in stomach; *2,* jejunum; *3,* ileum; *3′,* ileocolic junction; *4,* cecum; *5, 6,* and *7,* ascending, transverse and descending colon; *8,* rectum; *L,* left; *R,* right.

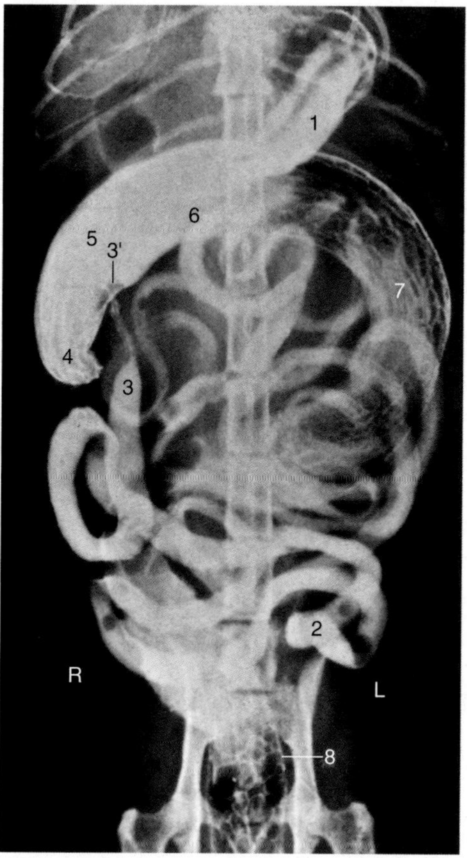

Fig. 14.20 Ventrodorsal radiographic view of the feline abdomen after administration of a barium suspension. *1,* Residue of barium in stomach; *2,* jejunum; *3,* ileum; *3′,* ileal papilla; *4,* cecum; *5–7,* colon—the long descending part *(7)* has curved far to the right in this animal; *8,* rectum; *L,* left; *R,* right.

Several colic *lymph nodes* lie within the curvature of the ascending and transverse colon. The more prominent jejunal nodes lie high in the root of the mesentery. One of the nodes, which is surprisingly large (perhaps 10 cm in the beagle), accompanies the jejunal arteries (Fig. 14.18/*5*). Several smaller caudal mesenteric nodes lie within the descending mesocolon, scattered about the branches of the caudal mesenteric artery.

THE LIVER

The liver (see also pp. 125-128) is relatively large, weighing about 450 g on average, and accounts for 3% to 4% of the body weight. It is almost entirely intrathoracic, occupying a central position with only a slight bias to the right side (Figs. 14.10/*2*, 14.23, 14.25 and 14.26). The modest asymmetry is caused by the enlargement of the caudate process beneath the last ribs, where it makes contact with the right kidney (Fig. 14.13/*9*). The ventral border extends across the costal arches and would be palpable were it not for the fat within the falciform ligament and the taut rectus muscles. Even so, it may be appreciated when significantly enlarged. The liver in dogs and cats is deeply divided by fissures extending from the ventral margin; the pattern, the relative extents, and the names of the lobes may be obtained from Fig. 3.53.

The cranial surface conforms to the curvature of the diaphragm with which it is in extensive contact and to which it is secured by the caudal vena cava embedded in the dorsal border (Fig. 14.25 and 14.26). The attachment to the tendinous center of the diaphragm is completed by right and left coronary ligaments caudolateral to the vein. Most of the liver can therefore be retracted during surgery to expose the diaphragm. The gallbladder is sunk deeply between the lobes, just to the right of the median plane opposite the eighth intercostal space. It usually makes contact with

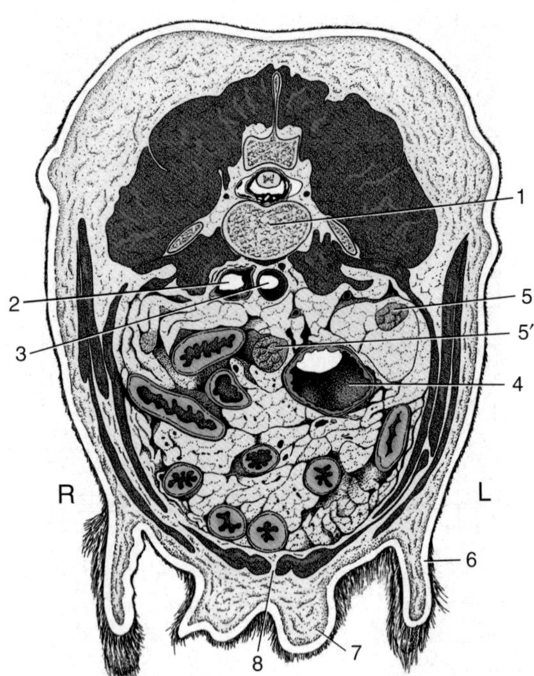

Fig. 14.21 Transverse section of the canine abdomen at the level of the fourth or fifth lumbar vertebra. *1,* Lumbar vertebra; *2,* caudal vena cava; *3,* aorta; *4,* descending colon; *5* and *5′,* right and left uterine horns; *6,* flank fold; *7,* mammary gland; *8,* linea alba; *L,* left; *R,* right.

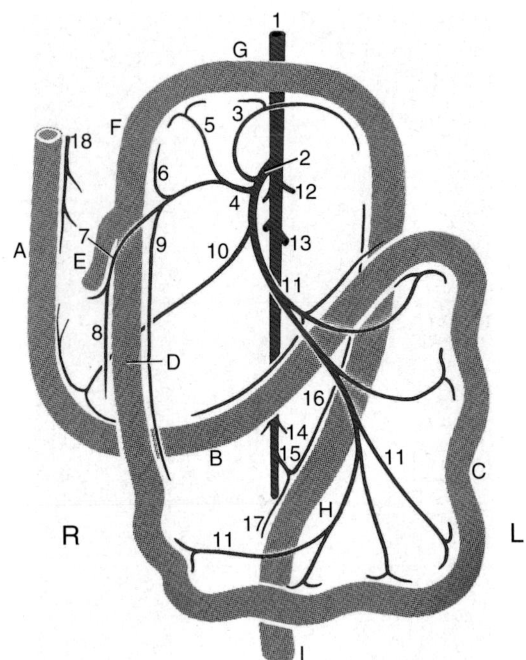

Fig. 14.22 The blood supply of the intestinal tract, ventral view; schematic. *A,* Descending duodenum; *B,* ascending duodenum; *C,* jejunum; *D,* ileum; *E,* cecum; *F,* ascending colon; *G,* transverse colon; *H,* descending colon; *I,* rectum; *1,* abdominal aorta; *2,* cranial mesenteric artery (a.); *3,* middle colic a.; *4,* ileocolic a.; *5,* right colic a.; *6,* colic branch of ileocolic a.; *7,* cecal a.; *8,* antimesenteric ileal branch; *9,* mesenteric ileal branch; *10,* caudal pancreaticoduodenal a.; *11,* jejunal arteries (aa.); *12,* phrenicoabdominal aa.; *13,* renal aa.; *14,* testicular (ovarian) aa.; *15,* caudal mesenteric a.; *16,* left colic a.; *17,* cranial rectal a.; *18,* cranial pancreaticoduodenal a.

the diaphragm and always appears at the visceral surface, although it is too short to reach the ventral border (Fig. 14.26/8).

The visceral surface, though concave, is made irregular by various visceral impressions. The largest of the impressions is made by the body of the stomach to the left of the median plane, and the pyloric part and duodenum produce a narrower impression leading away to the right (Fig. 14.13/7). The other prominent impression, involving the right lateral lobe and caudate process, is made by the right kidney. Other organs that may touch the liver, especially when the stomach is empty, leave no mark, except the pancreas, which attaches near the porta.

The attachments on the visceral surface are larger but looser and are part (as mentioned earlier) of the lesser omentum. The hepatogastric ligament contains the bile duct as well as the hepatic artery, the portal vein, lymphatic vessels, and nerves. Once the hepatic ducts receive the cystic duct from the gallbladder, the duct is known as the common bile duct (ductus choledochus). In dogs, it runs from the hilus to the duodenum. Its terminal portion continues for some 2 cm within the duodenal wall before opening by the side of the pancreatic duct on the major duodenal papilla, a small elevation 2 to 3 mm high, caudally directed, and located about 3 to 6 cm from the pylorus in both dogs and cats.

Biopsy samples of liver tissue may be obtained by puncture caudal to the xiphoid process; the instrument is directed toward the large left lobe to avoid the gallbladder (Fig. 14.5).

In survey radiographs of the abdomen the liver appears as a large, uniformly dense shadow from which its size, relative to the species norm, may be crudely assessed. When such an assessment is made, it is necessary to be mindful that the liver is more or less completely "intrathoracic" in large, deep-chested breeds, whereas a more appreciable portion projects beyond the costal arch in dogs of less extreme conformation. In overindulged cats the liver may be displaced dorsally and away from the abdominal floor owing to the deposition of excessive fat within the falciform ligament.

The liver is a soft organ with very little fibrous tissue. This characteristic makes ligation of the blood vessels very difficult in hepatic surgery.

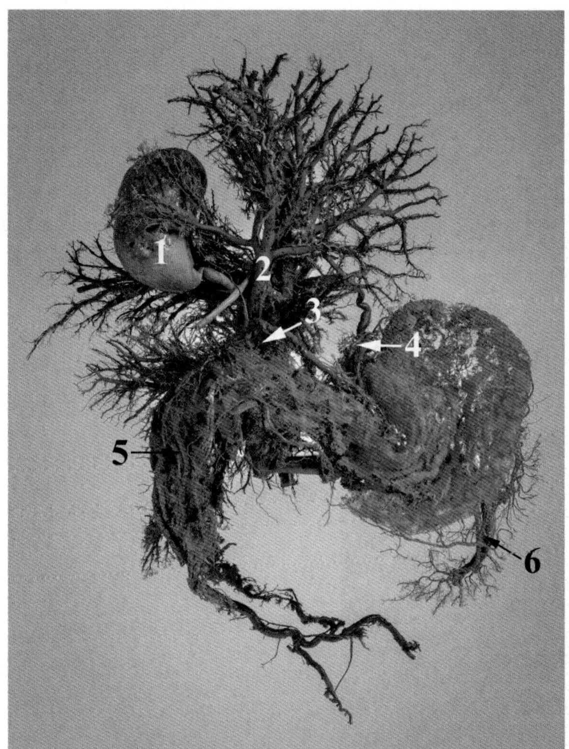

Fig. 14.23 Corrosion cast of the celiac artery and the caudal vena cava of the dog. *1,* Gallbladder; *2,* Hepatic vein; *3,* Hepatic artery; *4,* Left gastric artery and vein; *5,* Cranial pancreaticoduodenal artery and vein; *6,* Splenic artery and vein.

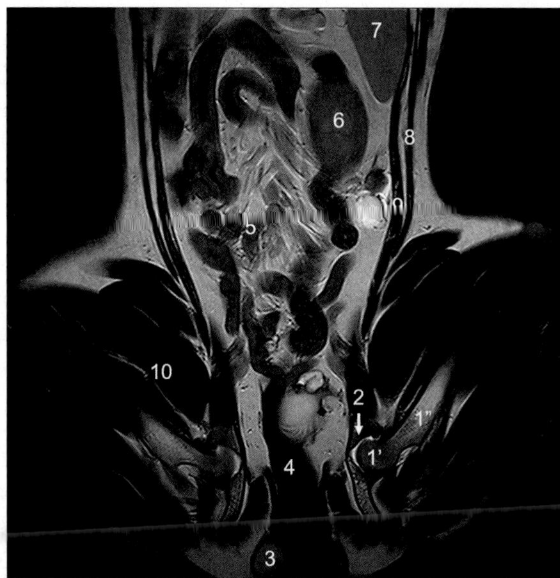

Fig. 14.24 A frontal section of a dog at the level of femur head; Magnetic Resonance Imaging (MRI). Notice the femur head (1′) and shaft (1″), acetabulum (2), anal sacs (3), rectum (4), jejunal loops (5), left kidney (6), spleen (7), external oblique (8) and internal oblique (9) abdominal muscles, and quadriceps muscles (10) of the thigh.

THE PANCREAS

The slender pancreas (see also pp. 129-131) consists of two limbs or lobes that diverge from the vicinity of the pylorus. The left lobe is directed caudomedially and crosses the median plane behind the stomach to end against the left kidney (see Fig. 3.56/*5*). It divides the branches of the celiac artery from those of the cranial mesenteric artery and is enclosed within the deep leaf of the greater omentum where the latter passes dorsal to the transverse colon. The dorsal surface of the left lobe is crossed by the portal vein where the lobe makes contact with the hilus of the liver to the right of the median plane.

The longer right lobe is directed caudodorsally and follows the dorsal surface of the descending duodenum within the mesoduodenum. It is related dorsally to the visceral surface of the liver and, behind it, to the ventral surface of the kidney (Fig. 14.27/*9*). The lobe lies lateral to the ascending colon and dorsal to the small intestine.

Two secretory ducts open into the duodenum where the two lobes diverge. The smaller and inconstant pancreatic duct joins the bile duct just before the latter opens on the major duodenal papilla, 3 to 6 cm distal to the pylorus. The accessory pancreatic duct, the main channel, opens on the minor duodenal papilla 3 to 5 cm farther down the gut. Both papillae can be detected with the unaided eye. The duct systems of the two lobes communicate internally. In the cat the main duct is the pancreatic duct. In a minority of cats (around 20%) an accessory duct can also be found that, as in dogs, opens onto the minor duodenal papilla, some 2 cm distal to the major papilla.

The major part of the pancreas is supplied by two of the *three branches of the celiac artery*. Only the caudal part of the right limb of the pancreas receives blood from the *cranial mesenteric artery*. The left lobe is entered by branches of the *splenic artery* whereas branches from the *hepatic artery* supply the body of the pancreas (gastroduodenal artery) and the cranial half of the right lobe (cranial pancreaticoduodenal artery). Duodenal branches are given off from cranial pancreaticoduodenal artery and course through the pancreatic tissue to supply the gut itself. Anastomoses between these various vessels occur within the gland. Lymphatics are abundant and drain into the duodenal lymph node, if present, or into the mesenteric lymph nodes.

Pancreatic Tumor: One of the most encountered problems in the pancreas of the dog is the presence of an insulin-producing tumor, an insulinoma. Thorough inspection for metastases must be performed in the liver, the duodenum, the mesentery, and the hepatic, splenic, gastric, duodenal, and cranial mesenteric

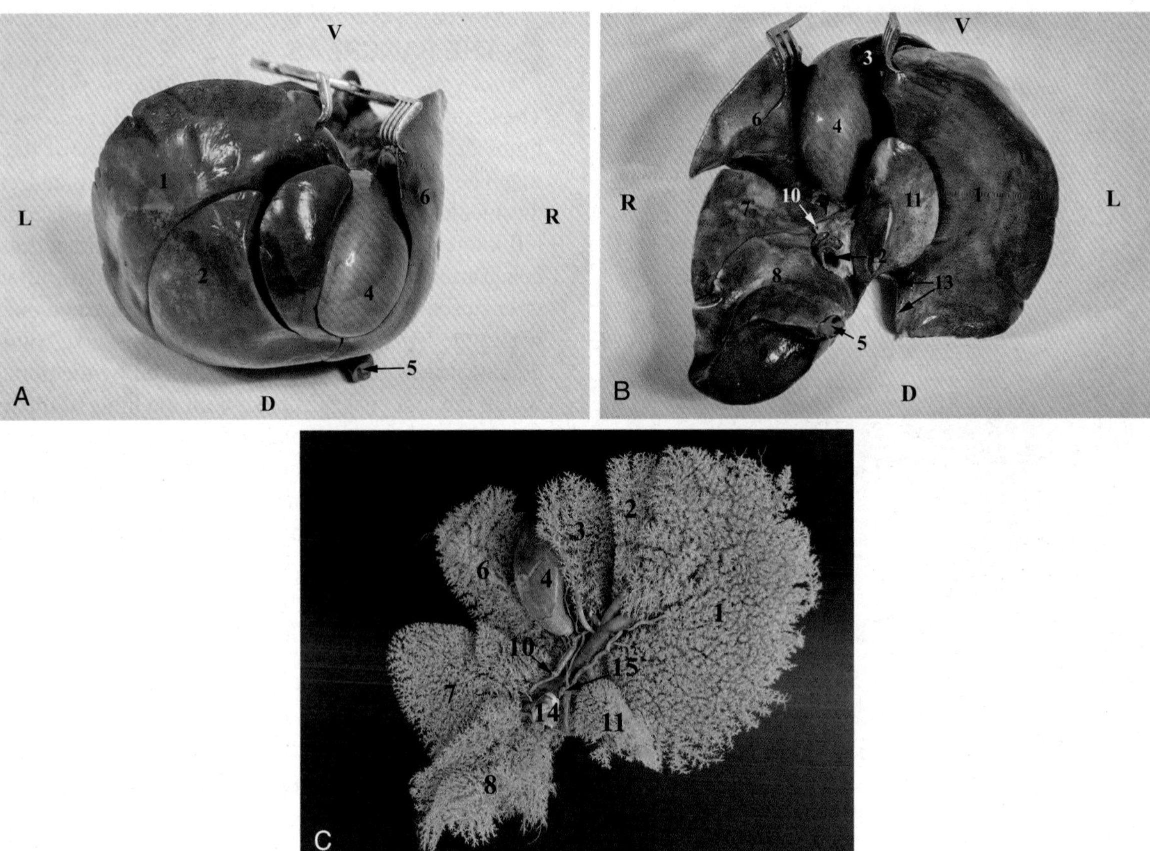

Fig. 14.25 Liver of the dog, diaphragmatic surface (A), visceral surface (B), a corrosion cast (C): *1.* Left lateral lobe; *2.* Left medial lobe; *3.* Quadrate lobe; *4.* Gallblader; *5.* Caudal vena cava, intrathoracal part; *6.* Right medial lobe; *7.* Right lateral lobe; *8.* Caudate process of the caudate lobe; *9.* Renal impression at the caudate process; *10.* Bile duct; *11.* Papillary process of the caudate lobe; *12.* Portal vein (on the fixed specimen); *13.* Esophageal impression; *14.* Portal vein (on the corrosion cast); *15.* Hepatic artery

lymph nodes. Resection of the part of the pancreas is difficult because it shares blood supply with the duodenum and the spleen. Removal of the spleen is indicated when the splenic artery cannot be preserved.

THE ADRENAL GLANDS AND KIDNEYS

The yellowish white *adrenal glands* (see also pp. 207–208) (Fig. 14.28/7 and 7′) of the dog are dorsoventrally flattened, about 2 to 3 cm long and 1 cm wide. Each occupies the retroperitoneal space medial to the kidney, cranial to the renal vessels, and dorsolateral to the aorta (the left gland) or the caudal vena cava (the right one). The capsule of the right adrenal gland may be continuous with the tunica externa of the vena cava. The right adrenal gland is located ventral to the transverse process of the last thoracic vertebra, with its cranial two thirds covered by the caudate process of the liver. The left adrenal gland, which has a somewhat dorsoventrally flattened oval cranial portion and a cylindrical caudal projection, is positioned ventral to the transverse process of the second lumbar vertebra, just caudal to the origin of the cranial mesenteric artery and adjacent to the origin of the phrenicoabdominal artery. This paired artery courses on the dorsal surfaces of both left and right glands. The ventral surfaces are crossed and indented by the phrenicoabdominal veins; on the left, this surface is also related to the pancreas.

The glands are diffusely supplied by branches from adjacent vessels: the aorta and the renal, phrenicoabdominal, lumbar, and cranial mesenteric arteries. The right and left adrenal veins enter the vena cava directly and the left renal vein, respectively.

The nerve supply is derived from a dense network on the dorsal surface of the glands that appears continuous with the nearby celiac and mesenteric plexuses. The fibers that actually enter the glands are preganglionic and are provided by the splanchnic nerves that enter the abdominal cavity close by.

In cats the adrenal glands are shorter and similar to oval disks. The adrenal glands of older cats are occasionally calcified and if so are visible on radiographs. The topography is the same in both species.

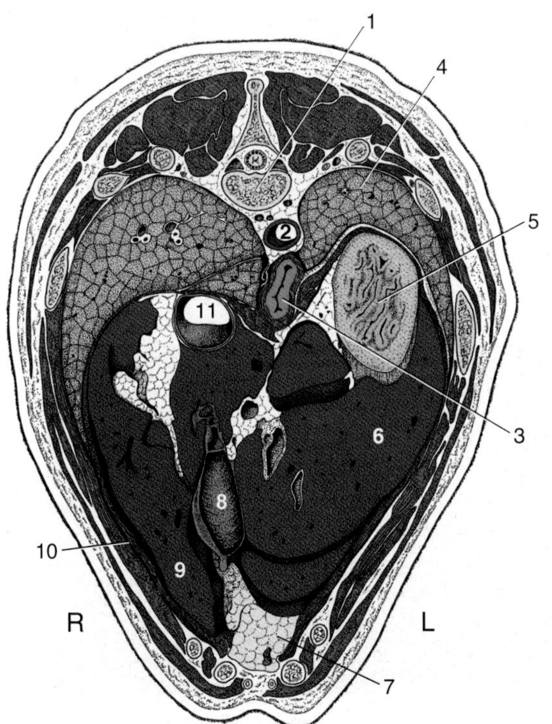

Fig. 14.26 Transverse section of the canine trunk at the level of the 11th thoracic vertebra. *1,* 11th thoracic vertebra; *2,* aorta; *3,* esophagus; *4,* left lung; *5,* fundus of stomach; *6,* left lateral lobe of liver; *7,* fat-filled falciform ligament; *8,* gallbladder; *9,* right medial lobe of liver; *10,* diaphragm; *11,* caudal vena cava; *L,* left; *R,* right.

The Kidneys

The account of the kidneys presented here concentrates on their positions and relations. The rest of the anatomy is considered in Chapter 15.

The kidneys in the dog are bean shaped and retroperitoneally positioned against the sublumbar muscles. The usual position of the right kidney is below the first three lumbar vertebrae, and that of left is below the second to fourth (Fig. 14.25, 14.28, 14.29 and 14.30), although they may be found a full vertebral length more caudally. The right kidney is more restricted by being deeply recessed within the liver and is related medially to the right adrenal gland and caudal vena cava, laterally to the last rib and abdominal wall, and ventrally to the liver and pancreas (Fig. 14.30). The left kidney is related cranially to the spleen (or stomach when enlarged), medially to the left adrenal gland and aorta, laterally to the abdominal wall, and ventrally to the descending colon.

The cat's kidneys are relatively large and are given a distinctive appearance by capsular veins converging over the surface toward the hilus (Fig. 14.31). They are more mobile than the kidneys of the dog Fig. 14.27 and a call out especially the left one, which can be displaced cranially or caudally from its usual position below the second to fifth lumbar vertebrae; it has been taken for a pathologic swelling. In cats, both kidneys are readily palpable.

The Major Vessels

The abdominal aorta and caudal vena cava run the length of the abdomen, partly recessed between the right and left sublumbar muscles.

The abdominal aorta gives rise to paired dorsal lumbar arteries; the last pair originates from the median sacral artery. Near the second lumbar vertebra in the dog, the phrenicoabdominal trunk emerges branches into the caudal phrenic artery and the cranial abdominal artery, which is also the origin of the adrenal arteries. In the cat the caudal phrenic artery originates from the celiac artery as a single artery. The deep iliac circumflex artery branches off the aorta near the sixth vertebra but may split off the external iliac artery in the dog.

The ventral branches of the aorta are the celiac artery, the cranial and caudal mesenteric, the renal arteries, and the ovarian/testicular arteries; sometimes paired adrenal arteries also branch off the aorta. The *celiac artery* branches off directly after the passage of the aorta through the diaphragm and divides into *the hepatic, splenic, and left gastric arteries*. The hepatic artery courses to the right of the midline before dividing into three to five branches, which supply the individual liver lobes. After giving off the hepatic branches, the hepatic artery bifurcates into the right gastric and gastroduodenal arteries. The gastroduodenal artery in turn divides into the right gastroepiploic and pancreaticoduodenal arteries.

The *cranial mesenteric artery* originates one vertebra behind the celiac artery and forms the base of the mesentery. It gives rise to the ileocolic, pancreaticoduodenal, and jejunal arteries in the dog and cat. The *renal arteries* branch off in the dog ventral to the first and second lumbar vertebrae and in the cat ventral to the third and fourth , and directly [illegible] the gonadal arteries split off. Ventral to the fifth lumbar vertebrae is the origin of the *caudal mesenteric artery*, and one to two vertebral bodies more caudal, the *external iliac arteries* split off to supply the hindlimbs. The abdominal aorta terminates opposite the seventh lumbar vertebra by bifurcating into right and left *internal iliac and middle sacral arteries* (Fig. 14.3). The aorta lies in the furrow formed by the left and right iliopsoas muscles.

Aortin Thrombus: In both dog and cat, but especially in the cat, the terminal segment of the aorta is commonly the location of a large thrombus, often known as a *"saddle" thrombus* from its disposition across the division, which may partially or wholly block the three terminal branches. The origin of the thrombus, the degree of obstruction it causes, and the rate at which it developed determine the severity of the clinical signs, which may include complete paralysis of the hindlimbs. Surgical removal of the thrombus has very poor survival rates.

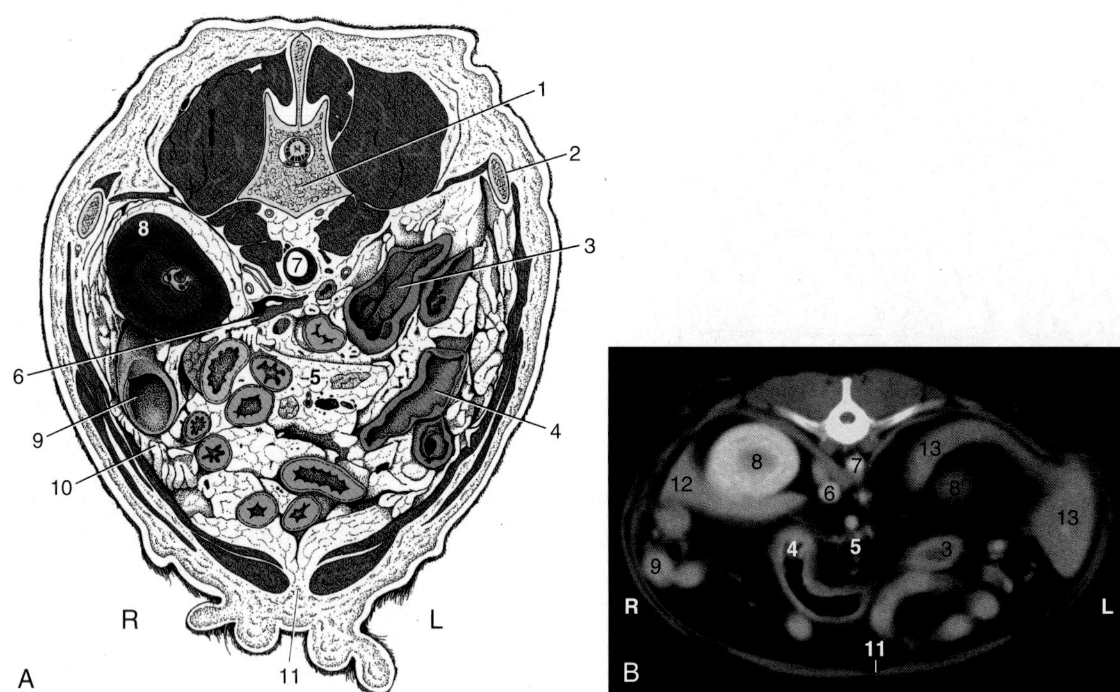

Fig. 14.27 (A) Transverse section of the canine abdomen at the level of the first lumbar vertebra. (B) Corresponding computed tomography (CT) image slightly more caudal than (A); the dog was lying on its back during the CT procedure. *1,* First lumbar vertebra; *2,* last rib; *3,* descending colon; *4,* transverse colon; *5,* lymph nodes and blood vessels in mesentery; ventral to them is the jejunum; *6,* caudal vena cava; *7,* aorta, between crura of diaphragm; *8,* right kidney; *8′,* cranial pole of left kidney; *9,* descending duodenum and pancreas; *10,* greater omentum; *11,* linea alba; *12,* liver; *13,* spleen; *L,* left; *R,* right.

The *portal vein* results from the confluence of the cranial mesenteric, caudal mesenteric, and gastrosplenic veins. In dogs, the portal vein is additionally fed by the gastroduodenal vein, which originates from the merger of the right gastric, right gastroepiploic, and cranial pancreaticoduodenal veins. It has been reported that the contributions to the portal vein in cats are variable and cannot be described on the basis of a common pattern.

Venography of the portal vein (see Fig. 7.45) is occasionally employed to ascertain the existence (and condition) of portosystemic connections. A small intestinal tributary is chosen for the injection. The shunts most commonly revealed connect the portal system with both the caudal caval tributaries at the abdominal roof and the azygos vein within the thorax.

LYMPHATIC STRUCTURES

The lymph nodes of the abdomen can be divided into a parietal group and a visceral group (Table 14.2). The *lumbar aortic* lymph nodes, when present, are located along the aorta and vena cava. They supply the cisterna chyli or the caudal lumbar aortic nodes. The paired *hypogastric* lymph nodes are small and are located in the angle of the internal iliac and median sacral artery, ventral to the body of the seventh lumbar vertebra. They receive lymph from the thigh, the pelvic viscera, the tail, and a portion of the lumbar region and have efferent vessels to the cisterna chyli. The *sacral* lymph nodes are positioned ventral to the body of the sacrum but are often not present. They receive afferent vessels from the adjacent musculature and send off efferent vessels to the hypogastric nodes. The *deep inguinal* or *iliofemoral* lymph nodes can be found on the ventral surface of the tendon of the psoas minor at its insertion and receive lymph from the pelvic limb. The *medial iliac* lymph nodes lie between the deep circumflex iliac and the external iliac artery, ventral to the bodies of the fifth and sixth lumbar vertebrae, and they can be 4 cm long in the dog. They receive lymph from all parts of the dorsal half of the abdomen, the pelvis, and the pelvic limb, including that from the genital system and the caudal part of the digestive and urinary system. They also receive lymph from the deep and superficial inguinal, the left colic, sacral, and hypogastric lymph nodes and supply the cisterna chyli. The lymph nodes at the

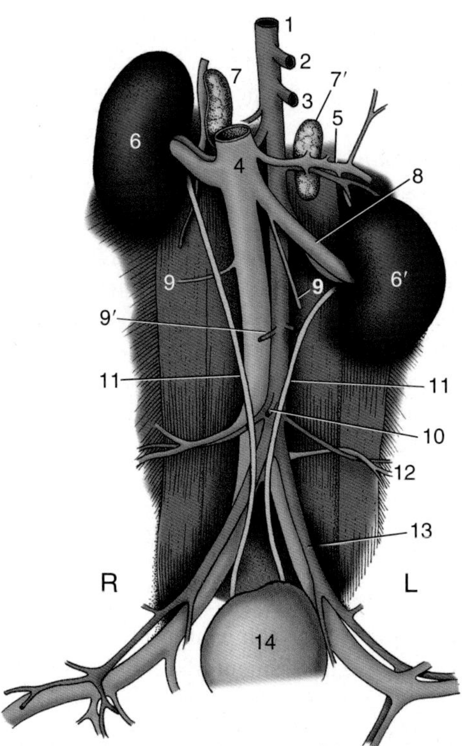

Fig. 14.28 The canine urinary organs and adjacent blood vessels in situ. *1,* Aorta; *2,* celiac a.; *3,* cranial mesenteric a.; *4,* caudal vena cava; *5,* phrenicoabdominal vessels; *6* and *6′,* right and left kidneys; *7* and *7′,* right and left adrenal glands; *8,* left renal vessels; *9,* ovarian veins.; *9′,* ovarian arteries; *10,* caudal mesenteric artery; *11,* ureters; *12,* deep circumflex iliac vessels; *13,* external iliac vessels; *14,* bladder; *L,* left; *R,* right.

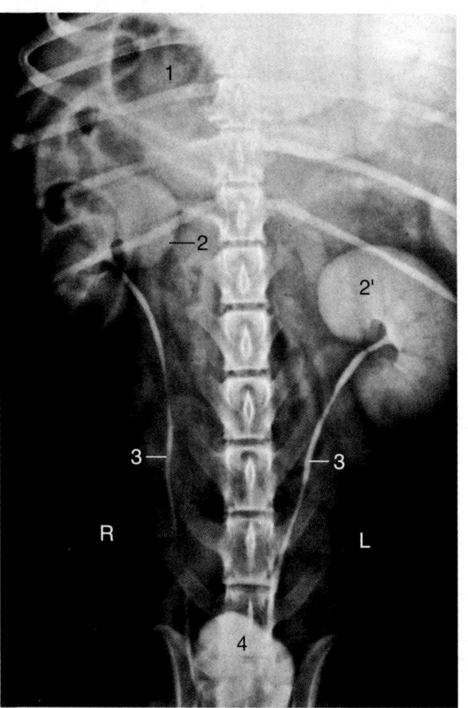

Fig. 14.29 Urogram of a dog. *1,* Gas in stomach; *2* and *2′,* right and left kidneys; *3,* ureters; *4,* bladder; *L,* left; *R,* right.

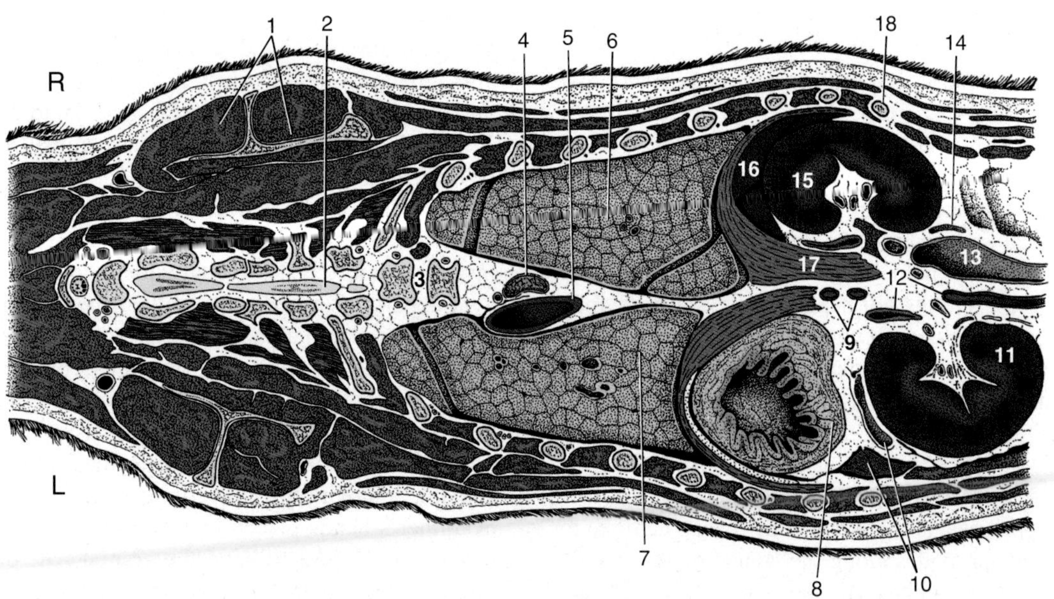

Fig. 14.30 Dorsal section of the canine trunk at the level of the kidneys. *1,* Supraspinatus muscle and scapula; *2,* spinal cord; *3,* sixth and seventh thoracic vertebrae; *4,* right azygous vein; *5,* thoracic aorta; *6, 7,* right and left lungs; *8,* fundus of stomach; *9,* celiac and cranial mesenteric arteries; *10,* splenic vessels and spleen; *11,* left kidney; *12,* left adrenal gland and abdominal aorta; *13,* caudal vena cava; *14,* right ureter; *15,* right kidney (the right adrenal gland is shown medial to the cranial pole); *16,* liver; *17,* right crus of diaphragm; *18,* last rib; *L,* left; *R,* right.

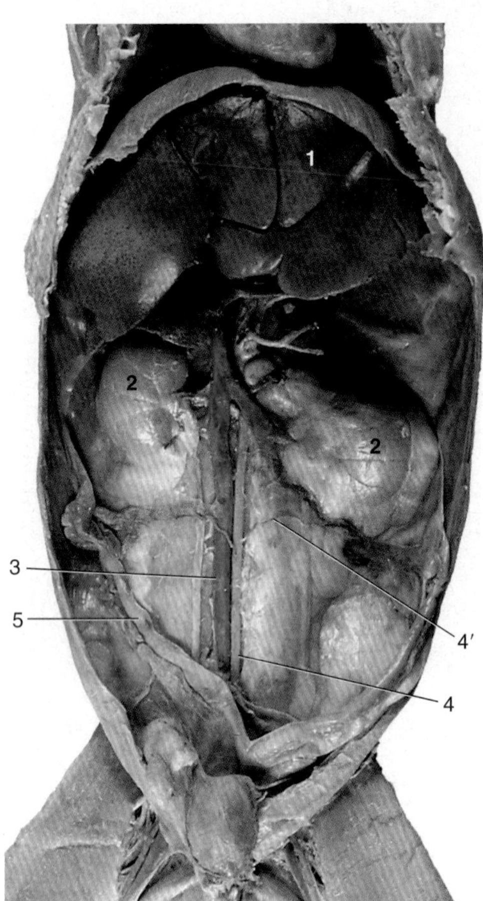

Fig. 14.31 Ventral view of feline abdominal roof. *1,* Liver; *2,* kidneys (with stellate veins); *3,* caudal vena cava (injected); *4,* aorta; *4′,* ovarian artery (injected); *5,* uterus.

bifurcation of the aorta can be palpated rectally in larger individuals (Fig. 14.32/*3*).

The visceral lymph nodes are those directly related to the abdominal organs. The *gastric* lymph node in the lesser omentum near the pylorus is very small and receives lymph from the esophagus, the stomach, the liver, the diaphragm, the mediastinum, and the peritoneum and sends its efferent vessels to the left hepatic or the splenic lymph nodes. The *pancreaticoduodenal* lymph node is also small, receives lymph from the duodenum, the pancreas, and the omentum, and sends its vessels to the right hepatic or right colic lymph nodes. The *hepatic* lymph nodes are situated on each side of the portal vein, at 1 to 2 cm from the hilus of the liver. They receive lymph from the stomach, the duodenum, the pancreas, and of course the liver. The three to five *splenic* lymph nodes along the course of the splenic artery can be 4 cm long in the dog and receive afferent vessels from the esophagus, the stomach, the pancreas, the spleen, the liver, the omentum, and the diaphragm. The *cranial mesenteric* lymph nodes are the largest nodes of the abdomen, can be found along the root of the mesojejunum, and receive lymph from the jejunum, the ileum, and the pancreas. The *colic* lymph nodes in the mesocolon receive afferent vessels from the ileum, cecum, and colon (Table 14.2).

The *cisterna chyli* is an elongated saccular reservoir receiving lymph from the lumbar and mesenteric lymphatic trunks. The cisterna chyli in the dog is located ventral to the first four lumbar vertebrae and dorsal, at the right side, to the aorta and is related to the crura of the diaphragm. The cisterna chyli in cats has a large saccular part dorsal to the aorta and a plexiform part ventral to the aorta and the last thoracic and first three lumbar vertebrae, and it is also closely associated with the diaphragmatic crura.

PALPATION

Abdominal palpation is an important diagnostic tool in the examination of companion animals as it allows identification and assessment of a number of abdominal organs.

> **Abdominal palpation** is an important skill and competency for the veterinarian. Abdominal palpation can be reliably used to identify the masses in 20%–50% of dogs with intestinal tumors.

The system of reference to abdominal regions that is preferred by clinicians divides the abdomen into 18 compartments. Epigastrium, mesogastrium, and hypogastrium are visualized as being defined by two transverse planes:

1. The cranial plane is situated just caudal to the last rib.
2. The caudal plane is situated just cranial to the thigh musculature.

The depth of the abdomen, between the lumbar muscles and the abdominal floor, is then visualized as divided into three, more or less equal parts—dorsal, middle, and ventral parts—yielding nine compartments to each side of the median plan. Palpation of these compartments is performed in a systematic way, generally commencing with the dorsal epigastrium, continuing ventrally, and proceeding from superficial (muscle tension, overfilled intestines) to deep. Palpation is usually performed with the subject standing and with the converging extended fingers of the examiner's hands placed over the flanks. For some purposes it is helpful to have the cranial part of the body raised, allowing the intrathoracic abdominal organs to slide caudally, and for other purposes to have the subject laterally recumbent or supine. A one-handed approach, with the converged fingers opposed to the thumb, is useful with cats and small dogs. Whatever the technique, it is important to allay anxiety so that the animal relaxes its

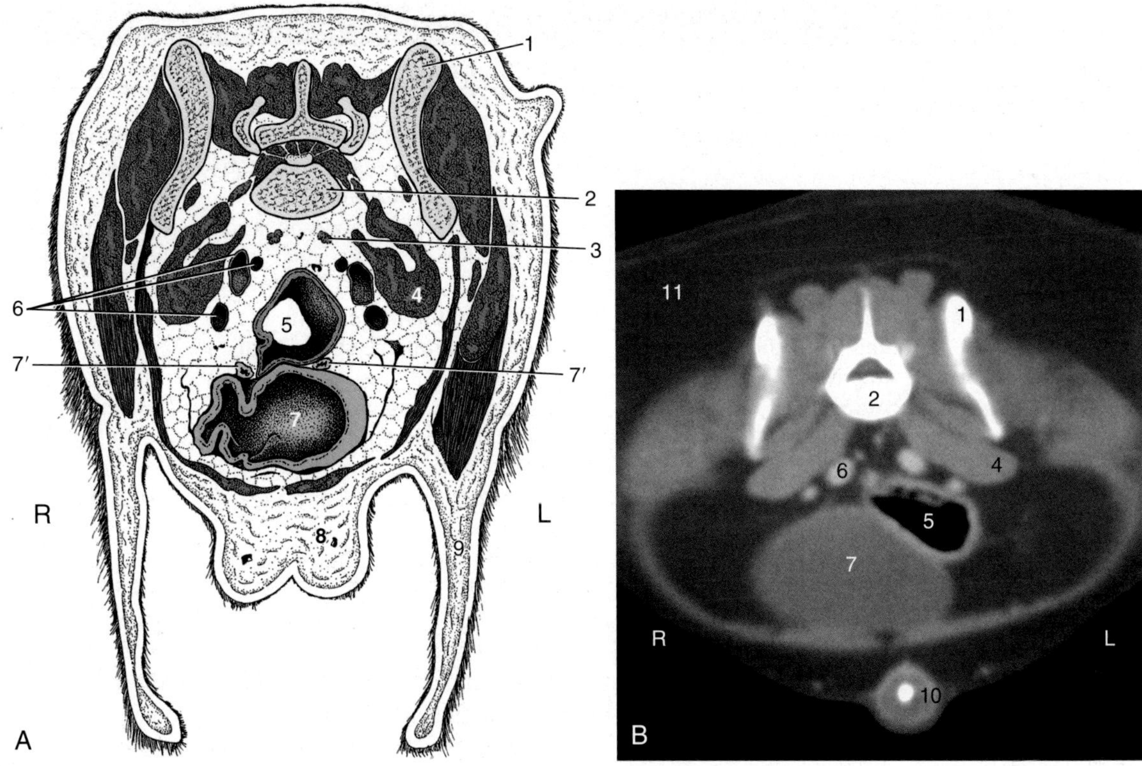

Fig. 14.32 (A) Transverse section of the canine abdomen at the level of the seventh lumbar vertebra. (B) Corresponding computed tomography image at about the same level. *1,* Wing of ilium; *2,* seventh lumbar vertebra; *3,* sacral lymph nodes; *4,* iliopsoas; *5,* descending colon; *6,* internal iliac artery (most dorsal), external iliac vein, and external iliac artery; *7,* bladder; *7′,* uterine horns; *8,* mammary gland; *9,* flank fold; *10,* penis with os penis; *11,* fat; *L,* left; *R,* right.

TABLE 14.2 ABDOMINAL LYMPH STRUCTURES

Lymph Node	Location	Areas Drained	Efferent Flow
Parietal abdominal lymph nodes:			
Lumbar aortic	Under the pleura at dorsal end of 5th or 6th intercostal space	Dorsal thoracic wall	Cisterna chyli or caudal lumbar aortic lymph nodes
Hypogastric	the angle of the internal iliac and median sacral artery, ventral to the body of the seventh lumbar vertebra	the thigh, the pelvic viscera, the tail, and a portion of the lumbar region; and from sacral lymph nodes when present	Cisterna chyli
Deep inguinal or iliofemoral lymph nodes	Ventral surface of the tendon of the psoas minor	Pelvic limb	Medial iliac lymph nodes
Medial iliac lymph nodes	between the deep circumflex iliac and the external iliac artery, ventral to the bodies of the fifth and sixth lumbar vertebrae	all parts of the dorsal half of the abdomen, the pelvis, and the pelvic limb, including that from the genital system and the caudal part of the digestive and urinary system; also receive from the deep and superficial inguinal, the left colic, sacral, and hypogastric lymph nodes	Cisterna chyli

TABLE 14.2 Cont'd

Lymph Node	Location	Areas Drained	Efferent Flow
Visceral abdominal lymph nodes:			
Gastric	Lesser omentum	the esophagus, the stomach, the liver, the diaphragm, the mediastinum, and the peritoneum	Left hepatic or splenic lymph nodes
Pancreaticoduodenal lymph node		the duodenum, the pancreas, and the omentum	right hepatic or right colic lymph nodes
Hepatic lymph nodes	Each side of the portal vein near the hilus of the liver	the stomach, the duodenum, the pancreas, and of course the liver	Cisterna chyli
Splenic lymph nodes	Along the splenic artery	the esophagus, the stomach, the pancreas, the spleen, the liver, the omentum, and the diaphragm	Cisterna chyli
Cranial mesenteric lymph nodes	The root of mesojejunum	the jejunum, the ileum, and the pancreas	Cisterna chyli
Colic lymph nodes	Mesocolon	the ileum, the cecum, and colon	Cisterna chyli

abdominal muscles. The procedure is most rewarding in cats and small dogs and least rewarding in large, well-muscled, or obese dogs.

The normal *liver* projects only slightly, and variably, behind the costal arches and is difficult if not impossible to recognize when the bilateral approach is used. Greater success may be obtained if the fingertips are insinuated deep to the costal arch, a maneuver possible only during full relaxation of the flank muscles. It may then be possible to identify the sharp free margin and narrow adjoining strip of the liver. Homogenous enlargement of the liver can first be palpated in the ventral epigastrium (on superficial palpation) and, following further enlargement, in the medial epigastrium, especially when one places the fingers within the costal arch. The liver can be more easily reached at the left than at the right side.

The empty *stomach* is tucked under the ribs, out of reach on the left side, but when full of ingesta or distended with gas, it projects behind the costal cartilages. It is more easily found in narrow, deep-chested dogs than in barrel-chested breeds. The stomach, when empty, does not contact the abdominal wall, but when moderately filled, it lies against the wall ventrally and to the left. The completely filled stomach, especially in pups, lies largely in contact with the ventral body wall, toward a transverse plane just caudal to the umbilicus. The *spleen* occupies the same region against the left flank, but its soft and deformable consistency does not make it easy to palpate unless the organ is considerably enlarged and firmed. Normally the spleen is located to the left in the epigastrium, close to the major curvature of the stomach (completely within the costal arch in the dog). In the case of enlargement the spleen moves ventrally and caudally, and can be felt in the ventral and medial mesogastrium.

Success in locating the *kidneys* is rather unpredictable in the dog. Most often, only the caudal pole of the left kidney is within reach, and it may be identified by its firm, rounded contours. The right kidney is commonly inaccessible. In some dogs, generally of the larger breeds, the left kidney is pendulous and "floats" at a more ventral level than usual; this is the normal condition for both kidneys in the cat, and both may be steadied through the abdominal wall for biopsy puncture. The entire surface of a "floating" kidney, including the depression at the dorsally facing hilus, may be examined. The left kidney contacts the dorsal part of the left lateral abdominal wall.

The fluctuating *intestinal mass* occupies a large part of the abdomen, extending from the roof to the floor and from one flank to the other. Identification of most individual parts is problematical. The descending duodenum may sometimes be identified on the right side if the fingers are first pressed against the abdominal roof and then drawn laterally. There is no difficulty in finding the jejunum, whose coils may be made to slip between the hands. In the dog the only part of the large intestine that may be sought with confidence is the descending colon on the left side. It is most readily identified when occupied by a column of hard or granular feces. The ascending colon and cecum may sometimes be identified, most readily when gas-distended, but the transverse colon is too deeply tucked under the ribs to be within reach. All parts of the large intestine are more readily found in cats, in which a useful guide to the positions of the cecum and ascending colon is provided by the firmness at the ileocecocolic junction. The lymph nodes associated with the intestine evade detection unless enlarged.

COMPREHENSION CHECK

1. Using cadavers and available imaging modalities (radiographs or CT scans), develop a thorough understanding of the topography of the abdominal organs.
2. Explore the inguinal canal and its contents, and gain an understanding of the process of inguinal hernia.

15 The Pelvis and Reproductive Organs of the Dog and Cat

GENERAL ANATOMY OF THE PELVIS AND PERINEUM (see also pp. 49-50)

The bony pelvis is formed by the pelvic girdle, sacrum, and first few caudal vertebrae; of course the caudal limit of the roof is, as always, difficult to define precisely. Because the bones and their surface landmarks are described in Chapters 2 and Chapter 17, respectively, only a few general features of the anatomy of the pelvis are recapitulated here.

The *pelvic cavity* is smaller than might be supposed from examination of the intact animal or the isolated girdle. The discrepancy is due to the shallowness of the caudal part of the abdomen and to the acute angle (about 20 degrees) formed between the ilia and the vertebral column (Fig. 15.1). The pronounced obliquity of the inlet places the pubic brim level with, or even behind, the caudal limit of the sacrum. The iliac shafts are not quite parallel, and the inlet is widest in its middle part and narrowest dorsally. The pelvic outlet is less confined than the inlet and possesses a considerable capacity for further enlargement through elevation of the tail behind the very short sacrum. Only a small part of the lateral wall is bony, as neither the ischial spine nor the ischial tuber rises to any great height. In the dog the sacrotuberous ligament is reduced to a narrow cord (under cover of the superficial gluteal muscle) extending between the ischial tuber and the caudolateral corner of the sacrum (Fig. 15.1A).

The pelvic girdle of the cat shows some differences. Cranially, the ilia diverge slightly, producing a somewhat funnel-shaped entrance to the pelvis from the abdominal cavity. The wings of these bones are relatively smaller and shallower, easing the transition. The ischial tubers stand closer together than in the dog, a feature that gives the pelvis a more rectangular appearance in the ventrodorsal view and a more confined exit (Fig. 15.2). In consequence of the last feature the perineum is narrow. *There are no sacrotuberous ligaments in this species.*

The almost straight axis of the short pelvic canal appears to be well adapted for easy parturition. Sexual dimorphism is not pronounced, and pelvic measurements have not been given much attention in small animal obstetrics. An ill match of the proportions of the fetus and the dam is most common in cases in which the litter is small (and the individual fetus relatively large) in toy dogs as well as in those breeds in which a measure of achondroplasia is a feature of the conformation. On rectal examination the pelvic canal of young dogs is shaped like an hourglass, which may mistakenly suggest a pelvic fracture.

The *perineum* slopes somewhat ventrocaudally and is largely concealed when the tail is carried low. When the tail is raised, it exhibits a shield of naked integument about the anal orifice and, at some distance ventral to this, the vulva or root of the penis. The *ischiorectal fossa* between the anus and the ischial tuber naturally varies in prominence with the character of the coat and the degree of obesity. The fossa is bounded by the sacrotuberous ligament and the deep face of the superficial gluteal muscle laterally and by the superficial face of the coccygeus medially. It is traversed by the large caudal gluteal vessels that run against the lateral wall and by the main trunks and certain branches of the internal pudendal vessels and pudendal nerve placed more medially, toward the floor (Fig. 15.3/*2* and *3*).

The *pelvic diaphragm* has the usual composition. The lateral muscle, *the coccygeus,* has a tendinous origin from the ischial spine and inserts on the lateral aspect of the tail between the second and fifth vertebrae (Figs. 3.48 and 15.3). The deeper and thinner *levator ani* (Fig. 3.48/*2*) has a wider origin, which extends from the iliac shaft onto the pelvic floor along which it runs, directly to the side of the symphysis (Fig. 15.4/*7*). The part arising from the pelvic floor closely embraces the pelvic viscera in its passage to its insertion on the tail, reaching as far caudally as the seventh vertebra. The fibers of the levator ani run more obliquely than those of the coccygeus, and part of the levator ani emerges superficially behind the other muscle. The levator ani has only a passing fascial connection with the external sphincter of the anus, and like the coccygeus, it is primarily a depressor of the tail. However, its fascial attachment enables it to help fix the position of the anus during defecation.

The **perineal hernia** is the escape of the pelvic viscera, due to weakness or atrophy of the muscles of the pelvic diaphragm, into the perineal area. This displaced pelvic organ causes a swelling to the side of the anus. Surgical repair of this condition involves suture of the external sphincter to the coccygeus and internal obturator muscles, and the sacrotuberous ligament about the margins of the space.

The *pelvic blood vessels and nerves* are sufficiently described in the general accounts (pp. 236 and 313).

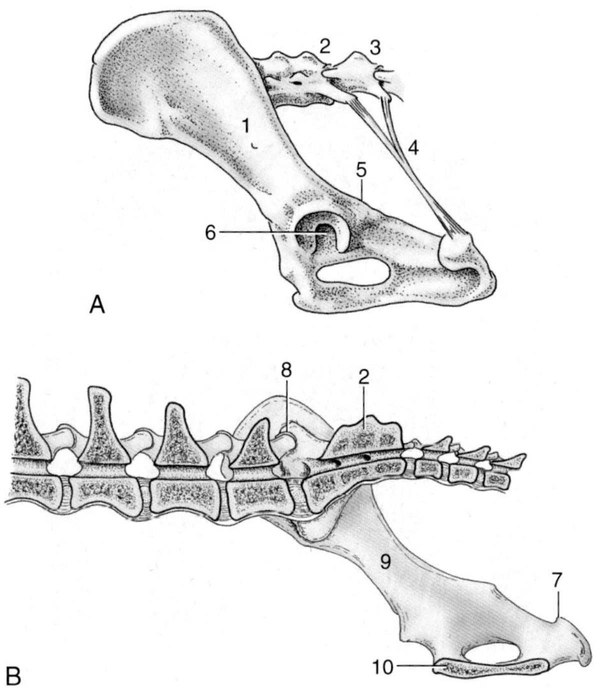

Fig. 15.1 (A) Canine sacrotuberous ligament, left lateral view. (B) Right half of canine bony pelvis, medial view. *1,* Ilium; *2,* sacrum; *3,* caudal vertebra(e); *4,* sacrotuberous ligament; *5,* ischial spine; *6,* acetabulum; *7,* ischial tuber; *8,* sacroiliac joint; *9,* shaft of ilium; *10,* symphysis.

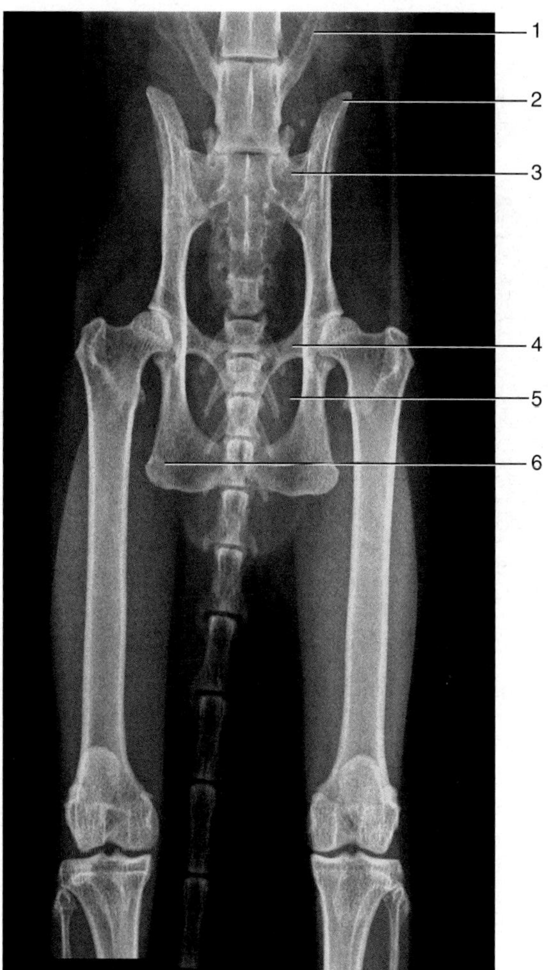

Fig. 15.2 Radiograph of the feline pelvis. *1,* Transverse process of last lumbar vertebra (L7); *2,* iliac crest; *3,* sacrum; *4,* pecten of the pubis; *5,* obturator foramen; *6,* ischial tuber.

Because there are only three sacral spinal nerves, the origins of the pudendal, caudal rectal, and pelvic nerves are rather compressed; variations in the branching patterns of the first two are common. The pudendal and caudal rectal nerves supply afferent and efferent fibers to the perineum, and their integrity is necessary for the execution of the perineal reflex that provides a means of gauging the depth of narcosis. The modified skin about the anus is especially sensitive, and even a gentle touch evokes a brisk contraction of the anal sphincter of the conscious or lightly anesthetized animal.

THE RECTUM AND ANUS (see also pp. 124 and 125)

The *rectum* joins the anal canal ventral to the second or third caudal vertebra. Although the intraperitoneal cranial part is joined to the pelvic roof by a short mesorectum (Fig. 15.4/*4*), the caudal part becomes entirely retroperitoneal once the serous covering is reflected onto the pelvic walls and the dorsal surface of the reproductive tract (bitch) or prostate (dog). The rectum is related dorsally to the ventral muscles of the tail and certain smooth muscle bundles (rectococcygeus) that run caudally from the rectal wall to the undersurface of the tail; these bundles probably help draw the anus caudally when a column of feces descends from the colon. The ventral relations of the rectum of the bitch are the cervix and, possibly, the body of the uterus in addition to the vagina; in the male dog they are the prostate and urethra. Laterally, the rectum is bounded by the levator ani muscle and crossed by the internal pudendal vessels (Fig. 15.3) and the sciatic, pelvic, pudendal, and caudal rectal nerves. The rectum has some freedom to deviate from its usual median course because of its mesorectum and its cushioning by fat.

The mucosa of the short (about 7 mm) initial columnar portion of the *anal canal* is fashioned by underlying vessels into a series of longitudinal ridges whose interdigitation helps maintain continence (Fig. 15.5). These ridges end on a line that represents the junction between the columnar intestinal epithelium and the stratified cutaneous epithelium. The outer cutaneous zone is of variable extent; the modified skin that lines this last part of the passage may be everted to appear as a purplish patch on the perineal surface, especially when defecation impends. At this time

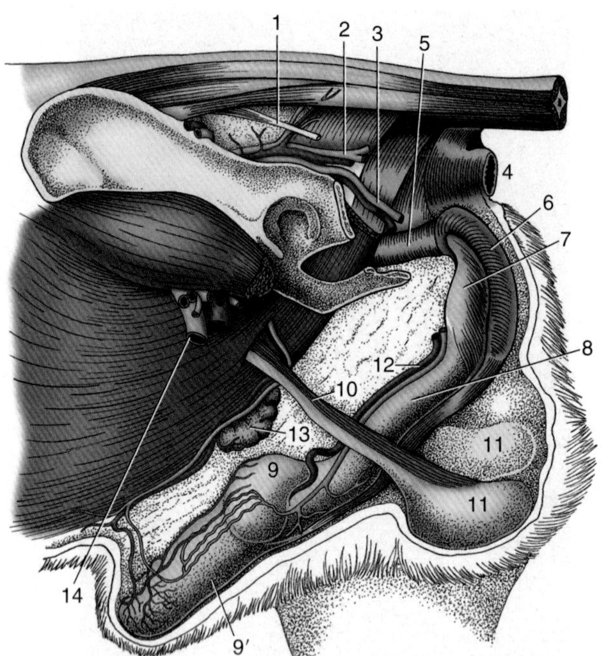

Fig. 15.3 Deep dissection of the external reproductive organs of the dog. *1,* Sacrotuberous ligament; *2,* caudal gluteal vessels; *3,* internal pudendal vessels; *4,* anus; *5,* pelvic urethra; *6,* bulb of penis enclosed by bulbospongiosus; *7,* ischiocavernosus over left crus; *8,* body of penis; *9* and *9′,* bulbus and pars longa glandis; *10,* spermatic cord; *11,* testes in scrotum; *12,* dorsal artery and vein of the penis; *13,* superficial inguinal lymph nodes and caudal superficial epigastric vessels; *14,* femoral vessels.

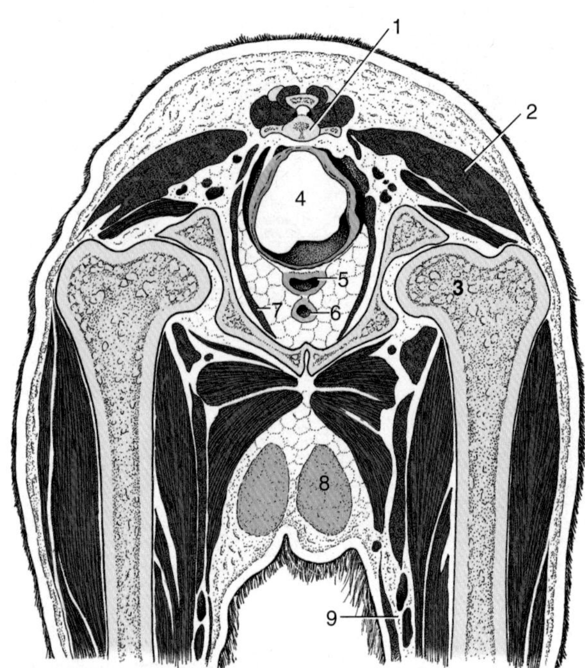

Fig. 15.4 Transverse section of the canine pelvis at the level of the hip joint. *1,* Caudal vertebra; *2,* superficial gluteal muscle; *3,* head of femur in acetabulum; *4,* rectum suspended by a short mesorectum; *5,* vagina; *6,* urethra; *7,* levator ani; *8,* inguinal mammary gland; *9,* femoral artery and vein.

the anal orifice takes on a triangular form in place of the transverse slit generally displayed (see Fig. 10.29A).

Developmental errors lead to an imperforate anus, which results from the persistence of an unusually thick anal membrane, or to the absence of a longer portion of patent bowel, which results from the failure of the rectum to make proper connection with the anal pit.

All fissiped carnivores (other than bears) possess paired *anal sacs* (sinus paranales) enclosed between the external and internal anal sphincters. In the dog, each is about 1 cm in diameter and discharges through a short duct that opens ventrolateral to the anal orifice at the level of the anocutaneous line, concealed or exposed on the perineal surface according to the physiologic condition (see Fig. 3.47/*1*). In cats, the ducts of the anal sacs open on small projections some distance lateral to the anus and not at the mucocutaneous junction as in dogs. Modified sweat glands are located beneath the epithelium and discharge into the lumen of the sac. In the cats, only apocrine glands are found, but in dogs both sebaceous and apocrine sweat glands are present. Because occlusion of the duct of the anal sac is frequently encountered in dogs but is rare in cats, it is thought that the lipid component of these sebaceous secretions is responsible for the difference. The evil-smelling content of the anal sacs, normally expressed in the later stages of defecation, serves as a marker that identifies the animal to other members of its species.

The impaction of anal sacs due to accumulation of secretions, generally secondary to inflammation of the sacs, is commonly seen in dogs. The anal sacs of dogs and bitches develop the malignant tumors of the apocrine glands. These tumors produce a parathormone-like hormone that raises the blood calcium levels.

The lymphatics of the anal sac drain to the sacral, hypogastric, and medial iliac lymph nodes.

There are, in addition, small anal glands within the columnar zone and much larger and more numerous circumanal or perianal glands within the cutaneous zone. In dogs, the circumanal glands are lobulated, modified sebaceous glands located in a ring about the anus, extending outward for a distance of perhaps 3 cm from the anocutaneous junction. These glands can be identified shortly after birth and increase in size throughout adult life in response to androgens. In older male dogs, slow-growing, generally benign tumors of these glands commonly develop near the anus.

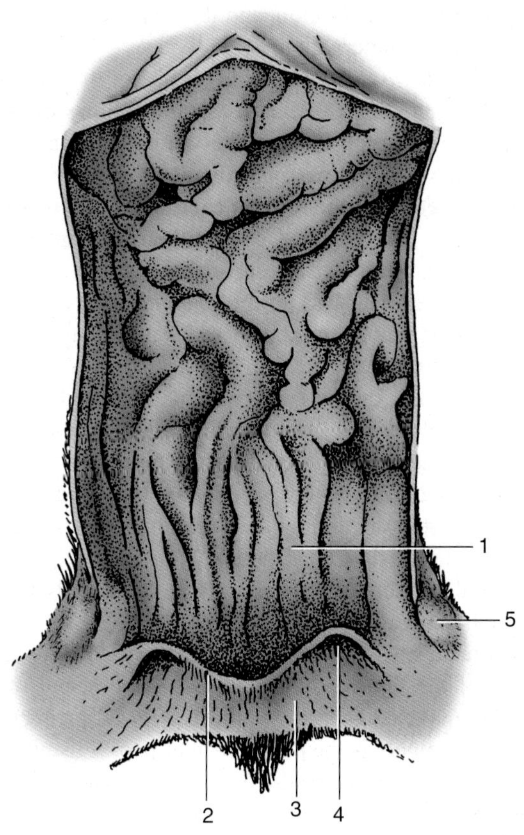

Fig. 15.5 Feline anal canal opened dorsally. *1,* Columnar zone; *2,* anocutaneous line; *3,* cutaneous zone; *4,* opening of the right anal sac; *5,* right anal sac.

The Kidneys

The positions and relations of the kidneys were described in the previous chapter.

The right kidney usually lies below the first three lumbar vertebrae, and the left one lies below the second to fourth, although both may be found a full vertebral length more caudally. In the bitch the caudal poles of both kidneys reach close to, or make contact with, the fat-filled mesovaria. Although described as unipyramidal (p. 165), the canine kidney retains clear evidence of a number of previous separate pyramids. The renal arteries, direct branches from the aorta, usually divide before entering the kidneys. The renal veins pass directly to the caudal vena cava (see Fig. 14.28). There are no features of major specific interest in the sympathetic and parasympathetic nerve supply.

The kidneys of the cat are relatively larger, shorter, and thicker than those of the dog and obtain a distinctive appearance from the capsular veins that converge toward the hilus, where they enter the renal vein (Fig. 15.6). The cut surface of the kidney is red to yellowish red because of a large amount of intracellular fat stored in the proximal convoluted tubules; the fat content is greatest in castrated males and pregnant females. There are fewer vestiges of

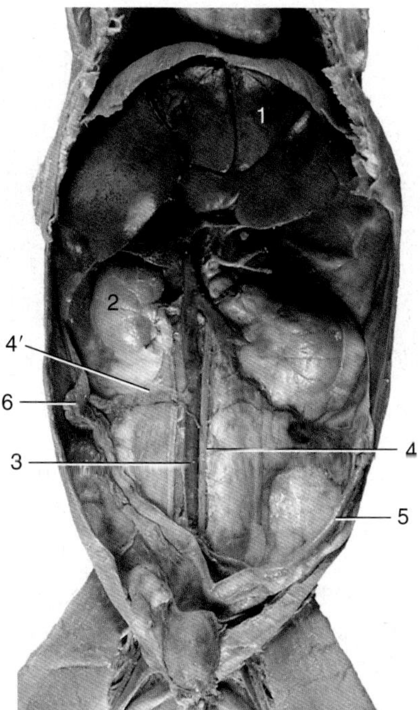

Fig. 15.6 Ventral view of feline abdominal roof. *1,* Liver; *2,* kidneys (with stellate veins); *3,* caudal vena cava (injected); *4,* aorta; *4′,* ovarian artery (injected); *5,* uterine horn; *6,* ovary.

the multipyramidal stage of development. The kidneys, especially the left one, can be displaced rather far cranially or caudally from its usual position (see Fig. 14.15); it has been mistaken for a pathologic swelling. In cats, both kidneys are readily palpable.

In the dog (if not the cat) it is more prudent to perform kidney biopsy by laparotomy rather than by a blind puncture.

The muscle of the renal pelvis is strongest at the transition to the ureter, presumably to impel urine into the narrower tube. The abdominal part of the ureter runs retroperitoneally close to the aorta or vena cava (see Figs. 14.21, 14.29/*3,* and 15.6), passing over the dorsal (lateral) surface of the gonadal vessels before crossing the ventral face of the deep circumflex iliac vessels and the terminal branches of the aorta (and corresponding veins). It is carried into the pelvis in the base of the broad ligament or genital fold, which brings it to the dorsal surface of the bladder; in the male the ureter crosses above the deferent duct toward the end of its course. It penetrates the bladder wall very obliquely. The inclusion of the ureter within the genital fold places it at some risk in the common spay operation.

The kidneys that are enclosed in fat are visible on the abdominal radiographs. (Deficiency of fat occurs in very young pups and in emaciated older subjects.) However, a series of timed radiographs taken following intravenous injection of an appropriate contrast material shows general opacification of the cortex and medulla (see Fig. 14.29), renal pelvic morphology (see Fig. 5.29), and, later, the status

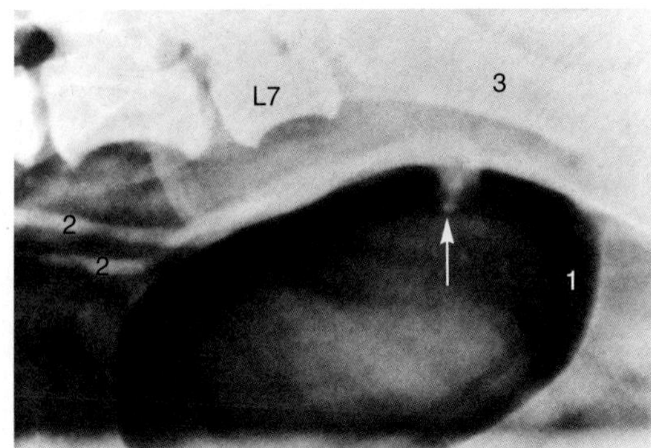

Fig. 15.7 The canine bladder made visible by the introduction of air. The *arrow* indicates the terminations of the ureters in the dorsal wall of the bladder, superimposed here on the air-filled lumen. *1,* Caudal end of bladder; *2,* ureters; *3,* shaft of ilium; *L7,* seventh lumbar vertebra.

of the ureters and bladder. Because the passage of urine is assisted by peristaltic contraction, a single radiograph does not usually depict a healthy ureter along its entire length.

The Bladder and Female Urethra (see also pp. 171-173)

The bulk of the bladder is visible as soon as the floor of the abdomen is removed because it is not covered by the greater omentum (Fig. 15.7). Its size varies greatly, and when excessively distended, it may reach to or even beyond the umbilicus (Fig. 15.27). Given freedom, dogs urinate frequently as a social (scent-marking) as well as eliminative function.* The bladder may be identified on abdominal palpation when moderately (or more greatly) distended. Unless handled with care, a grossly distended bladder may rupture when compressed through the abdominal wall to induce micturition. Although the oblique passage of the ureters through the bladder wall normally affords protection against reflux of urine to the kidneys, even gentle but prolonged compression may push the urine into the kidneys. A moderately expanded bladder is not accompanied by increased tension, and radiographs using contrast medium show its contours molded to those of adjacent organs (see Fig. 5.30). The organ is globular when the thick detrusor muscle is fully contracted.

The peritoneal covering, which extends onto the cranial part of the urethra, is reflected into the usual lateral and ventral folds.

The bladder receives its blood supply through the *cranial vesical artery,* a branch of the umbilical artery, and the *caudal vesical artery,* an indirect branch of the internal iliac artery. The *hypogastric nerve* supplies the sympathetic innervation, the pelvic nerve (S1–S3) supplies the parasympathetic innervation, and the *pudendal nerve* (S1–S3), the somatic innervation.

The *female urethra* is relatively long. It originates within the cranial part of the pelvis and follows the symphysis to open on the floor of the vestibule, immediately caudal to the vestibulovaginal junction. In the bitch, the orifice is raised on a tubercle that continues some way over the vestibular floor, flanked by well-marked depressions. Although blind catheterization is difficult in small subjects, the procedure is less troublesome in larger bitches, in which a finger may be introduced to locate the tubercle and guide the instrument.

The bladder of the cat is more cranially placed than that of the dog and lies wholly within the abdomen at all times. As a result, the urethra is unusually long (Fig. 15.8). The urethra of the queen is more or less uniformly wide (unlike its counterpart in the tom) and makes a more discrete entry into the vestibule than that in the bitch.

The male urethra of both species is considered with the reproductive organs.

The urachus, which connects the bladder with the allantoic sac of the fetus, normally closes at birth, but sometimes there is leakage at the umbilicus for a time. A more important anomaly is the persistence of part of the urachus as a diverticulum of the bladder, which seems to predispose to recurrent bladder infections.

Congenital *urinary incontinence* in dogs and cats is most often caused by ectopic ureters—those that terminate at a site other than the normal one at the trigone of the bladder. Sometimes ureters take an unusual course through the bladder wall, and sometimes they bypass the organ to enter a more distal part of the urogenital tract.

Acquired urinary incontinence occurs most often after the spaying of bitches and is caused by urethral sphincter incompetence, for which a number of explanations, some more likely than others, have been suggested: low urethral pressure, a short urethra, estrogen deficiency, and an intrapelvic position of the bladder. This type of incontinence is most often associated with relaxation or recumbency, particularly at night. Several surgical techniques have been developed to relocate the bladder neck to an intraabdominal position with the use of the prepubic tendon as an anchor.

THE FEMALE REPRODUCTIVE ORGANS

The Ovaries and Uterine Tubes (see also pp. 184-186)

The ovary projects and is entrapped in a bursa created by the fusion of the distal mesovarium and the mesosalpinx (see Fig. 5.60). The bursa contains enough fat in bitches to conceal the ovary (Fig. 15.9), which is a firm, flattened, ellipsoidal structure measuring about 15 × 10 × 6 mm. Its contours are obviously less regular in phases of the estrous

* In addition to marking, ostentatious cocking of the leg by a male dog when passing urine may assert superiority. Cats also make a social use of micturition (see later).

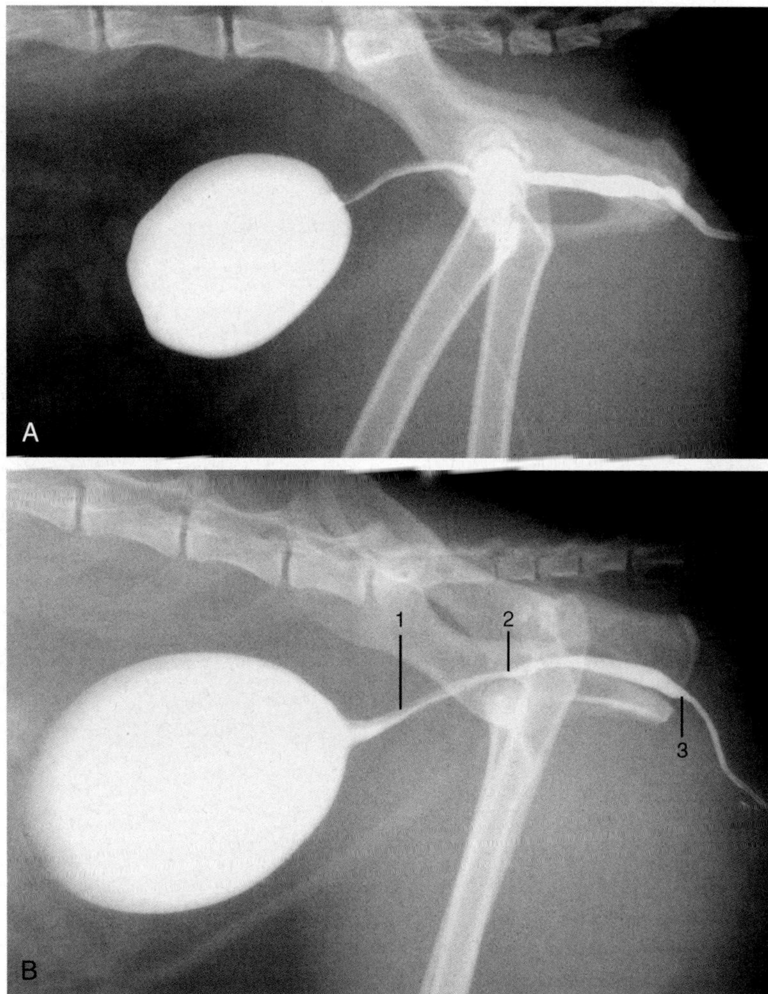

Fig. 15.8 Radiographs of the feline bladder when (A) moderately and (B) markedly full. *1,* Preprostatic urethra: the upper gray part is the urethral crest, the lower white part is the lumen filled with contrast medium; *2,* slight dorsal dip marks the seminal colliculus; *3,* isthmus, narrowing of lumen.

cycle in which large follicles or corpora lutea are present (Fig. 15.10). The wall of the ovarian bursa of the cat commonly contains conspicuously less fat than that of the bitch and covers only the lateral surface of the ovary to make it more visible.

The close proximity or even contact of the ovaries (within the bursae) with the caudal poles of the kidneys makes their position correspondingly asymmetrical. Although most spay procedures (the removal of ovaries and [parts of] the uterine horns; ovariectomy/ovariohysterectomy) are now performed by midline incision, an alternative lateral approach is quite often used in cats. The flank incision is made midway between the iliac crest and the last rib in the confident expectation that the ovary will be within easy reach. The right ovary is usually found dorsal or dorsolateral to the ascending colon, and the left one is found between the dorsal extremity of the spleen and the descending colon. Lengthening of the attachments in parous animals allows the ovaries a greater mobility. The laparoscopically assisted ovariectomy can be done through the placement of two laparoscopic ports 3–5 cm cranial to the umbilicus and the pubis.

The ovary is fixed additionally by suspensory and proper ligaments. The former is a peritoneal fold, thickened along its free margin, that attaches to the transverse fascia close to the last rib in the dog (Fig. 15.11/*6*). It is prolonged caudally as the proper ligament, which extends beyond the ovary to merge with the tip of the uterine horn. The anchorage provided by the suspensory ligament makes surgical exteriorization of the ovary difficult. The suspensory ligament in the cat reaches the diaphragm and allows the ovary greater mobility.

The entrance to the canine bursa is reduced to a slit in the medial wall, usually made obvious by the protrusion of a few reddish infundibular fimbriae. The infundibulum is continued by the narrower part of the uterine tube, which is not obviously divided between ampulla

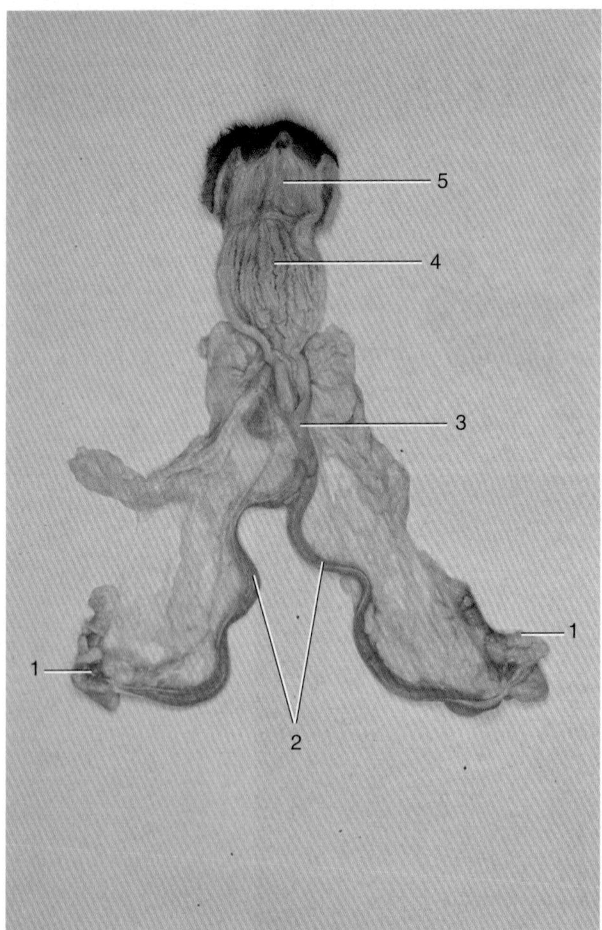

Fig. 15.9 Overview of canine female reproductive tract. Vagina has been opened. *1,* Ovaries; *2,* uterine horns; *3,* uterus body; *4,* vagina; *5,* vestibulum.

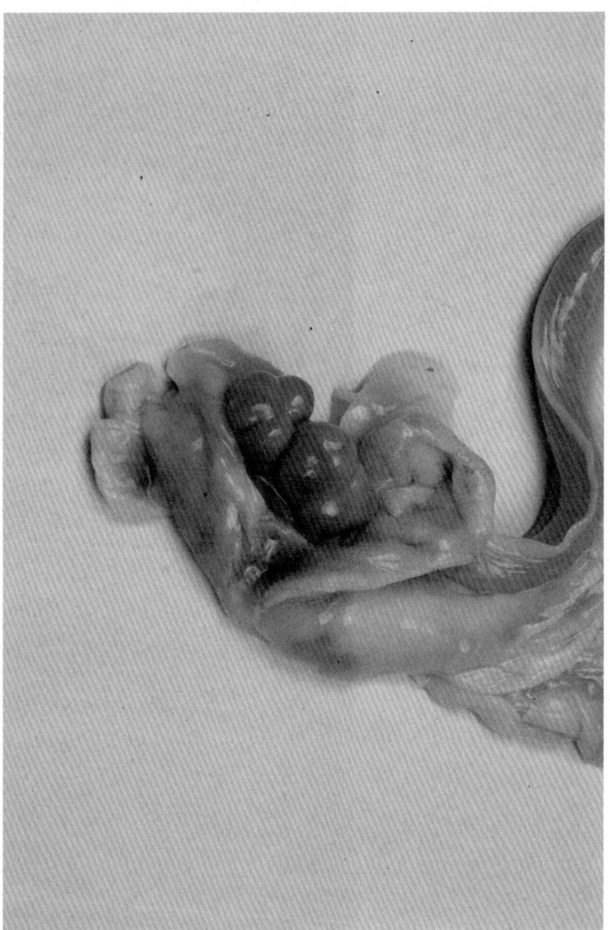
Fig. 15.10 Ovarian bursa opened to expose the ovary (bitch).

and isthmus. These parts follow a tortuous course within the walls of the bursa; disregarding minor kinks and bends, the tube runs in a broad sweep that first passes forward in the distal mesovarium before crossing cranial to the ovary to continue caudally in the mesosalpinx (see Fig. 5.60). It ends in an abrupt junction with the horn of the uterus. Although in most subjects much of the tube is concealed by fat deposits, the terminal part is usually visible. The infundibulum may transmit bacteria into the bursa (or abdominal cavity) in the case of pyometra.

Parovarian cysts originate from remnants of either mesonephric or paramesonephric ducts. They are more frequently encountered during ovariohysterectomy in dogs than in cats and are located between the ovary and uterine horn.

The Uterus (see also pp. 186-187)

The uterus, which lies mainly dorsal to the small intestine, consists of a very short (about 2 to 3 cm) body and two long and slender (about 12 × 1 cm) divergent horns (Figs. 15.11/*7* and *8* and 15.12). The body is near the pubic brim but may be abdominal or pelvic in position. It is, in fact, even shorter than external inspection suggests because a short internal septum continues caudally from the junction of the horns. The cervix is also very short—the canal is barely 1 cm long—but the tissue thickening extends beyond the external ostium as a fold on the roof of the vagina (Fig. 15.12/*3* and *3'*). Transverse grooves frequently divide this fold into cranial, middle, and caudal tubercles; they become very swollen at certain stages of the cycle. The ostium of the cervix generally faces caudoventrally, and this orientation, combined with the asymmetry of the fornix and the fissuration of the cervical prolongation, may make its identification rather difficult, even with the aid of an endoscope.

The feline cervix feels like a hard oval knot at the uterovaginal junction and, although small, is readily distinguished from the adjoining parts by the thickness of its wall. As in the bitch, the cervical mucosa is smooth, without conspicuous folds.

The *broad ligaments* also commonly contain much fat. They are wider in their middle parts than toward their extremities and allow the horns of the uterus considerable mobility. An unusual feature is the detachment from the

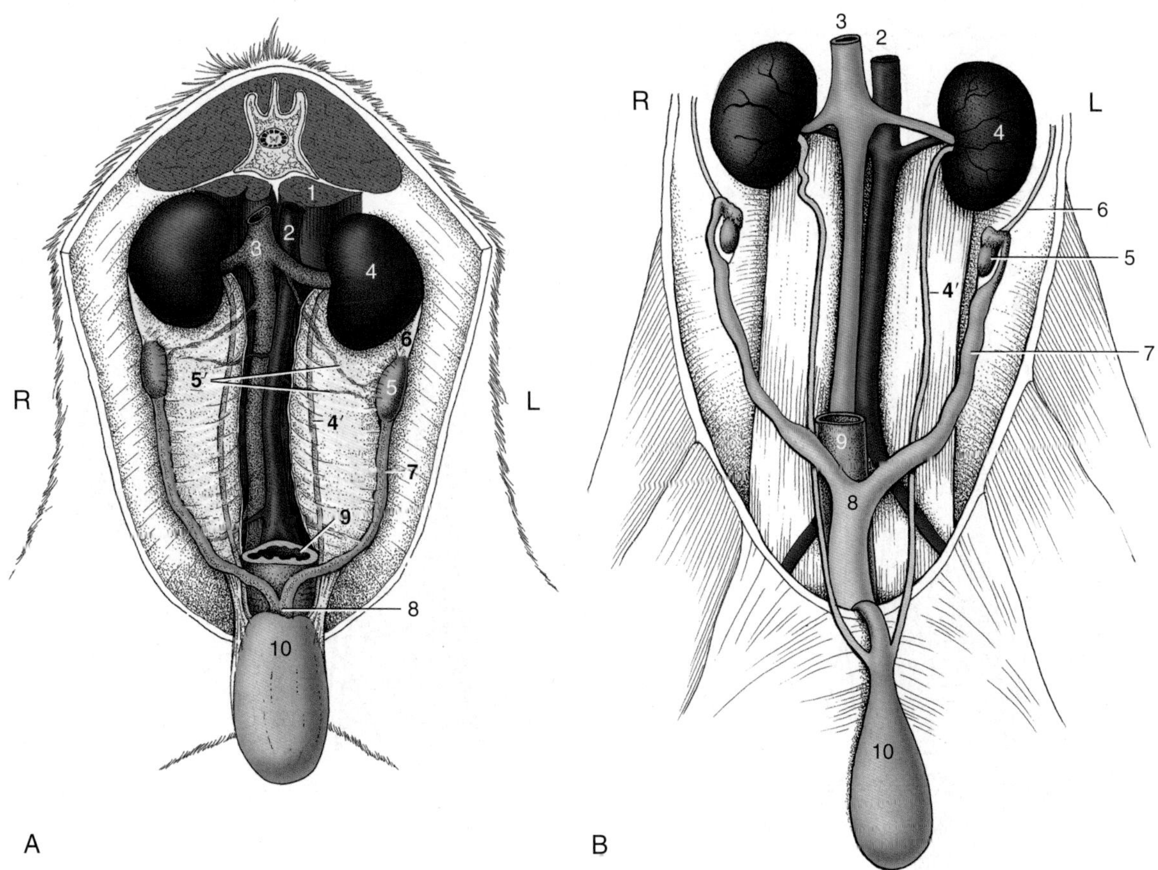

Fig. 15.11 (A) Canine and (B) feline ovaries and uterus in situ, ventral view. *1,* Psoas muscles; *2,* aorta; *3,* caudal vena cava; *4* and *4',* left kidney and ureter; *5,* ovary; *5',* ovarian vessels; *6,* suspensory ligament of ovary; *7,* uterine horn; *8,* body of uterus; *9,* rectum; *10,* bladder, reflected caudally; *L,* left; *R,* right.

lateral surface of a peritoneal fold that extends toward, and in the bitch through, the inguinal canal to end variously between the groin and the vulva. The fold is thickened at its free margin *(the round ligament),* slightly dilating the canal and predisposing to inguinal hernia, an almost male prerogative in other species. The most likely herniation is of the uterine horn, which may result in its subcutaneous entrapment of the pregnant uterus and may require a separate procedure to deliver the fetus.

The vascularization of the uterus depends on the uterine branch of *the ovarian artery and the uterine artery,* a branch of the vaginal artery (Fig. 15.13/*1* and *5*). The two vessels anastomose within the broad ligament and must be ligated when ovariohysterectomy is performed. These vessels lie close to the extremities of the uterus but swing away in the intermediate part of the broad ligament. The proximity of the uterine artery to the cervix allows an arterial ligature to be securely anchored to the uterine stump to prevent slippage when the bulk of the uterus is removed surgically. The uterus is drained by left and right uterine veins that empty into the renal vein and the caudal vena cava, respectively. The ovarian artery and vein do not closely accompany each other within the mesovarium.

The lymphatic drainage of the ovary and uterus passes to the medial iliac and aortic lumbar nodes.

The Vagina, Vestibule, and Vulva (see also pp. 187-189)

The vagina of the bitch is very long (about 12 cm) and extends horizontally through the pelvis before dipping beyond the ischial arch to join the vestibule (see Fig. 5.35/*5* and *9*). Apart from the prominent dorsomedian fold that continues the cervix for a short distance, the interior of the undistended organ is obstructed by the irregular folds that end at the junction with the vestibule (Figs. 15.12 and 15.13). The vestibule continues the downward slope of the vagina, requiring that a vaginal speculum or other instrument be passed in a craniodorsal direction to clear the ischial arch before it can be advanced horizontally (see Fig. 5.2). During such examinations the dorsal fold combines with the lateral and ventral vaginal walls to simulate a cervix (pseudocervix).

The cranial part of the vestibular floor (of the bitch) displays the tubercle and flanking depressions associated with the opening of the urethra, and the caudal part presents the fossa into which the glans of the clitoris projects

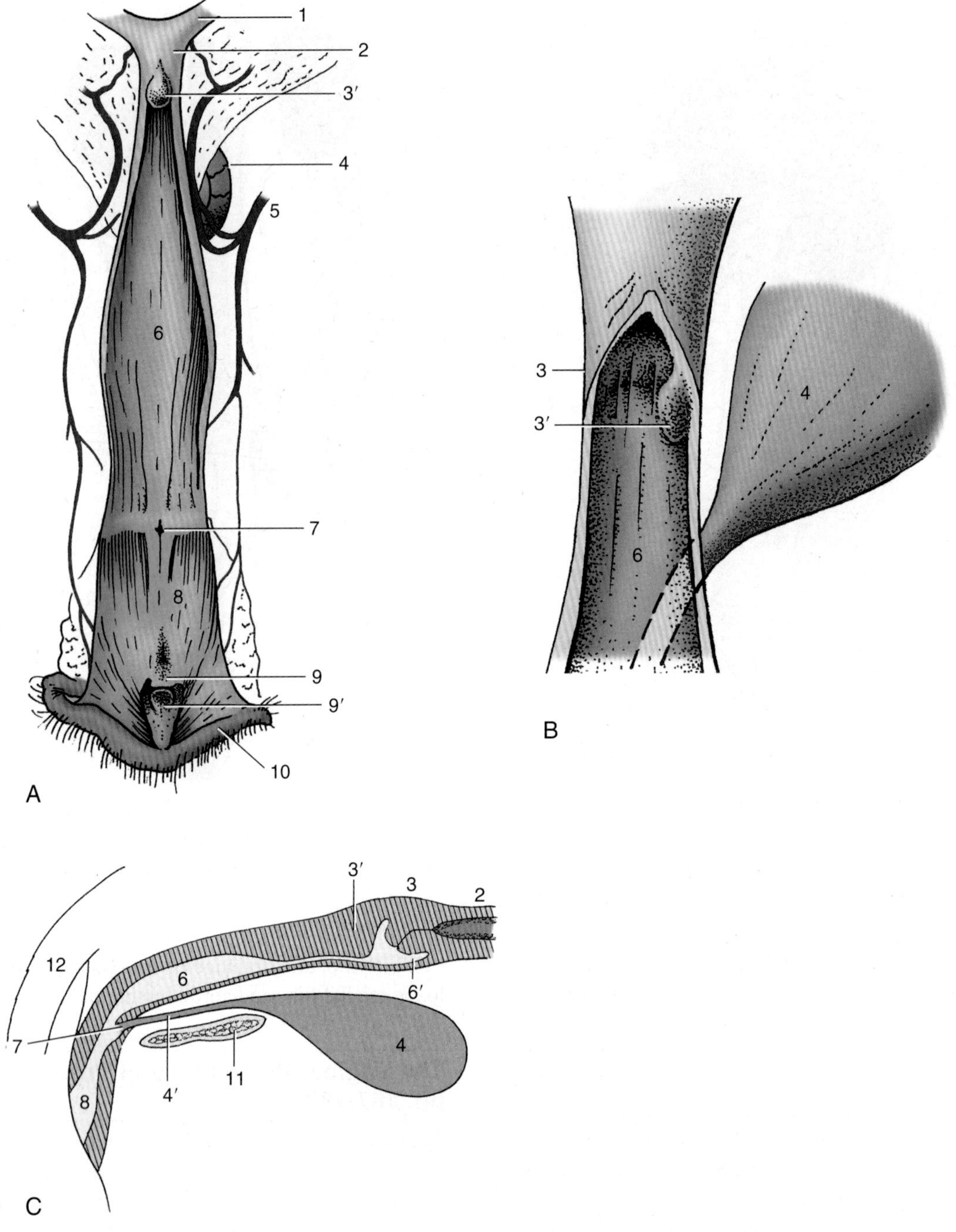

Fig. 15.12 (A) Canine vagina, vestibule, and vulva, opened dorsally. (B) Enlarged view of the cervix. (C) Schematic median section of the organs shown in (A). *1*, Right uterine horn; *2*, body of uterus; *3*, cervix; *3′*, dorsal fold, which may extend a considerable distance into the vagina; *4*, bladder; *4′*, urethra; *5*, vaginal artery; *6*, vagina; *6′*, fornix; *7*, external urethral orifice; *8*, vestibule; *9*, clitoris; *9′*, clitoral fossa; *10*, right labium of vulva; *11*, pelvic symphysis; *12*, tail.

(Fig. 15.12/*9* and *9′*). The functional significance of the urethral tubercle is not known. Darker patches of the lateral walls betray the positions of the vestibular bulbs in the bitch, but the cat has slighter and more diffuse (even insignificant) version. Vestibular glands are present only in the cat.

The thick labia of the vulva meet in a dorsally rounded and ventrally pointed commissure. More lateral folds that are sometimes apparent are believed to be homologous with the labia majora of human anatomy. The crura and body of the clitoris possess a little erectile tissue; the glans

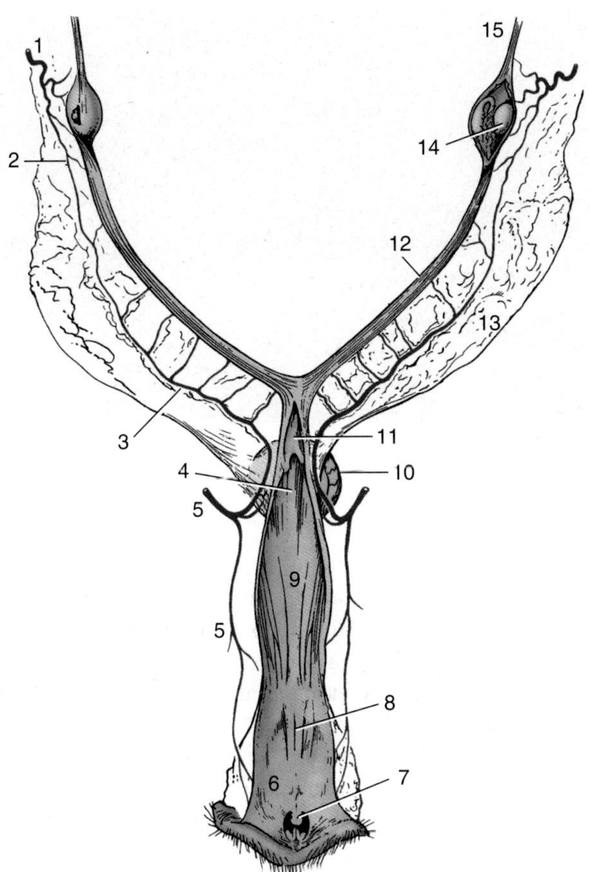

Fig. 15.13 Blood supply of the reproductive organs of the bitch, dorsal view. The right ovarian bursa and the caudal parts of the tract have been opened. *1,* Ovarian artery; *2,* uterine branch of ovarian artery; *3,* uterine artery; *4,* dorsomedian fold continuing the cervix; *5,* vaginal artery; *6,* vestibule; *7,* clitoris; *8,* external urethral orifice; *9,* vagina; *10,* bladder; *11,* cervix; *12,* right uterine horn; *13,* broad ligament; *14,* right ovary; *15,* suspensory ligament of ovary.

is largely of fatty fibrous tissue but sometimes contains a small bone, the os clitoridis. The queen has only a corpus cavernosum clitoridis and not a glans clitoridis.

Functional Changes

It is often stated that bitches come in heat twice a year, in spring and autumn. In fact, three heats are not uncommon, although even in bitches with three heats, the greater part of the year is occupied by periods of anestrus. Cats may even have four cycles in place of the usual two. The first heat occurs at the age of 6 to 9 months in bitches and at 6 to 12 months in young queens, depending on the season of their birth.

The reproductive organs, quiescent during anestrus, develop rapidly in proestrus, when over a period of a week, a batch of follicles enlarges. The uterus now increases in length and in thickness, its endometrium proliferates, and the entire reproductive tract becomes hyperemic. A thickened, edematous vulva discharges the blood-tinged serous uterine secretion. Estrus also lasts about a week and can be distinguished from proestrus by the female's readiness to accept a male. The endometrial hypertrophy and hyperemia continue, but the discharge gradually becomes less bloodstained. Ovulation, which occurs about the second day of estrus, is succeeded by very rapid formation of corpora lutea, which may be mature by the end of estrus.* The separation of diestrus and metestrus is difficult to determine because there is often a period (2 to 8 weeks) of pseudopregnancy, during which the bitch exhibits the usual physical and behavioral signs of pregnancy even though fertilization has not occurred; pseudopregnancy can perhaps be likened to a greatly extended period of diestrus. The cervix is tightly closed during diestrus and metestrus, and secretions that would have been utilized for embryo nutrition then accumulate in amounts that may distend the uterus. Sometime infection of the uterus (pyometra) may necessitate hysterectomy.

In comparison with other domestic species, the bitch's vaginal epithelium responds in a more pronounced manner to changes in hormonal levels, and the vaginal smears provide evidence of the stage within the cycle. Both cornified epithelial cells and erythrocytes are present in large numbers during proestrus. The cornified epithelial cells persist in estrus, but the erythrocytes gradually become fewer and leukocytes appear. The stages of the cycle are also reflected in the gross appearance of the vaginal lining, including that covering the dorsomedian fold. In proestrus the lining becomes edematous, and forms prominent soft folds. As estrogen levels drop rapidly during estrus, the vaginal wall becomes less edematous, and the lining wrinkles until about 4 days after ovulation, when the surface is said to resemble crepe paper. A few days later the mucosa becomes flat and patchy; with the desquamation of the cornified superficial layer of epithelium the blood vessels are able to shine through once more.

Ova enter the uterus about the sixth day after ovulation. The fertilized ova implant after another 10 days. The initially established omphalovitelline (yolk sac) is later replaced by the definitive chorioallantoic placenta (Fig. 15.14/*6*). The placenta develops through the invasion of the endometrium by villi growing from a broad band of the chorion encircling the trunk of the fetus and is a continuation of the erosion that started in the nonvascular *(chorioamniotic)* regions and about the yolk sac attachment. The erosion leads to the interdigitation of thin plates of fetal tissue, and endometrial lamellae are reduced to little more than the maternal capillary endothelium (see Fig. 5.70E–H). The tissue barrier of this basically *chorioendothelial placenta* is further reduced at the margins of the zonary band, where blood extravasated from maternal vessels directly bathes the fetal tissue. Hemoglobin breakdown in these marginal hematomas is responsible for

*Ovulation is not spontaneous in the cat; it is induced by coitus.

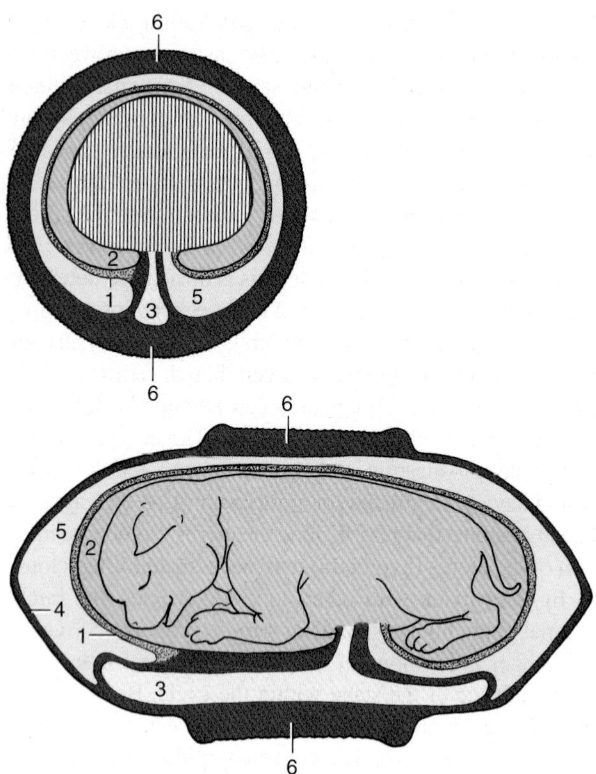

Fig. 15.14 The feline fetal membranes in transverse and longitudinal section, schematic. *1,* Amnion; *2,* amniotic cavity; *3,* yolk sac; *4,* chorioallantois; *5,* allantoic cavity; *6,* zonary placenta.

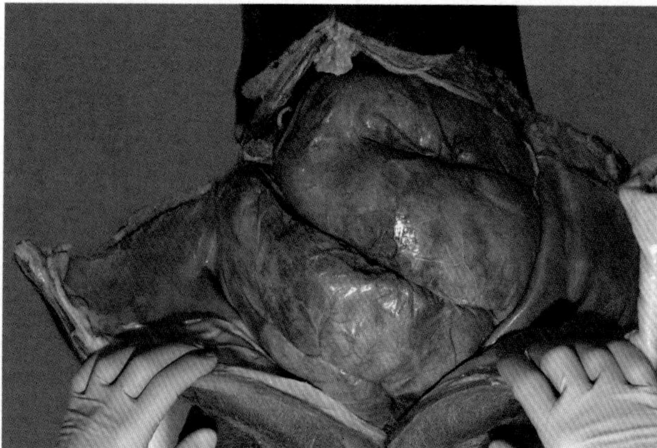

Fig. 15.15 Pregnant uterus of bitch, dominating the abdominal topography.

the brilliant green pigmentation that contrasts with the deep red of the major part of the placenta (see Fig. 5.67A). In short, this type of placenta consists of three zones: a transfer zone (around the embryo for nutrient transfer), a pigmented zone at either end of the transfer zone (maternal hematomas, probably important for iron transport from dam to fetus), and a relatively nonvascular zone, the allantochorion, which is thought to be responsible for resorption from the uterine lumen. Only a certain proportion of the antibodies the pup receives from the dam penetrates the placenta; the greater share (about 75%) of the passive immunization of the newborn depends on the colostrum.

Initially the uterus enlarges locally, and each conceptus is confined within a globular swelling that is bounded by regions of constriction. The separate ampullae persist until about the 40th day (in a gestation that averages 63 days, measured from the date of ovulation*), when there begins a gradual relaxation of the constrictions, eventually creating an almost uniformly expanded uterus. The positions of the individual fetuses are still obvious on inspection of the exposed organ because the whole thickness of the uterine wall is very vascular at the placental sites. The uterine horns are relatively fixed at their extremities, and when they lengthen, they are forced into loops that first bend cranially from the ovarian attachment before sweeping ventrally, then caudally, to join the body (Fig. 15.15). The pattern of coiling is even more complicated when the litter is large, and radiographs obtained in late pregnancy (when there is mineralization of the fetal skeletons) sometimes show the puppies arranged in a confusing jumble (Fig. 15.16B).

Pregnancy can be diagnosed through abdominal palpation of round swellings that are approximately 1 cm in diameter from 18 to 21 days of gestation and 2.5 to 4 cm in diameter between 24 and 32 days. From 35 to 45 days of gestation, the swellings enlarge, elongate, and become flaccid and are found ventrally in the abdomen. For a few days starting from about the 50th day, it is no longer possible to palpate individual swellings, but from the 55th day of gestation individual fetuses are easily palpable.

In the later stages of pregnancy abdominal radiographs serve to determine the number of pups in the litter and provide a means of assessing fetal age, thus predicting the date of parturition. Mineralization commences in the axial skeleton by about the 45th day and soon progresses to that of the appendicular skeleton in proximodistal sequence (see Fig. 5.74; Table 15.1). Mineralization of the skeleton of kittens follows the same pattern, but each element makes its appearance a few days earlier than in pups.

Ultrasonography provides an alternative or additional means of diagnosing pregnancy and predicting term. Claims have been made for its success in recognizing uterine enlargement at a very early stage, but confident diagnosis requires a longer wait (perhaps 28 days). Even then, exact litter size cannot be determined. In cats, a gestational

*Successful service may precede or follow ovulation by an interval of several days, and gestation measured from the date of service consequently has the inconveniently wide range of 58 to 68 days. The practice—generally unavoidable—of measuring gestation in days after service explains the difficulty of precisely specifying the period of change in the form of the uterus or of specific development of the fetus. Prediction of the date of parturition in days subsequent to the appearance of certain features of skeletal mineralization is more exact.

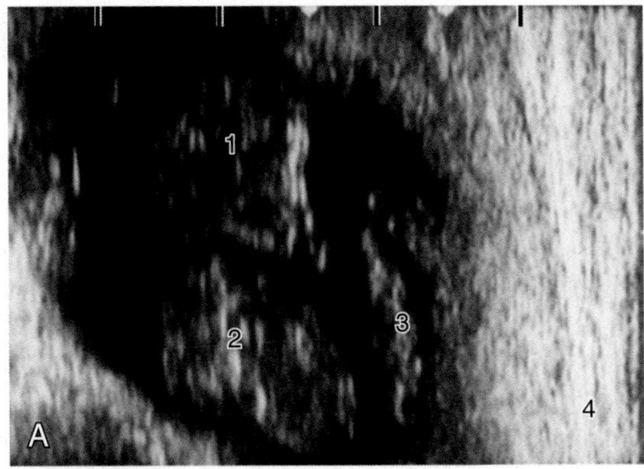

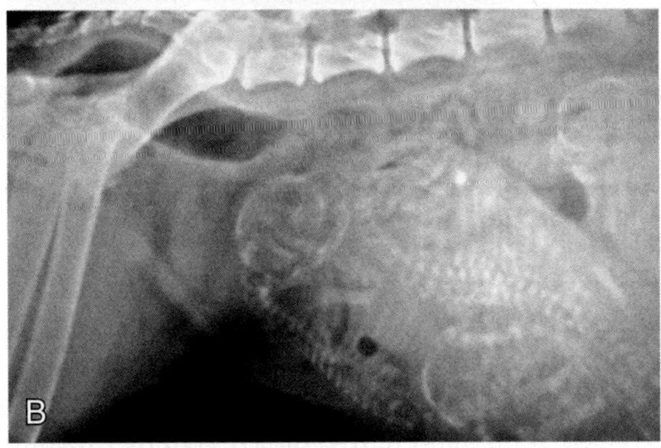

Fig. 15.16 (A) Ultrasonographic (transabdominal) view of a 33-day (after a single mating) Beagle fetus in its ampulla; the scale at *top* is in centimeters. *1,* Head of fetus; *2,* thorax of fetus; *3,* yolk sac; *4,* uterine wall. (B) Radiograph (lateral view) of pregnant bitch with several almost full-term fetuses. Note the gas in the rectum.

TABLE 15.1 GUIDE TO THE MINERALIZATION OF DOG FETUSES

Days	Skeletal Elements
45	Skull, vertebrae, and ribs
48	Proximal long bones of limbs
52	Distal long bones of limbs
54	Pelvis
60	Minor bones of limbs

Modified from Concannon P, Rendano V: Radiographic diagnosis of canine pregnancy: onset of fetal skeletal radiopacity in relation to times of breeding, preovulatory luteinizing hormone release, and parturition, *Am J Vet Res* 44:1506–1512, 1983; and Yaeger AE, Mohammed HO, Meyers-Wallen V, et al: Ultrasonographic appearance of the uterus, placenta, fetus and fetal membranes throughout accurately timed pregnancy in beagles, *Am J Vet Res* 53:324–329, 1992.

sac is visible about days 11 to 14, and fetal cardiac activity is present at day 14.

Parturition is facilitated by pelvic rotation at the sacroiliac joints and by elevation of the tail to significantly increase the dimensions of the pelvis. In both dogs and cats some 60% to 80% of fetuses present the head toward the cervix at term. Fetuses tend to be delivered from each horn in alternation, and when each is delivered, the emptied segment of the uterus contracts and brings those littermates left behind closer to the exit. When expelled, each fetus is still attached to its placenta, from which it is freed by the dam's biting through the umbilical cord. The "afterbirth," with which considerable maternal tissue is shed, is normally consumed.

Although less often useful to the clinician, some information on the development of certain external features of fetuses can be found in Tables 15.2 and 15.3.

The cat is sexually mature at 6 to 9 months of age. The proestrus stage, the nonacceptance of a male, lasts 12 to 48 hours. In cats, pea-sized swellings can be palpated at 21 days of gestation. By 28 days, the swellings are firm and are about 2.0 to 2.5 cm in diameter. The uterus is evenly distended during days 35 and 50 and may be difficult to differentiate from pyometra.

Potentially embarrassing mistakes in the determination of the sex of newborn kittens are relatively easily made. The difficulty arises from the orientation of the penis. The orientation brings the anal and genital openings relatively close together in the tom, and the spacing is inconveniently similar to that in the female.

THE MALE REPRODUCTIVE ORGANS

The Scrotum and Testes (see also pp. 173-180)

The rather pendulous scrotum of the dog is globular and placed in a position intermediate between the perineum and the groin (Fig. 15.3/*11*). It is most easily inspected from behind, and because it is sparsely haired, its close molding on the testes is obvious. A deep groove defines the boundary between the internal compartments occupied by the generally asymmetrical testes. The thin scrotal skin and underlying fasciae do not impede palpation, which normally allows recognition of the body and tail of the epididymis, the deferent duct, and the spermatic cord in addition to the testis itself. The scrotal skin of dogs is richly supplied with sweat glands. The scrotum of the cat is perineal, sessile, and commonly concealed by a dense covering of hair.

The testes are relatively small in both species. They are carried horizontally in dogs but with their caudal extremities tipped toward the anus in cats. Each testis is roughly oval in outline, laterally compressed, and related to the epididymis along its dorsal (in cats, craniodorsal) margin. The head and tail of the epididymis adhere to the testis, but the body is partly free, creating a testicular bursa. The constituents of the compact spermatic cord disperse at the internal inguinal ring. Because of the very caudal position of the scrotum, the spermatic cord in the tom is unusually long. Perhaps that length explains why the cremaster muscle of the cat is very weak. The striated cremaster muscle

TABLE 15.2 GUIDE TO THE AGING OF DOG FETUSES

Weeks	Crown–Rump Length (cm)	External Features
3	≈1	Embryo C-shaped; limb buds forming
4	≈2	Hand plate present; shallow grooves between digits
5	≈3	Eyelids partly cover eye; pinna covers acoustic meatus; external genitalia differentiated; digits separated distally
6	≈7	Eyelids fused; hair follicles present on body; digits widely spread; claws formed
7	≈11	Hair almost completely covering body; color markings present; full term: on average 63–64 days

From Evans HE, Sack WO: Prenatal development of domestic and laboratory animals: growth curves, external features and selected references, *Anat Histol Embryol* 2:11–45, 1973.

TABLE 15.3 GUIDE TO THE AGING OF CAT FETUSES

Weeks	Crown–Rump Length (cm)	External Features
3	≈1	Acoustic meatus forming; eye well formed and pigmented; forelimb hand plate notched
4	≈3	All digits widely spread; pinna almost covers acoustic meatus; claws forming; eyelids partly cover eyes
5	≈5	Eyelids fused; tactile hairs present on face
6	≈7	Fine hairs appearing on body; claws begin to harden
7	≈10.5	Fine hairs cover body; claws white and hard; color markings present; full term: on average 65 days (counted from first mating)

From Evans HE, Sack WO: Prenatal development of domestic and laboratory animals: growth curves, external features and selected references. *Anat Histol Embryol* 2:11–45, 1973.

originates from the iliac fascia on the ventral aspect of the psoas muscles just craniomedial to the caudal border of the internal oblique muscle, inserts on the internal spermatic fascia, and is innervated by the genitofemoral nerve.

The Urethra and Accessory Reproductive Glands (see also pp. 180-182)

The very short first part of the male dog's urethra is completely surrounded by the prostate (Fig. 15.17 and Fig. 5.1/*9*). It presents a lumen indented by a dorsal ridge, locally raised to form a seminal colliculus that is perforated to each side by the narrow opening of the deferent duct and the numerous pores that drain the prostate. The remaining part of the pelvic urethra is provided with a thin sleeve of spongy tissue within the striated urethralis muscle. The urethral lumen widens caudal to the prostate but narrows again as it leaves the pelvis at the ischial arch. In the tom, the prostate is located 3 to 4 cm caudal to the bladder neck, and the preprostatic part of the urethra has sometimes been described as an elongated bladder neck. The striking radiographic appearance of the feline urethra is shown in Fig. 15.8/*1–3*.

The ampullary glands and prostate provide the entire complement of accessory sex glands in the dog. In dogs, sometimes remnants of the paramesonephric duct (vagina masculine) are present in the genital fold, covered dorsally by the prostate.

The cat, which lacks ampullary glands, has small bulbourethral glands located on the urethra, level with the ischial arch. These glands are important landmarks in perineal urethrostomy (removal of the penis in chronic urethral obstruction). The pudendal nerve courses over the ventral part of the bulbourethral glands.

In both species the prostate contributes the bulk of the seminal fluid. In the dog, it comprises a large compact mass about the urethra and neck of the bladder and a small disseminate part spread within the urethral mucosa. The compact part varies greatly in size, and the variation obviously affects its position and relations. It may be within the pelvic cavity when small, but more usually, and especially in mature and older dogs, it is mainly if not entirely intraabdominal (Fig. 15.18/*2*). A dorsal groove and internal septum divide it into right and left lobes, which are subdivided into lobules by finer septa that radiate outward to the capsule. The right and ventral lobes do not join ventral to the urethra in cats.

The prostate is extremely sensitive to hormonal influences, and it is difficult to suggest normal dimensions because hyperplasia of the parenchymatous part commonly develops in early middle age and fibrosis and shrinkage are common senile changes. The hyperplasia

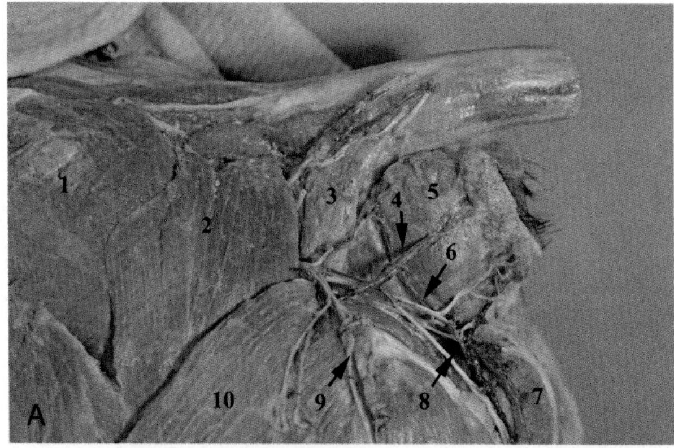

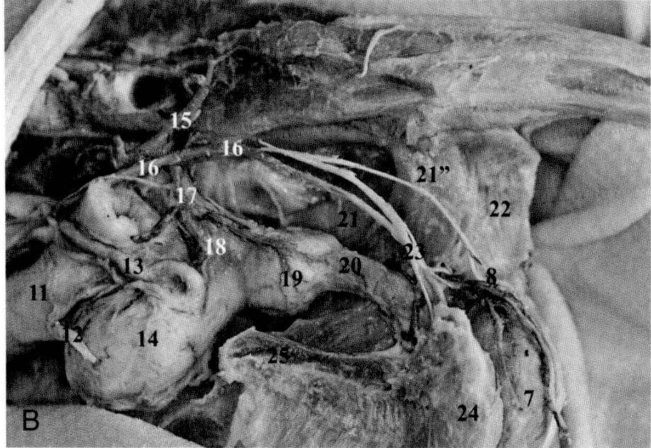

Fig 15.17 (A) Gluteal and perineal region of the dog. (B) Pelvic cavity after removal of the rectum and the anus. *1,* Gluteus medius muscle; *2,* superficial gluteus muscle; *3,* coccygeus muscle; *4,* caudal rectal vessels and nerve; *5,* sphincter ani externus muscle; *6,* superficial perineal vessels; *7,* bulbospongiosus muscle; *8,* perineal nerve, cutaneous branch; *9,* caudal cutaneus femoral nerve; *10,* biceps femoris muscle; *11,* rectum; *12,* deferent duct; *13,* ureter; *14,* urinary bladder; *15,* cranial gluteal artery; *16,* internal pudendal artery; *17,* prostatic artery; *18,* caudal vesical artery; *19,* prostate gland with the prostatic artery; *20,* pelvic urethra with the urethral branch of the prostatic artery; *21,* levator ani muscle (pars iliocaudalis); *21′,* pars pubocaudalis; *22,* superficial part of the sphincter ani externus muscle; *23,* pudendal nerve (branches to the penis); *24,* ischiocavernosus muscle; *25,* symphysis pelvis (cut).

sometimes affects the different lobes unequally. An enlarged prostate may press on the large intestine, producing constipation and difficulties in defecation; however, in contrast to the human experience, interference with micturition is unusual unless the condition is very gross. The state of the prostate—its size, firmness, and regularity of form—may be assessed by digital examination per rectum, a procedure facilitated by pushing the bladder toward the pelvis with pressure applied through the abdominal wall. The proportions of parenchyma and supporting tissue may be estimated from gross sections of autopsy specimens: connective tissue normally predominates in the prostate of the very young, glandular tissue predominates in those from animals in their prime, and the relationship is inconstant in the glands of aged dogs. It has been reported that the prostate is proportionately much larger (by a factor of four) in the Scottish terrier than in other breeds.

Enlargement of the prostate is sometimes treated by castration. Alternatively, or if castration fails, surgical removal may be performed. It is then relevant to note that generally only the craniodorsal aspect of the gland has a peritoneal covering. The trunk of the prostatic artery continues over the lateral aspect of the gland as the supply to the bladder after detaching prostaticovesical and prostaticourethral branches. The other structure at risk is the plexus formed by the pelvic and hypogastric autonomic nerves.

Beyond the prostate, the urethra widens before narrowing on leaving the pelvis and becoming incorporated in the penis. It is narrowest just before opening to the exterior at the tip of the glans, where urinary calculi, a frequent affliction of male cats, are often held up. Little is known of age changes to the prostate of this species, in which enlargement is a much less frequently encountered problem (Fig. 15.22/*8*).

The Penis and Prepuce (see also pp. 182-184)

The penis of carnivores has several unusual features, and additional differences between the organs of the dog and cat make separate description necessary.

The penis of the dog is slung between the thighs, where it may be palpated along its whole length. The root is formed of two slender crura that arch forward from their ischial attachments to combine in a common body that is little stouter than either contributor (Fig. 15.19/*4′*). The urethra is incorporated at the same level and runs forward on the ventral surface of the body (Fig. 15.19/*3*). At the level of the ischial arch the corpus spongiosum (which there surrounds the urethra) expands to form the paired bulbus penis (covered by the bulbospongiosus muscle, a continuation of the urethralis muscle); further distally, the corpus spongiosum expands to form the glans penis, which is unusually extensive and clearly divided, both externally and internally, into a proximal expanded part (bulbus glandis; Fig. 15.19/*7*) and a distal cylindrical part (pars longa glandis; Fig. 15.19/*7′*), which provides the apex. About half the bulbus and the whole pars longa project into the preputial cavity, where they may be palpated. The cavernous parts of both crura combine within the proximal part of the body to form a single corpus cavernosum (Fig. 15.19/*4*) with a tough outer fibrous covering and a substantial median septum; these are connected by radial trabeculae that divide and enclose relatively meager cavernous spaces. The corpus cavernosum comes to a premature end because its distal part is converted into a bone, the os penis, within the core of the organ (Fig. 15.19/*5*). This

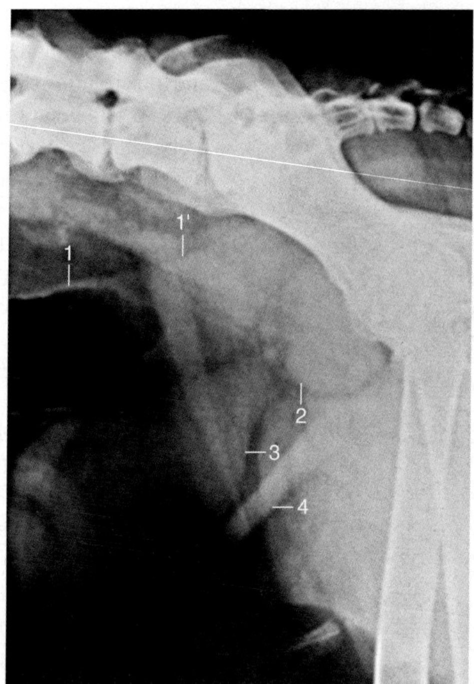

Fig. 15.18 Lateral radiographic view of the canine caudal abdomen to show the position of the prostate. *1 and 1′*, Descending colon containing gas and feces; *2*, prostate; *3*, bladder; *4*, abdominal floor.

bone is grooved ventrally for the reception and protection of the urethra within its spongy covering; the bone tapers toward its distal extremity, which is prolonged by a short, ventrally deflected rod of fibrocartilage that reaches almost to the very apex of the penis. The fibrocartilage remains unossified even in aged animals. The partial enclosure of the urethra within the groove of the os penis impedes the passage of urethral calculi, which therefore tend to lodge at the caudal end of the bone.

The caudal (or proximal) part of the glans penis, the bulbus glandis (Fig. 15.19D), is considerably expanded, even in the quiescent state. It is firmly anchored to the bone and considerably overlapped by the elongated distal division, which presents the urethral orifice toward its tip. The pars longa is more loosely attached to the bone. Both contain large blood spaces enclosed by relatively weak trabeculae.

The structure and connections of the various erectile bodies and their relationships to the supplying and draining vessels require close attention if the mechanism of erection is to be understood (Figs. 15.20 and 15.21). The penis is supplied by the continuation (beyond the origin of its perineal branch) of the *internal pudendal artery,* which now becomes the artery of the penis (Fig. 15.20/*1′*). The *artery of the penis* divides into three. One division, the artery of the bulb (Fig. 15.20/*2*), supplies the bulb (of the penis) and then runs distally within the organ to supply the corpus spongiosum about the urethra and later, on approaching the apex of the penis, the elongated portion of the glans. The second, the *deep artery of the penis* (Fig. 15.20/*3*), supplies several branches to both the tissues and the blood spaces of the corpus cavernosum. The third, the *dorsal artery of the penis* (Fig. 15.20/*4*), may be regarded as the direct continuation of the main trunk. It first runs on the dorsal aspect of the penis before sinking to the side and dividing close to the caudal limit of the bulbus. A superficial branch runs almost to the tip of the organ below the skin over the ventral aspect of the glans; a deep branch penetrates the bulbus to run apically on the os penis to enter the pars longa; and a preputial branch forks into a division that runs over the dorsal aspect of the bulbus to supply the dorsal aspect of the pars longa and the prepuce.

Internal pudendal artery
Artery of the penis
- Artery of the bulb: *Supplies the bulb, the corpus spongiosum, and the elongated part of the glans*
- Deep artery of the penis: *Supplies the tissue and the caverna of the corpus cavernosum*
- Dorsal artery of the penis: *Supplies the caudal parts of the bulbus, the skin over ventral aspect of the glans, and the pars longa and prepuce*

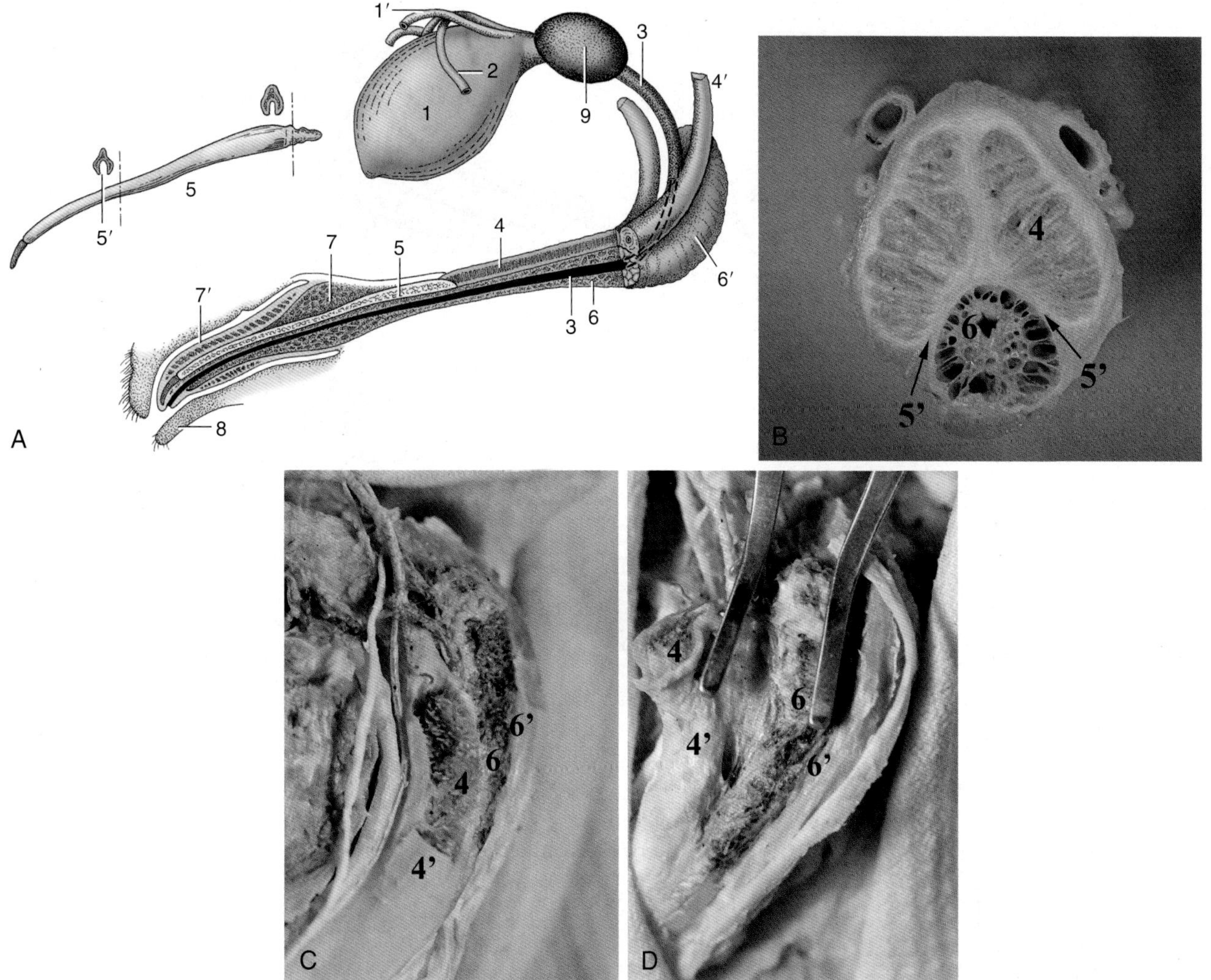

Fig. 15.19 Canine bladder, urethra, and penis (in section) schematic (A), transected (B), root of penis (C), and bulbus penis (D). *1,* Bladder; *1′,* left ureter; *2,* left deferent duct; *3,* urethra; *4,* corpus cavernosum; *4′,* left crus; *5,* os penis; *5′,* urethral groove; *6,* corpus spongiosum; *6′,* bulb of penis; *7,* bulbus glandis; *7′,* pars longa glandis; *8,* prepuce; *9,* prostate.

The *veins* are broadly satellite to the arteries. The *dorsal vein* leaves the lateral aspect of the bulbus and runs caudally, gradually shifting toward the dorsal aspect of the penis, where it is joined by a common trunk formed of the veins corresponding to the deep artery and the artery of the bulb. The augmented dorsal vein then bends around the ischial arch to enter the pelvis, where it provides the main radicle of the internal pudendal vein. Other veins assist in the drainage of the glans. A superficial vein leaves the pars longa to wind around the fornix of the prepuce before joining the external pudendal vein. A deep vein within the glans drains blood from the pars longa to the bulbus; it is valved so that reflux of blood is impossible and is so arranged that it may either provide a through passage to the dorsal vein or open into the blood spaces of the bulbus, from where the blood then enters the dorsal vein.

The usual muscles are present. The *retractor penis*, largely composed of smooth muscle, loops to the side of the anal canal before converging on its fellow to form a band that runs along the urethral aspect of the penis to a termination by the preputial fornix. A few small fascicles are detached to the scrotum. Short but powerful *ischiocavernosus* muscles cover the crura. The *bulbospongiosus* forms a transverse covering over the urethra from the bulb to its incorporation in the penis. A small *ischiourethralis* passes from the ischial tuber to a fibrous ring that encloses the dorsal veins at their entry to the pelvis. The two large muscles at the root of the penis can be identified on palpation (Fig. 15.3/*6* and *7*).

The prepuce of the dog is rather pendulous toward its cranial extremity, where it is suspended below the abdomen by a fold of skin. It has a simple arrangement, and the parietal part of its lining is studded with lymph nodules, which give it a rather irregular appearance. There are also small scattered preputial glands. Paired preputial

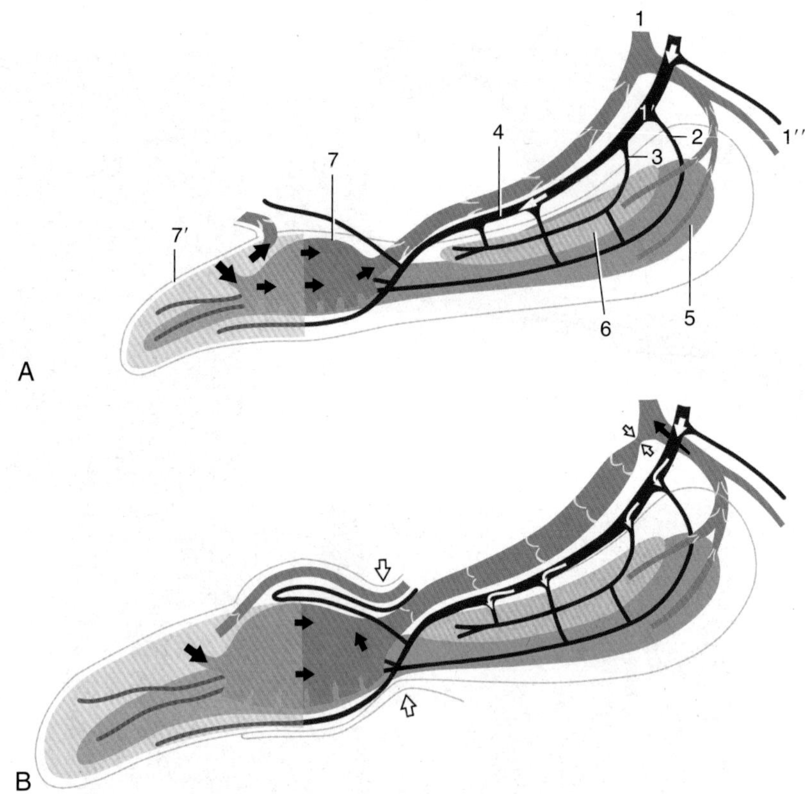

Fig. 15.20 Schematic representation of the blood supply and the blood spaces of the (A) quiescent and (B) erect canine penis. *1,* Internal pudendal vessels; *1',* artery of the penis; *1'',* perineal branches; *2,* artery of the bulb; *3,* deep artery of the penis; *4,* dorsal artery of the penis; *5,* corpus spongiosum; *6,* corpus cavernosum; *7,* bulbus glandis; *7',* pars longa glandis.

muscles, detachments from the cutaneous muscle of the trunk, run over the abdominal floor to meet and partially decussate in the skin of the prepuce caudal to the T-shaped orifice.

Phimosis and Paraphimosis: Congenital or acquired narrowing of the preputial orifice is rare and may prevent protrusion of the penis (phimosis). Those acquired cases that are due to scar formation after an earlier inflammation may be treated surgically. The wisdom of surgical intervention may be questioned when the defect is congenital and possibly hereditary. Paraphimosis, in which the erect penis is unable to subside and cannot be withdrawn into the prepuce, requires more urgent attention because the interruption of the circulation may cause tissue death within hours. The surgical intervention, called phallopexy, is required to create an attachment between the shaft of the penis and the mucosa of the prepuce.

At birth, the epithelial surface of the prepuce and penis adhere through a frenulum. Separation of the prepuce from the penis is under androgenic influence and usually occurs at puberty.

The *penis of the cat* is unique (among domestic species) in retaining the embryonic position: the apex is directed caudoventrally and the urethral surface is uppermost (Figs. 15.22/*6* and 15.23). Relatively much shorter than the penis of the dog, that of the cat has a similar construction, including the transformation of the distal part of the corpus cavernosum into bone. Kittens lack the os penis until 3 months of age. The existence of an apical ligament extending between the os penis and the proximal part of the corpus cavernosum appears to be responsible for the ventral deflection of the penis that occurs with erection. The dorsal artery supplies only the prepuce and not the penis. The glans is small, and its free surface is generously ornamented with small, keratinized spines in the tom; these spines develop during the first few months of postnatal life and regress to a very insignificant state in castrated animals (Figs. 15.23 and 15.24). Approximately 120 in number, they lie flat against the surface of the glans in the nonerect state but rise, as a result of the congestion of the blood spaces at their bases, on erection. The stimulus they provide to the queen is believed to be important in inducing ovulation.

The cat's prepuce is thick but short and often much obscured by hair; its orifice faces caudally, and urine is ejected in this direction. The spraying of urine by the tom is a social gesture marking territory (Fig. 15.25). The sites are not

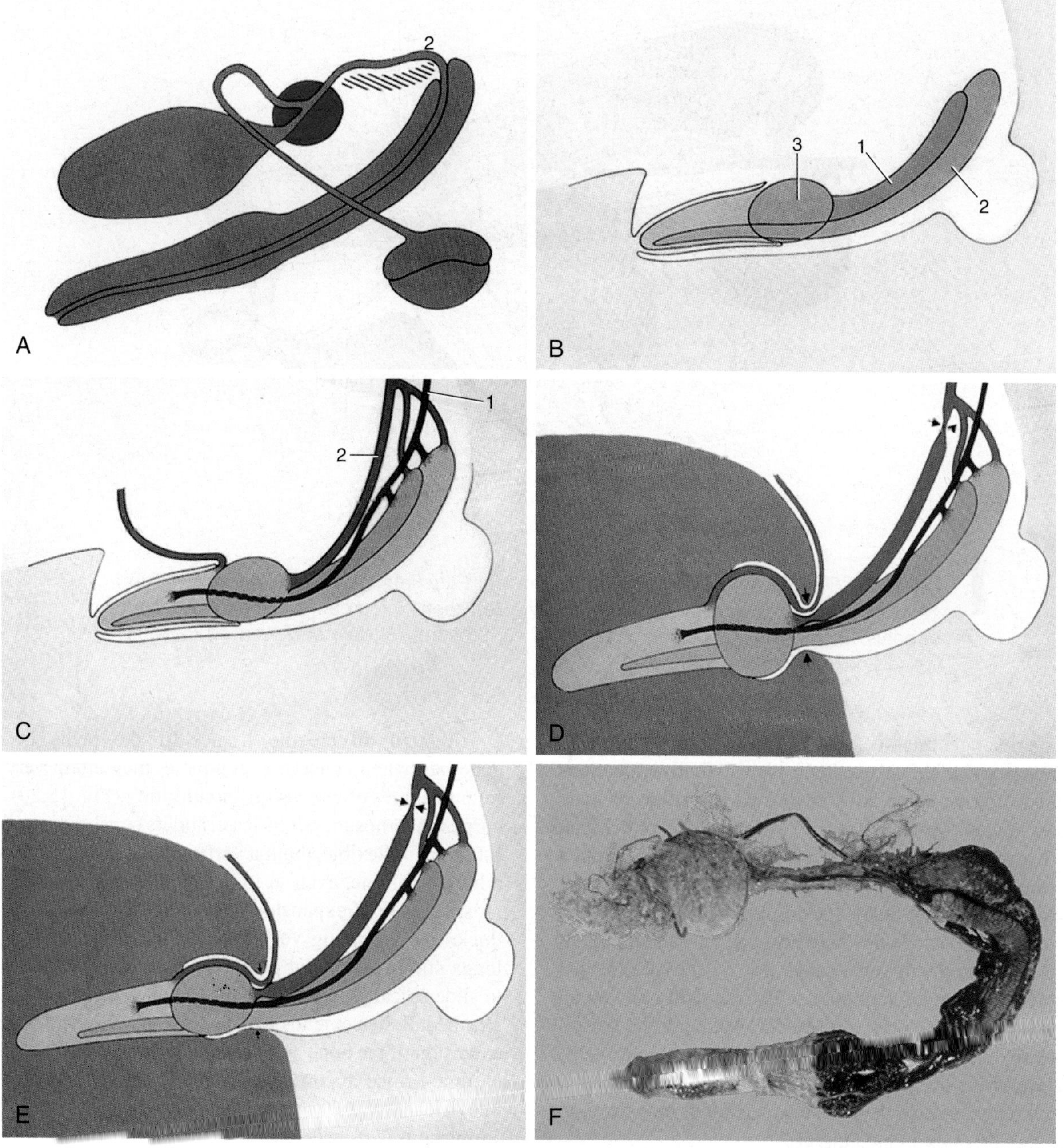

Fig. 15.21 (A) Schematic representation of canine male reproductive organs. (B) Major vascular parts of canine penis. *1*, Corpus cavernosum; *2*, corpus spongiosum; *3*, bulbus glandis. (C), (D), and (E) Stages in the erection process. *1*, Penile artery; *2*, dorsal penile vein. (F) Corrosion cast of the arterial supply to the prostate and penis.

always discretely chosen and are often inconvenient to the owner, one reason for the common practice of castration.*

*Queens also sometimes spray, though generally they squat when passing urine, which they then seek to conceal by scratching dirt over it. It seems that spraying by females is most often performed far from home, at the bounds of a territory disputed with other cats; it is, in consequence, less commonly objectionable to the householder. In both sexes, the practice may have sexual connotations.

Age and Functional Changes

Although there has been little detailed study of the postnatal development, it is known that the testes most often remain within the abdomen until about the third day after birth. Their descent through the inguinal canal then commences, and although it is completed within a couple of days, another 4 or 5 weeks is required before the testes occupy their definitive positions within the scrotum. The seminiferous tissue increases markedly in volume during this time,

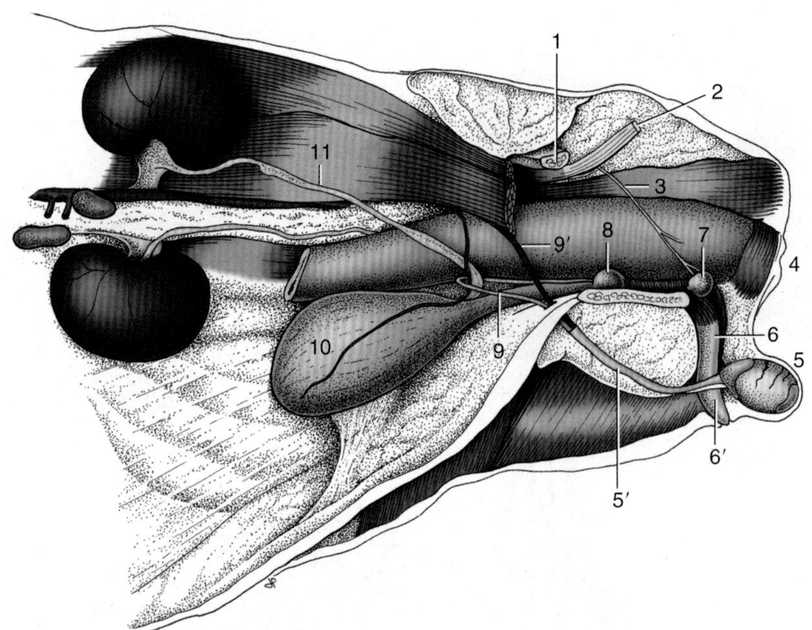

Fig. 15.22 The reproductive organs of the tomcat in situ, left lateral view. *1,* Shaft of ilium; *2,* sciatic nerve; *3,* pudendal nerve; *4,* anus; *5,* left testis in scrotum; *5′,* spermatic cord; *6,* penis; *6′,* prepuce; *7,* bulbourethral gland; *8,* prostate; *9,* deferent duct; *9′,* testicular vessels; *10,* bladder; *11,* left ureter.

but spermatogenesis does not begin until about the sixth month. Because the testes attain their definitive locations so precociously, some have advocated castration of male kittens at much younger ages—6 to 14 weeks—rather than the 5 or 6 months conventionally adopted. It is claimed that the operation is well tolerated by these very young animals.* If descent fails—the cryptorchid condition—the testis may be located anywhere between the caudal pole of the kidney and the inguinal canal. It is most easily located by following the deferent duct, which is readily picked up at the lateral ligament of the bladder. Although the germinal epithelium fails to develop normally at the core temperature of the body, Leydig cells produce androgens, and the full range of secondary sex characteristics may develop in bilaterally cryptorchid animals.

The mating behavior of dogs is most unusual. The dog mounts the bitch in the usual way, but shortly after intromission he drops to her side and reverses so that the pair stand rear to rear during the remainder of the "tie," which may last for a further 45 minutes or even longer. There has been surprisingly little consideration of the anatomy of this process.

*It is also claimed that female kittens can be spayed at the same early age without unacceptably greater risk. Humane societies tend to be the strongest advocates of early neutering, before kittens are adopted by their permanent owners, because it avoids unwanted pregnancies with the inevitable consequence of abandoned animals' contributing to feral populations.

Although all erectile tissues of the penis become engorged when erection is complete, they attain very different degrees of expansion and turgidity (Fig. 15.20). The corpus cavernosum swells least, and its construction allows it to remain flexible about a vertical axis, though not about a horizontal one, even in this state. The bulbus glandis is most capable of expansion and swells to twice its resting thickness, becoming very tense in the process. The pars longa stiffens least but elongates considerably, causing it to slide apically on the os penis to which it is only loosely attached. It then extends well beyond the fibrocartilaginous extension of the bone and presents an indentation about the urethral orifice in consequence of the tighter anchorage of this part.

Intromission necessarily occurs before the penis is markedly enlarged (Fig. 15.21D and E). The labia thrust the prepuce caudally when the dog mounts and introduces the glans into the vagina. The slope of the female passage requires a dorsocranial penetration, and the relatively soft tip of the glans is diverted ventrally by its impingement (through the soft tissues) on the pelvic roof. This deflection allows the penis to be advanced toward the fornix and perhaps explains the necessity for the softer nature of the pars longa and the early termination of its bony support. When the stud dog dismounts and turns through 180 degrees, the body of the penis is bent laterally and then caudally; withdrawal of the penis is prevented by the swollen bulbus glandis and the grip exerted on it by the engorged vestibular bulbs and muscles associated with the

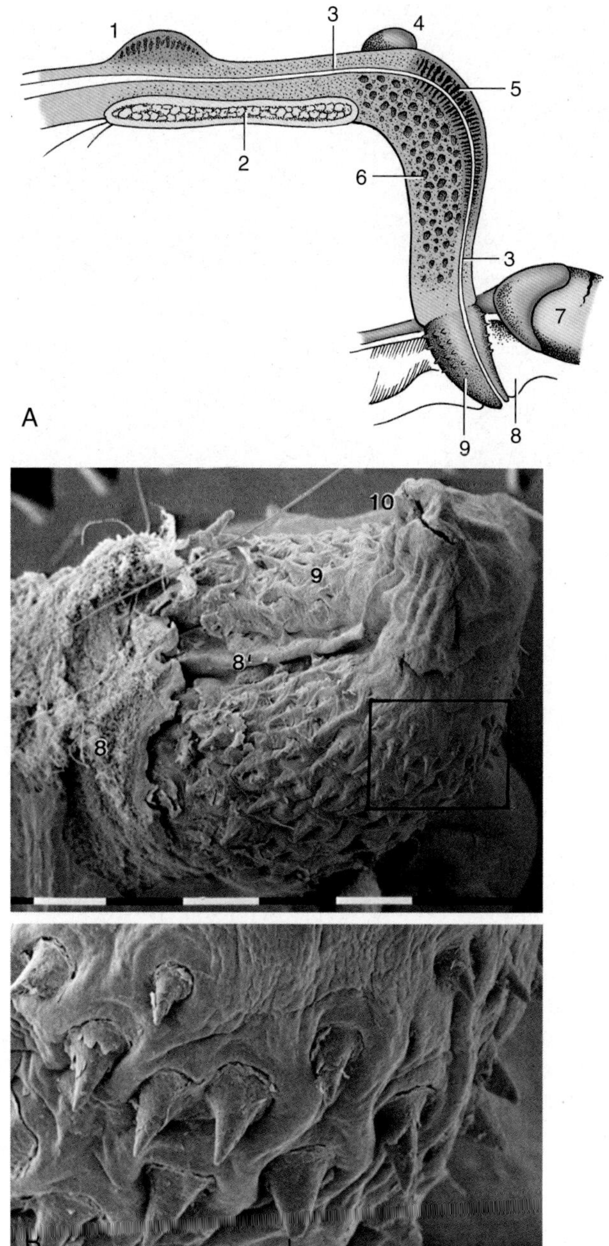

Fig. 15.23 (A) Median section of the feline penis, left lateral view. (B) Scanning electron micrograph of a feline glans and enlargement of the marked area (bar = 1 mm). *1,* Prostate; *2,* pelvic symphysis; *3,* urethra; *4,* right bulbourethral gland; *5,* corpus spongiosum; *6,* corpus cavernosum; *7,* right testis; *8,* prepuce; *8′,* preputial frenulum; *9,* glans (with spines); *10,* external urethral orifice.

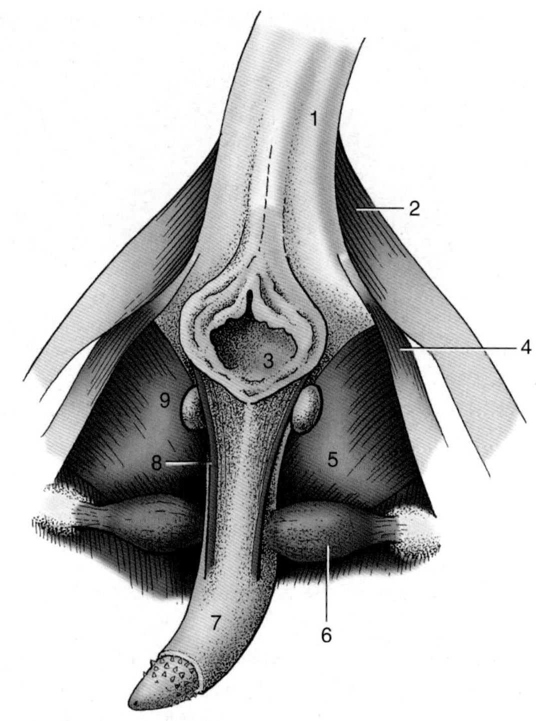

Fig. 15.24 Feline penis in situ, caudal view. *1,* Tail (raised); *2,* gluteofemoralis muscle; *3,* anus; *4,* coccygeus muscle; *5,* internal obturator muscle; *6,* ischiocavernosus muscle; *7,* penis; *8,* left retractor penis; *9,* left bulbourethral gland.

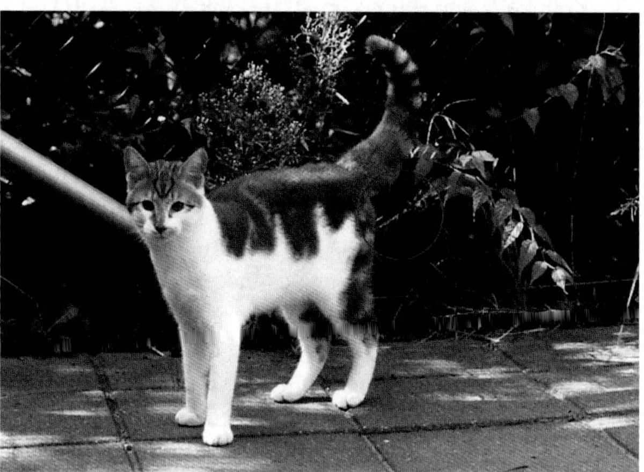

Fig. 15.25 Tomcat spraying.

female tract. The reversal of position twists the prepuce, tightening the preputial muscles into a cord that presses on the veins draining the glans. The dorsal veins of the penis, buckled by the flexion of the penis, are further obstructed by being pressed against the ischial arch by the contraction of the ischiourethralis. Detumescence is probably eventually achieved by relaxation of the bulbospongiosus, which allows the spaces within the corpus spongiosum to provide alternative channels for the escape of blood from the engorged penis.

The initial, sperm-rich fraction of the ejaculate is discharged during the first stage of coitus when the dog is mounted in the fashion conventional for quadrupeds. The second stage is occupied in pumping out the much larger fraction—perhaps 30 mL—provided by the prostate; the tide sweeps the sperm-rich part through the cervix into the body of the uterus. It is known that short matings—in which only first-stage coitus occurs—may be fertile. The

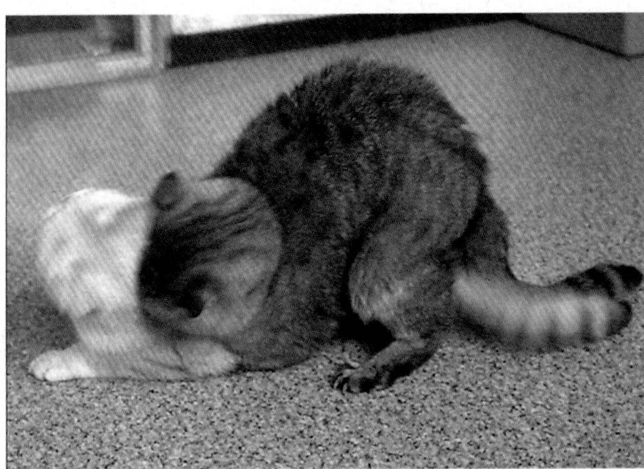

Fig. 15.26 Mating posture.

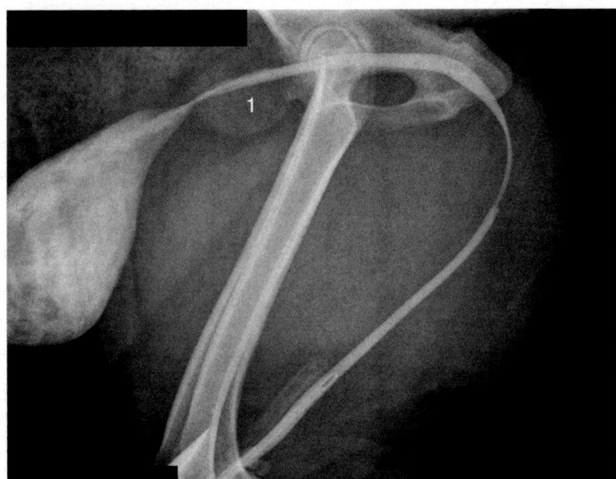

Fig. 15.27 Contrast medium in the male canine bladder and urethra. The prostatic urethra appears to be less distensible. *1,* Prostate.

purpose of the second-stage coitus may encourage uterine rather than vaginal insemination. Turning around discourages detumescence of the penis and therefore maintains high intravaginal pressure.

The *penis of the cat* increases considerably in length on erection and then curves downward and forward. This change in orientation, allied to a ventral flexion of the pelvic region, enables coitus to be performed in a fashion not greatly different from that usual in quadrupeds (Fig. 15.26).

THE ANATOMY OF ABDOMINAL AND RECTAL PALPATION

In the previous chapter the process of abdominal palpation was described, together with the examination of most abdominal organs. The remaining organs are now considered, together with the information that may be obtained from digital examination via the rectum.

Although the right kidney cannot be found in most dogs, the caudal pole of the left one is generally identifiable. Indeed, in some dogs, generally of the larger breeds, the left kidney "floats" as both kidneys normally do in cats.

The dog's *bladder* can be found extending forward from the pubic brim. The grossly distended bladder lies on the abdominal floor. Micturition may be induced by gentle compression through the abdominal wall, a procedure not free of risk if performed poorly. The bladder of the cat is located more cranially than that of the dog, well forward of the pubic brim. The *prostate,* notoriously variable in size and position, may sometimes be palpated between the pubic brim and the bladder (Fig. 15.27).

The empty *uterus* cannot normally be palpated. The gravid uterus is readily identified at certain stages of pregnancy by its beaded form or general enlargement or by the recognition of individual fetuses. The separate loculi within which the embryos initially develop are largest about the beginning of the sixth week (bitch), but this stage is soon followed by uniformly swollen horns. A little later, individual fetuses may be palpated, but it may not be possible to make an exact count in large litters. The gravid uterus may affect the position of other abdominal organs markedly. It always occupies the most ventral position in the abdomen because it contains no gas; therefore it is heavier than most freely movable abdominal organs. In advanced pregnancy it may almost fill the ventral half of the abdominal cavity.

Digital examination per rectum, a procedure possible only in subjects of a certain size, may provide additional information. In addition to revealing the tone of the anal sphincter and the condition of the rectum and its mucosa, digital examination may be used to explore the pelvic skeleton for evidence of fracture or deformity. The anal sacs may be palpated and their content expressed with the aid of a finger within the rectum. The only other visceral organs that can usually be examined are the urethra and the prostate in the male and the vagina in the female. Evaluation of the prostate requires consideration of its size, consistency, and symmetry. In large dogs the gland may be out of reach, but the prostate and the neck of the bladder may be made more accessible by coordinating the rectal examination with manipulation of the abdomen to press the caudal abdominal contents toward the pelvic entrance.

Palpation of the abdominal wall of the laterally recumbent animal reveals the position of the *superficial inguinal ring,* from which the spermatic cord may then be traced toward the scrotum in the male. The location of the ring is determined by recognition of its tense medial crus, which may be traced over the abdominal wall from the origin of the pectineus muscle (which forms the conspicuous swelling on the medial surface of the thigh). The superficial inguinal lymph nodes lie a little cranial to the ring. They are contained within the fold of skin that supports the prepuce in the male but are more difficult to find in the bitch, especially the parous bitch, because they lie deep to the inguinal mammary gland.

Main Vessels in the Pelvis

The *internal iliac artery* supplies blood to the pelvic wall and the pelvic organs. The *sacral median artery* courses over the ventral surface of the sacrum and continues as the median caudal artery in the tail. The internal iliac artery divides into the *caudal gluteal artery* (wide) and *internal pudendal artery* (smaller), after detaching the umbilical artery. In the mature dog and cat internal iliac artery gives off branches to the bladder, after which it becomes the ligament in the cranial edge of the lateral bladder ligament. The internal pudendal artery courses at the inside of the pelvic wall and branches off the *prostatic artery or the vaginal artery,* which continues cranially as the *uterine artery*. Internal pudendal artery also detaches branches to the rectum, bladder, and urethra. Near the anus the internal pudendal artery detaches the *ventral perineal artery* before continuing as the artery of the penis or clitoris.

COMPREHENSION CHECK

1. Relate the topography of the pelvic viscera observed in a cadaver to the two-dimensional radiographic and ultrasonographic images.
2. Develop a flow chart of the branches of the internal iliac artery and the specific areas of the urogenital tract they supply. Describe the changes in the vascular supply necessitated by the pregnancy.

16 The Forelimb of the Dog and Cat

Fractures and luxations resulting from traffic accidents contribute a large part of the clinical work on the forelimbs of dogs and cats. Among younger dogs, a second sizable contingent presents with various disorders of skeletal development, mostly due to anomalous endochondral ossification within an epiphysis or directly affecting a growth plate, leading to premature or delayed fusion. It is clear that a sound knowledge of the surface and radiologic anatomy of the region is necessary whether the abnormality has a traumatic or developmental origin. Knowledge of the courses of the major vessels and nerves is also important to preserve their functional and anatomic integrity during direct surgical access to a bone or joint.

Details of the development of the forelimb skeleton of both dogs and cats are summarized in Table 16.1. There is considerable variation in the ages at which events occur and a tendency for development to be more precocious in smaller breeds. The figures used in the text generally refer to dogs of medium size, such as the Beagle.

THE SHOULDER REGION AND UPPER ARM (SEE ALSO PP. 68–70 AND 73–75)

The scapula and humerus form the basis of the shoulder and upper arm, including the shoulder joint. Whereas the acromion on the distal end of the scapular spine and the greater tubercle are easily recognized on visual inspection, the following anatomic features may be located on palpation: the full length of the spine; the cranial border, angle, and dorsal border of the scapula; the tendon of origin of the biceps; the deltoid tuberosity; and the medial and lateral surfaces of the shaft of the humerus (these are revealed by grasping the bone between the fingers of one hand). The attachment of the *pectoral muscles* to cranial parts of the bones near the shoulder joint prevents palpation of the medial surface of both the joint and the upper part of the humerus.

The superficial cervical lymph nodes cranial to the scapula are most easily palpated with the limb retracted (see Fig. 2.55/*4*), whereas the axillary lymph nodes, located on the thoracic wall caudal to the shoulder joint, can be palpated with the limb protracted—but only when they are enlarged. Both these groups drain the forelimb. An accessory axillary lymph node draining local skin and muscles and the thoracic mammary glands is inconstantly present on the thoracic wall dorsal to the olecranon (see Fig. 2.55/*10*).

The scapula is covered laterally by the *trapezius, supraspinatus,* and *infraspinatus* (Fig. 16.1), with the tendons of the latter two muscles crossing the joint to attach to the humerus. The belly of the infraspinatus is suitable for intramuscular injections. The flexor aspect of the joint is covered by the deltoideus, which connects the scapular spine with the deltoid tuberosity (Table 16.2).

The shaft of the humerus is overlain laterally by the *long head of the triceps,* cranially by the *biceps* (itself partly covered by the brachiocephalicus), and on different aspects by the *brachialis* as it winds around the bone and by other heads of the triceps. In contrast, the medial surface, once free of the pectoral muscles, is relatively uncovered, which allows the brachial vessels and the nerve trunks heading for the distal portion of the limb to lie close to the bone (Fig. 16.2).

In craniocaudal radiographs of the extended shoulder joint, the supraglenoid tubercle overlaps the head of the humerus; in lateral radiographs this tubercle is superimposed on the greater tubercle of the humerus (Fig. 16.3A, C, and C′/*2*). In dogs younger than 3 to 5 months the supraglenoid tubercle is still separated from the rest of the scapula by cartilage. The proximal epiphysis for the tubercles and head of the humerus commonly fuses with the shaft at about 10 months (but several months later in larger breeds). In the cat the coracoid process, on the medial aspect of the supraglenoid tubercle, is a pronounced cylindric swelling with a separate ossification center. The flat *coracobrachial muscle* originates from the coracoid process and passes over the subscapularis insertion tendon, from which it is separated by a bursa, before running caudodistally over the medial aspect of the shoulder joint to end on the proximal part of the humerus. It adducts the arm and rotates the shoulder joint outward. The feline acromion is broadened by a flat, caudally directed (suprahamate) process (see Fig. 2.45D), which overhangs the infraspinatus muscle slightly. In the cat, an extra ossification center is also present for the lesser tubercle. The clavicle of the dog is represented by a small ossicle cranioventral to the shoulder joint. In the cat the vestigial clavicle takes the form of a slender rodlet, roughly 2 cm long, in the corresponding location; it is regularly depicted in radiographic films and may be palpated against the cranial aspect of the joint (Fig. 16.3C′/*5*).

In both cats and dogs, the capsule of the *shoulder joint* extends a diverticulum that invests the biceps tendon of origin, including the part that is secured in the intertubercular groove of the humerus by a transverse ligament extending between the greater and lesser tubercles. The lack of collateral ligaments on the spheroidal shoulder joint is partly compensated by the minor local thickenings of the capsule (glenohumeral ligaments) in addition to the

TABLE 16.1 DEVELOPMENT AND MATURATION OF THE FORELIMB SKELETON

	Approximate Age at Growth Plate Closure Observed on Radiographs	
Ossification Centers Present at Birth (After Birth)	**Dog**	**Cat**
	Scapula	
Body	—	—
Supraglenoid tubercle (7 weeks)	3–7 months[2,5]	3.5–4.0 months
	Humerus	
Prox. epiphysis (head and tubercles) (1–2 weeks)	10–15 months[2,5]	18–24 months
Diaphysis	—	—
Distal epiphysis	5–8 months[2,5]	4 months
Lat. part of condyle (2–3 weeks)	5 months[4]	3.5 months
Med. part of condyle (2–3 weeks)	5 months[4]	3.5 months
Med. epicondyle (6–8 weeks)	5–6 months[4,6]	4 months
Lat. epicondyle	At birth	3.5 months
	Radius	
Prox. epiphysis (3–5 weeks)	5–11 months[2,5]	5–7 months
Diaphysis	—	—
Distal epiphysis (2–4 weeks)	6–12 months[2,5]	14–22 months
	Ulna	
Olecranon tubercle (6–8 weeks)	5–10 months[2,4,5,6]	9–13 months
Diaphysis	—	—
Anconeal process (12 weeks)	3–5 months[7]	—
Distal epiphysis (6–8 weeks)	6–12 months[2,5,6]	14–25 months
	Carpus	
Radial carpal (3–4 weeks)	—	—
Three centers	3–4 months[1–3]	—
Accessory carpal	—	—
Diaphysis (3 weeks)	—	—
Epiphysis (7 weeks)	3–6 months[1,2,4,5]	4 months
Other carpal bones	—	—
One center each	—	—
	Metacarpus	
Metacarpal I	—	—
Prox. epiphysis (5 weeks)	6–7 months[3]	—
Diaphysis	—	—
Metacarpals II–V	—	—
Diaphysis	—	—
Distal epiphysis (4 weeks)	5–7 months[2,4,5]	7–10 months
	Digit	
Phalanges I and II	—	—
Prox. epiphysis (4–5 weeks)	5–7 months[1,2,5,6]	4.0–5.5 months
Diaphysis	—	—
Phalanx III	—	—
One center	—	—

Lat., Lateral; *Med.*, medial; *Prox.*, proximal.

[1]Based on Chapman WL: Appearance of ossification centers and epiphyseal closures as determined by radiographic techniques, *JAVMA* 147:138–141, 1965.

[2]Based on Hare WCD: The age at which epiphyseal union takes place in the limb bones of the dog, *Wien Tierärztl Monatsschr* 9:224–245, 1972.

[3]Based on Pomriaskynski-Kobozieff N, Kobozieff N: Étude radiologique de l'aspect du squelette normal de la main du chien aux divers Stades de son évolution de la naissance à l'âge adult, *Rec Med Vet* 130:617–646, 1954.

[4]Based on Smith RN, Allcock J: Epiphyseal fusion in the Greyhound, *Vet Rec* 72:75–79, 1960.

[5]Based on Sumner-Smith G: Observations on the epiphyseal fusion of the canine appendicular skeleton, *J Small Anim Pract* 7:303–311, 1966.

[6]Based on Ticer JW: Radiographic technique in small animal practice, Philadelphia, 1975, Saunders, p. 101.

[7]Based on Van Sickle D: The relationship of ossification to elbow dysplasia, *Anim Hosp* 2:24–31, 1966.

From de Lahunta A and Habel RE: Applied veterinary anatomy, Philadelphia, 1986, Saunders.

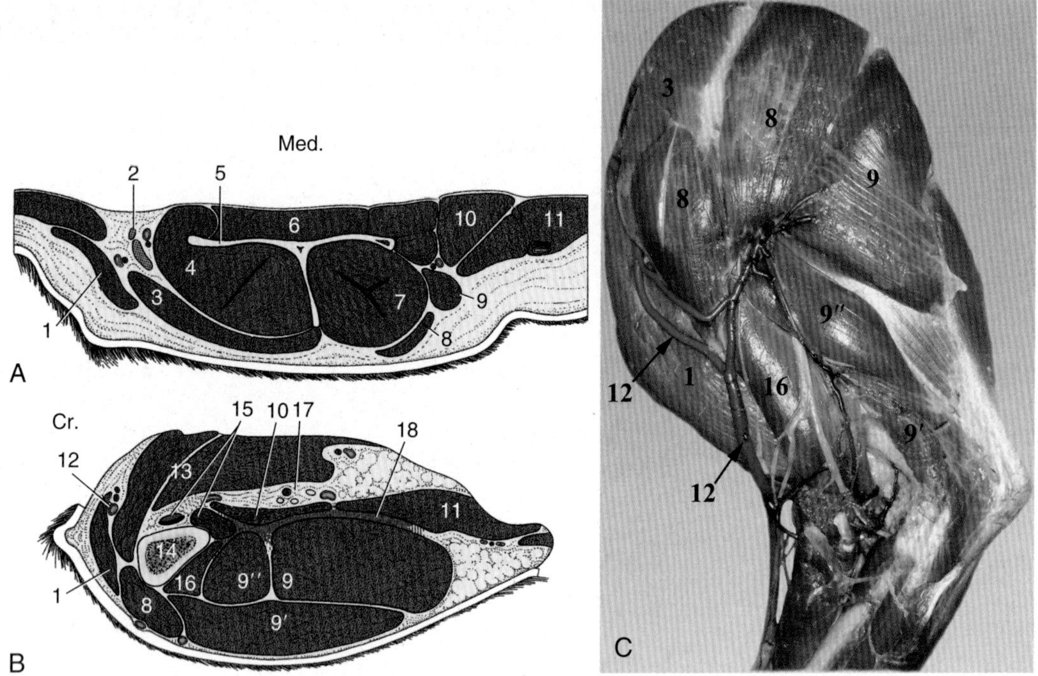

Fig. 16.1 Transverse sections of the left canine forelimb at the level of the scapula (A) and just distal to the shoulder joint (B) and lateral view (C). *1,* Brachiocephalicus; *2,* superficial cervical lymph nodes; *3,* omotransversarius; *4,* supraspinatus; *5,* scapula; *6,* subscapularis; *7,* infraspinatus; *8,* deltoideus; *9, 9',* and *9",* long, lateral, and accessory heads of triceps, respectively; *10,* teres major; *11,* latissimus dorsi; *12,* cephalic vein; *13,* pectoral muscles; *14,* humerus; *15,* biceps tendon and coracobrachialis; *16,* brachialis; *17,* brachial vessels and nerve trunks; *18,* heavy intermuscular fascia. *Cr.,* Cranial; *Med.,* medial.

transverse ligament already mentioned. The swellings of the shoulder joints are difficult to detect because of the overlying muscles.

The luxations of the shoulder joint occur when structures that support the joint are broken as a result of trauma. Most of the luxations occur medially or laterally. The rupture of the transverse ligament that restrains the biceps tendon in the bicipital groove lets the tendon slip over the lesser tubercle when the shoulder is flexed. This is a painful condition with the shoulder joint in a permanently extended state.

It is useful to remember, for purposes of orientation, that the distal end of the acromion is opposite the joint space. The glenoid concavity is considerably smaller than the head of the humerus, which considerably increases the range of movement. The relative looseness of the joint permits abduction of the humerus in sedated or anesthetized dogs and cats; it is then possible to puncture the capsule midway between the acromion and the greater tubercle by passing a needle mediocaudally through the deltoideus.

The *teres minor* muscle, deep to the deltoid muscle on the flexor aspect of the shoulder, runs between the distal part of the caudal margin of the scapula and the teres minor tuberosity. In the cat teres minor is covered by the infraspinous and triceps muscles and becomes stronger and more effective by fusing with the tendon of the latissimus dorsi. The flat tensor fasciae antebrachii muscle located over the medial surface of the triceps muscle arises by means of a broad aponeurosis from the latissimus dorsi and radiates into the forearm fascia. It acts as a tensor of the fascia and an extensor of the elbow joint. The triceps muscle has already been described (p. 77).

Luxation of the joint and fractures of the scapula are both relatively rare. Because the clavicle lacks a functional connection with the trunk, the entire joint appears to "ride with the blow" when subjected to a sudden external force. Fractures of the humerus are much more common and mostly occur at midshaft level. Malignant tumors of the proximal humerus and the distal radial

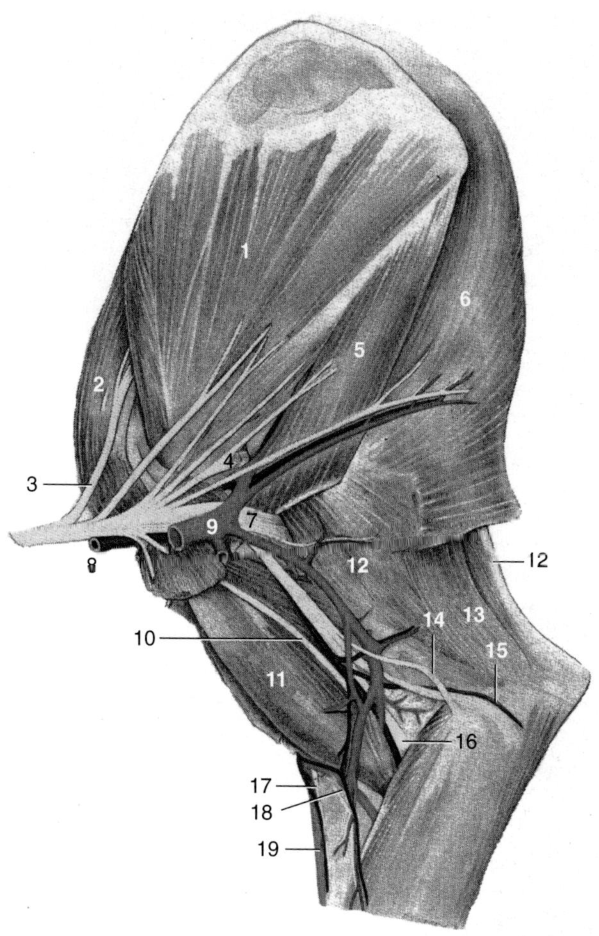

Fig. 16.2 Medial surface of the right canine shoulder and arm. *1,* Subscapularis; *2,* supraspinatus; *3,* suprascapular nerve; *4,* axillary nerve; *5,* teres major; *6,* latissimus dorsi; *7,* radial nerve; *8,* axillary artery; *9,* axillary vein; *10,* musculocutaneous nerve; *11,* biceps; *12,* long head of triceps; *13,* tensor fasciae antebrachii; *14,* caudal cutaneous antebrachial nerve; *15,* ulnar nerve and collateral ulnar artery; *16,* median nerve and brachial artery; *17,* medial branch of superficial radial nerve; *18,* median cubital vein; *19,* cephalic vein.

metaphyses are relatively more common in the large and the so-called giant breeds of dog compared to small dogs and cats.

THE ELBOW AND FOREARM (SEE ALSO PP. 70-71, 74, AND 78-80)

Both the medial and lateral aspects of the elbow joint are conveniently accessible because the arm is relatively free and the axillary fossa is deep. The most prominent feature of the region, the summit of the olecranon, is located just below the ventral end of the fifth intercostal space in a dog standing square. The medial and lateral epicondyles and adjacent parts of the humerus are all easily palpated. The bundle composed of the brachial vessels and median nerve can be palpated against the medial surface of the bone, between the biceps and triceps. The smaller bundle formed by the collateral ulnar vessels and ulnar nerve may be located against the triceps tendon and olecranon (see Fig. 16.13/*5* and *6*). The collateral ligaments arising from the epicondyles are also easily palpated. Although the condyle of the humerus projects forward and is offset from the long axis of the bone, a considerable covering of muscle makes it less accessible.

The entire medial border of the *radius* is subcutaneous. However, the cranial surface is palpable distally, where it is only thinly covered by the extensor carpi obliquus and the tendons of the other extensors (Fig. 16.4/*6*). The *ulna* is more deeply placed except at its distal end, where its styloid process connects with the carpal bones. A deep depression behind this process is bounded by the prominent tendon of the flexor carpi ulnaris and the accessory carpal bone.

The median vessels (Fig. 16.4/*3*) (continuations of the brachial) and nerve are embedded among the carpal and digital flexor muscles, close to the medial border of the radius (Fig. 16.5).

Arteries: Axillary → Brachial → Median → Radial
Veins: Cephalic; Median → Brachial → Axillary

The *cephalic vein* (Fig. 16.4/*1*), the most popular choice for intravenous injections, follows the cranial border of the forearm, where it can be palpated when raised by pressure over the elbow; it often produces a visible ridge even when not occluded in this way. Because it is connected (by the median cubital vein) to the deep system of veins at the elbow before it continues over the lateral surface of the arm, it is best compressed distal to this anastomosis (Fig. 16.6/*2*). The vein lies on the extensor carpi radialis in the forearm, accompanied by sensory branches of the radial nerve.

In cats, the distal end of the humerus is distinguished by a prominent medial (supracondylar) foramen (Figs. 2.46C/*14* and 16.7), which transmits the brachial artery and median nerve in the caudocranial direction. These structures are therefore vulnerable in fractures and surgery of this part.

Lateral *radiographs* show the humeral condyle deeply seated in the trochlear notch of the ulna (Fig. 16.8A). The prominent medial epicondyle (Fig. 16.8/*1*) is superimposed on the olecranon, while the anconeal process, at the proximal end of the notch (Fig. 16.8/*4*), is superimposed in turn on the medial epicondyle. In some breeds the anconeal process may have its own ossification center that fuses with the rest of the bone at 3 to 5 months of age. If it fails to do so (un-united anconeal process or elbow dysplasia), as

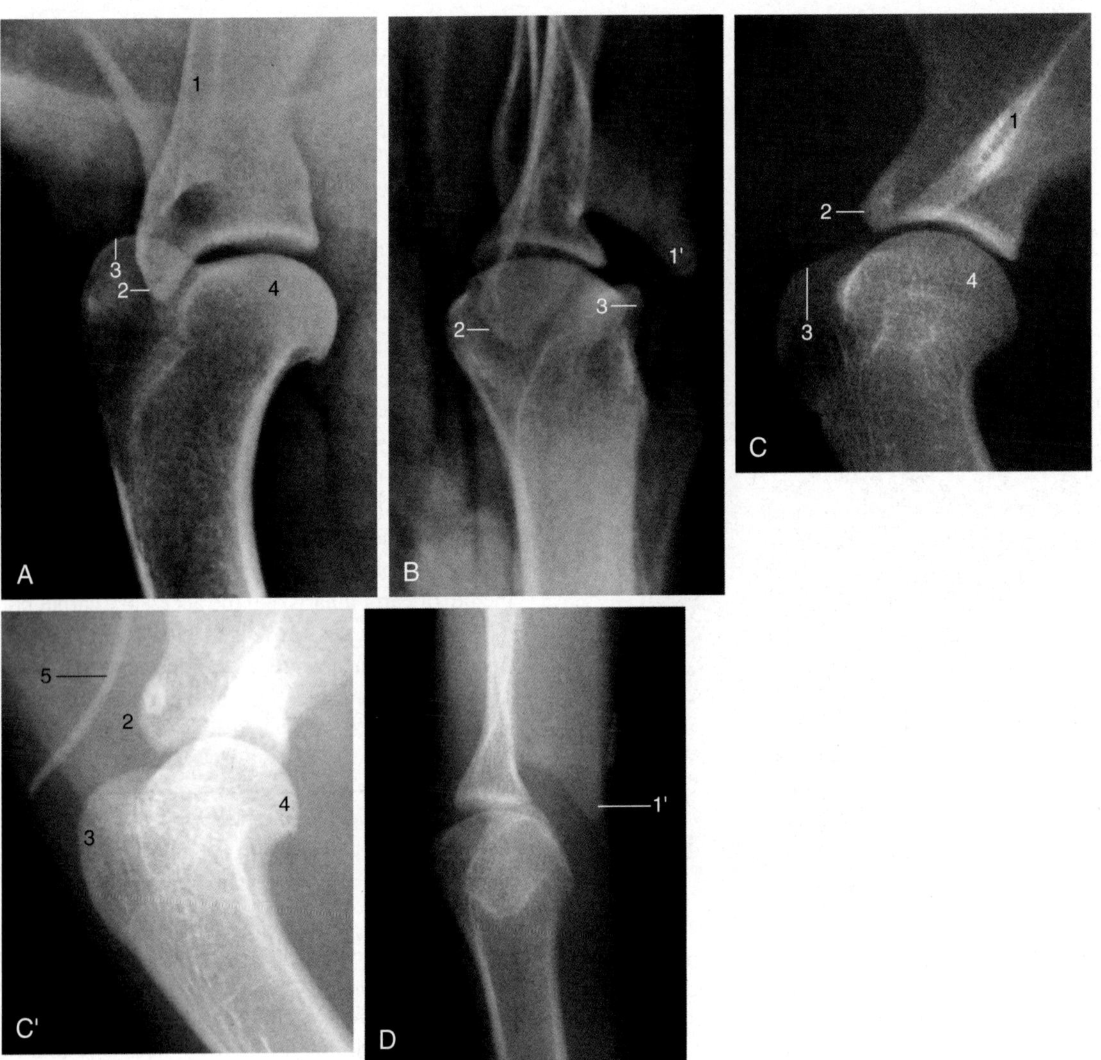

Fig. 16.3 Lateral (A, C and C′) and craniocaudal (B and D) radiographic views of the canine (A and B) and feline (C, C′, and D) shoulder joints; C and D were taken from specimens. *1*, Scapular spine; *1′*, acromion; *2*, supraglenoid tubercle; *3*, greater tubercle of humerus; *4*, head of humerus; *5*, vestigial clavicle.

occurs in fast growing large breed dogs, or if, having fused, it later becomes detached, the loose piece causes severe lameness. The medial coronoid process at the distal end of the trochlear notch (Fig. 16.8/*5*) is not formed from a separate ossification center, and its separation is therefore not due to a developmental failure but to another cause, such as osteochondrosis or fracture resulting from overloading. The medial coronoid process is superimposed on the proximal end of the radius in lateral radiographs of the normal joint.

The distal epiphysis of the humerus fuses with the shaft at 5 to 8 months, which is considerably earlier than closure at the proximal end. The proximal epiphyseal cartilage of the radius and that of the tuber olecrani generally disappear about the same time; the larger distal cartilages of the forearm bones disappear a little later, usually at about 6 to 9 months. Fully two-thirds of the lengthening of the radius is due to growth at its distal cartilage. The lengthening of the ulna (distal to the elbow joint) is almost equally dependent on growth of its V-shaped distal cartilage. The deformation that follows unequal elongation of these bones results from "premature fusion" of one of the distal growth cartilages; the most prominent effect is deviation of the paw, which tenses several interosseous connective tissue structures, most notably the distal part of the radioulnar ligament. Differences in growth velocity between the radius and ulna may also be responsible for incongruity at the elbow joint, which causes a step to develop between the normally level articular surfaces of the radius and ulna.

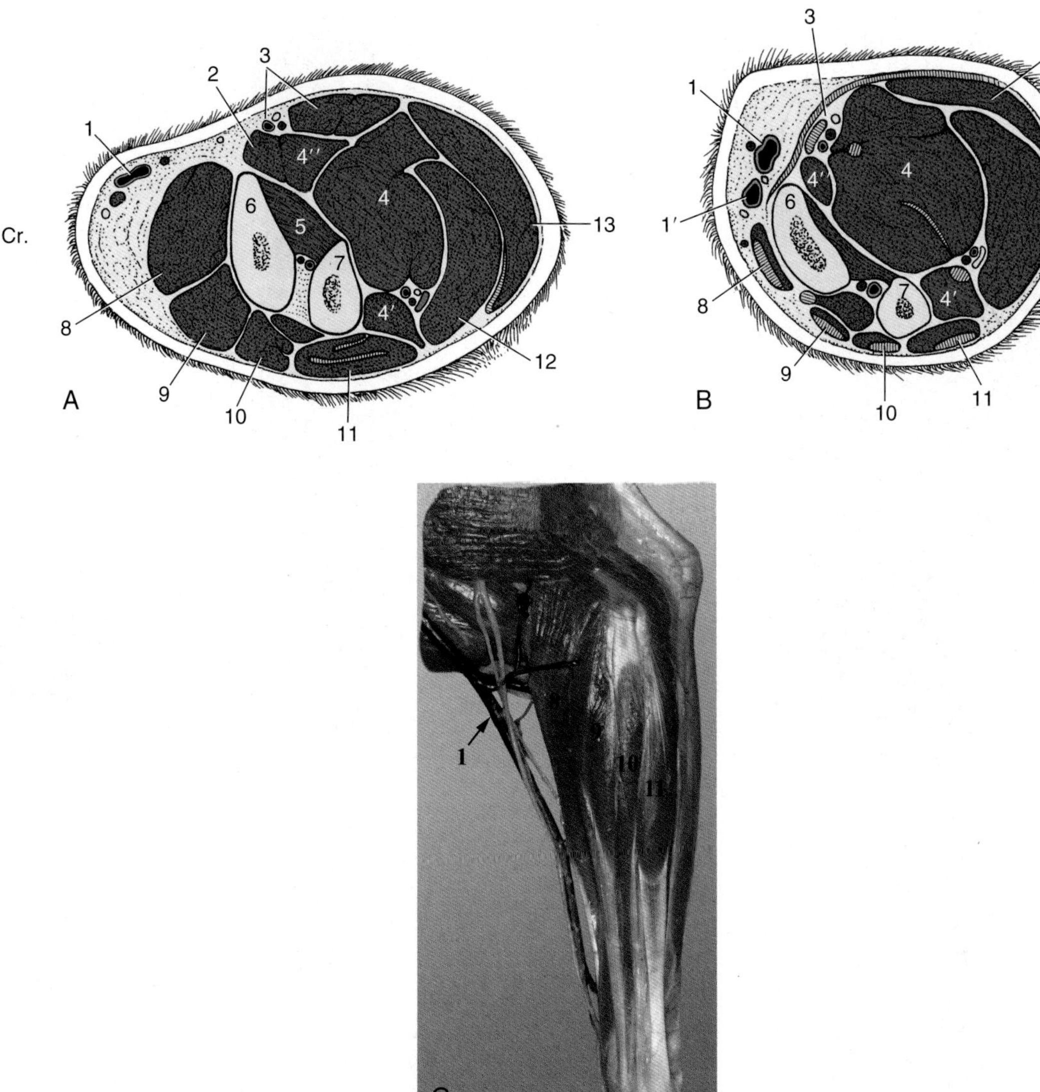

Fig. 16.4 Transverse sections of the left canine forelimb just distal to the elbow joint (A) and just proximal to the carpus (B) and lateral view (C). *1*, Cephalic vein and branches of superficial radial nerve; *1′*, accessory cephalic vein; *2*, pronator teres; *3*, median vessels and nerve and flexor carpi radialis; *4*, *4′*, and *4″*, humeral, ulnar, and radial heads of deep digital flexor, respectively; *5*, pronator quadratus; *6*, radius; *7*, ulna; *8*, extensor carpi radialis; *9*, common digital extensor; *10*, lateral digital extensor; *11*, ulnaris lateralis; *12*, flexor carpi ulnaris—its small ulnar head lies on its caudal aspect, and the ulnar vessels and nerve lie on its cranial aspect; *13*, superficial digital flexor; *Cr.*, cranial.

In the dog, the distal part of the humerus presents three ossification centers: that for the capitulum, the trochlea, and the medial epicondyle. The latter is reported to be liable to separate in young dogs of the larger breeds, which causes relocation of the origin of the flexor carpi radialis muscle. In the cat an additional ossification center is found in the lateral epicondyle.

Forearm fractures are relatively common. They occur most often in the distal half of the forearm and, as would be anticipated, generally involve both bones. Fracture of the olecranon is also fairly common.

Flexion of the elbow is accomplished by the brachialis and biceps brachii. The *brachial muscle* originates from the caudal part of the proximal humerus and winds over the lateral surface to gain the medial aspect of the elbow before inserting on the radial and ulnar tuberosities. The biarticular *biceps* arises from the supraglenoid tubercle and in the dog divides its insertion between the medial

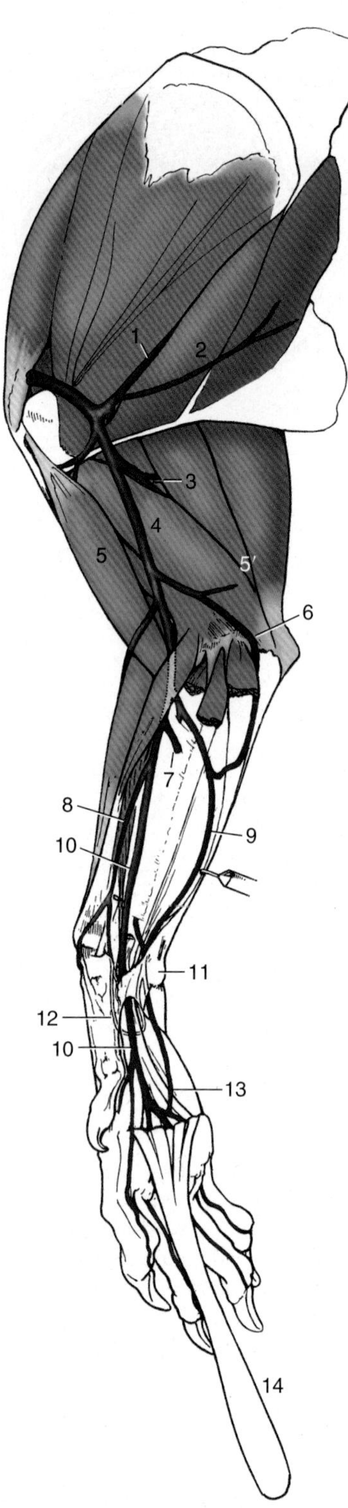

Fig. 16.5 The topography of the major arteries of the right canine forelimb, medial view. The caudomedial muscles of the forearm have been removed. *1,* Subscapular artery; *2,* teres major; *3,* deep brachial artery; *4,* brachial artery; *5,* biceps; *5′,* triceps; *6,* collateral ulnar artery; *7,* deep antebrachial artery; *8,* radial artery; *9,* ulnar artery; *10,* median artery; *11,* accessory carpal bone; *12,* deep palmar arch; *13,* superficial palmar arch; *14,* superficial digital flexor, reflected.

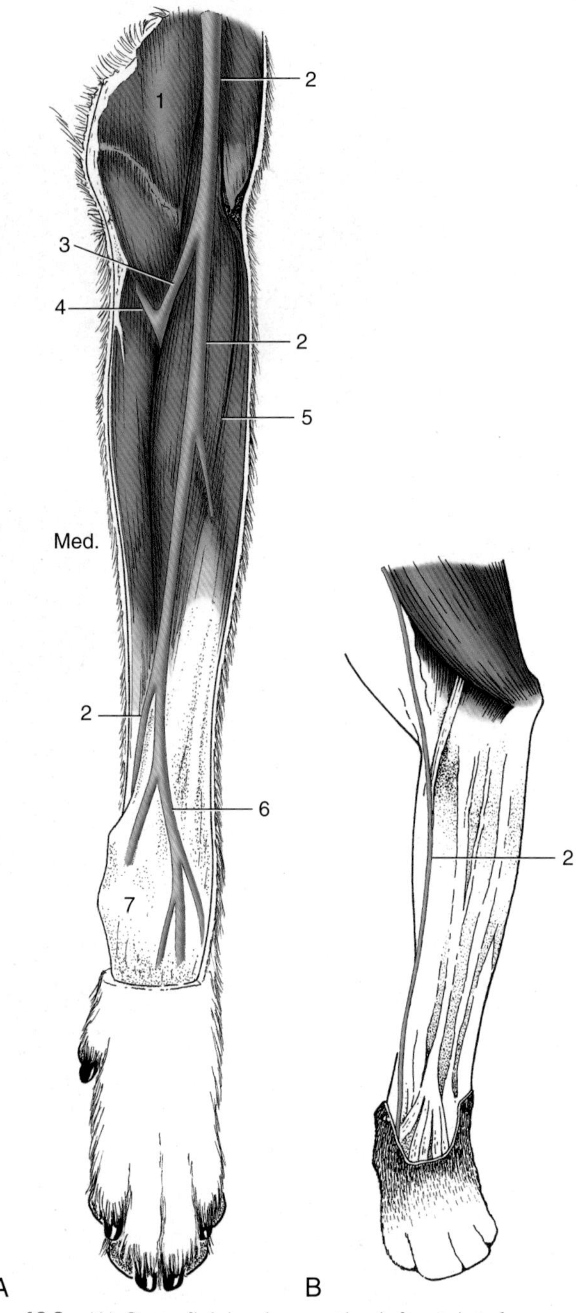

Fig. 16.6 (A) Superficial veins on the left canine forearm. (B) The course of the cephalic vein on the left feline forearm. *1,* Brachiocephalicus; *2,* cephalic vein; *3,* median cubital vein; *4,* brachial vein; *5,* extensor carpi radialis; *6,* accessory cephalic vein; *7,* carpus; *Med.,* medial.

coronoid process of the ulna and the radial tuberosity. A tendon strap of no obvious functional significance is sometimes present between the biceps and the extensor carpi radialis muscle. The biceps of the cat inserts only on the radial tuberosity. This muscle has some supinator capacity. The extensor group comprises the triceps, tensor, and anconeus (to be mentioned shortly).

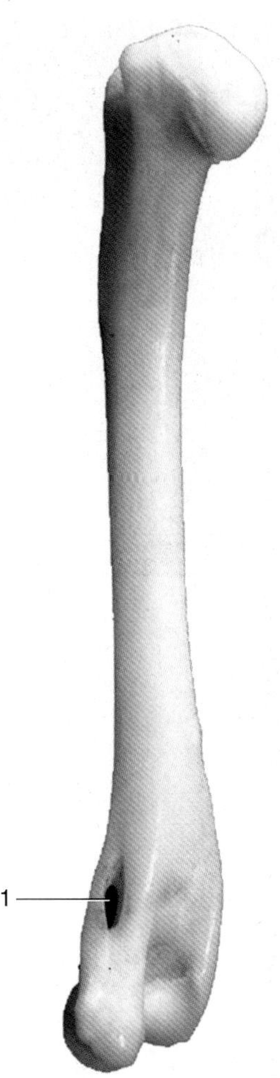

Fig. 16.7 Feline humerus exhibiting the supracondylar foramen *(1)*.

The movements of supination, in which the dorsal surface of the paw is turned outward, and pronation, in which it is turned inward, are primarily the task of a small group of dedicated muscles: two supinators and two pronators. The essential movement is of course rotation of the radius within the embrace of the ulna. The *supinator* is a small, flat, fusiform muscle that lies deep to the extensor muscles in the forearm. It originates from the lateral epicondyle of the humerus and adjacent structures and inserts on the dorsal surface of the proximal quarter of the shaft of the radius, reaching close to the medial border of this bone. The *second supinator, the brachioradialis,* is very weak or even absent in the dog and constant but hardly important in the cat, in which it forms a thin ribbon running close to the cephalic vein. The *pronator teres* comes from the medial epicondyle of the humerus and converges on the supinator; the two muscles insert close together. The pronator teres is stronger in the cat than in the dog. The *pronator quadratus* lies medial to the interosseous membrane that joins the radius and ulna along the length of their shafts, and, like this membrane, it runs between the two bones.

The *elbow joint capsule,* common to the joint between the humerus and the radius and ulna and to the proximal joint between the forearm bones, extends three pouches: craniolaterally beneath the common digital extensor, craniomedially beneath the biceps, and caudally between the lateral epicondyle and the olecranon. The last is used for injections in cats, whereas the first site is more often preferred in dogs. The caudal part of the capsule is closely related to the small, flat anconeus muscle, usually assigned to the extensors of the elbow but probably more important as a tensor of the capsule, preventing redundant folds of synovial membrane from being nipped between the bones.

Luxation of the elbow joint is relatively common. The joint is most easily luxated through lateral displacement of the radius and ulna when it is flexed because the anconeal process withdraws from the olecranon fossa of the humerus. Lateral luxation may also occur following trauma, which may rupture or avulse the collateral ligaments. Medial luxation is less frequent, probably because it is more difficult for the anconeal process to snap over the larger medial epicondyle. It follows that dislocations will be most easily reduced if the joint is first strongly flexed to disengage the anconeal process.

In both dogs and cats the collateral ligaments of the elbow present both radial and ulnar divisions, and there are differences in the relative strength of the parts in the two species. The differences influence the relative degrees of pronation and supination. The cat actively enjoys 100 degrees or more of movement, whereas the passive excursions in the dog are limited to about 50 degrees of supination and 20 degrees of pronation. The annular ligament that completes the ring within which the head of the radius rotates inserts on the cranial part of the medial coronoid process, which is consequently subjected to considerable tensile stress. A small sesamoid bone is occasionally associated with the lateral collateral ligament.

The muscles of the forearm conform in broad outline to the common pattern previously described (pp. 78–80), and any differences in their arrangements are not of functional significance. The extensors of the carpus and digit, lying cranial to the shaft of the radius, are separated from the flexors caudal to the bone by the palpable border of the radius medially and by the attachment of the most lateral extensor, the ulnaris lateralis, to the salient and easily identified accessory carpal bone laterally. Apart from acting as an abductor of the carpus, the ulnaris lateralis appears to support extension of an already extended carpal joint or flexion of one already flexed. The existence of a bridge (interflexorius) crossing

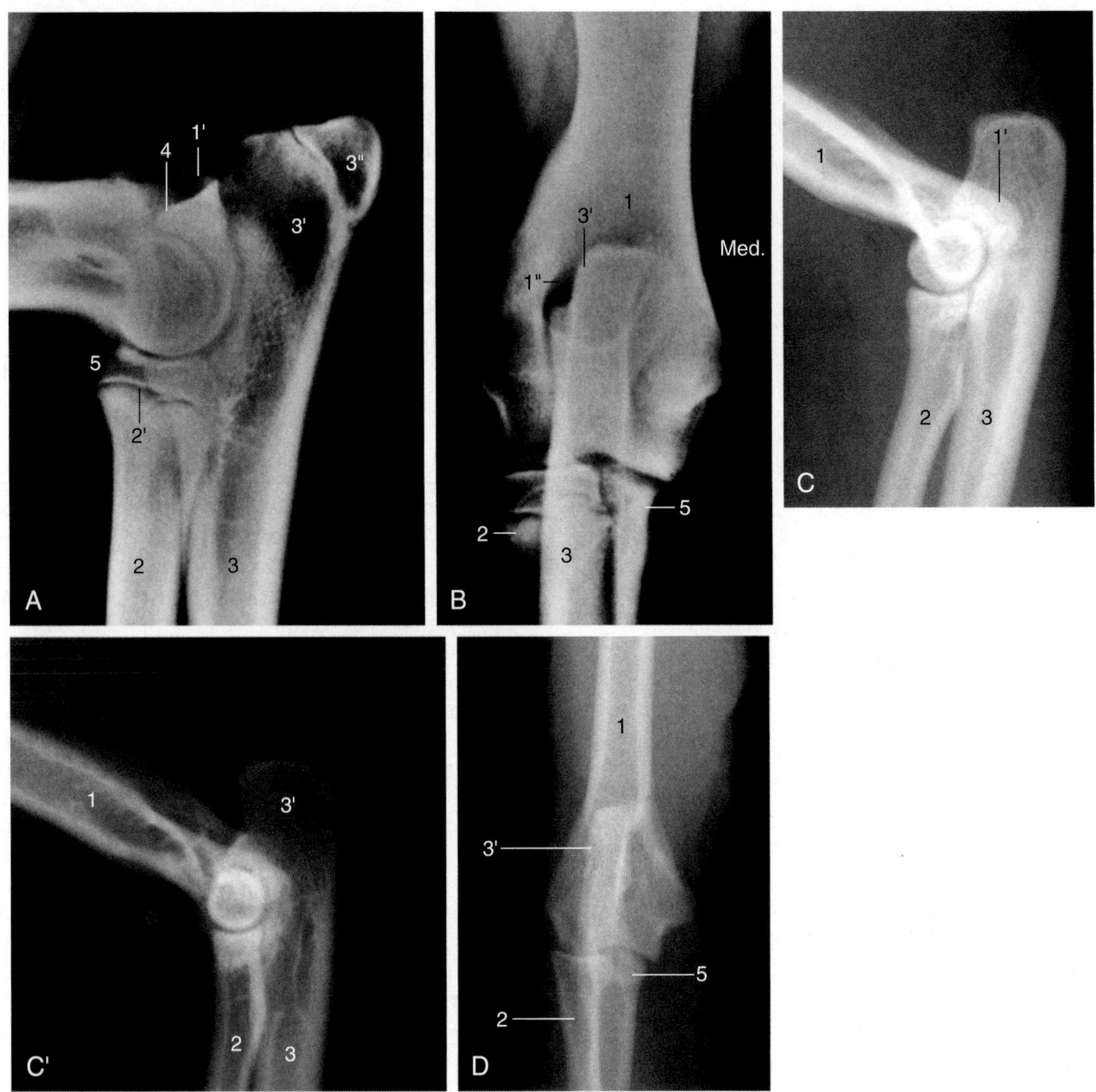

Fig. 16.8 Lateral (A) and craniocaudal (B) radiographic views of the elbow joint of a young dog (A and B) and of a cat (C, C′, and D). The (feline) supracondylar foramen is depicted in Fig. 16.7. *1,* Humerus; *1′,* medial epicondyle; *1″,* supratrochlear foramen; *2,* radius; *2′,* proximal epiphyseal cartilage; *3,* ulna; *3′,* olecranon; *3″,* apophysis of tuber olecrani; *4,* anconeal process; *5,* medial coronoid process; *Med.,* medial.

from the deep to the superficial digital flexor muscle in the distal forearm may be mentioned as a distinctive feature of carnivores, among the domestic species.

THE CARPUS AND FOREPAW (SEE ALSO PP. 71–75 AND 80)

The carpal and metacarpal bones and the phalanges should be studied principally with a view to becoming familiar with their radiographic appearances.

The most obvious external features are the digital, metacarpal, and carpal pads and the claws. At birth, a reduced first digit, or "dewclaw," is generally present below the carpus on the medial side of the paw. It is often removed routinely, even in city dogs, although the presumed purpose of this mutilation is to avoid the risk of injury should the dewclaws catch in scrub. It must be retained in puppies of certain breeds if there is a possibility that they will later be shown. The carpal pad, just distal to the palpable accessory carpal bone, is normally denied contact with the ground except in animals cornering at speed; it is occasionally injured in this way in racing Greyhounds (see Fig. 10.15/*4*). The metacarpal (Fig. 16.9/*8*) and digital (Fig. 16.9/*7*) pads over flexor surfaces of the metacarpophalangeal and the distal

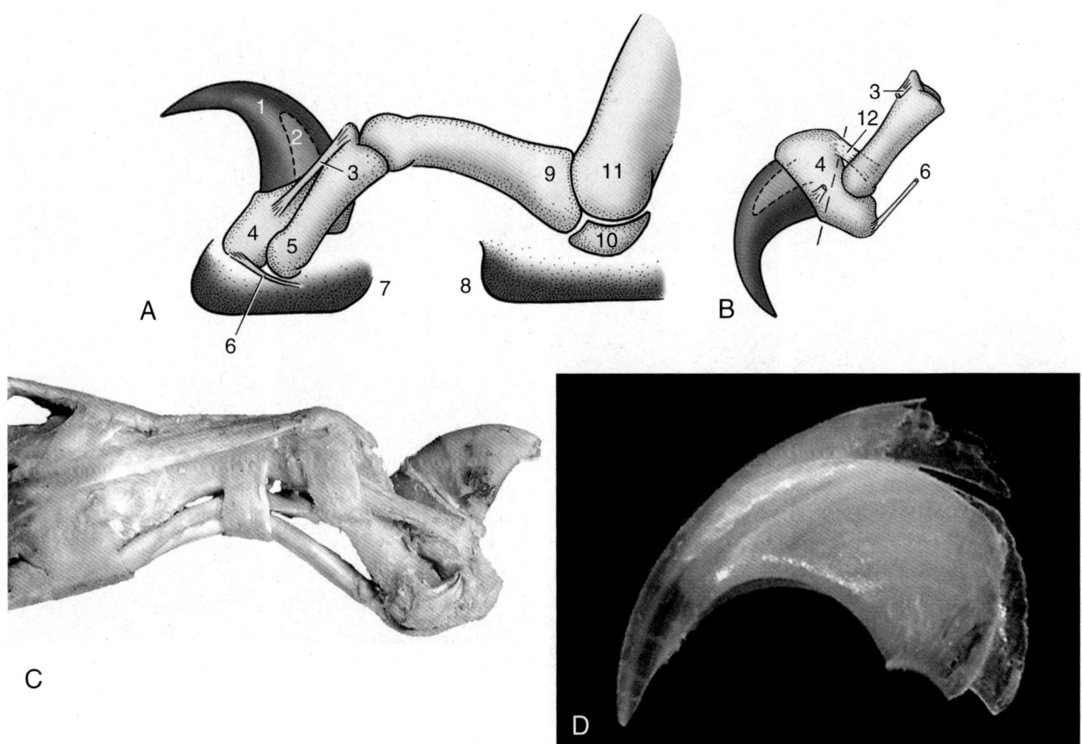

Fig. 16.9 The feline claw (A) fully retracted and (B) protruded, showing the division *(broken line)* of the distal phalanx in declawing. The arrangement of the elastic ligaments has been greatly simplified. (C) Claw of a tiger showing the same ligaments somewhat more clearly. (D) Outer layer of horn shed from cat claw. *1,* Claw; *2,* unguicular process of distal phalanx; *3,* medial dorsal elastic ligament; *4,* distal phalanx; *5,* middle phalanx; *6,* deep digital flexor tendon; *7,* digital pad; *8,* metacarpal pad; *9,* proximal phalanx; *10,* proximal sesamoid bone; *11,* metacarpal bone; *12,* lateral dorsal elastic ligament.

interphalangeal joints, respectively, make ground contact, and the small papillae that normally roughen their surfaces may be worn smooth in dogs regularly walked on pavement. The webs of skin connecting the digits proximal to the pads are common sites of interdigital infections and cysts.

Dorsopalmar radiographs show the carpal bones with a minimum of overlapping (Fig. 16.10). The large radial carpal bone (Fig. 16.10/*3*), which incorporates the intermediate element in both dogs and cats, lies distal to the radius; the oddly shaped ulnar carpal bone (Fig. 16.10/*4*) next to it extends distally (on the palmar surface) to be superimposed on the fourth carpal bone (and even on the corresponding metacarpal bones). The accessory carpal bone (Fig. 16.10/*5*) is superimposed on the junction of the radius, ulna, and ulnar carpal bone. On the medial side, carpals 1 and 2 are superimposed, and a sesamoid in the extensor carpi obliquus may also be seen opposite the midcarpal joint. Another two sesamoid bones may be visible on the palmar aspect between the proximal and distal carpal rows. The carpal pad produces a fainter shadow.

The distal radial epiphysis has occasionally been mistaken for a carpal bone. A wide space seen between the distal extremities of the radius and ulna in slightly oblique projections of the cat's carpus may be misinterpreted as a subluxation.

The proximal row of carpal bones includes the fused radial, intermediate, and central bone, the ulnar carpal bone, and the accessory carpal bone (see Fig. 2.48). The radial carpal bone exhibits three ossification centers that fuse 3 to 4 months after birth in dogs, although not until the seventh month in the cat. Although the ulnar carpal bone has a large distally protruding process, it possesses only a single ossification center. The epiphysis of the accessory carpal bone closes between 3 and 6 months of age. The distal carpal row is composed of four bones, the smallest of which is medial and the largest of which is lateral.

The antebrachiocarpal joint is an ellipsoid joint allowing flexion, extension, abduction, and adduction. In dogs and cats the collateral ligaments do not extend the length of the carpus but are limited to the

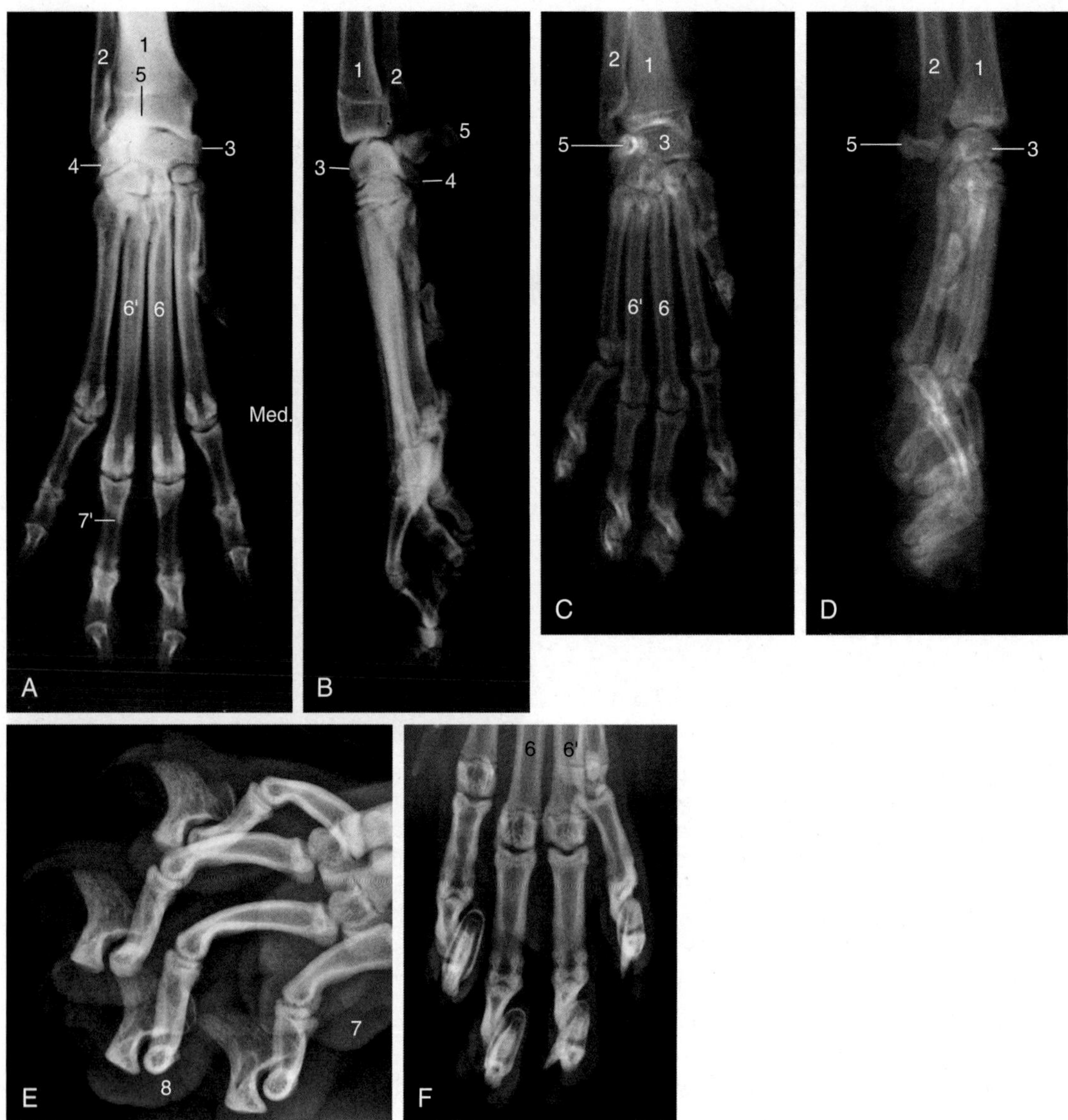

Fig. 16.10 (A to D) Dorsopalmar and lateral radiographic views of the canine (A and B) and feline (C and D) forepaws. (E) and (F) Oblique and dorsopalmar views of feline digits, respectively; note how the distal phalanges slide next to the middle phalanges when the claws are retracted. *1,* Radius; *2,* ulna; *3,* radial carpal; *4,* ulnar carpal; *5,* accessory carpal; *6* and *6′,* third and fourth metacarpals, respectively; *7,* metacarpal pad; *7′,* distal border of metacarpal pad, *8,* digital pad; *Med.,* medial.

proximal joint. Short carpal ligaments bridge the chief joints vertically, connect neighboring bones in the same row horizontally, and connect the accessory carpal bone to the ulna, the ulnar and fourth carpal bones, and the fourth and fifth metacarpal bones. Only the two distal joint spaces communicate, while the independent proximal (antebrachiocarpal) compartment may be punctured most readily by passing the needle between the palpable radial carpal and common digital extensor tendons when the joint is flexed. Flexion of the joint widens the dorsal gap at the antebrachiocarpal level and facilitates appreciation of the tendons of the extensor carpi radialis and common digital extensor. Except for the accessory, the individual carpal bones cannot be distinguished by palpation. The bones distal to the carpus are all readily identified by palpation because the metacarpals, though crowded together proximally, diverge distally. The extensor tendons can be rolled against the metacarpal bones, and the digital flexors and the interossei together form a soft package on the palmar aspect.

The distal epiphyses of the principal metacarpal bones fuse with the shafts at about 5 to 7 months. (The proximal metacarpal epiphyses fuse prenatally.)

The *paired sesamoid bones* on the palmar surface of the metacarpophalangeal joints are embedded in the metacarpal pad (Fig. 16.9/*8* and *10*). The sesamoid bones at the metacarpophalangeal joint are associated with the same complex of ligaments—straight, oblique, and so forth—as in the horse but without these possessing corresponding importance. Distal to the proximal sesamoid bones, the branches of the superficial tendon are split for the passage of the deep tendon, and at the metacarpophalangeal and proximal and distal interphalangeal joints, these are retained by annular ligaments. The functional digits (numbers 2 to 5) are equipped with interosseous muscles on the palmar aspects of the metacarpal bones, where their presence may be appreciated on deep palpation. In addition, digits 1, 2, and 5 each contain several small individual muscles of restricted functional and minimal clinical importance.

The *claws* are shaped to the dorsal and lateral surfaces of the curved unguicular processes of the distal phalanges to which they are connected by the laminar dermis (Fig. 16.11B and C). The sole of each claw (Fig. 16.11/*4*) covers the ventral surface of the process and appears as a crumbly whitish material between the lower edges of the wall. The claws, especially those of heavy city dogs, are generally worn level with the digital pads; they must be trimmed when there is insufficient wear because, if left unchecked, they would grow around to penetrate the pads. Special clippers should be used because the lateral pressure exerted by scissors or human nail clippers causes pain. The claw should be trimmed level with the ground surface of the pad but not so short that the vascular and sensitive dermis is damaged (Fig. 16.11B). The pink dermis may be recognized in nonpigmented claws, but when one is denied this guide, a warning sign is provided by the appearance of a black dot on the cut surface just distal to the dermis.

Elastic dorsal ligaments (Fig. 16.11/*5*) extend from the proximal ends of the middle phalanges to the unguicular crests of the distal phalanges to keep the claws elevated. The deep digital flexor opposes the ligaments and protrudes the claws for scratching or digging.

The *claws of the cat* are laterally compressed, strongly curved, and drawn out to sharp points. They can be fully retracted into the fur of the paw, which enables cats to walk silently and without blunting the claws through ground contact. The elastic dorsal ligaments are of unequal length; long ones extend from the proximal interphalangeal joint to the sides of the distal phalanx, and a single short ligament extends between the distal end of the middle phalanx and the top of the unguicular crest (Fig. 16.9/*3* and *12*). This disposition, combined with the obliquity of the articular surfaces, allows the base of the claw to be drawn lateral to the corresponding middle phalanx (Fig. 16.10F).

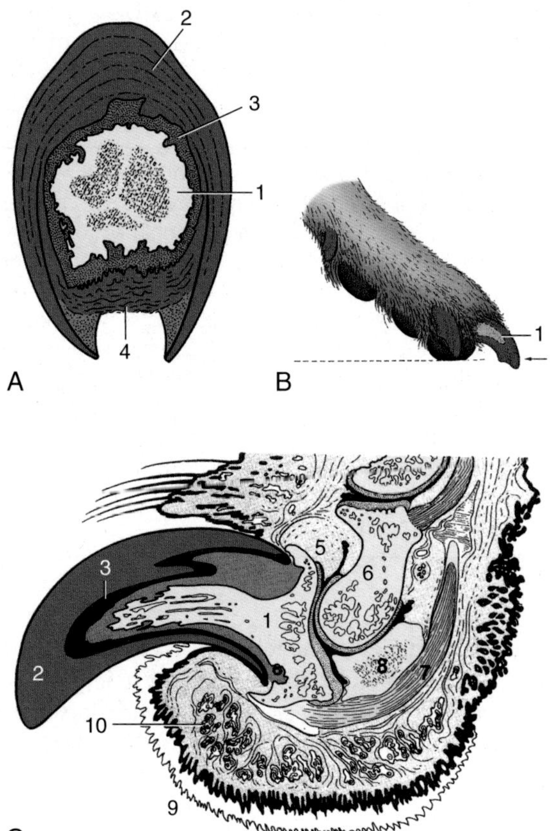

Fig. 16.11 (A) Transverse section of canine claw. (B) Correct trimming of canine claws. (C) Axial section of the canine digit. *1,* Unguicular process of distal phalanx; *2,* wall of claw; *3,* laminar dermis; *4,* crumbly sole of claw; *5,* dorsal elastic ligament; *6,* middle phalanx; *7,* deep digital flexor tendon; *8,* distal sesamoid (cartilaginous); *9,* digital pad; *10,* sweat glands.

The ligaments keep the claws strongly retracted so that the digital flexors move only the metacarpophalangeal and proximal interphalangeal joints. The claws are protruded by simultaneous contraction of the deep digital flexor, which flexes the distal interphalangeal joints, and the digital extensors, which stabilize the more proximal joints of the paw. Cats use their protrusible claws for climbing trees and for initial prey contact; dogs, however, use their jaws for prey contact. The characteristic "clawing" of cats on logs, rugs, or furniture, commonly thought to be performed to sharpen the claws, is actually related to territorial marking by sweat from the glands concentrated in the digital pads. Forceful scraping of the ground by dogs after defecation or urination may have a similar marking purpose that utilizes the secretion of the sweat glands of their pads. Clawing also promotes shedding of an outer, worn-out layer of a claw (Fig. 16.9D).

Onychectomy is the surgical procedure to remove P3 (the third digital phalanx) in destructive cats to prevent them from scratching furniture or people or to remove an infected nail or a nail tumor. The elective procedure is typically done between 3 and 12 months. The base of the bone with the attachment of the deep digital flexor is left in place while the unguicular crest, enclosing the base of the claw, is removed (Fig. 16.9B). The surgery is performed under general anesthesia and with nerve blocks. An alternative procedure, simpler and causing less postoperative pain, consists of deep digital flexor tenectomy. These procedures are forbidden in many European countries.

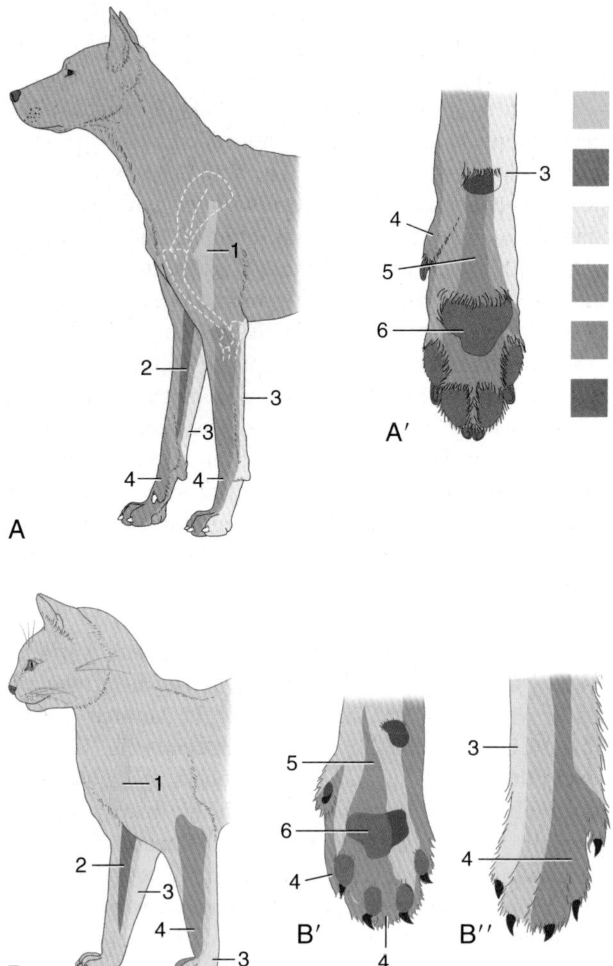

Fig. 16.12 The autonomous zones of the cutaneous innervation of the canine (A and A′) and feline (B, B′, and B″) forelimb. *1,* Axillary nerve *(green)*; *2,* musculocutaneous nerve *(red)*; *3,* ulnar nerve *(yellow)*; *4,* radial nerve *(blue)*; *5,* median nerve *(orange)*; *6,* mixture of median and ulnar nerves *(brown)*.

The main arteries of the forelimb have been described (pp. 231–232); their relations are shown in Fig. 16.5. A branch of the radial artery found on the dorsomedial aspect of the distal carpus may be used for taking the pulse of cats.

THE MAJOR NERVES OF THE FORELIMB

This description is concerned only with the nerves distal to the shoulder. Because the main features conform closely to the common pattern (pp. 309–311), it is sufficient to concentrate attention on their relations and cutaneous distribution. The brachial plexus originates from C6 to T1 in about 60%, from C5 to T1 in 20%, from C6 to T2 in about 20%, and from C5 to T2 in a very small proportion (<3%) of dogs. The origins of the individual nerves are therefore subject to considerable variation; those described later refer to the most common arrangements. There is also considerable overlap between their cutaneous territories, which can be indicated only approximately. Fig. 16.12 shows the much smaller autonomous zones used for testing the integrity of *individual* nerves. The courses and distributions of the nerves within the paw have little clinical application and can be dealt with summarily.

The *musculocutaneous nerve* (C6–C7) innervates the biceps, brachialis, and coracobrachialis. It descends on the medial surface of the arm between the biceps and the brachial artery and, at the elbow, detaches a communicating branch to the more caudally placed median nerve. It is continued into the forearm by a cutaneous branch (medial cutaneous antebrachial nerve), which passes between the biceps and brachialis to become subcutaneous craniomedial to the elbow, before supplying skin over the medial surface of the forearm (Figs. 16.12/*2* and 16.13/*1* and *11*). Although *dysfunction* of the nerve causes little change in gait, an affected animal is unable to respond to the invitation to "offer a paw" because flexion of the elbow requires activity of at least one of the biceps and brachialis muscles.

The *axillary nerve* (C7–C8) supplies the prime flexors of the shoulder joint. It leaves the axillary space by disappearing dorsal to the teres major (Fig. 16.2/*4* and *5*) and then winds around the caudal aspect of the joint to reach the deltoideus; the branches that continue beyond this point supply skin over the craniolateral region of the arm and a part of the forearm (Fig. 16.12/*1*). Paralysis of the nerve has little effect because the latissimus dorsi and the long

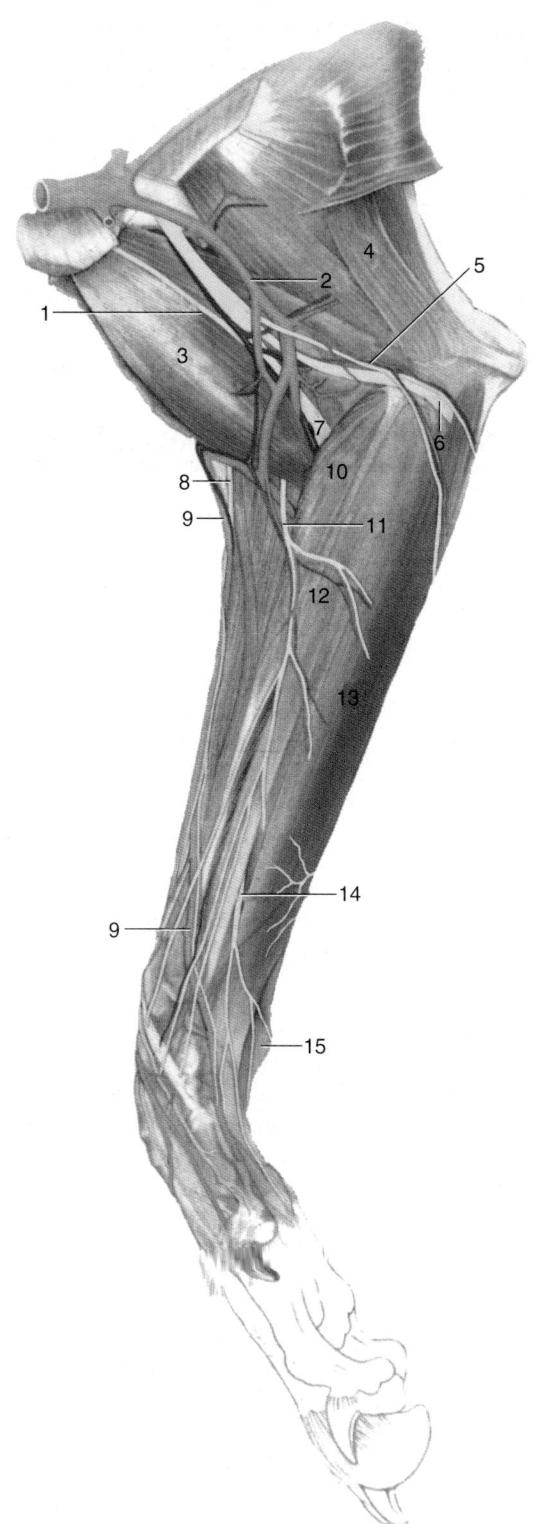

Fig. 16.13 Superficial dissection of the right canine forelimb, medial view. *1,* Musculocutaneous nerve; *2,* brachial vein; *3,* biceps; *4,* tensor fasciae antebrachii; *5,* caudal cutaneous antebrachial nerve and collateral ulnar vessels; *6,* ulnar nerve; *7,* median nerve and brachial artery; *8,* medial branch of superficial radial nerve; *9,* cephalic vein; *10,* pronator teres; *11,* medial cutaneous antebrachial nerve; *12,* flexor carpi radialis; *13,* superficial digital flexor; *14,* inconstant cutaneous branch of ulnar nerve; *15,* accessory carpal bone.

head of the triceps are available to compensate for the loss of most shoulder flexors.

The *median nerve* (C8–T1) innervates most flexors of the carpus and digits. It descends on the medial surface of the arm just caudal to the brachial artery and passes the elbow cranial to the medial collateral ligament before dipping under the pronator teres and flexor carpi radialis muscles (Fig. 16.13/*7*). It detaches most of its muscular branches here and then continues under the flexor carpi radialis near the medial border of the radius as a mainly sensory nerve. It goes through the carpal canal along with the digital flexor tendons and the median artery before dividing to supply the medial and palmar aspects of the paw in collaboration with the ulnar nerve. Dysfunction has little effect on the gait, but the carpus may become overextended when the dog is standing, which results in the claws being slightly raised from their normal posture.

The *ulnar nerve* (C8–T1) innervates the remaining carpal and digital flexors. It first descends with the median nerve, but in the distal half of the arm it seeks a more caudal course over the medial epicondyle of the humerus (where it is palpable), accompanied by the collateral ulnar vessels (Fig. 16.13/*6*). A cutaneous branch (caudal cutaneous antebrachial nerve; Fig. 16.13/*5*) that becomes subcutaneous on the medial aspect of the olecranon supplies the caudal surface of the forearm. The main trunk dives into the caudomedial forearm muscles and, after supplying some of these, it reemerges on the lateral side, where it joins the ulnar artery and vein before descending caudal to the ulna. It divides into dorsal and palmar branches in the distal half of the forearm. The *dorsal branch* comes to the surface in the large depression between the ulnaris lateralis and the flexor carpi ulnaris and innervates the skin on the lateropalmar aspect of the paw. The *palmar branch* crosses the carpus with the flexor tendons and median nerve to supply the palmar aspect of the paw. Paralysis of the nerve has no obvious effect on gait or posture.

The important *radial nerve* (C7–T1) [illegible] the extenso[illegible], carpal, and digital joints. It leaves the axilla by plunging into the triceps, about the middle of the arm (Fig. 16.2/*7*). After detaching branches to the triceps, it accompanies the brachialis muscle around the lateral aspect of the humerus to gain the flexor surface of the elbow, where it is eminently vulnerable in fractures and from the tumors that commonly affect the humerus. It divides into deep and superficial branches before leaving the arm. The deep branch continues distally, first between the brachialis and extensor carpi radialis and then between the supinator and the joint capsule, to supply the carpal and digital extensors in the upper part of the forearm. The superficial branch splits into medial and lateral branches that emerge from the cranial border of the lateral head of the triceps to run subcutaneously, one to each side of the cephalic vein, and enter the paw with the accessory cephalic vein (Fig. 16.4/*1* and *1′*). The superficial branch supplies skin on the dorsal surface of the forearm and paw, sharing the most proximal part of this region with the axillary nerve (Fig. 16.12/*4*).

If the radial nerve is seriously injured proximal to the origin of the tricipital branches, the elbow cannot be fixed, and the limb, unable to bear weight, is carried in the flexed position with the toes knuckled over and presenting their dorsal surfaces to the ground. More distal injury is less serious because the dog soon learns to compensate for loss of the digital extensors by flicking the raised paw forward so that it lands on the pads.

COMPREHENSION CHECK

Before dissecting the limb, clip the hair from the shoulder, elbow, and carpal joints, and practice injection of dyes into these joints.

Palpate the major anatomic landmarks on the forelimb of the dog and the cat.

The carpal canal is formed by the accessory carpal bone (laterally), the palmar carpal ligament and carpal bones (dorsally), and the flexor retinaculum (palmar). What is contained in it?

TABLE 16.2 MUSCLES OF THE FORELIMB, THEIR FUNCTION AND INNERVATIONS*

Name	Origin	Insertion	Function
Extrinsic Muscles of the Forelimb			
Superficial pectoral	First two sternebrae and raphe between two muscles	Greater tubercle of humerus	Adduct when not bearing weight Prevent abduction when bearing weight **Supplied by** cranial pectoral nerves (C7, C8)
Deep pectoral	Ventral sternum and raphe between two muscles	Lesser and greater tubercles of humerus	Limb advanced-fixed: pull trunk cranially and extend shoulder Draw limb caudally when not bearing weight; to adduct limb **Supplied by** caudal pectoral nerves (C8, T1)
Brachiocephalicus: cleidobrachialis and cleidocephalicus (pars mastoidea and pars cervicalis)	Distal end of humerus	Mid-dorsal raphe (cleidocervicalis) Mastoid part of the temporal bone	Advance limb; extend shoulder joint; draw head and neck to side **Supplied by** accessory nerve and ventral branches of cervical spinal nerves
Sternocephalicus	First sternebra	Mastoid part of temporal bone and nuchal crest of occipital bone	Draw head and neck to side **Supplied by** accessory nerve and ventral branches of cervical spinal nerves
Omotransversarius	Distal end of spine of scapula	Wing of atlas	Advance limb; flex neck laterally **Supplied by** accessory nerve
Trapezius	Median raphe of the neck; supraspinous ligament from third cervical to ninth thoracic vertebra	Spine of scapula	Elevate and abduct limb **Supplied by** accessory nerve
Rhomboideus	Nuchal crest of occipital bone; medial raphe of neck; spinous process of thoracic vertebrae 1–7	Dorsal border and adjacent surface of scapula	Elevate limb; draw scapula against the trunk **Supplied by** ventral branches of cervical and thoracic spinal nerves
Latissimus dorsi	Thoracolumbar fascia from lumbar and last 7 thoracic vertebrae; muscular attachment to last two ribs	Teres major tuberosity of humerus and teres major tendon	Retracts the limb and flexes the shoulder; draws trunk forward over a fixed limb **Supplied by** thoracodorsal nerve (C7, C8, T1)

TABLE 16.2 **MUSCLES OF THE FORELIMB AND THEIR INNERVATIONS*—cont'd**			
Name	**Origin**	**Insertion**	**Function**
Serratus ventralis cervicis; serratus ventralis thoracis	Transverse processes of last 5 cervical vertebrae; ribs 1–7 ventral to their middle	Dorsomedial third of scapula	Support trunk and depress scapula **Supplied by** ventral branches of cervical spinal nerves and long thoracic (C7)
Lateral Muscles of Scapula and Shoulder: deltoid and teres minor supplied by axillary nerve; supraspinatus and infraspinatus supplied by suprascapular nerve			
Deltoid	Spine and acromion of scapula	Deltoid tuberosity of humerus	All flex shoulder except supraspinatus extends and stabilizes; Infraspinatus and Teres minor rotate arm; Infraspinatus adducts
Infraspinatus	Infraspinous fossa	Greater tubercle of humerus	
Supraspinatus	Supraspinous fossa		
Teres minor	Distal third of caudal border: scapula	Teres minor tuberosity of humerus	Flex shoulder; rotate arm laterally
Medial Muscles of Scapula and Shoulder			
Subscapularis	Subscapular fossa	Lesser tubercle of humerus	Adduct/extend/stabilize shoulder; **Supplied by** subscapular nerve
Teres major	Caudal border of scapula	Teres major tuberosity of humerus	Flex shoulder; rotate arm medially; **Supplied by** axillary nerve
Coracobrachialis	Coracoid process of scapula	Lesser tubercle of humerus	Adduct/extend/stabilize shoulder; **Supplied by** musculocutaneous nerve
Caudal Muscles of Forelimb (brachium): all supplied by the radial nerve			
Tensor fasciae antebrachii	Fascia on lateral side: latissimus dorsi	Olecranon	Extend elbow Long head also flexes shoulder
Triceps brachii	Long: caudal border of scapula Lateral: tricipital line: humerus Accessory: neck of humerus Medial: lesser tubercle		
Anconeus	Lateral and medial epicondyles of humerus	Lateral surface of proximal end of ulna	
Cranial Muscles of Forelimb: all supplied by the musculocutaneous nerve			
Biceps brachii	Supraglenoid tubercle	Ulnar and radial tuberosities	Both flex elbow; Biceps brachii also extends shoulder
Brachialis	Proximal third of lateral surface: humerus		
Cranial and Lateral Muscles of Forelimb: all supplied by the radial nerve			
Extensor carpi radialis	Lateral supracondylar crest: humerus	Dorsal surface of metacarpals II and III	All extend carpus and/or digits depending upon insertion
Common digital extensor	Lateral epicondyle of humerus	Distal phalanges of digits II–V	
Lateral digital extensor		Phalanges (mainly distal) of digits III–V	
Extensor carpi ulnaris/Ulnaris lateralis		Lateral surface of digit V and accessory metacarpal	
Supinator		Cranial surface of proximal end of radius	Rotate forearm laterally

Continued

TABLE 16.2 MUSCLES OF THE FORELIMB AND THEIR INNERVATIONS*—cont'd

Name	Origin	Insertion	Function
Caudal and Medial Muscles of Forelimb: all supplied by the median nerve except flexor carpi ulnaris and ulnar head of deep digital flexor, which are supplied by the ulnar nerve			
Pronator teres	All from medial epicondyle of humerus except ulnar heads of flexor carpi ulnaris and deep digital flexor from ulna	Medial border of proximal third of radius	Rotate forearm medially
Flexor carpi radialis		Palmar side of metacarpals II and III	All flex carpus and/or digits depending upon insertion
Flexor carpi ulnaris		Accessory carpal bone	
Superficial digital flexor		Middle phalanges of digits II–V	
Deep digital flexor		Distal phalanges of each digit	

*The information in this table pertains to major muscles of the limbs of the dog. However, the information is broadly true for the horse and the cow as well.

The Hindlimb of the Dog and Cat

17

THE CROUP, HIP, AND THIGH (SEE ALSO PP. 83, 85–87, AND 89.)

The habitual stance varies among breeds. The major differences are well illustrated by the German Shepherd, which tends to crouch with the back and croup sloping down toward the tail (and the hip, stifle, and hock joints markedly flexed), and the Boxer, which favors a stiffer, more upright posture (with the major joints, particularly the hock, significantly straighter). The more upright limb appears to predispose to several common stifle disorders. In the Greyhound and other lean, short-coated dogs, the gluteal muscles such as the superficial gluteal create the croup contour. However, such details are more often obscured by subcutaneous fat or a thick coat. The major skeletal landmarks are always palpable and reveal the small angle the ilium makes with the vertebral column.

The dorsal and ventral spines of the ilium are very prominent and easily palpated. The convex (iliac) crest joining these points can also be followed in its length and provides a convenient site for bone marrow biopsy in larger breeds, but is too thin to serve this purpose in smaller animals. A narrow strip of the pelvic floor bordering the ischial arch can usually be palpated between the salient tubers. In the dog the cordlike sacrotuberous ligaments, which are lacking in cats, can also be palpated. The greater trochanter of the femur is found cranial to the ischial tuber, and because its summit is very nearly level with the femoral head, it provides a good guide to the position of the joint, which is not itself palpable.

The luxation of the femur (coxofemoral) from the acetabulum is due to trauma. The symmetry of the ilium, ischial tuber, and femur may reveal luxation of the femur. This is a relatively frequent mishap with the femoral head most often displaced dorsocranially (which widens the ischiofemoral gap), but it may pass dorsocaudally or, though rarely, ventrocaudally when it engages within the obturator foramen. The ligament of the head of the femur is especially likely to be ruptured or avulsed in full luxation but may survive subluxations. Luxation may be confirmed by rotating the thigh outward while the thumb is pressed between the trochanter and the tuber; the movement normally forces the thumb from the recess, but a luxated femur is unable to exert the necessary leverage.

The hip joint possesses greater range and versatility of movement in the dog and cat than in other domestic species. The enhanced potential for abduction allows dogs to cock their legs when urinating, while the general versatility combined with the suppleness of the trunk enables both species to reach most parts of the head, neck, and thorax with the hindpaw. The articular surfaces reflect these abilities. The femoral head is an almost perfect hemisphere, marred only by the small central fovea where the intracapsular ligament (of the femoral head) inserts. It is deeply seated within the acetabular cup, which is only slightly extended by a labrum about its rim (see Fig. 2.58). There are no peripheral ligaments to limit movement, although some capsule reinforcements can be identified. The intracapsular ligament may be hypertrophied in preexisting dysplasia of the joint. In normal hips, the ligament checks the movements that endanger stability of the hip joint. The joint capsule also maintains the femoral head within the socket and prevents overextension and flexion. The fit of the femoral head within the acetabulum can be estimated from a ventrodorsal radiograph of the pelvis by measuring the Norberg angle, that is, the angle between the line connecting the centers of the femoral heads and that connecting the center of a femoral head with the cranial part of the related acetabular rim. An angle of less than 105 degrees indicates displacement and suggests dysplasia.

The blood supply to the joint capsule, the femoral neck, and the proximal epiphysis arises from an extracapsular ring formed by the lateral and medial circumflex femoral arteries, and the caudal gluteal artery. The branches from the ring ascend the femoral neck and provide the epiphyseal arteries of the femoral head. Arteries demonstrable in the ligament of the femoral head are thought to be of little significance in the dog but make a major contribution to the supply of the femoral head of the kitten. Trauma to the femoral neck often leads to its resorption because of the limited blood supply.

The most convenient access to the joint, for puncture and in surgery, is from the craniolateral direction. An approach between the tensor and biceps muscles exposes the proximal part of the vastus lateralis (whose origin runs from just below the greater trochanter) and the gluteal muscles that clothe the joint directly. The procedure may create a minor danger of damage to the sciatic nerve and the caudal gluteal vessels.

The radiologic anatomy is very relevant to the diagnosis of the two conditions that commonly affect the joint: luxation and dysplasia. For the standard ventrodorsal radiograph (Fig. 17.1A), the supine animal must be placed with its hindlimbs drawn uniformly backward to ensure symmetrical depiction of bilateral structures. Although most features of the pelvis are too obvious to require comment, attention may be drawn to the slight lateral bowing of the canine ilia (in contrast to their parallel course in the cat). The relationship between the rim of the acetabulum and the femoral head on which it is superimposed is of the greatest importance in determining the integrity of the joint (Fig. 17.1/*3*). Attention is also directed to the relative radiolucency of the region (corresponding to the trochanteric fossa) between the greater and lesser trochanters of the femur, because it is sometimes misinterpreted. The less useful lateral view reveals the position of the hip joints below the first two caudal vertebrae (Fig. 17.1D).

A special position, in which the hindlimbs of the supine animal are rotated inward until the femoral trochleae and patellae face directly upward, is used for the better depiction of the contours of the femoral head when hip dysplasia is suspected. In this view it is easier to gauge the congruence of the femoral head with the acetabulum and to recognize any flattening or distortion of its contours. Progressive deformation of the head and worsening of fit characterize the progress of the condition.

The etiology of hip dysplasia, which is very common in certain larger breeds, is uncertain, but hereditary factors may be the primary drivers. It is believed that the dysplasia, which inevitably leads to osteoarthritic changes, is a consequence of the instability permitted by abnormally lax soft articular tissues. The synovitis also may lead to the accumulation of fluid in the joint and reduce the stability of the joint associated with the suction of the thin layer of the synovium between the surfaces of the head of the femur and the acetabulum.

The maturation of the skeleton can be followed in radiographs obtained from young animals. In puppies there are primary ossification centers for the bodies of the ilium, ischium,

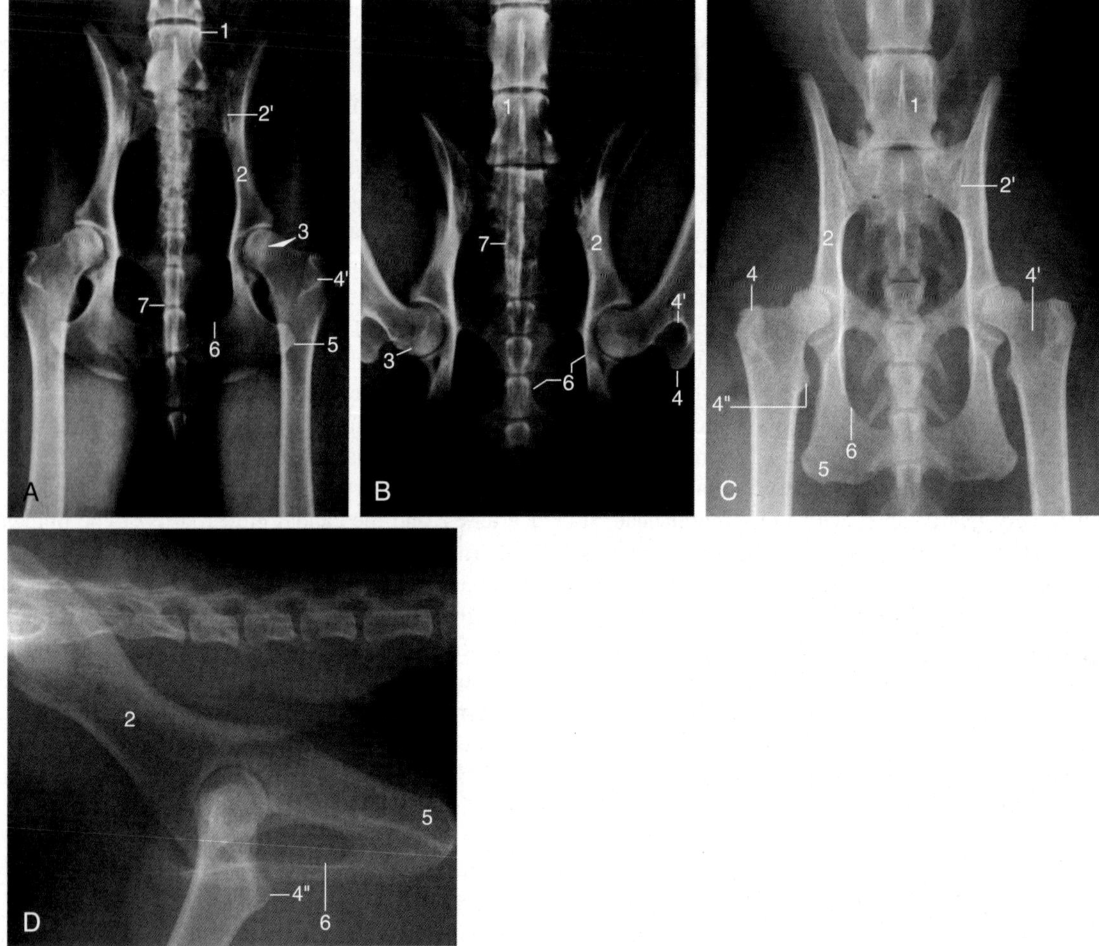

Fig. 17.1 (A) and (B) Ventrodorsal radiographic views of the canine pelvis with (A) extended and (B) flexed hip joints. (C) and (D) Radiographs of the feline pelvis in (C) ventrodorsal and (D) lateral views; D is taken of a specimen. *1,* Last lumbar vertebra (L7); *2,* shaft of ilium; *2′,* sacroiliac joint; *3,* dorsal border of acetabulum superimposed on the femoral head; *4,* greater trochanter; *4′,* trochanteric fossa; *4″,* lesser trochanter; *5,* ischial tuber; *6,* obturator foramen; *7,* os penis superimposed on vertebrae.

and pubis and for the acetabular bone and secondary centers for the iliac crest, ischial tuber, and the border of the ischial arch. The acetabular bone is the first to lose its independence, but this is followed by the merger of the other primary centers at a comparatively early age (4–6 months). The secondary centers remain distinct until much later (15 months to 5 years for the iliac crest and 8–14 months for the ischial tuber). Fusion at the proximal extremity of the femur is completed between the 6th and 12th month (Table 17.1; see Fig. 5.74).

The shaft of the femur is so deeply embedded among the muscles of the thigh that only a general impression of its presence may be obtained on palpation (Fig. 17.2/*9*). Despite this protection, the femur is the most commonly fractured bone, and most breaks occur about or below midshaft level. Such fractures are often complicated by considerable overriding because the lower fragment is commonly displaced caudally by the pull of the gastrocnemius. They are often repaired by intramedullary pinning, a procedure usually requiring direct exposure of the break, which is easily achieved through a lateral approach. The incision of the fascia lata followed by reflection of the biceps, whose cranial margin is often palpable through the skin, exposes the vastus lateralis and opens a path to the bone (Fig. 17.2/*8–10*).

Although the caudal thigh muscles appear to lend themselves to intramuscular injection, they should be avoided for this purpose because of possible damage to the sciatic nerve; a better alternative is injection into the muscles of the back.

The gluteal muscles have been described (Table 17.2). Caudal to these, the cat presents the gluteofemoral, a long and relatively strong muscle that arises from the second to fourth caudal vertebrae and runs caudal to the superficial gluteal muscle and cranial to the biceps to insert lateral to the patella in the fascia lata. It retracts the hindlimb and may also draw the tail to the side. The biceps femoris covers the abductor cruris caudalis, a small, thin muscle strap that emerges over the lateral head of the gastrocnemius in the lower leg.

The most important palpable structure of the thigh is the femoral artery (Fig. 17.2/*2*), which is subcutaneous on the medial aspect of the limb toward the groin. It lies within the femoral triangle, a pyramidal space whose base lies toward the vascular lacuna (the passage to and from the abdomen for the femoral artery and vein) and whose tip is closed distally by the convergence of the sartorius and pectineus muscles that form its cranial and caudal walls. The pectineus muscle forms so obtrusive a fusiform swelling that it immediately guides the fingers to the femoral artery, which is the first choice for taking the pulse. The femoral artery's name changes to the popliteal artery once it reaches

TABLE 17.1 **DEVELOPMENT AND MATURATION OF THE HINDLIMB SKELETON**

Ossification Centers Present at Birth (After Birth)	Approximate Age at Growth Plate Closure Observed on Radiographs	
	Dog	**Cat**[3]
Os coxae (hip bone)		
Ilium	4–6 months[1,2,6]	
Ischium	4–6 months[1,2,6]	
Pubis	4–6 months[1,2,6]	
Acetabular bone (7 weeks)	4–6 months[1,2,6]	
Iliac crest (4 months)	15 months–5.5 years[2]	
Ischial tuber, caudal border of ischium (3 months)	8–11 months[2,6]	
Caudal pelvic symphysis, interischiadic bone (7 months)	15 months–5 years[2,6]	
Pelvic symphysis closure (cranial to caudal)	2.5–6.0 years[2]	
Femur		
Lesser trochanter (8 weeks)	8–13 months[1,2,6]	8–11 months
Greater trochanter (8 weeks)	6–9 months[2,5]	7–10 months
Head (2 weeks)	6–9 months[2,5]	7–10 months
Diaphysis		
Distal epiphysis (3 weeks)	6–12 months[2-5]	13–19 months
Trochlea (3 weeks)	3 months[6]	
Patella (9 weeks)		
Tibia		
Tibial tuberosity (8 weeks)	8–10 months[2,6]	
Proximal epiphysis (3 weeks)	6-15 months[2,5]	12–18 months
Diaphysis		
Distal epiphysis (3 weeks)	5–11 months[2,5]	10–13 months
Medial malleolus (3 months)	4–5 months[2,6]	
Fibula		

Continued

TABLE 17.1 **DEVELOPMENT AND MATURATION OF THE HINDLIMB SKELETON—cont'd**

	Approximate Age at Growth Plate Closure Observed on Radiographs	
Ossification Centers Present at Birth (After Birth)	**Dog**	**Cat[3]**
Proximal epiphysis (9 weeks)	6–12 months[2,6]	13–18 months
Diaphysis		
Distal epiphysis (2–7 weeks)	5–13 months[2-5]	10–14 months
Sesamoids		
Gastrocnemius (3 months in dog; 2.5–4.0 months in cat)		
Popliteus (3 months in dog; 4–5 months in cat)		
Tarsus		
Calcaneus		
Calcanean tuber (6 weeks)	3–8 months[2,4-6]	7–13 months
Diaphysis		
Other tarsal bones (2–4 weeks), 1 center each		
Metatarsus		
Diaphysis		
Distal epiphysis (4 weeks)	5–7 months[2,5]	8–11 months
Digit similar to forelimb		

[1]Based on Chapman WL: Appearance of ossification centers and epiphyseal closures as determined by radiographic techniques, *J Am Vet Med Assoc* 147:138–141, 1965.
[2]Based on Hare WCD: The age at which epiphyseal union takes place in the limb bones of the dog, *Wien Tierärztl Monatsschr* 9:224–245, 1972.
[3]Based on Smith RN: Fusion of ossification centers in the cat, *J Small Anim Pract* 10:523–530, 1969.
[4]Based on Smith RN and Allcock J: Epiphyseal fusion in the Greyhound, *Vet Rec* 72:75–79, 1960.
[5]Based on Sumner-Smith G: Observations on the epiphyseal fusion of the canine appendicular skeleton, *J Small Anim Pract* 7:303–311, 1966.
[6]Based on Ticer JW: Radiographic technique in small animal practice, Philadelphia, 1975, Saunders, p. 101.
From de Lahunta A and Habel RE: Applied veterinary anatomy, Philadelphia, 1986, Saunders.

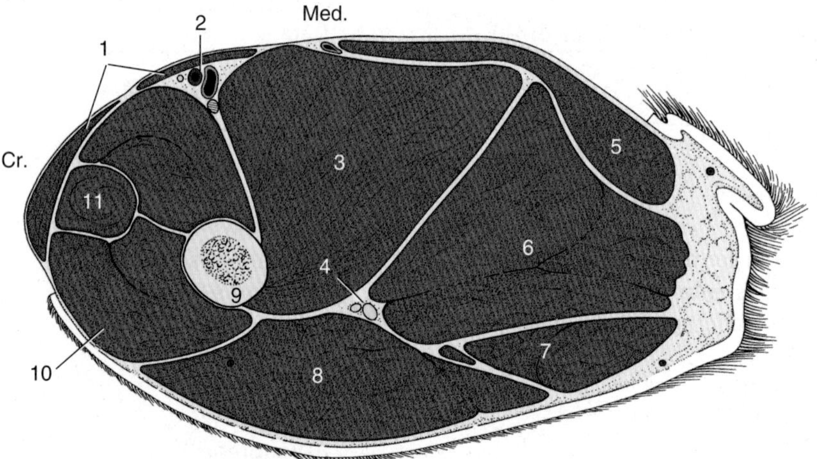

Fig. 17.2 Transverse section of the canine left thigh. *Cr.*, Cranial; *Med.*, medial. *1*, Sartorius; *2*, femoral vessels; *3*, adductor; *4*, sciatic nerve; *5*, gracilis; *6*, semimembranosus; *7*, semitendinosus; *8*, biceps; *9*, femur; *10*, vastus lateralis (of quadriceps); *11*, rectus femoris.

the popliteal fossa on the medial aspect of the femur (Fig. 17.3/*1* and *2*). The femoral vein is less conspicuous but is easily found along the caudal border of the artery and is convenient for intravenous injection in the supine, anesthetized subject. The saphenous artery (Fig. 17.3/*4*) branches from the concealed part of the femoral artery but soon becomes subcutaneous and runs over the medial aspect of the thigh toward the stifle. Both it and a large, more proximal branch (running caudally toward the gracilis) may be palpated.

Unlike the larger species, the dog and cat have no subiliac lymph nodes. However, the popliteal lymph node is usually palpable within the popliteal fossa, between the distal parts of the biceps and semitendinosus as they diverge toward their insertions at the stifle (Figs. 17.4/*10* and 17.5/*6*).

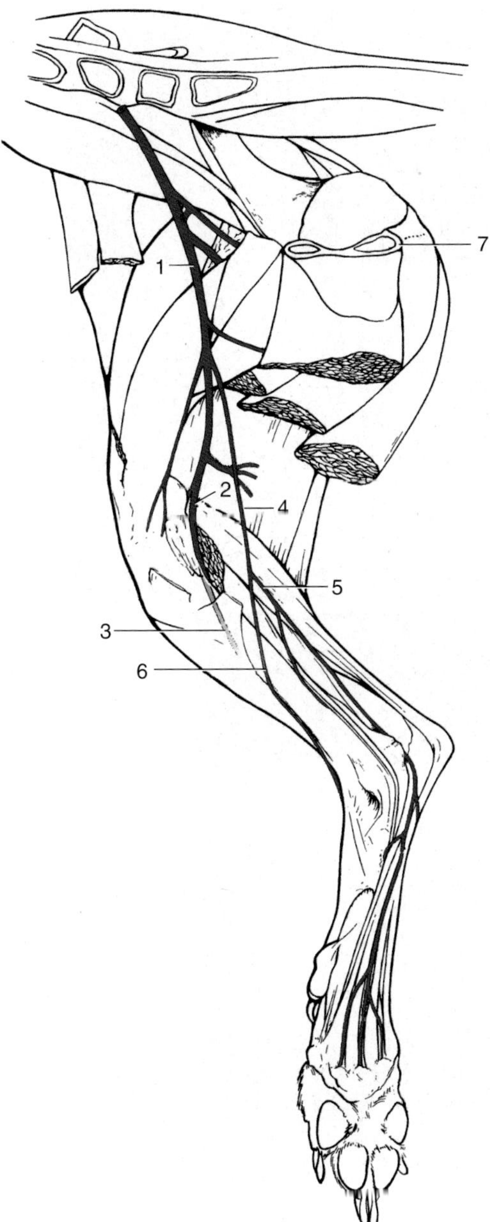

Fig. 17.3 The principal arteries of the canine right hindlimb, medial view. *1,* Femoral artery (a.); *2,* popliteal a.; *3,* cranial tibial a. passing between tibia and fibula; *4,* saphenous a.; *5* and *6,* caudal and cranial branches of saphenous a.; *7,* pelvic floor.

THE STIFLE JOINT AND LEG (SEE ALSO PP. 83–85 AND 89–90.)

The stifle joint is flexed in the standing posture. Although it is more fully extended in certain phases of locomotion, the femur and tibia are never brought into line, and the caudal angle of the joint does not open beyond 150 degrees or so in dogs; considerably greater extension is permitted in the cat. Some lateral or medial angulation of the joint may often be observed when the limb is viewed from the front or behind. In the "bowlegged" version common in certain toy breeds, the pull of the quadriceps does not coincide with the axis of the femoral trochlea and there is a tendency to medial luxation of the patella. The luxation, which may be intermittent or permanent, causes the limb to be carried and, if left uncorrected, leads to deformity of other parts. The trochlea can be brought into alignment with the axis of the tibia by translation of the tibial tuberosity. The same procedure can be used to correct any medial or lateral patellar luxation, whatever its origin.

Palpation of the stifle joint reveals the following features of the skeleton: the patella; the ridges of the trochlea and the outer surfaces of the condyles of the femur; the sesamoid bones within the origin of the gastrocnemius; the head of the fibula; the edge of the lateral condyle adjacent to the fibula; the tuberosity; the extensor groove; and the medial surface of the tibia. The single patellar ligament and the medial and lateral collateral ligaments may also be distinguished; however, the femoropatellar ligaments cannot be distinguished because they are overlain by the aponeuroses of the sartorius and semimembranosus on the medial side and by that of the biceps laterally.

The most distinctive internal feature of the joint is the free communication of the various synovial compartments, which ensures that a single injection will reach all parts of the cavity. The most convenient entry is from the lateral side, caudal to the thick pad of fat interposed between the patellar ligament (and adjoining retinaculum) and the synovial membrane. The lateral femorotibial joint has two pouches: one is under the tendon of the long digital extensor muscle at its origin from the extensor fossa, and the other invests the tendon of origin of the popliteal muscle, which contains a sesamoid bone close to the lateral tibial condyle.

The *cruciate ligaments* are set well back (see Fig. 2.63/*15* and *16*) and assist the collateral ligaments in opposing rotation and medial or lateral deviation of the leg; they are most susceptible to injury when tautened. The cranial cruciate ligament, named for the relative position of its tibial attachment (see Fig. 2.63/*16*), is therefore at greatest risk during overextension of the joint, and its rupture allows abnormally free forward displacement of the tibia in relation to the femur (the "cranial drawer" sign). A short cranial drawer movement (1–3 mm) brought to an abrupt stop is normal in young dogs. A deterioration in the strength of this ligament is correlated with age and is due to fiber bundle disruption and metaplastic cellular changes; the central part of the ligament is most affected. The changes are more pronounced and appear at earlier ages in larger dogs.

Cruciate Ligaments: The cruciate ligaments also have nerve endings and receptors for sensing mechanical forces. These nerves and receptors provide proprioceptive feedbacks to check the abnormal or excessive flexion or extension of the joint. Rupture of the cruciate ligaments is common in older dogs, and that may suggest an underlying degenerative process. Of course, mechanical trauma also is a major cause of rupture of the cruciate ligaments.

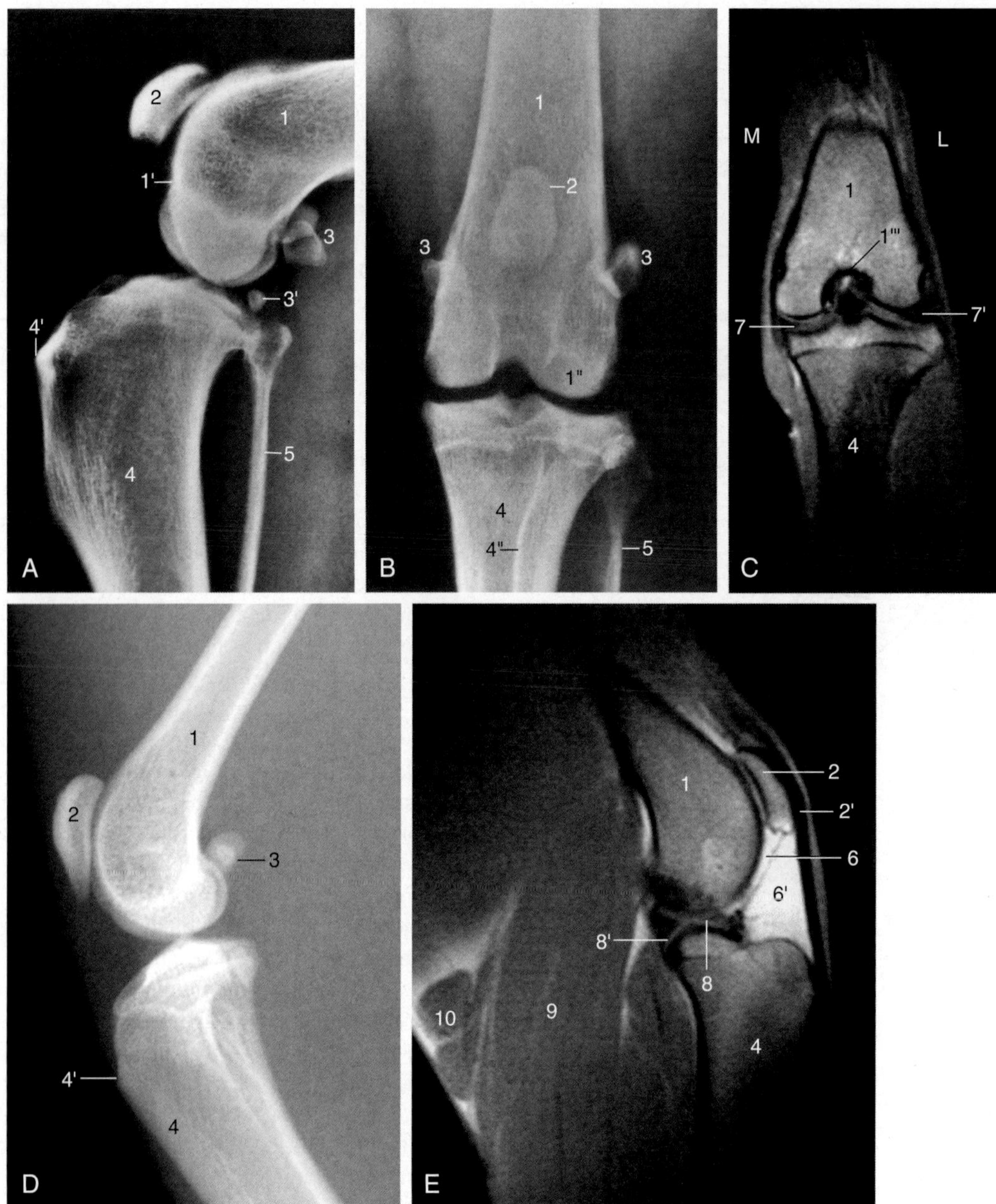

Fig. 17.4 (A) Lateral and (B) craniocaudal radiographic views of canine stifles. (D) Lateral radiographic view of feline stifles. (C) Frontal (*M*, medial; *L*, lateral) and (E) axial 4-mm-thick T1-weighted spin-echo magnetic resonance slices of the left canine stifle. *1,* Femur; *1′,* extensor fossa; *1″,* lateral condyle; *1‴,* intercondylar fossa; *2,* patella; *2′,* patellar ligament; *3,* sesamoid bones in gastrocnemius; *3′,* popliteal sesamoid bone; *4,* tibia; *4′,* tibial tuberosity; *4″,* tibial crest; *5,* fibula; *6,* femoropatellar joint cavity; *6′,* infrapatellar fat; *7* and *7′,* medial and lateral menisci, respectively; *8* and *8′,* cranial and caudal cruciate ligaments, respectively; *9,* gastrocnemius; *10,* popliteal lymph nodes.

The caudal cruciate ligament is at greatest risk in the flexed position of the joint, and its rupture allows excessive caudal displacement of the tibia (the "caudal drawer" sign). Various surgical techniques for the restoration or replacement of the cranial and caudal ligaments use fascial or artificial substitutes. The lateral collateral ligament can be used as a substitute for the cranial cruciate ligament after transposition of the head of the fibula cranially.

The *menisci*, joined cranially (also caudally, in the cat) by an intermeniscal ligament, provide additional restraints and are also prone to injury. They are most vulnerable when torsion is imposed on a limb in which the stifle is extended and the foot fixed—a combination of circumstances found

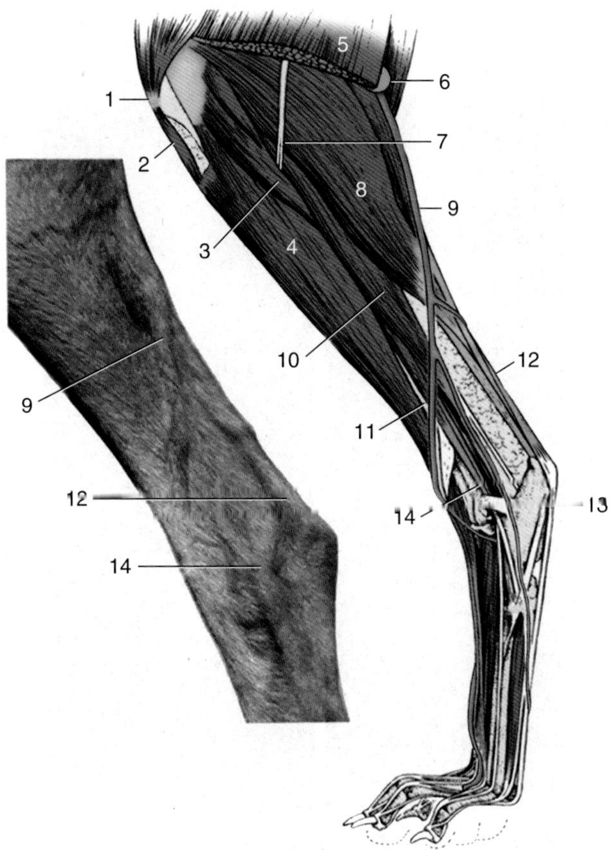

Fig. 17.5 Left canine hindlimb; the *inset* shows the actual appearance of the lateral saphenous vein *(9);* lateral view. *1,* Patella; *2,* patellar ligament; *3,* peroneus longus; *4,* tibialis cranialis; *5,* biceps femoris; *6,* popliteal lymph node; *7,* common peroneal nerve; *8,* lateral head of gastrocnemius; *9,* lateral saphenous vein; *10,* deep digital flexor; *11,* superficial peroneal nerve; *12,* calcanean tendon; *13,* calcaneus; *14,* peroneus longus tendon.

when an abrupt change in direction is attempted by a dog traveling at speed. Most often a meniscal tear is found in combination with a rupture of the cranial cruciate ligament. The meniscal horns are more richly supplied with blood vessels and nerves in comparison with the more central parts. The involved portion, or sometimes the whole meniscus, is often removed after injury; an imperfect replacement may ultimately be formed from granulation tissue produced by the capsule at the site of the original attachment. The medial meniscus has an additional restraint imposed by a connection with the medial femorotibial ligament by way of the joint capsule. This may limit the range of its excursions compared with those of the lateral meniscus and may thus be a factor in determining the incidence of injuries.

Both lateral and craniocaudal radiographic projections are commonly used in the diagnosis of stifle injuries (Fig. 17.4). In the craniocaudal view the patella is superimposed on the distal end of the femur, where it is flanked by the ridges of the trochlea, which appear as thin radiodense lines. The tibial condyles are relatively flat because they are not separated by the conspicuous intercondyloid tubercles found in the larger species. The head of the fibula falls short of the extremity of the tibia. In the lateral view the femoral and tibial condyles are seen to have only limited, rather caudal contact and the joint appears unstable because the menisci that maintain its congruence are not revealed. The patellar ligament, the most prominent soft tissue shadow, runs at some distance from the femur, and the space behind it is occupied by the infrapatellar fat cushion. Displacement of this fat may be evident in radiographs and may suggest either thickening of the capsule or effusion into the joint cavity. The same view best depicts the associated sesamoid bones. The pair within the heads of the gastrocnemius are large and well defined (Fig. 17.4/*3*). They articulate with small facets on the upper parts of the corresponding femoral condyles. The sesamoid within the popliteus tendon is smaller, less sharply outlined, and occasionally duplicated; it is related to the margin of the tibia (Fig. 17.4/*3′*). A relatively radiolucent area between the trochlea and lateral femoral condyle indicates the position of the extensor fossa (Fig. 17.4/*1′*) and has occasionally been mistaken for an osteolytic lesion.

In dogs, both the distal femoral and proximal tibial epiphyses generally fuse with their respective shafts between the 6th and 12th months. The wide and irregular cartilage line between the center for the tibial tuberosity and the shaft, which fuse between the 8th and 10th months, simulates avulsion of the tuberosity. The onset and completion of these fusions are somewhat delayed in cats.

Few features of the leg require further comment. The subcutaneous surface of the tibia divides the cranial and caudal crural muscles medially, while the fibula makes the same division laterally (Fig. 17.6). In lean dogs the fibula may be palpated along its length, but in fatter and particularly well-muscled animals only the head and the distal half of the shaft may be felt with certainty. The superficial flexor and gastrocnemius components of the common calcanean tendon may be identified separately, distal to the belly of the latter. The *lateral saphenous vein* is a very conspicuous surface feature of the lateral aspect (Fig. 17.5/*9*). It runs proximocaudally over the lower part of the leg before following the gastrocnemius on the caudal border to join the femoral vein within the popliteal fossa. The proximal part of the vein is relatively fixed and straight, making it more suitable for intravenous injections. The distal part undulates, dipping between the caudal crural muscles and the common calcanean tendon.

The vascularization of the leg and more distal parts depends on the cranial tibial and saphenous arteries because the caudal tibial artery is quite insignificant (Fig. 17.3/*3* and *4*). The cranial tibial artery continues the popliteal artery, which runs deep to the popliteal muscle on the caudal aspect of the stifle. The artery then passes between the tibia and fibula in the proximal part of the leg before penetrating

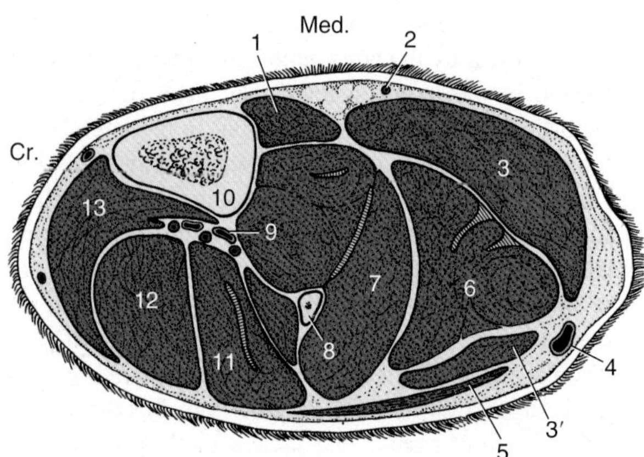

Fig. 17.6 Transverse section of the canine left leg. *Cr.*, Cranial; *Med.*, medial. *1*, Popliteus; *2*, saphenous artery; *3* and *3′*, medial and lateral heads of the gastrocnemius, respectively; *4*, lateral saphenous vein; *5*, biceps femoris; *6*, superficial digital flexor; *7*, deep digital flexor; *8*, fibula; *9*, cranial tibial vessels; *10*, tibia; *11*, peroneus longus; *12*, long digital extensor; *13*, tibialis cranialis.

the dorsal muscles. It reappears toward the hock and then follows the long extensor tendon across the joint into the paw. The saphenous artery, which broadly serves the territory assigned to the caudal tibial artery in many species, crosses the medial aspect of the stifle before dividing into cranial and caudal branches. The cranial branch (Fig. 17.3/*6*) remains superficial and continues into the paw, where it supplements the cranial tibial artery in supplying dorsal structures; the caudal branch (Fig. 17.3/*5*) accompanies the tibial nerve and, after supplying caudal crural muscles, follows the flexor tendons into the plantar aspect of the paw.

THE HOCK AND HINDPAW (SEE ALSO PP. 85, 89–90.)

Inspection of the distal part of the limb reveals the distinctive conformation of the hock; when it is taken apart, there is little external difference between the forepaws and hindpaws beyond the absence of any analogue of the carpal pad. A dewclaw is commonly present at birth in dogs but is routinely removed at an early age in puppies of many breeds. Duplication of this digit is known to occur in the French Shepherd breeds. Dewclaws of the hindlimb are not found in cats.

Although the hock skeleton is complete—there is no suppression or fusion of the standard elements—most bones cannot be individually identified on palpation. The most distinctive feature is the long, rather slender *calcaneus*, which provides the leverage for the effective extension of the hock. The bone is occasionally fractured by the force exerted by the powerful muscles attaching to its slightly swollen tip. The calcaneus extends a medial process, the *sustentaculum tali*, over the plantar aspect of the talus, where it may be felt despite being covered by the

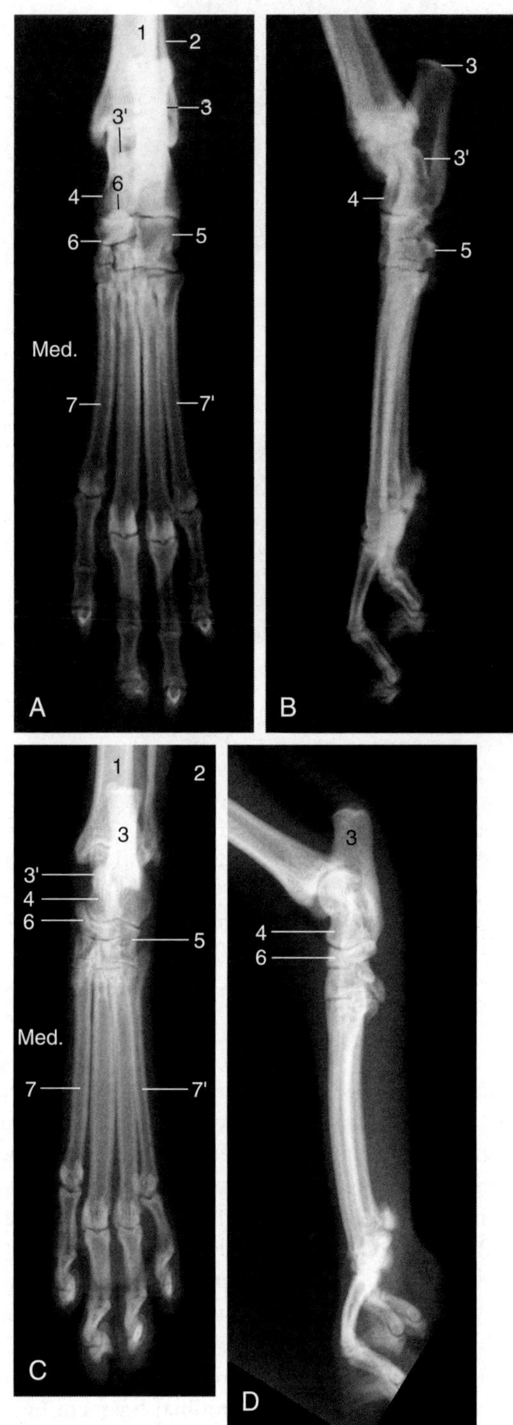

Fig. 17.7 (A) Dorsoplantar (*Med.*, medial) and (B) lateral radiographic views of the canine hocks and hindpaws. (C) Dorsoplantar (*Med.*, medial) and (D) lateral radiographic views of the feline hocks and hindpaws. *1*, Tibia; *2*, fibula; *3*, calcaneus; *3′*, sustentaculum tali; *4*, talus; *5*, fourth tarsal bone; *6*, central tarsal bone; *7* and *7′*, second and fifth metatarsal bones, respectively.

deep flexor tendon (Fig. 17.7/*3'*). The more distal tarsal bones lack identifying surface features, but their locations and extents may be deduced after reference to a skeleton or to radiographs. The other prominent surface features of the region are the projections of the tibial and fibular malleoli at the lower limit of the leg and the equally prominent swellings at the proximal ends of the second and fifth metatarsal bones. A long collateral ligament may be traced from the malleolar to the metatarsal thickening on each side of the limb. The extensor tendons can be followed over the dorsal surface of the hock; the retinacula that hold them in place over the distal tibia and again at the proximal end of the metatarsus can also be appreciated in many dogs.

Only the tarsocrural joint is large enough to be punctured in the live animal. This is done on the lateral side just distal to the malleolus; the needle is directed distally toward the lateral surface of the palpable lateral trochlear ridge of the talus.

Similar impressions of the bones and soft structures are obtained on palpation of the hindpaw as on palpation of the forepaw.

Although a complete *radiographic examination* of the hock calls for exposures in dorsoplantar, mediolateral, and oblique projections, the most useful general picture is obtained from the dorsoplantar view because it permits identification of all the bones, of which some are more easily identified than others because there is considerable superimposition (Fig. 17.7A). Both the talus and the calcaneus are well outlined despite the overlap of the sustentaculum tali. The two bones in the subjacent tier, the fourth and central tarsals (Fig. 17.7/*5* and *6*), are also generally well outlined, although the mediodistal part of the fourth is superimposed on the third. The second tarsal is clearly shown with the smaller first tarsal superimposed on it. The distal extremities of the tibia and fibula appear closely related in this projection; the gap between them is unexpectedly wide in slightly oblique projections obtained of the cat's hock and is a feature that is occasionally misinterpreted as evidence of luxation.

The lateral projection (Fig. 17.7B) depicts the calcaneus and talus clearly, although they overlap toward the center of the field. The more distal bones are less easily identified in this view, apart from the fourth tarsal bone, which is betrayed by a protuberance on its plantar aspect (Fig. 17.8/*4'*). Because the central tarsal bone is occasionally dislocated, it is important to note the normal alignment of the dorsal borders of the bones of successive tiers. Two previously unrecorded sesamoid bones have recently been described in the Greyhound at the plantar aspect of the hock about the level of the tarsometatarsal joint. Similar to other sesamoids, these can potentially be misinterpreted as chips fractured from the major bones.

There are no distinctive features of the radiological anatomy of the metatarsal bones and phalanges. The short digital muscles are comparable with those in the front limb.

THE MAJOR NERVES OF THE HINDLIMB

It is only necessary to deal briefly with the course, relations, and distribution of those nerves that extend substantially into the free limb because a general account of the lumbosacral plexus (usually formed by the nerves L4–S2) and its divisions has been presented (pp. 311-313) (Fig. 17.9 and Table 17.2).

The *femoral nerve* (L4–L6) has a very short course within the thigh before it ends by ramifying within the quadriceps femoris, the principal extensor of the stifle and an ancillary flexor of the hip. Shortly before disappearing into this muscle, it detaches the saphenous nerve, which descends subcutaneously over the medial aspect of the limb accompanied by the palpable saphenous artery. Although the *saphenous nerve* supplies the sartorius, it is largely sensory, serving the skin of the medial surface of the thigh, stifle, leg, and hock (Fig. 17.10). Dysfunction of the femoral nerve *paralyzes the quadriceps,* resulting in the collapse of the stifle and disabling the entire limb. Compensation is not available. The skin of the medial surface of the limb is deprived of sensation.

The *sciatic nerve* (L6–S1) crosses the dorsal border of the hip bone to enter the limb together with the caudal gluteal vessels. After passing the dorsocaudal aspect of the hip joint deep to the greater trochanter, where it is susceptible to injury in trauma or surgery of the joint, the nerve and accompanying vessels supply branches to the hamstring muscles. The nerve then continues distally in a central position within the thigh, caudal to the femur and cushioned between the biceps laterally, the adductor, and later the semimembranosus medially (Fig. 17.2/*4*). At a rather variable point it divides into the common peroneal and tibial nerves that continue the course of the parent trunk until they diverge caudal to the stifle. The sciatic nerve and its peroneal and tibial branches collectively supply the skin of the entire limb distal to the stifle with the exception of the medial strip claimed by the saphenous nerve.

The *common peroneal nerve,* the more lateral of the terminal divisions of the sciatic nerve, can be palpated in lean dogs where it passes over the lateral head of the gastrocnemius (Fig. 17.5/*7*). It then dives deeply among the dorsal crural muscles (the extensors of the digits and flexors of the hock), which it supplies. It is continued by superficial and deep (peroneal) branches that enter the paw over the dorsal aspect of the hock; they supply the skin of the dorsal surface. *Paralysis of the common peroneal nerve produces slight overextension of the hock and inability to extend the digits,* which may be rested on their dorsal surfaces. In time, affected dogs learn to flick their paws forward before putting them down, enabling their limbs to support weight. The dorsal surface of the paw is without sensation.

The *tibial nerve* passes between the two heads of the gastrocnemius, where it detaches branches to the muscles behind the tibia (the flexors of the digits and extensors of

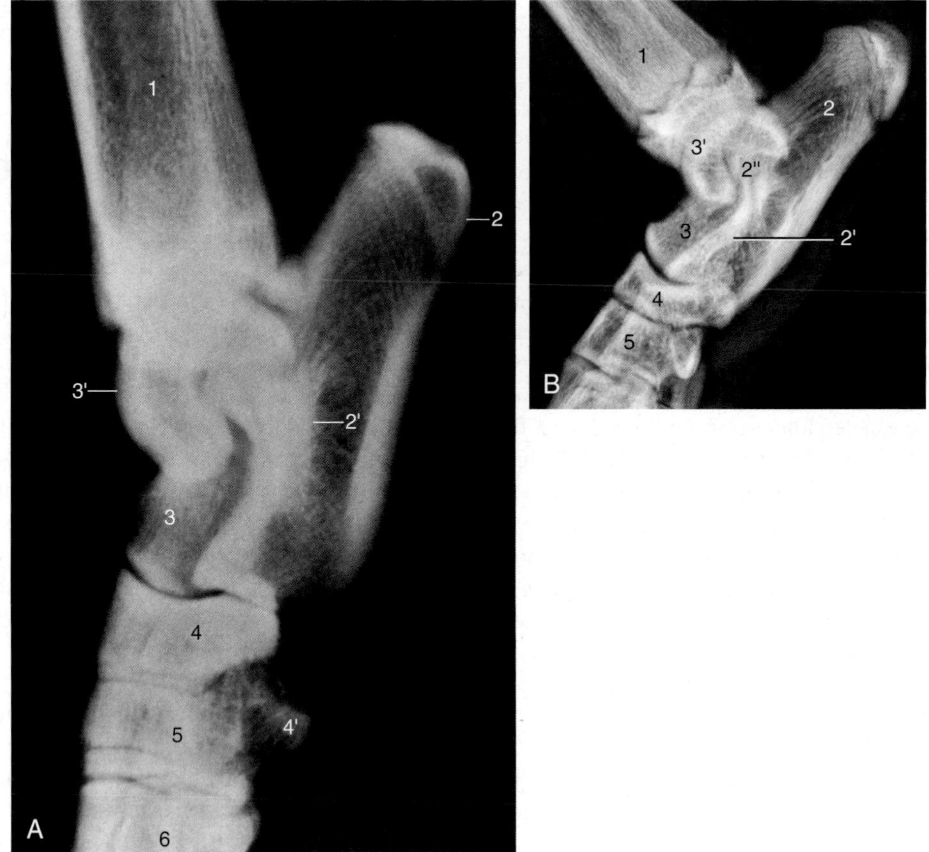

Fig. 17.8 Lateral radiographic views of the (A) canine and (B) young feline hocks. *1,* Tibia and fibula; *2,* calcaneus; *2′,* sustentaculum tali; *2″,* coracoid process; *3,* talus; *3′,* trochlea of talus; *4,* superimposed fourth and central tarsal bones; *4′,* plantar tubercle on fourth tarsal bone; *5,* distal row of tarsal bones; *6,* metatarsal bones.

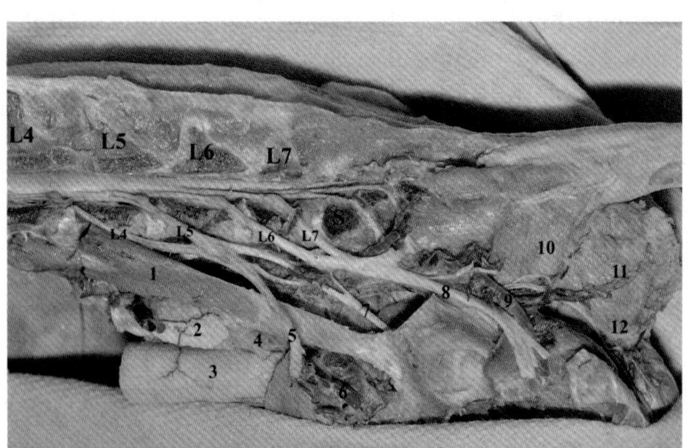

Fig. 17.9 Lumbal plexus. The lumbar vertebral arches and the iliopsoas muscle have been removed. 1. Psoas minor muscle. 2. Medial iliac lymph node. 3. Rectum. 4. External iliac artery. 5. Femoral nerve (Iliopsoas muscle removed). 6. Femoral artery. 7. Obturator nerve. 8. Ischiatic nerve. 9. Caudal gluteal artery and vein. 10. Coccygeus muscle. 11. Caudal rectal artery and vein on the external anal sphincter muscle. 12. Superficial perineal nerve

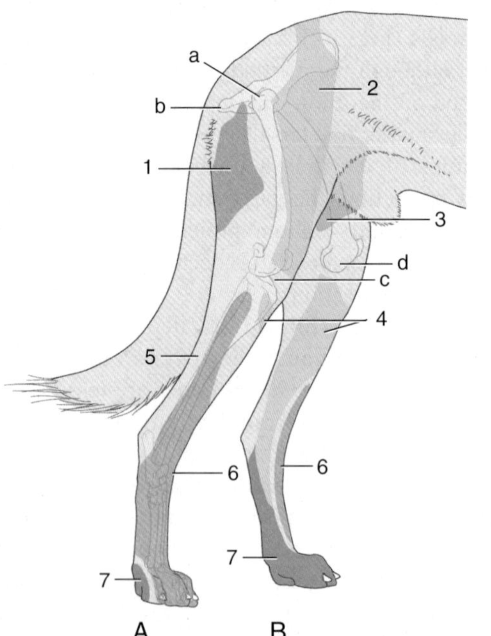

Fig. 17.10 Autonomous zones of the cutaneous innervation on the lateral (A) and medial (B) surfaces of the canine hindlimb. 1, Caudal cutaneous femoral nerve (purple); 2, lateral cutaneous femoral nerve (green); 3, genitofemoral nerve (teal); 4, saphenous nerve (blue); 5, sciatic nerve (yellow); 6, pero-neal nerve (orange); 7, tibial nerve (red). a, Position of greater trochanter; b, ischial tuber; c, lat-eral tibial condyle; d, medial tibial condyle.

the hock). The depleted nerve, now largely sensory but retaining a small motor component for the intrinsic muscles of the paw, continues distally within the web of skin between the caudal crural muscles and the common calcanean tendon. It crosses the hock beside the deep flexor tendon before branching to supply the plantar structures of the paw. *Tibial nerve injuries cause the hock to be flexed and lowered closer to the ground when the limb bears weight.* The paralysis of the digital flexors elevates the toes; their plantar aspect is without sensation.

COMPREHENSION CHECK

Describe the anatomy of the hip joint and the anatomic structures that prevent its luxation. Use the cadaver to practice the most efficient surgical approach to the hip joint.

Reviewing the nerve supply to the hindlimb of the dog, describe the impact of dysfunction of each nerve on the stability and locomotion of the limb along with any compensatory mechanisms.

TABLE 17.2

Name	Origin	Insertion	Function
Caudal Muscles of the Thigh and the Hip: all supplied by Sciatic nerve except * by the obturator nerve			
Biceps femoris	All from the ischiatic tuberosity BF has additional origin from sacrotuberous ligament	Patella, Tibia	All extend the hip BF and ST extend hock BF extends stifle while ST flexes the stifle
Semitendinosus		Medial side of tibia	
Semimebranosus		Medial side of femur Prox end of tibia	
Internal obturator	Dorsal pelvic symphysis	Tronchanteric fossa	Rotate the pelvic limb laterally
Gemelli	Ischium caudal to acetabulum		
Quadratus femoris	Caudal ventral ischium		
*External obturator	Ventral pelvic symphysis		
Medial Muscles of theThigh: All supplied by Obturator except * by the femoral nerve			
Gracilis	Pelvic symphysis	Cranial side of tibia	Adduct the limb
Pectineus	Cranial pubic ligament	Medial surface of femur	
Adductor	Pelvic symphysis	Caudal medial of femur	
*Sartorius	Cranial part: crest of Ilium Caudal part: Ilium	Patella Cranial side of tibia	Flex hip; cranial: extend stifle Caudal: flex stifle
Lateral Muscles of the Rump: all supplied by Cranial Gluteal nerve except * by the caudal gluteal nerve			
*Superficial Gluteal	Sarcum and Cranial Iliac Spine	3rd Trochanter	Extend and abduct the hip
Middle Gluteal	Crest of ilium	Greater Tronchanter	
Deep Gluteal	Body of ilium and ischiatic spine		
Quadriceps femoris: All heads from proximal femur and extend stifle except Rectus femoris from ilium which flexes hip. *Femoral nerve.* **Psoas major and Iliacus** insert at lesser tronchanter; Flexes hip; *Femoral nerve*			
Craniolateral Muscles of the Leg: all supplied by the peroneal nerve			
Cranial tibial	Lateral condyle of tibia	Plantar surface of metatarsal I-II	All flex tarsus plus LDE extending digits; Cranial tibial rotates paw laterally Peron longus rotates paw medially
Long digital extensor	Extensor fossa of femur	Distal phalanges of II-V digits	
Peroneus longus	Lateral condyle of tibia	4th tarsal + plantar of meta-tarsals	
Caudal Muscles of the Leg: all supplied by the tibia nerve			
Gastrocnemius	Medial & lat supracondylar tuberosities of femur	Tuber calcanei	Extend tarsus; flex stifle
Superficial digital flexor	Lat supracondylar tub:femur	Tuber calcanei and middle phalanges of II-V digits	Extend tarsus; flex digits
Deep digital flexor	Tibia and fibula; proximal caudo-lateral	Distal phalanges	
Popliteus	Lateral condyle of femur	Prox caudal border of tibia	Rotate leg medially
Arteries: Internal and external iliacs; deep femoral; femoral-popliteal-cranial tibial; saphenous; **Veins:** Medial and lateral saphneous; cranial tibial; femoral			

Part III

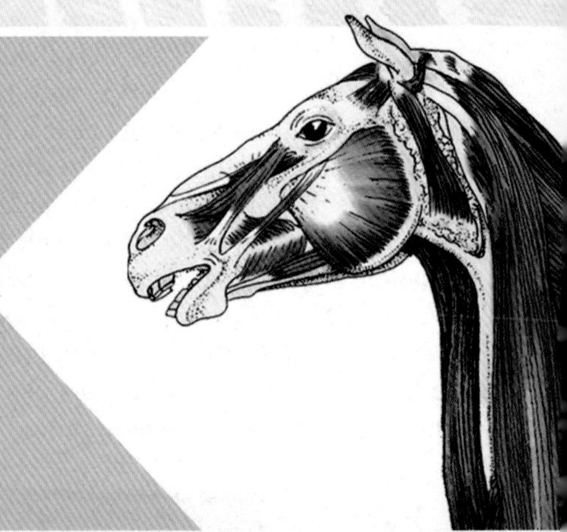

Horses

18 The Head and Ventral Neck of the Horse

CONFORMATION AND EXTERNAL FEATURES

The age, the sex, and the breed of a horse influence the morphology of the head. The cranial vault of the skull in young foals is shaped to accommodate the brain and projects above the face (Fig. 18.1). The age-related changes in complement of teeth and expansion of paranasal sinuses alter the conformation of the skull, including lengthening of the face. The enlargement of the frontal sinus smoothes the dorsal profile at the junction of the face and cranium. A longer face is a characteristic of the adult compared with the juvenile, the stallion with the mare, and the heavy draft horse with the pony. The other very obvious breed difference concerns the dorsal profile; a relatively straight profile is generally preferred but some convexity ("ram's head") is characteristic of certain heavy breeds, whereas concavity ("dishing") is the rule in Arabians and common in horses with admixture of Arabian blood (Fig. 18.1). As part of the normal developmental process, sometimes the root of an unerupted permanent cheek tooth may create rounded swellings on the ventral margin of the lower jaw (p. 505).

The skin of the face is thinner and more firmly bound down than that over most other parts of the body and is especially tight where it lies directly on bone. The coat is generally short, but a forelock continuing the mane may be prominent; a "mustache" is a feature of some animals, especially the larger breeds. Tactile hairs are numerous and widely scattered on the lips and chin and about the margins of the nostrils.

The *nostrils* are large and widely spaced, especially in the Thoroughbred (Fig. 18.2), which is largely due to the supporting alar cartilages (Fig. 18.3B/*1′* and *2′*). The upper part of the opening leads to a blind nasal diverticulum (Fig. 18.3/*1″*) that occupies the nasoincisive notch (Fig. 18.3/*6*) and is without counterpart in other domestic species.* The lower part leads directly to the nasal cavity and provides a passage for the stomach tube. The flexibility of the margins of the nostrils allows them to dilate during strenuous breathing or clinical procedures. The dilated nostril is rounded, and the change in form is achieved by apposition of the walls of the diverticulum. The pliancy of the tissues facilitates examination of the nasal vestibule and exposure

* The barbaric custom of splitting the lateral wall of this diverticulum is known from pharaonic times and may still be encountered in the Middle East. It is of course completely without the intended effect on the efficiency of respiration. However, vigorous inspiration may induce some inward movement of the wall of the nasal passage where it is unsupported by bone, with an adverse effect on respiratory efficiency and therefore performance. To counteract this, an adhesive strip designed to be fixed across the nose a few centimeters above the nostrils is now marketed. It is claimed that when fitted to horses required to race or undergo other especially strenuous tasks, it significantly improves performance and reduces the severity of exercise-induced pulmonary hemorrhage. Corresponding benefits were previously reported of the use of a similar device by human athletes.

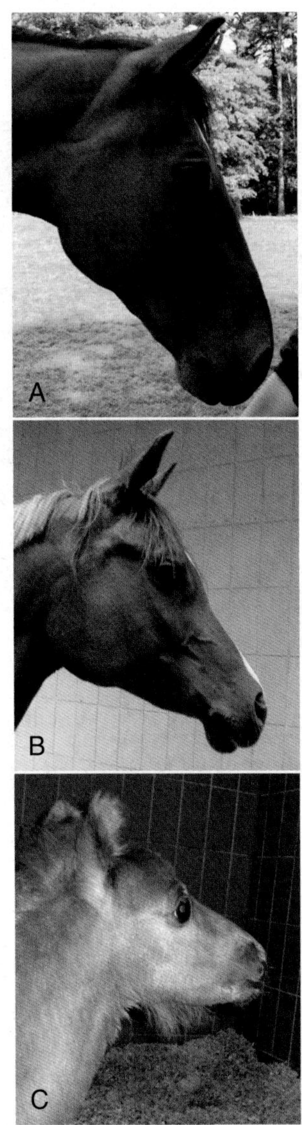

Fig. 18.1 Variations in the profile of the equine head. (A) The common straight profile. (B) The dished Arabian profile. (C) The domed contour of the foal.

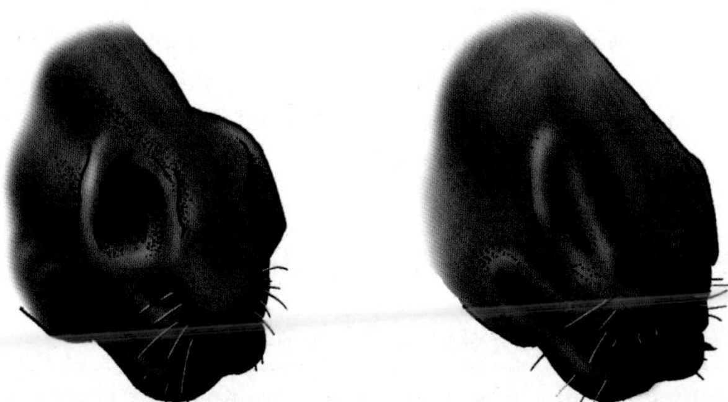

Fig. 18.2 Functional variations in the form of the nostril.

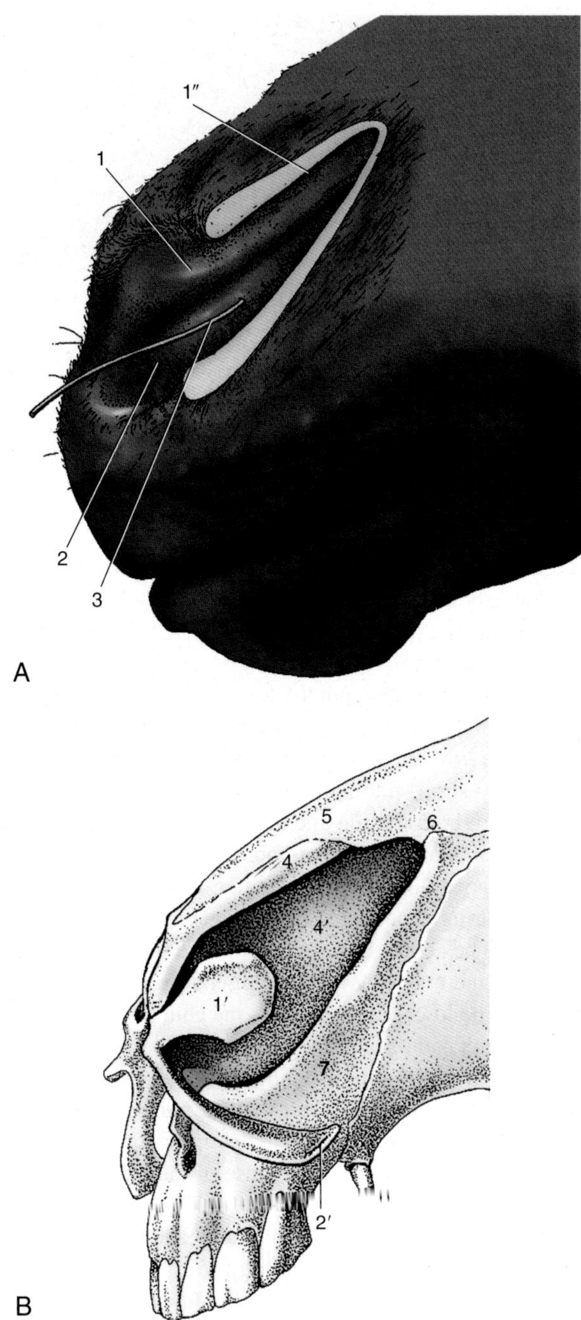

Fig. 18.3 (A) Left nostril opened laterally to expose nasal diverticulum. (B) Nasal cartilages. *1,* Alar fold, supported by the lamina *(1′)* of the alar cartilage; dorsal to the alar fold is the nasal diverticulum *(1″)*; *2,* floor of nostril supported by the cornu of the alar cartilage *(2′)*—the floor leads into the nasal cavity; *3,* probe in nasolacrimal duct; *4,* dorsal lateral nasal cartilage; *4′,* nasal septum; *5,* nasal bone; *6,* nasoincisive notch; *7,* incisive bone; *8,* canine tooth.

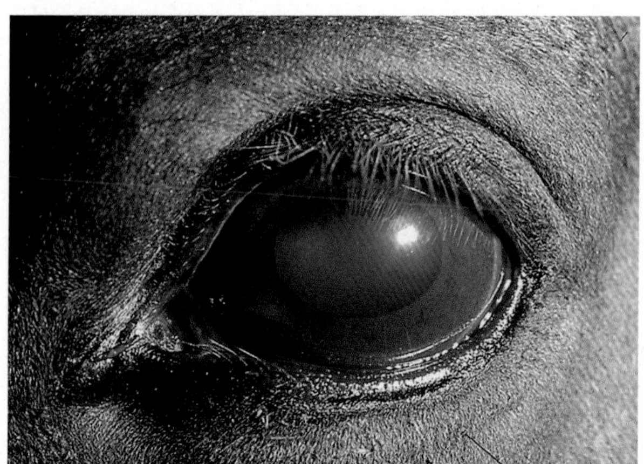

Fig. 18.4 Left equine eye; note implantation of eyelashes on lateral side of upper eyelid.

of the opening of the *nasolacrimal duct,* which is found on the floor about 5 cm internal to the entrance and near the mucocutaneous junction. Occasionally the duct has more than one opening.

The entrance to the mouth is small, and the commissure is a short distance in front of the first cheek teeth (P2). The skin of the *lips* and adjacent part of the muzzle is sparsely covered by short, fine hairs that impart a velvety texture. The lips are both mobile and sensitive and are used in the selection and prehension of food. The sensitivity of the upper lip is exploited when a twitch is applied to control a horse during procedures (e.g., injections) elsewhere on the body. The acupressure created by the twitch lowers the heart rate and may cause release of endorphins that diminish pain. The lower lip surmounts the chin swelling, which is based on a pad of fatty fibrous tissue.

The *eyes* are prominent and placed to each side of the head, providing the horse with a panoramic field of vision. This ability to survey widely—perhaps through 330 degrees—is obtained at the expense of the binocular field, which is limited to some 65 degrees. The field of overlap is further reduced by the length and shape of the muzzle, which creates a blind area directly to the front (see Fig. 9.1).

The upper and lower *eyelids* and adjacent skin carry a few scattered tactile hairs. The palpebral skin is thin and, being loosely attached, is thrown into folds when the eye is open. The lid margins carry numerous lashes, longer and more prominent on the upper than on the lower lid (Fig. 18.4). The *tarsal glands,* which open at the junction of the skin with the conjunctiva, number about 50 in the upper lid and rather fewer below and are clearly visible in palisade formation when the lids are everted. The palpebral conjunctiva is well vascularized, the bulbar part less generously. The bulbar conjunctiva is strongly pigmented toward the corneoscleral region. The third eyelid (Fig. 18.5/*1*) in the medial angle can be exposed in the usual way by pressing on the eyeball through the upper eyelid; a small accessory

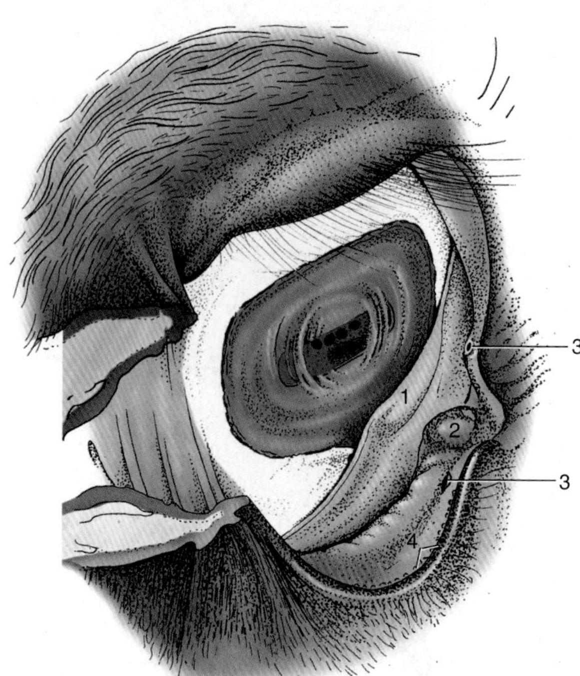

Fig. 18.5 The right conjunctival sac. *1,* Third eyelid; *2,* lacrimal caruncle; *3,* lacrimal puncta; *4,* openings of the tarsal glands.

lacrimal gland is associated with it. The lacrimal caruncle is prominent. The features of the eyeball are considered later (p. 516).

A depression caudal to the eye (behind the palpable postorbital bar of bone) is prominent in the animal at rest. It disappears and reappears during feeding in rhythm with the movements of the jaws; these effects are due to the displacement of a pad of fat interposed between the temporalis and the periorbita. The fat is depleted in horses in poor condition, and exaggeration of the hollow contributes significantly to the haggard appearance.

Deposition of fat above the upper eyelid may produce a conspicuous swelling seen in animals suffering from Cushing disease.

Little need be said concerning the external ears, which are prominent and capable of being swiveled when attempts are made to locate the origin of a sound. Their carriage is also very expressive of emotion.

SUPERFICIAL STRUCTURES

The Muscles of Facial Expression

Many clinically important features are revealed as soon as the skin is removed. Large areas of the skull are not covered by any considerable thickness of soft tissue and are therefore vulnerable to injury. These areas include the dorsal aspect of the nose, the forehead, and part of the temple,

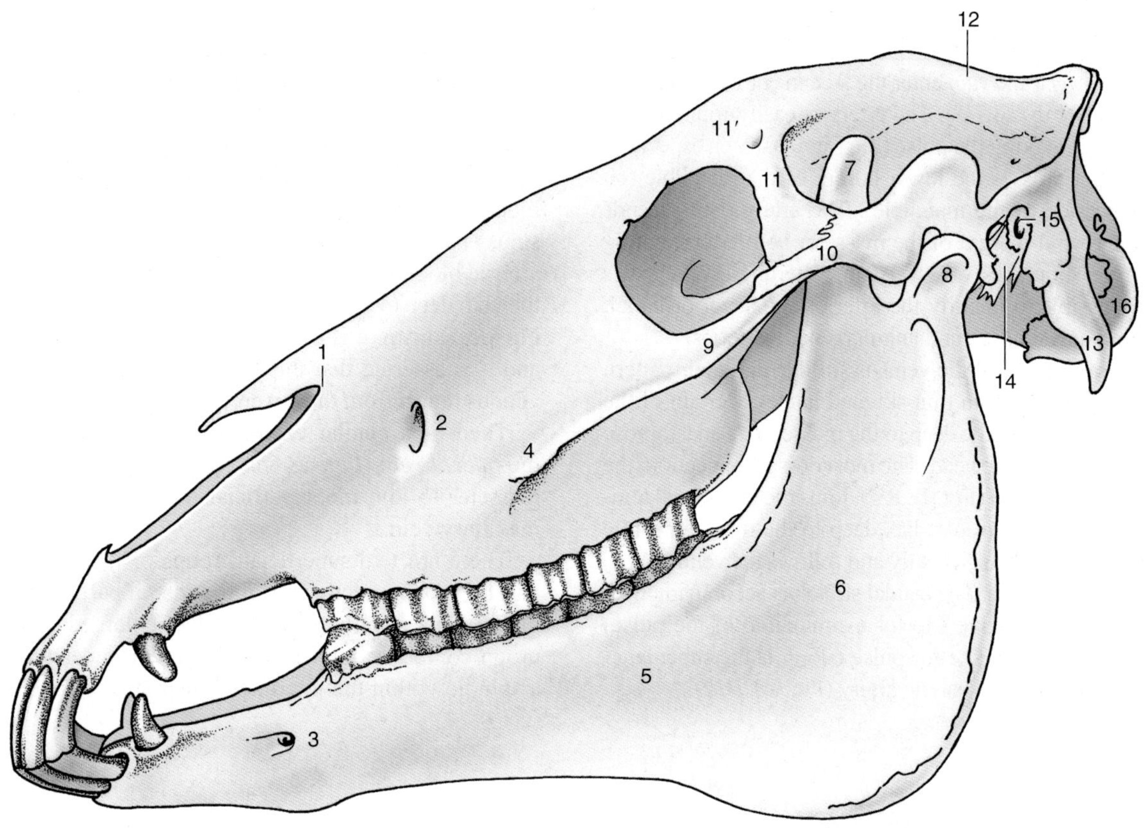

Fig. 18.6 Lateral view of the skull. *1,* Nasoincisive notch; *2,* infraorbital foramen; *3,* mental foramen; *4,* facial crest; *5,* body of mandible; *6,* ramus of mandible; *7,* coronoid process; *8,* condylar process; *9,* temporal process of zygomatic bone; *10,* zygomatic process of temporal bone; *11,* zygomatic process of frontal bone; *11′,* supraorbital foramen; *12,* external sagittal crest; *13,* paracondylar process; *14,* styloid process; *15,* external acoustic meatus; *16,* occipital condyle.

in addition to much of the mandible. Prominent landmarks include the facial crest, which runs parallel to the dorsum of the nose. It begins above the rostral margin of the fourth cheek tooth; continues into the zygomatic arch, which forms the lower margin of the orbit, and extends to the temporomandibular joint (Fig. 18.6/*4*). The joint itself is easily located by the salience of the lateral aspect of the condyle, directly before the palpable caudal margin of the mandible. The identification becomes more certain if the animal can be induced to perform chewing movements. The ventral margin of the mandible is also prominent, particularly the half that lies rostral to the masseter muscle. A shallow notch in the bone directly in front of the muscle conveys the facial vessels and parotid duct from the intermandibular space to the face.

The incomplete sheet of cutaneous muscle over the lateral aspect of the head is best developed where it merges with the orbicularis oris around the opening of the mouth.

A few individual mimetic muscles deserve notice. The *levator labii superioris* arises over the maxilla and runs dorsorostrally to form a common tendon with its fellow of the other side (Fig. 18.7/*7*). The tendon of this muscle is enclosed in a synovial sheath, travels between the nostrils, and splays out within the upper lip. This muscle is responsible for the lip curl (flehmen) seen in certain circumstances, including sexual excitement. The levator belly is easily palpated, and because it covers the infraorbital foramen, it must be pushed dorsally to locate the emergent infraorbital nerve. This foramen lies along the line joining the nasoincisive notch to the rostral end of the facial crest.

The *depressor labii inferioris* (Fig. 18.7/*5*) arises with the buccinator from the alveolar margin and adjacent part of the mandible under cover of the masseter. It can be identified as a rounded cord running rostrally over the body of the bone. The tendon covers the mental foramen, located about 2 to 3 cm caudal to the angle of the mouth, and this is readily palpable when the muscle is slid aside. The *buccinator* (Fig. 18.7/*3*) has a well-marked herringbone structure and is partly covered by the masseter. It is important in returning food to the central cavity of the mouth, preventing its accumulation in the oral vestibule.

Superficial Vessels

The *facial artery* and *vein* enter the face in company with the parotid duct (Fig. 18.7/*8*). The artery is easily found and is convenient for taking the pulse (see Fig. 18.40/*7*), especially just before it crosses the lower border of the mandible (on the medial side of the mandible). The artery then ascends along the rostral margin of the masseter before terminating in divergent branches with varying pattern. However, it is usually possible to identify the inferior and superior labial, lateral and dorsal nasal, and angularis oculi arteries.

The arrangement of the veins is similar, and their pattern may be visible in life in thin-skinned horses. Certain of the tributaries turn caudally, deep to the masseter, to anastomose with other veins of the head. The most dorsal connection, the *transverse facial vein* (Fig. 18.8/*4*), joins the superficial temporal vein. The rostral part lies deep to the masseter while the caudal part lies superficially and follows the ventral edge of the zygomatic arch. The caudal stretch is accompanied by an artery (an alternative site for examination of the pulse) and a nerve. Another site for pulse taking is the subcutaneous segment of the masseteric artery (Fig. 18.7/*12*).

The second connection, the *deep facial vein* (Fig. 18.8/*5*), burrows below the masseter and perforates the periorbita before passing through the orbital fissure to join the cavernous venous sinus within the cranial cavity. Two features of this vein are believed to possess functional significance. The cavernous sinus contains relatively cool blood drained from the hard palate and nasal cavity. The sinus envelops the internal carotid artery and may cool the arterial blood flowing to the brain. Second, an expansion of the vein deep to the masseter may form the basis of a pumping mechanism. It is liable to compression by the masseter, and it is asserted that this helps prevent stagnation of the venous return from the lowered head of the grazing animal.

There is a similar expansion on the third connection, the *buccal vein* (Fig. 18.8/*6*), which also runs deep to the masseter to join the superficial temporal tributary of the maxillary vein.

There are two superficial groups of *lymph nodes*. The parotid group under cover of the rostral part of the parotid gland is not usually palpable unless enlarged. The second group comprises numerous mandibular nodes arranged in a spindle within the intermandibular space. Together with

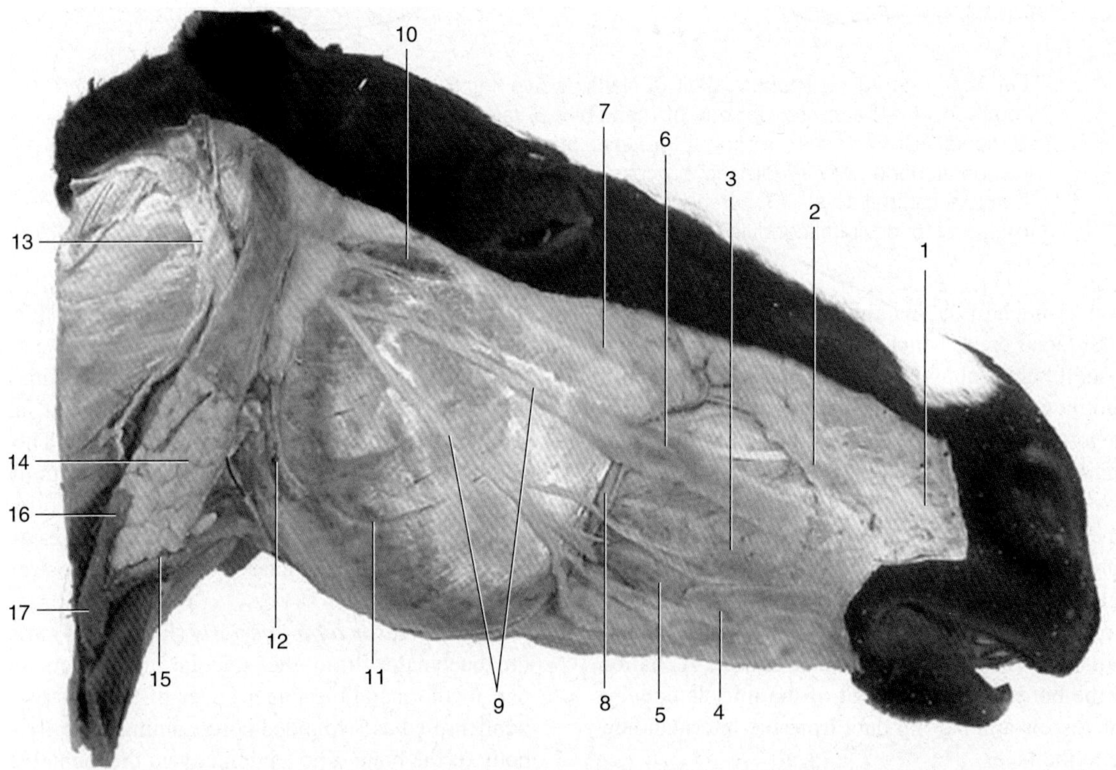

Fig. 18.7 Superficial dissection of the head. *1,* Caninus; *2,* levator nasolabialis; *3,* buccinator; *4,* stump of cutaneous muscle joining orbicularis oris; *5,* depressor labii inferioris; *6,* zygomaticus; *7,* levator labii superioris; *8,* facial artery and vein; *9,* buccal branches of facial nerve; *10,* transverse facial artery and vein and transverse facial branch of auriculotemporal nerve; *11,* masseter; *12,* masseteric artery and vein; *13,* great auricular nerve (C2); *14,* parotid gland; *15,* linguofacial vein; *16,* maxillary vein; *17,* external jugular vein.

their contralateral fellows, these nodes form a forward-pointing "V" shape that is always very distinctly palpable (see Fig. 18.39/*2*). The course of the lymph flow is dealt with later (pp. 520-521).

Superficial Nerves

Only a few features of the superficial nerves require notice. The *facial nerve* detaches its *auriculopalpebral branch* before it enters the face (see Fig. 18.36/*24*). This branch then takes an independent course across the zygomatic arch (where it is palpable), which leads it between the eye and the ear. The branch may be blocked by injection between the caudal end of the arch and the base of the ear to facilitate eye examination because it eliminates blinking and closure of the lids (p. 331).

The facial trunk divides into *dorsal* and *ventral buccal branches* before or, more commonly, shortly after emerging from under the protection of the parotid gland (Fig. 18.7/*9*). These branches and the smaller divisions into which they soon assort run forward over the masseter, where they are palpable and sometimes even visible through the skin. Blows over the masseter or pressure in prolonged recumbency may damage some or all of the divisions. The asymmetry of the face that results when the muscles of the lips, cheek, and nose are paralyzed is usually more striking than in other species. Because the auriculopalpebral branch is detached proximally, such trauma generally spares the muscles of the eyelids and external ear; their involvement points to injury at a more proximal level, which suggests a more sinister causation (Fig. 18.9).

The *trigeminal nerve* and its principal branches—the supraorbital, infraorbital, and mental nerves—provide sensory innervation of the face (Table 18.1). These are easily located at their emergence from the corresponding foramina. The supraorbital nerve to the upper eyelid and the adjacent part of the forehead skin leaves the supraorbital foramen within an easily located dimple in the root of the zygomatic process of the frontal bone. Directions for location of the infraorbital and mental nerves have already been given (p. 495). Anesthetic deposited about the infraorbital nerve at its emergence will desensitize the skin of the upper lip, nostril, and much of the nose extending well caudal to the foramen. Blockage of the mental nerve desensitizes the skin of the lower lip and chin region. During blockage of either of these nerves, it is possible to insert the tip of the needle through the foramen into the bony canal within the jaw to desensitize the more rostral teeth (from P2 forward).

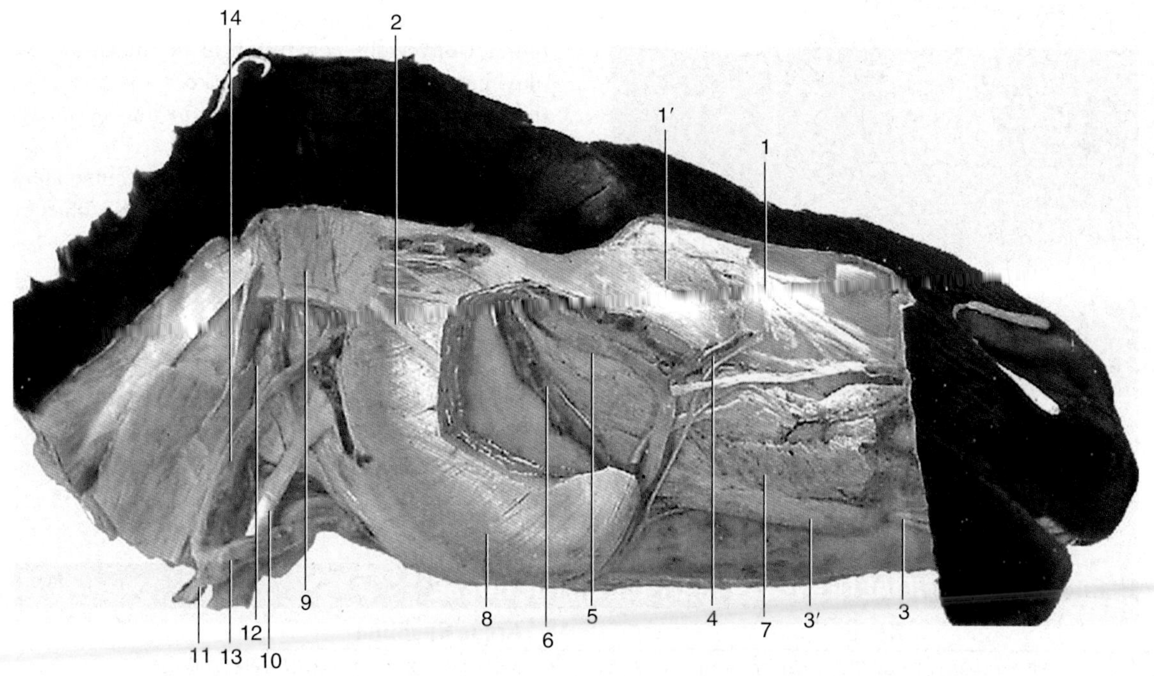

Fig. 18.8 Deeper dissection of the head. Parts of the superficial muscles, masseter, and parotid gland have been removed. *1,* Infraorbital nerve; *1′,* levator labii superioris; *2,* dorsal buccal branch of facial nerve; *3,* mental nerve; *3′,* depressor labii inferioris; *4,* facial vein; *5,* deep facial vein; *6,* buccal vein; *7,* buccinator; *8,* masseter; *9,* occipitomandibularis; *10,* sternocephalicus; *11,* external jugular vein; *12,* mandibular gland; *13,* linguofacial vein; *14,* maxillary vein.

THE NASAL CAVITY AND PARANASAL SINUSES

The Nasal Cavity

Some features of the external nose have been described (p. 492). The ventral part of the nostril leads through a constricted vestibule into a nasal cavity considerably less roomy than might be supposed from the exterior. Although the factors that determine this are common to all species, their importance is exaggerated in the horse by the reserve portions of the cheek teeth and the extensive development of the paranasal sinus system (see Fig. 3.14).

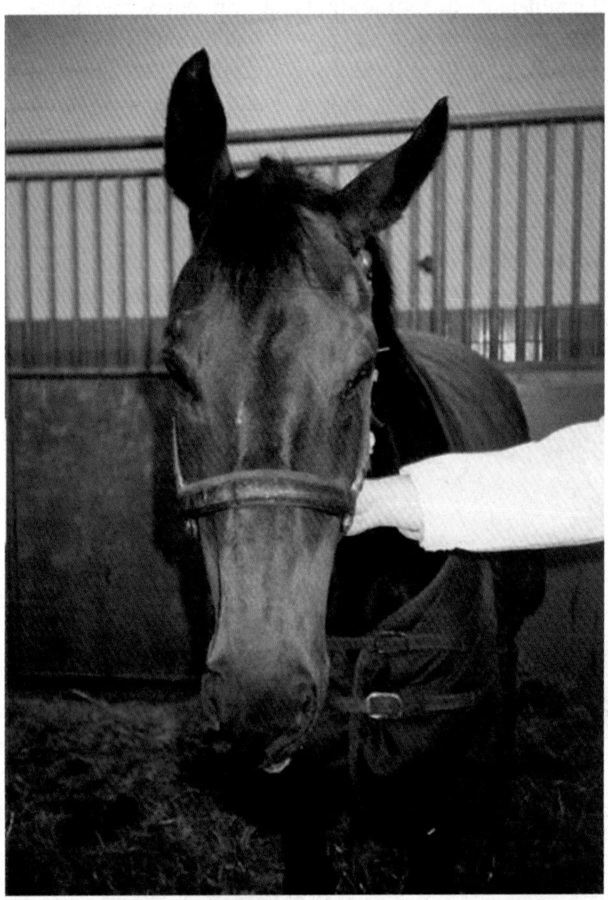

Fig. 18.9 Injury to the facial nerve. Note pronounced drooping of ear, moderate drooping of upper eyelid of affected side, and distortion of the nose, which is drawn toward the sound side.

The dorsal and ventral *conchae* form delicate scrolls that coil in opposite directions from their lateral attachments (Fig. 18.10). The space enclosed within each is divided into two compartments by an internal septum. The caudal part of the dorsal concha is occupied by a rostral extension of the frontal sinus, with which it enjoys free communication. The caudal space within the ventral concha communicates with the rostral maxillary sinus. The space within the rostral part of each major concha is in direct communication with the nasal cavity. Numerous small ethmoidal conchae projecting into the fundus serve to enlarge the olfactory area (Fig. 18.11/*3*).

The major *conchae* divide the cavity into the usual pattern of meatuses (Fig. 18.10). It may be presumed that air moves from the dorsal meatus to the olfactory mucosa and from the middle meatus to the sinuses, while the ventral and common meatuses supply the principal respiratory passage. The conjunction of the last two provides the widest and most convenient route for the introduction of a stomach tube, endoscope, or other instrument. The fragility of the ventral concha and the vascularity of the covering mucosa require that the procedure be performed with care.

Because breathing through the mouth is impossible for the horse, augmentation of the air intake in conditions of stress depends on reduction of the obstruction offered by the nose itself. The nostrils may be greatly widened by obliteration of the nasal diverticulum (Fig. 18.2), and contraction of the mucosal venous plexuses thins the membrane. Conversely, congestion of the mucosal vessels, as may happen in infections, thickens the mucosa around the entrance to the sinus system to impede air flow and obstruct the drainage.

The *vomeronasal organ* does not communicate with the mouth in the horse but maintains the usual connection with the nasal cavity (Fig. 18.12/*2*).

The Paranasal Sinuses

The extensive sinus system possesses considerable clinical interest because it is susceptible to infection that may spread from the nose or from an alveolar abscess. It also provides a means of access to the unerupted portions of the caudal cheek teeth (Fig. 18.13).

TABLE 18.1 SUPERFICIAL NERVES OF THE FACE OF THE HORSE

	Nerve	Areas Supplied
Facial	Auriculopalpebral branch	Muscles of eyelid and external ear
	Dorsal and ventral buccal branch	Muscles of lip, cheek, and nose
Trigeminal	Supraorbital nerve	Upper eyelid and the adjacent skin on forehead
	Infraorbital nerve	Skin of the upper lip, nostril, and nose extending caudal to the foramen
	Mental nerve	Skin of the lower lip and chin

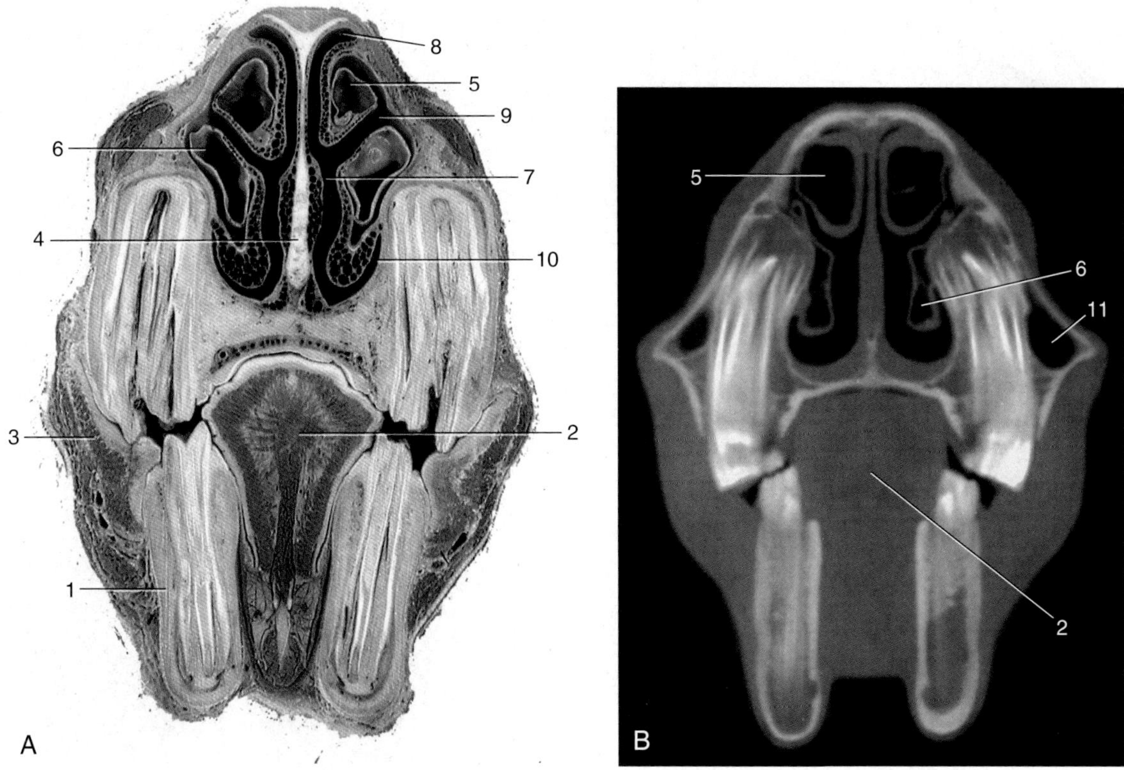

Fig. 18.10 (A) Transverse section of the head at the level of the rostral maxillary sinus. (B) Computed tomographic scan (bone window) at about the same level. *1,* P4; *2,* tongue; *3,* buccinator; *4,* nasal septum; *5,* dorsal nasal concha; *6,* ventral nasal concha; *7,* common nasal meatus; *8,* dorsal nasal meatus; *9,* middle nasal meatus; *10,* ventral nasal meatus; *11,* rostral maxillary sinus.

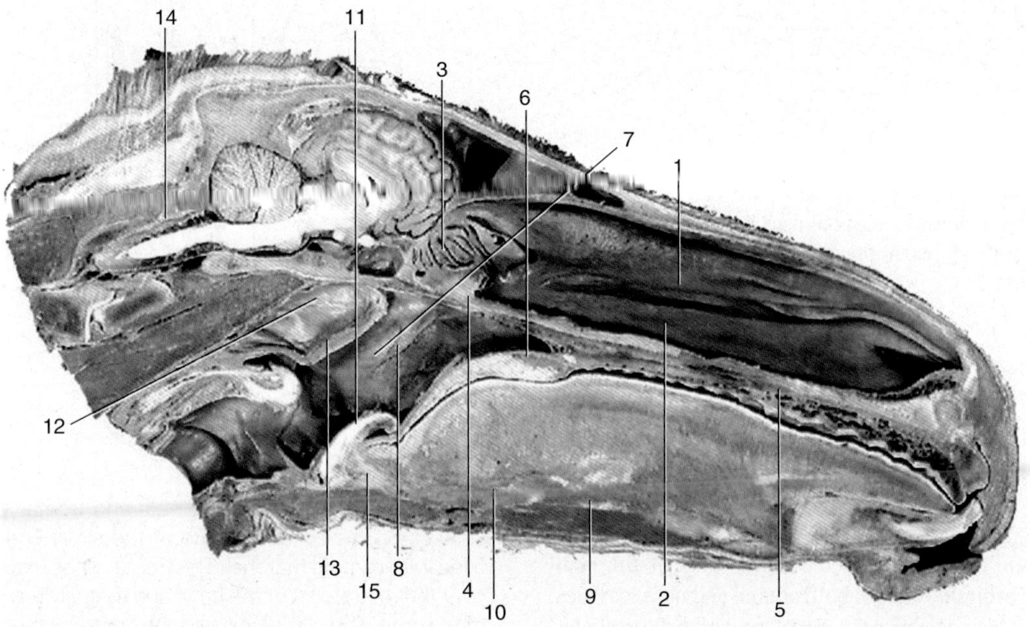

Fig. 18.11 Median section of the head; most of the nasal septum has been removed. *1,* Dorsal nasal concha; *2,* ventral nasal concha; *3,* ethmoidal conchae; *4,* right choana; *5,* hard palate with prominent ridges (rugae); *6,* soft palate; *7,* nasopharynx; *8,* pharyngeal opening of auditory tube; *9,* geniohyoideus; *10,* genioglossus; *11,* epiglottis; *12,* medial wall of guttural pouch; *13,* pharyngeal muscles; *14,* cerebellomedullary cistern; *15,* basihyoid.

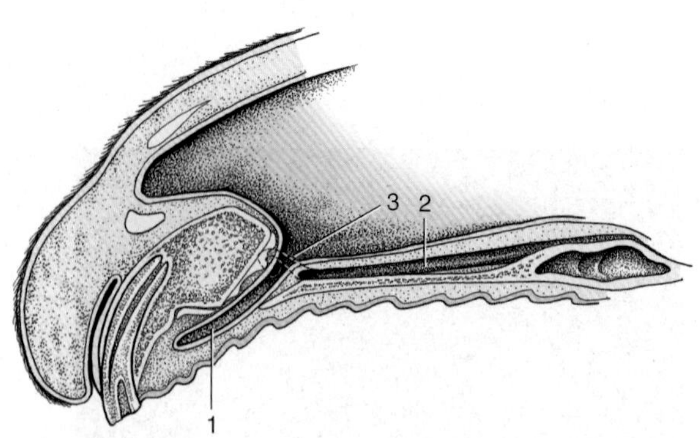

Fig. 18.12 Paramedian section of the rostral end of the nose. *1,* Incisive duct; *2,* vomeronasal organ; *3,* opening of the incisive duct into the nasal cavity and opening of the vomeronasal organ into the incisive duct.

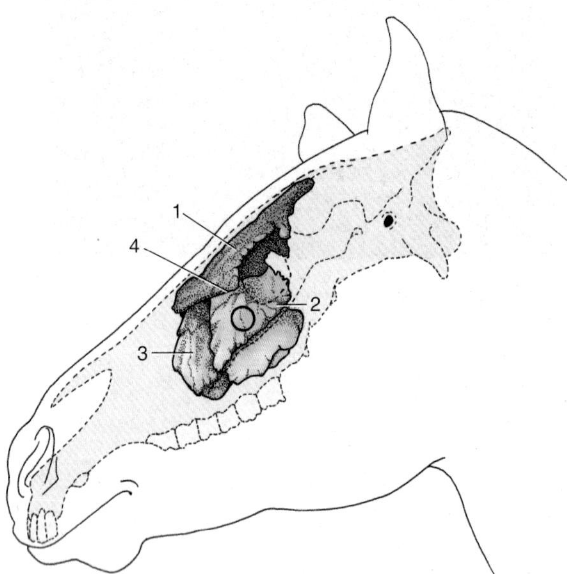

Fig. 18.13 Topography of the conchofrontal and maxillary sinuses, which are filled with casting material. The *circle* indicates where the caudal maxillary sinus can be trephined. *1,* Conchofrontal sinus; *2,* caudal maxillary sinus; *3,* rostral maxillary sinus; *4,* position of frontomaxillary opening between *1* and *2*.

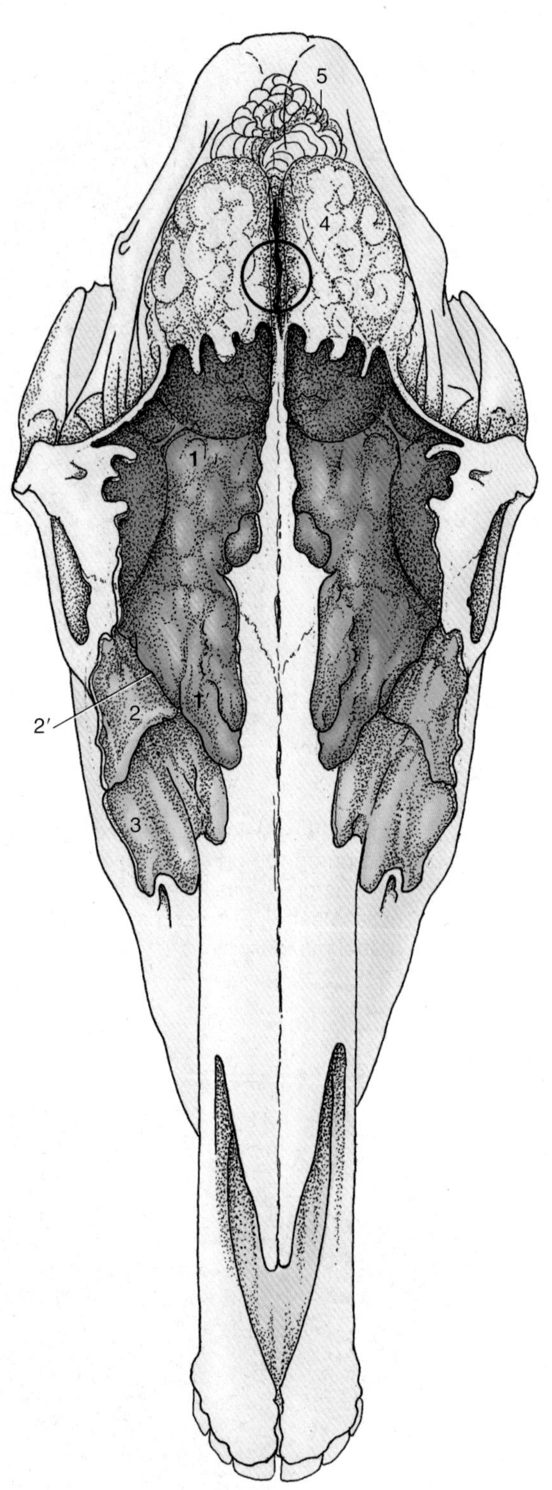

Fig. 18.14 Projection of the brain and frontal and maxillary sinuses on the dorsal surface of the skull. The sinuses are filled with casting material. The frontal sinus extends caudally over the rostral part of the brain and rostrally beyond the level of the orbit. The *circle* indicates the center of the brain and the location where a horse may be shot. *1* and *1′,* Conchofrontal sinus: frontal part (*1*) and dorsal conchal part (*1′*); *2,* caudal maxillary sinus; *2′,* position of frontomaxillary opening; *3,* rostral maxillary sinus; *4,* cerebrum; *5,* cerebellum.

On each side there are frontal, caudal maxillary, and rostral maxillary sinuses of importance and sphenopalatine and ethmoidal spaces of less account. The layout is complicated and, in one important respect, unique (among domestic species): the frontal sinus communicates with the nasal cavity indirectly via the caudal maxillary sinus.

The *frontal sinus* occupies the dorsal part of the skull medial to the orbit. It overlaps both cranial and nasal cavities, and because it also occupies the closed part of the dorsal concha, it is more correctly known as the *conchofrontal sinus.* Its extent is shown in Fig. 18.14/*1* and *1′*. From this it will be seen that the interior of the frontal part is incompletely divided by several bony lamellae. The floor of this part is molded over the ethmoidal labyrinth, and rostrolateral to these areas of unevenness, it displays the large oval communication (frontomaxillary opening) with the caudal maxillary sinus. The opening normally allows easy natural drainage.

Trephining: A window may be opened, usually by trephination, in the roof of the frontal sinus to allow for irrigation or for removal of a molar by repulsion, when a punch introduced through the frontomaxillary opening is brought to bear on the appropriate alveolus. Such a window also allows introduction of a fiberoptic endoscope to inspect the interior of this large sinus.

The two *maxillary sinuses* together occupy a large part of the upper jaw, where they have a critically important relationship to the embedded portions of the caudal cheek teeth. They share a slitlike communication (nasomaxillary opening) with the middle meatus of the nasal cavity but are otherwise completely divided by an oblique septum. This is variable in position but most commonly located about 5 cm caudal to the rostral end of the facial crest. The ventral part of each sinus is also divided into medial and lateral spaces by an upright longitudinal plate supporting the infraorbital canal and fused in young animals to the alveoli containing the roots and unerupted portions of the cheek teeth. The medial part of the caudal sinus continues into the irregular sphenopalatine sinus. The corresponding part of the rostral sinus extends into the ventral concha.

It is impossible to define the exact extent and projections of the maxillary sinuses, which enlarge considerably after birth as the teeth are extruded (Fig. 18.15). Their relationship to the teeth is also affected by the forward migration of the teeth as they develop and come into wear. As Fig. 18.15 shows, the relationship is confined to the last premolar and first molar tooth in the newborn foal; it later extends to involve the last four teeth but finally retains contact only with the three molars. There is much variation, and attention to the varying inclination of the embedded parts of different teeth is required.

Entering the Maxillary Sinus: Entry to the sinus may be required either to effect drainage (because the natural route, the nasomaxillary opening, is placed high in the wall) or to give access to certain teeth. Although factors such as the routes followed by the very vulnerable nasolacrimal duct and infraorbital nerve limit the safe surgical area of maxillary sinuses, the potential operating area is defined by the following boundaries: (1) the vertical line tangential to the rostral limit of the orbit; (2) the facial crest; (3) the oblique line joining the rostral limit of the crest to the infraorbital foramen; and (4) the line parallel to the facial crest that intersects the infraorbital foramen.

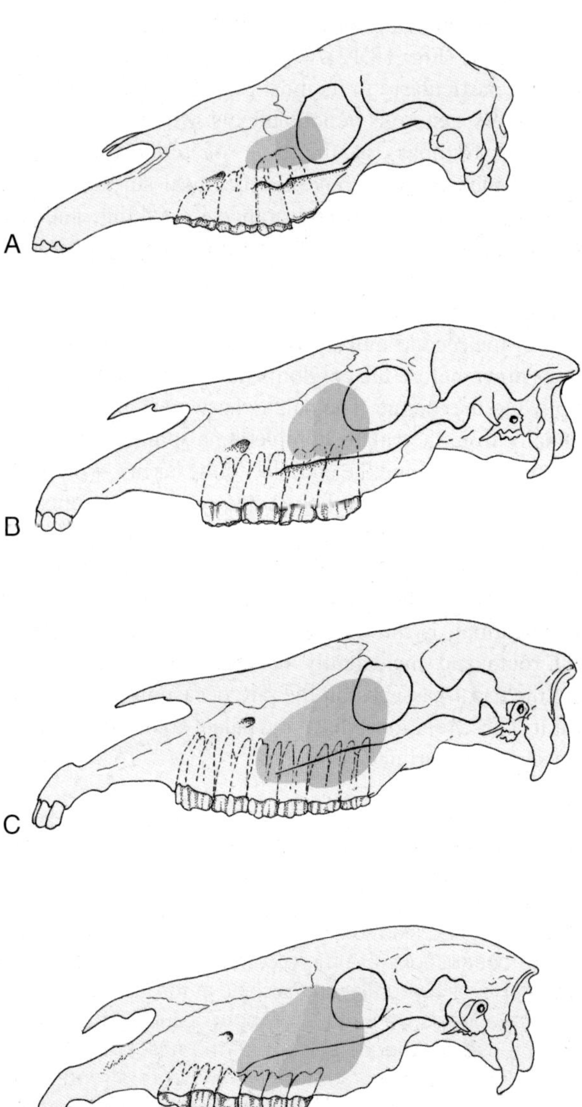

Fig. 18.15 Projection of the maxillary sinuses at various ages. In older horses the cheek teeth are more rostrally placed. (A) 1 month. (B) 1 year. (C) 4 to 6 years. (D) Older than 12 years.

THE MOUTH

The small size of the entrance makes it impossible to open the mouth wide; this limitation, coupled with the great depth of the cavity, severely hampers clinical inspection.

The *vestibule* communicates with the mouth cavity proper only between the incisor and cheek teeth (where the diastema may be interrupted by the canine teeth) and by small gaps behind the last molars. The *hard palate* is therefore largely bounded by the alveolar processes and teeth. It is almost uniformly broad and is marked by two more or less symmetrical series of ridges (Fig. 18.11/5). The incisive papilla is found directly behind the central incisors; grooves that flank the elevation end blindly and do not communicate with the nasal cavity and vomeronasal organs (Fig. 18.12). The mucosa of the hard palate is thick, particularly in its most rostral part, and incorporates a very generous venous plexus, which may become engorged (lampas) at the time of tooth replacement when it may project above the occlusal surfaces of the neighboring teeth. The appearance is striking, and laypeople are sometimes alarmed by this purely physiologic phenomenon.

The *soft palate* continues the hard palate beyond the level of the second molar tooth. It is remarkably long and hangs down before the epiglottis; its free margin is closely applied to the tongue. The palatopharyngeal arches extend caudally from the palate, completing a sphincter about the structures that bound the entrance to the larynx, which thus projects some way into the nasopharynx. The application of the palate to the tongue is so firm that an airtight seal is created that closes the oropharynx, which then provides a barrier between the mouth and the pharynx. This ensures that breathing is through the nose, precluding use of the oral route and incidentally resulting in ingesta passing into the nasal passages on the rare occasions when horses vomit. These relationships of the palate are normally maintained except during deglutition.

The obstructions of the upper respiratory tract commonly recognized in horses worked at a fast pace are often due to anomalous position and relations of the soft palate and lead to diminished physical performance. There obstructions are more common at the palatopharyngeal level in younger animals and at the laryngeal level in older animals, and frequently both occur together.

The use of videoendoscopy of the nasopharynx and larynx of affected horses while they were strenuously exercised on a treadmill has helped to identify two abnormal conditions of the soft palate. These apparently occur after admission of air into the oropharynx breaks the seal that normally maintains the parts in close apposition. In the less severe form, there is abnormal movement of the caudal part of the palate, aptly described as "billowing." In the more severe form, of which billowing is probably a precursor, the soft palate is displaced dorsally, losing contact with the ventral side of the epiglottis and narrowing the nasopharyngeal airway. At endoscopy the epiglottis is no longer visible. Both forms may be accompanied by abnormal respiration sounds.

Some of the factors that may break the seal include the following: the extreme negative pressure developed in the rostral nasopharynx at one stage of the respiratory cycle; dysfunction of the palate musculature weakening the contact between tongue and palate; overactivity of those ventral cervical muscles that attach to the larynx and hyoid, drawing the larynx caudally and freeing the palate from entrapment by the epiglottis; and abnormal activity of the hyoepiglottic muscle, tilting the epiglottis caudally with the same effect.

The mucosa on the oral surface of the soft palate is marked by numerous pits where the palatine glands open. It also exhibits a rostral median tonsillar swelling.

The *tongue* is long, conforming to the shape of the cavity, and is spatulate at its apex, which is incompletely restrained by a narrow frenulum. Its upper surface is thickly strewn with delicate filiform papillae that confer a velvet-like texture; the larger papillae with gustatory function are less widely spread (Fig. 18.16/*9–11*). A scattering of lymphoid tissue over the root constitutes a diffuse lingual tonsil. Each of two low mucosal folds beneath the apex of the tongue carries a fleshy sublingual caruncle where the mandibular duct opens.

THE DENTITION AND MASTICATORY APPARATUS

The Dentition

The dentition of the horse is admirably suited to a diet of grass, a surprisingly abrasive material. The masticatory area is increased by the enlargement of the premolars and their assimilation to the molars, with which they present a continuous grinding surface. Both cheek teeth and incisors have high crowns, which ensure a long working life, despite the considerable attrition that takes place at the occlusal surfaces. Delayed formation of the roots also allows the cheek teeth to grow for some years after they come into wear. Attrition wastes the cheek tooth by 2 to 3 mm each year; to allow for this the greater part of the crown is initially embedded within the jaw and only gradually extruded to compensate for this loss. The enamel casing of the incisor and cheek teeth is also folded, although in different ways in the incisor, upper cheek, and lower cheek teeth series. The folding increases the area of the durable enamel presented at the working surface, where it stands proud of the neighboring dentine; the alternation of harder and softer tissues provides efficient grinding instruments (see Fig. 18.19).

The formula of the temporary dentition is

$$\frac{3-0-3}{3-0-3}$$

and that of the permanent dentition is

$$\frac{3-1-3\,(4)-3}{3-1-3-3}.$$

The *incisor teeth* are ranked together to form a continuous arch in each jaw and are so implanted that their roots converge (Fig. 18.17). Each is curved lengthwise, presenting a labial convexity. When in occlusion, the upper and lower incisors of the young animal form a continuous arch when viewed in profile. Later, as they wear,

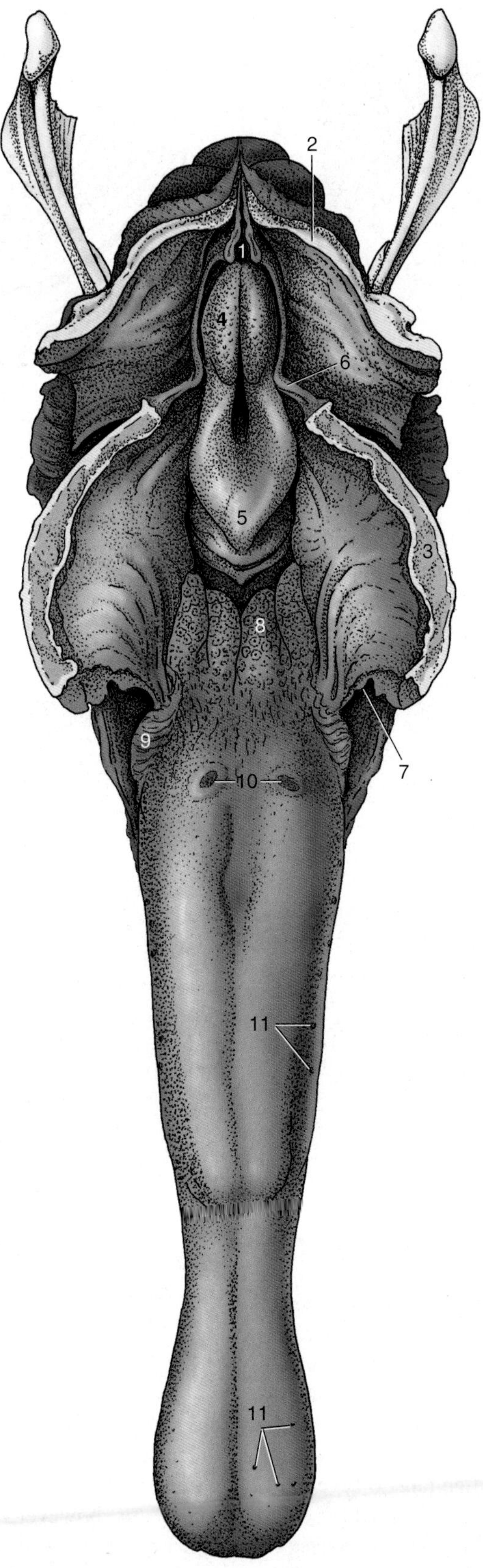

Fig. 18.16 The tongue and pharynx; the latter has been opened dorsally to expose the entrance to the larynx. *1,* Entrance into esophagus; *2,* dorsal wall of nasopharynx (split in median plane); *3,* soft palate (split in median plane); *4,* corniculate process of arytenoid cartilage; *5,* epiglottis; *6,* free border of soft palate, continued caudally by palatopharyngeal arch; *7,* palatoglossal arch; *8,* lingual tonsil; *9,* foliate papillae; *10,* vallate papillae; *11,* examples of fungiform papillae.

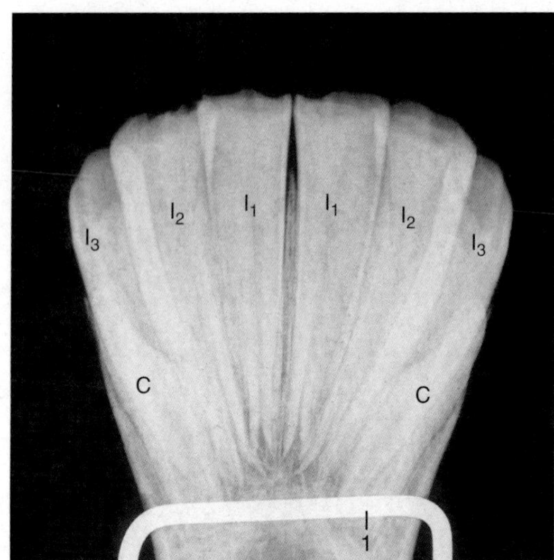

Fig. 18.17 Root convergence of permanent lower incisors; radiograph of a bone specimen from a 5-year-old (estimated) horse. Note the funnel-shaped infundibulum visible in each of the first and second incisors. I_1, I_2, and I_3, Lower first, second, and third incisors; *C,* lower canine tooth, present only in the male; *1,* mounting wire of specimen.

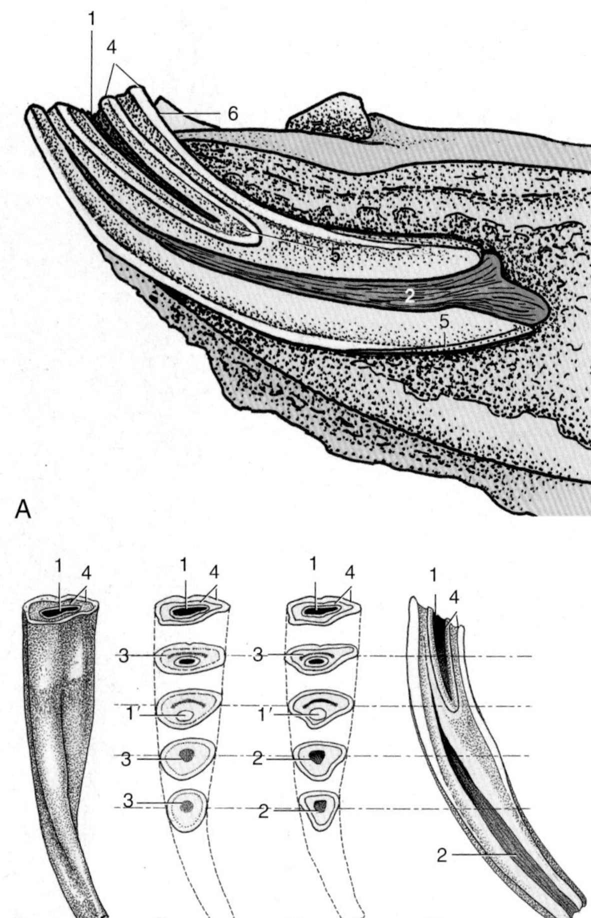

Fig. 18.18 Structure of a lower incisor. (A) In situ, sectioned longitudinally; the clinical crown is short in relation to the embedded part of the tooth. (B) Caudal view; the junction between the clinical crown and the rest of the tooth is not marked. (C) As a result of wear the occlusal surface changes; the cup gets smaller and disappears, leaving, for a time, the enamel spot; the dental star appears and changes from a line to a large round spot. (D) These are sawn sections of a young tooth for comparison. (E) Longitudinal section of incisor, showing the relationship between the infundibulum and dental cavity; the latter is rostral. *1,* Cup, black cavity in center of infundibulum; *1',* enamel spot, proximal end of infundibulum; *2,* dental cavity; *3,* dental star, changing in shape from a linear to a rounded form; *4,* outer and inner enamel rings; *5,* cement; *6,* lingual surface.

the upper and lower teeth meet at an increasingly pronounced angle. The occlusal surface recently brought into use is a broad transverse oval (Fig. 18.18B) and presents an outer enamel casing and an inner enamel ring lining the infolding known as the *infundibulum;* this is partially filled with cement, leaving a small cavity, the cup (Fig. 18.18/*1*). Because the enamel lining is more resistant, it projects above the surrounding dentine. Changes in the appearance of the occlusal surface provide the information principally used in aging older horses. The points to note are the depth of the infundibulum and its overlap with the dental cavity. Although it may appear that wear would eventually expose the pulp, this is prevented by the timely formation of secondary dentine, distinguishable from primary dentine by its darker color; this secondary dentine provides the feature known as the *dental star* (Fig. 18.18/*3*).

Although *canine teeth* generally form in both sexes, they are rudimentary and commonly fail to erupt in mares. In male animals they are low, laterally compressed cones placed within the diastemas rather closer to the corner incisors than to the cheek teeth. The embedded portions are disproportionately large in relation to the exposed crowns.

The *first premolar* ("wolf" tooth) often fails to develop, and when present, it is vestigial and almost invariably confined to the upper jaw. Although it is without functional significance, it does have a potential nuisance value because it may shift under the pressure of the bit and so irritate the gum. It is easily extracted.

The remaining *premolars* (P2–P4) form a continuous row with the *molars*. The first and last of the six cheek teeth are somewhat triangular in section and the others rectangular; nonetheless, each is so like its neighbors that only an expert may distinguish isolated teeth (see Fig. 18.21). There are, however, important differences between the upper and lower sets; the upper teeth are much wider and exhibit a more complicated enamel folding, which creates two infundibula that fill with cement before eruption. The enamel of the lower teeth is also much folded but forms no infundibula (Fig. 18.19B). Most teeth occlude with two members of the opposing set along a relatively narrow area

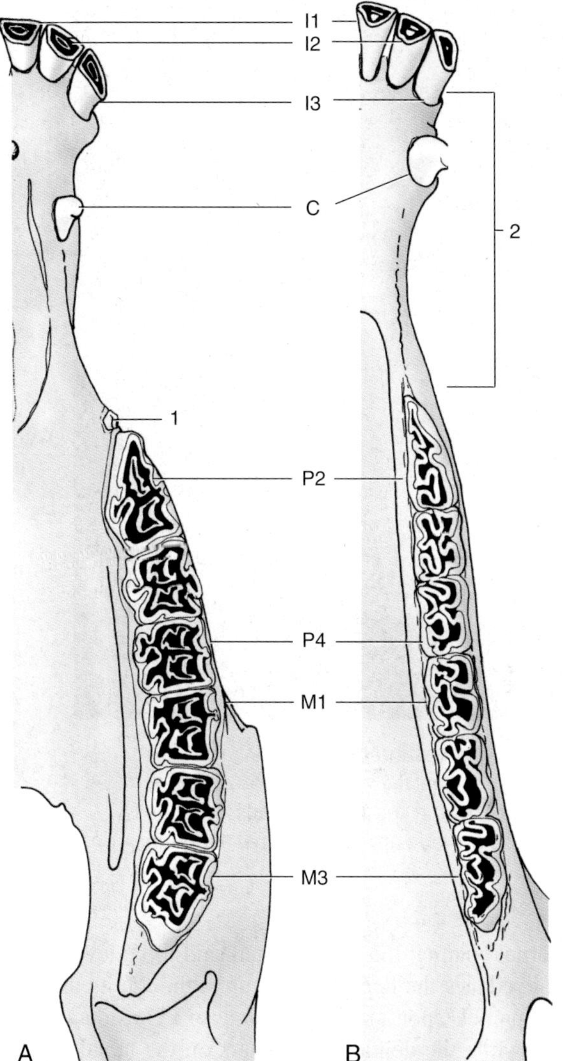

Fig. 18.19 The permanent teeth of the (A) upper and (B) lower jaws. *1,* "Wolf" tooth (P1); *2,* diastema.

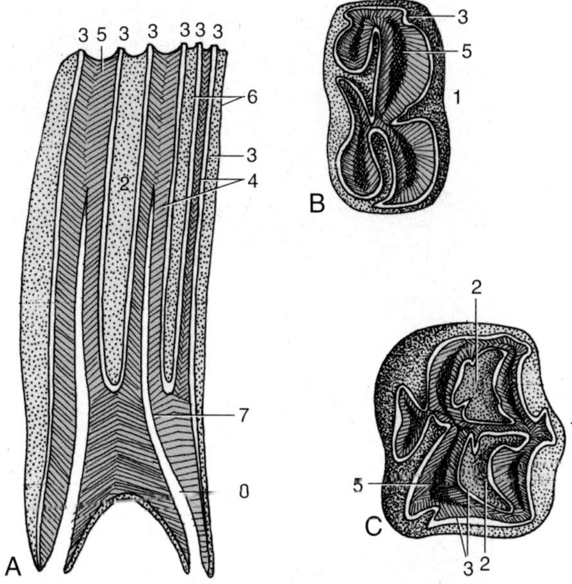

Fig. 18.20 Structure of the cheek teeth shown in sagittal section (A) and by views of the occlusal surface of lower (B) and upper (C) molars. *1,* Buccal (labial) surface; *2,* infundibulum; *3,* enamel; *4,* dentine; *5,* secondary dentine; *6,* cement; *7,* dental cavity; *8,* root canal.

of contact that follows the lingual edge of the upper teeth and buccal edge of the lower teeth. The occlusal plane slopes ventrobuccally (Fig. 18.10). Irregular or incomplete chewing movements may cause the buccal edge of the upper cheek teeth and the lingual edge of the lower cheek teeth to escape wear (sharp teeth); the resulting protrusions must be filed down (floated) to prevent injury to cheeks and tongue.

The structure of the cheek teeth is shown in Fig. 18.20. The upper teeth are anchored by three or four roots and are so implanted that the reserve portions slope caudally at varying angles (Fig. 18.21). The relationship to the maxillary sinuses and other features of the skull is very helpfully revealed in radiographs. Only a thin plate of alveolar bone separates the molars from the sinus; in consequence, infection may easily spread to the sinus from tooth or alveolar abscesses. The relationship changes with age, partly because gradual extrusion lowers the alveolar floor, enlarging the sinus, and partly because the teeth migrate rostrally (Fig. 18.15).

The transitory swellings occasionally seen on the ventral margin of the mandible of 2- to 4-year-old horses are produced by modeling of the mandible to accommodate the formation of the roots of permanent teeth, which are prevented from rising within the jaw by remnants (caps) of deciduous predecessors blocking the way (Fig. 18.22). When the remnants are shed, their successors can move into place. Further modeling of the mandibular border erases the swellings.

Simple extraction of cheek teeth is more or less impossible. Their length, curvature, and close fit would hamper any effort to draw one out past its neighbor(s), even were the attempt permitted by the small size of the opening between the lips and the depth of the oral cavity (Fig. 18.23). Instead, they must be removed by expulsion, that is, by means of a punch brought to bear over the root in an operation of some severity and difficulty involving the opening of a window through bone. Accurate determination of the position of the root of the tooth involved is essential, and for this it is necessary to be mindful of how the dispositions of the teeth change with age. The approach to a caudal member of the upper cheek teeth series is made via the caudal maxillary sinus or the frontal and caudal maxillary sinuses when M^3 is involved.

The deciduous teeth generally resemble the permanent teeth but are much smaller and significantly shorter in relation to their breadth. The deciduous incisors are constricted

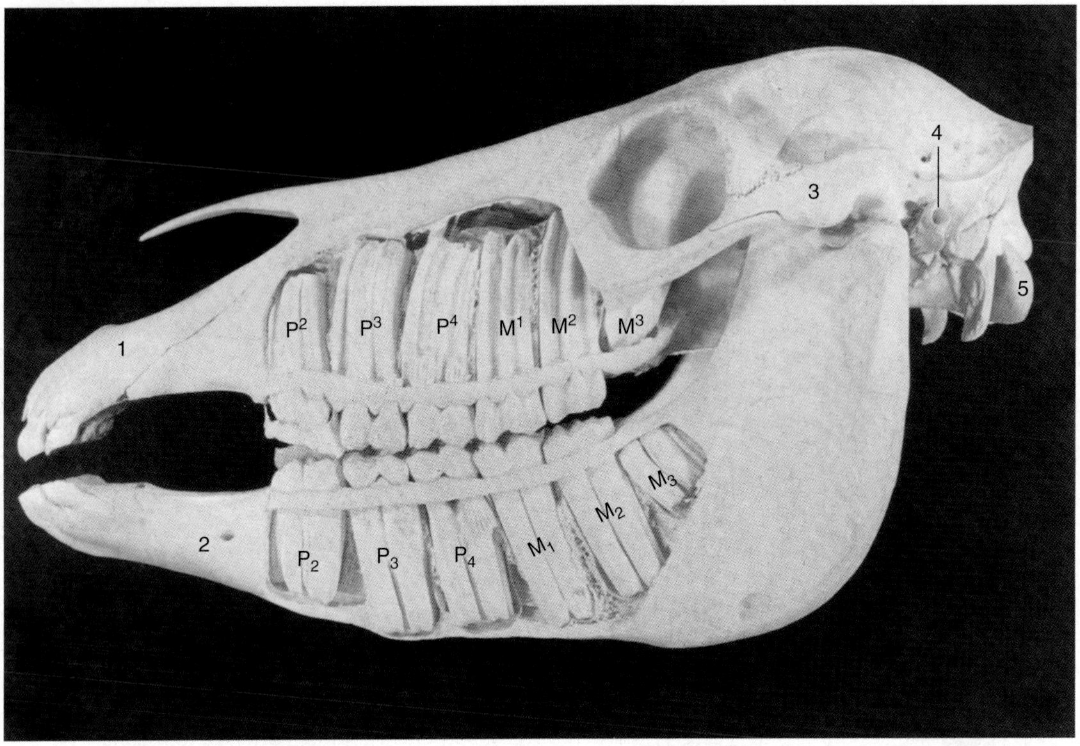

Fig. 18.21 Exposed cheek teeth of a horse 2½ years old (estimated). *Upper jaw:* The deciduous premolars are still present, p^2 in the form of a cap; M^3 has not yet erupted. *Lower jaw:* The deciduous premolars 3 and 4 are still present in the form of caps; M_3 has not yet erupted. *1,* Incisive bone; *2,* mental foramen; *3,* zygomatic arch; *4,* external acoustic meatus; *5,* occipital condyle.

at the neck and are much whiter than their replacements because the porcelain-like enamel is unobscured by the cement encrustation that gives permanent teeth a slightly yellow and porous appearance. Some longitudinal striation is apparent on the temporary incisor crown.

The Estimation of Age From the Teeth

Examination of the teeth provides the traditional and sole convenient means of estimating age. Because there is copious specialist literature, the subject is treated very briefly here (Table 18.2). The eruption dates and changes in appearance of the occlusal surfaces, specifically those of the lower incisors, are the main criteria. Neither is wholly dependable but the first is more reliable, although limited in application to younger animals; the second may be used throughout the life span but becomes increasingly inaccurate.

The initially oval occlusal surface of the incisors becomes rounded and finally forms a triangle elongated in the labiolingual direction. The enamel casing is intact when the tooth erupts, and the occlusal surface then presents a central depression *(cup)* that is soon stained by food debris. Wear first abrades the labial edge but quickly extends all around, isolating the infundibular from the external enamel; the tooth is then said to be level. Further wear reduces the depth of the cup, although its thick base (the enamel "spot") resists attrition for a considerable time. Meanwhile the dental star appears on the labial aspect of the cup and persists after the cup and the enamel spot have been entirely lost.

Less reliable criteria are a "hook" on I^3 (see Table 18.2) and Galvayne's groove on the labial surface of the same tooth. The hook is present when the horse is about 7 years old; unfortunately it may recur at 11 years. The appearance, progression, and disappearance of Galvayne's groove are also depicted in Table 18.2. Although unreliable by themselves, both features may enhance accuracy when combined with the appearance of the occlusal surfaces and the profile of the incisors (Figs. 18.24 and 18.25).

It must be emphasized that the variation in these (and in other undescribed) features is extremely large, and in a horse more than 8 years old the assessment may be at fault by several years.

The Muscles of Mastication and the Temporomandibular Joint

The muscles of mastication are well developed. The *masseter* takes origin along the whole length of the facial

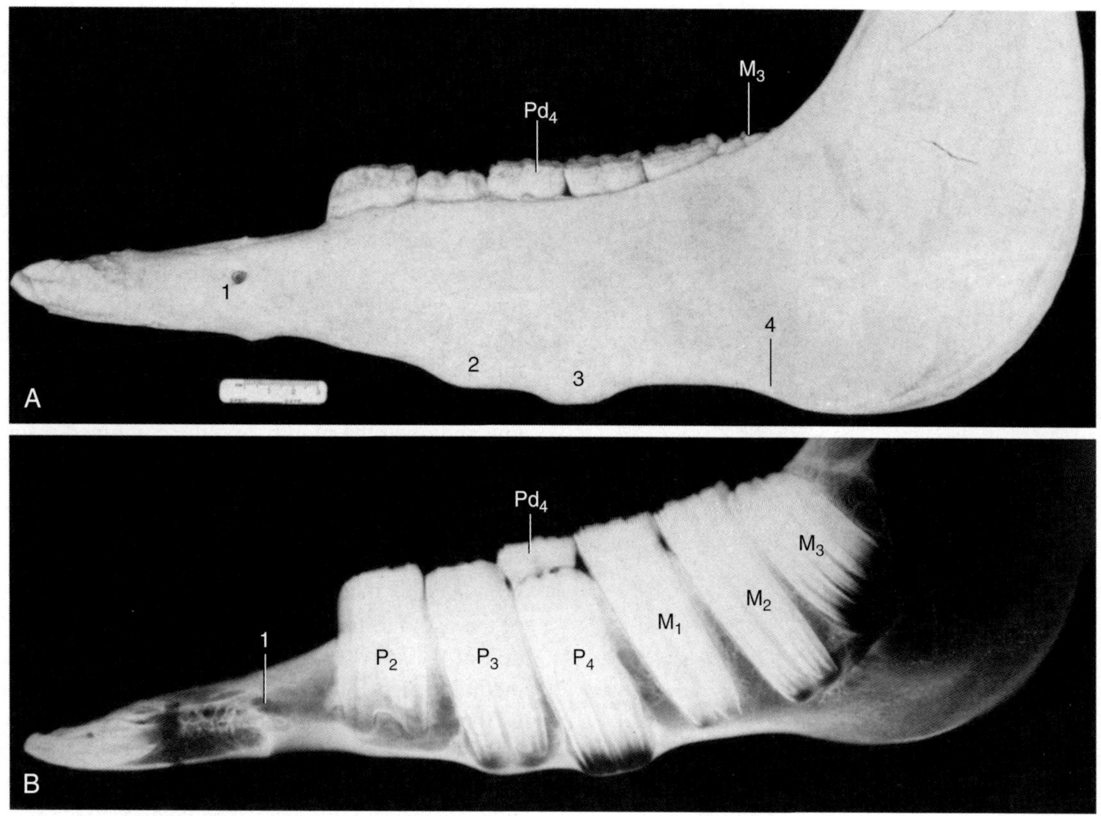

Fig. 18.22 (A) Photograph and (B) radiograph of the left half-mandible of a horse 3 years old (estimated). Note the transitory tubercles on the ventral border and the wedged-in cap (Pd_4) that retards the advance of P_3 and P_4. *1,* Mental foramen; *2* and *3,* tubercles over the proximal ends of P_3 and P_4, respectively; *4,* notch for facial artery and vein.

crest and zygomatic arch and inserts on the mandible between the vascular notch and condyle (Fig. 18.7/*11*). It is a multipennate muscle constructed so that the fibers of the superficial strata run caudoventrally, while those more deeply placed are nearly vertical. Its cranial margin produces a very prominent surface contour that serves as a guide to the location of the facial vessels and parotid duct. Its caudodorsal part is overlain by the parotid gland but to a variable depth and extent, which affect the accessibility to palpation of the parotid lymph nodes. Laterally, the masseter is traversed by buccal branches of the facial nerve.

The *temporalis* almost fills the temporal fossa, where it is easily palpated despite the partial covering of thin muscles concerned with the movement of the external ear (Fig. 18.23/*1*). It arises from the wall of the fossa and from the sagittal crest that forms its median margin, and it envelops the coronoid process of the mandible. On contraction it raises the mandible.

The *pterygoideus medialis* and *lateralis,* deep to the mandible, broadly correspond to the masseter in position, orientation, and attachments (Fig. 18.23/*2* and *3*). The medial muscle, always the larger, extends from the pterygoid process to the mandibular margin. The lateral muscle runs more horizontally to insert close to the condyle. The masseter and contralateral pterygoid muscles act together to produce the horizontal shifts that supply the principal grinding movement.

The *digastricus* and *occipitomandibularis* (strictly a part of the digastricus; Fig. 18.23/*4* and *4'*) are responsible for active opening of the mouth. Despite its much greater bulk, the latter may be regarded as a detachment from the caudal belly of the digastricus. It extends between the paracondylar process of the occipital bone and the caudal border of the mandible. The much more slender digastricus has a similar origin. It presents an intermediate tendon that passes through a split in the insertion of the stylohyoideus. The rostral belly attaches to the ventromedial part of the molar region of the mandible. When the mouth is closed, contraction of the digastricus raises the hyoid apparatus (by virtue of its association with the stylohyoideus) and thus the root of the tongue (Fig. 18.23B).

A thick intra-articular disk is interposed between the expanded and rather flat facets of the mandibular

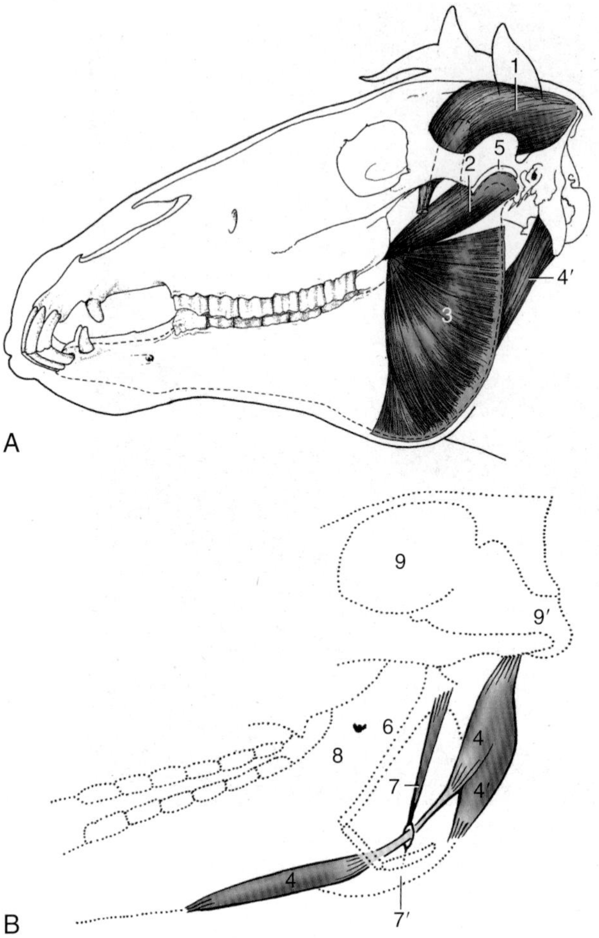

Fig. 18.23 (A) The deep masticatory muscles of the left side have been exposed by removal of the left mandibular ramus *(stippled)*. (B) Medial view of the right digastricus and some related structures. *1*, Temporalis; *2*, pterygoideus lateralis; *3*, lateral surface of pterygoideus medialis; *4*, digastricus; *4′*, occipitomandibularis; *5*, left temporomandibular joint; *6*, stylohyoid; *7*, stylohyoideus; *7′*, insertion of stylohyoideus on thyrohyoid; *8*, medial surface of right mandible and mandibular foramen; *9*, cranial cavity; *9′*, foramen magnum.

condyle and articular tubercle of the temporal bone (Fig. 18.23A/*5*). Hinge movements occur at the lower level, which is supported by a tight capsule; the lateral and slight protrusive movements occur at the upper level where the joint cavity is more capacious. The whole joint is supported by a fibrous lateral ligament and an elastic caudal one.

THE SALIVARY GLANDS

The *parotid gland* is clearly lobulated and has a firm texture and a yellow-gray or yellow-pink color. It is the largest salivary gland and extends ventrally from the base of the ear and wing of the atlas into the angle formed by the convergence of the maxillary and linguofacial veins and may possibly extend beyond this angle because the maxillary vein frequently tunnels through the gland substance (Fig. 18.7/*14*). The cranial margin is largely contained by the caudal border of the mandible, but a thin flange extends some distance over the masseter directly ventral to the jaw joint, where it covers the parotid lymph nodes. The lateral surface is overlain by a well-developed fascia that gives attachment to the parotidoauricularis muscle. The deep surface is related to the guttural pouch, the stylohyoid, the muscles that run to the corner of the jaw and open the mouth, and the combined insertion tendon of the brachiocephalicus and sternocephalicus, which separates it from the more deeply placed mandibular gland (Fig. 18.8).

The serous secretion of the parotid is drained by several sizable ducts that come together at the rostroventral angle of the gland to form a single channel. This crosses the tendon of the sternocephalicus before turning forward to run medial to the ventral border of the mandible. Accompanied by the facial vessels, it turns onto the face, where it ascends along the rostral margin of the masseter. It first lies caudal to the artery and vein but later shifts rostral to them. It ends by opening into the vestibule opposite the third upper cheek tooth. The duct is relatively exposed in the last part of its course and may be damaged in superficial wounds. Leakage is most profuse when feeding stimulates the flow of saliva.

The much smaller and crescentic *mandibular gland* extends from the basihyoid to the atlantal fossa and is thus partly under cover of the mandible (Figs. 18.8/*12* and 18.26/*5*). The superficial relations include the parotid gland and the medial pterygoid, sternocephalic, digastric, and occipitomandibular muscles. Its deep location puts it out of reach on palpation. The mandibular duct is formed along the concave rostral margin of the gland by the confluence of several ductules. It runs rostrally, covered by the mylohyoideus, and follows the medial aspect of the sublingual gland until it opens on the floor of the mouth at the small sublingual caruncle. The secretion is mixed.

The *sublingual gland* lies directly below the oral mucosa, between the body of the tongue and the medial surface of the mandible, extending as a thin strip from the symphysis to the level of the fifth cheek tooth (Fig. 18.26/*1*). It drains through numerous small ductules that open below the tongue.

Two rows of *buccal glands* are scattered along the dorsal and ventral margins of the buccinator. The glands of the dorsal series are more considerable and clump together caudally. Small salivary glands are found in the lips, soft palate, and tongue.

TABLE 18.2 A ROUGH GUIDE FOR THE AGING OF THE HORSE BY ITS TEETH

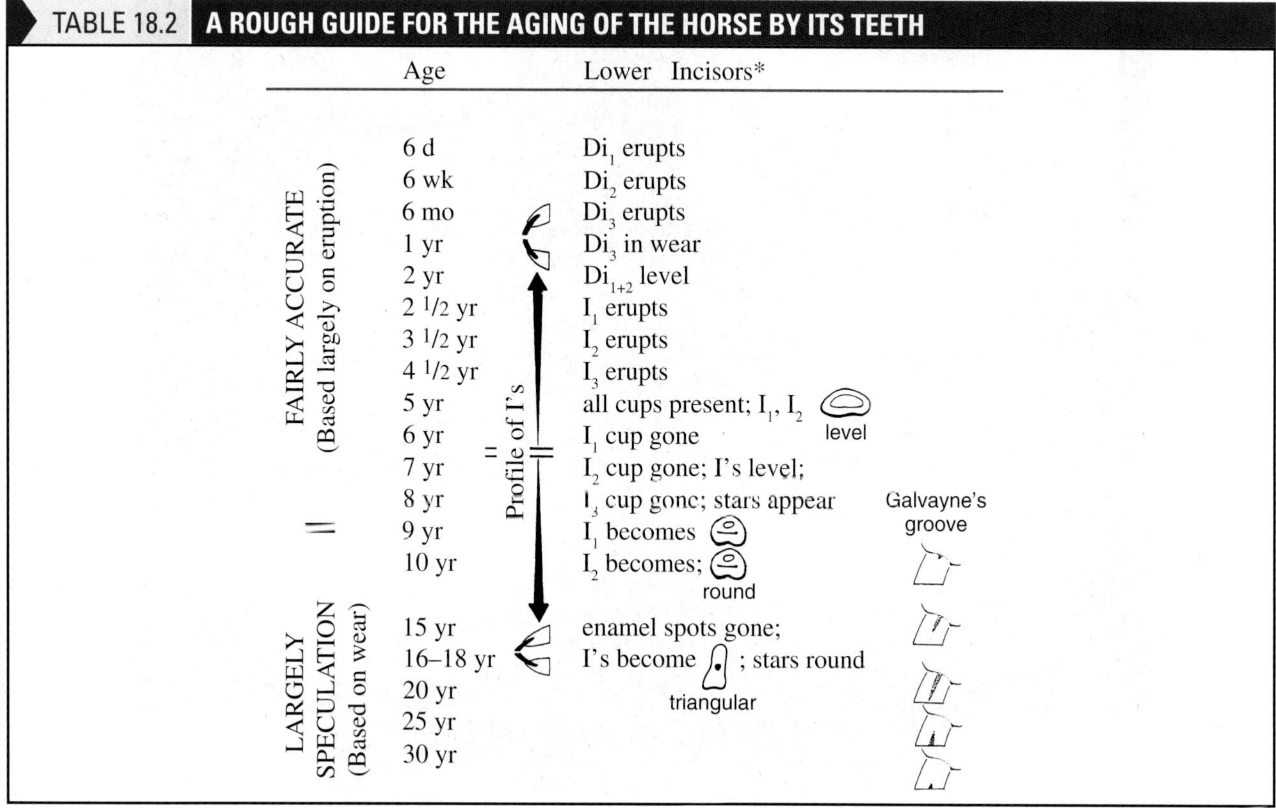

	Age	Lower Incisors*
FAIRLY ACCURATE (Based largely on eruption)	6 d	Di_1 erupts
	6 wk	Di_2 erupts
	6 mo	Di_3 erupts
	1 yr	Di_3 in wear
	2 yr	Di_{1+2} level
	2 1/2 yr	I_1 erupts
	3 1/2 yr	I_2 erupts
	4 1/2 yr	I_3 erupts
	5 yr	all cups present; I_1, I_2 level
	6 yr	I_1 cup gone
	7 yr	I_2 cup gone; I's level;
	8 yr	I_3 cup gone; stars appear
	9 yr	I_1 becomes round
	10 yr	I_2 becomes; round
LARGELY SPECULATION (Based on wear)	15 yr	enamel spots gone;
	16–18 yr	I's become triangular; stars round
	20 yr	
	25 yr	
	30 yr	

*It takes about 6 months for an erupted tooth to reach the height of its neighbors.
Di, deciduous incisor; *I*, incisor; *I's*, incisors.

THE PHARYNX AND GUTTURAL POUCH

The Pharynx

The pharynx lies wholly beneath the skull, to which the rostral third of its roof is directly applied. The remaining part of the roof and the lateral walls are enveloped by the guttural pouches (see further on). The lumen is clearly divided into upper and lower compartments by the soft palate and the palatopharyngeal arches, which extend over the lateral walls to meet directly above the entrance to the esophagus (Fig. 18.11). The most prominent features of the *nasopharynx* are the flaps guarding the entrances to the auditory tubes. Each tube is about 3 cm long and is pressed against the pharyngeal wall, presenting an oblique and rather sinuous ventral free edge (Fig. 18.27A). It is stiffened by a flange of cartilage, the expansion of the medial cartilage that supports the auditory tube. The slitlike opening lateral to the flap is normally held closed but becomes patent during swallowing to equalize the pressure on the two sides of the tympanic membrane. The maneuver, which can be observed endoscopically, involves the flap swinging medially while the soft palate rises and momentarily narrows the lumen of the nasopharynx (Fig. 18.28).

Endoscopy: The flap to the auditory tubes can also be elevated passively. It is a relatively simple matter to introduce an endoscope to examine, or a catheter to drain or irrigate, the guttural pouch. The entrance to the tube lies in the transverse plane of the lateral angle of the eye, which is a useful external guide to its position. The instrument encounters resistance during passage through the ventral meatus and nasopharynx. The firm support offered to its tip by the vertical lamina of the pterygoid bone is lost only a short distance rostral to the opening. Advancement of the instrument to this level generally provokes a swallowing movement when deflection of the cartilage flap facilitates entry to the pouch. Even when performed blindly, the absence of resistance to deeper penetration indicates that the pharyngotubal opening has been successfully passed.

The lower compartment of the pharynx is divided between the oropharynx and the laryngopharynx (Fig. 18.29/*4* and *5*). The narrow *oropharynx* extends between the attachment of the palatoglossal arches to the tongue and the epiglottis. Its lateral walls and floor contain

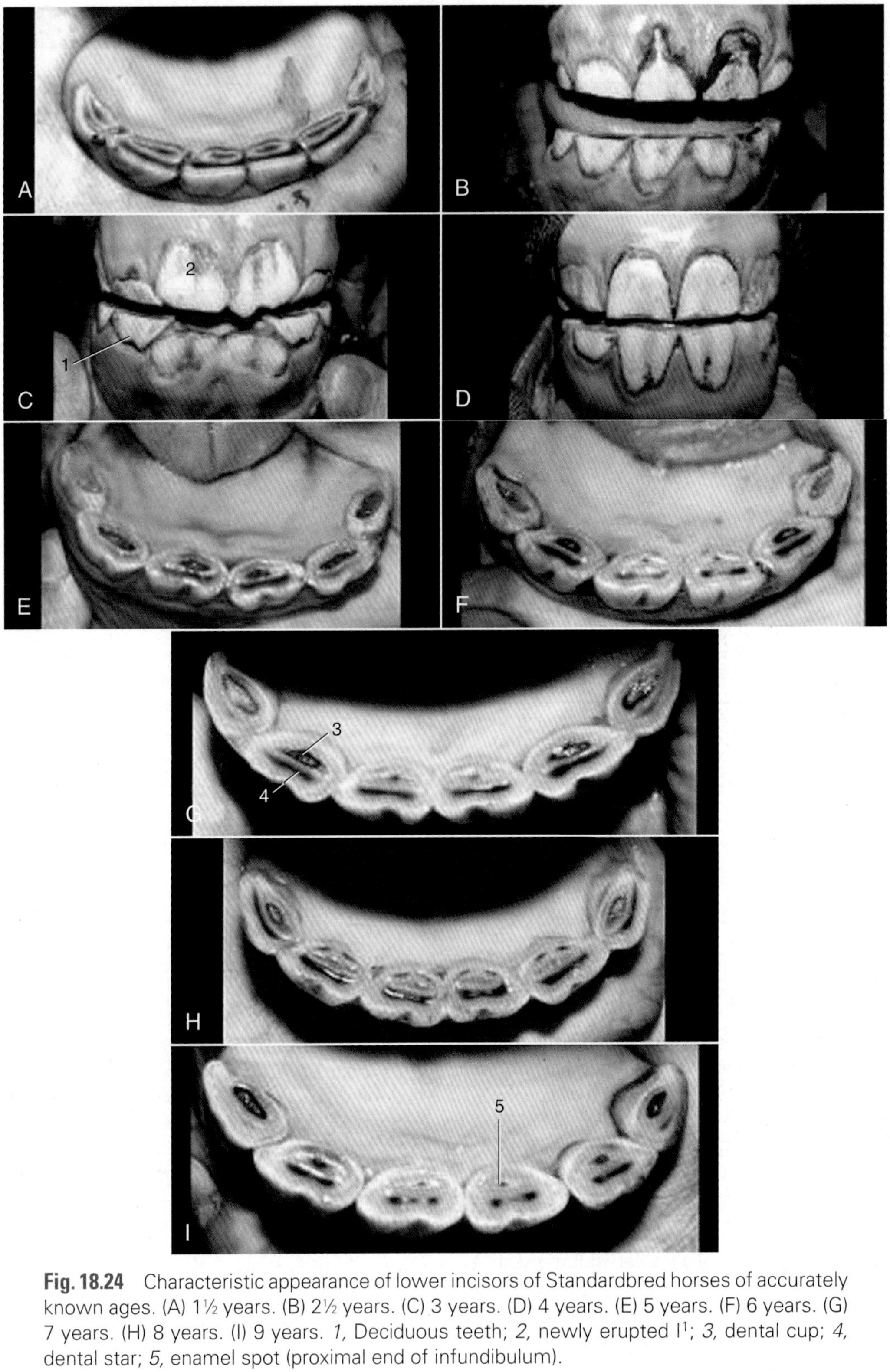

Fig. 18.24 Characteristic appearance of lower incisors of Standardbred horses of accurately known ages. (A) 1½ years. (B) 2½ years. (C) 3 years. (D) 4 years. (E) 5 years. (F) 6 years. (G) 7 years. (H) 8 years. (I) 9 years. *1,* Deciduous teeth; *2,* newly erupted I^1; *3,* dental cup; *4,* dental star; *5,* enamel spot (proximal end of infundibulum).

much diffuse tonsillar tissue, including the long palatine tonsil (see Fig. 3.26A). The *laryngopharynx* is largely occupied by the projection of the larynx, and its floor is reduced to the narrow flanking piriform recesses. The laryngopharynx narrows abruptly to the origin of the esophagus.

The structure and musculature follow the common pattern (Fig. 18.30). Difficulties in swallowing sometimes

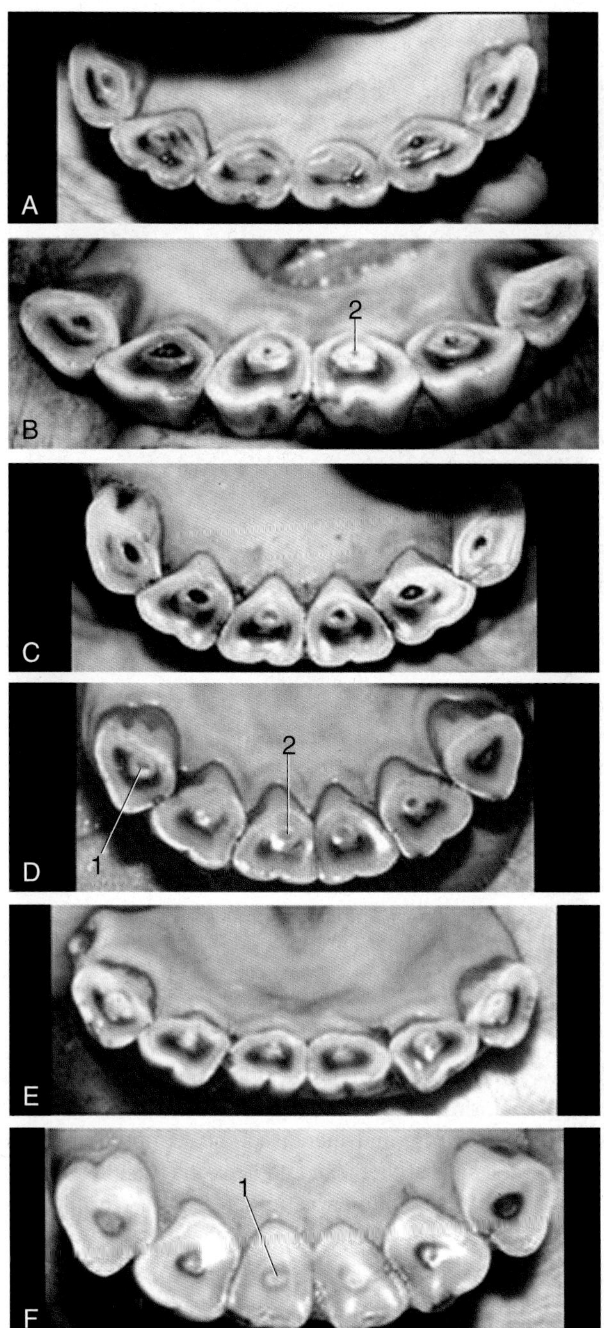

Fig. 18.25 Characteristic appearance of lower incisors of Standardbred horses of accurately known ages: (A) 11 years. (B) 12 years. (C) 14 years. (D) 16 years. (E) 17 years. (F) 20 years. Note particularity of the changes in form of the occlusal surface from round to triangular. *1*, Dental star; *2*, enamel spot.

arise from malfunction of the palatine and pharyngeal muscles. The cause frequently lies in involvement of the relevant glossopharyngeal and vagus nerves in infections of the guttural pouch; because the nerves run together, they are equally susceptible (Fig. 18.26/*7* and *14*).

The Guttural Pouch

The guttural pouch, a diverticulum of the auditory tube, is found in the horse and other Perissodactyla* (Fig. 18.31/*9*). It is formed by the escape of the mucosal lining of the tube through a ventral slit between medial and lateral supporting cartilages and attains a capacity of some 300 to 500 mL. It lies between the base of the skull and atlas dorsally and the pharynx and commencement of the esophagus ventrally; it is covered laterally by the pterygoid muscles and parotid and mandibular glands. Medially, the dorsal parts of the right and left sacs are separated by the ventral straight muscles of the head, but below this they meet, forming a thin median septum. The floor lies mainly on the pharynx but also covers and is molded to the stylohyoid, which raises a ridge that incompletely divides the medial and lateral compartments (Fig. 18.32).

More detailed relations include several cranial nerves and arteries that lie directly against the pouch as they pass to and from foramina in the caudal part of the skull. The glossopharyngeal, vagus, accessory, and hypoglossal nerves; the continuation of the sympathetic trunk beyond the cranial cervical ganglion; and the internal carotid artery are closely related for a stretch and together raise a mucosal fold that indents the medial compartment from behind. This is a conspicuous feature when the interior of the pouch is viewed endoscopically (Fig. 18.33/*4*). The facial nerve has a more limited contact with the dorsal part of the pouch. The large external carotid artery passes ventral to the medial compartment before crossing the lateral and then rostral walls of the lateral compartment (Fig. 18.33/*6*) in its approach (as the maxillary artery) to the alar canal. The pouch also directly covers the temporohyoid joint.

Function of the Guttural Pouch: The data now identify the pouch as a mechanism for cooling the cerebral blood supply, a mechanism that is peculiar to the horse (at least among domestic species) and additional to other devices found in mammals generally. The extensive contact between the extracranial part of the internal carotid artery and the exceedingly thin pouch wall cools the major (internal carotid) contribution to the cerebral blood supply. No local differences in blood temperature were registered in the resting animal, but a significant drop in temperature (of about 2°C) at the distal end of the artery was demonstrated in horses engaged in 15 minutes of strenuous exercise.

*It is also found in a small, strangely eclectic band of other species, including hyraxes, certain bats, and a South American mouse.

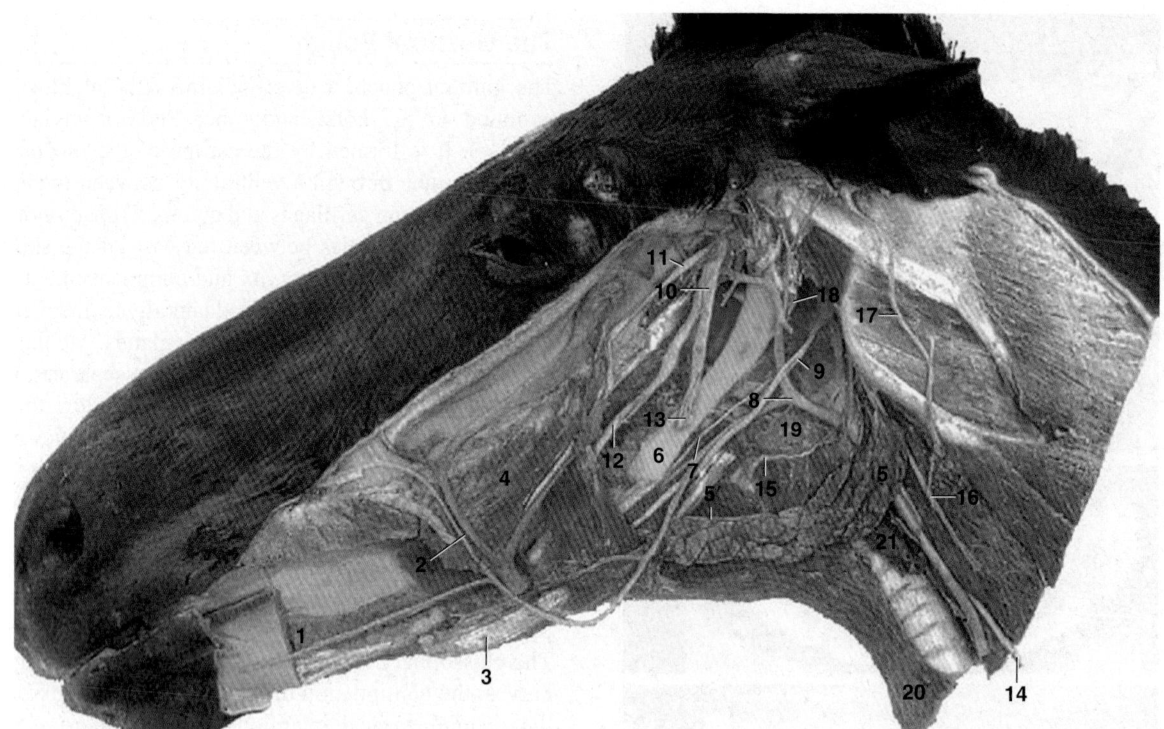

Fig. 18.26 Deep dissection of the head. The mandible and masticatory muscles have been removed. *1,* Sublingual gland; *2,* facial artery and vein; *3,* rostral belly of digastricus; *4,* buccinator; *5,* mandibular gland; *5′,* mandibular duct; *6,* stylohyoid; *7,* glossopharyngeal nerve (n.); *8,* linguofacial artery; *9,* hypoglossal n.; *10,* mandibular n.; *11,* masseteric n.; *12,* lingual n.; *13,* inferior alveolar n., cut where it enters the mandibular foramen; *14,* vagus and sympathetic trunk; *15,* cranial laryngeal n.; *16,* dorsal branch of spinal accessory n.; *17,* great auricular n.; *18,* guttural pouch; *19,* medial retropharyngeal lymph nodes; *20,* sternohyoideus; *21,* thyroid gland.

Clinical Conditions of Guttural Pouch

The mucous secretion of the lining normally drains into the pharynx through the pharyngotubal opening (Fig. 18.11/*8*) placed at the rostral end of the pouch, the most dependent part when the head is lowered. The connection opens when the horse swallows, and grazing normally promotes drainage. When the exit is blocked or the secretion accumulates for any reason, the pouch distends, producing a palpable, often visible swelling behind the jaw (Fig. 18.34). The guttural pouch may be infected with bacteria such as *Streptococcus equi equi* from the neighboring retropharyngeal lymph nodes. Mycotic infections of the guttural pouch also occur. The clinical signs include painful swelling of the parotid region, abnormal carriage of the head and neck, and nasal discharge. More frequent possible sequelae include inflammation of the middle ear (by extension of infection along the auditory tube), epistaxis (nasal bleeding) from erosion of the internal carotid artery, difficulty in swallowing following involvement of the glossopharyngeal and vagus nerves (or their pharyngeal branches), and laryngeal hemiplegia ("roaring") following vagus involvement. Other signs such as nasal congestion, drooping of the upper eyelid, pupillary constriction, sweating, and increased skin temperature over the affected side of the head and neck that result from the involvement of the sympathetic nerve form Horner syndrome. The facial and hypoglossal nerves and the external carotid artery are usually spared.

The pouch can be inspected or drained via the pharyngotubal opening or approached by open surgery through the Viborg triangle, which is an area bounded by the caudal border of the mandible (more deeply, the occipitomandibularis), the tendon of the sternocephalicus, and the linguofacial vein. The distance between the triangle and the pouch is greatly reduced when the pouch is enlarged. An alternative, more dorsal approach, involving reflection of the parotid gland is also employed.

Hemorrhage from the internal carotid artery is frequently fatal unless treated promptly by closure of the vessel on each side of the leak. A proximal ligature is easily applied, but direct access to a site distal to the lesion may be impossible. Recourse may then be had to a balloon-tipped

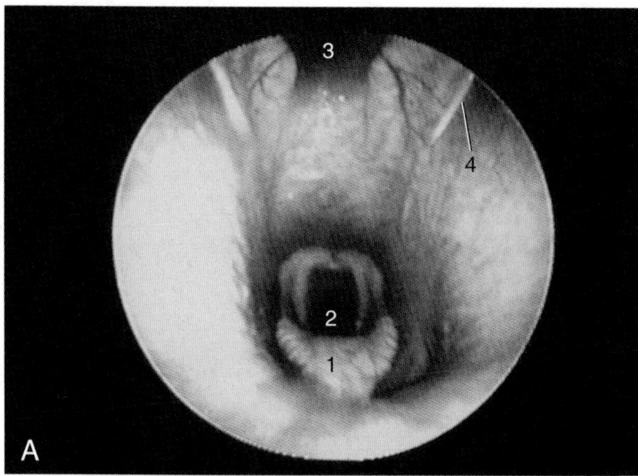

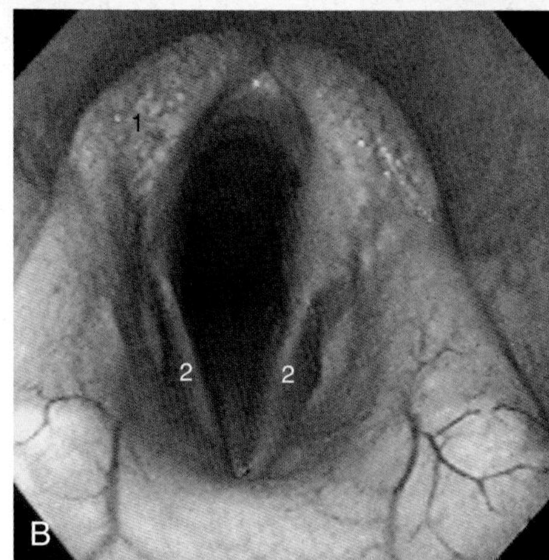

Fig. 18.27 (A) Endoscopic view of equine nasopharynx. *1,* Epiglottis; *2,* laryngeal entrance; *3,* pharyngeal recess; *4,* entrance to auditory tube. (B) Endoscopic view of larynx. *1,* Arytenoid cartilage; *2,* left and right vocal folds.

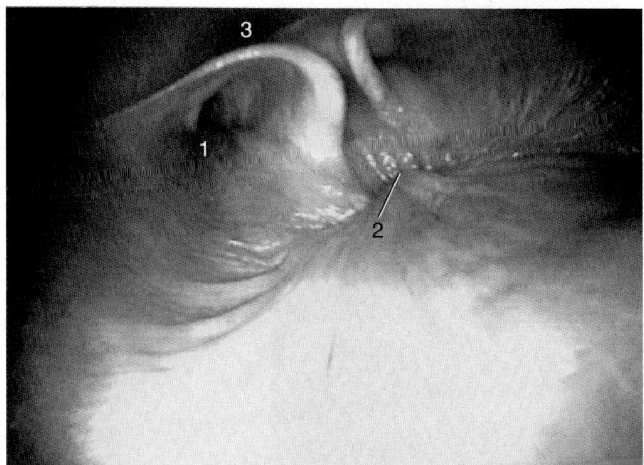

Fig. 18.28 Endoscopic view of the caudal part of equine nasopharynx (foal). *1,* Entrance to auditory tube; *2,* closure of the intrapharyngeal ostium between the nasopharynges and laryngopharynges (during swallowing); *3,* cartilage flange supporting the auditory tube.

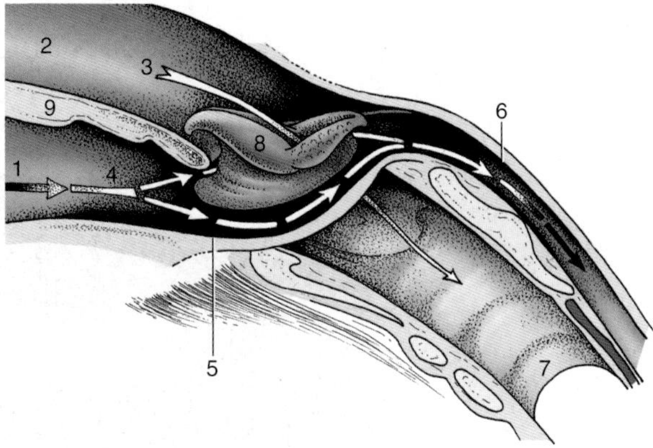

Fig. 18.29 The communications of the pharynx, rostrally with the oral and nasal cavities and caudally with the esophagus (schematic). The *broken arrows* mark the digestive pathway; the *unbroken arrow* marks the respiratory pathway. *1,* Oral cavity; *2,* nasal cavity; *3,* nasopharynx; *4,* oropharynx; *5,* laryngopharynx; *6,* esophagus; *7,* trachea; *8,* epiglottis, laryngeal entrance; *9,* soft palate.

catheter, which is introduced beyond the proximal ligature and advanced into the siphon-like formation that the artery displays immediately before entering the cranial cavity. The catheter is left in place until it is judged that thrombosis will have sealed the damaged segment of the artery.

In foals, malfunction of the pharyngotubal opening may result in the pouch becoming distended with air to the extent that a swelling is visible externally (Fig. 18.34). It appears that in some horses there may be a redundancy of the mucosal fold (plica salpingopharyngea) that is normally present at the entry of the tube. In these individuals the excess mucosa creates a one-way valve that allows air to be drawn into the pouch but not expelled from it. Unilateral tympany may be relieved by forcing an opening in the median septum so that both pouches communicate with the pharynx through a single opening. When swelling is bilateral, an alternative surgical method has to be used.

THE LARYNX

The larynx is suspended by the hyoid apparatus and is partly contained within the intermandibular space (see Fig. 4.8). Although few distinguishing features of the cartilages are important, attention must be drawn to the deep notch in the ventral part of the thyroid cartilage because this provides very convenient access to the interior after incision of the cricothyroid ligament. A prominence rostral to the notch and the ventral part of the cricoid arch provide the necessary landmarks (see Fig. 4.13/*7*), but the basihyoid may also be used to confirm the site of the initial skin incision. The normally retrovelar position of the leaf-shaped epiglottis has been pointed out (Fig. 18.11/*11*).

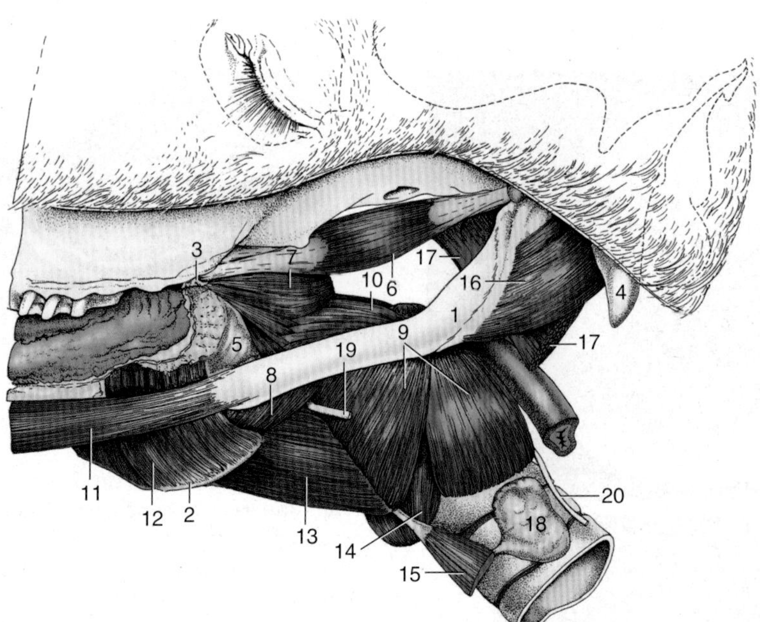

Fig. 18.30 Muscles of the pharynx, soft palate, and hyoid apparatus. *1,* Stylohyoid; *2,* thyrohyoid; *3,* hamulus of pterygoid bone; *4,* paracondylar process; *5,* buccopharyngeal fascia; *6,* tensor veli palatini; *7,* rostral pharyngeal constrictor; *8,* middle pharyngeal constrictor; *9,* caudal pharyngeal constrictor (thyropharyngeus and cricopharyngeus); *10,* stylopharyngeus caudalis; *11,* styloglossus; *12,* hyoglossus; *13,* thyrohyoideus; *14,* cricothyroideus; *15,* sternothyroideus; *16,* occipitohyoideus; *17,* longus capitis (stump); *18,* thyroid gland; *19,* cranial laryngeal nerve; *20,* caudal (recurrent) laryngeal nerve.

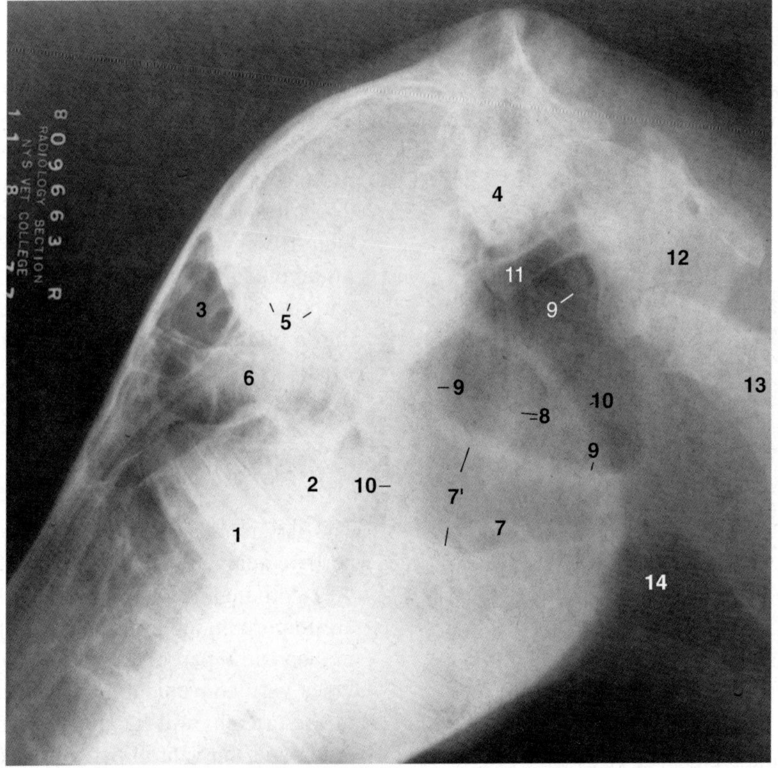

Fig. 18.31 Lateral radiographic view of the head to show the position of the guttural pouches *(9)* in a horse 1½ years old (estimated). *1,* M^1; *2,* unerupted M^2; *3,* frontal sinus; *4,* petrous temporal bone; *5,* caudal border of orbit; *6,* ethmoid labyrinth; *7,* epiglottis; *7′,* nasopharynx; *8,* stylohyoid bones; *9,* borders of guttural pouches; *10,* rostral and caudal borders of mandible; *11,* base of skull; *12,* atlas; *13,* axis; *14,* larynx.

The mucosa forms outpouchings (ventricles) that pass laterally between the vocal and vestibular folds but remain within the protection of the thyroid laminae. The ventricular entrance is sufficiently large to admit the bur that is used to evert the sac in one of the "roaring" operations (Fig. 18.35/*1*).

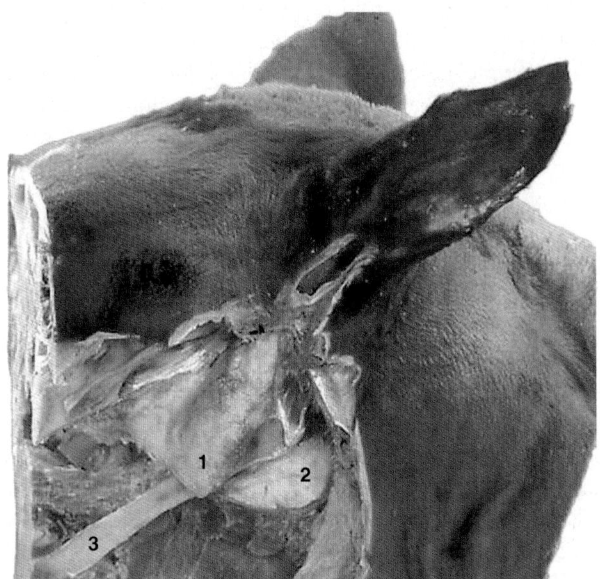

Fig. 18.32 Position of the guttural pouch in relation to the skull and stylohyoid. *1,* Lateral compartment of guttural pouch; *2,* medial compartment of guttural pouch; *3,* stylohyoid.

The interference with the normal dilation of the glottis during inspiration diminishes the respiratory efficiency. The condition known as *roaring,* from the strident sound emitted at inspiration, is commonly seen in high-performance horses. In its severe form it is characterized by unilateral adduction of the arytenoid cartilage and vocal cord; in less severe forms it is identified by limited abduction of these structures. The abnormal sound is produced by passive vibration of a lax vocal cord in the airstream as a result of dysfunction or even atrophy of part of the intrinsic laryngeal musculature. The pathology is almost always on the left side and is initially seen in the cricoarytenoideus dorsalis, the abductor muscle of the cartilage, before involving other adductors in the larynx (see Fig. 4.15/*5*). The asymmetry in incidence may be due to differences in the course of the right and left recurrent laryngeal nerves. The change in the contour of the larynx resulting from loss of function of the cricoarythenoideus dorsalis can be appreciated with palpation. The hollowed space above the arytenoid cartilage makes the muscular process of the cartilage more prominent.

The roaring can be relieved through the reinforcement of the wasted dorsal cricoarytenoideus muscle by a suture tightened to fix the arytenoid cartilage in permanent abduction. An older alternative was the eversion and excision of

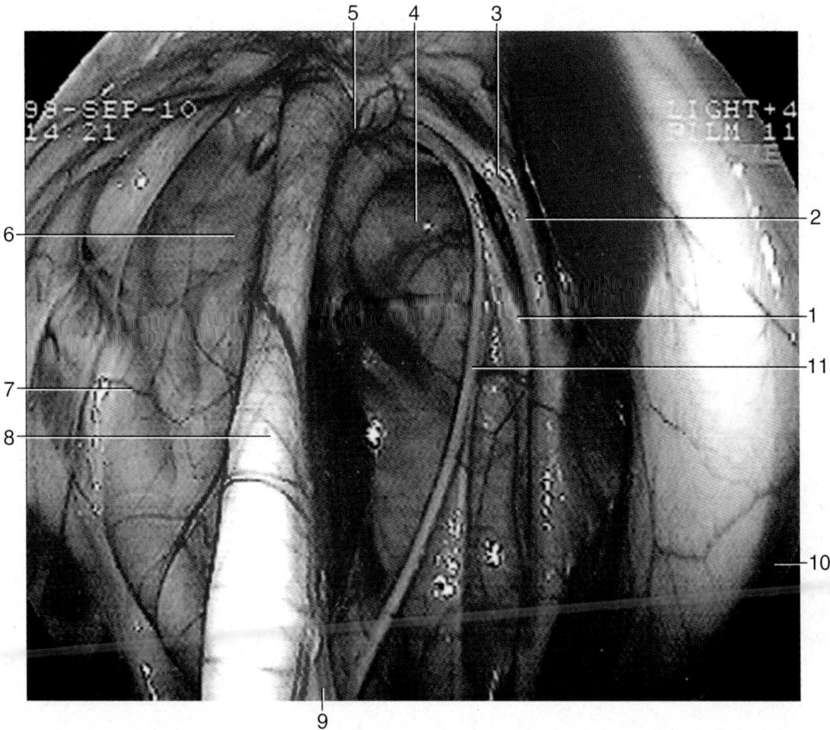

Fig. 18.33 Endoscopic view of the interior of the guttural pouch. *1,* Hypoglossal nerve; *2,* vagus nerve; *3,* internal carotid artery; *4,* medial compartment; *5,* articulation of the stylohyoid and petrous temporal bone; *6,* lateral compartment; *7,* external carotid artery; *8,* stylohyoid bone; *9,* stylopharyngeus muscle; *10,* longus capitis muscle; *11,* glossopharyngeal nerve.

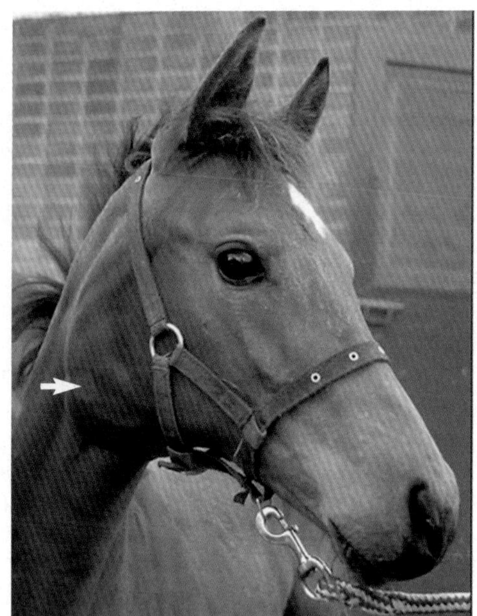

Fig. 18.34 Tympany of the guttural pouch *(arrow).*

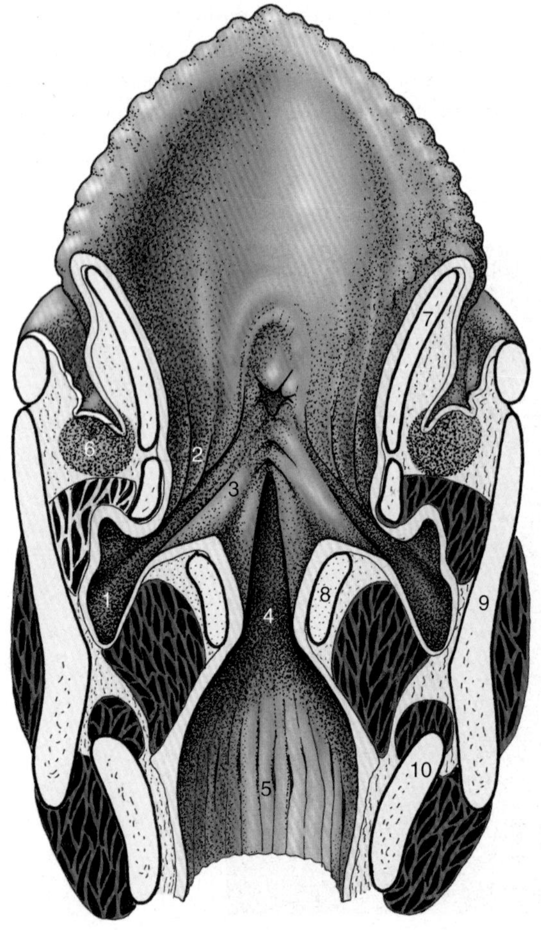

Fig. 18.35 Dorsal section of the larynx. *1,* Laryngeal ventricle; *2,* vestibular fold with ventricularis; *3,* vocal fold with vocalis; *4,* glottic cleft; *5,* infraglottic cavity; *6,* caudal end of palatine tonsil; *7,* epiglottic cartilage; *8,* arytenoid cartilage; *9,* thyroid cartilage; *10,* cricoid cartilage.

the lateral laryngeal ventricle in the expectation that the resulting scar tissue would bind this cartilage to the thyroid cartilage. Both operations result in tightening of the vocal fold and widening of the glottic cleft. Neither operation effects a cure of the condition, which has human and canine parallels. Other defects, such as partial collapse of an arytenoepiglottic fold or prolapse of the cricotracheal membrane, may also cause obstruction. It is noteworthy that multiple defects, possibly involving nasal, pharyngeal, and laryngeal levels, are quite common. Recently a syndrome of deformities that may afflict the derivates (the pharynx, larynx, and upper esophagus) of the fourth branchial arch has been described.

THE EYE

Some account has been given of the external features of the eye (p. 494). The adnexa call for little comment. The *lacrimal gland* is relatively large and placed over the dorsolateral aspect of the bulbus, where it is protected by the adjacent part of the orbital rim (Fig. 18.36/*1*). A small accessory lacrimal gland is associated with the deep part of the cartilage of the third eyelid.

The *nasolacrimal duct,* already mentioned in relation to surgical access to the maxillary sinus, provides a conspicuous feature where it opens on the floor of the nostril (Fig. 18.3). The extraocular muscles show little that is distinctive; as is common in ungulates, the retractor bulbi is relatively large (see Fig. 9.19/*7*).

The eyeball shows significant departure from the spheroidal form—it is compressed from front to back and is higher than it is wide—which is relevant to the concept of the ramp retina (see further on). It is constructed of the usual layers. The *sclera* is relatively thin toward the equator, where it obtains a bluish tint from the pigmentation of the underlying choroid. The *cornea* is relatively small and ovoid; its pointed end is lateral.

The *choroid* exhibits a triangular green or bluish-green tapetum dorsal to the optic disk (Fig. 18.37). The ciliary muscle is poorly developed; a second point is adduced in support of the theory of the ramp retina as the means of accommodation. The iris is generally dark brown; in the absence of pigmentation (a rather uncommon anomaly) it is a rather unattractive bluish color ("walleye") (see Fig. 9.10B). Both the iris and the pupillary opening within it are oval (with the long axes horizontal), but the pupil becomes rounder when contracted. The pupil of the newborn is almost round. Both margins of the pupil, but particularly the upper one, carry irregular granular excrescences interpreted as "shades" that limit the entry of light (see Fig. 9.9/*3*).

The *optic disk,* very prominent on ophthalmoscopic examination of the fundus, is placed ventral to the tapetum and ventrolateral to the posterior pole of the bulb (Fig. 18.37). The macula is said to comprise both round and

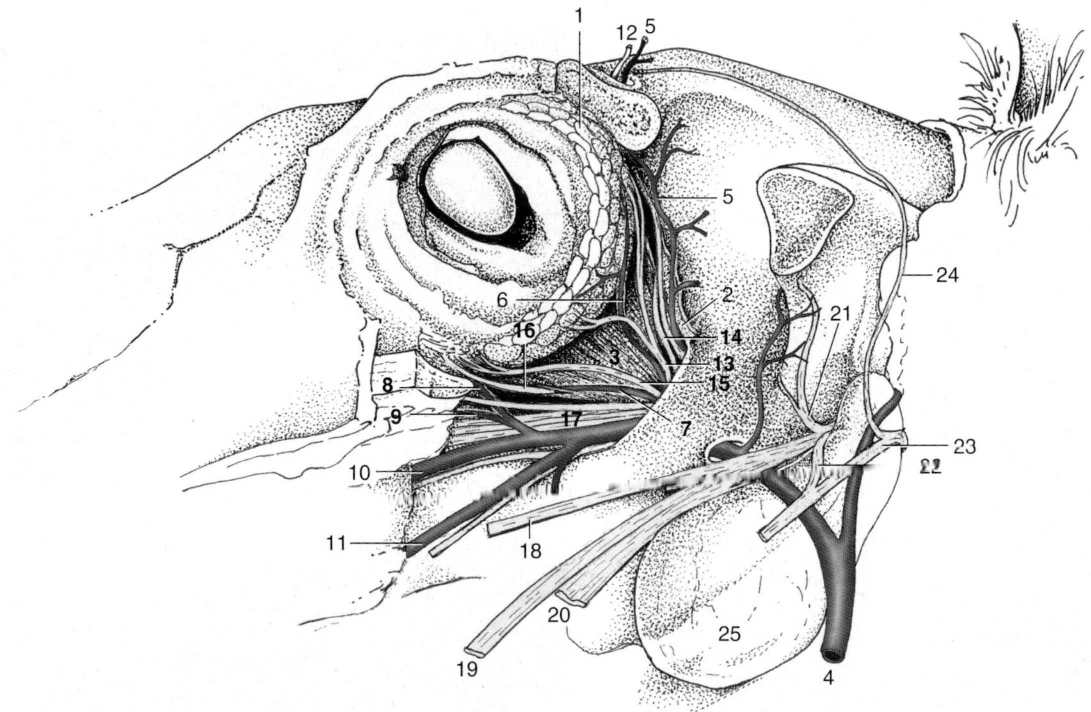

Fig. 18.36 Dissection of the orbit; the zygomatic arch and periorbita have been removed. *1,* Lacrimal gland; *2,* periorbita; *3,* lateral rectus; *4,* maxillary artery (a.); *5,* supraorbital a.; *6,* lacrimal a.; *7,* muscular branch of external ophthalmic a.; *8,* malar a.; *9,* infraorbital a.; *10,* major palatine a.; *11,* buccal a.; *12,* supraorbital nerve (n.); *13,* lacrimal n.; *14,* trochlear n.; *15,* zygomatic n.; *16,* oculomotor n.; *17,* rostral branches of maxillary n.; *18,* buccal n.; *19,* lingual n.; *20,* inferior alveolar n.; *21,* masticatory n.; *22,* auriculotemporal n.; *23,* facial n.; *24,* auriculopalpebral n.; *25,* guttural pouch.

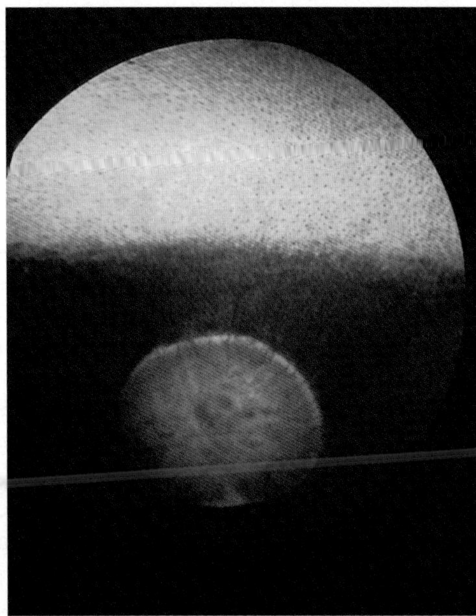

Fig. 18.37 Fundus of eye of horse.

elongated parts; it is asserted that the former is concerned with binocular vision, the latter with monocular vision. The central artery of the retina is poorly developed, and the few straight branches that radiate from the margins of the disk soon fade. Much the larger part of the retina is nourished by the vessels of the middle tunic. There is nothing noteworthy in the refractive media.

It is believed that the poor development of the ciliary muscle compels the horse to rely on the distorted form of the bulb for accommodation. The upper part of the retina, which is at a greater distance from the lens, serves for near vision; the lower part, closer to the lens, serves for distance vision. The animal therefore adjusts the carriage of the head—and thereby the location of the image on the retina—as a means of focusing. The technique is sometimes well illustrated by a horse approaching and jumping an obstacle.

THE VENTRAL PART OF THE NECK

The ventral part of the neck contains the visceral space occupied by the esophagus, trachea, and other structures passing

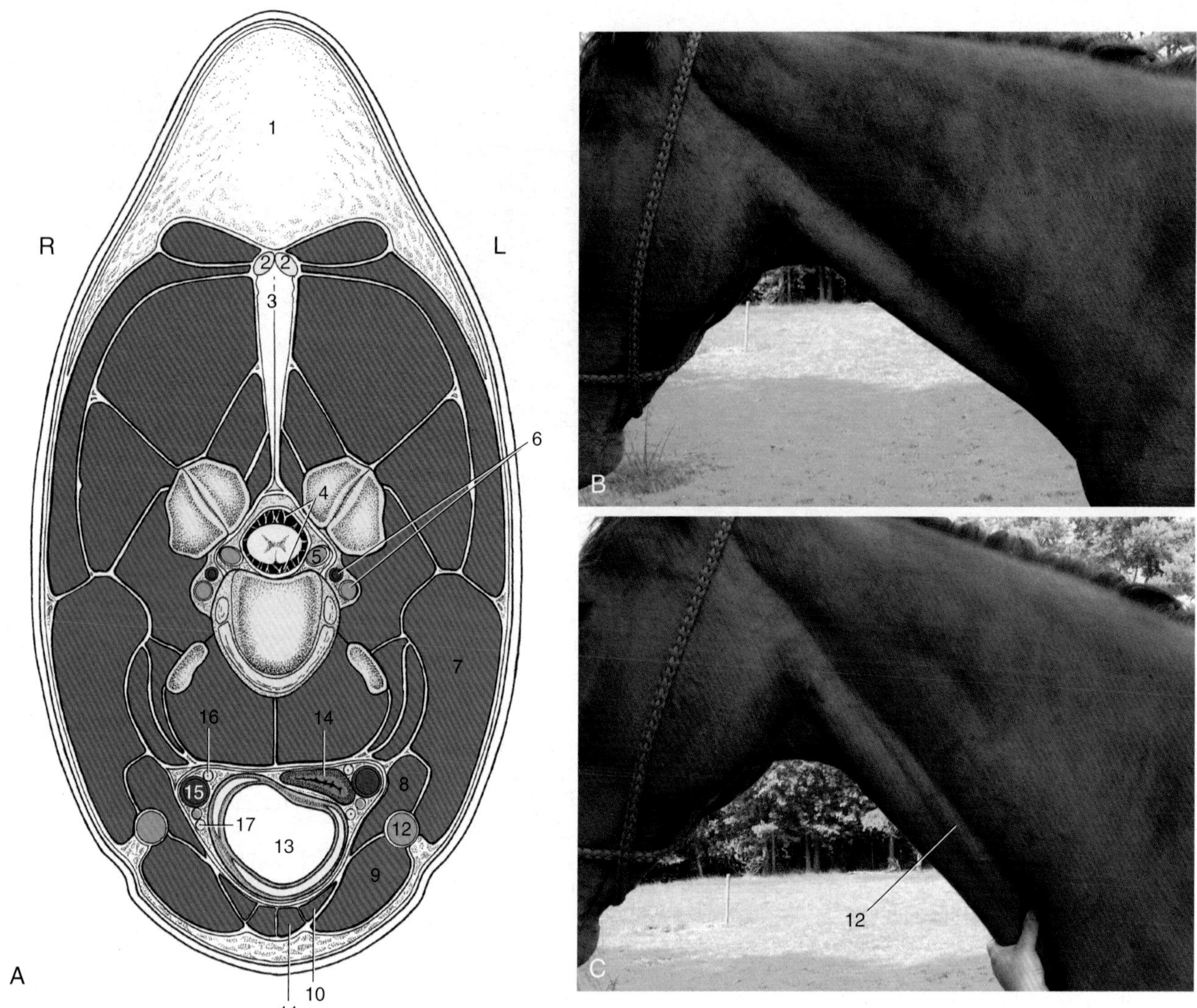

Fig. 18.38 (A) Transection of the neck at the level of the fourth cervical vertebra. *L,* Left side; *R,* right side. (B) and (C) The external jugular vein is not visible (B), but it is raised (C) when occluded in the jugular groove. *1,* Crest; *2* and *3,* funicular and laminar parts of nuchal ligament, respectively; *4,* subarachnoid space; *5,* internal vertebral venous plexus; *6,* vertebral artery and vein; *7,* brachiocephalicus; *8,* omohyoideus; *9,* sternocephalicus; *10,* sternothyroideus; *11,* sternohyoideus; *12,* external jugular vein; *13,* trachea; *14,* esophagus; *15,* common carotid artery; *16,* vagosympathetic trunk; *17,* recurrent laryngeal nerve.

between the head and the thorax. This space is bounded dorsally by the muscles below the vertebrae and laterally and ventrally by flatter muscles united by stout fasciae. The foremost lateroventral muscles are the brachiocephalicus and sternocephalicus, which bound the groove occupied by the (external) jugular vein (Fig. 18.38/*12*). The caudal part of this groove is covered by the cutaneous muscle of the neck, which radiates from a manubrial origin; the muscle thins as it passes from its origin, which increases the prominence of the cranial part of the vein, the obvious target when the vein is raised for puncture (Fig. 18.39/*9* and *11*). The brachiocephalicus is described on p. 574.

The right and left *sternocephalicus muscles* arise from the manubrium side by side but diverge toward their mandibular insertions (Fig. 18.39/*8*). This leaves a median space through which the trachea may be palpated, although it is still covered by the thin *sternothyroideus* and *sternohyoideus* (Fig. 18.39/*6*). These are combined at their origin from the sternum but branch into slips that diverge to attach to the thyroid cartilage and the basihyoid. The omohyoideus (Fig. 18.39/*7*), which extends between the medial aspect of the shoulder and the basihyoid, forms the floor of the jugular groove. It is said, unconvincingly, to protect the more deeply placed

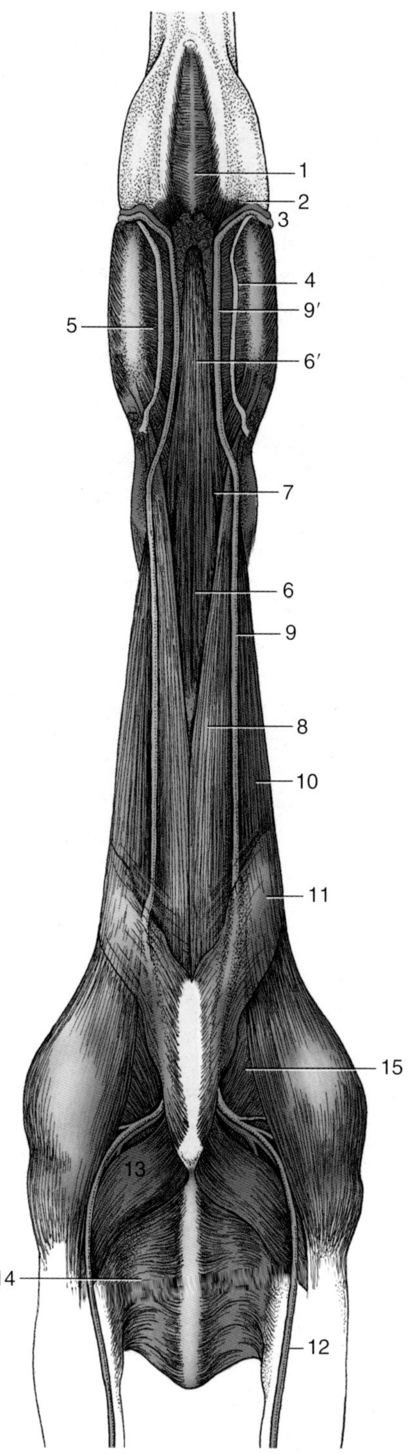

Fig. 18.39 Ventral view of the neck and intermandibular space. *1,* Mylohyoideus; *2,* mandibular lymph nodes; *3,* facial artery and vein; *4,* parotid duct; *5,* medial pterygoid; *6,* sternohyoideus and sternothyroideus; *6′,* combined sternohyoideus and omohyoideus; *7,* omohyoideus; *8,* sternocephalicus; *9,* external jugular vein; *9′,* linguofacial vein; *10,* brachiocephalicus; *11,* cutaneous colli; *12,* cephalic vein; *13,* pectoralis descendens; *14,* pectoralis transversus; *15,* subclavius.

common carotid artery in unskillful venipuncture (Fig. 18.38/*15*). The muscles ventral to the trachea constitute the "strap muscles" that are resected in Forsell's operation for cribbing, which is a condition of stabled horses in which a horse hangs onto the crib with its teeth and dilates the pharynx to swallow air.

The *trachea* occupies a median position in the visceral space. Its size bears no constant relation to that of the body, which is an important point when selecting an endotracheal tube because the generous size of the glottis is not a limiting factor. The tracheal lumen is slightly flattened dorsoventrally and is of course maintained patent by the tracheal rings. It is therefore customary to completely transect as few cartilages as possible to avoid collapse of the wall in tracheotomy operations.

The *esophagus* begins dorsal to the trachea but slips to the left side by the middle of the neck (Fig. 18.38/*14*). It then slowly creeps back toward a median position, though it is often ventral to the trachea just before it enters the chest. It takes a more direct course when the neck is extended. The esophagus is too soft to identify easily on palpation, but its position is revealed when the animal swallows.

The *common carotid artery* lies ventral to the trachea at the base of the neck but gradually ascends to a more dorsal position (Fig. 18.38/*15*). It divides above the pharynx into the occipital, internal carotid, and external carotid arteries. The internal carotid supplies the brain, and the occipital supplies the region of the poll. The overall pattern of distribution of the external carotid artery is shown in Fig. 18.40. Pulsations of the common carotid may sometimes be felt in the middle of the neck when the artery is pressed against the subvertebral muscles. Nowadays, puncture at this site may be employed for the provision of a sample of arterial blood. The artery is enclosed in a thick fascial sheath shared with the vagosympathetic trunk, which follows its dorsal border. The recurrent laryngeal nerve lies ventral to it in the tracheal fascia (Fig. 18.38/*16* and *17*).

The *deep cervical lymph nodes* are scattered in packets—cranial, middle, and caudal—along the course of the tracheal lymph duct. The caudal group receives the outflow from the superficial cervical nodes (Fig. 18.41).

The *external jugular vein* is supplemented by the vertebral vein and the plexus within the vertebral canal in the drainage of the head. It is formed at the caudoventral angle of the parotid gland by the confluence of maxillary and linguofacial veins. It stands out very prominently and very conveniently for injection and sampling when raised by pressure over the jugular groove.

The lobes of the *thyroid gland* can be recognized on palpation as soft ovoid structures placed dorsolateral to the first part of the trachea (Fig. 18.26/*21*). They are joined ventrally by a narrow isthmus.

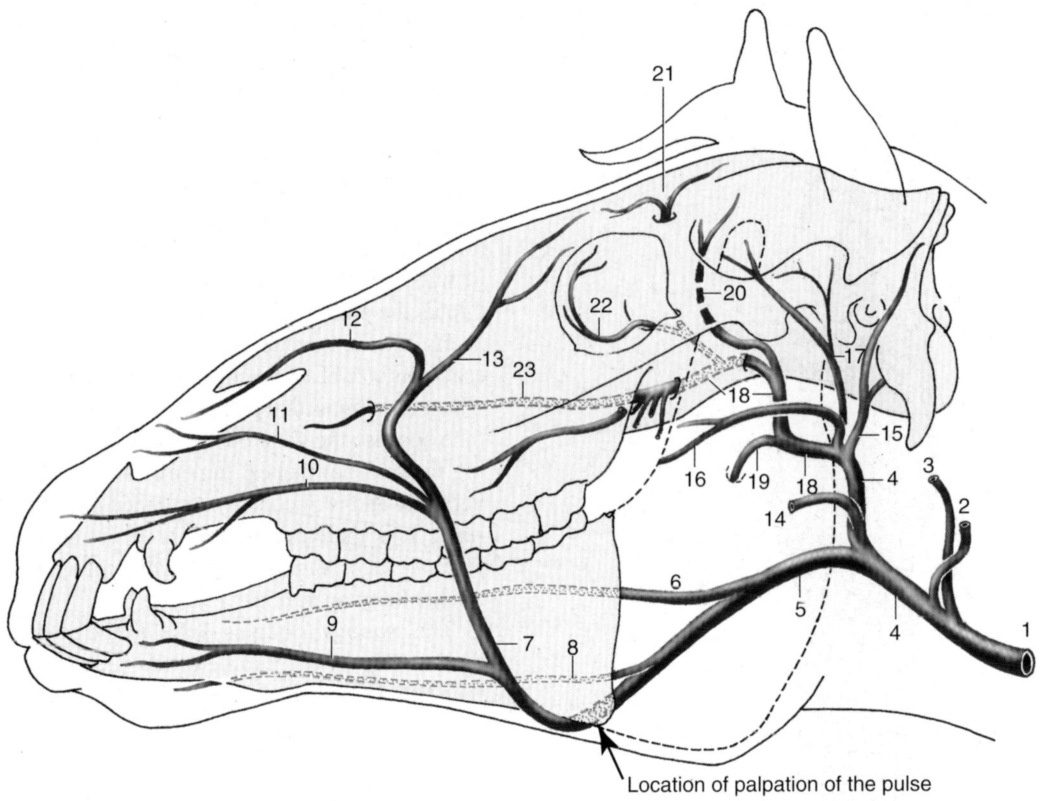

Fig. 18.40 Principal arteries of the head (schematic). *1,* Common carotid artery (a.); *2,* occipital a.; *3,* internal carotid a.; *4,* external carotid a.; *5,* linguofacial a.; *6,* lingual a.; *7,* facial a.; *8,* sublingual a.; *9,* inferior labial a.; *10,* superior labial a.; *11,* lateral nasal a.; *12,* dorsal nasal a.; *13,* angularis oculi a.; *14,* masseteric a.; *15,* caudal auricular a.; *16,* transverse facial a., displaced ventrally for clarity; *17,* superficial temporal a.; *18,* maxillary a.; *19,* inferior alveolar a.; *20,* caudal deep temporal a.; *21,* supraorbital a.; *22,* malar a.; *23,* infraorbital a.

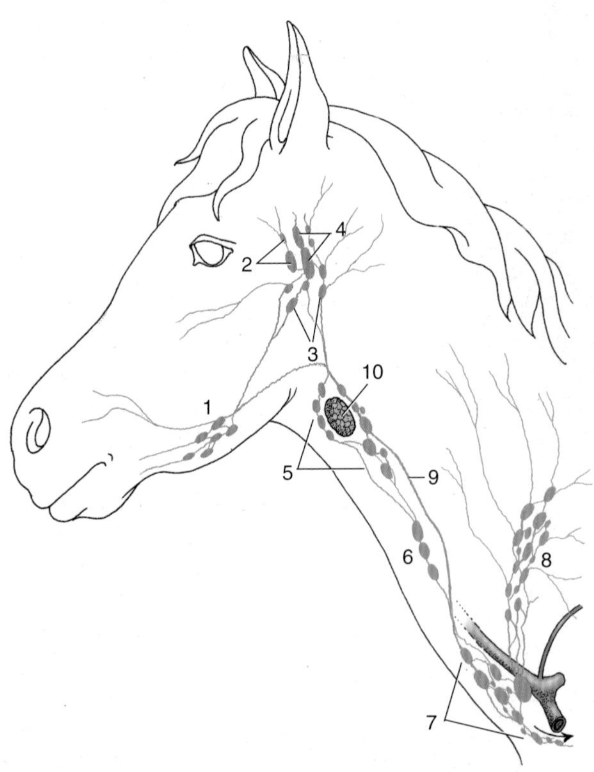

Fig. 18.41 Lymphatic structures of the head and neck (schematic). *1,* Mandibular lymph nodes; *2,* parotid lymph nodes; *3,* medial retropharyngeal lymph nodes; *4,* lateral retropharyngeal lymph nodes; *5, 6,* and *7,* cranial, middle, and caudal deep cervical lymph nodes, respectively; *8,* superficial cervical lymph nodes; *9,* tracheal duct; *10,* thyroid gland.

Although rarely as well developed as in the calf, a cervical part of the *thymus* may extend beside the trachea in the caudal part of the neck of the foal. It is often separated from the thoracic part and may be broken into several masses.

THE LYMPHATIC STRUCTURES OF THE HEAD AND NECK

The parotid, mandibular, and deep cervical lymph nodes have been encountered (p. 520). The superficial cervical nodes are described on page 607.

The *retropharyngeal nodes* are arranged in clumps on the pharyngeal wall (Fig. 18.26/*19*). The lateral group is also related to the guttural pouch, lying caudal to it within the atlantal fossa. Infection of these nodes, frequently leading to abscess formation (strangles), may be followed by contamination of the guttural pouch with the potential sequelae already mentioned (p. 512). The pattern of drainage is such that the medial retropharyngeal nodes serve as the collecting center for all lymph emanating from the upper part of the head (Fig. 18.41/*3*).

COMPREHENSION CHECK

Describe the anatomic basis of "roaring," a condition seen in the horse.

Use the equine skull to understand the arrangement of paranasal sinuses and describe the methods to access their interior.

Describe the anatomic relationships of the guttural pouch.

19 The Neck, Back, and Vertebral Column of the Horse

This chapter is concerned with the dorsal part of the neck, the back, the loins, and the tail. The ventral part of the neck was considered with the head; the croup is considered with the hindlimb.

CONFORMATION AND SURFACE FEATURES

The neck and back vary considerably in conformation according to breed, sex, age, and condition. The dorsal contour of the back and loins closely reflects the course of the vertebral column, but that of the neck, where the vertebrae are more deeply buried, depends largely on the nuchal ligament and crest (see further on).

The neck may be arched, straight, or hollowed in the natural standing posture. The arched form, known to horsemen as a *swan neck* or *peacock neck,* is characteristic of certain breeds, including the Lipizzaner. The concave form, or ewe neck, is not prized, and for most breeds it is the straight neck that is held in greatest esteem. The transition between the neck and withers may be smooth or marked by a dip. In saddle horses the neck deepens considerably toward the chest, but the change is usually less marked in the heavier draft breeds. Viewed from above, the neck is relatively narrow and of even width, except immediately before the shoulder where the mergence with the trunk is eased by the presence of the subclavius, which fills out the hollow along the cranial margin of the scapula. The heavy neck of the stallion is mainly due to the strong development of the fatty fibrous tissue (crest) dorsal to the nuchal ligament (see Fig. 18.38/*1* and *3*).

The course of the cervical vertebrae may not be evident on simple scrutiny, although the wing of the atlas is almost always a visible and palpable landmark. The positions of the transverse and articular processes of the third to sixth neck vertebrae may be visible in animals that are lean or in poor condition. These features are usually detectable on palpation, although in fat or particularly well-muscled horses, it may be impossible to gain more than a general impression of the course of the vertebrae (Fig. 19.1). In thin-skinned horses certain of the superficial muscles (especially the trapezius and rhomboideus) stand out as individual surface features when tensed (Fig. 19.2/*1* and *8*).

The characteristic prominence of the withers is due to the great length of the spinous processes of the second to ninth thoracic vertebrae, the scapular cartilages, and associated muscles. The high and long withers of moderate width are preferred in saddle animals because excessive narrowness may make a proper fit of the saddle difficult.

Behind the withers the line of the back is more or less straight, and though it slopes up somewhat toward the croup, this is only occasionally so exaggerated that the horse can be said to be "croup high." There is, however, a tendency for the back to sag in older animals, in those in poor condition, and in mares advanced in pregnancy. The cranial part of the back merges smoothly with the lateral chest and abdominal wall.

The caudal part (the loins) tends to be broader and flatter and merges with the flanks without the sharp change in contour that is so striking in ruminants. The transverse processes of the lumbar vertebrae are not palpable. The spinous processes of the lumbar and caudal thoracic vertebrae may be palpated, though rarely so easily that they can be separately identified and counted. A median groove between the muscles of the loins and croup is most marked in draft animals.

The dorsal contour of the croup is convex and slopes toward the root of the tail, sometimes—commonly in the Lipizzaner and Belgian breeds—so steeply as to merit the description "goose rump."

THE VERTEBRAL COLUMN

The vertebral column comprises 7 cervical, 18 thoracic, 6 lumbar, 5 sacral, and about 20 caudal vertebrae. Variations in number are not uncommon, with the most frequent being the reduction of the lumbar vertebrae to 5, especially in the Arabian. The impression of shortness in the loins in other breeds is more often due to a marked caudal inclination of the last ribs.

The vertebral column inclines ventrally below the withers to reach its lowest point at the cervicothoracic junction, although the external elevation creates a contrary impression. It then changes direction abruptly, and as it ascends toward the poll, it shifts closer to the dorsal contour (Fig. 19.1).

The cervical vertebrae are individually long. Those behind the axis have rudimentary spinous processes, large divided transverse processes, and broad articular surfaces. The thoracic vertebrae are unremarkable apart from the great length of the spinous processes that form the basis of the withers. Independent centers of ossification develop for the summits of the first 12 or so spinous processes, and these may not fuse until comparatively late (10 or more

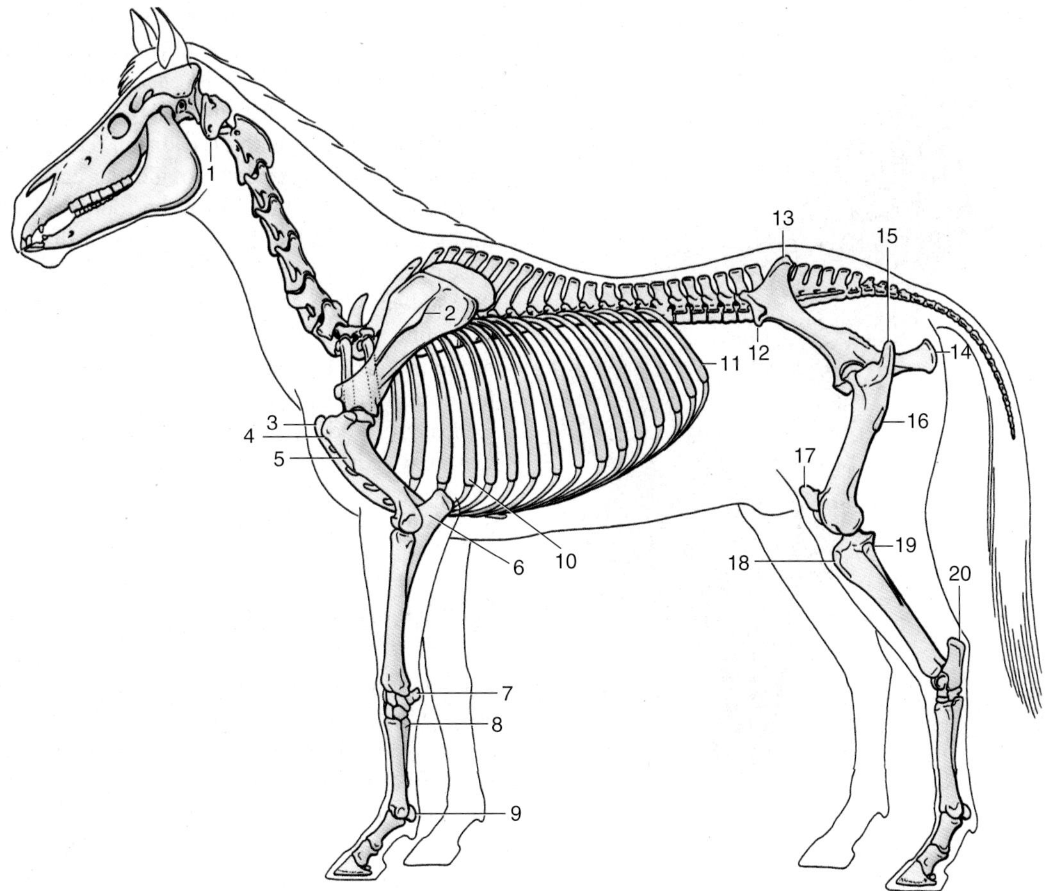

Fig. 19.1 The equine skeleton. The features labeled are among those normally palpable. *1,* Wing of atlas; *2,* tuber of scapula; *3,* manubrium; *4,* greater tubercle; *5,* deltoid tuberosity; *6,* olecranon; *7,* accessory carpal bone; *8,* proximal end (base) of lateral splint bone; *9,* proximal sesamoid bone; *10,* sixth rib; *11,* last (18th) rib; *12,* coxal tuber; *13,* sacral tuber; *14,* ischial tuber; *15,* greater trochanter; *16,* third trochanter; *17,* patella; *18,* tibial tuberosity; *19,* head of fibula; *20,* calcanean tuber.

years), if at all. The lumbar vertebrae have long horizontal transverse processes; synovial joints sometimes develop between those of the fourth and fifth bones and are constant between the fifth and sixth bones and between the sixth bone and the wings of the sacrum. In saddle horses exostoses sometimes develop on the summits of the thoracic spinous processes (mostly 14th–17th), bringing these into painful contact with their neighbors ("kissing spines") and resulting in minor local deflections of the vertebral axis.

The *intervertebral disks* are relatively thin, collectively accounting for only 10% to 11% of the length of the vertebral column. Each consists of a peripheral anulus fibrosus and a central nucleus pulposus, but the boundary between these parts is less distinct than in many species. Age changes include dehydration and fragmentation of the outer fibrous part but rarely calcification of the center. The disks most severely affected tend to be those of the neck and that between the last lumbar vertebra and the sacrum, which are the regions where movement is greatest. The clinical importance of these changes is not clear.

The *nuchal ligament,* which divides the dorsal cervical muscles into right and left groups, is massively developed and supports much of the burden of the head without interfering with the ability to lower the neck when grazing (Fig. 19.3). It consists of two clearly defined parts, each paired. The dorsal (funicular) part is a thick cord extending between the highest spines of the withers and the external occipital protuberance of the skull. It is flattened at its cranial attachment, becomes rounded shortly behind this, and flattens again as it nears the withers, where it forms a broad flange extending almost to the scapular cartilage. It is continued behind the withers as the narrower supraspinous ligament. The second (laminar) part forms a fenestrated sheet closely applied to its fellow. It fills the space between the funicular part and the cervical vertebrae and consists of bundles of elastic fibers that run cranioventrally from the funicular part and the spines of T2 and T3 to attach to C2 to C7. Synovial bursae are interposed between the funicular part and certain bony prominences to minimize pressure. One, the cranial nuchal bursa, is constantly present above

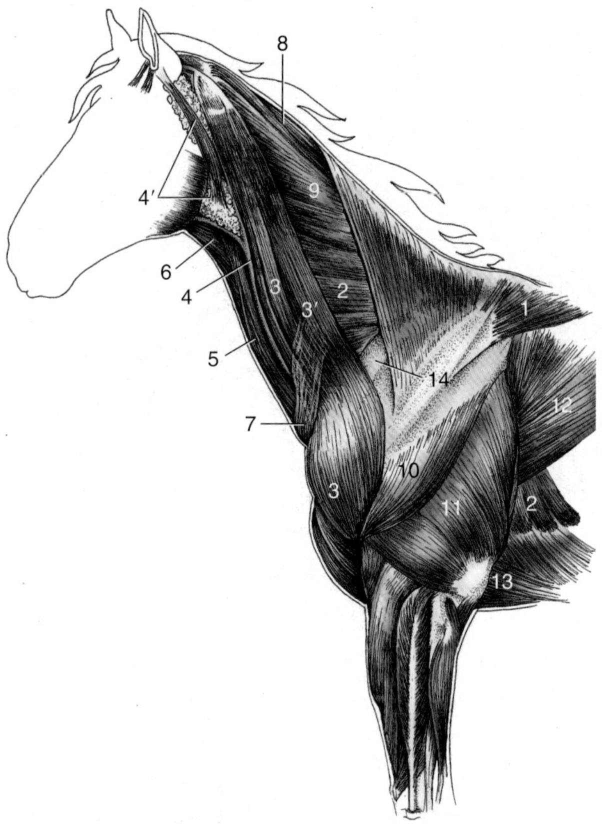

Fig. 19.2 Superficial dissection of the neck and shoulder region. *1,* Trapezius; *2,* serratus ventralis; *3,* brachiocephalicus; *3′,* omotransversarius; *4,* external jugular vein; *4′,* parotid gland; *5,* sternocephalicus; *6,* omohyoideus; *7,* cutaneous colli; *8,* rhomboideus cervicis; *9,* splenius; *10,* deltoideus; *11,* triceps; *12,* latissimus dorsi; *13,* pectoralis ascendens; *14,* subclavius.

the dorsal arch of the atlas; a second, the caudal nuchal bursa, is sometimes found above the spine of the axis; and a third, the supraspinous bursa, is constantly present over the most prominent processes of the withers (Fig. 19.3/*2, 2′,* and *2″*). Infections of the first and third bursae, leading to conditions known as "poll evil" and "fistulous withers," respectively, were formerly frequent and required extensive surgery for their eradication.

The complicated arrangement of the powerful epaxial muscles of the back and neck conforms, but only in a general way, to the account given in Chapter 2 (pp. 43–44). The many features of difference are fortunately not of clinical importance, and illustration of their arrangement in transverse sections of the neck and back will suffice for a description (see Fig. 18.38). One specific feature of the associated deep fascia does, however, require notice. In the horse this thoracolumbar fascia possesses, opposite the scapula, an additional superficial lamina of importance. This, the *dorsoscapular ligament* (Fig. 19.3/*5* and *5′*), has an origin, in common with the deeper layers, from the supraspinous ligament over the highest spines of the withers. In its ventral passage it is applied to the deep surface of the rhomboideus and gradually transforms from a purely fibrous to a largely elastic nature. It detaches a number of side branches that insert on the deep face of the scapula, alternating with divisions of the serratus ventralis muscle. The arrangement provides an elastic mechanism that helps absorb shock when the foot strikes the ground, limiting the dorsal shift of the scapula that would otherwise occur.

As always, the cervical part of the vertebral column is so mobile and flexible that the mouth may reach the flank or the pasture. The latter movement is not always so easy for draft animals, which have relatively short necks that lead them to adopt a spreading posture of the forelimbs; they may lean forward when grazing. Only small movements are permitted to the back and loins except at the very mobile lumbosacral joint.

THE VERTEBRAL CANAL

The relationships of the segments and cervical and lumbar enlargements of the spinal cord to the vertebrae are shown in Fig. 8.15. The first three sacral segments lie within the last lumbar vertebra, and the spinal cord terminates within the cranial quarter of the sacrum of the adult (Fig. 19.4).

The meninges remain separate to a more caudal level than in other species, and there is still a substantial subarachnoid space at the lumbosacral level. A communication exists in this species between the lumbar part of the space and a local widening (ventriculus terminalis) of the central canal of the spinal cord.

Epidural Anesthesia: Both lumbosacral and caudal sites of injection are commonly employed to obtain epidural anesthesia. The procedure at the former level utilizes the divergence of the spinous process of the last lumbar and first sacral vertebrae for identification of the injection site (Fig. 19.4). Although the interarcuate space is quite large, its distance (8–10 cm) from the skin makes it relatively easy to miss. "Low" epidural anesthesia is performed between the first and second caudal vertebrae, where the site for injection is readily discovered by "pumping" the tail up and down. The needle is inserted with a cranial inclination so that its point enters the canal within the first tail vertebra.

The vascularization of the spinal cord is mainly through spinal branches of the vertebral artery and appears to be relevant to the etiology of a relatively frequent form of ataxia ("wobbles") that occurs in foals and young horses. This may have its origin in congenital malformation and subsequent exostoses of the cervical articular processes that narrow the cervical vertebral canal at the intervertebral levels. This narrowing exerts pressure on the cord,

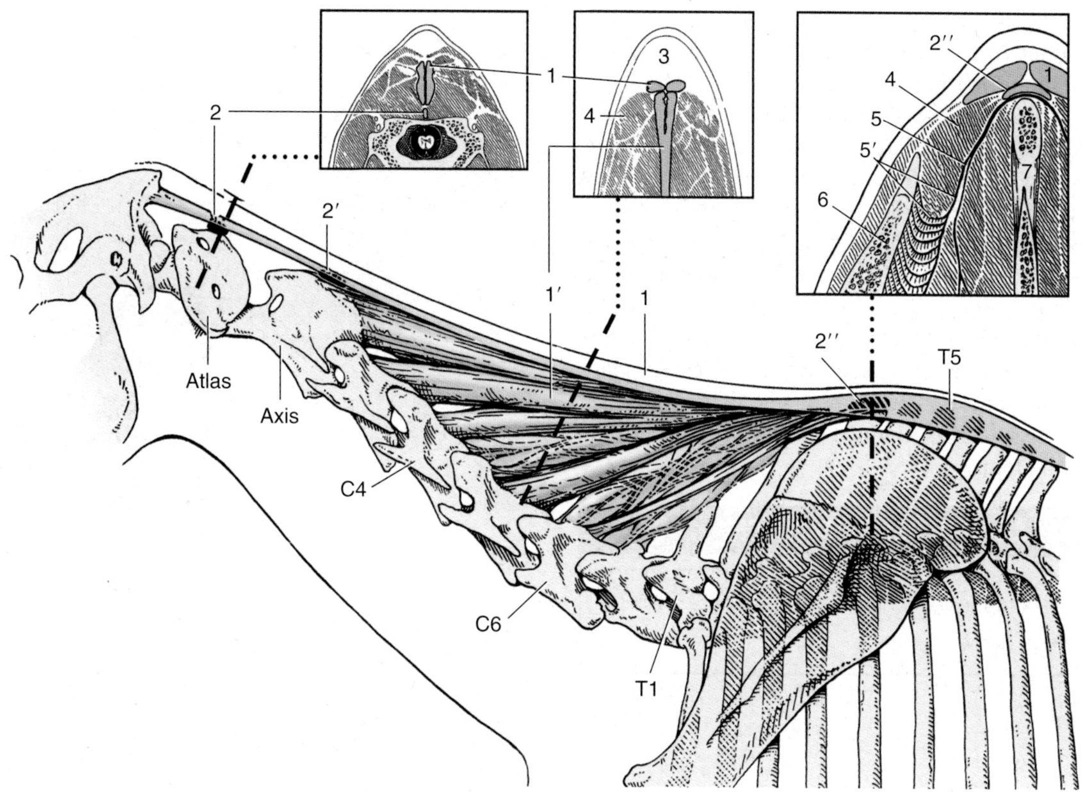

Fig. 19.3 The nuchal ligament and associated bursae in lateral view and in three transverse sections. *1* and *1′*, Funicular and laminar parts of nuchal ligament, respectively; *2*, *2′*, and *2″*, cranial nuchal, caudal nuchal (inconstant), and supraspinous bursae, respectively; *3*, fatty "crest" dorsal to nuchal ligament; *4*, rhomboideus; *5*, dorsoscapular ligament connecting spinous processes of the withers with the scapula; *5′*, elastic part of dorsoscapular ligament; *6*, scapula; *7*, spinous processes.

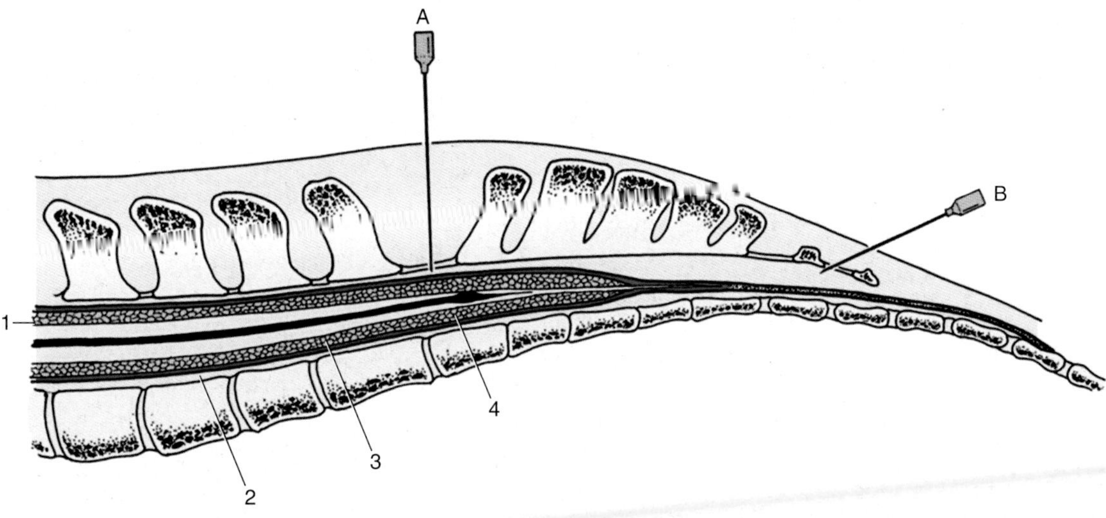

Fig. 19.4 Median section of the equine vertebral canal and spinal cord. The lumbosacral interarcuate space and the space between the first and second caudal vertebrae are indicated by hypodermic needles placed (A) for lumbosacral fluid collection and (B) for epidural anesthesia. *1*, Pia mater; *2*, dura mater; *3*, arachnoid; *4*, ventriculis terminalis.

although it is said that the cord lesions might be secondary to interference with the venous drainage. In this context, it should be known that the spinal arteries and veins are arranged in two sets, connected by relatively ineffectual anastomoses. One set of arteries and veins enters the cord by way of the ventral fissure and supplies (and drains) the central gray matter and a thin surrounding shell of white matter. The second set of arteries and veins passes over the lateral aspect to detach branches at intervals; these enter periodically to supply (and drain) the bulk of the white matter (Fig. 19.5). It is the veins of the second set that are supposedly compressed, leading to venous congestion and subsequent degeneration of the nervous tissue. It is claimed that the condition may develop in the fetus.

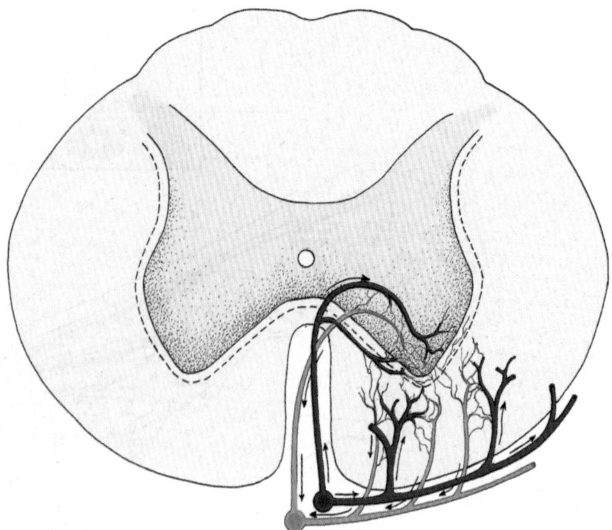

Fig. 19.5 Blood circulation in the ventral part of the spinal cord (schematic). The blood supply to the gray matter and to the adjacent layer of the white is more or less independent of that to most of the white matter.

COMPREHENSION CHECK

Review the anatomy of the vertebral column, and determine with scientific reasoning the appropriate sites for epidural injections.

The Thorax of the Horse

20

CONFORMATION AND SURFACE ANATOMY

The height of the withers and the caudal prolongation of the rib cage make it difficult to obtain a reliable impression of the thoracic cavity from simple inspection of the exterior. The narrow cranial part of the thorax is completely covered by the shoulder and arm. Some variation in the projection of the limb bones on the thoracic skeleton is due to the inconstant slope of the scapula. As a general guide, the caudal angle of this bone lies over the upper end of the seventh rib, while the supraglenoid tubercle projects in front of the first rib, a little above the manubrium of the sternum (Figs. 20.1 and 20.2). The humerus forms a lesser angle with the horizontal plane than in the smaller species, and this moves the elbow up within the skin of the trunk such that the summit of the olecranon is nearly level with the lowest part of the fifth rib or succeeding intercostal space. The triangle between the scapula and humerus is completely occupied by the massive triceps muscle, which severely restricts clinical access to the cranial part of the thorax.

There are 18 pairs of ribs. Those caudal to the seventh rib and lying behind the triceps are individually identifiable on palpation even though they are covered in varying degree by certain muscles: cutaneus trunci, latissimus dorsi, serratus ventralis, and obliquus externus abdominis. The most caudal ribs may even provide visible landmarks. For example, the upper part of the last rib prominently marks the cranial limit of the flank. Palpation of the ribs reveals their changing orientation. The last two or three, which are relatively short, have a pronounced caudal inclination; the half-dozen or so (R9–R15) in front of these are longer and of equal length and curvature. The more cranial ribs are both shorter and less strongly curved. The first rib, the shortest of all, is almost vertical. The increasing slope of the ribs as the series is followed caudally brings the last rib remarkably close to the coxal tuber (see Fig. 19.1).

Between the forelimbs the thorax is covered by the powerful pectoral muscles that form paired swellings separated by a prominent groove along the line of the sternum (see Fig. 23.4). The cranial part of this bone, the manubrium, projects as a readily found landmark. The caudal xiphoid process is also palpable, although it is not quite so easily found as the manubrium. It is broad and flexible and is enclosed between the converging costal arches. External inspection does not convey the reduced depth of the cranial part of the thoracic cavity because of the upward sloping of the sternum toward the manubrium and the ventral slope of the cranial thoracic vertebrae. An exact appreciation of the position of the diaphragm is essential for the clinician. The vertex is level with the sixth intercostal space (or even the sixth rib) and thus comes to within a short distance of the point of the elbow in an animal standing square (Fig. 20.3).

There are naturally considerable breed and individual variations in conformation. Without considering these in detail, it may be said that a deep chest is generally favored. In saddle horses it is desirable that the ribs slope caudally without excessive lateral bowing because too pronounced a "barrel" makes for an uncomfortable seat.

THE THORACIC WALL

Removal of the forelimbs exposes the contrasting form of the cranial and caudal parts of the thorax. The cranial part (formed by the sternal ribs) is narrow and bilaterally compressed and shows little movement. The caudal part (formed by the asternal ribs) is conspicuously wider and more rounded and makes a substantial contribution to the respiratory excursions (see Fig. 20.8). In comparison with the bovine chest, the ribs are narrow and the intercostal spaces markedly wide, especially in their ventral parts. The arrangement of the structures within the spaces follows the usual pattern.

The short, stout first rib is almost immobile because it is stabilized by tight joints with the vertebral column and sternum and by anchorage to the cervical vertebrae through the scalenus muscle. The brachial plexus divides this muscle into ventral and (small) middle parts, while the axillary vessels emerge ventral to it. These vessels wind around the cranial margin of the first rib, where the axillary artery may be palpated against the bone. Previously, the artery was punctured at this site when a sample of arterial blood was required (Fig. 20.3/*1′*), but currently the carotid artery is preferred.

In conformity with the length of the thorax, the diaphragm is more oblique than in other domestic species but has the same general form. It bulges forward from its peripheral attachments to the lumbar vertebrae, ribs, and sternum. Its most cranial part, the vertex, is situated directly above the sternum and projects on the lower part of the sixth space or preceding rib. The dorsal part of the diaphragm is molded to present right and left elevations between which the median portion is retracted by the crura

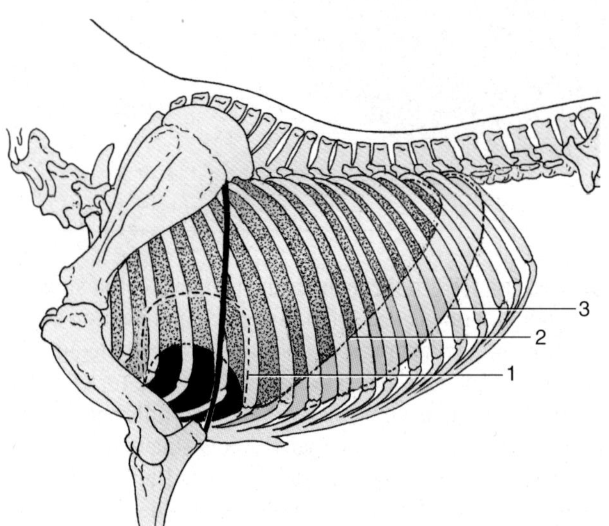

Fig. 20.1 Projections of the heart and lung on the left thoracic wall. The *heavy line* indicates the caudal border of the triceps. *1,* Outline of heart; *2,* basal border of lung; *3,* line of pleural reflection.

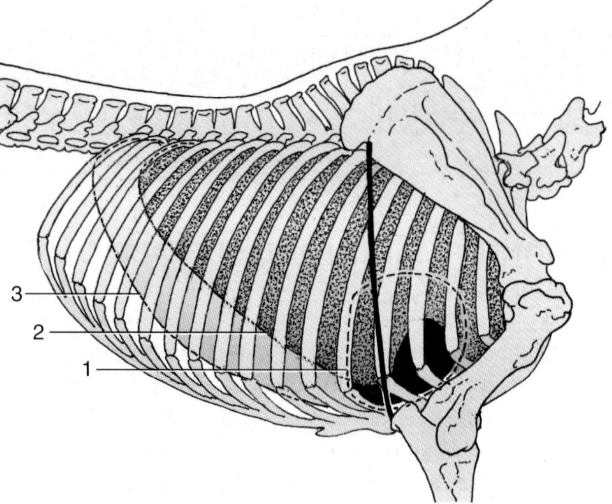

Fig. 20.2 Projections of the heart and lung on the right thoracic wall. The *heavy line* indicates the caudal border of the triceps. *1,* Outline of heart; *2,* basal border of lung; *3,* line of pleural reflection.

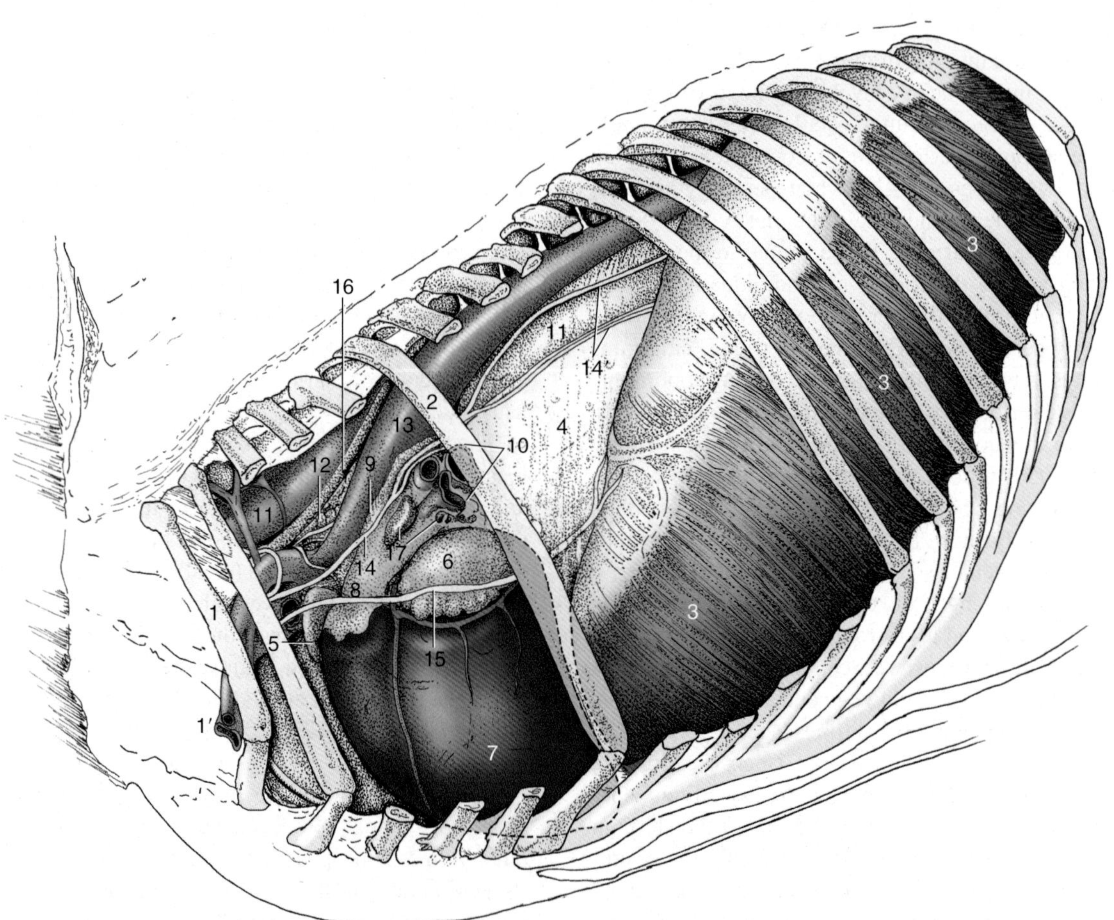

Fig. 20.3 Structures within the mediastinum. The mediastinal pleura cranial to the heart has been removed, which exposes the cranial lobe of the right lung. *1,* First rib; *1′,* axillary vessels; *2,* sixth rib; *3,* diaphragm; *4,* caudal mediastinum covering right lung; *5,* right auricle; *6,* left auricle; *7,* left ventricle; *8,* pulmonary trunk; *9,* ligamentum arteriosum; *10,* root of lung; *11,* esophagus; *12,* trachea; *13,* aorta; *14,* vagus nerve; *14′,* dorsal and ventral vagal trunks; *15,* phrenic nerve; *16,* thoracic duct; *17,* tracheobronchial lymph nodes.

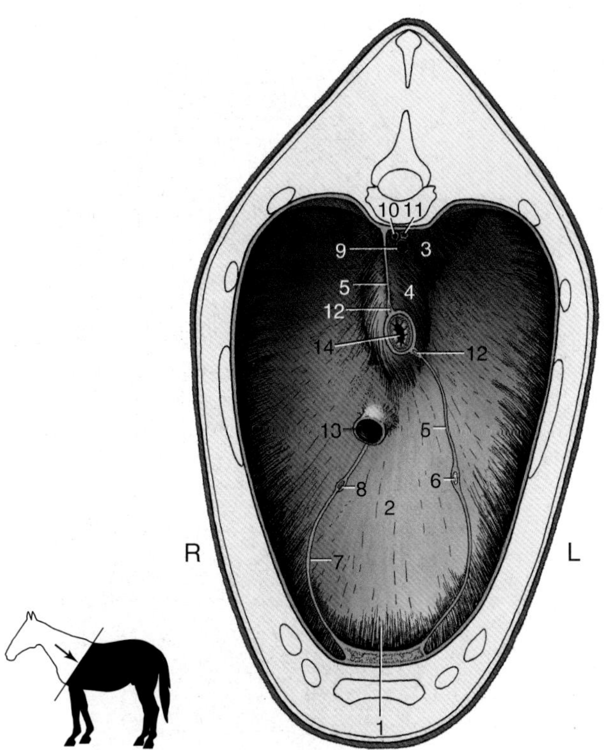

Fig. 20.4 Cranial surface of the diaphragm. *1*, Sternal and costal parts of diaphragm; *2*, tendinous center; *3*, left crus; *4*, right crus; *5*, caudal mediastinum; *6*, left phrenic nerve; *7*, plica venae cavae; *8*, right phrenic nerve; *9*, aorta; *10*, right azygous vein; *11*, thoracic duct; *12*, dorsal and ventral vagal trunks; *13*, caudal vena cava; *14*, esophagus; *L*, left side; *R*, right side.

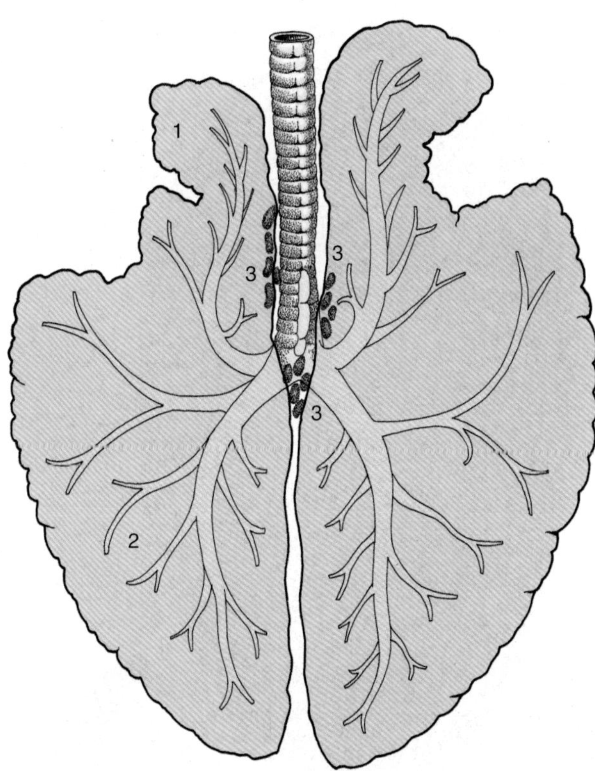

Fig. 20.5 Dorsal view of the lungs and bronchial tree (schematic). *1*, Apex (cranial lobe) of left lung; *2*, base (caudal lobe) of left lung; *3*, tracheobronchial lymph nodes.

to form a recess. The middle and ventral parts are uniformly curved from side to side. The openings within the diaphragm show no important specific features (Fig. 20.4).

THE PLEURAL CAVITIES

The arrangement of the pleura follows the usual pattern in that the thoracic interior is divided into two pleural cavities by an intermediate septum, the mediastinum. The mediastinum is weak because of poorly developed subpleural connective tissue.

The projection of the pleural cavities on the chest wall is always a matter of clinical significance. The mediastinal pleura is reflected onto the thoracic wall within the costovertebral gutter, and the costal pleura thus extends above the ventral border of the vertebral bodies. The ventral limit of the costal pleura follows an irregular line that passes over the costal cartilages. Cranially, the pleural sac extends medially to the first rib and beyond this on the right side for several centimeters into the neck (cupula pleurae), where it may be punctured by penetrating wounds that appear to spare the thorax. The caudal reflection of the costal pleura onto the diaphragm begins at the vertebral end of the 17th rib and is then deflected caudally to reach the middle of the last rib before turning forward. It then follows a more conventional course that intersects successive ribs at progressively lower levels until it continues along the eighth rib cartilage to the sternum. This line traces a slight dorsocranial concavity (Figs. 20.1/*3* and 20.2/*3*).

As always, the pleural cavities are considerably larger than the lungs, even when there is maximal inflation. There thus exist potential spaces (the costomediastinal and costodiaphragmatic recesses) along the ventral and caudal margins of the lung that are never utilized and vary with phase of respiration. The costodiaphragmatic recess lies over the intrathoracic part of the abdomen and provides a potential route for the puncture of certain abdominal organs. Obviously the risk of injury to the lung is minimized if the needle is introduced during full expiration (see Fig. 20.8/*13'*).

THE LUNGS

The lungs are elongated and shallow, corresponding to the general form of the pleural cavities. The right and left lungs are more nearly equal in size than in other species (Fig. 20.5), and because the difference lies mainly in the greater thickness of the right lung, the asymmetry may

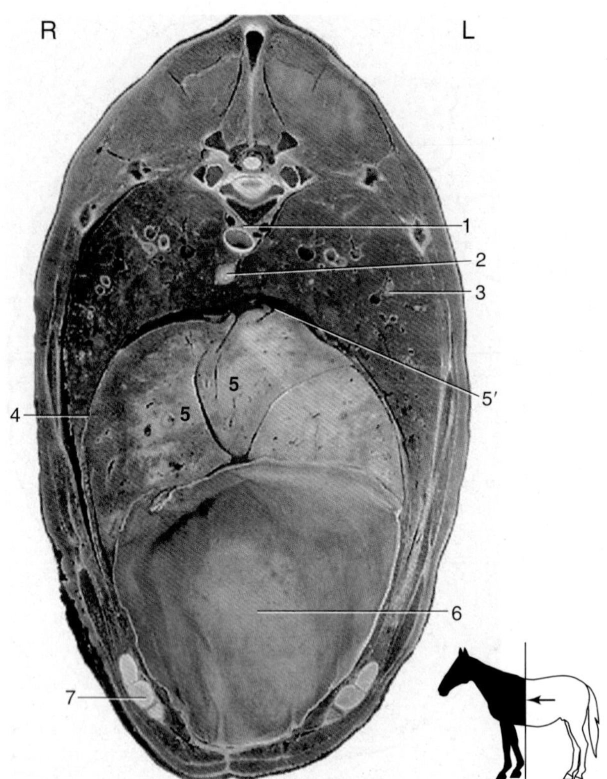

Fig. 20.6 Transverse section of the trunk at the level of T12 and the middle of the ninth rib. *1,* Aorta; *2,* esophagus; *3,* lung; *4,* diaphragm; *5,* liver; *5′,* caudal vena cava; *6,* diaphragmatic flexure of the ascending colon; *7,* costal arch; *L,* left side; *R,* right side.

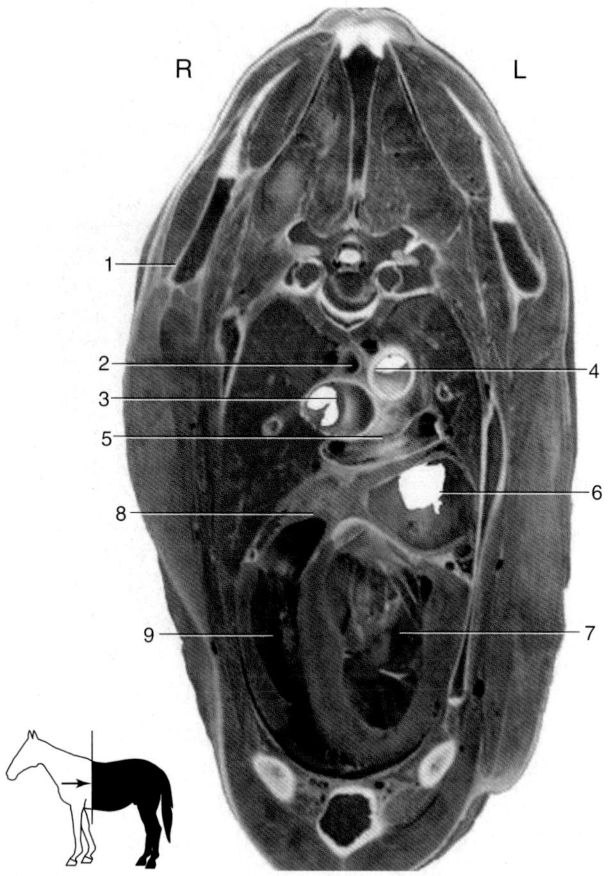

Fig. 20.7 Transverse section of the thorax at the level of T5. *1,* Caudal angle of scapula; *2,* esophagus; *3,* bifurcation of the trachea; *4,* aorta; *5,* bifurcation of the pulmonary trunk; *6,* left atrium; *7,* left ventricle; *8,* right atrium; *9,* right ventricle; *L,* left side; *R,* right side.

easily escape notice (Fig. 20.6). There is no external evidence of lobation other than the presence of the accessory lobe at the base of the right lung and some separation of the cranial part of each lung (see Figs. 4.26 and 20.1). The two lungs are extensively joined by connective tissue caudal to the bifurcation of the trachea.

The left lung exhibits a deep cardiac notch that allows the pericardium extensive contact with the chest wall between the third and sixth ribs (Fig. 20.1). The notch is margined by a thinned region so that the lung provides little cover to the pericardium over a much larger area (Fig. 20.7). The arrangement on the right side is similar, although the asymmetry of the heart reduces the size of the cardiac notch from the third rib to the fourth intercostal space (Fig. 20.2). When moderately expanded, the base of each lung reaches to a line passing through the upper part of the 16th, the middle of the 11th, and the costochondral junction of the 6th rib; the upper part of this line is almost vertical, and the lower part sweeps cranioventrally. This margin of the lung is separated from the line of pleural reflection by about 5 cm dorsally and ventrally but by as much as 15 cm in its middle part (Figs. 20.1 and 20.2). In young foals the extent of the lung is more restricted, and the caudal limit is at about the 13th rib.

Clinical Examination: The projection of the lung on the chest wall is considerably larger than the clinically useful area for percussion and auscultation, because examination of the thin margins of the lung will not provide useful information. The area for such examination is triangular and is defined by the caudal angle of the scapula, the point of the elbow, and the upper end of the 16th rib. Two sides of this triangle are more or less straight, but the caudoventral side is slightly bowed.

Centesis for collection of pleural fluid is most safely performed in the lower part of the seventh intercostal space, ventral to the margin of the lung. Care is required to avoid puncturing the superficial thoracic ("spur") vein that crosses the site (see Fig. 23.3/*11′*).

The lobulation of the lungs can be detected on careful examination of the expanded or sectioned lung but is less obvious in the collapsed state when the covering pleura is wrinkled. Because of incomplete septa, the possibility of collateral ventilation between neighboring lobules exists.

The chief bronchus, the pulmonary artery, and the pulmonary vein combine to form the root of the lung before entering at the hilus in a region deprived of pleura and directly adherent to the same part of the other lung. The chief bronchus separates within the lung into a small cranial division to the cranial lobe and a larger caudal division that attends to the ventilation of the remainder of the organ. Detailed knowledge of division of the bronchi of lower orders is not of great importance at the present time because lung surgery is rarely performed in horses.

In standing animals, the ventilation and perfusion of different regions and lobes of the lungs are reasonably well matched, although in larger species, such as the horse, there must be some tendency for gravity to favor the perfusion of more ventral parts. The spatial relationship of ventilation and perfusion is disturbed in animals placed in dorsal or lateral recumbency, and the disturbance becomes significant when the recumbent posture is long maintained—as during major surgery. In these circumstances there is compression of whichever part of the lung is at the bottom. This reduces the tensile forces that ordinarily hold airways open in that part of the lung. The ensuing airway closure permits complete collapse of the alveoli served by such airways; blood perfusing these alveoli cannot take part in respiratory gas exchange.

The pattern of division of the pulmonary artery corresponds to that of the bronchi. A separate bronchial artery attends to the supply of the bronchial and peribronchial tissue, but the blood is returned by the single set of pulmonary veins.*

The lymphatic drainage leads first through very small pulmonary nodes embedded in the substance of the organ and then to larger tracheobronchial nodes about the bifurcation of the trachea (Fig. 20.3/*17*). From here most lymph is drained via the cranial mediastinal nodes.

The nerves that enter at the hilus derive from the pulmonary plexus, to which both sympathetic and parasympathetic fibers contribute.

*The hemorrhage from the pulmonary vasculature that is induced by severe exercise is a major concern of the horse-racing industry. Although the existence of the condition is rarely made evident by loss of blood externally or by abnormal distress during or immediately after a race, tracheobronchial endoscopy at the latter time reveals hemorrhage in the lungs of most (some would say all) Thoroughbreds subjected to the extreme demands of racing. There is some dispute concerning the origin of the blood leakage—whether it is from branches of the bronchial or the pulmonary arteries and whether it results from preexisting structural abnormality of the vessel wall. The condition impairs performance, worsens progressively, and is responsible for the premature retirement of many horses from racing. It often occurs incidental to other problems such as laryngeal hemiplegia in horses exposed to more moderate stress. Similar exercise-induced hemorrhage is recognized in racing Greyhounds, camels, and some elite human athletes.

THE MEDIASTINUM

The heart divides the mediastinum into the familiar parts (Fig. 20.8/*4* and *4'*). The *cranial part* is markedly asymmetrical; it attaches to the left first rib and gradually shifts to reach a more or less median situation directly in front of the heart. The dorsal part is thick, the ventral part much thinner, especially after the thymus has regressed. The dorsal part occupies about half the transverse diameter of the thorax and includes the esophagus and trachea, the brachiocephalic trunk and cranial vena cava with their respective branches and tributaries, the cranial mediastinal lymph nodes, the thoracic duct, and the phrenic, vagus, and sympathetic nerves. The interstices between these structures are occupied by fat, sometimes present in large amounts. The thymus is the sole content of the ventral portion.

The *ventral part* of the middle mediastinum is very broad because it contains the heart and pericardium (Fig. 20.7). The dorsal part is paper thin except where it contains the esophagus, the continuation of the trachea to its bifurcation, the aorta, and certain nerves (including vagal branches).

In lateral view the *caudal mediastinum* is triangular (Fig. 20.3/*4*). It is divided into two parts by adhesion between the lungs about and caudal to their roots. The ventral part, whose sole occupant is the left phrenic nerve, is diverted far to the left before it merges with the pleura covering the diaphragm (Fig. 20.4/*6*). The dorsal part is thin except where it encloses the esophagus and aorta.

Except in foals, small openings in the mediastinum place the two pleural cavities in communication. The mediastinum is very fragile, and exposure during dissection inevitably increases the number of visible openings, which leaves it unclear whether any were present when the thorax was intact and suggests that the mediastinum might be an ineffectual partition. However, small openings in the thoracic wall such as are made for the purpose of thoracoscopy (when the influx of air can be controlled) result in incomplete unilateral pneumothorax and are survived without obvious adverse effects.

THE HEART

The heart lies in the ventral part of the middle mediastinum, directly cranial to the diaphragm and largely covered by the forelimbs (Fig. 20.1). It forms an irregular and laterally compressed cone. The larger part of the heart lies left of the median plane and is so disposed that the axis slopes caudoventrally and to the left (Fig. 20.3). The heart of a Thoroughbred obviously is conspicuously larger, both relatively and absolutely, than that of other horses of comparable body weight. The

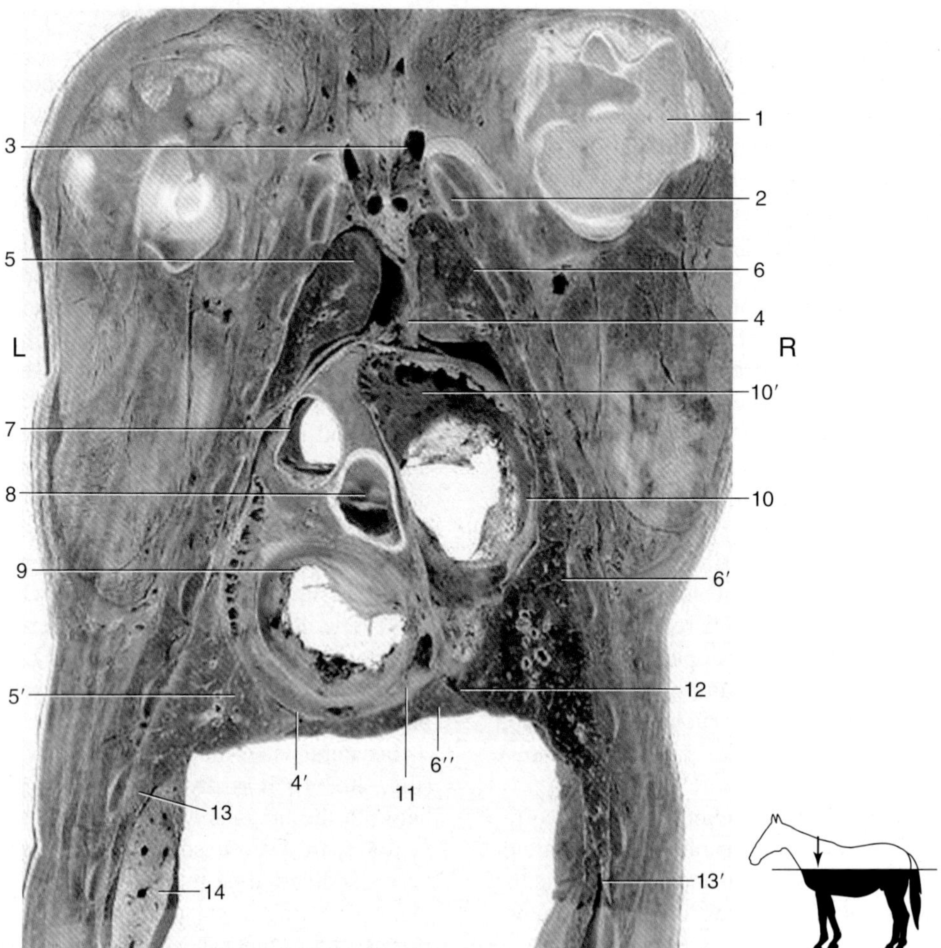

Fig. 20.8 Dorsal section of the thorax at the level of the atrioventricular valves. *1,* Head of humerus; *2,* first rib; *3,* formation of cranial vena cava; *4* and *4′,* cranial and caudal mediastinum, respectively; *5* and *5′,* cranial and caudal lobes of the left lung, respectively; *6, 6′,* and *6″,* cranial, caudal, and accessory lobes of the right lung, respectively; *7,* pulmonary valve; *8,* aortic valve; *9,* left atrioventricular valve; *10,* right atrioventricular valve; *10′,* right auricle; *11,* coronary sinus; *12,* plica venae cavae; *13,* diaphragm; *13′,* costodiaphragmatic recess; *14,* part of the liver; *L,* left side; *R,* right side.

difference is mostly inherited and partly conditioned by training and affects the topography. Most commonly the heart extends between the planes of the second to sixth intercostal spaces, which places the apex directly caudal to the level of the point of the elbow. The cranial margin is strongly curved and is arranged with its upper part vertical, and its lower part follows the dorsal surface of the sternum. The caudal border, though sinuous in profile, is more or less upright (Fig. 20.3). The flattened lateral surfaces are related through the pericardium to the mediastinal surfaces of the lungs, except where the cardiac notches allow direct contact, greater on the left side, with the thoracic wall. A strong sternopericardiac ligament attaches the pericardium to the sternum, and this, with the anchorage of the great vessels, limits the displacement allowed to the heart. A slight shift, however, does occur with the movement of the diaphragm.

Apart from the general form, there is little of significance to distinguish the heart of the horse. Mention should be made, however, of two features of the aortic and pulmonary valves, especially of the former. The cusps commonly develop nodules at the free margins, and these can be quite striking in older animals. In addition, fenestrations may appear in the middle region of the cusps. Neither development appears to have much, if any, functional significance. The puncta maxima, the sites at which the valve sounds are most clearly heard, do not correspond exactly to the projections of the openings on the chest wall.

Auscultation: The left atrioventricular valve is auscultated to most advantage in the fifth intercostal space, a little caudodorsal to the point of the elbow; the aortic valve at a somewhat higher level in the fourth space; and the pulmonary valve lower within the third space—all of course on the left side. The right atrioventricular valve is best heard in the lower parts of the third and fourth right intercostal spaces.

It is important to remember that the skeletal topography is not always easy to appreciate in practice. It may be more useful to remember that the puncta lie within a band of a few centimeters' depth about midway between the horizontal planes that intersect the points of the shoulder and the elbow. Within this band the punctum maximum of the left atrioventricular valve is at the intersection of the vertical line that falls a couple of fingerbreadths behind the point of the elbow. The approach to the other valves follows from the relative positions indicated and requires the introduction of the stethoscope between the limb and the chest wall.

The coronary arteries share the supply of the heart wall in more equal fashion than in many other species because the right one ends by descending within the right (subsinuosal) interventricular groove (see Fig. 7.19/*2'*).

THE ESOPHAGUS, TRACHEA, AND THYMUS

Although the *esophagus* still lies partly to the left on entering the chest, it quickly regains a position dorsal to the trachea; thereafter, it pursues a median course, apart from slight deflections as it passes the aortic arch and again just before the esophageal hiatus. The striated muscle of the cranial part of the esophagus is gradually replaced by smooth muscle as the heart is approached; the color change makes the transformation obvious. The muscle is somewhat thicker immediately before the diaphragm, and this part of the tube is commonly contracted in the dead specimen. There is no evidence that the diaphragm embraces the esophagus tightly at the hiatus, as sometimes alleged. Indeed, the free movement of the diaphragm over the esophagus is facilitated by the peritoneum pouching through the hiatus on the right and ventral side of the esophagus.

The *trachea* becomes median soon after entering the thorax. It then lies against the longus colli muscles but soon diverges to run lower within the mediastinum. After passing over the left atrium, it bifurcates at about the level of the fifth rib (or space) (Fig. 20.7/*3*). The bifurcation is not symmetrical; the right bronchus is larger.

Tracheotomy is needed as an emergency procedure to alleviate an upper airway obstruction. It can be performed in standing or recumbent horses, and it requires going through the cutaneous colli muscle and separation of the sternothyrohyoideus muscle bellies. Because of the potential for tracheal collapse, the trachea is opened with an incision parallel to the direction of the tracheal rings.

The *thymus* is prominent in early life but soon regresses. Its formation from right and left parts is not obvious because they are closely applied together. In the young foal it completely fills the ventral part of the mediastinum cranial to the heart and may even extend over the left side of the pericardium. The thymus may also pass into the neck beside the trachea, very occasionally reaching the thyroid gland. At this stage the thymus is clearly lobulated and bright pink. It is largest about 2 months after birth and thereafter regresses, although the rate is variable. Usually little remains after 3 years, when the vestige consists largely of fatty fibrous tissue. At its apogee the thymus makes contact with most structures within the cranial mediastinum.

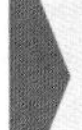

THE GREAT VESSELS AND NERVES WITHIN THE THORAX

The pattern of arterial branching of the aortic arch is shown in Fig. 7.37 and need not be further described because details are of no clinical significance. Rupture of the aortic wall in the sinus region or at the origin of the brachiocephalic trunk may occur and with fatal consequences in horses. It appears to indicate inherent weakness at these sites because pathologic change is rarely evident.

The presence of a single right azygous vein may be used to distinguish the equine from the bovine heart.

The formations, the courses, and the ramifications of the phrenic, sympathetic, and vagus nerves conform to the usual pattern. The relationship of the *left recurrent laryngeal nerve* to the aortic arch, though not specific to the horse, deserves emphasis because intermittent stretching of the nerve with the pulsation of the vessel has been postulated as a factor in the etiology of laryngeal hemiplegia ("roaring"). The closer association of the left nerve to the tracheobronchial lymph nodes is a second factor of alleged but unproven significance.

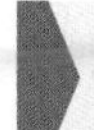

THE LYMPHATIC STRUCTURES OF THE THORAX

There are numerous lymph nodes within the thorax. Although most are collected in groups, these are sometimes less discrete than is often suggested. The following are the principal groups.

Small *intercostal nodes* lie in the dorsal part of some intercostal spaces. They receive lymph from the vertebrae and the adjacent muscles, the dorsal part of the diaphragm, and the local costal and mediastinal pleura. The efferent flow is to the thoracic duct.

The *cranial mediastinal nodes* are numerous and scattered about the esophagus, trachea, and vessels at the entrance to the thorax; usually some form a discontinuous chain that joins the caudal deep cervical nodes within the neck. The most caudal members reach the pericardium, where they overlap the nodes about the tracheal bifurcation that are assigned to the tracheobronchial and caudal mediastinal groups. Most efferent vessels pass to the thoracic duct; those from the most cranial nodes in the series may first perfuse deep cervical nodes.

The *tracheobronchial group* is scattered about the caudal part of the trachea and the chief bronchi (Fig. 20.5/*3*); left, middle, and right subdivisions are commonly distinguished. Small nodes within the peribronchial tissue of the lung may be regarded as members of this series. Most lymph passing through this group has origins within the lungs, but some comes from the pericardium, the heart, and the caudal mediastinal nodes. The efferent vessels are divided between those that go directly to the thoracic duct and those that first perfuse the cranial mediastinal nodes.

A number of small *caudal mediastinal nodes* lie directly in front of the diaphragm and between the esophagus and aorta. Lymph is received from the esophagus, the diaphragm, the liver, the mediastinal and diaphragmatic pleura, and, apparently, the lungs. The efferent lymph flow is divided between the thoracic duct and the tracheobronchial and cranial mediastinal lymph nodes.

The few ventral mediastinal lymph nodes are without significance.

The thoracic duct drains into one or another of the large veins at the entrance to the thorax, most commonly the cranial vena cava.

COMPREHENSION CHECK

Delineate areas of cardiac and pulmonary auscultation and percussion on an equine skeleton or a cadaver, followed by practice on a live animal.

List the abdominal organs that may be within the rib cage.

Practice tracheotomy on the cadaver.

21 The Abdomen of the Horse

CONFORMATION AND SURFACE ANATOMY

The horse has a capacious gastrointestinal tract and a correspondingly bulky abdomen. However, the extent of the abdomen is not immediately apparent because a large part is concealed within the rib cage. The olecranon and the lower end of the sixth rib are handy guides to the most cranial extent of the diaphragm (see Fig. 20.3). The flank is reduced in size by the caudal inclination of the ribs, the last of which may be within a few fingerbreadths of the coxal tuber (see Fig. 22.23A/*1″* and *3*).

Abdominal conformation varies much with age, condition, and the amount and nature of the rations. The ventral contour is especially variable; it slopes gradually between the sternum and the pubic brim in animals in hard condition but dips to reach its lowest point behind the xiphoid process in those in softer condition, in pregnant mares, and in ponies generally. In the latter groups the most caudal part of the floor ascends very steeply. These differences are not always visible because the most caudal part of the abdomen is covered laterally by the fold of skin that passes between the flank and the thigh (see Fig. 22.23A/*6*) and ventrally by the prepuce or udder.

The trunk is broadest at the last ribs. The upper part of the flank sinks in to form a paralumbar fossa, but it is much less obvious than in cattle. The lower part of the belly is rounded from side to side, except in foals, in which the whole abdomen is slab-sided and shallow (see Fig. 23.2). The usual symmetry may be disturbed in late pregnancy or by accumulation of gas in parts of the gastrointestinal tract.

The position of the last rib is often visible, but most other skeletal boundaries of the flank and floor are less easily found. The transverse processes of the lumbar vertebrae are usually too deeply buried under muscle to be palpable. The dorsal part of the coxal tuber is very conspicuous, but the ventral part, which gives origin to the internal oblique and tensor fasciae latae muscles, is not visible, although it is easily palpable.

Soft features that may be recognized include the internal oblique muscle, which raises a ridge along the caudoventral boundary of the paralumbar fossa (Fig. 21.1B/*5*), and the superficial thoracic ("spur") vein, which runs over the ventral part of the abdominal wall toward the axilla, following the dorsal border of the deep pectoral muscle. One can identify and palpate the subiliac lymph nodes arranged in a spindle at the cranial margin of the thigh, midway between the coxal tuber and patella. They are more easily found if drawn forward. The superficial ring of the inguinal canal can be found on deep palpation of the groin, which is a procedure sometimes resented by the horse and therefore to be performed with care (Fig. 21.1A/*3*).

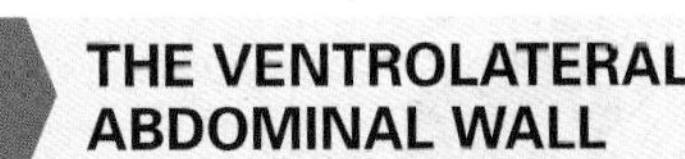

THE VENTROLATERAL ABDOMINAL WALL

Structure

The skin is thick over the flank but thins ventrally, particularly in heavy draft animals. It is especially thin in the cleft between the abdomen and thigh, where it is sparsely haired and glistens with the secretion of the sebaceous glands concentrated here. In contrast, sweat glands are most abundant over the flank.

A large subcutaneous bursa, a postnatal development, is present over the coxal tuber. Elsewhere the skin is closely adherent to the cutaneous trunci, which cover most of the flank, though not the abdominal floor. The upper border of the cutaneous muscle follows a line drawn from the withers to the stifle. The muscle is thickest cranially where it extends into the fascia over both the lateral and the medial aspects of the shoulder and arm. Caudally, it continues within the flank fold to end on the lateral femoral fascia. The cutaneous muscle is employed to twitch the skin to dislodge flies and other irritants. No detached bundles are associated with the prepuce, as in many species.

The loose fascia deep to the muscle conveys the cutaneous nerves and superficial vessels and encloses the subiliac lymph nodes. The deeper fascia consists largely of elastic tissue and, being yellowish, is also known as the tunica flava. It is well adapted to the passive support of the viscera and is thickest ventrally, where the burden is greatest. The dorsal part is easily dissected from the underlying muscle, but its ventral part exchanges fibers with the aponeurosis of the external oblique and is more tightly adherent. Bands detached from the deep fascia help support the prepuce or the udder. Careful suturing of this layer is necessary after abdominal surgery because its elastic nature tends to evert and draw apart the edges of a wound in the underlying muscle.

The linea alba, the prepubic tendon, and the associated structures have a particular importance in the horse. The

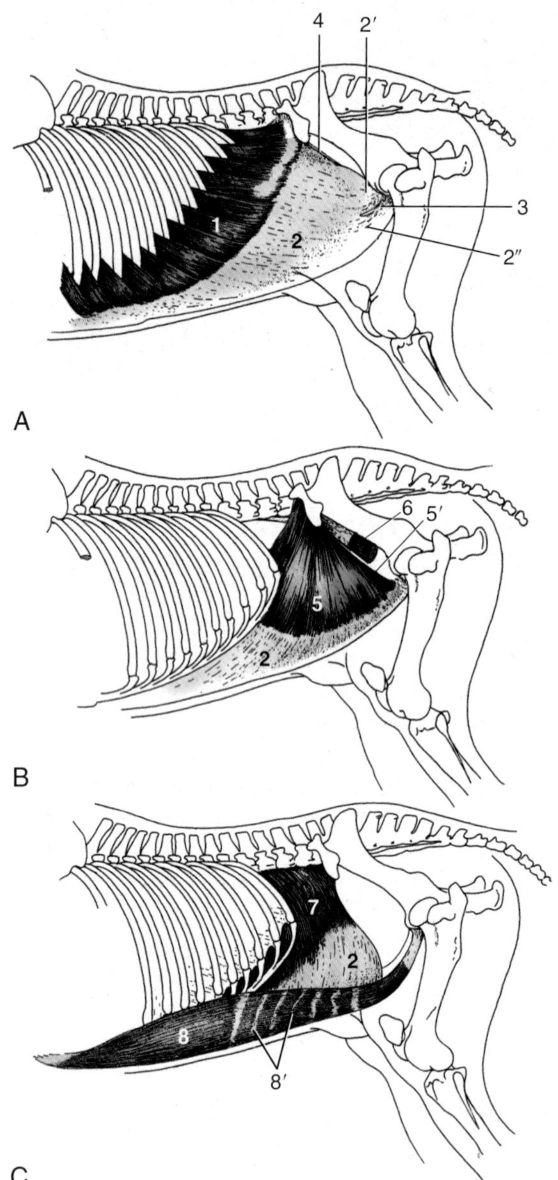

Fig. 21.1 The abdominal muscles and their skeletal attachments. *1,* External abdominal oblique, muscular part; *2,* aponeurotic parts of *1, 5,* and *7; 2′* and *2″,* pelvic and abdominal tendons of aponeurotic part, respectively; *3,* superficial inguinal ring; *4,* attachment of pelvic tendon of external oblique aponeurosis on iliopsoas and sartorius ("inguinal ligament"); *5,* internal abdominal oblique, muscular part; *5′,* free caudal border forming the cranial margin of the deep inguinal ring; *6,* iliopsoas, partly enclosed by iliac fascia; *7,* transversus abdominis, muscular part; *8,* rectus abdominis; *8′,* tendinous inscriptions.

linea alba, mainly formed from the aponeuroses of the flank muscles, is considerably strengthened by longitudinal fibers. It is unequally developed along its length, being widest where it carries the umbilical scar (Fig. 21.2/*d*). It finally combines with the insertion tendons of the right and left rectus abdominis muscles to form a broad plate.

The *prepubic tendon** attaches abdominal muscles to the pelvic skeleton (Fig. 21.3/*5*). Once formed, the tendon ascends almost vertically toward the pelvic brim, but before reaching this, it is augmented by a strong transverse thickening. This thickening is mainly formed by the tendons of origin of the pectineus muscles (of the thighs), which arise from both the ipsilateral and contralateral pubic bones (from and medial to the iliopubic eminences) and which thus partly decussate across the midline. The caudal margins of the oblique abdominal muscles and the cranial part of the gracilis also contribute to the prepubic tendon. An important feature, peculiar to the horse, is the detachment from the caudolateral aspects of the prepubic tendon of the stout rounded cords that furnish accessory ligaments to the hip joints (Fig. 21.3/*5′* and Fig. 21.2). Each accessory ligament crosses the ventral surface of the pubis, enters the acetabulum through the notch in the rim, and inserts on the head of the femur beside the intracapsular ligament (of the head of the femur). Each accessory ligament is predominantly composed of fibers from the two rectus muscles, and many fibers have decussated from the contralateral side. The ligaments appear to be the principal insertions of these muscles, which partly explains the restrictions on the movements permitted at the equine hips. It is postulated that the accessory ligaments are tensed by the weight of the abdominal contents and that this tension helps secure the femoral heads in place.

Because the main weight of the abdominal organs is carried by the prepubic tendon, it follows that its rupture has the most dire consequences. This mishap, fortunately rare, is for obvious reasons most common in heavily pregnant mares.

The *external abdominal oblique* (Fig. 21.1/*1*) is the most extensive muscle of the flank. It arises from the thoracolumbar fascia and also from the lateral aspect of the thoracic wall (from the fifth rib caudally) by a series of digitations that engage with those of the serratus ventralis. The majority of its fascicles run caudoventrally to a broad aponeurosis that succeeds the fleshy part of the muscle along a line that sweeps from the coxal tuber toward the ventral end of the fifth rib.

Before insertion, the aponeurosis splits into (1) a large abdominal tendon that continues over the rectus to reach and insert on the linea alba and (2) a small pelvic tendon that inserts on the coxal tuber, the fascia over the iliopsoas and sartorius muscles, and the prepubic tendon (see Fig. 21.3).

* Although all agree that the prepubic tendon is the means by which the abdominal muscles obtain a principal attachment to the pelvic skeleton, opinions are divided on what constitutes the essential elements of this structure (and what are to be regarded as secondary augmentations). We adhere to the view that it is primarily formed of the linea alba and rectus tendons and secondarily by the incorporation of other elements, especially the decussation of the pectineus tendons. Others have regarded it as primarily a transverse structure attaching to and lying in front of the right and left pubic bones and strengthened by giving attachment to the linea alba and recti (and other components). However, the details are not of major relevance to most of the readers of this book.

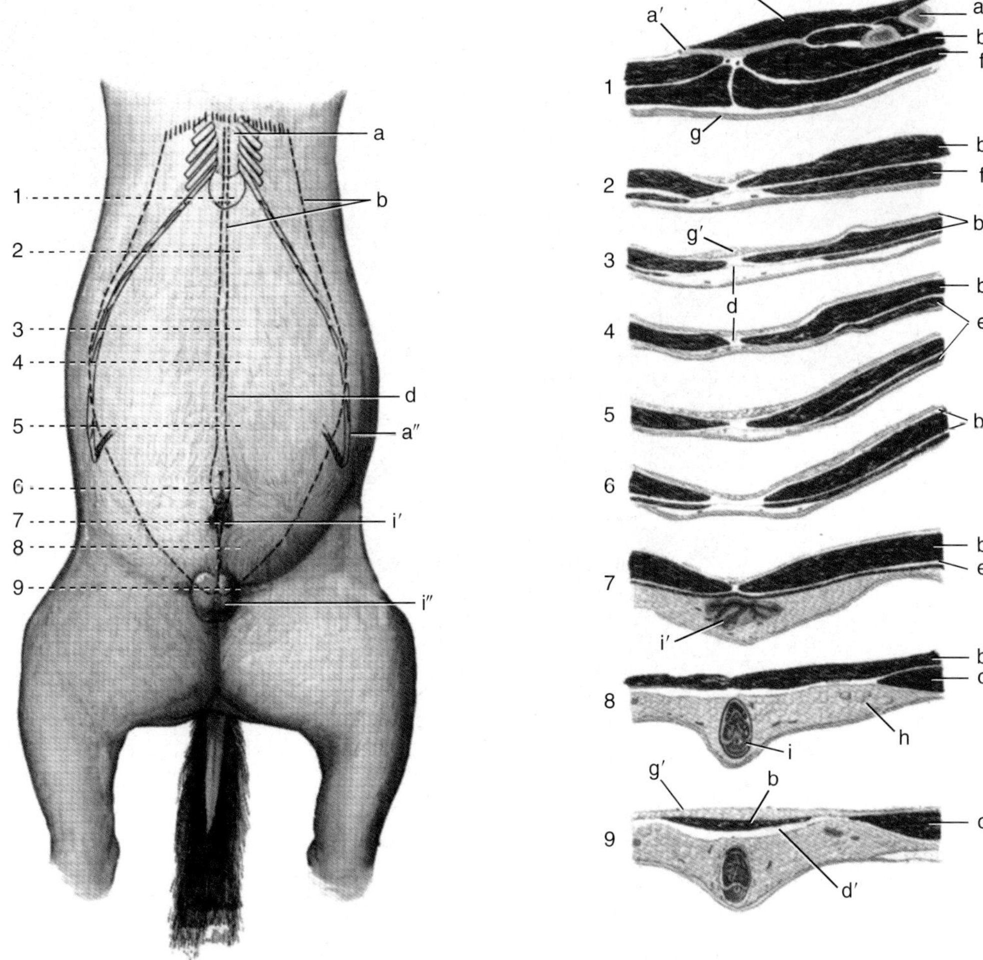

Fig. 21.2 Changes in the structure of the abdominal floor shown by means of a series of transverse sections *(1–9)* of a gelding. *a,* Sternum; *a′,* xiphoid cartilage; *a″,* costal arch; *b,* rectus abdominis; *b′,* rectus sheath; *c,* internal oblique; *d,* linea alba; *d′,* prepubic tendon; *e,* cutaneous trunci; *f,* pectoralis ascendens; *f′,* diaphragm; *g,* skin; *g′,* fat; *h,* superficial inguinal lymph nodes; *i,* penis; *i′,* prepuce; *i″,* scrotum.

The split between the two tendons constitutes the superficial ring of the inguinal canal (Fig. 21.1/[illegible]). (The margins of the tendons are known as *crura* where they bound the opening, but the term is often misapplied to the tendons themselves.) The unnecessary term *inguinal ligament,* sometimes applied to the thickened caudodorsal edge of the pelvic tendon, confuses many descriptions of these structures. In fact, the prominence of this edge (Fig. 21.1/*4*) owes less to thickening than to tension through its connection with the fascia covering the iliopsoas and sartorius.

The *internal oblique muscle* (Fig. 21.1/*5*) radiates from an origin concentrated on the coxal tuber but extending onto the dorsocaudal edge of the pelvic tendon of the external oblique. Most bundles run cranioventrally to insert on the last costal cartilages or, via an aponeurosis that fuses with that of the external oblique, into the linea alba. Some pass ventrally and caudoventrally, and these cover the superficial inguinal ring on its internal aspect (Fig. 21.4/*4*). A caudal slip provides the cremaster, which passes onto the spermatic cord. The junction of the fleshy and aponeurotic parts of this muscle occurs more than halfway down the abdominal wall.

The *transversus abdominis* (Fig. 21.1/*7*) takes origin from the lumbar vertebrae and the medial aspect of the last ribs, ventral to the origin of the diaphragm. The fleshy part is continued by an aponeurosis that passes deep to the rectus abdominis to reach the linea alba. The transversus, the least extensive of the three muscles of the flank, does not extend caudal to the level of the coxal tuber; the internal lamina of the rectus sheath is thus deficient caudally.

The *rectus abdominis* (Fig. 21.1/*8*) arises from the fourth to ninth costal cartilages and the adjacent part of the sternum. It inserts by way of the prepubic tendon and accessory ligaments. The muscle, relatively narrow over the thorax, widens considerably over the abdomen before again narrowing toward its insertion (see Fig. 21.2/*b*).

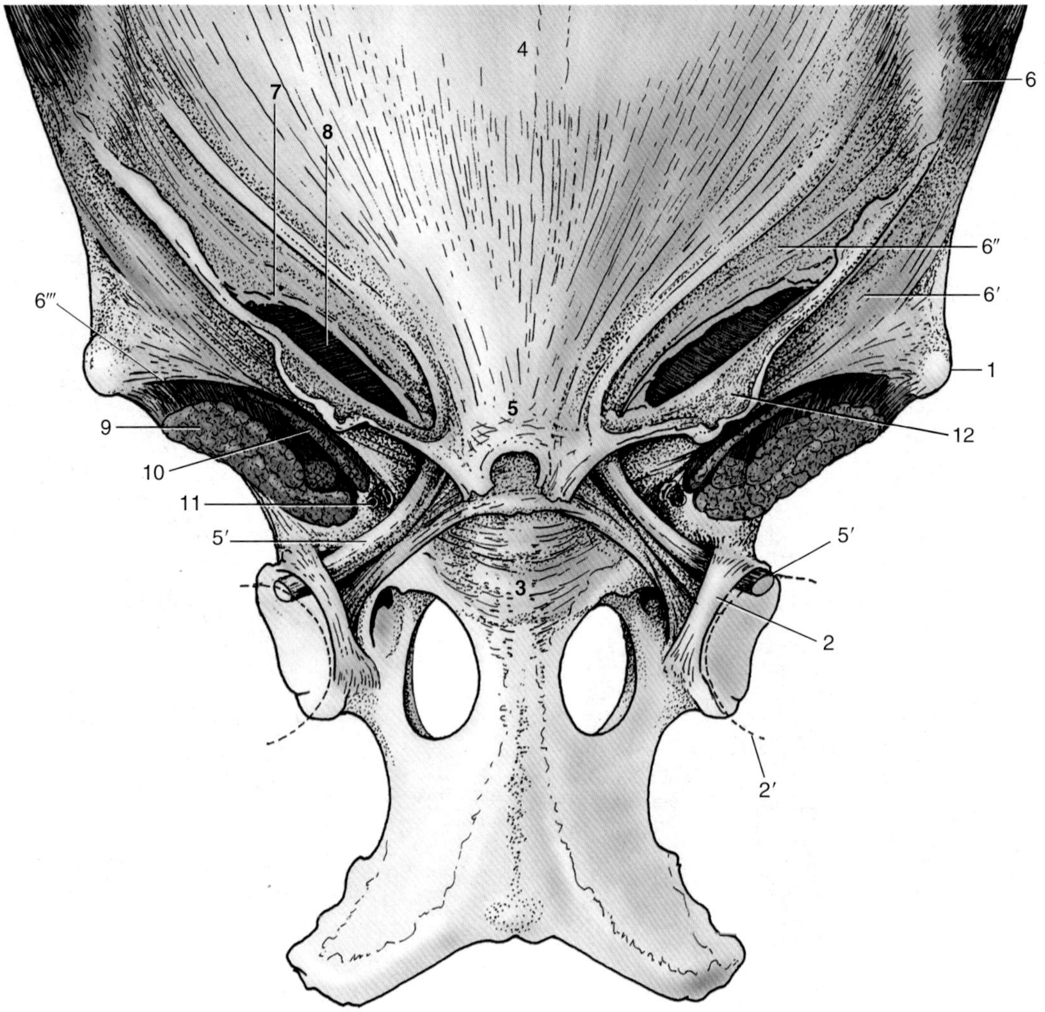

Fig. 21.3 The attachment of the abdominal muscles on the pelvis and the prepubic tendon. *1,* Coxal tuber; *2,* transverse acetabular ligament; *2′,* femoral head; *3,* pubis; *4,* tunica flava over linea alba; *5,* prepubic tendon; *5′,* accessory ligament; *6,* external abdominal oblique; *6′* and *6″,* pelvic and abdominal tendons of external oblique aponeurosis, respectively; *6‴,* attachment of pelvic tendon of external oblique aponeurosis on sartorius and iliopsoas ("inguinal ligament"); *7,* superficial inguinal ring; *8,* internal abdominal oblique; *9,* iliopsoas; *10,* sartorius; *11,* vascular lacuna containing femoral vessels; *12,* femoral fascia (lamina).

Although the functions of the abdominal muscles are the same in all species, the expiratory role is relatively more important in the horse because the elasticity of the lungs is frequently reduced in older horses. Contraction of the abdominal musculature is then more necessary to return the viscera, and thus the diaphragm, from the inspiratory position. In this action the junction between the fleshy and aponeurotic parts of the external oblique muscle becomes visible as the so-called heave line.

The fascia that supports the peritoneum is often heavily but unequally infiltrated with fat. This layer, which may be 6 cm or more thick in horses in good condition, must be taken into account when making and closing a surgical incision.

The Inguinal Canal

The inguinal canal follows the general pattern but merits a full description because of its relevance to castration, which is performed on the vast majority of male horses. It is the opening in the caudal part of the abdominal wall through which the testis travels in its descent into the scrotum, which is a process usually completed shortly before or shortly after birth in this species. The canal contains the spermatic cord of the colt and stallion; a stump frequently remains in the gelding. In addition, the external pudendal artery and the genitofemoral nerve travel through the canal.

The term *inguinal canal* suggests a roomier passage, but the canal is no more than a potential space between the flesh

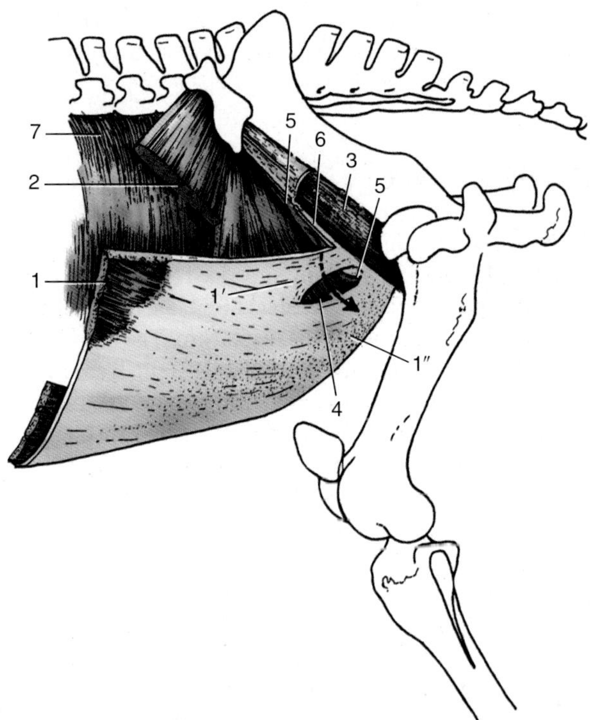

Fig. 21.4 The muscles of the inguinal region. The *arrow* passes through the inguinal canal. *1,* External abdominal oblique; *1′* and *1″,* pelvic and abdominal tendons of external oblique aponeurosis, respectively; *2,* internal abdominal oblique; *3,* iliopsoas partly enclosed by iliac fascia; *4,* superficial inguinal ring; *5,* cranial border of deep inguinal ring; *6,* attachment of pelvic tendon of external oblique aponeurosis on iliopsoas and sartorius ("inguinal ligament"); *7,* transversus abdominis.

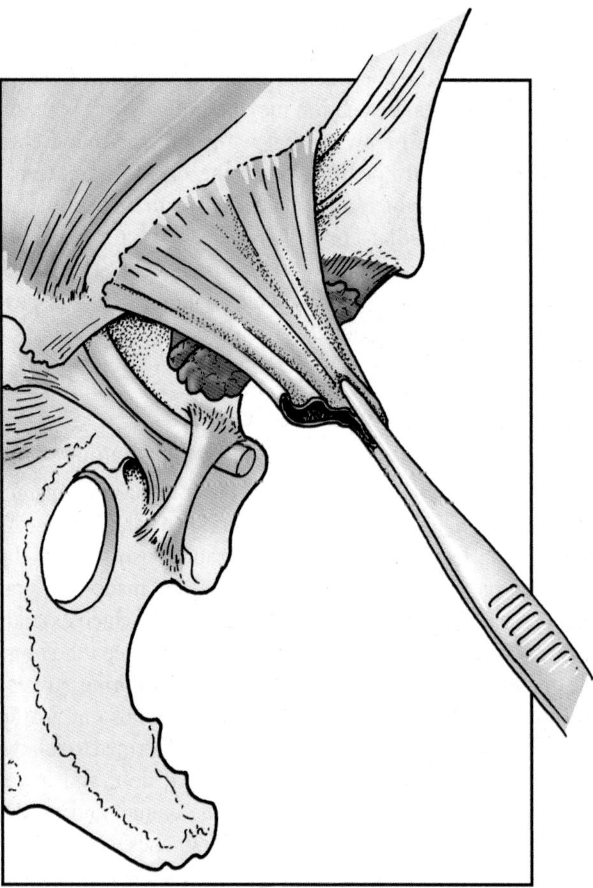

Fig. 21.5 The origin of the external spermatic fascia and femoral lamina from the margin of the superficial inguinal ring. (See Fig. 21.3 for orientation.)

of the internal abdominal oblique and the aponeurosis of the external abdominal oblique muscles. The entrance *(deep inguinal ring)* lies along the free caudal edge of the internal abdominal oblique muscle, which determines its oblique orientation (Fig. 21.4/*5*); the origin of the internal abdominal oblique from the external abdominal oblique and the convergence of the two muscles on the lateral edge of the prepubic tendon determine its length (generally about 15 cm).

The exit *(superficial inguinal ring)*, between the two tendons into which the external oblique aponeurosis splits, is more or less horizontal (Fig. 21.4/*4*). It is limited laterally by the exchange of fibers between the two tendons where they part company and medially by the tendons meeting and fusing with the edge of the prepubic tendon. The margins of the opening are less clearly defined than many accounts suggest. The lateral (dorsal) crus gives origin to the external spermatic fascia and femoral lamina, which appear to continue the lateral crus directly (Fig. 21.5). The medial (ventral) crus is somewhat frayed but can be identified on palpation through the skin. This is best performed by placing the palm against the belly and advancing the fingers into the cleft between the thigh and abdominal wall. The lateral crus is passed unnoticed, but the medial crus is recognized as a firm edge. The fingers pass into the outer part of the canal most readily with the thigh abducted (when the femoral fascia [lamina] draws the lateral crus outward). It follows from the orientation of the deep and superficial rings that the canal has a triangular outline. It is relatively long cranially and very short caudally where the two openings butt against the prepubic tendon (see Fig. 21.4).

The peritoneal sheath *(vaginal tunic)* of the spermatic cord contains a cavity that places the space about the testis in free communication with the peritoneal cavity of the abdomen. The communication occurs through the vaginal ring (≈3 cm long) situated midway in the deep inguinal ring (see Fig. 22.19A/*10* and Fig. 22.24A and B) and identifiable per rectum in the stallion because of the constituents of the spermatic cord converging on it. The vaginal cavity provides a possible route for the herniation of intestines that may even reach the scrotum. This occurrence (indirect inguinal hernia) is a comparatively common sequel to castration. Direct inguinal hernia, in which a loop of intestine forces an entry into the canal beside the vaginal tunic, is rare in horses.

Incomplete descent of one or both testes *(cryptorchidism)* is common in the horse (p. 567). The testis may be retained within the abdomen or may enter but fail to leave the canal. Surgical correction may be indicated. It is therefore necessary to be aware that while the spermatic cord occupies a central position within the canal, the external pudendal artery, which must be treated with respect, occupies the caudomedial corner. The artery is accompanied by the genitofemoral nerve and a small vein. The larger (accessory) external pudendal vein makes a separate passage between the pectineus and gracilis muscles.

Innervation and Vascularization

The segmental innervation of the abdominal wall corresponds to the common pattern, and the minor variations are of little importance because paravertebral anesthesia is rarely practiced in the horse. The vascularization also follows the common pattern primarily. Mention may be made of a cranial branch of the deep circumflex iliac artery, which extends forward from the region of the coxal tuber between the muscles of the flank and is susceptible to injury during surgery in this region. The artery of the right side is also at risk in trocarization, which may be occasionally performed to relieve tympany of the cecal base. The abdominal floor and lower flank are served in the usual way by the cranial and caudal epigastric arteries and their superficial branches. No warning of the exact position of the vessels is available, and should vascular damage occur, control of the resulting hemorrhage may be troublesome and time consuming. It is said that the caudal epigastric artery is the vessel most often traumatized. The superficial thoracic or spur vein runs toward the axilla in the superficial fascia at the ventral edge of the cutaneous muscle. Connections with tributaries of the external pudendal vein make it available as an alternative drainage route from the prepuce or udder.

GENERAL ASPECTS OF ABDOMINAL TOPOGRAPHY

The influences on abdominal topography common to all species have been discussed (pp. 113-114). The horse is prone to adhesions of the peritoneum, especially after abdominal surgery.

Except in advanced pregnancy, when the uterus has an even greater influence, the topography of the equine abdomen is dominated by the large intestine. The cecum and ascending colon are the seat of the microbial fermentation that makes the cellulose constituents of the diet available, and their significance is therefore comparable to that of the chambers of the ruminant stomach. The large intestine is so voluminous that it is almost always encountered immediately when the abdomen is opened, whether the incision is made in the flank or in the floor. Its disposition is complicated, and although it is necessary to give a systematic account of each individual part, a first impression may be obtained from such illustrations as Figs. 21.6, 21.7, and 21.10.

THE SPLEEN

The spleen lies within the left dorsal part of the abdomen where it is largely, if not wholly, protected by the most caudal ribs. Although the spleen is separated from the ribs by the diaphragm, it is not attached to the diaphragm. The broad dorsal base lies under the last three ribs, although a small corner may project against the flank. The pointed ventral apex reaches forward to about the 9th or 10th rib, a handbreadth above the costal arch (Fig. 21.6/*4*). The cranial margin is concave, the caudal margin is convex, and the organ is thus approximately sickle shaped. The parietal surface is generally smooth, though sometimes marked by depressions that may even perforate to the visceral surface. The visceral surface presents three parts. A small dorsal region fits against the left crus of the diaphragm and left kidney and is bound to these by phrenicosplenic and renosplenic ligaments (Fig. 21.8/*6* and *7*). The remainder of the visceral surface is divided by a ridge along which the splenic artery runs and to which the greater omentum attaches. The narrow strip cranial to the ridge, the gastric surface, is applied to the greater curvature of the stomach (Fig. 21.9). The larger area caudal to the ridge, the intestinal surface (Fig. 21.9/*1*), is related to various parts of the intestinal mass.

The position of the spleen naturally varies with respiration. Usually only the caudal margin is within reach on rectal exploration (see Fig. 22.23B/*10*); a greater part becomes accessible when the stomach is distended.

The thick capsule of spleen contains a considerable amount of smooth muscle, which relaxes to allow the engorgement of the spleen. This occurs in certain diseases and is very obvious in animals that have succumbed to anthrax. The organ is steel blue on first removal from the fresh carcass but turns reddish brown on exposure to the air. This color is derived from the red pulp that forms the bulk of the parenchyma. The white pulp that flecks the red is not normally visible to the naked eye. In addition to being a reservoir for red blood cells, the spleen is a major part of the immune system.

THE STOMACH

The most remarkable feature of the stomach is its small size (5- to 15-L capacity) in relation to the animal and to the volume of fodder consumed. It is relatively larger in the unweaned foal.

The equine stomach lies mainly within the left half of the abdomen (Fig. 21.10/*2*). Like other simple stomachs, it consists of two limbs that meet at a ventral angle. The left limb comprises the fundus (unusually large and often

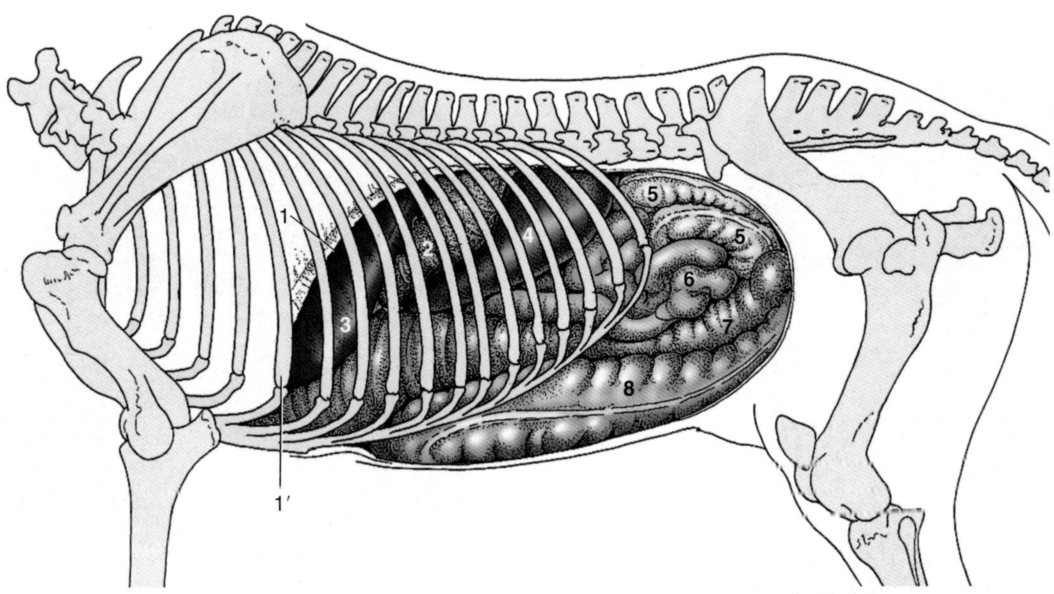

Fig. 21.6 Visceral projections on the left abdominal wall (including the diaphragm). *1,* Cut edge of diaphragm; *1′,* rib 6; *2,* stomach; *3,* liver; *4,* spleen; *5,* descending colon (banded); *6,* jejunum (smooth); *7,* left dorsal colon; *8,* left ventral colon.

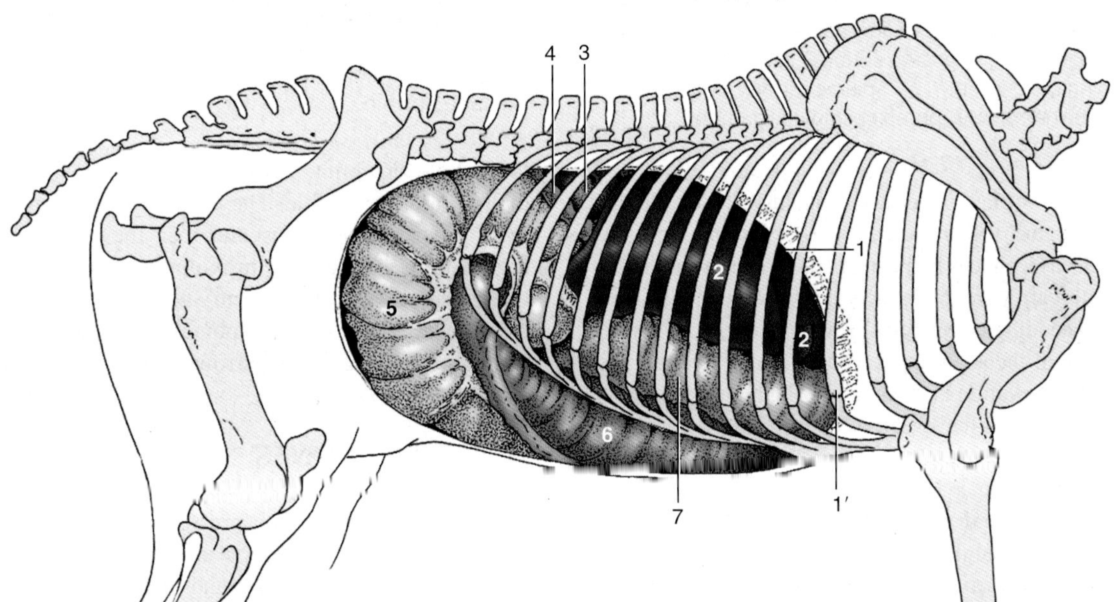

Fig. 21.7 Visceral projections on the right abdominal wall (including the diaphragm). *1,* Cut edge of diaphragm; *1′,* rib 6; *2,* liver; *3,* right kidney; *4,* descending duodenum; *5,* body of cecum; *6,* right ventral colon; *7,* right dorsal colon.

termed the *saccus cecus* [blind sac] in this species) and the body; the right limb or pyloric part is much narrower and extends across the midline to join the duodenum (Fig. 21.11A). It mostly lies within the rib cage and is inaccessible through the flank or the rectum even when grossly distended. Gross overdistention may be revealed by a raising of the overlying ribs on the left side, which destroys the normal symmetry of the trunk.

Stomach Surface Projections: When moderately distended, the fundus extends under the upper part of the 15th rib (or thereabouts), and the lowest part of the body reaches the ventral parts of the 9th and 10th ribs. The cardia provides a relatively fixed point, opposite the upper part of the 11th rib, and enlargement after feeding is therefore mainly downward and forward (Fig. 21.6/*2*).

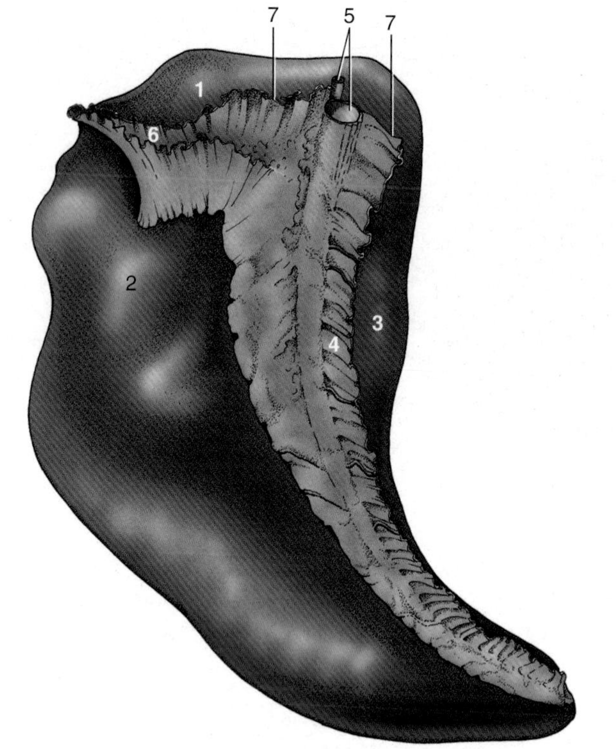

Fig. 21.8 Visceral surface of the spleen. *1,* Renal surface; *2,* intestinal surface; *3,* gastric surface; *4,* greater omentum (gastrosplenic ligament); *5,* splenic artery and vein; *6,* renosplenic ligament; *7,* phrenicosplenic ligament.

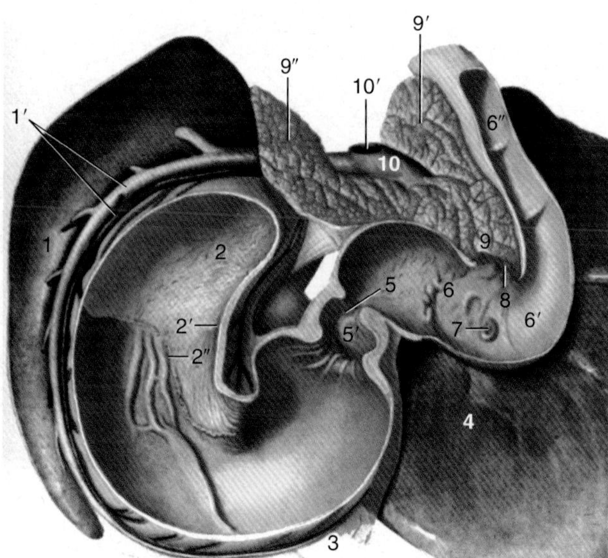

Fig. 21.9 Topography of spleen, stomach, pancreas, and liver, caudoventral view. *1,* Intestinal surface of spleen; *1′,* splenic artery and vein; *2,* fundus (blind sac) of stomach; *2′,* cardia; *2″,* margo plicatus; *3,* greater omentum; *4,* liver; *5,* pyloric orifice; *5′,* pyloric antrum; *6,* S-shaped cranial part of duodenum; *6′,* cranial flexure of duodenum; *6″,* descending duodenum; *7,* major duodenal papilla; *8,* minor duodenal papilla; *9,* body of pancreas; *9′* and *9″,* left and right lobes of pancreas, respectively; *10,* portal vein; *10′,* stump of cranial mesenteric vein.

The cranial surface is directed against the diaphragm above and against the left lobe of the liver more ventrally. The caudal surface faces in the opposite direction and makes contact with various viscera, including coils of small intestine and descending colon dorsally and the dorsal diaphragmatic flexure of the ascending colon ventrally. The left part of the greater curvature is followed by the hilus and adjoining gastric surface of the spleen (see Fig. 21.9).

A stepped edge (margo plicatus; Fig. 21.9/*2″*) divides the interior between a large nonglandular region, occupying the fundus and part of the body, and a glandular region. The nonglandular part resembles the mucosa of the esophagus and is dirty white and harsh to the touch (see Fig. 21.11). The softer glandular region consists of cardiac, proper gastric, and pyloric glandular zones. Although the borders between these zones are ill defined, the zone occupied by the proper gastric glands is somewhat darker and redder than the yellowish cardiac and pyloric zones in the fresh specimen. Both the cardiac and pyloric regions are incidentally parasitized by botfly *(Gasterophilus)* larvae, which may leave the mucosa densely pocked by small focal ulcerations. These, when semihealed, can be misinterpreted as normal features (Fig. 21.11B).

The cardiac sphincter is exceptionally well developed, and this, coupled with the oblique entrance of the esophagus, is held responsible for the horse's reputed inability to eructate or vomit. However, eructation and vomiting, though rare, is possible. The canal or distal portion of the pyloric part is more muscular than the remainder of the organ and is bounded by proximal and distal thickenings that converge at the lesser curvature. Even when the second of these, the pyloric sphincter, is fully relaxed, the actual exit is remarkably narrow (Fig. 21.9/*5*).

THE INTESTINES

The intestines occupy the greater part of the abdominal cavity. The small intestine is unremarkable, but the large intestine is greatly modified and enlarged. It provides the reservoir for microbial fermentation and assumes a form and disposition that make it difficult to recognize the homologies of its parts with those of the gut of other species. However, these may be deduced from the attachments and arterial supply and confirmed by reference to the development.

The Small Intestine

The small intestine measures about 25 m in the carcass, although it is probably much less in life. The *duodenum* is relatively short, and because it is closely tethered, it is more or less constant in position. It commences ventral to the liver where the initial (cranial) part forms a sigmoid

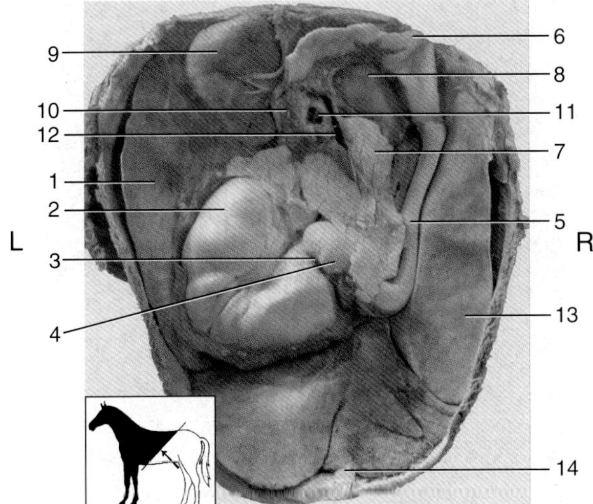

Fig. 21.10 The organs in the craniodorsal part of the abdominal cavity of a young horse, caudoventral view (see *inset*). *1,* Spleen; *2,* stomach; *3,* pylorus; *4* and *5,* cranial and descending parts of duodenum, respectively; *6,* caudal flexure of duodenum; *7,* pancreas; *8,* right kidney; *9,* left kidney; *10,* left adrenal gland; *11,* cranial mesenteric artery and vein; *12,* portal vein; *13,* liver; *14,* falciform ligament; *L,* left side; *R,* right side.

flexure of which the first curve is convex dorsally, the second convex ventrally. The second (descending) part then runs caudally, still below the liver, until it reaches the lateral margin of the right kidney, which it follows to the caudal pole followed by a turn medially behind the root of the mesentery (Figs. 21.10/*6* and 21.12/*2* and *3*). The descending duodenum is also related to the right lobe of the pancreas and crosses above the last part of the right dorsal colon and the base of the cecum, to which it is attached (see Fig. 21.15). This relationship permits the formation of a temporary duodenocecal anastomosis in the treatment of gastroduodenojejunitis, obviating the reflux of fluid and consequent overloading of the stomach that characterizes this condition. The third (ascending) part runs forward against, and adherent to, the left face of the mesentery. It bends ventrally below the left kidney to continue as the jejunum. The caliber of the duodenum is uniform except at its commencement, where the first bend of the sigmoid flexure is somewhat widened. The bile and pancreatic ducts open here. The bile and major pancreatic ducts discharge through a single papilla within an enclosure (ampulla hepatopancreatica) bounded by a circular mucosal rampart. This is situated on the convex margin of the flexure, while the accessory pancreatic duct opens on a small papilla on the facing margin (see Fig. 21.9/*7* and *8*). The position and restricted mobility of the duodenum make its access difficult through the usual surgical exposures, which fortunately are not commonly needed.

The remainder of the small intestine lies within the free margin of the great mesentery, which is sufficiently long to allow the coils considerable latitude in position. Most are piled into the left dorsal part of the abdomen, where they mingle with those of the descending colon. However, some insinuate themselves between the large intestine and the flanks, while others may reach the abdominal floor between the body of the cecum and the ventral parts of the ascending colon. The ileum (according to the convention we employ [pp. 119-120]) is very short, and in most circumstances it is distinguished from the remainder of the small intestine by its much thicker wall and firmer consistency. It approaches the left side of the cecal base from below and ends by protruding into the cecal interior, raising a papilla on which it opens.

The mobility of the small intestine may be blamed for the incarceration of a part within one of several openings such as the epiploic foramen, the vaginal ring, or even a rent in the mesentery. Intussusception is also relatively common, especially in the young horse. A form peculiar to the horse involves the passage of the terminal part of the small intestine into the interior of the cecal base. Necrosis of the intruded part follows quickly unless surgical correction is undertaken.

Surgical Approaches to the Abdomen: The abdomen may be approached through ventral midline, ventral paramedian, inguinal, or flank incisions. The most common is the ventral midline approach because it allows the surgeon to pull 75% of the intestinal tract out of the abdomen, leads to minimal hemorrhage, and contains resilient fibrous tissue.

The Large Intestine

In addition to its enormous capacity, the large intestine is also characterized by having a sacculated form. The sacculations or haustra result from the shortening of the taeniae, bands formed by the concentration of the external longitudinal muscle and elastic fibers at certain (from one to four) positions on the circumference. Semilunar folds project internally where grooves divide adjacent haustra externally (see Fig. 21.12). The haustral segmentation is not constant but is constantly modified in life by gradual "haustral flow" and by intermittent disappearance of the contractions followed by their re-formation in a different pattern. The arrangement of the large intestine of the horse predisposes to various forms of obstruction and displacement, conditions collectively known as *colic* (although this term is widely used to include any painful abdominal disorder).

The Cecum

The cecum incorporates an initial portion of the ascending colon as is revealed by its extension distally beyond the entrance of the ileum. It follows that the so-called cecocolic

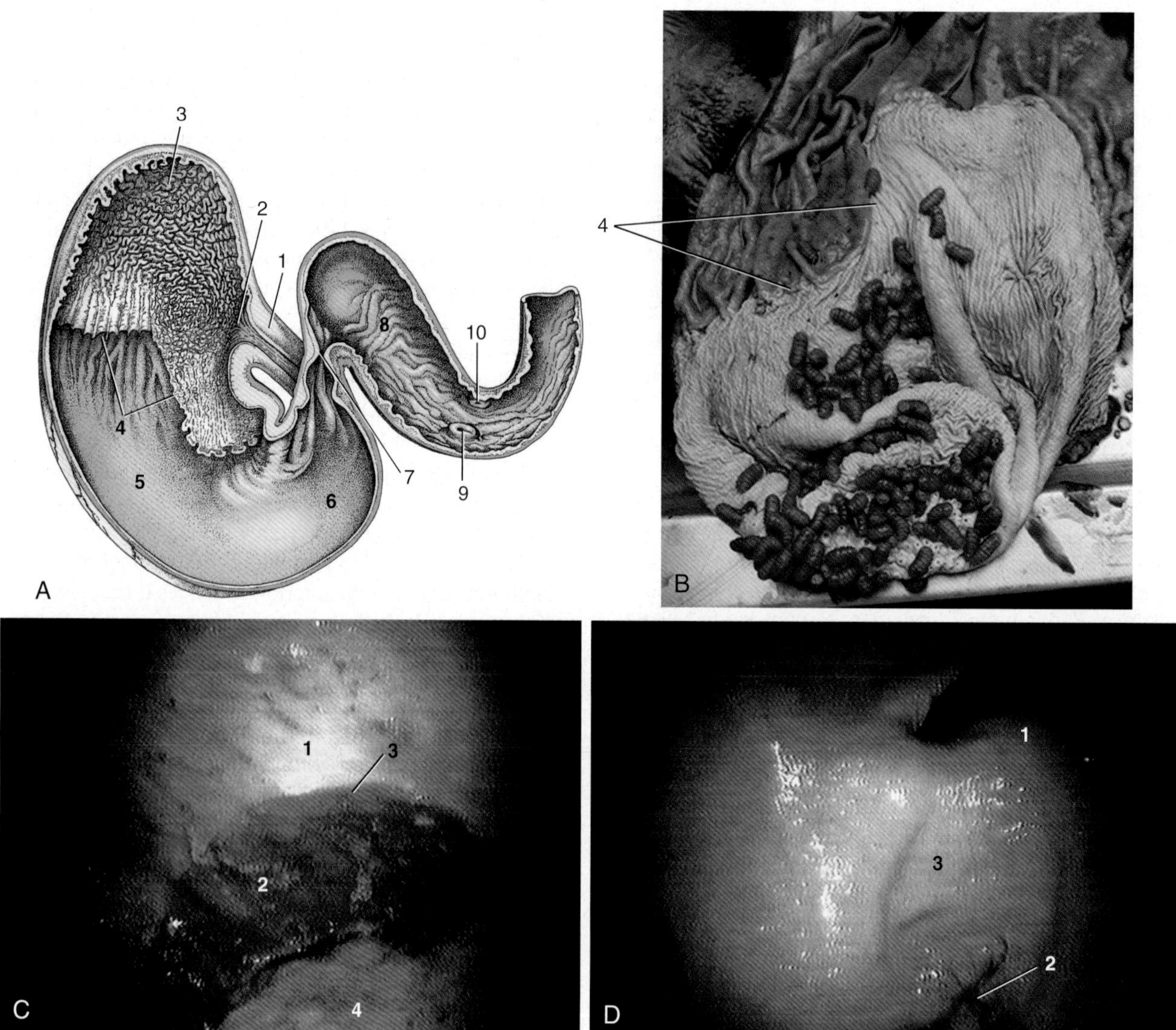

Fig. 21.11 (A) Interior of the stomach and cranial part of the duodenum. *1,* Esophagus; *2,* cardiac opening; *3,* fundus (blind sac); *4,* margo plicatus; *5,* body; *6,* pyloric part; *7,* pylorus; *8,* cranial part of duodenum; *9,* major duodenal papilla within hepatopancreatic ampulla; *10,* minor duodenal papilla. (B) Notice the white mucosa of the fundus. The *Gasterophilus* larvae are an incidental finding in this part of the stomach. *4,* Margo plicatus is clearly visible. (C) Endoscopic view of stomach. *1,* Nonglandular mucosa; *2,* glandular mucosa; *3,* margo plicatus; *4,* ingesta. (D) Endoscopic view of stomach. *1,* Fiberoptic cable of endoscope entering through cardia; *2,* pylorus; *3,* lesser curvature.

orifice is actually a constriction of the ascending colon set some distance distal to its true origin. However, the conventional terminology pays no regard to such considerations and is based entirely on the form of the adult organ (Fig. 21.13).

The cecum consists of an expanded dorsal base, a curved tapering body, and a blind ventral apex; these parts merge smoothly, and the organ is often likened to a comma (Fig. 21.14). In large horses it may have a capacity in excess of 30 L and may measure a meter or more between extremities. The base lies in the right dorsal part of the abdomen, partly against the flank and partly under cover of the ribs. It has an extensive contact with the abdominal roof and sublumbar organs from the 15th rib (or thereabouts) to the coxal tuber, but the direct dorsal adhesion is confined to the region of the pancreas and right kidney. This retroperitoneal attachment extends caudally to the level of the second lumbar vertebra. The base also fuses with the root of the mesentery medially and with the right dorsal colon cranially. The cranial part of the base forms an overhanging enlargement that at first sight appears to be blind (Fig. 21.15) but a closer inspection reveals the origin of the colon from the middle of the caudal wall of this overhang.

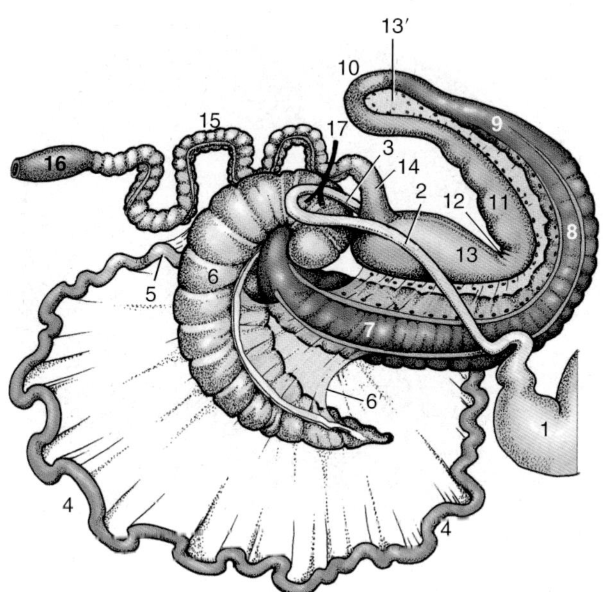

Fig. 21.12 The intestinal tract seen from the right (schematic). The caudal flexure of the duodenum and the cranial mesenteric artery *(17)* have been displaced to the right of the animal to lie over the base of the cecum. *1,* Stomach; *2* and *3,* descending and ascending duodenum, respectively; *4,* jejunum; *5,* ileum; *6,* cecum; *6′,* cecocolic fold; *7,* right ventral colon; *8,* ventral diaphragmatic flexure; *9,* left ventral colon; *10,* pelvic flexure; *11,* left dorsal colon; *12,* dorsal diaphragmatic flexure; *13,* right dorsal colon; *13′,* ascending mesocolon; *14,* transverse colon; *15,* descending (small) colon; *16,* rectum; *17,* cranial mesenteric artery.

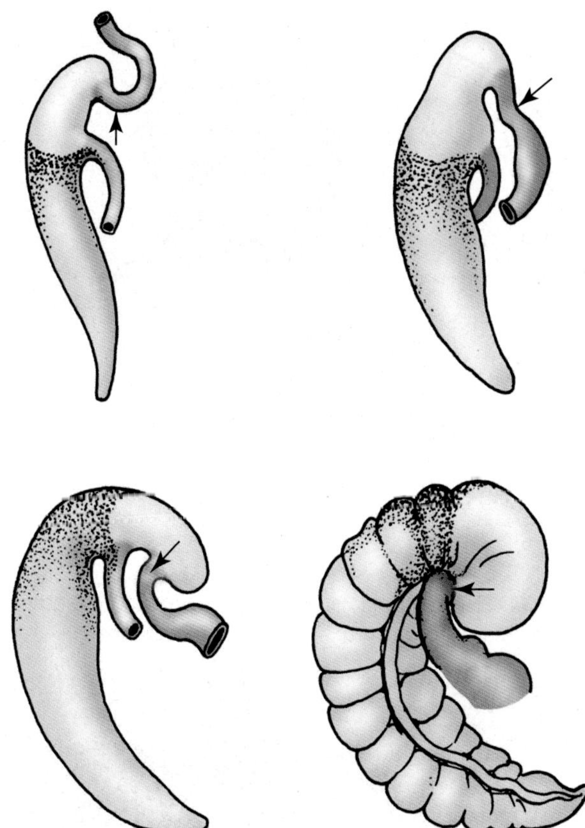

Fig. 21.13 Development of the equine cecum (schematic). The stippled part of the cecum is homologous with the cecum of other species. The nonstippled part is the annexed first part of the colon. The cecocolic orifice is a constriction of the ascending colon *(arrows).*

The caudal part of the base merges imperceptibly with the body of the cecum.

The body runs ventrally before turning cranially (Fig. 21.14/*2*). At first it lies against the right flank, following the caudal border of the right ventral colon, but as it sinks within the abdomen, it is displaced medially. When it reaches the abdominal floor, it lies between the ventral parts of the ascending colon. It terminates in the apex, close to the xiphoid cartilage. There are four taeniae over most of the organ, but the number diminishes toward the apex. Retroflexion of the apical part of the cecum is occasionally encountered in apparently healthy subjects.

The interior is marked by numerous folds corresponding to the external divisions of the haustra. These folds are impermanent, but a larger and more persistent fold at the level of the ileal papilla partially separates the cranial expansion from the remainder of the base (Fig. 21.16). The ileal papilla is variable in form. In most postmortem specimens it is a low conical projection whose summit carries a slitlike opening bounded by lax folds of mucosa (Fig. 21.16/*1*). In life, it is usually much more salient and more cylindrical and has a rounded orifice circumscribed by a firm and thickened rim. The erection of the papilla is caused by the tonus of the muscle and engorgement of a mucosal venous plexus.

Although the exit from the cecum near the cecocolic orifice (Fig. 21.16/*2*) lies at some distance from the ileal papilla, the curvature of the cecal base brings it more or less into the same transverse plane. In the dead specimen it is a transverse slit that scarcely admits a few fingers, but in life it generally allows the passage of a hand.

Microbial fermentation within the cecum produces gas that is normally discharged at intervals into the right ventral colon. Occasionally, gas is produced excessively, causing the overhanging part of the base to press on the origin of the right ventral colon, interfering with the normal mechanism. The resulting tympany of the base can only be relieved by needle decompression through the paralumbar fossa or possibly the transrectal approach. The apex and a part of the body of the cecum can be approached via the midventral celiotomy. The base may need a paracostal approach through the area of the 18th rib.

The Colon

The colon consists of the usual ascending, transverse, and descending parts (see Fig. 3.45). The first two together constitute the "large colon" of common usage, and the third constitutes the "small colon" (Fig. 21.12/*15*). The ascending

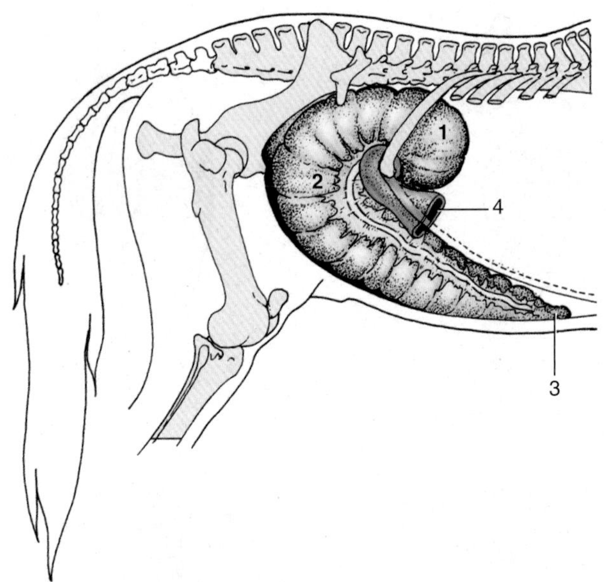

Fig. 21.14 The cecum in situ. *1,* Base of cecum; *2,* body of cecum; *3,* apex of cecum; *4,* right ventral colon.

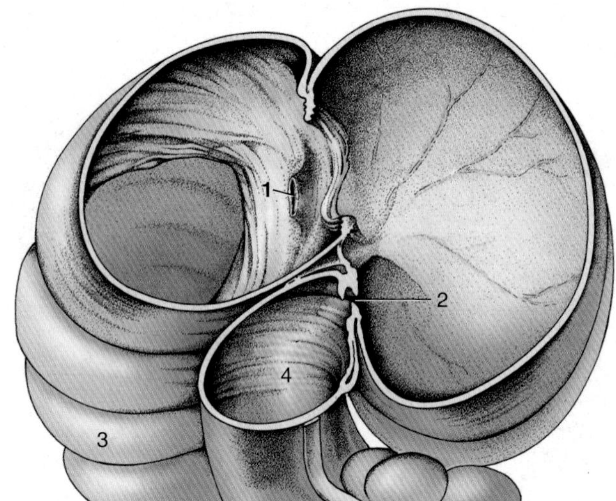

Fig. 21.16 The interior of the base of the cecum, right lateral view. *1,* Termination of ileum at ileal papilla; *2,* cecocolic orifice; *3,* body of cecum; *4,* right ventral colon.

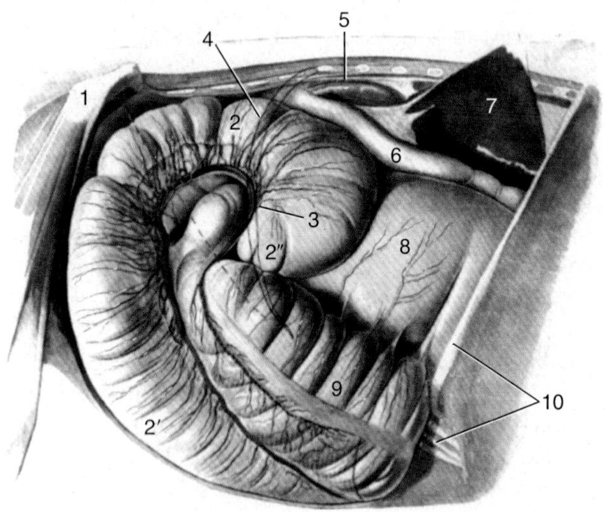

Fig. 21.15 Cecum and related organs lying against the right abdominal wall and flank. The *broken line* indicates the position of the cranial branch of the deep circumflex iliac artery crossing the flank. *1,* Coxal tuber; *2* and *2′,* base and body of cecum, respectively; *2″,* overhanging part of cecal base; *3,* position of cecocolic orifice; *4,* position of last rib; *5,* right kidney; *6,* descending duodenum; *7,* right lobe of liver, elevated; *8,* right dorsal colon; *9,* right ventral colon; *10,* tenth rib and costal arch.

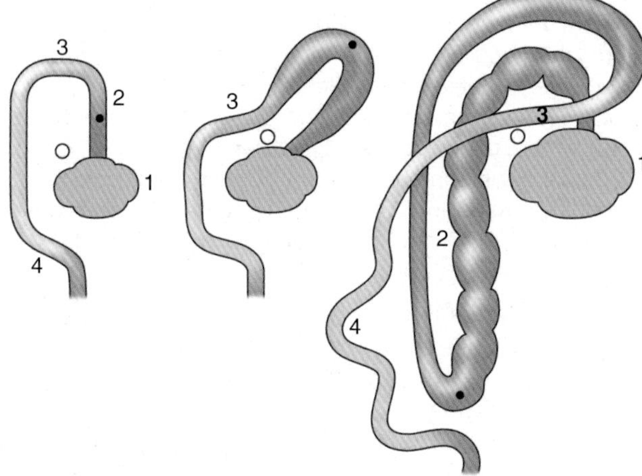

Fig. 21.17 The development of the ascending colon, dorsal view. The *dot* indicates the position of the pelvic flexure, the *circle* that of the cranial mesenteric artery. *1,* Cecum; *2,* ascending colon; *3,* transverse colon; *4,* descending colon.

colon is arranged in four parallel limbs separated by three flexures, each separately named. The sequence runs as follows: right ventral colon (Fig. 21.12/*7*), ventral diaphragmatic flexure, left ventral colon, pelvic flexure, left dorsal colon, dorsal diaphragmatic flexure, and right dorsal colon (Fig. 21.12/*13*). The right dorsal colon leads to the short transverse colon (Fig. 21.12/*14*), which is followed by the long and coiled descending colon (Fig. 21.12/*15*).

The *cecocolic transitional region* forms a sigmoid flexure: the convexity of the first bend (provided by the overhanging part of the cecal base) is directed ventrally, and that of the second bend (provided by the first part of the colon) is directed dorsally (Figs. 21.15 and 21.17). This conformation appears to be caused by the looser attachment of the medial and lateral taeniae at this level as they run as chords across the arcs into which the bowel is drawn. The *right ventral colon* is narrow when it emerges from this siphon-like arrangement but soon expands to continue, first ventrally and then cranially on the abdominal floor, as a wide (≈20-cm) tube of uniform caliber (see Fig. 21.7). It is deflected across the midline on reaching the diaphragm (ventral diaphragmatic flexure) and then becomes known

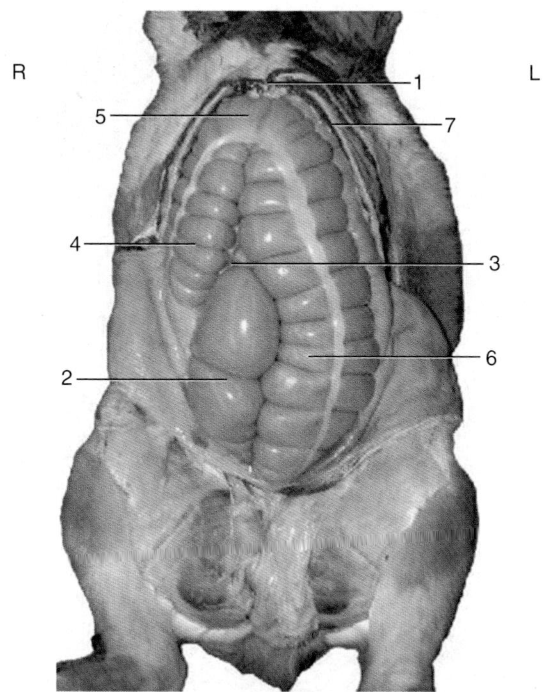

Fig. 21.18 Visceral projection on the ventral abdominal wall. The position of the apex of the cecum is variable. *1,* Xiphoid cartilage; *2,* body of cecum; *3,* apex of cecum; *4,* right ventral colon; *5,* ventral diaphragmatic flexure; *6,* left ventral colon; *7,* dorsal diaphragmatic flexure; *L,* left; *R,* right.

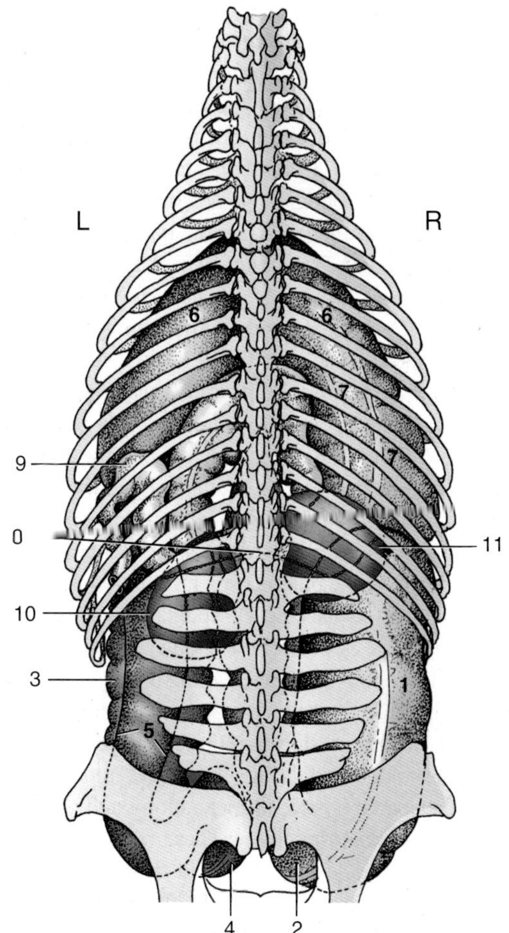

Fig. 21.19 Position of the large intestine and the kidneys, dorsal view. *1,* Base of cecum; *2,* body of cecum; *3,* left ventral colon; *4,* pelvic flexure; *5,* left dorsal colon; *6,* dorsal diaphragmatic flexure; *7,* right dorsal colon; *8,* transverse colon; *9,* proximal part of descending colon, cut; *10,* left kidney; *11,* right kidney; *L,* left; *R,* right.

as the left ventral colon (Fig. 21.18/*6*). The *left ventral colon* runs toward the pelvis, still on the abdominal floor (see Fig. 21.6/*8*), until a sharp flexure through 180 degrees marks its junction with the following left dorsal part. The *pelvic flexure* is also distinguished by a reduction in caliber (see Fig. 21.12/*10*) and by the disappearance of three of the four bands found on the ventral parts, of which the consequence is the loss of the haustrations. Although there is no evidence of a conventional sphincter, the pelvic flexure marks the boundary between two distinct functional units of the colon. The decrease in the fluidity of the ingesta, the [illegible] alteration in course, and the reduction in caliber explain why impaction is common at this level. The location of the flexure varies with the fullness of the rectum, bladder, and uterus, but because it is usually just within or in front of the pelvic cavity, it is easily found on rectal examination especially if impacted.

The *left dorsal colon* is narrow and smooth-walled where it emerges from the pelvic flexure, but it gradually widens, the taeniae increase from one to three, and the sacculations return. It runs cranially above the left ventral colon, below the coils of small intestine and descending colon, to reach the liver, where it continues as the right dorsal colon at the dorsal diaphragmatic flexure. Toward its termination it is related to the spleen and the stomach (Fig. 21.6/*7*). The *right dorsal colon* is both the shortest and, at its termination, by far the widest (≈30 cm) part of the ascending colon (Fig. 21.19/*7*). It ascends below the liver to meet the cranial part of the cecal base by which it is deflected medially to become the transverse colon (Fig. 21.19/*8*). The right dorsal colon is also the best-fixed part and is adherent to the abdominal roof, the cecal base, and the root of the mesentery. It carries three bands.

The *transverse colon* is very short and is situated according to the common mammalian pattern, passing from right to left in front of the root of the mesentery. It carries two bands and rapidly funnels to the much smaller caliber of the descending colon (Fig. 21.19/*9*) by which it is succeeded in the region of the left kidney. The transverse colon also has a direct retroperitoneal attachment to the abdominal roof.

Except at its origin and termination, the ascending colon is free within the abdomen, although its great bulk ensures that it does not change much in position. The folding it undergoes in development transforms the original mesentery into a short peritoneal sheet (ascending mesocolon) passing between adjacent portions of the dorsal and ventral limbs (Fig. 21.12/*13'*).

Through continuity with the cecum and transverse colon, it is anchored by the retroperitoneal attachments of these parts. The loose attachment between the left limbs allows the dorsal part to slip some way to the side (generally the right side) of the ventral part as a common and probably temporary variant of the usual topography. When the rotation of these parts about their common axis is pronounced, there arises the condition known as *twist* (torsio), which is one of the most severe abdominal catastrophes to which the horse is subject. A torsio coli initially narrows the lumen, but more important is the interruption of the blood flow in the capillaries of the bowel wall and in the vessels that follow the bowel. Recently, the lodgment of the left limbs above the spleen has also been recognized. Although the cause of this painful condition is not known with certainty, it is postulated that the accumulation of gas raises the left limbs against the abdominal wall until they pass over the base of the spleen to be trapped on the shelf formed by the phrenicosplenic and renosplenic ligaments (left dorsal displacement). Spontaneous restoration of normal topography is possible, but quicker restoration may be achieved by rolling and maneuvering the recumbent (anesthetized) animal. If the rolling procedure is failing, surgical intervention (decompression) is required.

The *descending colon* (Fig. 21.12/*15*), much narrower than the other parts, is several meters long and alone hangs within a conventional mesentery. These features account for its alternative names, *small colon* and *floating colon.* It lies mainly within the dorsal, caudal, and left part of the abdomen, largely dorsal to the small intestine, and ends in the rectum (Fig. 21.6/*5*). The distinction between the descending colon and rectum is based entirely on the pelvic location of the latter, and no immediate change in structure or appearance occurs. The descending colon is drawn by two prominent bands into a linear series of sacculations occupied by the familiar dry fecal balls. The rectum is considered with the pelvic organs.

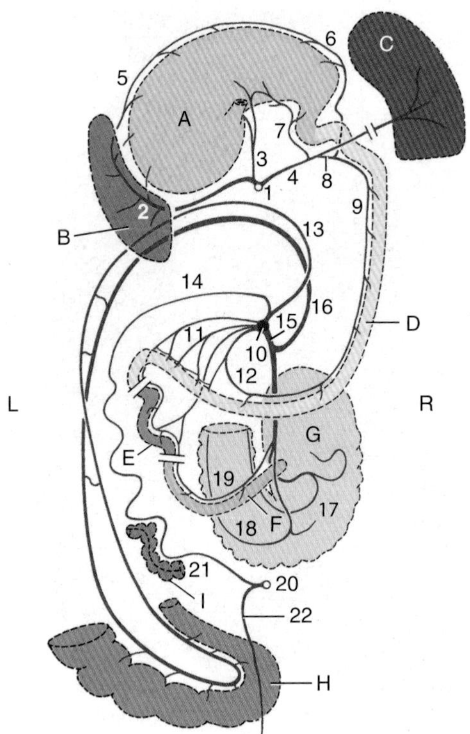

Fig. 21.20 The major arteries of the gastrointestinal tract (schematic), dorsal view. The structures have been stretched craniocaudally for clarity. (A) Stomach; (B) spleen; (C) liver; (D) duodenum; (E) jejunum; (F) ileum; (G) cecum; (H) pelvic flexure; (I) descending colon. *1,* Celiac artery (a.); *2,* splenic a.; *3,* left gastric a.; *4,* hepatic a.; *5,* left gastroepiploic a.; *6,* right gastroepiploic a.; *7,* right gastric a.; *8,* gastroduodenal a.; *9,* cranial pancreaticoduodenal a.; *10,* cranial mesenteric a.; *11,* jejunal arteries; *12,* caudal pancreaticoduodenal a.; *13,* right colic a.; *14,* middle colic a; *15,* ileocolic a.; *16,* colic branch of ileocolic a.; *17,* lateral cecal a.; *18,* medial cecal a.; *19,* mesenteric ileal a.; *20,* caudal mesenteric a.; *21,* left colic a.; *22,* cranial rectal a.; *L,* left; *R,* right.

VASCULARIZATION, LYMPH DRAINAGE, AND INNERVATION OF THE GASTROINTESTINAL TRACT

The vascularization of the equine abdominal viscera was of special clinical importance in the past because of the occurrence of migrant nematode larvae in the blood vessels. The pathology caused by the larvae is often more serious in the cranial mesenteric artery and its major branches and includes formation of aneurysms and connective tissue reaction. The caudal mesenteric artery, specifically concerned with the descending colon, may also be affected. The fact that these lesions are not often fatal is a testament to the extensive anastomoses between the major arteries supplying successive parts of the gastrointestinal tract. However, smaller arteries have poor anastomoses, and their closure has more serious consequences.

The branching and distribution of the two mesenteric arteries are shown in Fig. 21.20. The celiac artery has essentially the same distribution to the stomach, liver, and spleen as in other species. The venous drainage parallels the arterial supply, in that the portal vein is ultimately formed by the union of the caudal mesenteric, cranial mesenteric, and splenic tributaries.

Lymph from the regional nodes of the stomach, spleen, liver, pancreas, and diaphragm drains to a lymph center about the celiac artery and thence to the cisterna chyli via a celiac trunk.

The very numerous nodes that receive lymph from the intestines (with the exception of the caudal part of the descending colon) are scattered at the root of the mesentery and along the arteries of the cecum and colon. Lymph is collected and conveyed to the cisterna chyli by an intestinal trunk. The nodes scattered along the remainder of the descending colon send lymph to a center at the root of the colic mesentery and then to the lumbar trunk; this route is also followed by most of the lymph draining the rectum and anus.

The abdominal viscera are supplied by nerves that pass through plexuses associated with the mesenteric ganglia (see Fig. 21.24/*18* and *20*). The nervous structures about the celiac and cranial mesenteric arteries may be involved in the reaction provoked by the nematode larvae and are difficult to display satisfactorily except in juvenile animals. It is often asserted, although it remains unproven, that the "colic" pain and functional disturbance associated with helminth infestations are caused by secondary involvement of the nerves rather than by the primary vascular lesions.

THE LIVER

The liver is quite variable in form and size but on average weighs about 5 kg in a saddle horse. At about 1.5% of the body weight, it is a much smaller proportion than in carnivores.

It is situated in the most cranial part of the abdomen directly against the diaphragm. It is markedly asymmetrical in the healthy young subject, in which about two-thirds lies to the right of the median plane (see Fig. 21.7/*2*). The most caudal part, which is also the most dorsal, lies ventral to the vertebral extremities of the 16th and 17th ribs of the right side; the most cranial and most ventral part lies against the left part of the vertex of the diaphragm (Fig. 21.6/*3*). The long axis thus runs obliquely. In the newborn foal the liver is more symmetrical and relatively much larger and extends onto the abdominal floor behind the costal arch. In older subjects atrophy of the liver is common and is most obvious in the right lobe, probably resulting from chronic pressure from the right dorsal colon and cecal base. Less often, the left lobe atrophies, perhaps under pressure from the stomach.

The parietal surface is joined to the diaphragm by a complicated system of ligaments. The visceral surface lies against and is impressed by the stomach, duodenum, dorsal diaphragmatic flexure of the colon, and cecal base (see Fig. 21.10). The porta is central, within an area made rough by the direct attachment of the pancreas. The dorsal fixed margin of the liver extends between the right and left triangular ligaments and is very irregular (Fig. 21.21). Its right part is thick and excavated to receive the cranial pole of the right kidney; a sulcus medial to this transmits the caudal vena cava. Its left part is much thinner and does not extend nearly so far dorsally. It carries the impression of the esophagus close to the midline. The long free margin is much sharper and is interrupted by a series of fissures, the largest of which divide named lobes. The current nomenclature recognizes left, quadrate, right, and caudate lobes. The first two are separated by the fissure carrying the round ligament of the liver (vestige of the umbilical vein), but

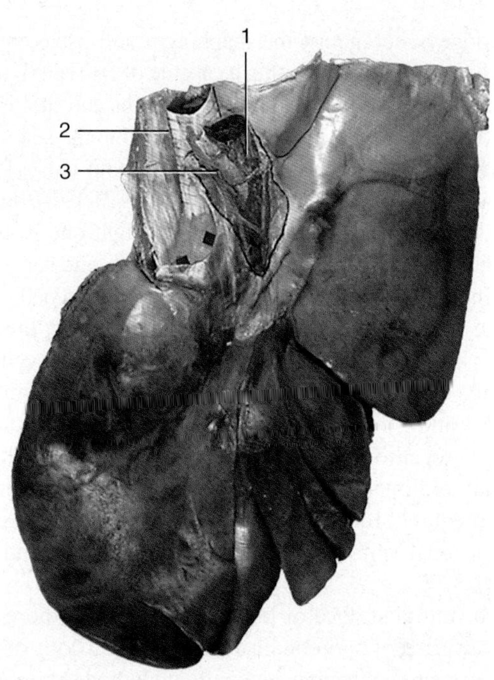

Fig. 21.21 Visceral surface of the liver. *1,* Portal vein; *2,* caudal vena cava; *3,* hepatic artery.

the boundaries of the others are more arbitrary and are of doubtful morphologic significance.

The duct system is remarkable for the absence of a gallbladder, but its wide caliber compensates for this. The bile duct opens into the cranial duodenum on the papilla shared with the major pancreatic duct (see Fig. 21.9/*7*). The oblique passage of the duct through the duodenal wall serves as a sphincter and prevents the influx of ingesta.

THE PANCREAS

The pancreas lies largely to the right and is pressed against the abdominal roof and sublumbar organs (Fig. 21.10/*7*). It is triangular in outline, and its apex is fitted into the second concavity of the duodenal sigmoid flexure. The right border follows the descending duodenum. The left border passes obliquely toward the left kidney. The portal vein (Fig. 21.9/*10*) perforates the pancreas close to the caudal border. The ventral surface is directly bound to the right dorsal colon and cecal base, the dorsal surface to the right kidney and liver. The openings of its two ducts (Fig. 21.9/*7* and *8*) are described with the duodenum.

THE KIDNEYS AND ADRENALS

The kidneys lie against the diaphragm and psoas muscles dorsally, each enclosed within a capsule of fat. The right kidney lies ventral to the last two or three ribs and first lumbar transverse process; the left one lies ventral to the last rib and first two or three processes and is thus about half a kidney length caudal to the level of its fellow (Fig. 21.19/*10* and *11*). Each kidney weighs about 700 g. The right one is shaped like the heart on a playing card, but the left one has a more conventional form. Both are dorsoventrally flattened.

The cranial pole of the right kidney fits into the renal impression of the liver; caudal to this it is ventrally attached to the pancreas and the base of the cecum (Fig. 21.15/*5* and *2*). The duodenum winds around the lateral margin and adjoining part of the ventral surface, which is the only region sometimes covered with peritoneum. The short medial border is indented by the hilus and is related to the caudal vena cava and the right adrenal gland (Fig. 21.22).

The ventral surface of the left kidney has a more complete covering of peritoneum and is related to coils of small colon and small intestine, generally including the duodenojejunal junction. Cranioventrally it lies against the spleen and may make contact with a distended stomach (see Fig. 21.10). The medial border is related to the aorta and the left adrenal gland (see Fig. 21.22).

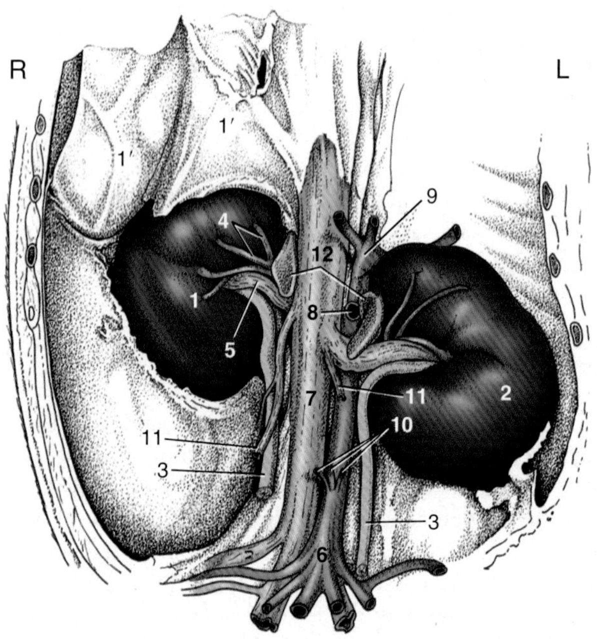

Fig. 21.22 Kidneys and adrenal glands in situ, ventral view. *1*, Right kidney; *1′*, liver; *2*, left kidney; *3*, ureter; *4*, renal artery; *5*, renal vein; *6*, aorta; *7*, caudal vena cava; *8*, cranial mesenteric artery; *9*, celiac artery; *10*, caudal mesenteric and testicular arteries; *11*, testicular veins; *12*, adrenal glands; *L*, left; *R*, right.

The kidneys are of a modified unipyramidal type; the numerous constituent pyramids are completely fused, and their former boundaries are revealed only by the arrangement of the interlobar arteries. A clearer indication of the lobation, with some external fissuration, is common in the foal. The structure is best revealed in section (Fig. 21.23). The strong external fibrous capsule can normally be easily stripped away, except within the renal sinus, where it merges with the adventitia of the structures entering and leaving. The division of the parenchyma between cortex and medulla is indicated by a color change and by the sectioned arcuate arteries. The cortex is brownish red and granular. The peripheral part of the medulla is dark red, the inner part pale; both show radial striations. The apices of the fused medullary pyramids form a common renal crest that projects into the pelvis. This has a curious form consisting of a central expansion (Fig. 21.23/*4*) at the origin of the ureter and two terminal recesses toward the poles (Fig. 21.23/*5*); most papillary ducts open into the recesses. The pelvic mucosa produces a mucous secretion, and as a result the unfiltered urine normally contains some protein (physiologic albuminuria).

The renal vessels are short and wide. The artery often splits before reaching the hilus, and a number of branches may enter the ventral surface independently (Fig. 21.23/*8*).

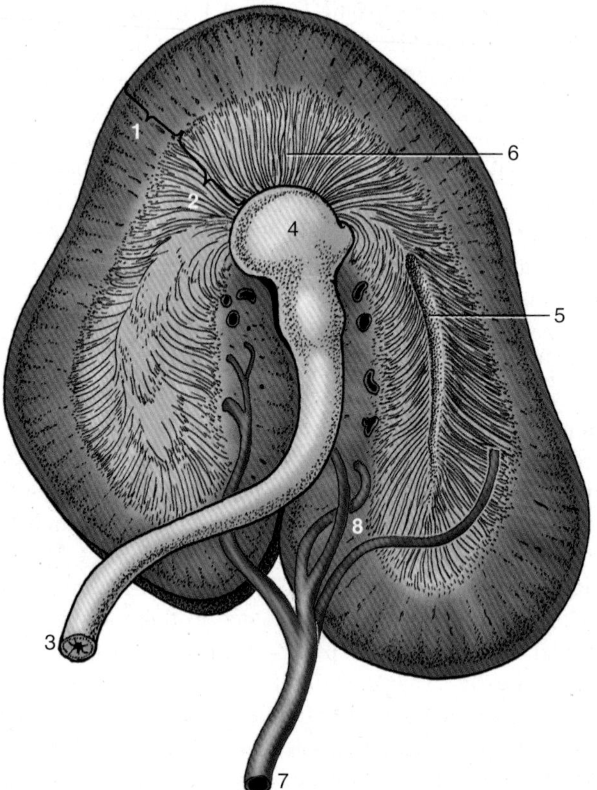

Fig. 21.23 Dorsal section through a kidney (semi-schematic). *1*, Renal cortex; *2*, renal medulla; *3*, ureter; *4*, pelvis; *5*, terminal recess; *6*, papillary ducts; *7*, renal artery; *8*, interlobar arteries.

For biopsy or complete removal (nephrectomy), the kidneys may be accessed through the 15th or 16th intercostal space or via resection of the 16th or 17th rib.

The ureters are wide at their origins but soon reduce to narrow, more uniform calibers. They bend caudally on emerging from the renal sinus and thereafter pursue a tortuous course over the roof of the abdomen to reach the pelvis. Here they follow the lateral parts of the broad ligaments (genital fold in the male) before inclining medially to pierce the bladder wall close to its neck.

The elongated and irregular *adrenal glands* lie against the cranial parts of the medial borders of the corresponding kidneys (Fig. 21.22/*12*). Each consists of an outer bright yellow cortex and an inner brownish red medulla. The glands are relatively large in juvenile animals.

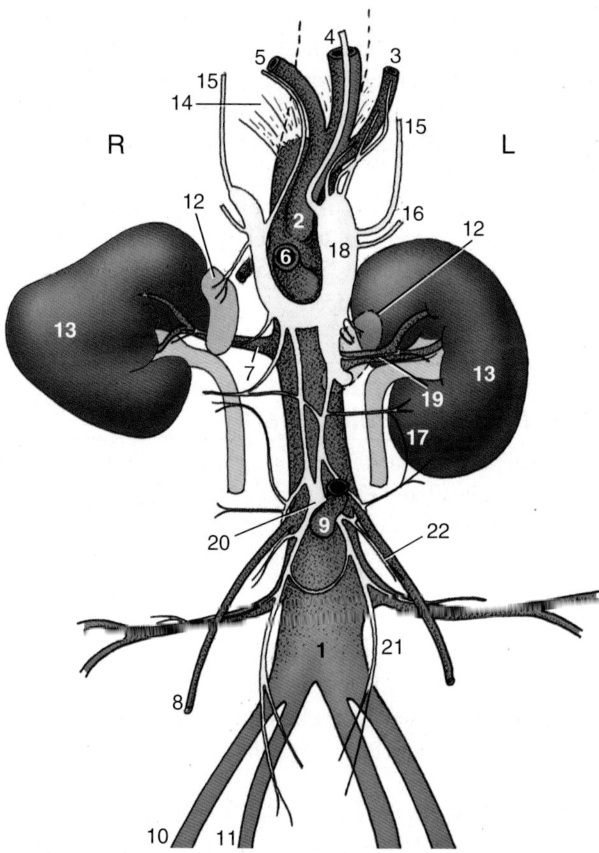

Fig. 21.24 Schema of the abdominal autonomic nerves and branches of the abdominal aorta, ventral view. *1,* Aorta; *2,* celiac artery (a.); *3,* splenic a.; *4,* left gastric a.; *5,* hepatic a.; *6,* cranial mesenteric a.; *7,* renal a.; *8,* testicular (ovarian) a.; *9,* caudal mesenteric a.; *10,* external iliac a.; *11,* internal iliac a.; *12,* adrenal glands; *13,* kidneys; *14,* crus of diaphragm; *15,* major splanchnic nerves; *16,* minor splanchnic nerves; *17,* lumbar splanchnic nerves; 18, combined celiac and cranial mesenteric ganglia; *19,* renal plexus; *20,* caudal mesenteric ganglion; *21,* hypogastric nerve; *22,* testicular (ovarian) plexus; *L,* left; *R,* right.

THE ROOF OF THE ABDOMEN

The bodies of the lumbar vertebrae, the sublumbar muscles, and the diaphragm furnish the roof of the abdomen. The aorta and caudal vena cava lie to the left and the right within the cleft between the two psoas minor muscles (Fig. 21.22/*6* and *7*). The branches of the aorta and the tributaries of the vein are, in principle, the same as in other species.

The autonomic nerves and ganglia show some equine-specific features, although not of much substance. The general pattern is shown in Fig. 21.24. The fused celiac and cranial mesenteric ganglia lie ventral to the aorta, to each side of the celiac and cranial mesenteric arteries. The right and left ganglia are joined by bridges cranial and caudal to the latter artery. They are sizable structures, 5 cm or so long, and are generally unequal, with the left being larger and more regular (Fig. 21.24/*18*). Each is joined by a major splanchnic nerve and, in varying fashion, by parasympathetic fibers from the dorsal vagal trunk. The nerves that leave the ganglia follow the branching pattern of the arteries and form a dense plexus in which the sympathetic and parasympathetic contributions mingle. The whole plexiform arrangement that radiates from the major ganglia is known as the *celiacomesenteric* (solar) *plexus*. Additional small renal ganglia occur on the nerves about the renal arteries.

The celiacomesenteric complex is joined to the caudal mesenteric plexus by a plexus on the aorta and an additional trunk that runs at a more ventral level within the colic mesentery. The caudal mesenteric ganglion lies cranial to the origin of the like-named artery (Fig. 21.24/*9* and *20*). It gives rise to nerve plexuses that follow this vessel and the gonadal vessels to the small colon and reproductive organs, respectively, and to the hypogastric nerves (Fig. 21.24/*21*) that pursue a retroperitoneal course on the roof of the pelvis. Lumbar splanchnic nerves join the major ganglia and the aortic plexus in an erratic fashion.

There is usual direct detachment of preganglionic fibers from the splanchnic nerves to the medullary parts of the adrenal glands.

COMPREHENSION CHECK

Working in a group, discuss and demonstrate the embryologic origins of the arrangement of the gastrointestinal tract of the horse. Develop a model to demonstrate the arrangement of the large intestine of the horse.

22 The Pelvis and Reproductive Organs of the Horse

This chapter is concerned with the pelvic cavity and its contents and with the extrapelvic parts of the reproductive organs of both sexes. It also includes a brief account of the udder. The general conformation of the region and the surface landmarks created by the pelvic skeleton are dealt with in Chapter 24.

GENERAL ANATOMY OF THE PELVIS AND PERINEUM

The pelvic cavity is roofed by the sacrum and first two or three caudal vertebra, and it is difficult to define the boundaries precisely. The roof narrows from front to back and is slightly concave in its length. The ischial tuber and spine are both less prominent than in cattle, and the contribution of the substantial sacrosciatic ligament to the lateral wall is therefore relatively greater (Fig. 22.1/*7*). The floor of the pelvic cavity is solid because the symphysis is firmly fused in mature animals, but the floor is more or less horizontal and flat in its length and somewhat hollowed from side to side. The pubic region presents a median swelling or ridge in young animals, and it retains this conformation in the stallion; however, the bone thins and the upper surface becomes markedly excavated in mares, especially those that have carried several foals.

The entrance to the pelvic cavity faces cranioventrally, and the pubic brim is below the third, or even fourth, sacral vertebra in the mare but only the second in the stallion. Viewed from the front, the inlet to the female pelvis is wide and rounded compared to the more angular and cramped inlet, particularly ventrally, in the stallion (Fig. 22.2B). In both sexes, the outlet from the cavity is much smaller than the inlet; it is bounded by a caudal vertebra, the free edges of the sacrosciatic ligaments, and the ischial tubers and arch.

The cavity has the approximate form of a truncated cone, and the longitudinal axis is almost straight between the entrance and the exit (Fig. 22.3). The pelvis of the mare is thus more favorably disposed for parturition than that of the cow: the entrance is wide, the exit less confined, the cavity generally more capacious, the axis without marked deflection, and a greater part of the lateral walls composed of soft tissue.

The reader is referred to page 40 for a general account of the structure of the pelvis and to Figs. 22.8 and 22.19 for an indication of the topography and peritoneal relationships of the viscera.

The most distinctive feature of the perineum is its confinement between the semimembranosus muscles, which extend ventrally from their vertebral heads of origin. These muscles cover the ischial tubers and also the ischiorectal fossae, which therefore do not contribute to the surface contour. Because the muscles bury the caudal borders of the sacrosciatic ligaments, they hamper recognition of the softening that is an indication of approaching parturition in cattle.

The thin, sparsely haired, and deeply pigmented perineal skin glistens from the secretion of sebaceous glands. It is raised over the caudal part of the anal canal, forming a projection whose shape and salience vary with the functional state. The unusual outline of the vulva and its variable position are the subject of a later comment (p. 561). In the male the urethra may be palpated where it bends around the ischial arch.

The deeper structures of the perineum closely resemble their bovine counterparts, to which reference may be made (Chapter 29); differences in detail, though numerous, are not of practical significance.

Innervation, Vascularization, and Lymph Drainage of the Pelvic Walls

The branches of the *lumbosacral plexus* that traverse the pelvis are considered in detail on page 311, and only a few features are mentioned here. The obturator nerve follows the usual course over the medial aspect of the shaft of the ilium to reach the obturator foramen, and this exposes it to risk of injury in fractures of the bone or by compression during parturition (Fig. 22.4/*15*). The point of origin of the cranial gluteal, sciatic, and caudal gluteal nerves is exposed to similar risk where it lies against the ventral aspect of the sacrum, en route to the greater sciatic foramen (Fig. 22.4/*13*).

The *pudendal nerve* (Fig. 22.4/*12*) arises from the middle sacral nerves (S[2]3–S4) and heads in the direction of the ischial tuber. The nerve first runs internal to the sacrosciatic ligament but later becomes embedded within its substance. As the nerve passes the lesser sciatic foramen, it exchanges fibers with the caudal cutaneous nerve of the thigh through the opening. With the main trunk continuing to the clitoris or the penis, the most important among its branches is the deep perineal nerve, which supplies the striated musculature of the perineum (Fig. 22.4/*12′*). The superficial branch is sensory to the anus, vulva, and perineal skin as far ventrally as the udder (or scrotum and prepuce).

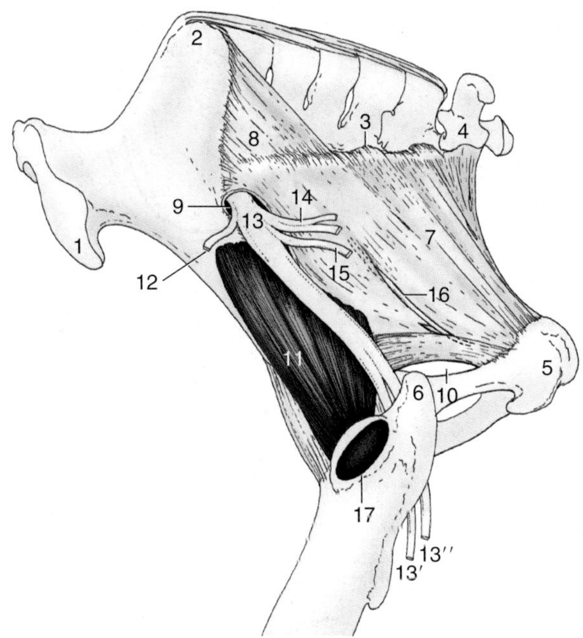

Fig. 22.1 Lateral view of the bony pelvis and sacrosciatic ligament. *1,* Coxal tuber; *2,* sacral tuber; *3,* lateral border of sacrum; *4,* caudal vertebra 1; *5,* ischial tuber; *6,* caudal part of greater trochanter; *7,* sacrosciatic ligament; *8,* dorsal sacroiliac ligament; *9,* greater sciatic foramen; *10,* lesser sciatic foramen; *11,* gluteus profundus; *12,* cranial gluteal nerve; *13,* sciatic nerve; *13′,* common peroneal nerve; *13″,* tibial nerve; *14,* caudal gluteal nerve; *15,* caudal cutaneous femoral nerve; *16,* pudendal nerve; *17,* trochanteric bursa.

The caudal rectal nerve (Fig. 22.4/*11*), which arises from the same sacral nerves (S[2]3–S4), is motor to the striated muscles of the dorsal part of the perineum and sensory to the rectum, the wall of the anal canal, and adjacent skin.

The pelvic nerves (Fig. 22.4/*14*) are deployed in the usual fashion and are composed of parasympathetic fibers from the second, third, and fourth sacral nerves.

The *blood supply* to the pelvic contents and walls is attended to by the *internal iliac arteries,* terminal branches of the abdominal aorta (Fig. 22.4). The very short internal iliac artery passes below the wing of the ilium and soon divides into internal pudendal and caudal gluteal arteries. The *internal pudendal artery* has a mainly visceral distribution. It runs caudoventrally on the deep face of the sacrosciatic ligament, close to the pudendal nerve, before swinging medially to divide about the level of the ischial spine. Its branches include the *umbilical artery,* which conveys a little blood to the vertex of the bladder (and the adjacent part of the deferent duct in the male), and a much more important branch that supplies the bulk of the intrapelvic reproductive organs. This is known as the *vaginal artery* in the female, in which it supplies the greater part of the bladder, the urethra, the caudal part of the uterus, the vagina, and, by way of the middle rectal artery, a substantial part of the rectum. The homologous *prostatic artery* supplies the bladder, the urethra, the accessory genital glands, and the corresponding part of the rectum. End branches of the internal pudendal artery (Fig. 22.4/*12′*) include the *caudal rectal artery* to the rectum and anus, a (ventral) *perineal artery* for the tissues between the anus and vulva, and branches to the vestibule and the vestibular bulb; the male counterpart of the last named is the *artery of the penis,* which anastomoses with divisions of the obturator.

The *caudal gluteal artery* passes caudally in the dorsolateral wall of the pelvis; it branches off the obturator and cranial gluteal arteries. The trunk pierces the sacrosciatic ligament before supplying the hamstring muscles and the tail. The obturator artery leaves the pelvis through the obturator foramen, and the cranial gluteal artery exits through the greater sciatic foramen.

The veins largely mirror the patterns of the arteries.

The *lymph nodes* associated with the pelvic walls display the usual species characteristics, comprising numerous, closely packed, and individually small nodes that aggregate to form sizable masses. The major groupings are related to the termination and parietal branches of the aorta. Sacral nodes lie between the divergent internal iliac arteries, medial iliac nodes lie at the origin (from the external iliac) of the deep circumflex iliac arteries, and lateral iliac nodes lie at the terminal division of the latter.

Other (anorectal) nodes lie over the caudal part of the rectum. In the horse the deep inguinal nodes (Fig. 22.4/*4*) lie outside the pelvic cavity, within the femoral triangle and at no great distance from the superficial inguinal nodes. The latter are interposed between the prepuce and scrotum (or udder) and the trunk. They drain lymph from the external reproductive organs (and udder) and from the skin and deeper structures over a considerable part of the ventral trunk. This lymph is then channeled to the deep inguinal nodes, which also receive most lymph from the hindlimb, of which a part has already been filtered through the nodes in the popliteal fossa. The outflow goes to the medial iliac nodes, which constitute the collecting center for lymph emanating from the caudal abdominal and pelvic walls and from the pelvic viscera. Much of this lymph has already passed through anorectal, sacral, or lateral iliac nodes. The outflow is either to the aortic lumbar nodes of the abdominal roof or directly to an erratically formed lumbar trunk.

THE RECTUM AND ANAL CANAL

The principal features of visceral topography and peritoneal disposition are shown in Figs. 22.5, 22.6, and 22.7.

The rectum continues the descending colon beyond the pelvic inlet. Initially it resembles the colon in structure and in relationship to the peritoneum, but as it proceeds caudally the mesentery shortens and the peritoneal covering is

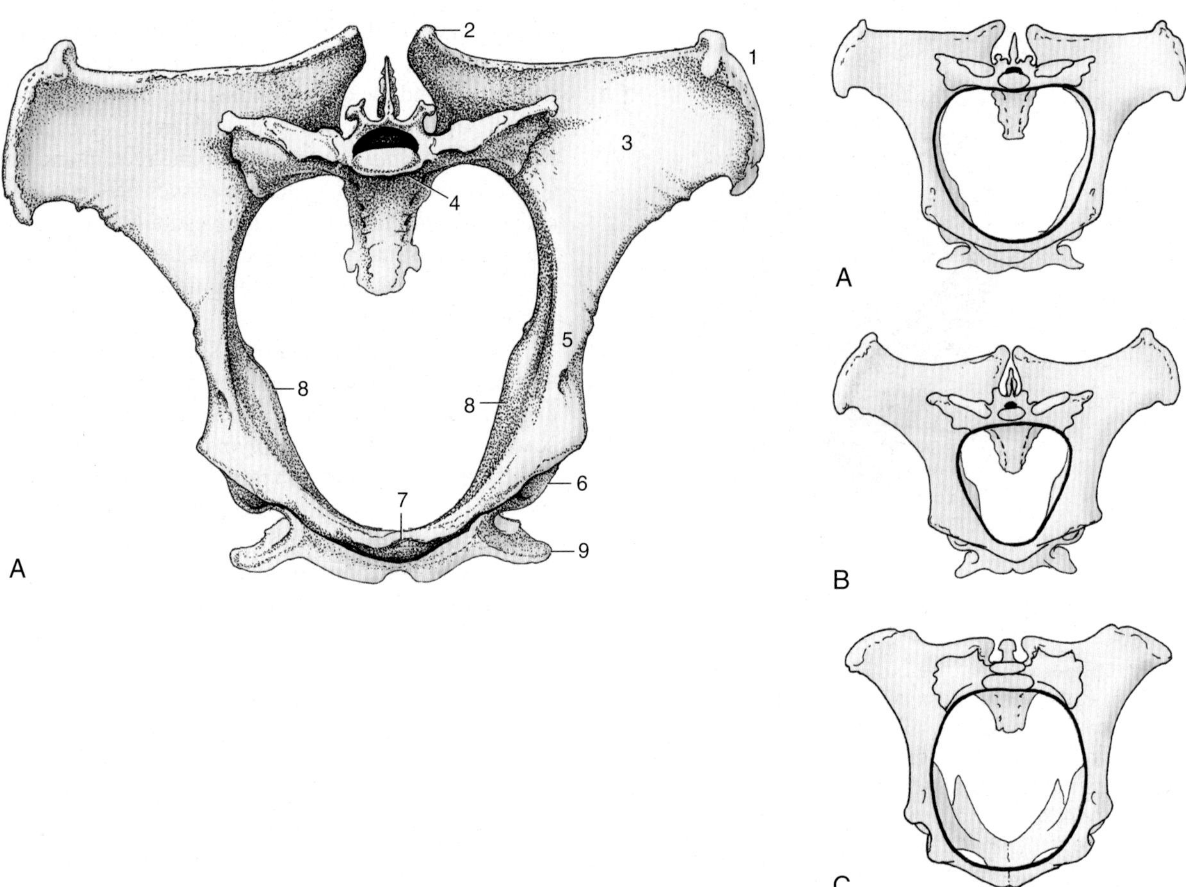

Fig. 22.2 Cranial view of the pelvis of the mare (A), stallion (B), and cow (C). The *terminal line* is emphasized in the smaller pictures; observe the differences in the shape of the pelvic inlet and position of the ischial spines. *1*, Coxal tuber; *2*, sacral tuber; *3*, wing of ilium; *4*, promontory; *5*, shaft of ilium; *6*, acetabulum; *7*, brim of pubis; *8*, ischial spines; *9*, ischial tuber.

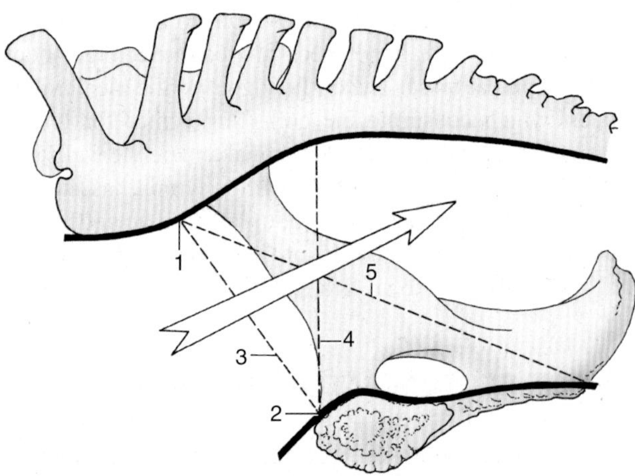

Fig. 22.3 Schematic median section of the mare's pelvis illustrating certain obstetric terms. *1*, Promontory; *2*, cranial end of the pelvic symphysis; *3*, conjugata; *4*, vertical diameter; *5*, diagonal conjugata. The *arrow* indicates the axis of the pelvic canal.

gradually lost (commencing with the dorsal aspect); finally, the rectum is wholly retroperitoneal and embedded in a fat-rich connective tissue. The proportion of the rectum that is retroperitoneal appears to vary between individuals and is among to the perforations of the wall of the rectum that may occur during clinical procedures. The terminal part of the rectum loses the sacculated character and forms a wide flask-like expansion (ampulla) just before it joins the anal canal. The ampulla stores feces before evacuation. The regrouped dorsal and lateral longitudinal muscle bundles break free, pass above the anus, and anchor the rectum to the fourth or fifth caudal vertebra; these bundles constitute the smooth rectococcygeus (Fig. 22.4/9).

The relations of the rectum depend on its fullness and on the sex. In the mare, the rectum lies on the uterus and vagina unless, as often happens, these are displaced to one side and the rectum is enabled to make contact with the bladder. In male animals the ventral surface lies on the bladder, the urethra, and the accessory reproductive glands; the extents of the individual contacts depend on the state of

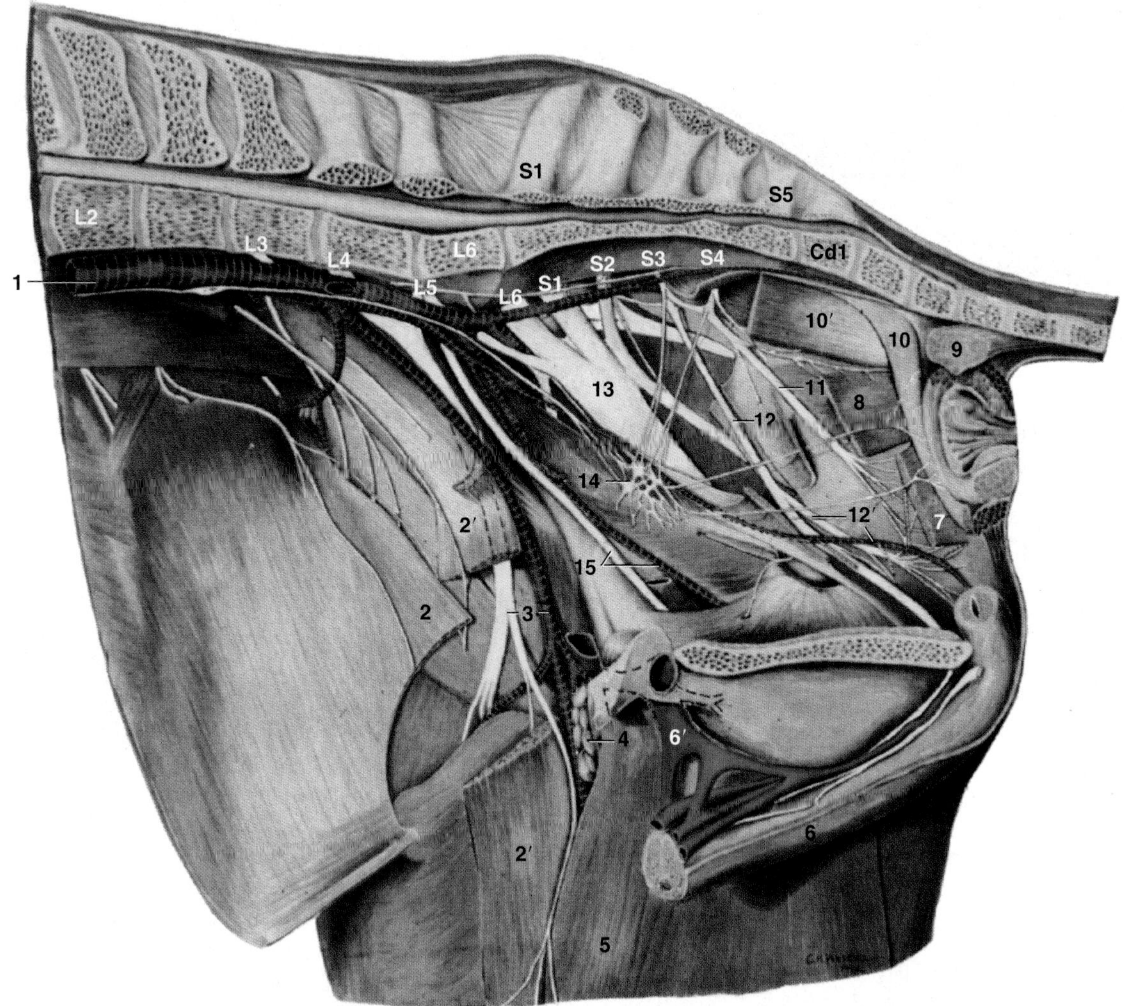

Fig. 22.4 Dissection of the pelvic wall, medial view. *1,* Aorta; *2,* internal abdominal oblique; *2′,* sartorius, resected; *3,* femoral artery and nerve (n.); *4,* deep inguinal lymph nodes; *5,* gracilis; *6,* penis; *6′,* (accessory) external pudendal vein; *7,* levator ani, resected; *8,* coccygeus; *9,* rectococcygeus; *10,* retractor penis; *10′,* ventral tail muscle; *11,* caudal rectal n.; *12,* [illegible]; *12′,* deep perineal n. and internal pudendal artery; *13,* sciatic n.; *14,* pelvic plexus; [illegible] n. and vessels. *Cd1,* caudal vertebra 1; *L2–L6,* second through sixth lumbar [illegible] *S1–S5,* first through fifth sacral vertebrae.

the bladder and the development of the glands, which are naturally smaller in the gelding.

The anal canal continues the rectum but, unlike this, is generally empty of feces. It is closed by the apposition and interdigitation of longitudinal mucosal folds and by the contraction of the internal and external anal sphincters. The extent of the canal is sharply defined by anorectal and anocutaneous lines marking the limits of epithelial specialization. The canal is embraced by the pelvic diaphragm (Fig. 22.4/*7* and *8*); the part caudal to the pelvic diaphragm projects as a cylindrical eminence within the perineal region.

THE BLADDER AND FEMALE URETHRA

The neck region of the bladder lies directly on the pelvic floor, and when the organ is fully contracted it forms a firm, globular swelling about the size of a clenched fist in the pelvic cavity and becomes wholly retroperitoneal. As the bladder fills, it gradually assumes a more ovoid form and extends cranially into the abdomen.

The relations of the bladder depend on the degree of filling and on the sex. When empty, its vertex is generally in contact with the pelvic flexure of the colon, but as the bladder enlarges, the vertex and adjacent parts obtain a more extensive and more varied relationship to the intestine. In the mare the dorsal surface is in contact with the cranial part of the vagina, the cervix, a variable part of the body of the uterus, and sometimes the rectum (Fig. 22.8). The corresponding relations in the male are the genital fold, the deferent ducts, the vesicular glands, the prostate, and the rectum.

The relatively large neonatal bladder is entirely intra-abdominal and adjusts to adult proportions and position with the postnatal development of the pelvis and the

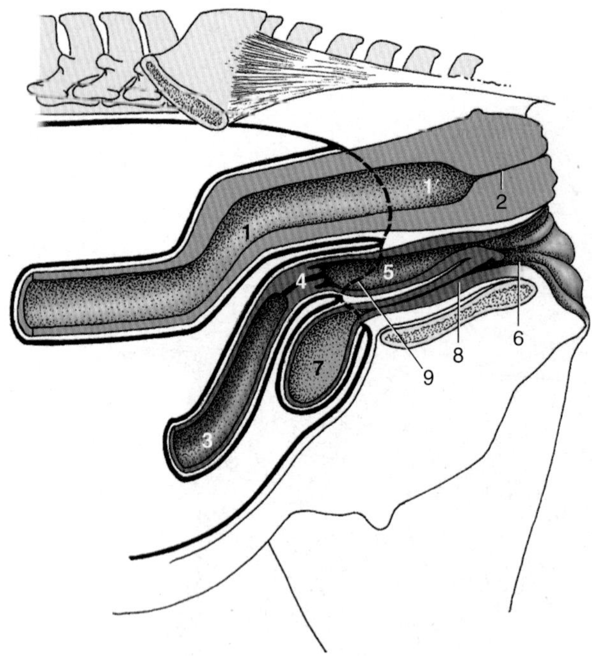

Fig. 22.5 Median section of the pelvis of the mare (schematic). *1* and *1'*, Peritoneal and retroperitoneal parts of the rectum, respectively; *2*, anal canal; *3*, uterus; *4*, cervix; *5*, vagina; *6*, vestibule; *7*, bladder; *8*, urethra; *9*, caudal extent of peritoneum.

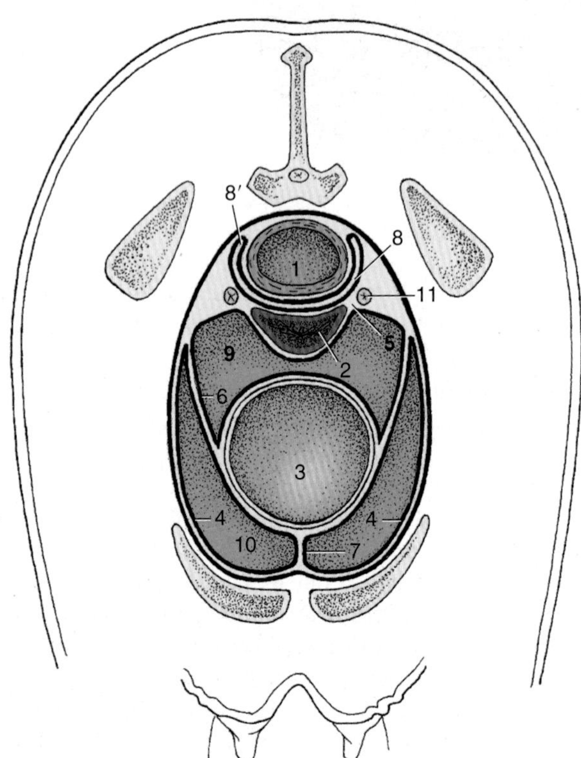

Fig. 22.6 The disposition of the peritoneum in the pelvis of the mare (transverse section). *1*, Rectum; *2*, vagina; *3*, bladder; *4*, parietal peritoneum; *5*, broad ligament; *6*, lateral ligament of bladder; *7*, median ligament of bladder; *8*, rectogenital pouch; *8'*, pararectal fossa; *9*, vesicogenital pouch; *10*, pubovesical pouch; *11*, ureter.

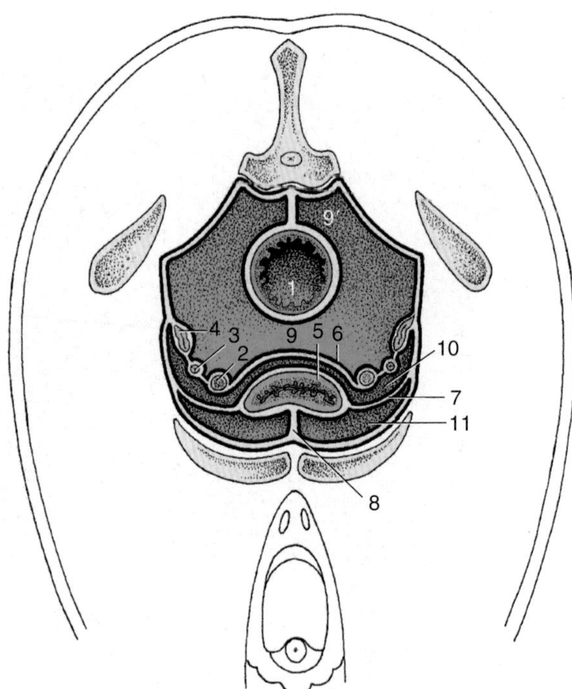

Fig. 22.7 The disposition of the peritoneum in the pelvis of the stallion (transverse section). *1*, Rectum; *2*, deferent duct; *3*, ureter; *4*, vesicular gland; *5*, bladder; *6*, genital fold; *7*, lateral ligament of bladder; *8*, median ligament of bladder; *9*, rectogenital pouch; *9'*, pararectal fossa; *10*, vesicogenital pouch; *11*, pubovesical pouch.

Surgical access to the urinary bladder is needed for removal of urinary calculi (cystotomy), to repair a disrupted bladder (cystorraphy), and to repair a patent or persistent urachus (cystoplasty). In the mare, an incision of 6 to 8 inches is made beginning slightly cranial to the umbilicus and extending caudally. In the male, the incision goes paramedially around the prepuce.

intestines. Leakage at the navel from a still-patent urachus is not uncommon in the first period after birth and provides a potential portal for infection.

The female urethra is very short (only 6 cm or thereabouts) and opens into the vestibule, immediately caudal to the transverse fold of the hymen. It wide enough to admit one finger without difficulty, and a small hand by gentle manipulation and low epidural anesthesia, which is convenient when returning a bladder prolapse or removing a urolith from the bladder. The shortness, wide caliber, and dilatable nature of the urethra permit occasional prolapse of the bladder into the vestibule.

The male urethra is described with the reproductive organs.

THE FEMALE REPRODUCTIVE ORGANS

The anatomy of the female reproductive organs is strongly influenced by age, present status, and previous reproductive

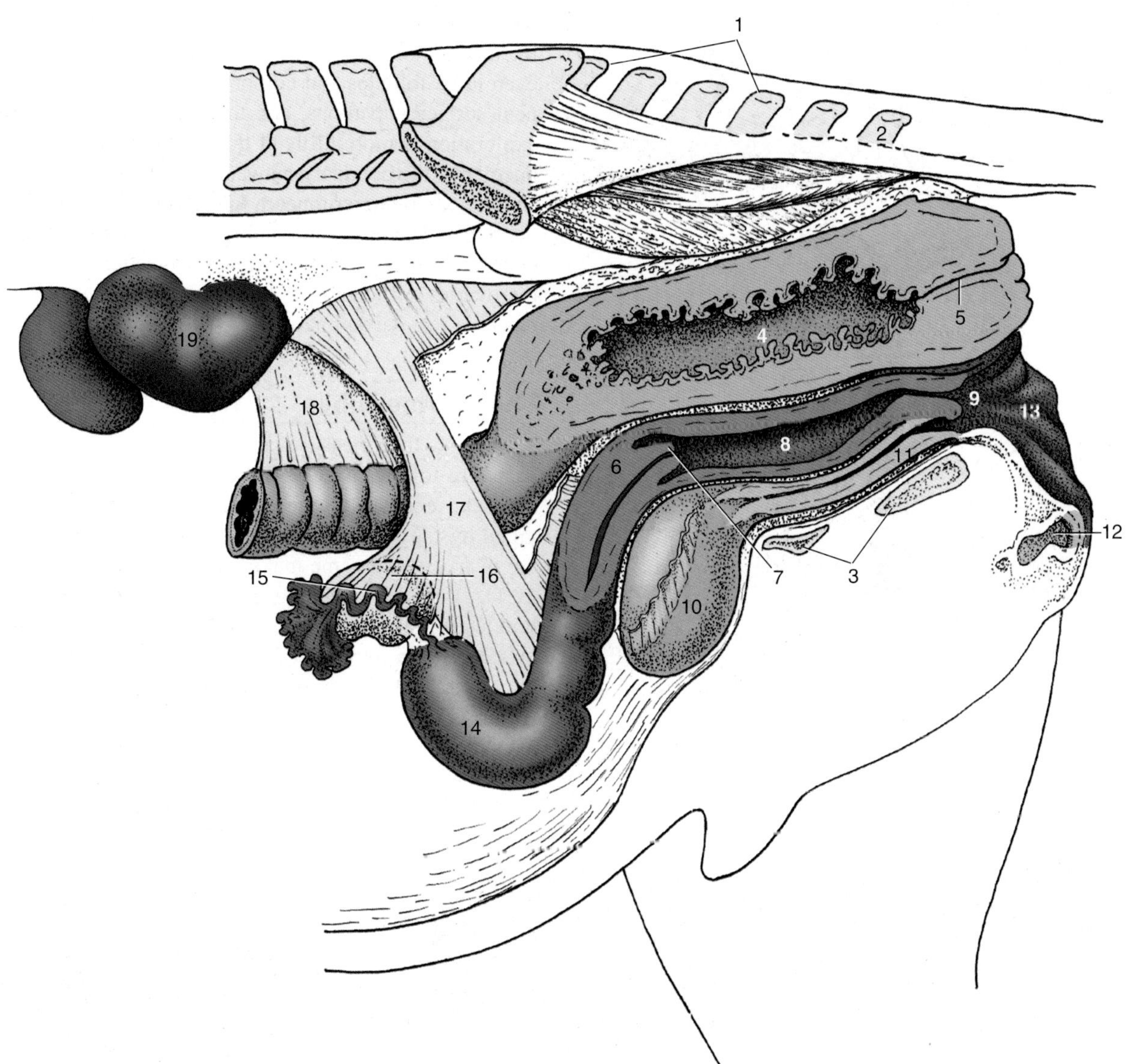

Fig. 22.8 Caudal abdominal and pelvic organs of the mare in situ; the organs have been sectioned in a paramedian plane with the pelvis. Because of the absence of the intestines, the ovaries hang much lower than they would in the intact animal. *1,* Sacrum; *2,* caudal vertebra 2; *3,* floor of pelvis; *4,* rectum; *5,* anal canal; *6,* cervix; *7,* vaginal part of cervix; *8,* vagina; *9,* vestibule; *10,* bladder; *11,* urethra; *12,* clitoris; *13,* vulva; *14,* left uterine horn; *15,* uterine tube; *16,* ovary; *17,* broad ligament (largely cut away); *18,* descending mesocolon; *19,* left kidney.

history. The initial description refers to the mature, parous but nongravid mare (Fig. 22.9).

The Ovaries

The ovaries commonly lie in the dorsal part of the abdomen, cranioventral to the iliac wings, approximately in the plane of the fifth lumbar vertebra—the site of their initial development. Each is suspended by a thick mesovarium that allows the ovary considerable latitude in position (Fig. 22.8/*16*). The length of the mesovarium is such that the ovary may generally be brought into, but not through, a flank incision.

In comparison with those of other species, the ovaries of the mare are conspicuously large; indeed, in a large draft mare they may measure as much as 8 to 10 cm along the major axis. They are also remarkable for their shape because the free border is deeply indented to form an "ovulation fossa," the site of rupture of the mature follicles (Fig. 22.10). The internal structure also shows a departure from the usual arrangement. The follicles and corpora lutea are scattered within the central part of the organ and toward the ovulation fossa. They are enclosed within a dense, richly

The ovaries can be accessed for surgical procedures such as **ovariectomy** by making an incision through the vaginal wall about 2 inches caudal to the cervix (colpotomy) or through the abdominal wall (laparotomy) via ventral (midline, paramedian, or diagonal paramedian) or flank approaches.

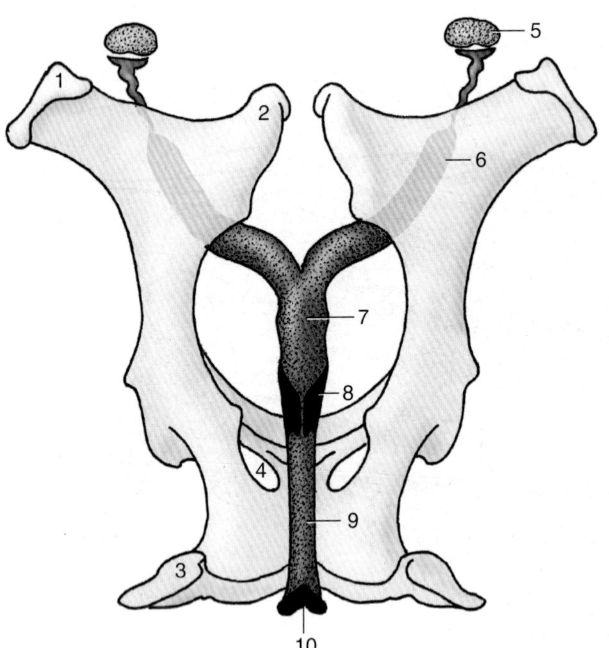

Fig. 22.9 The female reproductive organs in relation to the pelvis, dorsal view. *1,* Coxal tuber; *2,* sacral tuber; *3,* ischial tuber; *4,* obturator foramen; *5,* ovary; *6,* uterine horn; *7,* body of uterus; *8,* cervix; *9,* vagina; *10,* vulva.

vascularized connective tissue casing that corresponds to the medulla of the ovary of other species. Because of this, even large follicles and corpora lutea do not form prominent surface elevations, and their identification on rectal exploration is more difficult than in the cow. A change in hue marks the boundary between the covering of the fossa and the common peritoneum that clothes the remainder of the organ. The position, the form, the consistency, and the general absence of marked surface projections characterize the ovaries sufficiently to allow them to be easily recognized on rectal examination.

The Uterine Tubes

The uterine tube measures about 20 cm when extended but in nature follows a tortuous course that brings its beginning and end close together. The infundibulum is margined by ragged fimbriae that spread over the surface of the ovary, where some make permanent attachment (Fig. 22.11/*2*). A small opening in the depth of the infundibulum leads to the ampulla (Fig. 22.11/*3*), which is approximately 10 cm long and about 6 mm wide; its caliber at all stages of the cycle is greater than that of the isthmus, which is only half as wide. The isthmus (Fig. 22.11/*4*), also about 10 cm long, opens into the apex of the uterine

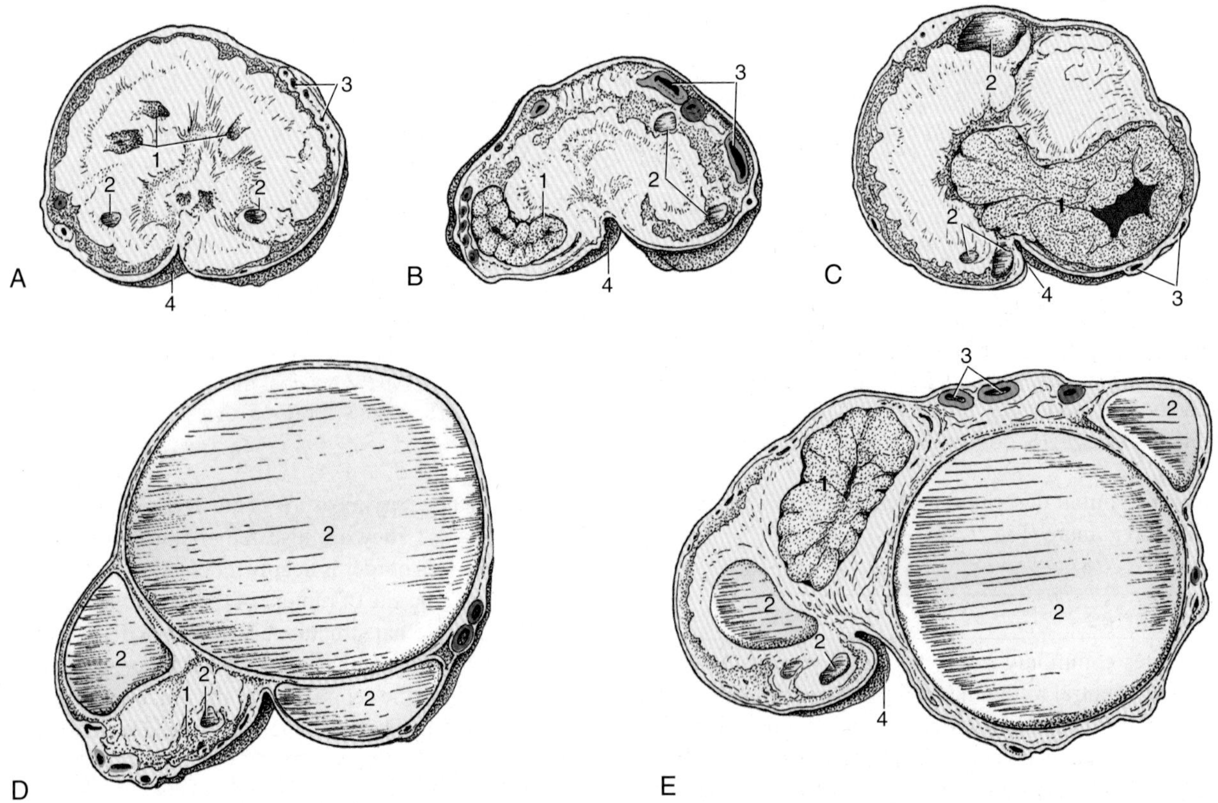

Fig. 22.10 Sections of ovaries in various functional states. (A) Ovary with corpora lutea and small follicles. (B) Ovary with developing corpus luteum. (C) Ovary with fully developed corpus luteum. (D) Ovary with mature follicle. (E) Ovary with follicles of various sizes and a rather large corpus luteum. The corpus luteum of the mare does not protrude from the ovary as in other species. *1,* Corpora lutea; *2,* follicles; *3,* blood vessels; *4,* ovulation fossa.

horn through a small orifice on the summit of an eccentrically placed papilla. Strangely, this uterotubal junction is able in some way to distinguish between fertilized and infertile ova to allow entry to only fertilized eggs. The tubal mucosa is plicated, especially within the ampulla, where the elaborate major folds carry secondary and even tertiary ridges. The mesosalpinx, which supports the tube, branches from the lateral surface of the mesovarium and, with this, encloses a large but shallow ovarian bursa (Fig. 22.11/*9* and see Fig. 5.60B/*5*).

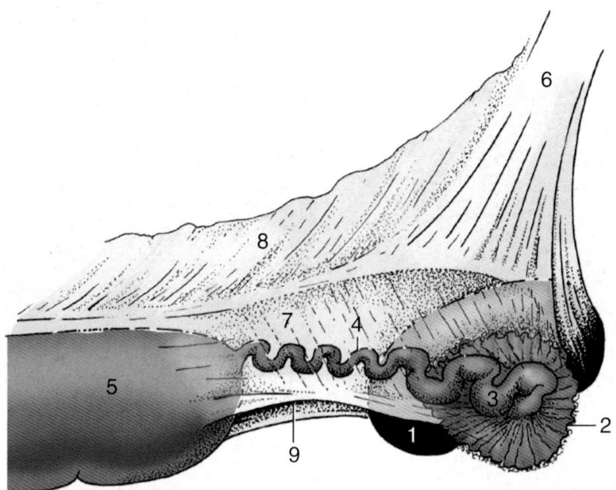

Fig. 22.11 The right ovary, uterine tube, and uterine horn; lateral view. *1*, Ovary; *2*, infundibulum with fimbriae; *3*, ampulla of uterine tube; *4*, isthmus of uterine tube; *5*, uterine horn; *6*, mesovarium; *7*, mesosalpinx; *8*, mesometrium; *9*, entrance to the ovarian bursa.

The Uterus

The uterus has a large body and two divergent horns. The horns, which are about 25 cm long, lie wholly within the abdomen and diverge sharply from each other. They are suspended from the abdominal roof by the broad ligaments, whose width varies such that the extremities of each horn are more tightly tethered than the intermediate part (Fig. 22.8/*14*). However, in life, the horns are usually raised toward the abdominal roof on the mass of intestines. The body of the uterus is a little shorter (≈20 cm) than the horns and lies partly within the abdomen and partly within the pelvis. Although its relations vary, they always include the terminal part of the descending colon and rectum dorsally and the bladder and various parts of the gut ventrally. The body is often displaced to one side by a distended bladder or by pressure from the gut. When the uterus is empty, both horns and body are flattened and the lumen is almost obliterated.

The cervix (Fig. 22.8/*6*) is rather short (≈6 cm). Although its position and extent are not readily distinguishable on visual inspection, they are at once revealed on palpation because the cervix has a somewhat firmer consistency. The difference is less pronounced at estrus. The caudal part of the cervix projects into the lumen of the vagina, where it is surrounded by an annular space (fornix) of more or less uniform depth. This intravaginal part (Fig. 22.8/*7*) has a lobed appearance created by the extension through the external ostium of the mucosal folds lining the cervical canal. These folds continue onto the vaginal wall, where

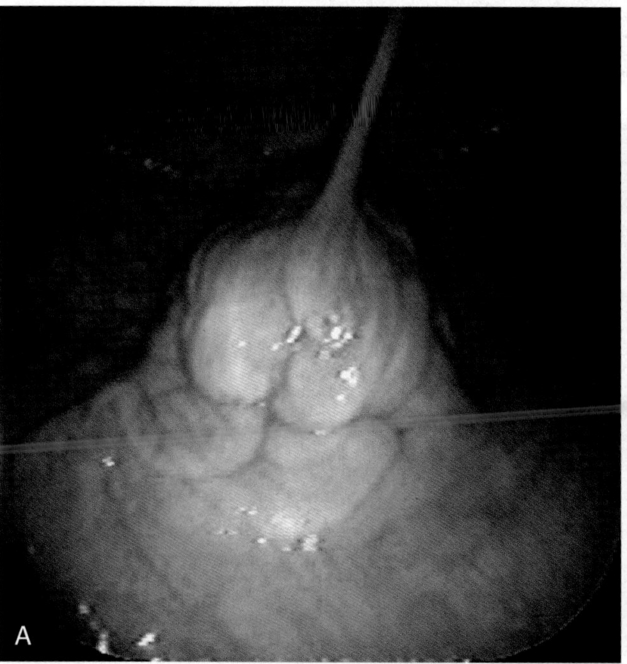

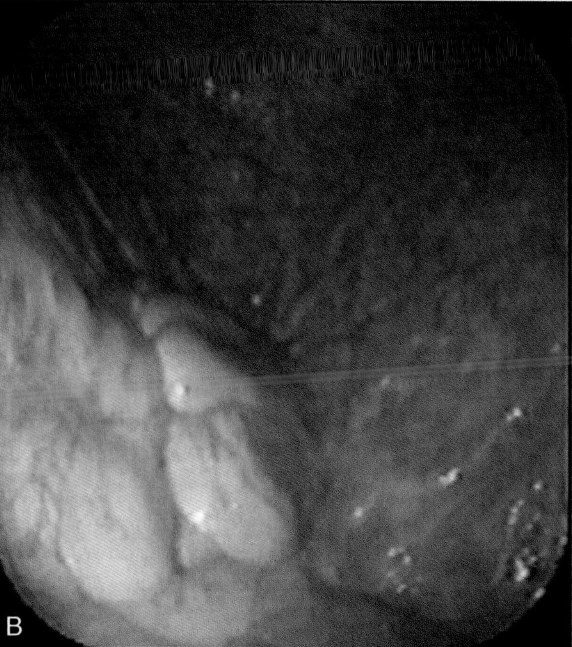

Fig. 22.12 The changing appearance of the cervix. (A) Diestrus. (B) Estrus.

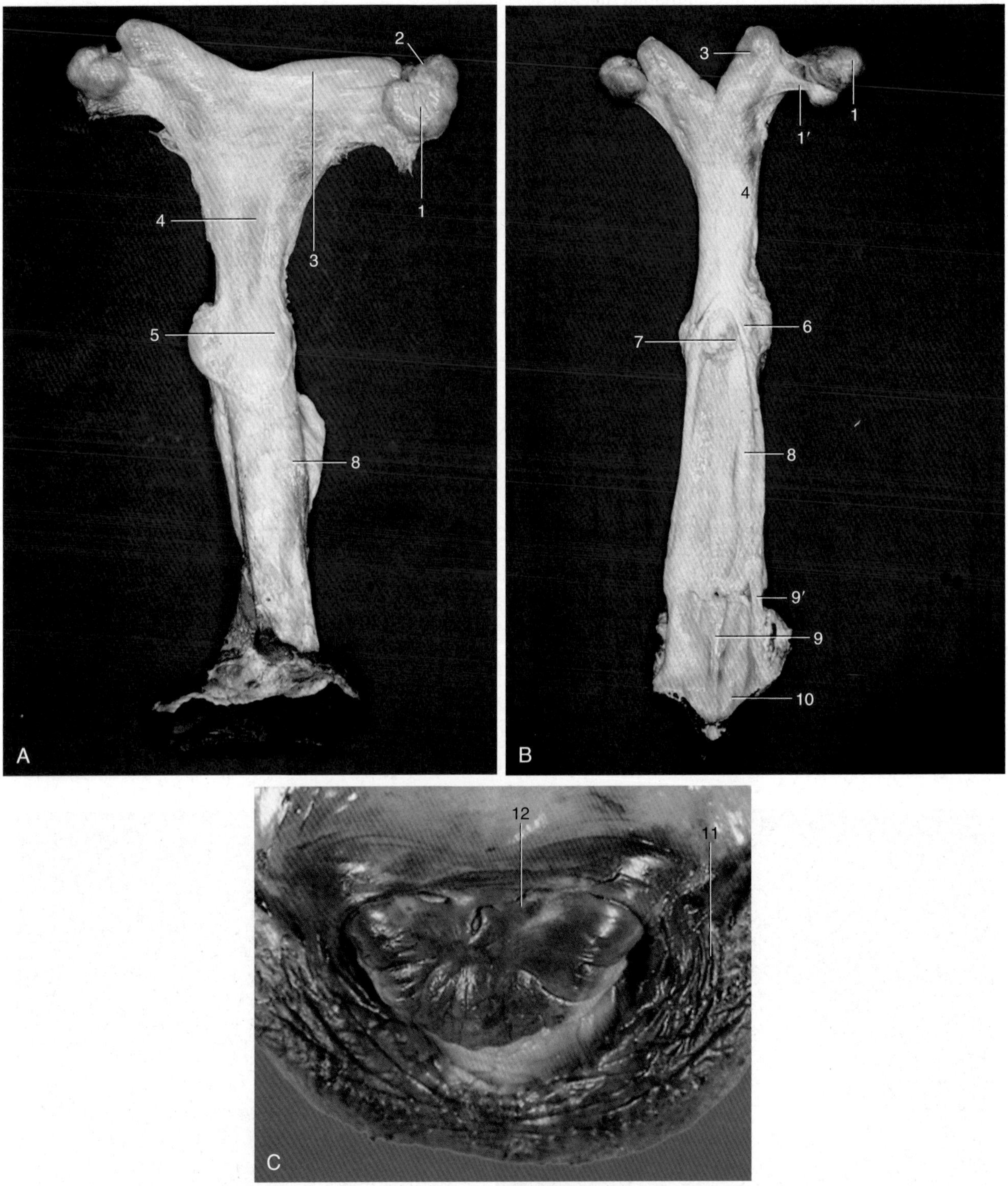

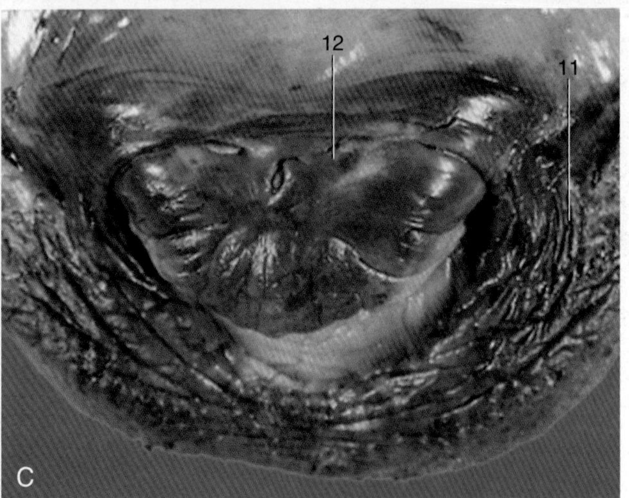

Fig. 22.13 (A) and (B) Dorsal view of the female reproductive organs. The dorsal wall of the caudal part of the tract has been opened in B. *1,* Right ovary; *1′,* proper ligament of ovary; *2,* uterine tube; *3,* horn of uterus; *4,* body of uterus; *5,* cervix; *6,* vaginal part of cervix; *7,* fornix; *8,* vagina; *9,* vestibule; *9′,* wall of vestibule; *10,* vulva. (C) An enlargement of the vulva, showing the glans of the clitoris within the ventral commissure. *11,* Right labium; *12,* glans of clitoris.

they gradually subside. Except at estrus and parturition the cervical canal is closed; however, it will still admit a finger on gentle probing (Fig. 22.12).

The Vagina

The vagina is about as long as the body of the uterus. It lies ventral to the rectum, dorsal to the bladder and urethra, and in lateral contact with the pelvic wall (Figs. 22.8 and 22.13/*8*). Although it is largely retroperitoneal, the extent of the covering depends on the degrees of filling of the bladder and rectum (Fig. 22.5). A small cranial part of the ventral aspect and a somewhat larger part of the dorsal aspect are always clad in peritoneum. This arrangement is useful because the dorsal part of the vaginal fornix provides a convenient approach to the peritoneal cavity for various procedures, including the recovery of ova.

The vagina is thin walled, and although its lumen is normally closed by the dorsal and ventral walls falling together, the organ is remarkably distensible in length and circumference. The vaginal mucosa is ridged lengthwise, although the ridges are readily effaced on distention. The mucosa is normally pale pink but darkens when suffused with blood, as tends to happen on prolonged exposure to air during vaginoscopy. A transverse fold cranial to the opening of the urethra represents the remains of the hymen; although variable, it is generally more prominent than in other domestic species.

The Vestibule and Vulva

The dorsal wall of the vestibule only gradually departs from the line of the rectum and anal canal; the longer ventral wall slopes more steeply downward beyond the ischial arch (Fig. 22.8/*9*). Noteworthy features are the urethral opening at the cranial limit and the clitoris within the ventral commissure of the vulva. The clitoris varies much in development and is largely covered by a transverse preputial fold that attaches to the dorsal surface of its glans (Fig. 22.13C/*12*). The fold and ventral commissure together constitute the prepuce. The clitoris is very prominent in mares in heat when exposed by "winking" movements of the labia. Laterally and ventrally it is separated from the labia by a clitoral fossa. Several sinuses of varying depth invade the glans. These may harbor the organism responsible for contagious equine metritis. Further mucosal recesses are present in the ventral parts of the clitoral fossa and labia. Although no major vestibular glands exist, numerous minor glands discharge within small depressions, ranked in ventral and dorsolateral rows. The mucosa overlying the vestibular bulb, situated in the lateral wall toward the vulva, is more darkly colored.

The vulva is unusual in having rounded ventral and pointed dorsal commissures, which is a reversal of the usual arrangement (Fig. 22.14/*3*). The relationship of the vulva to the pelvic skeleton varies considerably. Usually it is largely ventral to the pelvic floor with the cleft closed. Sometimes, and quite commonly in Thoroughbreds, the opening is more dorsal and closure is less effective; in this circumstance, air may

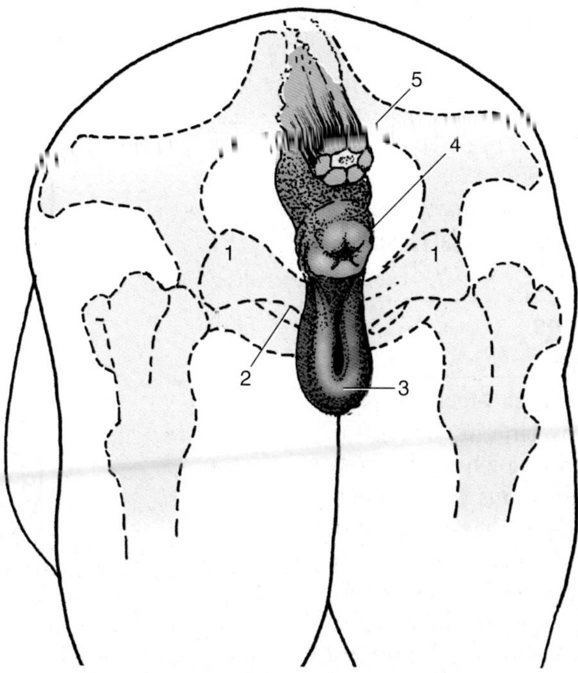

Fig. 22.14 The anus and vulva superimposed on the outline of the bony pelvis. Note the relationship of the ischial arch and tubers to the vulva. *1,* Ischial tuber; *2,* ischial arch; *3,* vulva; *4,* anus; *5,* tail (section).

be drawn into or expelled from the tract with each change in intra-abdominal pressure. Bacteria may be introduced, and the contamination may spread to the endometrium, which may result in sterility. The same fault ("wind-sucking") may be due to laceration of the vulva at a previous parturition.

Vascularization and Innervation

The reproductive organs are principally supplied by the *ovarian, uterine,* and *vaginal arteries.* The ovarian artery, a direct branch from the aorta, divides into uterine and ovarian branches. The ovarian branch pursues a tortuous course within the mesovarium before dividing into several branches that spread over the surface of the ovary; this contrasts with the arrangement in other species, in which the vessels penetrate the ovary immediately on arrival. The other branch passes to the cranial part of the horn. The corresponding vein is disproportionately large and drains much of the uterus in addition to the ovary. Little transfer of prostaglandins from venous to arterial blood occurs in the mare, which may be due to a less intimate relationship of the ovarian artery and vein compared to other species.

The *uterine artery*, a branch of the external iliac, is the foremost supply to the uterus (also see Fig. 7.43). It divides into several branches within the broad ligament, and these approach the mesometrial border of the horn and body separately. The antimesometrial aspect is reached only by small vessels, thus lending itself to relatively bloodless incision. Anastomoses with branches of the ovarian and vaginal arteries are present.

The *vaginal artery* takes origin from the internal pudendal in common with the middle rectal artery. It passes through the retroperitoneal tissue lateral to the vagina before bending forward to divide and supply the larger part of the vagina, the cervix, the caudal part of the body of the uterus, the bladder, and the urethra. The remaining part of the vagina and the vestibule are supplied from the vestibular branch of the internal pudendal artery.

The veins draining the genital organs are satellite to the arteries. The innervation displays no noteworthy special features.

Growth and Cyclical Changes in the Reproductive Organs

At midgestation the fetal ovaries are much larger than those of the dam but they later regress by birth to one-tenth of their greatest fetal size. They then grow slowly until puberty when a sudden spurt occurs. The first estrus is generally at the beginning of a breeding season, and the age of first estrus varies with the date of the individual's birth as well as with breed and nutrition. It usually occurs sometime between the 18th and 27th months. The neonatal ovary is ellipsoidal but develops into the peculiar indented adult form during the first 2 or 3 years (Fig. 22.15). In the mature ovary the larger follicles are concentrated near the ovulation fossa to which they migrate as they enlarge (Fig. 22.10/*2*). Two or three (perhaps spread between the two ovaries) reach full size of about 5 cm in each cycle, but usually only one ruptures. After rupture, the cavity contains some blood, and for a time the soft clot may be appreciated on rectal examination. It then gradually fills with luteal cells, but even when mature the corpus luteum hardly projects above the surrounding surface. The corpus luteum is initially brick red but becomes ocherous as it matures. Its regression begins about the 10th day and is more or less complete when its successor forms. The cycle averages 22 days. The left ovary is generally the more active; despite this the right uterine horn is slightly more favored by conceptuses. Transuterine migration by a conceptus must be common.

Ultrasonography may be used to follow follicular development, to detect the occurrence of ovulation, and to trace the fate of the resulting follicular cavity. It successfully determines the course of events a little before this is possible by palpation per rectum. It may allow the prediction of ovulation by about a day because it can reveal the change in form, from spherical to pyriform, of the ripening follicle. A further advantage lies in its success in recognizing the parallel maturation of multiple follicles that may result in twin pregnancy.

The juvenile reproductive tract is small, symmetrical, and thin walled. The endometrium is pale, and the layers of the

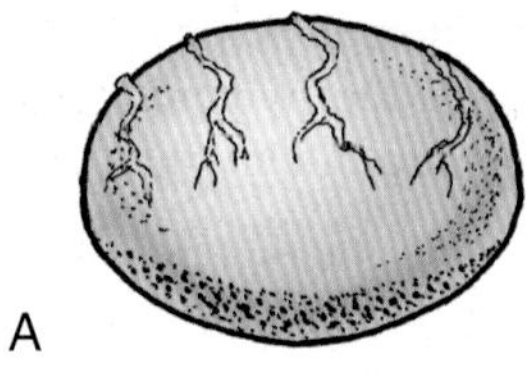

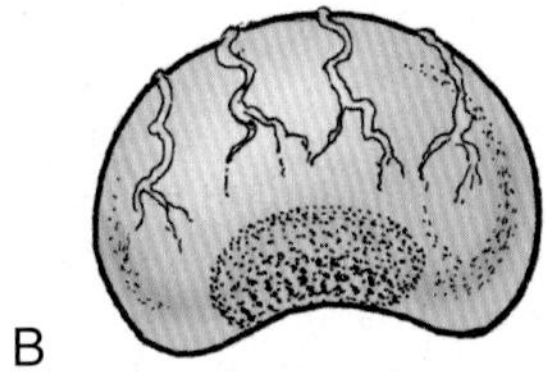

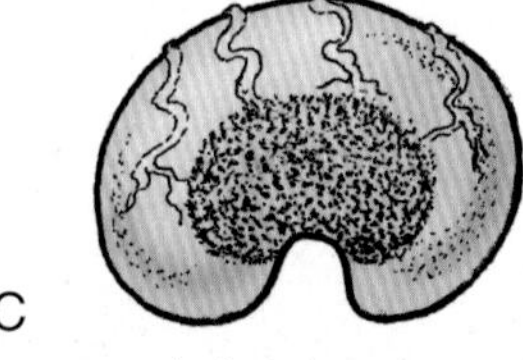

Fig. 22.15 The postnatal development of the ovary. The more rapid growth at the poles confines the germinal epithelium *(stippled)* to a small central area. (A) At birth; the germinal epithelium is widespread over the surface. (B) At 6 months of age. (C) Adult; the germinal epithelium surrounds an indentation known as the *ovulation fossa*.

uterine wall are difficult to differentiate with the naked eye. The broad ligaments are thin and transparent, and the blood vessels are narrow and relatively inconspicuous. Growth is initially isometric—it keeps pace with growth of the body as a whole—until a prepubertal acceleration occurs. Cyclical changes in the uterus, including increased retention of water, a greater blood flow, and activation of the glands thickening the wall in preparation for the reception of the blastocyst, broadly resemble those in other species. If pregnancy does not result, these changes recede with the regression of the corpus luteum. Cyclical changes in muscular tonus are the subject of some controversy, but most authorities hold that tonus is greatest about a week after ovulation.

The cervix softens during estrus when the intravaginal part droops so that its orifice is lost to view on vaginoscopic examination (Fig. 22.12B). When stimulated by handling, it becomes firmer, returns to the horizontal, and may exhibit rhythmic contractions. It is also moist, swollen, and pink at this time. It is paler in appearance and firmer during metestrus and diestrus when the lumen is closed by a plug of thick mucus (Fig. 22.12). Although the vaginal wall is pink and moist during estrus, its liability to change color on prolonged exposure to air denies diagnostic significance to its appearance. Cytologic changes in the vaginal epithelium are slight and also of little diagnostic value.

The Reproductive Tract During Pregnancy

The ovaries, continue to show cyclical activity during the first months of pregnancy. Although the first corpus luteum does not persist beyond the usual term, it is replaced by a succession of other corpora over the next 5 months; some are formed after rupture of follicles, others apparently by direct luteinization. The accessory corpora lutea survive longer than the original one and are a rich source of progesterone. The growth, ripening, and luteinization of the new follicles are controlled by gonadotropic hormones derived from the endometrial cups that are so distinctive a feature of the species. After 5 months the accessory corpora lutea also regress and pregnancy is then maintained by progesterone of placental origin. The enormous enlargement of the fetal gonads, peculiar to the horse among domestic species, reaches a peak between 6 and 8 months. Despite assertions that fetal hypophyseal luteinizing hormone is responsible for the enlargement, the endometrial gonadotropins also contribute (see Fig. 22.18B). The temporary enlargement of the fetal testes influences the timing and the success of their descent, which is normally completed about full term.

Early Pregnancy Diagnosis: The pregnancy is mainly diagnosed through careful internal examination per rectum, supplemented by ultrasonography (Fig. 22.16). The rectal examination will reveal a closed cervix as early as 16 to 18 days post ovulation. The uterine walls show tone under the influence of progesterone between 12 and 25 days and become soft after 48 to 50 days. The conceptus of 30 to 40 mm between 17 and 30 days is within the part of a uterine horn adjacent to the junction with the body of the organ and creates a slight bulge of the ventral aspect of the gravid horn. It increases to a length of 8 to 10 cm and a diameter of 6 to 8 cm by day 50.

Ultrasonic examination may detect a conceptus as early as day 10 post ovulation. The smaller size of the conceptus at this stage requires very systematic examination to distinguish it from a fluid-filled structure such as an endometrial cyst. The early conceptus enjoys considerable mobility, which also distinguishes it from any pathologic lesion, before adopting a fixed location within the uterus. Most of the equine conceptuses are located within the body of the uterus about the 10th day and settled in a horn a week or so later. Ultrasonography may be employed after 55 days of pregnancy to determine the sex of the fetus, which is revealed by the location of the genital tubercle close to the umbilical cord in the male and nearer the tail in the female.

The proliferative changes of the endometrium that occur with each cycle continue and intensify if pregnancy has occurred. The early diagnosis of pregnancy and, because of the prevalence of early embryonic death, the confirmation of its continuation through the critical early stages have

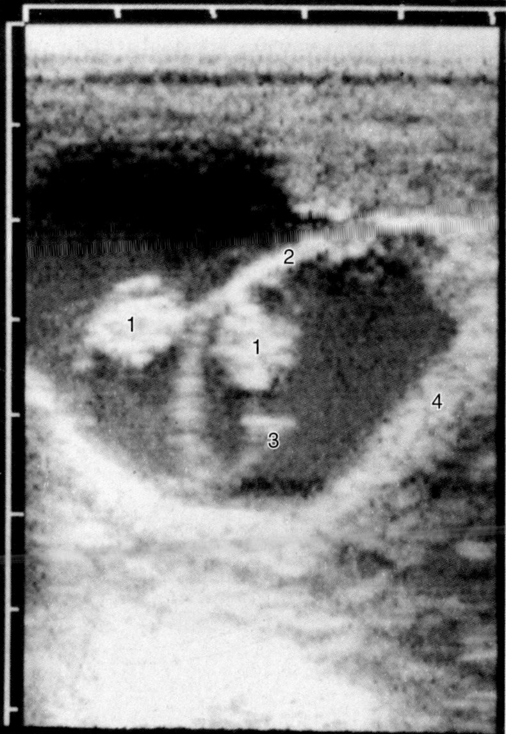

Fig. 22.16 Ultrasonographic view of 31-day equine twin embryos. The scale is in centimeters. *1*, Twin embryos; *2*, junction of the two conceptuses; *3*, developing allantoic membrane; *4*, uterine wall.

particular importance in equine practice. An additional significance is provided by the desirability of recognizing twin pregnancies at an early stage. Twin pregnancies are rarely completed successfully, and the clinician and client may choose to destroy one of the twins by manual crushing before the implantation to lessen the risk of losing a breeding season.

After the conceptus settles in the horn, the whole gravid horn (which is more commonly the right one) then gradually enlarges, followed by the body and, although to a lesser degree, the nonpregnant horn. As the uterus enlarges it sinks into the abdomen, dragging the body and the cervix out of the pelvis (Fig. 22.17). The broad ligaments exert constraint on the mesometrial margins, and the horns therefore enlarge asymmetrically and become more flexed on themselves; the ovaries are drawn ventrocranially. The uterine arteries, which are pulled in the same direction, develop a characteristic vibration (fremitus or thrill) in the pregnant mare. This feature may be appreciated on rectal examination, and its diagnostic value is greatest at that stage of pregnancy (between the third and fifth month) when the uterus has sunk out of reach. The position of the foal adapts to the form of the uterus; by midpregnancy it has come to lie with its back against the greater curvature of the horn (and thus ventrally) and with its head generally (99% of the time) raised toward the cervix. In the circumstances that most favor easy parturition, the bulky body of the foal is preceded into the cervix by the extended forelimbs, on which rest the relatively small head and slender neck. The foal is delivered with its back uppermost. Because of the general enlargement and considerable size of the body of the uterus, it is possible for the occasional fetus to lie transversely, extending from one horn into the other; clearly this bodes ill for parturition. Enlargement of the uterus displaces the other abdominal contents forward and upward; in later pregnancy the uterus dominates the entire abdominal topography, extending forward on the abdominal floor and under the rib cage; however, it generally remains to the left of the cecum.

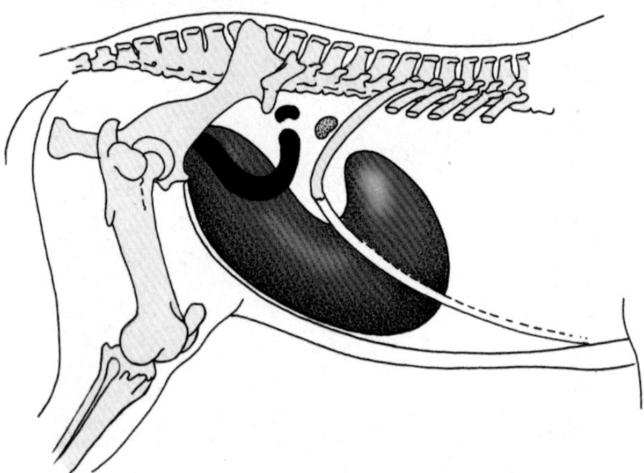

Fig. 22.17 Changes in the topography of the uterus and ovary between the beginning *(black)* and the end *(red)* of pregnancy.

A prominent feature of the uterus in early months of pregnancy is the presence of a ring or horseshoe formation of scablike structures, disfiguring the endometrium of the caudal part of the horn, the location where the young conceptus comes to rest. These so-called endometrial cups (Fig. 22.18B) are unique to Equidae and are the source of both equine chorionic gonadotropin (formerly known as pregnant mare's serum gonadotropin [PMSG]), the hormone responsible for the unusual activity of the ovary of the pregnant mare and the even more remarkable, though temporary, enlargement of the gonads of equine fetuses of both sexes. The cups have their origin in cells that invade the endometrium from a limited region of the chorion: the (allanto-) chorionic girdle that marks the boundary between the allantochorionic and omphalochorionic (yolk sac) portions of the embryonic vesicle and provides the area of initial adhesion of the conceptus to the uterus (Fig. 22.18A). The migration of chorionic cells begins about the 35th day, and the cups soon become visible as low endometrial elevations. They continue to grow, forming irregular centrally depressed prominences that reach their zenith about the 60th day, only to enter a process of degeneration and necrosis shortly thereafter. The process culminates in their separation and sloughing from the endometrium, which are events largely concluded by the 120th day (or thereabouts), although a few may persist much longer. The fetal (chorionic) cells penetrate some way into the endometrial stroma, and although they provide the essential endocrine components of the cups, they become admixed with connective tissue cells, blood vessels, and glandular debris and secretion contributed by the endometrium. Some detached cups come to lie between the endometrium and chorion; other detachments of this material push into the allantoic cavity, enclosed within pedunculated sacs of allantochorion, and these protrusions may be the origin of some of the hippomanes mentioned shortly.

The cervix of the pregnant mare is firm and closed by a plug of mucus (Fig. 22.12). The pale vaginal wall is also coated with mucus that becomes stickier and more inspissated as pregnancy progresses. The connective tissues of the cervix, vagina, and vulva and the sacrotuberal ligaments soften shortly before birth, which is generally speedily executed, facilitated by the generous dimensions of the pelvic cavity. It is necessary that it should be so, because rupture of the membranes with loss of fetal fluids allows separation of the loose attachment between the chorion and the endometrium, jeopardizing fetal respiration.

Puerperal changes follow the same pattern as in other species but run a rapid course. Involution of the uterus is completed sooner than in the cow, and because there is no endometrial

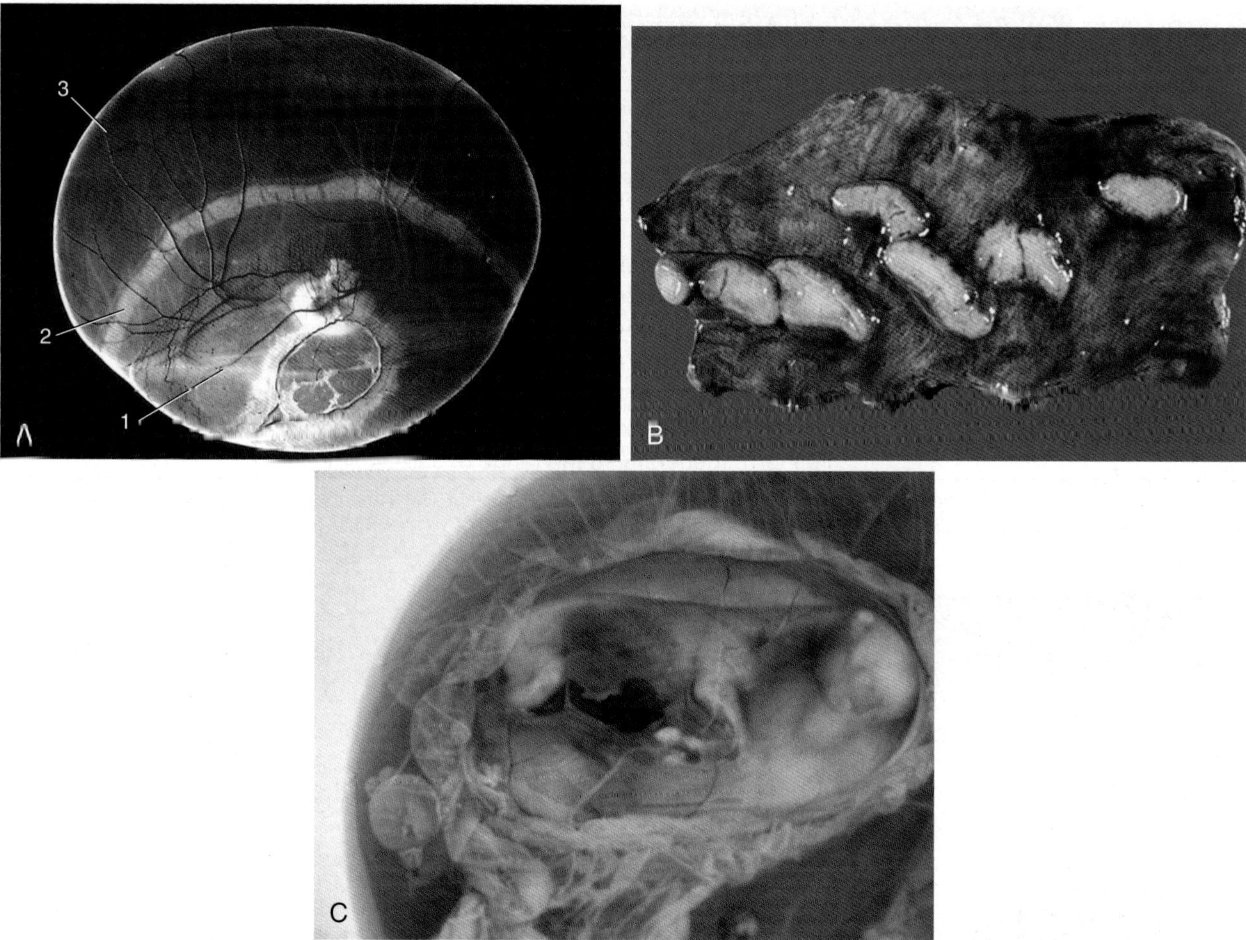

Fig. 22.18 (A) Young conceptus (horse). *1,* Yolk sac; *2,* chorionic girdle; *3,* allantochorion. (B) Endometrial cups (mare) during early pregnancy. (C) The placenta of the horse fetus is not very complex. The villi do not penetrate deep into the endometrium.

damage to repair, mares covered at the "foal heat"—about the 8th to 10th day after giving birth—often conceive.

Placentation and Prenatal Development

In the horse, unlike other domestic species, a choriovitelline placenta (or omphalochorion) provides the principal organ of exchange for the first third or so of intrauterine life. Thereafter, with the establishment of the chorioallantoic placenta, the yolk sac wanes. The definitive chorioallantoic placenta is of the epitheliochorial type and is commonly described as diffuse. The outer surface of the chorion carries innumerable branched villi that penetrate into crypts of the endometrial surface to form a loose attachment that is reinforced by the radial pressure exerted by the fetal fluids. Although the villi are widely spread, their distribution is not uniform, and they are clumped together in groups sometimes known as *microcotyledons* (because they resemble the cotyledonary arrangement in ruminants on a smaller scale). Small spaces between the microcotyledons face the openings of the uterine glands and fill with their secretions.

The capillaries of both fetal and maternal parts of the placenta reach directly below the corresponding epithelia, and only a thin tissue layer separates the two bloodstreams. Even so, the passage of large molecules, including antibodies, is impossible, and the passive transfer of immunity from mother to offspring is dependent on the foal ingesting colostrum.

A peculiar feature is the presence of so-called hippomanes in the allantoic (and, to a lesser extent, amniotic) fluid. Most of these soft brownish bodies are formed by the deposition of mucoproteins and calcium phosphate on nuclei provided by solid particles within the fluids, but some originate in material flaked from endometrial cups when these have completed their role. The latter are sometimes found anchored to the chorioallantoic membrane by attenuated stalks. Hippomanes have no known clinical (or residual physiologic) importance.

Although detailed information must be sought elsewhere, it may be useful to have a basic guide to the estimation of fetal age (Table 22.1). Crown–rump measurements are of limited value in this species because of its wide range of body size.

TABLE 22.1 GUIDE TO THE AGING OF HORSE FETUSES

Month	Crown–Rump Length	External Features
1	—	The embryo is about 1–1.5 cm long.
2	≈7 cm	The species is recognizable and the sex determinable from the external genitalia.
3	≈14 cm	The parts of the hoof are distinct.
4	≈25 cm	Some hair is present around the mouth.
5	≈36 cm	Hairs are present above the eyes.
6	≈50 cm	Eyelashes are present.
7	≈65 cm	Hair is present at the tail tip.
8	≈80 cm	Hair has appeared along the back and on the limbs.
9	≈95 cm	Fine hair covers most of the body (the belly excepted).
10	≈110 cm	The body is completely haired.
11		Full term (generally in the range of 330–345 days)

From Evans HE, Sack WO: Prenatal development of domestic and laboratory animals. Growth curves, external features and selected references, *Anat Histol Embryol* 2:11–45, 1973.

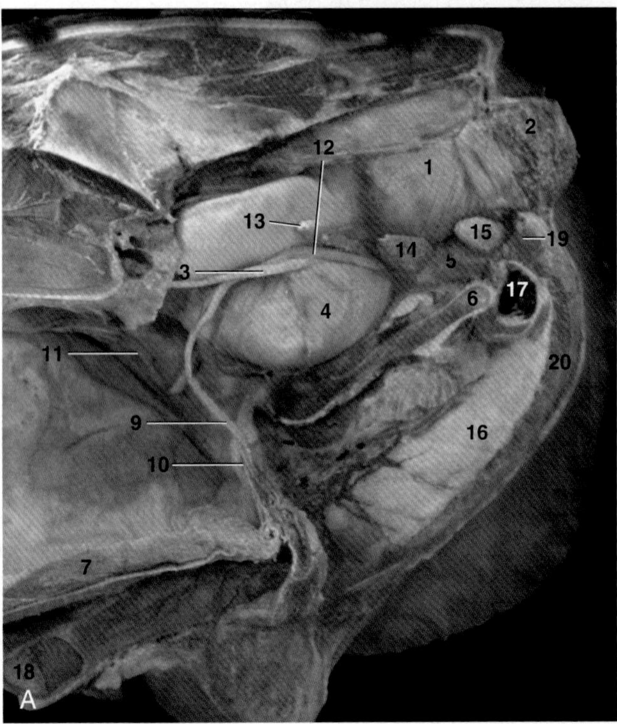

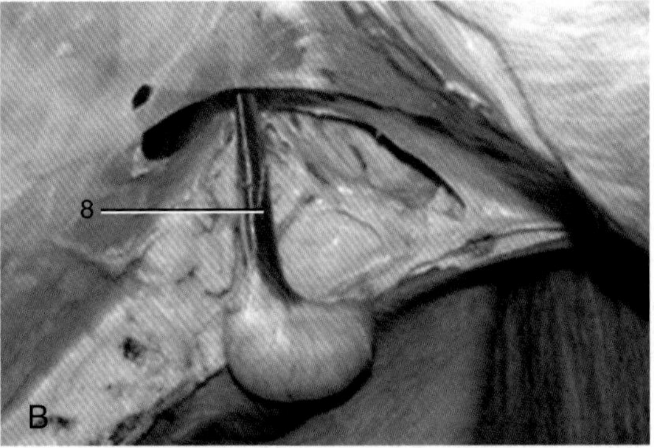

Fig. 22.19 (A) The reproductive organs of the stallion in situ. *1,* Rectum; *2,* external anal sphincter; *3,* ureter; *4,* bladder; *5,* urethra; *6,* floor of pelvis; *7,* floor of abdomen; *9,* left deferent duct; *10,* vaginal ring; *11,* right testicular artery and vein; *12,* ampulla of deferent duct; *13,* vesicular gland; *14,* prostate; *15,* bulbourethral gland; *16,* penis; *17,* left crus (in section); *18,* glans penis; *19,* ischiocavernosus; *20,* bulbospongiosus. (B) Testis and spermatic cord within exposed vaginal process. *8,* Cremaster.

THE MALE REPRODUCTIVE ORGANS

The Scrotum and Testes

The scrotum lies below the pubic brim, where it is concealed from lateral inspection by the thigh. It is broadly globular, commonly asymmetrical, and divided by an external raphe that extends cranially onto the prepuce and caudally onto the perineum. The scrotal skin is thin, supple, and sparsely haired and is usually deeply pigmented; it glistens from sebaceous secretion. The deeper layers of the scrotal wall are constructed in the usual fashion.

The *testes* are imperfectly ellipsoidal, being slightly compressed from side to side (Fig. 22.19 and see Fig.

5.41). They generally lie with their long axes horizontal but become almost vertical on strong contraction of the cremaster muscles that attach to the vaginal tunic near the cranial poles. The tunica albuginea is less thick than in ruminants, and the testes yield on gentle compression. The grayish pink parenchyma is contained under some pressure and bulges through any incision of the tunic. The septa that extend inward from the capsule do not join to form a visibly distinct mediastinum. The epididymis lies along the dorsal border and projects a little beyond the poles of the testis, where it is most firmly attached. It leaves a distinct testicular bursa that opens laterally. The ligament of the tail of the epididymis is quite thick and must be severed in castration by the "open" method. Wartlike growths (*appendices testis*) on the testis near the head of the epididymis are very common; they are remnants of the paramesonephric duct.

The *spermatic cord* is broad and thin where it attaches to the testis but rounds when followed toward the superficial inguinal ring. The cranial vascular part (see Fig. 5.41/5) is clearly distinguished from the caudal part that carries the deferent duct. The constituents diverge in the usual manner on entering the abdomen (Fig. 22.19 and see Fig. 22.24B). The course of the deferent duct then takes it across the dorsal face of the bladder, beside the medial border of the vesicular gland, before it penetrates the prostate to reach the urethra. The subterminal part (≈20 cm) of the duct is widened to form an ampulla, which is an inappropriate term because it is the wall and not the lumen that is enlarged. The ampulla is less distinct in geldings, particularly those castrated early.

The wide inguinal canal makes inguinal hernias a relatively common occurrence.

Although the process of testicular descent may be presumed to be governed by the same factors (p. 163) as in other species, it *is marked by* one circumstance unique among domestic mammals. The testes of the fetal colt exhibit an inordinate though temporary increase in size between the 100th and 250th days of gestation, attaining a peak on about the 215th day. (A comparable enlargement affects the ovaries of the fetal filly.) In consequence, although each testis arrives in the vicinity of the vaginal ring on about the 120th day, it is delayed here and does not resume its migration until it has shrunk to a fraction of its maximal size. It does not arrive in the scrotum until close to the time of birth and may even arrive after this event (probably within 2 weeks either way).

Not infrequently a testis fails to reach the scrotum even then and remains hidden within the abdomen or delayed within the inguinal canal. Retention may be temporary or permanent, confined to one side or bilateral, and if bilateral, the sites of lodgment may be asymmetrical. The condition, known as cryptorchidism, may resolve spontaneously, and the testis may make a delayed appearance in the scrotum at some time within the first year of postnatal life or possibly even later. In such cases it may be assumed that the testis was held up within the inguinal canal because the vaginal ring normally contracts shortly after birth, preventing a late entry to the canal from the abdomen. Testes that fail to make an appearance within a reasonable time require surgical removal, for which a variety of techniques is available depending on the location of the arrest. The diagnosis of cryptorchidism is sometimes less obvious than might be supposed. Cryptorchid animals that have changed hands may be presented in good faith as geldings, and suspicion may only arise when stallion characteristics of conformation and behavior develop. Moreover, in young horses of nervous disposition, successfully descended testes may initially escape detection by being withdrawn into the groins, against the superficial inguinal rings, when the scrotum and inguinal regions are palpated.

The Pelvic Reproductive Organs

The short (≈12 cm) pelvic urethra lies directly over the pelvic symphysis. Although generally remarkably wide (≈6 cm), its lumen is narrowed in two places: one level with the body of the prostate, and the other where the urethra crosses the ischial arch (Fig. 22.20). The *deferent ducts* (Fig. 22.20/2) penetrate

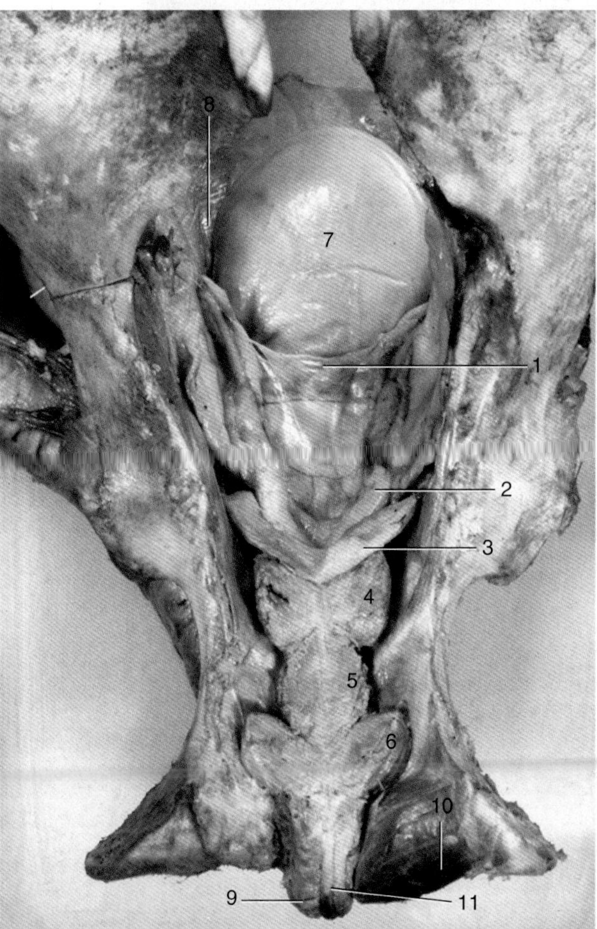

Fig. 22.20 Dorsal view of the pelvic urethra and accessory reproductive glands (in situ). *1,* Genital fold; *2,* ampulla of deferent duct; *3,* vesicular gland; *4,* prostate; *5,* urethralis; *6,* bulbourethral gland; *7,* bladder; *8,* lateral ligament of bladder; *9,* bulbospongiosus; *10,* ischiocavernosus; *11,* retractor penis.

the urethral wall close to the origin of the urethra from the bladder. Each combines with the duct of the neighboring vesicular gland to form a common passage, the ejaculatory duct. This is only a few millimeters long and opens into the urethra to the side of the dorsal thickening, the seminal colliculus.

The *vesicular glands* (Fig. 22.20/*3*) of the horse merit the alternative name *seminal vesicles* because they take the form of smooth-surfaced, pear-shaped bladders, approximately 12 cm long, with large central lumina. Each is contained within the genital fold.

The *prostate* (Fig. 22.20/*4*) is largely retroperitoneal and entirely compact. It consists of two lateral lobes joined by a narrow isthmus that crosses the dorsal aspect of the urethra close to the bladder neck. Each lateral lobe is pressed against the border of the urethra and extends cranially along the caudolateral edge of the adjacent vesicular gland. Because the prostate is firm and lobulated, the two glands are easily distinguished on rectal examination. Numerous ductules drain from the prostate to discharge into the urethra through tiny slits beside the colliculus (see Fig. 5.50/*7*).

The paired *bulbourethral glands* lie dorsolateral to the urethra at the pelvic outlet. They are thinly covered by striated muscle (bulboglandularis), about 4 cm long, and so oriented that their pointed caudal ends converge (Fig.

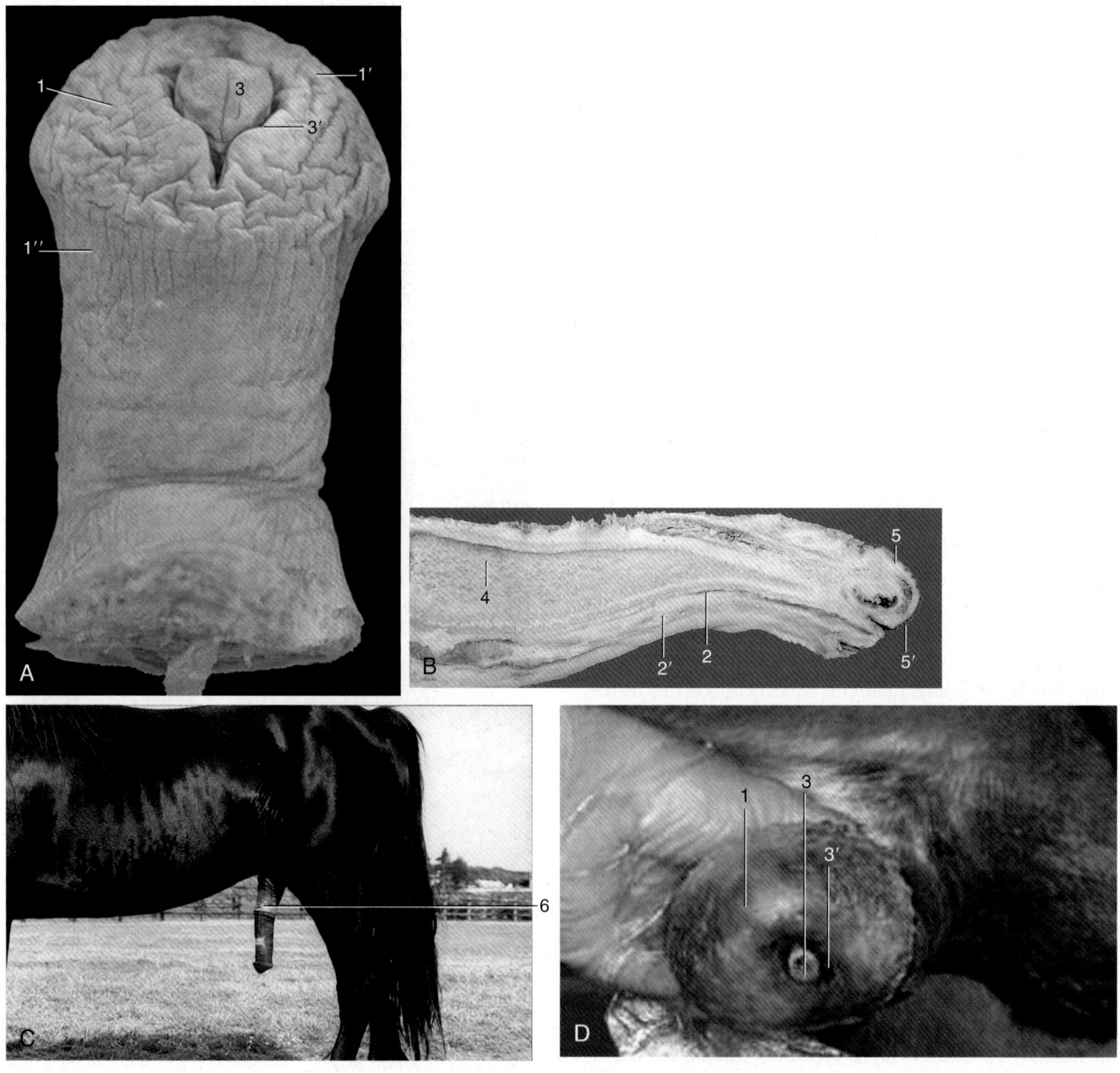

Fig. 22.21 (A) Extremity of penis exposed. (B) Enlarged glans penis. (C) Within prepuce in median section. (D) Enlarged glans penis. *1*, Glans; *1′*, corona glandis; *1″*, collum glandis; *2*, urethra; *2′*, corpus spongiosum; *3*, urethral process within fossa glandis; *3′*, urethral sinus; *4*, corpus cavernosum; *5*, preputial fold; *5′*, preputial ring; *6*, prepuce, forming preputial orifice with the body wall.

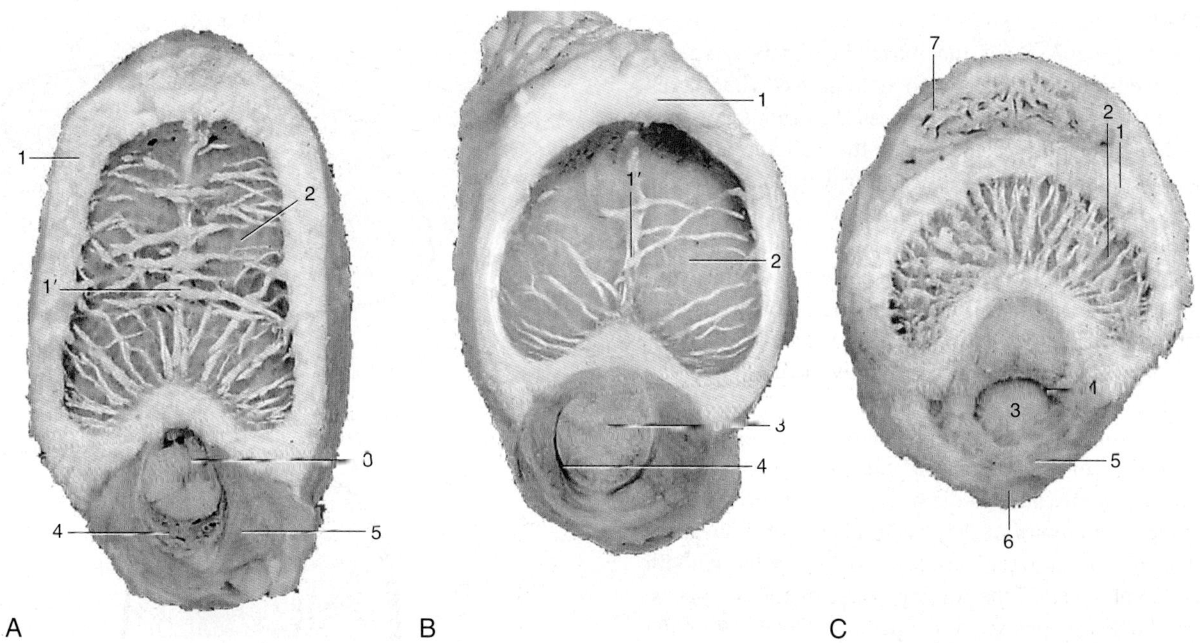

Fig. 22.22 Transections of the penis, (A) directly distal to the root, (B) midshaft, and (C) in its free part. *1,* Tunica albuginea; *1′,* incomplete septum penis; *2,* corpus cavernosum; *3,* urethra; *4,* corpus spongiosum; *5,* bulbospongiosus; *6,* retractor penis; *7,* dorsal process of glans.

22.20/*6*). These glands discharge through numerous small pores that open into the urethra where it leaves the pelvis.

All accessory reproductive glands are of course much reduced in geldings.

The Penis and Prepuce

The penis of the horse is composed of the usual triad of structures and is of the musculocavernous variety. The two dorsal elements, the crura penis, arise from the ischial arch, bend forward between the thighs, and soon unite in a single corpus cavernosum, which is divided in its proximal part by a median septum that reflects the compound origin (Fig. 22.21A/*3*). The septum fades and finally disappears when followed toward the apex. The corpus cavernosum is somewhat compressed laterally and carries ventrally a groove into which the third erectile body, the corpus spongiosum, fits.

The corpus spongiosum expands over the apex of the organ to form the distinctively shaped *glans* (Fig. 22.21A/*1*). This has a resemblance to a mushroom; the widest part, the corona, is some distance proximal to the apex, where the terminal part of the urethra protrudes into a central fossa (Fig. 22.21/*3*). The glans is constricted to form a neck behind the corona and is then prolonged in a tapering process over the dorsal aspect of the body; this feature is not visible externally (Fig. 22.22/*7*).

A considerable portion of the quiescent penis projects into the preputial cavity. The equine prepuce (sheath) is peculiar in being thrown into an additional fold that allows for the considerable lengthening of the penis on erection (Fig. 22.21C). The entrance (preputial ring; Fig. 22.21B/*5′*) to this inner sleeve lies just within the preputial orifice. Sometimes as a congenital defect, the ring is unduly tight and prevents protrusion of the penis (phimosis). The condition may be corrected by section of the responsible encircling band of muscle that is included within the ring. The preputial lining contains many glands and is commonly fouled by their secretion, the smegma. An inspissated mass of this dark material—the "bean" of the penis is the stable term—commonly fills a small (urethral) sinus above the urethral process (Fig. 22.21A and D/*3′*).

The penis of the horse obtains blood from the obturator and external pudendal arteries in addition to the usual internal pudendal source.

Unusually, the *bulbospongiosus* continues along the ventral aspect of the penis well beyond the point of incorporation of the urethra (Fig. 22.22/*5*). The muscle, which is the direct continuation of the urethralis, bridges the ventral groove of the corpus cavernosum and on contraction compresses the corpus spongiosum (and urethra), assisting in the expulsion of urine and semen. The *ischiocavernosus muscles* are powerful but in no way remarkable. The smooth *retractor penis muscles* loop around the rectum before passing onto the ventral surface of the penis (Fig. 22.22/*6*). They continue forward, gradually weaving through the transverse fibers of the bulbospongiosus, to find attachment on the glans.

Erection

Because the penis is of the musculocavernous type, it becomes considerably engorged with blood when erect. When erection is complete, a process requiring some time and achieved by the relaxation of the helicine arteries* and the pumping action of the ischiocavernosi, the organ is much enlarged in both length and girth (Fig. 22.21C). A very considerable pressure, perhaps as much as 3700 mm Hg, is attained within the blood spaces of the corpus cavernosum, and as in other species, this occasionally results in rupture of the fibrous capsule. The ejaculate is relatively large (≈65 mL on average) and is mainly the product of the vesicular glands.

Dismounting after service is often followed by a remarkable "flaring" or enlargement of the glans, in which the corona may briefly attain a diameter of 12 cm or so before it subsides. The return of the flaccid penis to the sheath is effected by the retractor muscles assisted by the smooth muscle component of the walls of the cavernosal spaces. Indeed, the resting posture of the penis is dependent on the tonus of this muscle. If this is reduced or lost—a relatively common occurrence in horses that are fatigued or in poor condition—the penis limply droops from the prepuce. It is vulnerable to injury when exposed in this way. The resistance of the muscle may also be overcome by sustained traction when it is necessary to expose the organ for clinical examination or for washing as part of routine stable hygiene.

THE ANATOMY OF RECTAL EXPLORATION

Exploration per rectum is an important diagnostic technique in the horse. A hand can very easily be introduced into the rectum and descending colon and then be passed in various directions to examine the pelvic and caudal abdominal wall, the pelvic contents, and a variable amount of the abdominal contents (Fig. 22.23/*7*). *Rectal examinations are not free from risk of injury to the mucosa or even, in extreme cases, of perforation of the intestinal wall—a mishap most likely to occur when invasion of the rectum induces straining. The novice should not attempt the procedure without appropriate supervision.*

Some organs can always be identified with certainty and others less consistently, because the results of the investigation depend not only on the relative sizes of the investigator and patient but also on the condition of the organs. It is one thing to palpate an organ through the gut wall and quite another to recognize enough of its nature

*These are terminal arteries that open directly into the cavernosal spaces of the erectile tissue of the penis. Their myoepithelial walls cause them to be coiled (helicine) and closed in the flaccid penis. Sexual stimulation relaxes them, which allows blood to engorge the erectile tissue.

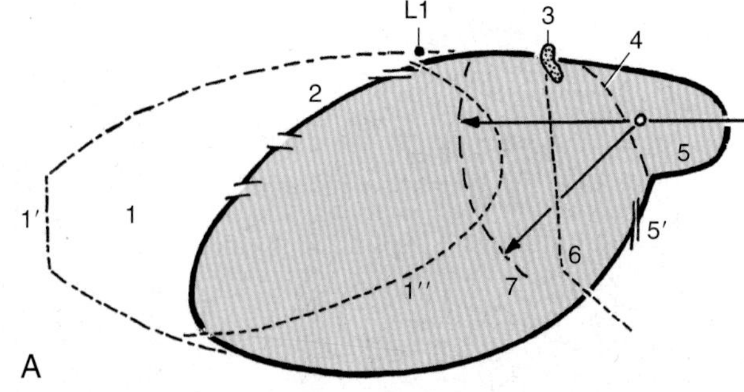

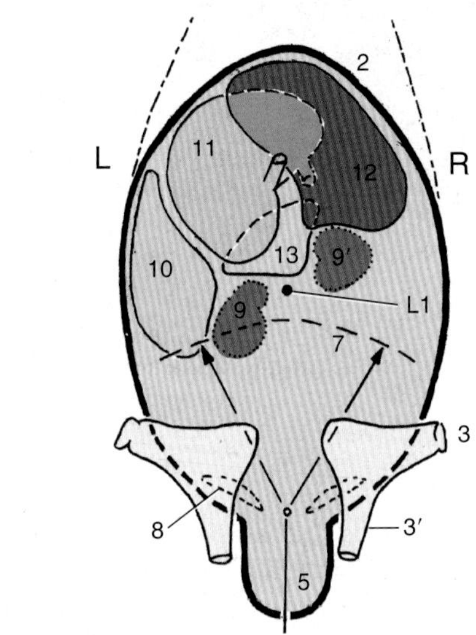

Fig. 22.23 Drawings of the abdominal and pelvic cavities in (A) left lateral and (B) dorsal outline, indicating the scope of rectal exploration. The dorsal outline encloses a ring of the relatively fixed organs (*9, 9′, 10, 11,* and *12*) with the pancreas (*13*) in the center. *1,* Thoracic cavity; *1′,* thoracic inlet; *1″,* costal arch; *2,* diaphragm; *3,* coxal tuber; *3′,* shaft of ilium; *4,* terminal line; *5,* pelvic cavity; *5′,* inguinal canal; *6,* thigh and stifle; *7,* approximate range in rectal palpation in the median plane (A) and directly ventral to the kidneys (B); *8,* deep inguinal ring; *9* and *9′,* left and right kidneys, respectively; *10,* spleen; *11,* stomach; *12,* liver; *13,* pancreas; *L,* left side; *R,* right side.

to be confident of identification. The greater part of the pelvic skeleton can be identified with absolute certainty, although the part of the floor about the symphysis may be made inaccessible by overlying organs. The caudal part of the abdominal wall is also within reach, although it rarely reveals much of interest other than the caudal margin of the internal oblique muscle bordering the deep inguinal ring and the vaginal ring (Fig. 22.24/*1*) within that opening. The vaginal ring can be recognized most easily in the stallion, in which the deferent duct may be picked up where it lies on the bladder and traced to its disappearance.

The *small colon* is the most easily recognized because of the chain of sacculations usually filled with firm feces;

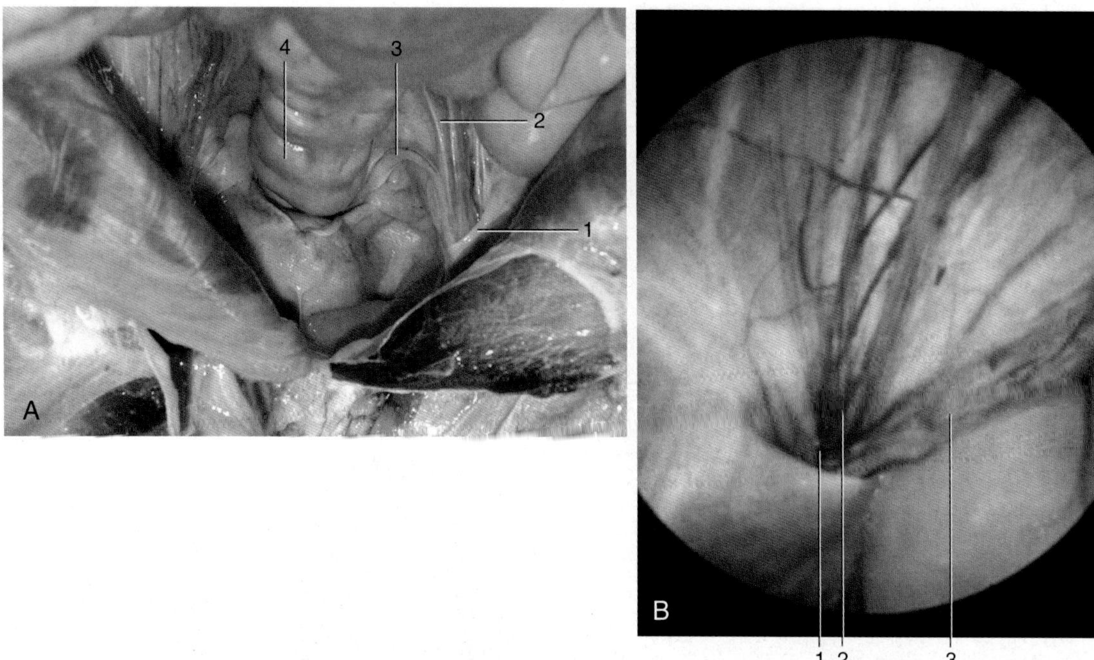

Fig. 22.24 (A) Dissection showing the vaginal ring. (B) Endoscopic view of the ring. *1,* Vaginal ring; *2,* testicular artery and vein; *3,* deferent duct; *4,* descending colon.

even when empty, this part of the gut can be distinguished by a single taenia following the free border (the taenia along the opposite mesenteric border is not normally palpable). Although the small colon has a mobile disposition, a mass of coils is generally found just in front of the pelvic inlet and mainly to the left. The pelvic flexure, the part of the ascending colon most easily identified, is usually found immediately before or even within the pelvic cavity. Most often it lies just to the left of the median plane but it may cross to the right. The adjoining parts of the left ventral and dorsal parts of the ascending colon can be followed for some distance. They are most easily recognized when gas filled, because this emphasizes the contrast between the sacculations of the wide ventral part and the smooth surface of the narrower dorsal part. Although the names of these parts are indicative, it must not be assumed that they necessarily lie directly one above the other. The dorsal diaphragmatic flexure and right parts of the colon are out of reach of even the longest arm, although sometimes it is just possible for the fingertips to touch and trace the junction of the ascending and transverse parts of the colon. The base and the dorsal part of the body of the cecum are consistently within reach. The cranial mesenteric artery, adherent to the left face of the cecal base, may sometimes be identified when thickened by reaction to nematode larval invasion. Even in the most favorable circumstances it is barely within reach.

Although much of the *small intestine* is accessible, it is usually impossible to identify it with certainty other than the firmer terminal part of the ileum, which may be picked up as it approaches the medial aspect of the cecal base. Identification is easiest when it is impacted. When distended with gas, the caudal flexure of the duodenum may be identified as it crosses the root of the mesentery.

A small horse and a long arm are the prerequisites if many of the contents of the cranial part of the abdomen are to be touched. The caudal pole of the left kidney may usually be felt. It is theoretically possible to trace both ureters over the abdominal roof, but in practice healthy ureters cannot be identified. The caudal margin of the spleen is also accessible, although it may not always be appreciated except when the stomach is distended.

An emergency means of euthanasia, of little relevance today, is available in transection of the abdominal aorta per rectum.

The *bladder* is invariably identifiable, regardless of its degree of filling and despite the fact that it is partly overlain by reproductive organs. In the mare, the vagina is distinguishable as a rather lax organ interposed between the rectum and the bladder; if followed forward, it leads to the somewhat firmer cervix. Beyond the cervix, the body of the uterus may be traced to its bifurcation, and the horns may then be followed laterally toward the ovaries. The dimensions and the texture of the uterus vary greatly with its state, and the experienced equine clinician can

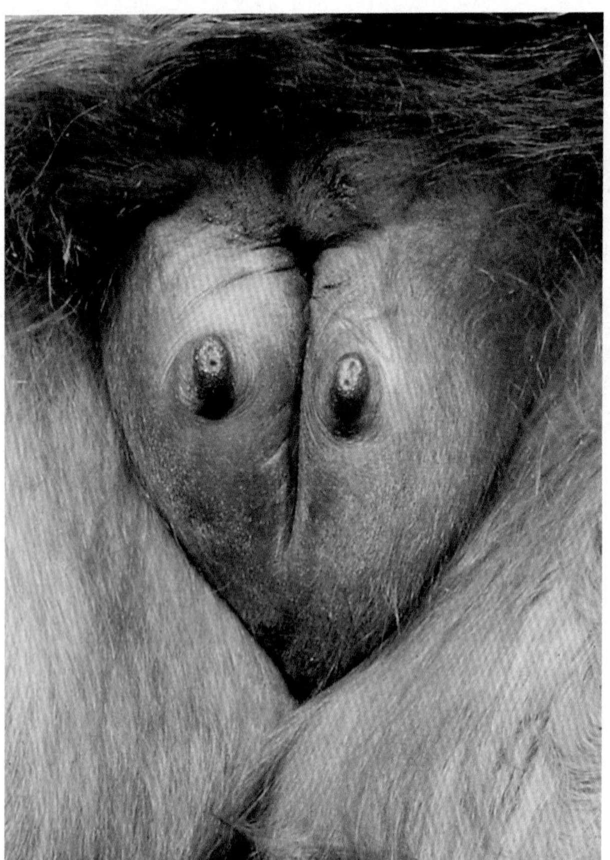

Fig. 22.25 The udder is consolidated from right and left halves. The apices of the teats are perforated by the papillary ducts.

date an early pregnancy with quite remarkable precision by palpating the uterus. The ovaries are among the easiest organs to identify because they have a very characteristic shape and consistency. They are rather movable and are not always found exactly where expected. Only the largest follicles may be appreciated individually.

The *pelvic urethra of the stallion* is easily identified as a wide, slack tube, although its outline is partly concealed by the associated glands (Fig. 22.20). The bulbourethral glands at the pelvic exit, the smooth pear-shaped vesicular glands, the more knobby prostate, and the fusiform enlargements of the ampullae of the deferent ducts are almost always individually distinctive. Manipulation may stimulate the urethral muscle, which may firm the urethra and cause it to exhibit rhythmic contractions.

THE UDDER

The mammary glands are consolidated in a rather small udder situated below the caudal part of the abdominal floor and cranial part of the pelvis and concealed from casual inspection by the thigh (Fig. 22.25). The form and size of the udder vary with the present state and previous history of

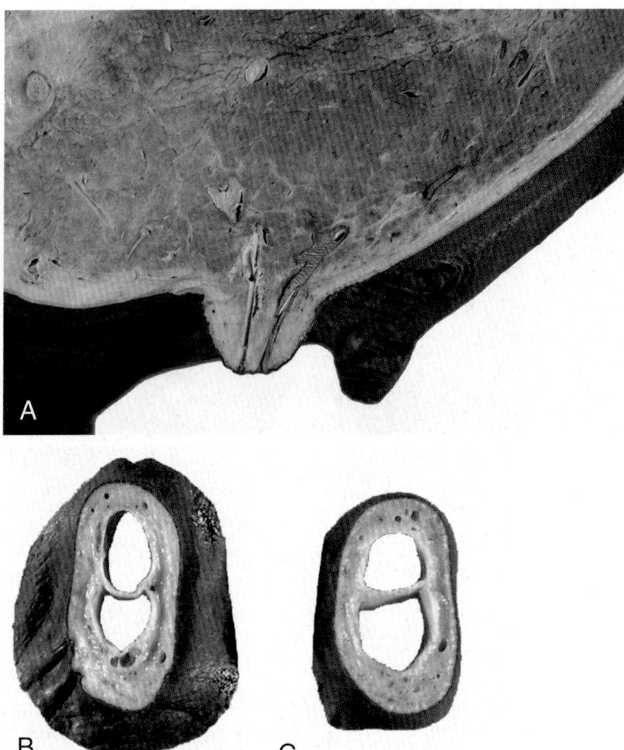

Fig. 22.26 (A) Sagittal section of the udder demonstrating the construction of the teat and the location of the lactiferous sinus. (B) and (C) Transected teats showing internal division.

the mare; the udder is very small in young virgin animals. A prominent external groove indicates its formation from right and left halves; each half has the form of a laterally compressed cone and, though carrying a single teat, is composed of two (occasionally three) separate duct systems.

The skin over the udder is thin, strongly pigmented, and sparsely haired. It glistens from the secretion of many sweat and sebaceous glands. The teat is small and cylindrical, except in the lactating mare, in which it is both larger and more conical. Two (or three) openings perforate the apex; each leads through a short papillary duct to a small lactiferous sinus spread between the teat and gland mass and associated with an independent set of lactiferous ducts (Fig. 22.26A–C). The tissues of the individual glands of each side interdigitate, and it is impossible to demonstrate their independence on dissection. Although much less developed, the suspensory apparatus resembles that of the cow's udder and combines medial elastic and lateral fibrous ligaments, which together encapsulate the udder and supply the lamellae that support the parenchyma. The medial ligaments provide a cleavage plane between the apposed surfaces of the udder halves.

The blood supply comes from the *external pudendal artery*, and the principal venous return is by the corresponding vein, which does not follow the usual course through the inguinal canal (p. 540). As in the cow, a

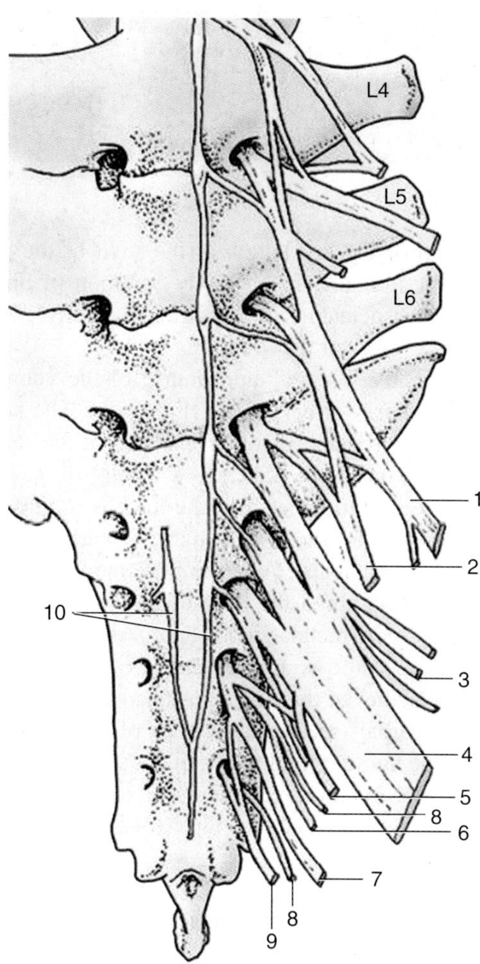

Fig. 22.27 Ventral view of sacrum and caudal lumbar vertebrae (L4–L6) with emerging ventral rami forming the lumbosacral plexus. *1,* Femoral nerve (n.); *2,* obturator n.; *3,* cranial gluteal n.; *4,* sciatic n.; *5,* caudal cutaneous femoral n.; *6,* caudal gluteal n.; *7,* pudendal n.; *8,* pelvic n.; *9,* caudal rectal n.; *10,* continuation of sympathetic cord.

subcutaneous venous connection with a superficial vein of the thoracic wall develops as an alternative drainage route during the first pregnancy. Lymph drains to the mammary (superficial inguinal) nodes. The cutaneous innervation is divided between the nerves of the flank and a descending (mammary) branch of the pudendal nerve; the contributing spinal nerves are thus those of cord segments L2–L4 and S2–S4 (Fig. 22.27). The substance of the gland is supplied by the genitofemoral nerve (L3–L4). The glands develop rapidly during the second half of the first pregnancy and commence secretion before birth. Sebaceous secretion, epithelial debris, and possibly colostrum that escape through the teat openings during the last days of pregnancy dry to give the apex a waxy covering, which is a useful indication that parturition impends.

COMPREHENSION CHECK

As a group, compare the anatomy of the equine and ruminant female and male reproductive tracts, including the structure of the pelvis.

23 The Forelimb of the Horse

In the Western world horses are now mainly bred for use in sport and recreation, pursuits that often make heavy demands on their speed and endurance and expose their limbs to continual strain and repeated risk of injury. Even relatively minor incapacity may unfit a horse for this work, and the importance of soundness of limb is crisply stated by the old adage "no foot, no horse." Considering the importance of lameness in equine medicine, a detailed knowledge of the anatomy of the limb is needed.

The limbs of the horse display extreme adaptations for fast running with a concomitant loss of versatility. The forelimbs carry the greater part (some 55%–60%) of the body weight at rest and supply the principal shock absorbers that are necessary in the faster gaits and especially when landing from a jump. The hindlimbs furnish the main propulsive thrust. Furthermore, the share of the load that is supported by each limb may be altered by varying the posture to shift the center of gravity. The most obvious maneuver is to raise or lower the head to displace the center caudally or cranially, respectively. The lame animal also lifts the head when a painful forelimb is placed on the ground and lowers it when the sound limb bears weight. Because the later movement is more obvious, a horse with forelimb lameness is said to "nod on the sound foot." When there is a painful condition of a hindlimb, the head is lowered as the affected limb assumes support.

A forelimb with good conformation is straight when viewed from the front. A line dropped from the point of the shoulder bisects the limb and passes through the center of the hoof; the digit continues the cannon (metacarpus) in a straight line, neither "toeing-in" nor "toeing-out" (Fig. 23.1). Much of the limb should also be straight when viewed from the side. A line dropped from the tuberosity of the scapular spine should bisect it to the fetlock and then pass just behind the hoof, whose slope should parallel that of the digit. Deviations from the normal conformation can result in abnormal movements, which in turn may cause interference between the feet, unequal and abnormal hoof wear, and development of lameness.

The more common deviations seen when viewing from the front are categorized as "base-wide," in which the limbs slope laterally, and "base-narrow," in which they slope medially. Deviations seen from the side include "standing under," in which the limbs slope caudally, and "camped," in which they slope cranially. Cranial, caudal, medial, and lateral deviations of the carpus are also recognized; the last two faults are "knock-knees" and "bowlegs."

Retention of the full length of the shaft of the ulna is a congenital anomaly that is fairly common in Shetland ponies. It is associated with a valgus deformity*—sometimes very severe—of the limb.

The distinctive "leggy" appearance of the young foal must be familiar to every reader (Fig. 23.2). The acquisition of the adult shape involves changes in the ratios of the lengths of the limbs (taken as a whole) to that of the trunk and in the ratios between the lengths of successive segments of the limbs—arm (thigh), forearm (leg), and metacarpus (metatarsus). According to one source, in the newborn Thoroughbred the ratio of the humerus (femur) to the metacarpus (metatarsus) is approximately 4:5 (4:5); in the adult the ratio is approximately 6:5 (6.5:5). These changes are achieved through a postnatal growth in length of the metacarpal (metatarsal) bones of about 20% and growth of the humerus and femur of about 100%.

The cutaneous features known as *chestnuts* and *ergots* are described on page 362 (see Fig. 10.17).

THE GIRDLE MUSCLES

The same muscles join the limb to the trunk as in other species, but there are certain differences in detail. The trapezius arises from the dorsal midline, extending almost from the poll to beyond the withers. Both cervical and thoracic parts insert on the spine of the scapula, and when they act in unison, they raise this bone against the trunk. The cervical part acting alone swings the scapula forward, which advances the limb, whereas the thoracic part acting alone swings it in the opposite direction. Both parts may be visibly outlined through the skin when contracted. The nerve supply is the accessory nerve.

The *brachiocephalicus* (Fig. 23.3/*4*) arises from the mastoid region of the skull and inserts on a ridge of the humerus that extends distally from the deltoid tuberosity. It is intimately joined in the neck to the *omotransversarius* (Fig. 23.3/*6*), which takes origin from the transverse processes of the more cranial cervical vertebrae and ends at the clavicular intersection that divides the brachiocephalicus into cervical (cleidomastoideus) and brachial (cleidobrachialis) parts. The dorsal edge of the omotransversarius is connected to the trapezius by the superficial fascia.

*A lateral deviation of a part of a limb distal to a joint. The opposite varus deformity is a similar deviation but is angled medially.

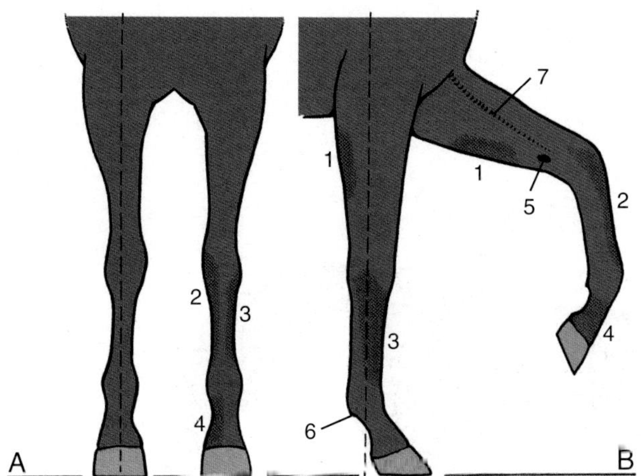

Fig. 23.1 Desirable conformation and autonomous zones of cutaneous innervation of the forelimb. (A) Cranial view; a *vertical broken line* dropped from the point of the shoulder bisects the limb. (B) Right lateral view; a *vertical line* dropped from the tuberosity of the scapular spine bisects the limb down to the fetlock. The autonomous zones *(shaded areas)* represent skin areas innervated solely by the nerves below. *1,* Caudal cutaneous antebrachial nerve (ulnar); *2,* medial cutaneous antebrachial nerve (musculocutaneous); *3,* ulnar nerve; *4,* median nerve; *5,* chestnut; *6,* ergot; *7,* cephalic vein.

The ventral edge of the brachiocephalicus is clearly delineated, at least in its cranial half, as it forms the upper margin of the jugular groove (see Fig. 18.38B).

The muscle is broadest over the shoulder joint, where it covers the origin of the biceps and the insertions of the supraspinatus and infraspinatus. Bilateral action flexes the neck ventrally when that part is free to move. Unilateral action in the same circumstances bends the neck toward the active side; when the neck is fixed and it is the limb that is free, unilateral action advances the limb. The innervation is shared by the accessory, cervical, and axillary nerves.

The *latissimus dorsi* (Fig. 23.3/[illegible]) arises from the supraspinous ligament and thoracolumbar fascia and converges to an insertion on the teres tuberosity of the humerus. The cranial strip covers the caudal angle of the scapula and holds it against the trunk. This muscle is commonly described as a retractor of the limb and thus is an antagonist of the brachiocephalicus; in fact, its most important role, especially in draft animals, may be to pull the trunk forward onto an advanced limb. It is supplied by the thoracodorsal nerve.

The superficial layer of girdle muscles is completed by the two superficial pectoral muscles supplied by pectoral branches of the brachial plexus. The cranial *pectoralis descendens* arises from the manubrium and divides its insertion between the humerus and fascia of the arm (Fig. 23.4/*4*). It is well developed and clearly outlined in life; a median groove separates it from its contralateral fellow. The lateral groove that marks its boundary with the brachiocephalicus is occupied by the cephalic vein. It is primarily an adductor.

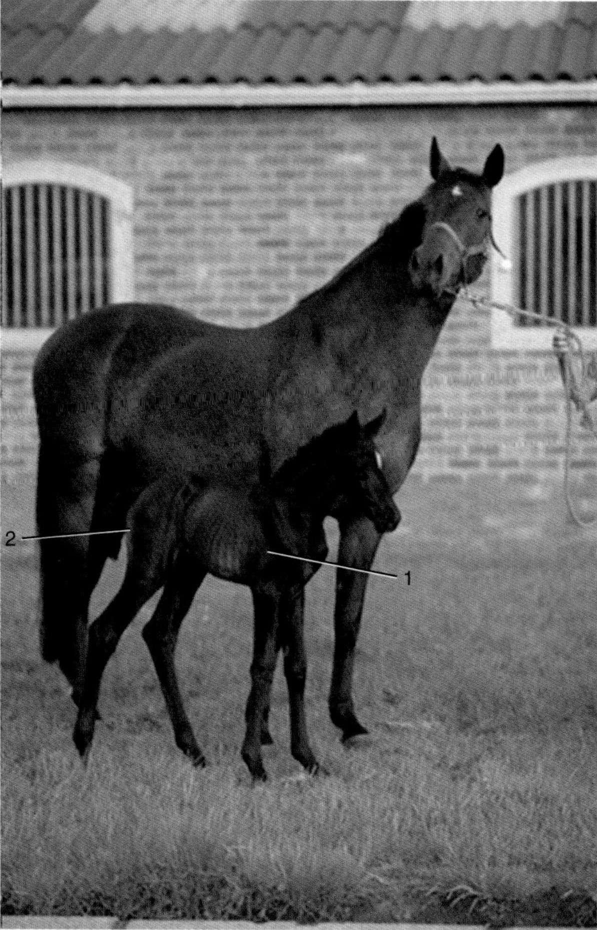

Fig. 23.2 This photograph of a 10-day-old foal with its dam illustrates the proportions of the limbs and trunk that account for the "leggy" appearance of the young foal. *1,* Flaccid long and medial heads of triceps; *2,* "poverty" line between biceps femoris and semitendinosus.

The caudal *pectoralis transversus* (Fig. 23.4/*5*) arises from the cranial sternebrae and inserts into the fascia over the medial aspect of the upper part of the forearm. The transverse course of its fibers makes it clear that it is essentially an adductor.

Although the *rhomboideus* lies deep to the trapezius, it may, when contracted, form a visible surface feature. Its origin from the nuchal and supraspinous ligaments extends between the second cervical and seventh thoracic vertebrae. The entire muscle inserts on the deep face and dorsal edge of the scapular cartilage (Fig. 23.5/*4*). It raises the scapula, and the thoracic fascicles rotate the bone so that the ventral angle is carried caudally. The innervation is by dorsal branches of caudal cervical nerves.

The *serratus ventralis* (Fig. 23.5/*1*) is very strong, both actively because of its extent and bulk and passively because it is covered and interlinked by stout connective tissue sheets. The origin spreads from the 4th cervical vertebra to the 10th rib. The insertion is confined

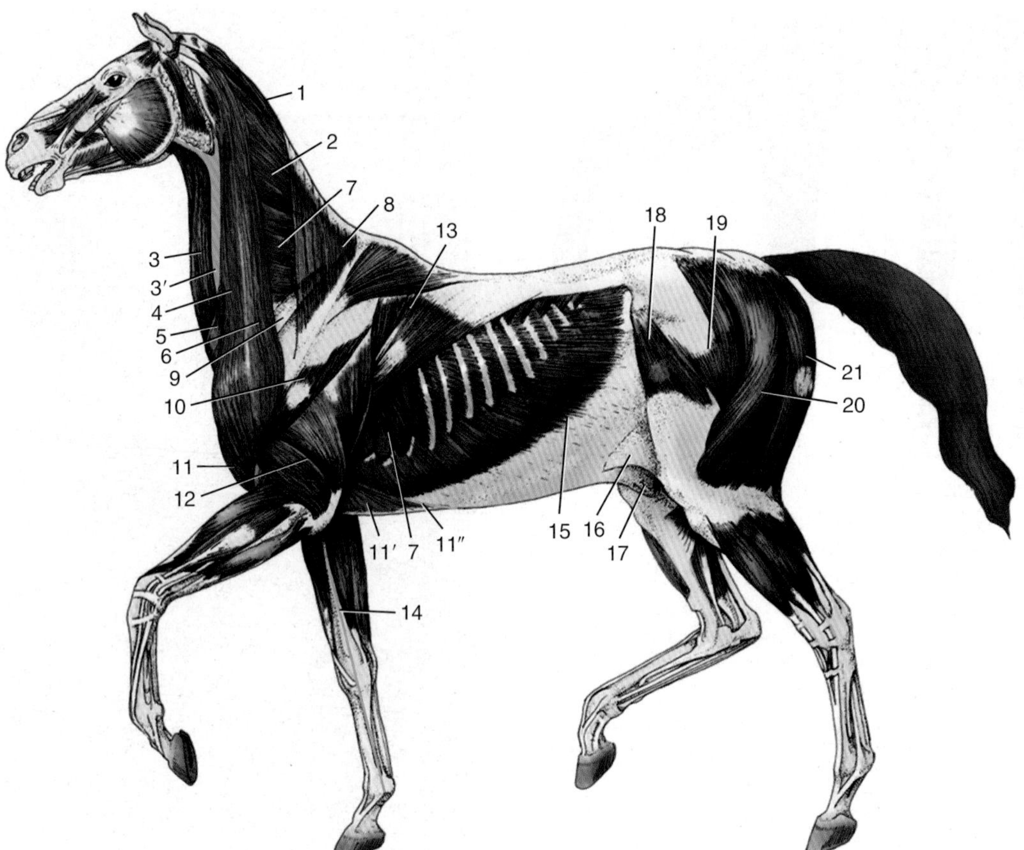

Fig. 23.3 The superficial muscles and veins. The cutaneous muscles, except for the cutaneous colli, have been removed. *1,* Rhomboideus; *2,* splenius; *3,* sternocephalicus; *3′,* jugular vein; *4,* brachiocephalicus; *5,* cutaneous colli; *6,* omotransversarius; *7,* serratus ventralis; *8,* trapezius; *9,* subclavius; *10,* deltoideus; *11,* pectoralis descendens; *11′,* pectoralis ascendens; *11″,* superficial thoracic vein; *12,* triceps; *13,* latissimus dorsi; *14,* cephalic vein; *15,* external abdominal oblique; *16,* stump of cutaneous trunci forming flank fold; *17,* sheath; *18,* tensor fasciae latae; *19,* gluteus superficialis; *20,* biceps femoris; *21,* semitendinosus.

to the scapular cartilage and to two triangular areas on the adjacent part of the medial surface of the scapula. The dominant function of the serratus is support of the trunk. However, the cervical and thoracic parts each have an additional (and antagonistic) function in rotating the scapula. The cervical part rotates the bone so that the ventral angle is carried caudally, thus retracting the limb; contraction of the thoracic part advances this angle and thus the limb. The serratus ventralis is supplied by the long thoracic nerve.

The *pectoralis profundus* has a widespread origin from the caudal part of the sternum and adjacent area of the abdominal floor (Fig. 23.5/*3*). The fascicles converge, and the muscle thickens as it passes craniolaterally to a restricted insertion on the greater and lesser tubercles of the humerus. Although the relative heights of the origin and insertion suggest that the deep pectoral muscle may assist the serratus in supporting the weight of the trunk, this capacity is highly limited (Fig. 23.5B). Its foremost uses are probably adduction, retraction of the limb when this is free to move, and advancement of the trunk onto an advanced and fixed limb. It is supplied by pectoral nerves.

The *subclavius* (Fig. 23.5/*2*), to the front of the deep pectoral, takes origin from the cranial part of the sternum. It then bends dorsally to follow the cranial surface of the supraspinatus, over which it tapers to an extended insertion on the epimysium. Its presence along the leading edge of the scapula helps smooth the transition from the narrow neck to the greater breadth between the shoulders. The actions of the subclavius complement those of the deep pectoral (of which it was formerly regarded as a part). It too is supplied by pectoral nerves (Table 23.1).

THE SHOULDER REGION AND UPPER ARM

The scapula and humerus form the bases of the shoulder region and both are wholly included within the skin of the trunk. The slope of the *scapula* varies considerably and is revealed by the

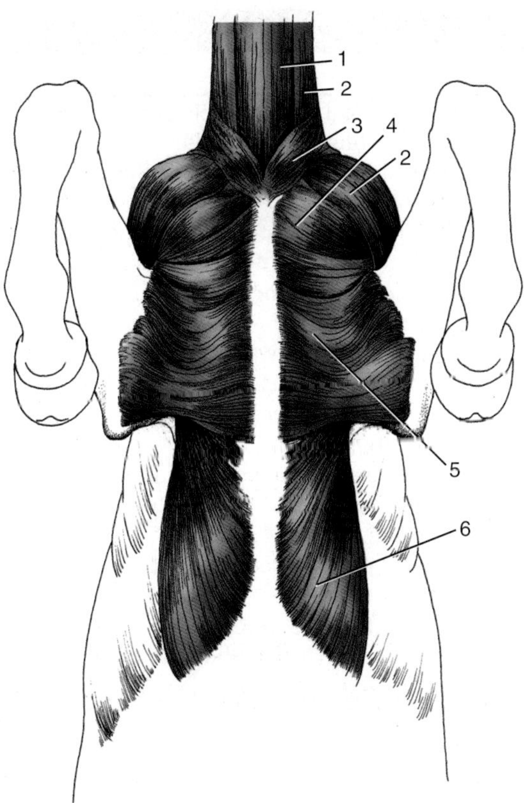

Fig. 23.4 Muscles on the ventral surface of the thorax. *1,* Sternocephalicus; *2,* brachiocephalicus; *3,* cutaneous colli; *4,* pectoralis descendens; *5,* pectoralis transversus; *6,* pectoralis profundus.

orientation of its spine. A more sloping shoulder is preferred in saddle horses. The thickened middle portion (tuber spinae) of the spine is readily recognized on palpation and may even provide a visible landmark (Fig. 23.6A/*3*). The distal part of the spine subsides gradually and does not form an acromion. The bone is extended beyond its dorsal border by a large scapular cartilage that is [illegible]. The [illegible] of the cartilage and the cranial and caudal angles of the bone may be palpated in most subjects. The caudal angle is often quite prominent, even though it is covered by the latissimus dorsi (Fig. 23.3/*13*).

The *humerus* forms a right angle with the scapula and slopes less steeply than in the smaller species. Its surface relief is marked, and many features may be felt through the skin and musculature. The greater and lesser tubercles of the proximal extremity are both well developed and are more nearly equal than those in most species. Each is divided into cranial and caudal parts. The cranial parts are separated by an intertubercular groove that is interrupted by an intermediate tubercle; there are thus five processes. Although both parts of the greater tubercle are easily palpated, its cranial division creates the "point of the shoulder" (Fig. 23.6A/*8*). Distal to this, the deltoid tuberosity furnishes another easily found landmark (Fig. 23.6A/*10*).

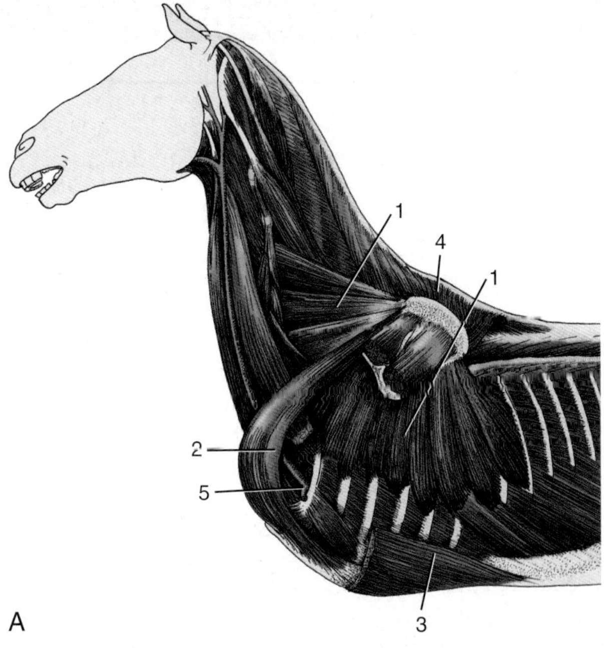

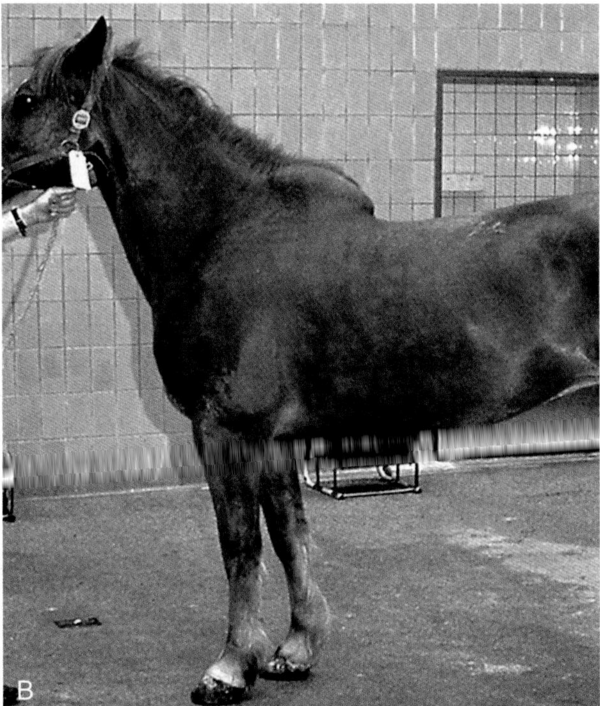

Fig. 23.5 (A) Deep muscles attaching the forelimb to the trunk. *1,* Serratus ventralis; *2,* subclavius; *3,* pectoralis profundus; *4,* rhomboideus; *5,* axillary vessels turning around first rib into limb. (B) Rupture of serratus ventralis muscle.

The *shoulder joint* has anatomic attributes of a spheroidal joint, but it acts as a hinge joint because of the restrictions imposed by the tendons of the muscles that closely surround the shoulder, notably the infraspinatus (and, to a lesser degree, the supraspinatus) laterally and

TABLE 23.1 GIRDLE MUSCLES

Muscle	Nerve	Action
Trapezius	Axillary	Both cervical and thoracic parts acting together raise the scapula Cervical part alone advances the limb while thoracic part alone swings the limb caudally
Brachiocephalicus	Accessory, cervical and axillary	Bilateral muscle action flexes the neck Unilateral actions advance the limb
Latissimus dorsi	Thoracodorsal	Commonly antagonistic of the brachiocephalicus Pulls the trunk forward on an advanced limb
Superficial pectorals	Pectoral	Pectoralis descendens: adducts Pectoralis transversus: adducts
Rhomboideus	Dorsal branches of caudal cervical nerve	Raises the scapula Rotates the scapula such that the ventral angle is carried caudally (retraction)
Serratus ventralis	Long thoracic	Supports the trunk Cervical part retracts the limb
Pectoralis profundus	Pectoral nerves	Adducts the limb Retracts the free limb Advances the trunk when the limb is fixed
Subclavius	Pectoral	Complements the deep pectorals

the subscapularis medially (Fig. 23.7). The relatively capacious joint cavity may be tapped by inserting a needle at the cranial margin of the palpable infraspinatus tendon about 2 cm proximal to the caudal part of the greater tubercle. The needle is directed ventromedially and must be introduced about 4 or 5 cm before its tip penetrates the capsule. The procedure requires some care because a cranial deflection may cause the needle to enter the bursa that protects the biceps tendon within the intertubercular groove. This intertubercular bursa corresponds to the diverticulum of the joint capsule found in the dog and sheep.

The muscles that act primarily on the shoulder may be considered as being arranged in lateral and medial groups, although they enclose the joint on all sides. The lateral group comprises the supraspinatus, infraspinatus, deltoideus, and teres minor (Fig. 23.6B).

The *supraspinatus* (Fig. 23.6B/*7*) arises from and occupies the supraspinous fossa of the scapula. It bulges beyond the bone cranially where its covering epimysium provides insertion to the subclavius. It splits into two short tendons that straddle the origin of the biceps before attaching to the cranial parts of the tubercles of the humerus. The muscle is placed to extend the shoulder joint, but its most important function may be stabilization of the joint.

The *infraspinatus* (Fig. 23.6B/*8*) is located in the infraspinous fossa, and its insertion crosses the lateral aspect of the shoulder joint before separating into deep and superficial tendons. The short deep tendon attaches to the edge of the caudal part of the greater tubercle. The superficial tendon crosses this projection to attach at a more distal level and is protected by a synovial bursa where it lies against the bone. Inflammation of the bursa may be painful and may cause the animal to stand with the affected limb abducted at the shoulder, which is a posture that relieves the pressure at the site. The infraspinatus is primarily a shoulder fixator whose tendon substitutes for a lateral collateral ligament. It has a secondary abductor action. Both the supraspinatus and the infraspinatus are supplied by the suprascapular nerve.

The *deltoideus* (Fig. 23.6B/*9*) arises from the caudal border and spine of the scapula; the latter origin is indirect and effected by way of an aponeurosis that covers the infraspinatus. The insertion is to the deltoid tuberosity, which is used as a landmark to trace the muscle proximally. It is partly recessed within a depression of the triceps, and the line between the muscles is sometimes visible in thin-skinned animals. The deltoideus is a shoulder flexor with a secondary role as abductor of the arm. Innervation is by the axillary nerve.

The unimportant *teres minor* is buried by the deltoideus over the caudolateral aspect of the shoulder joint.

The medial muscle group comprises the subscapularis, teres major, coracobrachialis, and capsularis, of which the last is of trivial significance. The *subscapularis* arises from and occupies the subscapular fossa (Fig. 23.8/*1*). It inserts on the lesser tubercle and, though primarily employed to stabilize the joint, may also function as an adductor of the arm. It is supplied by the subscapular nerve.

The *teres major* (Fig. 23.8/*3*) arises from the caudal angle of the scapula. It is contained between the subscapularis and the latissimus dorsi and inserts in common with the latter. It is chiefly a flexor of the shoulder but may also

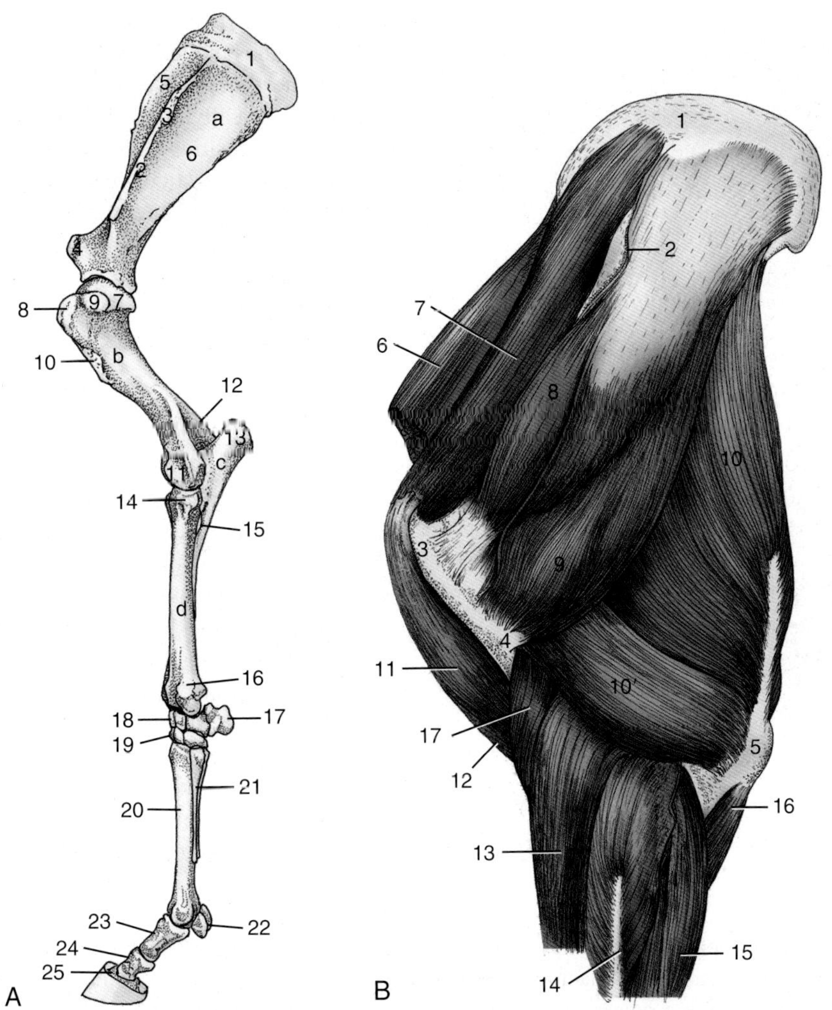

Fig. 23.6 (A) Skeleton of the left forelimb, lateral view. *a,* Scapula; *b,* humerus; *c,* ulna; *d,* radius; *1,* scapular cartilage; *2,* scapular spine; *3,* tuberosity of scapular spine; *4,* supraglenoid tubercle; *5* and *6,* supraspinous and infraspinous fossae, respectively; *7,* head of humerus; *8* and *9,* cranial and caudal parts of greater tubercle, respectively; *10,* deltoid tuberosity; *11,* condyle; *12,* olecranon fossa; *13,* olecranon; *14,* tubercle for lateral collateral ligament; *15,* interosseous space; *16,* lateral styloid process; *17,* accessory carpal; *18* and *19,* proximal and distal row of carpal bones, respectively; *20,* large metacarpal (cannon) bone; *21,* small metacarpal (splint) bone; *22,* proximal sesamoid bones; *23,* proximal phalanx; *24,* middle phalanx; *25,* distal phalanx. (B) Muscles associated with shoulder and elbow joints, lateral view. *1,* Scapular cartilage; *2,* scapular spine; *3,* greater tubercle of humerus; *4,* deltoid tuberosity of humerus; *5,* olecranon; *6,* subclavius; *7,* supraspinatus; *8,* infraspinatus; *9,* deltoideus; *10,* long head of triceps; *10′,* lateral head of triceps; *11,* biceps; *12,* lacertus fibrosus; *13,* extensor carpi radialis; *14,* common digital extensor; *15,* ulnaris lateralis; *16,* ulnar head of deep digital flexor; *17,* brachialis.

adduct the arm. It is supplied by the axillary nerve, as are all the true flexors of the shoulder.

The *coracobrachialis* (Fig. 23.8/*8*) arises from the coracoid process on the medial aspect of the supraglenoid tubercle and inserts on the proximal part of the shaft of the humerus. It is an adductor of the arm but is of little consequence. It is supplied by the musculocutaneous nerve (Table 23.2).

THE ELBOW JOINT AND THE MUSCLES OF THE ARM

The skeletal basis of the *elbow joint* is provided by the distal end of the humerus and proximal parts of the radius and ulna (Fig. 23.6A). Both epicondyles of the humerus may be palpated without much difficulty, but the medial one is especially prominent and projects to the inner aspect of the

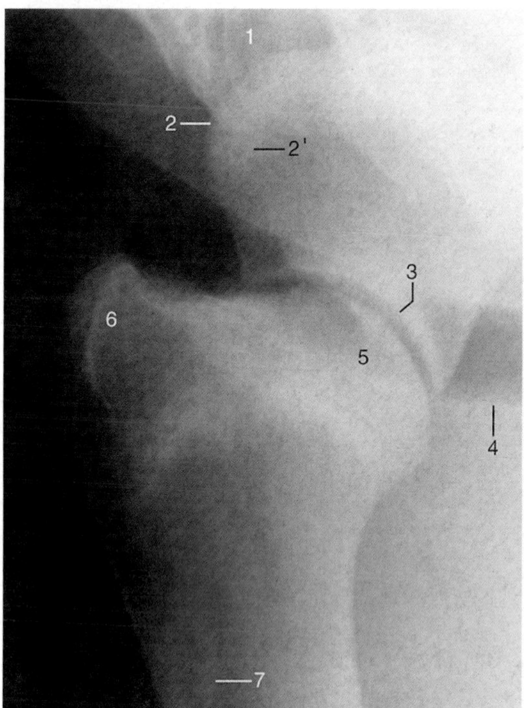

Fig. 23.7 Lateral radiograph of a shoulder joint. *1,* Sixth cervical vertebra; *2,* supraglenoid tubercle of scapula; *2′,* coracoid process; *3,* glenoid cavity; *4,* trachea; *5,* head of humerus; *6,* superimposed greater, lesser, and intertubercular tubercles; *7,* deltoid tuberosity.

olecranon. The condyle, identifiable more distally, presents a deep fossa for the anconeal process of the olecranon (Fig. 23.9/*4* and *6*). A shallow radial fossa occupies the corresponding site on the cranial aspect.

The powerful olecranon of the ulna rises high above the joint to project on the lower part of the fifth rib (or following space) and is therefore a less direct guide to the position of the articulation. The much reduced shaft of the ulna tapers distally to fuse and ultimately submerge with the shaft of the radius, but it leaves open an interosseous space in the proximal forearm. The proximal extremity of the radius is expanded and engages with the cylindrical humeral condyle. It also has medial and lateral eminences that furnish attachment to the collateral ligaments. The radial tuberosity is present to the front (Fig. 23.9/*8*). Both collateral ligaments may be palpated, although the medial one is covered by the relatively thick pectoralis transversus. A cranial division of this ligament represents a vestige of the pronator teres.

The shape of the articular surfaces and the presence of stout collateral ligaments restrict movement of the elbow joint to flexion and extension in a sagittal plane. The equine elbow is a good example of the "snap" joint, which abruptly moves from a stable to a more mobile position. This character depends on two features of its construction. The first is the unequal curvature of the humeral surface such that the radius of curvature of the central part is longer than those of the parts in front and behind, which are in contact with the radius in the more flexed and more extended positions of the joint. The second is that the collateral ligaments insert eccentrically on the humerus and are taut only in the intermediate position (Fig. 23.10).

The joint is most conveniently punctured by passing a needle between the lateral epicondyle and the olecranon into a caudal pouching of the joint capsule within the olecranon fossa.

The muscles of the arm that operate the elbow joint are arranged in flexor and extensor groups.

The Flexor Muscles

The flexor muscles comprise the biceps brachii and brachialis. Although largely under cover of the brachiocephalicus, the belly of the *biceps* is palpable as it lies against the cranial face of the humerus. The biceps takes origin from the supraglenoid tubercle of the scapula by means of a short, broad, and largely fibrocartilaginous tendon that is molded on the intertubercular groove. The intertubercular bursa that protects the tendon spreads from the groove onto the cranial aspect of the humerus. It may be a cause of shoulder lameness when inflamed. The bursa may be reached, certainly if overdistended, by inserting a needle between the muscle and the bone, slightly above the level of the deltoid tuberosity, and then directing it proximally (Fig. 23.11/*3*).

The biceps inserts mainly on the radial tuberosity, but a branch of the attachment passes beneath the medial collateral ligament to the adjoining parts of the radius and ulna. A more important peculiarity is the existence within its belly of a fibrous strand (internal tendon; Fig. 23.10/*5′*) that joins the tendons of origin and insertion; a part splits away to emerge on the surface and blend more distally with the epimysium of the extensor carpi radialis. The bridging band, known as the *lacertus fibrosus,* is easily found as a firm structure crossing the flexor aspect of the elbow (Fig. 23.10/*5″* and see Fig. 23.8/*12*). It is taut in the standing animal but slackens as the joint is flexed. The internal tendon and the lacertus help maintain the carpal joint in extension when the biceps resists collapse of the shoulder under the weight of the trunk (see Fig. 23.38A/*2* and *6*).

The bicep is a fixator and, potentially, an extensor of the shoulder; the construction and form of the tendon of origin suggest its particular fitness for the first task. Although it is regarded as the most important flexor of the elbow, the fibrous arrangements imply that its passive role may also be more significant at this joint. Research has shown that the central tendon allied to the bipennate construction of the muscle enables it to store energy when stretched during the support phase of the stride and that this energy is later very rapidly released to accelerate the forward movement of the limb. Its nerve supply comes from the musculocutaneous nerve.

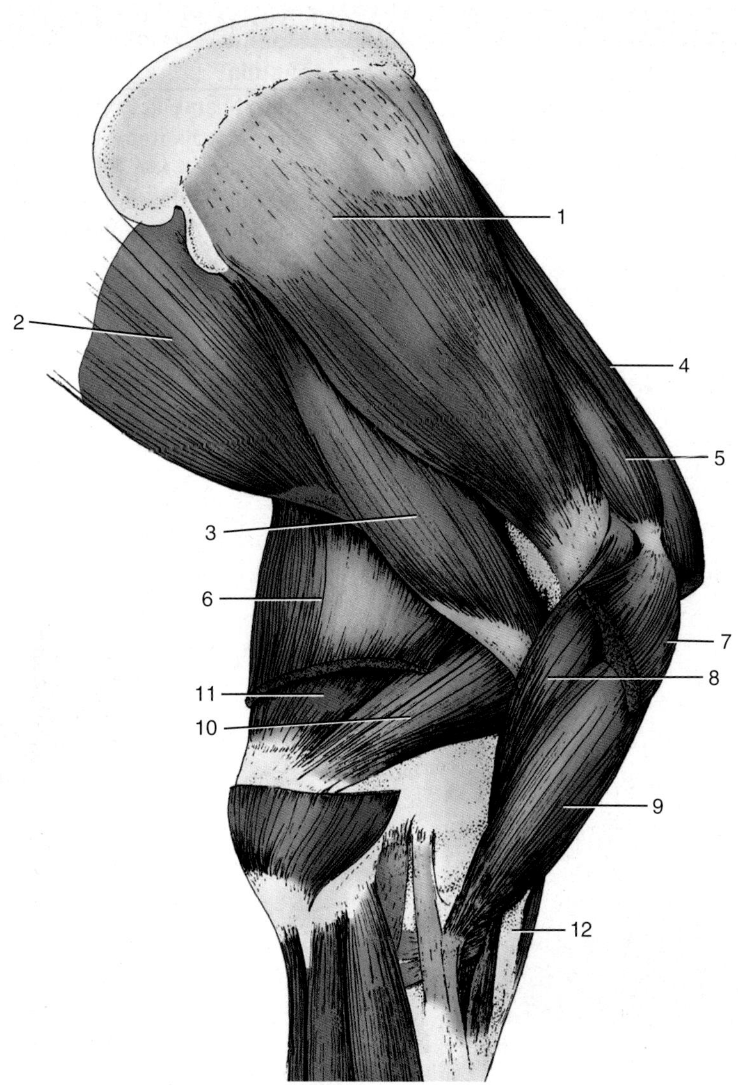

Fig. 23.8 Muscles on the medial surface of the right shoulder and arm. *1,* Subscapularis; *2,* latissimus dorsi; *3,* teres major; *4,* subclavius; *5,* supraspinatus; *6,* tensor fasciae antebrachii; *7,* deep pectoral; *8,* coracobrachialis; *9,* biceps; *10,* medial head of triceps; *11,* long head of triceps; *12,* lacertus fibrosus.

The *brachialis* is purely fleshy and crosses only one joint, the elbow. It arises from the caudoproximal part of the humerus, winds laterally within a spiral groove, and then crosses the flexor aspect of the elbow to insert on the craniomedial part of the proximal radius (Fig. 23.12/*3*). Proximally, the muscle is covered by the triceps, but its distal part is superficial and may be palpated. The brachialis is purely an elbow flexor. It is supplied by the musculocutaneous nerve with, rather surprisingly, a contribution from the radial nerve (Table 23.3).

The Extensor Muscles

The extensor muscles constitute a large mass that fills the triangle between the scapula and humerus. The group comprises the triceps, tensor fasciae antebrachii, and anconeus and is supplied by the radial nerve.

The *triceps* is by far the most important extensor of the elbow. It presents three heads (Fig. 23.6B/*10* and *10'*). The long head arises from the caudal border of the scapula by a short aponeurosis, and the lateral and medial heads arise from the shaft of the humerus. Together they insert on the olecranon where a small bursa is inserted between the tendon and the bone. The division between the long and lateral heads is sometimes visible in thin-skinned animals. A second, acquired (adventitious) bursa is commonly found subcutaneously, over the triceps insertion and expanded part of the olecranon tuber ("capped elbow" between the long and lateral heads; Fig. 23.11/*5*).

TABLE 23.2 MUSCLES ACTING ON THE SHOULDER JOINT

Muscle	Nerve	Action
Supraspinatus	Suprascapular	Mainly stabilizes the joint
Infraspinatus	Suprascapular	Primary: fixates; secondary: abducts the joint
Deltoideus	Axillary	Primary: flexes; secondary: abducts
Subscapularis	Subscapular	Stabilizes the joint
Teres major	Axillary	Mainly flexes but may adduct the joint
Coracobrachialis	Musculocutaneous	Minor adduction of the arm

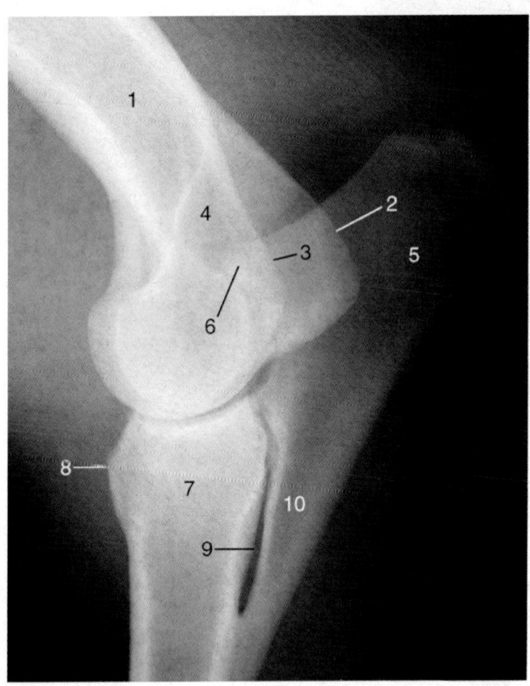

Fig. 23.9 Lateral radiograph of an elbow joint. *1,* Humerus; *2,* medial epicondyle; *3,* lateral epicondyle; *4,* olecranon fossa; *5,* olecranon; *6,* anconeal process of olecranon; *7,* radius; *8,* radial tuberosity; *9,* interosseous space; *10,* ulna.

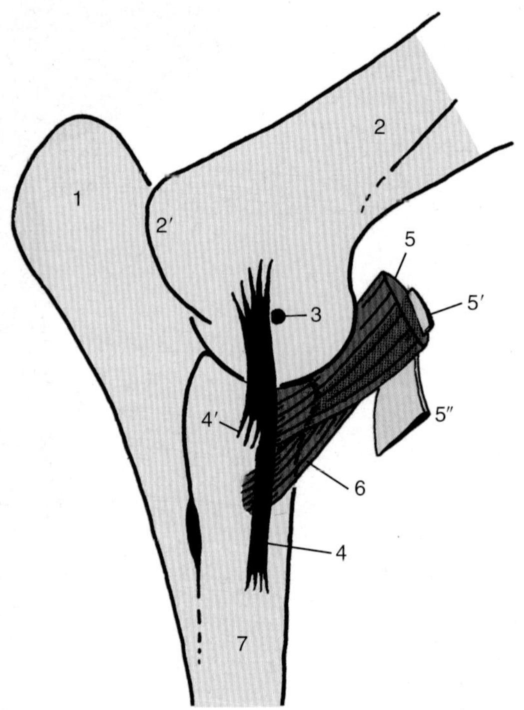

Fig. 23.10 Medial view of left elbow joint to show the eccentrically placed collateral ligament and the insertions of the biceps and brachialis. The internal tendon *(5)* of the biceps splits off the lacertus fibrosus *(5″)* from the surface of the muscle. *1,* Olecranon; *2,* humerus; *2′,* medial epicondyle; *3,* axis of rotation; *4* and *4′,* long superficial and short deep parts of medial collateral ligament, respectively; *5,* biceps; *5′,* internal tendon of biceps; *5″,* lacertus fibrosus; *6,* brachialis; *7,* radius.

The triceps is an extensor to the elbow. Because the long head spans the shoulder joint, it is theoretically available to flex this joint; however, it is probably little used for that purpose.

The *tensor fasciae antebrachii* (Fig. 23.8/*6*) is a broad, thin sheet covering the medial aspect of the triceps. Its origin is from the caudal border of the scapula and the tendon of the latissimus, while its insertion is spread between the olecranon and forearm fascia. Because it crosses both the shoulder and elbow joints, it must be considered as having a potential action at each; neither is likely to be of great importance.

The much smaller *anconeus* lies within the olecranon fossa, embedded within the deep face of the lateral head of the triceps and directly related to the capsule of the elbow joint. It may be supposed that its principal action is to tense the capsule, thus preventing it from being pinched between the humerus and ulna (Fig. 23.12/*4* and Table 23.4).

THE FOREARM AND CARPUS

The Skeleton and Carpal Joint

The shaft of the radius is flattened from front to back and is covered by muscle on all but its subcutaneous medial border. The distal extremity broadens to meet the expanded carpus (commonly known as the “knee”). On each side it carries a styloid process and, proximal to this, an eminence for the attachment of a collateral ligament. The cranial aspect is grooved for the passage of the extensor tendons. These tendons, the adjacent molding of the bone, the styloid processes, and the eminences for ligamentous attachment are all very distinctly palpable.

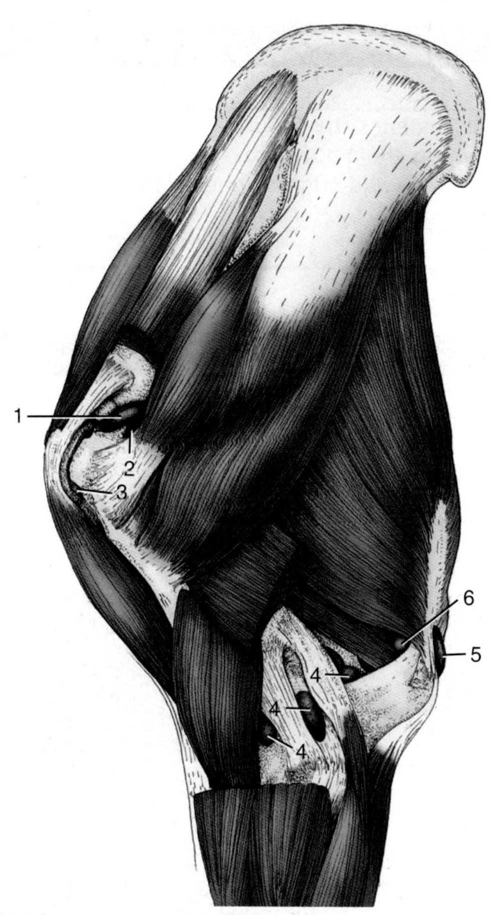

Fig. 23.11 Synovial structures of the left shoulder and elbow regions, lateral view. *1,* Shoulder joint capsule; *2,* infraspinatus bursa; *3,* intertubercular bursa (between biceps tendon and humerus); *4,* elbow joint capsule; *5,* subcutaneous olecranon bursa; *6,* subtendinous olecranon bursa. (For identification of the muscles, see Fig. 23.6B.)

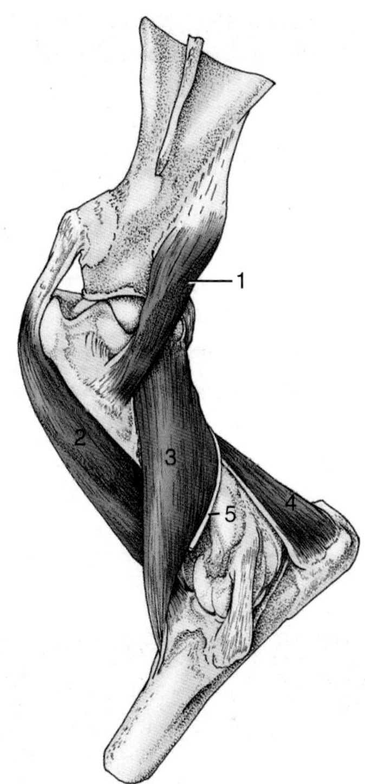

Fig. 23.12 Deep muscles of the left shoulder and elbow joints, lateral view. *1,* Teres minor; *2,* biceps; *3,* brachialis; *4,* anconeus; *5,* radial nerve.

The *carpal skeleton* is arranged in the usual two rows (see Fig. 23.20A). The proximal row comprises radial, intermediate, and ulnar carpal bones, concerned in weight-bearing, together with a laterally flattened, discoidal accessory bone that projects backward in a very conspicuous fashion. The accessory bone articulates with the lateral styloid process and the ulnar carpal but bears no weight. The distal row is also deep; in addition to three constant elements—second, third, and fourth carpal bones—there is often a pea-shaped first carpal. This bone is frequently isolated from the remainder of the skeleton, embedded in the palmar carpal ligament behind the second carpal; it may be mistaken for a bone fragment when shown in radiographs (Fig. 23.13/*6*).

Fractures of the carpal bones are mostly caused by repetitive loading and jumping. For example, the "slab fracture" commonly occurs in the frontal plane of the third carpal bone. Thoroughbred horses experience accessory carpal bone fracture during jumps over fences or collisions. Collision accidents or kicks may also cause multifragment fractures.

The *carpal joint* is maintained in full extension in the standing posture but is capable of very considerable flexion. It presents three levels of articulation. Movement is most free at the radiocarpal (antebrachiocarpal) level, where as much as 90 or 100 degrees of flexion is allowed. The midcarpal articulation is also mobile, allowing perhaps 45 degrees of flexion, but no significant movement is possible at the carpometacarpal level (Fig. 23.13B). The articular surfaces of the bones reflect these differences (Fig. 23.14A). The radial articular surface shows some demarcations corresponding to the three proximal carpal bones but overall presents a caudal hemicylindrical ridge and narrow cranial gutter. The upper surfaces of the proximal carpal bone row have the reciprocal conformation. Their lower surfaces are convex in front and concave behind. The surfaces at the distal joint are broadly flat. Fig. 23.15A illustrates these features and the two axes of rotation. The fronts of the bones are driven together in full extension of the joint and may splinter ("chip fractures"*) during the fast gaits.

The carpus is mainly supported by the cannon bone but also makes contact with the bases of the splint bones. Indeed, so large a part of the second carpal bone rests on the second metacarpal that it may tend to drive that bone away from the cannon bone, leading to painful acute inflammation known as "splints." This condition is more common at the medial intermetacarpal joint.

*Similar fractures also occur rarely on the palmar surface of these bones; they are given a poor prognosis.

TABLE 23.3 ARM MUSCLES: FLEXORS

Muscle	Nerve	Action
Biceps brachii	Musculocutaneous	Fixes and extends the shoulder May also flex the elbow Tendon stores and releases energy for rapid gait
Brachialis	Musculocutaneous and some contribution from radial	Flexes the elbow

TABLE 23.4 ARM MUSCLES: EXTENSORS

Muscle	Nerve	Action
Triceps brachii	Radial	Extends the elbow
Tensor fasciae antibrachii	Radial	Extends the elbow and shoulder but not of major importance
Anconeus	Radial	Prevents pinching of the elbow joint capsule

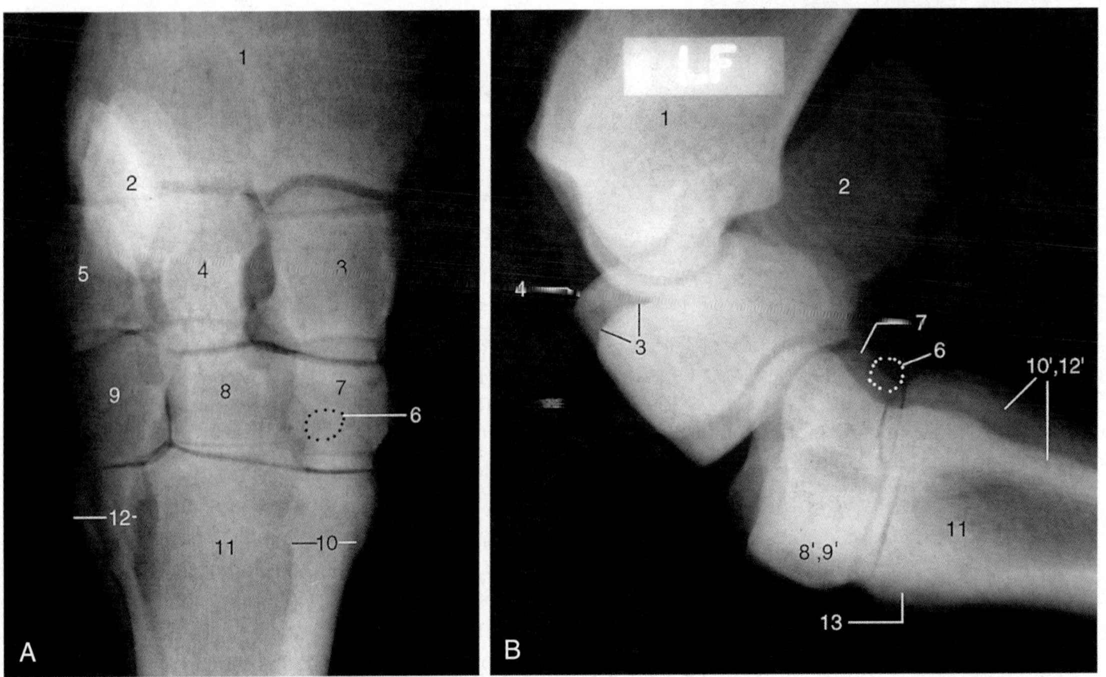

Fig. 23.13 (A) Dorsopalmar and (B) lateral radiographs of the carpus. *1,* Radius; *2,* accessory carpal (faint); *3,* radial carpal; *4,* intermediate carpal; *5,* ulnar carpal; *6,* position of first carpal, when present; *7, 8,* and *9,* second, third, and fourth carpals, respectively; *8′* and *9′,* superimposed third and fourth carpals, respectively; *10, 11,* and *12,* second, third, and fourth metacarpals, respectively; *10′* and *12′,* superimposed second and fourth metacarpals, respectively; *13,* metacarpal tuberosity.

The three levels of articulation share a common fibrous capsule, but the synovial compartments are separate except for a narrow communication between the middle and distal levels (Fig. 23.14). The fibrous capsule (Fig. 23.15A/*3*), which has extensive connections with all the bones involved in the joint, is of very unequal thickness. It is weakest dorsally, where it is rather loose in the extended position of the joint. It is much thicker over the palmar aspect (Fig. 23.15/*7*), where it opposes overextension. This part, the palmar carpal ligament, fills the irregularities of the bones and smooths the backward-facing aspect of the carpal skeleton. Medial and lateral collateral ligaments extend between the lower end of the radius and the upper part of the metacarpus. They have intermediate attachments to the carpal bones to restrict the joint movement to the sagittal plane.

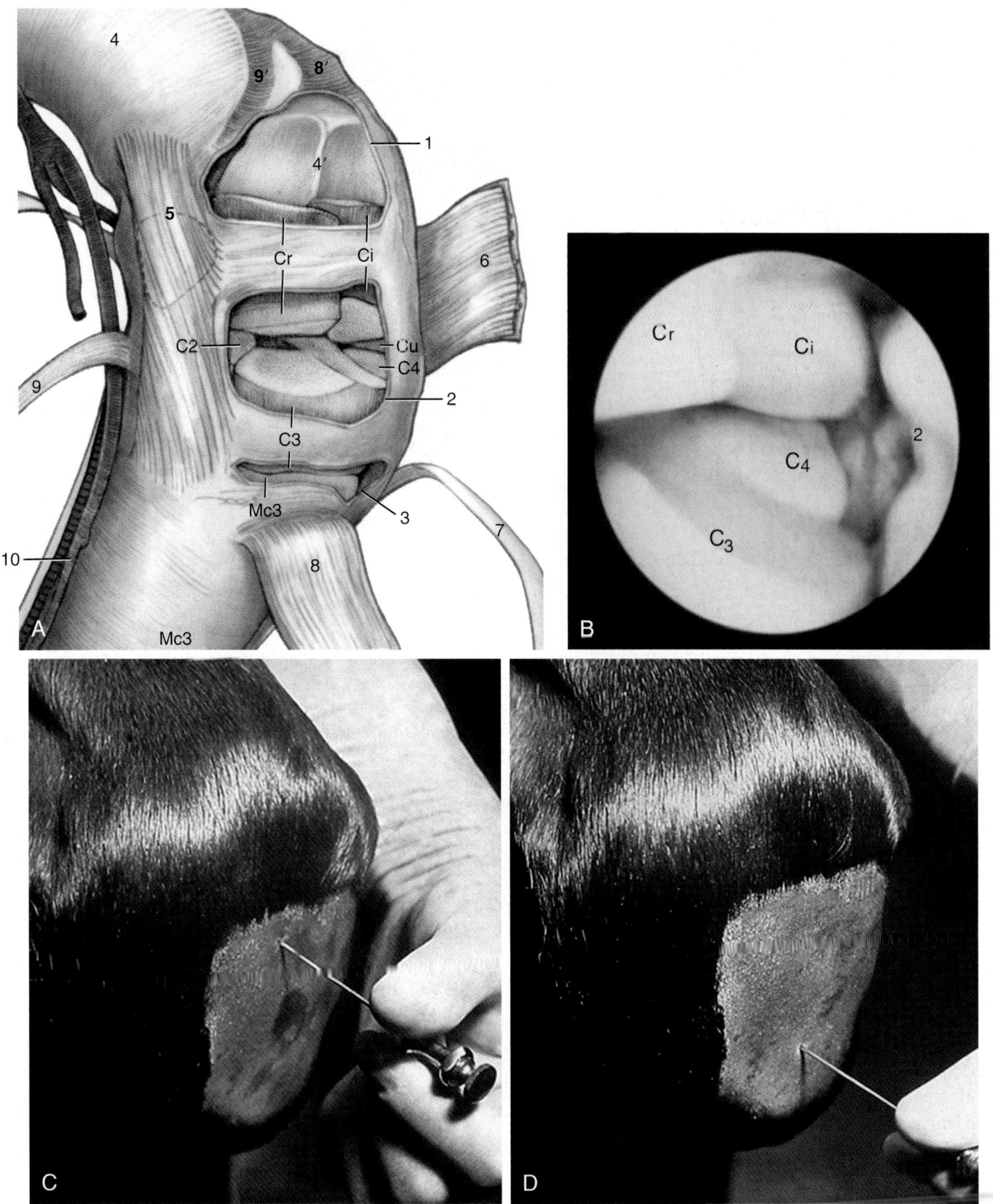

Fig. 23.14 (A) Flexed left carpus, dorsomedial view. The articular surfaces are *stippled.* (B) Arthroscopic medial-to-lateral view of the left midcarpal joint. *Cr, Ci,* and *Cu,* Radial, intermediate, and ulnar carpal bones, respectively; *C2, C3,* and *C4,* second, third, and fourth carpal bones, respectively; *Mc3,* third metacarpal (cannon) bone. *1,* Radiocarpal joint capsule, fenestrated; *2,* midcarpal joint capsule, fenestrated in A; *3,* carpometacarpal joint capsule, fenestrated; *4* and *4′,* radius and its distal articular surface, respectively; *5,* position of bursa between medial collateral ligament and extensor carpi obliquus *(9); 6,* extensor retinaculum, reflected; *7,* common digital extensor; *8* and *8′,* extensor carpi radialis and its groove on radius, respectively; *9* and *9′,* extensor carpi obliquus and its groove on radius, respectively; *10,* medial palmar nerve, artery, and vein. (C) Puncture of radiocarpal joint. (D) Puncture of midcarpal joint.

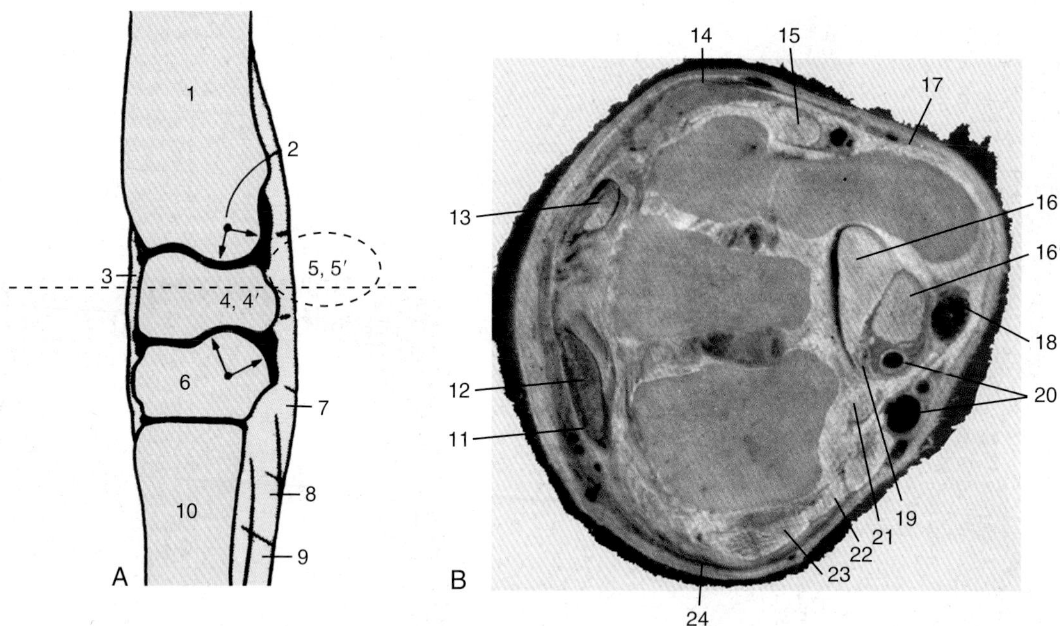

Fig. 23.15 (A) Axial section of the carpus. The *broken transverse line* indicates level of section in B. *1,* Radius; *2,* axis of rotation; *3,* fibrous joint capsule; *4* and *4′,* intermediate and radial carpal, respectively; *5* and *5′,* accessory and ulnar carpal, respectively; *6,* third carpal; *7,* palmar carpal ligament; *8,* accessory (check) ligament of deep digital flexor; *9,* interosseus; *10,* large metacarpal. (B) Transverse section of the right carpus, proximal surface. Both joints face to the left. *11,* Extensor retinaculum; *12,* extensor carpi radialis; *13,* common digital extensor; *14,* lateral digital extensor; *15,* long tendon of ulnaris lateralis; *16* and *16′,* deep and superficial flexor tendons in carpal canal, respectively; *17,* dorsal branch of ulnar nerve; *18,* palmar branch of median artery and lateral palmar nerve; *19,* median artery and medial palmar nerve; *20,* radial artery and vein; *21,* flexor carpi radialis; *22,* flexor retinaculum; *23,* medial collateral ligament; *24,* extensor carpi obliquus.

There are numerous additional ligaments that collectively stabilize the joint through joining of adjacent bones in the same row or distal bones to the metacarpus. Others secure the accessory bone, including one that runs obliquely from its distal edge to the metacarpus and forms a conspicuous ridge. A larger transverse ligament (flexor retinaculum; Fig. 23.15B/*22*) extends from the palmar edge of the accessory bone to attach at the mediopalmar aspect of the joint. It completes the enclosure of a space, *the carpal canal*, through which pass the flexor tendons and other structures en route from the forearm to the distal part of the limb.

Distention of the radiocarpal joint capsule is not uncommon (Fig. 23.16/*1*). The capsule pouches where support is weak, dorsally between the extensor tendons and proximally above the accessory bone, just caudal to the lateral digital extensor tendon. It may be punctured here, but a more convenient approach is from the dorsal aspect. Flexion of the carpus opens up the joint space, facilitating the entry of a needle between the extensor tendons. A similar approach may be made to the middle compartment (Fig. 23.14C and D).

The Muscles of the Forearm

The Extensor Group

With one exception—the extensor carpi obliquus—all carpal and digital extensors arise from the craniolateral aspect of the distal end of the humerus and occupy the craniolateral part of the forearm. Their insertion tendons begin a little above the carpus and are secured in their passage over the joint by condensed deep fascia known as the *extensor retinaculum* (Fig. 23.15B/*11*). Each is also individually protected by a synovial sheath, from just above to well below the carpus (Fig. 23.16).

Except for the ulnaris lateralis, all are extensor to the carpus, and the longer muscles also extend the joints of the digit. In addition, their origin provides them with some, albeit little used, capacity to flex the elbow. All are supplied by the radial nerve. They may each be identified on palpation, and several provide quite conspicuous visible features of the forearm of thin-skinned animals.

The *extensor carpi radialis* (Fig. 23.17/*5*), the most medial member of the group, runs directly to the front of the subcutaneous border of the radius. Its epimysial

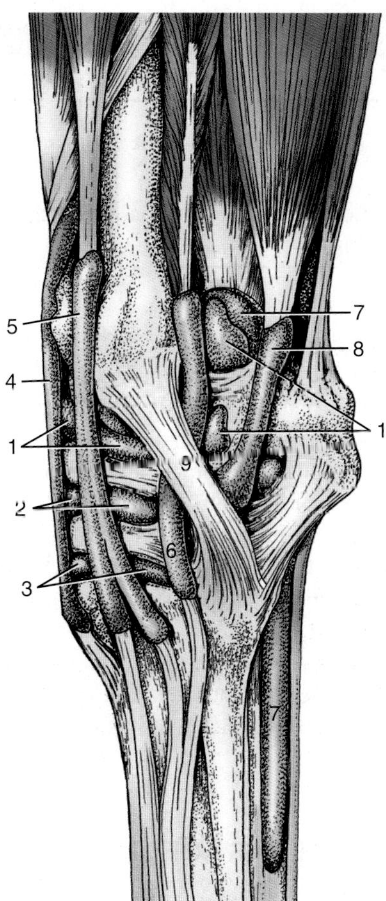

Fig. 23.16 Synovial structures of the left carpus, lateral view. *1,* Radiocarpal joint capsule; *2,* midcarpal joint capsule; *3,* carpometacarpal joint capsule; *4,* tendon sheath of extensor carpi radialis; *5,* tendon sheath of common digital extensor; *6,* tendon sheath of lateral digital extensor; *7,* tendon sheath of superficial and deep digital flexors (carpal sheath); *8,* tendon sheath of ulnaris lateralis; *9,* lateral collateral ligament.

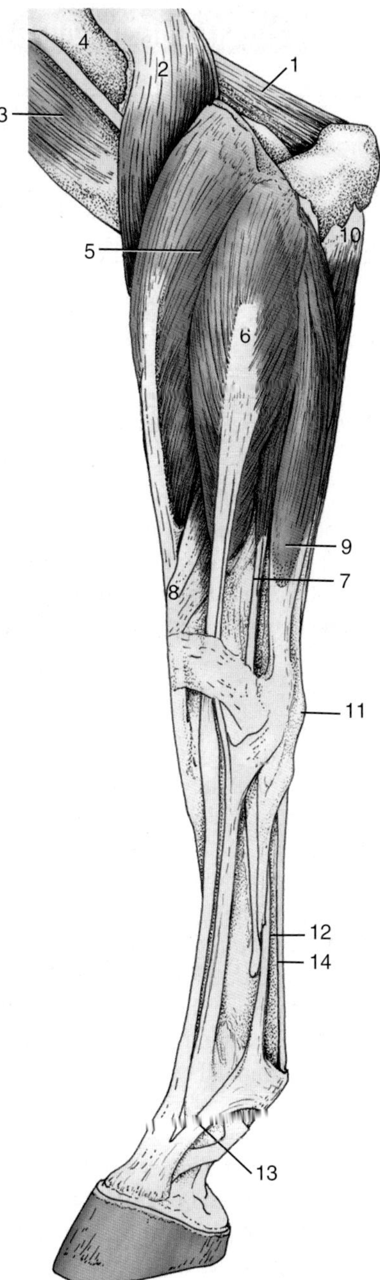

Fig. 23.17 Distal muscles of the left forelimb, lateral view. *1,* Anconeus; *2,* brachialis; *3,* biceps; *4,* deltoid tuberosity of humerus; *5,* extensor carpi radialis; *6,* common digital extensor; *7,* lateral digital extensor; *8,* extensor carpi obliquus; *9,* ulnaris lateralis; *10,* ulnar head of deep digital flexor; *11,* accessory carpal bone; *12,* interosseus; *13,* extensor branch of interosseus; *14,* flexor tendons.

covering is joined by the lacertus fibrosus that enables it passively to prevent flexion of the carpal joint when weight is on the limb.

The *common digital extensor* (Fig. 23.17/*6*) possesses a rather slight radial head in addition to the more substantial origin from the humerus. The radial head is never fully incorporated in the main mass and separates in the lower part of the forearm; its tendon joins that of the lateral digital extensor within the cannon. The main tendon continues down the dorsal aspect to the metacarpus and digit to insert on the extensor process of the distal phalanx. Just before this, it is joined by branches of the interosseus that wind around the sides of the digit from the palmar aspect (Fig. 23.17/*13*).

The slighter *lateral digital extensor* (Fig. 23.17/*7*) creates a prominent ridge on the lateral aspect of the forearm. It is joined by the contribution from the common extensor in the upper part of the cannon and then gently inclines toward the dorsal aspect of the limb to insert on the proximal end of the proximal phalanx.

The *ulnaris lateralis* (Fig. 23.17/*9*) runs down the caudal aspect of the forearm. Its short tendon of insertion splits above the accessory carpal bone; a part at once inserts on

TABLE 23.5 **MUSCLES OF FOREARM: EXTENSORS**

Muscle	Nerve	Action
Extensor carpi radialis	Radial	Flexes the carpus
Common digital extensor	Radial	Extends the carpus and digits
Lateral digital extensor	Radial	Extends the elbow
Ulnaris lateralis	Radial	Extends the elbow and shoulder but not of major importance
Extensor carpi obliquus	Radial	Prevents pinching of the elbow joint capsule

this bone, while a longer branch descends over the lateral aspect of the bone, tunnels under the collateral ligament, and ends on the head of the lateral splint bone. The longer division requires the protection of a synovial sheath (Fig. 23.16/*8*).

The *extensor carpi obliquus* is distinguished by arising from the shaft of the radius. It runs in a mediodistal direction to insert on the medial splint bone. Although largely covered by the other muscles, its tendon becomes superficial to that of the extensor carpi radialis (Fig. 23.17/*8* and Table 23.5).

The Flexor Group

The muscles of the flexor group also share several attributes. They arise from the caudomedial aspect of the humerus, occupy the caudal part of the forearm, obtain their innervation from the median and ulnar nerves, and are flexor to the carpal joint; those that proceed beyond this level are also flexor to the digital joints.

The *flexor carpi radialis* (Fig. 23.18/*8*) follows the subcutaneous border of the radius and covers the important median vessels and nerve. The tendon of insertion tunnels through the flexor retinaculum, where it obtains the necessary protection of a synovial sheath before attaching to the medial splint bone.

The *flexor carpi ulnaris* (Fig. 23.18/*9*) lies on the medial aspect of the forearm, partly under cover of the flexor carpi radialis. It arises by two heads—from the humerus and the ulna—and inserts on the proximal margin of the accessory carpal bone by means of a short tendon that has no need of synovial protection.

The *superficial digital flexor* occupies a central position within the flexor group, between the larger mass of the deep flexor and the flexor carpi ulnaris (Fig. 23.19/*9*). A purely tendinous head, usually known as an *accessory or check ligament* (Fig. 23.19/*4*), arises from the caudal surface of the radius to join the main tendon in the lower part of the forearm; it is a component of the passive stay apparatus (see further on). The superficial and deep flexor tendons share a common synovial sheath, the carpal sheath, in their passage through the carpal canal.

The tendon is superficial to that of the deep tendon in the metacarpus, but at the fetlock it obtains the deeper position necessary for its insertion on neighboring parts of the proximal and middle phalanges (Fig. 23.18/*13*).

The *deep digital flexor* is by far the largest of the flexors, although this is not apparent without dissection (Fig. 23.19/*9′*). In addition to the humeral head, there are lesser heads of origin from the upper parts of the radius and ulna. The common tendon passes through the carpal canal and continues down the palmar aspect of the limb to find insertion on the palmar surface of the distal phalanx. In the metacarpus the tendon is joined by a stout tendinous band that arises from the thick fibrous joint capsule on the palmar aspect of the carpal joint (Fig. 23.18/*14* and *14′*). This is almost invariably known as an *accessory* or *check ligament*; it provides an important element of the passive stay apparatus that is of far greater significance than the analogous contribution to the superficial tendon (Table 23.6).

THE DISTAL PART OF THE LIMB

The more distal structures of the limb not only have the greatest propensity to injury but also show many and important specific differences.

The Skeleton and Joints

The skeleton comprises the metacarpal bones and the proximal, middle, and distal phalanges. The metacarpophalangeal and the proximal and distal interphalangeal joints linking these bones are commonly referred to as the fetlock, pastern, and coffin joints. A pair of proximal sesamoid bones enlarges the concavity of the fetlock joint, and a single distal sesamoid bone enlarges that of the coffin joint.

The metacarpal skeleton comprises second, third, and fourth *metacarpal bones.* The third bone, the cannon bone, is much stronger than the other two and is the functional element. It carries a prominent tuberosity on its dorsal surface just distal to the joint. The bones to each side, generally known as the *splint bones,* are much reduced in size. Each has a small proximal base that continues into a tapering shaft. In young animals the splint and cannon bones are joined by fibrous tissue; this generally later ossifies, and the upper parts of the shafts are then fused together. The process is often accompanied by an acute inflammation (a condition known as "splints"), which leaves a palpable—and often visible—blemish on the dorsal surface.

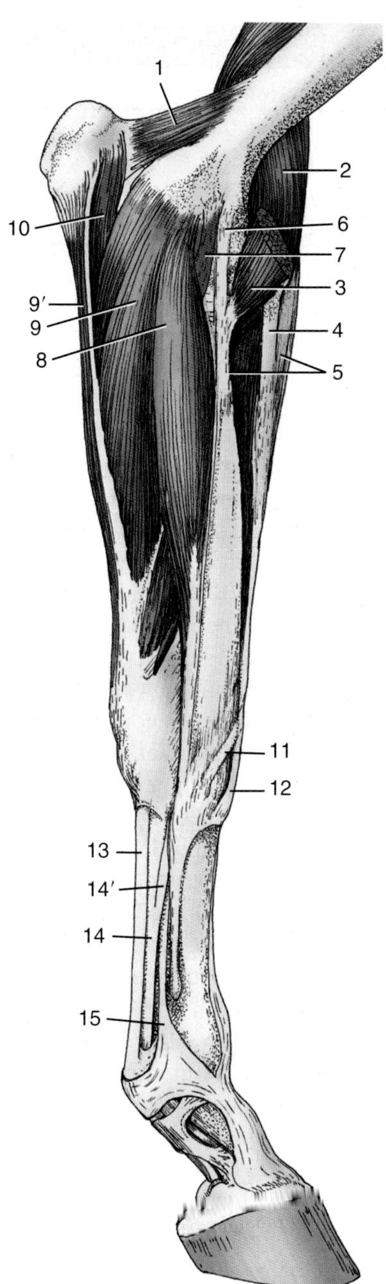

Fig. 23.18 Distal muscles of the left forelimb, medial view. *1,* Anconeus; *2,* brachialis; *3,* biceps; *4,* lacertus fibrosus; *5,* extensor carpi radialis; *6,* long part of medial collateral ligament (pronator teres); *7,* short part of medial collateral ligament; *8,* flexor carpi radialis; *9* and *9′,* humeral and ulnar heads of flexor carpi ulnaris, respectively; *10,* ulnar head of deep digital flexor; *11,* tendon of extensor carpi obliquus; *12,* tendon of extensor carpi radialis; *13,* tendon of superficial digital flexor; *14,* tendon of deep digital flexor; *14′,* accessory (check) ligament; *15,* interosseus.

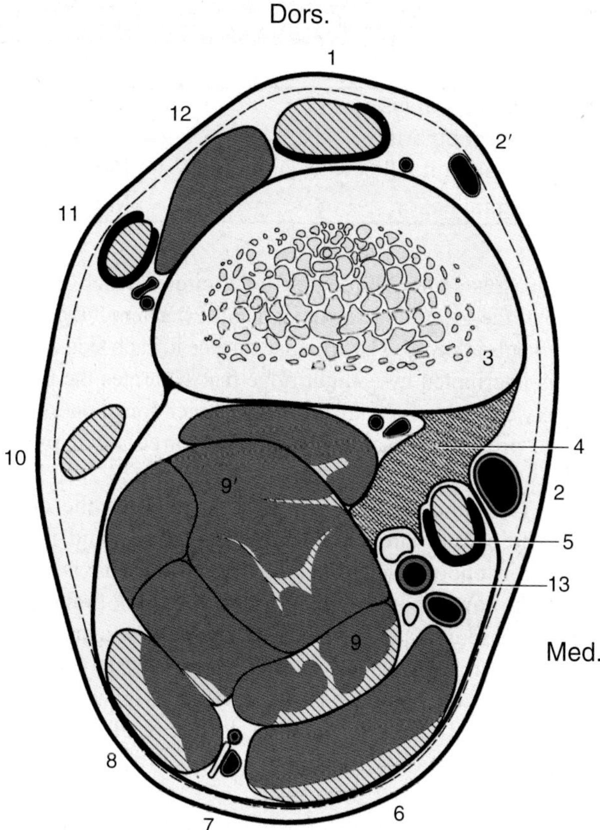

Fig. 23.19 Transverse section of the right forearm 6 cm proximal to the proximal border of the accessory carpal, to demonstrate the topography of the accessory (check) ligament of the superficial digital flexor; looking distally. The *hatched blue areas* are tendons or tendinous tissue, and the *dark pink areas* are muscle tissue. *1,* Extensor carpi radialis; *2* and *2′,* cephalic and accessory cephalic veins, respectively; *3,* radius; *4,* accessory (check) ligament of superficial digital flexor; *5,* flexor carpi radialis; *6,* flexor carpi ulnaris; *7,* ulnar nerve and collateral ulnar vessels; *8,* ulnaris lateralis; *9* and *9′,* superficial and deep digital flexors, respectively; *10, 11,* and *12,* lateral, common, and oblique extensors, respectively; *13,* median artery, medial and lateral palmar nerves; *Dors.,* dorsal; *Med.,* medial.

The tapering second and fourth metacarpals end in slight but easily palpable buttons three-quarters of the way down the cannon (see Fig. 2.49B). The lower parts of their shafts are free, and when a break occurs, it is a simple matter to remove the fragment below the fracture line.

The *third metacarpal bone* is exceptionally robust. It is oval in cross section (which distinguishes it from the longer but more rounded cannon bone of the hindlimb), and its thick compacta attests to its tremendous strength; it is in fact one of the strongest elements of the skeleton (see Fig. 23.46/*1*). Despite the obvious strength of the cannon bone, longitudinal fractures of the distal extremity are common racing injuries, more often involving the lateral than the medial side and the forelimb rather than the hindlimb. The degree of involvement of the joint surface is an important factor in prognosis.

The distal extremity presents an axially keeled condyle that articulates with the proximal phalanx and the paired sesamoid bones. When viewed from the side, the condyle

TABLE 23.6 MUSCLES OF FOREARM: FLEXORS

Muscle	Nerve	Action
Flexor carpi radialis	Median	Flexes the carpus
Flexor carpi ulnaris	Ulnar	Flexes the carpus
Superficial digital flexor	Median	Flexes the carpus and digits
Deep digital flexor	Median and ulnar	Extends the elbow

encompasses some 220 degrees of a circle, which is evidence of the great range of flexion and extension—the only movements allowed. The articular surface to each side of the keel is interrupted by a slight ridge that separates the more strongly curved palmar area from the larger dorsal one.

The proximal sesamoid bones are three-sided pyramids whose bases face distally (Fig. 23.20/*10*). The dorsal (articular) surface of each lies against the condyle, the palmar (flexor) surface tilts axially and faces the flexor tendons that ride over it, and the abaxial surface is hollowed for the reception of the thick branch of the interosseous (see further on). The palmar aspects of the bones are converted by thick fibrous tissue (palmar ligament) into a single bearing surface over which the flexor tendons change direction. Although close to the proximal phalanx, the sesamoid bones do not articulate with it.

The proximal sesamoids fracture, commonly at the apical surface, most often of all the bones in the forelimb, followed in frequency by the metacarpal and carpal bones. These fractures are known in racetrack practice as "the big three" for which, when serious, horses pay with their lives. Fractures of proximal sesamoids are largely because of excessive pressure from the deep digital flexor tendon.

The strong *proximal phalanx* (also called PI) is compressed from front to back and is wider proximally than distally. Its proximal extremity is hollowed and deepened axially by a groove that allows it to conform to the condyle of the large metacarpal bone. Palpable tubercles to each side receive the collateral ligaments of the fetlock joint. The distal end is shaped as two condyles separated by a shallow axial groove and presents similar but smaller tubercles for the collateral ligaments of the pastern joint. The palmar surface of the bone is roughened for the attachment of several ligaments; a large triangular area and various smaller ones to each side stand out (Fig. 23.20B/*11, 11′, 11″,* and *11‴*).

The *middle phalanx* (PII) is generally similar to PI but, being only half as long, is proportionately very robust. Both extremities are of equal width. The proximal articular surface—hollowed with a slight axial ridge—is the reciprocal of the lower end of PI, whereas the distal one—two condyles separated by a groove—mimics that of PI. The distal articular surface extends onto the palmar aspect, where it articulates with the distal sesamoid bone. There are proximal collateral tubercles on PII for the collateral ligaments of the pastern joint; the corresponding distal sites from which the collateral ligaments of the coffin joint arise are excavated. The proximopalmar border presents a smooth area (Fig. 23.20/*12″*) that is enlarged in the natural state by a complementary fibrocartilage that forms a bearing surface for the deep flexor tendon (see further on). The fibrocartilage enlarges the articular surface of the pastern joint and gives attachment to several ligaments. Fractures of the middle phalanx are seen more in Quarter horses and more commonly in the hindlimb.

The *distal phalanx* (PIII, coffin bone) generally conforms to the interior of the hoof in which it resides, "as in a coffin." It is wedge shaped: sharp distally and to the sides and blunt proximally and toward the back. The dorsal (parietal) surface is convex from side to side and lies against the dermis that unites it to the inner surface of the hoof wall. It tapers caudally into medial and lateral palmar processes that are notched (or perforated) and grooved for the dorsal terminal branches of the digital arteries and accompanying nerves (Fig. 23.20/*13″*). Depressions for the collateral ligaments of the coffin joint are present proximodorsal to the processes. The palmar (sole) surface is slightly concave to fit the domed sole of the hoof. Both parietal and sole surfaces are very porous to allow the passage of numerous small arteries from the interior of the bone into the overlying dermis. The articular surface, consisting of two fossae separated by an axial ridge, faces proximally. Its dorsal border tapers to an extensor process, the highest point of the bone, where the common digital extensor tendon is attached. The palmar border is extended by a narrow articular zone for the distal sesamoid bone, which, in contrast to the proximal sesamoids, articulates with both middle and distal phalanges. Just distal to this, two prominent foramina lead to a U-shaped canal within the bone that contains the anastomosis of the terminal palmar branches of the digital arteries. The deep flexor tendon ends on the semilunar crest just distal to the foramina (Fig. 23.20/*15*).

The flat cartilages (of the hoof), which surmount and continue the palmar processes, lie mainly against the inner wall of the hoof, but their proximal borders are free, subcutaneous, and palpable to each side of the pastern joint (Fig. 23.20B/*14*).

The *distal sesamoid (navicular) bone* (Fig. 23.21/*3*) is boat shaped with straight proximal and convex distal borders. Its dorsal (articular) surface contacts the distal end of PII; a narrow distal facet touches PIII. The palmar (flexor)

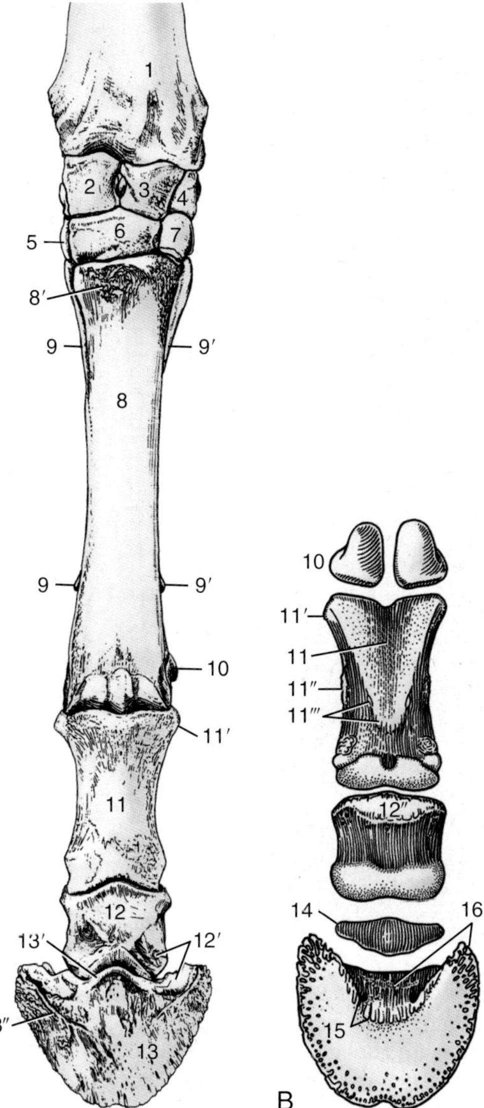

Fig. 23.20 Skeleton of the distal part of the forelimb. (A) Left limb, dorsal view. (B) Palmar view. *1*, Radius; *2*, radial carpal; *3*, intermediate carpal; *4*, ulnar carpal; *5*, *6*, and *7*, second, third, and fourth carpals, respectively; *8*, large metacarpal bone; *8′*, metacarpal tuberosity; *9* and *9′*, medial and lateral splint bones, respectively; *10*, proximal sesamoid bones; *11*, proximal phalanx; *11′*, proximal tubercle; *11″*, attachment of distal digital annular and abaxial palmar ligaments; *11‴*, attachment of axial palmar and oblique sesamoidean ligaments; *12*, middle phalanx; *12′*, attachments of collateral ligament of coffin joint; *12″*, bearing surface for deep flexor tendon; *13*, distal phalanx; *13′*, extensor process; *13″*, parietal groove; *14*, navicular bone; *15*, sole foramen and semilunar crest for attachment of deep flexor tendon; *16*, palmar process and attachment of distal navicular ligament.

surface faces the wide tendon of the deep flexor, providing it with yet another bearing surface as it bends toward its attachment at the semilunar crest on the undersurface of PIII. The navicular bone enlarges the distal articular surface of the coffin joint (see Fig. 23.24/*7′* and *7″*).

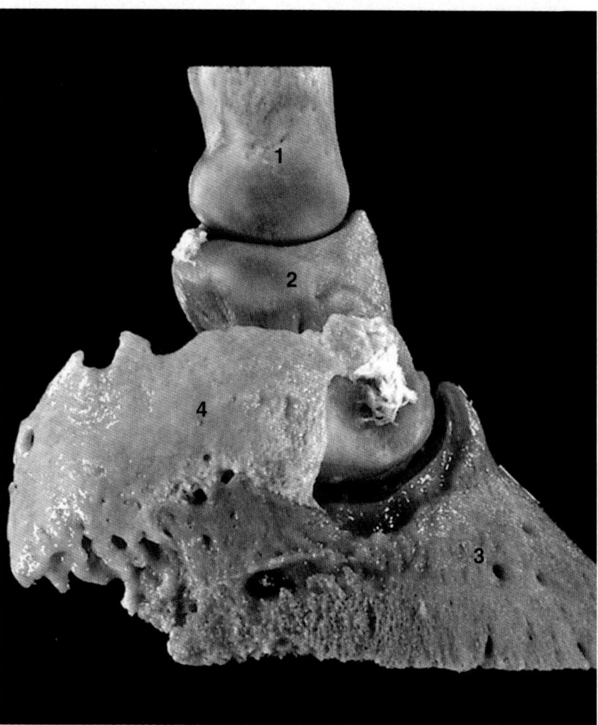

Fig. 23.21 Hoof cartilage attached to palmar process of distal phalanx. *1*, *2*, and *3*, Proximal, middle, and distal phalanges, respectively; *4*, hoof cartilage.

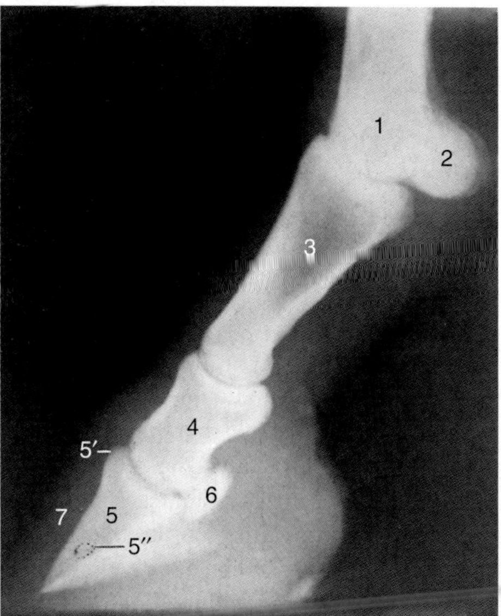

Fig. 23.22 Lateral radiograph of fetlock joint and digit. *1*, Large metacarpal bone; *2*, proximal sesamoid bones; *3*, proximal phalanx; *4*, middle phalanx; *5*, distal phalanx; *5′*, extensor process; *5″*, canal containing terminal arterial arch; *6*, navicular bone; *7*, wall of hoof.

The *fetlock joint* is formed between the large metacarpal bone (PI) and the proximal sesamoid bones (Fig. 23.22). The large bones are connected by medial and lateral collateral ligaments, while additional smaller and triangular (collateral) ligaments anchor the sesamoid bones to the

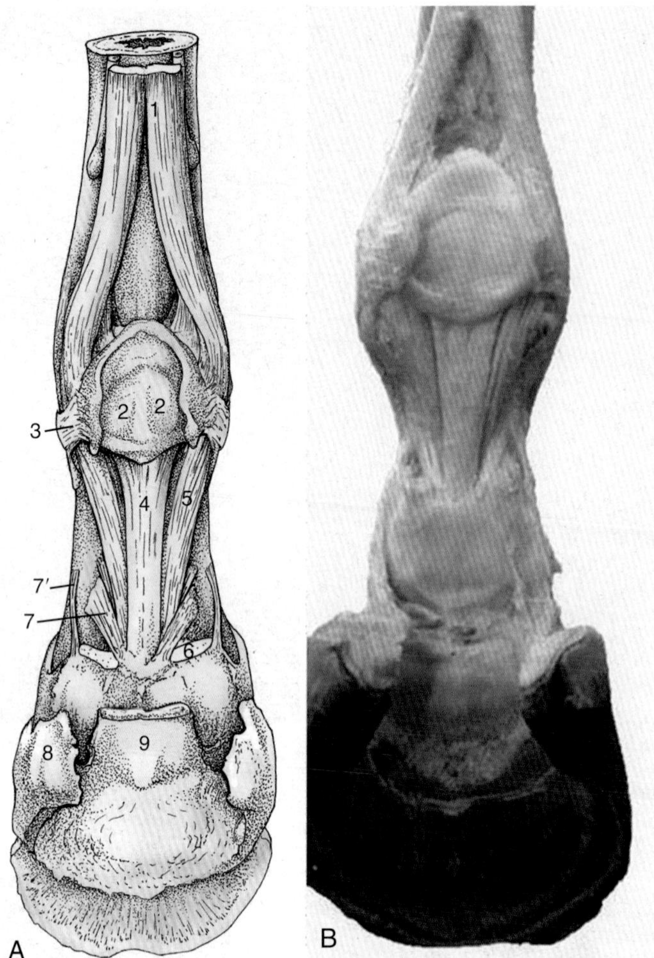

Fig. 23.23 (A) Structures supporting the fetlock joint (schematic). *1,* Interosseus; *2,* proximal sesamoid bones connected by thick palmar ligament; *3,* collateral sesamoidean ligament; *4,* straight sesamoidean ligament; *5,* oblique sesamoidean ligament; *6,* stump of superficial flexor; *7* and *7′,* axial and abaxial palmar ligaments of pastern joint, respectively; *8,* hoof cartilage; *9,* stump of deep flexor. (B) Real specimen.

sides of the metacarpal condyle and the proximal tubercles of PI. A series of sesamoidean ligaments connects the bases of the sesamoid bones to the first phalanx and ensures that the sesamoids move against the metacarpal condyle in unison with PI. The series includes short and deepest ligaments to the proximopalmar border overlain by rather longer cruciate ligaments that end a little more distally, and these in turn are overlain by oblique ligaments that attach broadly to the central triangular area of the palmar surface of PI. Finally, an additional straight sesamoidean ligament, arising from the bases of the sesamoids, connects with the complementary fibrocartilage of PII (Fig. 23.23/*4*).

The sesamoid bones are connected to each other by a thick palmar ligament that extends the bearing surface for the flexor tendons proximally by about 2 cm (Fig. 23.23/*2*). This extension supports the tendons when the sesamoids themselves slip below the condyle in maximal overextension of the fetlock joint (when the dorsal angle can be as small as 90 degrees). When the joint is fully flexed, the sesamoid bones lose contact with the condyle and ride up on the back of the metacarpal bone, where bone-to-bone contact is prevented by the proximal extension of the palmar ligament.

The joint capsule is capacious, and to allow for the fetlock's mobility, it extends large dorsal and palmar pouches proximally (see Fig. 23.26/*7* and *7″*). These lie against the shaft of the metacarpal bone and are easily punctured from the side; the end of the splint bone, the interosseus, and the sesamoid bone are convenient (almost visible) landmarks for entry into the palmar pouch. Another perhaps better place in the bowed limb is between the sesamoid bone and the metacarpus, directly through the collateral ligament of the flexed joint (see Fig. 23.27B *(arrow)* and C). Distentions of the joint known as *wind puffs* or *galls* manifest themselves at this site. The interior of the dorsal pouch contains a so-called capsular fold (see Fig. 23.26/*7′*).

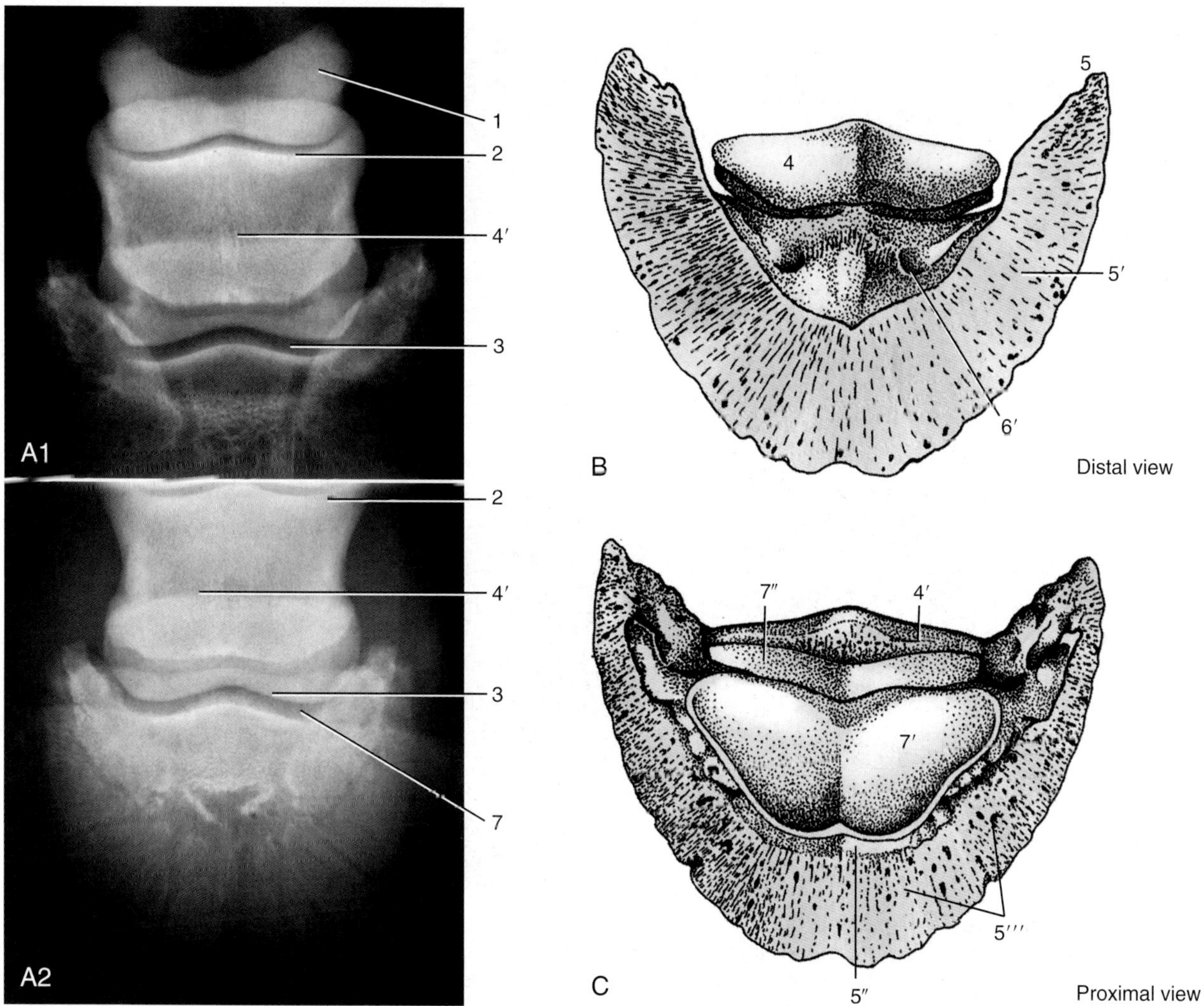

Fig. 23.24 (A1) and (A2) Dorsopalmar radiographs of hoof. (B) and (C) Palmar and dorsal surfaces of distal phalanx (PI) and navicular bone. *1,* Proximal phalanx; *2,* proximal contour of middle phalanx; *3,* distal contour of middle phalanx; *4,* navicular bone (its flexor surface in B); *4′,* proximal border of navicular bone; *5,* palmar process of PIII; *5′,* palmar (sole) surface of PI; *5″,* extensor process and dorsal (parietal) surface of PI; *5‴,* dorsal surface; *6,* sole foramen; *7,* coffin joint; *7′,* articular surface of PI; *7″,* articular surface of navicular bone.

This arises from the shaft of the metacarpal bone and projects distally into the center of the pouch; its inflammation and enlargement can cause lameness. Short distal palmar pouches are palpable as small depressions in the angles between PI and the bases of the sesamoid bones.

The movement of the *pastern joint* is much more restricted. Paired (axial and abaxial) palmar ligaments connect the palmar aspect of PI with the complementary fibrocartilage of PII (Fig. 23.23/*7* and *7′*); together with the straight sesamoidean ligament (Fig. 23.23/*4*) they limit overextension. The capsule is similar to that of the fetlock joint, but the pouches are smaller and only the dorsal one is accessible for puncture, again from the side. The radiographic appearance of the pastern and coffin joints is shown in Fig. 23.24(A1 and A2).

The *coffin joint* allows flexion and extension to about the same degree as the pastern joint. The collateral ligaments are short and thick and are solidly anchored at both ends to depressions in the bones. The navicular bone, an integral part of the joint, is suspended from the distal extremity of PI by the collateral navicular ligaments (Fig. 23.25/*2*) that cross the medial and lateral borders of PII and attach to the ends and proximal border of the navicular bone in a U-shaped fashion. A very short but wide distal navicular ligament (Fig. 23.25/*3*) connects the distal border of the navicular bone with PIII, attaching proximal to the prominent sole foramina. The capsule attaches to the articular margins of the three bones and resembles those of the other digital joints in having dorsal and palmar pouches. The pouches are

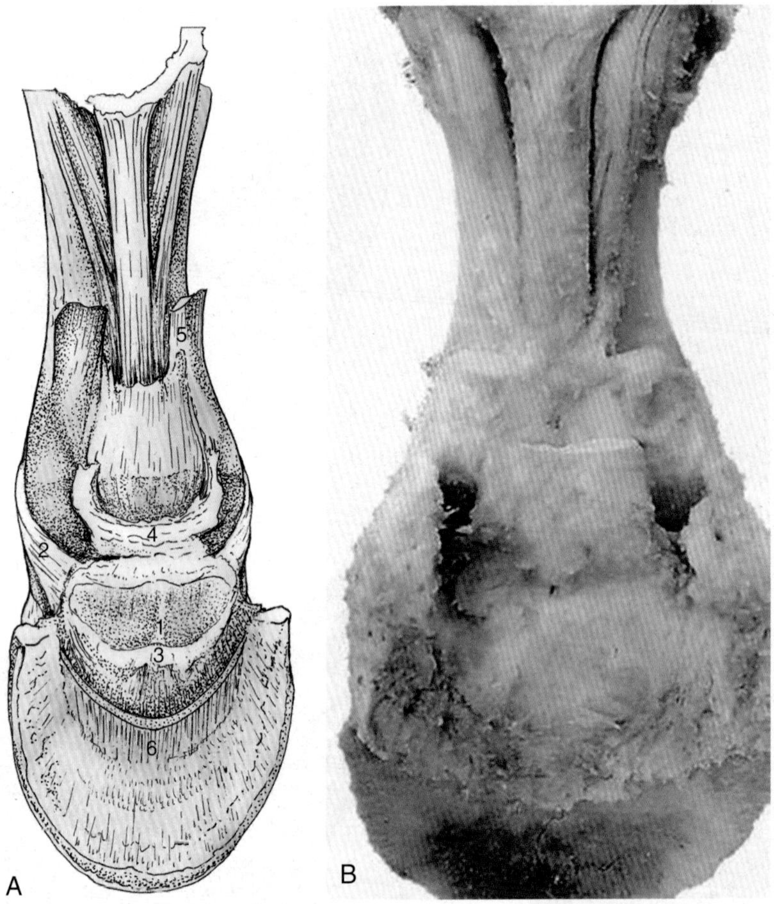

Fig. 23.25 (A) Ligaments of the navicular bone, palmar view (schematic). *1,* Navicular bone; *2,* collateral ligament of navicular bone; *3,* distal navicular ligament; *4,* connective tissue between coffin joint, digital sheath, and navicular bursa (see Fig. 23.26/*15*); *5,* stump of superficial digital flexor; *6,* stump of deep digital flexor. (B) Real specimen.

small, and only the dorsal one is accessible for puncture (at the proximal border of the hoof); the procedure is not easy (Fig. 23.26C and D).

The incorporation of sesamoid bones in the fetlock and coffin joints divides the weight pressing onto the lower part of each joint over the phalanx and sesamoid bones. The elasticity of the sesamoid ligaments and the flexor tendons behind them allows the joint to yield slightly during foot impact. This is but one of several mechanisms designed to dissipate the concussion generated by so heavy and swift an animal. The concussive effects may be accentuated by poor conformation: upright pasterns and small feet (in relation to body size) are a combination encountered frequently in animals afflicted with navicular disease, a relatively common cause of lameness. This condition is characterized by erosion at the margins of the navicular bone, where its ligaments attach, and by inflammation and degeneration of the navicular bursa (Fig. 23.26/*10*) and the related part of the deep flexor tendon (Fig. 23.26/*13*). However, the exact pathogenesis is still debated, and different authorities give quite contradictory explanations.

The Tendons, Annular Ligaments, and Interosseus Muscle

The tendons of the common and lateral digital extensors enter the foot to the front of the metacarpal bone; those of the superficial and deep flexors enter behind it. A third very important element in the support of the fetlock, the *tendinous interosseus muscle*, is situated on the palmar aspect, between the bone and the flexor tendons. The structures on the palmar surface of the cannon are enclosed within a deep fascia that extends from one splint bone to the other. The fascia is thickest immediately below the carpus but gradually thins when followed distally, and toward the fetlock it offers little hindrance to the palpation of deeper structures.

The *common digital extensor tendon* is protected by a synovial bursa as it passes over the dorsal pouch of the fetlock joint. Broadening, it makes limited attachments at the proximal borders of PI and PII before receiving the extensor branches of the interosseus that wind around the digit. It ends on the extensor process of PIII (Figs. 23.27/*1* and 23.26/*17*).

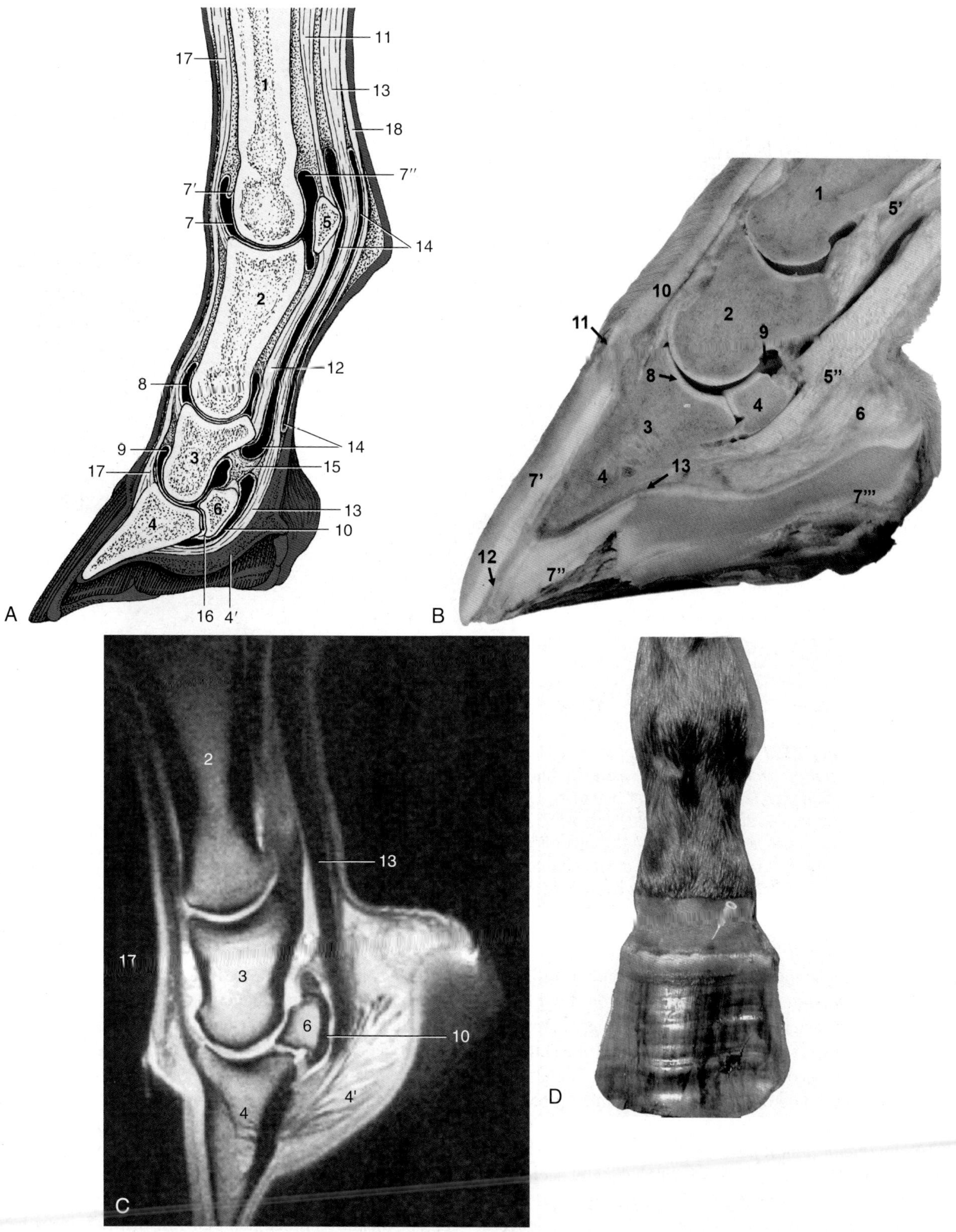

Fig. 23.26 (A) Axial section of digit (semi-schematic). (B) Axial section of digit with latex-injected fetlock, pastern, and coffin joints. (C) Corresponding magnetic resonance image. (D) Puncture of coffin joint. *1,* Large metacarpal bone; *2,* proximal phalanx; *3,* middle phalanx; *4,* distal phalanx; *4′,* digital cushion; *5,* proximal sesamoid bone; *6,* distal sesamoid (navicular) bone; *7,* dorsal pouch of fetlock joint; *7′,* capsular fold; *7″,* palmar pouch of fetlock joint; *8* and *9,* dorsal pouches of pastern and coffin joints, respectively; *10,* navicular bursa; *11,* interosseus; *12,* straight sesamoidean ligament; *13,* deep flexor tendon; *14,* digital sheath; *15,* connective tissue bridge; *16,* distal navicular ligament; *17,* common digital extensor tendon; *18,* superficial flexor tendon.

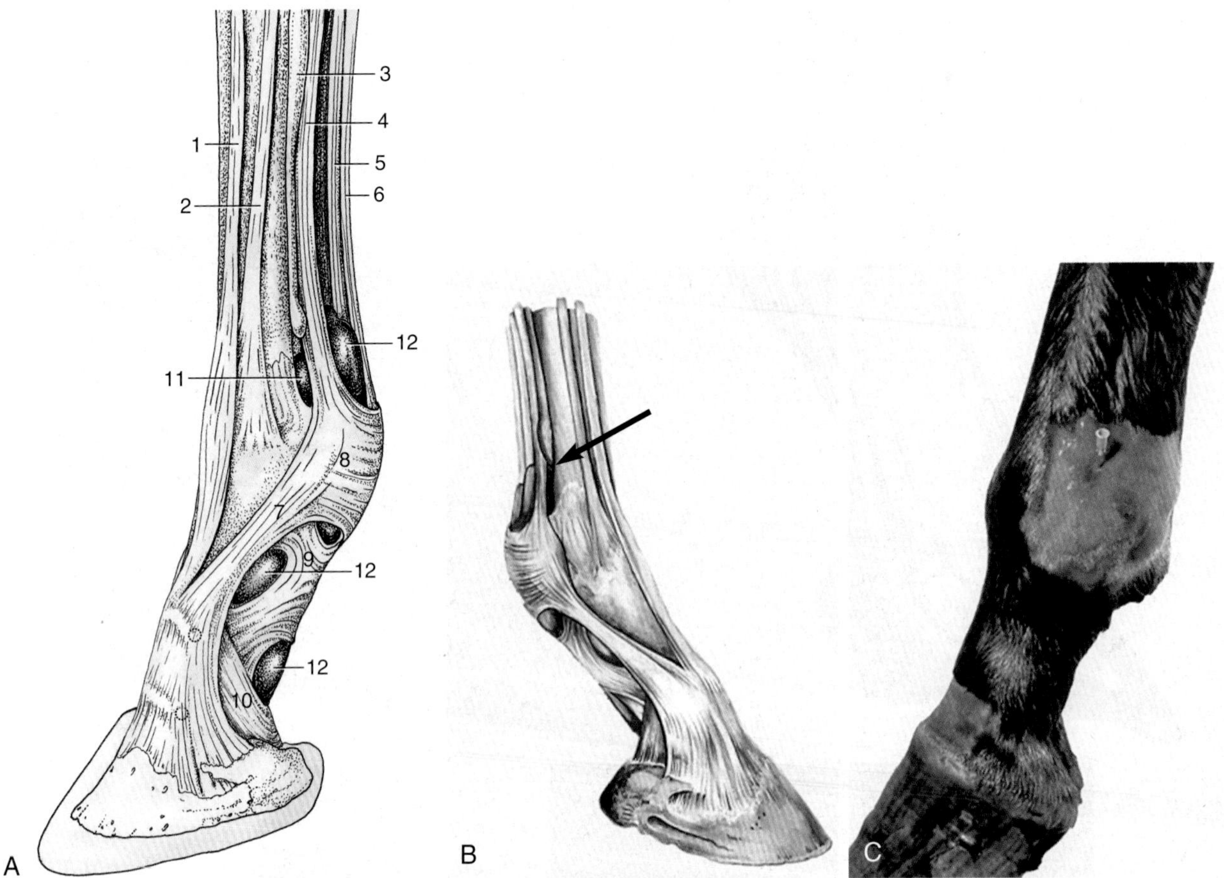

Fig. 23.27 (A) Tendons and annular ligaments of the left digit, dorsolateral view. The two *dotted circles* indicate the sites for injecting the pastern and coffin joints. *1,* Common digital extensor; *2,* lateral digital extensor; *3,* lateral splint bone; *4,* interosseus; *5,* deep digital flexor; *6,* superficial digital flexor; *7,* extensor branch of interosseus; *8,* palmar annular ligament; *9,* proximal digital annular ligament; *10,* distal digital annular ligament; *11,* palmar pouch of fetlock joint; *12,* digital sheath. (B) Schematic drawing of right digit showing digital sheath *(green)* and palmar pouch of fetlock joint *(arrow).* (C) Puncture of fetlock joint.

The *lateral digital extensor tendon* descends on the metacarpal bone lateral to the common tendon, crosses the fetlock joint, and ends on a roughening on the dorsal aspect of PI. Both extensor tendons, though easily palpated in the metacarpus, evade recognition beyond the fetlock joint, where they become broader and thinner. The extensor branches of the interosseus are more prominent below the skin.

The *superficial digital flexor tendon* becomes subcutaneous (except for the fascial investment of distally decreasing thickness) after emerging from the carpal canal and provides the caudal border of the cannon. It forms a sleeve around the deep flexor tendon at the level of the proximal sesamoid bones (Fig. 23.28B). The deep part of the sleeve splits opposite the middle of PI to allow the superficial flexor to attach to the distal tubercles of PI and the adjacent complementary fibrocartilage of PII. The palmar part of the sleeve ends at about the same level to allow the deep flexor tendon to gain the superficial position, where it is palpable for a few centimeters before it enters the hoof.

Only the medial and lateral borders of the *deep digital flexor tendon* can be palpated above the fetlock. The tendon is most easily separated and distinguished from that of the superficial flexor muscle when the fetlock joint is flexed to relieve tension, but even in these circumstances, it is usually impossible to identify the very strong *accessory (check) ligament* that arises from the palmar carpal ligament to join the deep face of the tendon toward the middle of the cannon (Fig. 23.18/*14'*). The tendon then passes the fetlock in the sleeve formed by the superficial tendon, and beyond the middle of PI it rides over the bearing surface provided by the complementary fibrocartilage of PII. It then widens before passing over the navicular bone to terminate on PIII.

Lameness: Recent data obtained with magnetic resonance imaging and computed tomography have shown that inflammation of the deep digital flexor tendon is the most common soft tissue injury that leads to lameness in the horse.

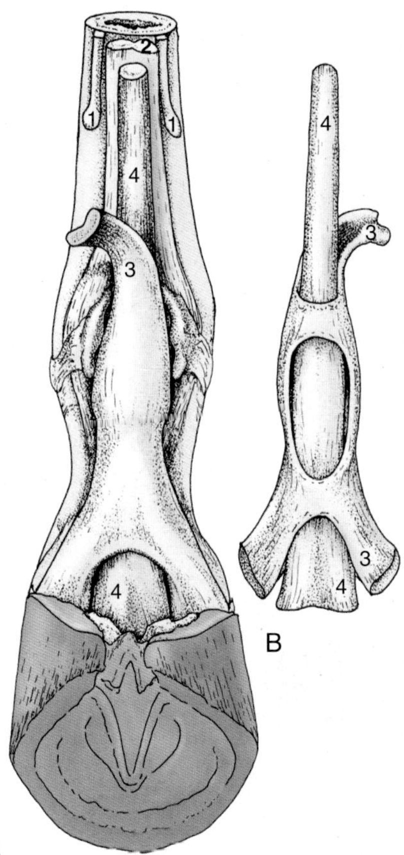

Fig. 23.28 Relations and topography of the superficial and deep flexor tendons. (A) Palmar view, in situ. (B) Dorsal view, isolated. *1,* Splint bones; *2,* interosseus; *3,* superficial digital flexor; *4,* deep digital flexor.

The flexor tendons are held in place by three *annular ligaments,* which are local thickenings of the deep fascia. The first, the *palmar annular ligament,* arises from the abaxial borders of the proximal sesamoid bones. Because the ligament adheres to the superficial flexor tendon, the potential for movement between the tendon and the sesamoids is clearly restricted. The second, the *proximal digital annular ligament,* resembles an X when viewed from behind (Fig. 23.29/*6*). The proximal margin of the X and the four corners, which attach near the proximal and distal tubercles of PI, are most easily distinguished because the body and the distal margin fuse with the superficial tendon. The third, the *distal digital annular ligament,* arises from the medial and lateral borders of PI together with the abaxial palmar ligaments of the pastern joint. It provides a sling that fuses with the palmar surface of the deep tendon, continuing to the insertion on PIII within the hoof, and separates the tendon from the digital cushion. Usually, only its free upper border can be demonstrated (Fig. 23.29/*7*).

The repetitive excessive strain or external trauma may cause pathology of flexor tendons. The navicular (podotrochlear) bursa protects the deep flexor tendon from excessive friction and pressure against the navicular bone (Fig. 23.26/*10*). Nonseptic inflammation of the navicular bursa or its adhesions with the deep digital flexor tendon can occur in navicular disease. More proximally, the tendon shares a complex synovial (digital) sheath (Fig. 23.26/*14*) with the superficial flexor tendon. The sheath begins a few centimeters proximal to the fetlock joint and ends level with the middle of PII (Fig. 23.26B). It lubricates the passage of the tendons over the bearing surfaces and under the free parts of the annular ligaments and facilitates their movements against each other where they exchange position. It is a common site of inflammation and, when distended, bulges most noticeably above the proximal sesamoid bones. Although the sheath is in close proximity to the fetlock, pastern, and coffin joints and to the navicular bursa, these cavities do not communicate, except for a connection between the sheath and the coffin joint in the foal. Despite this, anesthetics injected into the coffin joint of adult horses reach the navicular bursa by diffusion.

The *interosseus muscle* is a strong, flat, predominantly tendinous band, better known as the suspensory ligament. The small contingent of muscle fibers in the interosseous plays an important role in dampening the concussion and consequent heat generation in this tendinous structure. The interosseus arises from the palmar carpal ligament and adjacent part of the large metacarpal bone, descends between the splint bones, and divides a short distance above the fetlock. The two divisions are substantial—and easily palpable—and insert on the abaxial surface of the proximal sesamoid bones. Each detaches a weak (extensor) branch that winds around PI to join the common extensor tendon at the level of the pastern joint (Figs. 23.23/*1* and 23.27/*7*).

A functional continuation of the interosseus beyond the sesamoid bones is provided by *the cruciate, oblique, and straight sesamoidean ligaments* as described earlier (Fig. 23.23/*4* and *5*). These support the normally overextended fetlock joint, and the sesamoids permit frictionless movement over the flexor aspect of the joint (Fig. 23.26/*5, 11,* and *12*). Energy, stored within the apparatus (and in the flexor tendons) by stretching on hoof impact, is released at the end of the stride, which allows the joint to flex and impart forward impetus.

The Hoof

The distal extremity of the limb is protected by the hoof, which is formed by epithelial keratinization over a greatly modified dermis,* which is continuous with the common dermis of the skin at the *coronet* (the term applied to the junction between skin and hoof). The hoof is conveniently divided into wall, periople, sole, and frog; the last is an integral part of the hoof capsule, although homologous with the digital pad of other species (see Fig. 10.18).

The *wall* is the part of the hoof visible in the standing animal (see Fig. 10.20). It is highest at its dorsal segment (toe) and decreases in height over the sides (quarters) until

* Formerly, and still occasionally, termed the *corium.*

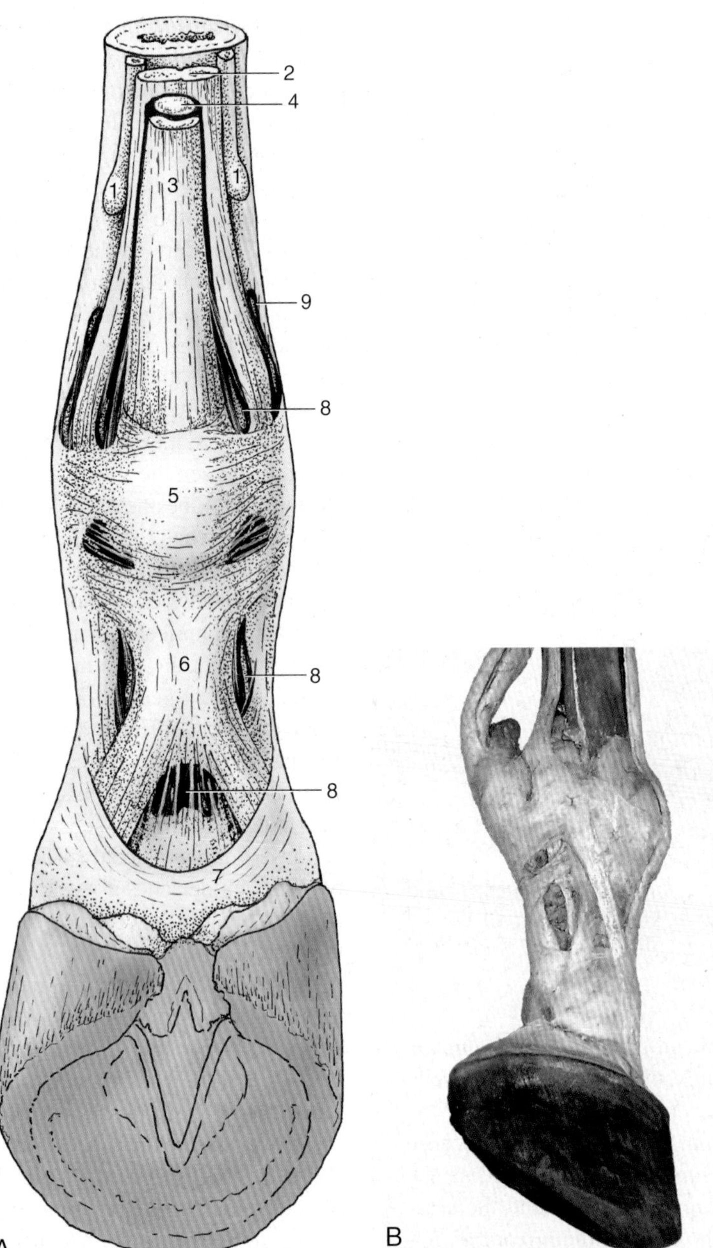

Fig. 23.29 (A) Annular ligaments of the digit. *1*, Splint bones; *2*, interosseus; *3*, superficial digital flexor; *4*, deep digital flexor; *5*, palmar annular ligament; *6*, proximal digital annular ligament; *7*, distal digital annular ligament; *8*, digital sheath; *9*, palmar pouch of fetlock joint. (B) Digital sheath injected with pink latex, fetlock joint with red latex.

it is reflected on itself, forming the rounded heels at the back of the hoof. The inflected parts continue forward for a short distance as the bars that are visible beside the frog when the hoof is raised (Fig. 23.30/*1‴*). The angle that the toe makes with the ground is about 50 degrees in the forelimb and slightly more in the hindlimb. The quarters descend toward the ground more steeply, especially on the medial side. The wall is thickest at the toe and gradually thins toward the bars, which is an important point for farriers to bear in mind when rasping or driving nails.

The wall grows from the epithelium covering the coronary dermis (Fig. 23.31/*2*) (which almost surrounds the digit at the coronet). It consists of horn tubules embedded in less structured intertubular horn and slides over the dermis covering the coffin bone and hoof cartilages to be worn away by contact with the ground. The greater part forms the generally pigmented stratum medium. The deeper, nonpigmented stratum internum comprises about 600 (horny) laminae that interdigitate with the sensitive laminae of the underlying laminar dermis (Fig. 23.31/*5*). Trauma affecting

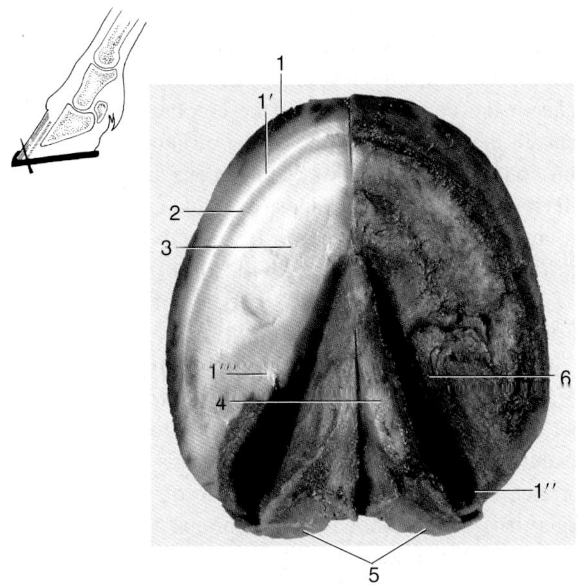

Fig. 23.30 Ground surface of the hoof. The *inset* shows the direction of hoof nails started at the white line. *1,* Wall; *1′,* unpigmented part of wall; *1″,* heel; *1‴,* bar; *2,* white line (union of wall and sole); *3,* sole; *4,* frog; *5,* bulbs of the heels; *6,* paracuneal groove.

the coronary dermis causes horn defects that descend with the wall, reaching the ground in about 8 months (a rate of growth of less than 1 cm per month). Weakness of the horn or trauma may lead to formation of cracks in the hoof wall.

The *periople* contributes the stratum externum of the wall (Fig. 23.31/*6* and *6′*). It consists of a band of soft, rubbery horn a few millimeters thick near the coronet but dries to a thin glossy layer distally. The band widens toward the palmar aspect, where it covers the bulbs of the heels and blends with the base of the frog. The periople, which also consists of an admixture of tubular and intertubular horn, is produced over the narrow perioplic dermis (Fig. 23.31/*1*) directly proximal to the coronary dermis.

The *sole* fills the space between the wall and frog and forms most of the undersurface of the hoof (see Fig. 23.33). It is slightly concave so that only the distal edge of the wall and the frog make contact on firm ground. The parts between the bars and quarters, known as the *angles of the sole,* are the seat of "corns," blood-soaked flecks resulting from trauma to the underlying dermis. Sole horn, though softer than that of the wall, again consists of an admixture of tubules and intertubular horn; it tends to

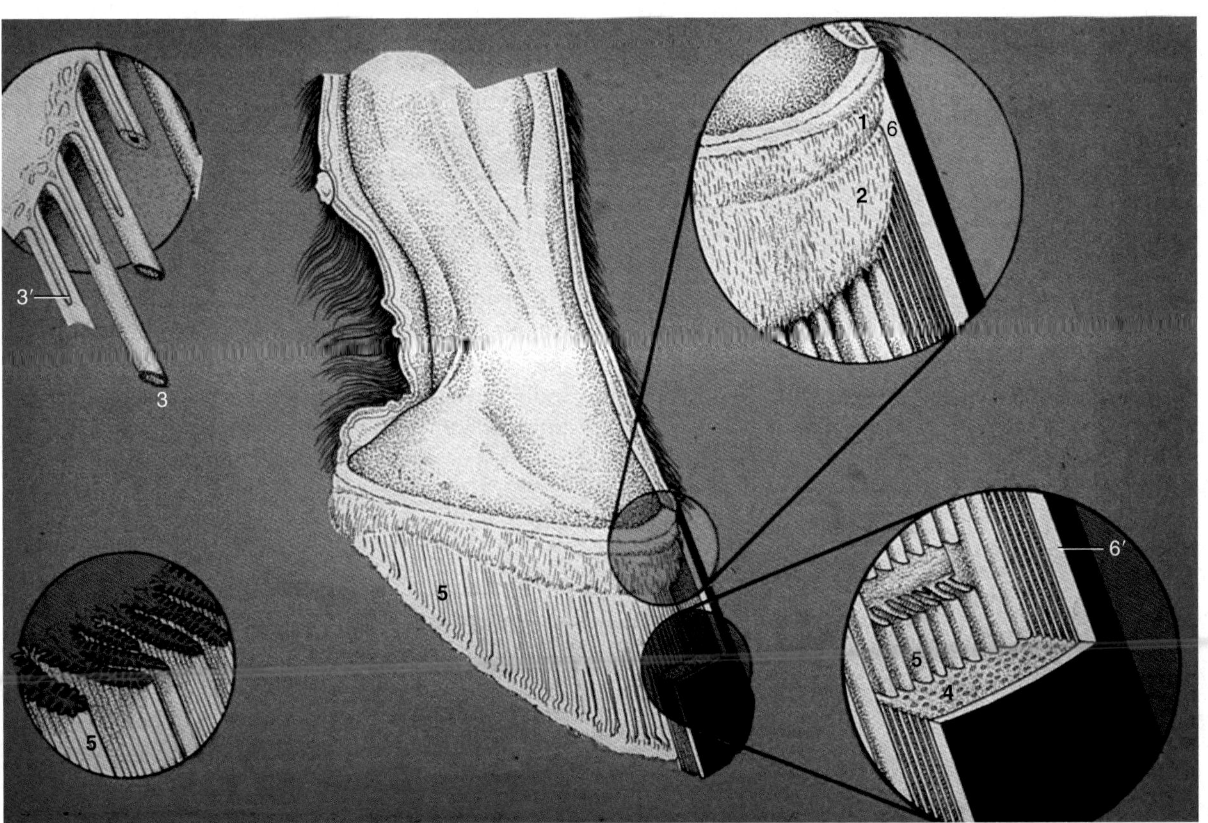

Fig. 23.31 The structure of the hoof wall and of the underlying laminar dermis. *1,* Perioplic dermis; *2,* coronary dermis; *3,* horn tubules growing from epithelium over papillae *(3′)* of the coronary dermis (enlarged in *left inset*); *4,* stratum medium of wall consisting of horn tubules embedded in less structured intertubular horn; *5,* dermal laminae that interdigitate with the horny laminae of the hoof wall (see also *insets* to the right); *6,* periople; *6′,* stratum externum of wall (dried periople).

become spongy and to flake in animals required to stand on soiled bedding.

The junction between the sole and the wall is known as *the white line* (zona alba; Figs. 23.30 and 23.32A). It includes some of the nonpigmented stratum medium of the wall, the distal ends of the horny laminae (stratum internum), and, between these, pigmented horn produced over the terminal papillae of the laminar dermis (these project distally, level with the dermal papillae above the sole) (Fig. 23.33/*3*). The startlingly white streak within the broad, so-called white line is provided by "cap horn" produced over the distal third of the dermal laminae. The internal rim of the white line is where farriers place nails when shoeing; the nails pass obliquely through the wall to emerge a few centimeters above the shoe, where they are cut and clinched (Fig. 23.30).

The wedge-shaped *frog* (cuneus ungulae) projects into the sole from behind. Its wide base closes the gap between the heels, where it furnishes the palmar part of the hoof (Fig. 23.30/*4*) and spreads upward to end in thickenings—the bulbs of the heels—that overhang the heels of the wall. Its external surface is marked by a central groove to which corresponds an internal spine (frog-stay) that juts proximally into the digital cushion (see further on). The frog is separated from the bars and the sole by deep (paracuneal) grooves (Fig. 23.30/*6*) that accentuate its medial and lateral borders. The grooves are convenient for the application of hoof testers (large "pincers" used to detect soreness in deeper structures). The projection of these structures is shown in Fig. 23.33.

Thrush is a term applied to a necrotic infectious disease of the frog. The foot emits a foul smell and leads to softening of the horn and resulting puncture wounds. This largely occurs in horses housed on wet or damp bedding.

The frog horn is tubular and fairly soft and elastic, being kept pliable by the fatty secretion of glands in the underlying digital cushion. Though horses can be shod with the "frog off the ground" (as were city draft horses formerly), a sound hoof requires the frog pressure that is obtained through ground contact.

The *dermis* deep to the hoof capsule can be divided into five parts: perioplic, coronary, and laminar dermis and those of the sole and frog that are associated with the like-named segments of the hoof. Both the coronary and laminar dermis are associated with the wall.

The entire dermis (other than the laminar part) carries papillae that run parallel to each other and to the dorsal surface of the hoof, directed toward the ground. It is richly supplied with vessels and nerves, and an ill-directed farrier's nail that penetrates the dermis ("quick") therefore draws blood and causes pain. Because nerves are absent from the hoof capsule, the apposing dermal and epidermal tissues are often designated sensitive and insensitive, respectively.

The *subcutis,* generally thin, attaches the dermis to such deeper structures as the coffin bone, the hoof cartilages, and the tendons. It is greatly thickened in two places: beneath the coronary dermis (the coronary cushion) and beneath the frog dermis (the digital cushion). These cushions consist of a feltwork of collagenous and elastic fibers interspersed with small islands of fat and cartilage.

The narrow, raised *perioplic dermis* embraces the digit at the coronet. Studded with short papillae, it widens caudally where it covers the bulbs of the heels (Fig. 23.34/*1*).

The wider elevation of the coronary dermis (Fig. 23.34/*2*) is separated from the perioplic dermis by a shallow groove. Its prominence is due to the rounded underlying coronary cushion. The coronary dermis also follows the coronet, but like the hoof wall, it folds on itself above the heels. It is widely known as the coronary band, although many clinicians interpret this term more widely to include the (external) coronet. The epithelium over most of its surface produces the bulk of the wall; that over the tucked-in distal margin produces most of the unstructured horn of the horny laminae.

The *laminar dermis* is composed of about 600 sensitive (dermal) laminae that interdigitate with the insensitive (horny) laminae on the deep surface of the wall (Fig. 23.32/*5–7*). Both sets bear numerous secondary laminae that further secure the wall to the dermis, and ultimately to the coffin bone, while leaving it possible for the horn to slide over the bone.

Normally the epithelium covering the sensitive laminae proliferates just sufficiently to allow the wall to slide past. However, it has the capacity to produce additional amounts of (scar-) horn when a defect in the wall must be closed. This potential is utilized even more dramatically in chronic laminitis (founder), a disease in which the normal attachment is loosened and the coffin bone rotates away from the wall. The space in front of the bone becomes filled with irregular horn produced over a new set of sensitive laminae that form near the dorsal surface of the bone.

The *dermis of the sole* is firmly attached to the undersurface of the coffin bone.

The *dermis of the frog* lies between the frog and the digital cushion, which occupies the space below the deep flexor tendon and between the cartilages of the hoof (Fig. 23.35/*6*).

The *blood supply* of the dermis comes from three sets of vessels, all branches of the digital arteries that descend into the hoof to each side of the flexor tendons. Those that arise at the level of the coronet supply the perioplic and coronary dermis, and those that arise opposite the pastern joint supply branches to the digital cushion and the dermis of the caudal aspect of the hoof, including the frog; the vessels of the third set arise from the dorsal and palmar terminal branches (mentioned in connection with the sole foramina of PIII) and go to the laminar and sole dermis. Veins do not accompany the arteries but instead

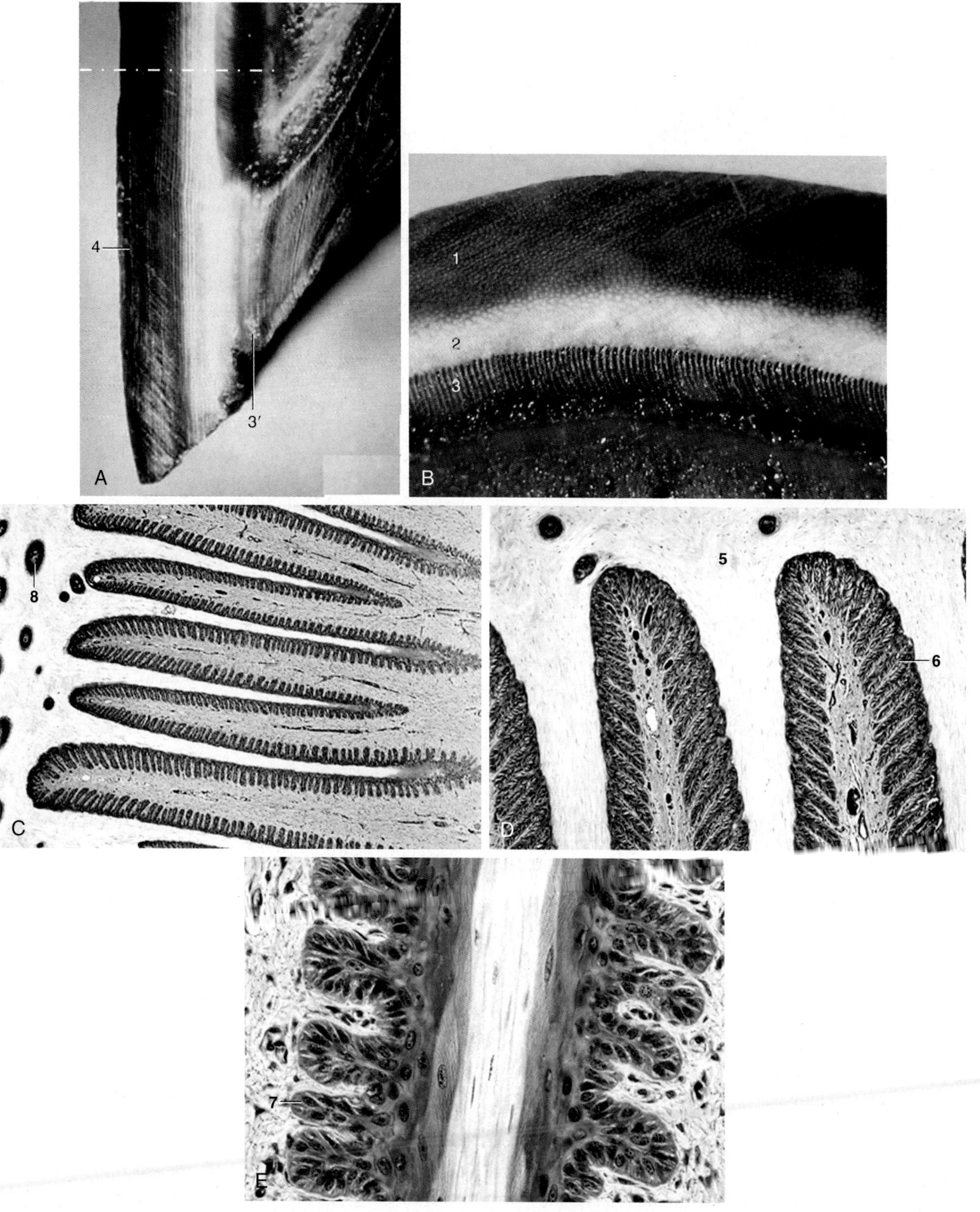

Fig. 23.32 (A) Section of the hoof. (B) Transverse section of the part of the hoof at level indicated in A. (C) Dermal lamellae that interdigitate with the horny lamellae of the hoof wall. (D) Enlargement of the dermal lamellae. (E) The small secunduring lamellae of the dermal lamellae are shown. *1*, Stratum externum; *2*, stratum medium; *3*, stratum internum; *3′*, white line; *4*, wall; *5*, primary horny laminae; *6*, primary dermal laminae; *7*, interdigitating secondary laminae; *8*, horn.

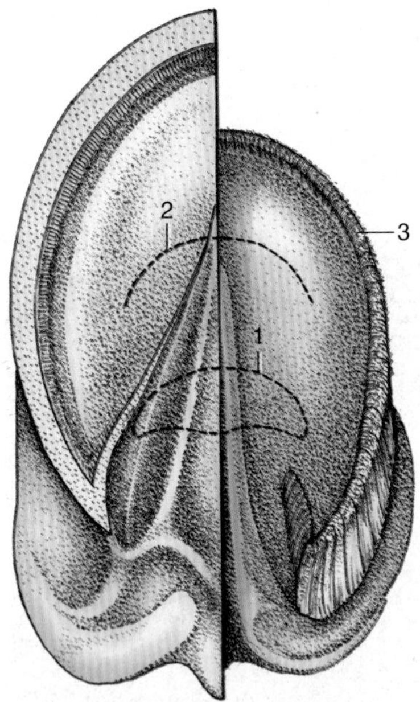

Fig. 23.33 Ground surface of the hoof. Half of the hoof has been removed to expose the dermis. *1,* Position of navicular bone; *2,* position of the insertion of the deep flexor tendon; *3,* terminal papillae.

form extensive interconnected networks in the dermis* and underlying subcutis, particularly in the coronary band, in the laminar dermis, and under the palmar aspect of the hoof (the coronary, dorsal, and palmar plexuses, respectively). They combine to form medial and lateral digital veins that become satellites to the arteries at the level of the pastern joint.

The hoof is a flexible structure, yielding under pressure on impact with the ground and so dissipating much of the attending concussion. The load that presses on the coffin joint is split between PIII and the navicular bone. The force on PIII is transmitted by the interdigitating laminae to the wall of the hoof, whose distal border is thus a principal weight bearer, especially in horses shod with the frog off the ground. The force retracts the slanted toe while the heels are spread by the distortion of the wall. The force exerted on the navicular bone presses into the yielding "sling" provided by the deep flexor tendon, which in turn compresses the digital cushion and frog (see Fig. 23.26). These redirect the force sideways: the cushion presses against the cartilages and the frog presses against the bars and sole, thus assisting the outward movement of the heels (Fig. 23.34C).

The to-and-fro movement of the heels is not obvious to the eye, but as any farrier can verify, it polishes the upper surface of the related parts of the shoe. It is to avoid interfering with this mechanism that farriers do not nail these parts of the shoe to the wall; if this precaution is neglected, the horse develops "contracted heels" and eventually goes lame (Fig. 23.34D).

The mechanism explains why the coffin bone is continued caudally by cartilage rather than by bone (Fig. 23.21/*4*). Progressive calcification of the cartilage with subsequent replacement by bone is a common aging process known as *sidebone,* which is yet another cause of lameness.

The movements of the heels have a further benefit, aiding venous return. The dense plexuses on both sides of the cartilages (Fig. 23.35/*7*) are compressed at each step and deliver blood into the valved digital veins. This has been shown experimentally by cannulating a digital vein under local anesthesia; blood is squirted at every step the horse takes. (In other species, contractions of striated muscles within the foot compress the veins and assist the venous return.)

Apart from minor differences in conformation, the forehoofs and hindhoofs are identical (Fig. 23.36). In conformity with its larger weight-bearing role, the forehoof is somewhat wider and therefore more rounded in outline than the narrower, more pointed hindhoof (Fig. 23.36C and D). However, the distinction is less than the adjectives suggest, and the provenance—fore or hind—of a single specimen is not always obvious.

When the hoof capsule first forms early in fetal life, it consists of horn that is soft, unpigmented, and of uniform composition. Later, new hard and more structured horn is produced that pushes the soft horn distally, where it becomes a rather misshapen mass covering the entire ground surface of the hoof and (thinly) an adjoining strip of the hoof wall. When exposed to air at term, the soft mass soon dries and sloughs away. The soft mass over the hard horn of the fetal hoof is said to prevent injury to the fetal membranes and birth canal (Fig. 23.37).

THE PASSIVE STAY APPARATUS

It is well known that horses can remain on their feet for much longer than other domestic animals. In fact, they are thought by many to sleep while standing. This is not quite true: they may rest or doze standing, but for a refreshing sleep they lie down, often only at night when unobserved. When horses stand quietly, most weight is carried by the tendons, ligaments, and deep fascia of the stay apparatus, which do not tire, while expending a minimum of muscular energy.

*It is known that certain regions of the hoof dermis are generously provided with epithelioid arteriovenous anastomoses (of a rather unusual character). It has been postulated that these anastomoses may be affected by vasoactive peptides released in certain pathologies of various organs remote from the limbs. According to the theory, the resulting dilation of these channels, when prolonged, may prejudice the normal capillary circulation, and this may sometimes be a predisposing factor in the development of acute laminitis.

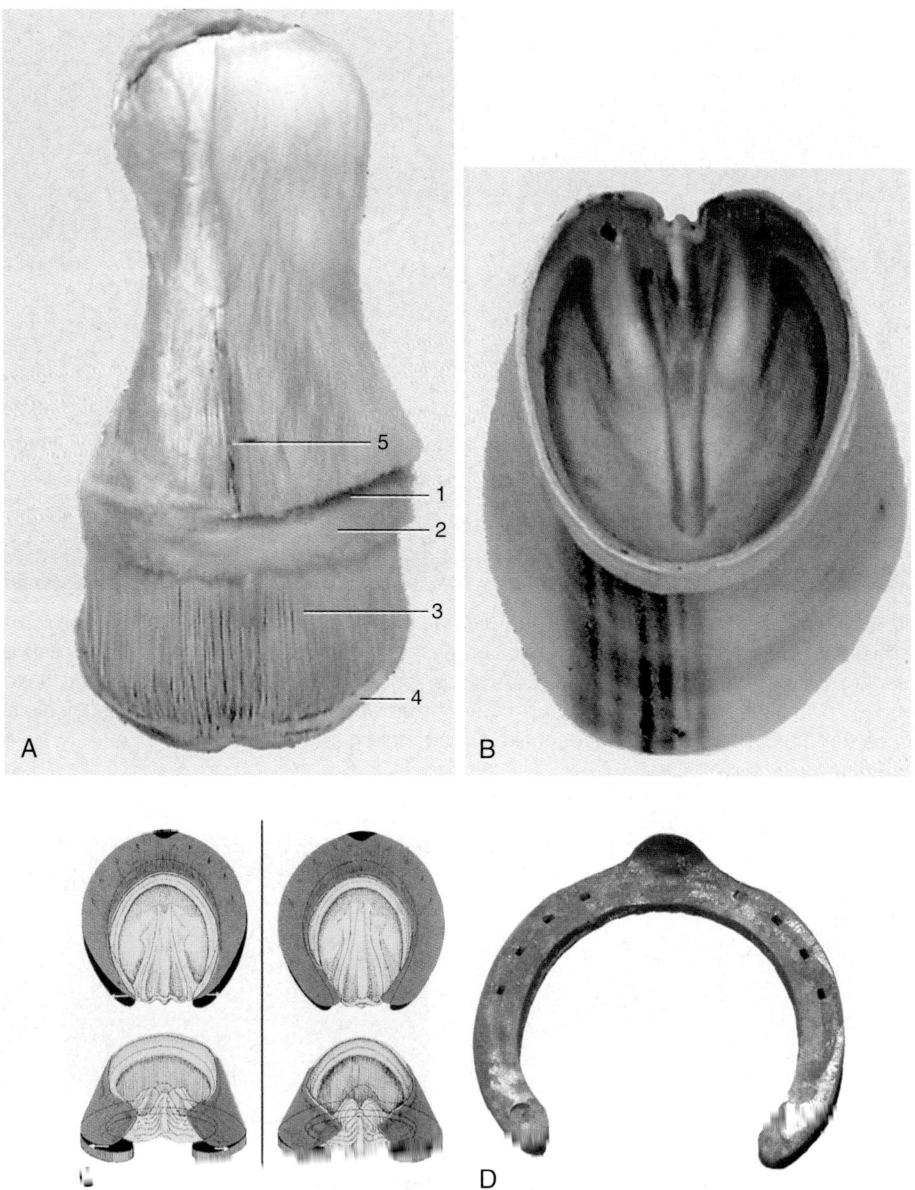

Fig. 23.34 (A) Dermis exposed by removal of the hoof. *1*, Perioplic dermis; *2*, coronary dermis; *3*, laminar dermis; *4*, terminal papillae on the ends of the dermal laminae; *5*, cut edge of skin. (B) Hoof shoe removed from specimen A. (C) Changes in the form of the hoof during locomotion. (D) Shoe showing the heel part polished by movement of the hoof heel.

The bony column of the forelimb supports the cranial end of the trunk at the attachment of the serratus ventralis muscle to the medial surface of the scapula (Fig. 23.38A/*1*). A vertical line dropped from the center of this attachment passes caudal to the shoulder, through the elbow, through or slightly cranial to the carpal joint, and cranial to the fetlock and pastern joints. If unsupported, the column would collapse by flexion of the shoulder and elbow joints, by overextension (or possibly flexion [buckling forward]) of the carpal joint, and by overextension of the fetlock and pastern joints. (The coffin joint actually flexes when the fetlock sinks under weight and can be disregarded in this discussion.)

The *shoulder joint* is prevented from flexion by the strong internal biceps tendon (Fig. 23.38/*2*) that connects the supraglenoid tubercle of the scapula with the radius. The latter attachment can be regarded as fixed because it is very close to the axis of rotation of the elbow joint (Fig. 23.38/*5*), which is stabilized by the weight on the limb. Tension in the wide biceps

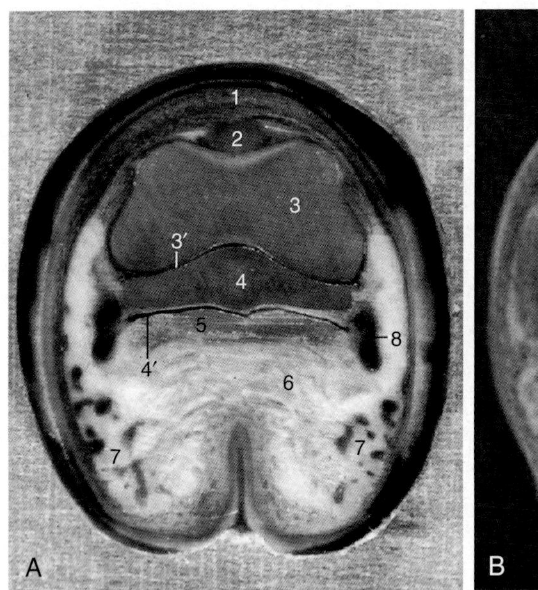

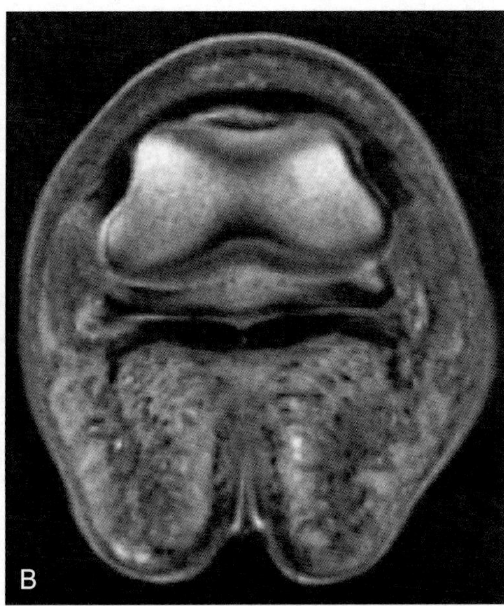

Fig. 23.35 (A) Transverse section of the digit at the level of the navicular bone, proximal surface. *1,* Coronary dermis; *2,* extensor process of distal phalanx (PIII); *3,* distal end of middle phalanx (PII); *3′,* coffin joint; *4,* navicular bone; *4′,* navicular bursa; *5,* deep flexor tendon; *6,* digital cushion; *7,* cartilage of hoof and venous plexus; *8,* position of digital vessels and nerve. (B) Magnetic resonance image taken at the same level as in A.

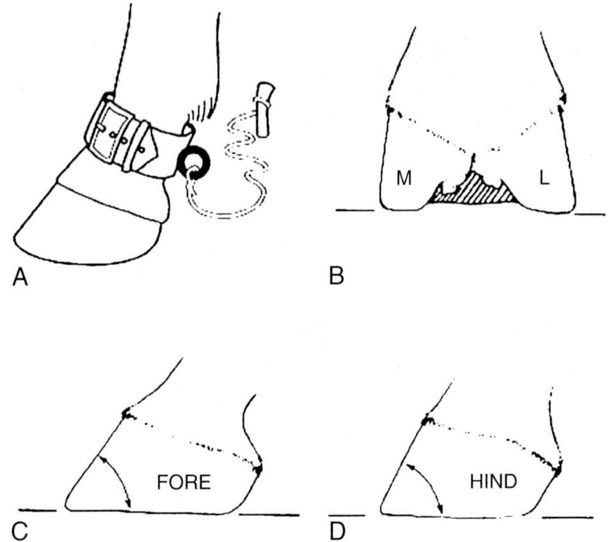

Fig. 23.36 (A) In former days horses at pasture were hobbled with a "pastern"; this is why the narrow part of the limb above the hoof is known today as the pastern. (B) Palmar (plantar) view of the foot; the lateral *(L)* angle of the wall (with the ground) is more acute than the medial *(M).* (C) and (D) The angle at the toe is more acute in the forelimb (C) than in the hindlimb (D).

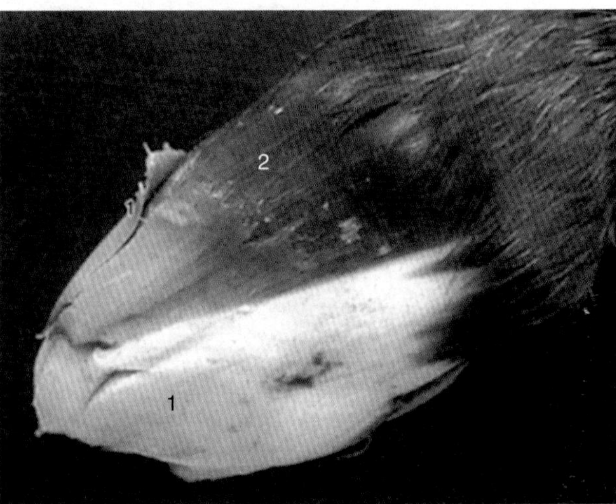

Fig. 23.37 Hoof of a newborn foal. *1,* Mass of soft, primary horn covering the ground surface and distal half of the hard, permanent hoof wall; *2,* pigmented permanent hoof wall.

tendon puts great pressure on the intertubercular groove of the humerus. Indeed, some believe that the molding of the tendon to the intermediate tubercle actually causes the joint to lock. At its other end, the pull of the biceps is transmitted via the lacertus and extensor carpi radialis (Fig. 23.38/*6* and *10*) to a second fixed point at the upper end of the large metacarpal bone. This pull augments the action of the extensors of the carpal joint and prevents that joint from buckling forward and collapsing the limb. Any tendency toward overextension is prevented by close packing of the carpal bones in front and by the strong palmar carpal ligament behind (Fig. 23.15A and B/*7*).

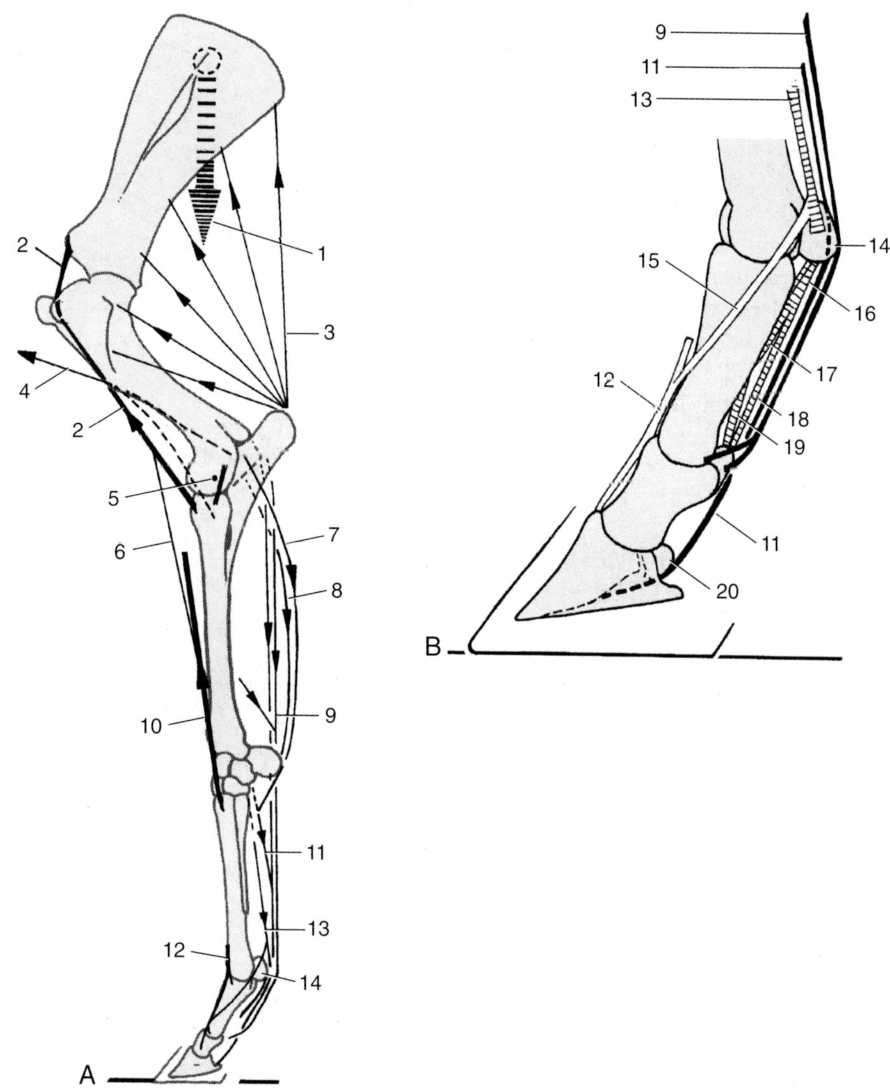

Fig. 23.38 (A) The stay apparatus of the left forelimb, lateral view. (B) Detail of digit, lateral view. *1,* Weight of trunk; *2,* internal biceps tendon; *3,* triceps; *4,* brachiocephalicus and brachial fascia to elbow joint; *5,* axis of elbow rotation, next to eccentric collateral ligament; *6,* lacertus fibrosus; *7,* ulnaris lateralis; *8,* flexor carpi ulnaris; *9,* superficial digital flexor and accessory (check) ligament; *10,* extensor carpi radialis; *11,* deep digital flexor and accessory (check) ligament; *12,* common digital extensor; *13,* interosseus; *14,* proximal sesamoid bones; *15,* extensor branch of interosseus; *16, 17,* and *18,* cruciate, oblique, and straight sesamoidean ligaments, respectively; *19,* axial palmar ligament; *20,* navicular bone.

The *fetlock joint* is prevented from overextension principally by *the suspensory apparatus (comprising the interosseus, proximal sesamoid bones, and distal sesamoidean ligaments)*, which is tensed under load (Fig. 23.38/*13, 14,* and *16–18*). The effect is reinforced by tension in the accessory (check) ligaments and distal parts of the superficial and deep flexor tendons (Fig. 23.38/*9* and *11*). Tension in the deep flexor tendon tends to flex the coffin joint, which causes the toe of the hoof to dig into the ground. The extensor branches of the interosseus (Fig. 23.38/*15*), pulling on the extensor process of the bone at impact, counteract this and keep the hoof level.

Overextension of the pastern joint is opposed by the axial and abaxial palmar and straight sesamoidean ligaments (Fig. 23.38/*18* and *19*), which span its palmar aspect. The taut deep flexor tendon gives additional support. (Buckling forward is prevented by the superficial flexor that attaches on the palmar aspect of the joint.)

With the shoulder joint fixed (by the biceps tendon), the weight of the trunk rests on the upper end of the nearly vertical radius. Therefore, unless the horse sways markedly forward, only small forces are required to prevent the elbow joint from flexing. These are mainly supplied by passive tension of the tendinous components of the carpal and digital flexors (the superficial digital flexor especially) and the eccentrically placed collateral ligaments (Fig. 23.38/*5* and *7–9*). Recent information indicates that because of their muscle fiber composition—characteristic of postural muscles—the anconeus and the medial head of the triceps may also oppose flexion of the elbow joint. The large mass of the long and lateral heads of the triceps—the principal extensor of the elbow joint—remains flaccid even when the other forelimb is picked up to make the horse stand three-legged (see Fig. 23.2/*1*, and the effects of radial paralysis on page 609).

THE BLOOD VESSELS AND LYMPHATIC STRUCTURES OF THE FORELIMB

The *axillary artery,* the main supply of the limb, enters the axillary space after crossing the cranial border of the first rib, where it may be punctured (p. 528). It descends on the medial aspect of the arm in company with the median and ulnar nerves and shortly becomes known as the *brachial artery.* The trunk releases several branches to the muscles of the shoulder and arm, the most prominent being the subscapular artery, which follows the caudal border of the scapula, and the deep brachial artery, which disappears between the heads of the triceps (Fig. 23.8). Just proximal to the elbow joint, lesser cranial and caudal branches (transverse cubital and collateral ulnar arteries, respectively) are detached for the muscles in the forearm (Fig. 23.39/*11* and *12*). The brachial artery crosses the elbow cranial to the medial collateral ligament, where it can be palpated and the pulse evaluated, through the pectoralis transversus (Fig. 23.40/*5*). Together with the median nerve it dips under the flexor carpi radialis caudal to the radius and soon gives off the common interosseous artery, which passes through the interosseous space to reach the craniolateral muscles of the forearm.

The main trunk, now redesignated the *median artery* (Fig. 23.41/*12*), gradually works its way to the caudal surface of the forearm before dividing into three branches above the carpus. The lesser branch (palmar branches of the median and radial artery) contributes the small palmar metacarpal arteries that accompany the interosseus muscle, while the main trunk passes through the carpal canal with the digital flexor tendons (Fig. 23.15B/*19*). It continues with these in the cannon where it becomes *the medial palmar artery, the main artery to the digit and hoof.* This inclines axially before splitting into the medial and lateral digital arteries above the fetlock. The digital arteries pass over the abaxial surfaces of the sesamoid bones (where they are palpable) and continue into the digit on each side

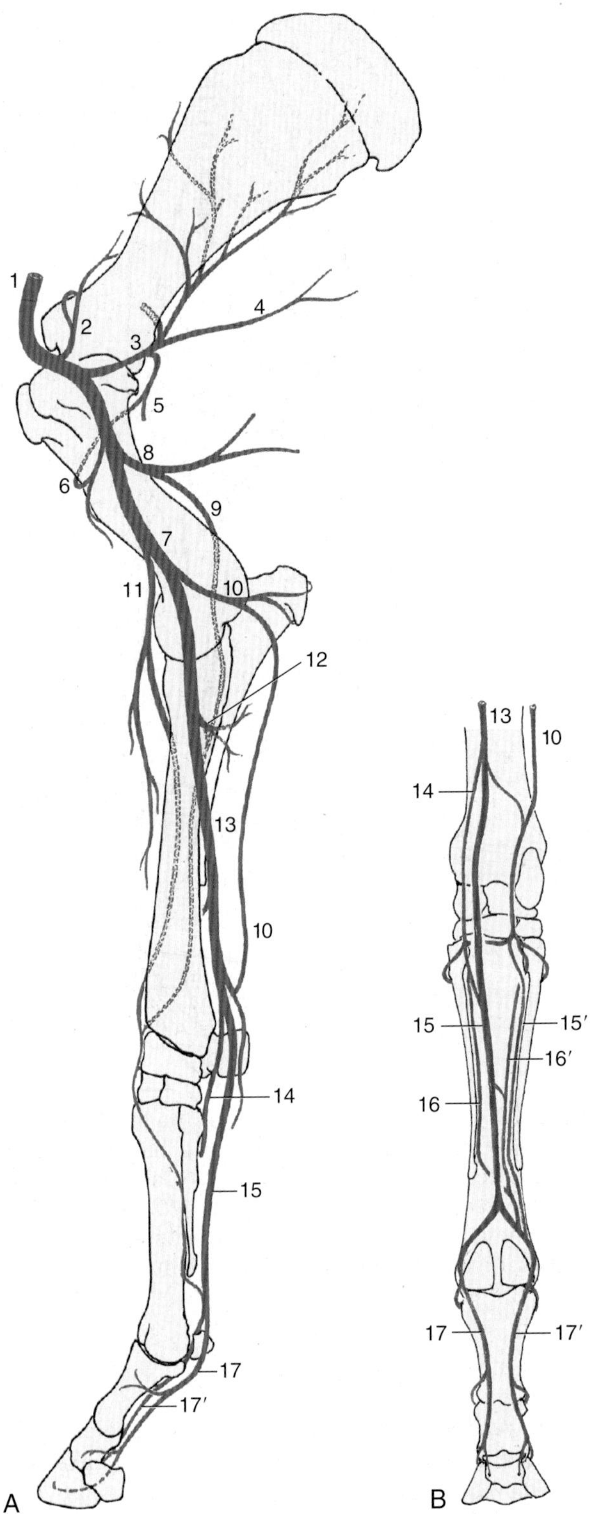

Fig. 23.39 The major arteries (aa.) of the right forelimb: (A) medial view; (B) palmar view. *1,* Axillary artery (a.); *2,* suprascapular a.; *3,* subscapular a.; *4,* thoracodorsal a.; *5* and *6,* caudal and cranial circumflex humeral aa., respectively; *7,* brachial a.; *8,* deep brachial a.; *9,* collateral radial a.; *10,* collateral ulnar a.; *11,* transverse cubital a.; *12,* common interosseous a.; *13,* median a.; *14,* radial a.; *15* and *15′,* medial and lateral palmar aa., respectively; *16* and *16′,* medial and lateral palmar metacarpal aa., respectively; *17* and *17′,* medial and lateral digital aa., respectively.

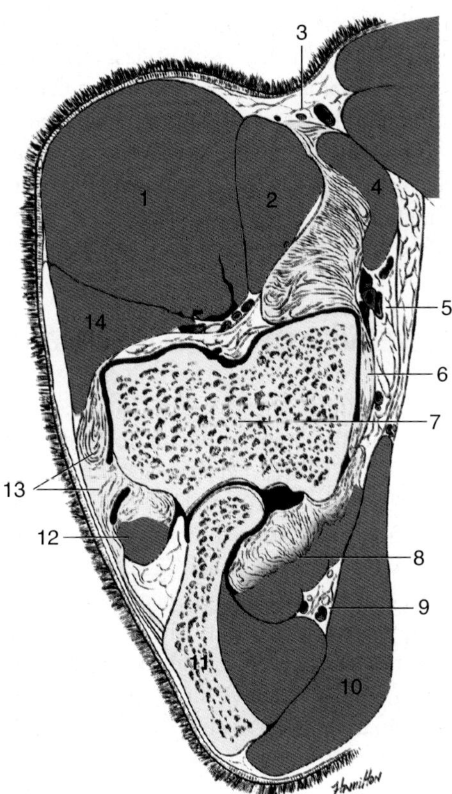

Fig. 23.40 Transverse section of the left elbow. *1,* Extensor carpi radialis; *2,* brachialis; *3,* medial cutaneous antebrachial nerve and cephalic vein lying on lacertus fibrosus; *4,* biceps; *5,* brachial vessels and median nerve; *6,* medial collateral ligament; *7,* humerus; *8,* flexors arising from medial epicondyle of humerus; *9,* ulnar nerve and collateral ulnar vessels; *10,* tensor fasciae antebrachii; *11,* olecranon; *12,* ulnaris lateralis; *13,* lateral collateral ligament; *14,* common digital extensor.

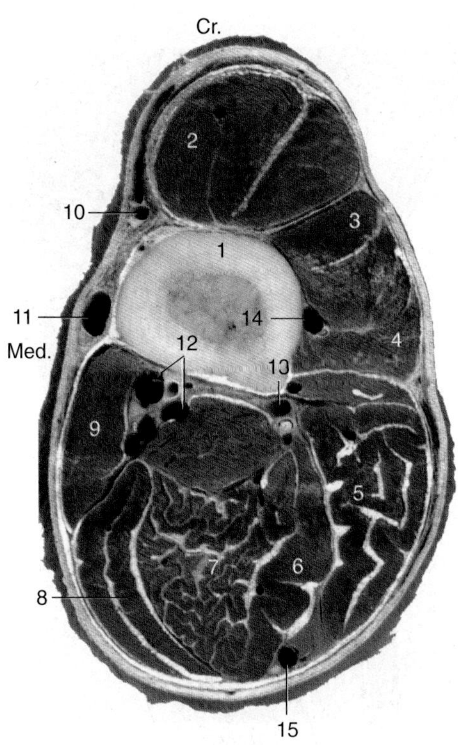

Fig. 23.41 Transverse section of the right forearm at the level shown in Fig. 23.42. *Cr.,* Cranial; *Med.,* medial; *1,* Radius; *2,* extensor carpi radialis; *3,* common digital extensor; *4,* lateral digital extensor; *5,* ulnaris lateralis; *6,* deep digital flexor; *7,* superficial digital flexor; *8,* flexor carpi ulnaris; *9,* flexor carpi radialis; *10,* accessory cephalic vein and medial cutaneous antebrachial nerve (from musculocutaneous); *11,* cephalic vein; *12,* median artery, veins, and nerve; *13,* muscular branches of median vessels; *14,* cranial interosseous vessels; *15,* ulnar nerve and collateral ulnar vessels.

of the flexor tendons. The lateral artery is reinforced by the small metacarpal arteries that join above the sesamoid bone (Fig. 23.39/*18′*). The branches of the digital arteries distal to the fetlock are symmetrical. Dorsal and palmar branches are given off opposite PI, and these supply adjacent structures while forming a circle about the bone. A branch to the digital cushion is detached level with the pastern joint before the digital artery disappears by passing deep to the hoof cartilage. Dorsal and palmar branches detached opposite the middle of PII comport themselves similarly to the branches about PI but also take part in the supply of the dermis of the hoof. The dorsal and palmar terminal branches (to PIII) have been described (pp. 590 and 600); the palmar branches anastomose to form a terminal arch within the bone.

Most veins of the forelimb are satellite veins, although they are often duplicated or further replicated where they accompany the larger arteries (Fig. 23.42/*1*). Some superficial veins seek independent courses, and those coming from the hoof have already been mentioned. The superficial veins include the *cephalic and accessory cephalic veins,* which are prominent and palpable in the forearm (Fig. 23.42/*10* and *10′*). The cephalic vein is joined to the brachial vein via the median cubital at the elbow and continues to ascend in the groove between the brachiocephalicus and pectoralis descendens, where it is at risk in "staking" injuries. It joins the external jugular vein at the base of the neck.

Two clusters of *lymph nodes* drain the free part of the limb. The cubital nodes lie on the medial aspect of the humerus just proximal to the elbow joint. They drain more distal parts of the limb and channel their outflow to the axillary nodes. These lie medial to the shoulder joint in the angle between the axillary and subscapular arteries and drain the arm and shoulder, together with a part of the thoracic wall caudal to the limb. Their efferent vessels go to the caudal deep cervical nodes, and thence the lymph flows directly or indirectly to the veins at the thoracic inlet. The superficial cervical nodes are arranged in a long chain that crosses the deep surface of the

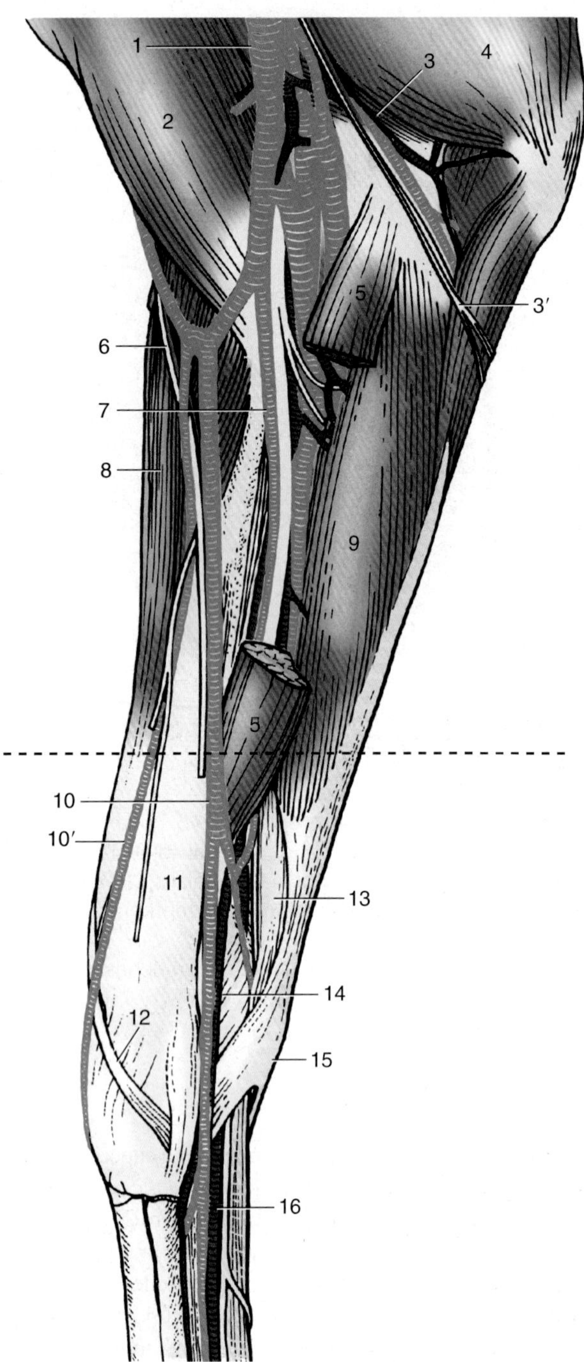

Fig. 23.42 Dissection of the medial surface of the right forearm. (The *broken transverse line* indicates level of section in Fig. 23.41.) *1,* Multiple brachial veins; *2,* biceps; *3,* ulnar nerve and collateral ulnar vessels; *3′,* caudal cutaneous antebrachial nerve; *4,* triceps; *5,* flexor carpi radialis, resected; *6,* medial cutaneous antebrachial nerve; *7,* median nerve and vessels; *8,* extensor carpi radialis; *9,* flexor carpi ulnaris; *10* and *10′,* cephalic and accessory cephalic veins, respectively; *11,* radius; *12,* extensor carpi obliquus; *13,* superficial digital flexor; *14,* radial artery and vein; *15,* accessory carpal bone; *16,* medial palmar nerve and vessels.

omotransversarius and brachiocephalicus (see Fig. 18.41/*8*). The group consists of many small nodes, and because these are embedded in fat and do not form a firm compact mass, the group is not always easily located. Palpation should be directed to drawing the nodes forward, away from the subclavius against which they lie. The superficial cervical nodes mainly drain skin over the upper part of the limb but also receive some lymph from deeper structures.

THE NERVES OF THE FORELIMB

With few exceptions, the structures of the forelimb are innervated from the brachial plexus formed by contributions from the last three cervical and first two thoracic nerves (C6–T2). The plexus reaches the axilla as a broad band that emerges between the parts of the scalenus, but this soon divides into the usual dozen or so trunks. The major trunks, of clinical interest because of their vulnerability to injury or availability for nerve-blocking techniques, are described even though there are few specific features of significance above the carpus.

The *suprascapular nerve* (C6–C7) leaves the axilla by sinking between the subscapular and supraspinatus muscles. It then winds around the neck of the scapula before expending itself in the supraspinatus and infraspinatus (Fig. 23.43/*2*). A direct relationship to bone always carries a risk of injury, and the suprascapular nerve may be damaged where it lies against the scapula likely through the pulling on the nerve as the animal stumbles with the limb stretched back. Even serious damage to the nerve may have little immediate effect, although an observer stationed in front of an affected horse may notice a lateral deviation of the shoulder joint at each stride. After a time, atrophy of muscles supplied by the nerve markedly alters the conformation of the shoulder region, causing the scapular spine to project above the wasted muscles. Suprascapular paralysis is commonly known as *sweeny* or *shoulder slip.*

The *musculocutaneous nerve* (C7–C8) (Fig. 23.43/*3, 3′,* and *3″*) first runs craniolateral to the axillary artery before turning below the vessel to unite with the median nerve. A branch to the coracobrachialis and biceps is detached before the union. The part incorporated in the median trunk separates in the distal arm to supply the brachialis and give medial cutaneous antebrachial nerve that crosses the lacertus fibrosus, where it is easily palpated, and then is distributed to the skin over the cranial and medial aspects of the forearm and carpus. Although uncommon, damage to the musculocutaneous nerve and associated loss of activity by the principal elbow flexors is unlikely to greatly affect the gait.

The *axillary nerve* (C7–C8) (Fig. 23.43/*5*) has the usual course and distribution—to the principal flexors of the shoulder and the skin over the lateral aspect of the arm and forearm. There appear to be no records of traumatic damage

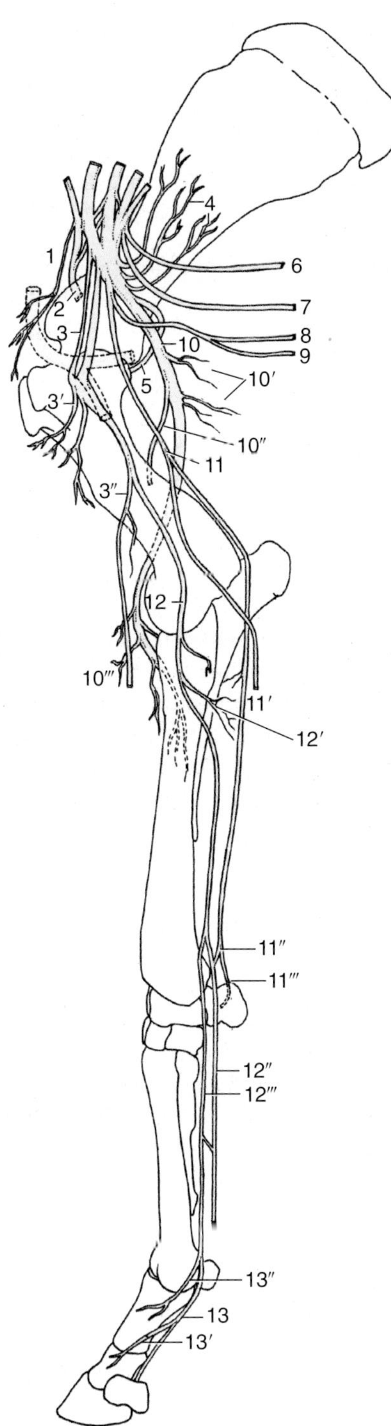

Fig. 23.43 Distribution of the nerves in the right forelimb, medial view. The axillary artery at the shoulder joint is *stippled*. *1,* Cranial pectoral nerves; *2,* suprascapular nerve (n.); *3,* musculocutaneous n.; *3′,* proximal branches; *3″,* distal branches with medial cutaneous antebrachial n.; *4,* subscapular n.; *5,* axillary n.; *6,* long thoracic n.; *7,* thoracodorsal n.; *8,* lateral thoracic n.; *9,* caudal pectoral nerves; *10,* radial n.; *10′,* proximal muscular branches (triceps); *10″,* lateral cutaneous antebrachial n.; *10‴,* distal muscular branches; *11,* ulnar n.; *11′,* caudal cutaneous antebrachial n.; *11″,* palmar branch; *11‴,* dorsal branch; *12,* median n.; *12′,* muscular branches; *12″,* lateral palmar n.; *12‴,* medial palmar n.; *13,* medial palmar digital n.; *13′* and *13″,* dorsal branches.

to this nerve in the horse. It is known that in other species section of the nerve does not impair the gait because other muscles are potentially able to flex the shoulder.

The *radial nerve* (C8–T1) is one of the larger branches of the plexus (Fig. 23.43/*10*). It follows the caudal border of the brachial artery in the upper arm and later sinks between the medial and long heads of the triceps, rounding the caudal surface of the humerus to gain the lateral aspect of the limb. The nerve detaches branches to the triceps group in the proximal part of the arm; more distally, where it is covered by the lateral head of the triceps, it detaches other branches to the extensor muscles of the carpus and digit. A purely sensory continuation (lateral cutaneous antebrachial nerve) supplies skin over the lateral aspect of the forearm, and contrary to the pattern in other species, this branch fades at the carpal level.

The *radial nerve* is the sole supply to the extensor muscles of all joints distal to the shoulder; the effects of damage are therefore proportionately severe. When injury is proximal to the origin of the tricipital branches, the animal is unable to support weight on the affected limb. It stands with the joints uncharacteristically flexed such that the angle between scapula and humerus is enlarged, and the elbow is dropped in relation to the trunk. The hoof is rested on its dorsal aspect. High radial paralysis may arise from injury to or disease of the humerus or from damage to the brachial plexus itself. If other components of the plexus are affected, the signs may be complicated by simultaneous paralysis of the flexor muscles of the distal joints.

The results of injury distal to the origin of the tricipital branches are naturally less severe. Normal stances of the shoulder and elbow are maintained (Fig. 23.44). The animal may rest the dorsal surface of the hoof on the ground but supports weight on the limb if the hoof is first restored to the normal position. Many horses learn to compensate for this disability by setting the hoof down before the impetus—gained when the limb is swung forward during the stride—is lost. The gait may appear almost normal when the terrain is flat, but unevenness quickly brings an affected animal into difficulties. Low radial paralysis may be simulated by the ischemia that sometimes results from prolonged lateral recumbency.

The *median nerve* (C8–T2) is the largest branch of the brachial plexus (Fig. 23.43/*12*). It follows the cranial border of the brachial artery for most of its course through the arm but shifts to the caudal margin on approaching the elbow. Although it is covered by the pectoralis transversus as it crosses the elbow, the nerve and artery together still form a palpable cord (Fig. 23.42/7). The two structures continue together as they descend the forearm, buried within the flexor mass of muscle. They divide at the same level, a little above the radiocarpal joint. The end branches, known as the *medial* and *lateral palmar nerves,* are described in the next section. After detaching the muscular branches to

Fig. 23.44 Lower radial paralysis.

the flexor muscles of the carpus and digit in the very proximal part of the forearm, the nerve becomes purely sensory.

The *ulnar nerve* (T1–T2) follows the caudal border of the brachial artery in the proximal part of the arm (Fig. 23.43/*11*). It then diverges caudally, detaches the caudal cutaneous antebrachial nerve (for the caudal aspect of the forearm), and passes over the medial epicondyle of the humerus before entering the forearm. As it does so, it releases branches to the flexor muscles. The much depleted and now purely sensory nerve follows the ulnar head of the deep flexor at the caudal margin of the limb, under cover of deep fascia (Fig. 23.41/*15*). A few centimeters above the carpus it divides into dorsal and palmar branches. The dorsal branch comes to the surface a short distance proximal to the accessory carpal bone and can be palpated against the ulnaris lateralis tendon attaching here. It passes over the lateral aspect of the carpus to expend itself in the skin over the lateral surface of the metacarpus. The palmar branch passes the carpus within the flexor retinaculum, where it exchanges fibers with the lateral palmar nerve, one of the terminal branches of the median nerve.

The overlap of the median and ulnar nerves in their motor distribution makes it unlikely that damage restricted to either one would much affect the gait.

Innervation of the Forefoot

Four nerves attend to the innervation of most of the structures distal to the carpus: *the medial and lateral palmar nerves from the median nerve, and the palmar and dorsal branches of the ulnar nerve.* All but the dorsal branch of the ulnar lie palmar to the large metacarpal bone.

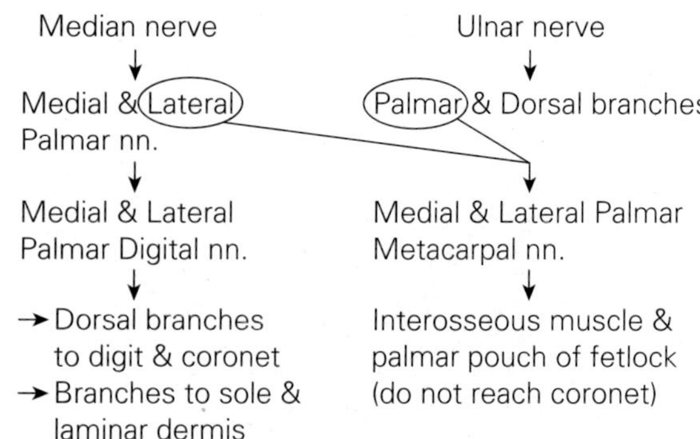

The *medial palmar nerve* lies in the groove between the interosseus and the flexor tendons. In midcannon it detaches a communicating branch that crosses obliquely over the superficial flexor tendon (where it is palpable) to join the lateral palmar nerve. A little above the fetlock the medial palmar becomes the medial digital nerve, which immediately gives rise to one or two dorsal branches that ramify over the dorsomedial aspect of the digit and coronet. The main trunk of the digital nerve continues with the like-named artery over the outer aspect of the proximal sesamoid bone, passes under the ligament of the ergot (Fig. 23.45), and then disappears into the hoof. The neurovascular bundle may be palpated against the sesamoid bone. Small branches supply the structures caudal to the phalanges. The nerve ends by supplying the laminar and sole dermis.

The *lateral palmar nerve*, it will be recalled, exchanged fibers with the palmar branch of the ulnar nerve at the carpus. It emerges from the short (1- to 2-cm) union and takes a course and has a distribution similar to that of the medial palmar nerve, including the ramifications in the digit. The first branch of this composite nerve arises at the carpus and soon splits into thin medial and lateral palmar metacarpal nerves that descend, deeply embedded, along the axial surface of the splint bones. These nerves supply the interosseus and the palmar pouch of the fetlock joint before becoming subcutaneous at the distal ends of the splint bones. They now supply the dorsal pouch of the joint before mingling with the dorsal branches of the digital nerves and stop short of the coronet.

All of these nerves can be blocked at various levels—mainly for the diagnosis of lameness. The rationale of the procedure is that a lame horse temporarily becomes sound when the area that contains the undetected lesion is desensitized. A sequence of injections, in which increasingly larger territories are desensitized, is therefore required. The details of the nerve blocks will be encountered later in the veterinary medical program. However, four sites commonly used for nerve blocks are presented here:

1. The *palmar digital blocks* have as their targets the digital nerves, level with the pastern joint and just proximal to the hoof cartilage (the digital artery lies next to the

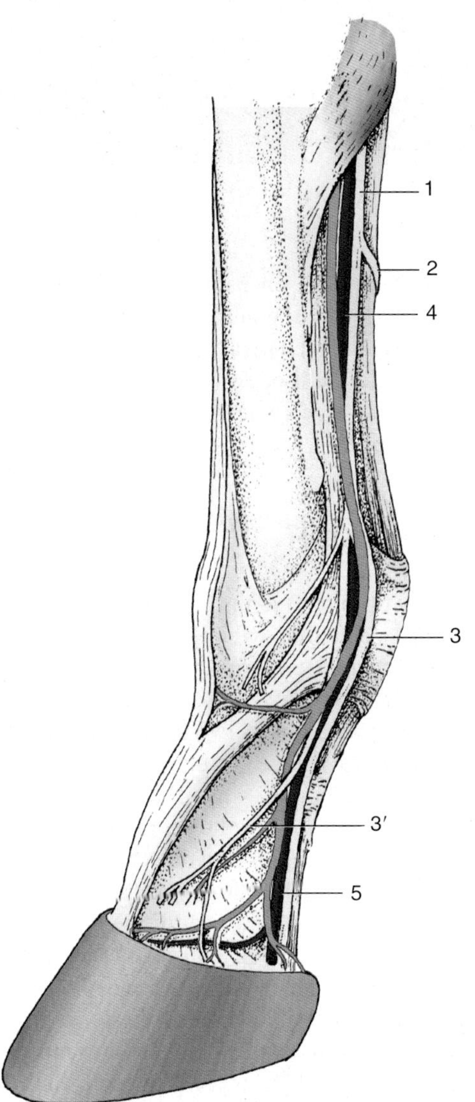

Fig. 23.45 Distribution of the medial palmar nerve. *1,* Medial palmar nerve; *2,* communicating branch; *3,* medial digital palmar nerve; *3′,* dorsal branch; *4,* medial palmar artery and vein; *5,* medial digital artery and vein.

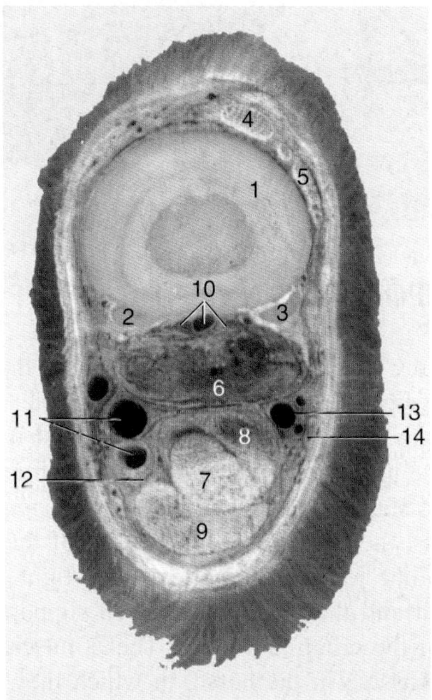

Fig. 23.46 Transverse section of the middle of the right metacarpus. *1, 2,* and *3,* Large *(1)* and small (*2* and *3*) metacarpal bones; *4,* common digital extensor; *5,* lateral digital extensor; *6,* interosseus; *7,* deep digital flexor; *8,* accessory (check) ligament; *9,* superficial digital flexor; *10,* palmar metacarpal vessels and nerves; *11,* medial palmar artery and vein; *12,* medial palmar nerve; *13,* lateral palmar artery; *14,* lateral palmar nerve.

nerve). The block desensitizes all structures in the hoof, except the dorsal part of the coronary band.

2. Blocks at the level of the proximal sesamoid bones have as their targets the digital nerves and their dorsal branches (the digital artery and vein lie dorsal to the nerve adjacent to the dorsal branches). The block desensitizes the digit, except the dorsal aspect of the pastern.
3. In the *distal metacarpal block* the injections are made level with the distal extremities of the splint bones. The target combines the palmar nerves (the palmar vein lies dorsal to the nerve; the artery lies deep to it) and branches of the palmar metacarpal nerves (subcutaneous, distal to splint bone; deep, between splint bone and interosseus; Fig. 23.46). The block desensitizes the digit, including the fetlock joint, with the possible exception of its dorsal pouch.
4. In the *proximal metacarpal block* the injections are made on the axial surface of the proximal end of the splint bones. The targets are the medial and lateral palmar nerves and the origin of the metacarpal nerves from the latter (large vessels accompany especially the medial palmar nerve). The block desensitizes the digit, including the fetlock joint (with the possible exception of its dorsal pouch), and most structures in the caudal metacarpus; because of distopalmar outpouchings of the nearby carpometacarpal joint, this and the midcarpal joint may also be desensitized.

The *autonomous zones of skin innervation* are shown in Fig. 23.1. A skin prick in the center of a zone tests for the integrity of the particular nerve.

COMPREHENSION CHECK

Using a cadaver, practice arthrocentesis in various joints of the forelimb. Make use of a colored dye to determine the accuracy of the injection.

Develop a model or discussion to demonstrate the integration of functions of various muscles and tendons that provide stability while standing or walking.

24 The Hindlimb of the Horse

CONFORMATION OF THE CROUP

Although the hindlimbs support little more than 40% of the body weight, they supply by far the greater part of the forward impetus in locomotion. This thrust is delivered through the hip and sacroiliac joints, which are intrinsically more stable than the shoulder and scapulothoracic synsarcosis, the corresponding "joints" of the forelimb. The sacroiliac joint is strengthened by tight ligaments, and both it and the hip joint are well supported by the muscles of the croup and thigh. These muscles are particularly massive in the horse, in which they round the contours in a distinctive fashion. In consequence, it is more difficult to appreciate the features and orientation of the pelvis of the horse than those of the pelves of other domestic species.

The coxal tuber is a conspicuous landmark that is palpable in its whole extent and visible in its upper part (Fig. 24.1/*2*). The sacral tuber (Fig. 24.1/*2′*), difficult to palpate in most animals, rises a little above the level of the adjacent spinous processes. The ischial tuber (Fig. 24.1/*3*) is also not always easy to appreciate, although its location and a general impression of its form may be obtained on deep palpation over the muscles that form the caudal contour of the croup and thigh. The slope of the pelvis may be estimated by visualizing the line joining the coxal and ischial projections. In the standard, generally approved conformation, this line forms an angle of about 30 degrees with the horizon, and the sacrum more or less horizontal. When the angle is significantly smaller—and the two tubers come close to sharing the same horizontal plane—the tail appears to be set high. When the angle is significantly greater, the animal is said to be goose rumped. The croup is short in such animals, and leverage and length of the hamstring muscles are reduced. Although this is clearly disadvantageous, some compensation is obtained from the more stable support the limbs afford the trunk, and many horsemen and horsewomen find a gently sloping croup acceptable in a saddle horse. Undue prominence of the sacral tubers ("hunter's bumps") sometimes develops, especially in show jumpers and other horses subjected to similar repeated stress. The deformity is commonly ascribed to subluxation of the sacroiliac joints.

The position of the hip joint may be deduced from its relationship to the greater trochanter of the femur. This protuberance is divided into low cranial and high caudal parts, separately identifiable on palpation (Fig. 24.1/*5* and *5′*). At more distal levels, the third trochanter (prominent only in this species) and the lateral epicondyle are easily distinguished and may be used to reveal the orientation of the femur. This bone is more nearly vertical than is often supposed (see Fig. 19.1).

THE HIP JOINT

The stability of the hip joint owes much to the depth and extent of the acetabulum, which is considerably increased by a fibrocartilaginous rim embracing a large part of the femoral head (Fig. 24.1/*4*). The head is additionally secured against luxation by two ligaments. One, the *ligament of the femoral head,* is short and stout but is not peculiar in any important way. The other, the *accessory ligament,* is unique to the horse (and donkey) among domestic species. It begins as a detachment from the prepubic tendon and reaches the joint by following a shallow groove on the ventral aspect of the pubis and passes through the acetabular notch to insert on the head (see Fig. 21.3/*5′*). The two ligaments together place severe restrictions on rotation and abduction of the joint. In practice, movement is almost confined to flexion and extension in a sagittal plane, which is a much more limited range than the geometry of the articular surfaces suggests. The stability of the joint is partly dependent on the tension exerted by the weight of the abdominal viscera pulling on the prepubic tendon and thus on the accessory ligament (p. 536).

Although the joint capsule is quite capacious, its deep location makes it relatively difficult to access. To puncture, the needle is introduced between the two parts of the greater trochanter and is directed horizontally and craniomedially, at an angle of about 40 degrees to the transverse plane.

THE MUSCLES OF THE HIP AND THIGH

These muscles are conveniently regarded as comprising gluteal, hamstring, medial, and cranial groups.

The Gluteal Muscles

The superficial and deep fasciae of the croup and thigh continue the corresponding coverings of the loins. The

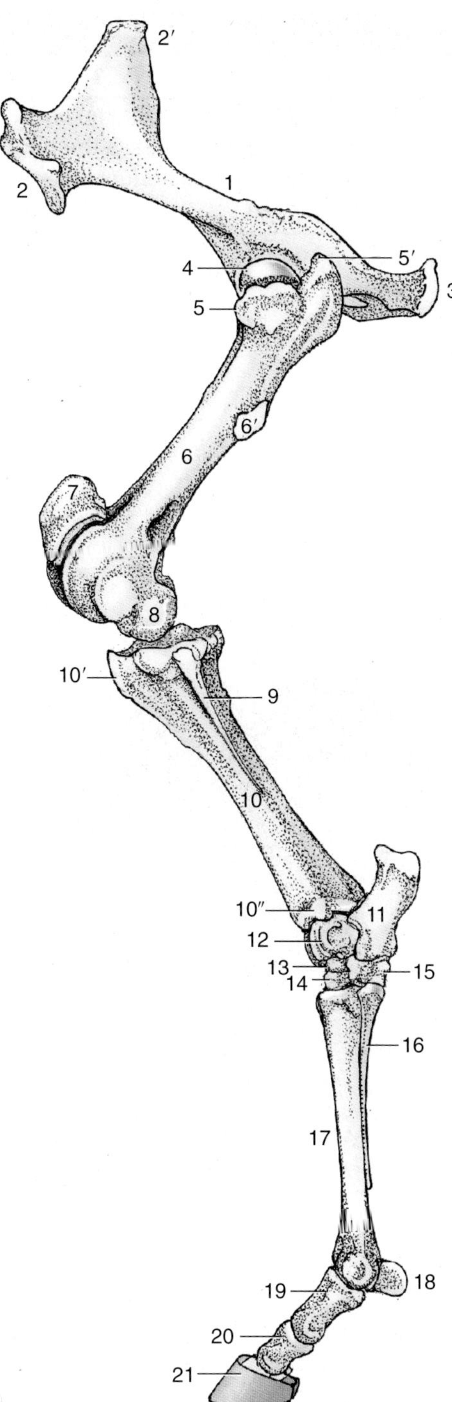

Fig. 24.1 The skeleton of the left hindlimb, lateral view. *1,* Hip bone (os coxae); *2,* coxal tuber; *2′,* sacral tuber; *3,* ischial tuber; *4,* head of femur; *5* and *5′,* cranial and caudal parts of greater trochanter, respectively; *6,* femur; *6′,* third trochanter; *7,* patella; *8,* femoral condyle; *9,* fibula; *10,* tibia; *10′,* tibial tuberosity; *10″,* lateral malleolus; *11,* calcaneus; *12,* talus; *13,* central tarsal; *14,* third tarsal; *15,* fourth tarsal; *16,* metatarsal IV (lateral splint bone); *17,* metatarsal III (cannon bone); *18,* proximal sesamoid bones; *19, 20,* and *21,* proximal, middle, and distal phalanges, respectively—the last within the hoof.

deep fascia detaches various septa that find anchorage on the pelvic girdle and the caudal edge of the sacrosciatic ligament after passing between certain muscles. The most substantial of these separate the gluteus superficialis and biceps femoris, the biceps and semitendinosus, and the semitendinosus and semimembranosus, thus molding the muscles so that their individual contours are often clearly visible through the skin, especially in animals in "hard" training and when the muscles are contracted. The inner surface of this fascia itself, including the sides of the septa, gives origin to many fascicles of the muscles it covers.

The *tensor fasciae latae* (Fig. 24.2/*3*) radiates from its origin on the coxal tuber to end by a broad aponeurosis (fascia lata) that inserts on the patella, the lateral patellar ligament, and the cranial border of the tibia. The cranial border of the fleshy part is related to the subiliac lymph nodes. The tensor is a flexor of the hip that helps to advance the limb during the swing phase of the stride. It is supplied by the *cranial gluteal nerve.*

The *gluteus superficialis* lies between the tensor and biceps (Fig. 24.2/*4*), with separate origins from the coxal tuber and the gluteal fascia but a single insertion on the third trochanter. Occasionally, the third trochanter is broken off and pulled dorsally by the attaching muscle. The gluteus superficialis is potentially a flexor of the hip and abductor of the thigh. Its two parts are separately supplied by the *cranial* and *caudal gluteal nerves.*

The *gluteus medius* is a muscle of exceptional size and power (Fig. 24.2B/*2′*). Its wide origin spreads from a depression scooped in the surface of the longissimus dorsi, over the coxal tuber and iliac wing, to the sacrum and adjacent part of the sacrosciatic ligament. The principal insertion is to the caudal part of the greater trochanter, but a deep division—the gluteus accessorius—has a [illegible] aponeurotic attachment to the intertrochanteric line of the femur. This aponeurosis passes over the cranial part of the trochanter, where its passage is eased by the interposition of a synovial (trochanteric) bursa. This bursa may become inflamed. Horses so afflicted obtain relief by standing with the affected limb somewhat abducted and, when moving, by adopting an oblique doglike gait, swinging the limb in an arc.

This muscle is primarily an extensor of the hip, but it has a secondary use as an abductor of the thigh. Its association with the longissimus dorsi makes it an effective participant in rearing. It is supplied by the *cranial gluteal nerve.*

The *gluteus profundus* lies deep to the caudal part of the gluteus medius. It arises from and around the ischial spine and passes more or less transversely to insert on the cranial part of the greater trochanter. An abductor of the thigh, it is supplied by the *cranial gluteal nerve* (Table 24.1).

TABLE 24.1 GLUTEAL MUSCLES

Muscle	Nerve	Action
Tensor fasciae latae	Cranial gluteal	Flexes the hip to advance the limb
Superficial gluteal	Cranial and caudal gluteal	Flexes the hip and abducts the thigh
Middle gluteal	Cranial gluteal	Extends the hip and abducts the thigh
Deep gluteal	Cranial gluteal	Abducts the thigh

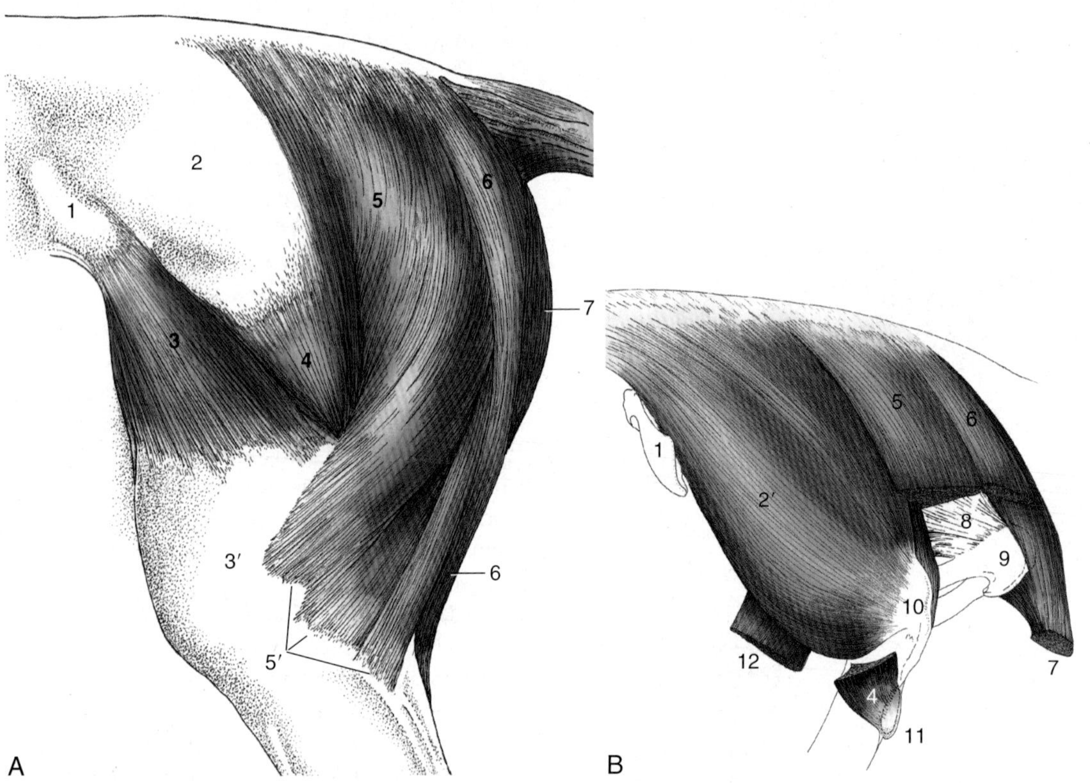

Fig. 24.2 (A) Muscles of the croup and thigh, lateral view. (B) Croup muscles, resected to expose the ischial tuber; lateral view. *1,* Coxal tuber; *2,* deep gluteal fascia; *2′,* gluteus medius; *3,* tensor fasciae latae; *3′,* fascia lata; *4,* gluteus superficialis; *5,* vertebral head of biceps; *5′,* the three distal divisions of the biceps; *6,* semitendinosus; *7,* semimembranosus; *8,* sacrosciatic ligament; *9,* ischial tuber; *10,* caudal part of greater trochanter; *11,* third trochanter; *12,* stump of rectus femoris.

The Caudal (Hamstring) Muscles

In the horse, the three muscles of this group possess well-developed vertebral heads of origin (in addition to the usual pelvic heads) that account for the characteristic filling and rounding of the croup (Fig. 24.2/*5* and *6*). The vertebral head of the *biceps* arises from the sacrum and adjacent part of the sacrosciatic ligament. It descends behind and partly covers the gluteal muscles before it crosses the ischial tuber to be joined by the smaller pelvic head that arises from that process. The muscle inserts by three divisions (Fig. 24.2/*5′*): the first in the fascia lata and on the patella, the second on the lateral patellar ligament and tibial crest, and the third, the tarsal tendon, on the common calcanean tendon. *The vertebral head is supplied by the caudal gluteal nerve, and the pelvic head is supplied by the sciatic nerve.*

The origin of the vertebral head of the *semitendinosus* (Fig. 24.2/*6*) is near that of the biceps. After merging with the pelvic head, the muscle travels to insert on the medial aspect of the tibia and the crural fascia and contributes a tarsal tendon to the common calcanean tendon. *The vertebral and pelvic heads are supplied by the caudal gluteal and sciatic nerves, respectively.*

The *semimembranosus* (Fig. 24.2/*7*) is included in the hamstring group, but topographically it is a muscle of

TABLE 24.2 HAMSTRING MUSCLES

Muscle	Nerve	Action
Biceps femoris	Vertebral head by the caudal gluteal and pelvic head by the sciatic	All can extend the hip. Extend the stifle when the limb is bearing weight, and flex the stifle when the hoof is raised. Biceps and semitendinosus extend the hock through contributions to the common calcanean tendon.
Semitendinosus	Vertebral head by the caudal gluteal and pelvic head by the sciatic	
Semimembranosus	Sciatic	

the medial aspect of the thigh. The vertebral head is relatively weak, and the pelvic head is more substantial. The combined muscle is largely covered by the gracilis and follows the caudal margin of the adductor, to which it is closely bound. It inserts by two divisions. The cranial division inserts on the medial epicondyle of the femur and the medial collateral ligament of the stifle joint; the caudal division proceeds distally to the medial condyle of the tibia. The principal nerve supply is from the *sciatic nerve* (Table 24.2).

The actions and uses of the three hamstring muscles are complicated and in certain respects enigmatic. It is clear that all three units are well placed to extend the hip. The actions of the hamstring muscles on the stifle can be better understood by dividing them into two functional units: one that inserts proximal to the axis of rotation of the joint and the other distal to it. The "proximal unit" comprises parts of the muscles that are potentially extensor, because they may straighten the stifle by drawing the femur caudally when the limb bears weight. The "distal unit" will flex the stifle when the hoof is raised from the ground but will extend it when the hoof is firmly planted. Through their contributions to the common calcanean tendon, the biceps and semitendinosus extend the hock.

Some of these actions are clearly incompatible because the movements of the stifle and hock joints are linked in their actions by the reciprocal mechanism (see p. 626). It follows that the entire hamstring group, which includes parts that may flex the stifle, cannot always contract en masse.

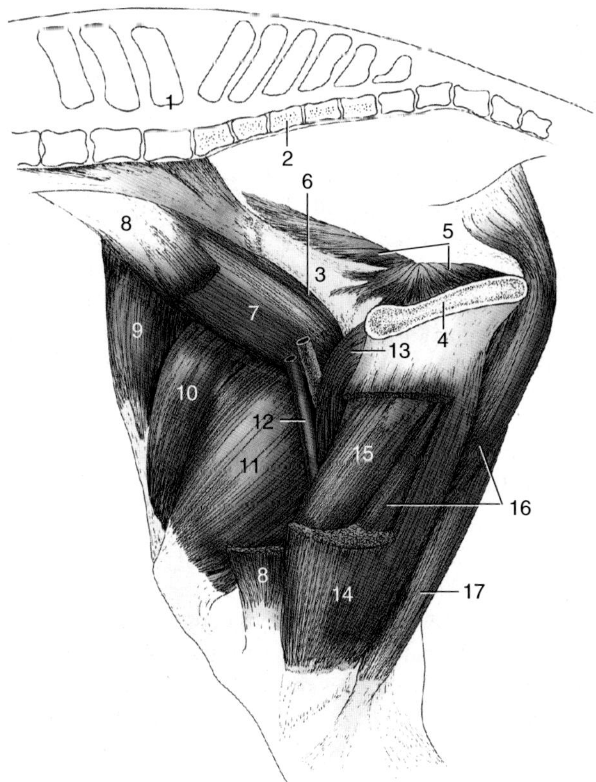

Fig. 24.3 Muscles of the thigh, medial view. *1,* Last lumbar vertebra; *2,* sacrum; *3,* shaft of ilium; *4,* pelvic symphysis; *5,* internal obturator; *6,* psoas minor; *7,* iliopsoas; *8,* sartorius, resected; *9,* tensor fasciae latae; *10,* rectus femoris; *11,* vastus medialis; *12,* femoral vessels in femoral triangle; *13,* pectineus; *14,* gracilis, fenestrated; *15,* adductor; *16,* semimembranosus; *17,* semitendinosus.

The Medial Muscles

The medial muscles are disposed in the same three layers as in other species. The superficial layer comprises the *gracilis* and *sartorius* (Fig. 24.3/*8* and *14*). The sartorius arises from the psoas fascia and the insertion tendon of the psoas minor and gains the thigh by passing through the gap between the caudal margin of the flank and the ilium. It is related to the deep inguinal lymph nodes, where it forms the cranial margin of the *femoral triangle.* The sartorius inserts on medial structures of the stifle joint, including the condyle of the tibia. Both muscles may adduct the thigh, but the sartorius is probably more important as a hip flexor. *The gracilis and the sartorius are supplied by the obturator nerve and the saphenous nerve, respectively.*

The pectineus and adductor constitute the middle layer. The *pectineus* (Fig. 24.3/*13*) is a small fusiform muscle that arises from the margin of the pubis and inserts on the medial surface of the femur. A part of the tendon of origin is from the contralateral side, and the resulting decussation

TABLE 24.3 THE MEDIAL THIGH MUSCLES

Muscle	Nerve	Action
Gracilis	Obturator	Adducts the thigh
Sartorius	Saphenous	Adducts the thigh and flexes the hip
Pectineus	Obturator	Adducts the thigh and flexes the hip
Adductor	Cranial gluteal	Adducts the thigh

The quadratus femoris, gemelli, and obturator internus (supplied by the sciatic nerve) and the obturator externus (supplied by the obturator nerve) are of minor significance.

contributes a transverse strengthening to the prepubic tendon (p. 536). The pectineus is placed to flex the hip and adduct the thigh. It is supplied by the *obturator nerve.*

The much larger *adductor* (Fig. 24.3/*15*) fills the space between the pectineus and semimembranosus. It arises from the floor of the pelvis and symphyseal tendon and inserts on the caudal surface and medial epicondyle of the femur and the medial collateral ligament of the stifle. Although adduction of the thigh is the primary function, a subsidiary extensor action is possible. Innervation is from the *obturator nerve* (Table 24.3).

The Cranial Muscles

This group comprises the *quadriceps femoris,* which possesses the usual four individually named heads of origin, and the insignificant capsularis.

The four heads of the quadriceps combine in a common insertion on the patella, and the intermediate patellar ligament (Fig. 24.4/*8*) supplies the functional continuation to the tibial tuberosity. The rectus femoris is a potential flexor of the hip, but the principal action of the group is extension of the stifle. Extension, of course, embraces stabilization of the joint to prevent its collapse when the limb bears weight during the support phase of the stride. It can be observed (and confirmed by palpation) that the muscle appears relaxed when the animal stands quietly. This suggests that, once the patella has been brought into its resting position, no considerable further effort is required of the quadriceps. Quadriceps paralysis is a very severe handicap. The animal is unable to stabilize the stifle and the hock joint, whose movements are interlinked by the reciprocal mechanism. The group is supplied by the *femoral nerve.*

THE STIFLE JOINT

Although generally conforming to the common pattern, the equine stifle also exhibits several important features of distinction. The most remarkable provide the means of "locking" the joint so that one hindlimb may support a disproportionate part of the body weight while standing

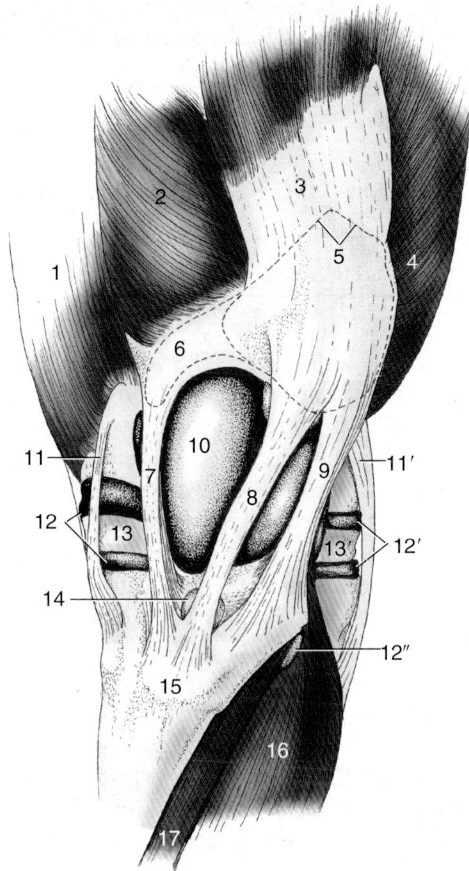

Fig. 24.4 The left stifle joint, cranial view. *1,* Adductor; *2,* vastus medialis; *3,* rectus femoris; *4,* vastus lateralis; *5,* outline of patella; *6,* outline of patellar fibrocartilage; *7, 8,* and *9,* medial, intermediate, and lateral patellar ligaments, respectively; *10,* joint capsule over medial ridge of femoral trochlea; *11* and *11′,* medial and lateral collateral ligaments, respectively; *12* and *12′,* medial and lateral femorotibial joint capsules, respectively; *12″,* recess of *12′* under combined tendon of peroneus tertius and long digital extensor; *13* and *13′,* medial and lateral menisci, respectively; *14,* distal infrapatellar bursa; *15,* tibial tuberosity; *16,* long digital extensor; *17,* tibialis cranialis.

and allow the other to be rested. The arrangement is a major component of the passive stay apparatus (p. 625).

The locking mechanism relies on certain peculiarities of the articular surfaces. The *femoral trochlea* is markedly asymmetrical. The medial ridge is larger than the lateral one and is prolonged proximally to a terminal protuberance that is easily identifiable on palpation (Figs. 24.4/*10,* 24.5/*4,* and 24.6/*2*). The trochlear surface comprises two distinct areas. The larger one, known as the *gliding surface,* corresponds to the whole trochlea of most species and faces in a predominantly cranial direction; the smaller one, known as the *resting surface,* forms a narrow shelf above the gliding surface, from which it is sharply angled to face proximally (Fig. 24.7/*18*). The *patella* is broadly diamond

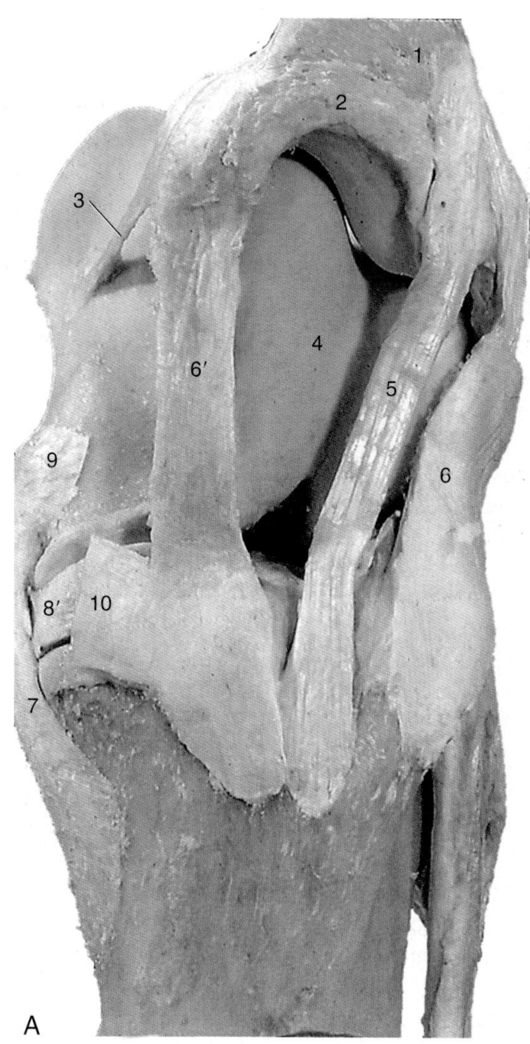

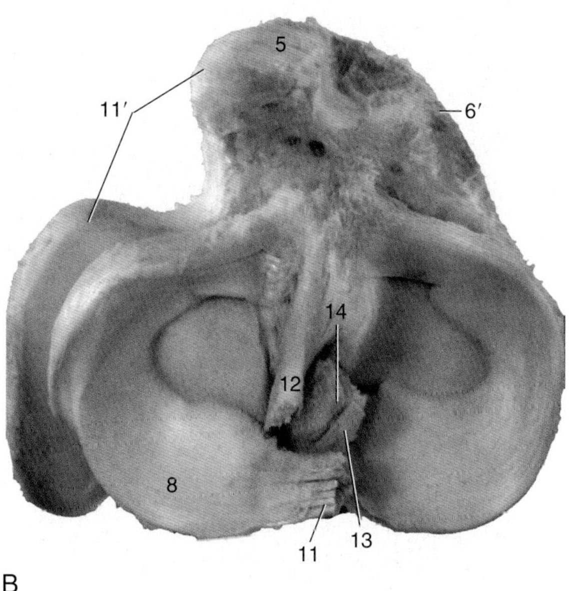

Fig. 24.5 The ligaments of the left stifle joint. (A) Medial view. (B) Proximal view of the left tibia and the menisci. *1,* Patella; *2,* patellar fibrocartilage; *3,* medial femoropatellar ligament; *4,* medial ridge of trochlea; *5,* intermediate patellar ligament; *6* and *6′,* lateral and medial patellar ligaments, respectively; *7,* lateral collateral ligament, respectively; *8* and *8′,* lateral and medial menisci, respectively; *9,* insertion of semimembranosus; *10,* insertion of gracilis and sartorius; *11,* meniscofemoral ligament; *11′,* tendon of popliteus; *12* and *13,* cranial and caudal cruciate ligaments, respectively; *14,* intercondylar eminence.

shaped when viewed from in front (Fig. 24.7B/*2*). In the fresh state it is extended medially by a *parapatellar fibrocartilage* (Fig. 24.7/*3*). The articular surface of the patella is also divided. The more extensive backward-facing area engages with the trochlea during the greater part of the normal range of movement; a narrow strip at the apex is directed distally and makes contact with the femur only at the limit of extension.

The horse has three *patellar ligaments* joined by a retinaculum in which the insertion tendons of several thigh muscles merge. The intermediate ligament (Fig. 24.4/*8*), the homologue of the single structure of the smaller species, runs from the apex of the patella to the tibial tuberosity. The lateral and medial ligaments run from the angles of the patella or, more accurately where the medial one is concerned, from the parapatellar cartilage. The three ligaments are thus quite widely separated at their origins but converge distally and insert close together. The gap between the proximal parts of the medial and intermediate ligaments is especially wide and is occupied by the medial ridge of the trochlea (Fig. 24.4/*10*).

The patella slides up and down over the femoral trochlea during the greater part of the normal movement of the joint. Only in extreme extension, as momentarily during the support phase of a walking stride, do the resting surfaces engage. The resting position is also adopted when the animal is standing squarely with its weight evenly distributed over the two hindlimbs. This is easily verified on

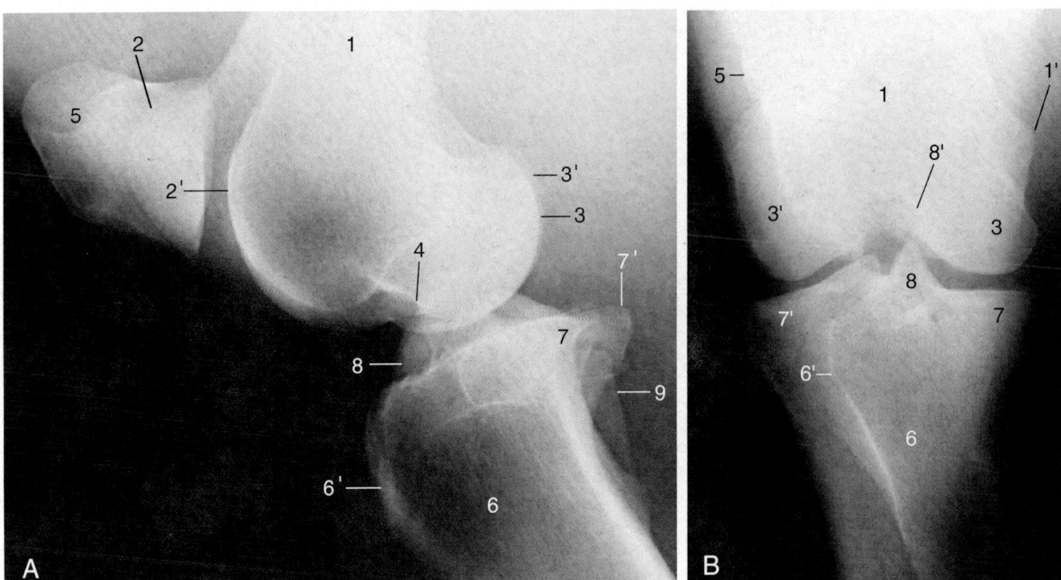

Fig. 24.6 (A) Lateral and (B) caudocranial radiographs of the stifle joint. *1*, Femur; *1'*, medial epicondyle; *2* and *2'*, medial and lateral ridges of the trochlea, respectively; *3* and *3'*, medial and lateral condyles, respectively; *4*, extensor fossa; *5*, patella; *6*, tibia; *6'*, tibial tuberosity; *7* and *7'*, medial and lateral condyles, respectively; *8*, intercondylar eminence; *8'*, intercondylar fossa; *9*, fibula.

palpation, and it can be found that the medial ligament then runs even with the edge of the corresponding ridge of the trochlea. This position is maintained without the assistance of the main extensor (quadriceps femoris) of the stifle but does require some effort on the part of the muscles that converge on the medial and lateral patellar ligaments: the biceps and tensor fasciae latae laterally and the gracilis and sartorius medially. The position is unstable and the patella is easily dislodged; it then slips back onto the gliding surface of the trochlea.

The stifle joint cavity is capacious, and its division into compartments is relatively complete. The extensive femoropatellar compartment is mainly contained between the femur, the patella, and the quadriceps. The part distal to the patella is more accessible, though separated from the patellar ligaments (and retinaculum) by a thick cushion of fat. It communicates with the medial femorotibial compartment in the large majority of horses but with the corresponding lateral compartment in far fewer (perhaps 25%). The partition between the medial and lateral compartments is almost always imperforate. The inconstancy of these arrangements should lead to an assumption that any infection spreads readily among the three compartments, while therapeutic substances should be separately injected into each.

The injections into the stifle joint require familiarity with the disposition of the ligaments and the ability to recognize them on palpation. The medial collateral ligament can be picked out close to its origin from the femoral epicondyle and provides a convenient landmark in puncture of the *medial femorotibial compartment.* The needle is introduced close to its cranial border, between it and the medial patellar ligament (Figs. 24.4/*7* and *11* and 24.5/*6'* and *7'*). The lateral collateral ligament is palpable along its whole length but is most easily found close to its insertion on the head of the fibula. The *lateral femorotibial compartment* is punctured between the lateral patellar ligament and the more cranial, and also palpable, tendon of origin of the long digital extensor (Fig. 24.4/*11'* and *16*). The *femoropatellar compartment* is also easily entered from the cranial side between the middle and the medial or the middle and the lateral patellar ligaments (Fig. 24.4/*9*). Alternatively, this compartment can be approached from the lateral side by inserting a needle behind the lateral patellar ligament.

Stifle Joint: Osteochondrosis, a developmental cartilaginous disease, is the most common disease of the stifle joint. Osteoarthritis may develop secondary to some other pathology of the stifle or may be a primary manifestation. Meniscus tears are the most common soft tissue injury in the stifle.

THE SKELETON OF THE LEG AND HOCK: THE HOCK JOINT

The *tibia* is the only functional component of the skeleton of the leg. Its shaft is thickly covered by muscle on its craniolateral and caudal aspects but is subcutaneous medially

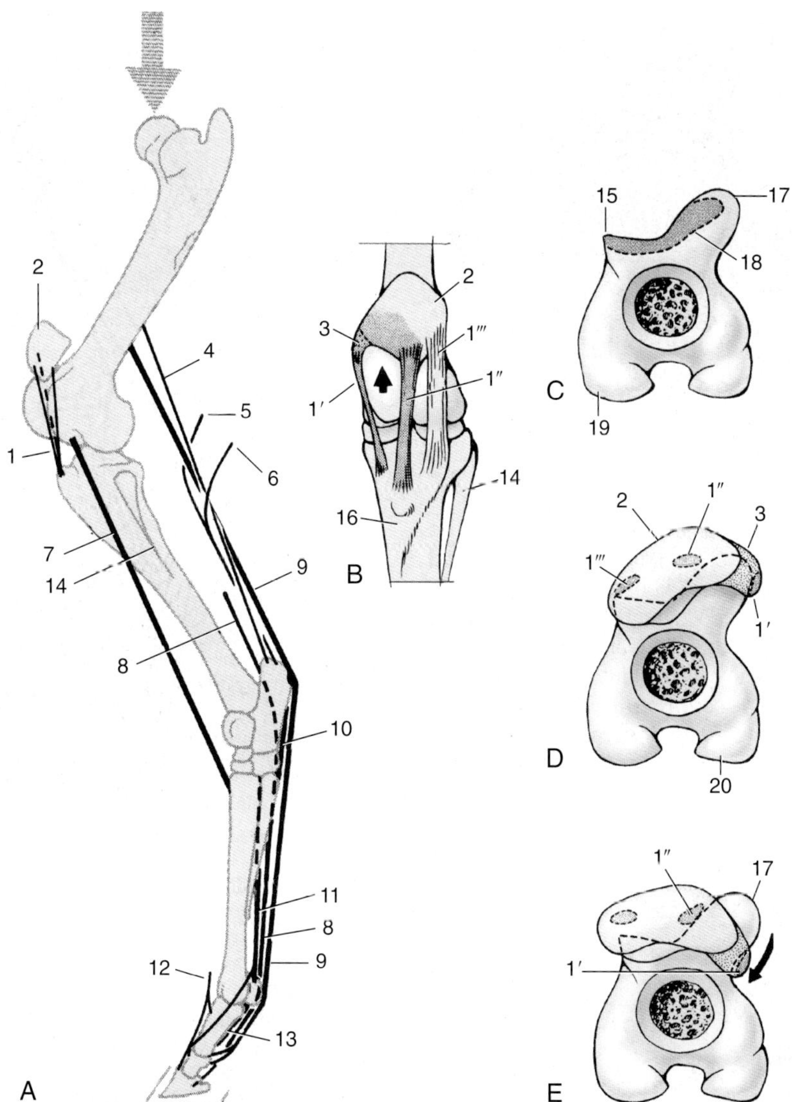

Fig. 24.7 (A) Stay apparatus of the left hindlimb, lateral view. (B) Left stifle joint, cranial view. (C to E) Distal end of left femur, looking distally; in D, position of patella in horse standing square; in E, the stifle is locked. *1,* Patellar ligaments: *1′* [medial], *1″* intermediate, and *1‴*, lateral; *2,* patella; *3,* parapatellar fibrocartilage; *4,* fibrous [illegible] with gastrocnemius; *5,* tarsal tendon of semitendinosus; *6,* tarsal [illegible] biceps; *7,* peroneus tertius; *8,* deep digital flexor; *9,* superficial digital flexor; *10,* [long plantar] ligament; *11,* interosseous; *12,* long digital extensor; *13,* sesamoidean ligaments; *14,* fibula; *15,* lateral trochlear ridge; *16,* tibia; *17,* tubercle on proximal end of medial trochlear ridge; *18,* resting surface on proximal end of trochlea; *19,* lateral condyle; *20,* medial condyle.

(Fig. 24.8/*1*). The distal articular surface, known as the *cochlea,* comprises two grooves separated by a ridge, all with a craniolateral inclination. The cochlea is flanked by medial and lateral malleoli (Fig. 24.9/*2* and *2′*).

The *fibula* is much reduced. The proximal extremity or head forms a tight articulation with the lateral condyle of the tibia (Fig. 24.1/*9*). The head usually continues into a short and rodlike shaft, but sometimes a band of soft tissue intervenes; this may simulate a fracture when depicted in a radiograph. In later embryonic life the isolated distal extremity of the fibula becomes assimilated within the tibia, to which it furnishes the lateral malleolus (see Fig. 2.59D and E/*6′*). The independence of the malleolar center of ossification is clearly evident in radiographs of young animals, and the line of union may be evident in the adult bone. The hock (Fig. 24.9) comprises the following elements: talus and calcaneus in the proximal row, a central tarsal bone in the intermediate row, and fused first and second bones and separate third and fourth bones in the distal row. The proximodorsal surface of the talus (Fig. 24.9/*3*) carries an oblique trochlea corresponding to the cochlea of the tibia. The distal surface is more or less flat

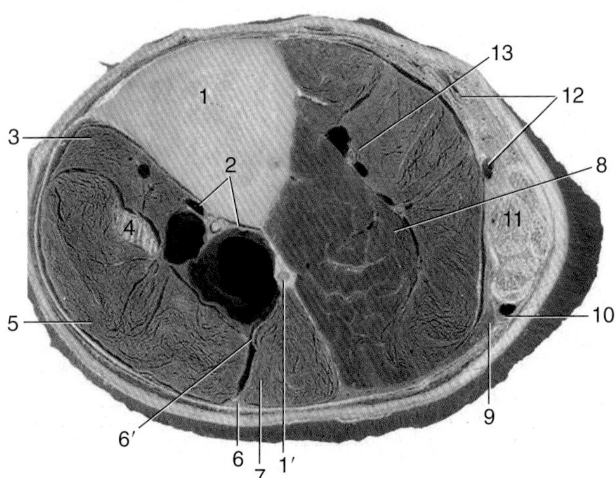

Fig. 24.8 Transverse section of the left leg slightly above its middle. *1,* Tibia; *1′,* fibula; *2,* cranial tibial vessels; *3,* tibialis cranialis; *4,* peroneus tertius; *5,* long digital extensor; *6* and *6′,* superficial and deep peroneal nerves, respectively; *7,* lateral digital extensor; *8,* deep digital flexors; *9,* soleus; *10,* lateral saphenous vein and caudal cutaneous sural nerve; *11,* superficial digital flexor surrounded by the other components of the common calcanean tendon (gastrocnemius and tarsal tendons of semitendinosus and biceps); *12,* caudal branch of medial saphenous vein, tibial nerve, and saphenous artery; *13,* caudal tibial vessels.

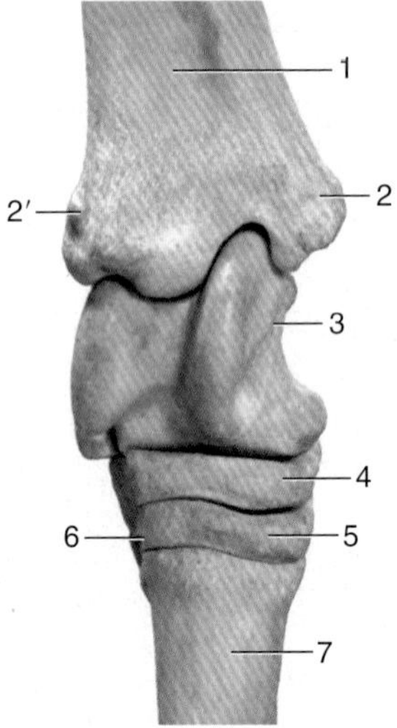

Fig. 24.9 Dorsal view of the right hock. *1,* Tibia; *2,* medial malleolus; *2′,* lateral malleolus; *3,* talus with trochlea; *4,* central tarsal bone; *5,* third tarsal bone; *6,* fourth tarsal bone; *7,* third metatarsal (cannon) bone.

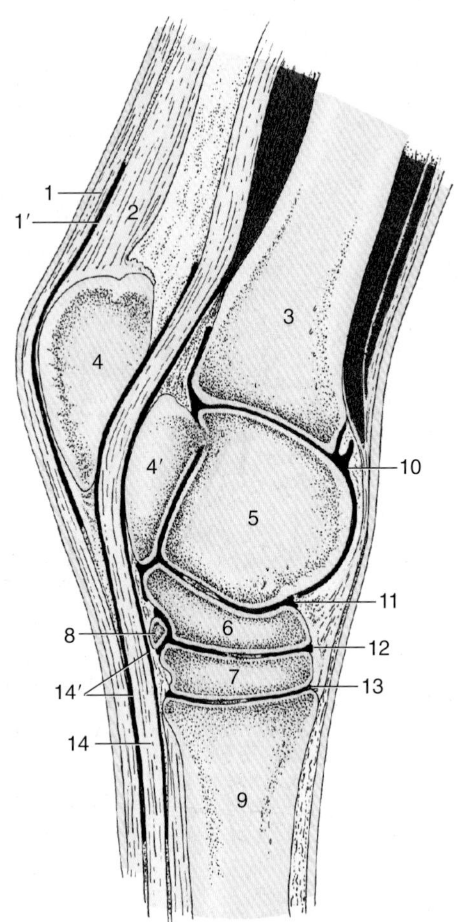

Fig. 24.10 Sagittal section of the hock joint. *1,* Superficial digital flexor; *1′,* subtendinous calcanean bursa; *2,* gastrocnemius; *3,* tibia; 4, calcaneus; *4′,* sustentaculum tali; *5,* talus; *6,* central tarsal; *7,* third tarsal; *8,* fourth tarsal (mainly on lateral side); *9,* large metatarsal (cannon) bone; *10,* tarsocrural joint; *11,* proximal intertarsal joint (communicates with *10*); *12,* distal intertarsal joint; *13,* tarsometatarsal joint; *14,* deep digital flexor; *14′,* tarsal sheath.

and rests on the central bone. The calcaneus (Fig. 24.10/*4* and *4′*) lies largely to the plantar aspect of the talus, and its tuber rises about 5 cm above the tarsocrural joint space. The composite bone formed by the first and second tarsal bones is relatively small and lies mainly behind the much larger, wedge-shaped third tarsal (Fig. 24.9/*5*). The fourth bone (Fig. 24.9/*6*; on the lateral side) is cuboidal, unlike the other bones in the distal row, which are flattened; its greater depth causes it to occupy both the intermediate and the distal tiers. The bones of the distal row articulate with the metatarsal bones—that is, the third (cannon) bone centrally and the much smaller second and fourth (splint) bones to the sides.

Even cursory examination of the tarsal skeleton is sufficient to make it plain that, although free movement is allowed at the tarsocrural joint, there can be almost no motion at any other level. The obliquity of the articular surfaces of the tibia and talus ensures that the distal part of the limb is carried outward as well as forward when the hock joint is flexed.

The fibrous layer of the joint capsule extends from the tibia to the metatarsus. It is firmly attached over various parts of the skeleton but is free elsewhere and then varies considerably in strength, with bulging of weaker parts when the synovial sac is distended. Numerous ligaments are associated with the hock, but the majority are short and are conveniently regarded as mere local thickenings of the capsule. Three that are larger and more discrete are of greater importance. *Paired collateral ligaments* extend from the malleoli to the corresponding splint bones and may be palpated along their whole lengths (Fig. 24.11D/*9* and *9'*). They have intermediate attachments to the bones they cross, and these help ensure that movements of the hock are restricted to flexion and extension at the tarsocrural level. A *long plantar ligament* (Fig. 24.11D/*10*) follows the plantar aspect of the calcaneus, passes over the fourth tarsal, and then continues distally onto the proximal part of the metatarsus. It is largely covered by the tendon of the superficial digital flexor but may be palpated to each side of this. It is commonly strained about the middle of its length, and in lateral view the resulting thickening gives a convex profile to the plantar aspect of the hock. The condition is known as a *curb,* from the French *courbe* (curve, contour).

The hock is a compound joint with *three joint sacs*: one common to the tarsocrural and proximal intertarsal levels, one for the distal intertarsal level, and one for the tarsometatarsal level (Fig. 24.10/*10–13*). The tarsometatarsal and the distal intertarsal joints have been found to communicate with each other. However, for diagnostic and therapeutic purposes both joints should be injected separately. The distal intertarsal sac may be punctured from the medial side, while access to the tarsometatarsal sac may be gained between the fourth tarsal and the head of the splint bone (Fig. 24.12). The novice will find neither technique very reliable. The proximal part of the talocrural sac is capacious and is prone to overdistention and pouching at its weakest points. There are three such pouches. One, at the dorsomedial aspect of the hock, is bounded by the tendon of the peroneus tertius, the medial collateral ligament, the medial malleolus, and the medial branch of the tendon of the tibialis cranialis (Figs. 24.11D/*8* and 24.11A–C). The sac is easily punctured here, even when it is not distended, but care must be taken to avoid the cranial branch of the medial saphenous vein at this site. The second and third pouches are on the plantar aspect. One is found between the medial collateral ligament and the deep flexor tendon at the level of the medial malleolus; the other is behind the lateral collateral ligament, between the calcaneus and the lateral malleolus. Unless the joint sac is considerably distended, puncture at either of these sites may prove difficult.

Swelling of the joint sac may be confused with swelling of the synovial (tarsal) sheath around the deep flexor tendon (Fig. 24.11/*3''*). The differential diagnosis is simple. When the joint sac is distended, pressure applied to either plantar pouch is transmitted to the dorsal pouch (and vice versa). Swelling of the tarsal sheath is transmitted from plantaromedial to plantarolateral (or vice versa) but not to the dorsal aspect upon application of local pressure.

Osteoarthritis is the most diagnosed disease of the tarsus, and it occurs in three forms. The one that involves the distal tarsal joints is called *spavin,* and the second occurs between the talus and the calcaneus. The last form is called *high spavin* and occurs at the tarsocrural joint. The changes most commonly begin on the medial aspect, near the meeting of the third and central tarsal and third metatarsal bones. This region, the *seat of spavin,* is crossed by the medial branch of the tibialis cranialis tendon (the cunean tendon of clinical authors) (Fig. 24.11/*7*) en route to its insertion on the combined first and second tarsal bones. The tendon is a useful reference point because it is palpable. A portion is sometimes resected for the purposes of reducing pressure over the lesion and eliminating movement between the distal tarsal elements. The treatment is often effective in reducing pain, although obviously it does not cure the condition. Moreover, the swelling of the tendon sheath is evident about 5 cm proximal to the plantar swelling of the joint.

THE MUSCLES OF THE LEG

The leg is enveloped by three layers of fascia. The superficial layer continues the corresponding fascia of the thigh. The middle layer is formed by the aponeuroses of the tensor fasciae latae, biceps, semitendinosus, gracilis, and sartorius. Its lateral and medial parts combine on the caudal aspect to form a stout plate that bridges the space between the deep flexor and the common calcanean tendon. The plate receives the tarsal tendons of the biceps and semitendinosus and attaches to the calcaneus as part of the common calcanean tendon formation. The saphenous artery, medial and lateral saphenous veins, and lateral and caudal sural nerves are enclosed between the superficial and middle fasciae. The deep fascial layer extends septa that pass between the muscles to attach to the tibia. It thus divides the leg into a number of osteofascial compartments.

The Craniolateral Muscles

This group comprises the tibialis cranialis, peroneus tertius, and long and lateral digital extensors. All are flexors of the hock, and those that proceed farther are extensors of the digit. The *tibialis cranialis* arises from the lateral condyle and tuberosity of the tibia and continues distally, closely applied to the bone (Fig. 24.8/*3*). The insertion tendon begins just above the level of the hock and passes through a split in the tendon of the peroneus tertius before dividing itself. The larger dorsal branch continues to the metatarsal tuberosity. The smaller medial branch diverges to cross the medial collateral ligament before inserting on the combined first and second tarsal bones (Fig. 24.11). When the muscle contracts, it presses on the seat of spavin. Although the tibialis cranialis appears to be a flexor of the hock, it is difficult to be certain of its function. According

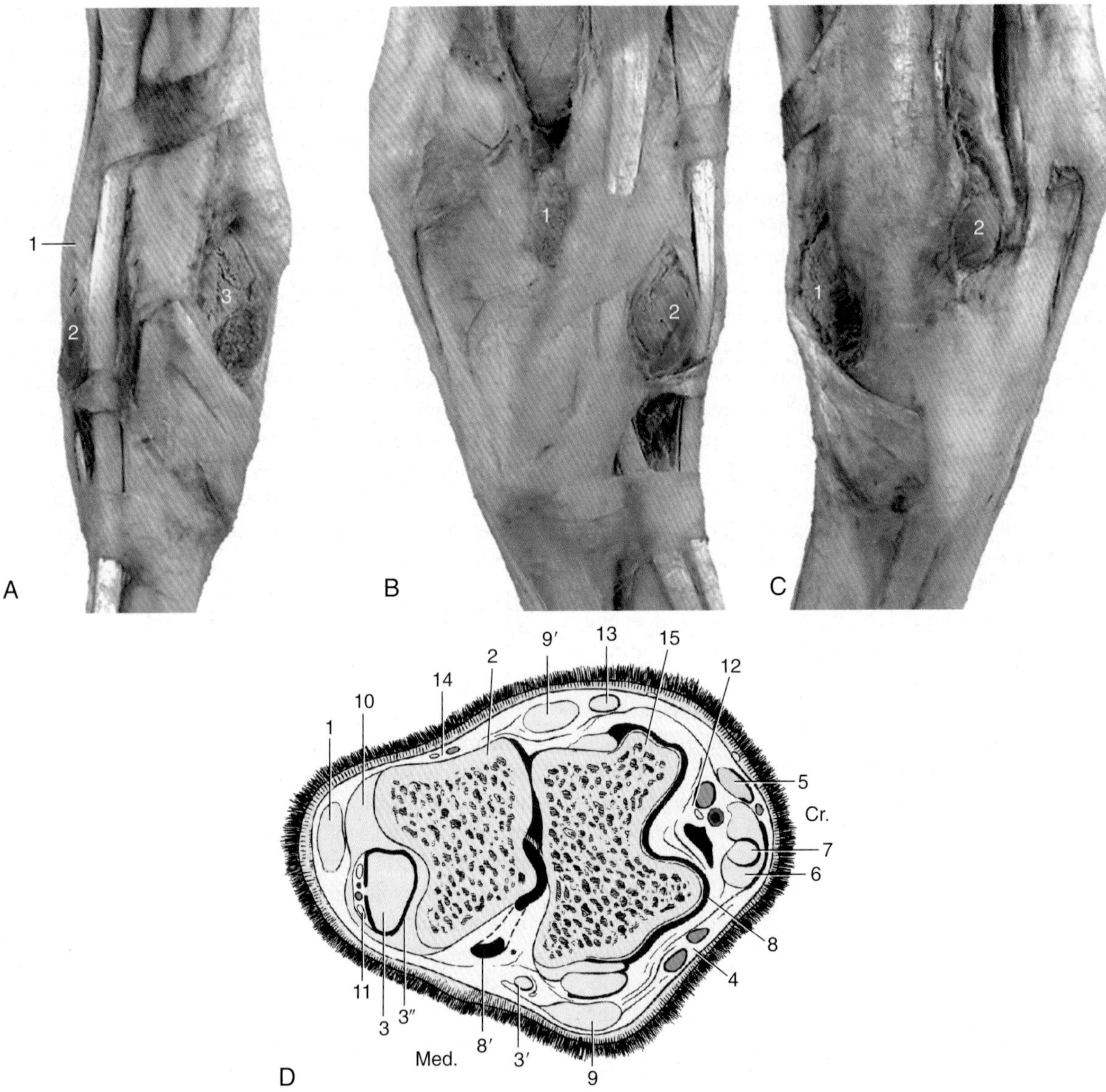

Fig. 24.11 (A to C) Illustrations of hock. (A) Dorsal view of right hock. *1,* Long digital extensor; *2* and *3,* laterodorsal and mediodorsal pouches of tarsocrural joint, respectively, filled with latex. (B) Lateral view of right hock. *1* and *2,* Lateral plantar and laterodorsal pouches of tarsocrural joint, respectively, filled with latex. (C) Medial view of right hock. *1* and *2,* Mediodorsal and medioplantar pouches of tarsocrural joint, respectively. (D) Bursae, tendon sheaths, and joint pouches of the left hock. *1,* Superficial digital flexor; *2,* calcaneus; *3,* lateral deep digital flexor and tibialis caudalis (combined tendon in B); *3′,* tendon of medial deep digital flexor; *3″,* tarsal sheath; *4,* cranial branch of medial saphenous vein; *5,* long digital extensor; *6,* peroneus tertius; *7,* tibialis cranialis and underlying bursa; *8* and *8′,* dorsal and medioplantar pouches of tarsocrural joint, respectively; *9* and *9′,* medial and lateral collateral ligaments (superficial parts), respectively; *10,* long plantar ligament; *11,* plantar nerves and saphenous vessels; *12,* cranial tibial vessels and deep peroneal nerve; *13,* lateral digital extensor; *14,* caudal cutaneous sural nerve and lateral saphenous vein; *15,* talus; *Cr.,* cranial; *Med.,* medial.

to one view, its prime role is to counteract the bending moment applied to the tibia by the action of other muscles and by gravity.

The *peroneus tertius* is almost exclusively tendinous (Fig. 24.8/*4*). It arises from the lower end of the femur together with the long extensor, and for much of its course it is recessed in the deep surface of that muscle. It bifurcates at the hock with the lateral branch inserting on the calcaneus and fourth tarsal bone, and the dorsal one on the proximal part of the third tarsal and third metatarsal

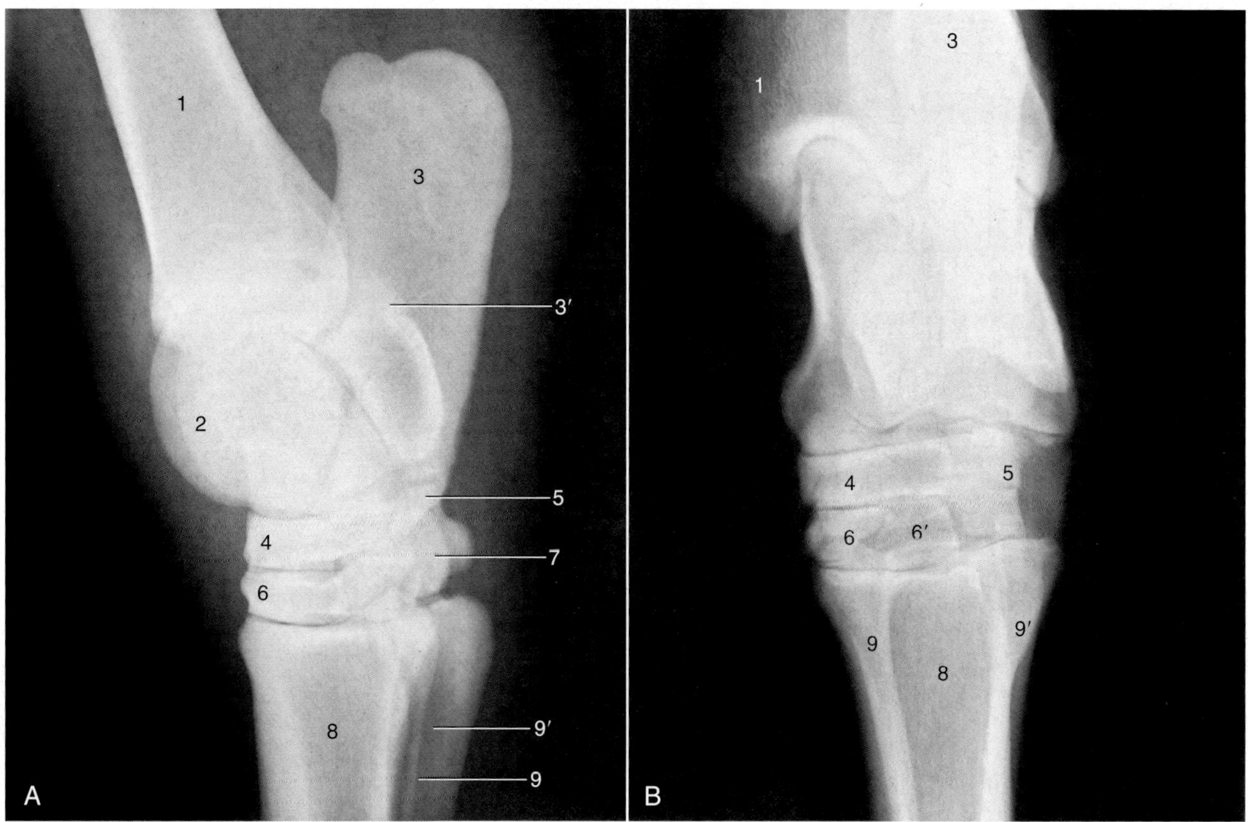

Fig. 24.12 (A) Lateral and (B) dorsoplantar radiographs of the hock joint. *1,* Tibia; *2,* talus; *3,* calcaneus; *3′,* sustentaculum tali; *4,* central tarsal; *5,* fourth tarsal; *6,* third tarsal (in B, superimposed on tarsal 1 and 2); *6′,* plantar projection of third tarsal; *7,* tarsals 1 and 2; *8,* large metatarsal bone; *9* and *9′,* medial and lateral splint bones, respectively.

bones (Fig. 24.13/*1*). The tendon links the actions of the stifle and hock joints. Rupturing of this muscle (see Fig. 24.16A) enables extension of the hock while retaining a flexed stifle, which is a combination of movements normally impossible.

The *long digital extensor,* the largest muscle of the group, arises in common with the peroneus tertius by a short tendon. This is soon succeeded by a broad belly that covers the tibialis cranialis (Fig. 24.14/*5*). The insertion tendon begins in the lower leg and continues to the extensor process of the distal phalanx, with passing attachments to the proximal and middle phalanges. It is joined by the smaller tendon of the lateral digital extensor (Fig. 24.14/*6*) near the middle of the cannon. As it descends on the dorsal surface of the limb, it is surrounded by a synovial sheath from retinacula where it crosses the hock. This muscle is capable of flexion of the hock and extension of the digit.

The *lateral digital extensor* runs between the long extensor and the deep flexor on the lateral aspect of the limb. It arises from the lateral collateral ligament of the stifle and adjacent parts of both tibia and fibula and ends by joining the long extensor tendon. Its tendon is also held down by retinacula and protected by a synovial sheath where it crosses the hock. A very small, short digital extensor muscle (extensor digitalis brevis) occupies the angle between the converging tendons of the larger muscles (Fig. 24.14/*10*). It is of no importance (Table 24.4).

All muscles of the craniolateral group are supplied by the *peroneal nerve.*

The Caudal Muscles

This group comprises the popliteus, whose action is confined to the stifle, and the gastrocnemius, soleus, and superficial and deep digital flexors, which all extend the hock with the last two also flexing the digit.

The *popliteus* is a relatively small triangular muscle placed directly over the caudal aspect of the stifle joint (Fig. 24.15B/*7*). It arises from the lateral condyle of the femur and inserts on the caudomedial border of the tibia. The popliteus flexes the stifle and rotates the leg inward.

The *gastrocnemius,* the most superficial and largest muscle of the group, arises by two heads from the supracondylar tuberosities of the femur (Fig. 24.15/*1*). The heads, which are first covered by the hamstring muscles, soon unite in a single strong tendon that is a major component of the calcanean tendon. The gastrocnemius tendon inserts on the point of the hock where it is covered by the tendon of the superficial flexor. To attain this deep

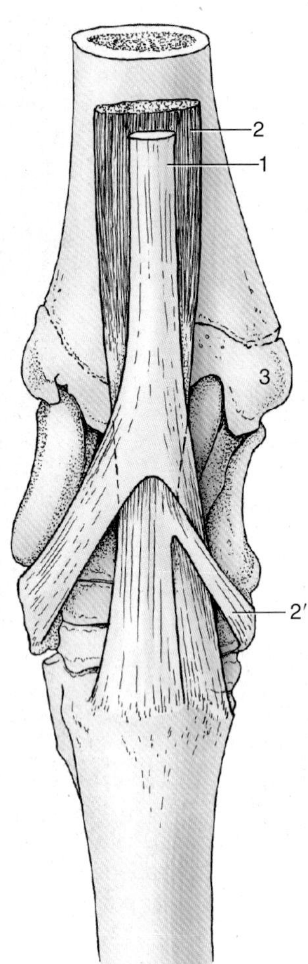

Fig. 24.13 The insertion of the flexors of the right hock, dorsal view. *1,* Peroneus tertius, splitting into dorsal and lateral branches; *2,* tibialis cranialis, splitting into dorsal and medial (cunean, *2′*) branches; *3,* medial malleolus.

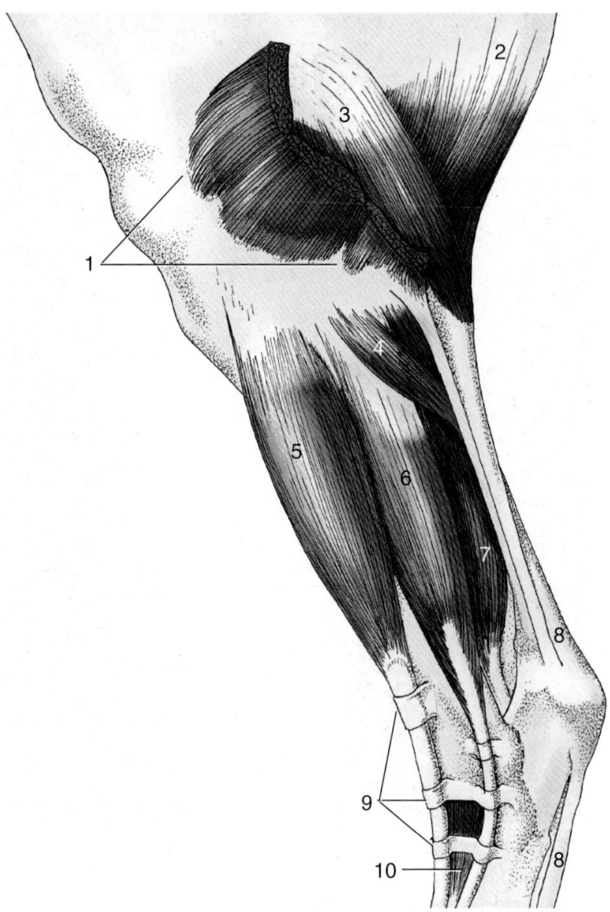

Fig. 24.14 The stifle and leg, lateral view. *1,* Distal divisions of biceps; *2,* semitendinosus; *3,* gastrocnemius; *4,* soleus; *5,* long digital extensor; *6,* lateral digital extensor; *7,* deep digital flexors; *8,* superficial digital flexor; *9,* proximal, middle, and distal extensor retinacula; *10,* extensor digitalis brevis.

position, it must first wind around the lateral border of the flexor tendon, where it is cushioned by the interposition of a synovial bursa (see later). Theoretically, the gastrocnemius is a flexor of the stifle and extensor of the hock, but because the tendons of the peroneus tertius and superficial flexor ensure that these joints extend or flex together, it is difficult to envisage its action. It has been asserted that its prime function is comparable to that of the tibialis cranialis—that is, adjustment of the load on the tibia. A ribbon-like soleus runs from the head of the fibula to the gastrocnemius tendon but is of no importance.

The *superficial digital flexor* (Fig. 24.15B/*3*) is largely tendinous, although it has a slightly greater content of flesh than the peroneus tertius. The highly diminished muscle fibers dampen the vibrations in the tendinous part to prevent overheating and tissue damage. It arises from the supracondylar fossa of the femur under cover of the gastrocnemius and, twisting around the medial surface of the tendon of that muscle, passes toward the calcanean tuber, where it expands to form a cap. The medial and lateral edges attach at the tuber, and the main part continues over the plantar aspect of the hock to enter the cannon, followed by insertion on the first and second phalanges in similar fashion to the superficial flexor of the forelimb. A considerable synovial bursa protects the expanded tendon where it caps the tuber, and also extends proximally between the flexor and gastrocnemius tendons, where they wind around each other (Fig. 24/10/*1′*). A second, smaller, subcutaneous bursa may form over the expanded tendon where it caps the calcaneus ("capped hock"). Both bursae usually communicate and are liable to inflammation and distention. The proximal part of the muscle is a main constituent of the so-called reciprocal mechanism (p. 626). The distal part supports the fetlock and pastern joints in similar fashion to the superficial flexor of the forelimb (Table 24.5).

The *deep digital flexor* arises by three separate and individually named heads—lateral digital flexor, medial digital flexor, and tibialis caudalis—which later unite to form a single stout tendon of insertion. The medial flexor arises from the lateral condyle of the tibia but soon swings to the

TABLE 24-4 THE CARIOLATERAL MUSCLES OF THE LEG

Muscle	Nerve	Action
Tibialis cranialis	Peroneal	Flexes the hock; may counter the gravity and muscular actions on the tibia
Peroneus tertius	Peroneal	Links the hock and stifle actions as part of the reciprocal apparatus
Long digital extensor	Peroneal	Flexes the hock and extends the digits
Lateral digital extensor	Peroneal	Flexes the hock and extends the digits

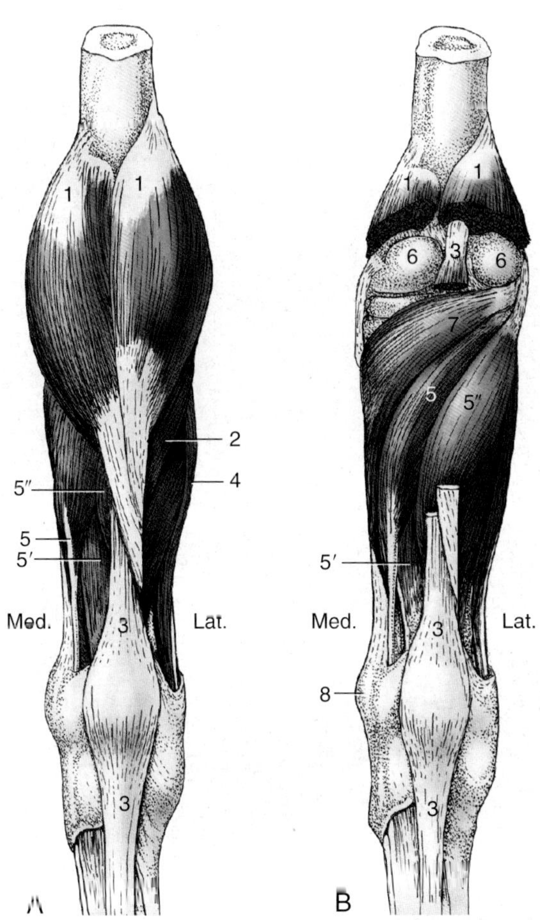

Fig. 24.15 (A) Superficial and (B) deep muscles of the right leg, caudal view. *1,* Gastrocnemius; *2,* soleus; *3,* superficial digital flexor; *4,* lateral digital extensor; *5, 5′,* and *5″,* medial and lateral deep digital flexors and tibialis caudalis, respectively; *6,* femoral condyles; *7,* popliteus; *8,* medial malleolus; *lat.,* lateral; *Med.,* medial.

medial side of the leg (Fig. 24.15/*5*). The narrow tendon passes the hock, resting within a groove on the medial malleolus and medial collateral ligament, where it is protected by a synovial sheath. Once past the hock, the tendon unites with the tendon common to the other two bellies.

The lateral flexor and the tibialis caudalis have extensive origins from the caudal surface of the tibia, distal to the attachment of the popliteus (Fig. 24.15/*5′* and *5″*). They are difficult to separate, and there is little merit in attempting the distinction because the tendons combine in the lower part of the leg. The common tendon crosses the plantar aspect of the hock over the sustentaculum tali of the calcaneus. A synovial (tarsal) sheath invests the tendon from the distal part of the leg to its junction with the tendon of the medial flexor in the upper part of the cannon (Fig. 24.11D/*3″*). A further tendinous slip (the *accessory ligament*) that passes from the joint capsule to join the common tendon is analogous to the forelimb formation but is usually less developed and may even be absent. The distal part of the tendon comports itself similarly to the corresponding part of the deep digital flexor of the forelimb.

The deep plantar metatarsal fascia resembles the corresponding forelimb fascia and offers the same obstruction to palpation of the flexor tendons in the proximal half, and more, of the cannon.

The *tibial nerve* supplies all muscles of the caudal group.

The remaining structures of the metatarsus and digit closely resemble the corresponding parts of the forelimb. Certain quantitative differences have been mentioned (p. 574 and 588 and see Fig. 23.36).

THE PASSIVE STAY APPARATUS

The caudal end of the trunk rests on the head of the femur. A vertical line dropped from the center of the support passes caudal to the stifle joint and cranial to the hock, fetlock, and pastern joints before intersecting the hoof (Fig. 24.7A/*arrow*). If unsupported, the bony column of the hindlimb would collapse by flexion of the stifle and hock and overextension of the fetlock and pastern joints. The tendons and ligaments of the passive stay apparatus enable the horse to prevent this collapse using only a minimum of muscular effort.

The supportive mechanisms below the hock are very similar to those of the forelimb (pp. 602-606). However, the accessory ligament of the deep digital flexor tendon, which arises from the caudal aspect of the hock, is weak and occasionally absent. This is compensated by the firm, intermediate attachment of the superficial digital flexor tendon to the point of the hock, which is broadly comparable in function to the accessory ligament of the corresponding

TABLE 24-5 THE CAUDAL MUSCLES OF THE LEG

Muscle	Nerve	Action
Popliteus	Tibial	Flexes the stifle and inwardly rotates the leg
Gastrocnemius	Tibial	Theoretically, flexes the hip and extends the hock, but major function is adjustment of load on the tibia
Superficial digital flexor	Tibial	Flexes the digits
Deep digital flexor	Tibial	Flexes the digits

tendon of the forelimb. The part of the superficial flexor tendon between its attachments proximal and distal to the fetlock joint is tensed when weight is on the limb and assists the interosseous muscle in supporting the fetlock.

Fixation of the stifle and hock joints depends on the locking mechanism of the former joint and the existence of the so-called reciprocal mechanism, which associates the movements of the two joints. For the horse to "lock" the stifle, the patella is first brought into the resting position (by extending the joint) and then fixed by being rotated medially through about 15 degrees (Fig. 24.7E/*arrow*). This hooks the parapatellar cartilage and medial patellar ligament securely over the protuberance of the medial trochlear ridge (Fig. 24.7/*17*) and places the medial ligament more caudally, as much as 2 cm behind the crest of the medial ridge, than before. The patella now firmly resists displacement, and a larger part of the body weight can be lowered onto the locked joint, which enables the other hindlimb to be rested with only the toe of the hoof on the ground. The "unlocking" is effected quite briskly with lateral rotation of the patella to snap it back into its usual place.

The *reciprocal mechanism* is provided by two tendinous cords—the peroneus tertius and the superficial digital flexor—that pass between the distal end of the femur and the hock, one on the cranial and the other on the caudal aspect of the tibia (Fig. 24.7/*7* and *9*). (Fig. 24.16A demonstrates the result of the rupture of the peroneus tertius.) These ensure that the two joints flex or extend in unison. However, some looseness in the system renders it unnecessary for the angular changes at the two joints to be exactly the same, especially during fast gaits when large forces must be absorbed by the tendons.

When the stifle is locked, the weight of the hindquarters tends to flex the hock joint; this is opposed by tension in the superficial flexor caudal to the tibia. The peroneus tertius is not involved at this time, and it seems that it is superfluous in the animal standing quietly.

The stifle joint is fully locked only when the horse takes most of the weight on that limb and rests the other on the toe of the hoof. It should be emphasized that although the arrangement conserves energy, it does not eliminate

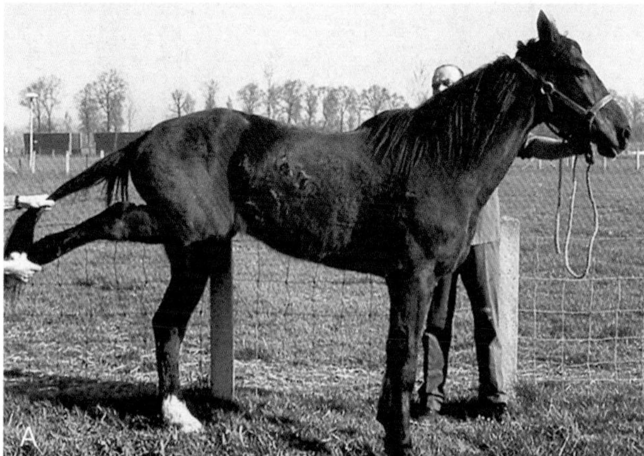

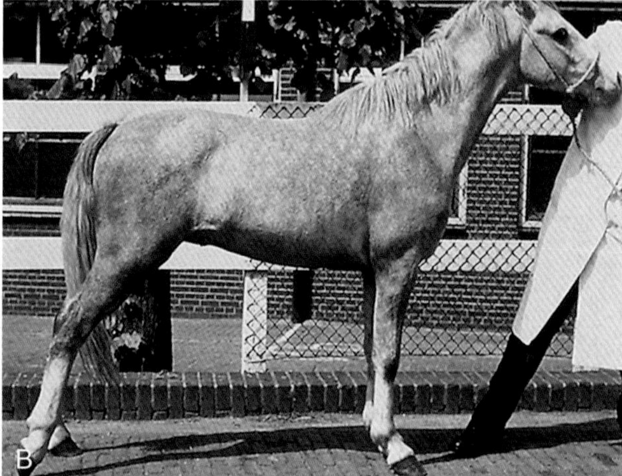

Fig. 24.16 (A) Rupture of peroneus tertius. (B) Locked patella.

muscular effort; every few minutes the animal shifts its support from one side to the other as muscles tire or, perhaps, as tension in the passive supporting structures becomes uncomfortable.

Sometimes a neuromuscular disorder makes unlocking of the stifle difficult or even impossible (Fig. 24.16B). A temporary "lock" may be broken by startling a horse into sudden movement; a persistent "lock" may be alleviated by surgical section of the medial patellar ligament to break the retention loop (Fig. 24.7B/*1'*). The operation is easily

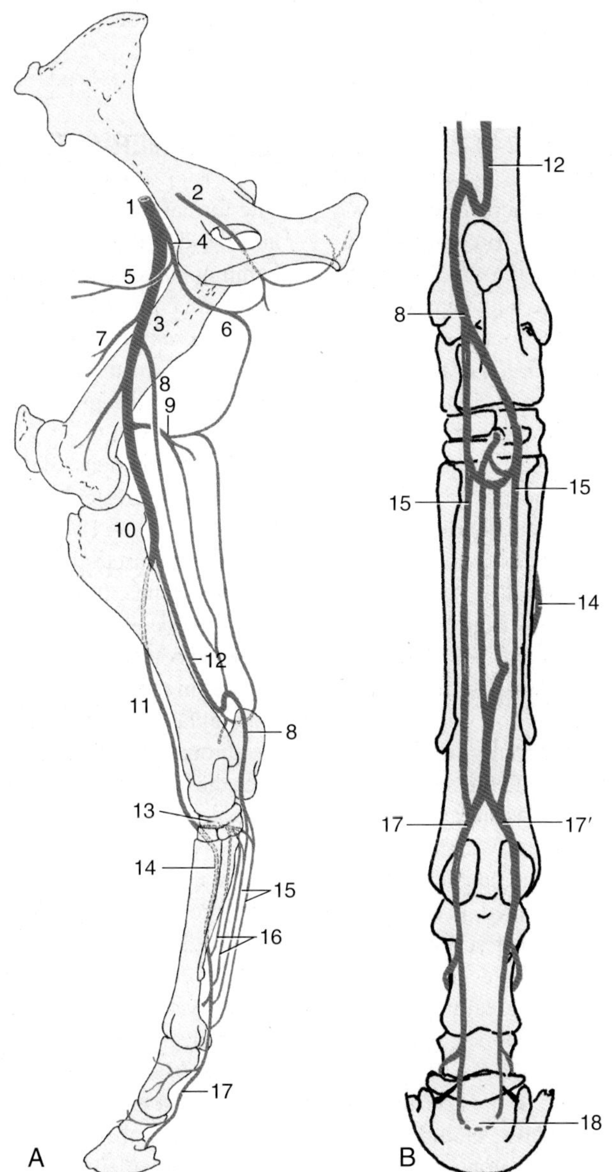

Fig. 24.17 The principal arteries (aa.) of the right hindlimb: (A) medial view; (B) caudal view. *1*, External iliac artery (a.); *2*, obturator a.; *3*, femoral a.; *4*, deep femoral a.; *5*, pudendoepigastric trunk; *6*, medial circumflex femoral a.; *7*, lateral circumflex femoral a.; *8*, saphenous a.; *9*, caudal femoral a.; *10*, popliteal a.; *11*, cranial tibial a.; *12*, caudal tibial a.; *13*, perforating tarsal a.; *14*, dorsal metatarsal a.; *15*, medial and lateral plantar aa.; *16*, medial and lateral plantar metatarsal aa.; *17* and *17′*, medial and lateral digital aa., respectively; *18*, terminal arch, anastomosis of digital aa. within the distal phalanx.

and safely performed because a considerable thickness of fat lies deep to the ligament, protecting the synovial membrane.

VASCULARIZATION OF THE HINDLIMB

The chief artery of the limb, the *femoral artery*, directly continues the external iliac artery (Fig. 24.17/*1* and *3*). It reaches the femoral triangle, traveling in company with the femoral vein and nerve and almost at once detaches the saphenous artery and several larger muscular branches. The saphenous artery (Fig. 24.17/*8*) pursues a superficial course down the medial aspect of the limb, where it may be traced almost to the hock.

The muscular branches include *deep and caudal femoral arteries* (Fig. 24.17/*4* and *9*) that anastomose with each other and with other more proximal and more distal arteries, forming an alternative pathway available when the chief trunk is obstructed. The femoral artery then passes obliquely over the femur to gain the caudal aspect of the stifle, where it passes between the heads of the gastrocnemius. The segment at the stifle, known as the popliteal artery, divides into cranial and caudal tibial arteries in the upper part of the leg.

The larger *cranial tibial artery* (Fig. 24.17/*11*) passes through the interosseous space between the fibula and tibia to gain the dorsolateral aspect where it turns distally between the muscles and the bone. It comes to the surface at the hock and continues as the *dorsal pedal artery* and then, on entering the groove between the cannon and lateral splint bones, as the dorsal metatarsal artery. A perforating branch (Fig. 24.17/*13*) of the dorsal pedal artery passes between the tarsal bones to reach the plantar aspect of the limb, where it anastomoses with branches of the saphenous artery. The dorsal metatarsal artery, the major supply to the foot, is well placed at the proximal end of the cannon for evaluation of the pulse. Toward the fetlock, it passes under the free end of the splint bone to gain the plantar aspect of the cannon, where it is reinforced by small branches from the saphenous. It ends by dividing into medial and lateral digital arteries (Fig. 24.17/*17* and *17′*) that replicate the pattern of the forelimb vessels.

The *caudal tibial artery* first runs distally in the deep flexor (Fig. 24.17/*12*). Toward the hock it enters the space before the calcanean tendon and sends a short S-shaped anastomosis to the nearby saphenous artery and a longer branch that reascends the leg to join the caudal femoral artery. The saphenous artery, thus reinforced, divides into *medial and lateral plantar arteries* that descend toward the fetlock (Fig. 24.17/*15*). These and the deeper plantar metatarsal arteries are individually of no great importance and may eventually fade away or join the dorsal metatarsal artery or its digital divisions.

The deep *veins* are largely satellite to the arteries. As in the forelimb, certain superficial trunks, including the medial and lateral saphenous veins, run alone. A branch of the former is often prominent where it crosses the dorsal aspect of the hock, and its swelling ("blood spavin") may occasionally be mistaken for a distention of the dorsal joint pouch (Fig. 24.11/*4* and *8*). Within the leg, the saphenous veins run between the calcanean tendon and the caudal muscle mass, one to each side (Fig. 24.8/*10* and *12*). The medial vein later crosses the medial aspect of the thigh to open into the femoral vein. The lateral vein joins the caudal femoral vein at the stifle.

Lymph draining from the distal part of the limb passes mainly to the group of *popliteal nodes* tucked within the popliteal fossa between the biceps and semitendinosus. Efferent vessels from this group and additional vessels that arise within the thigh proceed mainly to the *deep inguinal nodes* within the femoral triangle. Some lymph from superficial structures passes to the *subiliac nodes,* which drain into the lateral and medial iliac nodes. The courses of certain lymphatic vessels may be manifested as cords visible through the skin in some lymph-borne infections.

THE NERVES OF THE HINDLIMB

The formation and ramification of the lumbosacral plexus and the distribution of its peripheral branches follow the common pattern in broad outline; important species differences are confined to the innervation of the foot.

The *cranial and caudal gluteal nerves* attend to the innervation of the lateral muscles of the croup, including the vertebral heads of the hamstring muscles; the details have been given.

The distributions of the femoral, obturator, and sciatic nerves have greater clinical relevance. The *femoral nerve* (L4–L6) (Fig. 24.18/*1*) passes through and also supplies the sublumbar muscles before entering the thigh by way of the vascular lacuna. It then splits into several branches, most of which at once enter the quadriceps. The one branch of more extended course, the *saphenous nerve* (Fig. 24.18/*1′*), continues within the femoral triangle before penetrating the medial femoral fascia to obtain a more superficial position. It continues through the thigh, leg, and upper cannon, supplying skin over the medial aspect of the limb from thigh to fetlock. It also supplies the sartorius. Extensive damage to the femoral nerve is uncommon, but when it does occur, the consequences are paralysis of the quadriceps, inability to fix the stifle and therefore inability to support weight on the affected limb, In addition, skin sensibility is lost over a considerable area.

The *obturator nerve* (L4–L6) (Fig. 24.18/*2*) leaves the pelvis by way of the obturator foramen and innervates the adductor muscles (pectineus, gracilis, adductor, and obturator externus). Injury, which generally follows foaling or a pelvic fracture, results in partial or complete inability to adduct the limb. The severity of the dysfunction is rather unpredictable depending on the weight of the animal, the nature of the terrain, and the extent of the lesion.

The *sciatic nerve* (L6–S2) (Fig. 24.18/*4*) leaves the pelvis by the greater sciatic foramen and, after a short course over the sacrosciatic ligament, turns distally caudal to the hip joint to enter the thigh under cover of the biceps. It divides about the level of the joint into *tibial and peroneal nerves* that initially run together. They part company a little above the stifle, when the peroneal nerve moves laterally to pass between the biceps and the lateral head of the gastrocnemius. The tibial nerve holds its course and runs between the two heads of the gastrocnemius. Both divisions detach cutaneous branches while still within the thigh. That from the peroneal (lateral cutaneous sural nerve; Fig. 24.18/*5′*) becomes subcutaneous by piercing the biceps and then spreads to supply skin over the lateral aspect of the leg. The corresponding tibial branch (caudal cutaneous sural nerve; Fig. 24.18/*6′*) descends in the fascial plate between the calcanean tendon and deep flexor, following the lateral

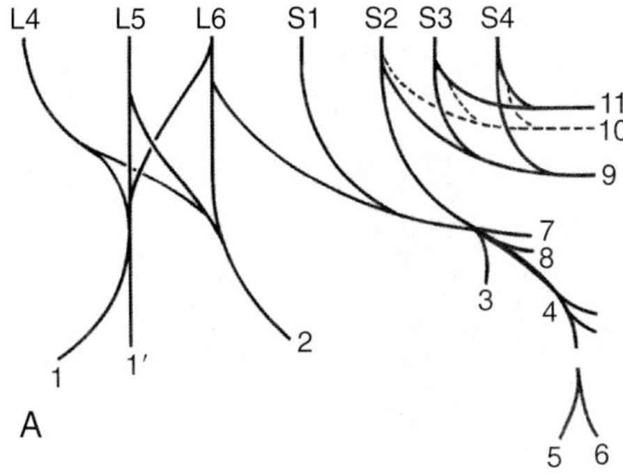

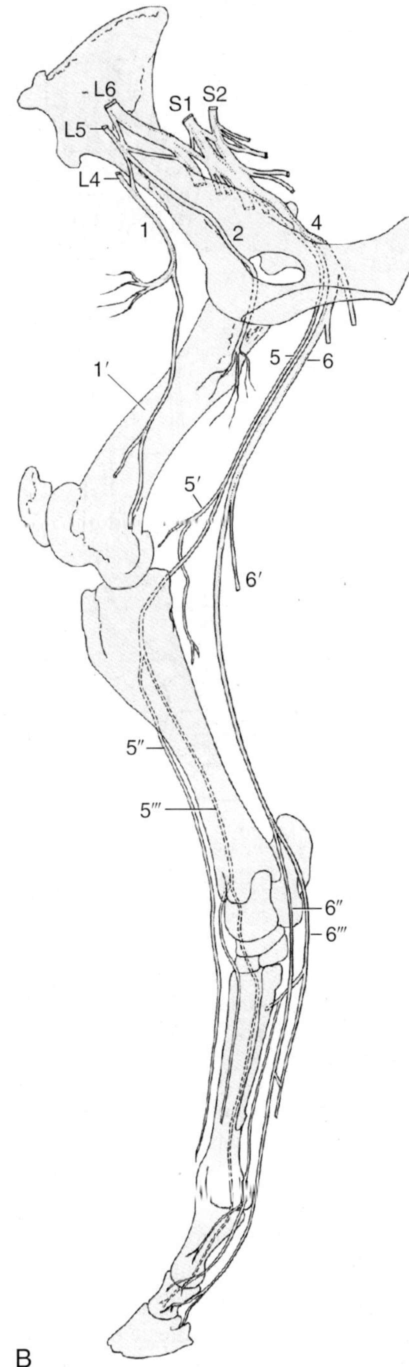

Fig. 24.18 The nerves of the hindlimb. (A) The lumbosacral plexus, schematic. *L*, Lumbar; *S*, sacral. (B) The principal nerves, medial view. *1*, Femoral nerve (n.); *1′*, saphenous n.; *2*, obturator n.; *3*, cranial gluteal n.; *4*, sciatic n.; *5*, common peroneal n.; *5′*, lateral cutaneous sural n.; *5″* and *5‴*, superficial and deep peroneal nerves, respectively; *6*, tibial n.; *6′*, caudal cutaneous sural n.; *6″* and *6‴*, medial and lateral plantar nerves, respectively (the lateral nerve gives rise to the plantar metatarsal nerves); *7*, caudal gluteal n.; *8*, caudal cutaneous femoral n.; *9*, pudendal n.; *10*, pelvic n.; *11*, caudal rectal n.

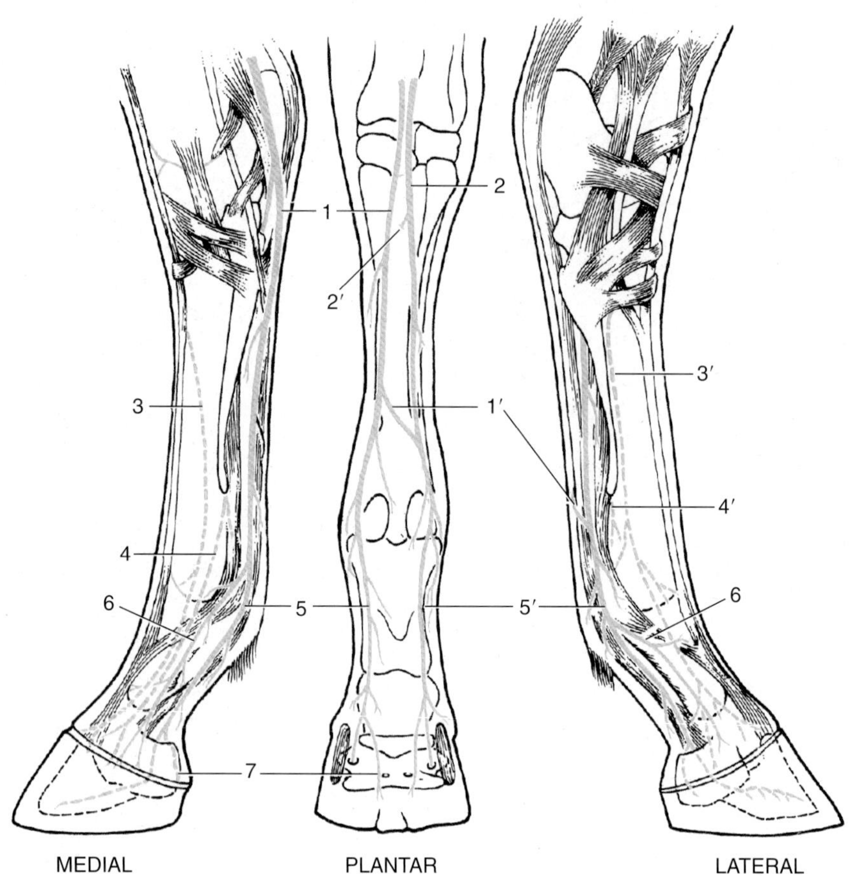

Fig. 24.19 The nerves (nn.) of the right hindfoot. *1* and *2,* Medial and lateral plantar nn. (from tibial), respectively; *1′,* communicating branch; *2′,* deep branch (for plantar metatarsal nn.), cut; *3* and *3′,* medial and lateral dorsal metatarsal nn. (from deep peroneal), respectively; *4* and *4′,* medial and lateral plantar metatarsal nn. (from lateral plantar, *2′*), respectively; *5* and *5′,* medial and lateral digital nn., respectively; *6,* dorsal branch of digital nerve; *7,* branch to digital cushion.

saphenous vein for part of its course. It supplies branches to the skin over the plantarolateral aspect of the hock and cannon, reaching to the fetlock.

The *peroneal nerve* divides caudal to the lateral collateral ligament of the stifle into deep and superficial branches. The *superficial branch* (Fig. 24.18/*5″*) continues down the leg, slightly sunken within the groove between the long and lateral extensors, where it can be palpated below the middle of the leg. It supplies the lateral extensor, the skin over the lateral aspect of the leg, and more distal segments of the limb. The *deep branch* takes a parallel course after sinking deeply between the same two muscles to follow the cranial face of the intervening septum (Figs. 24.18/*5‴* and 24.8/*6′*). It supplies branches to the remaining muscles of the dorsolateral group and then continues under cover of the long extensor tendon as a purely sensory nerve that splits into medial and lateral branches over the hock. These, the *medial and lateral dorsal metatarsal nerves,* edge toward the grooves between the cannon and splint bones (Fig. 24.19/*3* and *3′*). The lateral nerve follows the palpable dorsal metatarsal artery (Fig. 24.20/*8*). After detaching twigs to the skin and the fetlock and pastern joints, both finally fade within the hoof.

Complete section of the peroneal nerve results in inability to extend the digit actively. The hoof rests on its dorsal surface unless the ground surface is passively set down. The posture invites comparison with that which occurs in radial paralysis. Afflicted animals may learn to compensate by flicking the foot forward and planting the hoof before the impetus is lost. In addition to the motor disability, skin sensation is lost over the dorsolateral aspect of the lower part of the limb. Peroneal lesions are most frequent in two circumstances: intrapelvic damage to the sciatic nerve (which is likely also to involve the tibial division) and trauma in the region of the fibula, where the nerve is superficial (see Fig. 31.13, shown on a cow).

The *tibial nerve* dives between the two heads of the gastrocnemius and crosses the stifle on the surface of the popliteus. It detaches branches to these muscles and to other muscles of the caudal group before continuing as a sensory

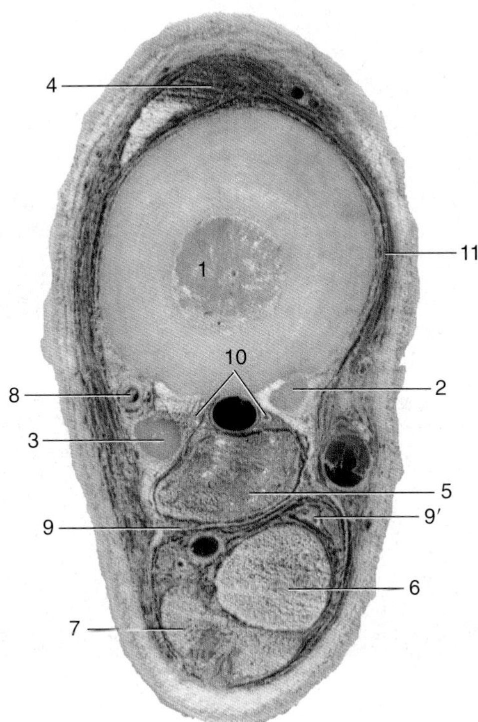

Fig. 24.20 Transverse section of the middle of the left metatarsus. *1–3,* Large and small metatarsal bones; *4,* long digital extensor; *5,* interosseous; *6,* deep digital flexor; *7,* superficial digital flexor; *8,* dorsal metatarsal artery and lateral dorsal metatarsal nerve; *9* and *9′,* lateral and medial plantar vessels and nerve; *10,* plantar metatarsal vessels and nerves; *11,* medial dorsal metatarsal nerve.

trunk in the space between the calcanean tendon and the deep flexor, where it is easily palpated (Fig. 24.8/*12*). When level with the calcaneus, it divides into medial and lateral plantar nerves that pass over the sustentaculum tali beside the deep flexor tendon. The lateral nerve diverges laterally, and just distal to the hock, it detaches the common trunk of the *medial and lateral plantar metatarsal nerves* (Fig. 24.19/*2′*). These supply the interosseous muscle and associated structures and the plantar pouch of the fetlock joint (Fig. 24.19/*4* and *4′*). The medial plantar nerve follows the line of the parent trunk. Although the plantar nerves generally resemble the palmar nerves of the forelimb, the communicating branch is relatively slight or even absent; when present, it can usually be palpated as it slopes in a laterodistal direction over the superficial aspect of the flexor tendons (Fig. 24.19/*1*).

There is one other difference. The dorsal and plantar metatarsal nerves play a larger role in the sensory innervation of the hoof contents than do the corresponding forelimb trunks—the dorsal branch of the ulnar nerve and the palmar metacarpal nerves—which commonly fail to reach the coronet.

Tibial paralysis is manifested by a slight sagging of the hock when weight is borne on the affected limb. Despite the inability to flex the distal joints, the gait is not seriously disturbed. The sensory deficit is very considerable.

Lesions that affect the sciatic trunk involve the hamstring as well as the leg muscles. Despite this, the consequences are less disastrous than might well be supposed. *Retention of activity by the quadriceps enables the animal to fix the stifle and, through the reciprocal apparatus, the hock.* It is thus able to support weight on the limb. Cutaneous and deep sensations are lost below the stifle, except in the province of the saphenous nerve.

The tibial nerve may be blocked on the lateral side of the limb approximately 10 cm above the point of the hock.

Both superficial and deep branches of the peroneal nerve can be blocked by injecting, subcutaneously and then deeply from the same point of entry, between the long and lateral extensors a handbreadth or so proximal to the tarsocrural joint (Fig. 24.8/*6* and *6′*). Apart from this, the local anesthetic techniques for surgical and diagnostic purposes generally resemble those prescribed for the forelimb; the one distinction of relevance is the distal extension of the dorsal metatarsal nerves. It is possible to block the undivided tibial nerve (level with the point of the hock) as an alternative to the plantar nerves (Fig. 24.8/*12*).

COMPREHENSION CHECK

Demonstrate the anatomy and mechanics of the reciprocal apparatus.

Compare the core neuromuscular components that ensure the stability of the hindlimb with similar components in the forelimb.

Part IV

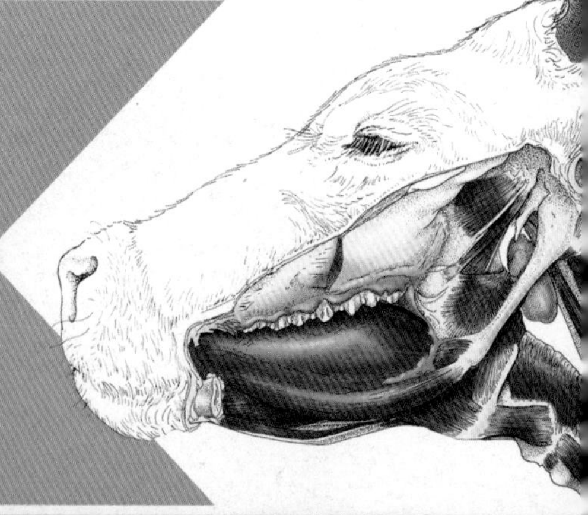

Ruminants

25 The Head and Ventral Neck of the Ruminant

The description contained in this and the following chapters (Chapters 26–31) is predominantly of bovine anatomy. Sheep and goats differ from one another and, more obviously, from cattle in many features of their anatomy, but it seems unnecessary to include any but the most significant and clinically relevant distinctions.

CONFORMATION AND EXTERNAL FEATURES

Conformation and External Features in Cattle

The features of the bovine head that first attract notice are the angular, pyramidal form, the bare muzzle, and the horns (when these are present). The form owes much to the late development of the frontal sinuses that invade the bones of the cranial vault, transforming the domed contours of the calf's head into the broad, flattened forehead and upright nuchal surface of the adult (Figs. 25.1, 25.2, and 25.3). The proportions are also much altered after birth by the greater growth of the facial part than of the neurocranium.

The modified skin around the nostrils extends to the margin of the upper lip, forming the slightly cobbled, naked *nasolabial plate.* This is kept moist by the watery secretion of a thick subcutaneous layer of eccrine glands.

The naked integument continues through the large oval nostril into the nasal vestibule, where it blends with the mucosa. The opening of the nasolacrimal duct is placed just caudal to the mucocutaneous junction. It is concealed on the ventromedial side of the fold that prolongs the ventral concha rostrally but may be uncovered for cannulation by bending the wing of the nostril outward.

The lips are thick, relatively immobile, and insensitive. They take little part in prehension of food. The upper one is the larger and overlaps the lower lip to the front and sides when at rest.

The size and conformation of the *horns* depend on breed, age, and sex. The horns are based on much smaller cornual processes that grow from the frontal bones at the caudolateral angles of the forehead. The cornual process has a ridged and porous surface and is covered by a papillated dermis that also serves as periosteum. The specialized dermis blends with that of the surrounding skin at the base of the projection. The major part of the horn wall or sheath grows from the epithelium that covers the dermis over the horn process. The softer outermost layer (epiceras) is produced by an irregular epithelial strip at the base that is transitional to the ordinary epidermis. The horn sheath represents a modification of the cornified stratum of the epithelium and consists chiefly of tubules formed over the dermal papillae. The tubules run lengthwise and are welded together by irregular, intertubular horn produced by the interpapillary regions of the epithelium. Because the entire epithelial surface is productive and the older horn is thrust apically by that of more recent origin, it follows that the horn sheath increases in thickness toward the tip (Fig. 25.4). Although horn growth is continuous, the rate of production is affected by physiologic stress such as calving,

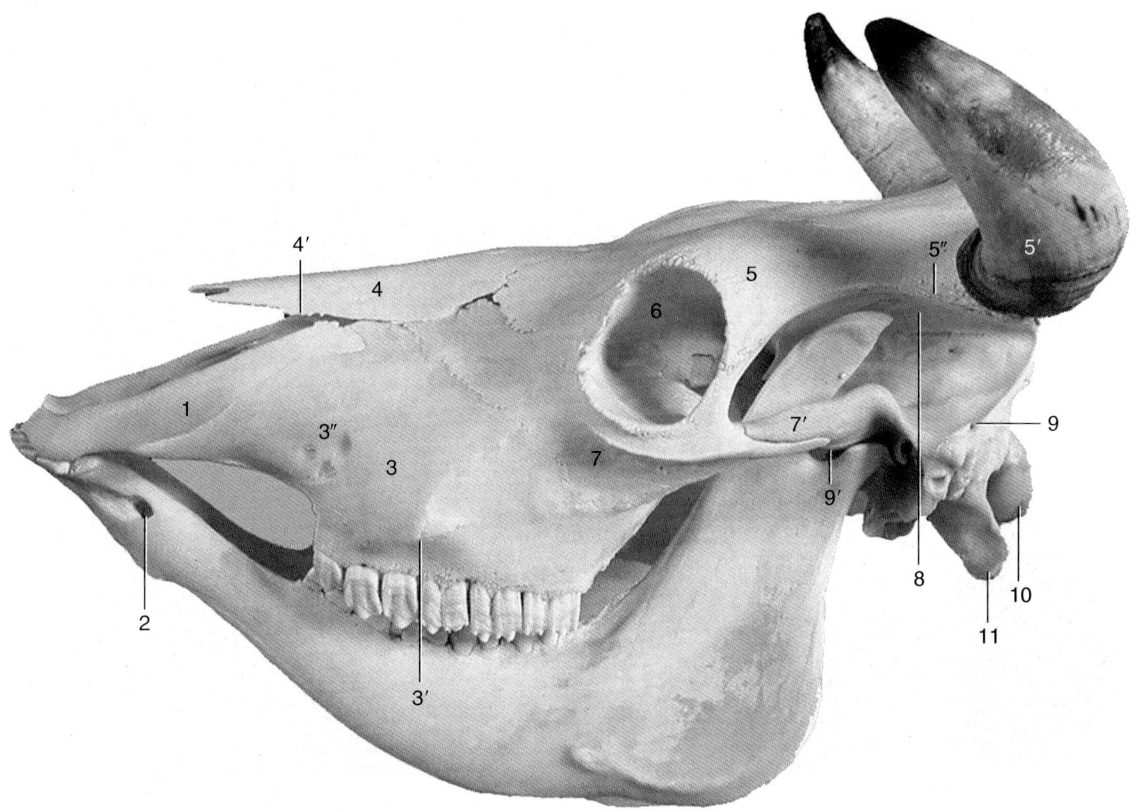

Fig. 25.1 Lateral view of bovine skull. *1,* Incisive bone; *2,* mental foramen; *3,* maxilla; *3′,* facial tuberosity; *3″,* infraorbital foramen; *4,* nasal bone; *4′,* nasoincisive notch; *5,* frontal bone; *5′,* horn surrounding cornual process of frontal bone; *5″,* temporal line; *6,* orbit; *7,* zygomatic bone; *7′,* zygomatic arch; *8,* temporal fossa; *9,* temporal bone; *9′,* temporomandibular joint; *10,* occipital condyle; *11,* paracondylar process.

and it is usual to find the horns marked by alternating rings of greater and lesser thickness. The latter represent periods of lower production and softer horn, which is more prone to wear. Because the first calf is generally born when the cow is about 2 years of age and subsequent calves are born at yearly intervals thereafter, the number of rings is commonly one fewer than the animal's age in years (Fig. 25.5).

The sensitive dermis of the horn is supplied mainly by the cornual nerve (Fig. 25.6/*1*), a branch of the zygomaticotemporal division of the maxillary nerve. The cornual nerve arises within the orbit and then passes backward through the temporal fossa under the shelter of the prominent ridge of the temporal line. The nerve later divides into two or more branches that wind around this ridge and approach the horn separately under cover of the thin frontalis muscle. The *cornual nerve* is often blocked for dehorning operations where it crosses the ridge, roughly midway between the postorbital bar and the horn (Fig. 25.6/*1*). The anesthetic technique is not always successful because of variation in the relationship of the nerve to the bony ridge, precocious division into divergent branches, and the existence of unusually substantial contributions from the supraorbital or infratrochlear nerves. Because the nerve to the frontal sinus may extend to the diverticulum within the horn, even infiltration around the horn base does not ensure complete loss of sensitivity.

The cornual nerve is accompanied by a considerable artery and vein that branch from the *superficial temporal vessels* within the temporal fossa. The artery ramifies before it reaches the horn. Its smaller branches run in the grooves and canals of the cornual process and retract when severed so that they cannot be easily grasped with hemostats. Because of this, dehorning is accompanied by spurting arterial hemorrhage unless the cut is made close to the skull where the arteries are still embedded in soft tissue.

The horns are barely indicated in the newborn calf, and their development can be prevented by cauterization of the germinal epithelium at an early age (2 to 4 weeks). The epidermis, which spreads to heal the wound, lacks the specialized inductive capacity of the original covering. An extension from the frontal sinus invades the cornual process when the calf is about 6 months old.

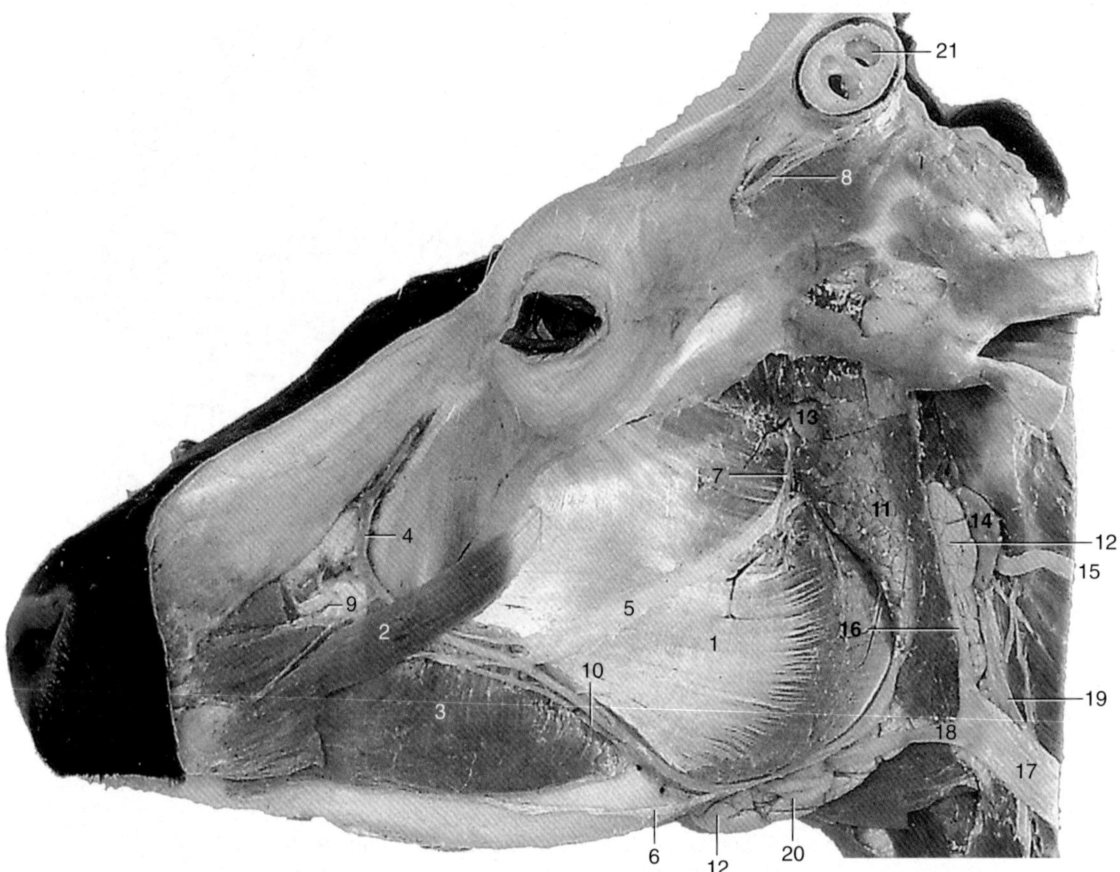

Fig. 25.2 Superficial dissection of the head. *1,* Masseter; *2,* zygomaticus; *3,* buccinator; *4,* facial vein; *5* and *6,* dorsal and ventral buccal branches of facial nerve, respectively; *7,* auriculotemporal nerve; *8,* cornual nerve; *9,* infraorbital nerve; *10,* parotid duct and facial artery and vein; *11,* parotid gland; *12,* mandibular gland; *13,* parotid lymph node; *14,* lateral retropharyngeal lymph node; *15,* spinal accessory nerve; *16,* maxillary vein; *17,* external jugular vein; *18,* linguofacial vein; *19,* common carotid artery; *20,* mandibular lymph node; *21,* cornual diverticulum of frontal sinus.

Conformation and External Features in Sheep and Goats

The shape and appearance of the head show many characteristics specific to breed, sex, and age, but they are for the most part of no great clinical interest. It is, however, important to note that the dorsal profile of the skull, unlike that of adult cattle, is domed over the cranial cavity and slopes caudally toward the nuchal plane; this feature is commonly masked by the location and size of the horns (Fig. 25.7).

The goat's head has a fairly long coat of hair, but that of sheep is shorter, and in some breeds wool extends considerably onto the face. The nasal plate resembles that of the dog but has a more limited extent, particularly in goats. It is confined to a narrow strip to each side of the deep median philtrum, with lateral prolongations along the upper edges of the long, slitlike nostrils.

The horns arise close behind the orbits in a parietal position (see Fig. 26.2). Each is based on a separate ossification center that makes a secondary fusion to a projection of the skull quite close to its contralateral fellow. In both sheep and goats the frontal sinus later excavates the horn core at the base but does not reach so far toward the tip as in cattle. Polled breeds are common, but when horns occur they are generally present in both sexes, although those of males are more strongly formed. In a few rare breeds, two (in rams occasionally three) pairs may exist. The multiple-horn (polycerate) condition is frequently associated with defects of cranial sutural closure and also of the eyelids.

The horns of goats generally have an oval section and grow caudally over the skull. Those of sheep are triangular in section and pursue a helical course that carries them first caudally, then successively ventrally, rostrally, and dorsally in a form of increasing complexity. This growth sometimes carries the inner surface of the horn close to the skin of the face, which may suffer from pressure necrosis if contact is made. Often a surface slice from the horn is removed in treatment or in prevention. The operation can be performed

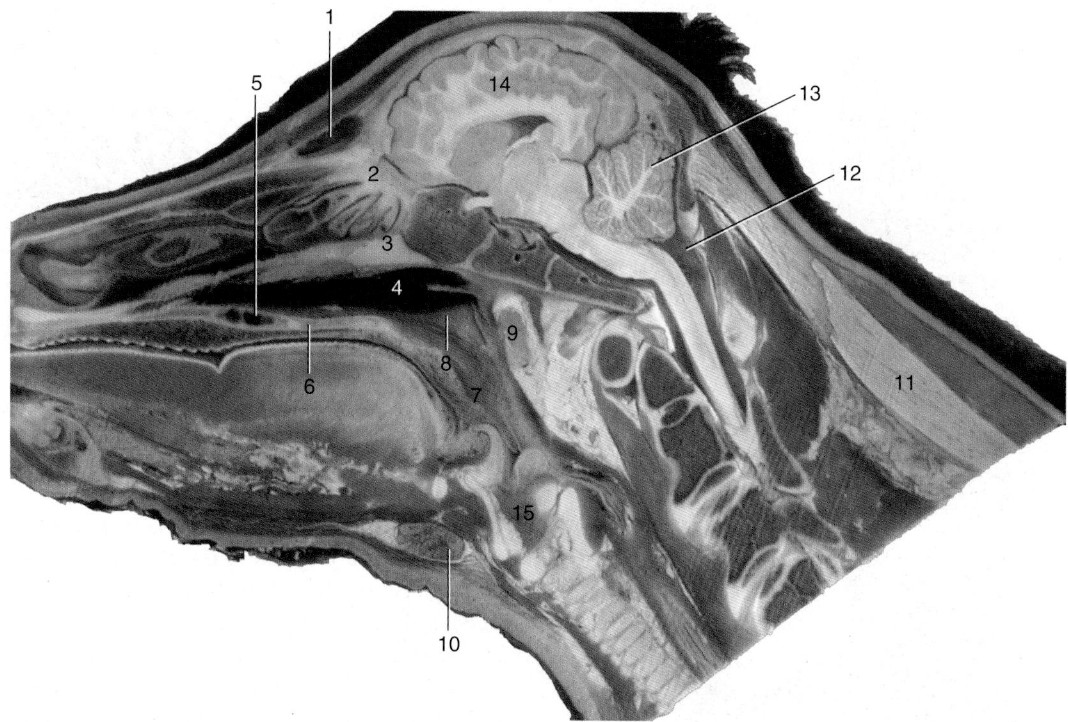

Fig. 25.3 Paramedian section of the head of a 2-week-old calf. Note the rounded vault. *1,* Frontal sinus; *2,* ethmoidal conchae; *3,* vomer; *4,* pharyngeal septum; *5,* palatine sinus; *6,* hard palate; *7,* soft palate; *8,* nasopharynx; *9,* medial retropharyngeal lymph node; *10,* mandibular gland; *11,* nuchal ligament; *12,* cerebellomedullary cistern; *13,* cerebellum; *14,* cerebrum; *15,* larynx.

without anesthetic if only "horn" is sawn away; on occasion sensitive dermis and bone must also be removed.

The horns of the sheep and goat are placed so close to the orbit that the supplying structures ascend directly behind the zygomatic process, where the nerve may be blocked. The horn of the goat receives a subsidiary supply through branches of the infratrochlear nerve, which require a separate injection at the dorsomedial margin of the orbit.

Certain glands of the skin of the heads of sheep and goats are mentioned in Chapter 10.

SUPERFICIAL STRUCTURES

Other organs that are visible or palpable in life may be identified with the assistance of Fig. 25.2. Relatively little of the skull lies directly below the skin, but large areas have thin coverings of fascia and cutaneous muscle, making it easy to palpate the broad forehead, dorsum of the nose, temporal line, zygomatic arch, facial tuberosity, nasoincisive notch, and ventral border. The supraorbital, infraorbital, and mental foramina can also be identified (Figs. 25.1, 25.2, and 25.7).

Few specific features of the mimetic musculature are important. It is supplied by the *facial nerve* (VII), which divides into its principal terminal branches under cover of the parotid gland. The *auriculopalpebral nerve* supplies muscles of the external ear and eyelids. It reaches these by crossing the zygomatic arch directly in front of the temporomandibular joint, where its superficial position makes it vulnerable (Fig. 25.6/*3*). Damage to the nerve may be evidenced by drooping of the ear and sagging of the eyelids, particularly the lower one. Paralysis of the orbicularis makes it impossible to close the eye. It is therefore clear that it may be advantageous to block the nerve to eliminate the blink reflex when examining the eye. It is most easily palpated where it passes over the zygomatic arch.

The *dorsal buccal branch* continues the parent trunk, crossing the masseter muscle in an exposed position that carries considerable risk of injury. The effects of such injury include loss of innervation to the muscles of the nose and upper lip and to the buccinator. The first loss leads to slight distortion of the face, which is drawn toward the unaffected side; the second allows food to collect in a wad within the oral vestibule. The *ventral buccal branch* takes a more protected course caudomedial to the ramus of the mandible and reaches the face in company with the facial artery and vein. It has a limited distribution, and the visible effects of injury are minimal (Fig. 25.2/*5* and *6*).

The distribution of the *cutaneous nerves* is shown in Fig. 25.8. Specific "blocks" of certain of these nerves are occasionally attempted. The large *infraorbital nerve* can be

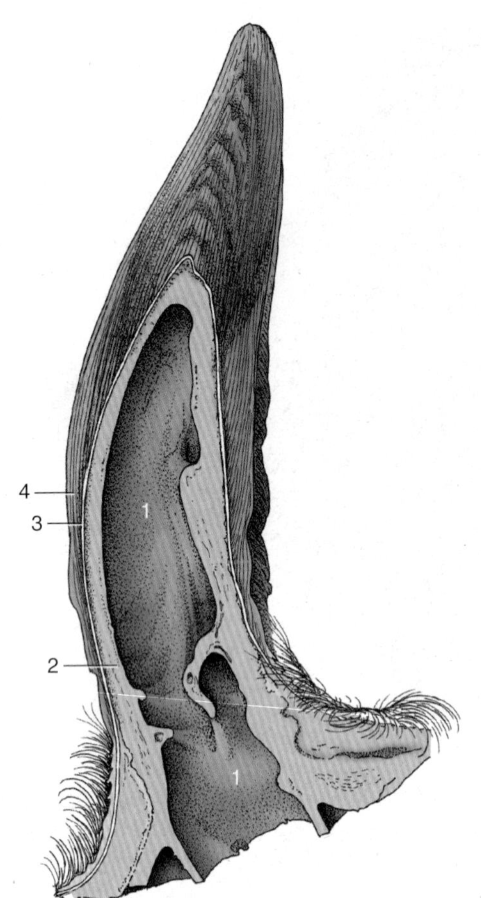

Fig. 25.4 Longitudinal section of a bovine horn. *1,* Cornual diverticulum of frontal sinus; *2,* cornual process; *3,* periosteum, dermis, and epidermis; *4,* horn tubules.

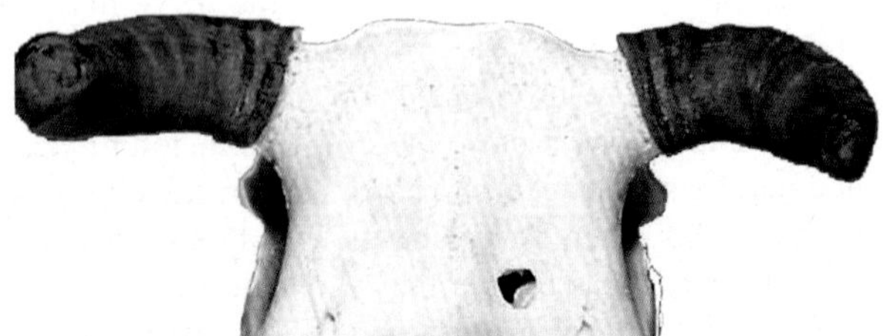

Fig. 25.5 Horn rings resulting from variation in horn production and wear in cattle.

palpated where it leaves the infraorbital foramen, about 3 cm dorsal to the first cheek tooth. The mental nerve is found where it leaves the mental foramen of the mandible, about 3 to 4 cm caudal to the lateral incisor tooth (Table 25.1).

The *facial artery* and *vein* are the most important superficial vessels. They cross the ventral margin of the mandible in front of the masseter muscle and are distributed to the lips, cheeks, muzzle, and periocular structures. The pulse may be examined where the artery lies on the side of the bone; it is less easily located in the notch of the ventral border.

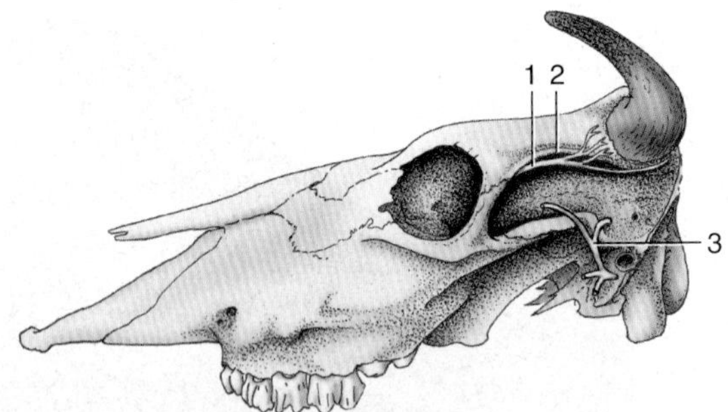

Fig. 25.6 Cornual nerve *(1)* follows the temporal line *(2)* on bovine skull. The auriculopalpebral nerve *(3)* is palpable where it crosses the zygomatic arch.

The position of the *frontal vein* should also be noted because this fair-sized vessel is at some risk in trephination of the caudal frontal sinus. The vein takes a caudorostral course in a palpable groove over the frontal bone to enter the supraorbital foramen; it then traverses a canal in the lateral part of the sinus. The foramen is located about 2 cm medial to the temporal line and about 2 cm caudal to the lateral angle of the eye (see Fig. 25.12/*4*). A system of veins on the external surface of the pinna becomes engorged and prominent when a tourniquet is applied around the base of the ear. The central member of the set is sometimes used as an alternative to the jugular vein for the placement of an indwelling catheter. Neither site is free from problems.

The ventral end of the *mandibular gland* forms a conspicuous swelling in the intermandibular space. When palpated, this gland is often mistaken for the adjacent *mandibular lymph node* (Fig. 25.2/*20*) but is identified based on its larger size, softer consistency, and more medial and more rostral extent. The lymph node can be separately identified on the medial aspect of the sternomandibularis tendon. Normally the parotid lymph node is also palpable rostroventral to the temporomandibular joint.

In the last part of its course along the rostral margin of the masseter, the *parotid duct* accompanies the facial vessels and ventral buccal nerve. The duct penetrates the cheek opposite the fifth upper cheek tooth.

THE NASAL CAVITY AND PARANASAL SINUSES

The nasal cavity is much smaller than would be supposed from the exterior because its walls are widened and hollowed by air sinuses, while much of the internal space is occupied by the conchae. Caudally, the nasal septum fails to reach the floor, which results in the formation of a single median channel that continues the paired nasal passages into the nasopharynx (Figs. 25.9 and 25.10).

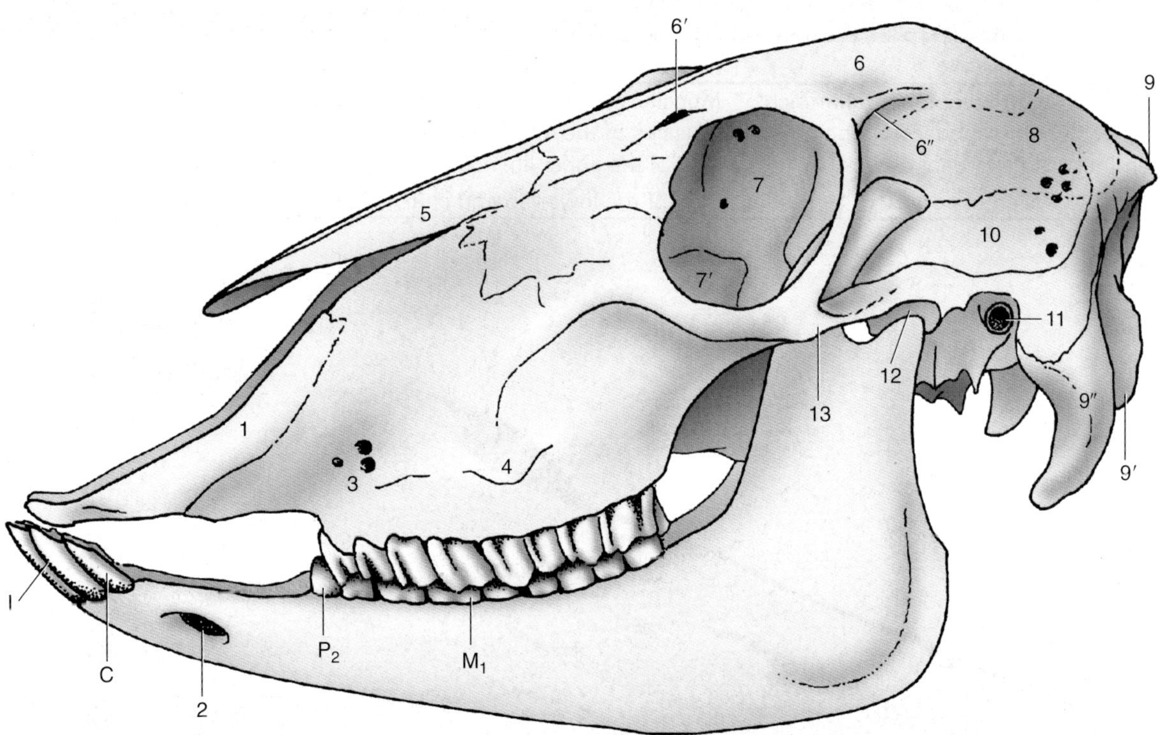

Fig. 25.7 Lateral view of the skull of a sheep. *I,* Incisor; *C,* canine; M_1, first lower molar; P_2, second upper premolar; *1,* incisive bone; *2,* mental foramen; *3,* infraorbital foramina; *4,* facial tuberosity; *5,* nasal bone; *6,* frontal bone; *6′,* supraorbital foramen and groove; *6″,* temporal line; *7,* orbit; *7′,* lacrimal bulla; *8,* parietal bone; *9,* external occipital protuberance; *9′,* occipital condyle; *9″,* paracondylar process; *10,* temporal fossa; *11,* external acoustic meatus; *12,* temporomandibular joint; *13,* zygomatic arch.

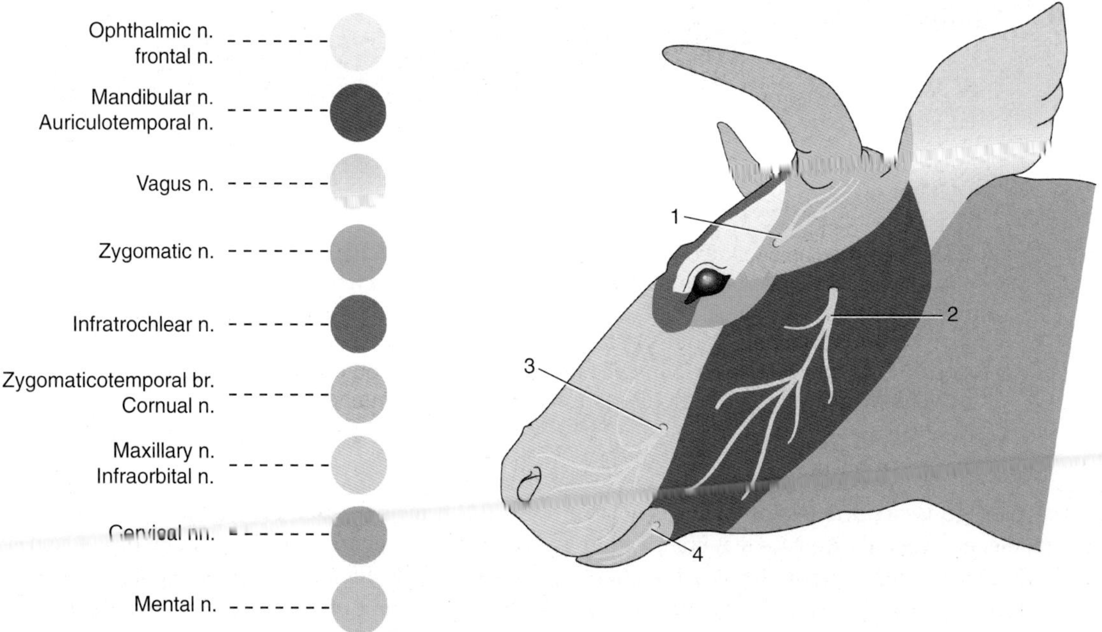

Fig. 25.8 Skin innervation of the head. *1,* Cornual nerve (n.); *2,* auriculotemporal n.; *3,* infraorbital n.; *4,* mental n; *Br.,* branch; *nn.,* nerves.

TABLE 25.1 FACIAL AND TRIGEMINAL NERVES

	Nerve	Areas Supplied
Facial	Auriculopalpebral branch	Muscles of the eyelid and external ear
	Dorsal buccal branch	Muscles of the upper lip, cheek, and nose
Trigeminal	Infraorbital nerve	Skin of the upper lip, nostril, and nose extending caudal to the foramen
	Mental nerve	Skin of the lower lip and chin

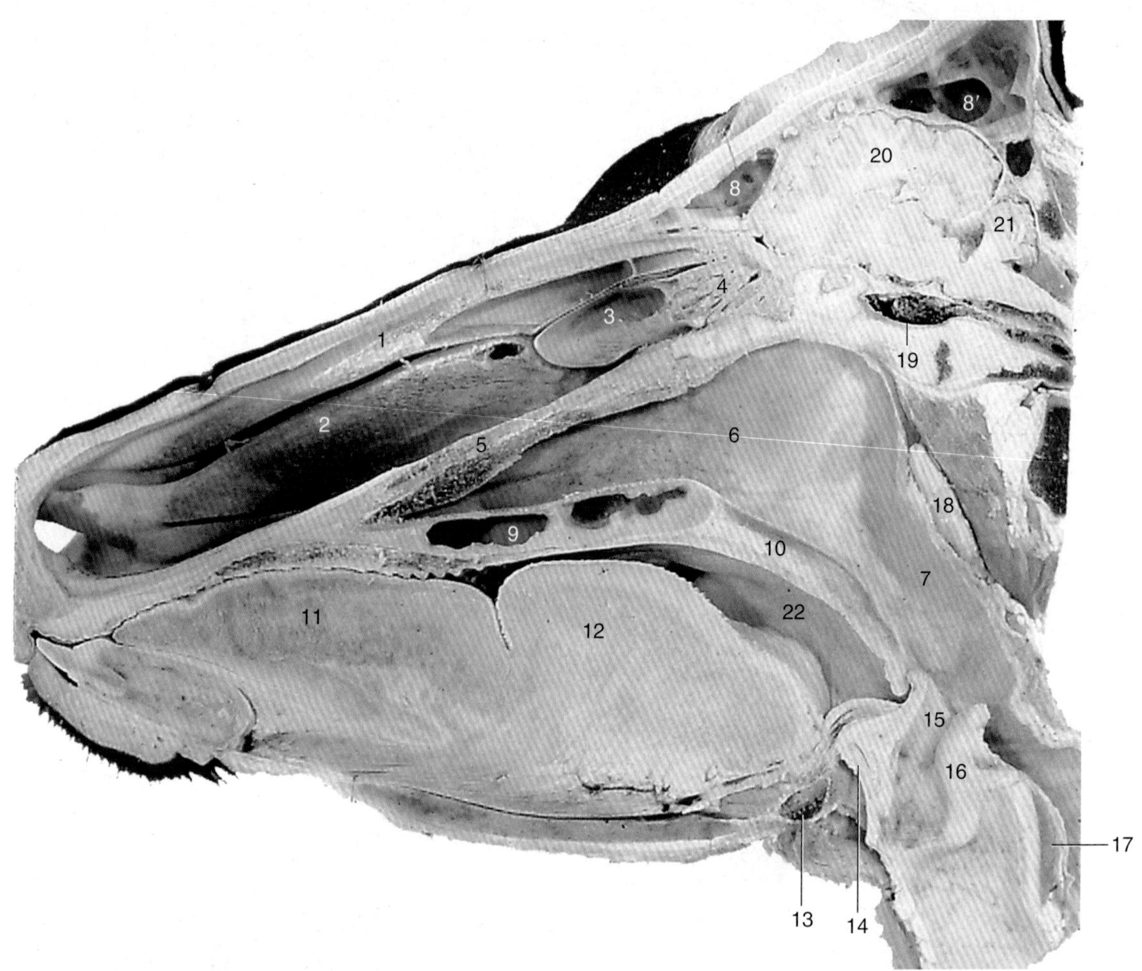

Fig. 25.9 Paramedian section of the head. *1,* Dorsal nasal concha; *2,* ventral nasal concha; *3,* middle nasal concha; *4,* ethmoidal conchae; *5,* vomer; *6,* choana; *7,* nasopharynx; *8,* rostral frontal sinus; *8',* caudal frontal sinus; *9,* palatine sinus; *10,* soft palate; *11,* apex of tongue; *12,* torus linguae; *13,* basihyoid; *14,* thyroid cartilage; *15,* epiglottis; *16,* arytenoid cartilage; *17,* cricoid cartilage; *18,* medial retropharyngeal lymph node; *19,* venous plexus surrounding hypophysis; *20,* cerebrum; *21,* cerebellum; *22,* entrance to tonsillar sinus.

Each nasal passage is divided by the major conchae into dorsal, middle, and ventral meatuses that branch from the common meatus located against the nasal septum. The deeper part of the cavity is further subdivided by the numerous ethmoidal conchae; the largest of these projects rostrally and is known as the middle concha. The dorsal meatus leads to the ethmoidal meatuses; the middle meatus communicates with certain sinuses; and the ventral meatus is the principal respiratory pathway. The nasal route is occasionally chosen for the passage of a sound when the instrument is directed to follow the largest space, formed at the junction of the ventral and common meatuses (Fig. 25.10/*9*).

The wall of each nasal passage is clothed by a thick, generously vascularized mucous membrane that ventrally encloses the *vomeronasal organ.*

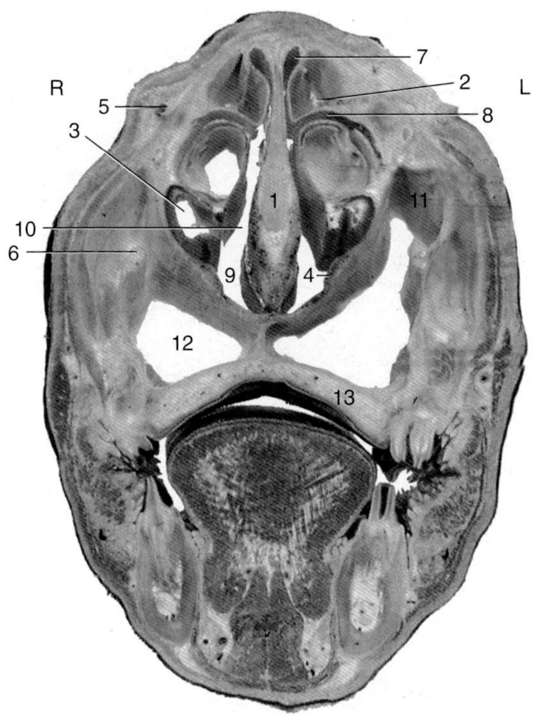

Fig. 25.10 Transverse section of a bovine head at the level of the last premolars. *1,* Nasal septum; *2,* dorsal nasal concha; *3,* ventral nasal concha; *4,* thick nasal mucosa containing venous plexus; *5,* nasolacrimal duct; *6,* infraorbital canal with infraorbital nerve; *7,* dorsal nasal meatus; *8,* middle nasal meatus; *9,* ventral nasal meatus; *10,* common nasal meatus; *11,* maxillary sinus; *12,* palatine sinus; *13,* hard palate; *L,* left side; *R,* right side.

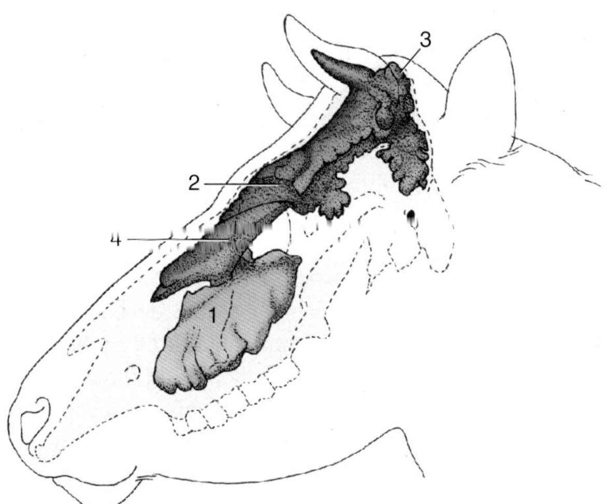

Fig. 25.11 Topography of the paranasal sinuses, which are filled with casting material. *1,* Maxillary sinus; *2,* rostral frontal sinuses; *3,* caudal frontal sinus; *4,* dorsal conchal sinus.

The paranasal sinus system is very poorly developed in the young calf, and several years must elapse before it attains full size. Even in the mature animal, the maxillary compartment continues to adjust to extrusion of the cheek teeth (Figs. 25.3/*1* and *5* and 25.11).

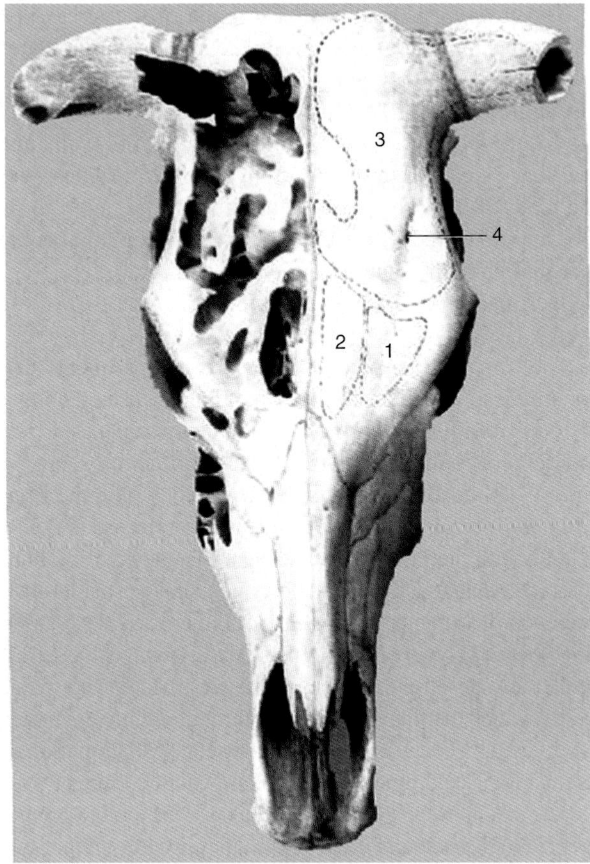

Fig. 25.12 Dorsal projection of the frontal sinuses. *1,* Lateral rostral frontal sinus; *2,* medial rostral frontal sinus; *3,* caudal frontal sinus with cornual diverticulum; *4,* supraorbital foramen.

The complete set of sinuses is very complicated. It comprises frontal compartments within the bones of the cranial roof and side walls; a palatomaxillary complex within the caudal part of the hard palate and the face, both before and below the orbit; a lacrimal sinus within the medial orbital wall, sphenoidal sinuses that extend past the orbit into the rostral part of the cranial floor; and conchal sinuses within the nasal conchae. Any of these may be infected or otherwise become an object of clinical interest, but in practice attention is concentrated on the maxillary and caudal frontal sinuses. The surface projections over which these spaces may be percussed are illustrated in Figs. 25.11 and 25.12.

Sinuses of Cattle: The maxillary, lacrimal, palatine, and conchal sinuses open into the middle nasal meatus, whereas the frontal and its various compartments, the sphenoidal and the middle conchal, open into the ethmoidal meatuses in the caudal part of the nasal cavity.

Paranasal sinuses, typically the frontal and maxillary, get inflamed most commonly in cattle and may do so in sheep and goats as well. The frontal sinusitis is typically associated with dehorning and the maxillary sinusitis with infected teeth. In addition, some fungal, bacterial, or viral infections may extend into the sinuses.

The *maxillary sinus* occupies much of the upper jaw above the alveoli of the cheek teeth. It communicates with the nasal cavity via a large nasomaxillary opening, but natural drainage of pus or other fluid is hindered by the location of this opening high in the medial wall. The maxillary sinus is continuous with the palatine sinus over the plate of bone that carries the infraorbital nerve in its free margin (Fig. 25.10/*6*). It also extends caudally (as the lacrimal sinus in front of the orbit) and within the fragile lacrimal bulla that intrudes into the ventral part of the orbit.

The *frontal sinus* comprises several compartments that communicate separately with ethmoidal meatuses. The two or, occasionally, three small rostral compartments are of little clinical interest. The caudal compartment, by far the largest and most important, spreads mainly within the frontal bone. It covers the dorsal part of the braincase and also extends into the lateral and nuchal walls and into the horn core. It is separated from its fellow and from the smaller ipsilateral compartments by partitions of rather variable position (Fig. 25.12). The openings in these partitions, visible in dry skulls, are closed by mucosa in the fresh state. The major cavity, which continues to increase throughout life, is further subdivided by irregular and perforate septa. Inflammation of its mucosa is a common sequel to surgical dehorning.

The extent of the frontal sinus makes it difficult to predict the size of the *cranial cavity*. The cranial cavity is in fact surprisingly small, rather globular, and so tilted that its rostral extremity is placed above as well as behind the nasal cavity (Fig. 25.9). It is protected above, behind, and to the sides by the pneumatized bones of the cranial vault. The topography is relevant to the usual humane slaughter technique. The target spot is defined by the intersection of the diagonals joining the lateral angles of the eyes to the nearest parts of the opposite horn bases (or equivalent points in polled breeds). The bolt or bullet then has to pass through the shallowest part of the frontal sinus en route to the brain.

The maxillary sinus is shallower and simpler in the sheep and goat. It does not communicate with the lacrimal sinus, which may open into the nasal cavity separately or via the lateral frontal sinus. The frontal sinus comprises separate medial and lateral compartments in both these species. They lie medial to the orbit (and extend slightly beyond this, both rostrally and caudally) and are of irregular form. The lateral compartment corresponds to the caudal sinus of cattle and provides the extension into the horn core. Sheep and goats do not have a sphenoidal sinus.

Fly Larvae in Sinuses of Sheep: The most common clinical involvement of the sinuses of sheep is that caused by invasion of the frontal sinus by larvae of oestrid flies. Treatment involves surgical puncture, and the preferred sites are rostral to the horn or medial to the middle of the orbital rim, where there is no risk of injury to the frontal vein.

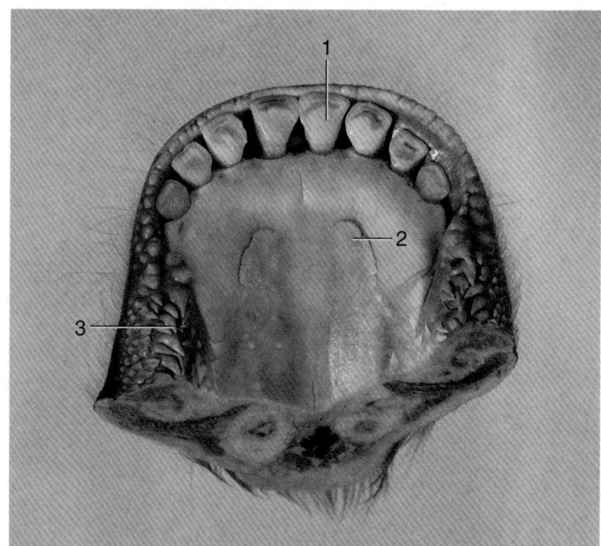

Fig. 25.13 Floor of the bovine mouth. *1,* Central incisor; *2,* sublingual caruncle; *3,* buccal papillae.

THE MOUTH

Because cattle do not ingest large mouthfuls, the small size of the oral opening is no disadvantage to the animal. However, it is a considerable hindrance to clinical inspection of the mouth parts and pharynx. The vestibule between the cheeks and the margin of the jaws is surprisingly roomy; the inner surface of the lips and cheeks bears large, backward-pointing papillae that are most prominent toward the corners of the mouth (Fig. 25.13/*3*).

The mouth cavity proper is long and narrow and is largely occupied by the tongue. The hard palate is most constricted directly in front of the cheek teeth. It is sculpted to display a dozen or more transverse ridges that progressively decrease in prominence and at last fade out toward the back of the mouth; their crests carry numerous papillae (Fig. 25.14). The region occupied in other species by the upper incisor teeth here carries the paired dental pads; these are crescentic elevations that are pliant when compressed, though cornified on the surface (Fig. 25.14/*2*). Cattle do not graze by edge-to-edge biting but, after drawing a tuft into the mouth with the assistance of the tongue, their main organ for prehension, sever it by pressing the incisor blades against these pads. The highly mobile lips of the small ruminants are main organs for prehension and allow them close cropping of the pasture. The pads are protected from injury by their tough but pliant covering and by the procumbent arrangement and rather loose implantation of the incisors (Figs. 25.15 and 25.16). The incisive papilla behind the pads is flanked by the small openings of the incisive ducts.

In cattle the caudal part of the pointed *tongue* is raised to form a large torus that has a transverse lingual fossa on its rostral side. The delicate epithelium in the fossa may be pricked by sharp particles in the food and become a portal

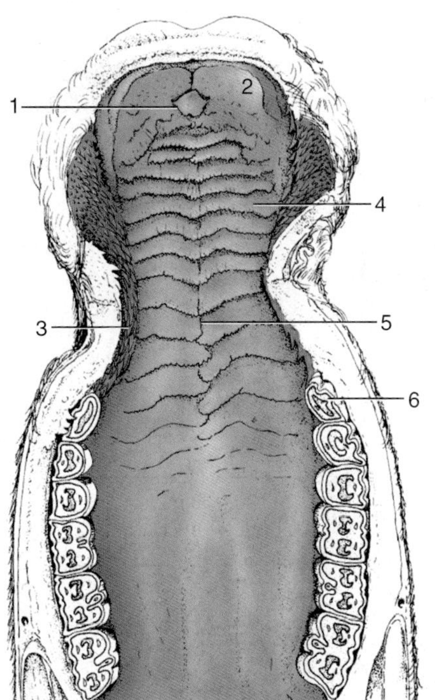

Fig. 25.14 The roof of the bovine oral cavity. *1,* Incisive papilla; *2,* dental pad; *3,* buccal papillae; *4,* palatine ridges; *5,* palatine raphe; *6,* first upper cheek tooth (P^2).

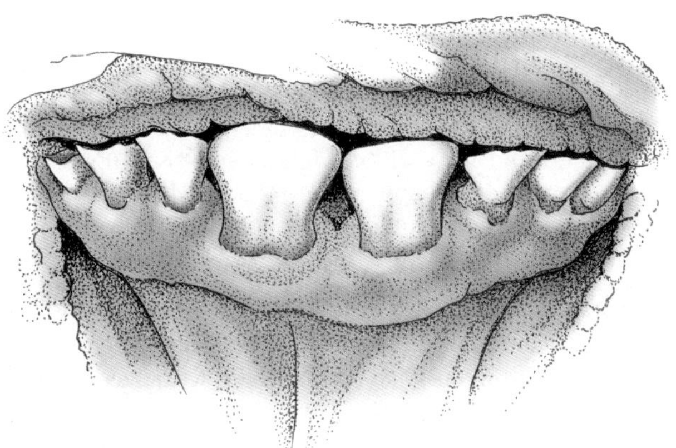

Fig. 25.15 Front view of the incisors of a 2-year-old cow. The central incisors are permanent, the others deciduous.

for infection (Fig. 25.17/*5*). The papillae that give the surface of the tongue a characteristic roughness are concentrated over the dorsum and toward the apex. Harsh, caudally directed, filiform papillae are freely spread over the apex in the area rostral to the fossa, while the conical and lenticular papillae populate the torus (Fig. 25.17/*4′* and *4″*); all of these have a purely mechanical function. As usual, the fungiform papillae scattered on and along the edges of the apex and the vallate papillae (8–12 in cattle, 18–24 in sheep, and 12–18 in the goat on each side of the tongue) (Fig. 25.17/*3*) present caudal to the torus perform the sensory function. Foliate papillae are usually absent in the ruminants. Although the mechanical nature and direction of the papillae make it

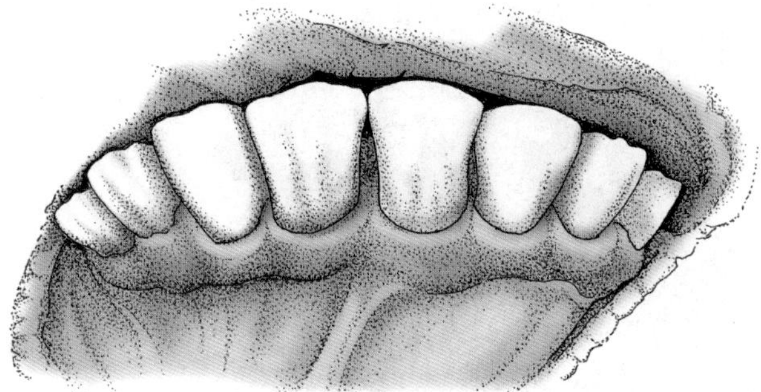

Fig. 25.16 Front view of the incisors of a 4½- to 5-year-old cow. The fourth incisors have reached the height of their neighbors and are coming into wear.

easier for cattle to prehense and swallow food, it also makes it difficult for them to expel undesirable food items such as nails from their mouth. An accumulation of lymphoid tissue toward the root constitutes the diffuse lingual tonsil.

The oral floor below the apex of the tongue presents a fleshy sublingual caruncle to each side; the ducts of the mandibular and monostomatic sublingual glands open beside this (Fig. 25.13).

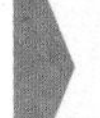

THE DENTITION AND MASTICATORY APPARATUS

The most unusual features of the dentition are the absence of incisor and canine teeth in the upper jaw and the assimilation of the canines to the incisors in the lower one. Because both upper and lower first premolar teeth fail to develop, the dental formulae read

$$\frac{0-0-3}{3-1-3}$$

for the temporary set, and

$$\frac{0-0-3-3}{3-1-3-3}$$

for the permanent set. It is customary to refer to the canine tooth as the fourth or corner incisor.

The eight *incisor teeth* toward the front of the lower jaw are arranged in a continuous crescent that is opposed to the dental pads when the mouth is closed. Each tooth presents a wide spatulate crown abruptly joined to a narrow, peglike root. The crown is asymmetrical, and in young animals

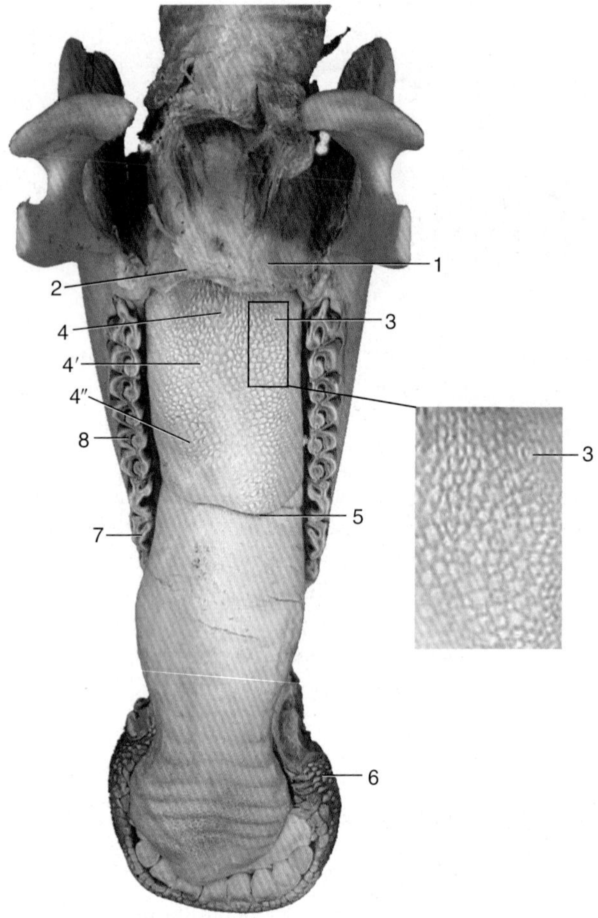

Fig. 25.17 Bovine tongue and lower jaw. *1,* Soft palate, cut; *2,* palatoglossal arch; *3,* vallate papillae; *4, 4′,* and *4″,* filiform, lenticular, and conical papillae, respectively; *5,* lingual fossa; *6,* buccal papillae; *7,* first lower cheek tooth (P_2); *8,* first lower molar (M_1).

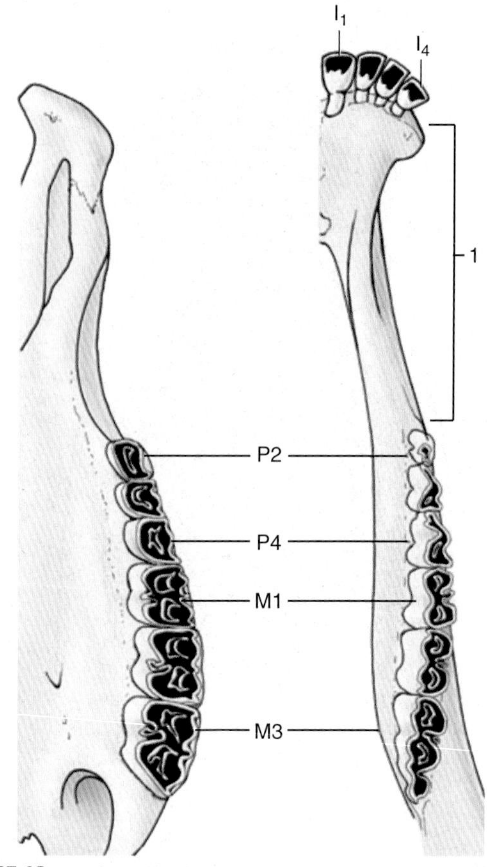

Fig. 25.18 Left half of upper and right half of lower jaw of cow. Note the different shapes of the upper and lower cheek teeth and the large diastema *(1)*. I_1 and I_4, First and fourth incisors; *M1* and *M3,* fourth and sixth upper and lower cheek teeth, respectively; *P2* and *P4,* first and third upper and lower cheek teeth, respectively.

it overlaps the lingual aspect of its medial neighbor (Fig. 25.15). The convex labial and concave lingual surfaces initially meet at a ridge, but this becomes increasingly broadened and the dentine increasingly exposed with continuing use (Fig. 25.16 and see Fig. 25.19 D and E). The crowns are sometimes wholly eroded in old animals, and then only narrow but widely spaced roots remain in the margin of the jaw. Often the incisors are shed before this state is reached.

The wide gap or diastema that separates the front teeth from the cheek teeth makes it easy to grasp the tongue to force the animal to permit examination of its mouth. The six *cheek teeth* in each jaw increase in size from front to back and are so arranged that most occlude with two opponents. The upper tooth rows are more widely separated than those of the lower jaw; consequently, only narrow strips of opposing teeth are in contact when the mouth is closed in central occlusion (Fig. 25.10). The tables slope transversely; the buccal edge is raised on the maxillary teeth, and the lingual edge is raised on those in the mandible. The masticatory surfaces of unworn teeth bear a series of crescentic enamel cusps arranged in two rows parallel to the axis of the jaw: the premolars have one pair of these cusps, and the molars have two. Once wear has exposed the dentine, the alternation of softer and more resistant tissues creates an uneven surface that is a very efficient shredding mechanism when the lower teeth are swung inward across their upper counterparts (Fig. 25.18). Attrition of the crowns is compensated by their continuing growth for a time; when growth eventually ceases, the roots are formed, and the height of the exposed part is then maintained only by gradual extrusion of the embedded portion. Eventually the crowns completely erode in animals that survive to very advanced age.

Most *temporary teeth* closely resemble their replacements, but the temporary premolars, which initially bear the full burden of mastication, are larger and more complicated than those that succeed them. The eruption dates of the teeth are given in Table 25.2.

Estimation of age is based on these dates and on the state of wear of the incisors. Neither factor is very reliable. The dates of eruption are influenced by breed and

TABLE 25.2 ERUPTION DATES OF THE TEETH OF CATTLE

	Temporary Tooth (wks)	Permanent Tooth (mos)
Incisor 1	Birth–2	18–24
Incisor 2	Birth–2	24–30
Incisor 3	Birth–2	36–42
Incisor 4	Birth–2	42–48
Premolar 2	Birth–1	24–30
Premolar 3	Birth–1	18–30
Premolar 4	Birth–1	20–36
Molar 1		6
Molar 2		12–18
Molar 3		24–30

reflect differences in the general rate of maturation. The rate of wear provides a somewhat more useful criterion, though it obviously depends on the nature of the fodder. Wear converts the cutting edge into a surface that gradually broadens. The lingual edge of this surface is originally jagged (because of the ridging of the distal part of the lingual surface of the crown) but becomes smooth when the tooth is worn down; the change in character occurs at 6 years on the first incisor and at 7, 8, and 9 years on the second, third, and fourth incisors, respectively. The teeth are then said to be "level." Exposure of the root coincides with this alteration in the crown (Fig. 25.19E). The changes at later ages are too unreliable to be of value.

The dentition of the *small ruminants* broadly resembles that of cattle. The teeth of sheep are often exposed to very rough wear, and tooth loss ("broken mouth") is a frequent reason for culling older animals. The dates of tooth eruption and replacement in sheep and goats are given in Table 25.3.

Because of the unequal width of the upper and lower dental arcades, mastication is unilateral, and although both sides are used in alternation, most animals tend to favor one. The usual action comprises three phases. In the first, the jaw is dropped and carried laterally; in the second, it is raised while displaced farther to the side; and in the third, which is performed much more swiftly and vigorously, it is carried upward and medially so that the tooth crescents of the lower row engage between those of the upper row as the jaw is returned to its resting position.

The pterygoids of the active side and the masseter of the passive side are the most important muscles in the work stroke.

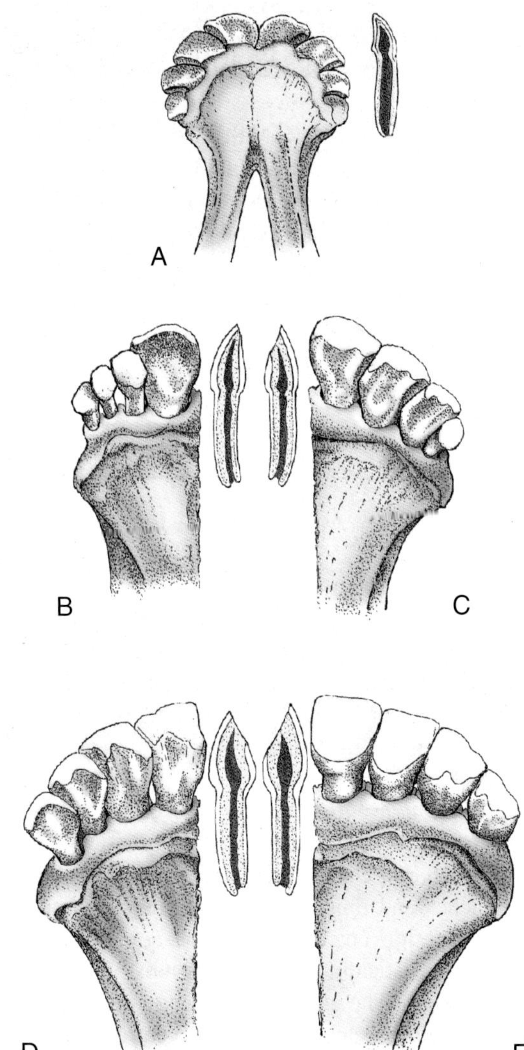

Fig. 25.19 Changes in the bovine incisors with increasing age. (A) Deciduous incisors in the newborn calf. In the longitudinal section of the first incisor *(I_1)* the enamel still surrounds the crown. (B) Two years: I_1 has been replaced. The other incisors are deciduous. The distal border of I_1 is slightly worn, and the dentine is exposed. (C) Three and one-half years: I_1, I_2, and I_3 (the first, second, and third incisors, respectively) are permanent; the fourth incisor *(I_4)* is deciduous. The occlusal surface of I_2, wider than that of I_3, is shown in the longitudinal section. (D) Five years. (E) Eight years. Note the size of the occlusal surface in the longitudinal section. The lingual edge of the occlusal surfaces of I_1 and I_2 is smooth; these two teeth are said to be "level."

THE SALIVARY GLANDS

Cattle produce an enormous volume of saliva—perhaps as much as 100 L a day—which contributes to the fermentation medium within the forechambers of the stomach, where it helps to buffer the fatty acids that are produced. Interference with the normal flow to the stomach results in serious depletion of the electrolytes that are normally reabsorbed and recycled.

Although the *parotid gland* is almost continuously active, it is smaller than might be expected. It lies ventral to the ear along the caudal border of the masseter, where

TABLE 25.3 ERUPTION DATES OF THE TEETH OF SHEEP AND GOATS

	Temporary Tooth (wks)	Permanent Tooth (mos)
Incisor 1	Before birth–1 (at birth)	12–18
Incisor 2	Before birth–1 (at birth)	18–24
Incisor 3	Before birth–1 (at birth)	30–36
Incisor 4	Birth–1 wk (1–3)	36–48
Premolar 2	Birth–4 wk (3)	18–24
Premolar 3	Birth–4 wk (3)	18–24
Premolar 4	Birth–4 wk (3)	18–24
Molar 1		3 (3–4)
Molar 2		9 (8–10)
Molar 3		18 (18–24)

From Habermehl KH: *Altersbestimmung bei Haus- und Labortieren*, ed 2, Berlin, 1975, Blackwell Wissenschafts-Verlag.

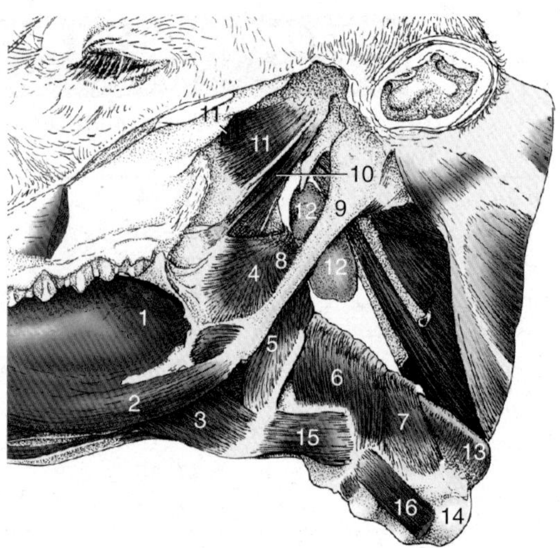

Fig. 25.20 Connections of the pharynx and larynx with the base of the skull and the tongue. *1,* Root of tongue; *2,* styloglossus; *3,* hyoglossus; *4,* rostral pharyngeal constrictor; *5,* middle pharyngeal constrictor; *6* and *7,* caudal pharyngeal constrictors (thyropharyngeus and cricopharyngeus, respectively); *8,* stylopharyngeus caudalis; *9,* stylohyoid; *10,* tensor and levator veli palatini; *11,* pterygoideus lateralis; *11',* remnants of pterygoideus medialis; *12,* medial retropharyngeal lymph node; *13,* esophagus; *14,* trachea; *15,* thyrohyoideus; *16,* sternothyroideus.

it partly covers the parotid lymph node. It touches the temporomandibular joint dorsally. A spurt in its growth is coordinated with the initiation of ruminant digestion by the calf. The duct, included in the description of the face (Fig. 25.2/*10*), opens on the parotid papilla opposite the fifth upper cheek tooth.

The *mandibular gland* is considerably larger and attains a length of 18 to 20 cm and a width of 8 to 10 cm. The gland has lateral relationships with the external jugular vein branches and those of the facial nerve. It produces a mixed secretion but only when the animal is actually feeding or remasticating; the flow is most copious when the fodder is dry. The gland extends in an arc on the inner aspect of the lower jaw. Its palpable ventral end projects below the mandible and often almost meets its fellow in the midline; its dorsal end is within the atlantal fossa. The duct runs below the oral mucosa to open by the sublingual caruncle (Fig. 25.13/*2*).

The *sublingual gland* has the usual two divisions and is seromucous in nature. The polystomatic part lies in the mouth floor, lateral to the tongue, and drains through many small openings beside the frenulum. It is overlapped by the more compact rostral monostomatic part, whose single duct formed through the union of many smaller ducts opens close by or together with that of the mandibular gland on the sublingual caruncle.

Many minor salivary glands are scattered below the labial, buccal, palatine, and lingual mucosae; those in the cheeks are particularly well developed. In the aggregate, these lesser glands must contribute a considerable volume of secretion.

THE PHARYNX

The pharynx is divided in the customary fashion.

The *nasopharynx* extends the nasal cavity caudally. In the ruminants it is incompletely divided by a median membranous fold (pharyngeal septum) that prolongs the nasal septum to the dorsal pharyngeal wall (Fig. 25.9/*7*). The caudal end of this septum is thickened by a mass of lymphoid tissue, the pharyngeal tonsil. Other lymphoid aggregations are found around the slitlike entrances to the auditory tubes on the lateral pharyngeal walls (see Fig. 3.25).

The *oropharynx* is narrow, and this significantly restricts the size of the morsels that can be swallowed. It contains within each lateral wall the palatine tonsil, which projects away from the lumen around a deep, branching tonsillar sinus. The entrance to this sinus (Fig. 25.9/*22*), not the tonsil itself, is visible on the surface.

The *laryngopharynx* tapers caudally before joining the esophagus, and its lumen is normally held closed by the investing muscles; the muscle principally involved, the cricopharyngeus (Fig. 25.20/*7*), is sometimes described as the cranial sphincter of the esophagus. The piriform recesses to each side of the entrance to the larynx allow a continuous dribble of saliva to reach the esophagus without need for active swallowing.

The pharynx may be examined by palpation, externally or through the mouth, and its interior may also be inspected with the use of an oral speculum. Swelling of lymphoid tissue in the pharyngeal wall may intrude on the food and air pathways. The pharynx may also be compressed when the adjacent medial retropharyngeal lymph nodes are inflamed (Fig. 25.20/*12*).

The pharynx receives and transmits the regurgitated cud to the mouth. It also receives the gas that is eructated from the stomach in large amounts; some of this gas is lost to the exterior, but a significant portion is directed to the lungs when the communication with the nasopharynx is shut off. The significance of this phenomenon is not fully understood; in animals on certain rations, absorption of eructated gas may lead to tainting of the milk and to pathology of the lung.

THE LARYNX

The larynx is largely situated between the mandibular rami but extends into the upper part of the neck, where it may be felt. The appreciation of its palpable features requires the correct identification of three midline skeletal structures: the basihyoid and the thyroid and cricoid cartilages. Those familiar with the surface anatomy of the horse may experience an initial uncertainty when first examining cattle. The different spacing of the ventral prominences is due to the shape of the bovine thyroid cartilage, which is complete ventrally and most salient toward its caudoventral point.

The bovine larynx shows few other peculiarities of note. The *entrance,* which may be inspected with the assistance of a laryngoscope, is bounded by the low, curled margin of the epiglottis and the prominent corniculate extensions of the arytenoid cartilages (Fig. 25.9/*15* and *16*). Intubation is made difficult by a slight caudal deflection of the entrance (see Fig. 25.*9*).

The *vestibule* possesses neither median nor lateral ventricles, and its side walls shelve smoothly to the glottis. The size of the *glottic cleft* varies with the phase of respiration, but the changes are not pronounced during quiet breathing. It is narrower than might be supposed, and this limits the caliber of the endotracheal tube that may be passed. The relationship to the medial retropharyngeal lymph nodes is important; when much enlarged, these may seriously compress the larynx as well as the pharynx (Fig. 25.9/*18*).

THE EYE

The orbital rim projects above the surrounding surfaces. The *orbital cavity* is capacious, although reduced ventrorostrally by the fragile, thin-walled swelling of the lacrimal bulla into which the maxillary sinus extends. The orbital axes diverge upward, outward, and forward and together subtend an angle of approximately 120 degrees. It is therefore clear that, as is usual in ungulates, the field of monocular vision is large and that of binocular vision is small.

The *eyelids* are supported by dense fibrous plates or "tarsi." The skin adheres tightly over the orbicularis muscle but is loose elsewhere, leading to a furrowed lid when the eye is open. The lashes are long and are more densely spread on the upper lid. The muscles of the lids include the *frontalis,* which extends from the forehead into the upper lid, and the *malaris,* which radiates from the lower lid onto the face. These are supplied by the facial nerve, mainly through the auriculopalpebral nerve. *The levator*, supplied as always by the oculomotor nerve, remains active in facial paralysis, which mitigates the effects of this injury.

The conjunctiva contains considerable scattered lymphoid accumulations in its palpebral part. The usual glands are present within the eyelids. The largest, the *tarsal (meibomian) glands,* occupy the deeper layers of the tarsi; they may be visible through the conjunctiva of the everted lid.

Infectious bovine keratoconjunctivitis (pink eye) is caused by *Moraxella bovis.* This disease causes significant economic losses to the dairy industry through treatment and management costs. The initial mucous and pus discharge is followed by a corneal ulcer.

The medial corner of the palpebral opening forms a bay containing the fleshy lacrimal caruncle. The *third eyelid* covers a variable part of the bulb. The supporting cartilage sinks medial to the eyeball, where it is associated with superficial and deep accessory lacrimal glands. Only a small part of the third eyelid is normally visible. A larger part is brought into view when the eyeball is withdrawn or pressed into its socket; this displaces the retrobulbar fat, which in turn pushes the cartilage and therefore the fold outward.

The lobulated, bipartite *lacrimal gland* lies dorsolaterally on the eyeball. It drains by numerous ducts of varying caliber into the upper conjunctival fornix. The tears collect by the lacrimal caruncle before entering the slitlike puncta lacrimalia that lead to the lacrimal sac. The sac lies within a depression of the cranial part of the orbital wall. It tapers to the nasolacrimal duct, which first traverses the maxillary sinus and then runs on the lateral nasal wall to discharge within the nasal vestibule.

The *extrinsic muscles,* which exhibit no especially notable features, are shown schematically in Fig. 9.19.

The eyeball is small in relation to the orbit. The *sclera* is thin and locally obtains a bluish tinge from the dark underlying choroid. Some pigmentation is common, especially toward the junction with the cornea, and tends to increase with age. The cornea is ovoid, and its pointed end is lateral. It is rather thick, especially toward its margin.

The bovine pupil is widened from side to side when constricted but becomes circular on dilation. Its upper and lower margins are broken by irregular projections, the iridic granules, which are smaller than in the horse; they are more prominent along the upper margin. The ciliary muscles are poorly developed, and the capacity for accommodation is limited accordingly. The vascular and choroidocapillary layers of the choroid are separated in the caudal part of the bulb by the brilliantly colored reflective *tapetum* (Fig. 25.21).

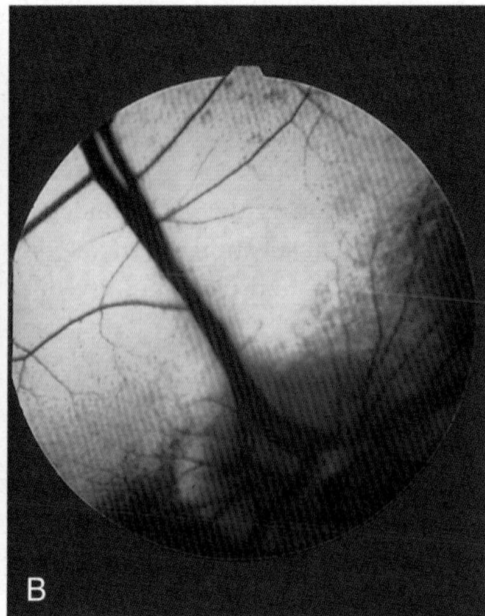

Fig. 25.21 (A) Fundus of eye of cow. (B) Fundus of eye of goat.

The tapetum is triangular, and its base is directly above the optic disk. Its peripheral parts are most colorful and display an array of metallic blues and greens, while the area close to the optic disk is reddish, especially in the calf. Ophthalmoscopic examination of the tapetum reveals scattered dark flecks, where capillaries enter, and larger vessels, which appear as red lines. Four pairs of arteries and veins radiate in cruciate fashion from the optic disk, which is lateroventral to the posterior pole of the eye. The dorsal vein is especially large and is entwined by a spiraling artery. A clear spot in the center of the disk indicates the vestige of the hyaloid artery; as would be expected, the remnant is more obvious in the newborn calf. The macula of the retina consists of two rather ill-defined parts: a rounded area placed dorsolateral to the optic disk is concerned with binocular vision, and a horizontal strip below the tapetum is concerned with monocular vision. Their extents are suggested by their relatively poor vascularization.

Evisceration of the orbit is sometimes performed under local anesthesia. The anesthetic technique, though simple, is exacting because it requires the deposit of anesthetic solution deep in the orbit, precisely by the single foramen (orbitorotundum) through which emerge the nerves that supply the structures within the periorbita. The nerves are thus blocked where bundled together before dispersing to their scattered destinations. Movement of the eyelids may be prohibited in the usual way—that is, by blockage of the palpebral branch of the facial nerve where it crosses the zygomatic arch (Fig. 25.6/*3*).

THE VENTRAL PART OF THE NECK

Dorsal cervical structures are described with the vertebral column (Chapter 26). The skin of the ventral aspect

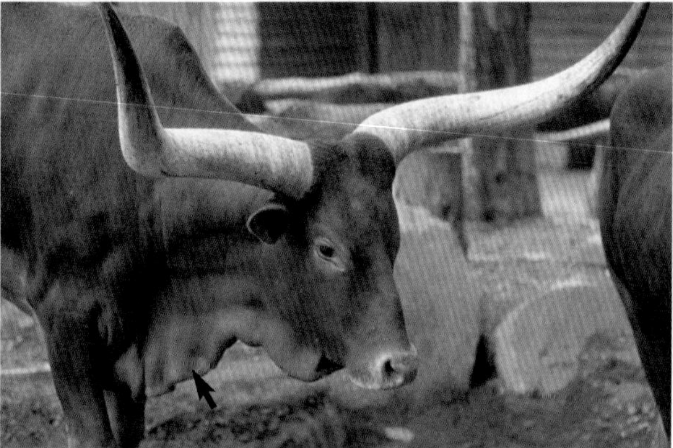

Fig. 25.22 Large median skinfold (dewlap, *arrow*) at the caudal end of the neck of a Watusi cow.

is freely movable and redundant in amount; it becomes folded and creased when the head is lowered to the ground. In addition, the caudal part of the neck carries the large dewlap that continues onto the brisket (breast) between the forelimbs (Fig. 25.22). There is scant evidence for the belief that this increase in surface area is important in heat dissipation as is sometimes claimed, for the Zebu in particular. Zebu cattle do possess, here and elsewhere, more numerous, larger, and more saclike sweat glands than are found in cattle of European origin.

The *groove* over the course of the external jugular vein is generally obvious, at least in cows. It is bounded dorsally by the brachiocephalicus (cleidomastoideus) extending from the arm to the skull and ventrally by the part (sternomandibularis) of the sternocephalicus that runs between the manubrium of the sternum and the angle of the jaw. Except in the most caudal part of the neck, a second part of the sternocephalicus (sternomastoideus) forms the floor of the groove and provides a substantial separation between

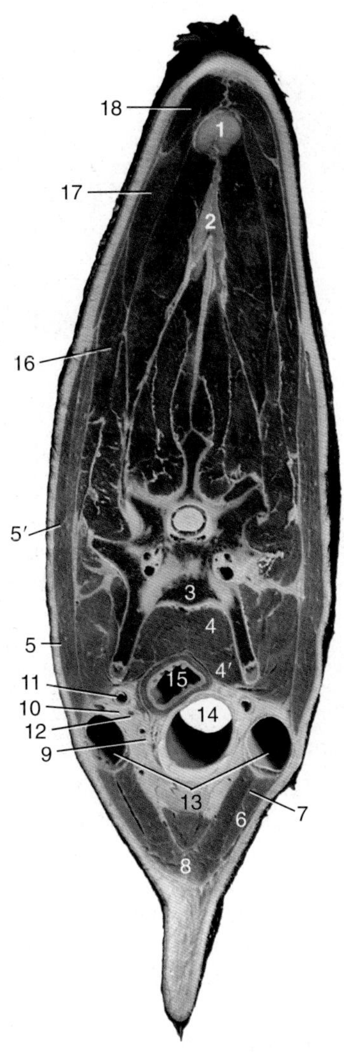

Fig. 25.23 Transverse section through the middle of the bovine neck. *1* and *2,* Nuchal ligament (funiculus and lamina nuchae, respectively); *3,* vertebra; *4,* longus colli; *4′,* longus capitis; *5* and *5′,* parts of the brachiocephalicus: *5,* cleido-occipitalis, and *5′,* cleidomastoideus; *6* and *7,* parts of the sternocephalicus: *6,* sternomandibularis, and *7,* sternomastoideus; *8,* combined sternohyoideus and sternothyroideus; *9,* thymus and internal jugular vein; *10,* recurrent laryngeal nerve; *11,* common carotid artery; *12,* vagosympathetic trunk; *13,* external jugular vein; *14,* trachea; *15,* esophagus; *16,* omotransversarius; *17,* trapezius; *18,* rhomboideus.

the vein and the common carotid artery (Fig. 25.23/*7*). The external jugular vein is easily raised for injection and blood sampling because only the caudal part is covered by the cutaneous muscle, and even this is rather weak. The vein is formed caudal to the parotid gland by the confluence of maxillary and linguofacial radicles (Fig. 25.2). It is the principal drainage of the head and neck but is assisted by the internal jugular vein, the vertebral vein, and the internal vertebral plexus. Variation in the prominence of the vein may reflect conditions within the thorax. Gentle undulation in time with respiration is due to a change in intrathoracic pressure. Pulsation in time with the heartbeat in healthy cattle indicates the recurrence of atrial systole; in other animals it points to atrioventricular valvular incompetence. The normal jugular pulse does not persist after compression of the cranial part of the vein, but the pathologic pulse does.

The superficial muscles enclose the space that contains the cervical viscera and the vessels and nerves that make their way between the thorax and the head (Fig. 25.23). All of these organs are invested by tough fascia and are joined by looser tissue.

The *trachea,* composed of 48 to 60 cartilages, may be identified on deep palpation and is most easily appreciated toward the upper end of the neck, between the diverging sternocephalic muscles; even here it is not directly subcutaneous because the thin straplike sternothyrohyoid muscles follow its whole length. The trachea (Fig. 25.23/*14*) is small in section and slightly deeper than it is wide. Its form makes it susceptible to narrowing by local pressure. The symmetry of its relations is disturbed by the devious course of the esophagus. Its structure is mainly remarkable for the concentration of lymphoid tissue in the dorsal retromucosal space (external to the tracheal muscle but within the cartilage rings).

Although the *esophagus* cannot be identified by palpation, its position is made evident by the swift movement along its track when the animal swallows. In its cervical course the esophagus gradually slips to the left of the trachea, only to creep back to a more dorsal position as the thorax is approached. However, its position varies with posture; its course is considerably straightened when the neck is extended. The relations in the middle of the neck are shown in Fig. 25.23.

The ruminant esophagus is very distensible, but its wide appearance in the cadaver gives a misleading impression of the usual condition in life. The mucosa is remarkably insensitive, which is one reason why cattle rarely appear to be distressed by the passage of a stomach tube or probang. Although transport is normally rapid in both directions, chunks of food quite commonly become lodged in the esophagus. The sites with a predilection for lodgment are at the origin from the pharynx, at the thoracic inlet, and level with the tracheal bifurcation.

The *thyroid gland* is almost completely divided into two lobes, each shaped like an inverted pyramid and placed laterally over the cricoid cartilage. They are tenuously joined by an isthmus that crosses the second tracheal ring ventrally. They are finely granular and brick red in the adult but paler in the calf (see Fig. 6.4C).

The *parathyroid glands* are small (≈8–10 mm) and, because they are irregular in shape and inconstant in position, frequently difficult to find. They may be embedded in other structures—usually the thyroid, thymus, or mandibular gland. The external parathyroid most often lies cranial to the thyroid but caudal to the carotid bifurcation; the internal one is perhaps most often embedded in the thyroid or located

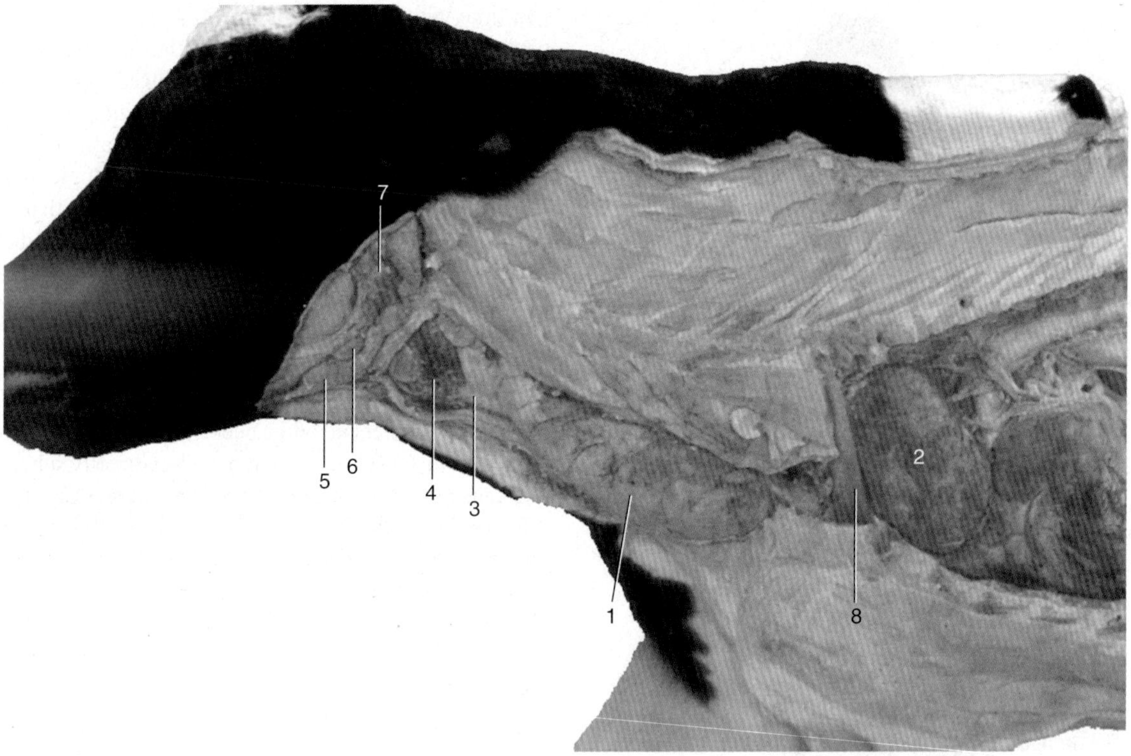

Fig. 25.24 The thymus in the newborn calf. *1,* Cervical part of thymus; *2,* thoracic part of thymus; *3,* trachea; *4,* thyroid gland; *5,* mandibular gland; *6,* mandibular lymph node; *7,* parotid gland; *8,* first rib.

between this and the trachea. They have been confused with lymph nodes, which they resemble superficially.

The *thymus* is large and lobulated and extends from the larynx to the pericardium in young animals (Fig. 25.24/*1* and *2*). Its cervical part is connected to the thoracic thymus by a narrow isthmus ventral to the trachea. The cervical part comprises two horns that taper over the lateral aspects of the trachea, possibly reaching the larynx. The cranial tip may be, or may appear to be, detached and fragmented and more closely associated with the medial retropharyngeal lymph node and the mandibular and parathyroid glands. The thymus grows rapidly during the first 6 or 9 months of postnatal life, although it attains its greatest relative size much earlier. Indeed, involution may begin as early as the eighth week after birth. The tempo of regression varies, and the thymus, particularly its thoracic part, may still be quite large in animals several years old. Ultimately the isthmus and neck part disappear almost completely. The thymus of young calves is bright pink or even red, but the organ lightens with age; its consistency also firms as the active tissue is progressively replaced by fatty fibrous tissue.

The *common carotid artery* runs dorsolateral to the trachea within a fascial sheath shared with the vagosympathetic trunk. The internal jugular vein and the recurrent laryngeal nerve are closely related to the sheath on the right side; the esophagus intervenes on the left. The artery detaches a small occipital artery over the lateral pharyngeal wall and continues as the external carotid artery. In the fetus an internal carotid artery arises with the occipital artery, but the part proximal to the rete mirabile (see Fig. 7.35) begins to close even before birth. Complete obliteration is usually achieved a few months after birth, although a residual lumen sometimes persists for a year or two (Fig. 25.25/*4*). Pulsation in the common carotid may sometimes be detected when the artery is pressed against the transverse processes of the vertebrae.

The brain is supplied by a combination of vessels that feed very intricate arterial plexuses within the cranial cavity, external to the dura mater and submerged within the cavernous and associated venous sinuses. These plexuses, the retia mirabilia, are formed by many closely wound, anastomosing arteries. The retia are entered on their peripheral aspect from several sources (see Fig. 7.35); on the distal or cerebral side the network narrows to one emissary trunk that pierces the dural membrane to form the cerebral arterial circle with its fellow. The circle lies on the ventral aspect of the brain and gives off branches according to the conventional pattern. The *basilar artery,* which runs caudally over the medulla and continues down the spinal cord, is a contributor to the circle in cattle but leads blood from it in sheep. Although difficult to explain on hemodynamic grounds, all parts of the bovine brain are supplied by a mixture of carotid and vertebral blood, whereas in sheep the vertebral blood is

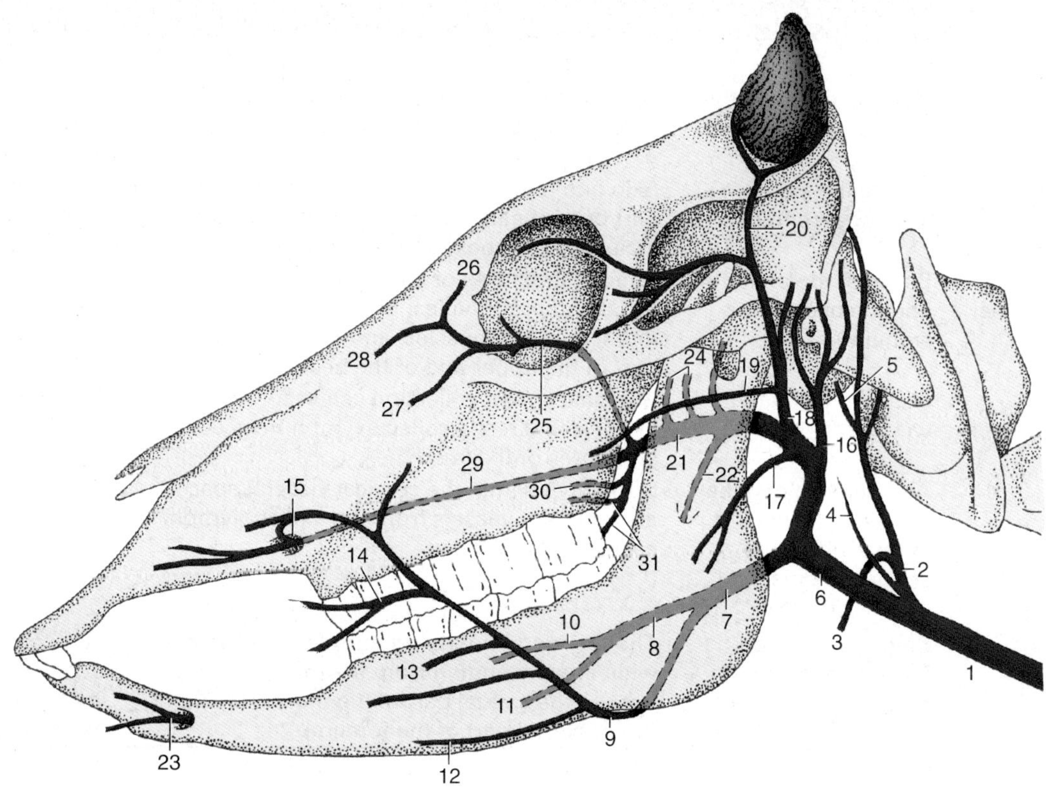

Fig. 25.25 Branching of the left common carotid artery (a.). *1,* Common carotid a.; *2,* occipital a.; *3,* ascending palatine a.; *4,* remnant of internal carotid a.; *5,* medial meningeal a.; *6,* external carotid a.; *7,* linguofacial trunk; *8,* lingual a.; *9,* facial a.; *10,* deep lingual a.; *11,* sublingual a.; *12,* submental a.; *13,* inferior labial arteries; *14,* superior labial a.; *15,* infraorbital foramen; *16,* caudal auricular a.; *17,* masseteric branch; *18,* superficial temporal a.; *19,* transverse facial a.; *20,* cornual a.; *21,* maxillary a.; *22,* inferior alveolar a.; *23,* mental a.; *24,* rostral and caudal branches to rete mirabile; *25,* malar a.; *26,* angular a. of the eye; *27,* caudal lateral nasal a.; *28,* dorsal nasal a.; *29,* infraorbital a.; *30,* sphenopalatine a.; *31,* major and minor palatine arteries.

restricted to the caudal part of the brainstem. These differences are germane to the ritual slaughter technique in some religions because the vertebral arteries are spared when the common carotid trunks are severed. The suggestion that abrupt reduction of the pressure within the cerebral arteries produces almost immediate loss of consciousness has been questioned.

The *vagosympathetic trunk* exhibits no particular features of note. The vagus and sympathetic components loosen their association and part company before entering the thorax. Their further courses and connections are described elsewhere. The recurrent laryngeal nerves resemble those of other species.

THE LYMPHATIC STRUCTURES OF THE HEAD AND NECK

The most important lymph nodes of the head were mentioned in their topographic contexts; other smaller nodes that are usually found medial to the ramus of the mandible are of slight practical concern.

The *parotid node* (Fig. 25.2/13) receives lymph from the skin covering most of the head, especially the more dorsal areas. It also collects from the upper jaw, temporomandibular joint, masticatory muscles, nasal cavity, hard palate, orbit, and the region about the external ear. The efferent vessels pass to the lateral retropharyngeal node (Table 25.4).

The territory of the *mandibular node* (Fig. 25.2/20) overlaps those of the parotid and medial retropharyngeal nodes. The chief afferent vessels come from the skin and underlying structures of the ventral part of the head and from the rostral part of the mouth, including the apex of the tongue. The efferent vessels pass to the lateral retropharyngeal node.

The large *medial retropharyngeal node* lies embedded in fat between the pharynx and the muscles below the cranial base (Figs. 25.9/18 and 25.20/12). It collects lymph from most of the deeper structures of the head, including the nasal

TABLE 25.4 LYMPH NODES OF THE HEAD AND NECK

Lymph Node	Location	Areas Drained	Efferent Flow
Parotid	Partly covered by the parotid salivary gland	Skin on head, temporomandibular joint, masticatory muscles, hard palate, orbit	To lateral retropharyngeal lymph node
Mandibular	Beside the sternum at level of second rib	Skin and underlying structures of the ventral part of the head, the rostral part of the mouth, including the apex of the tongue	To lateral retropharyngeal lymph node
Medial retropharyngeal	Between the pharynx and the base of the cranium	Deeper structures of the head, including the nasal and oral cavities, pharynx, larynx, cranium, and jaw muscles, and from the ventral part of the upper end of the neck	To lateral retropharyngeal lymph node
Lateral retropharyngeal	Near the atlantal wing	Regional lymph collection center for entire head; also directly collects lymph from deeper structures of the head	To tracheal duct
Deep cervicals	As a series along the course of tracheal duct; divided into cranial, middle, and caudal clusters	Structures within the cervical visceral space; also efferent vessels from the axillary lymph center of the forelimb	To tracheal duct
Superficial cervical	Single large node located in the lower part of the neck and cranial to the scapula	The skin and underlying muscles over a very wide area extending from the middle of the neck to the caudal part of the thorax, including the proximal part of the forelimb	Compartmentalized flow to major venous and lymph trunks

and oral cavities, pharynx, larynx, cranium, and jaw muscles, and from the ventral part of the upper end of the neck. The efferent vessels once again drain into the *lateral retropharyngeal node,* which is the collecting center for the entire head (Fig. 25.26/*4*). This lateral node, which is placed below the atlantal wing (Fig. 25.2/*14*), also acts as a primary center for additional lymph vessels draining deeper structures of the head. It channels its outflow into a single large vessel, the tracheal duct, that runs down the neck within the fascia covering the lateral aspect of the trachea. The duct ends by joining the thoracic duct or by opening into one or another vein at the thoracic inlet; most usually the left tracheal duct opens into the thoracic duct while the right one drains directly into a major tributary of the cranial vena cava (Fig. 25.26/*9*).

A series of small *deep cervical lymph nodes* is spread along the course of each tracheal duct. These are supposedly divided into cranial, middle, and caudal clusters and receive lymph from the structures within the cervical visceral space. They transmit this lymph to the tracheal duct, sometimes directly and sometimes after serial passage through several nodes within the group. Usually one or more of the most caudal of these nodes receive the efferent vessels of the axillary lymph center of the forelimb, as well as smaller trunks coming directly from the brisket.

A single, much larger node lies in the lower part of the neck in front of the scapula. This is the *superficial cervical* (prescapular) *node* (Fig. 25.26/*6*), which rests on the deep muscles over the cervical vertebrae; it is easily palpated, though covered by the omotransversarius. It collects from the skin and underlying muscles over a very wide area extending from the middle of the neck to the caudal part of the thorax, including the proximal part of the forelimb. The flow through the node is compartmentalized; particular portions of the node are related to different parts of the drainage field. The large efferent vessels open variously into the major lymph and venous trunks in the vicinity.

Any of the major nodes may be duplicated.

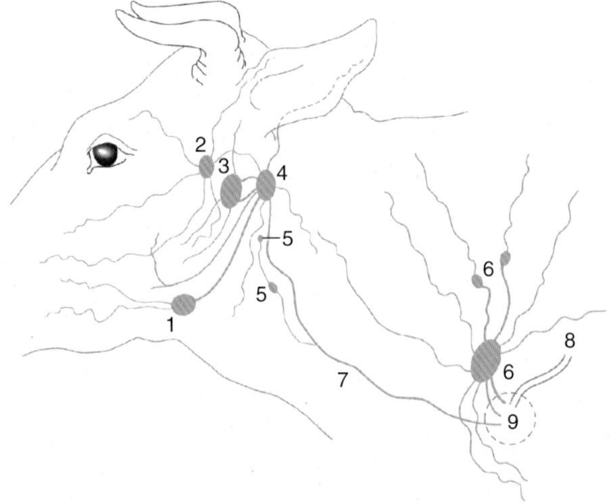

Fig. 25.26 The lymph drainage of the head and neck. *1,* Mandibular lymph node; *2,* parotid lymph node; *3,* medial retropharyngeal lymph node; *4,* lateral retropharyngeal lymph node; *5,* deep cervical lymph nodes; *6,* superficial cervical lymph nodes; *7,* tracheal duct; *8,* thoracic duct; *9,* area within which lymphatic vessels enter veins.

COMPREHENSION CHECK

Examine the teeth of the cadavers in the laboratory, and estimate the age of the animals.

Sketch the location of various lymph nodes in the head and neck of cattle, and show the path of lymph drainage.

Use bovine skull, intact and sectioned in various planes, to understand the location and extent of various paranasal sinuses.

26 The Neck, Back, and Tail of the Ruminant

CONFORMATION AND SURFACE FEATURES

The back and loins are shaped over the framework of the thoracic and lumbar vertebrae. The loins are sharply divided from the flanks by the prominent tips of the lumbar transverse processes, but the boundaries of the back cannot be defined so precisely because the back blends smoothly with the lateral thoracic wall and incorporates the upper line of the shoulder blades with their cartilages and covering muscles. It is convenient to include in this chapter the few observations that are necessary regarding the dorsal sacral region, which merges with the quarters and root of the tail.

In the animal standing quietly, the dorsal contour is slightly raised over the withers, but otherwise it follows a fairly straight line from immediately behind the skull to the tail root (Fig. 26.1).* The line of the neck, which is based on the funicular part of the nuchal ligament, of course varies with the carriage of the head.

The dorsal contour of the trunk is prescribed by the summits of the spinous processes of the vertebrae, many of which can be palpated separately. Identification of individual bones is most reliable if begun at the wide space between the upright process of the last lumbar vertebra and the sloping cranial margin of the median sacral crest. The sacral crest can be followed caudally until it is succeeded by the separate projections of the spinous processes of the caudal vertebrae; any doubt about the identity of these processes may be resolved by pumping the tail up and down to discover the very mobile joint between the first and second tail bones. Certainty in identifying the first intercaudal space has a special importance because this is the site for injection of local anesthetic when producing "low" epidural anesthesia (p. 655). The tail root is sometimes elevated, especially in cows during estrus.

Working cranially from the lumbosacral space, the lumbar spinous processes are easily distinguished in lean animals. Enumeration becomes more difficult over the caudal part of the chest where several processes converge, and the count is completely lost where the vertebrae become enclosed between the scapular cartilages. The first thoracic spine lies cranial to the scapulae, where it can be felt only on deep palpation. The cervical vertebrae cannot be reached from above, but their general position is detectable on palpation from the side. The transverse processes are well developed and divided into two parts, of which the ventral one is quite large; this is very obvious at the sixth cervical vertebra. Despite this, the individual identification of these bones is difficult until the wing of the atlas provides an unmistakable landmark.

Additional features that may be picked out in the region of the hindquarters include the salient sacral tubers of the pelvis, which lie to each side of the lumbosacral space, and the strong iliac crests, which join these projections to the coxal tubers. The crests are raised above their surroundings and are crossed by cranial prolongations of the gluteal musculature.

The head is carried higher in sheep and goats; these species also slope at the croup (Fig. 26.2).

THE VERTEBRAL COLUMN

The vertebral axis runs parallel to the surface of the back in the loins and caudal part of the back; in the thoracic region, it is deflected ventrally. It reaches its most ventral level at the entrance to the thorax; an abrupt flexure there gradually returns the vertebral axis closer to the dorsal border of the neck as it ascends toward the skull (Fig. 26.1).

The vertebral skeleton and articulations follow the usual pattern, and few features need be mentioned. For the cervical (C), thoracic (T), lumbar (L), sacral (S), and caudal (Cd) vertebrae, the formula is C7, T13, L6, S5, Cd18–C20 in cattle. The formula for sheep and goats is C7, T13, and L6(7), S4 in sheep or S5 in goats, and Cd16–C18 in both small ruminants. The great mobility of the neck allows the animal to raise and lower its head and to reach its side with its tongue. Most cervical movements represent the summation of small changes at several joints, but the adoption of the grazing position requires a considerable straightening at the cervicothoracic joint, where the cervical vertebrae are brought into line with those of the thorax. Although movements of the thoracic region are limited by the presence of the rib cage, the greatest flexibility of the trunk is found cranial to the level of the diaphragm. Behind this, movement is greatly restricted, especially in the lateral direction, by the close fit of the articular processes and the tightness of the joint capsules that embrace them. Greater mobility is again found at the lumbosacral joint.

*This description refers to cattle of European origin. The pronounced hump in cattle of the Zebu *(Bos indicus)* line (and their crosses) is mainly due to enlargement of the rhomboideus muscles.

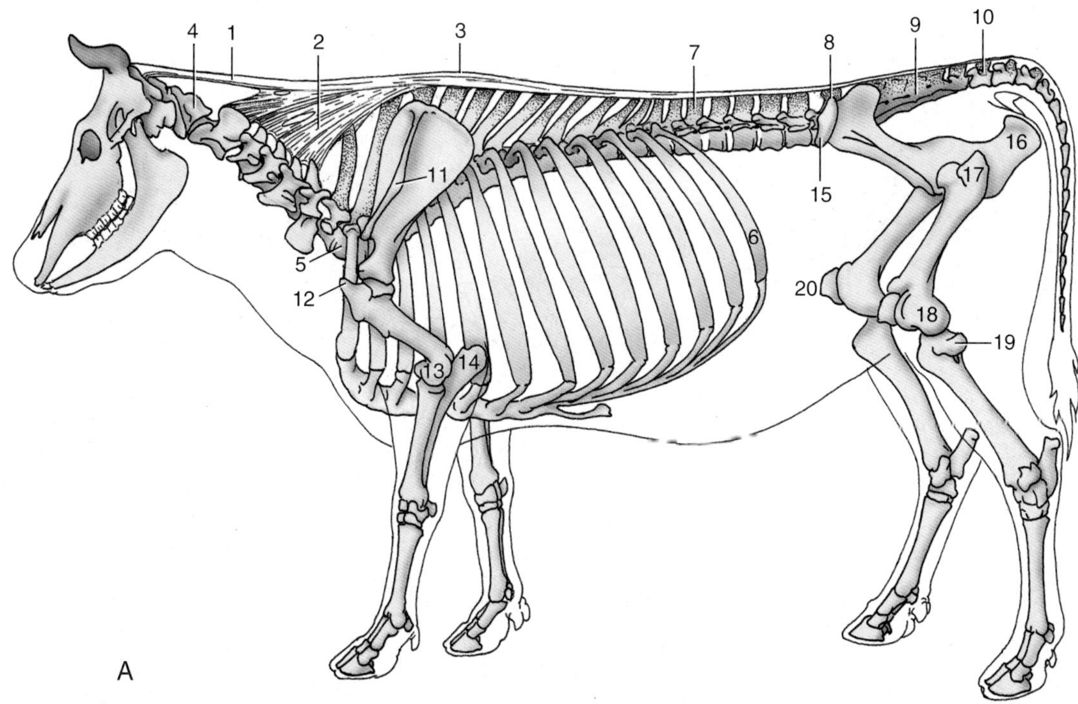

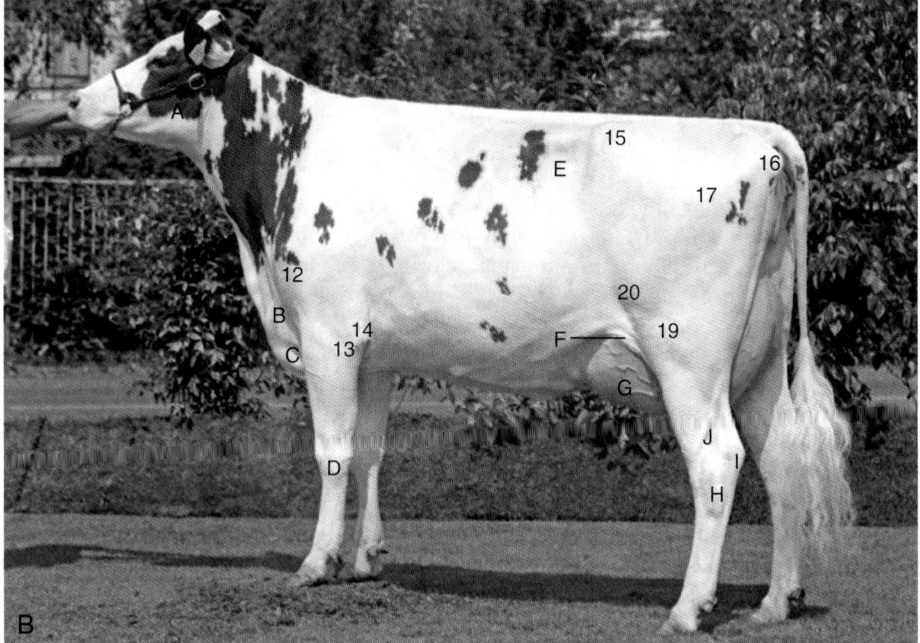

Fig. 26.1 (A) Skeleton with nuchal and supraspinous ligaments; most labeled parts are palpable. (B) Cow in good condition. *1* and *2,* Nuchal ligament: *1,* funiculus nuchae, and *2,* lamina nuchae; *3,* supraspinous ligament; *4,* atlas; *5,* last cervical vertebra (C7); *6,* 13th rib; *7,* first lumbar vertebra (L1); *8,* last lumbar vertebra (L6); *9,* sacrum; *10,* first caudal vertebra; *11,* spine of scapula; *12,* greater tubercle; *13* and *14,* palpable features at elbow joint: *13,* lateral epicondyle, and *14,* olecranon; *15,* coxal tuber; *16,* ischial tuber; *17,* greater trochanter; *18, 19,* and *20,* palpable features of stifle joint: *18,* lateral condyle of femur, *19,* lateral condyle of tibia and remnant of fibula, and *20,* patella. *A,* Masseter; *B,* jugular vein; *C,* brisket; *D,* carpus; *E,* paralumbar fossa; *F,* flank fold; *G,* udder; *H,* hock joint; *I,* calcaneus (point of the hock); *J,* lateral saphenous vein.

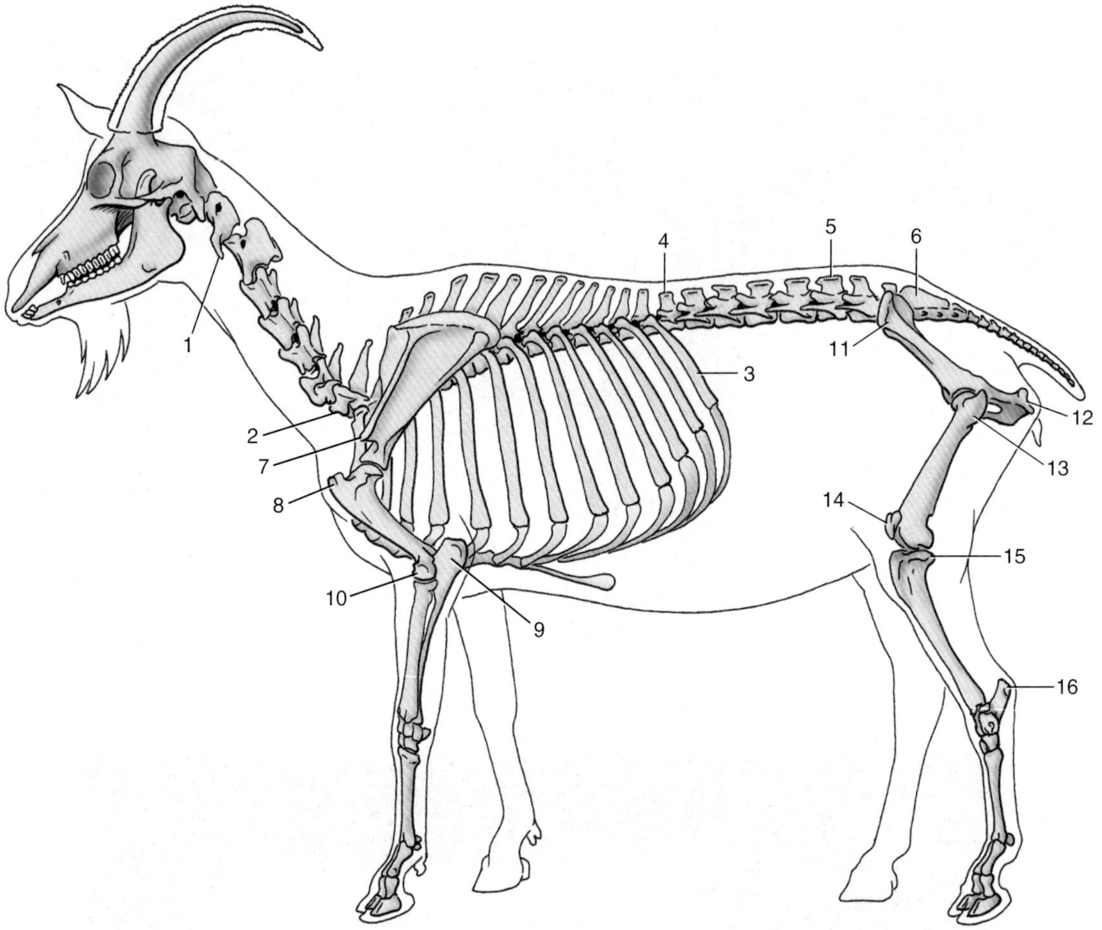

Fig. 26.2 The skeleton of the goat. Most labeled parts of the skeleton are palpable. *1*, Atlas; *2*, last cervical vertebra (C7); *3*, last rib; *4*, first lumbar vertebra (L1); *5*, last lumbar vertebra (L7); *6*, sacrum; *7*, acromion; *8*, greater tubercle; *9*, olecranon; *10*, lateral epicondyle; *11*, coxal tuber; *12*, ischial tuber; *13*, greater trochanter; *14*, patella; *15*, lateral condyle of tibia; *16*, calcaneus.

The generally rather limited flexibility of the spine is consistent with the relative shortness of the intervertebral disks, which in cattle contribute only 10% of the length of the column. The disks are of similar composition and are subject to the same degenerative changes as those in other species. The lumbosacral disk is most commonly grossly damaged because of the greater stress to which it is subjected by the special mobility of the lumbosacral articulation. Disk lesions are sometimes accompanied by changes in the lumbosacral synovial articulations and by the formation of abnormal bony outgrowths (osteophytes) from the ventral margins of the vertebral bodies. Certain of these common changes have a particular importance in bulls because they may lead to an inability to serve.

The elastic *nuchal ligament* (Fig. 26.1/*1* and *2*) consists of two parts, as in the horse. The funicular part, which runs between the occiput and the highest spines of the withers, is a paired cord that is rounded in cross section at its occipital attachment but widens as it passes caudally. It attaches to the sides of the first few thoracic spines, close to their summits; caudal to this, it approaches and fuses with its fellow laminar part to form the supraspinous ligament that caps the bone processes. The rhomboideus and trapezius muscles cover the funicular part of the ligament, in contrast to the arrangement in the horse (see Fig. 25.23/*1*). The laminar part is divided into a cranial paired web that extends between the funicular part and the second to the fourth cervical bones and an unpaired sheet that fills the triangle between the first thoracic and last one or two cervical spinous processes. In addition to relieving the cervical muscles, the nuchal ligament has an occasional significance in determining the track followed by infection. No cranial nuchal bursa exists, but a supraspinous bursa frequently is present between the ligament and the first few thoracic spinous processes.

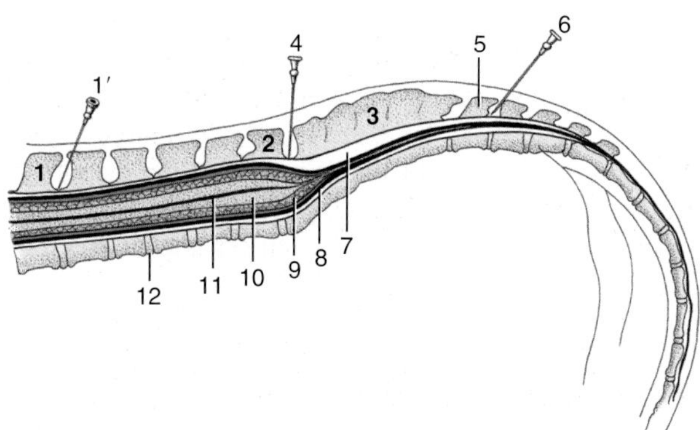

Fig. 26.3 Caudal part of the bovine vertebral canal and its contents (schematic). Epidural injection sites are indicated by the *needles*. *1*, First lumbar vertebra; *1′*, *needle* in position for flank anesthesia; *2*, last lumbar vertebra (L6); *3*, sacrum; *4*, *needle* in lumbosacral space; *5*, first caudal vertebra; *6*, *needle* between first and second caudal vertebrae (tail block); *7*, epidural space; *8*, dura mater; *9*, subarachnoid space; *10*, spinal cord; *11*, central canal; *12*, intervertebral disk.

THE VERTEBRAL CANAL

The vertebral canal is widest within the atlas and tapers rapidly within the sacrum; in between, it is most expanded where it contains the cervical and lumbar enlargements of the spinal cord that give rise to the nerves that form the limb plexuses. Access to the vertebral canal is frequently necessary to withdraw cerebrospinal fluid from the subarachnoid space or to introduce local anesthetic into the epidural space. Therapeutic agents are also occasionally injected into these spaces. Examination of the skeleton shows that, although entry is theoretically possible through any of the interarcuate spaces, it is easiest at the wider gaps between the atlas and the skull, at the lumbosacral joint, and between the first two caudal vertebrae of the tail (Fig. 26.3). The first intercaudal space is conveniently large, measuring about 2 × 2 cm. Most other interarcuate spaces measure only a few millimeters in each direction, and because they lie at a considerable depth below the skin, they are not easily located. The cranialmost interlumbar interarcuate spaces are occasionally used to perform epidural injections to obtain local anesthesia of the flank. A slightly oblique approach, from a point of entry a little lateral and caudal to the target space, gives the least risk of having the needle impinge on bone.

The cord reaches to the first sacral vertebra in adult cattle and considerably farther in young calves, perhaps into the caudal half of the sacrum. It may occupy almost the whole sacrum in the small ruminant species.

The spinal cord is divided into 8 cervical, 13 thoracic, 6 lumbar, 5 sacral, and (usually) 5 caudal segments. The 8 cervical segments are accommodated within the 7 cervical vertebrae, while each of the thoracic and cranial lumbar segments shows an almost exact correspondence with the vertebrae of the same designation. The cranial shift of the more caudal part of the cord leaves the canal within the last lumbar vertebra occupied by the 5 short sacral segments (Fig. 26.4). The *subarachnoid space* extends well into the sacrum, and its dimensions are sufficiently generous to make subarachnoid puncture a relatively simple procedure at the lumbosacral level (Fig. 26.3/*4*).

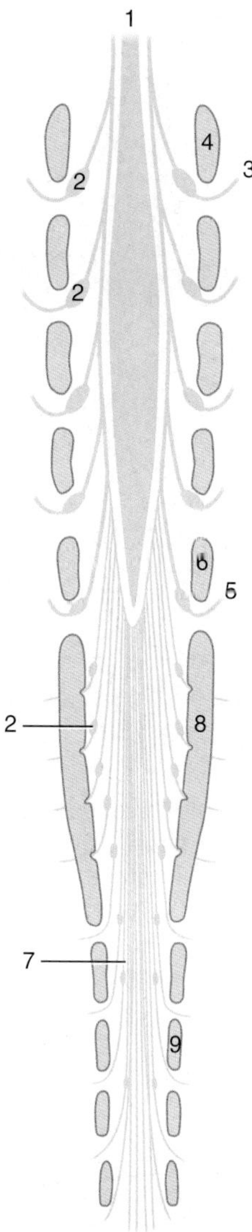

Fig. 26.4 The relationship to the vertebrae of the caudal end of the spinal cord and its branches (schematic dorsal view). Note the position of the spinal ganglia (*2*). The schema indicates the situation in adult cattle. The cord extends to the second or even third sacral vertebra in the newborn calf and in adult sheep and goats. *1*, Spinal cord; *2*, spinal ganglia; *3*, second lumbar spinal nerve; *4*, section of arch of second lumbar vertebra; *5*, sixth lumbar nerve; *6*, section of arch of sixth lumbar vertebra; *7*, cauda equina; *8*, section of sacrum; *9*, section of arch of second caudal vertebra.

The *internal vertebral plexus* of the vertebral column (Fig. 26.5/1) presents two features of potential interest.

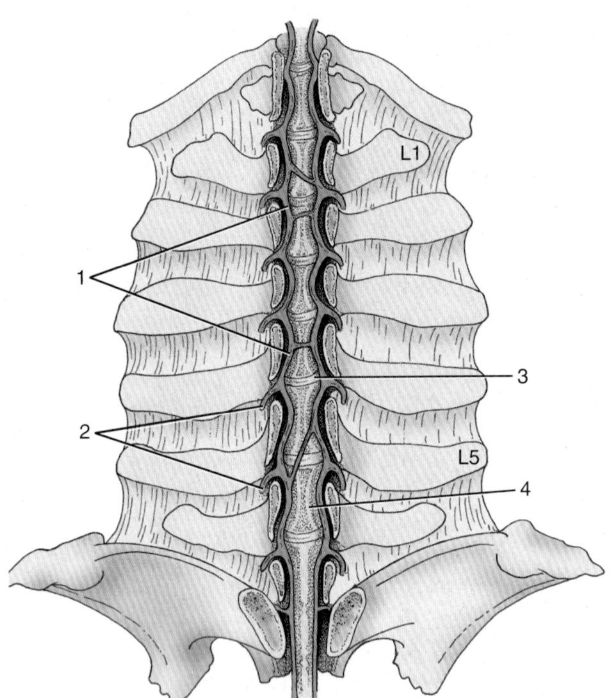

Fig. 26.5 Dorsal view of the venous drainage in the bovine vertebral canal. The internal vertebral plexus, with its internal connections and its lateral segmental branches, has been exposed. *1,* Internal vertebral plexus; *2,* intervertebral veins; *3,* intervertebral disk; *4,* vertebral body; *L1,* first lumbar vertebra; *L5,* fifth lumbar vertebra.

The first involves the possibility of the plexus conveying blood diverted from the caudal vena cava when this is narrowed or obstructed by ruminal tympany; compression of the vena cava may be direct or exerted indirectly by a shearing displacement of the liver against the diaphragm (Fig. 26.6). The second significant feature involves the risk of hemorrhage in the performance of subarachnoid or epidural puncture.

THE VESSELS OF THE TAIL

The median artery and vein of the tail require brief notice. The artery, which continues the median sacral, is ventral to the vein for most of the length of the tail and is commonly used for pulse taking, usually about 18 cm from the root of the tail. The vessels lie side by side in the proximal part of the tail (Cd2 or Cd3), where both artery and vein are available for obtaining blood, although this site is an unwise choice because of the inevitable fecal contamination (Fig. 26.7B). At this level both vessels lie against the ventral aspect of the caudal vertebrae, where they are protected by the hemal processes (Fig. 26.7A), arches on the first few vertebrae (see Fig. 2.12E/9). The vessels are thus accessible only at intervertebral levels. It is usual to dock the tail of lambs.

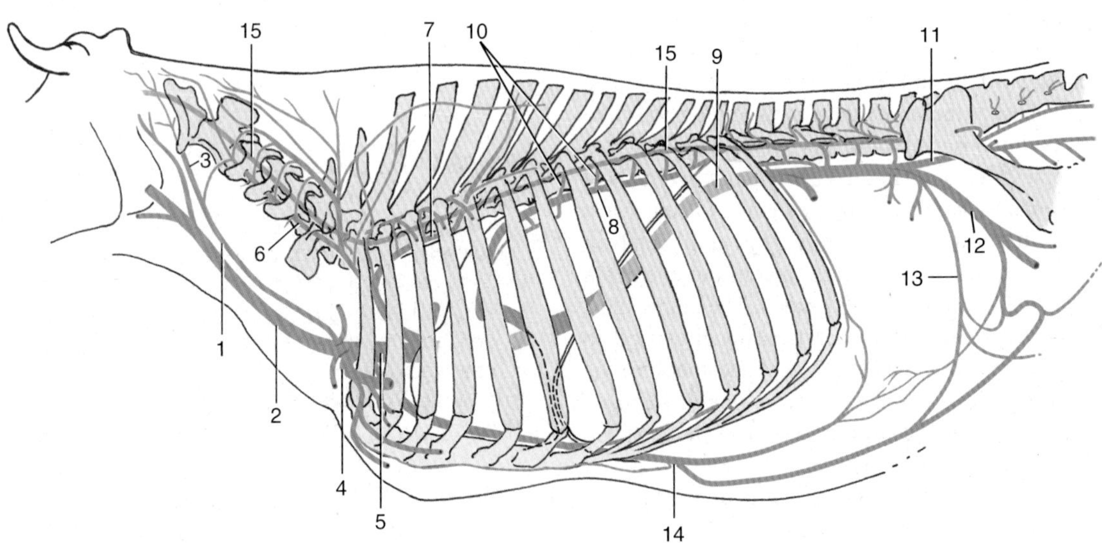

Fig. 26.6 The connections of the major veins with the vertebral plexus–azygous system. Note specifically the connections between the internal vertebral plexus *(15)* and the intercostal veins *(10)* and between the plexus and the branches of the vertebral vein *(6)*. *1,* Internal jugular vein (v.); *2,* external jugular v.; *3,* occipital v.; *4,* axillary v.; *5,* cranial vena cava; *6,* vertebral v.; *7,* supreme intercostal v.; *8,* left azygous v.; *9,* caudal vena cava; *10,* intercostal veins; *11,* internal iliac v.; *12,* external iliac v.; *13,* deep circumflex iliac v.; *14,* cranial epigastric v.; *15,* internal vertebral plexus *(red)*.

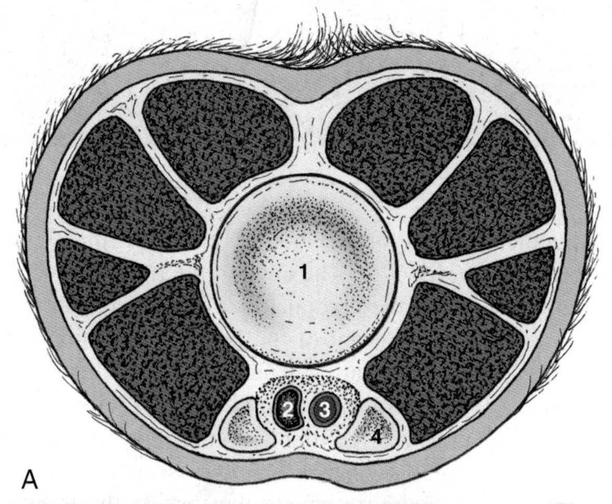

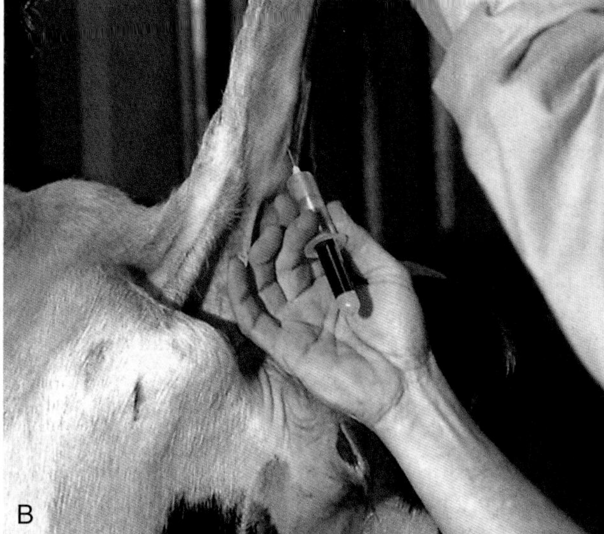

Fig. 26.7 (A) Transverse section of the bovine tail between Cd3 and Cd4. *1,* Intervertebral disk; *2,* median caudal vein; *3,* median caudal artery; *4,* hemal process. (B) Collection of blood from a median caudal vessel.

COMPREHENSION CHECK

Review the anatomic boundaries of the flank, and determine the reasons for its suitability for surgical access to the abdomen.

27 The Thorax of the Ruminant

The extent and dimensions of the thoracic cavity are not apparent on inspection of the live animal. Features such as the narrowness of the cranial part of the thorax or the part of the abdomen enclosed by the rib cage are not appreciated from the external viewpoint (Fig. 27.1). Certain features of the limb skeleton provide helpful guides to the location of deeper parts: the point of the shoulder projects a few centimeters in front of the lower part of the first rib, the caudal angle of the scapula lies over the vertebrae dorsal to the sixth rib, and the point of the elbow lies over the fifth intercostal space, just above the costochondral joints, and just a short way cranial to the vertex of the diaphragm (Fig. 27.2A and B).

The thoracic wall of cattle, unlike that of sheep or goats, is mainly remarkable for the great breadth of the ribs that hampers access to the thoracic cavity through the intercostal space for any rarely indicated thoracic surgery. The intercostal vessels follow both margins in the ventral parts of the spaces, which is a point relevant to pleurocentesis, which is best performed by puncture of the 6th or 7th space directly above the level of the costochondral joints. The ribs from the 5th to the 13th may generally be identified with ease, though possibly not palpated along their entire lengths. The ribs become more oblique and bowed while the cartilages gain more forward slope as the series is followed caudally. The cartilages of the last five (asternal) ribs combine to form the costal arch that defines the cranial limit of the flank. The sternal ribs join the sternum via their cartilages. Compared to the rigid cranial part of the chest wall, the wider caudal part makes more contributions to the respiratory movements; but the activity of the diaphragm still predominates. Despite this, cattle survive diaphragmatic paralysis; however, they suffer greater distress than is usual in smaller species.

THE PLEURA AND THE LUNGS

The lungs are very unequal in that the right one is the larger by a ratio of 3:2. The asymmetry affects the disposition of the pleural sacs; the most obvious consequence is the deviation of both the cranial and the caudal mediastinum far to the left. The cranial mediastinum actually attaches to the left wall of the thorax, while the caudal part meets the diaphragm in a sagittal plane that, when projected into the abdomen, bisects the reticulum, which exposes the two pleural sacs to almost equal chance of involvement when foreign bodies penetrate the thorax from that organ (p. 675). The apex of the right sac, which contains the tip of the cranial lobe of the lung, projects a few centimeters in front of the first rib, exposing it to risk of injury in penetrating wounds that are apparently confined to the base of the neck. The caudal reflection of the costal pleura onto the diaphragm is more important. It follows a cranially concave line that ascends steeply in its caudal part, tracing a course that passes through the 8th costochondral junction and the middle of the 11th rib before reaching the 12th rib just below the edge of the iliocostalis (see Fig. 27.2). Behind this line the diaphragm is directly attached to the thoracic wall, and the abdomen may be approached without risk of injury to the pleural sac. A space in front of this line, the costodiaphragmatic recess, is never fully exploited by the lung. Its extent may be considerably exaggerated after death, when the lung is collapsed.

Apart from their asymmetry, the lungs of cattle are distinguished by their pronounced lobation and very evident lobulation.

The left lung possesses cranial and caudal lobes (see Fig. 27.2), and the former is divided into two parts: one extends forward toward the apex of the pleural sac, and the other descends ventrally over the pericardium. The notch between the two extends from the 3rd intercostal space to the 5th rib and defines the area in which the heart is in direct contact with the thoracic wall (Fig. 27.3). The basal border changes position with the phase of respiration; as a compromise between the inspiratory and expiratory positions, it may be described as following an almost straight line from the 6th costochondral joint to the upper part of the 11th rib. The thin marginal strip of lung does not provide useful clinical information, and the major area for *percussion and auscultation is reduced to the surprisingly small triangle bounded by the triceps, the edge of the muscles of the back, and as the hypotenuse, the line joining the point of the elbow to the upper part of the 11th rib.* A second (prescapular) area, extending a few centimeters in front of the ventral half of the cranial border of the scapula, is of minimal clinical significance.

The right lung possesses four lobes—cranial, middle, caudal, and accessory (Fig. 27.4). The cranial lobe is independently ventilated by a bronchus detached from the trachea shortly before the bifurcation. The cardiac notch, smaller than that on the left side, is restricted to the lower parts of the 3rd and 4th spaces and is

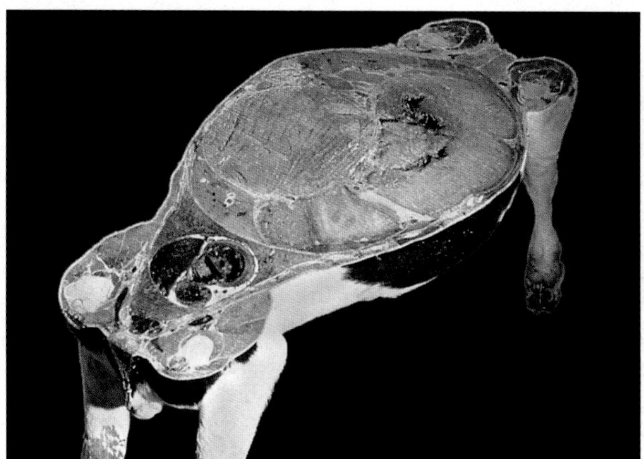

Fig. 27.1 Horizontal section at the level of the shoulder and stifle joints. Note the relative volumes of the thoracic and abdominal cavities.

wholly under cover of the arm. The major area for clinical examination is a little larger on this side because it is free from the pressure exerted on the diaphragm by the rumen. Percussion toward the basal border is also more accurately performed because there is a sharp transition from the hollow lung sound to the duller note over the liver.

Respiratory diseases cause significant economic losses to the cattle industry. Bronchial pneumonia occurs when infectious agents gain access to the lung through the airways. This occurs during physiologic stress induced by factors such as inclement weather and nutritional deficiencies, which lead to compromised immune defenses. The common pathogens include bovine herpesvirus, *Mycoplasma* spp., and *Mannheimia hemolytica.* Thick connective tissue septa divide the lung substance and mark the surface where they impinge on the pulmonary pleura (see Fig. 4.27). These septa may help to localize infection, leading to a diseased part of the lung next to a normal part. This pattern is distinct from the diffuse pattern of the disease in the lungs of dogs.

The capacity for respiratory exchange is limited by a relatively low total alveolar surface area and a lesser capillary density when compared with that of other species. A large part is required for basal needs, and little is held in reserve.

The lungs of the small ruminants are similar in gross form but show a lesser and usually patchy lobulation.

Although the circulation through the lungs is maintained by pulmonary and bronchial arteries, all the blood returns through a single set of veins. Two lymphatic plexuses drain the lungs. One lies directly below the pleura and drains this and the adjoining connective tissue. The other follows the peribronchial tracts and may be interrupted by

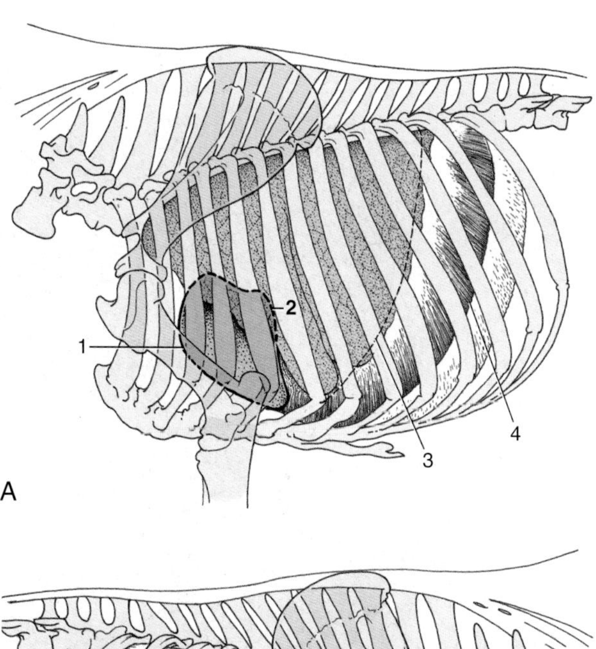

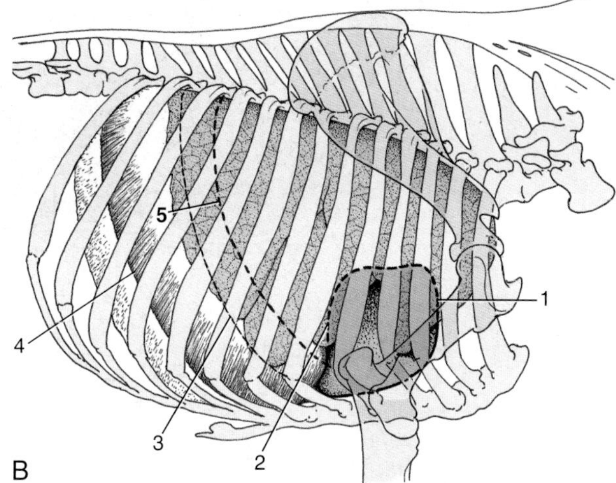

Fig. 27.2 (A) Left and (B) right projections of the bovine heart and lungs on the thoracic wall. The basal border of the lung and the line of pleural reflection are also shown. *1,* Cranial extent of heart; *2,* caudal extent of heart; *3,* basal border of lung; *4,* line of pleural reflection; *5,* caudal border of lung percussion area, shown on right side.

the interposition of peribronchial nodes (though these are never conspicuous and cannot always be found). Both sets enter the tracheobronchial nodes placed about the origins of the principal bronchi.

THE MEDIASTINUM AND ITS CONTENTS

The thick dorsal part of the cranial mediastinum contains the esophagus and trachea, the vessels passing to and from the neck and forelimbs, an assembly of lymph nodes, the thoracic duct, and various nerves. In older animals the ventral part is thin, containing only the internal thoracic vessels and a vestige of the thymus. The difference in thickness is less striking in younger animals, in which the thymus has yet to regress (Fig. 27.5).

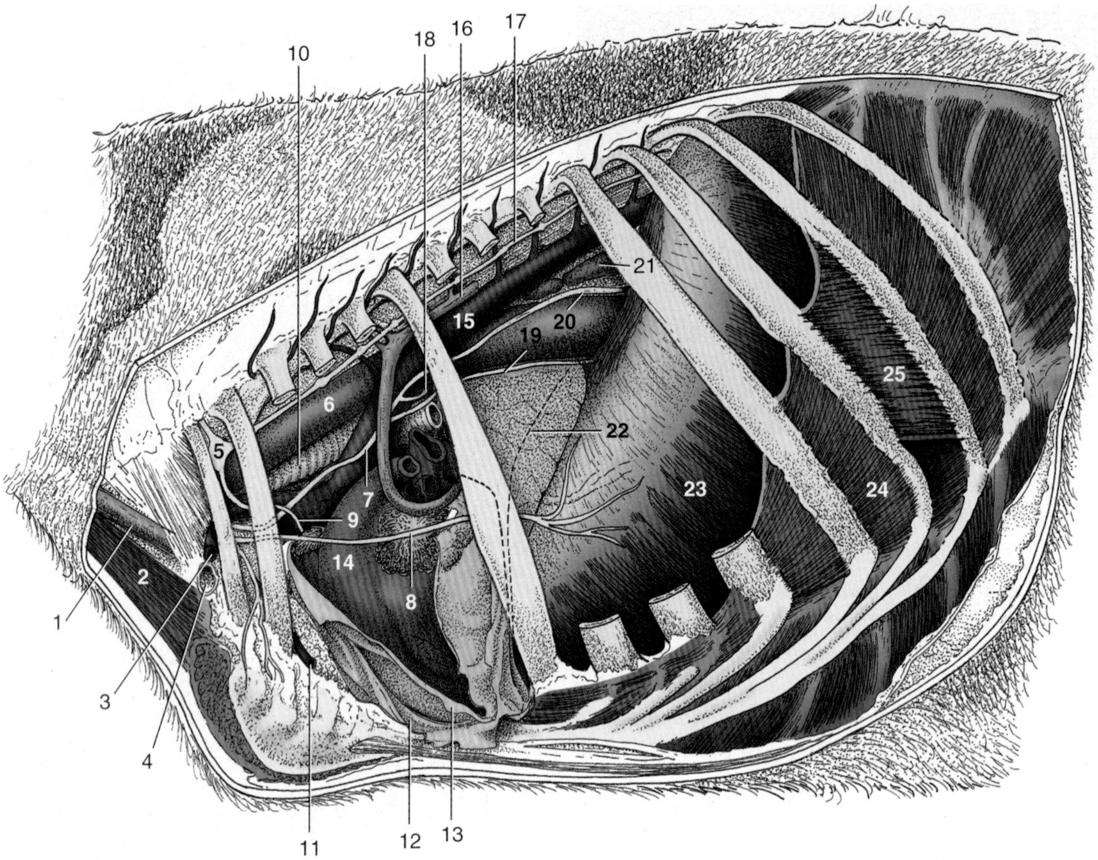

Fig. 27.3 Left lateral view of the bovine thoracic cavity. The left lung and part of the mediastinal pleura have been removed. *1,* External jugular vein; *2,* sternocephalicus; *3,* axillary artery; *4,* axillary vein; *5,* cervicothoracic ganglion; *6,* esophagus; *7,* vagus; *8,* phrenic nerve; *9,* one of the cardiac nerves; *10,* trachea; *11,* internal thoracic artery; *12,* mediastinal pleura; *13,* pericardium, reflected; *14,* pulmonary trunk; *15,* aorta; *16,* left azygous vein; *17,* sympathetic chain; *18,* recurrent laryngeal nerve; *19,* ventral vagal trunk; *20,* dorsal vagal trunk; *21,* caudal mediastinal lymph nodes; *22,* cranial extent of diaphragm; *23,* diaphragm; *24,* internal intercostal muscle; *25,* external intercostal muscle.

The middle mediastinum is occupied by the heart (within the pericardium) ventrally, and the esophagus, the termination of the trachea, the aortic arch, pulmonary vessels, left azygous vein, various lymph nodes, and the vagal trunks dorsally (Fig. 27.6). It is thus of very irregular thickness, being reduced in places to apposed pleural sheets. Ventral to the heart, it widens to contain the pericardiosternal ligament.

The caudal mediastinum is generally thin. The dorsal part contains the esophagus, aorta, vagus trunks, and caudal mediastinal nodes (Fig. 27.7). The septum is very short and level with the base of the heart but, below this, lengthens where it deviates to the left (Fig. 27.5).

The Heart

The heart is placed asymmetrically, 60% or more being to the left of the midline, and extends from the second intercostal space (or following rib) to the fifth space. It thus lies mainly under cover of the limbs in an animal standing square. *The base lies in the plane of the last costochondral joint and the apex opposite the sixth cartilage, a few centimeters above the sternum; its long axis inclines somewhat caudally and to the left.* Direct contact with the thoracic walls is restricted to the areas described with the lungs. The upright caudal border is related to the diaphragm and, through this, to the reticulum and liver; the sloping cranial border is related to the thymus in the young. The relations of the base include the trachea and principal bronchi, the pulmonary vessels, and lymph nodes (Fig. 27.5).

The bovine heart is constructed according to the general mammalian plan. The right atrium receives a left azygous vein, by way of the coronary sinus. It occasionally retains communication with the left atrium through an open foramen ovale; this is usually only probe patent and without significance. Two ossicles are found in the connective tissue related to the cusps of the aortic valve; they

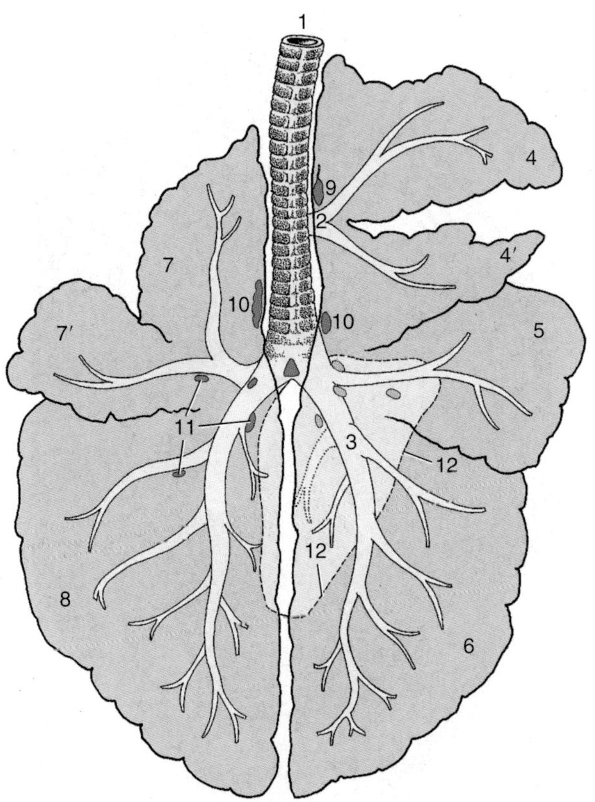

Fig. 27.4 Lobation and bronchial tree of the bovine lungs, dorsal view (schematic). *1,* Trachea; *2,* tracheal bronchus; *3,* right principal bronchus; *4* and *4′,* divided right cranial lobe; *5,* middle lobe; *6,* right caudal lobe; *7* and *7′,* divided left cranial lobe; *8,* left caudal lobe; *9,* cranial tracheobronchial lymph node; *10,* tracheobronchial lymph nodes; *11,* pulmonary lymph nodes; *12,* outline of accessory lobe of right lung.

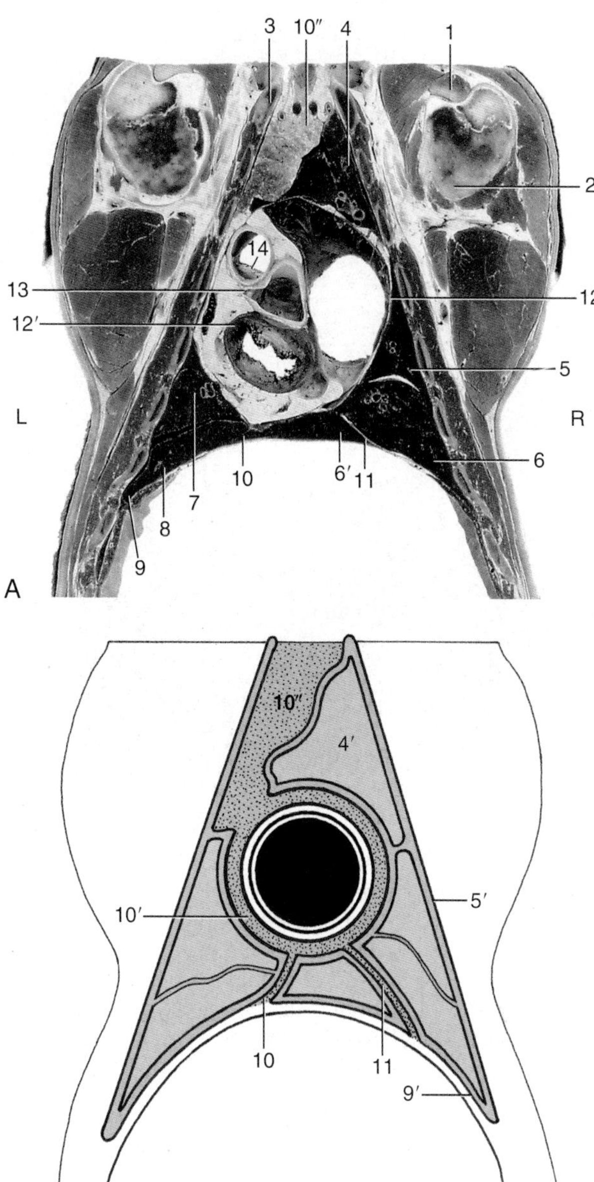

Fig. 27.5 Dorsal section of the bovine thorax directly ventral to the shoulder joint. (A) Actual. *L,* Left side; *R,* right side. (B) Schematized to show the asymmetry of the cranial and caudal parts of the mediastinum *(stippled). 1,* Biceps tendon; *2,* humerus; *3,* first rib; *4,* cranial lobe of right lung; *4′,* pulmonary pleura; *5,* middle lobe of right lung; *5′,* costal pleura; *6* and *6′,* caudal and accessory lobes of right lung, respectively; *7,* caudal part of cranial lobe of left lung; *8,* caudal lobe of left lung; *9,* diaphragm; *9′,* diaphragmatic pleura; *10, 10′,* and *10″,* caudal, middle, and cranial mediastinum, respectively, the last occupied by the thymus; *11,* plica venae cavae; *12* and *12′,* right and left atrioventricular valves, respectively; *13,* left coronary artery arising from aortic valve; *14,* pulmonary valve.

are not unique to cattle, as often supposed, but do appear to develop precociously in this species. The left coronary artery is dominant, with the right one restricted to a circumflex course. It is worth mentioning that the isthmus of the aorta (the segment between the origin of the brachiocephalic trunk and the junction with the ductus arteriosus) is greatly constricted in the newborn calf, which is an appearance that may falsely suggest the aorta arising from the right ventricle. The heart attains usual proportions in neonates within a few days of the birth.

The projections of the heart valves on the thoracic wall, or more accurately the puncta maxima, are obviously of much greater significance. The pulmonary and aortic valves may be regarded as being placed under the 3rd rib and following space and the 4th rib, respectively. These valves are about 10 cm above the costochondral junctions, although the slope of the heart raises the aortic valve a little above and lowers the pulmonary valve a little below the suggested level. The left atrioventricular valve lies under the 4th space and 5th rib, and the right one lies under the 4th rib and space;

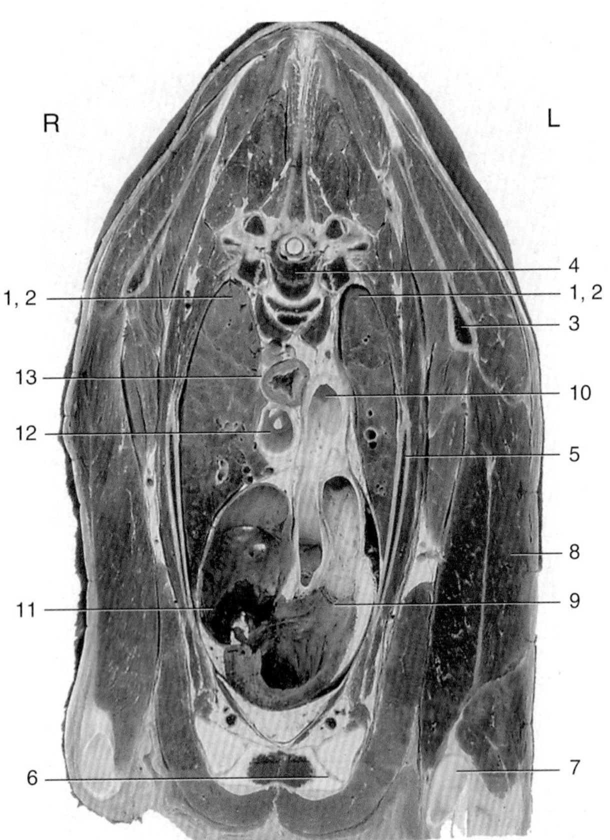

Fig. 27.6 Transverse section of the bovine thorax at the level of the fourth thoracic vertebra. Note the asymmetry of the lungs. *1* and *2,* Cranial lobes of right and left lungs; *3,* scapula; *4,* fourth thoracic vertebra; *5,* third rib; *6,* sternum; *7,* olecranon; *8,* long head of triceps; *9,* pulmonary valve; *10,* aortic arch; *11,* right atrioventricular valve; *12,* trachea; *13,* esophagus; *L,* left side; *R,* right side.

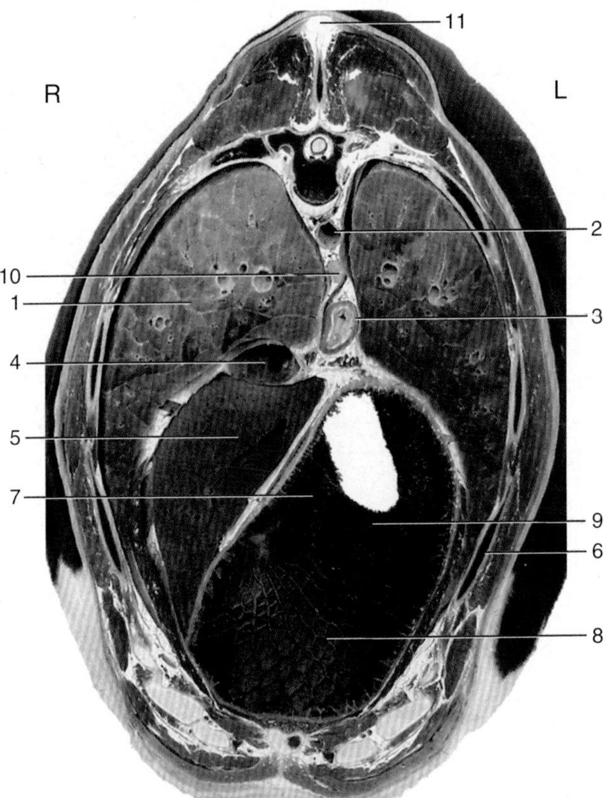

Fig. 27.7 Transverse section of the bovine trunk at the level of the eighth thoracic vertebra. Note the cover to abdominal viscera provided by the ribs. *1,* Caudal lobe of right lung; *2,* aorta; *3,* esophagus; *4,* caudal vena cava; *5,* liver; *6,* seventh rib; *7,* reticular groove; *8,* reticulum; *9,* ruminoreticular fold; *10,* caudal mediastinal lymph node; *11,* supraspinous ligament; *L,* left side; *R,* right side.

each is at a slightly more ventral level than the associated arterial valve. It is of course only the right atrioventricular valve sound that is sought on the right side (Fig. 27.5).

Pericardiocentesis is most safety performed in the 5th intercostal space of the left side, directly dorsal to the costochondral joints.

The Esophagus, Trachea, Thymus, and Vagus Nerves

The *esophagus* and trachea enter the thorax surrounded by a loose fascia that continues the connective tissue of the neck and provides a pathway for the spread of fluids and infection that is most relevant in connection with leaking wounds of the esophagus. At this level the esophagus lies dorsolateral to the trachea on the left side but soon obtains a median position. Its relations include the cranial mediastinal lymph nodes and the vagus and sympathetic nerves when still close to the thoracic entrance and the aorta, thoracic duct, azygous vein, and tracheobronchial and middle mediastinal nodes more caudally. In its final thoracic stretch, it has the important relations of the vagal trunks and the caudal mediastinal nodes.

Post mortem, the esophagus is seen relaxed, providing no evidence of the prediaphragmatic sphincter that is sometimes alleged to exist. The part embraced by the diaphragm may be found constricted, which may not be the case in life.

The *trachea,* deep and compressed from side to side, first lies dorsal to the veins combining to form the cranial vena cava. It continues this relationship to its bifurcation above the right atrium, shortly after detaching the bronchus that serves the right cranial lobe. Its relations at different levels include the principal nerves within the thorax, the aorta and thoracic duct, and the tracheobronchial nodes.

The *thymus* has previously been described in the neck (p. 648 and Fig. 25.24). The thoracic part fills the ventral part of the cranial mediastinum, extending at its apogee over the cranial surface of the pericardium and reaching the origin of the pulmonary trunk and the aortic arch. Involution is rarely complete, and some vestige, consisting mainly of fat and fibrous tissue, persists even in aged animals.

The sympathetic and phrenic nerves are unremarkable. The *vagus nerves* exhibit no special features before their division into dorsal and ventral branches that unite with their partners of the other side to form the trunks that follow the borders of the esophagus. A connection over the left face of the esophagus before entry into the abdomen may be relevant to the inconsistent effects of nerve sections on gastric function. The connection sometimes suggests reinforcement of the ventral trunk at the expense of the dorsal one and sometimes the reverse. The relationship to the caudal mediastinal lymph node(s) is of importance.

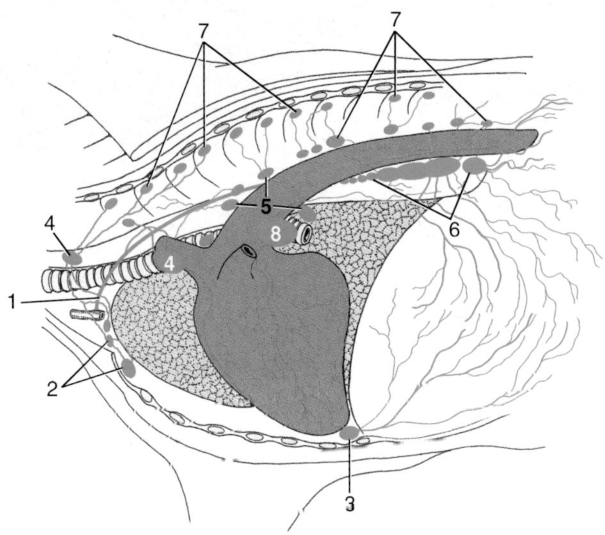

Fig. 27.8 Lymph drainage of the bovine thoracic wall and mediastinum. *1,* Thoracic duct; *2,* cranial sternal lymph nodes; *3,* caudal sternal lymph node; *4,* cranial mediastinal lymph nodes; *5,* middle mediastinal lymph nodes; *6,* caudal mediastinal lymph nodes; *7,* intercostal and thoracic aortic lymph nodes; *8,* tracheobronchial node.

THE LYMPHATIC STRUCTURES WITHIN THE THORAX

The lymphatic drainage of the thorax is complicated and variable. Not every node is present in every animal, and some may be placed so that it is difficult to assign them to a particular group. A series of small intercostal nodes is present directly below the pleura in certain spaces, and these are supplemented by a scattering of nodes along the aorta (Fig. 27.8). Both sets drain lymph from structures about the vertebral column and within the dorsal mediastinum. Most of their outflow is directed toward the cranial mediastinal nodes (Table 27.1).

The *thoracic duct,* into which most of the lymph eventually flows, inclines ventrally over the left face of the trachea to end by opening into the cranial vena cava or one of its tributaries of the left side. The duct is often duplicated for all or part of its course.

COMPREHENSION CHECK

Demarcate the area of auscultation of the lungs, and practice auscultation on live animals.

Compare the gross and subgross anatomy of the lungs of cattle with those of the horse, and discuss the functional implications of differences in structure.

TABLE 27.1 LYMPH NODES OF THE THORAX

Lymph Nodes	Location	Areas Drained	Efferent Flow
Caudal sternal	Below the transverse thoracic muscle on the thoracic floor	Ventral parts of the thoracic and cranial abdominal floors and overlying muscles of the forelimb	To cranial mediastinal group
Cranial sternal	In front of the caudal sternal lymph nodes		
Cranial mediastinal	Near the entrance to the thorax	Drain adjacent mediastinal structures, plus from caudal and cranial sternal lymph nodes	To thoracic duct or one or two tracheal ducts
Middle mediastinal	To the right of the aortic arch	Mediastinal structures and from some of the tracheobronchial lymph nodes	To tracheal duct
Tracheobronchial	Directly on the trachea and the bronchi	Lung	Various mediastinal lymph nodes
Caudal mediastinal: 1–2; could be 20 cm long	Dorsal to the hiatus over the esophagus	Adjacent structures	To thoracic duct; enlargement can compress the esophagus to cause bloating

28 The Abdomen of the Ruminant

CONFORMATION AND SURFACE ANATOMY

The form of the abdomen varies with age, obesity, and physiologic condition. In adult animals it is both deep and wide, and the floor, which dips behind the sternum, ascends very steeply in its caudal part to join the pubic brim. This marked steepness is not obvious on first inspection because the caudal part of the abdomen is covered by the thighs and the skinfolds that pass between the flanks and stifle joints and is overlain ventrally by the udder or the prepuce. The considerable extent of the abdomen under cover of the ribs follows from the curvature of the diaphragm (see Fig. 27.3). The abdomen is usually bilaterally symmetrical, although advanced pregnancy or excessive distention of the rumen may cause one side to bulge more markedly (Table 28.1). The upper part of the flank is dished, forming the paralumbar fossa beside the loins (see Fig. 26.1/*B* and *E*), while the lower convex part merges with the floor.

In the younger calf the abdomen is shallower and laterally compressed, and the floor slopes more gradually to the pelvis. The spreading of the caudal ribs, the deepening of the trunk, and the depressions beside the vertebral column develop with growth of the rumen.

The lateral and ventral abdominal walls are bounded by the last rib and costal arch, the extremities of the lumbar transverse processes, the coxal tuber, and the terminal line of the pelvic inlet (see Fig. 26.1A). Not all of these are palpable, although identification of the margin of the thoracic cage, the coxal tuber, and most lumbar transverse processes normally presents no problem. The correct identification of the bones with palpation is important in certain anesthetic techniques. Out of the six lumbar vertebrae in cattle, the second to fifth vertebrae are easy to recognize and may even be identifiable without palpation in lean cattle. The first process, however, cannot always be located because it is short, tucked into the angle between the last rib and the spine, and generally overlain by a pad of fat. The last one always eludes the fingers because it lies medial to the coxal tuber below a thick covering of muscle (see Fig. 26.5). There are occasionally seven lumbar vertebrae in sheep and goats.

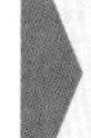

THE VENTROLATERAL WALL OF THE ABDOMEN

Structure

The ventrolateral wall of the abdomen is composed of as many as 9 or 10 layers, although not all cover the entire extent. The skin is freely movable except over the coxal tuber. The *cutaneous muscle* is thick over the lower parts of the flank but thins dorsally and does not extend over the paralumbar fossa. It also leaves the abdominal floor bare except for detached fascicles that supply the male animal with cranial and caudal muscles of the prepuce. The cutaneous muscle extends through the flank fold to end in an aponeurosis over the lateral surface of the thigh (Fig. 28.1A).

The loose *superficial fascia* provides pathways for the cutaneous nerves and encloses certain lymph nodes. The elongated subiliac node is easy to palpate and lies vertically within the skinfold, pressed against the cranial margin of the thigh some distance above the patella. It drains the more superficial layers of the body wall as far forward as the caudal part of the thorax and also receives lymph coming from the skin and superficial muscles of the thigh and croup (see Fig. 29.46). A number of smaller nodes within the paralumbar fossa drain the surrounding parts but normally escape notice except when enlarged. The subcutaneous abdominal ("milk") vein runs forward over the abdominal floor from the udder (see Fig. 29.44).

The *deep fascia* is transformed into an elastic tunica flava, attached to the underlying muscle and sharing in supporting the viscera. Ventrally it gives origin to the external spermatic fascia or the medial lamina of the suspensory apparatus of the udder.

The *muscle layer* is broadly arranged as in other species. The flank has a triple layer of flat muscles (*external oblique, internal oblique,* and *transversus abdominis*) that take origin from the ribs, lumbar transverse processes, and ilium (Fig. 28.1). These are continued over the abdominal floor by aponeurotic tendons that enclose the rectus muscles to each side of the linea alba where the aponeuroses attach (see Fig. 1.37). The linea alba runs from the xiphoid process of the sternum to the center of the prepubic tendon, where it blends with the end tendons of the recti.

TABLE 28.1 ABDOMINAL CONTOURS AND ANIMAL STANCE IN RELATION TO MEDICAL CONDITION

Contour or Stance	Condition
Unilateral or bilateral ventral abdominal wall distention	Dilation of ventral rumen
Distention of the left flank	Ruminal tympany (accumulation of gas in dorsal chamber); abomasal displacement to the left
Right-sided abdominal distention	Dilation, displacement, and obstruction of abomasum or intestines
Arched back, tucked up abdomen, reluctance to move	Anterior abdominal pain (e.g., traumatic reticulopericarditis)

The most superficial muscle of the flank, the *external oblique,* arises by fleshy serrations from the outer surfaces of the last eight ribs. Its most dorsal fibers run more or less horizontally toward the coxal tuber, but the greater number slope caudoventrally to find attachment to the linea alba (Fig. 28.1B). The gap that intervenes between the dorsal border and transverse processes is closed by a sheet of fascia. The fleshy part is succeeded by an aponeurotic tendon, and the transformation occurs along a line that first drops vertically, from a point roughly level with the coxal tuber, before sweeping cranially. A split within the aponeurosis provides the superficial opening (ring) of the inguinal canal.

The second muscle, the *internal oblique,* has a tendinous origin from the coxal tuber and the pelvic tendon of the external oblique and several independent fleshy origins from the tips of the lumbar transverse processes. It radiates to insert on the last rib and into the linea alba. Most fibers run cranioventrally, but the thicker, most caudal fascicles pass slightly behind the plane of the tuber. The muscle–tendon junction slopes caudoventrally, and only the most caudal strip is fleshy where the muscle crosses the margin of the rectus (Fig. 28.1C). The aponeuroses of the two oblique muscles become increasingly interwoven where they pass ventral to the rectus and together furnish the external layer of the rectus sheath. The flesh of the internal oblique forms the inner wall of the inguinal canal.

The third, the *transversus abdominis,* arises from the last ribs and the extremities of the lumbar transverse processes. Its craniodorsal triangle is tendinous, but most of the part covering the flank is fleshy. Before reaching the edge of the rectus, the flesh gives way to an aponeurosis that crosses the dorsal face of the rectus to gain the linea alba to form the inner layer of the rectus sheath. Most fibers run transversely, and none passes behind the plane of the coxal tuber, thus leaving the dorsal surface of the rectus uncovered in its most caudal part (Fig. 28.1D).

The *rectus abdominis* muscle is interrupted in the usual way by several tendinous intersections (Fig. 28.1D/*3*). It arises from the outer surfaces of the lower ends of the last 10 ribs and continues as a wide band separated from its neighbor by the flattened linea alba. It narrows suddenly as it approaches the pubic brim, and the tendon that succeeds the flesh twists to form, with its fellow and the linea alba, a V-shaped trough that continues as the central part of the prepubic tendon. Before reaching the pubic brim, which it approaches almost vertically from below, the prepubic tendon is strengthened by joining the decussation formed by the contralateral parts of the pectineus muscles (each of which arises from both pubic bones) and by additional contributions from the aponeuroses of the abdominal oblique muscles. Ultimately, and after partial decussation, the rectus tendons end in common on the symphyseal crest of the pelvis and on the medial symphyseal tendon that arises here. A rounded median depression of the internal surface of the prepubic tendon is ascribed to the drag of the udder (see Fig. 29.40).

A thin fascia covers the abdominal muscles internally and supports the parietal peritoneum. The largest deposits of fat in the subperitoneal tissues are encountered toward the pelvic inlet. The wholly tendinous nature of a region of the abdominal wall, along the border of the rectus in front of the stifle, merits emphasis.

The *inguinal canal* resembles that of the horse (p. 538) so closely that a separate description is unnecessary. Inguinal hernias are infrequent in cattle but common in male sheep, although there are no obvious differences in the adult anatomy. It is probable that the frequent incidence in rams is connected with inherited anomalies in gubernacular development.

Innervation and Vascularization

The most important nerves of the abdominal wall are the last thoracic (T13) and the first and second lumbar nerves, although the floor ventral to the costal arch is served by continuations of the caudal intercostal nerves. A knowledge of the topography and distribution of the nerves to the flank is of practical importance in obtaining local anesthesia.

The skin is divided into bands (dermatomes) that encircle the trunk, and each is the territory of a particular spinal nerve. The peritoneal regions supplied by spinal nerves correspond very closely to the dermatomes. The skin of the abdomen is supplied by branches from both dorsal and ventral primary rami, but the muscles and other deep structures are supplied by ventral rami alone (see Fig. 1.37). The *dorsal rami* (Fig. 1.37/*4*) of the thoracic and lumbar nerves supply the epaxial muscles and the strip of skin extending from the dorsal midline

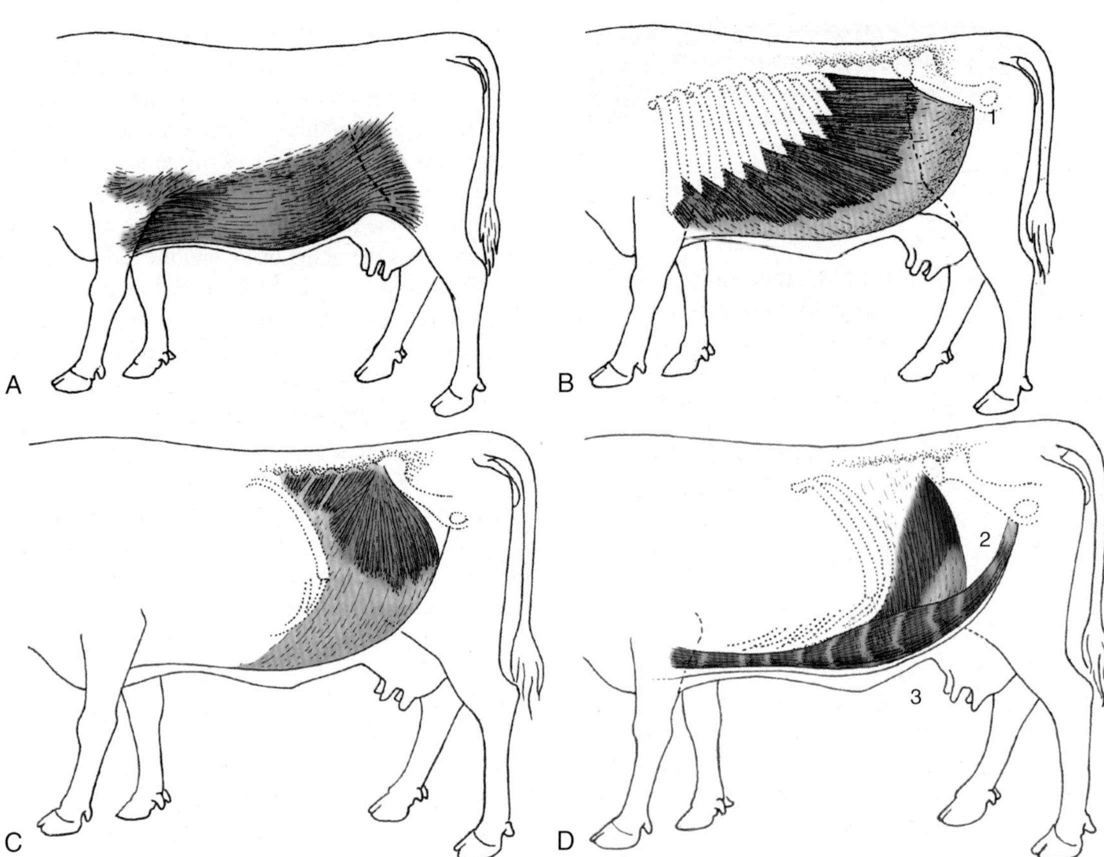

Fig. 28.1 Cutaneous trunci and abdominal muscles. (A) Cutaneous trunci, especially well developed ventrally. (B) External abdominal oblique with superficial inguinal ring *(1)* in its aponeurosis. (C) Internal abdominal oblique. (D) Transversus abdominis *(2)* and rectus abdominis *(3)*. Note the reduction in the thickness of the wall along the caudal part of the rectus margin.

roughly to the level of the patella. Below this line the skin is supplied by two tiers of branches from the ventral rami (Fig. 1.37/5).

The *ventral rami* are much widened where they enter the flank between the internal oblique and transverse muscles. Each possesses a rather constant relationship to the skeleton that is a useful guide for blocking the nerves with anesthetics. These nerves run obliquely, deviating in an increasingly caudal direction (Fig. 28.2). The last thoracic ventral branch usually passes below the tip of the first lumbar transverse process, the first lumbar branch *(iliohypogastric nerve)* passes below the tip of the second, and the second lumbar branch *(ilioinguinal nerve)* passes below the tip of the fourth (Fig. 28.3). Most variations affect the last of these three nerves, which sometimes passes below the transverse process of the third lumbar vertebra.

An exception to the general pattern of innervation of the abdominal wall is the nerve from the brachial plexus to the cutaneous muscle.

Incisions of the upper flank require blockage of both dorsal and ventral branches. Anesthesia is most conveniently obtained by paravertebral injection of the relevant nerves close to their foramina of emergence from the vertebral canal. Anesthesia of the lower flank and abdominal floor requires blockage of the ventral branches only, and these are most conveniently reached where they pass close to the tips of the lumbar transverse processes *(paralumbar block)*. Variation in topography requires wider diffusion of the anesthetic agent for reliable effects. Lumbar epidural injection provides an alternative procedure. The specific innervation of the cutaneous muscle must be kept in mind regardless of the method chosen.

The abdominal wall receives *blood vessels* from several sources. The ventral part obtains its supply through the cranial and caudal epigastric arteries, which are branches of the internal thoracic and external pudendal arteries, respectively. The flanks are supplied from parietal branches of the aorta, of which the most important surgically is the deep circumflex iliac artery, which comes from the external iliac to pierce the flank a little cranial to the coxal tuber. The veins are initially satellite, but in the parous cow the arrangement is modified with the formation of the "milk" vein (p. 710).

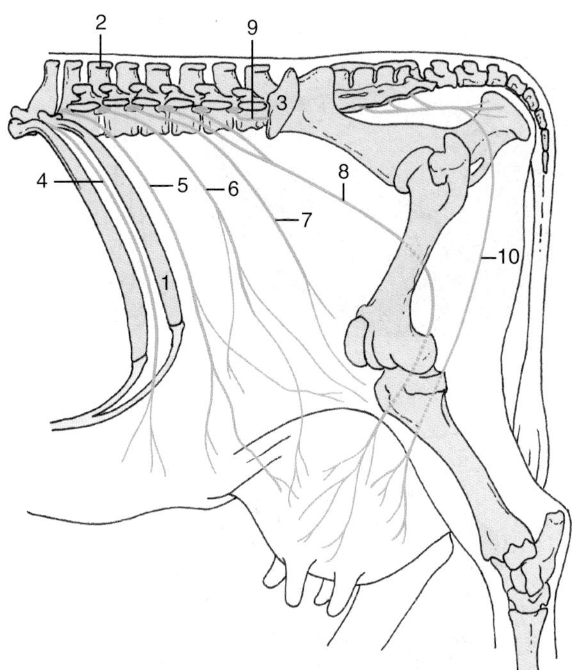

Fig. 28.2 Topography of the nerves to the flank and udder, simplified. The dorsal branches of the spinal nerves to the upper part of the flank are not shown. *1,* Last rib; *2,* spinous process of second lumbar (L2); *3,* coxal tuber; *4,* 12th thoracic (T12) (intercostal nerve [n.]); *5,* T13 (costoabdominal n.); *6,* L1 (iliohypogastric n.); *7,* L2 (ilioinguinal n.); *8,* L3 and L4 (genitofemoral n.); *9,* L5 (nerve); *10,* ventral perineal n.

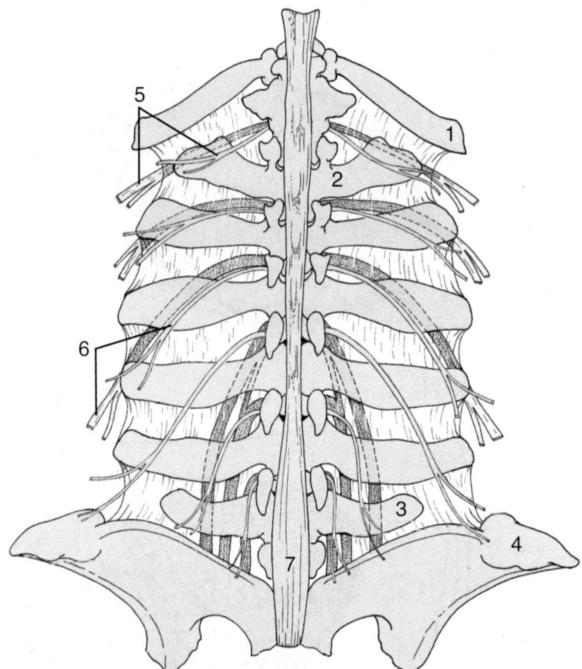

Fig. 28.3 Relationship of the lumbar spinal nerves to the transverse processes of the bovine lumbar vertebrae. *1,* Last rib; *2,* first lumbar vertebra; *3,* sixth lumbar vertebra; *4,* coxal tuber; *5,* dorsal and ventral branches of the 13th thoracic nerve (the ventral branch is *partly stippled*); *6,* dorsal and ventral branches of second lumbar nerve; *7,* supraspinous ligament.

THE SPLEEN

A general impression of the visceral topography should be obtained from Fig. 28.4 before the individual organs are considered.

The flat oblong spleen of adult cattle is about 45 cm long and 12 cm wide. It is situated over the craniodorsal part of the rumen, against the left half of the diaphragm, and is attached to both these organs by the gastrosplenic ligament and the phrenicosplenic ligament, respectively. Its upper end lies under the dorsal ends of the last few ribs, and its axis extends ventrally, with a slight cranial inclination, across the line of the ribs to end in the region of the seventh costochondral joint (Figs. 28.4A/2 and 28.5/6). In most animals the lower end passes onto the reticulum, which brings risk of involvement in the common abscesses and perforations of that organ. The upper part of the spleen is retroperitoneal: the line of serosal reflection runs cranioventrally over both parietal and visceral surfaces. The hilus is confined to the dorsocranial angle of the medial side, and to reach this site, the splenic vessels must first pass over the roof of the rumen.

The capsule contains little muscle, and physiologic variation in spleen size is therefore rather restricted. Occasionally an enlarged spleen may extend behind the last rib in the angle between this and the lumbar spine, but for practical purposes the spleen may be regarded as out of reach for palpation or percussion. Access for a biopsy is normally made through the upper end of the 11th intercostal space and involves little risk of injury to the lung, particularly if the needle is introduced during expiration.

The spleen has a relatively soft consistency. Its color varies considerably, tending to be steel blue in cows and more reddish in males and younger animals. The division of the pulp into red and white areas is very obvious. The white corpuscles are somewhat larger than pinheads.

The spleen is relatively small in *sheep* and *goats,* in which its form, position, and attachments resemble those of the dorsal extremity of the bovine organ. It is roughly triangular in sheep and quadrilateral in goats (Fig. 28.6B and C).

THE STOMACH

General Considerations

The stomach is composed of four chambers—rumen, reticulum, omasum, and abomasum—through which the food passes successively (Fig. 28.7). The first three, collectively known as the *forestomach* (proventriculus), are

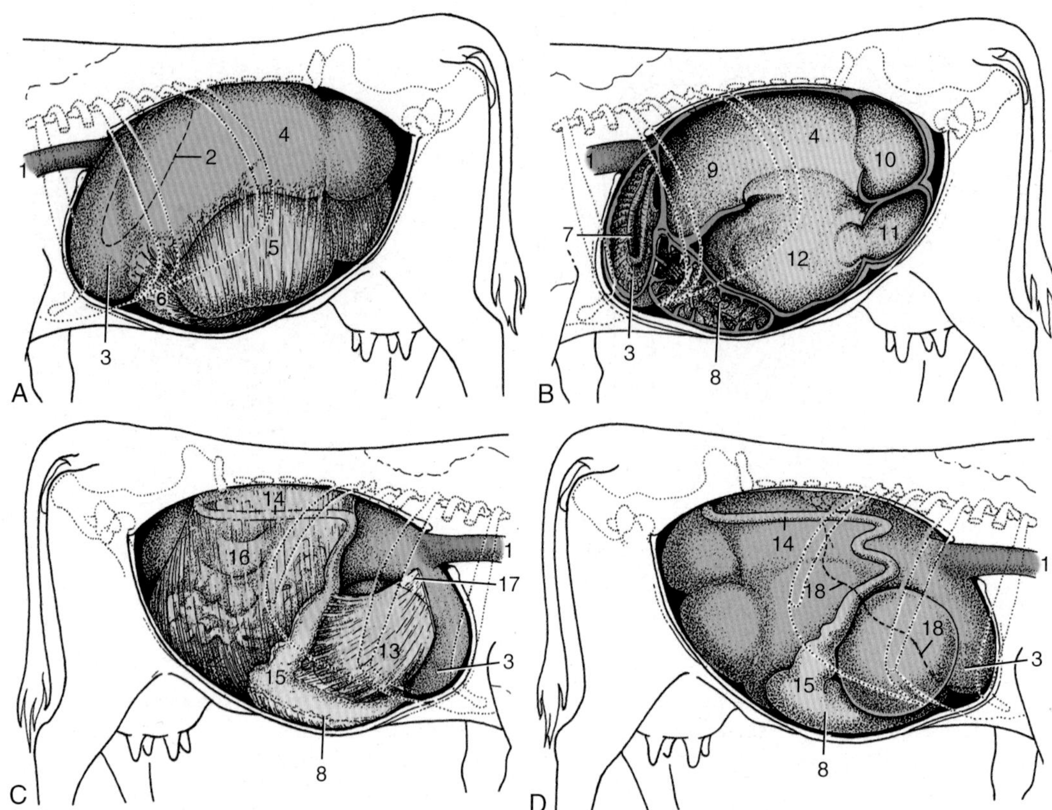

Fig. 28.4 Topography of the abdominal viscera. (A) Relationship of abdominal viscera to the left abdominal wall. (B) The interior of the stomach seen from the left. (C) Relationship of abdominal viscera to the right abdominal wall; the liver has been removed. (D) Position of the parts of the stomach seen from the right. *1,* Esophagus; *2,* outline of spleen; *3,* reticulum; *4,* dorsal sac of rumen; *5,* ventral sac of rumen, covered by superficial wall of greater omentum; *6,* fundus of abomasum, covered by superficial wall of greater omentum; *7,* reticular groove; *8,* body of abomasum; *9,* atrium ruminis; *10,* caudodorsal blind sac; *11,* caudoventral blind sac; *12,* ventral sac of rumen (opened); *13,* omasum, covered by lesser omentum; *14,* descending duodenum; *15,* pyloric part of abomasum; *16,* greater omentum covering the intestinal mass; *17,* lesser omentum cut away from the liver; *18,* position of caudoventral border of liver.

developed to cope with the complex carbohydrates that form so large a part of the normal diet of ruminants, and only the last chamber is comparable in structure and function to the simple stomach of most other species. All are derived, however, from the gastric spindle of the embryo (Fig. 28.8).

The topography of the ruminant abdomen is dominated by the enormous development of the stomach, which in adult cattle almost fills the left half of the cavity and occupies a substantial portion of the right (Figs. 28.9, 28.10, 28.11, and 28.12 and see Fig. 27.1). Its capacity measures about 60 L. This amount, which is much more modest than many estimates, may be apportioned between the various chambers as follows: rumen, 80%; reticulum, 5%; omasum, 8%; and abomasum, 7%. The proportions in small ruminants are somewhat different, being perhaps 75% rumen, 8% reticulum, 4% omasum, and 13% abomasum. The relative volumes are fairly constant in the short term because the enormous storage capacity of the first chambers and the more or less continuous passage of ingesta into the distal parts minimize the effects of intermittent feeding.

The different chambers are identifiable as expansions of the foregut spindle in the early embryo. They increase at unequal rates throughout the embryonic and fetal periods as first one takes the lead and then another. At one stage the fetal stomach has an almost adult configuration, but during the last months of intrauterine life the abomasum outstrips the others; at birth it accounts for more than half the weight and capacity of the entire organ—which is appropriate because it is the only part that has an immediate function to perform. The postnatal changes through which the adult proportions and topography are acquired are described later (p. 680).

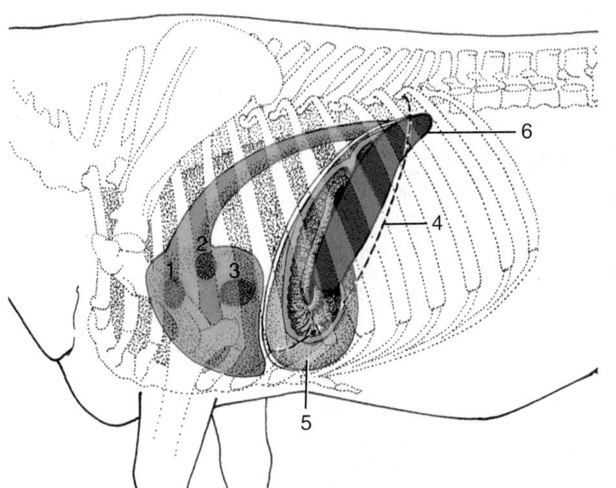

Fig. 28.5 Left lateral projection of certain organs on the bovine thoracic wall. *1*, Pulmonary valve; *2*, aortic valve; *3*, left atrioventricular valve; *4*, position of basal border of the lung, *5*, reticulum, opened (note position of reticular groove); *6*, spleen.

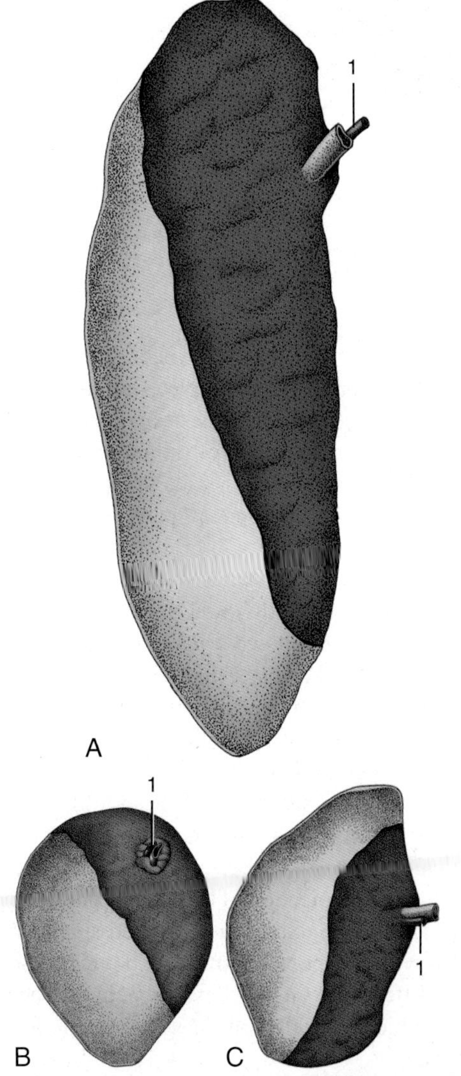

Fig. 28.6 The spleens of (A) cattle, (B) sheep, and (C) goats; visceral surface. The craniodorsal area is bare. *1*, Splenic artery.

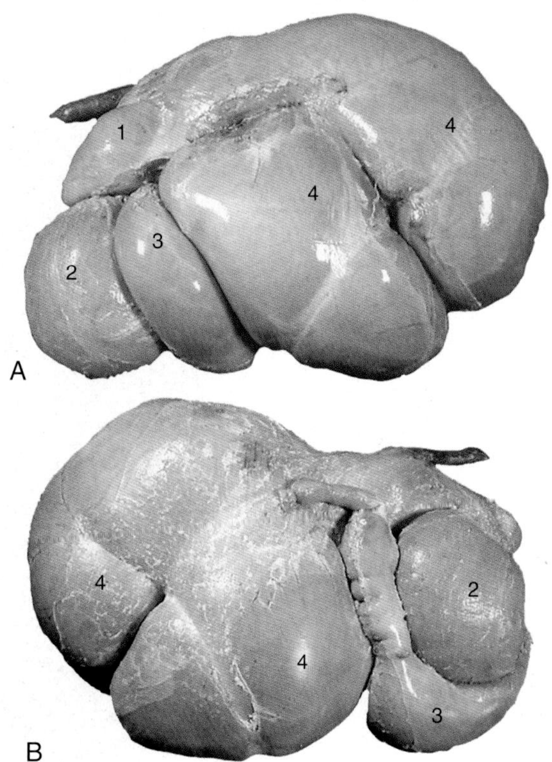

Fig. 28.7 (A) Bovine stomach, left side. (B) Bovine stomach, right side. *1*, Reticulum; *2*, omasum; *3*, abomasum; *4*, rumen.

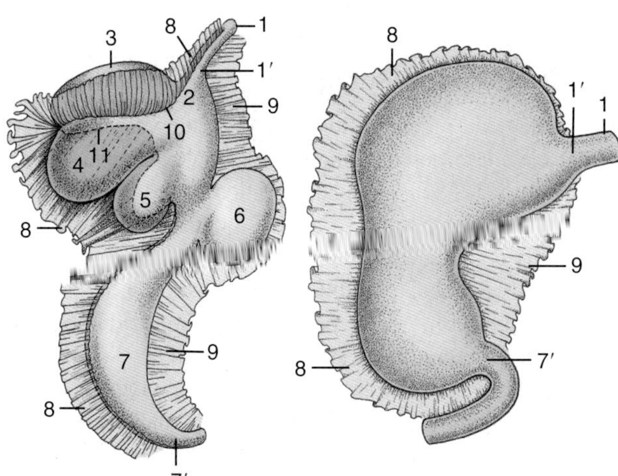

Fig. 28.8 The attachments of the greater and lesser omenta on the developing ruminant stomach. The simple stomach to the right shows the correspondence of its parts to the compartments of the ruminant stomach. *1*, Esophagus; *1′*, cardia; *2*, atrium ruminis; *3*, dorsal sac of rumen; *4*, ventral sac of rumen; *5*, reticulum; *6*, omasum; *7*, abomasum; *7′*, pylorus; *8*, greater omentum; *9*, lesser omentum; *10*, part of greater curvature corresponding to the right longitudinal groove of the rumen; *11*, part of greater curvature corresponding to the left longitudinal groove of the rumen.

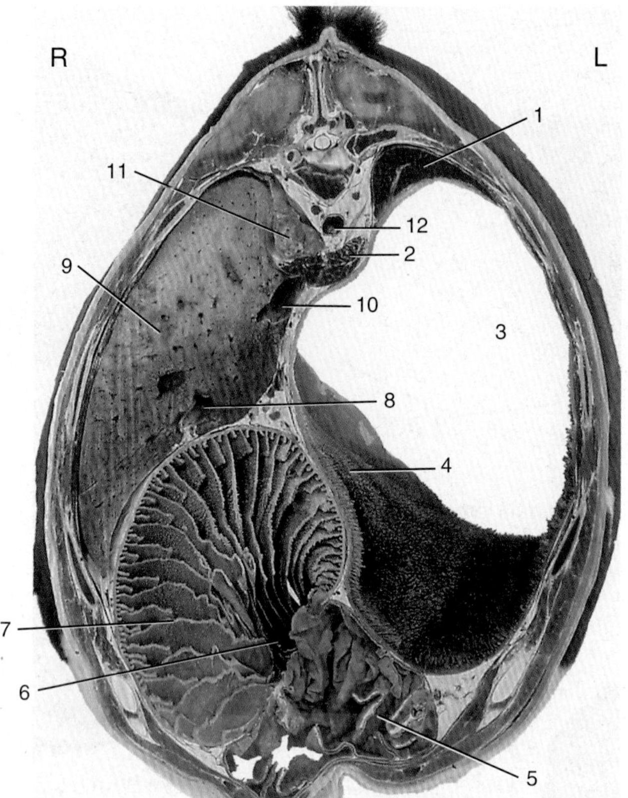

Fig. 28.9 Transverse section of the bovine trunk at the level of the 10th thoracic vertebra. *1,* Spleen; *2,* crura of diaphragm; *3,* atrium ruminis; *4,* cranial pillar; *5,* abomasum; *6,* omasoabomasal opening; *7,* omasum; *8,* portal vein; *9,* liver; *10,* caudal vena cava; *11,* right lung; *12,* aorta; *L,* left side; *R,* right side.

The Rumen and Reticulum

The rumen and reticulum together form the vessel that ferments and breaks down the incoming complex and rough food to prepare it for conventional digestion lower in the digestive tract while it also absorbs some nutrients. The rumen is laterally compressed and extends from the cardia—which lies a little way above the middle of the seventh intercostal space or eighth rib—to the pelvic inlet, from the abdominal roof to the floor, and from the left body wall across the midline, especially caudally and ventrally, where it may reach the lower right flank (Fig. 28.12). The much smaller reticulum lies cranial to the rumen under cover of the sixth to eighth ribs and mainly to the left of the median plane. It reaches from the cardia to the most forward part of the diaphragm and occupies the full height of this shallower part of the abdomen. The reticulum also crosses the midline, especially ventrally, where it lies above the xiphoid process of the sternum (Fig. 28.4/*3* and see Fig. 27.7/*8*). This position allows the application of external pressure in the expectation of eliciting pain when the reticulum is diseased.

Because of the integrated structure and function of the rumen and reticulum, many prefer to describe it as a combined ruminoreticular compartment. There is much in favor of this convention. The division of the rumen from the reticulum, though more complete, is achieved similar to the subdivisioning of the rumen—namely, by the inflection of the walls to form a series of pillars (pilae) that project internally (Fig. 28.4B). The whole thickness of the stomach wall, except the peritoneum, participates in these formations. The rumen and reticulum communicate over the U-shaped *ruminoreticular fold.* The principal *ruminal pillars* encircle the organ, dividing dorsal and ventral major sacs, while lesser *coronary pillars* mark off the caudal blind sacs. The *cranial pillar* has an oblique direction that partially divides the cranial extremity from the remainder of the dorsal sac, emphasizing the association of the former part *(atrium ruminis)* with the reticulum. External grooves correspond to the positions of all these folds. The relative proportions of the compartments vary among the domestic ruminants. The smaller size of the dorsal sac and the extensive caudal projection of the ventral blind sac give the rumen of sheep and goats an unbalanced appearance when compared with the more symmetrical bovine rumen. There are also differences in the development of the grooves that are visible externally, but these are altogether without significance.

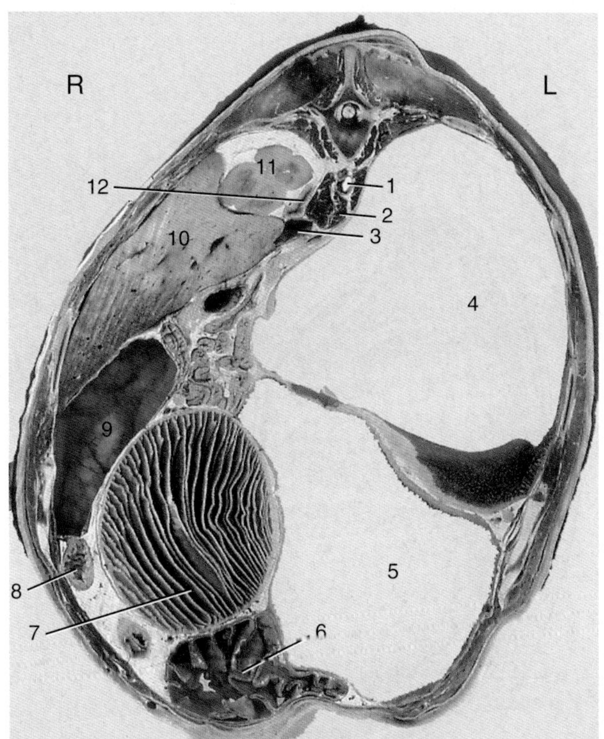

Fig. 28.10 Transverse section of the bovine trunk at the level of the 13th thoracic vertebra. *1,* Aorta; *2,* right crus of diaphragm; *3,* caudal vena cava; *4,* dorsal sac of rumen; *5,* ventral sac of rumen; *6,* abomasum; *7,* omasum; *8,* duodenum; *9,* gallbladder; *10,* liver; *11,* cranial pole of right kidney; *12,* right adrenal gland; *L,* left side; *R,* right side.

The serosa covers the entire surface of the rumen and reticulum, except dorsally where the ruminal wall is directly adherent to the abdominal roof from the esophageal hiatus of the diaphragm to the level of the fourth lumbar vertebra (Fig. 28.13/*12*), and over certain grooves where it is reflected to continue into the greater omentum. The limited attachment allows the ruminoreticulum the freedom necessary for the incessant and reciprocal contractions and enlargements of its various parts.

The *relationships* are most easily studied by reference to the illustrations (Figs. 28.4A and B, 28.7, and 28.10). The most important points are contact between the reticulum and the diaphragm and liver cranially; insinuation of the abomasum between the two chambers (ventral sac of rumen and reticulum) ventrally; relation of the right surface of the rumen to the intestinal mass, omasum, abomasum, pancreas, and kidneys; and intrusion of the superficial wall of the greater omentum between the ventral sac of the rumen and the abdominal wall. The rumen also has a variable relationship to the uterus and other organs at the entrance to the pelvis, where the dorsal sac may be palpated per rectum. The direct contact of the dorsal sac with the upper part of the left flank makes auscultation and palpation simple. It also facilitates trocarization for the relief of tympany.

The *interior* of the ruminoreticulum communicates with the esophagus and omasum through openings placed

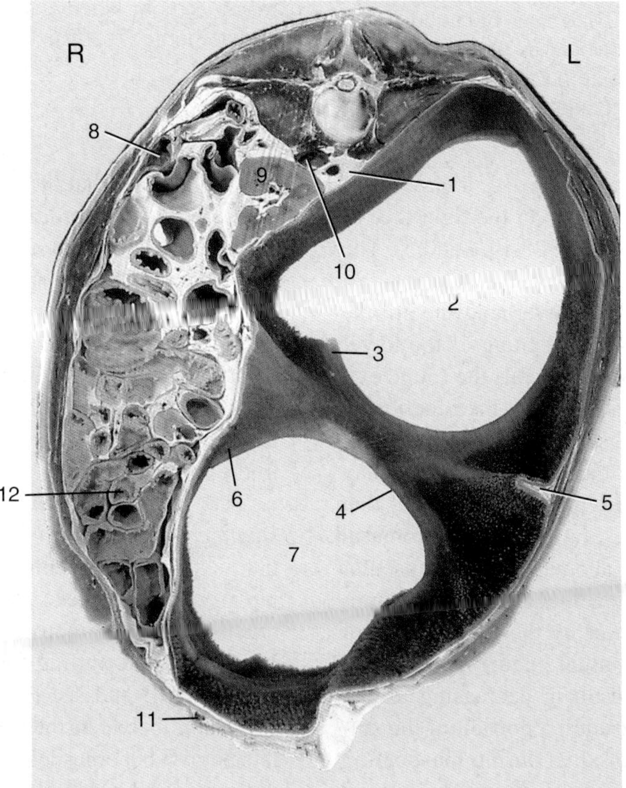

Fig. 28.11 Transverse section of the bovine trunk at the level of the 3rd lumber vertebra. *1,* Aorta; *2,* caudodorsal blind sac; *3,* dorsal coronary pillar; *4,* caudal pillar; *5,* left longitudinal pillar; *6,* ventral coronary pillar; *7,* caudoventral blind sac; *8,* descending duodenum; *9,* left kidney; *10,* caudal vena cava; *11,* milk vein; *12,* intestinal mass; *L,* left side; *R,* right side.

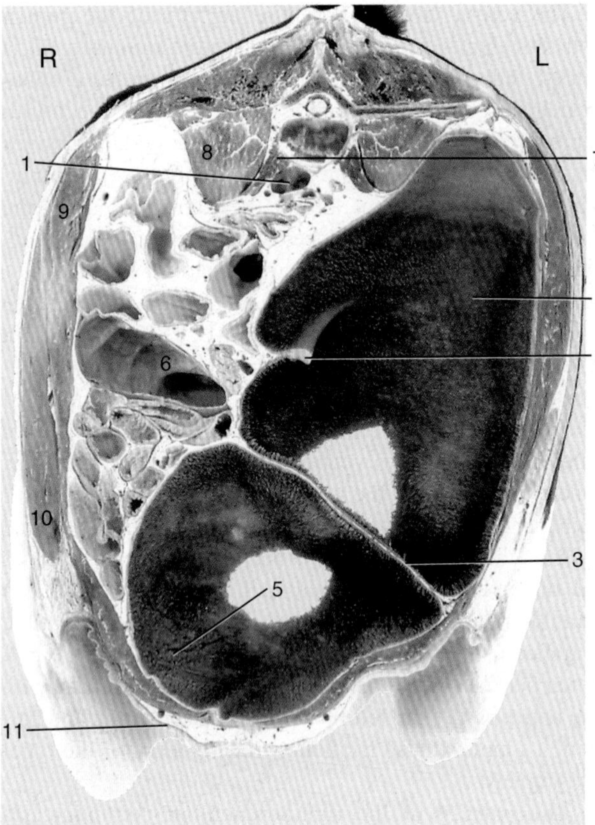

Fig. 28.12 Transverse section of the bovine trunk at the level of the 5th lumbar vertebra. *1,* Bifurcation of aorta and formation of caudal vena cava; *2,* right dorsal coronary pillar; *3,* caudal pillar; *4,* caudodorsal blind sac; *5,* caudoventral blind sac; *6,* colon; *7,* psoas minor; *8,* psoas major; *9,* internal abdominal oblique; *10,* external abdominal oblique; *11,* milk vein; *L,* left side; *R,* right side.

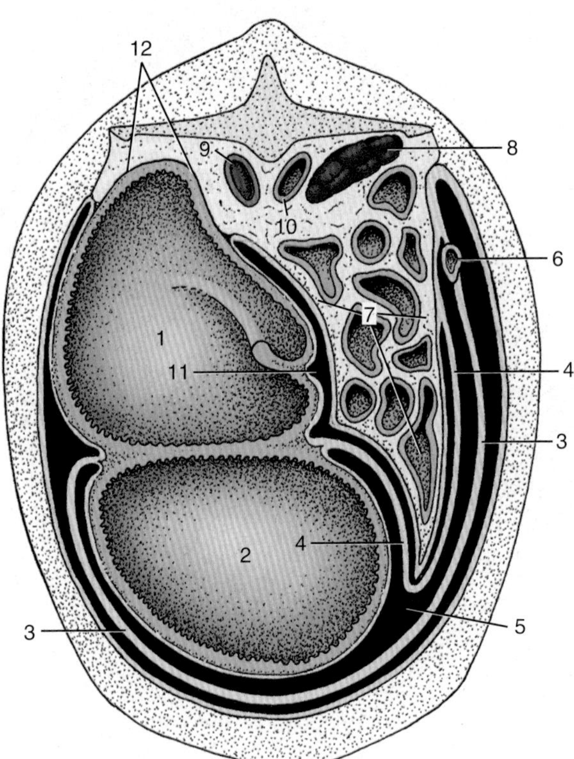

Fig. 28.13 Schematic transverse section of the abdominal cavity to show the disposition of the greater omentum. *1,* Dorsal sac of rumen; *2,* ventral sac of rumen; *3,* superficial wall of greater omentum; *4,* deep wall of greater omentum; *5,* omental bursa; *6,* descending duodenum; *7,* intestinal mass; *8,* right kidney; *9,* aorta; *10,* caudal vena cava; *11,* supraomental recess; *12,* retroperitoneal attachment of rumen.

at the extremities of the *reticular groove,* a prominent gutter that descends from the cardia over the right face of the reticulum toward the fundus (Fig. 28.14/*4* and *5*). The groove is bounded by spiral fleshy lips; the upper end of the left (cranial) lip is expanded to overhang the slitlike cardiac opening, while a similar thickening of the lower end of the right (caudal) lip partly conceals the round exit into the omasum. The cardia is placed at the junction of the rumen and reticulum and discharges into both chambers. In the unweaned animal the reticular groove may be converted into a closed tube, forming a channel that conveys milk directly from the esophagus to the omasal canal, whence it drops into the abomasum. The muscular contractions that draw the lips together are reflexly stimulated by sucking from the dam or by the presentation of suitable bucket feeds. As the animal matures, alterations in diet and feeding regimen result in decreasing use of this route, although even in the adult a portion of the soluble nutrients released into the saliva during mastication succeeds in bypassing the ruminoreticulum. The groove reflex is stimulated by antidiuretic hormone (ADH), which indicates that the reflex may have some function in adult life. ADH is produced in response to dehydration or an increase in plasma osmolality. ADH is associated with thirst, and its effect on the reticular groove may cause a portion of the water drunk by dehydrated animals to bypass the ruminoreticulum. Closure of the groove can be stimulated by certain chemicals (e.g., copper sulfate). This provides a useful strategy when it is desirable to introduce drugs to the abomasum without prior dilution in the forechambers.

The *ruminoreticular mucosa* is lined by a harsh *stratified cutaneous epithelium* (Fig. 28.15A and B) that is stained a greenish brown. The floor of the reticular groove, however, is smooth and pale. The reticular mucosa has a distinctive pattern formed by ridges about 1 cm high that outline four-, five-, and six-sided "cells" (Fig. 28.16B and see Fig. 27.7/*8*). These ridges and the cell floors between them carry low papillae. The reticulate pattern becomes less regular toward the junction with the rumen and gradually modifies to merge with the papillated surface of this chamber. The upper keratinized layer

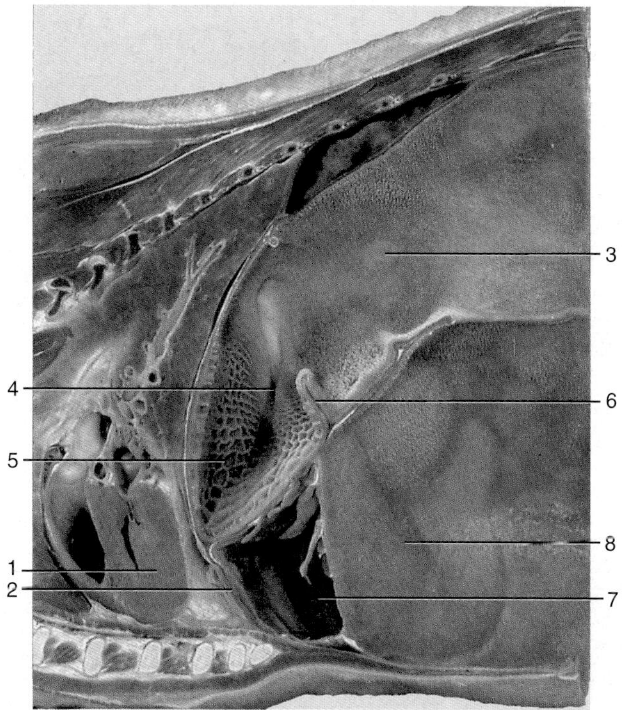

Fig. 28.14 Paramedian section of part of the trunk of a goat. *1,* Heart; *2,* diaphragm; *3,* atrium ruminis; *4,* reticular groove; *5,* reticulum; *6,* ruminoreticular fold; *7,* abomasum; *8,* ventral sac of rumen.

of the epithelium protects against abrasion by the rough, fibrous diet, whereas the deeper layers metabolize volatile short-chain fatty acids. Histologically, the epithelium shows many similarities with the epidermis. The *lamina propria–submucosa,* formed by a network of collagen and elastic fibers, includes bands of smooth muscle within the distal parts of the reticular ridges (Fig. 28.15A). The ruminal papillae vary in prominence according to age, diet, and location (Figs. 28.16A and 28.14). Normally they are largest and most densely strewn within the blind sacs, fewer and less prominent in the ventral sac, and least developed over the center of the root and toward the free margins of the pillars. Individual papillae vary from low rounded elevations through conical and tongue-like forms to flattened leaves about 1 cm long. The ruminal epithelium resembles that of the reticulum. A thick subepithelial *lamina propria* forms the core of the papilla through collagen, elastic, and reticular fibers and also contains a dense capillary network. There is no muscularis mucosae. The looser submucosa is located directly against the lamina propria and also contains a vascular network (Fig. 28.15B).

The rugose nature of the ruminoreticular lining was formerly interpreted as an adaptation for the mechanical disruption of the ingesta. Now it is regarded as a mechanism to increase the surface area for the absorption of the volatile fatty acids produced by microbial fermentation. Volatile fatty acids, especially butyric, stimulate papillary development, and their absorption is facilitated by the very rich subepithelial capillary plexus. In some wild ruminants but not in domestic species, striking changes in papillary prominence and size, and thus in the ruminal surface area (Fig. 28.16A), accompany seasonal changes in forage quality.*

The reticulum of the *small ruminants* is relatively larger than that of cattle. Although it extends farther caudally, its contact with the abdominal floor is subject to much functional variation (Fig. 28.14/5). There are conspicuous species differences in its lining. The ridges that bound the reticular "cells" are relatively much lower and have more prominently serrated margins. The papillated "ruminal" mucosa also extends over a larger part of the reticular wall.

The *smooth muscle of the ruminoreticular wall* is arranged in two coats that continue the striated muscle of the esophagus. The thin outer coat runs craniocaudally over the rumen but has an oblique course on the reticulum. Most bundles of the much thicker inner layer run more or less at right angles to the superficial coat and thus encircle the long axis of the rumen. They extend into the

*In wild ruminants, striking changes in the total mass of the salivary glands are correlated with the ruminal response to the fibrous content of the forage.

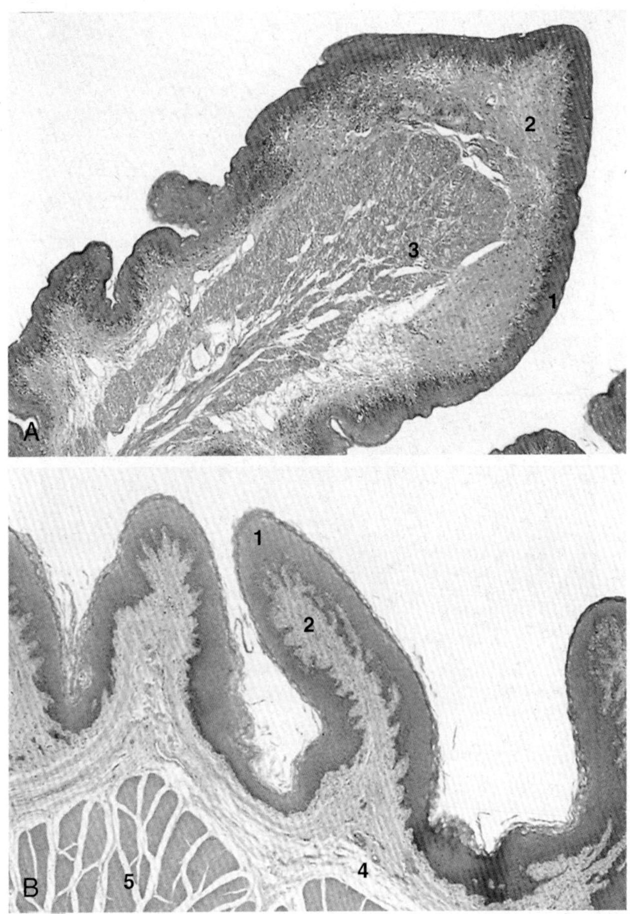

Fig. 28.15 (A) Reticulum of a goat (magnification ×28). (B) Rumen of a goat (magnification ×28). *1,* Stratified squamous epithelium; *2,* lamina propria; *3,* lamina muscularis mucosae; *4,* submucosa; *5,* muscularis interna.

pillars and form the bases of these structures. The thicker parts of the ruminoreticular muscle are sold for consumption as tripe.

The regular sequence of *ruminoreticular contractions* mixes and redistributes the stomach contents. The cycle consists of a biphasic reticular contraction (relaxation between contraction phases is more consistent in cattle than in sheep), which throws the reticular contents into the atrium ruminis, followed by contraction of first the dorsal and later the ventral rumen sacs. The wave of contraction passes over each in a craniocaudal direction. The process is centrally regulated, and the tempo and vigor are adjusted according to information supplied by intramural receptors that are stimulated by stretching of the wall and by contact with floating fragments. Both the sensory and the motor pathways travel within the vagus nerves.

Regurgitation of food for remastication requires the coordination of the stomach movements with those of the thoracic wall and throat. It is preceded by an additional reticular contraction that floods the cardiac region. The ingesta are drawn into the esophagus on expansion of the thorax with a closed upper airway and are then carried orally by an antiperistaltic wave. The heavy remasticated cud, now further sodden and divided, tends to drop from the cardia into the reticulum.

In eructation (the discharge of gas through the esophagus), ruminal contractions without the reticulum's participation substitute for the normal pattern of activity. These contractions originate in the ventral sac and generally spread to the dorsal sac, where they begin caudally and extend cranially. These contractions force the ruminal gas forward to the cardiac area whence it is aspirated into the esophagus, through which it is hurried orally by an antiperistaltic wave. It then passes through the relaxed pharyngoesophageal sphincter into the pharynx. Some escapes from the mouth, but part is directed to the lungs.

The content of the rumen shows some stratification, with the recent ingesta piled above the heavier, more sodden remasticated material. It is therefore the lighter material that is most liable to be regurgitated for further mastication and insalivation (Fig. 28.17).

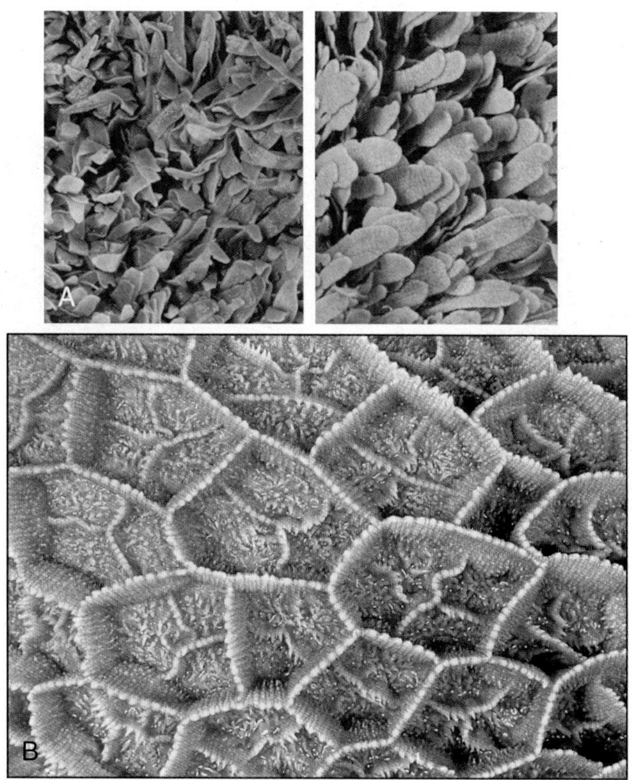

Fig. 28.16 (A) Rumen papillated mucosa taken from a Waterbuck *(left)* and a lesser Kudu. (B) Reticulum: mucosal ridges outlining "cells" characteristic of the reticular mucosa (cow).

Inflammation of the rumen and the reticulum in cattle can occur through mechanical or chemical (e.g., lactic acidosis) causes. Cattle are notoriously careless feeders and often ingest foreign bodies, especially pieces of wire and nails, with their forage. These bodies tend to collect within the reticulum and, when sharp, may be driven through the reticular wall by the contractions of this organ. This leads to inflammation of the reticulum at the site of the perforation (traumatic reticulitis, or "hardware disease") and peritonitis or pericarditis if the nail penetrates the diaphragm. The inflammation in the forestomach leads to pain in the anterior abdomen and a hunched posture with abducted elbows. Some of these bodies corrode, while others may be immobilized by introducing a magnet through the mouth (Fig. 28.18/*2* and inset).

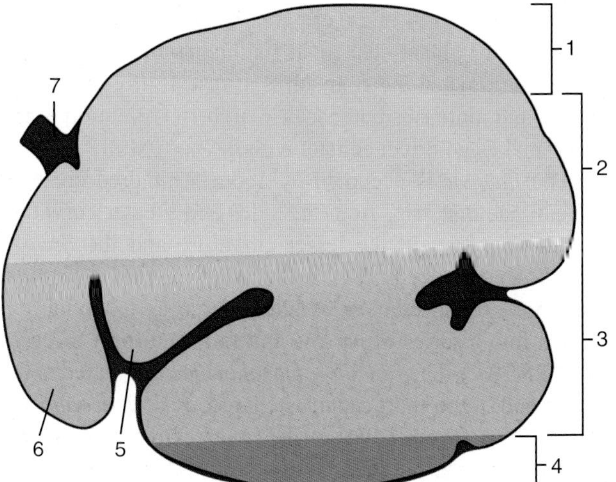

Fig. 28.17 Stratification of ingesta in the ruminoreticulum, left lateral view. *1,* Gas bubble; *2,* coarse forage ("floating mat"); *3,* more finely ground material with higher specific gravity than that in *2; 4,* liquid zone; *5,* atrium ruminis; *6,* reticulum; *7,* esophagus.

The Omasum

The omasum lies within the intrathoracic part of the abdomen to the right of the midline, between the rumen and reticulum to the left and the liver and body wall to the right (Figs. 28.7/*2* and 28.9/*7*). It is bilaterally flattened and displays a long convex border that faces dextrocaudally and a much shorter lesser curvature that faces in the opposite direction. The long axis is more or less vertical in the cadaver, but the position and orientation of the living organ alter constantly. Most of the omasum lies under cover of the 8th to 11th ribs, but in cattle the lower pole generally projects onto the abdominal floor below the costal arch (Fig. 28.19/*5*). Although its position places most of

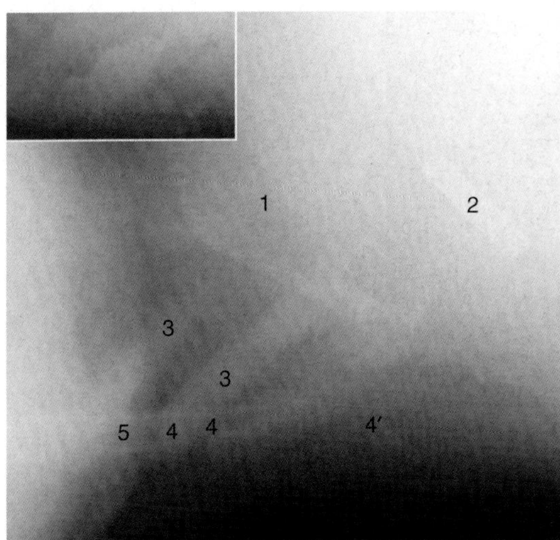

Fig. 28.18 Lateral radiograph of the vicinity of the reticulum of a young cow (cranial is to the *left*). The *inset* shows a close-up of a magnet with adhering metal objects. *1,* Cranial wall of reticulum with sediment in its "cells"; *2,* magnet; *3,* costal cartilages; *4,* sternebrae; *4′,* xiphoid cartilage; *5,* proximal epiphysis of ulna (olecranon).

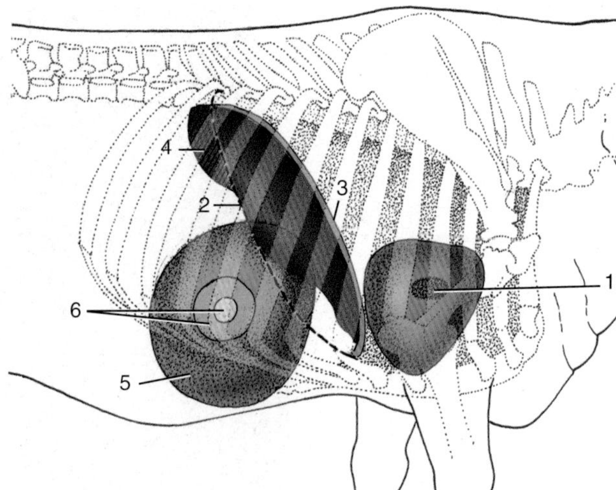

Fig. 28.19 Right lateral projection of certain organs on the bovine thoracic wall. *1,* Right atrioventricular valve; *2,* position of basal border of lung; *3,* cranial extent of diaphragm and liver; *4,* field of liver percussion; *5,* omasum; *6,* field for percussion and auscultation of omasum.

the omasum beyond direct manual reach, the organ may be examined by auscultation and percussion. The lower pole of the omasum has an extensive attachment to the fundic region of the abomasum around the omasoabomasal orifice. Much of its right surface is covered by and partly connected to the lesser omentum (Fig. 28.4C/*13*).

The omasum is relatively smaller in sheep and goats, in which it is bean shaped. It maintains an almost vertical position when the stomach is at rest. It projects on the eighth and ninth ribs but, because of the intervention of the liver, makes no direct contact with the body wall.

The *interior* is occupied by about a hundred crescentic laminae that arise from the sides and greater curvature and project toward the lesser curvature and the *omasal canal* (see Fig. 28.9). The laminae are of several lengths, and those of different sizes alternate so as to divide the lumen into a series of narrow and fairly uniform recesses (Fig. 28.10/*7*). The *reticulo-omasal orifice* is situated at the upper end of the short canal. The large, oval *omasoabomasal opening* (Fig. 28.9/*6*) at the other extremity is partly occluded by the prolapse of abomasal folds. The floor of the canal (known as the *omasal groove*) is smooth except for a few low ridges that run along its length and a scattering of clawlike projections that guard the upper opening.

The *keratinized stratified squamous epithelium* over the laminae is raised to cover numerous papillae. Most are small and lenticular, but there are a few larger, conical projections that point distally and perhaps promote the onward movement of the ingesta. The mucosa is further characterized by a *lamina propria* that includes a dense subepithelial capillary network and encloses a *thick muscularis mucosae* consisting of a thin outer longitudinal layer and a thicker inner circular layer. The inner layer is continuous with the muscle of the omasal wall. The contents of the omasal recesses are finely divided and rather dry, which make the organ firm and easy to recognize on palpation at laparotomy, directly, or from within the rumen after opening that chamber.

Omasal contractions are biphasic. The first phase squeezes ingesta from the omasal canal into the recesses between the laminae; the second phase is a mass contraction. The principal effect is to squeeze fluid from the material within the recesses, which is a process essential to the continuing movement of ingesta to the abomasum. These contractions occur at a much slower and more deliberate tempo than those of the ruminoreticulum. Although the rough surfaces and muscular cores of the laminae suggest that these folds triturate the food by rubbing against each other, there is no evidence of such activity. Absorption is continued in the omasum.

The Abomasum

The abomasum lies flexed on the abdominal floor, embracing the lower pole of the omasum from behind (Fig. 28.7/*3*). The larger of the two limbs forms a piriform sac that reaches forward to the left to make contact with the body wall between the reticulum and the atrium and ventral sac of the rumen (Fig. 28.4A/*6*). Analogous to the simple stomach but not as precisely, this limb is divided into *fundus* and *body*. In fact, the location of the omasoabomasal opening in the living animal is not known with certainty. Therefore, it is possible that the opening is terminal, and in that case no blind diverticulum and therefore no true fundus exists. The cranial part of the fundus is extensively connected to the reticulum, atrium, and ventral sac by muscle bundles.

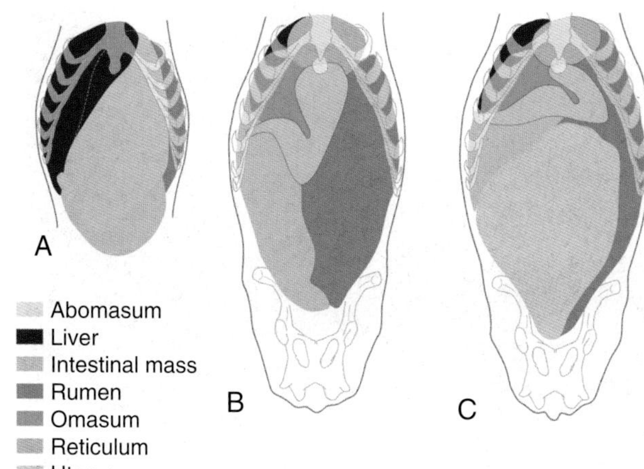

Fig. 28.20 Ventral views of the abdominal viscera of (A) a newborn calf, (B) a 5-year-old cow, and (C) a 6-year-old heavily pregnant cow based on reconstructions of transverse sections of animals frozen in the standing position.

The narrower and more uniform distal limb constitutes the *pyloric part* of the organ. It passes transversely, or with a slightly cranial inclination, toward the right body wall and ascends to terminate at the pylorus, caudal to the lower part of the omasum (Fig. 28.4D/*15*). The abomasum does not usually come into contact with the liver in adult cattle.

The abomasum of the sheep and the goat is relatively large. In contrast to the situation in adult cattle, it is usually allowed direct contact with the liver by the smaller size of the omasum.

The position and relations of the abomasum depend on the fullness of the different parts of the stomach, intrinsic abomasal activity, and, most important, the contractions of the rumen and reticulum to which the abomasum is attached. Age and pregnancy are also an influence (Fig. 28.20). Although it is difficult to specify abomasal relations exactly, it is vital to appreciate that there are limits beyond which deviations produce digestive disturbances and may endanger life. Abomasal displacement, which may be to the right or left, is a well-recognized disorder, particularly in dairy cows (see further on).

The abomasum is lined by a pink, slime-covered *glandular mucosa* that is in striking contrast to the harsh lining of the forestomach. At the omasoabomasal junction the *epithelium* changes abruptly to a simple columnar epithelium with occasional goblet cells. The *lamina propria* is less dense than that of the omasum, and solitary lymph nodules frequently are observed at the junction with the epithelium. The mucosa of the abomasum has all the characteristics of those of the simple stomach (Fig. 28.21A–C). The area is increased about sixfold by the presence of almost a dozen large folds that arise around the entrance and course over the walls of the fundus and body before subsiding as the flexure is approached (Fig. 28.22/*2*). Approximation of the proximal ends of these folds forms a mucosal valve or "plug" that discourages the reflux of ingesta into the omasum. The mucosa of the pyloric part is most remarkable for the large swelling or *torus* that projects from the lesser curvature to narrow the pyloric passage (Fig. 28.22/*6*). The vascular arrangements within the torus suggest that it is capable of a form of erection, but the possible functional significance of this (and of the entire structure, for that matter) is unknown. The dark mucosa of the body and fundus contains true peptic glands; the glands of the lighter pyloric part secrete mucus alone.

The abomasal wall is relatively thin. The serous covering is deficient only at the attachment to the other stomach chambers and along the origins of the omenta. The *muscle coat* consists of longitudinal and circular strata. The longitudinal muscle is confined to the curvatures of the fundus and body but forms a thicker and wider covering for the pyloric part. The circular fibers provide a more complete layer that is better developed over the pyloric part, especially distally.

The *movements* of the adult abomasum are rather sluggish. They consist of general contractions of the proximal limb and more forceful peristalsis confined to the pyloric part. The latter activity often appears to be prompted by the tipping of the ingesta toward the pylorus when the fundic region is elevated by reticular contraction. It is possible that these normal alterations in position facilitate morbid displacements. Atony, with the accumulation of gas in the fundus, is a constant finding in these cases, and it may be that a slight initial displacement is worsened because this gas is denied its usual escape through the omasoabomasal opening when this comes to lie below the gas bubble.

Abomasal Displacements: Displacements of the abomasum are commonly related to the high proportion of concentrates to roughage in the rations of stabled cows, which leads to atony of the abomasum and accumulation of liquid ingesta and gas. Pregnancy may be a predisposing factor (Fig. 28.20C). Because the abomasum is well fixed proximally to the heavy omasum and distally by the lesser omentum, it is its middle part that travels farthest from its usual position on the abdominal floor. Contractions of the ruminoreticulum may allow the abomasum, buoyed by the gas within, to work its way under the atrium of the rumen and up on the left side. The loop formed by the middle part of the abomasum eventually comes to lie between the rumen and the left abdominal wall, deep to the last three or four ribs, where it can be identified by simultaneous percussion and auscultation (left displacement of the abomasum). In right displacement of the abomasum, which is less common than the left displacement, the loop formed by the middle part of the abomasum slides to the right and lies between the right abdominal wall and the intestines and liver. Displacements to the right may result in the

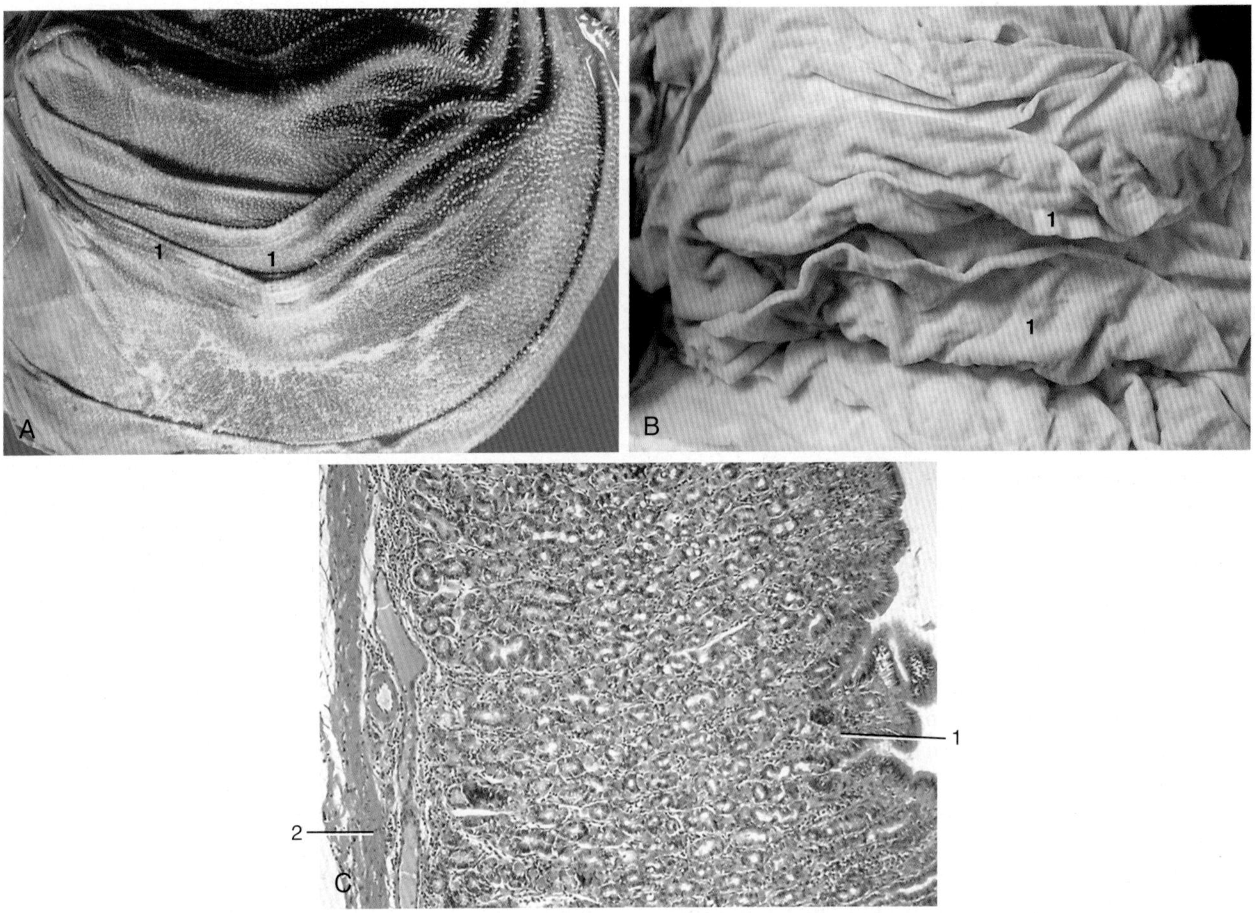

Fig. 28.21 (A) Internal surface of omasum of a cow. *1,* Omasal laminae. (B) Internal surface of abomasum of a cow. *1,* Abomasal folds. (C) Abomasum of a goat (magnification ×70). *1,* Gastric pit; *2,* lamina muscularis mucosae.

complete right torsion of the abomasum (abomasal volvulus), which requires emergency surgery. Treatment of uncomplicated displacements consists of returning the abomasum to its normal position by placing the cow on her back, by deflating the organ through a paramedian incision of the abdominal wall, and by including its muscular coat in the closing of the incision (abomasopexy).

The Omenta

The attachment of the *greater omentum* begins dorsal to the esophagus. The two serosal sheets of which it is composed pass directly onto the rumen but are so widely separated that the immediately postcardiac part of the rumen roof is enabled to attach directly to the abdominal roof (Fig. 28.13/*12*). This retroperitoneal space is closed caudally where the two serosal sheets come together halfway along the right longitudinal groove to form a conventional duplicature attaching to the stomach. The attachment of this fold may be traced along the right longitudinal groove, through the caudal groove between the caudal blind sacs, and then forward along the

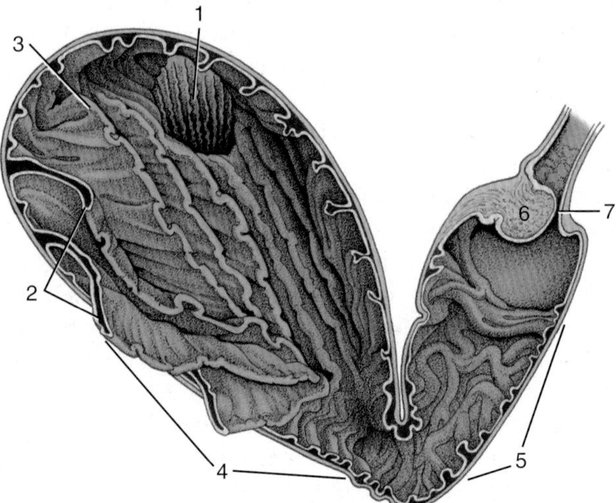

Fig. 28.22 Opened abomasum as seen from behind, above, and slightly from the left. *1,* Omasoabomasal opening through which the omasal laminae can be seen; *2,* abomasal folds; *3,* fundus; *4,* body; *5,* pyloric part; *6,* torus pyloricus; *7,* pylorus.

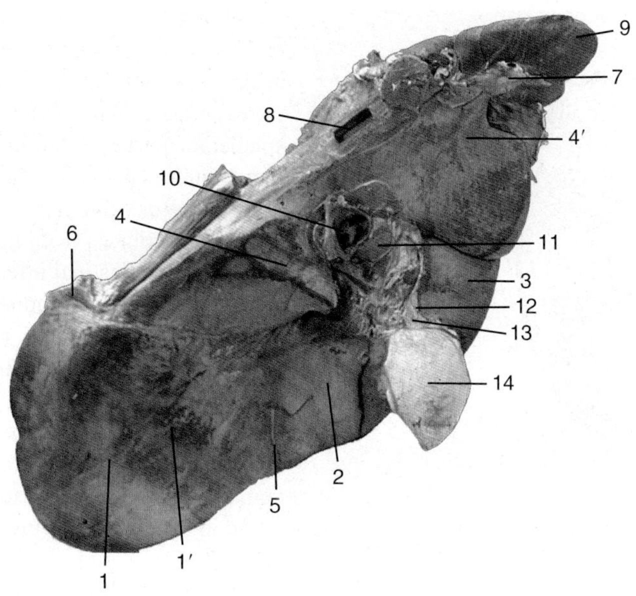

Fig. 28.23 Visceral surface of the bovine liver. *1,* Left lobe; *1′,* omasal impression; *2,* quadrate lobe; *3,* right lobe; *4* and *4′,* papillary and caudate processes of caudate lobe, respectively; *5,* round ligament; *6,* left triangular ligament; *7,* right triangular ligament; *8,* caudal vena cava; *9,* right kidney; *10,* portal vein; *11,* hepatic lymph node; *12,* bile duct; *13,* cystic duct; *14,* gallbladder.

left longitudinal groove. It now crosses the atrium ruminis and widens to make a broad attachment to the reticulum before bending sharply to the right, ventral to the ruminoreticulum, to reach the greater curvature of the abomasum (Figs. 28.4A and C and 28.8/*8*). It follows this to the pylorus and continues onto the caudal aspect of the first (vertical) part of the duodenum, from which it extends onto the descending duodenum and later the mesoduodenum. The omental attachment is reflected where the duodenum turns cranially, and it retraces its attachment along the descending duodenum until carried back to the cranial duodenal flexure at the porta of the liver. It then returns to the right face of the rumen via the pancreas.

The *lesser omentum* arises from the visceral surface of the liver, between the porta and the esophageal impression (Fig. 28.23), and passes to the region of the reticular groove, the right face of the omasum, and thence along the lesser curvature of the abomasum to the first part of the duodenum, which returns it to the liver (Fig. 28.4C).

The omental sheets enclose a space, the *omental bursa,* that is completely divided from the greater peritoneal cavity except at the epiploic foramen near the porta of the liver. The bursa is a mere capillary cleft in life, but it is simpler for descriptive purposes to envisage it as distended. A first impression of its topography may be obtained from the schema, in which it can be seen that the ventral sac of the rumen projects into it (Fig. 28.24B/*2′* and *6*). Of the omental sheets that run transversely across the abdomen, one lies against the abdominal wall and the other lies against the viscera (chiefly, the intestines) (Fig. 28.13/*3* and *4*). The superficial and deep sheets pass into each other caudally and, in this way, close the bursa behind (Fig. 28.24A). The omasum, abomasum, and lesser omentum provide most of the cranial bursal wall. The entrance to the bursal cavity, the epiploic foramen, is situated dorsocranially between the liver and the duodenum or, more precisely, between the caudal vena cava dorsally and the portal vein ventrally.

The greater omentum is an important store of fat that is first deposited along the small vessels that ramify between the peritoneal layers. Usually, the fat is present in such large amounts that the whole omentum becomes thick and opaque. (In many cows one such thickening forms a short offshoot near the pylorus known as a *pig's ear;* it can be palpated during surgery and marks the position of the pylorus.) The superficial sheet screens the ventral sac of the rumen from view when the lower left flank is opened, and both superficial and deep sheets intervene between the organs that lie ventral to the duodenum and the right flank (Fig. 28.4A and C). The intestines are closeted in the *supraomental recess,* the space above the bursa and to the right of the rumen. The recess is freely open behind and is often entered by the pregnant uterus (Figs. 28.13/*11* and 28.24/*7*).

Innervation and Vascularization

The principal gastric nerves, parasympathetic efferent and afferent, run in the trunks formed along the esophagus by the regrouping of vagal fibers (see Fig. 27.3/*19* and *20*). The sympathetic nerves that reach the stomach

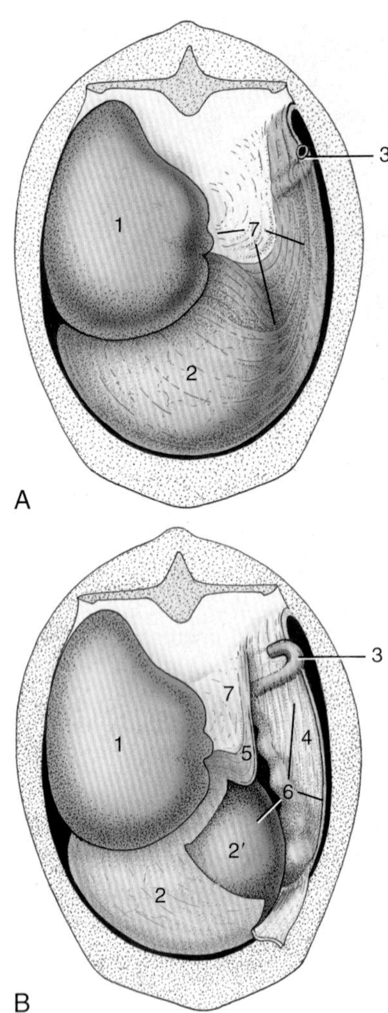

Fig. 28.24 Attachment of the greater omentum to the stomach and the dorsal body wall. (A) Caudal view of intact greater omentum. (B) Caudal view of greater omentum fenestrated to permit a view into omental bursa. *1,* Dorsal sac of rumen; *2,* ventral sac of rumen, covered by superficial wall of greater omentum; *2′,* ventral sac of rumen projecting into omental bursa; *3,* caudal flexure of duodenum; *4,* superficial wall of greater omentum; *5,* deep wall of greater omentum; *6,* omental bursa; *7,* supraomental recess.

through periarterial plexuses have a subordinate role. Section of both vagal trunks abolishes all motor activity of the forechambers (Hoflund syndrome). Section of the dorsal trunk alone results in almost complete but not necessarily permanent paralysis of the rumen, while the effect on the reticulum is generally less marked. The effects of loss of the ventral trunk are unpredictable and range from little or no discernible change to almost complete paralysis of the forechambers. These inconstant results may be due to differences in the regrouping of fibers during formation of the dorsal and ventral vagal trunks and by the later assumption of part of these functions by association neurons in the stomach wall.

Abomasal contractions are greatly reduced after bilateral vagal section but are not wholly interrupted, possibly because of some intrinsic control from a submucosal nerve plexus present in the wall of the abomasum. Division of the splanchnic nerves brings only slight alteration to the gastric movements. Clinically, disturbances of stomach function may follow involvement of the vagus nerves at any point along their courses from the brainstem; the most common causes are mediastinal infections and traumatic reticulitis.

The stomach is supplied by several branches of the *celiac artery.* The large right ruminal artery runs caudally in the right longitudinal groove and continues into the left groove by passing between the dorsal and ventral blind sacs. It supplies most of the rumen wall and ends in anastomosis with the left ruminal artery, which follows the cranial groove (between atrium and ventral sac) to supply adjoining parts of the rumen and reticulum. The omasum and abomasum are supplied by the left gastric and left gastroepiploic arteries that follow their curvatures.

The *veins* are mainly satellite to the arteries. The left ruminal vein joins the right ruminal and the one from the spleen to produce a major radicle (splenic vein) of the portal vein.

Many small *lymph nodes* are scattered over the stomach, particularly in the ruminal grooves and over the omasal and abomasal curvatures. Lymph from the forechambers leads, after serial passage through these peripheral nodes, to a number of large atrial nodes situated between the cardia and omasum and thence to the visceral root of the cisterna chyli. The nodes placed along the abomasal curvatures direct their efferent vessels to the hepatic lymph nodes.

Postnatal Development

At birth the ruminant stomach is prepared for the digestion of milk. The abomasum of the neonate is structurally mature and has more capacity than the combined capacity of the other chambers. Its full extent is apparent directly after the consumption of a generous feed, when it extends from the liver and diaphragm to the pelvic entrance, from one flank to the other, and from the floor well into the upper half of the abdomen (Figs. 28.20A and 28.25/*4*). Its capacity may already exceed 60% of the adult measure. The abomasum impinges on nearly all other abdominal organs but makes extensive contact only with the liver, which in the neonate reaches far across the median plane. The abomasal mucosa is at first not quite mature, and a few days elapse before the fundic glands become fully active, which actually benefits the host in protecting the colostral antibodies and keeping them in their native state for absorption in the intestine.

In contrast to the abomasum, the rumen and reticulum of the newborn calf are very small. They are confined to the left dorsal and cranial corner of the abdomen and are generally found crumpled and collapsed (Fig. 28.25/*2* and *3*). They are

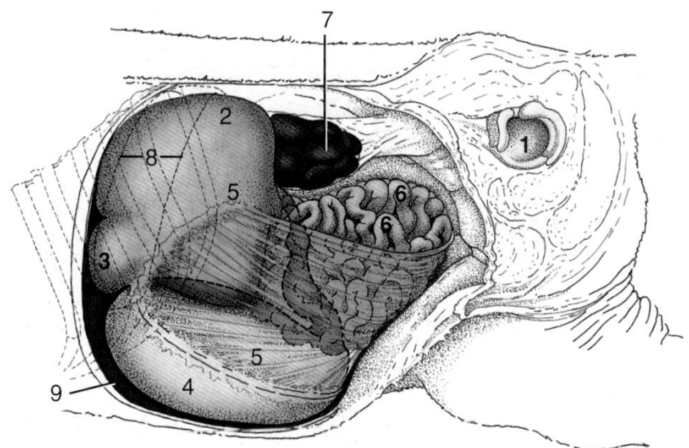

Fig. 28.25 Topography of the abdominal organs in a newborn calf, left lateral view. The left abdominal wall and the left hindlimb have been removed. *1*, Left acetabulum; *2*, rumen; *3*, reticulum; *4*, abomasum; *5*, greater omentum; *6*, small intestine; *7*, left kidney; *8*, position of spleen; *9*, liver.

bypassed by milk feeds and normally contain only a small amount of fluid from secretions of the respiratory tract (swallowed in utero) in the youngest animals and saliva in those a little older. The omasum is also retarded in development and forms a relatively inconspicuous bridge between the reticulum and the abomasal fundus. The walls of the forechambers are thin and deficient in muscle, and while their mucosae possess the characteristic adult features, these are present in subdued form.

No striking changes in proportions and structure of the chambers take place until the young calf is 2 to 3 weeks old and starts on solid food. Thereafter, the abomasum continues to increase at a slow but steady rate while the rumen and reticulum enter a period of spectacular growth. They have generally overtaken the abomasum by 8 weeks, and at 12 weeks they are more than twice as large. This unequal growth continues—but more slowly—till the definitive topography and proportions are established, which many contend [illegible] by [illegible] months but others think is not complete until 12 months.

Normal development depends on the availability of a normal diet of solid forage and other factors. Earlier it was thought that roughage stretched and stimulated the muscle of the stomach wall and also promoted the differentiation of the mucosa. Later it was shown that many gross and microscopic features of the mucosa develop only with exposure to certain end products of microbial fermentation, notably butyric acid. The full development requires exposure to these stimuli for some time because the return of a young, partly weaned calf to a wholly milk diet may result in the arrest and sometimes even reversal of the maturation processes.

The abomasum is initially the most vigorous chamber, but its activity diminishes as the ruminoreticulum, first inert and then only spasmodically active, establishes a regular cycle of contraction by the second month. The feeding habits, the structural changes, and the motor and chemical activities of the stomach, when taken in conjunction, define three phases of development. A neonatal period, in which milk forms the sole diet, may last for 2 or at most 3 weeks and may be followed by a transitional period when the stomach is adapting to solid food. From the eighth week onward the anatomy and the processes of digestion may be essentially those of the adult. The chronology will clearly be different in dairy and suckler calves.

In the newborn the liver is relatively large and lies across the midline, extensively related to the abomasum. The growing rumen and reticulum press the liver to the right and dorsally, and it rotates such that its left lobe comes to lie cranioventral to the right one and out of the reach of the abomasum. The intestines are simultaneously pushed away from the left flank and become confined to the right side. The expansion of the dorsal ruminal sac also displaces the left kidney, thrusting it across the midline until it comes to rest below and caudal to its fellow (Fig. 28.11/*9* and see Fig. 29.9/*10*).

THE INTESTINES

The intestines lie almost entirely to the right of the midline, packed mainly into the dorsal part of the abdomen and in part lying under cover of the ribs. Although they may measure up to 50 m in adult cattle, their capacity is relatively slight, which is a feature correlated with the efficiency of gastric digestion. Adhesion of the mesenteries of the small intestine and ascending colon during the fetal period leads to their sharing a common support in which they are flexed and coiled in a complex arrangement (Fig. 28.26) difficult to unravel in situ.

The *duodenum* takes origin below the ribs. Its first part rises almost vertically toward the visceral surface of the liver, followed by a run toward the pelvis as the descending duodenum, but it turns when almost level with the coxal tuber. The ascending part then returns toward the liver,

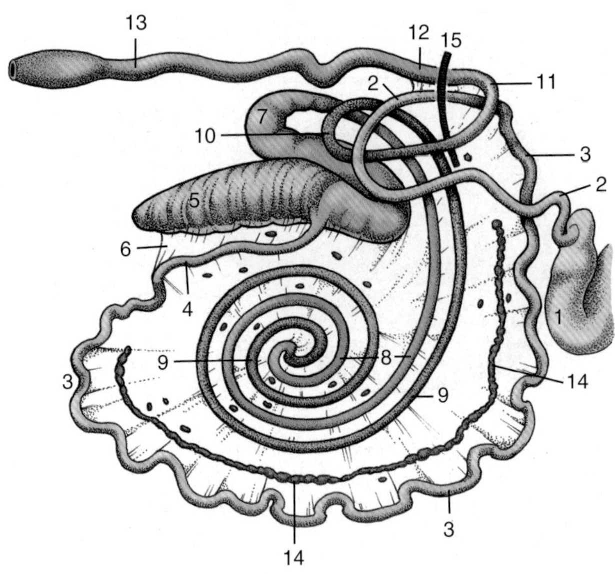

Fig. 28.26 Right lateral view of the bovine intestinal tract (schematic). *1,* Pyloric part of abomasum; *2,* duodenum; *3,* jejunum; *4,* ileum; *5,* cecum; *6,* ileocecal fold; *7–10,* ascending colon: *7,* proximal loop of ascending colon, *8,* centripetal turns of spiral colon, *9,* centrifugal turns of spiral colon, and *10,* distal loop of ascending colon; *11,* transverse colon; *12,* descending colon; *13,* rectum; *14,* jejunal lymph nodes; *15,* cranial mesenteric artery.

passing to the left of the cranial mesenteric artery, to enter the fringe of the mesentery to continue as the jejunum. The first part of the duodenum is joined to the liver by the lesser omentum. The other border of the first and descending parts gives attachment, directly or at slight remove, to both walls of the greater omentum (Figs. 28.4C and 28.24). Only the descending duodenum is immediately visible on opening the right flank. Recently, a new condition called *volvulus of the sigmoid flexure of the duodenum* has been reported.

The *jejunum* forms many short coils within the free margin of the mesentery. Their general course takes them ventrally, then caudally, and finally dorsally toward the large bowel. The position of these coils depends on the fullness of the rumen and the size of the uterus. Usually most lie within the supraomental recess, but some may insinuate themselves behind the rumen and so appear against the left flank. The extent of the short *ileum* is defined by the ileocecal fold (Fig. 28.26/*4* and *6*).

The *cecum* continues into the colon without obvious change in diameter. The junction is marked only by the entrance of the ileum. Its rounded blind tip projects caudally from the supraomental recess and floats high when filled with gas. When greatly distended with gas for protracted periods, it must be deflated surgically. Rotation of the cecum together with the proximal loop of the colon (Fig. 28.26/*7*) is common, compromises its function and blood supply, and requires surgical correction.

The *colon* is divided into the usual *ascending, transverse, and descending parts* (see Fig. 3.45/*Ru*). The first of these is wound in a very elaborate manner. On leaving the cecum, it forms a flattened sigmoid flexure (see Fig. 3.45/*11*) before narrowing and turning ventrally to trace a double spiral attached to the left side of the mesentery. Two centripetal turns are succeeded by two centrifugal turns that restore the colon toward the periphery of the mesentery, where it continues into a distal loop that carries it first toward and then away from the pelvis (see Fig. 3.45/*11′*). Beyond this it joins the short transverse colon that crosses the midline in front of the mesenteric artery and leads directly into the descending colon. This part runs toward the pelvic entrance within a mesentery that is thickened by fat and fused with neighboring parts of the gut. The mesentery of the descending colon is at first short but lengthens in front of the sacrum, where the colon forms a sigmoid flexure before continuing as the rectum. This looseness gives the hand of the veterinarian considerable range in rectal exploration (p. 707). The rectum is described with the pelvic viscera.

The ascending colon of *small ruminants* performs three or four turns in each direction. A more significant difference lies in the "pearl necklace" appearance of the centrifugal turns, in which the contents are already segmented into the pellets so characteristic of the feces. The string of these pellets in the ascending colon is replaced by their massing in a thicker column in the wider descending colon and rectum.

Volvulus: The large and small intestine are susceptible to volvulus around the root of the mesentery, seen more commonly in pre-ruminant calves. The condition causes abdominal pain, quickly leads to hypovolemic shock, and requires emergency surgery to correct the condition.

Few features of the *interior* of the intestines call for comment. In cattle the accessory pancreatic duct opens far down the descending duodenal limb; the bile duct opens more proximally, where the duodenum lies against the liver. In the small ruminants the greater pancreatic duct is usually present. The ileum projects into the cecum, and a low rampart is thus present around the ileal orifice. Lymphoid tissue is generously spread through the mucosa, especially in the small intestine, where both solitary and aggregated nodules occur. The aggregated nodules may reach lengths of 25 cm and are distinguished by their irregular cribriform surfaces. Usually one of these patches extends through the ileal orifice into the large gut.

The bulk of the intestines is supplied by the *cranial mesenteric artery;* however, the first part of the duodenum is supplied from the celiac artery, and the descending colon is supplied from the caudal mesenteric artery. The intestinal veins combine to form the cranial mesenteric radicle of the portal vein. Many jejunal lymph nodes are found within the mesentery, where they form a more or less continuous chain of giant nodes placed between the peripheral festoons of small intestine and the more central coils of the spiral colon (Fig. 28.26/*14*). The largest may be as much as a meter in length. In the small ruminants this chain of nodes lies central to the last centrifugal turn of the spiral colon. Other small nodes are scattered beside the cecum, colon, and rectum. The efferent stream from the mesenteric nodes joins the cisterna chyli. The nerves that reach the gut along the cranial mesenteric artery consist of both sympathetic and vagal fibers.* The parasympathetic nerves to the last part of the colon are derived from the sacral outflow.

THE LIVER

The liver of the adult animal lies almost entirely within the right half of the abdomen, related to the caudal face of the diaphragm and under cover of the ribs (Fig. 28.9/*9*). Its projection extends between the ventral third of the sixth intercostal space and the upper part of the last (Fig. 28.19/*4*). The visceral surface is related to the reticulum, atrium ruminis, omasum, duodenum, gallbladder, and pancreas, most of which leave impressions on the living organ. The impressions are retained by the specimen hardened in situ (Fig. 28.23). The thick dorsal border extends farthest caudally and is partly fashioned by the blunt caudate process; this is separated from the main mass by a recess into which fits the cranial pole of the right kidney. The medial (originally dorsal) border follows the midline rather closely; toward its lower end it is marked by an impression that gives passage to the esophagus, and below this a small part spreads across into the left half of the abdomen. The caudal vena cava (Fig. 28.23/*8*) tunnels through this edge of the liver and in its course receives its hepatic tributaries (Fig. 28.9/*10*).

The thin lateral border is marked by the fissure that divided the right and left "halves" of the fetal organ, and in most adult cattle this provides entrance for the round ligament, the remains of the umbilical vein (Fig. 28.23/*5*). The blind vertex of the piriform gallbladder (Fig. 28.23/*14*) projects beyond the lateral margin of the right lobe. It lies against the diaphragm opposite the ventral part of the 10th or 11th rib.

The liver is retained in position by certain ligaments attaching it to the diaphragm and, more important, by visceral pressure. Its position may be verified by dullness on percussion over an area centered on the dorsal part of the 11th rib and 11th intercostal space. The percussion area is small in relation to the size of the organ and corresponds to the area of direct contact with the body wall (Fig. 28.10/*10*). A detectable increase in its extent generally signifies a disproportionate enlargement of the organ.

The relationship of the liver to the right pleural sac should be noted to reduce the risk during collection of biopsy specimens (Fig. 28.19/*2* and *4*). The preferred site for taking a liver biopsy is to puncture through the 11th intercostal space in the plane of the lower part of the coxal tuber. The trocar is directed to meet the diaphragm and thus the liver at right angles so that a clean puncture is ensured and to avoid the larger vessels. The relatively larger size of the liver of the young calf may allow the organ to be palpated behind the last rib.

The ruminant liver has no significant species-specific features. It is enclosed within a tough fibrous capsule, but the extensions into the parenchyma do not outline obvious lobules as in the liver of the pig. The hepatic ducts join together in the portal region to form a single channel from which the cystic duct branches to the gallbladder. The continuation beyond this junction constitutes the bile duct, which enters the duodenum. The most superficial hepatic ducts may be visible through the covering liver tissue, especially when thickened by disease. The cattle liver may show fluke infestation (distomiasis) in many countries.

The liver receives blood from the *hepatic artery and portal vein,* which enter at the porta. Blood from both sources returns to the general circulation through the *hepatic veins,* which enter the embedded portion of the caudal vena cava. The openings of the major hepatic veins are arranged in two widely separated clusters. Intrahepatic anastomoses between the two sets provide a potential collateral pathway that becomes important when the intervening stretch of the caudal vena cava is obstructed.

The efferent lymphatic vessels pass mainly to the hepatic group of *nodes* scattered about the porta; the lymph

*There is evidence that the infective (prion protein) agents responsible for the transmissible spongiform encephalopathies (e.g., bovine spongiform encephalopathy) reach the central nervous system by transport from the gut along the splanchnic and vagal nerves.

thence drains into the visceral radicle of the cisterna chyli. Some lymph is routed via accessory hepatic (on the caudal vena cava) and caudal mediastinal nodes.

Although the livers of the *sheep* and the *goat* generally resemble that of cattle, size alone prevents confusion of the adult organs. They are distinguished from the liver of the calf by the much deeper umbilical fissure, narrower and less bluntly shaped caudate process, more elongated gallbladder, and absence of the sizable vestige of the umbilical vein that is evident on the liver of the young calf. An extensive contact with the abomasum is retained throughout life.

THE PANCREAS

The pancreas is of irregular form and pinkish yellow in color. The pancreas of the calf is consumed as a delicacy, together with the thymus, under the title of *sweetbread.* It has two lobes that join in a body located cranial to the portal vein, where the gland is adherent to the liver. The left lobe extends across the abdomen, insinuated between the liver, diaphragm, and great vessels dorsally and the intestinal mass and dorsal ruminal sac ventrally; it thus enters the retroperitoneal area above the rumen. The right lobe has a more complete peritoneal covering and follows the mesentery of the descending part of the duodenum, ventral to the right kidney and against the flank.

Although developed from dorsal and ventral primordia, the excretory system is usually reduced in cattle to a single (accessory) duct when the ventral outgrowth loses its direct connection to the gut. The surviving duct enters the descending duodenum about 20 to 25 cm past the entry of the bile duct. Its orifice is raised on a slight papilla.

The pancreas of *small ruminants* is very similar in form and topography to that of cattle. A single ventral duct is present, and it opens into the duodenum with the bile duct, usually by means of a common trunk.

THE KIDNEYS AND ADRENAL GLANDS

The kidneys of adult cattle retain much of their fetal lobation and are divided by surface fissures into about a dozen lobes (see Figs. 5.21 and 5.23). The right kidney has a flattened ellipsoidal form and lies in a conventional position with a dorsal retroperitoneal attachment to the sublumbar musculature. It is received cranially into the renal impression of the liver. The left kidney is less regular, being flattened at its cranial pole and thickened caudally. Its position below and behind its fellow is unusual and is the consequence of the postnatal growth of the rumen (see Fig. 29.9/*10*). Although surrounded by considerable accumulations of fat (capsula adiposa), both kidneys vary in position with the phase of respiration and according to the pressure exerted by other viscera. In the cadaver the right kidney is commonly found below the last rib and first two or three lumbar transverse processes, while the left one lies at a more ventral level under the second to fourth lumbar vertebrae. The left kidney is accessible on rectal exploration, but the right one usually is not. The left kidney may return to the left side when the pressure on it is relieved by fasting in life or after evisceration in the course of an autopsy.

The numerous relations of the right kidney need not be described at length. They include the liver, pancreas, duodenum, colon, and, in most animals, the adrenal gland. The hilus is widely open and lies ventromedially; the ureter runs from it, crossing the medial margin to follow a winding retroperitoneal course below the abdominal roof that carries it into the pelvis.

The left kidney is swung through about 90 degrees around the axis of the aorta in moving from its fetal (see Fig. 28.25) to its adult location against the right face of the dorsal sac. It hangs in a relatively long fold, rests on the intestinal mass, and is flattened by contact with the rumen. The left ureter crosses the dorsal aspect of the kidney to regain the left half of the abdomen. Its later course is similar to that of the right duct.

In *structure* the bovine kidneys are of the multipyramidal type (Fig. 28.27). The separate medullary pyramids are capped by a continuous cortex, which appears fragmented by fissures extending inward from its surface (Fig. 28.28). The cortex (Fig. 28.27/*4*) is clothed in a tough capsule that is easily stripped from the healthy organ, except toward the hilus, where it blends with the wall of the ureter. The cortical and medullary regions are distinguishable in gross sections by the much lighter color of the former and by the cut vessels that mark their mutual boundary. The glomerular vascular tufts scattered through the cortex may be visible to the naked eye. The apex (papilla; Fig. 28.27/*3*) of each medullary pyramid fits into a calyx or cup formed by one of the terminal branches of the ureter; these branches eventually unite to form two major channels that converge from the cranial and caudal poles to yield a single ureter (see Fig. 5.23). There is thus no large central expansion corresponding to a renal pelvis.

The *renal arteries* are derived from the aorta; the *renal veins* join the caudal vena cava. Lymphatic vessels lead to the renal nodes, enlarged members of the lumbar aortic series, and these in turn drain into the lumbar lymph trunk.

The kidneys of the *sheep* and *goat* are quite unlike those of cattle but conform closely in external appearance and internal structure to those of the dog (see Fig. 5.23). They are more regular in shape than the dog's, being protected from distorting pressures by enclosure in thick masses of fat. The fat cushion makes the left kidney less subject to displacement by the rumen.

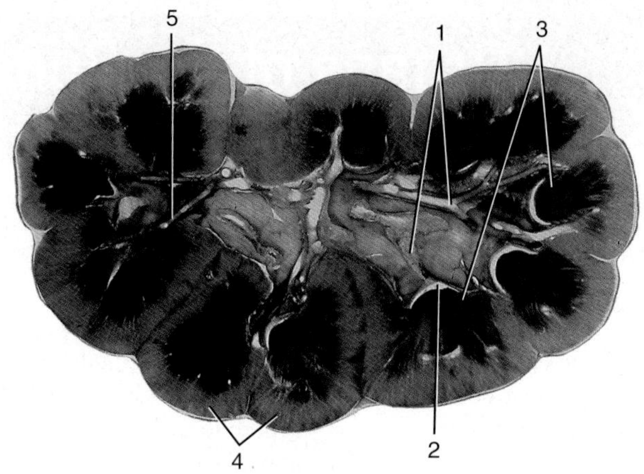

Fig. 28.27 Bovine kidney dissected to show its interior (semi-schematic). *1,* Principal branches of ureter; *2,* calyx; *3,* renal papillae; *4,* renal cortex; *5,* interlobular artery.

The *adrenal glands* are located close to the kidneys. The right gland is heart shaped and usually lies against the medial margin of the cranial extremity of the corresponding kidney (Fig. 28.10/*12*). The left one is less regular in form and less constant in position; generally it is found within the perirenal fat some centimeters cranial to the left kidney. The division into cortex and medulla is very evident in gross sections.

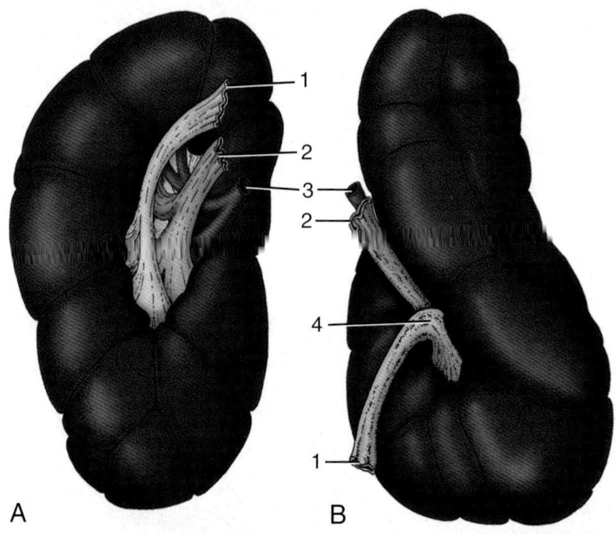

Fig. 28.28 Ventral views of the (A) right and (B) left bovine kidneys. *1,* Ureter; *2,* renal vein; *3,* renal artery; *4,* renal sinus.

THE LYMPH NODES OF THE ABDOMINAL ROOF

A number of important lymph nodes are scattered about the bifurcation of the aorta and between its terminal branches. Most belong to the *medial iliac group,* which collects lymph from the hindlimbs, pelvic walls, and pelvic viscera (see Fig. 29.4). The large *deep inguinal (iliofemoral) node,* in the angle between the external and deep circumflex iliac arteries, receives the flow from the udder; when enlarged it can be palpated per rectum near the cranial border of the ilium. The efferent stream forms the lumbar trunk, which runs forward over the aorta to enter the cisterna chyli. A few much smaller *(lumbar aortic)* nodes that are spread along the psoas musculature are concerned with the lymphatic drainage of the vertebrae and neighboring muscles. The renal nodes belong to this series.

COMPREHENSION CHECK

With the aid of diagrams, explain the anatomic relationships that arise in the bovine abdomen when the abomasum is normally situated, when it is displaced to the left, and when it is displaced to the right.

Review the innervation of the abdominal wall and the paravertebral nerve blocks to anesthetize the abdominal wall for laparotomy.

29 The Pelvis and Reproductive Organs of the Ruminant

This chapter is concerned with the pelvic cavity, the intrapelvic and extrapelvic reproductive organs of both sexes, and the udder.

THE PELVIC CAVITY

The pelvic cavity of the cow becomes progressively narrower between the entrance and the exit. There is a pronounced dip of the middle part of the floor resulting in a local increase in height before the caudal part slopes steeply upward to the shallow exit (Fig. 29.1).

The entrance faces ventrocranially at an angle that carries the pecten of the pubis below the second intersacral joint (Fig. 29.1/*15*). Behind the iliac shaft, the width is reduced by inflection of the high ischial spine, and it becomes further reduced by the encroachment of the massive ischial tuber on the exit (Fig. 29.2). The conspicuously cramped exit is roughly triangular; the third caudal vertebra and the tubercular ischial tubers are its corners. The lateral border is completed by the sacrotuberous ligament (the edge of the sacrosciatic ligament), while the caudal margin of the floor is cut away at the ischial arch. The strong development of the ischial crest and tuber combine to reduce the contribution to the lateral wall that is made by the sacrosciatic ligament (Fig. 29.2/*4*).

There are certain variations associated with age and gender. The entrance is almost uniformly wide in mature cows but considerably narrowed in its ventral part in heifers. In these younger animals the cranial part of the floor raises a ridge over the symphysis; in older cows, especially those that have carried several calves, the same region is level or sunken. The male girdle, despite being significantly more robust, encloses a cavity that is clearly less capacious. It is even more confined at the entrance, and beyond this the cranial part of the floor tends to be domed.

In sheep and goats the long, slender iliac shafts approach the vertebral column at an acute angle that, in combination with the shortness of the sacrum, places the pecten below the second joint of the tail (see Fig. 26.2).

The sacroiliac joints (Fig. 29.3) are complemented and rendered virtually immobile by strong ligaments between the two bones. About the time of parturition, hormones induce some slackening of the collagenous structures of the pelvis to allow modest but potentially significant mobility (p. 200). Ankylosis of these joints, accompanied by lumbar spondylosis, is common in aging bulls and, when severe, may disable the animal for service.

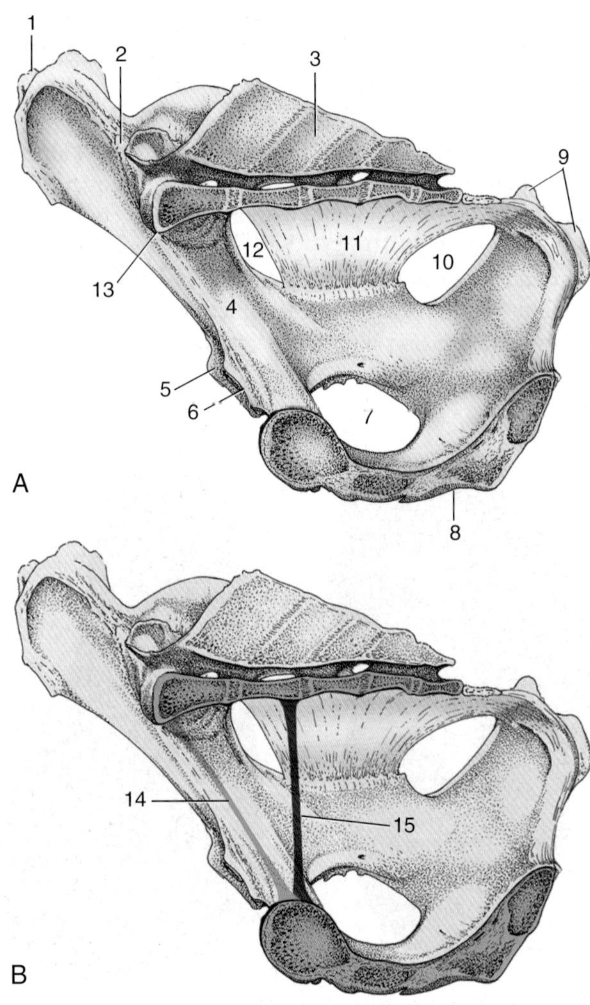

Fig. 29.1 (A) and (B), Median section of the bony pelvis of a cow. Certain obstetrical terms are illustrated in (B). *1*, Coxal tuber; *2*, sacroiliac joint; *3*, sacrum; *4*, shaft of ilium; *5*, cranial border of acetabulum; *6*, pecten pubis; *7*, obturator foramen; *8*, symphysis; *9*, ischial tuber; *10*, lesser sciatic foramen; *11*, sacrosciatic ligament; *12*, greater sciatic foramen; *13*, promontory; *14*, conjugate (the line connecting the promontory with the pecten); *15*, vertical diameter (the vertical line between the pectin and the pelvic roof).

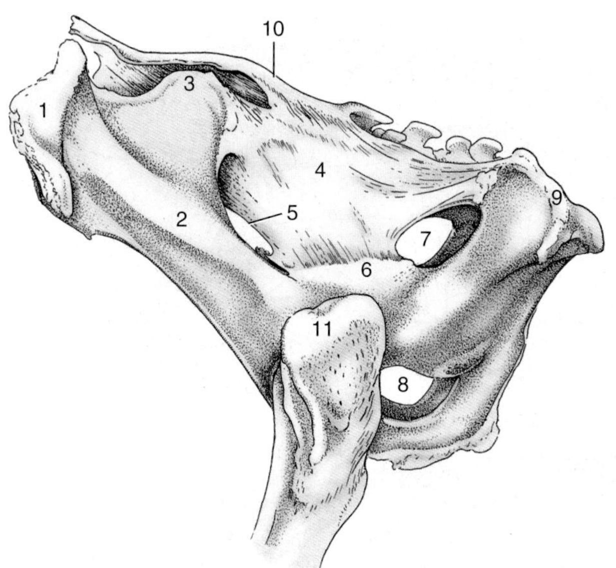

Fig. 29.2 Lateral view of the bony pelvis of a cow. *1,* Coxal tuber; *2,* shaft of ilium; *3,* sacral tuber; *4,* sacrosciatic ligament; *5,* greater sciatic foramen; *6,* ischial spine; *7,* lesser sciatic foramen; *8,* right and left obturator foramina; *9,* ischial tuber; *10,* sacrum; *11,* greater trochanter.

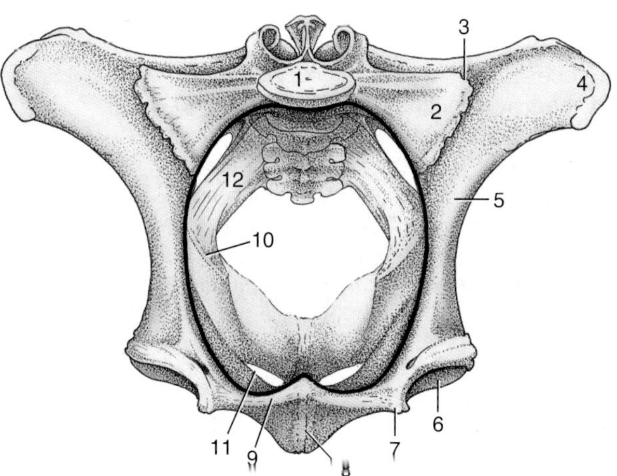

Fig. 29.3 Cranial view of the bony pelvis of a cow. The terminal line *(black)* is indicated. *1,* Body of first sacral vertebra; *2,* wing of sacrum; *3,* sacroiliac joint; *4,* coxal tuber; *5,* shaft of ilium; *6,* acetabulum; *7,* iliopubic eminence; *8,* symphysis; *9,* pecten pubis; *10,* ischial spine; *11,* obturator foramen; *12,* sacrosciatic ligament.

The perineal region is extensive because those parts of the hamstring musculature that in the horse provide it with very prominent lateral boundaries are lacking in cattle. By convention, the region is considered to extend ventrally to include the nearest part of the udder (or scrotum). The increase in breadth exposes the sacrotuberous ligaments, the ischial tubers, and the ischiorectal fossae as visible and palpable surface landmarks. The anus and vulva, the most obvious features of the dorsal and ventral perineal regions, respectively, are considered later (see Fig. 29.10).

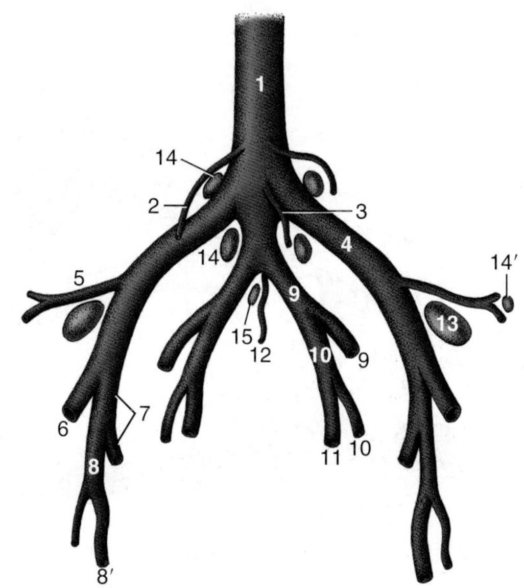

Fig. 29.4 Branching pattern of the caudal part of the bovine abdominal aorta. *1,* Aorta; *2,* ovarian artery; *3,* caudal mesenteric artery; *4,* external iliac artery; *5,* deep circumflex iliac artery; *6,* femoral artery; *7,* deep femoral artery; *8,* pudendoepigastric trunk; *8′,* external pudendal artery; *9,* internal iliac artery; *10,* umbilical artery; *11,* uterine artery; *12,* median sacral artery; *13,* deep inguinal (iliofemoral) lymph node; *14* and *14′,* medial and lateral iliac lymph nodes, respectively; *15,* sacral lymph nodes.

The *blood supply* to pelvic structures is delivered by the small *median sacral artery* and the much larger, paired *internal iliacs* (Fig. 29.4). The first or, more accurately, its continuation as the median caudal artery has already been encountered (p. 656). The *internal iliac artery* serves both parietal and visceral structures, contrary to the usual arrangement. It enters the pelvic cavity close to the sacroiliac joint and continues down the ilium to reach the vicinity of the lesser sciatic foramen (Fig. 29.1/*10*) before dividing into *internal pudendal and caudal gluteal arteries.* The latter, like other parietal branches, is of no present concern. The internal iliac's first visceral branch, detached close to the origin of the parent trunk, is the *umbilical artery.* This term, though appropriate to its role in the fetus, is misleading because the vessel is now almost exclusively concerned with supplying blood to the uterus through a large *uterine artery;* the continuation of the umbilical, reduced to a fibrous cord with a vestigial lumen, is better known as the round ligament of the bladder. The male homologue of the uterine artery is the deferential. (The distribution of the arteries to the viscera is considered with the organs they supply.) The second visceral branch, the *vaginal artery,* is detached close to the termination of the internal iliac trunk and supplies the bulk of the pelvic viscera. The male homologue is the *prostatic artery.* The *internal pudendal artery* supplies both parietal structures, including the muscles of

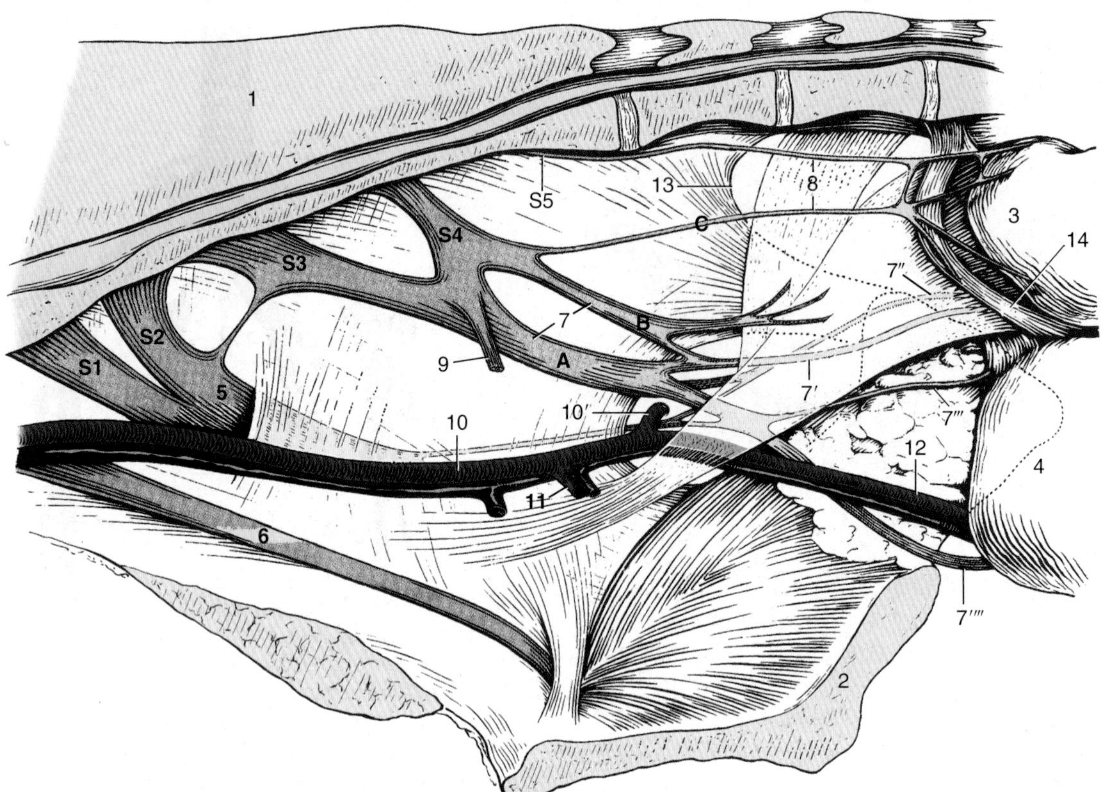

Fig. 29.5 Nerves and vessels on the medial surface of the bovine pelvic wall. Local anesthesia of the pudendal nerve (n.) can be obtained by injections at points *A* and *B;* anesthesia of the caudal rectal nerves is possible by an injection at point *C*. *1*, Sacrum; *2*, pelvic symphysis; *3*, rectum (reflected); *4*, vagina (reflected); *5*, sciatic n.; *6*, obturator n.; *7*, pudendal n.; *7′*, distal cutaneous branch of pudendal n.; *7″*, proximal cutaneous branch of pudendal n.; *7‴*, deep perineal n.; *7⁗*, continuation of pudendal n. to clitoris; *8*, caudal rectal nerves; *9*, pelvic n.; *10*, internal iliac artery (a.); *10′*, caudal gluteal a.; *11*, vaginal a.; *12*, internal pudendal a.; *13*, caudal border of sacrosciatic ligament; *14*, retractor clitoridis; *S1* to *S5*, sacral nerves 1 through 5.

the pelvic diaphragm, and viscera, including the female tract from the caudal vagina to the vestibule. The depleted trunk leaves the pelvis, through an opening in the fascia directly above the symphysis, to supply branches to the clitoris and labia and other branches to the perineum, some of which reach the caudal part of the udder (or scrotum and prepuce).

The *nerves* within the pelvis fall into two groups (Fig. 29.5). The first comprises the *obturator and sciatic nerves* that, despite their vulnerability to injury at parturition, will be described with the hindlimb. The second group comprises the *pudendal, caudal rectal, and pelvic nerves,* of which all are purely sacral in origin and concerned with the supply of the pelvic viscera and the perineum. The significant divisions of the pudendal nerve are the deep perineal and distal cutaneous branches and the continuation of the main trunk. The *deep perineal* supplies both visceral and somatic structures of the caudal pelvic region. The *distal cutaneous branch* supplies structures of the ventral perineum (before it becomes superficial by emerging from the ischiorectal fossa), crosses the medial process of the ischial tuber (where it may be palpated), and supplies the vulva and perineal skin; some branches extend as far as the nearest part of the udder. The depleted trunk passes ventral and leaves the pelvis in company with the internal pudendal artery; it supplies the *dorsal nerve of the clitoris/penis* and supplies other branches to the skin of the udder/scrotum and prepuce.

Pudendal nerve block is used in surgery of the prepuce in bulls and also in the management of chronic prolapse in cows. The block is instituted by locating the lesser sciatic foramen and the nerve that lies on the sacrosciatic ligament a bit craniodorsal to the foramen. The needle, inserted via the ischiorectal fossa, is guided close to the nerve followed by depositing of the anesthetic.

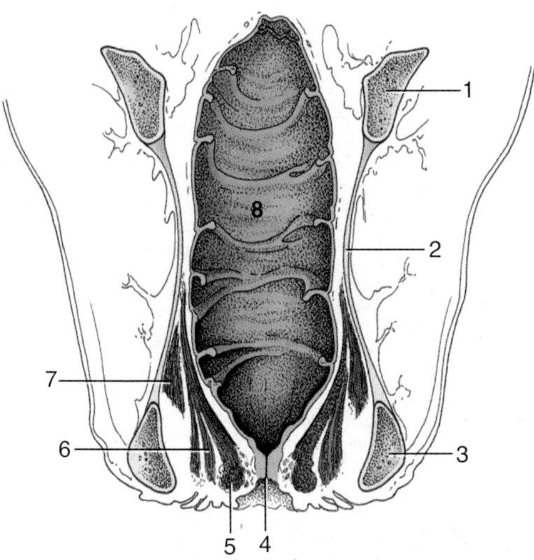

Fig. 29.6 Dorsal section of the bovine rectum and adjacent structures. Note especially the topography of the pelvic diaphragm (*6* and *7*). *1,* Shaft of ilium; *2,* sacrosciatic ligament; *3,* ischial tuber; *4,* anus; *5,* external anal sphincter; *6,* levator ani; *7,* coccygeus; *8,* rectum.

THE RECTUM AND ANUS

Although the origin of the rectum is arbitrarily defined, its most caudal part is distinguished from the colon by a wider caliber and more muscular wall. The interior, marked by impermanent transverse folds, is generally distended with feces (Fig. 29.6).

The colic mesentery continues as the mesorectum, which abruptly shortens to a mere 3 cm, before gradually decreasing further until it eventually disappears (Figs. 29.7 and 29.8), which brings the rectum into broad contact with the pelvic roof. In this process more and more of the rectal circumference becomes denuded of serosa until the last part is completely embedded in fat, which provides the cushion that allows the gut to adjust to changing circumstances. The close connection with the pelvic roof and walls is a handicap to rectal explorations, and for many purposes the hand must be carried forward into the more mobile colon (Fig. 29.9) (p. 707).

The anal canal is embraced by the pelvic diaphragm; the postdiaphragmatic part forms a low eminence presenting a short transverse slit through which the skin continues to provide the last stretch of the canal with a cutaneous epithelial covering. The anus is guarded by the usual two sphincters, and the striated external one exchanges fascicules with other muscles of the perineum (Fig. 29.10).

Most of the rectum is supplied from the *cranial rectal artery,* a branch of the caudal mesenteric, but the terminal section and the anal region are supplied by twigs from the *caudal rectal artery,* an indirect branch of the vaginal artery. The venous drainage is divided between the portal and systemic systems.

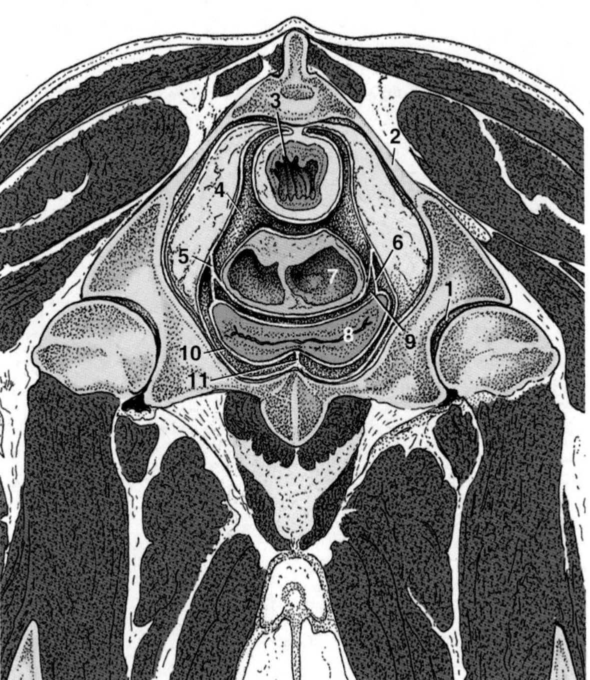

Fig. 29.7 Transverse section of the bovine pelvis at the level of the hip joint (cranial surface). Note the large amount of retroperitoneal fat in the pelvis. (See Fig. 29.11 for the level of this section.) *1,* Hip joint; *2,* sacrosciatic ligament; *3,* rectum; *4,* rectogenital pouch; *5,* broad ligament of uterus; *6,* lateral ligament of bladder; *7,* uterus sectioned where the two horns are conjoined; *8,* bladder; *9,* vesicogenital pouch; *10,* pubovesical pouch; *11,* median ligament of bladder.

THE BLADDER AND URETHRA

The bladder is intra-abdominal in the young calf. In the adult, the bladder is in the pelvic cavity when empty but extends over the abdominal floor when distended. The neck within the pelvis is without a peritoneal covering and is attached to the pelvic floor by fat and loose connective tissue (see Figs. 29.7 and 29.8). Urine escaping from a ruptured bladder—a relatively common mishap, especially in steers—may infiltrate this tissue or enter the peritoneal cavity according to the site of the tear. There are the usual lateral and median ligaments.

The relations of the bladder naturally vary. In the cow, it is always in contact with the cranial part of the vagina and the cervix and often with the body and horns of the uterus. Within the abdomen it makes contact with the dorsocaudal blind sac of the rumen and with the intestines (Fig. 29.11).

The urethra is much narrower than that of the mare and runs below the vagina, to which it becomes increasingly attached as it proceeds caudally. It opens into the vestibule through a median slit that is shared with the suburethral

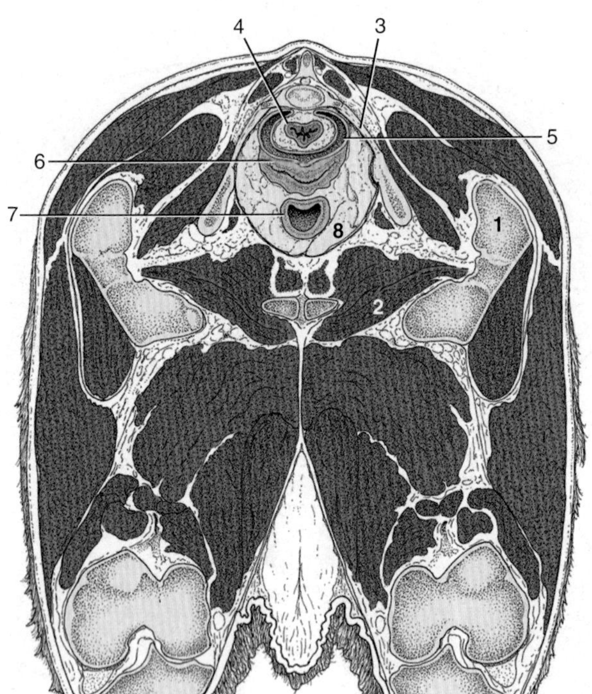

Fig. 29.8 Transverse section of the bovine pelvis at the level of the first caudal vertebra (cranial surface). The section passes through the obturator foramina. Note that the peritoneum covers only the dorsal surface of the vagina; the lateral and ventral surfaces are retroperitoneal at this level. (See Fig. 29.11 for the level of this section.) *1,* Greater trochanter; *2,* obturator foramen; *3,* sacrosciatic ligament; *4,* rectum; *5,* rectogenital pouch; *6,* vagina; *7,* neck of bladder; *8,* retroperitoneal fat.

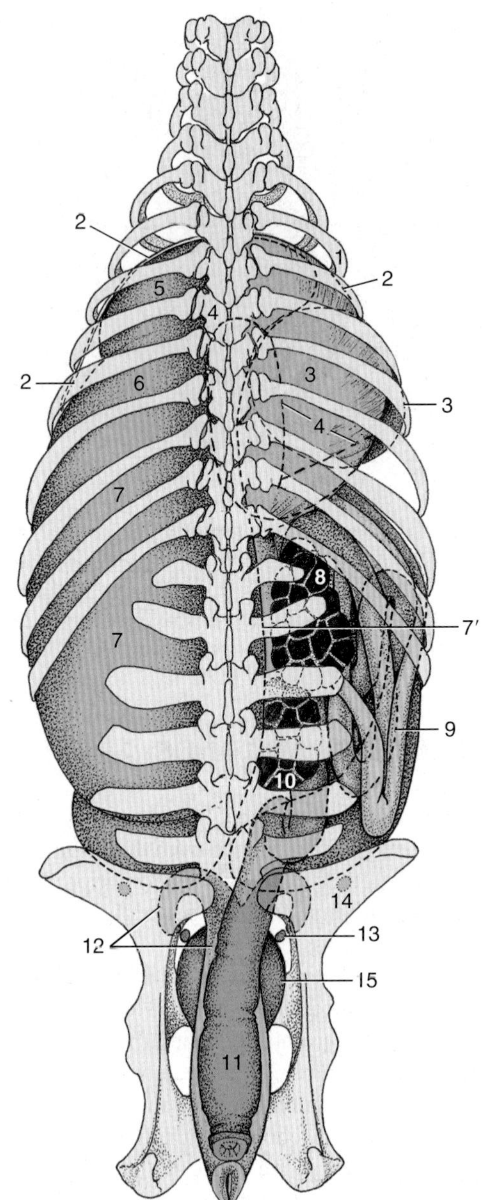

Fig. 29.9 Relationship of the principal abdominal and pelvic organs to the bovine skeleton, dorsal view. *1,* Sixth rib; *2,* cranial extent of diaphragm; *3,* omasum, most of it covered by the liver; *4,* outline of abomasum; *5,* reticulum; *6,* atrium ruminis; *7,* dorsal sac; *7′,* right face of rumen; *8,* right kidney; *9,* descending duodenum (ventral to it is the intestinal mass); *10,* left kidney; *11,* rectum; *12,* uterus; *13,* ovary; *14,* lateral iliac lymph node; *15,* bladder.

diverticulum (Fig. 29.11/*13*), a blind pouch extending cranially that is large enough to admit the end joint of a finger. The pouch can be a nuisance when catheterization is attempted. The urethralis muscle only covers the caudal part of the urethra, which more cranially is anchored to the floor by a short but strong ligament. The cranial fascicules of the urethralis muscle insert on a dorsal raphe that completes the encirclement of the urethra; the more caudal ones form a "U" shape that attaches to each side of the vagina and vestibule, enclosing both the diverticulum and the urethra.

The *blood supply* to these organs comes from the umbilical and vaginal arteries.

THE FEMALE REPRODUCTIVE ORGANS

The topographic peculiarities of the reproductive organs of the female ruminant are the consequence of the descent of the fetal ovaries to the most caudal part of the abdomen, which is a more considerable descent than in other domestic species. As a result, the horns of the uterus are drawn back toward their ovarian attachments and do not range far into the abdomen except in advanced pregnancy.

The following account refers primarily to the organs of the mature, nonpregnant cow.

The Ovary and Uterine Tube

The ovary is a firm, rather irregular ovoid body, small (4 × 2.5 × 1.5 cm) in relation to body size. Joined to the body wall and to the reproductive tract by inclusion in the broad

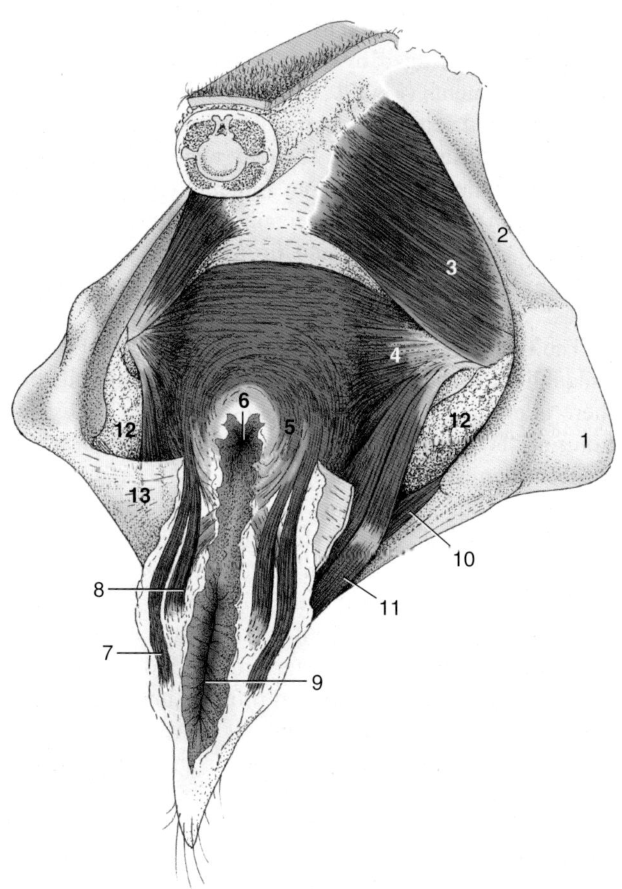

Fig. 29.10 The perineal muscles of a cow. *1,* Ischial tuber; *2,* sacrosciatic ligament; *3,* coccygeus; *4,* levator ani; *5,* external anal sphincter; *6,* anus; *7,* retractor clitoridis; *8,* constrictor vulvae; *9,* vulva; *10,* urogenital diaphragm; *11,* constrictor vestibuli; *12,* fat in ischiorectal fossa; *13,* perineal fascia (partly removed on the right side).

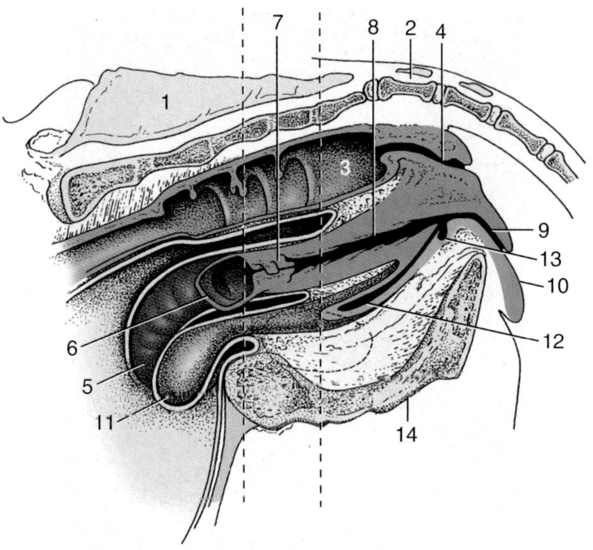

Fig. 29.11 Median section of the bovine pelvis. The *two vertical broken lines* indicate the levels of the transverse sections in Figs. 29.7 *(left line)* and 29.8 *(right line).* The position of the obturator foramen is indicated by a *broken outline. 1,* Sacrum; *2,* first caudal vertebra; *3,* rectum; *4,* anal canal; *5,* right uterine horn; *6,* left uterine horn, mostly removed; *7,* cervix; *8,* vagina; *9,* vestibule; *10,* vulva; *11,* bladder; *12,* urethra; *13,* suburethral diverticulum; *14,* symphysis.

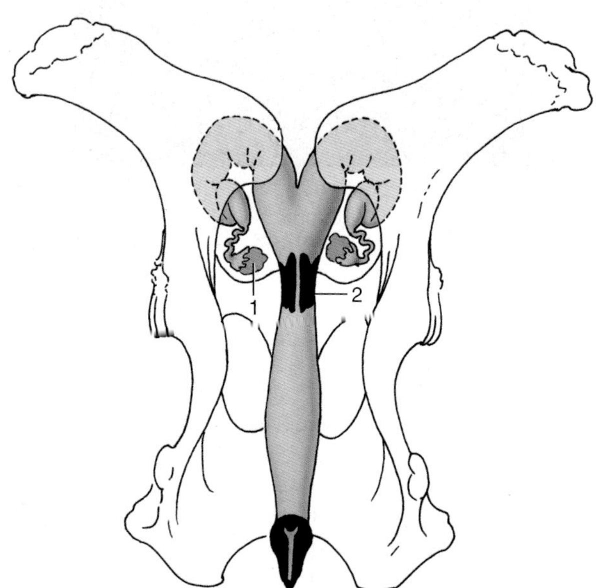

Fig. 29.12 Dorsal view of the bony pelvis and related (nongravid) bovine reproductive organs. Note the position of the ovaries in relation to the pecten pubis. *1,* Ovary; *2,* cervix.

ligament, it is related to the ventral part of the shaft of the ilium, level with the bifurcation of the uterus. Follicles and corpora lutea may project from any part of the surface (Figs. 29.12 and 29.13).

The largest follicles attain a diameter of 2 cm, but even those as small as 5 mm in diameter may be detected on palpation per rectum. Because the estrus cycle is short (generally 21 days), follicles and corpora lutea of some size may be present together.

Ovarian follicular cysts affect 10% of dairy cattle. Because cows are generally infertile until the cyst is treated, it increases the inter calving interval and causes significant economic losses to the dairy industry. There is some evidence as to the heritability of the cysts.

The uterine tube is rather long, but its flexuous course brings its beginning and end close together (Fig. 29.14A and B). The thin-walled infundibulum lies over the lateral wall of the ovary in the free margin of the mesosalpinx. The succeeding, narrower part of the tube winds within the lateral wall of the ovarian bursa to reach the tip of the uterine horn. It is divided into ampulla and isthmus, approximately in the ratio of 2:1, but the distinction is only

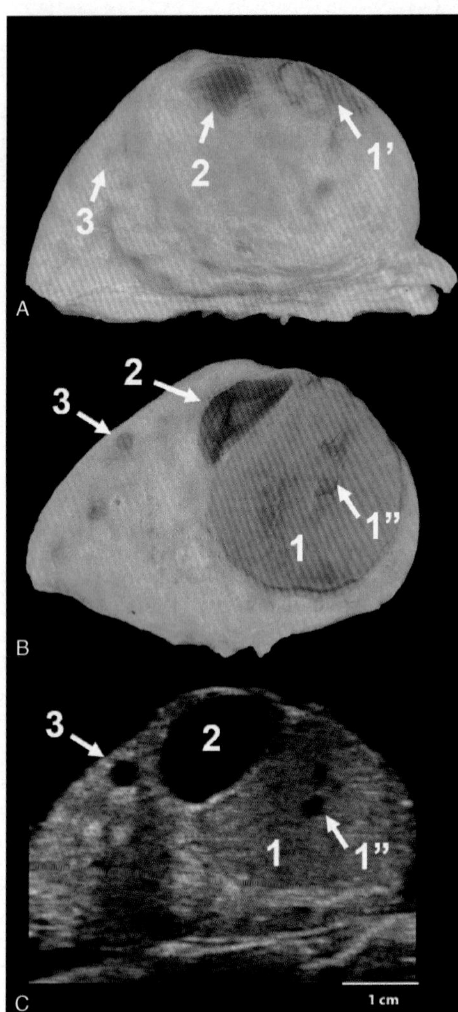

Fig. 29.13 Images showing the surface (A), a longitudinal cut view (B), and an ultrasound image (C) of the bovine ovary. Only a small part of the fully developed corpus luteum *(1')* projects above the surface while the majority of the glandular tissue structure *(1)* is embedded within the ovary. Irregular-shaped cavities *(1'')* are common in the corpus luteum and easily detectable by ultrasound imaging. Note a large *(2)* and a small *(3)* antral follicle in the cortex of the ovary. Fluid-filled antrum appears as an anechoic (dark) structure in ultrasound images.

obvious at certain stages of the cycle. The transition of isthmus to horn is gradual and marked by muscular thickening.

Apart from features associated with the frequency of twin and multiple pregnancies, the ovaries as well as the tubes of sheep and goats are very similar to those of cows.

The Uterus

The uterus gives a misleading impression of consisting of a relatively long body succeeded by two divergent, tapering horns coiled ventrally on themselves (Fig. 29.15). Actually the apparent body is furnished by the two horns lying within shared serosal and muscular coats, which is an arrangement suggested by a dorsal groove. The diverging horns are bridged by short dorsal and ventral intercornual ligaments (Fig. 29.14/*4*). The ligaments create a small pocket that allows placing of a finger to fix the organ during rectal examinations. The tight winding of the horns is not constant but results from stimulation of the muscle of the organ and of the broad ligament; the uterus appears to become more definite and firmer in the course of a rectal examination. The effect is most noticeable during estrus.

The firmness of the cervix permits recognition of the caudal limit of the body of the uterus during handling, but there is nothing to indicate its cranial limit. The dissection reveals that the body is a mere 3 cm in length while the cervix measures 8 to 10 cm. Each horn measures 35 cm or so, of which about one third is incorporated in the "pseudobody." The cervix begins at the constriction of the internal uterine ostium, beyond which the passage is occluded by the interlocking of projections from the walls; these consist of three or four circular folds in virgin animals, but these become broken and irregular in multipara. The most caudal fold projects into the vagina, where it is surrounded by an annular fornix. The cervical mucosa also shows longitudinal folds that, on reaching the external ostium, radiate in a fashion recalling the segments of an orange (Fig. 29.16A and B). Many irregular, originally circular folds project into the lumen, fitting closely together; the last one is sunken into a recess of the vaginal wall. In combination, these features make catheterization of the uterus very difficult if not impossible at most stages of the cycle for insemination or embryo transfer.

Most features that distinguish the uterus of the small ruminants are of little practical importance. The most characteristic feature of the interior of the uterus are the caruncles, the attachment sites of the fetal membranes in pregnancy. About 40 of these are arranged in four more or less regular rows in the wider parts of the horn, reducing to a double line toward the tip. The free surfaces of the caruncles are concave, most obviously in the ewe (Fig. 29.17).

Surgical Approach to the Uterus: The uterus can be approached for surgical procedures such as the cesarean section in the standing animal via the flank approach. In this approach the paralumbar fossa is desensitized through caudal epidural anesthesia or paravertebral nerve block.

The Vagina

The remaining part of the genital tract is divided between the vagina and vestibule, approximately in the ratio of 3:1; the boundary is a few centimeters cranial to the ischial arch (Fig. 29.11). Because the vagina is capable of great expansion, in length and in diameter, its passive dimensions are

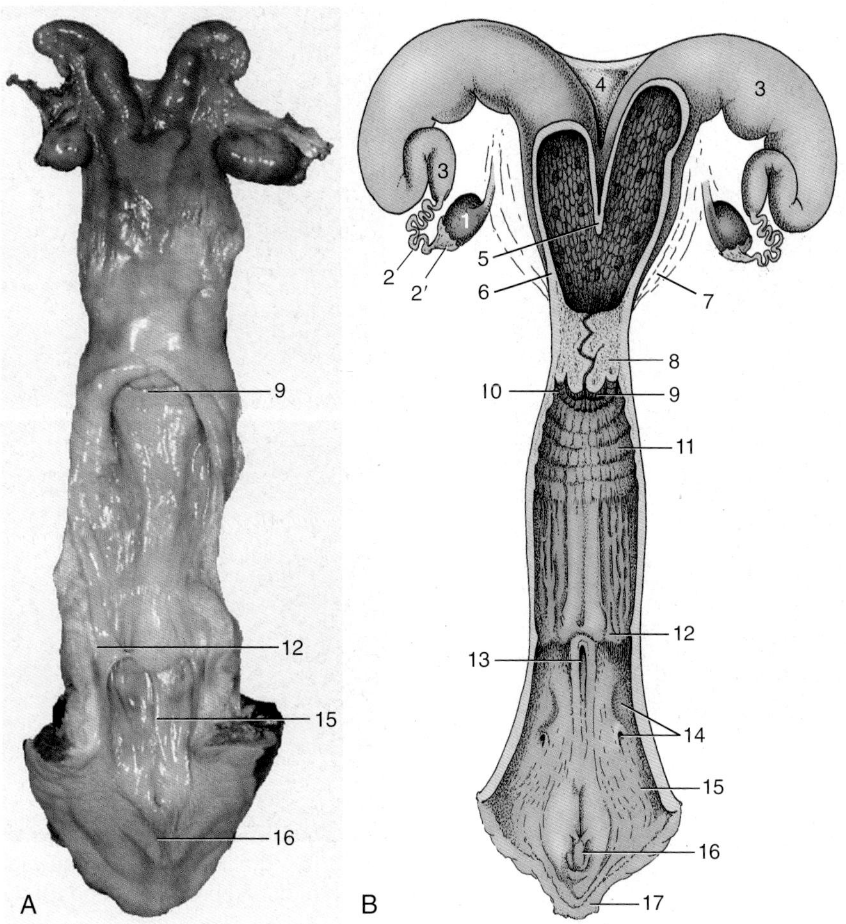

Fig. 29.14 The bovine reproductive organs, dorsal view. (A) The vagina and the vestibule have been opened in the specimen. (B) The greater part of the tract is shown opened in the schema. *1,* Ovary; *2,* uterine tube; *2′,* infundibulum; *3,* uterine horn; *4,* intercornual ligament; *5,* wall of uterus dividing the two horns; *6,* body of uterus with caruncles; *7,* broad ligament; *8,* cervix; *9,* vaginal part of cervix; *10,* fornix; *11,* vagina; *12,* position of former hymen; *13,* external urethral orifice and suburethral diverticulum; *14,* major vestibular gland and its excretory orifice; *15,* vestibule; *16,* glans of the clitoris; *17,* right labium.

not of great significance. The lining exhibits low folds, both circular and longitudinal, and the lumen is closed by the falling together of the roof and floor (Fig. 29.8). It is usual to find the caudal part ventrally narrowed, especially in young animals, because of the urethralis muscle.

The cranial two-thirds of the dorsal wall faces into the rectogenital pouch, but caudal to this the vagina and rectum are joined by a wedge of tissue (Fig. 29.11). The ventral surface has a less complete peritoneal covering and is related to the bladder and urethra and to the packing tissues about the urethra. The lateral walls are also largely without peritoneum, being cranially included in the broad ligament and more caudally sharing in the general retroperitoneal arrangement (Figs. 29.7 and 29.8). This limitation of the peritoneum is relevant to the prognosis of wounds to the vaginal wall. The peritoneal covering of the dorsal fornix region provides a convenient route for surgical access to the abdominal cavity, most often used for operations on the ovary; it has the additional advantage of avoiding the major vessels that pass below and to the sides of the vagina.

Vestiges of the mesonephric ducts may be found below the mucosa of the floor near the junction with the vestibule; they are sometimes the origin of cysts.

The vagina is almost absent in the freemartin (p. 701), whose abnormally short tract is evident on examination of the vestibule. Aplasia or constriction of the vagina also occurs in white heifer disease, another congenital anomaly. The freemartin is found after a twin pregnancy in which the female fetus is adversely affected by the male twin (Fig. 29.18).

The Vestibule and Vulva

The vestibule slopes ventrally to open between the labia (Fig. 29.11). It is less distensible than the vagina, and its

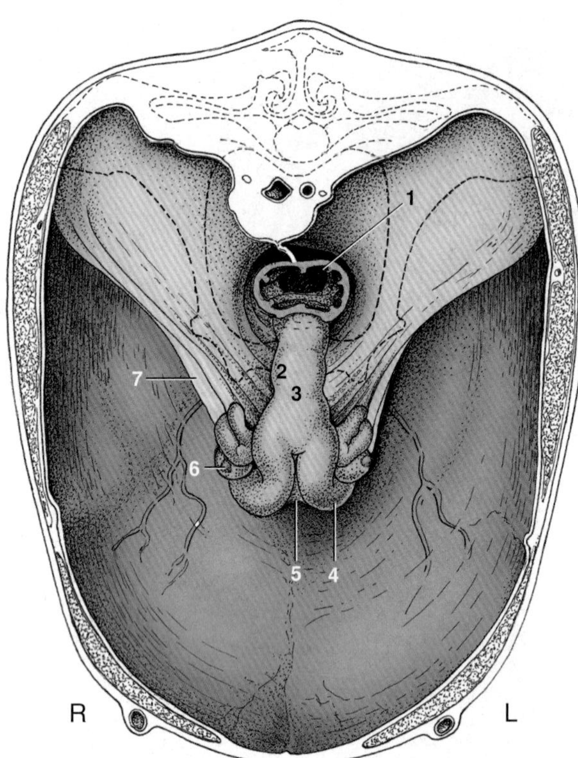

Fig. 29.15 The reproductive organs of a cow in situ, cranial view. The bony pelvis is indicated by *broken lines.* The uterus sags within this largely eviscerated abdomen. *1,* Rectum; *2,* cervix; *3,* body of uterus; *4,* left uterine horn; *5,* intercornual ligament; *6,* right ovary; *7,* broad ligament.

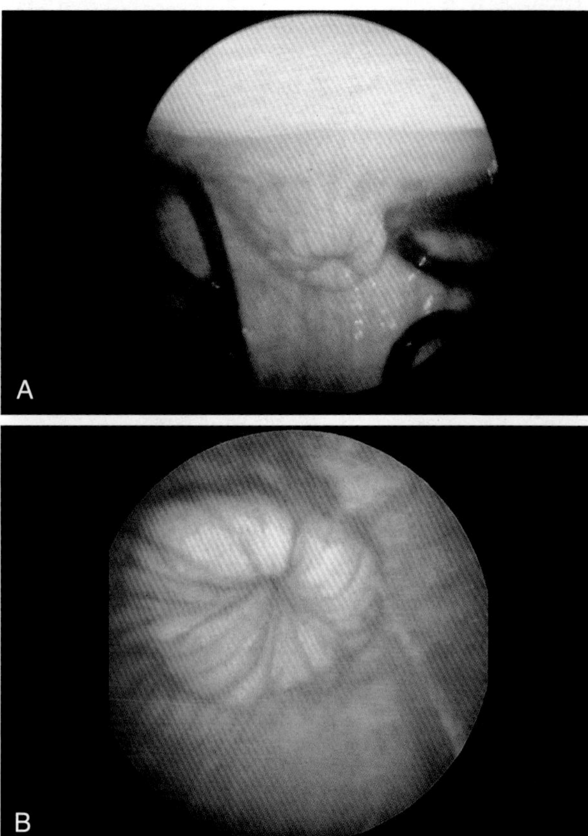

Fig. 29.16 The appearance of the vaginal part of the bovine cervix (A) during pregnancy and (B) during estrus.

side walls are normally in contact. When drawn apart, the opening of the urethra is exposed at the cranial end of the vestibule, and, at the other, the fossa containing the glans of the clitoris is exposed (Fig. 29.14). A large depression caudolateral to the urethral opening marks the location of the major vestibular gland, about 3 cm long, which is enclosed within the urogenital diaphragm. The vestibular mucosa is generally darkened over the gland.

The rounded, rather low labia are often marked by trauma sustained at previous calvings. Simple inspection exposes relatively little of the slender clitoris because the glans is fused with the prepuce. The vulva of the freemartin, abnormally small, is surrounded by unusually long hair.

The vestibule penetrates the urogenital diaphragm (perineal membrane), which fills the gap between the rectovaginal septum and the pelvic floor. The fascia of the diaphragm arises from the pelvic floor, bends around and attaches to the wall of the vestibule, and merges with the rectovaginal septum, the lower edge of the pelvic diaphragm, and the parietal pelvic fascia. One importance of the arrangement lies in its anchorage of the genital tract, opposing the drag of the gravid uterus as it sinks into the abdomen and the backward drag during calving.

The constrictor vestibularis and constrictor vulvae muscles are associated with the vestibule and vulva. The former, the more important, incorporates some fascicles that continue from the levator ani and form the perineal body. It runs over the wall of the vestibule caudal to the diaphragm and passes below the vestibule to join its fellow; on contraction it narrows the genital passage and raises a ridge in its floor. The constrictor vulvae, through its insertion to the vulva and adjacent skin, may cause the opening to gape.

Vascularization

The relatively small *ovarian artery,* a direct branch of the aorta in cattle, supplies the ovary, the uterine tube, and the adjoining part of the horn of the uterus. The ovarian artery is distinguished by an extraordinarily convoluted course within the cranial part of the broad ligament and has extensive contact with the plexiform ovarian vein (Fig. 29.19). These features facilitate the transfer of prostaglandins from venous to arterial blood. The *uterine artery* arises from the internal iliac and enters the pelvic cavity within the broad ligament. It is ostensibly a branch of the umbilical but appropriates virtually the entire flow of its parent (Fig. 29.4). It is the largest of the arteries to the female tract, and before reaching the uterus, it divides into cranial and caudal parts, each the source of about half a dozen stem vessels that reach the mesometrial border of the uterus. Branches from these run over the uterine walls following courses that appear to coincide with the locations of the

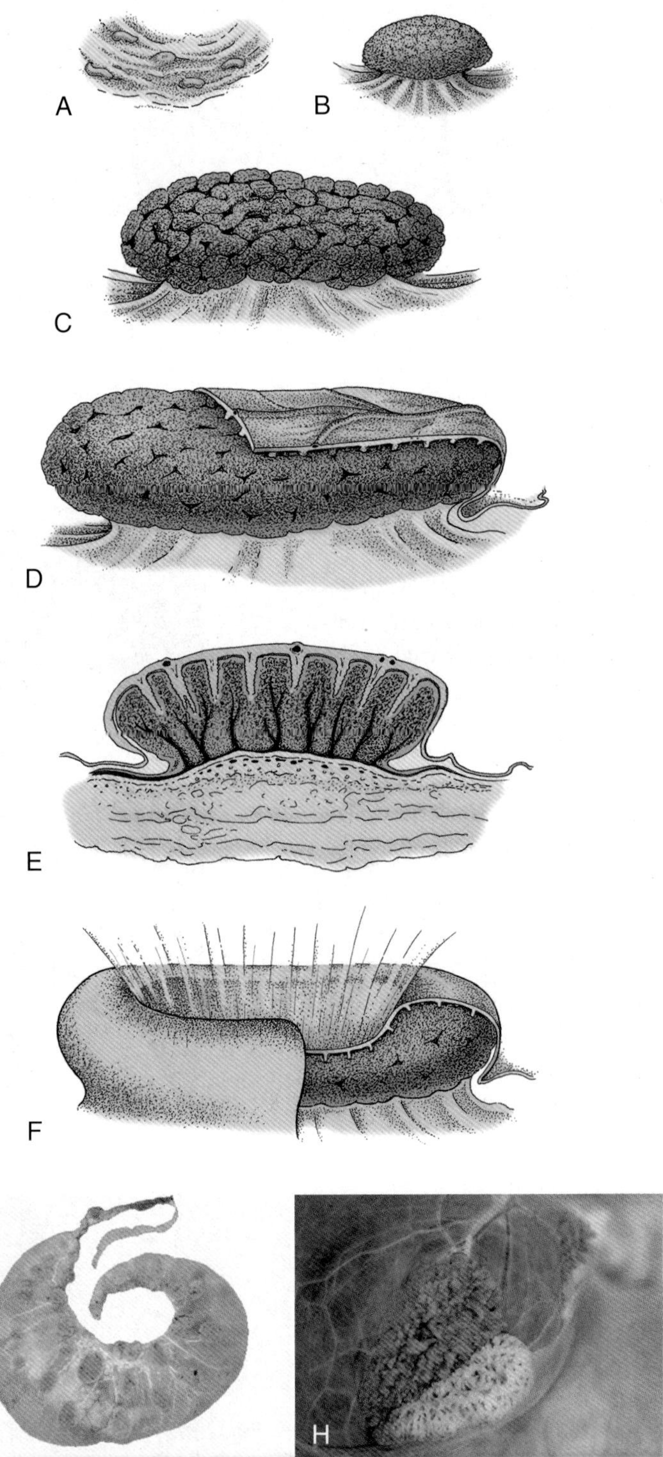

Fig. 29.17 Development of caruncles in the wall of the bovine uterus. (A) Caruncle in a nongravid uterus. (B) Caruncle in a 2-week gravid uterus. (C) Caruncle in a 6-month gravid uterus. (D) Caruncle near term, covered in part by a cotyledon (fetal tissue). (E) Section of a placentome. (F) Placentome of a sheep. (G) Cotyledonary placenta (ruminant). (H) Partial separation of maternal and fetal parts of placentome (cow).

caruncles internally. The arrangement leaves the antimesometrial border of the uterus less well supplied and thus less prone to bleeding when incised. The *vaginal artery,* branching from the internal iliac near the ischial spine, runs over the dorsolateral surface of the vagina before swinging forward over the lateral wall, where it risks involvement, with possibly fatal outcome, in vaginal rupture, a relatively common calving catastrophe in heifers. Various

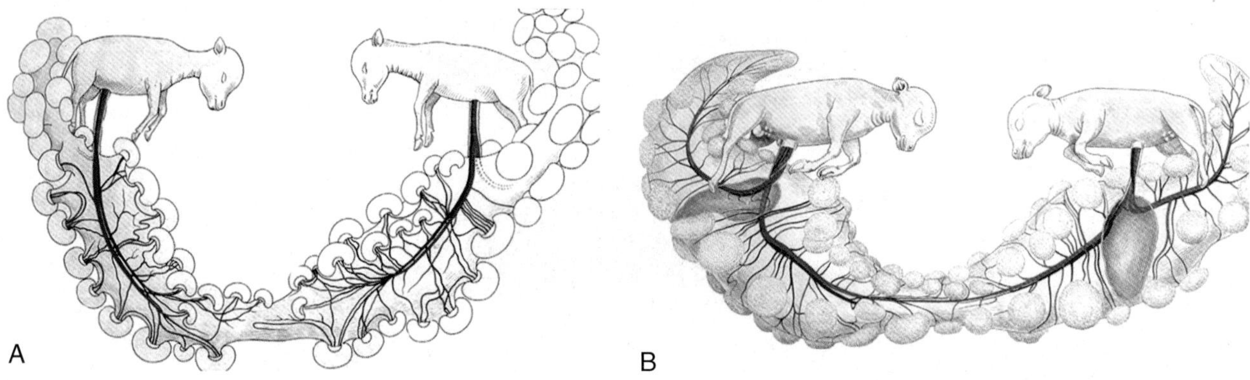

Fig. 29.18 (A) Twin bovine pregnancy showing separate circulations. (B) Twin bovine pregnancy showing conjoined circulations (freemartin development possible).

branches pass to the caudal genital tract and to the bladder and urethra.

A very large and conspicuous venous plexus lies in the parametrial tissues of the broad ligament and over the ventral surface of the uterus and vagina, partly covered by the outer layers of muscle. It constitutes a blood pool that can drain in several directions (Fig. 29.19). The ovarian vein, the largest emissary vessel, runs in the cranial part of the broad ligament; the vaginal veins, including a surprisingly small vein that corresponds to the large uterine artery, play a secondary role. Both sympathetic and parasympathetic nerves supply the genital tract.

Growth and Cyclical Changes

The growth of the reproductive organs, isometric in the very young, accelerates in response to the production of ovarian hormones after the initiation of the estrus cycle, generally when a heifer is about 8 to 10 months old. The cumulative effects of a few cycles produce a striking increase in the dimensions and a clearer differentiation of the component tissues of the tract.

The bovine estrus cycle is repeated at intervals of 21 days. The small ruminants are seasonally polyestrous, largely in the fall and early winter; the cycle lasts 16 or 17 days in sheep and 20 in goats.

In each cycle a follicle becomes identifiable on rectal examination about the 16th day and attains its full size a couple of days later. Its rupture is preceded by a reduction in internal pressure, recognizable on rectal palpation; the clot that succeeds the moderate ensuing hemorrhage is soon replaced by a corpus luteum. This reaches its maximal size, approximately that of the follicle it replaces, after about a week; regression then begins, and by the 21st day, the time of the next estrus, it has already shrunk by about two-thirds. It is eventually replaced by a scar. The waxing and waning of the corpus luteum are marked by color changes progressing from brown to ochre and then through orange, brick red, and dirty white in regression.

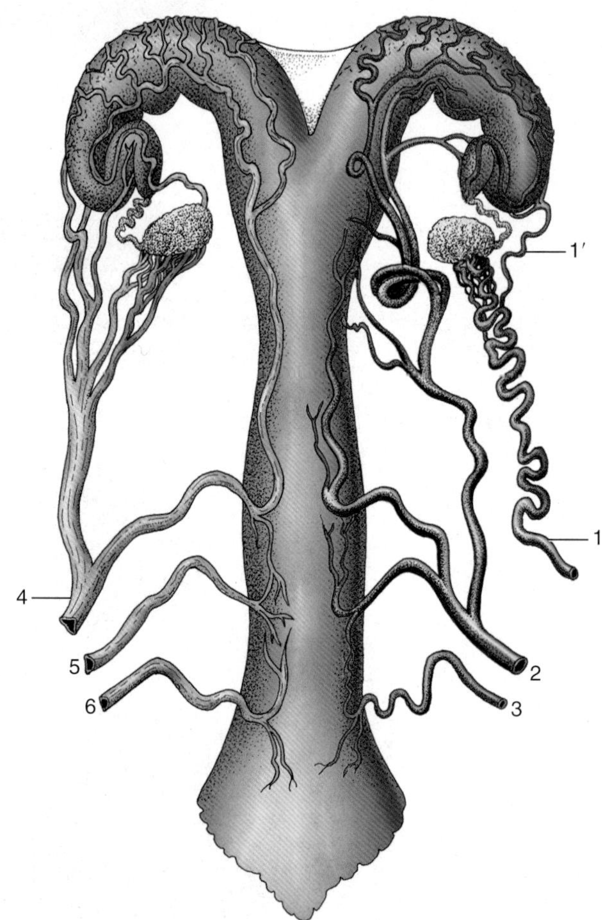

Fig. 29.19 Ventral view of the blood supply to the bovine reproductive tract (semischematic). The arteries are depicted on the right side, the veins on the left. *1,* Ovarian artery; *1′,* uterine branch; *2,* uterine artery; *3,* vaginal artery; *4,* ovarian vein; *5,* accessory vaginal vein; *6,* vaginal vein.

The ampulla becomes noticeably wider after ovulation, when the sphincter action of the isthmus delays the entry of the egg into the uterus. The uterine changes that commence in proestrus and continue into metestrus involve hyperemia and edema thickening the endometrium. The moderate

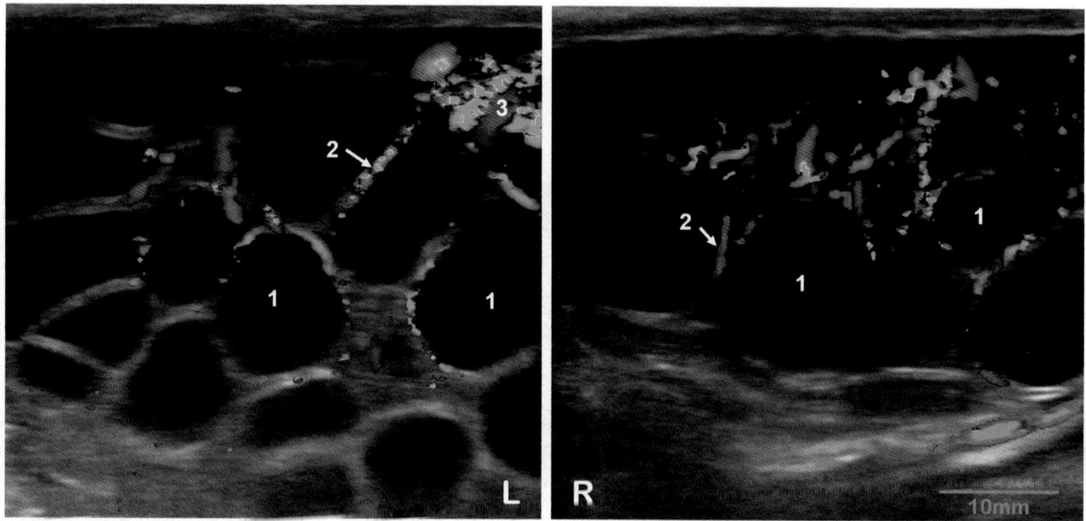

Fig. 29.20 Transrectal color Doppler ultrasonography of left (L) and right (R) ovaries of a 4-month old calf that was stimulated with gonadotropin to induce superovulation. The large black circular areas (1) represent the antral of preovulatory follicles, and colored areas (2) represent the blood flow in the wall of the follicle and ovarian stroma. Scale bar = 10 mm.

hemorrhage that sometimes accompanies their subsidence appears to be the origin of the increasing pigmentation of the uterine wall of older animals.

An increase in the size, complexity, and activity of the endometrial glands culminates a week or so after ovulation. The activity of the myometrium, whether spontaneous or in response to external stimuli, is greatest immediately before and during estrus.

The greater activity of the cervical mucosa during estrus spreads to the mucosa that lines the cranial part of the vagina. The transparent mucus of low viscosity that is produced is eventually discharged and may be tinged with blood when bleeding at metestrus is pronounced. There is no distinct cycle of cornification of the vaginal epithelium.

Gestation and Parturition

Gestation lasts 280 days in cattle, 147 days in sheep, and 154 days in goats. During this time every part of the reproductive system shows some changes, but obviously the most striking are in the uterus, which increases its weight 15-fold (100-fold when its content is included).

The ovary is distinguished by the presence of the corpus luteum of pregnancy, which persists beyond the life span of the infertile cycle. Its survival is not always accompanied by total suppression of follicular activity; a few cows come into heat and ovulate in early pregnancy. The corpus luteum is not necessary for the support of pregnancy during the past 3 months and usually begins to regress about a month before term (Figs. 29.20 and 29.21).

The progestational changes that are part of every cycle persist and intensify in the presence of an embryo.

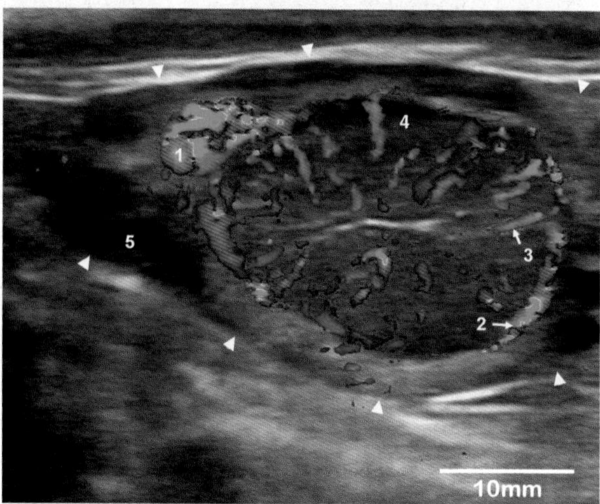

Fig. 29.21 Transrectal color Doppler ultrasonography of the ovary (outlined by *arrowheads*) showing corpus luteum in a cow on Day 65 of gestation. Notice the marked corpus luteum blood vessels *(color areas)* originate from main vessels at end one spot *(1)*, spread along the periphery of the corpus luteum *(2)* giving rise to radial vessels *(3)* that supply the glandular tissue *(4)*. Black areas *(5)* represent small antral follicles in the cortical area. Scale bar = 10 mm.

Although the blastocyst is initially confined to one horn, the membranes soon spread to the other; however, the embryo, and later the fetus, is almost invariably restricted unilaterally, and a developing asymmetry is one of the first detectable signs of pregnancy. The amniotic sac becomes palpable about the 30th day, the fetus itself about the 70th. The caruncles of the gravid horn gradually increase from low, smooth-surfaced bumps to become large, pedunculated swellings with surfaces pitted for the reception of the chorionic villi; by term the largest may attain the size of a clenched fist (Figs. 29.22 and 29.23 and see Fig. 29.17). Those in the nongravid horn later also enlarge but to a lesser degree.

The enlargement of the uterus does not affect all parts equally. The lesser curvature, being tethered by the broad ligament, most resists expansion, which causes the horn to alter shape: the greater curvature and adjacent parts grow

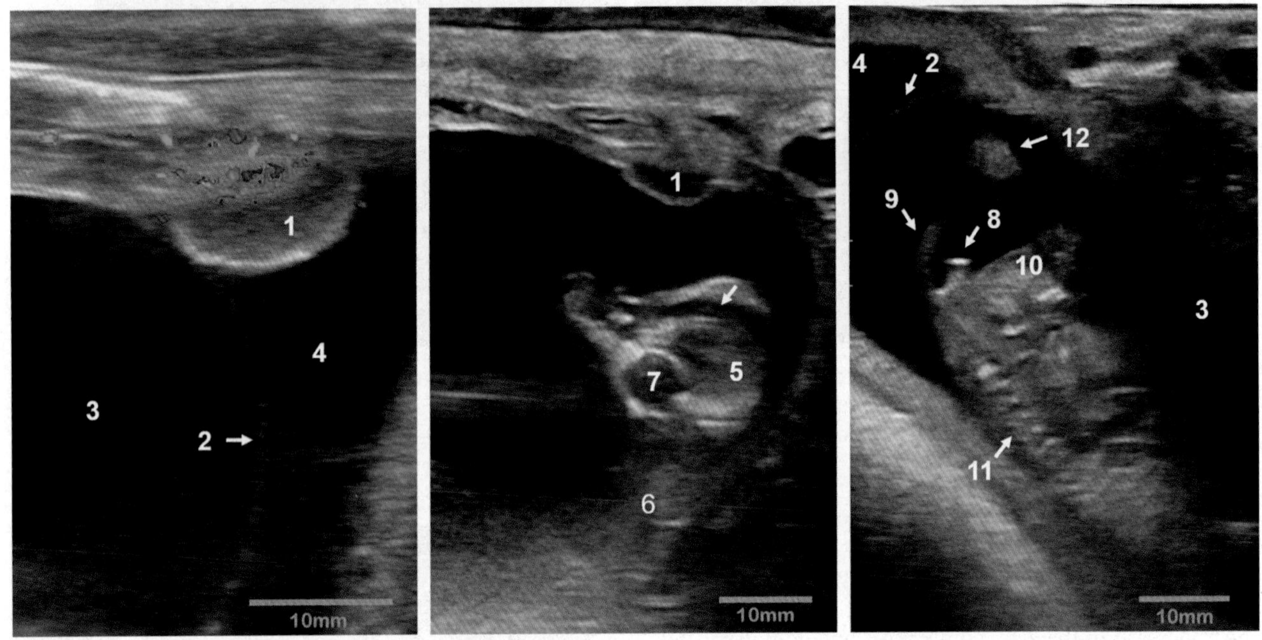

Fig. 29.22 Transrectal ultrasonographic sections of the the placentome *(left)*, fetal head *(middle)*, and caudal part of female fetus *(right)* at 65 days of gestation. Notice the rich blood flow *(color areas)* to the placentome *(1)* in the figure on the left. Amniotic membrane *(2)* separates the fluid-filled amniotic *(3)* and allantoic *(4)* cavities. If fetus is not easily accessible, fetal membranes and placentomes can be used to differentiate pregnancy from other fluid collections in the uterus. Notice the size of the placentome in comparison to the fetal head *(5)* and neck *(6)*. Fetal cranium is cartilaginous, showing clear demarcation *(arrow)* between the two halves. Eye sockets *(7)* are prominent. In the female fetus, genital tubercle *(8)* is located under the tail *(9)* and is used clinically to performed gender determination at 2 months of pregnancy (in male fetus, genital tubercle is present close to the attachment of umbilical cord). Notice part of the the hindlimb *(10)* and vertebral column *(11)* of the fetus and cross section of the umbilical cord *(12)*.

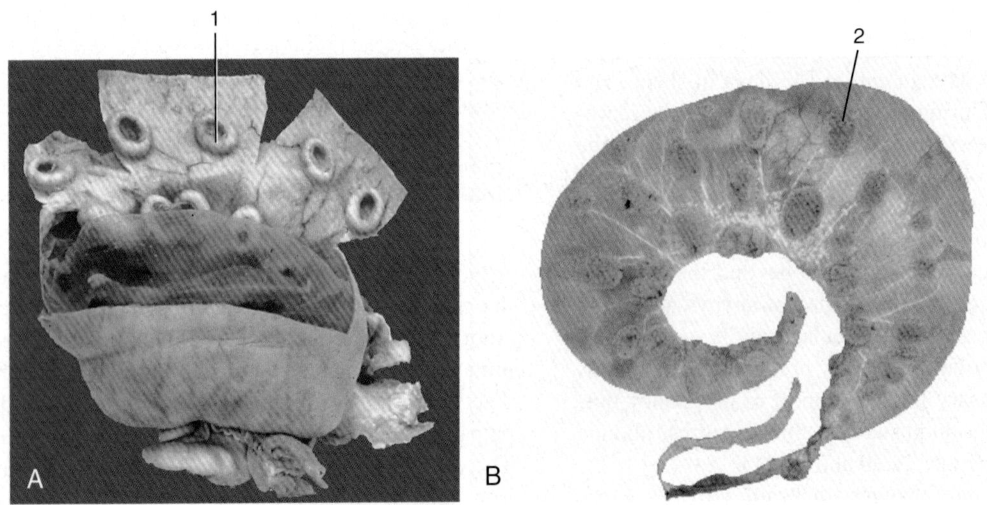

Fig. 29.23 (A) A gravid uterus, partly opened. (B) A bovine fetus within its membranes. The villi are mainly restricted to the cotyledons. *1*, Caruncle; *2*, cotyledon.

away from the attachment. Hypertrophy of the tissues of the broad ligament restrains the uterus from sinking into the abdomen for a time, but by the third month this resistance is overcome and the uterus begins to slip forward over the abdominal floor. The supply of blood to the gravid uterus by all vessels but especially the uterine artery, which expands from a few millimeters to a centimeter or more, is necessarily greatly increased. The uterine artery loses its flexuous character and now passes forward into the abdomen, where it is easily identified based on characteristic vibrations (fremitus) on palpation against the ilium.

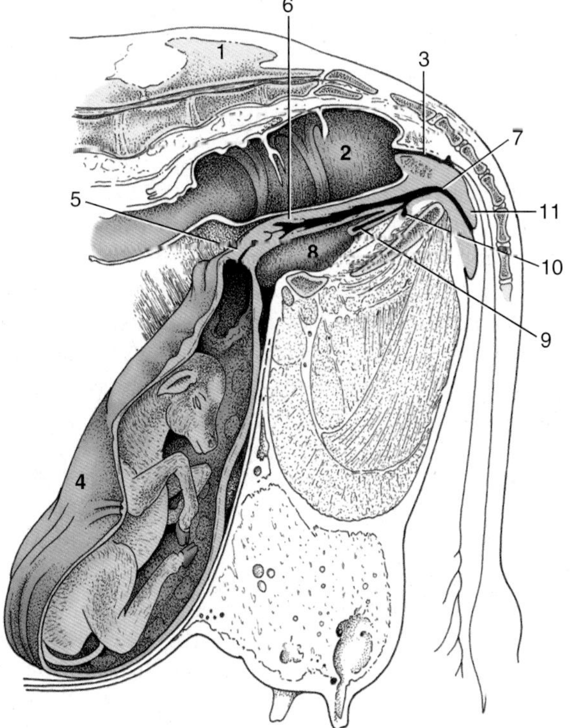

Fig. 29.24 Paramedian section of the caudal abdomen and pelvis of a pregnant cow. The section is not quite vertical because it cuts through the vertebral canal and an obturator foramen. Note the large placentomes. *1,* Sacrum; *2,* rectum; *3,* anal canal; *4,* uterus; *5,* cervix; *6,* vagina; *7,* vestibule; *8,* bladder; *9,* urethra; *10,* suburethral diverticulum; *11,* vulva.

The topography is not the same in every pregnancy. The enlarging uterus usually enters the supraomental recess but sometimes may slip forward against the right or the left flank. As it expands, it sinks within the abdomen and for a time passes out of reach of a hand within the colon; this inability to reach the uterus at about the fifth month is as diagnostic of pregnancy as its palpable enlargement at earlier and later times. The descent into the abdomen stretches the vagina and carries the cervix over the pubic brim. Toward term, the uterus occupies most of the ventral and right sections (in the common arrangement) of the abdomen, which raises the rumen dorsally and crushes the intestines upward (Fig. 29.24). It makes contact with the liver and diaphragm, on which it exerts increasing pressure. During the first months the calf enjoys freedom to move and adjust position within the amniotic fluid, but as pregnancy continues, it is forced to adapt to the form and dimensions of the uterine horn.

The cervical canal is closed by a mucous plug, developing from the first month and later projecting through the external cervical ostium. The first changes in the vagina are due to traction, but the wall later becomes increasingly elastic and the lumen potentially roomier. Enlargement of the vulva is evident by the end of the first trimester in animals carrying their first calf, but in multipara, in which the vulva tends to be permanently enlarged, there may be no obvious change until shortly before birth.

Changes that signal the approach of parturition include softening of the sacrosciatic ligament, with insinking beside the tail head (Fig. 29.25A and B); a similar loosening of other pelvic ligaments allows some relaxation of the sacroiliac joints. The connective tissues of the cervix and caudal reproductive tract and vulvar and perineal skin share in these changes that, though spread over several weeks, are much intensified in the last few days. When

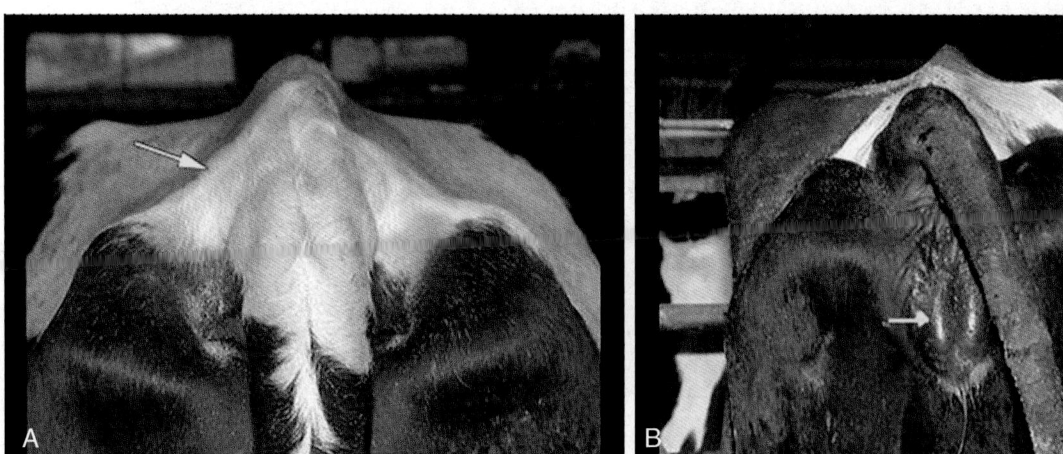

Fig. 29.25 Indications of impending parturition. (A) Relaxation of the sacrosciatic ligament *(arrow).* (B) Swelling of the vulva *(arrow).*

parturition actually impends, edema of the soft parts may cause the vulva to gape.

The bony pelvis of cows is not particularly favorable to easy parturition. Its dimensions are relatively small, and the axis of the birth canal is broken where it passes over the pubic brim and again where the floor changes direction to rise toward the exit. Some increase in the vertical diameter is possible if the pelvis can rotate about the relaxed sacroiliac joints, but this relief is clearly denied to the standing cow. The principal soft tissue impediments to easy birth are the cervix, the caudal end of the vagina, and the vulva. Normally these parts also loosen under hormonal influence.

The umbilical cord ruptures when the cow gives birth and, being relatively short, often before delivery is complete. Its constituents part at different levels.

The fetal membranes (the "cleansings" in lay speech) normally separate from the endometrium and are expelled shortly after delivery; it is a process hastened by suckling, which stimulates the release of oxytocin.

Retention of fetal membranes (placenta) in utero may require human intervention to accomplish their removal. The retention of fetal membranes may lead to inflammation of the uterus (metritis) or mammary glands (mastitis) and consequent economic losses. The major reason for the retention of the fetal membranes is the lack of breakdown of the complex that attaches the fetal cotyledons to the maternal caruncles.

After parturition, the tract tends to return to its former state, but first pregnancies leave a permanent legacy in the form of thickening and loss of symmetry (Fig. 29.26). The uterus contracts as soon as it empties, undergoing a very rapid atrophy in which a third of its weight is lost within a couple of days; the second third is lost before the week is out. The decline is slower thereafter, but should a cow remain "empty," a period of superinvolution (lactation atrophy) may follow in which the size of the uterus drops below the resting norm. Involution of the vagina, vestibule, and vulva is slower.

Some Aspects of Development

Only a few points need be raised to supplement the general account given in Chapter 5.

Most unusually, ovulation in cattle does not occur until some hours after the end of estrus. Cleavage commences in the uterine tube, where fertilized ova are detained for several days before being released by the isthmus into the horn of the uterus. The small, spherical blastocyst that is first formed undergoes very rapid elongation from about the 13th day, first extending as a threadlike structure through the entire length of that horn and then, by about the 18th day, passing through the body to invade the contralateral horn. In this way, a single embryo takes maximal advantage of the endometrium available for its support. When twins are present, each claims one horn, and because both usually derive from the same ovary, transuterine migration seems to be readily accomplished. Contact between the two chorionic sacs is inevitable and results in fusion and

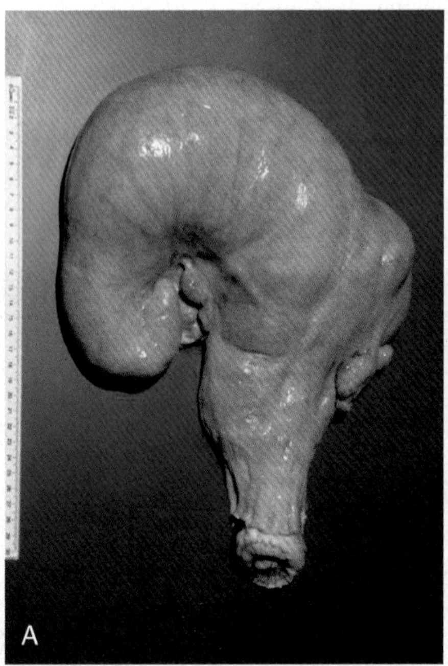

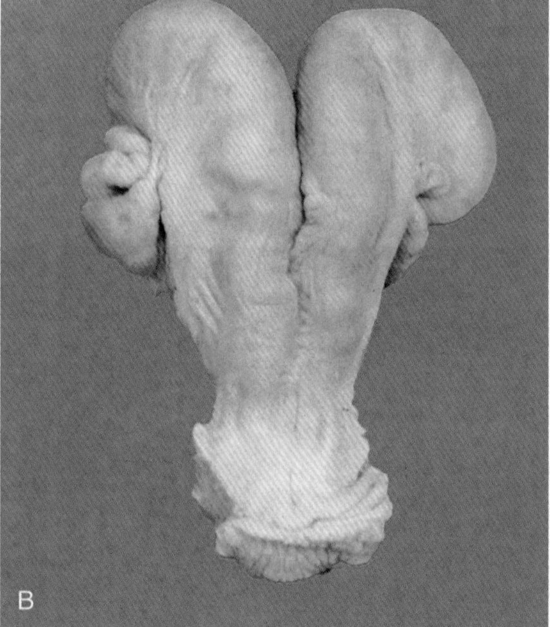

Fig. 29.26 Changes in the uterus. (A) Pregnancy involves mainly one horn, resulting in enormous asymmetry of the uterus. (B) After pregnancy, the uterus returns to its former state; some asymmetry usually remains.

anastomoses of the twin sets of vessels (with potentially unfortunate results; see Fig. 29.18).

The account of the development of the embryonic membranes and establishment of the cotyledonary placenta (Fig. 29.17) already given requires no amplification. The placenta is a barrier to the intrauterine exchange of immune bodies in utero in ruminant species, and the newborn relies on colostrum for its early immunologic protection.

Although the incidence of twin pregnancy in cattle is not high (1%–4% according to breed), twinning has attracted much attention because of the virtual certainty that the female partner of a male calf will exhibit intersex characteristics. The masculinization of the female, the so-called freemartin, is due to exchange between the two circulations. It was long thought that exposure to androgens was the causal factor, but this is now believed to be of little importance. In the prevailing view, what is significant is the transfer of antimüllerian hormone (causing regression of the müllerian ducts) and descending (causing gubernacular outgrowth) and the exchange of cells between the two embryos, which are in fact chimeras (Fig. 29.18). Support for the last point is obtained from the fact that most cattle twins, presumably those that shared a common placental circulation, accept grafts of their partner's skin in adult life, which indicates that cellular exchange had taken place when they were immunologically tolerant.

Twins and triplets are of course common in sheep and goats. The incidence varies with the breed and reflects the clemency or severity of the environment in which that breed evolved.

It is often convenient to be able to estimate the age of an aborted fetus in the field. There are many tables relating various measurements to age, but all suffer from the disadvantage of recording average values for parameters that vary considerably with breed, nutritional status, and other factors. One guide, easily memorized, allows 1-cm crown–rump length for each of the first 12 weeks' gestation and 2.5 cm for each week thereafter. Except with the youngest embryos, it is rarely more than 2 weeks off, and greater accuracy is hardly to be expected of any rule-of-thumb method. Qualitative methods that consider the external and internal anatomy are more accurate.

A few of the most obvious features are given in Tables 29.1 and 29.2.

TABLE 29.1 GUIDE TO THE AGING OF CATTLE FETUSES

Age (mo)	Crown–Rump Length (cm)	External Features
1	1	Head and limb buds are distinguishable
2	6	Digits are distinguishable
3	10	Scrotal (male) or mammary (female) swelling is distinct
4	20	First hairs appear about the eyes; horn buds are present
5	30–40	Hairs appear about the mouth; testes are within the scrotum
6	40–60	Hair is present on the tail extremity
7	50–70	Hair is present on the proximal parts of the limbs
8	60–80	The haircoat is general but still short and sparse over the belly
9	70–90	The appearance is mature, and the body is well haired; the incisors have erupted
Full term (270–290 days)		

From Evans HE, Sack WO: Prenatal development of domestic and laboratory animals. Growth curves, external features and selected reference. *Anat Histol Embryol* 2:11–45, 1973.

TABLE 29.2 GUIDE TO THE AGING OF SHEEP FETUSES

Age (mo)	Crown–Rump Length (cm)	External Features
1	2	Pinna triangular; eyelids forming; tactile hair follicles beginning to appear around eyes; principal forelimb digits prominent
1.5	6	Eyelids fused; external genitalia differentiated; teats present
2	11	Hair begins to cover the body
3	24	Tactile hairs appear on face; testes in upper part of scrotum
4	38	Woolly hair begins to grow; eyes open again
Full term (147–155 days)		

From Evans HE, Sack WO: Prenatal development of domestic and laboratory animals. Growth curves, external features and selected reference. *Anat Histol Embryol* 2:11–45, 1973.

Maturity in the sense of the capacity to make the integrated physiologic responses necessary for survival outside the uterus is not achieved until late in gestation. In lambs the mortality is 100% in those delivered at 135 days and is still very high in those delivered at 140 days. Unfortunately, reliable information on these matters for cattle is not readily available.

THE MALE REPRODUCTIVE ORGANS

The Scrotum and Testes

The pendulous *scrotum* is contained between the cranial parts of the thighs and may reach the level of the hocks. A constricted neck joins it to the trunk, just caudal to the superficial inguinal ring, while its lower part is molded on the testes (Fig. 29.27). A mass of fat ("cod fat") is commonly found about the cord stump of the castrate; when present in excess, it may dilate the inguinal canal and produce a pseudohernia inguinalis. Although the rudimentary teats often found on the cranial face of the scrotum possess little intrinsic interest, their number and spacing receive attention in dairy bulls because the corresponding characters are likely to be transmitted to their female offspring. The scrotal nerve supply is diffuse; it comes from the first two lumbar, the genitofemoral, and the pudendal nerves.

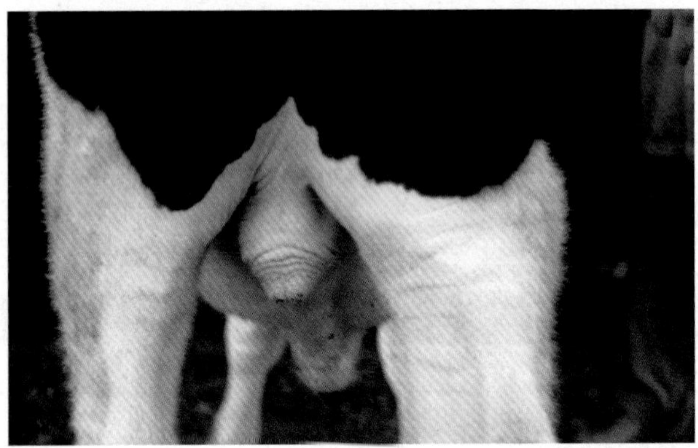

Fig. 29.27 Scrotum of bull. Musculature in tunica dartos has been contracted.

Wool covering the scrotum of the ram may cause infertility by impairing the dissipation of heat.

Each *testis* is ellipsoidal, is large in relation to body size (especially in the smaller ruminants), and hangs vertically in the scrotum, where it may be palpated (Fig. 29.28). It carries a large epididymis along the medial or caudomedial border that is turned to face its fellow. The epididymis is firmly attached to this border of the testis; the head extends a considerable distance down the free border, while the large, conical, and very distinctly palpable tail projects ventrally. The capsule of the testis displays a distinctive winding pattern of vessels and contains the parenchyma under slight pressure. The capsule also sends delicate partitions into the testicular tissue to form a prominent mediastinum (see Figs. 5.37 and 5.38).

After emerging from the tail, the deferent duct ascends along the medial border of the epididymis but is separated from this by the mesorchium, which is a relationship that

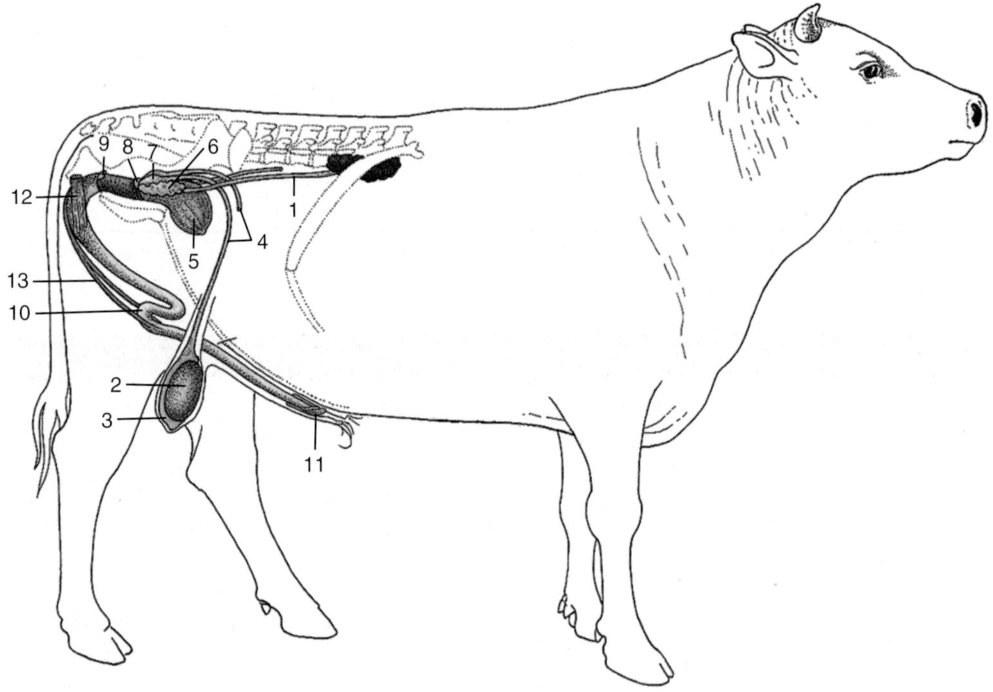

Fig. 29.28 Disposition of the urogenital organs of a bull. *1,* Ureter; *2,* right testis; *3,* epididymis; *4,* deferent duct; *5,* bladder; *6,* vesicular gland; *7,* ampulla of deferent duct; *8,* body of prostate; *9,* bulbourethral gland; *10,* sigmoid flexure of penis; *11,* glans penis; *12,* ischiocavernosus; *13,* retractor penis.

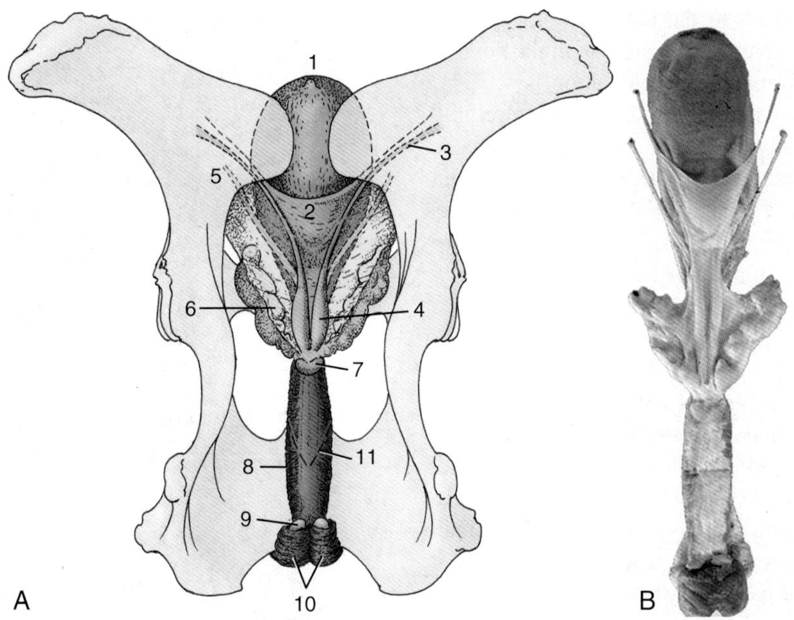

Fig. 29.29 Dorsal view of the bull's pelvis and related urogenital organs. (A) Schema. *1,* Bladder; *2,* genital fold; *3,* right deferent duct; *4,* ampulla of deferent duct; *5,* left ureter; *6,* vesicular gland; *7,* body of prostate; *8,* urethralis (surrounding urethra); *9,* bulbourethral gland; *10,* bulbospongiosus; *11,* caudal extent of the rectogenital pouch *(broken line).* (B) Specimen.

advises a cranial approach in vasectomy operations. The duct is easily recognized on palpation as a firm, narrow strand. The conical, dorsally tapering spermatic cord is largely composed of the exceptionally convoluted testicular artery embedded in the pampiniform plexus (see Fig. 5.43). The significance of the arteriovenous anastomoses found here remains obscure (see Fig. 5.46).

Castration is an important surgery in young bulls (1–3 months of age). The castration may be performed by crushing the spermatic cord as in the Burdizzo method (closed method of castration). In the open or surgical method of castration, both of the testes are removed usually without the application of any anesthetic; however, lidocaine may be applied locally for analgesia.

The lymphatic drainage of the testis is to the medial iliac nodes; that of the scrotum is to the superficial inguinal node by the scrotal neck.

The Pelvic Reproductive Organs

The constituents of the spermatic cord disperse at the vaginal ring, from whence the deferent duct may be traced over the dorsal surface of the bladder. It passes under the body of the prostate to reach the urethra, and in the last part of its course it is combined with the duct of the vesicular gland in a very short common passage. The subterminal stretch (≈10–12 cm) lies beside its fellow in the genital fold; the

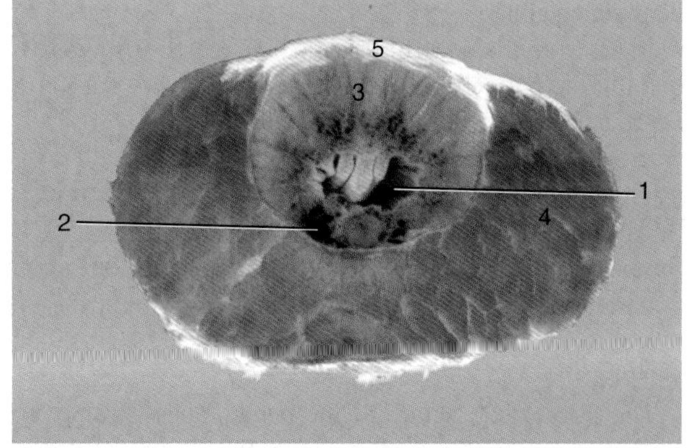

Fig. 29.30 Transverse section of the bovine pelvic urethra immediately caudal to the body of the prostate. *1,* Urethra; *2,* spongy tissue (stratum spongiosum); *3,* disseminate part of prostate; *4,* urethralis; *5,* dorsal aponeurosis of urethralis.

wall of this part is swollen to form the cylindrical ampulla or ampullary gland. A median vestige of the fused paramesonephric ducts is sometimes present between the two ampullae (Fig. 29.29).

The *urethra* runs over the pelvic floor from the bladder (Fig. 29.30) and leaves the pelvic cavity by bending around the ischial arch. Level with the arch, the lumen presents a dorsal diverticulum guarded at its entrance by a mucosal flap. The flap splits at its caudal extremity into two folds that constrict the urethral lumen by attaching to the walls. The tip of a catheter almost inevitably engages in this diverticulum, which makes catheterization of the bladder impossible if surgical access to the urethra is not gained first. (Even without the diverticulum, the sigmoid flexure of the penis presents a formidable complication.)

The pelvic urethra is encircled by the striated urethral muscle, completed dorsally by a stout aponeurotic plate. A thin sleeve of spongy tissue directly surrounds the lumen; when followed caudally, it expands to form the bulb of the penis. The penile urethra is narrower, especially at the sigmoid flexure, where calculi most often lodge, particularly in castrated animals.

The *vesicular glands* are very large (10 × 3 to 15 × 5 cm) and contribute the bulk of the seminal fluid. They are flexed on themselves, grossly lobulated with narrow branching lumina, and lie within the genital folds, mainly lateral to the ampullary glands (Fig. 29.29A and B). The *prostate* of the bull consists of a disseminate part stretching along the length of the urethra, largely dorsal to the lumen and diminishing in thickness when followed caudally, and a compact part (body) consisting of paired lobes that have broken through the urethral aponeurosis and together form a bar lying across the first part of the urethra (4 × 1 cm).

The small *bulbourethral glands*, located by the ischial arch, are flattened and covered by the bulbospongiosus muscle (Fig. 29.29B). Their watery secretion is discharged into the diverticulum and flushes the urethra in advance of the main ejaculate.

Apart from the body of the prostate, which is specific to the bull, the pelvic reproductive glands are very similar in the three domestic ruminants.

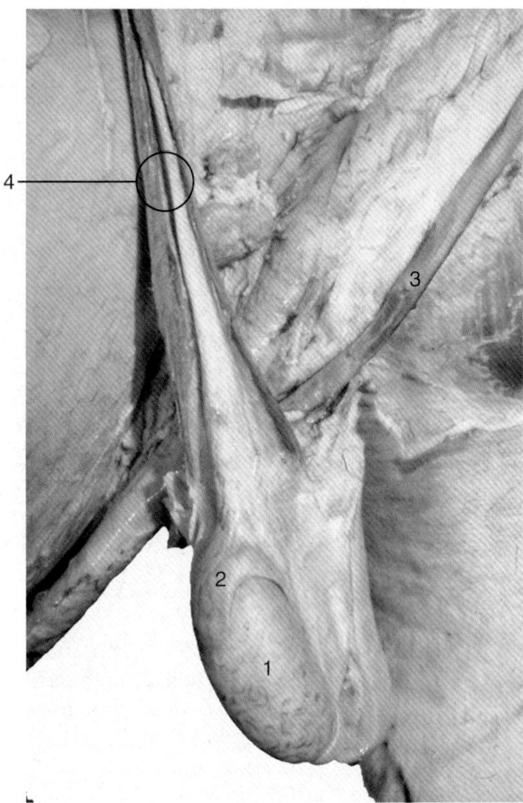

Fig. 29.31 Scrotum opened, and testis and epididymis exposed. Note tortuous veins on surface of the testis. *1,* Testis; *2,* epididymis; *3,* retractor penis muscle; *4,* spermatic cord.

The Penis and Prepuce

The penis of an adult bull is almost 1 m long, but about a quarter of its length is taken up by the sigmoid flexure located above and behind the scrotum (Figs. 29.31, 29.32, and 29.33).

The fibroelastic nature of the penis keeps it relatively rigid at all times. The rodlike, laterally compressed crura are almost surrounded by the powerful ischiocavernosus muscles and contain more generous cavernous spaces than are present in other parts of the organ. The construction of the body of the penis is not immediately evident because its constituents, the crura and the urethra, are enclosed within a common tunica albuginea (Fig. 29.34). Paired ligaments suspend the caudal part of the body from the symphyseal tendon; their occasional rupture causes the penis to sag. The extremity of the quiescent penis is capped by a cushion of softer tissue, forming an asymmetrical, ventrally bent, and slightly spiraled glans that is contained within the caudal part of the prepuce. The glans exhibits a raphe or seam over its right aspect; the urethra follows this to open on the summit of a low process (Fig. 29.35).

The prepuce shows the usual disposition and encloses a cavity that is both long and narrow. The prepuce droops behind the umbilicus, most obviously in beef bulls, which makes it vulnerable to injury by sharp grasses.

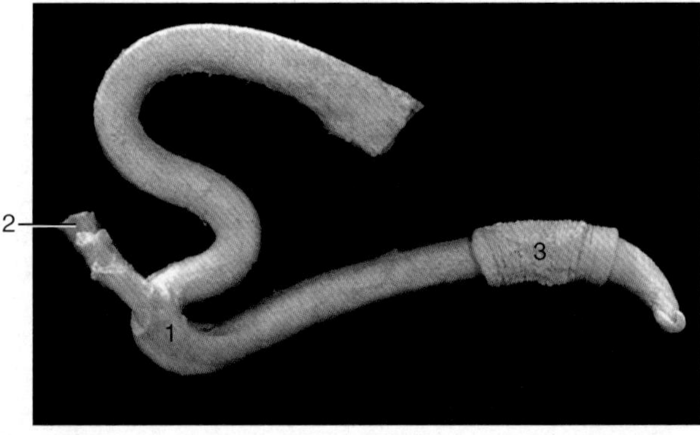

Fig. 29.32 The fibroelastic bovine penis and its retractor muscle. *1,* Sigmoid flexure; *2,* retractor penis muscle; *3,* preputial skin.

The penis obtains its *blood supply* from branches of the *internal pudendal artery* that are detached within the pelvis. One, the *artery of the bulb,* supplies the bulb and corpus spongiosum; a second, the *deep artery of the penis,* supplies the crus; and a third, the *dorsal artery,* travels along the upper border to reach the glans, detaching twigs to the prepuce en route. All three are

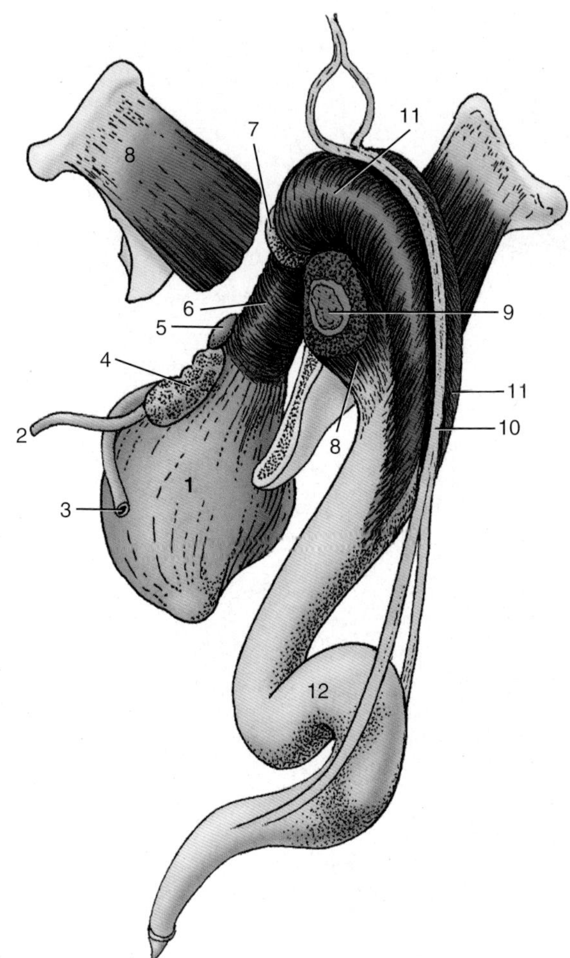

Fig. 29.33 The bovine penis and its muscles: caudolateral view. *1,* Bladder; *2,* ureter; *3,* deferent duct; *4,* vesicular gland; *5,* body of prostate; *6,* urethralis; *7,* bulbourethral gland; *8,* ischiocavernosus; *9,* crus of penis (in transverse section); *10,* retractor penis; *11,* bulbospongiosus; *12,* sigmoid flexure.

accompanied by satellite veins that drain both the tissues and the blood spaces within the spongy and cavernous bodies. The crura and corpus cavernosum constitute a single unit into which blood is transferred during erection. Venous blood leaving this unit reaches the systemic circulation via pelvic channels. The bulb, the corpus spongiosum, and the glans form a second unit that also drains via pelvic channels but possesses an additional more cranial outlet. Consequently, drainage of the spongiosus system is not completely arrested by contraction of the bulbospongiosus.

The paired *dorsal nerves,* which run with the dorsal arteries, overlap in their distribution. Because stimulation of the apex of the penis is necessary for the attainment of full erection, the integrity of these nerves is essential for reproductive competence. The preputial skin, including that over the penis, is supplied from the first two lumbar, the genitofemoral, and the pudendal nerves.

Cranial preputial muscles that arise in the xiphoid region and insert beside and behind the preputial orifice are able to draw the prepuce craniodorsally, which constricts its orifice. Anomalies of these muscles may prevent protrusion or impair the return of the penis to the prepuce. Caudal preputial muscles of inconstant occurrence appear to have little significance.

The usual suite of muscles is associated with the penis (Fig. 29.33). The well-developed *retractor penis* possesses particular interest because it must relax to allow exposure of the penis for examination or treatment. It arises from the caudal vertebrae, passes to the side of the rectum, and reaches the penis at the second bend of the flexure; some fibers attach here, but others continue to more distal and diffuse insertions. The local contractions of the retractor that help maintain the flexure are controlled by a sympathetic innervation that is conveyed within the pudendal and caudal rectal nerves; these must be blocked to allow withdrawal of the penis for examination. The administration of an antiadrenergic tranquilizer has the same effect. A low lumbar epidural block is additionally required when anesthesia is indicated.

The lymphatics from the prepuce pass to the superficial inguinal node.

The penis of the small ruminants is chiefly distinguished by the length of the slender, erectile urethral process, which projects 2 to 3 cm beyond the glans in bucks and 3 to 4 cm in rams (Fig. 29.35C and D). In former times, as in primitive societies today, amputation of the process was performed with the intention of depriving rams of their fertilizing capacity. The sheath is also relatively short in these species.

Growth and Functional Changes

The bovine testes have arrived in the scrotum by mid gestation, a surprisingly early period. They are very small at birth but grow more rapidly than the body as a whole from the first week and at an accelerated rate when the young bull approaches puberty. Growth for a time then keeps pace with general development; in older bulls some shrinkage is demonstrable. Libido may develop before spermatogenesis is achieved, which is generally about the 10th month. Epididymal growth lags a little behind that of the testes.

Progress in the development of the secondary reproductive glands is testosterone dependent and follows after testicular maturation. These glands are all initially small, but to varying degrees, and take some time to acquire their adult sizes and conformations.

Less than half its final length, the neonatal penis is very slender, without a sigmoid flexure, contains little erectile tissue, and is fused with the prepuce at its apex. The preputial cavity, which does not extend proximally beside the penis, is occupied by low folds. The characteristic bends

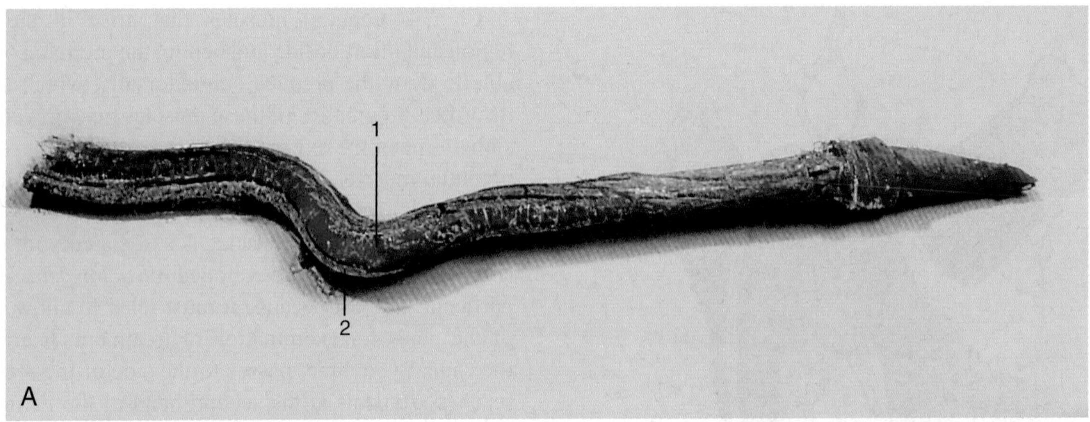

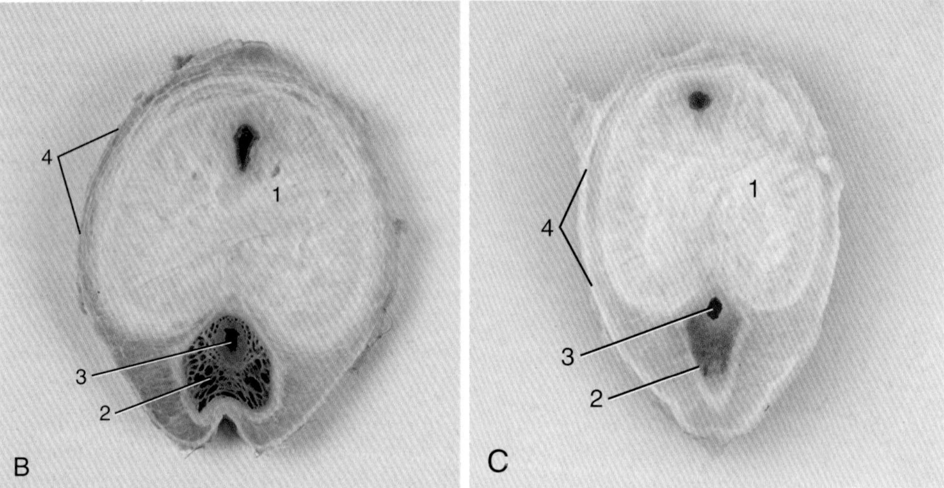

Fig. 29.34 Cast of the cavernous spaces of (A) the bovine penis and transverse sections (B) caudal and (C) cranial to the sigmoid flexure. *1,* Corpus cavernosum; *2,* corpus spongiosum; *3,* urethra; *4,* tunica albuginea.

begin to develop about the third month. Growth is slow, and, though it quickens from puberty, the final size is not attained until well into the second year. Separation from the sheath is first confined to the left side of the apex but later spreads around the whole circumference and extends proximally. A narrow frenulum persists for some time, and tags may remain until ruptured at first service. The occasional persistence of the frenulum may produce a ventral deflection of the apex.

Erection involves only a slight increase in length and diameter; protrusion results from effacement of the flexure. Relatively little extra blood is required to engorge the cavernous spaces; this is initially produced by relaxation of the supplying arteries, which increases the pressure within these spaces from the low resting level (5–16 mm Hg) to the arterial pressure (75–80 mm Hg). The apex protrudes at this stage. Contractions of the ischiocavernosi raise the pressure further and, by compressing the vessels against the ischial arch, occlude the venous drainage route. These contractions impel blood forward through certain thick-walled veins of the corpus cavernosum to discharge at the sigmoid flexure (Fig. 29.33). Effacement of this flexure now causes the apex to protrude considerably (25–40 cm); contact with the vaginal wall after intromission stimulates the completion of erection. For a short period, pressure within the corpus cavernosum rises to a remarkable level; it is asserted that it can be as much as 60 to 100 times the arterial pressure. Ejaculation follows, and the semen is rapidly impelled through the urethra by the coordinated activity of the urethralis and bulbourethralis muscles.

The free part of the penis spirals in the later stages of erection, following a left-hand thread around the raphe (Fig. 29.36). This is due to the apical ligament, a local concentration of collagen within the tunica albuginea. Because precocious or exaggerated spiraling makes intromission impossible, there are occasional indications for the surgical division of this ligament. Another problem, fortunately only of occasional occurrence, is rupture of a tunica albuginea unable to withstand the extreme pressure briefly developed in the late stage of erection; the weakest region appears to be the distal bend of the sigmoid flexure.

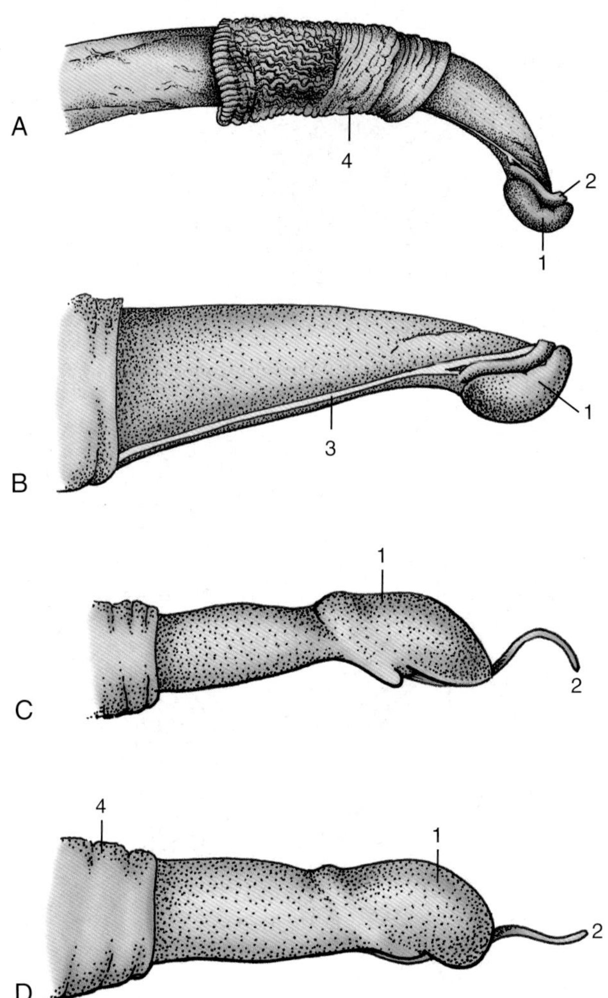

Fig. 29.35 Right lateral view of the distal end of the bull's penis, flaccid (A) and erect (B). The distal end of the ram's (C) and buck's (D) penis. *1,* Glans; *2,* urethral process; *3,* raphe; *4,* preputial skin.

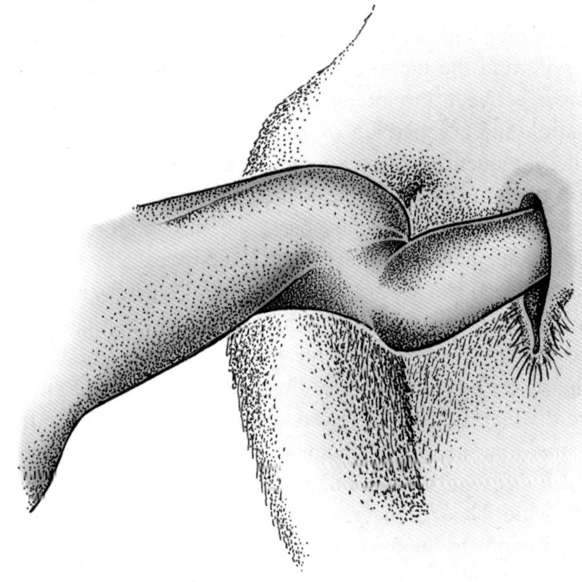

Fig. 29.36 Spiraling of the free part of the bovine penis in full erection.

THE ANATOMY OF RECTAL PALPATION IN CATTLE*

As in the horse, rectal exploration in cattle is not free from risk of injury to the mucosa or even, in extreme cases, perforation of the intestinal wall—a mishap most likely to occur when invasion of the rectum induces straining. Although rectal examinations of cows are most frequently performed to determine the health of the reproductive organs, it is also used to appreciate a much larger anatomic area once the hand is carried into the descending colon.

The parts of the pelvic and abdominal walls that are accessible include the bones bounding the pelvic cavity and the regions of the deep inguinal rings. Dorsally, the caudal segment of the aorta and its bifurcation are within reach, and, scattered about the vessels, the larger lymph nodes of the medial iliac and deep inguinal groups (Fig. 29.4/*13* and *14*) can be palpated. The deep inguinal nodes are particularly important in connection with mastitis. The caudal part of the rumen is very obvious directly before the pelvic inlet, and it can be confirmed that ventrally the rumen extends into the right half of the abdomen. The caudodorsal blind sac may even intrude into the pelvic cavity when distended with gas. However, much of the rumen and the remaining compartments of the stomach are inaccessible, as are the liver and the spleen. The one necessary qualification of this statement refers to the abomasum, part of which is brought into reach in certain displacements. The right dorsal quadrant of the abdomen is occupied by small intestine, cecum, and colon, which together form a soft, fluctuating mass in which individual parts are mostly not identifiable when normal; the most common exception is the rounded tip of the gas-filled cecum.

Most of the left kidney, pushed to the right by the rumen and suspended from the abdominal roof, may be palpated; only the caudal pole of the right kidney is within reach and then only in smaller subjects. Healthy ureters are not detectable unless the initial portion of the left one can be appreciated where it passes over the surface of the kidney. The impression made by the bladder varies greatly because it forms a firm mass over the most cranial part of the pelvic floor when contracted but extends well forward into the abdomen as a fluctuating structure when distended. The intervention of the female reproductive tract makes this organ far less accessible in cows than in male animals.

A systematic examination of the reproductive tract is best begun by locating the cervix, easily recognized by its firmness and dimensions, although its location varies

*Except for digital explorations, rectal palpation is not routinely performed in small ruminants.

greatly according to the present status and past history of the animal. The short body of the uterus lies forward of the cervix, and the uterus may be fixed by the insertion of a finger between the intercornual ligaments to allow examination and comparison of the horns that diverge to each side. Frequently, these manipulations stimulate contraction of the uterine muscle, which can sometimes be quite powerful. The uterus may pass into the abdomen. If not too much enlarged, it may be retrieved by passing the hand forward and downward into the ventral part of the abdomen on the right side and then withdrawing the hand with the fingers flexed toward the palm to enclose the uterus. The broad ligaments proceeding to the horns of the uterus are distinct, but the uterine tubes, which run near the free cranial margins of the ligaments, are less certainly discoverable because, although fairly firm, they are only about 2 mm wide. The free margins of the broad ligaments also provide a guide to the location of the ovaries, which lie on the floor of the pelvic cavity in the young virgin animal but are displaced cranially and ventrally into the abdomen in older, more sexually experienced cows. An indication has already been given of the features of the follicles and corpora lutea that may be appreciated by examination of the ovarian surface. The reader is also reminded that the forward and downward movement of the reproductive organs in pregnancy may carry them out of reach for a time (Fig. 29.37).

THE UDDER

The four mammary glands of the cow are consolidated in a single mass, the udder, placed below the caudal part of the abdomen and extending between the thighs. The udder is divided into quarters corresponding to the four glands, and each bears a principal teat. A median groove divides the udder into right and left halves, but the boundary between a forequarter and a hindquarter is rarely distinct. Most of the dorsal base is shaped to fit against the belly wall, but the part below the pelvis is narrower because it is compressed between the thighs (Fig. 29.38). The skin over the udder is thin, supple, and mobile, except over the teats, where it is tightly bound down and naked.

The udder is suspended by strong sheets of fascia that surround and enclose the gland substance and are continuous with the connective tissue framework that permeates the entire organ. The fascia forms a continuous investment over each half, but it is customary to describe medial and lateral laminae as though these were independent formations. The medial lamina arises mainly from the tunica flava and in small part from the symphyseal tendon and is largely composed of elastic tissue. The lateral lamina arises from the external crus of the inguinal ring and, behind this, from the medial femoral fascia and is composed of dense connective tissue (Figs. 29.39 and 29.40). Both laminae thin when followed ventrally, which is the result of their

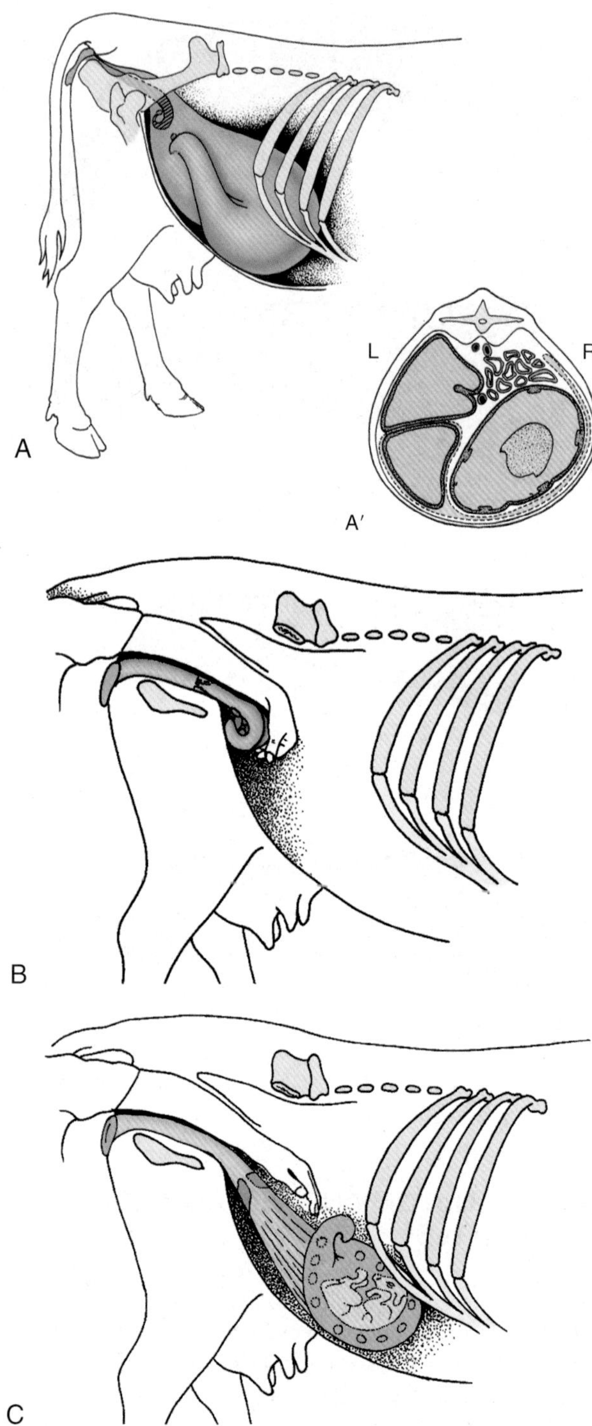

Fig. 29.37 The position of the nongravid uterus and various stages of the gravid uterus in lateral view. (A) Nongravid and 6-month gravid uterus. (A′) The topography of the 6-month gravid uterus in transverse section. L, Left side; R, right side. (B) At 2 to 3 months the gravid uterus has begun to slide down the caudal abdominal wall, but it can be scooped up by the hand in the colon. (C) At 5 months the gravid uterus is temporarily out of reach.

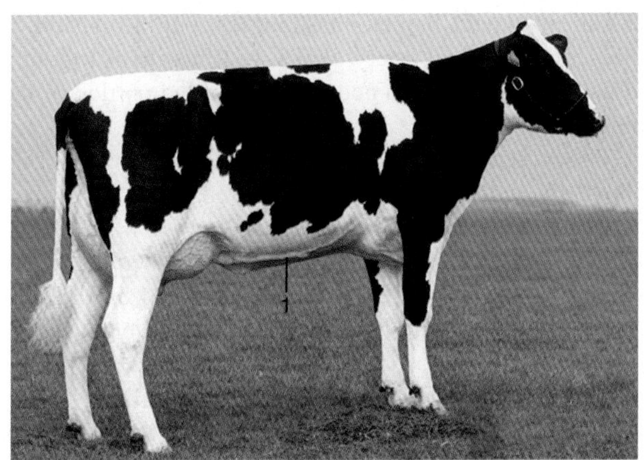

Fig. 29.38 Holstein cow with well-developed udder. *1,* Mammary vein.

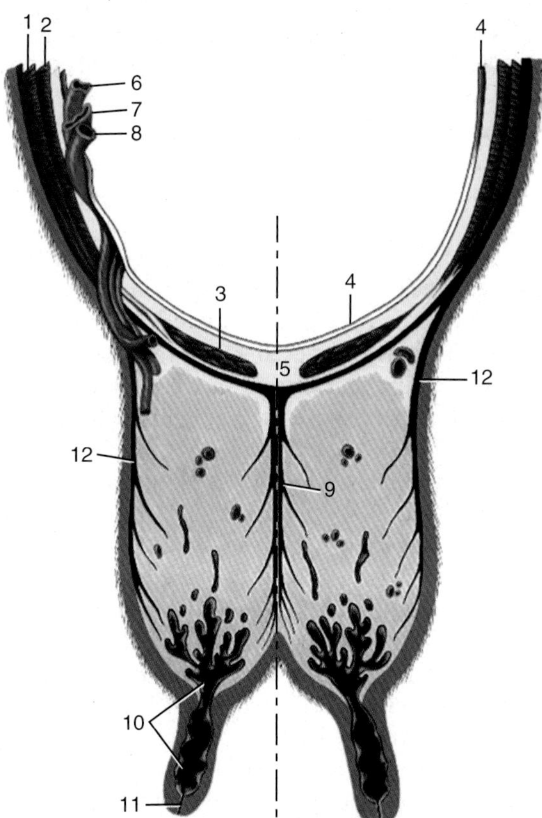

Fig. 29.39 Transverse section of the abdominal floor and cranial quarters of the bovine udder. *1,* External abdominal oblique; *2,* internal abdominal oblique; *3,* rectus abdominis; *4,* peritoneum; *5,* linea alba; *6,* lymph vessel; *7,* external pudendal vein; *8,* external pudendal (mammary) artery; *9,* medial laminae of suspensory apparatus; *10,* lactiferous sinus; *11,* papillary duct; *12,* lateral laminae of suspensory apparatus.

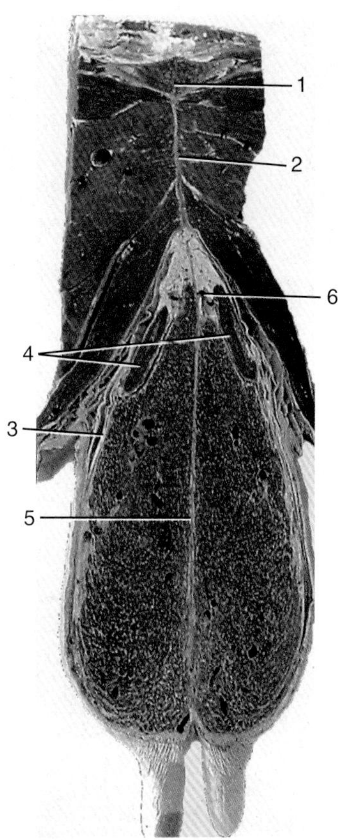

Fig. 29.40 Transverse section of the pelvic floor and caudal quarters of the bovine udder. *1,* Pelvic symphysis; *2,* symphyseal tendon; *3,* lateral suspensory laminae; *4,* mammary (superficial inguinal) lymph node; *5,* medial suspensory laminae; *6,* tributary of external pudendal vein.

detachment of numerous leaves that interdigitate with layers of glandular tissue. The different natures of the two laminae explain the sagging of the medial part of the heavily laden udder. Ever-increasing demands for milk production place a heavy and sometimes unsustainable burden on the suspensory apparatus, which occasionally ruptures—a disastrous outcome.

Each gland is constructed about a branching duct system, separated from its neighbors by connective tissue. The alveolar secretory units lead to small excretory ducts that combine with others until, after several successive unions, about a dozen wide lactiferous ducts are produced; these converge on a large sinus situated in the lower part of the quarter and extend into the teat (Fig. 29.41). The lactiferous ducts are unusual in demonstrating alternating wider and narrower sections. The more superficial dilations, which may be 3 cm or more in caliber, may be palpable when distended with milk and are then known as *milk knots.* Although the duct systems are independent, infection readily spreads between the quarters of the same side.

The lactiferous sinus has a capacity of several hundred milliliters and is divided by a mucosal fold into gland and teat parts. The fold, based on a submucosal ring of veins, varies in prominence; occasionally it may be sufficiently pronounced to impede milk flow.

The teats, though variable, are most often cylindrical and about 8 cm long. The teat wall, generally about 6 mm

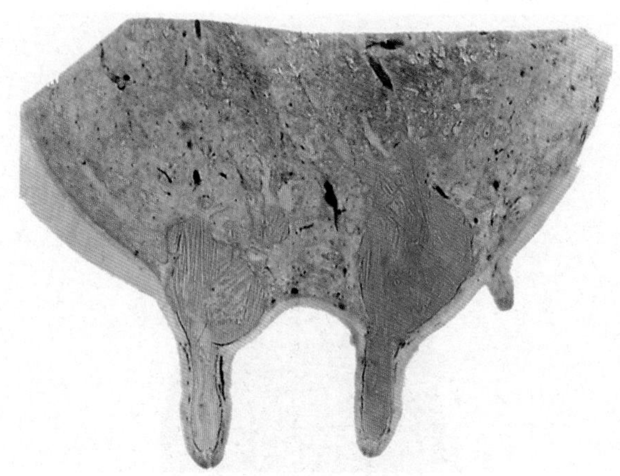

Fig. 29.41 Sagittal section of udder, showing teat and gland sinuses and lactiferous ducts filled with latex: cranial quarter *(green)*; caudal quarter *(blue)*.

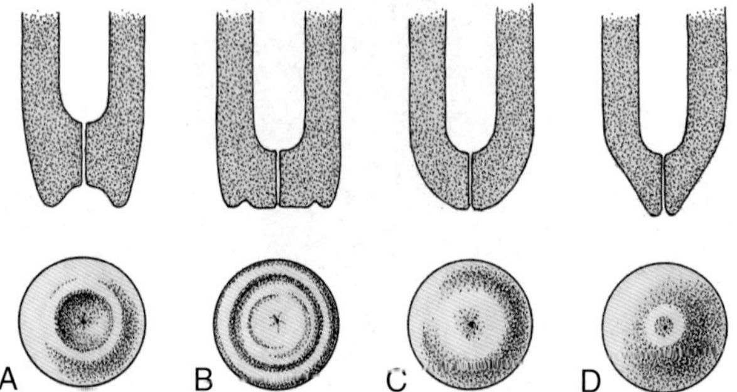

Fig. 29.42 Variations in the form of the bovine teat extremity. (A) Funnel shaped. (B) Dish shaped. (C) Rounded. (D) Pointed.

thick, increases to about 1 cm at the lower end, where it is traversed by the papillary duct (Fig. 29.42). The wall consists of a dry, outer skin, an intermediate layer that includes smooth muscle and many veins and constitutes a form of erectile tissue, and an inner mucosal layer marked by folds. The lining, generally yellowish, is white in the papillary duct, where it shows a pattern of low ridges; these, when followed proximally, are found to radiate from the upper opening, although it must be admitted that the arrangement is rarely as distinct as traditionally described (Fig. 29.43). Desquamation of the epithelium provides a bacteriostatic substance that helps occlude the passage. A more effective means of closure is provided by a sphincter muscle, reinforced by elastic tissue.

Accessory teats, sometimes associated with functional glandular tissue, are very common. They are undesirable because they may be a complication at milking.

The vascular arrangements are necessarily generous. The main supply, which continues the *external pudendal artery,* has a diameter that may exceed 15 mm where it passes through the inguinal canal accompanied by a satellite vein, lymphatics, and nerves (Fig. 29.39). On reaching the base of the udder, it divides into divergent branches, one passing cranially and the other caudally; both are partially or wholly embedded in the gland substance. The caudal mammary branch anastomoses with a division of the ventral perineal artery, which restricts its distribution to the mammary lymph nodes and a limited portion of the hindquarter.

The *pattern of the veins* is complicated. A venous ring above the udder is formed by paired veins connected across the midline by transverse vessels (Fig. 29.44). Drainage is effected by the external pudendal veins, which pass through the inguinal canals, and by the subcutaneous abdominal ("milk") veins, which pursue very flexuous subcutaneous courses over the abdomen before disappearing through palpable openings ("milk wells") in the body wall to discharge into the internal thoracic veins (Fig. 29.44).

Connections of the caudal part of the ring with ventral labial veins are of uncertain significance. The arrangement described is characteristic of the adult lactating cow and includes features that developed during the first pregnancy, a time when increased mammary blood flow led to venous congestion and dilation, followed by valvular incompetence and breakdown. This opened a continuous channel connecting the cranial and caudal superficial epigastric veins, which previously drained in opposite directions (Fig. 29.45).

The significance of the mature arrangement lies in its assurance of effective venous drainage should some channels be occluded in the recumbent cow. The milk vein is sometimes used for intravenous injection or blood sampling, but it is not a wise choice; its varicosed structure predisposes it to potentially troublesome leakage.

The teats and gland substance are permeated by a rich lymphatic plexus from which emerge larger vessels that run to the mammary lymph nodes situated above the caudal part of the udder. Many of these large lymphatic vessels reveal their positions through the skin and, running caudodorsally (Fig. 29.46), are readily distinguished from the subcutaneous veins that run craniodorsally. The *mammary lymph nodes*, generally two on each side—one large and one much smaller—lie deep to the lateral lamina of the suspensory apparatus, where the larger one may be reached on deep palpation from behind (Fig. 29.47). The efferent flow is to the deep inguinal node in the angle between the deep circumflex and external iliac arteries. This node may be palpated per rectum.

The *cutaneous innervation* of the udder is inconveniently diffuse; innervation is obtained from three sources: *ventral branches of the first two lumbar nerves, the genitofemoral nerve,* and *mammary branches of the pudendal nerve.* The gland substance and the deeper tissues of the teat wall are supplied by the genitofemoral nerve alone; this reaches the udder through the inguinal canal.

At full term, the mammary glands exhibit short but well-formed teats, small sinuses, and the first branches of the duct systems. The bulk of the udder consists of fat.

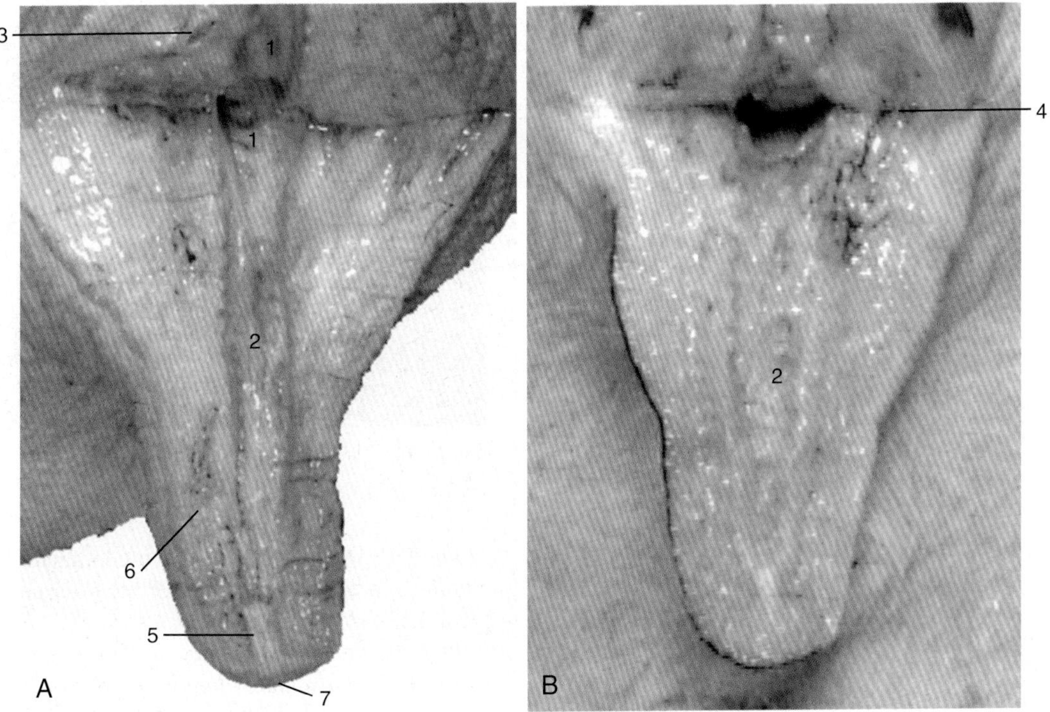

Fig. 29.43 (A) and (B) Sections of a cow's teat and lactiferous sinus. *1* and *2,* Lactiferous sinus: *1,* gland sinus, and *2,* teat sinus; *3,* openings of lactiferous ducts; *4,* submucosal venous ring; *5,* papillary duct; *6,* venous plexus in teat wall; *7,* teat orifice.

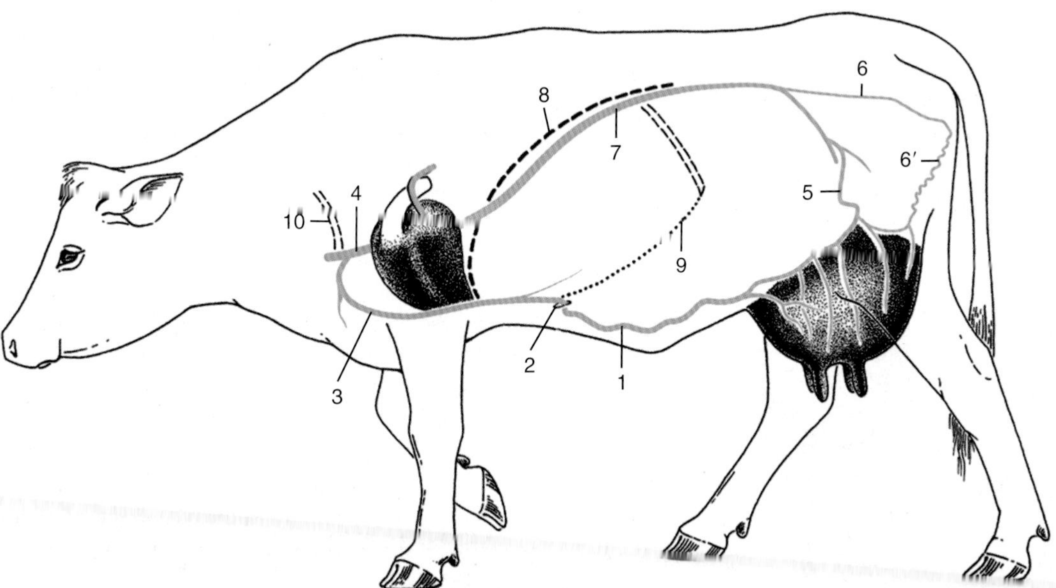

Fig. 29.44 The venous drainage of the udder. *1,* Subcutaneous abdominal ("milk") vein (v.); *2,* "milk well"; *3,* internal thoracic v.; *4,* cranial vena cava; *5,* external pudendal v.; *6,* internal pudendal v.; *6′,* ventral labial v. (connecting ventral perineal v. with caudal mammary veins); *7,* caudal vena cava; *8,* diaphragm; *9,* costal arch; *10,* first rib.

During the next few months growth keeps pace with the general growth of the body and is entirely due to deposition of fat. Thereafter, and thus commencing well before puberty, growth quickens; the rapid development of both the duct system and the gland tissue is probably due to the cyclical production of estrogen because spurts of activity occur directly before ovulation. Although a well-developed duct system is present by the time a heifer first conceives,

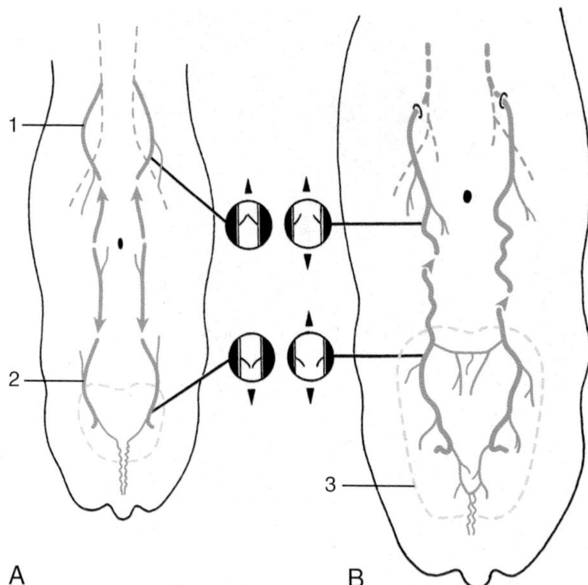

Fig. 29.45 Development of the subcutaneous abdominal veins (schematic dorsal view). (A) The region drained by the cranial superficial epigastric vein *(1)* is separated from that of the caudal superficial epigastric vein *(2)* in the calf and heifer. The valves in the cranial superficial epigastric vein direct blood cranially, while those in the caudal superficial epigastric vein direct blood caudally. (B) The subcutaneous abdominal vein is formed during pregnancy. The increased blood flow through the enlarging udder *(3)* causes the veins to distend, the valves to become inefficient, and the two drainage regions to unite, which allows blood to flow in both directions.

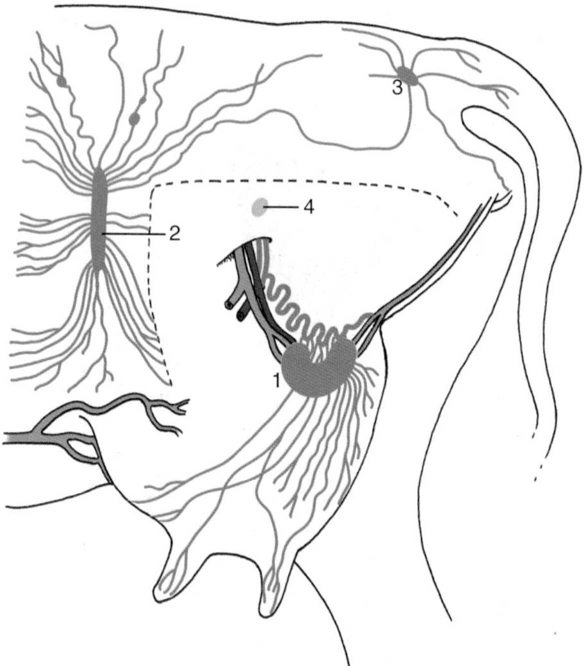

Fig. 29.46 Lymph drainage of the udder. The *broken line* indicates where the left limb was removed to expose the udder. *1,* Mammary (superficial inguinal) lymph node; *2,* subiliac lymph node; *3,* ischial lymph node; *4,* position of deep inguinal (iliofemoral) node.

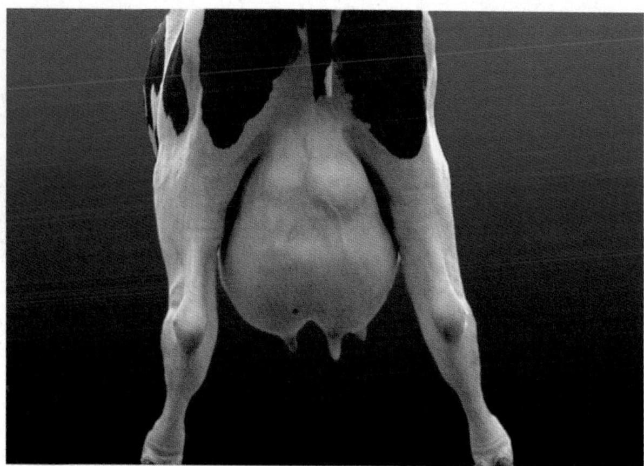

Fig. 29.47 Holstein cow with enlarged mammary lymph nodes.

additional growth of the ducts predominates in the first months of pregnancy, and the secretory tissue grows in the second half.

Growth in late pregnancy is dependent on prolactin and growth hormone of hypophyseal origin, in addition to progesterone and estrogen. Secretion of milk is later maintained by corticotropin, thyroid-stimulating hormone, and somatotropin. Regular milking is also necessary to maintain production. Because the act of milking stimulates the release of prolactin, oxytocin, and corticotropin, more frequent milking, within limits, increases the yield.

The mammary gland is composed of *tubuloalveolar secretory units* grouped to form lobules defined by connective tissue septa (Fig. 29.48A). The secretory alveoli are lined by a simple epithelium that changes markedly in height during the cycle of activity. The cells demonstrate maximal activity in those alveoli prepared to release milk when stimulated by suckling (or milking). After this the alveolar lumina are collapsed and irregular (Fig. 29.48B), and the epithelium is much reduced in height. All lobules within one gland do not necessarily exhibit the same stage of the secretory cycle, and both active and nonactive lobules may be present concurrently. The milk is forced from the secretory units into the duct system by contraction of surrounding myoepithelial cells (Fig. 29.49). The interlobular and intralobular connective tissue provides important structural support and conveys blood, lymph vessels, and nerves.

The udder of the small ruminants combines two glands that are more (goats) or less (sheep) distinctly demarcated externally. In milk goats the udder is large in relation to body size, deep, and conical (Fig. 29.50); in ewes it is smaller and more hemispherical, although inclining toward the caprine form in breeds used for cheese production. The teats are cylindrical in the young, but in older animals, especially in goats of high productivity, they tend to become conical and blend more smoothly with the contours of the gland (Fig. 29.51). Accessory teats are not uncommon in

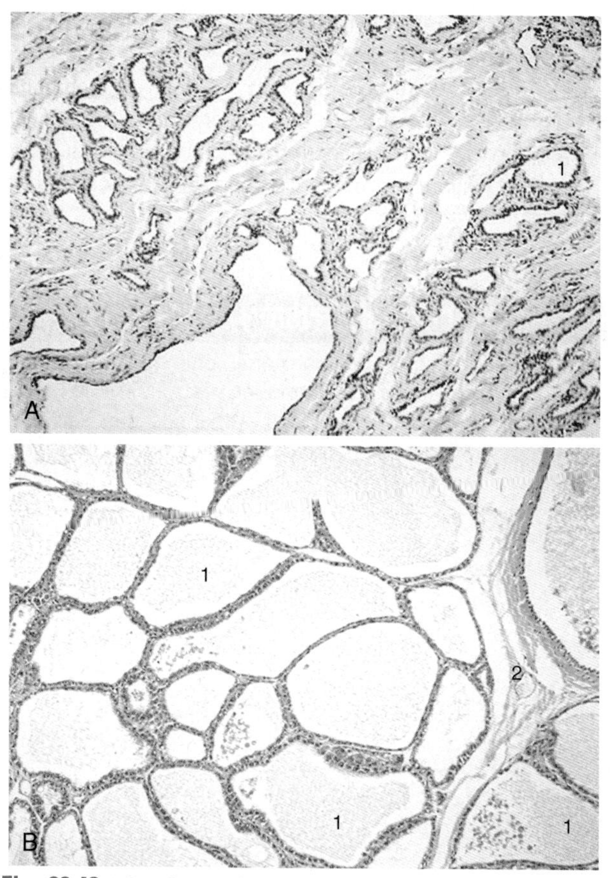

Fig. 29.48 Sections of (A) nonlactating and (B) lactating mammary glands; a compound tubuloalveolar gland (magnification ×70). *1,* Alveolus; *2,* interlobular septum.

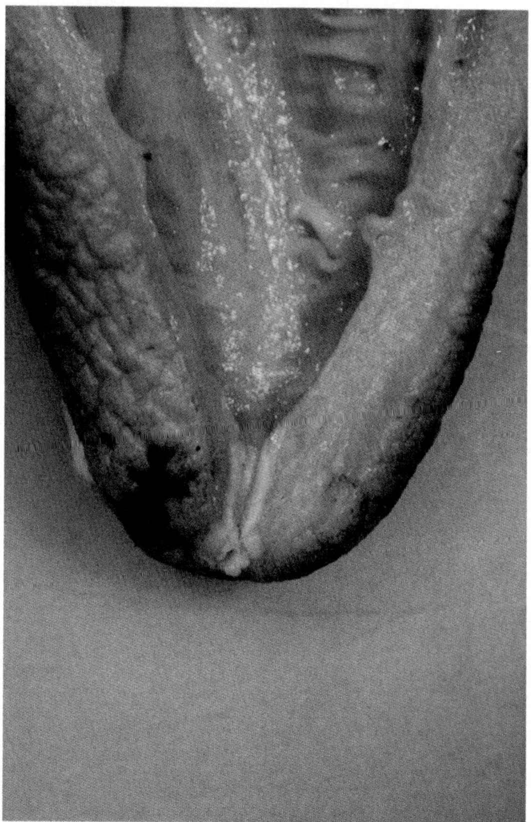

Fig. 29.49 Section of the teat extremity showing the smooth muscle encircling the papillary duct.

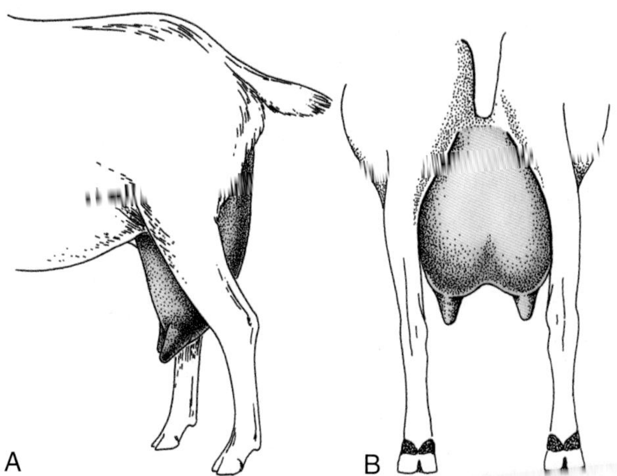

Fig. 29.50 (A) Lateral and (B) caudal views of the goat's udder.

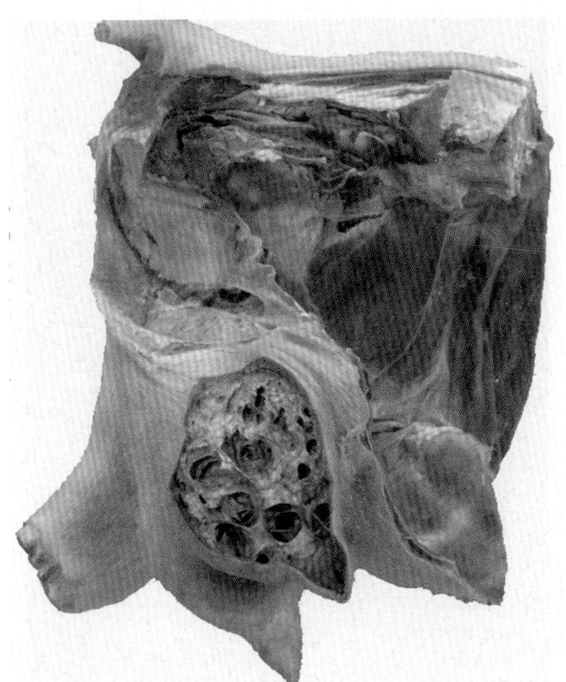

Fig. 29.51 Sagittal section of a young goat's udder and teat.

goats. The udder skin is finely haired in goats; in sheep the upper part may cover the fleece.

The structure, suspension, and vascular arrangements generally resemble those of the bovine udder. However, the teats are not wholly naked. In sheep, closure of the papillary duct is achieved without the presence of a sphincter muscle.

COMPREHENSION CHECK

Demonstrate how the hormonal changes influence the anatomic changes during an estrous cycle and gestation. Primarily focus on the changes that can be detected with an ultrasound examination or through rectal examination.

The Forelimb of the Ruminant 30

Cattle generally lead lives that do not expose them to frequent risk of injury to the proximal segments of the limbs, and there is less need for detailed knowledge of the anatomy of these parts than is required by the equine practitioner. Therefore, certain topics in this and the following chapter will receive only cursory treatment. Cattle, sheep, and goats are, however, frequently exposed to trauma and infections of the foot, and this part of the limb will receive greater attention.

THE SHOULDER AND THE ARM

The scapula and humerus, and the associated muscles, are enclosed within the skin of the trunk and held closely against the thoracic wall. Some cows, especially Jerseys, stand with their shoulder and elbow slightly abducted, which causes the humerus to angle away from the ribs. This "wing shoulder" defect, which seems to arise from inherited weakness of certain girdle muscles, looks awkward but is of little consequence (Fig. 30.1). It is not to be confused with "flying scapula," which is a serious myopathy observed in cattle turned out to pasture in the spring. In this condition, muscle tissue actually degenerates, which causes the dorsal border of the scapula to rise above the withers.

The position and slope of the bones can be determined by palpation of certain features: the cranial and caudal angles and the spine of the scapula and the greater tubercle and deltoid tuberosity of the humerus. The capacious shoulder joint may be punctured at the cranial border of the infraspinatus muscle, just proximal to its insertion on the greater tubercle.

Only those *muscles* that claim practical attention are discussed here (Fig. 30.2). The brachiocephalicus forms the dorsal border of the jugular groove and is joined along its upper margin by the omotransversarius extending between the acromion and the wing of the atlas. The latter muscle covers but does not prevent palpation of the large superficial cervical lymph node. The pectoral group is distinguished by the very rudimentary development of the subclavius. This explains the very abrupt transition from the narrow neck to the much greater breadth at the level of the shoulder joint—a striking difference in conformation between cattle and horses. The rhomboideus rarely attracts attention in cattle of European origin but makes the major contribution to the hump in Zebu stock. The hump varies in position (cervicothoracic or thoracic) and structure in animals of different breeds and strains. In some it is essentially a thickening of muscle, and in others it is a replacement of flesh by fat. The serratus ventralis, the principal supporter of the trunk, is adapted to this role by the inclusion of many tendinous strands and a stout aponeurotic covering. Its occasional rupture, a disaster of the first magnitude, is made very evident by the projection of the scapular cartilage above the dorsal contour of the thorax (see Fig. 26.1).

The superficial branch of the infraspinatus tendon is protected by a synovial bursa where it passes over the lateral face of the greater tubercle. The bursa is sometimes the seat of a painful inflammation made obvious by abduction of the arm. The tendon of the biceps brachii is also protected by a synovial (intertubercular) bursa on its deep face, and its role is assumed by a pouch of the shoulder joint capsule in sheep and goats. In the distal part of the arm, the biceps detaches a lacertus fibrosus that is palpable despite being much weaker than that of the horse. It descends in front of the elbow to blend with the covering of the extensor carpi radialis. Two other bursae are associated with the insertion of the triceps: one is interposed between the tendon and the olecranon, and the other, inconstant, is between the tendon and the skin over the point of the elbow.

THE ELBOW, FOREARM, AND CARPUS

The *elbow joint* projects onto the ventral ends of the fourth and fifth ribs. The olecranon, the medial and lateral epicondyles of the humerus, and the robust collateral ligaments are all easily palpable and provide the necessary orientation for joint puncture. This is performed from the lateral aspect with the needle directed between the lateral epicondyle and the olecranon to enter a considerable pouch of the capsule within the deep olecranon fossa.

Long Bone Fractures: Food animals experience a high incidence of fractures, mainly of the long bones. Among the long bone fractures, those of the metacarpus (III/IV) and metatarsus account for nearly half.

The ulna is complete but slender, and it is the massive radius that bears the weight. As always the subcutaneous medial border of the radius marks the division between

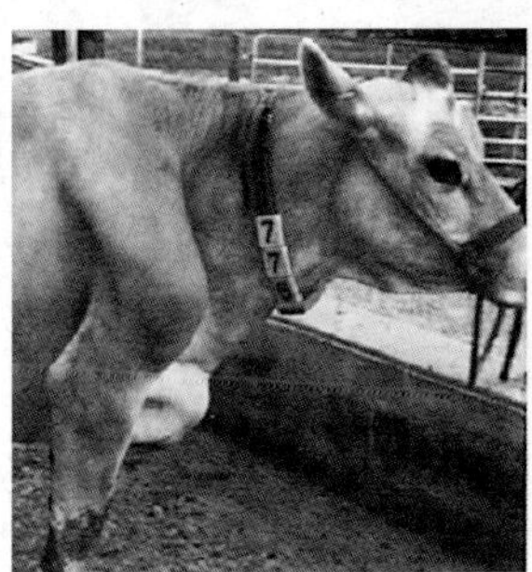
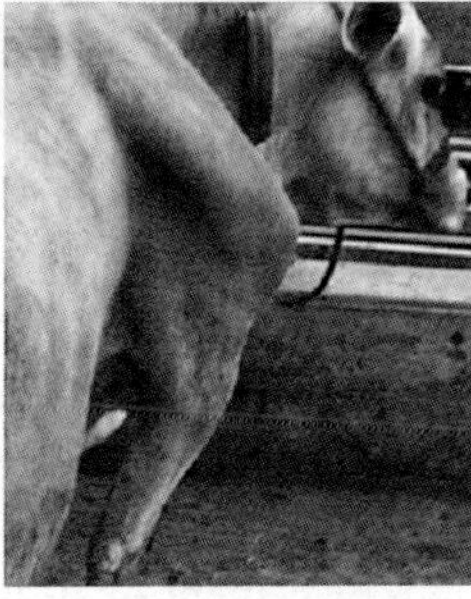

Fig. 30.1 "Wing shoulder" in a 6-year-old Jersey cow.

the cranial extensor and caudal flexor muscle groups (Fig. 30.3). The ulna is palpable only at its extremities, the olecranon and lateral styloid process. In most subjects the forearm inclines mediodistally to the carpus while the foot angles laterally, producing a "knock-kneed" stance. Although straight limbs are preferred, this inward bulging of the carpus does not appear to be a disadvantage.

The proximal row of *the carpal* skeleton comprises radial, intermediate, and ulnar carpal bones. The upper and lower borders of the accessory bone provide rough guides to the levels of the antebrachiocarpal and midcarpal joints. The distal row consists of only two bones: fused second and third carpals and the fourth carpal (see Fig. 2.48). In theory, movement is possible at all three levels, but most occurs between the forearm and carpus, a moderate amount takes place at the middle joint, and next to none occurs at the carpometacarpal level. Movements other than flexion and extension are largely prevented by the many ligaments, of which the collateral pair is most important. The cavities of the two distal joints always communicate; occasionally all three do so. Puncture is possible at the proximal and middle levels and is obviously most easily performed when the joint is flexed.

Irregularities of the palmar aspect of the carpal bones are covered and smoothed by the thick fibrous layer of the joint capsule (palmar carpal ligament), which combines with the accessory bone and flexor retinaculum to enclose the carpal canal. The joint capsule also bends dorsally with deep fascia to form the extensor retinaculum that binds the extensor tendons in place. An inconstant bursa between this retinaculum and the skin occasionally enlarges to form an unsightly but painless blemish (hygroma).

Hygromas of the carpus and tarsus result from repeated trauma or inadequate bedding and are manifested as fluid accumulation in subcutaneous tissue. These may require procedures such as drainage or surgical resection.

Only the digital extensors and flexors among the muscles of the forearm merit notice. The *common digital extensor* has two bellies: the larger medial one extends its tendon

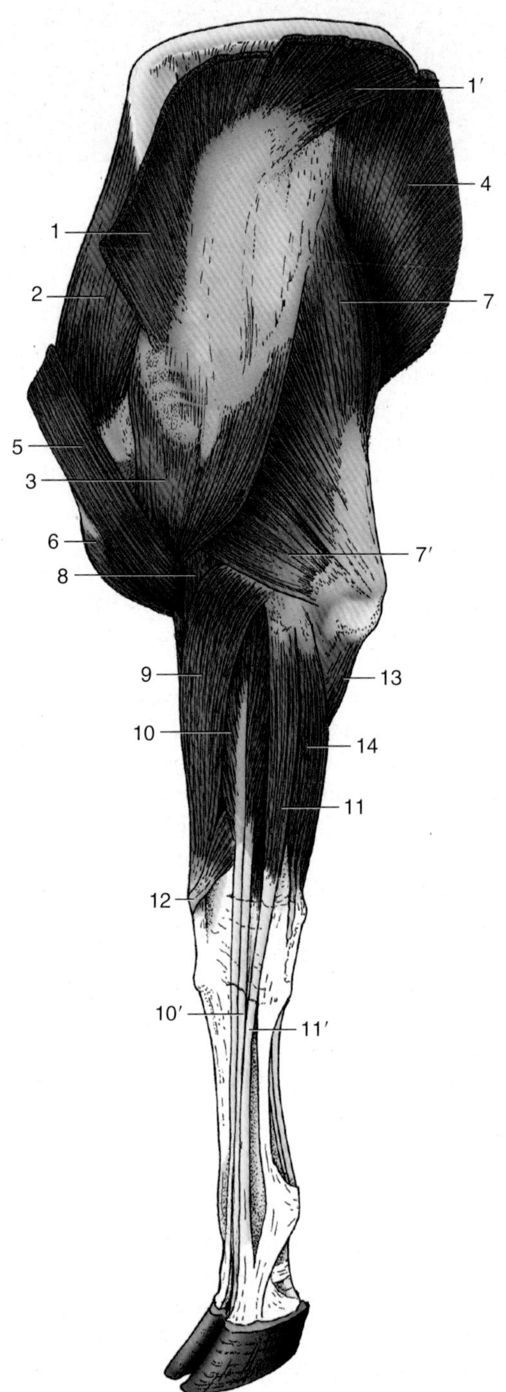

Fig. 30.2 Muscles of the bovine forelimb, lateral view. *1* and *1′*, Trapezius; *2*, supraspinatus; *3*, deltoideus; *4*, latissimus dorsi; *5*, brachiocephalicus; *6*, biceps; *7* and *7′*, long and lateral heads of triceps, respectively; *8*, brachialis; *9*, extensor carpi radialis; *10*, common digital extensor; *10′*, tendon of lateral belly; *11* and *11′*, lateral digital extensor and its tendon, respectively; *12*, extensor carpi obliquus; *13*, ulnar head of deep digital flexor; *14*, ulnaris lateralis.

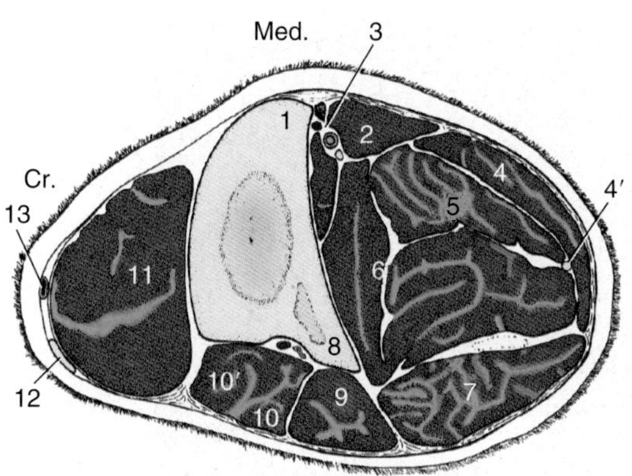

Fig. 30.3 Transverse section of the middle of the bovine left forearm. *Cr.*, Cranial; *Med.*, medial; *1*, radius; *2*, flexor carpi radialis; *3*, median vessels and nerve; *4*, flexor carpi ulnaris; *4′*, ulnar nerve; *5*, superficial digital flexor; *6*, deep digital flexor; *7*, ulnaris lateralis; *8*, ulna; *9*, lateral digital extensor; *10* and *10′*, common digital extensor; *11*, extensor carpi radialis; *12*, superficial branch of radial nerve; *13*, cephalic vein.

of insertion to the medial digit, and the smaller lateral belly has a tendon that splits at the fetlock to insert on both digits. The two tendons share a synovial sheath where they descend over the carpus. The *lateral digital* extensor comports itself like the medial belly of the common extensor (Fig. 30.2). The superficial digital flexor also possesses two bellies. The three bellies of the deep flexor give rise to a stout tendon that receives synovial protection during its passage through the carpal canal, while the superficial one remains outside the flexor retinaculum. Both are protected by long synovial sheaths that extend beyond the carpus into the cannon where the tendons merge. All these tendons receive further discussion later.

THE DISTAL PART OF THE LIMB

The distal part of the limb, loosely known as the foot, consists of the expanded lower end of the metacarpus, the two principal digits (toes or claws), and the dewclaws. The toes are enclosed in a common envelope of the skin that extends to the coronets so that the hooves alone are separated by the interdigital cleft. The dewclaws project behind the fetlock and do not come into contact with firm ground.

The Skeleton and Joints

The skeleton is reduced to the bones of the principal digits (III and IV) together with vestiges of those of the flanking ones (II and V) (Fig. 30.4). Although the principal metacarpal elements are fused to form a single cannon bone, this divides at its lower end into separate articular trochleae for the two proximal phalanges. All more distal bones are duplicated. Vestigial structures include the short, rodlike fifth metacarpal bone in articulation with the upper end of the cannon bone (see Fig. 2.48) and phalangeal rudiments isolated within the dewclaws.

The cannon bone is compressed from front to back and expanded to the sides at each end. A dorsal axial groove (presenting a vascular foramen at each end) and an incomplete internal septum (visible in radiographs) attest to the composite origin of the bone (see Fig. 30.8B/*4*). The proximal and middle phalanges are broadly alike, although the former are about twice the length of the latter. All four of these bones present proximopalmar tubercles, paired on the proximal phalanges and single and abaxial on the middle ones. Each has a distal surface that is grooved sagittally to fit the bifaceted surface of the bone with which it articulates. The distal phalanx is shaped like the hoof in which it is lodged and presents articular, axial, abaxial, and sole surfaces (Fig. 30.5). The extensor process is the highest point, and from it a crest runs to the apex of the bone, dividing the axial and abaxial surfaces. These surfaces are separated caudally by a thick transverse tubercle (Fig. 30.5/*4*) to which the deep flexor tendon attaches. Apart from the articular surface, the exterior displays numerous vascular foramina most conspicuously on the axial aspect of the extensor process and at the palmar end of the abaxial surface. (The proximal and distal sesamoid bones are described with the joints.)

As in the horse, the articulations linking the metacarpal and digital bones are commonly known as the fetlock, pastern, and coffin joints. The *fetlock joint,* the first duplicated joint of the limb, is slightly overextended when the animal stands at rest (Fig. 30.6/*3*). Its movements are confined to flexion and extension by reciprocally keeled and grooved articular surfaces and by strong collateral ligaments. The axial (interdigital) collateral ligaments of both joints have a common origin in the intertrochlear notch of the metacarpal bone (Fig. 30.4). The phalangeal articular surfaces are complemented on their palmar aspect by a row of four (proximal) sesamoid bones embedded within a continuous fibrocartilaginous bridge and joined by the interosseous muscle. These sesamoids are additionally secured by collateral and a complex suite of distal sesamoidean ligaments. The collateral sesamoidean ligaments connect each abaxial sesamoid to the metacarpal bone and proximal phalanx. The ligaments that arise from the distal surfaces pass to the prominent tubercles on the proximopalmar aspect of the related phalanges, crossing in passage to their destinations (cruciate sesamoidean ligaments); fibers of the axial pair also cross the interdigital space (interdigital phalangosesamoidean ligaments (Fig. 30.7C/*10*). The fetlock joints are mobile and capsules are large, with each extending proximally as a dorsal pouch between the metacarpal bone and extensor tendons and as a palmar pouch between the bone and the interosseous muscle (see Fig. 30.8/*9* and *9′*). Between the two, the larger palmar pouch is reached more easily by entering from the side, about 2 or 3 cm proximal

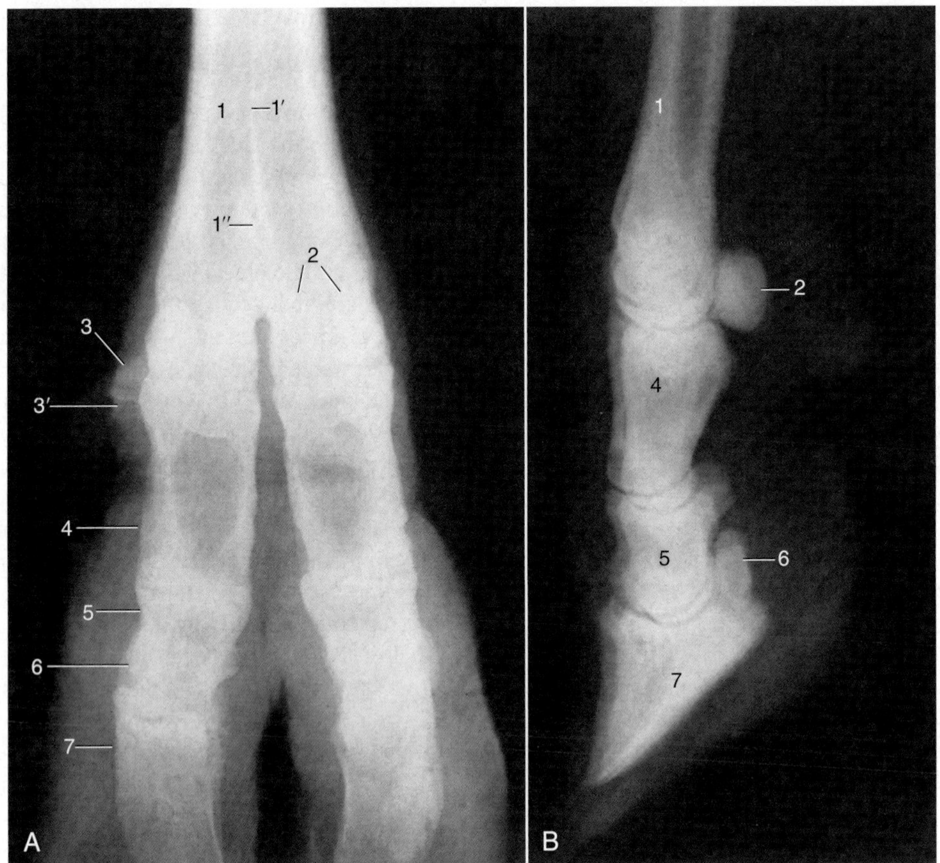

Fig. 30.4 (A) Dorsopalmar and (B) lateromedial radiographs of the bovine foot. *1,* Metacarpal bone; *1′,* median septum; *1″,* distal metacarpal canal; *2,* proximal sesamoid bones; *3,* dewclaw; *3′,* rudimentary phalanx within dewclaw; *4,* proximal phalanx; *5,* middle phalanx; *6,* navicular bone; *7,* distal phalanx.

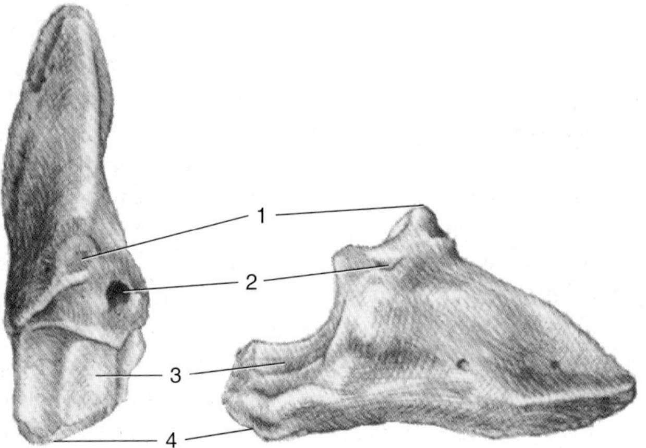

Fig. 30.5 The distal phalanx looking distally *(left)* and axial surface *(right). 1,* Extensor process; *2,* axial foramen for the principal artery to the hoof; *3,* articular surface; *4,* tubercle on which the deep digital flexor attaches.

to the joint space. Communication between the paired capsules allows infection or injected material to travel from one joint to the other.

The less mobile *pastern joints* also allow only flexion and extension. Each joint is supported by one pair of collateral ligaments. The better developed axial collateral ligament and an additional axial ligament extending to the distal phalanx may prevent the spreading of toes under the body weight. The joint obtains further support from a fibrocartilage that extends the palmar border of the articular

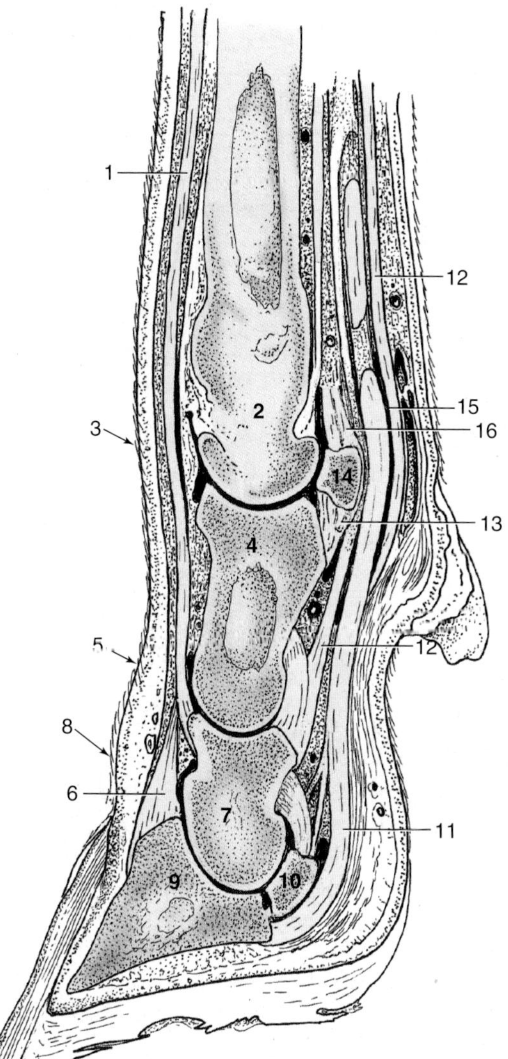

Fig. 30.6 Sagittal section of the bovine foot, splitting the lateral digit. *1,* Lateral digital extensor; *2,* metacarpal bone; *3,* fetlock joint; *4,* proximal phalanx; *5,* pastern joint; *6,* common digital extensor; *7,* middle phalanx; *8,* coffin joint; *9,* distal phalanx; *10,* navicular bone; *11,* deep digital flexor; *12,* superficial flexor; *13,* distal sesamoidean ligaments; *14,* proximal sesamoid bone; *15,* digital sheath; *16,* interosseous.

surface of the middle phalanx and from three palmar ligaments (Fig. 30.8A). The capsules of the two pastern joints are separate. Each forms dorsal and ventral pouches against the proximal phalanx; the dorsal one is said to be accessible to puncture from the side.

The *coffin joint* resembles the pastern in conformation and in the possession of collateral ligaments. It is entirely within the hoof, and because the small dorsal and ventral pouches barely reach beyond the coronet, puncture is difficult (Figs. 30.6 and 30.8). The distal articular surface is enlarged by the navicular bone located about 2 cm within the hoof (when measured abaxially). Its other end is above the axial wall of the hoof, which is lower. The bone is mainly related to the middle phalanx and is held in place by a complex set of distal and collateral ligaments, which pass to the adjacent phalanges and resist overextension. An elastic ligament spanning the axial surface of the joint prompts recollection of the ligament that retracts the claw in cats but appears not to have a comparable function. Interdigital ligaments are also present to prevent splaying of the digits. One connects the axial surfaces of the proximal phalanges (Fig. 30.7), and a second crosses the interdigital space level with the navicular bones, where it is related to the interdigital bridge of skin.

The Tendons

The *interosseous muscle,* morphologically a compound formation, is conventionally referred to in the singular (Fig. 30.7). This flat muscle is fleshy in the young but becomes increasingly fibrous as the animal matures and gains weight. In the adult it forms a strong, almost wholly tendinous band that continues distally from the capsule of the carpal joint (Fig. 30.8/*8*). In midmetacarpus it gives rise to five principal branches; four of these—all but the central one—appear to terminate on the proximal sesamoid bones but obtain a functional continuation from the distal (sesamoidean) ligaments that attach on the proximal phalanges. The arrangement forms a "sling" that is tensed when the foot bears weight and the fetlock joint is overextended. Thin slips from the interosseous join the extensor tendons. Two of these split from the abaxial branches already mentioned and wind around the abaxial surfaces of the proximal phalanges to merge with the proper extensor tendons. Two more are provided by the bifurcation of the fifth (central) branch. They pass through the interdigital space, wind around the axial surfaces of the phalanges, and merge in the same tendons. In midmetacarpus the interosseous muscle also releases from its palmar surface a strong band (Fig. 30.8A/*7*) that divides to join the branches of the superficial digital flexor tendon above the fetlock. (The band may be regarded as a check ligament of the superficial digital flexor.)

The three *extensor tendons* can be palpated where they lie side by side on the dorsal surface of the metacarpal bone. The middle tendon (from the lateral belly of the common digital extensor) bifurcates at the fetlock and the thin branches, each surrounded by an independent synovial sheath (Fig. 30.9/*2'*), follow the dorsal surface of the digits to insert on the extensor processes of the distal phalanges. The medial tendon (from the medial belly) widens as it passes over the dorsal pouch of the fetlock joint, where a subtendinous bursa facilitates its passage. This tendon receives the extensor branches from the interosseous muscle before it inserts on the proximal end of the middle phalanx (but with a secondary connection to the distal phalanx). The lateral tendon (lateral digital extensor;

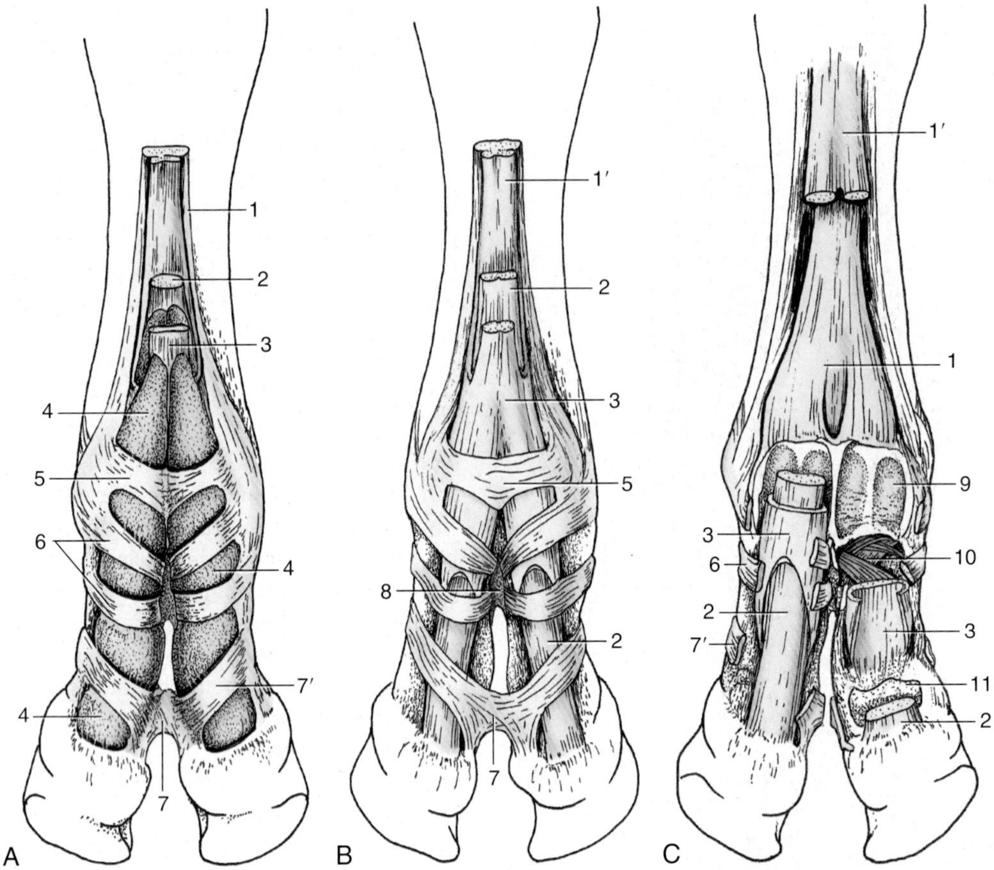

Fig. 30.7 Palmar view of the bovine forefoot. (A) Superficial dissection. (B) Tissues of the digital sheath have been removed. (C) Parts of the superficial and deep flexors have been removed. *1,* Interosseous; *1′,* band of interosseous to superficial flexor; *2,* deep digital flexor; *3,* superficial digital flexor; *4,* digital sheath; *5,* annular ligament of fetlock joint; *6,* digital annular ligaments; *7* and *7′,* distal interdigital ligament. *7,* deep part, and *7′,* superficial part; *8,* proximal interdigital ligament; *9,* proximal sesamoid bones; *10,* cruciate sesamoidean and interdigital phalangosesamoidean ligaments; *11,* navicular bone.

Fig. 30.9/*3*) comports itself identically in relation to the lateral digit.

The *superficial* and *deep flexor tendons* are separated from the metacarpal bone by the interosseous muscle (Fig. 30.8). Together they can be palpated as they emerge from the carpus medial to the accessory carpal bone, and they become individually distinguishable in the distal half of the cannon, where the deep fascia is thin. They are never so easily identified as the sharp-edged interosseous lying against the bone. The tendons are difficult to palpate in the digits.

The *superficial flexor tendon* splits above the fetlock joints (Fig. 30.7/*3*). Each branch receives a band from the interosseous muscle with which it forms a sleeve about the corresponding branch of the deep flexor when level with the proximal sesamoid bones. These bones provide bearing surfaces around which the combined tendons bend, secured in place by *annular ligaments* (Fig. 30.7/*5* and *9*). The palmar wall of the sleeve ends at the middle of the proximal phalanx, exposing the deep tendon that has now exchanged relative position with the superficial flexor. The dorsal wall of the sleeve continues the superficial flexor tendon and terminates on the proximal end and complementary cartilage of the middle phalanx. Two narrower (digital) annular ligaments strap the tendons to the proximal phalanx. The *deep flexor tendon* widens after leaving the confines of the sleeve and continues over the insertion of the superficial flexor tendon, which provides it with another bearing surface. The deep digital flexor tendon is protected by the navicular bursa during its passage over the navicular bone. It ends in a wide insertion on the hind end of the distal phalanx. The distal interdigital ligament binds the deep tendon down at the middle phalanx. The attachments of the superficial flexor tendon enable it to assist the interosseous muscle in preventing overextension of the fetlock joint.

A complex sheath (digital sheath; Fig. 30.7/*4*) that is independent of the digital joint capsules and the navicular bursae surrounds the two flexor tendons from the distal

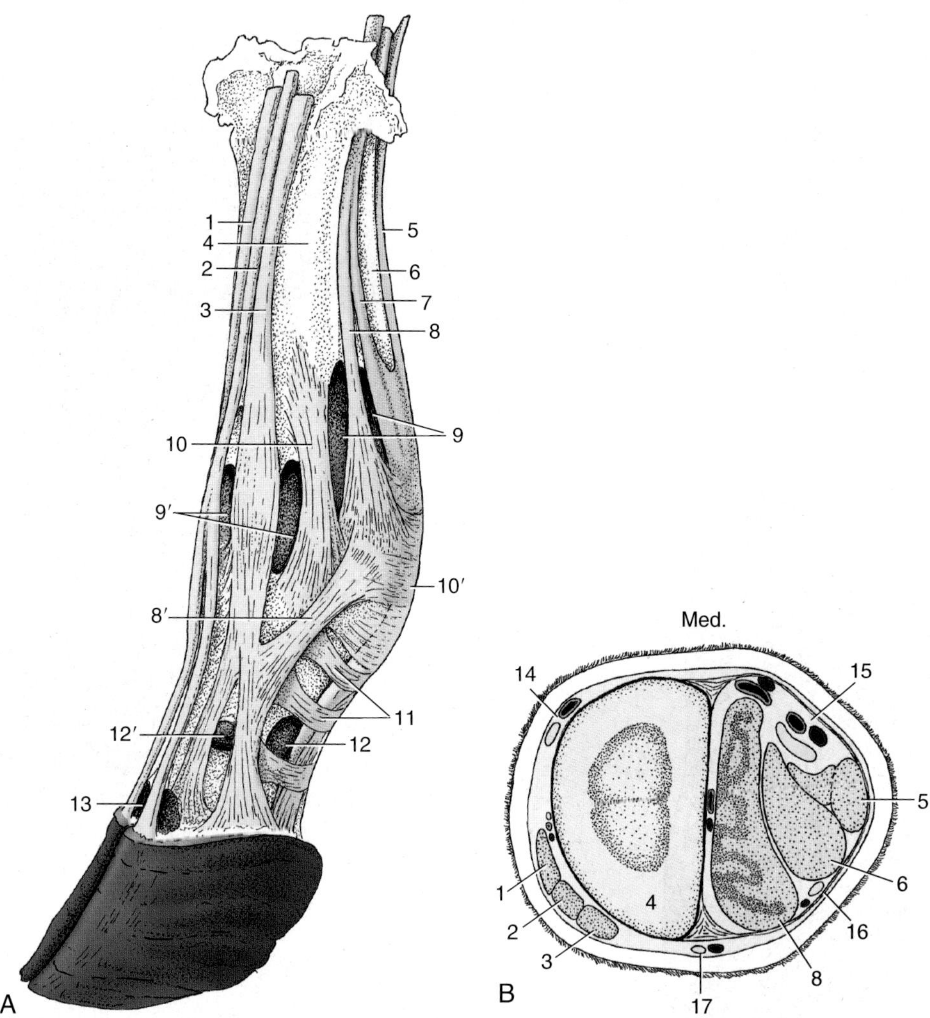

Fig. 30.8 (A) Bovine left forefoot, lateral view. (B) Transverse section of the left metacarpus. *Med.*, Medial; *1* and *2*, medial and lateral tendons of common digital extensor, respectively; *3*, lateral digital extensor; *4*, metacarpal bone; *5*, superficial digital flexor; *6*, deep digital flexor; *7*, band from interosseous to superficial flexor; *8* and *8′*, interosseous and its extensor branch, respectively; *9* and *9′*, palmar and dorsal pouches of fetlock joint, respectively; *10* and *10′*, lateral collateral and annular ligaments of fetlock joint, respectively; *11*, digital annular ligaments; *12* and *12′*, palmar and dorsal pouches of pastern joint, respectively; *13*, dorsal pouch of medial coffin joint; *14*, dorsal common digital vein III and superficial radial nerve; *15*, median vessels and nerve; *16*, palmar branch of ulnar nerve; *17*, dorsal branch of ulnar nerve.

third of the metacarpus almost to the navicular bone. It facilitates their passage against each other and against the various bearing surfaces and annular ligaments. The sheaths of the medial and lateral branches of the tendons touch locally and occasionally communicate. Distention of an infected sheath is possible where it is unsupported, namely, at its proximal end and between the annular ligaments below the fetlock. The sheath may be punctured from the side at the dorsal border of the flexor tendons, about 5 cm proximal to the dewclaw.

The following skeletal features may be palpated at the fetlock (Fig. 30.4): the dorsal and abaxial surfaces of the metacarpal trochleae, the corresponding parts of the proximal phalanges, the abaxial sesamoid bones, the abaxial tubercles of the proximal phalanges, and the gaps between the proximal phalanges and the neighboring sesamoids, which mark the level of the joint spaces (opposite the dewclaws). Except for its palmar surface, most of the proximal phalanx is easily appreciated, but its distal end and the pastern joint space are obscure even though the level is marked by the insertion of the flat extensor tendon (3 cm above the coronet) and the prominent abaxial tubercle of the middle phalanx; the joint space itself lies about 2 cm above the coronet. The narrow branches of

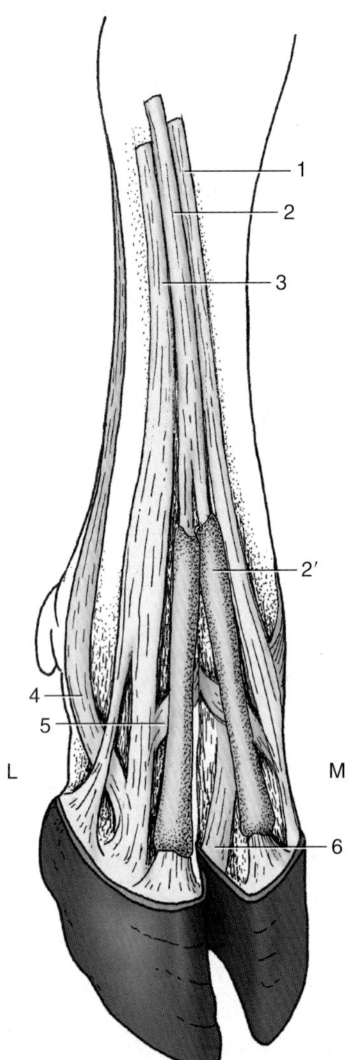

Fig. 30.9 Dorsal view of the bovine right forefoot. *L,* Lateral; *M,* medial; *1,* medial tendon of common digital extensor to the medial digit; *2* and *2′,* common digital extensor and its sheaths, respectively; *3,* lateral digital extensor; *4* and *5,* abaxial and axial extensor branches, respectively, of the interosseous to the lateral digital extensor; *6,* common axial collateral ligament.

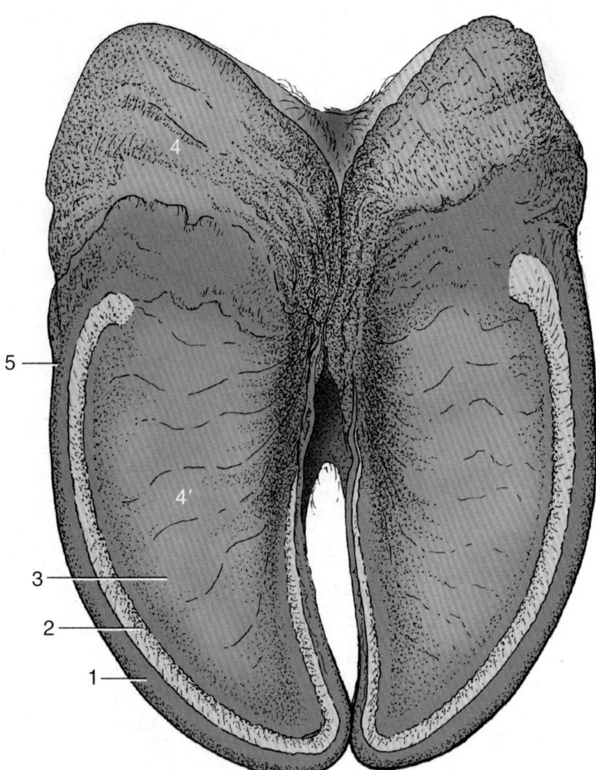

Fig. 30.10 Ground surface of the hooves of the bovine forefoot. *1,* Wall; *2,* white line; *3,* sole; *4,* bulb; *4′,* dorsal part of bulb; *5,* abaxial groove on the wall, dividing wall from bulb.

the common extensor are more easily appreciated than the wide but flat tendons of the proper extensors. The flexor tendons form a firm mass behind the bones. The dewclaws are attached to thickened deep fascia that forms two ligaments extending to the abaxial ends of the navicular bones; these ligaments become palpable when the dewclaws are raised.

THE HOOVES

The hooves of the principal digits curve toward each other at both ends, making contact behind and occasionally also at their apices (Fig. 30.10). The lateral hoof carries the greater share of weight and is larger than the medial one, although this is not always so in the hindfoot. Each hoof consists of periople, wall, sole, and bulb. The ground surface is formed by the distal border of the wall, the sole, and the dorsal part of the bulb (Fig. 30.10/*1, 3,* and *4′*); the parts visible in the standing animal are the wall to the sides and the bulb at the back of the hoof. The coronary border of the hoof is higher on the abaxial than on the axial side. The apical two thirds or so of the hoof are occupied by the distal phalanx and deep flexor tendon; the space behind is taken up by the digital cushion, the springy pad of fatty-fibrous tissue that also extends under the larger "half" of the bone (Fig. 30.11/*8*).

Laminitis: The most important clinical disease of the claw in dairy cattle is subclinical laminitis. The signs include claw horn deformities, soft sole horn, and widened white line.

The *periople* provides a narrow (≈1 cm) strip along the coronary border that widens at the back where it grades into the bulb and merges with the periople of the other

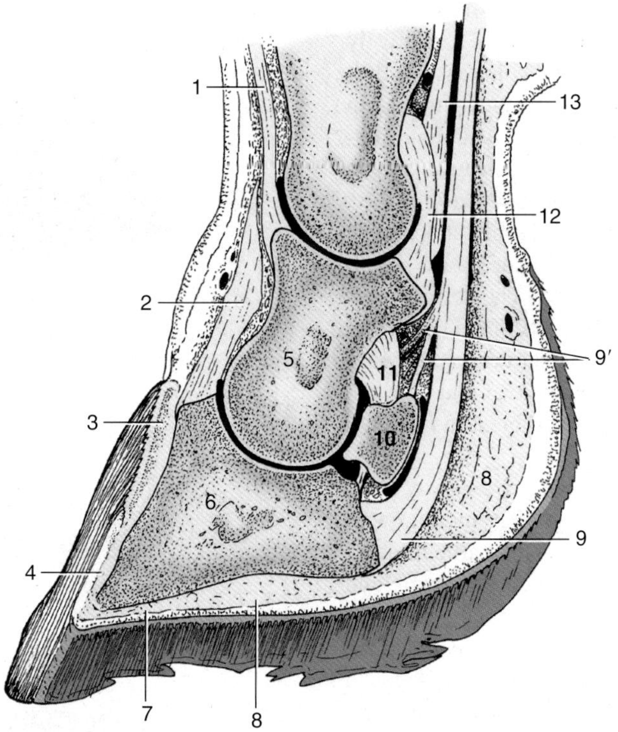

Fig. 30.11 Sagittal section of the medial digit of the bovine forefoot. *1,* Proper (medial) digital extensor; *2,* common digital extensor; *3,* coronary dermis; *4,* laminar dermis; *5,* middle phalanx; *6,* distal phalanx; *7,* sole dermis covered by sole; *8,* digital cushion; *9,* deep digital flexor; *9′,* fibers of deep digital flexor to the middle phalanx and navicular bone; *10,* navicular bone; *11,* collateral navicular ligament; *12,* palmar ligaments of pastern joint; *13,* superficial digital flexor.

hoof. It is partly hidden by hair. In consistency it is intermediate between the epidermis of the skin and the hard horn of the wall.

The *wall,* sharply flexed on itself, forms the greater part of both axial and abaxial surfaces (Fig. 30.10); the flexure produces a crest at the front that curves distally toward the tip or "toe" of the hoof. Both surfaces are bounded caudally by more or less distinct grooves (Fig. 30.10/*5*) that extend from the coronary border to the ground surface; the horn caudal to the grooves belongs to the bulb. The axial groove is more cranial and provides an area of weakness that is sometimes penetrated leading to injection of the coffin joint located only a few millimeters away. The wall is marked by prominent ridges, parallel to the coronary border, caused by uneven production of horn due to local or more general disturbances. Although the distal border normally makes contact with, the ground along the whole length of the abaxial wall, it does so only toward the toe on the axial side; the greater part of this margin bears weight only on softer ground. The wall is thicker near the apex and toward the ground, especially abaxially. It consists of both tubular and intertubular horn and is produced over the wide, flat coronary dermis. The horny laminae are short and low and form a weaker union with the laminar dermis than in the horse. This may be correlated with the greater extent of the weight-bearing surface in ruminants.

The *sole* (Fig. 30.10/*3*) is a relatively smooth area confined within the inflected angle of the wall from which it is separated by the softer so-called white line. This line, hardly lighter than the unpigmented horn to each side, is only a few millimeters wide and comprises the alternation of the distal ends of the horny laminae with the slightly darker horn produced over the terminal papillae of the sensitive laminae. Centrally, the sole blends imperceptibly with the apex of the bulb. The junction marks the extent of the digital cushion (Fig. 30.11/*7* and *8*).

Sole Hemorrhage: Sole dermis is richly vascularized, and sole hemorrhages are a high-incidence clinical manifestation. The hemorrhages are associated with laminitis and rapid weight gain.

The *bulb* provides both the caudal aspect and a considerable portion of the ground surface where its apex inserts into the V-shaped sole. It is the chief weight-bearing part. A large proportion of intertubular horn makes it relatively soft, but its considerable thickness may compensate. Bulbar horn tends to flake when allowed to build up (as in animals that have stood on fouled bedding), and the resulting fissures provide access to infection leading to abscesses that may destroy the dermis and deeper structures.

The hoof capsule is molded on a dermis attached to underlying structures by a modified subcutis, best developed where it forms the digital cushion. The dermis presents segments that correspond to the parts of the hoof (Fig. 30.12). The horn of the wall is produced over the coronary dermis (Fig. 30.12/*2*) and slides distally over and between the dermal laminae, where horn just sufficient to maintain adhesion is produced.

The horn of other parts of the hoof grows away from the dermis at a rate of about 5 mm per month, with growth occurring a little faster in calves. In cattle allowed free range, wear at the ground surface equals growth, and at the toe the angle with the ground is maintained at about 50 degrees. On soft surfaces, growth exceeds wear, and the hooves must be trimmed periodically if the toe is not to grow forward at a lesser angle. When this occurs, the coffin joint is gradually overextended, the deep flexor tensed, and greater weight placed on the (caudal) part of the hoof over the insertion of the deep flexor and navicular bone. This causes pain and therefore lameness.

In late fetal life the distal parts of the hoof are covered with soft horn, which is said to prevent injury to the fetal membranes and the birth canal. This soft cushion soon dries when exposed to air.

The dewclaws, miniatures of the principal hooves, consist mainly of wall and bulb; they have no practical importance.

THE BLOOD VESSELS AND LYMPHATIC STRUCTURES

The axillary artery, located with deep palpation as it winds around the first rib, is the main supply to the forelimb and is used occasionally as a source of arterial blood. The courses and branches of the arteries in the proximal segments of the limb follow the general pattern closely enough to make description unnecessary.

The account may commence where the median artery accompanies the deep digital flexor tendon through the carpal canal. It runs with a satellite vein and the median nerve where it enters the metacarpus to continue medial to the flexor tendons under cover of a thick deep fascia (Fig. 30.13) but becomes superficial and vulnerable at the fetlock joint. Its course now takes it over the palmar surface of the medial branches of the flexor tendons before diving into the interdigital space. The artery and accompanying vein bulge visibly at this level in thin-skinned animals, but though the artery may be palpated, a pulse cannot usually be perceived. It now bears a new title, *palmar common digital artery III,* and within the space it gives off a number of branches of minor importance

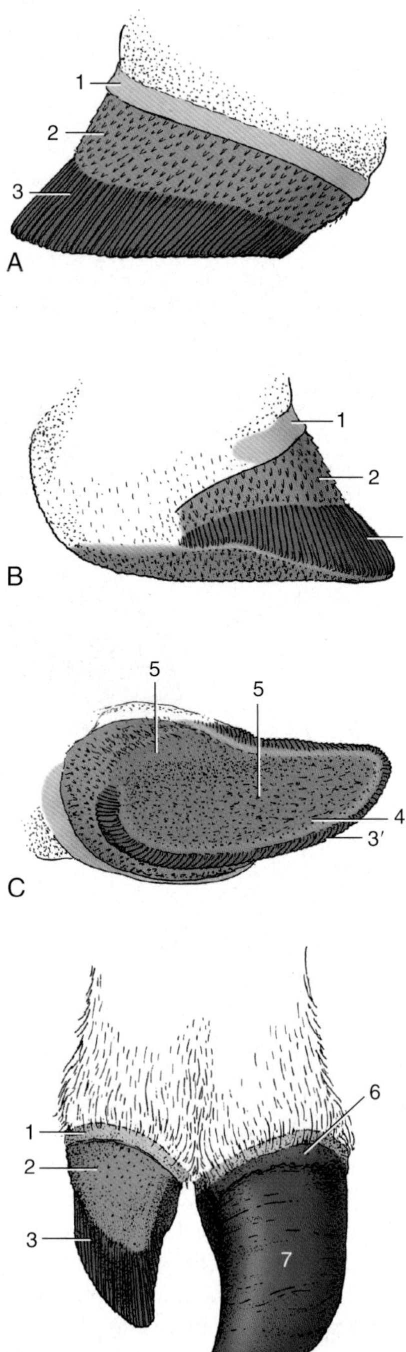

Fig. 30.12 Dermis over which the horn of the hoof is produced. (A to C), Abaxial, axial, and ground surface, respectively. (D) Dorsal surface of dermis and hoof. *1,* Perioplic dermis; *2,* coronary dermis; *3,* laminar dermis; *3′,* terminal papillae at the distal ends of the laminae; *4,* sole dermis; *5,* dermis of the bulb; *6,* periople; *7,* wall of hoof.

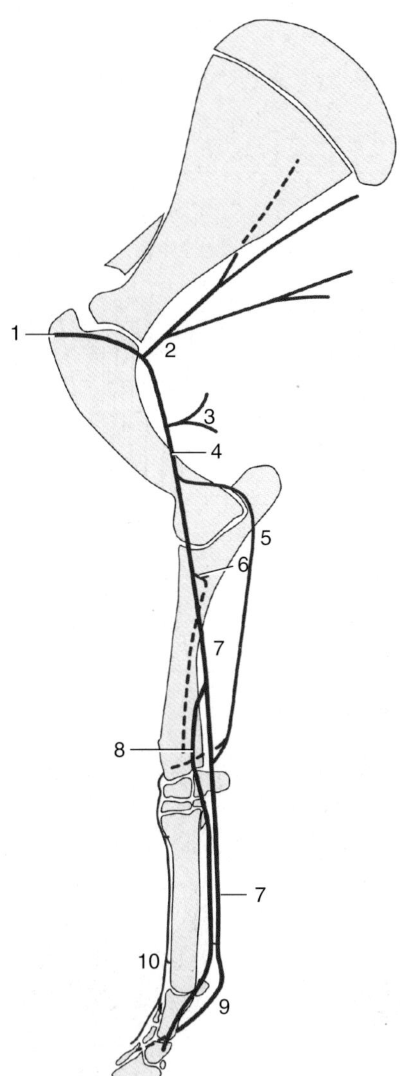

Fig. 30.13 The principal arteries on the bovine right forelimb; medial view. *1*, Axillary artery (a.); *2*, subscapular a.; *3*, deep brachial a.; *4*, brachial a.; *5*, collateral ulnar a.; *6*, common interosseous a.; *7*, median a.; *8*, radial a.; *9*, palmar common digital a. III; *10*, dorsal common digital a. III.

before dividing into the two axial palmar digital arteries. Each of these passes distally to reach and enter the distal phalanx through the large foramen located by the extensor process. Lesser *palmar abaxial digital arteries,* derived from arteries of the forearm, enter the distal phalanges at the palmar ends of their abaxial surfaces. Within the bone the axial and abaxial arteries anastomose to form a terminal arch from which numerous branches are released to the dermis. Other small arteries on the dorsal aspect of the digits are of little importance. All the arteries are severed when a digit is amputated; the stump of the axial palmar artery bleeds most profusely, and it, at least, must be ligated.

The limb veins are divided between a deep system, satellite to the arteries, and a quasi-independent superficial system. The two systems are connected by prominent anastomoses at the elbow, above the carpus, and in the foot and eventually join into one when the *cephalic vein* opens into the external jugular at the base of the neck. The superficial system comprises the *cephalic and accessory cephalic veins* and the tributaries of the latter in the foot (Fig. 30.14A). Most can be palpated, and especially in young, thin-skinned subjects, they may provide visible surface landmarks. Their positions are more certainly revealed when raised by a tourniquet. They are now much used for obtaining surgical anesthesia of the digits by retrograde intravenous injection. Those that lend themselves to the procedure are shown in Fig. 30.14B and C. The technique is simpler and more reliable than the alternative method, which requires the deposit of anesthetic solution over several nerves.

The *lymph nodes* of the forelimb comprise the large proper axillary node, which lies against the thoracic wall caudal to the shoulder joint, and a few small accessory nodes (lymphonodi axillares primae costae) placed over the first rib and adjoining intercostals space. The axillary node receives lymph from the deeper structures of the upper segments of the limb, including the ventral girdle muscles, and forwards it first to the accessory nodes and thence either to the caudal deep cervical nodes or directly to one or another of the veins at the thoracic inlet. This node may be inspected through an incision of the first intercostal space of the split carcass. The dorsal girdle muscles, the skin and subcutaneous fascia of the shoulder, arm, and forearm, and all structures distal to the carpus drain directly to the superficial cervical node, which may be palpated in front of the shoulder.

THE NERVES OF THE FORELIMB

The brachial plexus is formed by the last three cervical and first two thoracic nerves. Its branches generally conform to the common pattern, but some points merit repetition or amplification because of their clinical relevance.

The *suprascapular* (C6–C7) nerve winds around the cranial border of the scapula to reach the supraspinatus and infraspinatus muscles (Fig. 30.15). Destruction has little effect on the standing posture beyond producing occasional slight abduction of the arm. Walking is more severely affected, and the limb is advanced with a stiff, circumducted stride while the shoulder is abducted most obviously in the support phase. In chronic paralysis the muscles atrophy and the scapular spine becomes sharply defined.

The large *median nerve* (C8–T2) runs down the medial aspect of the arm, crosses the elbow joint (where

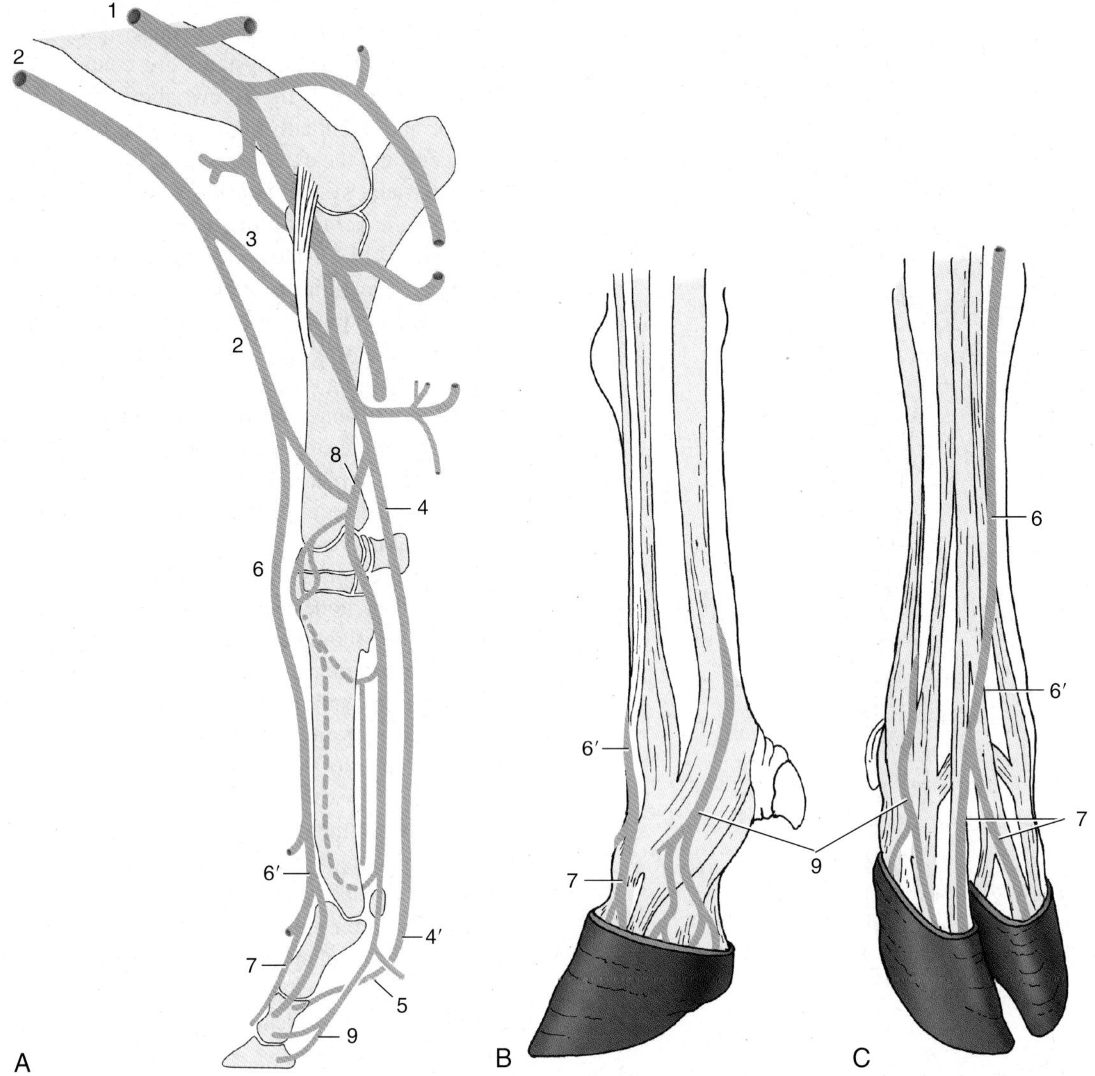

Fig. 30.14 The principal veins (vv.) of the bovine forelimb. (A) Right limb, medial view. (B) Left foot, lateral view. (C) Right foot, dorsal view. *1,* Brachial vein (v.); *2,* cephalic v.; *3,* median cubital v.; *4,* median v.; *4′,* palmar common digital v. III; *5,* axial palmar digital vv.; *6,* accessory cephalic v.; *6′,* dorsal common digital v. III; *7,* dorsal digital vv.; *8,* radial v.; *9,* abaxial palmar digital vv.

it is palpable in front of the brachial artery), and dips under the flexor muscles to which it sends branches. The much-reduced trunk then follows the median artery under cover of the flexor carpi radialis (Fig. 30.3/*2*) into the carpal canal before dividing in midmetacarpus into several branches that supply most of the palmar aspect of the foot.

The *ulnar nerve* (C8–T2) arises with the median nerve but diverges from this in midarm (Fig. 30.15/*15*). After releasing a branch to the skin, it passes toward the olecranon, where it dips between the origins of the flexor muscles. It detaches branches to these before continuing as a mainly sensory nerve (Fig. 30.3/*4′*) that divides a short distance above the accessory carpal bone. The *palmar branch* runs through the carpal canal lateral to the flexor tendons. The *dorsal branch* becomes superficial and may be palpated where it descends over the lateral aspect of the accessory carpal bone.

Because the median and ulnar nerves share in the supply of the carpal and digital flexors, destruction of either one has little effect on posture or gait. Even when both are sectioned, no immediate change in the appearance of the standing animal occurs, although overextension of the carpus develops later. Walking is affected by the double neurectomy and is performed with an exaggerated “goose-stepping” action in which the carpal and lower joints are

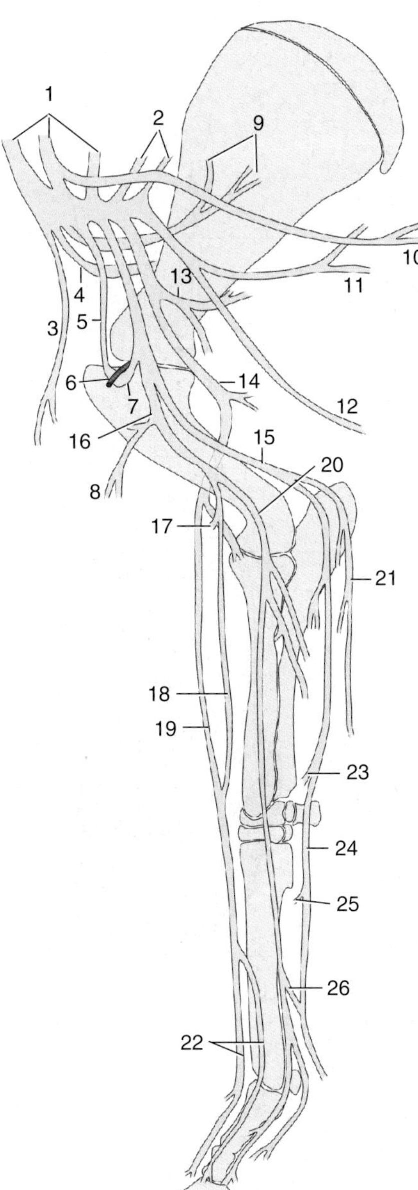

Fig. 30.15 Nerves of the bovine forelimb, medial view. *1* and *2,* Roots of brachial plexus; *3,* cranial pectoral nerve (n.), *4,* suprascapular n.; *5,* musculocutaneous n.; *6,* axillary artery; *7,* loop of musculocutaneous n. before joining median n.; *8,* proximal branch of musculocutaneous n.; *9,* subscapular n.; *10,* long thoracic n.; *11,* thoracodorsal n.; *12,* lateral thoracic n.; *13,* axillary n.; *14,* radial n.; *15,* ulnar n.; *16,* combined musculocutaneous and median nerves; *17,* distal branch of musculocutaneous n.; *18,* medial cutaneous antebrachial n.; *19,* superficial branch of radial n.; *20,* median n.; *21,* caudal cutaneous antebrachial n.; *22,* dorsal common digital nerves III and II; *23,* dorsal branch of ulnar n.; *24,* palmar branch of ulnar n.; *25,* deep branch of ulnar n. (to interosseous muscles); *26,* communicating branch.

overextended. However, the stride is not shortened, and the foot remains able to support weight.

The *radial nerve* (C7–T1) lies more caudally in the arm. It dives between the heads of the triceps before following the brachialis to reach the cranial surface of the elbow while furnishing muscular branches en route. The trunk is vulnerable as it passes over the sharp epicondyloid crest of the humerus deep to the lateral head of the triceps. In this position it divides into several branches that innervate the extensor muscles of the carpus and digits and a cutaneous branch that accompanies the cephalic and, more distally, the accessory cephalic vein. It is joined by a branch of the musculocutaneous nerve before crossing the carpus (Fig. 30.15/*18* and *19*). The radial nerve is the exclusive supply to the extensors of all joints distal to the shoulder, and the effects of injury in the proximal part of its course are correspondingly severe. The elbow is "dropped," and the limb appears to be abnormally long. The animal moves with difficulty, dragging the toes and taking no weight on the affected limb. It is unable to place the sole of the hoof on the ground and rests on the dorsal surfaces of the digits. If the damage is more distal, the animal can usually learn to compensate for the loss of carpal and digital extensor muscle function.

Nerve-blocking procedures, such as are widely used in equine practice, are not used for the differential diagnosis of lameness in cattle. Because the retrograde intravenous techniques used to secure anesthesia for the performance of digital surgery are now so popular, it seems unnecessary to supply detailed accounts of the digital nerves, which are available in reference texts.

In very brief summary, it may be stated that the dorsal aspect of the foot is the province of the radial nerve, the palmar aspect is the province of the median nerve, and the lateral aspect the province of the ulnar nerve (Fig. 30.16A–C).

COMPREHENSION CHECK

Compare the anatomy of the distal limb of the cow with that of the horse.

Does the loss of function of the radial nerve create deficits similar to those observed after resection of the ulnar and median nerves? Support your answer based on your knowledge of the anatomy.

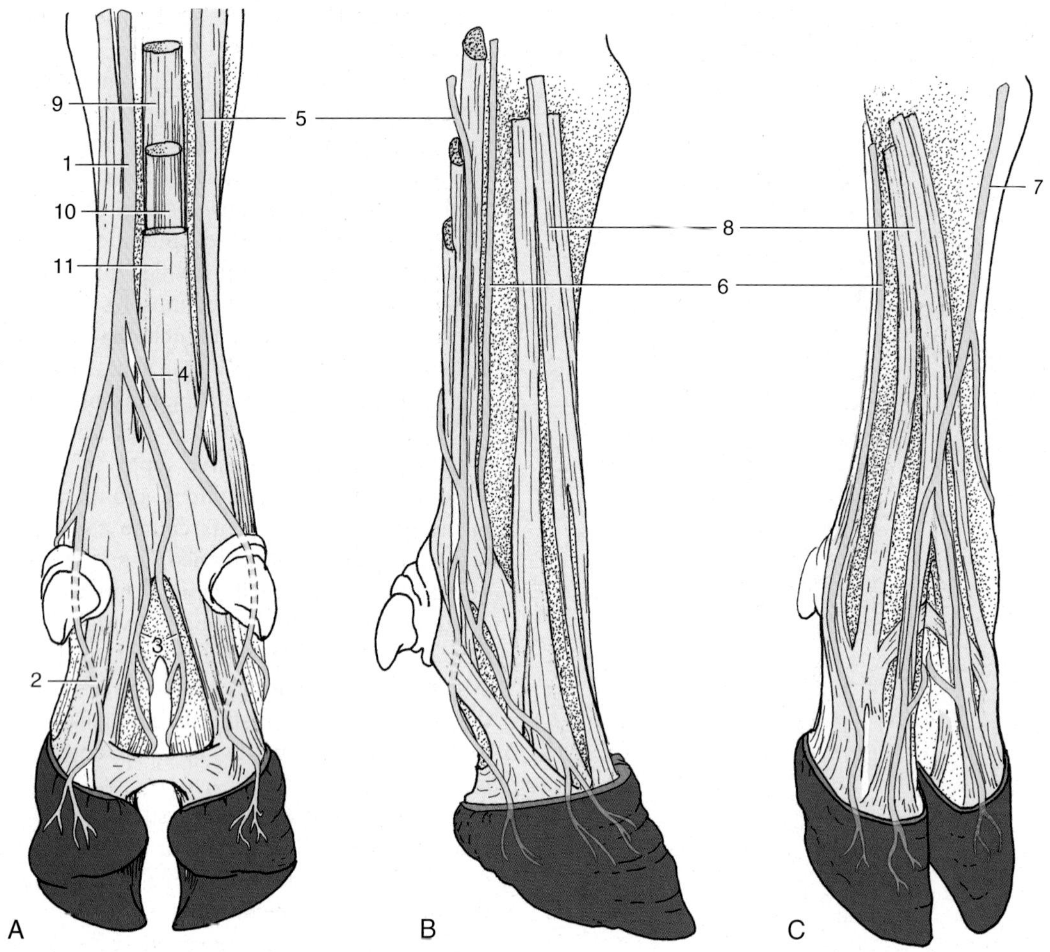

Fig. 30.16 The principal nerves of the bovine right forefoot in (A) palmar, (B) lateral, and (C) dorsal views. *1,* Median nerve (n.); *2,* palmar abaxial digital n.; *3,* palmar axial digital nerves; *4,* communicating branch; *5,* palmar branch of ulnar n.; *6,* dorsal branch of ulnar n.; *7,* superficial branch of radial n.; *8,* digital extensor tendons; *9,* interosseous muscle; *10,* deep flexor tendon; *11,* superficial flexor tendon.

The Hindlimb of the Ruminant

31

The angular appearance of the hindquarters of cattle is due in part to the robust formation of the *pelvic girdle,* much of which is outlined below the skin, and in part to the weak development of the muscles of the croup. The sacral tuber is palpable to the side of the lumbosacral space even though it fails to reach the height of the sacral crest. (Its occasional elevation above the crest prompts suspicion of sacroiliac dislocation.) This tuber is joined to the much more prominent coxal tuber ("hook bone") by the iliac crest, which is only thinly—and incompletely—covered by the gluteus medius (Figs. 31.1 and 31.2). The triangular ischial tuber ("pin bone") is raised considerably above the pelvic floor and projects largely or wholly above the vulva. Its subcutaneous dorsal angle is joined by the sacrotuberous ligament, which is readily palpable because of lack of muscle cover (Fig. 31.3/*1*).

The line connecting the coxal and ischial tubers reveals the slope of the pelvis. An angle larger than usual is associated with a more upright pelvic inlet. A smaller angle (flattened rump) makes the femur more vertical and may predispose to concussive trauma of the hip joint. The hip joint's position is deduced from the palpation of the greater trochanter situated lateral and slightly caudal to the femoral head, below the intertuberal line (Fig. 31.3/*2*). The disturbance of this relationship suggests fracture of the neck or dislocation of the head of the femur. Dislocation may occur in several directions and may be due to the relative weakness or occasional absence of the sole intra-articular ligament (ligamentum capitis). Most commonly the trochanter is displaced dorsocranially to project above the intertuberal line. This joint is nominally a ball-and-socket joint, but the extension of the femoral articular surface onto the semicylindrical neck makes it evident that flexion and extension must be the principal movements. However, the degree of outward rotation of the thigh that accompanies flexion ensures that the stifle is carried free of the abdomen. The cavity of the joint may be reached if a needle is inserted directly in front of the trochanter and is advanced medially and slightly cranially. The deep location and contractions of the muscle pierced en route make the procedure difficult to accomplish successfully.

Disorders of the Hip Joint: The hip joint may suffer from luxation, septic arthritis, or fracture of the head of the femur. Luxations occur more in a craniodorsal compared to a caudoventral direction; the latter will likely lodge the dislocated head of the femur in the obturator foramen.

The most striking features of the *regional muscles* are the relative weakness of the gluteal group and the absence of vertebral origins of the semitendinosus and semimembranosus. The gluteus superficialis is wholly incorporated within the biceps to form the combination sometimes known as *gluteobiceps.* The gluteus medius possesses a well-defined deep division (gluteus accessorius) with its own insertion tendon protected by a synovial bursa where it passes lateral to the greater trochanter. The *biceps* fills the caudolateral part of the thigh and has a wide insertion spread between the fascia lata, patella, lateral patellar ligament, and, via the crural fascia, the tibia and calcaneus. A large *bicipital bursa* intervenes between the lateral epicondyle of the femur and the part of the insertion proceeding to the patellar ligament. The bursa, which may communicate with the stifle joint cavity, is sometimes the site of a painful inflammation, most often encountered in cattle required to rest on bare concrete. The insertions of the semitendinosus and semimembranosus and the actions of the group follow the usual pattern.

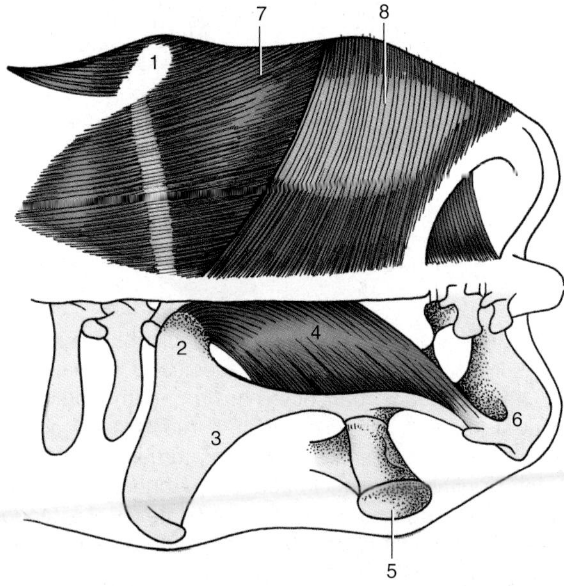

Fig. 31.1 Dorsal view of the bovine croup; the muscles on the left side have been removed. *1,* Coxal tuber; *2,* sacral tuber; *3,* ilium; *4,* sacrosciatic ligament; *5,* greater trochanter of femur; *6,* ischial tuber; *7,* gluteus medius; *8,* biceps.

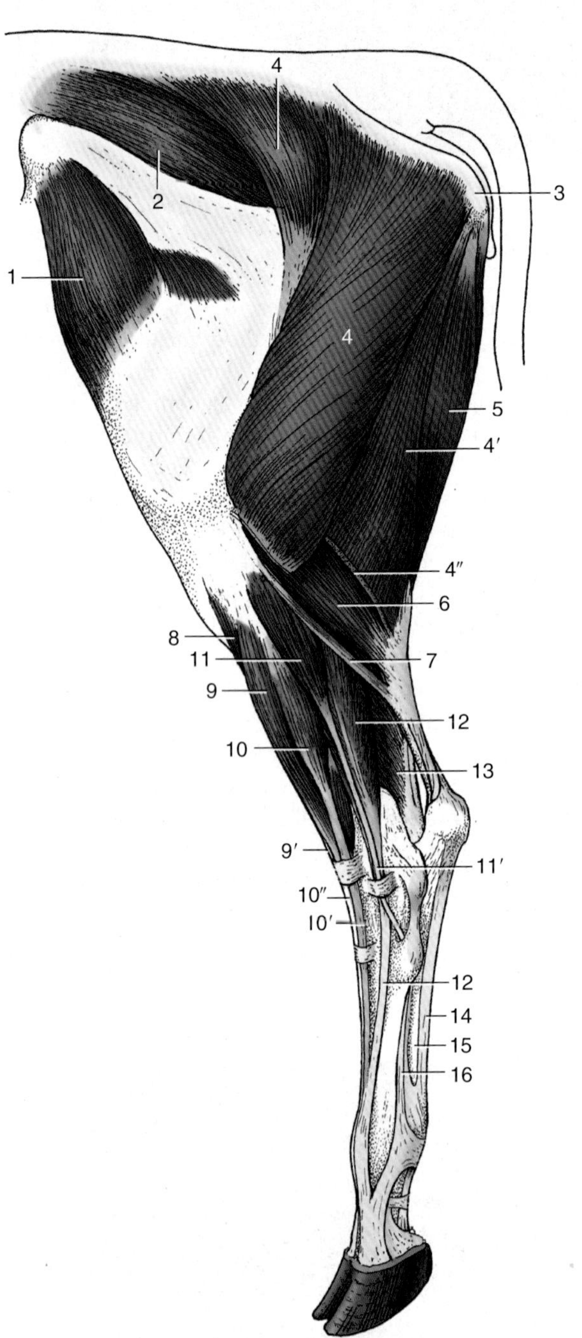

Fig. 31.2 Muscles of the bovine left hindlimb, lateral view. *1,* Tensor fasciae latae; *2,* gluteus medius; *3,* ischial tuber; *4, 4′,* and *4″,* biceps, transected at *4″*; *5,* semitendinosus; *6,* lateral head of gastrocnemius; *7,* rudimentary soleus; *8,* tibialis cranialis; *9* and *9′,* peroneus tertius; *10, 10′,* and *10″,* long digital extensor; *11* and *11′,* peroneus longus; *12,* lateral digital extensor; *13,* lateral digital flexor; *14,* tendon of superficial digital flexor; *15,* combined tendon of deep digital flexors; *16,* interosseous.

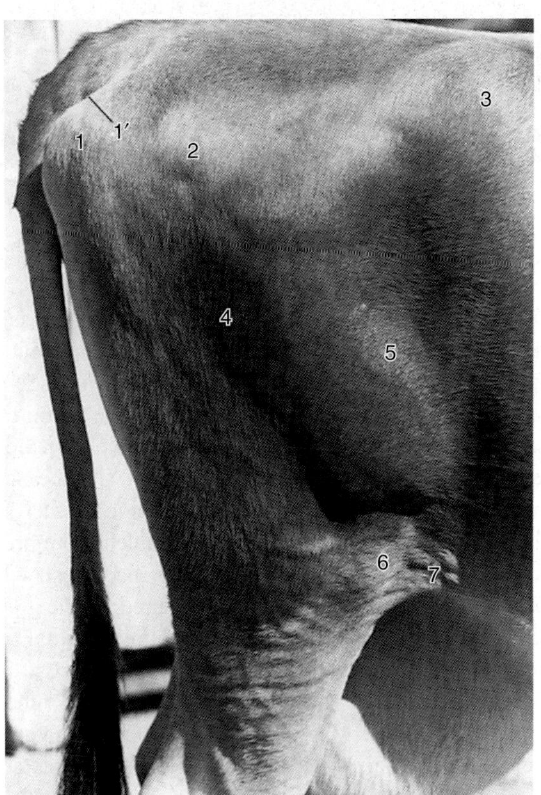

Fig. 31.3 Right bovine thigh. *1,* Ischial tuber; *1′,* sacrotuberous part of sacrosciatic ligament; *2,* greater trochanter of femur; *3,* coxal tuber; *4,* biceps; *5,* lateral vastus; *6,* patella; *7,* flank fold.

The adductor muscles of the medial thigh, the deep group about the hip joint, and the quadriceps femoris require no special notice. The tensor fasciae latae at the cranial margin of the thigh is a guide to the location of the subiliac lymph node.

THE STIFLE, LEG, AND HOCK

The stifle joint resembles that of the horse in possessing three patellar ligaments and an asymmetrical trochlea (Fig. 31.4B). The patella, patellar ligaments, and tibial tuberosity can be palpated on the cranial surface. Two palpable "dimples" at the proximal end of the tuberosity separate and conveniently identify the three ligaments. The prominent femoral epicondyle, collateral ligament (and its attachment to the rudimentary fibula; Fig. 31.4A/*9*), and, more cranially, the common origin of the long digital extensor and peroneus tertius (Fig. 31.4A/*5*) are palpable on the lateral aspect. As in the horse, the intermediate patellar ligament, the patella, a medial fibrocartilage, and the medial patellar ligament combine to form a loop that passes over the expanded proximal end of the medial ridge (Fig. 31.4B/*11*) of the femoral trochlea. Although relatively little muscular

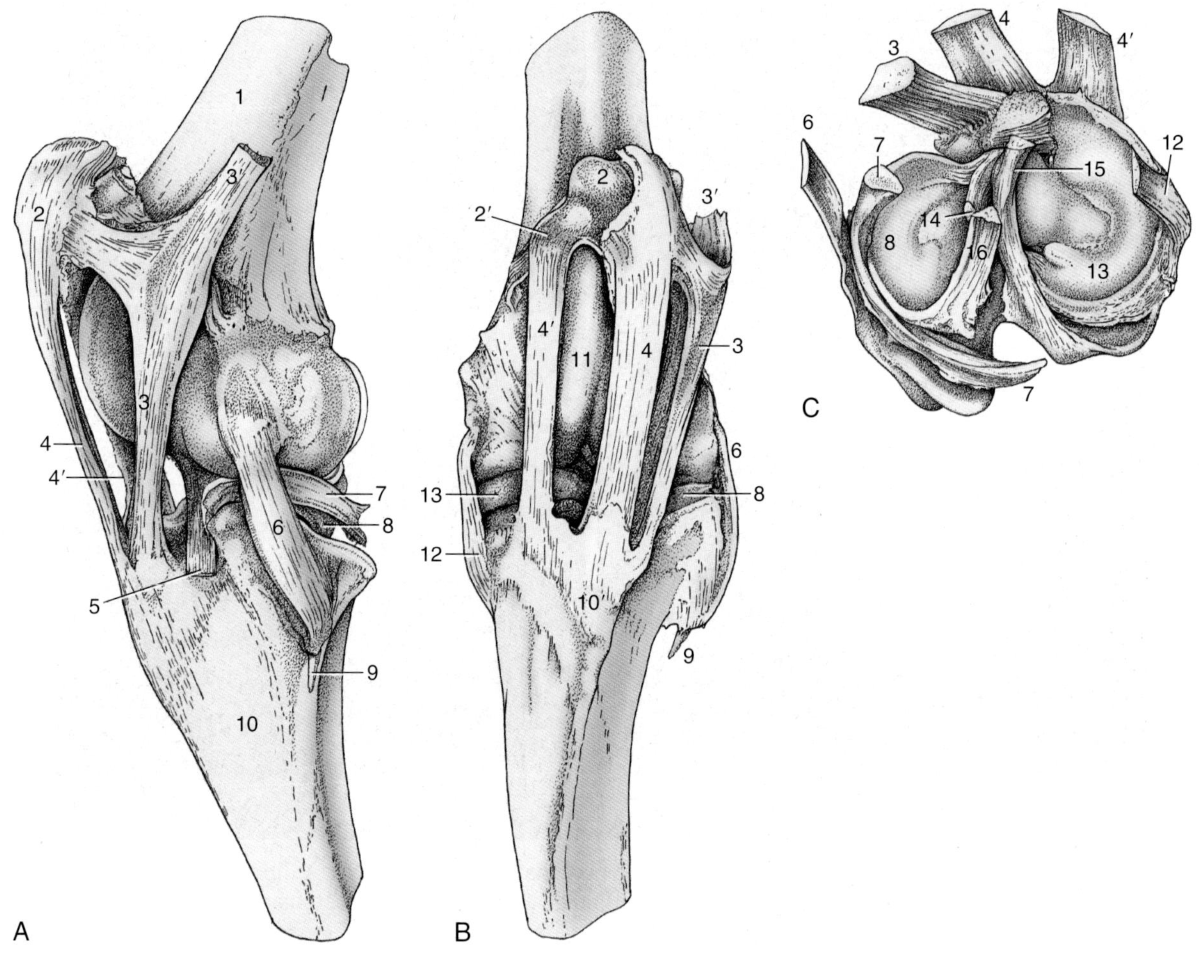

Fig. 31.4 The left bovine stifle joint. (A) Lateral view. (B) Cranial view. (C) The menisci and ligaments attaching on the proximal end of the left tibia. *1,* Femur; *2,* patella; *2′,* fibrocartilage of patella; *3,* lateral patellar ligament; *3′,* attachment of biceps; *4,* intermediate patellar ligament; *4′,* medial patellar ligament; *5,* combined tendon of long digital extensor and peroneus tertius; *6,* lateral collateral ligament; *7,* tendon of popliteus; *8,* lateral meniscus; *9,* fibula; *10,* tibia; *10′,* tibial tuberosity; *11,* medial ridge of femoral trochlea; *12,* medial collateral ligament; *13,* medial meniscus; *14,* cranial cruciate ligament; *15,* caudal cruciate ligament; *16,* meniscofemoral ligament.

effort keeps the loop in place (which prevents flexion of the stifle), the mechanism is by no means as efficient as that of the horse, in which the stifle can be fully locked. Lateral and medial luxations of the patella are occasionally reported.

Dorsal dislocation, better described as upward fixation of the patella, is rather common among working bullocks and water buffalo of the Indian subcontinent. The condition is usually intermittent, interferes with the gait, and, if not relieved spontaneously, may be treated by section of the medial patellar ligament.

The femoropatellar and medial femorotibial joint cavities always communicate, but the lateral femorotibial joint does not communicate with either of the other two. Two puncture sites are therefore in use. One, injection between the medial and intermediate patellar ligaments, a short distance proximal to the tibia, gives access to the femoropatellar space. The second site, in the extensor groove of the tibia, cranial to the common tendon of the long digital extensor and peroneus tertius, provides access to the lateral femorotibial compartment.

The *tibia* is the only weight-bearing bone of the leg (crus). Its medial surface, including the prominent medial malleolus, is subcutaneous, but the remaining surfaces are covered by muscle (see Fig. 31.6). The distal articular surface (cochlea) presents two sagittal grooves, each bounded by a malleolus, separated by a ridge. The *fibula* is much reduced. A proximal rudiment, generally drawn into a distal point, is fused with the lateral condyle of the tibia and

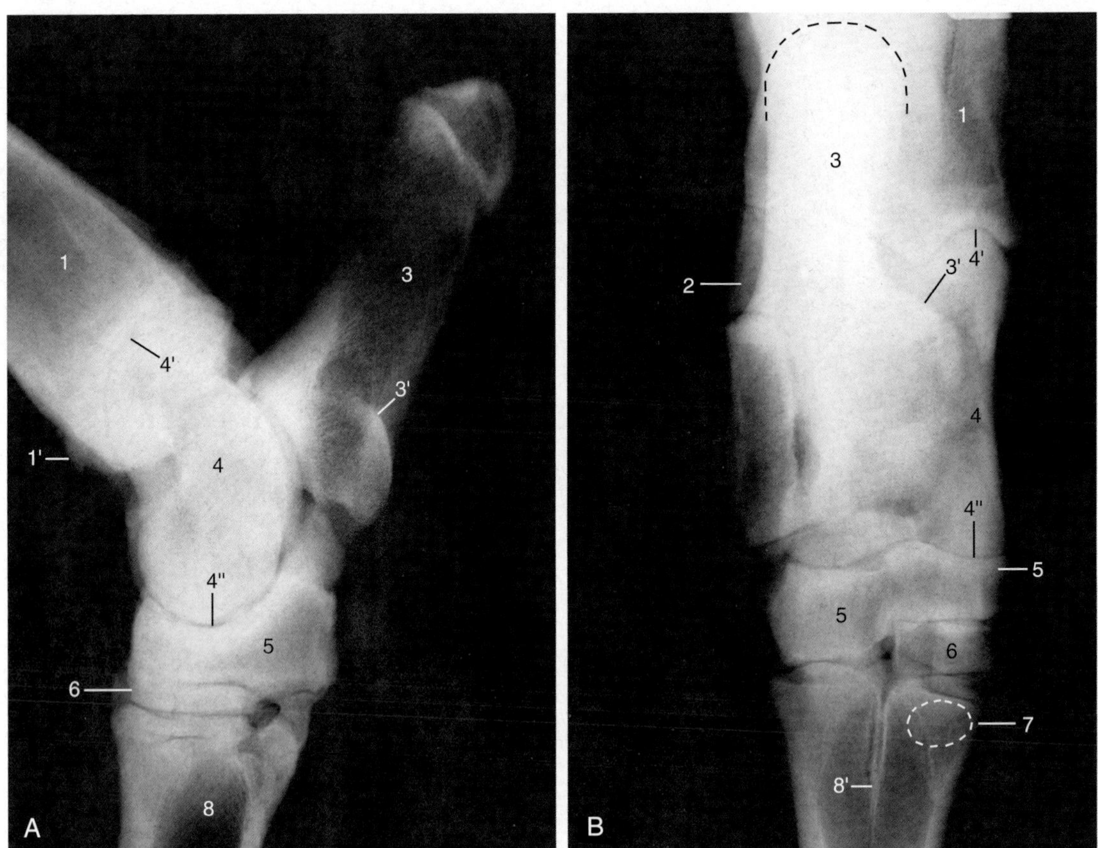

Fig. 31.5 (A) Lateral and (B) dorsoplantar radiographs of the bovine hock. *1*, Tibia; *1′*, medial malleolus; *2*, lateral malleolus (distal end of fibula); *3*, calcaneus; *3′*, sustentaculum tali; *4*, talus; *4′* and *4″*, proximal and distal trochleae of talus, respectively, *5*, fused central and fourth tarsal bones; *6*, fused second and third tarsal bones, in (B) superimposed on small first tarsal bone (not labeled); *7*, position of sesamoid bone in interosseous; *8*, metatarsal bone; *8′*, median septum.

receives the lateral collateral ligament of the stifle. The distal rudiment is a separate (and palpable) quadrilateral bone (lateral malleolus; Fig. 31.5/*2*) that articulates securely with the tibia by means of an interlocking spike and groove. It also takes part in the formation of the hock joint.

The *tarsal skeleton* is formed by the following elements: calcaneus and talus in the proximal row, fused central and fourth bones in the intermediate row, and fused second and third bones and a small independent first bone in the distal row (see Fig. 2.60). In marked contrast to that of the horse, the talus carries a trochlea at each end (as in artiodactyls generally; Fig. 31.5/*4′* and *4″*). The proximal trochlea articulates with the tibial cochlea and malleolar bone, forming the tarsocrural joint. The distal trochlea articulates with the calcaneus behind and the fused central and fourth tarsal bones distally, forming the proximal intertarsal joint. Both joints engage in flexion and extension as the principal movements at the hock, but the proximal joint has the greater excursions. The *calcaneus,* more slender than the equine bone, has an additional articulation with the lateral malleolus. The tuber calcanei (point of hock) is slightly expanded. The combined *central and fourth tarsals* (Fig. 31.5/*5*) span the breadth of the hock. The part provided by the fourth tarsal extends into the distal row and articulates with the metatarsal bone. It is related to the *fused second and third bones* on its medial side. The small *first tarsal* lies on the plantar aspect of the joint. The surfaces of the distal elements that concur in the formation of the distal intertarsal and tarsometatarsal joints are relatively flat and permit minimal movement. A small discoid sesamoid bone on the plantar surface of the metatarsal bone is embedded in the proximal part of the interosseous (Fig. 31.5B/*7*).

The tarsocrural and proximal intertarsal articulations share a common and relatively capacious cavity. When enlarged, the capsule pouches noticeably on the dorsomedial aspect of the hock, medial to the tibialis cranialis tendon and directly distal to the medial malleolus. It can be punctured more safely than in the horse because the pouch is not overlain by a vein. The other joints are rarely of clinical concern.

There are many ligaments of the hock joint, but only a few are individually important. The long and palpable collateral ligaments extend the respective malleolus to the metatarsus and facilitate hinge movement. The long plantar ligament (palpable on the plantaromedial aspect) follows the plantar border of the calcaneus and extends beyond this to the metatarsus. This ligament unites the bones on the plantar aspect that would otherwise be pulled apart by the powerful muscles attaching on the point of the hock.

The conformation of the hindlimb, particularly the hock, is important in the selection of animals for breeding. The points of the hock should be vertically below the ischial tubers in both lateral and caudal views. If they are too close the animal is said to be "cow-hocked", and its feet assume a wide stance. An adaptation to an overlarge udder is one cause of an exaggerated approximation of the points of the hocks. (The opposite bowlegged conformation brings the feet close together.) The normal angle of the hock joint (viewed from the side) is about 140 degrees, which gives the metatarsus a slightly forward inclination. When the angle is noticeably smaller, the hock sinks and the animal is said to be "sickle-hocked"; when it exceeds the normal, the animal is said to be "straight-hocked," a defect that may lead to "weak pasterns" because of the reduced angle at the fetlock joint. Abnormal postures of the hock cause faulty footing and risk damage to the tendons and synovial structures of the digits

The *muscles of the leg* are divided into the usual craniolateral and caudal groups. Among the former, the *tibialis cranialis* and *peroneus tertius* broadly resemble those of the horse (Fig. 31.2/*8* and *9*). The peroneus tertius, though largely tendinous, is yet significantly fleshier than its equine equivalent. The *long digital extensor* resembles the common extensor of the forelimb in possessing two bellies: one supplies the tendon proper to the medial digit, while the tendon of a second, smaller one splits to reach both digits. There is also a *lateral extensor* (Fig. 31.2/*12*), proper to the lateral digit. All extensor tendons are of necessity held in place by (two) stout, palpable retention bands and also protected by synovial sheaths where they descend over the flexor surface of the hock. The proximal retinaculum is easily palpated even in heavy, thick-skinned cows. The group is completed by a *peroneus longus* muscle (Fig. 31.2/*11*) that arises near the lateral collateral ligament of the stifle and descends on the lateral side of the leg. It then crosses over the tendon of the lateral digital extensor to wind around to insert on the plantar aspect of the hock. Some inward rotation of the foot is produced by its contraction.

The *gastrocnemius* (Fig. 31.2/*6*) arises by twin heads from the caudal surface of the femur and forms a muscular swelling at the upper end of the leg before narrowing abruptly to the strong tendon that inserts on the point of the hock.

The *superficial digital flexor,* though more muscular than that of the horse, is very tendinous and relatively inextensible (Fig. 31.6/*14*). It arises between the heads of the gastrocnemius, winds around the medial surface of that muscle's tendon, and spreads to cap the point of the hock. The edges of the cap attach here, but the bulk of the tendon continues down the plantar surface into the foot. The crural segment, acting in concert with the peroneus tertius, links the movements of the stifle and hock joints. (This needs to be kept in mind when attempting to correct the breech position of a fetus that presents the tail and flexed hocks.) An extensive subtendinous (calcanean) bursa protects the tendon both where it wraps around the gastrocnemius and again over the point of the hock. Occasionally a subcutaneous bursa (hygroma) develops over the tendon here.

The gastrocnemius and superficial flexor are in a continuous (reflex) state of contraction in calves with "spastic paresis." In these animals the hock and stifle are maximally extended, and the affected limb is used stiffly with only the toes of the hoofs touching the ground (Fig. 31.7). Section of the tendons (or of the [tibial] nerve branches to the

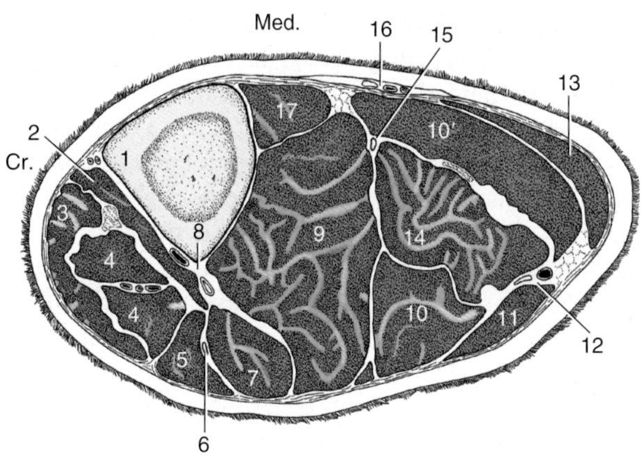

Fig. 31.6 Transverse section of the left bovine leg. *Cr.*, Cranial; *Med.*, medial; *1*, tibia; *2*, tibialis cranialis; *3*, peroneus tertius; *4*, long digital extensor; *5*, peroneus longus; *6*, peroneal nerve; *7*, lateral digital extensor; *8*, cranial tibial vessels; *9*, deep digital flexors; *10* and *10′*, lateral and medial heads of gastrocnemius, respectively; *11*, biceps; *12*, caudal cutaneous sural nerve and lateral saphenous vein; *13*, semitendinosus; *14*, superficial digital flexor; *15*, tibial nerve; *16*, saphenous vessels and nerve; *17*, popliteus.

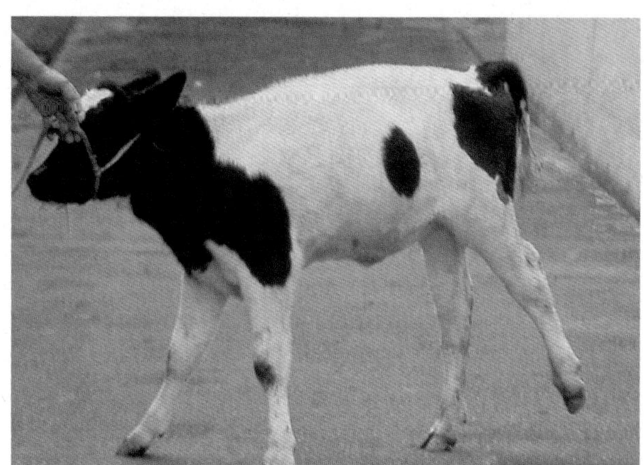

Fig. 31.7 Calf with spastic paresis.

gastrocnemius) gives relief. Although there is no proof of inheritance, it is generally agreed that it is unwise to breed from affected animals even after surgical "cure."

The *deep digital flexor* (Fig. 31.6/*9*) has three heads. Two come together in the leg to form a thick tendon that passes over the plantar surface of the hock medial to the calcaneus and is protected by the tarsal synovial sheath. The tendon is bound down by the flexor retinaculum and other deep fasciae so that, when distended, the sheath bulges only at its ends, proximal and distal to the joint. The thin tendon of the third head tunnels through the dense medial tarsal fascia, within its own synovial investment, to join the major tendon in the metatarsus. The *popliteus* has no special features.

Most locomotor and cutaneous structures of the hindfoot are very similar to their forelimb counterparts and need not be described. However, the metatarsal bone is noticeably longer than the metacarpal and is quadrilateral in transverse section, which gives the hind cannon a deeper appearance in lateral view (see Fig. 31.14). The higher incidence of disease in the digits of the hindlimb, especially the lateral one, has not been fully explained.

THE BLOOD VESSELS AND LYMPHATIC STRUCTURES OF THE HINDLIMB

The femoral artery continues the *external iliac artery* beyond the vascular lacuna. It passes between the medial muscles of the thigh to reach the flexor surface of the stifle, where it is renamed the *popliteal artery*. This soon divides into cranial and caudal tibial arteries (Fig. 31.8/*10* and *11*). One branch of the femoral, the *saphenous artery* (Fig. 31.8/*7*), runs on the surface of the gracilis and is often used for taking the pulse of cows by sliding the hand from behind, between the udder and thigh. This vessel is responsible for the vascularization of the caudal part of the leg and follows the common calcanean tendon to the hock, where it gives rise to medial and lateral plantar arteries.

The *cranial tibial artery* (Fig. 31.6/*8*), which may be regarded as the continuation of the femoral trunk, runs embedded between the crural muscles to reach the flexor (dorsal) surface of the hock joint under cover of the long digital extensor tendon. The caudal tibial artery is of minor local significance.

Renamed the *dorsal metatarsal artery* (Fig. 31.8/*12*), the main trunk now sends a perforating artery through the upper part of the metatarsal bone before continuing in the dorsal groove of this bone. A second perforating artery is released toward the fetlock. The perforating branches join the plantar arteries and are also connected by small deeper vessels. The *plantar arteries* resemble the corresponding forelimb vessels. One branch of the medial plantar artery crosses the plantar surface of the medial tendon of the superficial flexor proximal to the fetlock and is here liable to injury.

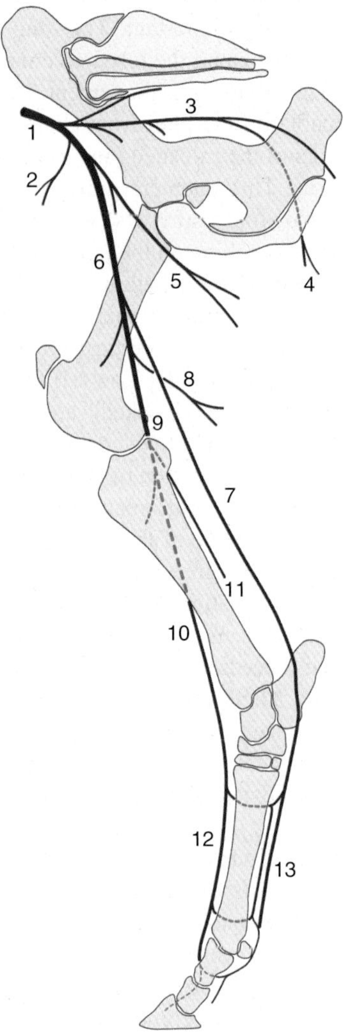

Fig. 31.8 The principal arteries of the bovine right hindlimb, medial view. *1,* External iliac artery (a.); *2,* deep circumflex iliac a.; *3,* internal iliac a.; *4,* caudal gluteal a.; *5,* deep femoral a.; *6,* femoral a.; *7,* saphenous a.; *8,* caudal femoral a.; *9,* popliteal a.; *10,* cranial tibial a.; *11,* caudal tibial a.; *12,* dorsal metatarsal arteries; *13,* medial and lateral plantar and metatarsal (closer to the bone) arteries.

This branch continues into the interdigital space, where it anastomoses with the main trunk. The anastomosis is substantial and winds around below the proximal interdigital ligament, where it is encountered in amputation of a digit. The axial surfaces of the digits are supplied by branches arising from the anastomosis. The abaxial surfaces are supplied by direct continuations of the plantar arteries. There are a large number of other anastomoses that do not merit description here.

The *veins* are divided between a deep system satellite to the arteries and a few superficial vessels that follow independent courses (Fig. 31.9). The superficial vessels comprise the medial and lateral saphenous veins and their tributaries. The larger *lateral saphenous vein* (Fig. 31.9A/*9*)

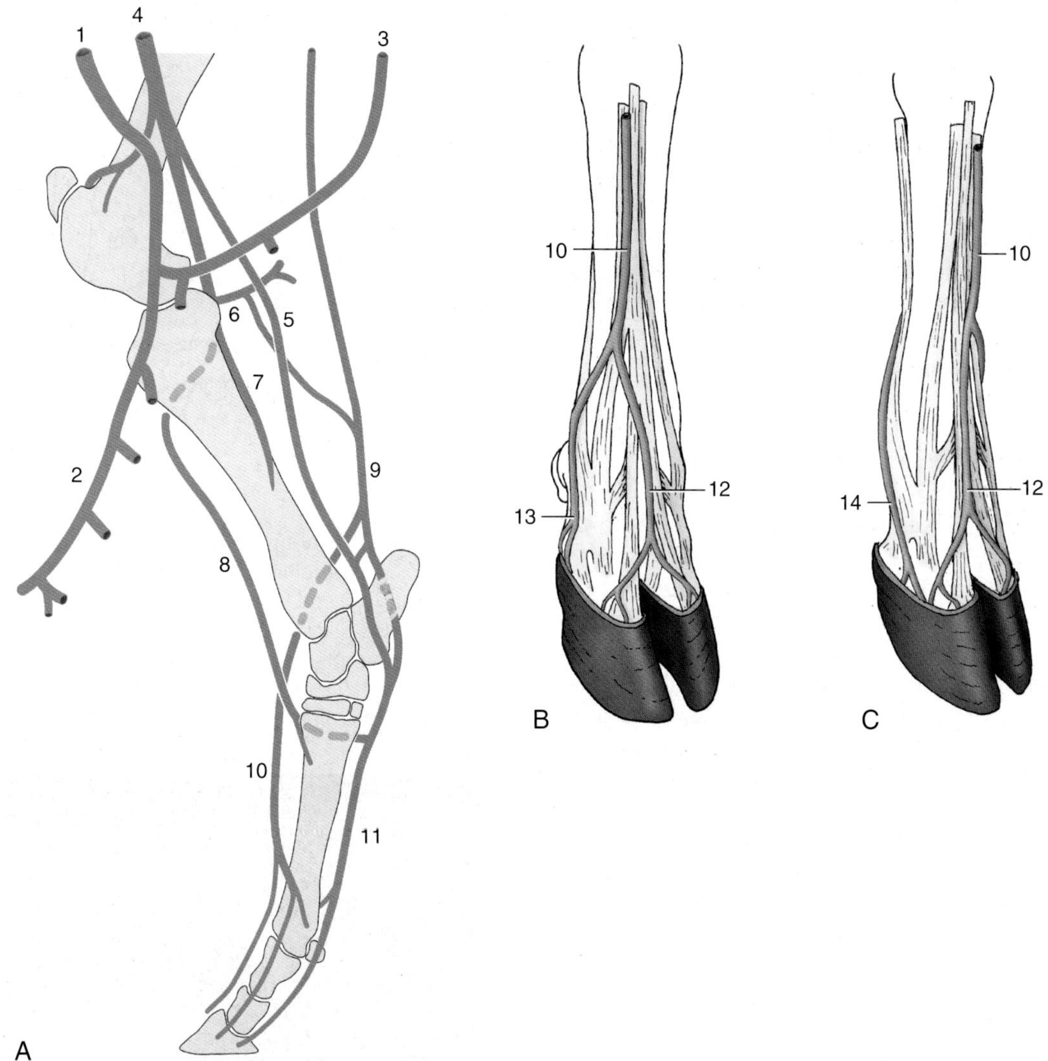

Fig. 31.9 The major veins of the bovine hindlimb. (A) Right limb, medial view. (B) Right hindfoot, dorsolateral view. (C) Left hindfoot, dorsomedial view. *1,* External pudendal vein (v.); *2,* mammary v.; *3,* ventral labial v.; *4,* femoral v.; *5,* medial saphenous v.; *6,* caudal femoral v.; *7,* caudal tibial v.; *8,* cranial tibial v.; *9,* lateral saphenous v.; *10,* cranial tributary of lateral saphenous v.; *11,* medial and lateral plantar veins; *12,* dorsal common digital v. III, *13,* plantar v. of lateral digit; *14,* plantar v. of medial digit.

arises from two tributaries: one ascends with the extensor tendons and superficial peroneal nerve and crosses on the dorsolateral aspect of the hock, and the other ascends with the lateral plantar artery from a subcutaneous origin on the lateral digit and follows the flexor tendons under cover of the deep fascia to cross the joint plantarolaterally. The lateral saphenous vein raises a ridge below the skin as it crosses to the caudal border of the leg and then follows the curvature of the gastrocnemius, eventually to open into the femoral vein. The *medial saphenous vein* (Fig. 31.9A/*5*) is also formed by two tributaries. The more important caudal one takes its origin from the abaxial aspect of the medial digit, ascends with the medial plantar artery, and passes the hock plantaromedially. The medial saphenous vein ascends together with the palpable saphenous artery on the medial aspect of the leg to dip between the gracilis and sartorius muscles to join the femoral vein.

The superficial veins (Fig. 31.9B and C) may be raised by application of a tourniquet below the hock for injection of local anesthetic so that the digits may be desensitized.

The *lymph nodes* include the *popliteal node* within the popliteal fossa and the very large *subiliac node* described with the abdominal wall (Fig. 31.10/*9* and *10*). A small *coxal node* ventral to the coxal tuber and a group of *gluteal nodes* on the lateral surface of the sacrosciatic ligament are also commonly present (Fig. 31.10/*2* and *5*). An *ischial node* (Fig. 31.10/*6*) that lies on the ligament just dorsal to the lesser sciatic foramen can be inspected in the split carcass by incision of the ligament from within the pelvis. A *tuberal node* (Fig. 31.10/*7*) lies medial to the ischial tuber within the ischiorectal fossa.

The *popliteal node* collects from the distal part of the limb, including most of the leg, and sends its efferent vessels along two routes: one follows the sciatic nerve to the ischial node, and the second accompanies the femoral vessels to the large, *deep inguinal node* (Fig. 31.10/*4*) at the side of the pelvic inlet. The *subiliac node* drains the skin over the thigh and stifle in addition to the flank; its efferents also go chiefly to the deep inguinal node. The smaller nodes are only of local significance.

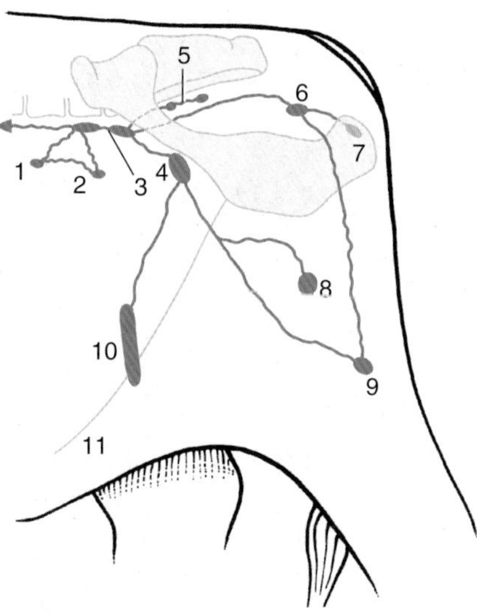

Fig. 31.10 The lymph nodes of the bovine pelvis and hindlimb. *1,* Lateral iliac lymph node; *2,* coxal lymph node; *3,* medial iliac and sacral lymph nodes; *4,* deep inguinal lymph node; *5,* gluteal lymph node; *6,* ischial lymph node; *7,* tuberal lymph node; *8,* superficial inguinal (mammary) lymph node; *9,* popliteal lymph node; *10,* subiliac lymph node; *11,* linea alba.

THE NERVES OF THE HINDLIMB

The lumbosacral plexus and its branches adhere to the common pattern. The *obturator nerve* (L4–L6) crosses the ventral surface of the sacroiliac joint, runs medial to the shaft of the ilium, and passes through the obturator foramen to reach the adductor muscles of the thigh. It is vulnerable where it lies against bone, and the most common cause of injury is compression during parturition. Conduction is rarely completely interrupted in this injury; cows can still stand and walk on rough ground even when both nerves have been damaged. However, they cannot prevent their feet sliding sideways on smooth floors and, once down, are often unable to rise (Fig. 31.11). The role of obturator nerve injury in postparturient paralysis (the "downer cow" syndrome) has probably been exaggerated; insufficient attention has been directed toward traumatic or ischemic injury to the adductor muscles ventral to the pelvis as alternative or aggravating causes. These muscles may suffer from direct compression or through constriction of their blood supply in prolonged recumbency.

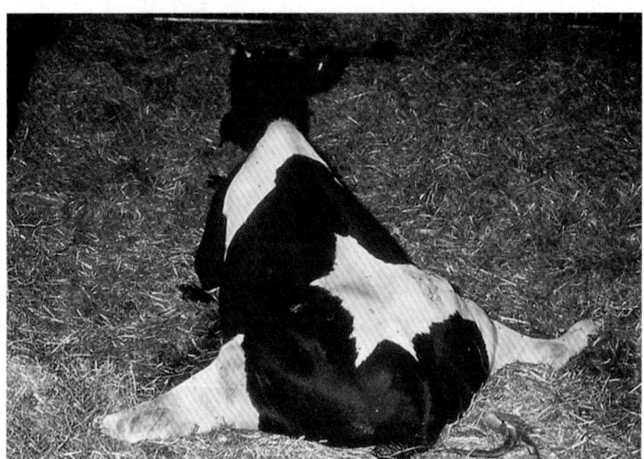

Fig. 31.11 Bilateral obturator paralysis.

The *femoral nerve* (L4–L6) (Fig. 31.12A) ramifies in the quadriceps after detaching the saphenous branch, which supplies skin over the medial aspect of the limb from midthigh to midmetatarsus. Damage to this nerve is occasionally encountered in newborn calves that were delivered by strong traction on the hindlimbs. An affected limb is unable to bear weight, and the diagnosis is confirmed by the loss of sensation in the appropriate area (Table 31.1).

Leaving the pelvis, the *sciatic nerve* (L6–S2) winds around the dorsal and caudal aspects of the hip joint before supplying the caudal muscles of the thigh. Its course between the biceps and semimembranosus, a few centimeters caudal to the femur, exposes it to risk of damage from careless intramuscular injection. Before reaching the gastrocnemius, it divides into tibial and common peroneal nerves, which share responsibility for the innervation of all structures below the stifle, except the medial skin territory of the saphenous nerve. The sciatic nerve may also be damaged at the birth of an overlarge or ill-positioned calf. When the injury is severe, the affected limb hangs loose, and the stifle and hock joints are extended, the digital joints flexed, and the foot knuckled. Cutaneous sensation is lost over most of the extremity.

The *tibial nerve* (L6–S2) passes between the heads of the gastrocnemius and at once detaches branches to the caudal muscles of the leg (Fig. 31.12A), including those that are severed in the treatment of spastic paresis (see earlier). Severe lesions of this nerve are manifested by overflexion of the hock and overextension of the fetlock, resulting in a vertical pastern. Because the digital extensors are not affected, the hooves are correctly set down as the animal walks, and they continue to bear their share of

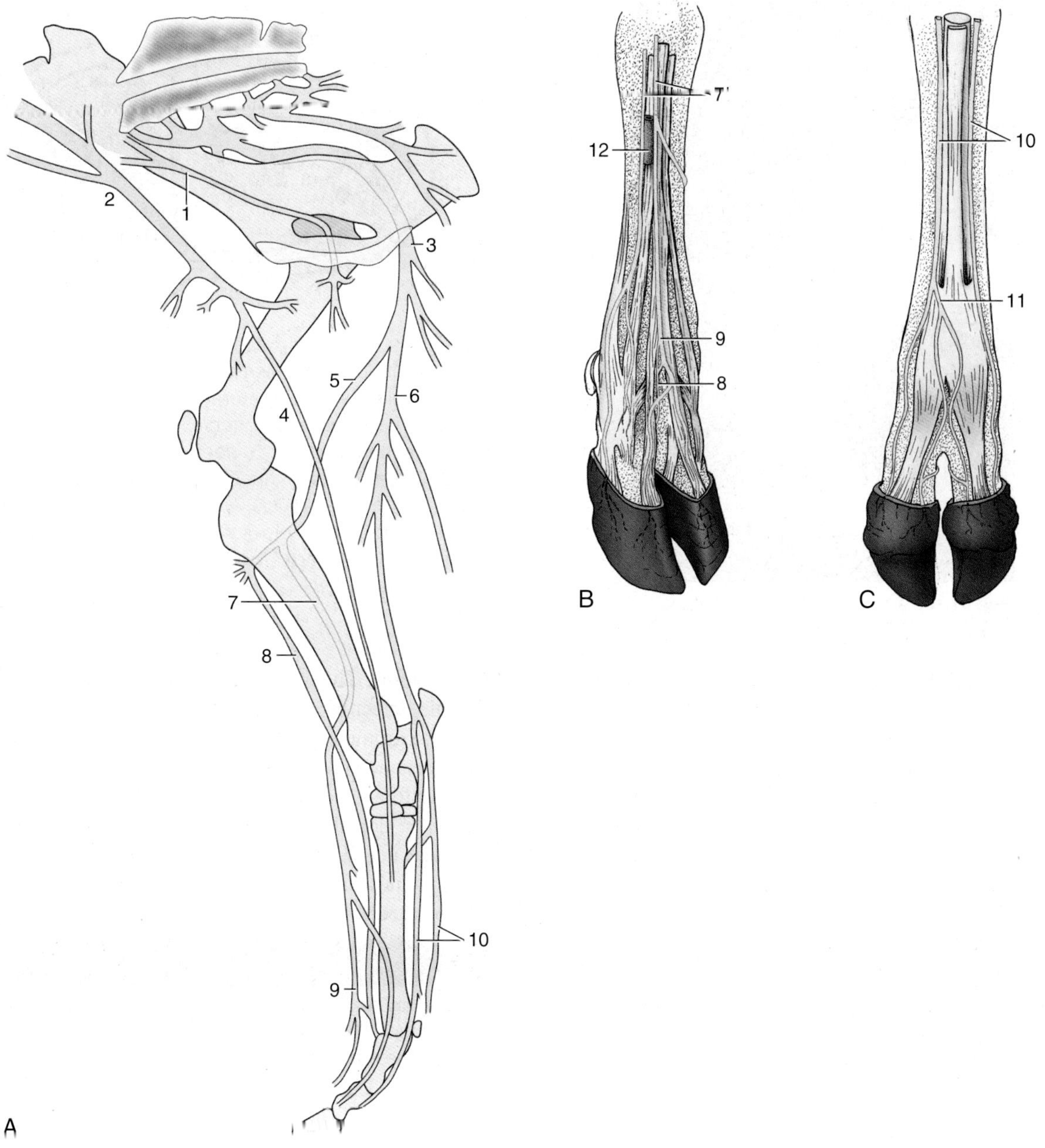

Fig. 31.12 Nerves of the right bovine hindlimb. (A) Medial view. (B) Right hindfoot, dorsolateral view. (C) Right hindfoot, plantar view. *1,* Obturator nerve (n.); *2,* femoral n.; *3,* sciatic n.; *4,* saphenous n.; *5,* common peroneal n.; *6,* tibial n.; *7,* superficial peroneal n.; *7',* lateral and middle branches of superficial peroneal n.; *8,* deep peroneal n.; *9,* dorsal common digital n. III; *10,* medial and lateral plantar nerves; *11,* plantar common digital n. III; *12,* cranial tributary of lateral saphenous vein.

TABLE 31.1 **DEFICITS RELATED TO INJURY TO HINDLIMB NERVES**

Nerve	Deficits if Damaged
Femoral nerve	Inability to bear weight
Sciatic nerve	If the injury is severe, the limb hangs loose; the stifle and hock joints are extended, the digital joints flexed, and the foot knuckled Loss of cutaneous sensation because the saphenous branch may be damaged
Tibial nerve	Overflexion of the hock and overextension of the fetlock, but digital extensors are affected, leading to the foot resting on its dorsal surface
Common peroneal nerve	Overextension of the hock and overflexion of the joints distal to the hock

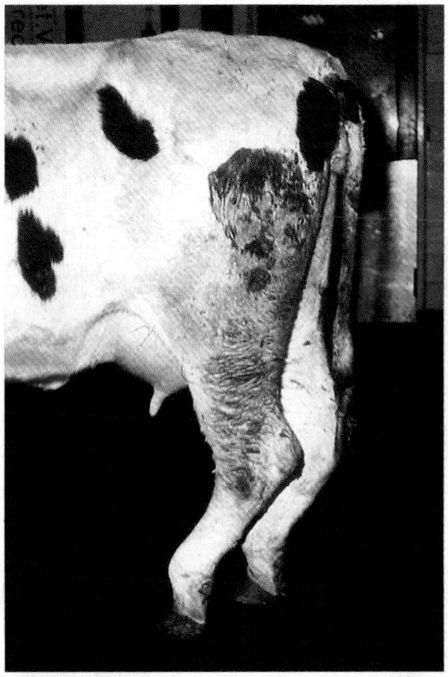

Fig. 31.13 Cow with peroneal paralysis.

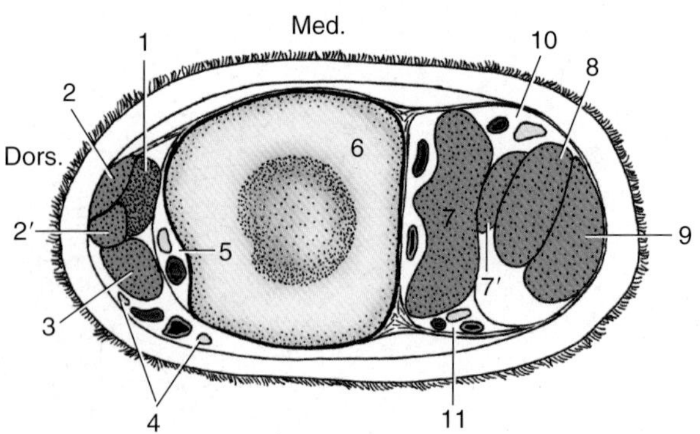

Fig. 31.14 Transverse section of the bovine left cannon. *Dors.*, Dorsal; *Med.*, medial; *1*, extensor brevis; *2* and *2′*, long digital extensor; *3*, lateral digital extensor; *4*, branches of superficial peroneal nerve and cranial tributary of lateral saphenous vein; *5*, deep peroneal nerve and dorsal metatarsal artery (continuation of cranial tibial); *6*, metatarsal bone; *7*, interosseous; *7′*, band from interosseous to superficial digital flexor; *8*, deep digital flexor; *9*, superficial digital flexor; *10* and *11*, medial and lateral plantar nerves and vessels.

weight at rest. The anomalous attitude of the joints is exaggerated at the walk.

The *common peroneal nerve* (L6–S2) crosses the gastrocnemius under cover of the biceps to become palpable (and vulnerable) where it passes behind the lateral collateral ligament of the stifle joint. It then sinks between the peroneus longus and the lateral digital extensor before dividing into *deep and superficial branches.* The larger superficial peroneal nerve crosses deep to the peroneus longus to enter the foot. The deep peroneal nerve supplies the dorsal crural muscles, among which it is embedded, and also enters the foot. Paralysis of the common peroneal is betrayed by overextension of the hock and overflexion of the more distal joints (Fig. 31.13). Unless passively set down correctly, the limb rests on the dorsal surface of the flexed digits. The animal eventually learns to compensate for this defect by flicking the foot forward before placing it on the ground.

The same considerations apply to the digital nerves of the hindfoot as to those of the forefoot. In very brief summary, the dorsal aspect of the foot is the province of the peroneal nerve, and the plantar aspect is the province of the tibial nerve; there is some overlapping to the sides (Fig. 31.14; see also Fig. 31.12B).

COMPREHENSION CHECK

Develop an integrated model to demonstrate the actions of the bones, muscles, and nerves that are critical to the stability of the stifle.

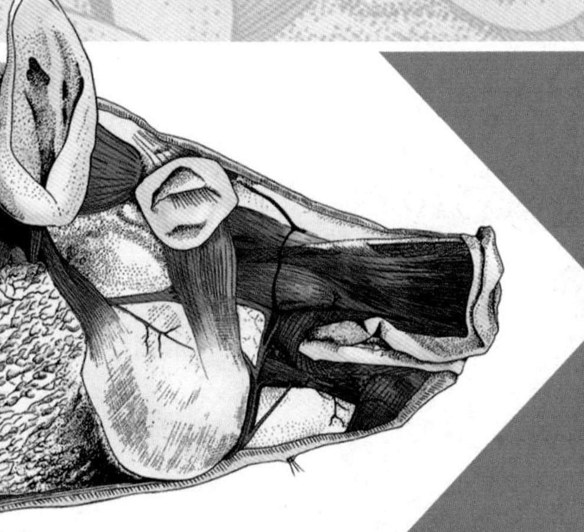

Part V

Pigs

32 The Head and Ventral Neck of the Pig

The way in which most pigs are reared today results in veterinary attention being concentrated on infectious diseases and other matters affecting the herd rather than on conditions affecting the individual animal. The short life span of usually 5 or 6 months generally allowed to pigs makes many interventions uneconomic. In addition, clinical examination of individual animals may be difficult because of the thick layer of subcutaneous fat (panniculus adipose) and the frequently aggressive disposition of older animals. A wide knowledge of the anatomy of the pig is therefore less necessary than it is for most other species. However, pigs are being increasingly used in biomedical research. Therefore, succinct description of their comparative anatomy is sufficient for the purpose of this book.

CONFORMATION AND SUPERFICIAL FEATURES

The head and neck together form a cone that blends with the trunk at the level of the forelimbs. The skull of primitive breeds, as of the ancestral wild form, is more or less pyramidal, but that of most improved breeds sweeps sharply upward to a prominence that rises well above the brain (Fig. 32.1). The dorsal surface of the cranium is bounded caudally by a thick nuchal crest and demarcated from the temporal fossa to each side by a prominent temporal line that continues into the zygomatic process of the frontal bone. This process, relatively short, fails to meet the zygomatic arch, which completes the margin of the small orbit (see Fig. 32.8). The arch is extremely sturdy and carries the wide, flat articular surface and, more rostrally, the depression from which the levator labii superioris arises.

On the basal surface, the cranial and choanal regions of the skull are dorsal to the plane of the palate. The large paracondylar processes and tympanic bullae are prominent features of the cranium. The body of the stout, rather rectilinear mandible is cut away in adaptation to the rooting habit. The mandibular symphysis ossifies at about 1 year.

The *most striking feature* of the head is the rostrum, or snout, the disklike and mobile tip of the muzzle that incorporates the middle part of the upper lip and is perforated by the rounded nostrils (Fig. 32.2). The snout is supported by a small rostral bone set against the end of the nasal septum that gives attachment to the levator labii superioris (Fig. 32.3/*3*), the muscle principally concerned with movements of the snout. Pigs allowed access to open ground are generally "ringed" through the upper margin of the snout to discourage the rooting habit, a practice more frequently required in former times than today. The lips are short and rather immobile; the upper one is notched to accommodate the projecting canine tooth (tusk).

The small *eyes* are deeply placed and, uniquely among domestic species, lack a tapetum lucidum and therefore are not reflective of light. A deep lacrimal gland is associated with the third eyelid in the ventromedial angle of the orbit. Together with the retrobulbar muscles, it is engulfed by an orbital venous sinus that may be punctured at the medial angle of the eye by directing a needle

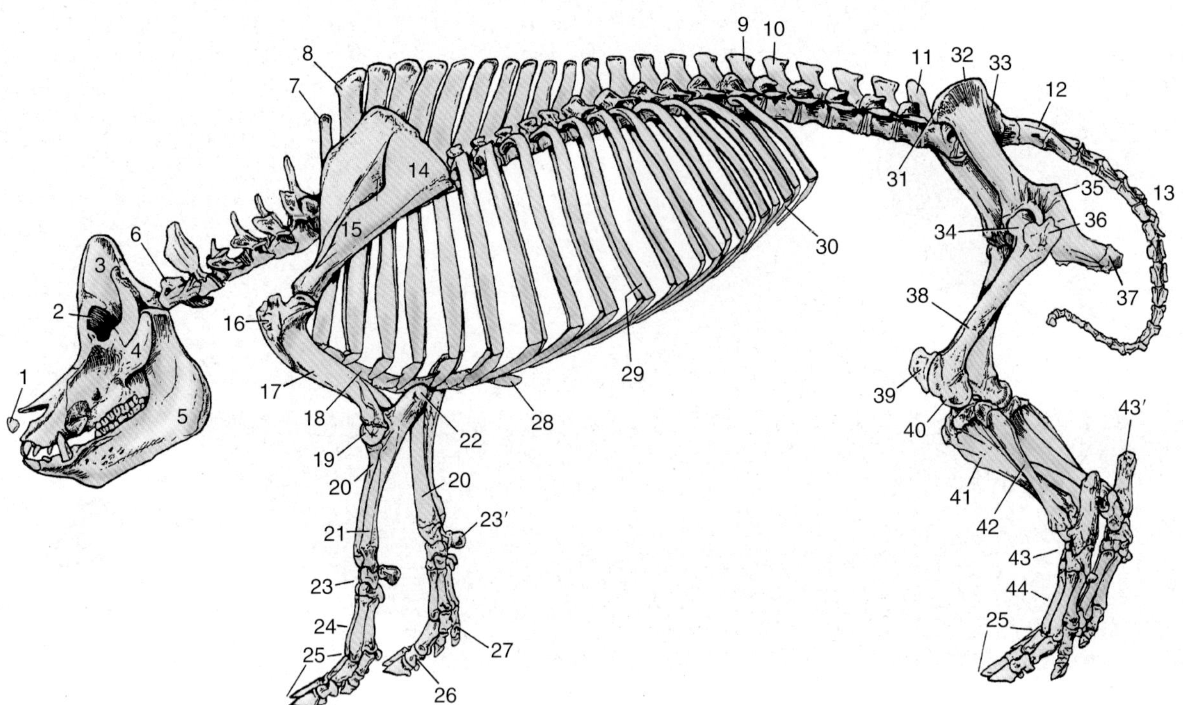

Fig. 32.1 Skeleton of a pig. *1,* Rostral bone; *2,* orbit; *3,* temporal fossa; *4,* zygomatic arch; *5,* mandible; *6,* first cervical vertebra; *7,* last cervical vertebra (C7); *8,* first thoracic vertebra; *9,* last thoracic vertebra (T16); *10,* first lumbar vertebra; *11,* last lumbar vertebra (L5); *12,* sacrum; *13,* caudal vertebrae; *14,* scapula; *15,* spine of scapula; *16,* greater tubercle of humerus; *17,* humerus; *18,* sternum; *19,* condyle of humerus; *20,* radius; *21,* ulna; *22,* olecranon; *23,* carpal bones; *23′,* accessory carpal bone; *24,* metacarpal bones; *25,* phalanges; *26,* phalanges of principal digit; *27,* phalanges of accessory digit; *28,* xiphoid cartilage; *29,* 10th pair of ribs; *30,* costal arch; *31,* coxal tuber; *32,* iliac crest; *33,* sacral tuber; *34,* head of femur in acetabulum; *35,* ischial spine; *36,* greater trochanter; *37,* ischial tuber; *38,* femur; *39,* patella; *40,* lateral condyle of femur; *41,* tibia; *42,* fibula; *43,* tarsal bones; *43′,* calcaneus; *44,* metatarsal bones.

medioventrally, between the globe and the third eyelid. The procedure is most likely to be performed in a research context. The sinus is said to be involved in thermoregulation of brain temperature by conveying cool blood from the nasal cavity.

The oval *ears* are attached to the high caudal part of the head and in lop-eared breeds hang down over the face. The external surface displays the only veins convenient for intravenous injection. These may be readily visible but, if not, are made so by application of a tourniquet at the base of the ear. The lateral vein of the set is most often used. Chewing of their companions' ears is a common vice among young pigs raised together in close quarters.

Subcutaneous injections are commonly made at a site just caudal to the ear; awareness of the proximity of the parotid gland is necessary (Fig. 32.3/*15*). The same site is used for injection into the muscle mass directly caudal to the skull; however, the orientation of the needle is different.

The *neck* is roughly cylindrical but with some lateral compression. It is remarkably short; the closeness of the angle of the mandible to the shoulder joint prevents the animal from turning its head to any great degree. The flabby lateroventral parts of the neck, the jowls, are common seats of abscesses.

The more important superficial structures of the head are shown in Fig. 32.3. They include the *buccal branches of the facial nerve* (Fig. 32.3/*19* and *20*); the ventral one follows a course around the lower margin of the masseter in company with the parotid duct and the facial artery and vein. The artery is short because the dorsal part of the face is supplied by the *infraorbital artery* that reaches the region through the infraorbital foramen together with the nerve of the same name. The *facial vein* is partly formed by a frontal tributary that becomes superficial by emerging through the foramen dorsomedial to the orbit. As would be expected, the *infraorbital nerve* is large because it supplies the sensitive snout.

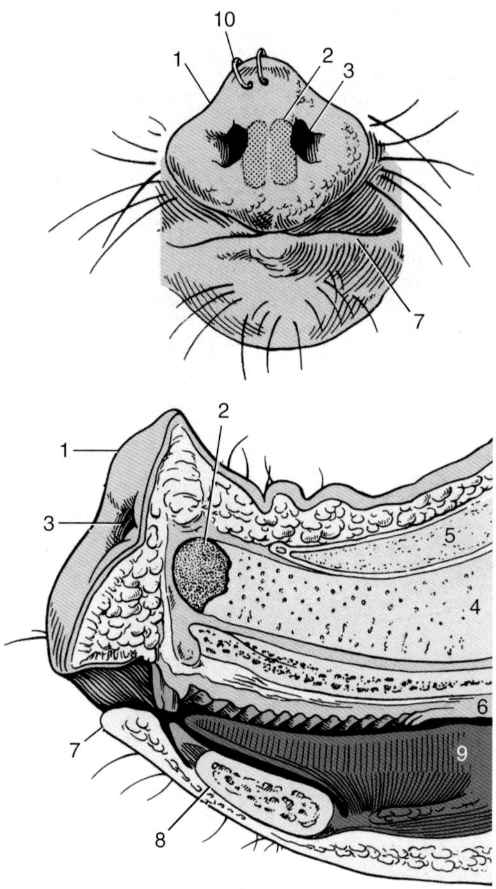

Fig. 32.2 The snout from the front and in median section. *1,* Rostral plate; *2,* rostral bone; *3,* nostril; *4,* nasal septum; *5,* nasal bone; *6,* hard palate; *7,* lower lip; *8,* mandible; *9,* tongue; *10,* nose rings to discourage rooting.

THE NASAL CAVITY AND PARANASAL SINUSES

The deep nasal cavities extend well behind the level of the orbits (Fig. 32.4). Despite the widening of the face, they remain narrow because they are separated from the lateral surface of the head by the thick muscles of facial expression and by fat, not by paranasal sinuses as in cattle and horses. Two conchae divide each cavity into the usual system of meatuses. The dorsal meatus leads to the fundus, which lies dorsal to the nasopharynx and is largely occupied by the ethmoidal conchae, which are covered by olfactory mucosa. This is extensive in a species endowed with a sense of smell sufficiently acute to be exploited in the search for buried truffles.

The dorsal concha is a thick plate projecting from the dorsolateral wall of the cavity. The ventral concha, though shorter, is more complicated and consists of upper and lower scrolls arising in common from a lateral plate. Familiarity with the conformation of these conchae is necessary if the deformity that develops in atrophic rhinitis, a common debilitating disease of young pigs, is to be recognized (Fig. 32.5).

The *paranasal sinus system* is complicated and comprises frontal, maxillary, lacrimal, sphenoidal, and conchal units, but not all of these merit attention (Fig. 32.4). The maxillary sinus, level with the orbit, extends into the base of the deep zygomatic arch. The frontal sinuses of the mature pig excavate the entire dorsal surface of the skull caudal to the nasal bones. They spread the outer and inner plates of the cranial roof so widely apart that all correspondence between the external form and the cranial cavity is lost (Fig. 32.4/7). The brain thus lies at a depth of about 5 cm below the skin, protected by two plates of bone. The consequence is that pigs cannot be reliably stunned by mechanical means (hammer or captive bolt), and humane slaughter requires the use of electrocution or carbon dioxide gas, which are the methods commonly employed today. When shooting is employed, the target site must be carefully chosen; for most pigs it is the intersection of the diagonal lines connecting the eyes with the bases of the opposite ears (Fig. 32.6). In particularly large pigs, it is more satisfactory to shoot through the occipital bone from behind.

THE MOUTH AND DENTITION

The animal's inability to open its mouth widely and problems with restraint make it difficult to examine the long and narrow mouth of the conscious animal. The ridges of the roof of the rostral part of the cavity end abruptly at the boundary of the soft palate, where the two discrete tonsils of the soft palate, which correspond to the tonsils embedded in the lateral walls of the oropharynx of other species, are found. These tonsils are cut in routine meat inspection.

The pointed tongue occupies the floor. In the newborn, the tongue is fringed with lacelike marginal papillae (Fig. 32.7/3), which persist for the first 2 or 3 weeks of life; because they swell visibly preparatory to contact with the teat, they are believed to help seal the mouth about the teat when sucking.

Pigs have the most complete dentition of any domestic animal (see Fig. 3.18); the formula for the permanent dentition is:

$$\frac{3-1-4-3}{3-1-4-3}$$

The straight lower incisors meet the curved upper incisors to provide a potential grasping action (Fig. 32.8). The curved canine teeth, or tusks, are firmly embedded in the jaws. In boars the roots remain open, and the tusks grow throughout life, providing these animals with formidable weapons; however, in sows growth ceases after

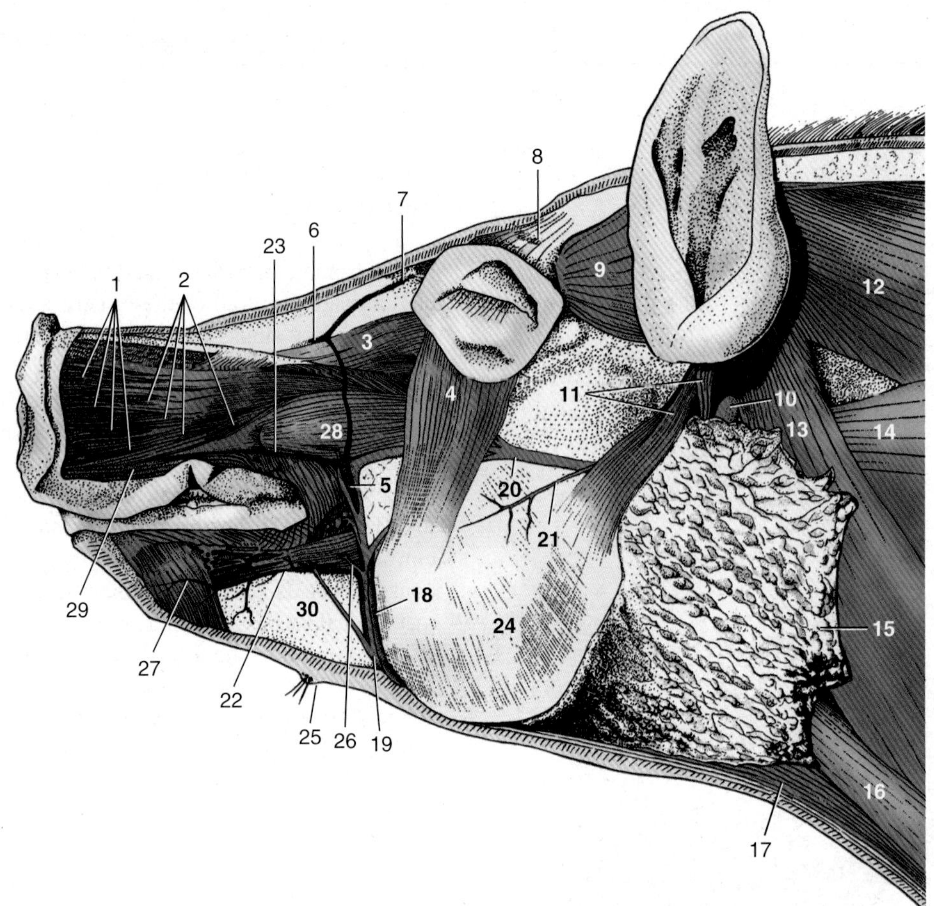

Fig. 32.3 Head, superficial dissection. *1,* Cut fasciculi of levator nasolabialis; *2,* caninus; *3,* levator labii superioris; *4,* malaris; *5,* facial vein; *6,* dorsal nasal vein; *7,* frontal vein; *8,* levator anguli oculi; *9,* frontoscutularis; *10,* lateral retropharyngeal lymph node; *11,* parotidoauricularis; *12,* trapezius; *13,* cleidooccipitalis; *14,* omotransversarius; *15,* parotid gland; *16,* sternocephalicus; *17,* sternohyoideus; *18,* parotid duct; *19* and *20,* ventral and dorsal buccal branches of facial nerve, respectively; *21,* transverse facial nerve; *22,* inferior labial vein; *23,* superior labial vein; *24,* masseter; *25,* mental hairs and gland; *26,* depressor labii inferioris; *27,* mentalis; *28,* depressor labii superioris; *29,* orbicularis oris; *30,* mandible.

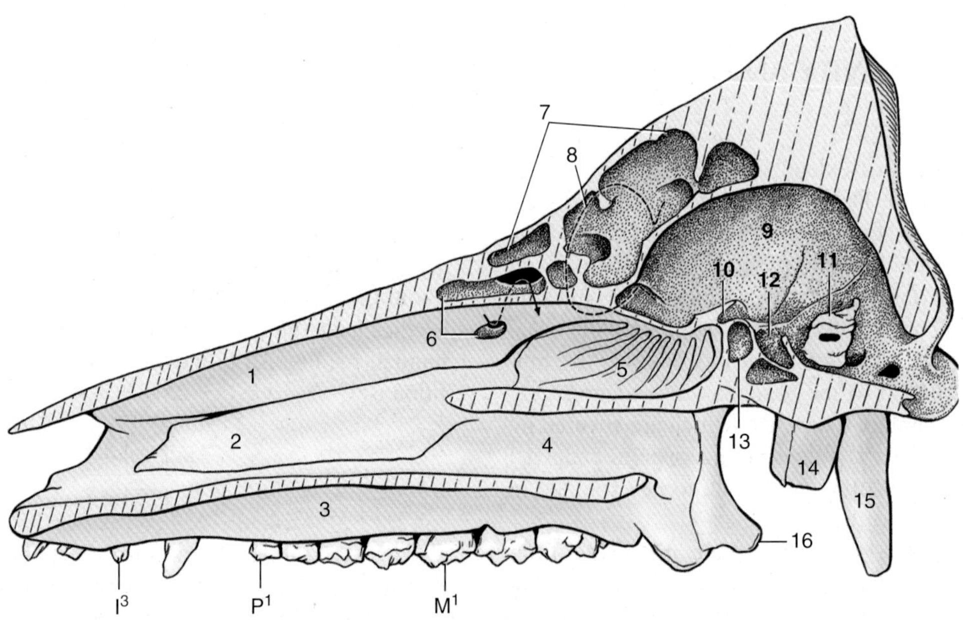

Fig. 32.4 Paramedian section of the skull. *1,* Dorsal turbinate bone, fenestrated at *6* to show conchal sinus; *2,* ventral turbinate bone; *3,* hard palate; *4,* choana; *5,* ethmoturbinates in fundus of nasal cavity; *6,* conchal sinus; *7,* portion of frontal sinus exposed by paramedian saw cut; *8,* position of orbit; *9,* cranial cavity; *10,* optic canal; *11,* petrous temporal bone; *12,* fossa for hypophysis; *13,* sphenoid sinus; *14,* tympanic bulla; *15,* paracondylar process; *16,* hamulus of pterygoid bone. I^3, third upper incisor; M^1, first upper molar; P^1, first upper premolar.

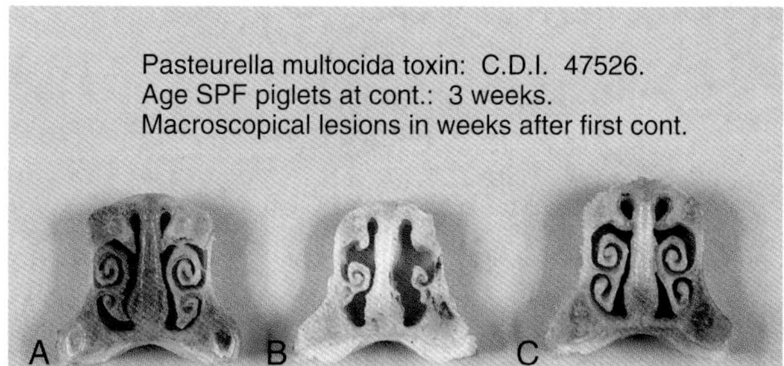

Fig. 32.5 Transverse sections of the nose of piglets treated with the toxin causing atrophic rhinitis. (A) The piglet is treated with a low dose. (B) The piglet is treated with an activated dose. (C) The piglet is treated with an inactivated dose.

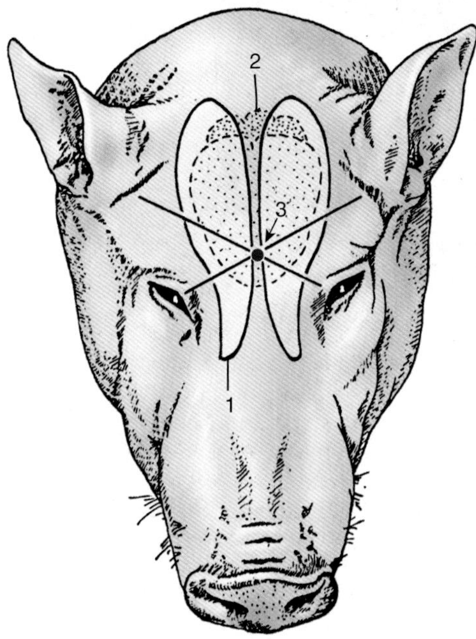

Fig. 32.6 Head of a 9-month-old pig. *1,* Outline of frontal sinuses; *2,* position of brain; *3,* point at which pig is best shot for stunning at slaughter.

2 years, and their smaller tusks do not project from the mouth. The tusks of boars are often cut short, sometimes without benefit of anesthesia. The crowns of the check teeth increase in both length and breadth from first to last in the series. The occlusal surfaces of the molars show many irregularities and are ideally adapted for crushing food.

Table 32.1 summarizes the ages at which different teeth erupt and are replaced. The deciduous incisors and canines with which the piglet is born are known as *needle teeth.* They project laterally from the gums and, being very sharp, may injure the mother's teat or any littermate in competition for this. They are therefore commonly nipped off within hours of birth; the procedure requires some care if the marginal lingual papillae are not to be injured. The dentition is normally complete by the age of 18 months, long after sexual maturity is reached.

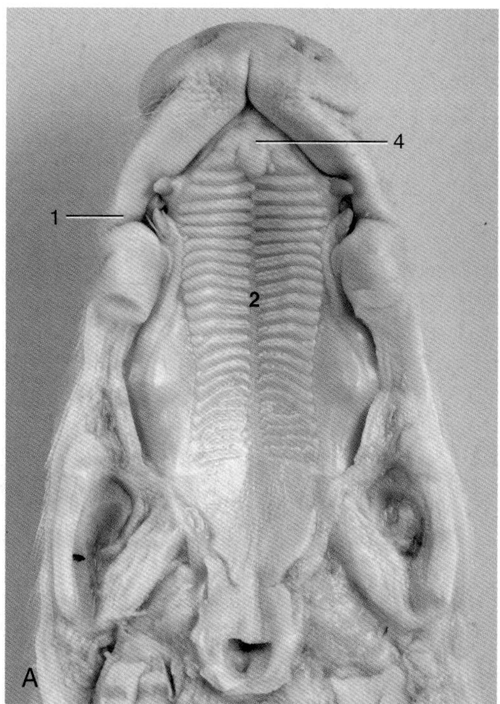

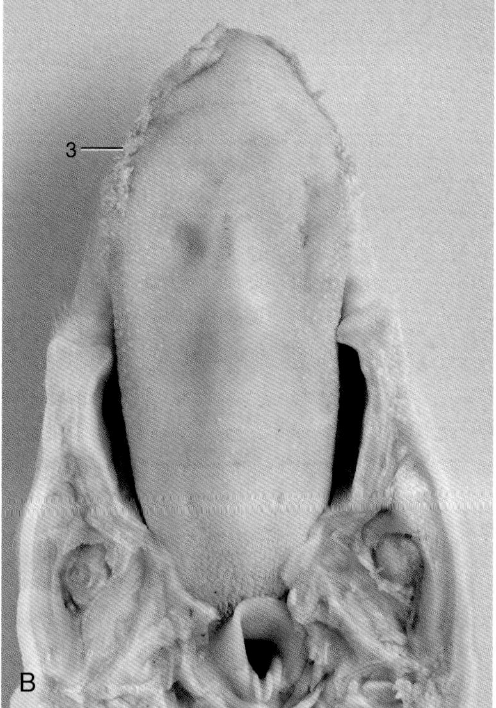

Fig. 32.7 (A) The roof and (B) the floor of the mouth of a newborn piglet. *1,* Permanent notch in upper lip opposite tusk; *2,* hard palate with ridges; *3,* lingual marginal papillae; *4,* incisive papilla.

The large *parotid gland* lies ventral to the base of the ear (Fig. 32.3/*15*). It extends only a little way over the masseter muscle rostrally, but its cervical angle reaches beyond the

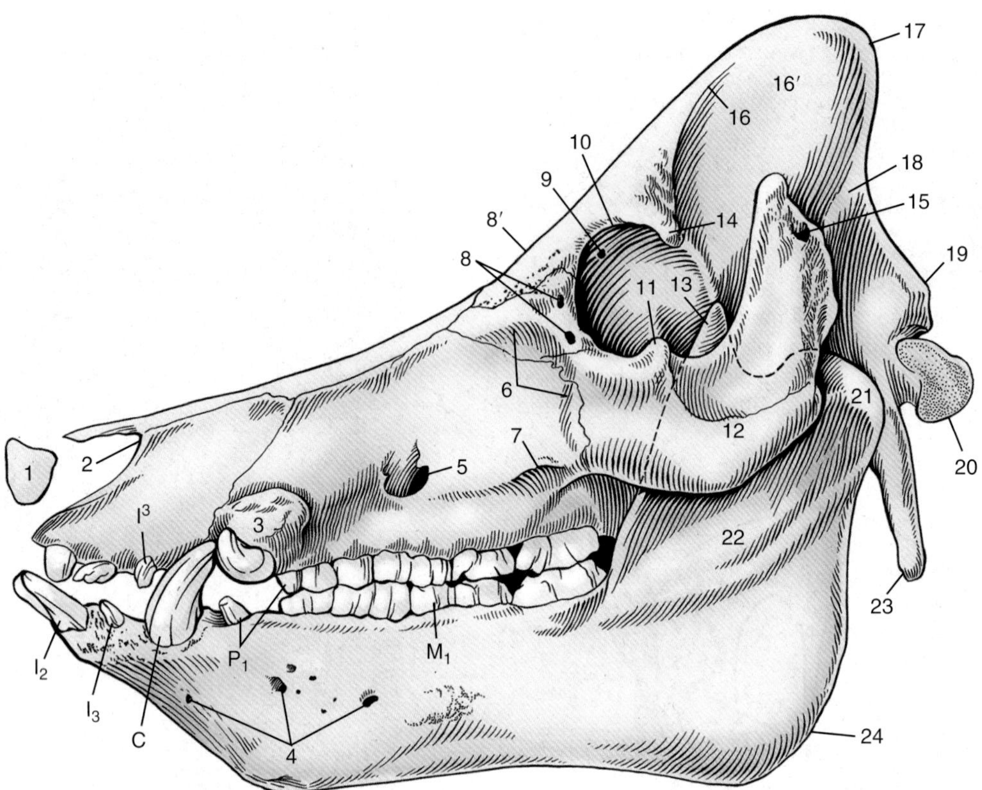

Fig. 32.8 Skull of a boar. *1,* Rostral bone; *2,* nasoincisive notch; *3,* canine eminence; *4,* lateral mental foramina; *5,* infraorbital foramen; *6,* fossa canina; *7,* facial crest; *8,* lacrimal foramina; *8′,* location of supraorbital foramen on dorsal surface; *9,* orbital end of supraorbital canal; *10,* orbital rim; *11,* frontal process of zygomatic bone; *12,* zygomatic arch; *13,* coronoid process of mandible; *14,* zygomatic process of frontal bone; *15,* external acoustic meatus; *16,* temporal line; *16′,* temporal fossa; *17,* nuchal crest; *18,* temporal crest; *19,* nuchal tubercle; *20,* occipital condyle; *21,* condylar process of mandible; *22,* ramus of mandible; *23,* paracondylar process; *24,* angle of mandible; *C,* canine teeth (tusks); I_2, I_3, and I^3, first and second lower and third upper incisors; M_1, first lower molar; P_1, first premolars.

TABLE 32.1 ERUPTION DATES OF PORCINE TEETH

	Temporary Tooth	Permanent Tooth
Incisor 1	1–3 weeks	11–18 months
Incisor 2	8–12 weeks	14–18 months
Incisor 3	Before birth	8–12 months
Canine	Before birth	8–12 months
Premolar 1	4–8 months	—
Premolar 2	6–12 weeks	12–16 months
Premolar 3	1–3 weeks	12–16 months
Premolar 4	2–5 weeks	12–16 months
Molar 1	—	4–8 months
Molar 2	—	7–13 months
Molar 3	—	17–22 months

middle of the neck under cover of the cutaneous muscle. It has numerous relations to the structures within the visceral space of the neck. Its duct crosses the *mandibular gland* and curves around the ventral border of the mandible to gain the face and open into the buccal cavity. The smaller rounded mandibular gland lies partly medial to the mandible and partly deep to the parotid. Its duct runs alongside the sublingual gland to open at the sublingual caruncle. Both parts of the sublingual gland are present; they drain in the usual way.

THE PHARYNX

The only feature of this organ to require notice is the presence of a diverticulum that burrows into the pharyngeal muscles dorsal to the entrance to the esophagus (Fig. 32.9/*13*). The diverticulum is about 1 cm long in the piglet and grows to about 3 or 4 cm in the adult. It appears to be without functional significance but is of practical importance because it is vulnerable to injury when a pig is dosed with a syringe. Should the diverticulum be perforated, the medication will be deposited in the tissues of the neck, with damaging effect. In the piglet of 4 weeks the diverticulum is level with the rostral part of the base of the ear, and about 2.5 cm caudal to the intended site of deposition

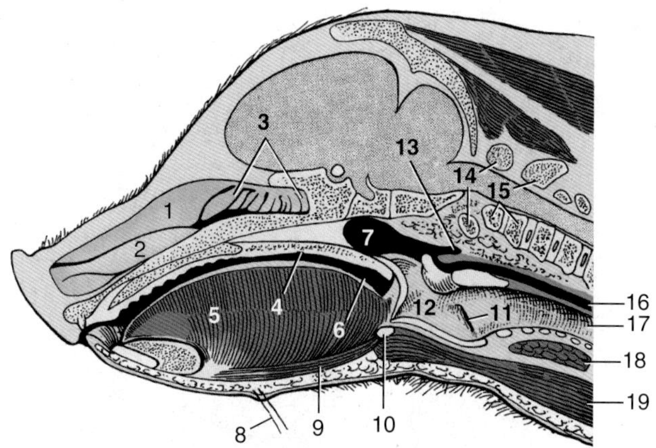

Fig. 32.9 Median section of the head of a 4-week-old pig; the nasal septum has been removed. *1,* Dorsal nasal concha; *2,* ventral nasal concha; *3,* ethmoidal conchae; *4,* soft palate; *5,* tongue; *6,* oropharynx; *7,* nasopharynx; *8,* mental hairs; *9,* geniohyoideus; *10,* basihyoid; *11,* laryngeal ventricle; *12,* larynx; *13,* pharyngeal diverticulum; *14,* atlas; *15,* axis; *16,* esophagus; *17,* trachea; *18,* thyroid gland; *19,* sternohyoideus.

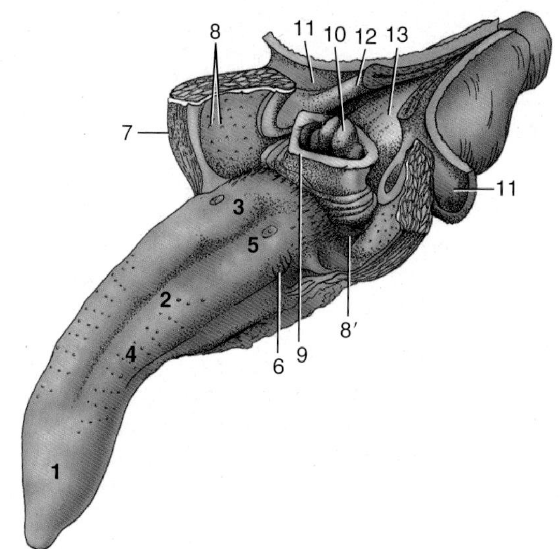

Fig. 32.10 Tongue and pharynx. The soft palate and the dorsal wall of the esophagus have been split in the midline. *1, 2,* and *3,* Apex, body, and root of tongue, respectively; *4,* fungiform papillae; *5,* vallate papillae; *6,* foliate papillae; *7,* palatoglossal arch; *8,* tonsil of the soft palate; *8′,* paraepiglottic tonsil; *9,* epiglottis; *10,* corniculate processes of the arytenoid cartilages; *11,* dorsal wall of nasopharynx; *12,* palatopharyngeal arch; *13,* entrance to esophagus.

is the oropharynx; a useful guide to the appropriate level is provided by the lateral angle of the eye.

The disposition of *tonsils* in the pig (Fig. 32.10) may appropriately be summarized here. A paraepiglottic tonsil is situated rostrolateral to the base of the epiglottis (Fig. 32.10/*8′*); a pharyngeal tonsil is found on the roof of the pharynx; tubal tonsils are associated with the pharyngeal openings of the auditory tubes; and there are the tonsils of the soft palate, already mentioned (Fig. 32.10/*8*). The first and last of these are sometimes examined at meat inspection, on the pluck (tongue, larynx, trachea, esophagus, heart, liver, and lungs) and on the cut surface of the head, respectively.

THE LARYNX

The most important feature of this organ is the obtuse angle it forms with the trachea (Fig. 32.9/*12* and *17*). Both this and the presence of lateral ventricles in the larynx (Fig. 32.9/*11*) have been cited as the causes of the difficulty that may be experienced when intubation is attempted for the induction of inhalation anesthesia; the procedure is most likely to be indicated in research settings. The larynx lies caudal to the intermandibular space, and its prominence may be palpated in the middle of the neck.

THE VENTRAL ASPECT OF THE NECK

The visceral space of the neck has the same contents as in other species and is similarly enclosed ventrolaterally by a series of thin, straplike muscles. The cutaneous muscle is thick at its origin from the manubrium but thins when followed cranially to merge with the cutaneous muscles of the face. A more important impediment to puncture of the external jugular vein is the thick subcutaneous fat.

The trachea and esophagus show no unusual features, nor do the vessels and nerves passing between head and thorax, apart from the internal jugular vein, which is considerably better developed than in most other species. The *thyroid gland* consists of two lobes, broadly connected ventral to the trachea (Fig. 32.11/*4*); because of the shortness of the neck, it lies close to the thoracic inlet (see Fig. 6.4D). The *thymus* lies to each side of the larynx and trachea (Fig. 32.11/*3*) and is particularly well developed. It does not attain its greatest size until the animal is about 9 months old and begins to regress a few months later. Its bulbous cranial extremity carries on its surface the minute (1- to 4-mm) external parathyroid glands. (The internal parathyroid glands are thought to disappear in the embryo.)

Cranial Vena Cava Puncture: The most common clinical procedure involving the neck is cranial vena cava puncture, which may be performed in the standing animal or in one suitably restrained on its back. The needle is inserted in the depression between the manubrium and the point of the right shoulder and advanced in the direction of the left scapula until it meets one or another of the large veins between or just in front of the first pair of ribs. Entry is best made from the right because the left phrenic nerve is more vulnerable to injury; the thoracic duct also lies more to that side (Fig. 32.12).

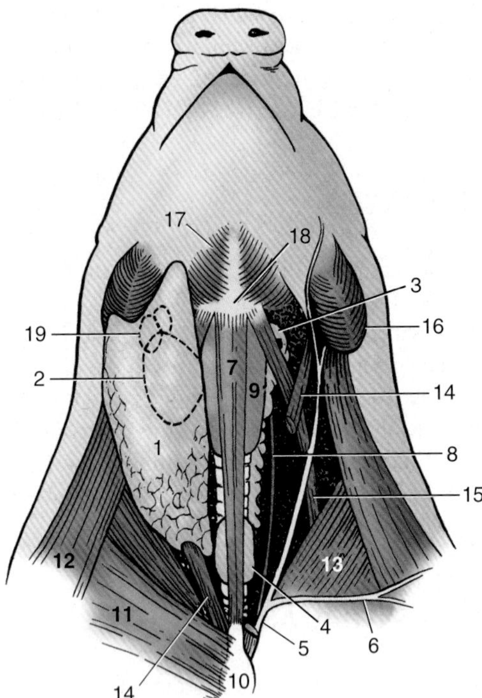

Fig. 32.11 Ventral view of the neck. Deep dissection to the right; superficial dissection, from which the cutaneous colli has been removed, to the left (semischematic). *1,* Parotid gland; *2,* mandibular gland; *3,* thymus; *4,* thyroid; *5,* external jugular vein; *6,* cephalic vein; *7,* sternohyoideus (drawn narrower than actual width); *8,* internal jugular vein; *9,* larynx; *10,* manubrium sterni; *11,* superficial pectoral muscle; *12,* brachiocephalicus; *13,* subclavius; *14,* sternocephalicus; *15,* omohyoideus; *16,* angle of mandible; *17,* mylohyoideus; *18,* basihyoid; *19,* mandibular lymph nodes.

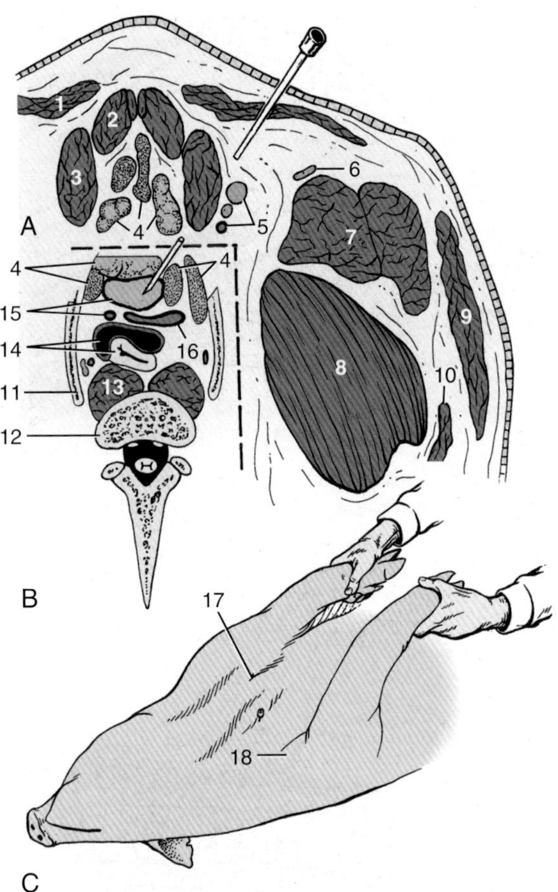

Fig. 32.12 (A) Transverse section of the ventral neck slightly cranial to the manubrium sterni. (B) The *area below and to the left of the broken lines* represents the topography at the slightly more caudal level of the first ribs. (C) Pig held on its back for cranial vena cava venipuncture (see needle in position). *1,* Cutaneous colli; *2,* sternohyoideus; *3,* sternocephalicus; *4,* lymph nodes and thymus; *5,* common carotid artery and external and internal jugular veins; *6,* cephalic vein; *7,* brachiocephalicus; *8,* subclavius; *9,* platysma; *10,* omotransversarius; *11,* first rib; *12,* body of C7; *13,* longus colli; *14,* trachea and esophagus; *15,* cranial vena cava and left subclavian artery; *16,* bicarotid trunk and right subclavian artery; *17,* palpable manubrium sterni; *18,* shoulder joint.

THE LYMPHATIC STRUCTURES OF THE HEAD AND NECK

Five lymph centers are located in the head and ventrolateral part of the neck (Fig. 32.13). The *mandibular center* comprises about six principal and four accessory nodes. The mandibular nodes lie behind the caudoventral border of the mandible, related to the mandibular gland and crossed laterally by the facial vein (Fig. 32.14/*1*). They drain the ventral half of the head and forward lymph to the accessory group and to ventral and dorsal superficial cervical nodes and are routinely examined in meat inspection. The accessory nodes (Fig. 32.14/*2*) are also located by the border of the mandible and under cover of the parotid gland. They drain the same part of the head and also the ventral part of the neck; their efferents also go to the superficial cervical nodes. The parotid nodes (Fig. 32.14/*3*) are located ventral to the temporomandibular joint covered by the parotid gland. They drain the head dorsal to the palate and send their efferents to the lateral retropharyngeal nodes (Fig. 32.14/*4*).

The *retropharyngeal center* consists of one medial and two lateral nodes (Fig. 32.14/*4* and *5*). The latter lie near the joint, again under the parotid gland and a few centimeters caudal to the parotid center. They drain superficial structures where the head joins the neck; their efferents go to the dorsal superficial cervical nodes. The medial node lies above the pharynx and drains deeper structures at the same level as the lateral nodes; its efferents join to form a tracheal duct.

The *superficial cervical center* consists of about 10 nodes, roughly arranged in a triangle and divided into dorsal, middle, and ventral groups (Fig. 32.14/*6–8*). Together, they correspond to the single group found deep

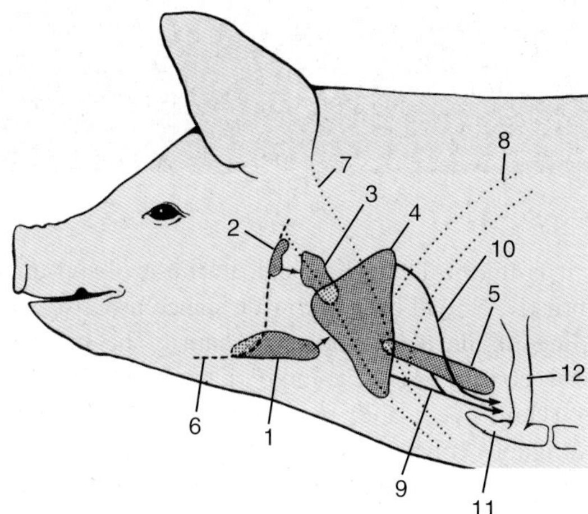

Fig. 32.13 The lymph centers of the head and neck (schematic). The *arrows* indicate lymph flow. *1,* Mandibular lymph center; *2,* parotid lymph center; *3,* retropharyngeal lymph center; *4,* superficial cervical lymph center; *5,* deep cervical lymph center; *6,* mandible; *7,* brachiocephalicus; *8,* subclavius; *9,* tracheal lymph trunk; *10,* lymph from dorsal superficial cervical nodes; *11,* manubrium sterni; *12,* first rib.

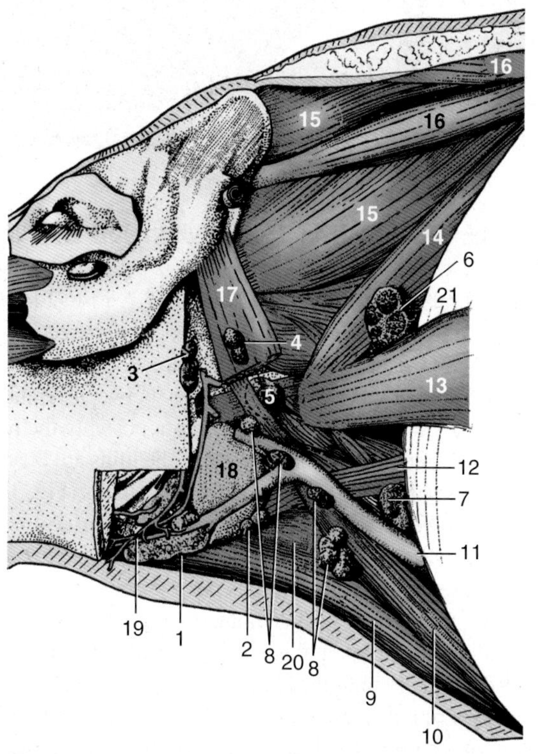

Fig. 32.14 Dissection of the neck to show the lymph nodes, left lateral view. *1,* Mandibular lymph nodes; *2,* accessory mandibular lymph nodes; *3,* parotid lymph nodes; *4,* lateral retropharyngeal lymph nodes; *5,* medial retropharyngeal lymph node; *6, 7,* and *8,* dorsal, middle, and ventral superficial cervical lymph nodes, respectively; *9,* sternohyoideus; *10,* sternocephalicus; *11,* external jugular vein; *12,* omohyoideus; *13,* omotransversarius; *14,* serratus ventralis cervicis; *15,* splenius; *16,* rhomboideus cervicis et capitis; *17,* cleidomastoideus; *18,* mandibular gland; *19,* facial vein; *20,* thyrohyoideus; *21,* subclavius.

to the omotransversarius in other species. The dorsal nodes drain the neck and neighboring parts of the thoracic wall and forelimb. They also receive lymph from the head nodes, other than the medial retropharyngeal, and pass it to veins at the thoracic inlet. The middle group is dorsal to the external jugular vein and drains the shoulder region; its efferents accompany or join those of the dorsal group. The ventral group is arranged in a chain and, like the middle nodes, lies deep to the brachiocephalic muscle. It drains superficial structures of the neck, the forelimb, the ventral thoracic wall, and the first two mammary glands. It also receives lymph from the mandibular and lateral pharyngeal nodes.

In theory, the many nodes of the *deep cervical center* are divided into several groups spread at intervals along the internal jugular vein. In practice, usually few are to be found. They drain directly to the large veins at the thoracic inlet.

COMPREHENSION CHECK

Develop a list of unique and comparative features of the head and ventral neck with particular focus on the features that are of importance in clinical work and meat inspection.

33 The Vertebral Column, Back, and Thorax of the Pig

THE VERTEBRAL COLUMN AND BACK

The vertebral formula is usually given as C7, T14–T15, L6–L7, S4, Cd20–C23, but variation outside this range is common and almost always affects the thoracolumbar region, where the total number of vertebrae vary between 19 and 23. An increase in number is more common, possibly the result of selective breeding for this character: the loins are the most valuable part of the carcass, apart from the hams (Fig. 33.1).

Among other features, the vertebrae of the cervical region are distinguished by a high spine on C2 and a very high one on C7. Because the neck is almost as deep as the cranial part of the thorax, the body of the first thoracic vertebra is located near the middle of the trunk at this level. The vertebrae behind the first rise gradually until those of the caudal thoracic and lumbar regions run close to, and almost parallel with, the dorsal contour of the back. The lack of spinous processes on the four units of the sacrum causes an abrupt drop in the height of the vertebral column at the lumbosacral junction. The iliac crest, which flanks the spinous process of the last lumbar vertebra, is the highest skeletal feature in this area (see Fig. 32.1/*32*).

The *lumbosacral space* is available, but rarely used, for the epidural administration of anesthetic (see Fig. 8.56C). It measures about 2 cm craniocaudally and 3 cm transversely and is situated between 2 and 5 cm caudal to the line connecting the coxal tubers, which are palpable in less fat animals. If this guide cannot be used, an indication of the location of the lumbosacral space is provided by the transverse plane of the flank fold. The space is 5 cm or more below the skin, and the arrival of the needle point at the interarcuate ligament is made known by the greater resistance encountered there. In young hogs, the spinal cord extends into the sacrum and is at risk in this procedure; in older animals the ascent of the cord carries it to safety within the lumbar part of the canal.

The most caudal vertebrae are incorporated in the curly tail, which carries the *median caudal vessels,* including the caudal artery, near its ventral surface. Blood may be collected most easily at the tail head (Cd4 or C5), but because the artery and accompanying veins run together, it cannot be predicted whether this blood will be of arterial, venous, or mixed origin. The tail is often removed when a piglet is a few days old to prevent the common vice of tail biting, which sometimes results in ascending infection. Trichinosis (occurring in some countries) may also be transmitted in this way. The cross section of the tail (Fig. 33.2) shows the arrangement of muscles around the caudal vertebra.

The contour of the back depends on breed and condition. In fat, old animals it may be flat, but in most modern hogs it is uniformly arched and, in those of top quality, also broad. A broad back and wide stance promisees good muscling of the trunk and thick hams. The muscles of the back conform to the common pattern, and the longissimus ("loin eye") and, most especially, psoas muscles (filet mignon) constitute particularly valuable parts of the carcass. Because subcutaneous fat has limited value, too thick a layer is undesirable; this indication of carcass quality may be measured by ultrasound. Fat deposited over the loins is especially well formed and thick, and, because it has to be trimmed, it represents a substantial loss to the producer. Some of it is rendered into lard, and some is cured to become the "pork" in the popular canned food "pork and beans." Selective breeding has markedly reduced to 3 cm or less the thickness of back fat; consequently, caution is needed when intramuscular injections are performed.

THE THORAX

The body of a pig does not widen appreciably where the neck joins the trunk: the subcutaneous layer of fat allows the forelimb to blend in unobtrusively, and only a slight depression between the flabby jowls and the shoulder joint marks the junction. There is a similar depression between the elbow joint and the thoracic wall. The "points" of both joints are palpable. The olecranon of the elbow projects onto the ventral end of the fifth rib (Fig. 33.3). The manubrium of the sternum is also easily found.

Most pigs have 14 or 15 pairs of ribs; asymmetry of number is common (see Fig. 32.1). The first seven pairs are sternal. The rib cage is smaller than the external dimensions suggest; it is especially narrow and shallow between the forelimbs but deepens caudally with the upward sweep of the thoracic vertebrae. It is relatively long, depending to some extent on the number of vertebrae. The line of pleural reflection follows the dorsal half of the last rib before descending in a gentle curve to cross the seventh costochondral joint (Fig. 33.3). The cranial mediastinum, like that of ruminants, attaches to the ventral parts of the left first and second ribs, but more dorsally it is separated from the thoracic wall by the cranial lobe of the left lung.

The left *lung* possesses a cranial lobe, divided by a cardiac notch, and a caudal lobe (Fig. 33.3/*5–7* and see Fig. 4.23). The right lung possesses cranial, middle, caudal, and accessory lobes; the cardiac notch separates the first two (see Fig. 4.23A). The cranial lobe of this lung is ventilated by a separate tracheal bronchus (see Fig. 4.24). The lobulation of the

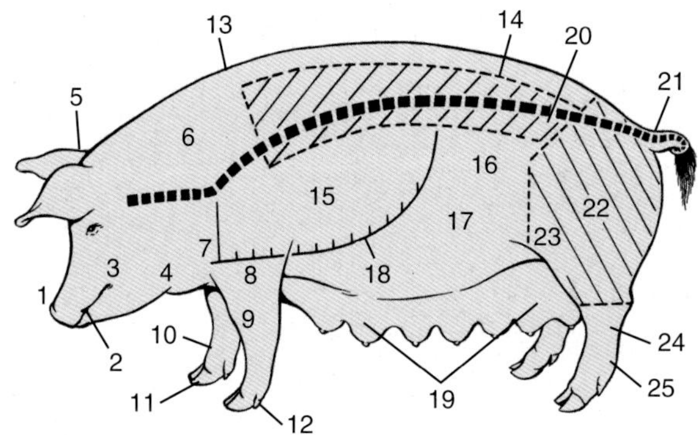

Fig. 33.1 Parts of the pig. The position of the vertebral column is indicated. The hatched areas show ham and loin of the meat trade. *1,* Snout; *2,* mouth; *3,* cheek; *4,* jowls; *5,* poll; *6,* neck; *7,* shoulder joint; *8,* elbow joint; *9,* carpus; *10,* fetlock joint; *11,* hoof; *12,* accessory digit; *13,* withers; *14,* loin (lumbar area); *15,* thorax; *16,* flank; *17,* abdomen; *18,* ventral extent of bony thorax; *19,* mammary glands; *20,* position of coxal tuber; *21,* tailhead; *22,* thigh; *23,* stifle joint; *24,* hock joint; *25,* metatarsus.

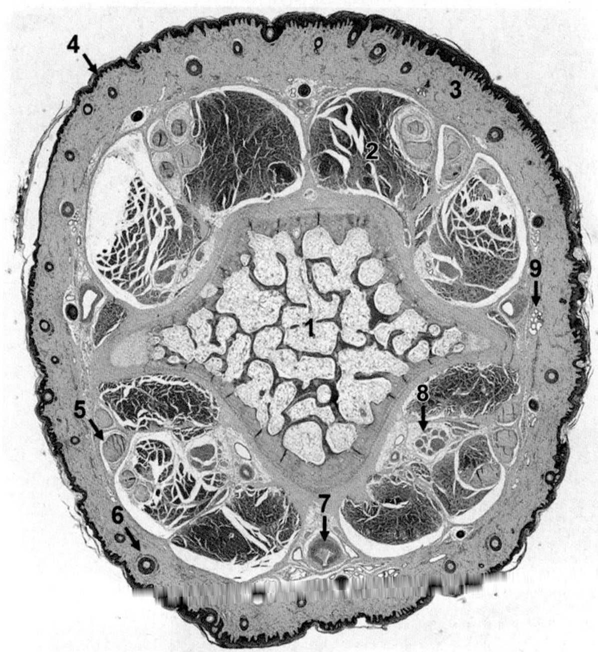

Fig. 33.2 Cross section of the pig tail, Masson's trichrome stain. *1,* Caudal vertebra; *2,* epaxial muscles; *3,* dermis and hypodermis; *4,* epidermis of skin; *5,* muscle tendon; *6,* hair follicle; *7,* caudal artery; *8,* nerve fascicles; *9,* sweat gland.

lungs is relatively distinct (Figs. 33.4 and 33.5). Fig. 33.6 shows the air in the mouth, pharynx, and lungs.

Lungs: The projection of the lungs onto the thoracic wall is small. The basal border of the left lung extends from the sixth costochondral junction to the upper end of the third last rib. This border of the right lung is less steep and reaches the penultimate rib. Auscultation and percussion of the lungs are usually reserved for young pigs of cooperative disposition.

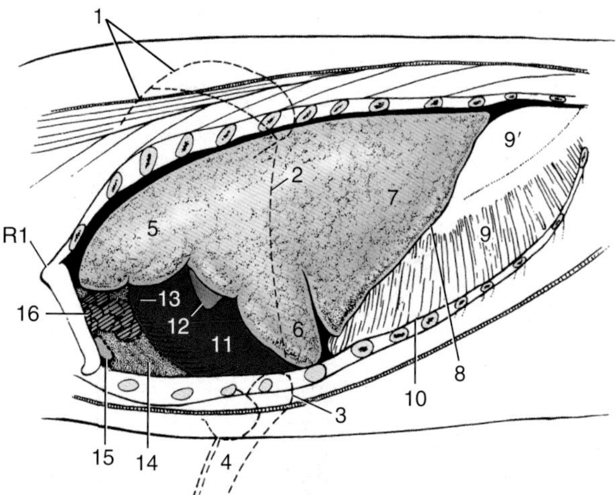

Fig. 33.3 The thoracic viscera in situ (semi-schematic). *1,* Scapula; *2,* caudal border of triceps; *3,* olecranon; *4,* radius and ulna; *5* and *6,* cranial and caudal parts of cranial lobe of lung, respectively; *7,* caudal lobe of lung; *8,* basal border of lung; *9* and *9′,* muscular and tendinous parts of diaphragm, respectively; *10,* line of pleural reflection; *11,* heart; *12* and *13,* left and right auricles, respectively; *14,* cranial mediastinum; *15,* sternal lymph node; *16,* thymus; R1, first rib.

The *heart* is small, providing as little as 0.3% of body weight (compared with 1.5% or more in athletic species such as the horse and dog), and this has been cited as a predisposing factor in the "sudden death syndrome" commonly occurring in pigs. Heart size has not kept pace with the much accelerated growth of modern, improved pigs, which reach a weight of 115 kg at 5 or 6 months; in striking contrast, 2 or 3 years was required to reach the much more modest weight of 40 kg in the year 1800 (Fig. 33.7). The heart occupies the ventral half of the thoracic cavity, extending between the second and fifth ribs (Figs. 33.8/*6* and 33.9/*1*). It is thus covered by the forelimb in the standing animal but can be made accessible by drawing the limb forward. It [illegible] no structural distinctions of note (see Fig. 7.7).

Paracentesis is best performed through the fifth left or the fourth right intercostal space; the needle is inserted about 5 cm dorsal to the olecranon (Fig. 33.3).

THE LYMPHATIC STRUCTURES OF THE THORAX

The thoracic lymph nodes, arranged in four centers (Fig. 33.8/*1–4*), collect lymph from the thoracic walls and contents and from adjacent structures and channel it to the thoracic duct or, where some more cranial nodes are concerned, directly into veins at the thoracic inlet.

The dorsal thoracic center comprises a variable number of small aortic nodes that receive lymph from the dorsal

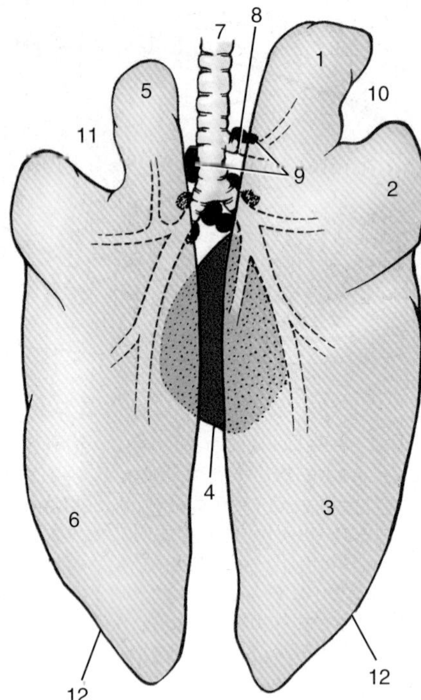

Fig. 33.4 The lungs, dorsal view (see also Fig. 4.23). *1,* Right cranial lobe; *2,* right middle lobe; *3,* right caudal lobe; *4,* accessory lobe of right lung; *5,* divided left cranial lobe; *6,* left caudal lobe; *7,* trachea; *8,* tracheal bronchus; *9,* tracheobronchial lymph nodes; *10,* right cardiac notch; *11,* left cardiac notch; *12,* basal border.

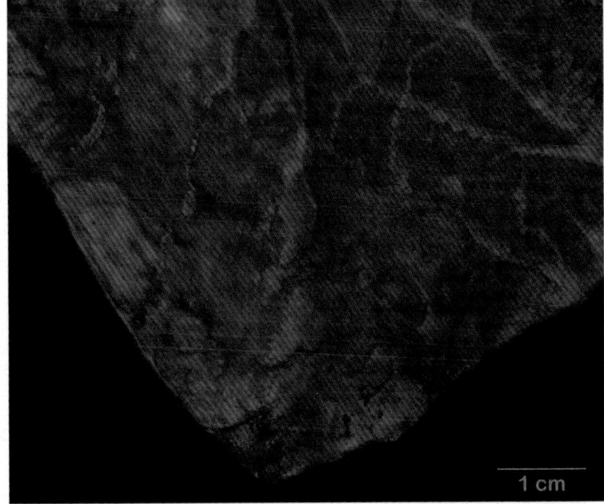

Fig. 33.5 Surface of pig lung showing lobulation.

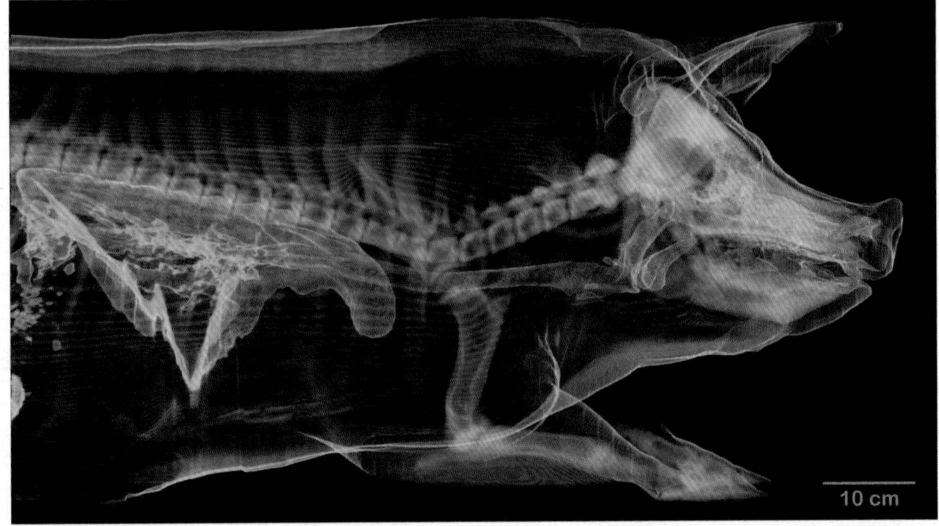

Fig. 33.6 Three dimensional projection generated from computed-tomographic imaging of gilt showing location of respiratory tract and lungs. Air in the nasal cavity, ethmoturbinates, larynx, trachea and lungs is shown in *yellow*. Skeleton is shown in *blue*.

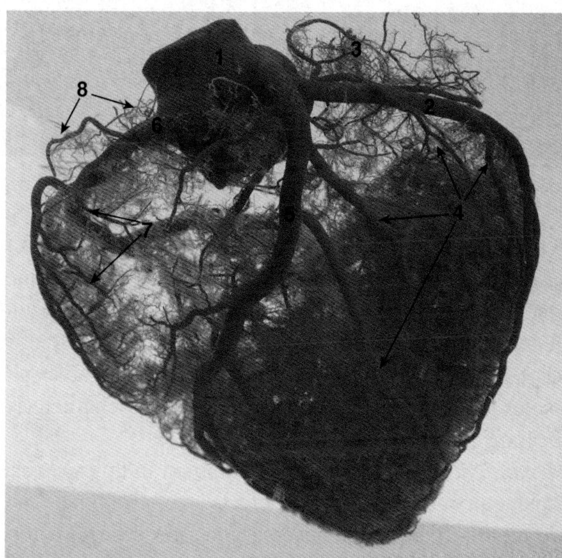

Fig. 33.7 Corrosion cast of the pig heart (auricular surface). *1,* Aorta; *2,* circumflex branch of the left coronary artery, also called the left circumflex artery (LCX); *3,* atrial branches of the LCX; *4,* ventricular branches for the left ventricle; *5,* paraconal interventricular branch of the left coronary artery, also called the left anterior descending branch (LAD); *6,* right coronary artery (RCA); *7,* ventricular branches for the right ventricle.

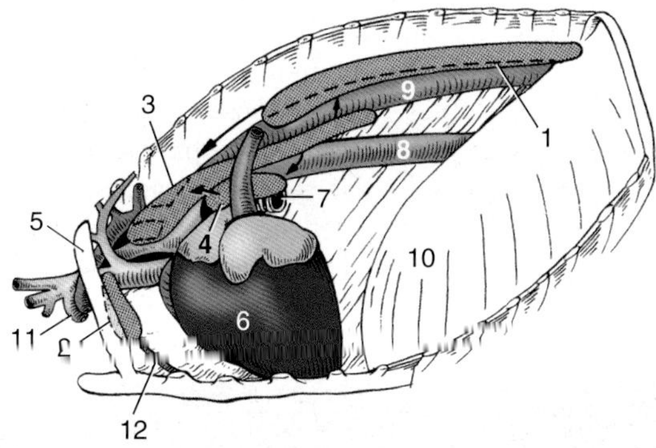

Fig. 33.8 The lymph centers of the thorax, left lateral view. *1,* Dorsal thoracic lymph center; *2,* ventral thoracic lymph center; *3,* mediastinal lymph center; *4,* tracheobronchial lymph center; *5,* first rib; *6,* heart; *7,* left bronchus; *8,* esophagus; *9,* aorta; *10,* diaphragm; *11,* axillary vein and artery; *12,* internal thoracic artery.

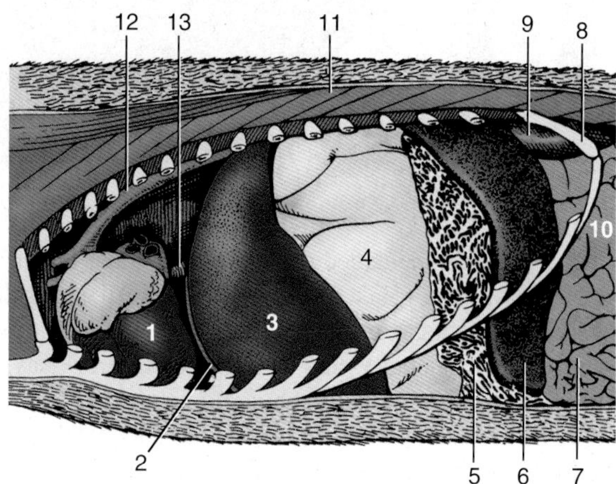

Fig. 33.9 The heart in situ, lateral view of dissected thorax. *1,* Heart; *2,* diaphragm; *3,* left lobe of liver; *4,* stomach, greatly dilated; *5,* greater omentum, gastrosplenic ligament; *6,* spleen; *7,* jejunum; *8,* last rib; *9,* left kidney; *10,* ascending colon; *11,* back muscles; *12,* aorta; *13,* caudal vena cava.

part of the thoracic wall, the mediastinum, and mediastinal nodes. The ventral center consists of fewer but larger sternal nodes concerned with the ventral part of the thoracic walls and the first two or three pairs of mammary glands.

Inconstant numbers of cranial and caudal mediastinal nodes form a chain above the base of the heart (Mediastinal lymph centre). The cranial nodes drain structures of the neck in addition to mediastinal contents, including the tracheobronchial nodes. Their efferents are divided into some that open into veins directly and others that lead to the thoracic duct. The caudal nodes are not always to be found. When present, they drain neighboring structures and send their efferents to the tracheobronchial and aortic nodes.

The *tracheobronchial centre* (Fig. 33.8/*4*) consists of a dozen or so tracheobronchial nodes arranged about the origin of the bronchi (Fig. 33.4/*9*). They drain the lungs, heart, and pericardium and in turn drain to the cranial mediastinal nodes or directly into the thoracic duct.

The thoracic duct runs from caudal to cranial between the aorta and esophagus, passing the trachea at its left side before joining the bloodstream.

COMPREHENSION CHECK

Indicate the sites for paracentesis of the thorax.

Describe the major lymph collection centers in the thorax, and list the areas/organs serviced by them.

34 The Abdomen of the Pig

A thick layer of subcutaneous fat obscures most underlying features of the trunk of the pig, making it generally impossible to recognize the extent of the flank on simple inspection. Occasionally, and then most often in heavily pregnant sows, there is a slight bulging behind the last rib. At the other limit, the thigh and flank fold conceal the caudal part of the abdomen where it tapers to its junction with the pelvis.

THE MAMMARY GLANDS

In sows the ventral contour of the abdomen is made irregular by the presence of the mammary glands, of which there are almost invariably seven pairs arranged in a double row extending from the thorax to the groin (Fig. 34.1; see also Fig. 33.1). Each gland is pendulous and, though confluent with its neighbors at its base, is otherwise clearly defined. Those at the caudal end of the series are generally the largest, but the cranial ones are the most productive.

The teats are elongated and cylindrical, with each having two openings at its tip (see Fig. 10.31B) leading to independent gland units. Some teats tend to project a little to the side, and because sows generally suckle while laterally recumbent, certain teats may not be readily accessible to the litter; this may cause some glands to be little used and regress early. On the other hand, when the litter is large some piglets may find it hard to obtain an adequate share of milk and may fail to grow normally.

The blood supply to the mammary glands is provided by local vessels: the *internal thoracic* and the *cranial and caudal superficial epigastric arteries.* The venous drainage is satellite. Lymph from the first two (or three) pairs of glands leads to ventral superficial cervical nodes, and that from the remainder leads to the superficial inguinal nodes.

THE ABDOMINAL WALL

The construction of the abdominal wall follows the common pattern in its essential features. The cutaneous muscle of the trunk is extensive as well as thick ventrally where it passes through the flank fold. It leaves the abdominal floor uncovered, except for cranial (and inconstant caudal) preputial muscles. The deep fascia is without the elastic component that in the larger species imparts the characteristic yellow color. The three muscles of the flank show few distinctions of importance. Because the fleshy parts of the three flank muscles tend not to hold sutures well, the favorite site for laparotomy is an almost wholly tendinous aponeurotic strip, about 10 cm long and barely 5 cm wide, situated along the lateral edge of the rectus muscle and deep to the flank fold. The alternation of the abdominal muscles with layers of fat accounts for the characteristic appearance of the bacon rasher.

Umbilical hernias used to be common in this species. If a satisfactory closure of these defects is to be obtained in the abdominal wall, it is first necessary to reflect the cranial part of the prepuce. This exposes the wide part of the linea alba that alone provides sufficient breadth of tissue to allow overlapping and suture of the margins of the hernia ring.

The other region of practical interest is provided by the *inguinal canal.* In principle, this conforms to the general arrangement of a potential space between the two oblique muscles (for details, see Fig. 34.2). The deep ring, the entry to the canal, is found between the caudal border of the internal oblique and the aponeurosis of the external oblique (see Fig. 2.27). The superficial opening is the split in the external aponeurosis that defines its division into pelvic and abdominal parts. The caudal part of the canal is very short, but it widens cranially because of the craniodorsal orientation of the deep ring compared to the slightly ventral and cranial angle of the superficial ring. Anomalies of gubernacular development are common in pigs. If the canal is dilated (Fig. 34.3), pigs are predisposed to inguinal hernia involving a loop of small intestine that stretches the vaginal ring and forces a passage into the tunica vaginalis, leading to a subcutaneous swelling between the thighs. These hernias require attention in the castration of affected animals.

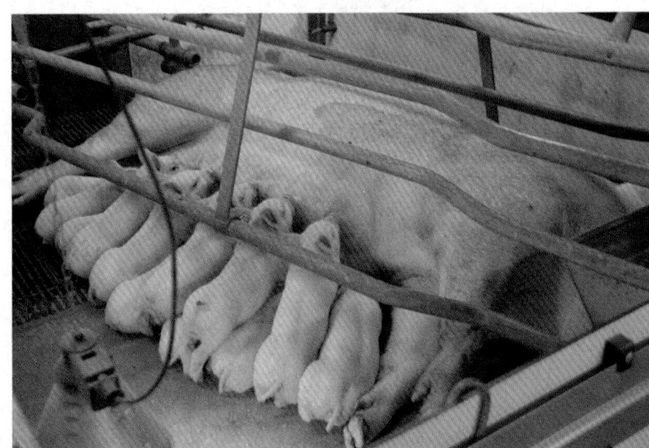

Fig. 34.1 The mammary glands of the sow extend from the pectoral to the inguinal region.

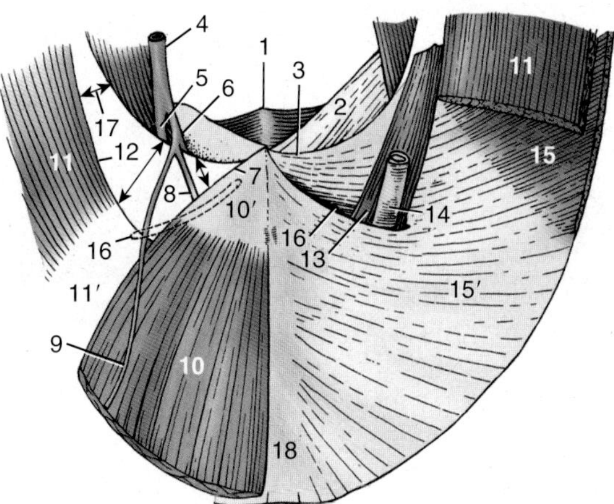

Fig. 34.2 Inguinal canal of the male made visible on the interior surface of the caudal abdominal wall; semi-schematic, cranial view. *1*, Pelvic symphysis; *2*, prepubic tendon; *3*, caudal border of external oblique aponeurosis ("inguinal ligament"); *4*, external iliac artery; *5*, femoral artery; *6*, deep femoral artery; *7*, lateral border of rectus tendon; *8*, external pudendal artery; *9*, caudal epigastric artery; *10*, rectus abdominis; *10′*, rectus tendon; *11*, muscular part of internal abdominal oblique; *11′*, aponeurotic part of internal abdominal oblique; *12*, caudal free border of internal abdominal oblique; *13*, cremaster; *14*, tunica vaginalis and spermatic cord; *15*, muscular part of external abdominal oblique; 15′, aponeurotic part of external abdominal oblique; *16*, superficial inguinal ring; *17*, deep inguinal ring *(arrows)*; *18*, linea alba.

THE ABDOMINAL ORGANS (FIGS. 34.4, 34.5, 34.6)

The Spleen

The bright red, elongated, and straplike spleen is oriented more or less vertically under the protection of the more caudal ribs on the left side (Fig. 34.5 and 34.7). It follows the greater curvature of the stomach, to which it is loosely attached by a gastrosplenic ligament that is sufficiently generous to make splenic torsion a relatively frequent mishap. Its parietal surface is in contact with the diaphragm. Its visceral surface is divided by a long hilus into cranial and caudal strips that relate to the stomach and the intestines, respectively. The dorsal extremity extends into the space between the stomach, left kidney, and pancreas, but it is usually prevented from making direct contact with these organs by the interposition of fat. The ventral extremity may emerge below the left costal arch and, exceptionally, may even cross the abdomen to the right side; although its position is determined by the degree of fullness of the stomach, it never wholly leaves the protection of the ribs. Its sectioned surface is patterned by the presence of very prominent splenic corpuscles.

The Stomach

The stomach is of the simple type, presenting fundus, corpus, and a pyloric part (Fig. 34.8/*2*). The first two are generally confined to the left side of the abdomen but may extend across the median plane when the stomach is grossly distended. They are cranially related to the liver and diaphragm. The pyloric part extends to the right and is

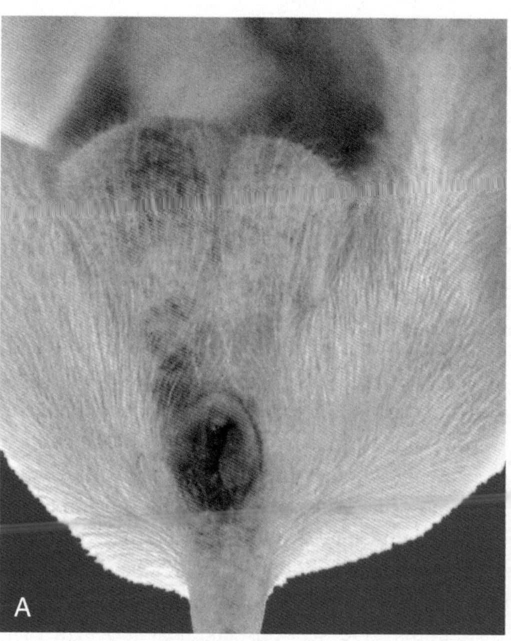

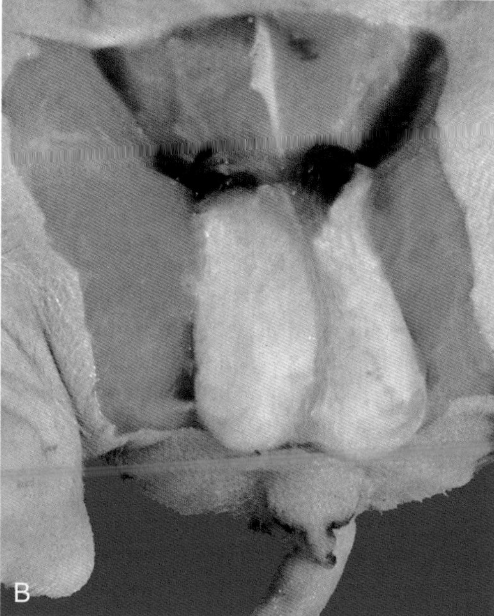

Fig. 34.3 A, Gubernacula in a freemartin piglet. B, Exposed.

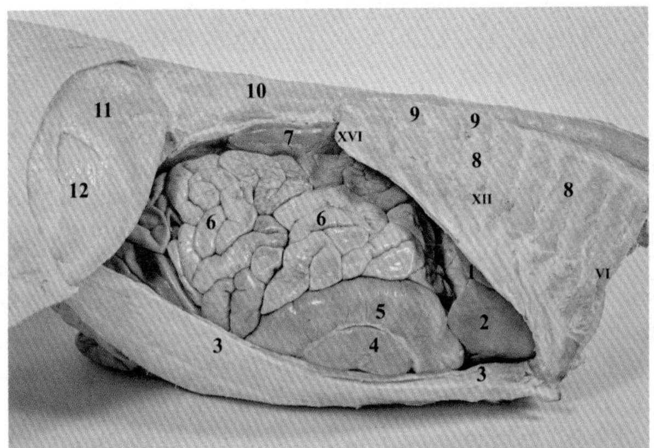

Fig. 34.4 Abdominal cavity of the pig from the right side. *1*, Liver, right lateral lobe; *2*, liver, right medial lobe; *3*, abdominal muscles (cut); *4*, ascending colon (gyri centrifugales); *5*, ascending colon (gyri centripetales); *6*, jejunal loops; *7*, right kidney; *8*, intercostal muscles; *9*, serratus dorsalis muscle (caudal part); *10*, epaxial muscles (iliocostalis lumborum and longissimus); *11*, tensor fasciae latae muscle; *12*, vastus lateralis muscle; VI, XII, XVI: ribs with respective numbers.

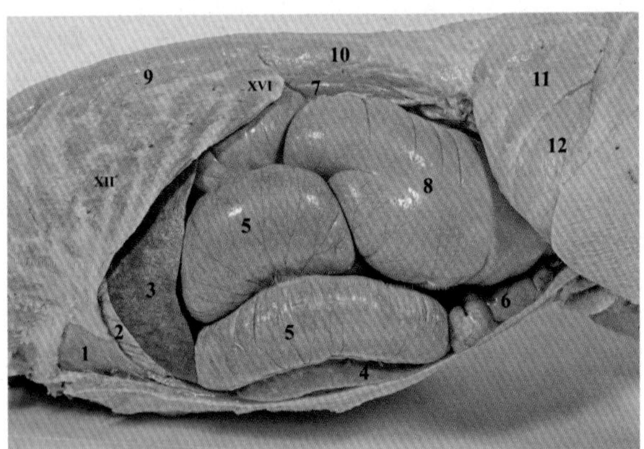

Fig. 34.5 Abdominal cavity of the pig from the left side. *1*, Liver, left lateral lobe; *2*, stomach; *3*, spleen; *4*, ascending colom (gyri centrifugales); *5*, ascending colon (gyri centripetales); *6*, jejunal loops; *7*, left kidney; *8*, cecum; *9*, serratus dorsalis muscle (caudal part); *10*, epaxial muscles (iliocostalis lumborum and longissimus); *11*, tensor fasciae latae muscle; *12*, vastus lateralis muscle XII, XVI: ribs with according numbers.

also in contact with the liver. All parts are related caudally to various parts of the intestinal mass, with the principal relation being to the ascending colic spiral. It is only when grossly distended that the stomach makes contact with the abdominal floor and, on the left, extends beyond the protection of the rib cage. A feature unique to the pig among domestic species is the presence of a conical diverticulum (Fig. 34.8/*2*) projecting caudally from the fundus.

The interior displays a narrow *nonglandular strip of mucosa* that extends into the diverticulum and follows the lesser curvature for some distance below the cardia (Fig. 34.9/*1*). The remainder of the mucosa is divided into the usual

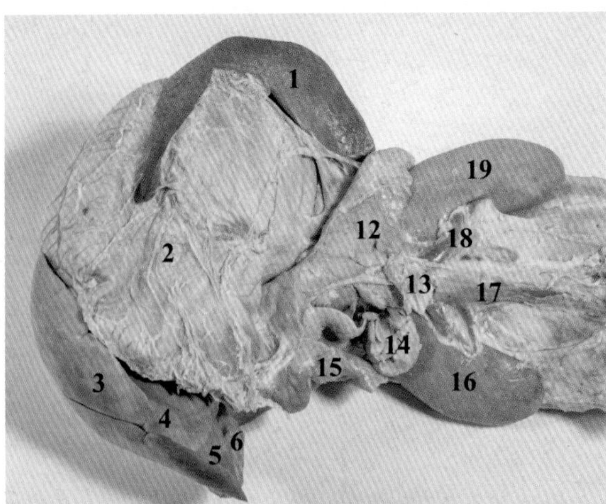

Fig. 34.6 Abdominal organs of the pig, after removal of the intestines. *1*, Spleen; *2*, stomach; *3*, liver, left medial lobe; *4*, liver, left lateral lobe; *5*, liver, quadrate lobe; *6*, gallbladder; *12*, pancreas, left lobe; *13*, cranial mesenteric artery (cut); *14*, pancreas, right lobe; *15*, descending duodenum; *16*, right kidney; *17*, caudal vena cava; *18*, renal artery and vein; *19*, left kidney.

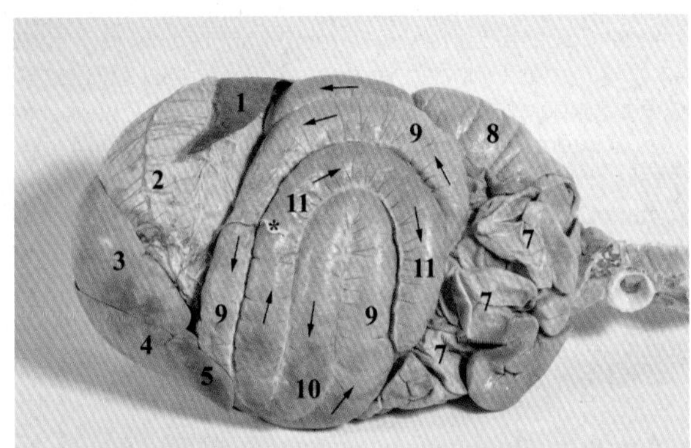

Fig. 34.7 Abdominal cavity of the pig (ventral view). *1*, Spleen; *2*, stomach; *3*, liver, left lateral lobe; *4*, liver, left medial lobe; *5*, liver, quadrate lobe; *7*, jejunal loops; *8*, cecum; *9*, ascending colon (gyri centripetales); *10*, ascending colon (flexura centralis); *11*, ascending colon (gyri centrifugales). Asterisk shows the teres hepatis ligament at the attachment to the adbominal wall at the navel.

three glandular regions, which are more clearly distinguished by color than in most species, although their borders are not always sharply defined (Fig. 34.9/*2a*, *2b*, and *2c*). A second feature of distinction is the *very prominent torus* narrowing the pyloric canal at the exit into the duodenum (Fig. 34.8/*10*).

Although the omenta are arranged much as in the dog, the greater one is less extravagantly developed, does not intervene between the intestines and the abdominal floor, and is therefore not encountered when the abdomen is first opened.

The arrangement of abdominal viscera is demonstrated in transverse sections taken at the 11th (Fig. 34.10) and 16th (Fig. 34.11) thoracic vertebrae.

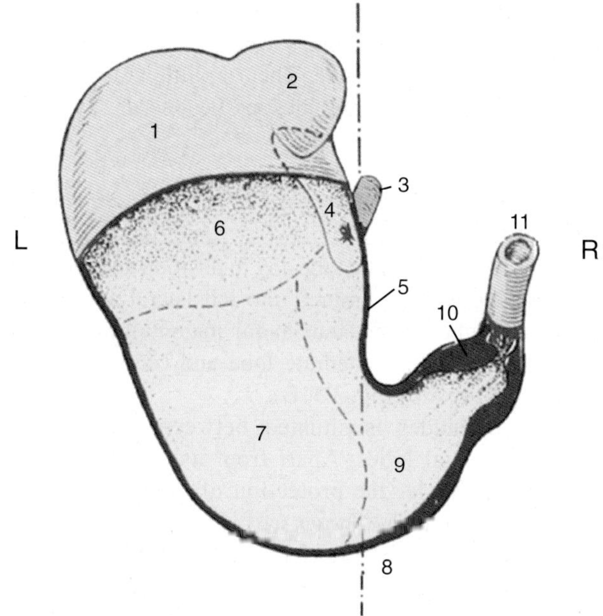

Fig. 34.8 Stomach partially opened, caudoventral view, semischematic. *1*, Fundus; *2*, diverticulum; *3*, esophagus; *4*, nonglandular mucosa; *5*, lesser curvature; *6*, cardiac gland region; *7*, region of proper gastric glands; *8*, approximate position of median plane; *9*, pyloric gland region; *10*, torus pyloricus; *11*, duodenum.

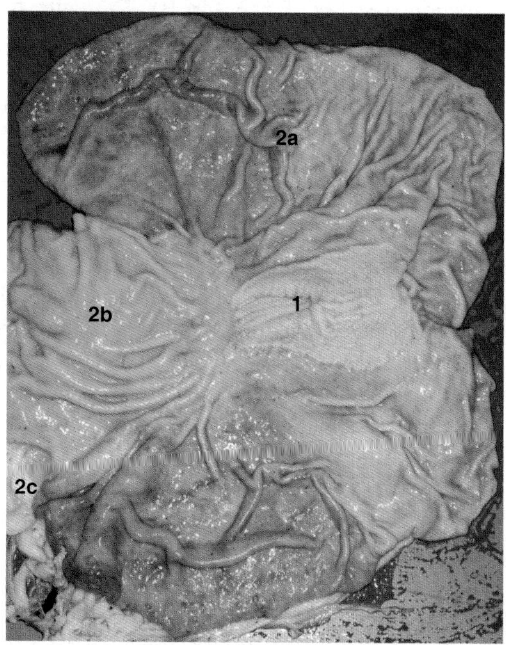

Fig. 34.9 The stomach laid open (cardia to the right). *1*, Nonglandular region; *2a*, region with cardiac glands; *2b*, region with proper gastric glands; *2c*, region with pyloric glands.

The Small Intestine

The *duodenum* is also arranged rather like that of the dog, descending toward the pelvis before turning to run forward to the left of the root of the mesentery before dipping

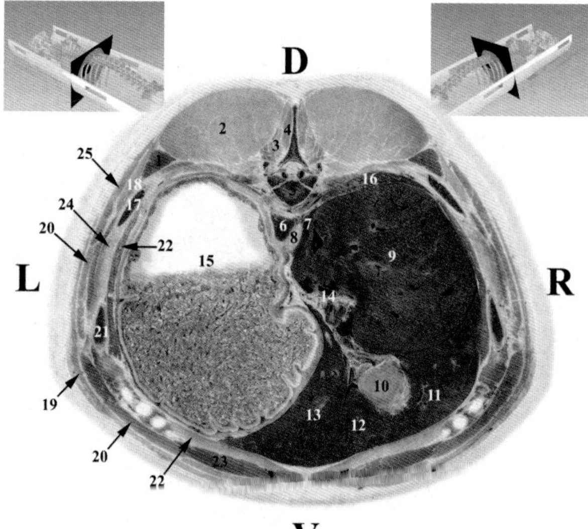

Fig. 34.10 Transverse section of the abdomen of the pig at the level of the 11th thoracic vertebra. *1*, Iliocostalis thoracis muscle; *2*, longissimus dorsi muscle; *3*, multifidi muscles; *4*, spinalis muscle; *5*, 11th thoracic vertebra; *6*, diaphragm, left crus; *7*, diaphragm, right crus; *8*, esophagus; *9*, liver (right lateral lobe); *10*, gall bladder; *11*, liver (right medial lobe); *12*, liver (quadrate lobe); *13*, liver (left medial lobe); *14*, porta hepatis; *15*, stomach; *16*, right lung, caudal lobe; *17*, 11th rib; *18*, serratus dorsalis muscle, caudal part; *19*, cutaneus trunci muscle; *20*, obliquus externus abdominis muscle; *21*, 10th rib; *22*, transversus abdominis muscle; *23*, rectus abdominis muscle; *24*, intercostalis muscles; *25*, latissimus dorsi muscle.

ventrally to be continued by the jejunum (Fig. 34.6 and 34.7). It is entered by the bile duct about 3 cm beyond the pylorus and by the single (accessory) pancreatic duct about 10 cm farther on. Both openings are raised on papillae.

The *jejunum* is arranged in many small loops (see Fig. 34.13) suspended by a mesentery that gives them much freedom of position. The greater part lies in the right half of the abdomen, ventrally and toward the pelvis, but some part may be in contact with the left flank behind the colic spiral. Like many other abdominal organs, the jejunum must accommodate its position to the condition of the stomach and, in sows, to that of the uterus.

The Large Intestine

The large intestine is capacious and, like that of the horse, is much sacculated, being drawn into a series of pouches by two (on the colon) or three (on the cecum) taeniae that run along its length. The peculiar disposition presented by the *cecum and ascending colon* in this animal, unique among domestic species, results from the greater than 360-degree rotation performed by the loop of bowel that is herniated into the umbilical cord early in development (see Figs. 3.64 and 3.65). This carries the caudal limb of the loop,

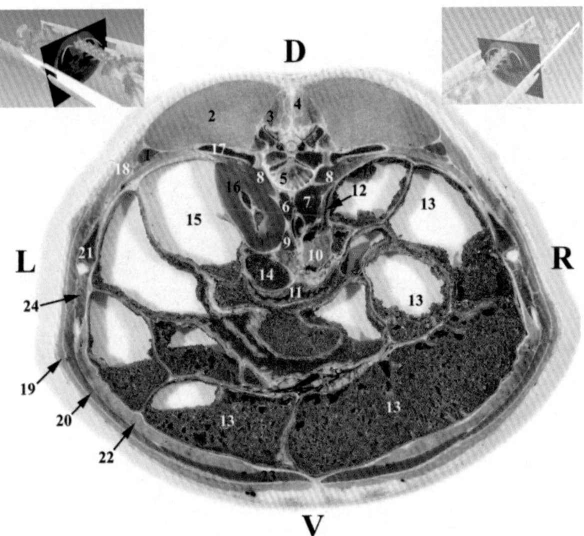

Fig. 34.11 Transverse section of the abdomen of the pig at the level of the 16th thoracic vertebra. *1*, Iliocostalis muscle; *2*, longissimus dorsi muscle; *3*, multifidi muscles; *4*, spinalis muscle; *5*, 16th thoracic vertebra; *6*, diaphragm, left crus; *7*, diaphragm, right crus; *8*, psoas minor muscle; *9*, left adrenal gland; *10*, pancreas, right lobe; *11*, dudodenum, caudal duodenal flexure; *12*, ascending duodenum; *13*, ascending colon; *14*, descending colon; *15*, cecum; *16*, left kidney; *17*, 16th rib; *18*, serratus dorsalis muscle, caudal part; *19*, cutaneus trunci muscle; *20*, obliquus externus abdominis muscle; *21*, 15th rib; *22*, transversus abdominis muscle; *23*, rectus abdominis muscle; *24*, intercartilaginei muscles.

including the cecocolic junction, to the left of the mesenteric axis, where it remains throughout later development and into adult life. The ascending colon thus commences on the left side and only gains its usual continuation into the transverse colon on the right side of the abdomen in consequence of the reversal of course described next.

The cecum and colon must be considered together because they combine in a conical, ventrally tapering mass suspended from the roof of the abdomen (Fig. 34.12). The *cecum,* which has a capacity of about 2 L, has its origin below the left kidney and extends ventrally or caudoventrally against the left flank to its rounded, blind apex. The *ascending colon* is arranged around its mesentery in a cone that points ventrally to reach the abdominal floor (with some deviation possible in any direction) (Fig. 34.12). The outer part of the cone is provided by the wide, sacculated portion continuing from the cecum; when viewed from above, it spirals ventrally, clockwise and centripetally, before reversing course at the apex of the cone to ascend in narrower, smoother, and tighter centrifugal coils concealed within the center of the cone. These carry it dorsally to emerge from the base of the cone, pass to the right of the root of the mesentery, and continue as the transverse colon. The cecocolic mass mainly occupies the middle third of the left side of the abdomen, leaving the caudal and right regions available to the jejunum. However, variation is common and, especially where the jejunum is concerned, can be considerable. There is little notable about the remainder of the large intestine beyond the existence of a rectal ampulla.

The Liver

The liver resembles that of the dog in position and lobation. It is divided by deep fissures into left lateral and medial lobes and right medial and lateral major lobes, supplemented by a smaller quadrate lobe and caudate process (Fig. 34.14; see also Fig. 3.51B).

The gallbladder is situated between the quadrate and right medial lobes. Apart from its ventral margin, the liver lies under the protection of the ribs (see Fig. 33.9/*3*); the somewhat larger part is situated to the right of the median plane (Fig. 34.4 and 34.5). The cranial surface is shaped to the diaphragm, and the caudal surface is indented by the stomach and duodenum; other contacts with the pancreas, jejunum, and colon leave less distinct or no impressions.

The two most notable features of the liver of this species are the lack of contact with (and molding by) the right kidney and the very well-developed fibrous tissue framework that prominently outlines the hepatic lobules on the surface and in section (see Fig. 3.52A and B). The latter feature is relevant to the clinician because surgery is required if a biopsy is indicated (aspiration is impossible with so fibrous a tissue) and is also relevant to the producer because it limits the price the consumer can be charged for a not very palatable foodstuff.

The Pancreas

The pancreas is related to the abdominal roof, largely on the left side. It is related ventrally to the gastric fundus, the spleen, and the left kidney (through fat) and, on the right, follows the duodenum. Other contacts are with the liver and right kidney. As happens in most mammals, it is penetrated by the portal vein traveling to the liver.

The Kidneys

The shape of the pig's kidneys is very distinctive. They are flattened (see Fig. 5.21C) against the abdominal roof (within a fatty capsule), extending from the level of the last rib to that of the fourth lumbar vertebra (Fig. 34.15/*5*). This symmetry of position is most unusual and deprives the right kidney of the expected contact with the liver. The left kidney is related ventrally to the colic spiral, the cecum, and the pancreas; the right one is related to the descending duodenum and also possibly to the pancreas.

The internal structure resembles that of the human kidney (Fig. 34.16). A central cavity with two recesses

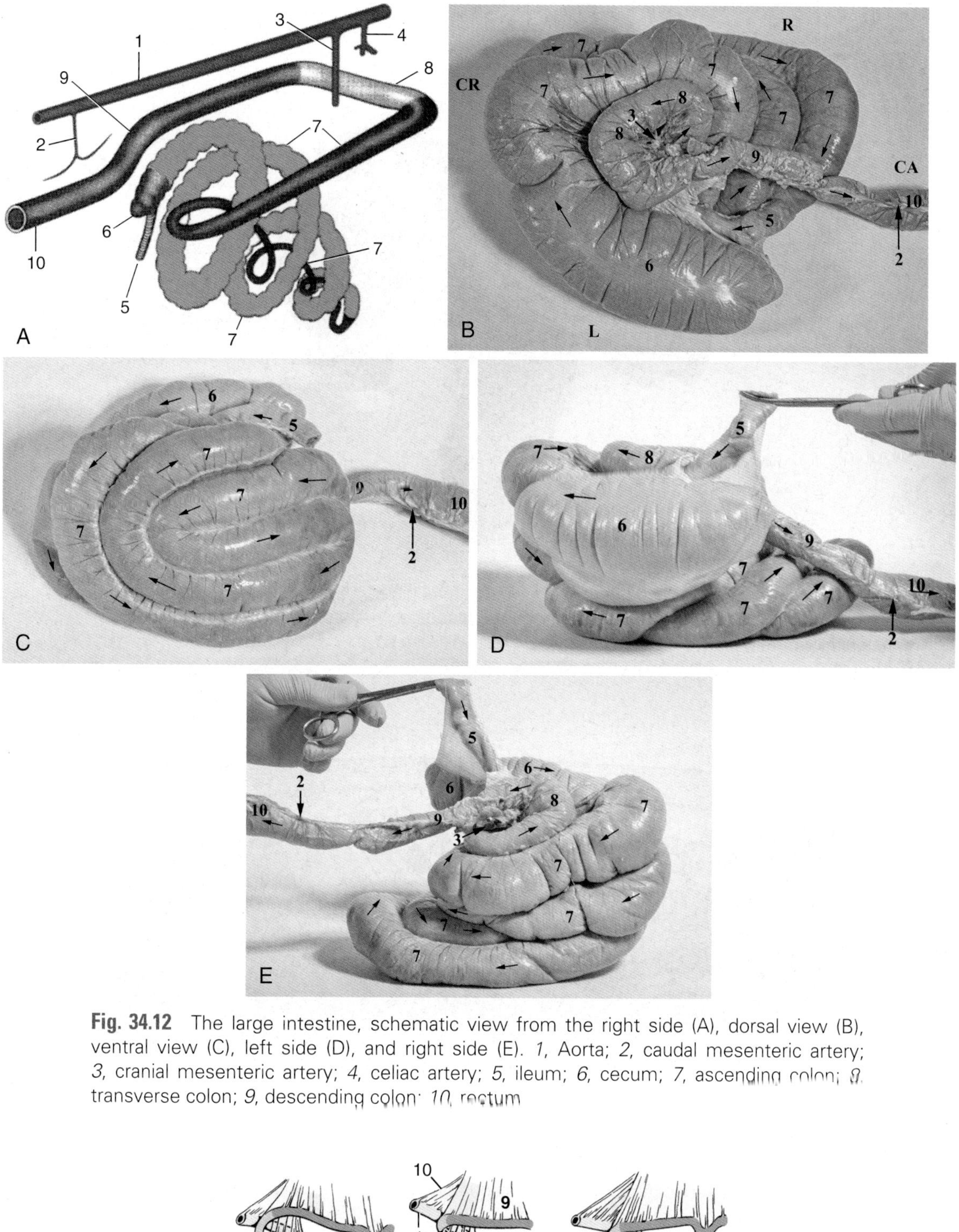

Fig. 34.12 The large intestine, schematic view from the right side (A), dorsal view (B), ventral view (C), left side (D), and right side (E). *1*, Aorta; *2*, caudal mesenteric artery; *3*, cranial mesenteric artery; *4*, celiac artery; *5*, ileum; *6*, cecum; *7*, ascending colon; *8*, transverse colon; *9*, descending colon; *10*, rectum

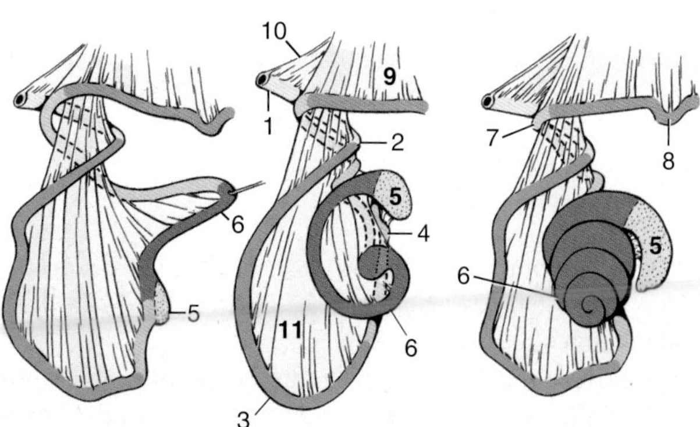

Fig. 34.13 The development of the ascending colon, left lateral view. *1*, Descending duodenum; *2*, caudal flexure of duodenum; *3*, jejunum; *4*, ileum; *5*, cecum; *6*, ascending colon; *7*, transverse colon; *8*, descending colon; *9*, descending mesocolon; *10*, mesoduodenum; *11*, mesentery.

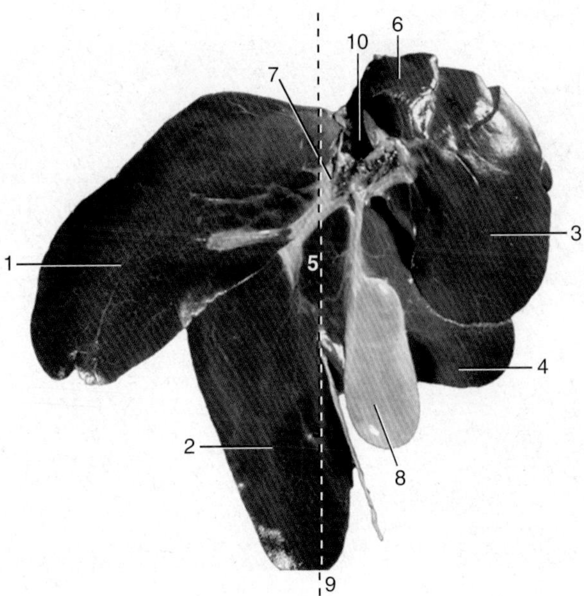

Fig. 34.14 Visceral surface of the liver. *1*, Left lateral lobe; *2*, left medial lobe; *3*, right lateral lobe; *4*, right medial lobe; *5*, quadrate lobe; *6*, caudate process; *7*, porta; *8*, gallbladder; *9*, approximate position of median plane; *10*, caudal vena cava.

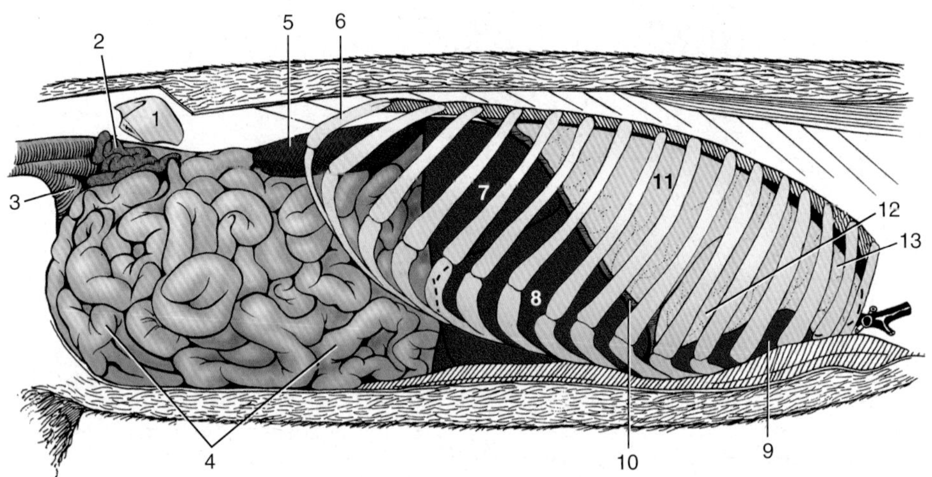

Fig. 34.15 Abdominal and thoracic viscera, right lateral view. *1*, Wing of ilium; *2*, uterine horns; *3*, bladder; *4*, jejunum; *5*, right kidney; *6*, last rib; *7* and *8*, right lateral and medial lobes of liver; *9*, heart in pericardium; *10*, diaphragm, cut; *11–13*, caudal, middle, and cranial lobes of right lung.

(major calices) directed toward the poles comprises the pelvis, which extends about a dozen minor calices, each embracing a renal papilla through which the papillary ducts discharge urine. The papillae correspond to renal pyramids, and because the number of these is reduced by fusions in the course of development, there is some inequality in the size of the units presented by the mature organ.

THE LYMPHATIC STRUCTURES OF THE ABDOMEN

The numerous abdominal lymph nodes fall into three groups: those of the abdominal roof, those associated with the mesogastric viscera (supplied by the celiac artery), and those associated with the viscera supplied by the two mesenteric arteries (Fig. 34.17).

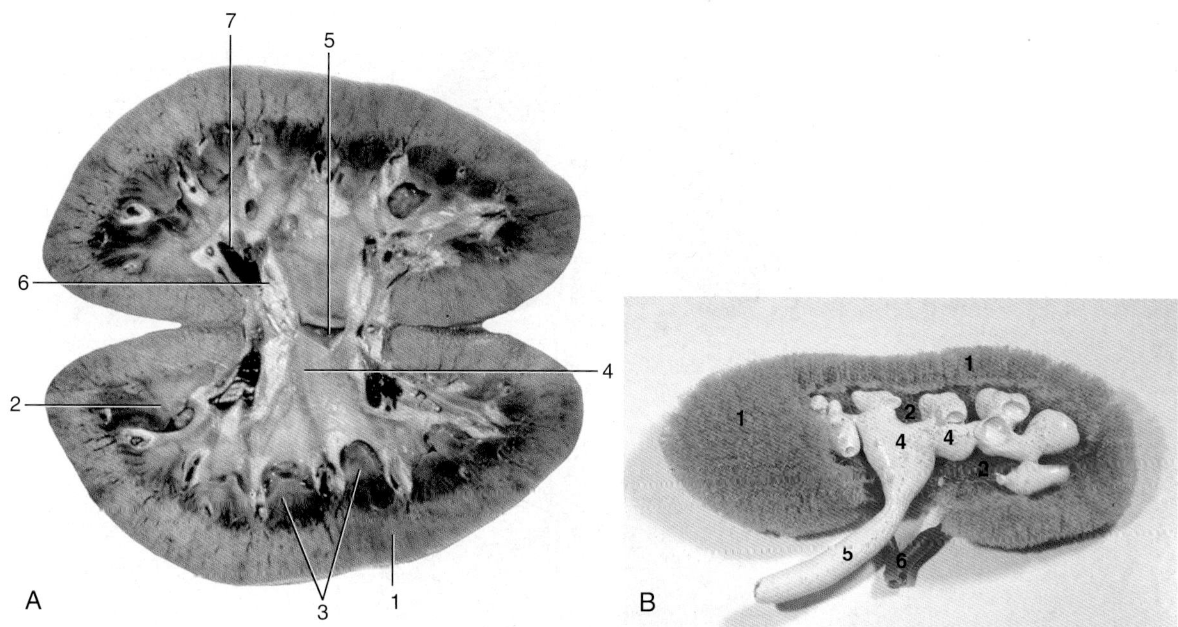

Fig. 34.16 Kidney sectioned through poles and hilus (A) and corrosion cast (B). *1*, Cortex; *2*, medulla; *3*, papilla; *4*, pelvis; *5*, ureter; *6*, renal artery; *7*, renal vein.

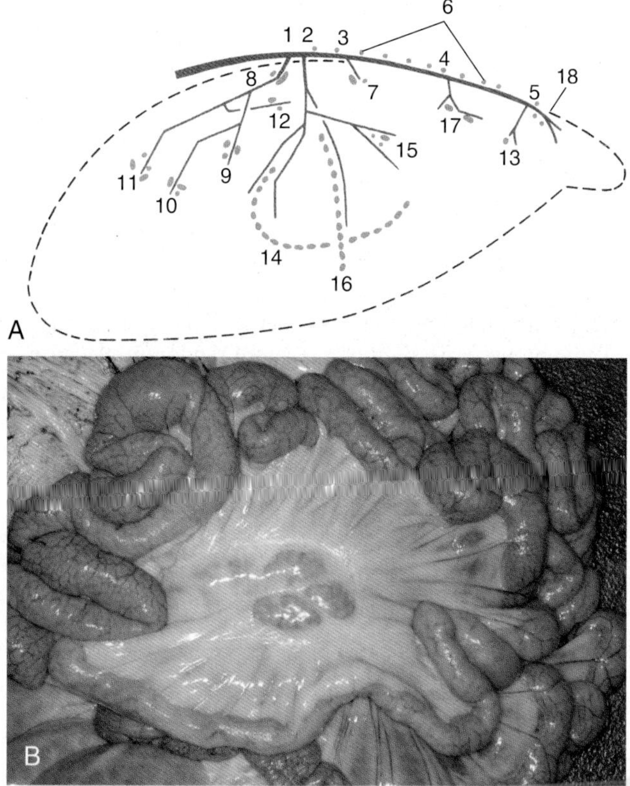

Fig. 34.17 (A) Schema of the major abdominal arteries and lymph nodes. *1*, Celiac artery; *2*, cranial mesenteric artery; *3*, renal artery; *4*, caudal mesenteric artery; *5*, deep circumflex iliac artery; *6*, lumbar aortic nodes; *7*, renal nodes; *8*, celiac nodes; *9*, splenic nodes; *10*, gastric nodes; *11*, hepatic nodes; *12*, pancreaticoduodenal nodes; *13*, lateral iliac nodes; *14*, jejunal nodes; *15*, ileocolic nodes; *16*, colic nodes; *17*, caudal mesenteric nodes; *18*, medial iliac nodes. (B) Part of the jejunum, showing the inclusion of jejunal lymph nodes in the mesentery.

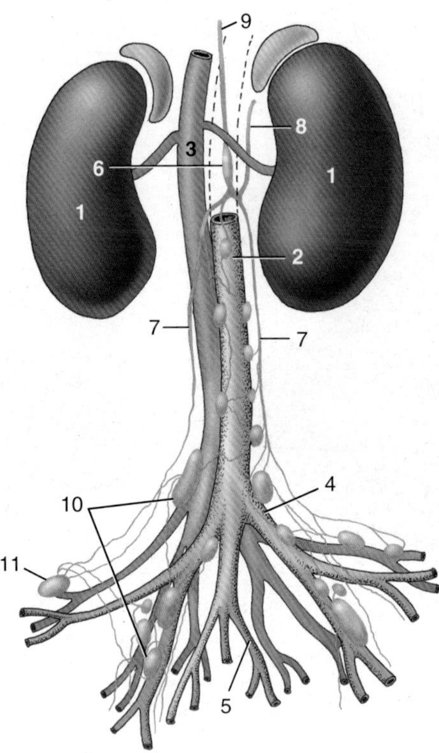

Fig. 34.18 The lymph nodes of the sublumbar area, ventral view. *1*, Kidneys; *2*, aorta; *3*, caudal vena cava; *4*, external iliac artery; 5, internal iliac artery; *6*, cisterna chyli; *7*, lumbar trunks and lumbar aortic nodes; *8*, intestinal trunk; *9*, thoracic duct; *10*, medial iliac nodes; *11*, lateral iliac node.

The *first group* includes aortic, renal, and iliac nodes whose disposition is illustrated in Fig. 34.18. The iliac assemblage receives lymph from structures of the hindlimb and pelvis and from part of the belly wall, including most mammary glands. Most nodes of this group drain lymph from structures of the back and forward it to the lumbar trunks or directly into the cisterna chyli.

The *second group of nodes* that are associated with the mesogastric viscera are mainly located close to where the arteries enter the individual organs; others, directly related to the celiac artery, provide an additional station on the drainage route, which ultimately joins the cisterna chyli. The *celiac nodes* also receive some lymph from caudal thoracic structures, including the caudal lobes of the lungs. The group that drains lymph from the small and large intestines includes a long chain in the mesentery of the jejunum, placed midway between its root and the gut, and a second set within the mesentery of the ascending colon; others are more randomly placed in relation to the remainder of the large intestine. All drain to the cisterna via an intestinal trunk. The nodes associated with the jejunum are of particular importance in meat inspection (Fig. 34.17B).

COMPREHENSION CHECK

Create a flow chart of the blood supply to the abdominal viscera of the pig.

The Pelvis and Reproductive Organs of the Pig

35

The thick layer of subcutaneous fat almost completely hides the junction between abdomen and pelvis, which is indicated only by a slight indentation above the fold of the flank. The landmarks of the pelvic skeleton are not immediately visible, but the positions of the coxal and ischial tubers is easily palpable, which reveals the small size of the girdle in relation to the overall dimensions of the hindquarters. The body and tuber of the ischium unite in very few pigs, and the unfused tuber is at risk of detachment by the pull of the powerful hamstring muscles that arise from it. Young sows are most commonly affected and are unable to rise when this happens; the very painful condition has no cure but slaughter.

From a lateral view, the pelvic floor and the iliac shaft meet at an angle that approaches 180 degrees (Fig. 35.1) and create a large and oval pelvic inlet. The "vertical diameter" is maintained caudally, to intersect the part of the sacrum composed of yet unfused bones to allow some mobility. The pelvic floor slopes caudoventrally. The pelvic canal is a little higher than it is wide (Fig. 35.1). The slight inward bending of the ischial spines and presence of soft tissue structures narrow the canal. The slackening of the sacrosciatic ligament, which completes the lateral wall of the pelvic cavity, and of the joints of the girdle helps during farrowing.

THE RECTUM AND ANUS

The shortness of its mesentery is the only additional point that need be made concerning the rectum. Congenital absence of the anus (atresia ani) once was of frequent occurrence; perhaps surprisingly, it may allow afflicted piglets to survive for 3 or 4 weeks without treatment. If the rectum ends blindly at no great distance from the skin, a passage may be created by simple surgery.

Prolapse of the rectum, encountered in somewhat older pigs, requires more sophisticated surgery, especially if the everted bowel has been mutilated by pen mates, as so often happens. The muscles of the anus are more or less as in other species (see Figs. 3.47 and 3.48): bundling together of the longitudinal muscle of the rectum creates the rectococcygeus, and thickening of the circular muscle creates the internal anal sphincter. There is a striated external sphincter. The levator ani runs between the sacrosciatic ligament and the lateral aspect of the anal canal, and the two retractor penis (or clitoridis) muscles form a sling below the rectum before continuing to the penis (or clitoris).

THE BLADDER AND FEMALE URETHRA

The empty bladder is a small, firm ovoid structure placed over the pubic pecten (Fig. 35.2/*5* and *5'*). When full, the bladder extends over the abdominal floor, sometimes up to the umbilicus. It becomes spherical when grossly distended. The bladder is wholly covered in peritoneum, which continues into paired recesses below the urethra. A small suburethral diverticulum (Fig. 35.2/*6*), associated with the opening of the urethra into the vestibule, may interfere with catheterization of the bladder.

THE FEMALE REPRODUCTIVE ORGANS

The Ovary and Uterine Tube

The ovaries, about 5 cm long, are distinguished by the many follicles and corpora lutea that project from the entire surface (Fig. 35.3). They are usually found hidden among the intestines, slightly ventrolateral to the pelvic inlet. The relatively long mesovaria commonly allow both ovaries to lie against the one flank, and consequently, both may be removed through a single incision.

The uterine tube (Fig. 35.4/*4*) is about 20 cm long, is carried in the wall of the cone-shaped ovarian bursa, and meets the horn of the uterus at a tapering junction. Obstruction of the tube (the origin of hydrosalpinx) can cause infertility in sows.

The Uterus

The sow's uterus is distinguished by its short body and long, tortuous horns (Fig. 35.4/*5* and *8*). The body, about 5 cm long, is deceptively short because the parts of the horns at their origin lie within common investments (as in ruminants). In the nongravid state each horn measures about 1 m, and a fairly generous broad ligament (Fig. 35.4/*6*) gives it freedom of position, relations, and arrangement; however, it fails to reach the abdominal floor. Some parts become mingled with coils of small intestine and can be confused with these. The cervix, which lies half within the abdomen and half within the pelvis, is peculiar for its length (≈25 cm). The cervix is about 20 cm in length and has rows of interdigitating mucosal prominences (Fig. 35.4/*11*) that project into the lumen and close the canal, except at estrus and parturition. The cervix has many goblet cells that produce mucus during the estrus. Its junctions with the uterine body and the vagina taper and are ill defined.

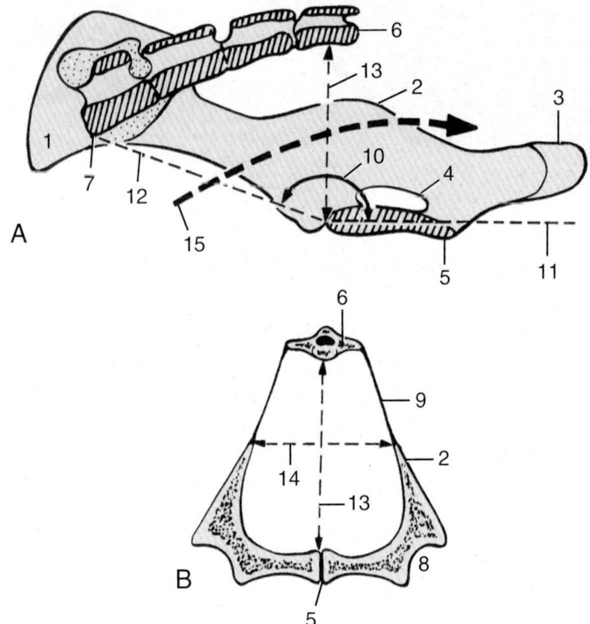

Fig. 35.1 (A) Median section of the sow's pelvis. (B) Transverse section of the pelvis near the level of the vertical diameter. *1,* Coxal tuber; *2,* ischial spine; *3,* ischial tuber; *4,* obturator foramen; *5,* pelvic symphysis; *6,* fourth sacral vertebra (S4); *7,* promontory; *8,* acetabulum; *9,* sacrosciatic ligament; *10,* angle between pelvic floor and conjugata; *11,* plane of pelvic floor; *12,* conjugata; *13,* vertical diameter; *14,* transverse diameter; *15,* pelvic axis.

The Vagina, Vestibule, and Vulva

The vagina is about 7 to 12 cm in length. It is unremarkable, and the vestibule is relatively long. The vestibule has openings for the minor vestibular glands and has solitary lymph nodes. The conical vulva slopes so that it faces rather obliquely upward (Fig. 35.2A/*7*); it is sometimes so upturned that the cleft is inaccessible to the boar. Gilts with an infantile vulva are common, and the defect hints at poor development of the reproductive organs and greater risk of infertility. The clitoris is normally barely visible (Fig. 35.4/*17*). Clitoral enlargement is common and is associated with intersexuality (female pseudohermaphroditism).

The *uterine artery,* the principal supply to the uterus, is supplemented by branches of the ovarian and vaginal arteries (Fig. 35.5/*2* and *7*). The ovarian vein, which drains most of the uterus in addition to the ovary, forms a plexus around the uterine and ovarian arteries that facilitates the transfer of luteolytic prostaglandins.

The examination of the reproductive tract is done to determine the reproductive health of the animals. Many times the reproductive tract is collected in the slaughterhouse to examine it for gross and histologic abnormalities to determine causes of reproductive failure. Therefore, the knowledge of the anatomy of the reproductive organs is of vital importance.

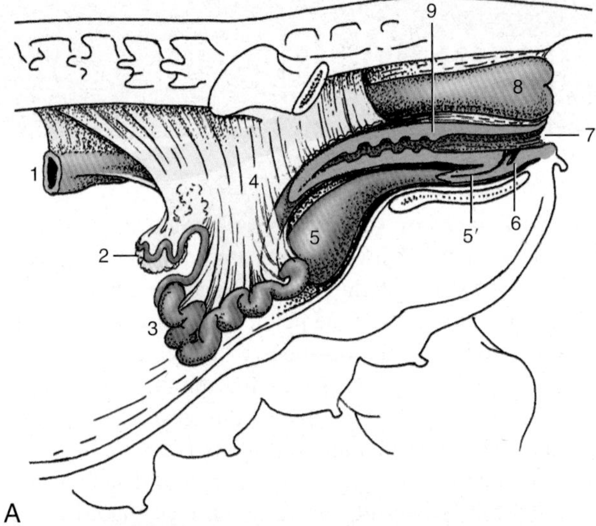

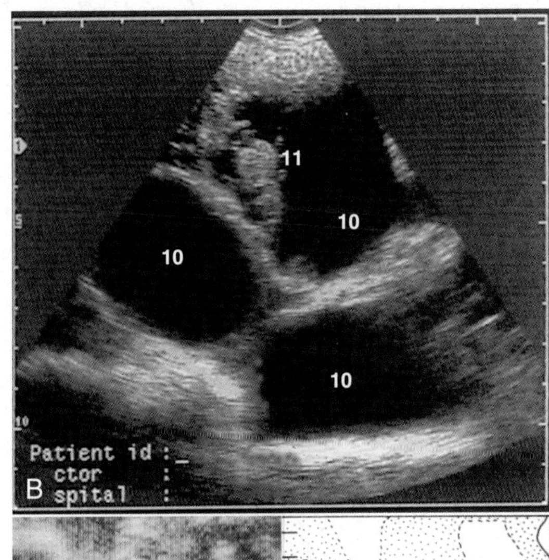

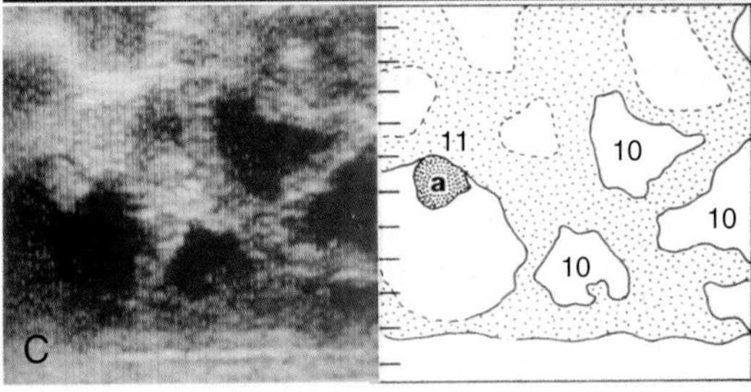

Fig. 35.2 (A), The reproductive organs of the sow in situ. (The presence of the intestines in the intact animal causes the ovaries and uterine horns to lie more dorsally than shown here.) *1,* Descending colon; *2,* ovary; *3,* uterine horns; *4,* broad ligament; *5,* bladder; *5′,* urethra; *6,* suburethral diverticulum; *7,* vulva; *8,* rectum; *9,* cervix. (B) Transrectal ultrasonographic image and (C) transabdominal ultrasonographic image and schematic of 30-day gravid porcine uteruses. (Scales in centimeters.) *10,* Allantoic fluid-filled spaces; *11* and *(a),* embryo.

Functional Aspects

Gilts attain puberty around 6 months. The species is polyestrous: the cycle repeats at intervals of about 17 to 25 days. Fertilization takes place in the ampullae, where

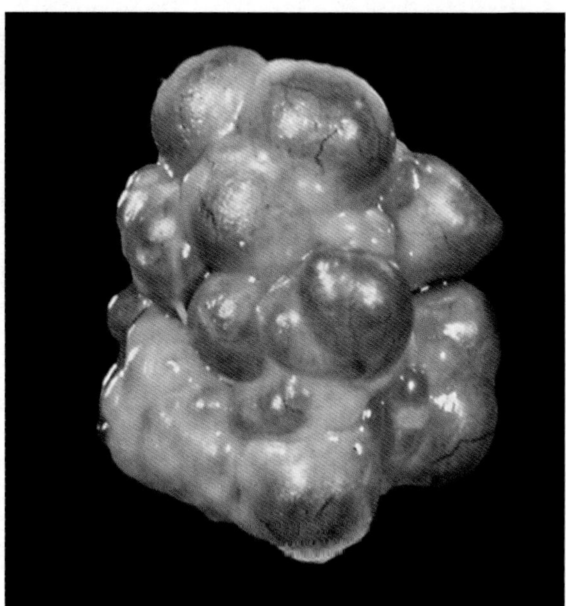

Fig. 35.3 Ovary (sow) exhibiting mature follicles.

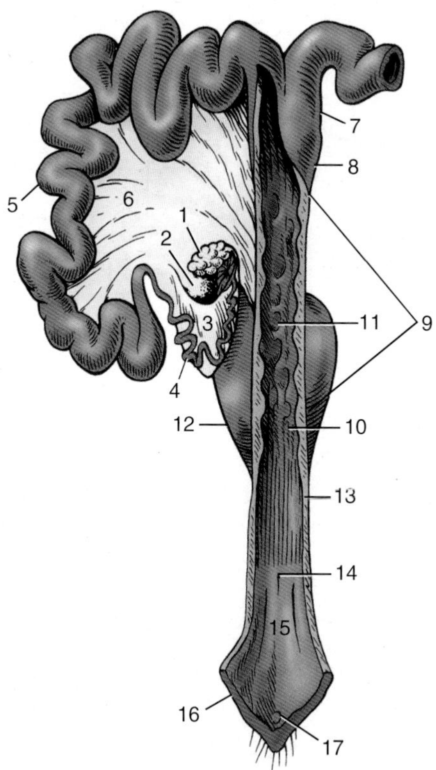

Fig. 35.4 The reproductive tract of the sow opened dorsally in part; the right uterine horn and ovary are not shown. *1,* Left ovary; *2,* ovarian bursa; *3,* mesosalpinx; *4,* uterine tube; *5,* uterine horn; *6,* broad ligament; *7,* parallel segments of uterine horns; *8,* body of uterus; *9,* cervix; *10,* external uterine orifice; *11,* mucosal prominences; *12,* bladder; *13,* vagina; *14,* external urethral orifice; *15,* vestibule; *16,* vulva; *17,* glans of clitoris.

the conceptuses are detained for a few days before being admitted to the uterus. Cleavage continues there, creating blastocysts that are initially spherical and randomly placed. By the end of 2 weeks they have become filamentous and greatly lengthened—up to 60 cm—and have adopted permanent, regularly spaced stations that make full use of both horns, which is an arrangement that may have required some conceptuses to migrate from one horn to the other. The conception rate is high, but so also is prenatal mortality—40% or more. The placenta is of the diffuse epitheliochorial type. Antibody transfer does not occur in utero, and the newborn is dependent on the ingestion of colostrum for its initial immunologic protection.

During pregnancy, the horns increase greatly in diameter, and their length may double. Growth of the tissues within the broad ligaments allows the horns to sink into the ventral half of the abdomen, where they push the intestines craniodorsally and make contact with the stomach and liver. The ovaries are carried forward and out of reach of a hand within the rectum. Confirmation of pregnancy at this stage is provided by the firmness of the cervix and, more reliably, by the characteristic fremitus of the enlarged uterine artery. Ultrasonography is a less troublesome method of pregnancy diagnosis (Fig. 35.2B and C).

Rectal palpation is used for pregnancy detection in the pig. It is highly accurate based on the examination of the cervix, uterus, and middle uterine artery. The accuracy is approximately 95% around day 30 and 100% after day 60 of the gestation.

Gestation averages about 114 days with a range of 111 to 117 days, and farrowing is preceded by the usual relaxation of the joints and tissues of the pelvic region, although this may not be apparent to an observer. The risk of simultaneous arrival of two fetuses from opposite horns at the entrance to the body is prevented by the circular muscle of the uterus, which very effectively closes the exit from one horn while simultaneously securing maximal enlargement of the exit from the other. The arrangement does not operate at all times; both horns open freely into the body of the atonic uterus, which allows fetuses to be transferred from one horn to the other at cesarean section. The expulsion of first piglets lubricates the passage for easier movement of the remaining fetuses.

Some criteria that may be used for estimating the age of pig fetuses are provided in Table 35.1.

THE MALE REPRODUCTIVE ORGANS

The Scrotum and Testes

The scrotum is perineal in position. The tail of the epididymis and the less salient associated pole of the testis point dorsocaudally by the anus and are readily palpable.

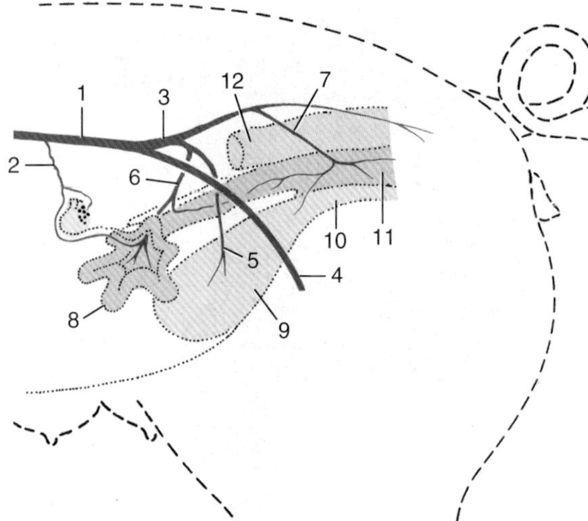

Fig. 35.5 The principal arteries supplying the left side of the female reproductive tract (schematic). *1,* Aorta; *2,* ovarian artery (a.) with cranial uterine branch; *3,* internal iliac a.; *4,* external iliac a. continued by femoral a. into left thigh; *5,* umbilical a.; *6,* left uterine a. crossing medial surface of external iliac a.; *7,* vaginal a. with caudal uterine branch; *8,* left uterine horn; *9,* bladder; *10,* urethra; *11,* vagina; *12,* rectum.

The free border of the testis faces caudoventrally, and the attached border is closely applied to the surface of the thigh (Fig. 35.6).

Castration: Male pigs are usually castrated within 2 weeks of their birth to prevent the development of the taint that characterizes the flesh of boars. It is now increasingly appreciated, in some countries at least, that the taint does not appear until after the usual age at slaughter and that castration is therefore pointless. Both the open and closed methods of castration are used with young pigs. In the former technique, which is preferred, the tunica vaginalis is incised, the ligament joining it to the epididymis divided, and the cord severed. This is the method employed with old boars. In the closed method (Fig. 35.7B), the scrotum is opened, the tunica vaginalis is left intact but freed from attachments, and the cord is transected close to the external inguinal opening. The situation of the scrotum explains the unusual length of the cord.

In pigs, descent of the testis commences about the 60th day of gestation, and regression of the extra-abdominal gubernaculum creates the conditions in which the testis is able to leave the inguinal canal by approximately the 90th day. After a period of uncertainty, when the testis may move back and forth between the canal and the groin, a permanent position in the scrotum is adopted by full term. Abnormalities of gubernacular development

TABLE 35.1 GUIDE TO THE AGING OF PIG FETUSES

Weeks	Crown–Rump Length (cm)	External Features
2.5	≈1	Limb buds forming
4	≈2	Tactile hair follicles appear; mammary primordium present
5	≈3.5	Palate fused; facial clefts closed
6	≈6.5	Prepuce and scrotum, or labia and clitoris present
7	≈9	Eyelids fused; intestines returned to abdomen
13	≈24	Eyelids separated
Full term		On average 114 days

From Evans HE, Sack WO: Prenatal development of domestic and laboratory animals. Growth curves, external features, and selected references. *Anat Histol Embryol* 2:11–45, 1973.

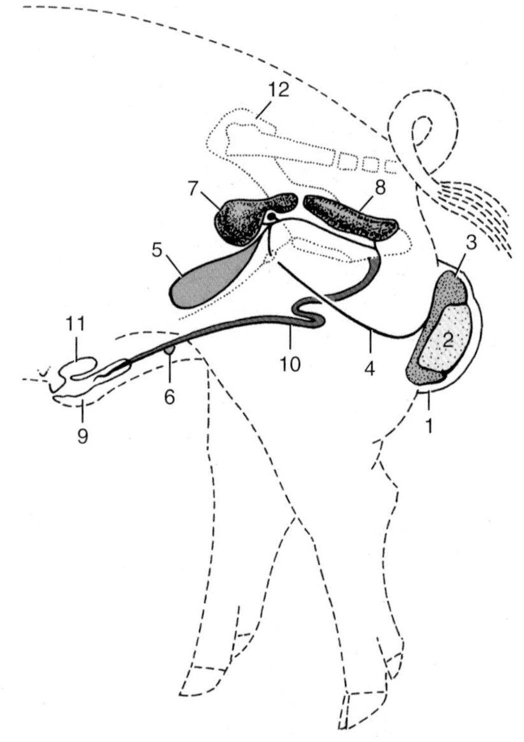

Fig. 35.6 Reproductive organs of the boar (schematic). *1,* Scrotum; *2,* left testis; *3,* tail of epididymis; *4,* deferent duct; *5,* bladder; *6,* rudimentary teat; *7,* vesicular gland covering the small body of the prostate; *8,* bulbourethral gland; *9,* prepuce; *10,* penis; *11,* preputial diverticulum; *12,* right hip bone.

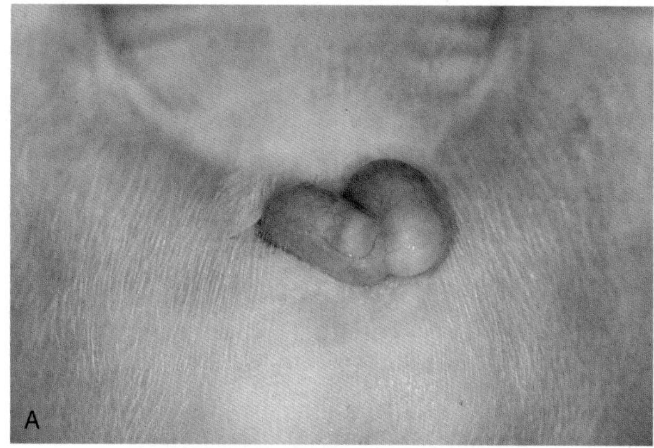

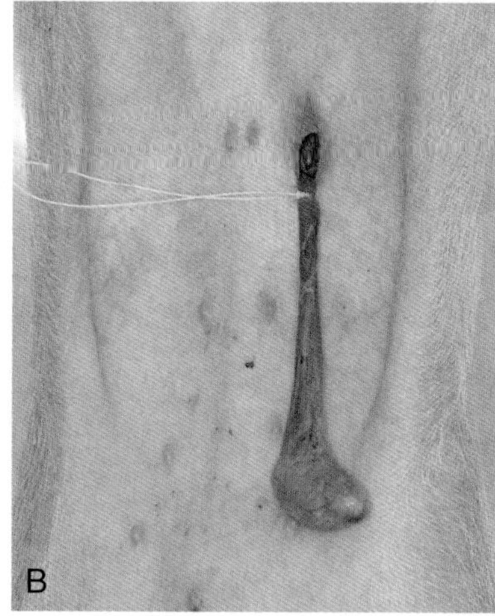

Fig. 35.7 (A) Open castration method of a newborn piglet. (Note: The parietal layer of vaginal tunic is still intact.) (B) The closed castration method in a 5-week-old piglet (also performed in case of an inguinal hernia).

and regression are common. Both excessive swelling and delayed regression may widen the canal abnormally, allowing a loop of intestine to slip into the vaginal cavity and thus creating an indirect inguinal or, should it reach so far, scrotal hernia. Surgical correction of this defect in [illegible] with castration by the closed method. (The inguinal hernias occasionally seen in young gilts are associated with abnormal genital tracts that resemble those of bovine freemartins.)

The Pelvic Reproductive Organs

The *deferent ducts* take their usual courses to penetrate the body of the prostate before opening into the urethra on the summit of a low papilla (Fig. 35.8/*5*). They do not expand to form ampullae and in the last part of their courses are covered by the very large *vesicular glands* that open beside them (Fig. 35.8/*7*). Only small parts of these glands are contained within the pelvic cavity; the bulk protrudes into the abdomen, beyond the neck of the bladder (Fig. 35.6/*7*), and is enclosed within the genital folds. In addition to a modest irregular body, the prostate (Fig. 35.8/*8*) possesses a large disseminate part spread within the wall of the pelvic urethra.

The *bulbourethral glands* are remarkable for their shape and size. They lie dorsolateral to the pelvic urethra and are sufficiently long to touch the vesicular glands (Fig. 35.8A/*11* and see Fig. 35.6/*8*). Each drains through a dilated, sometimes duplicated duct that opens onto the thickening that separates a dorsal diverticulum from the lumen of the urethra where this bends around the ischial arch. The glands are covered by the bulboglandularis muscles, whose contraction secures their evacuation (Fig. 35.8A/*12*). The caudal ends of the glands may be palpated per rectum. The ability to touch the urethra between them is diagnostic of the castrate (Fig. 35.8B); inability to do this in the absence of palpable testes suggests cryptorchidism.

The Penis and Prepuce

The penis, broadly similar to that of the bull, is relatively thin, exhibits a prescrotal sigmoid flexure, and is about 60 cm long (when flaccid) (Fig. 35.6/*10*). A thick tunica albuginea encloses the corpus cavernosum (Fig. 35.9/*1*). The corpus spongiosum lies first on the ventral surface of the corpus cavernosum, but more distally it is recessed in a deep groove that brings it to a central position (Fig. 35.9B/*6*). Apart from the sigmoid flexure, the shaft is twisted on its longitudinal axis a full turn counterclockwise (when viewed from behind). The direction of the twist is the same as that of the spiral of the apex (Fig. 35.9C).

The relatively long prepuce houses the free part of the penis in its narrow caudal half. The wider cranial half communicates with a dorsal diverticulum, a pouch containing an evil-smelling fluid consisting of cell debris soaked in urine (Fig. 35.6/*9* and *11*). The diverticulum is [illegible] preputial muscle, which empties it before copulation (Fig. 35.10A/*1*). The fluid contains a pheromone that encourages the sow to assume the immobile mating stance. If the contents of the diverticulum collect excessively, the appearance may mimic umbilical hernia. An infected diverticulum may be opened and drained through a dorsolateral incision that inevitably includes the muscle. The diverticulum is sometimes removed in boars used for artificial insemination so that contamination of the semen is reduced. Although the tip of the penis occasionally becomes entrapped in the diverticulum, it is readily freed.

Functional Aspects

The size of the accessory glands is related to the large volume of the ejaculate, at least 200 mL. Despite their great

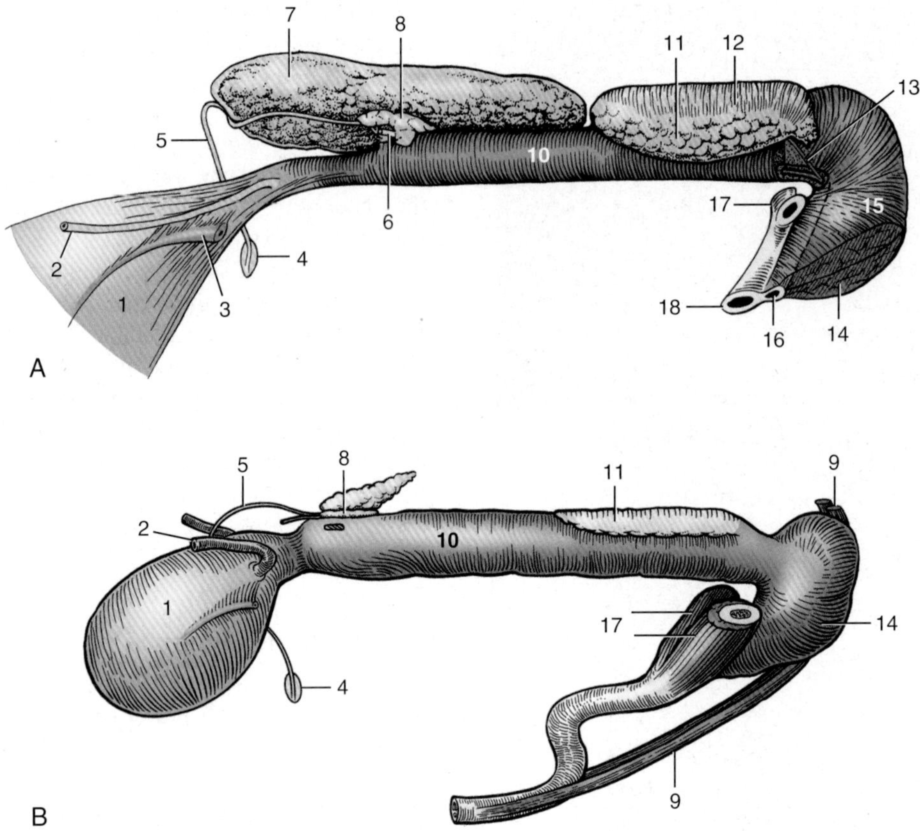

Fig. 35.8 Pelvic urethra and associated organs of (A) an 8-month-old boar and (B) a 6-month-old castrate, left lateral views. The left vesicular gland has been removed to expose the prostate. *1*, Bladder; *2*, left ureter; *3*, left umbilical artery; *4*, right vaginal ring; *5*, right deferent duct; *6*, left deferent duct, cut at prostate; *7*, right vesicular gland; *8*, body of prostate; *9*, retractor penis; *10*, pelvic urethra, surrounded by urethralis; *11*, left bulbourethral gland; *12*, bulboglandularis covering dorsal half of bulbourethral gland; *13*, excretory duct of left bulbourethral gland; *14*, bulbospongiosus; *15*, bulb of penis; *16*, urethra and corpus spongiosum; *17*, right and left crura, cut; *18*, corpus cavernosum.

size, the vesicular and bulbourethral glands together contribute somewhat less than half the seminal fluid; the bulk is provided by the prostate and urethral glands.

During erection the blood pressure in the cavernous spaces rises sharply, straightening the sigmoid flexure and increasing the length of the penis by about a quarter. The single longitudinal twist of the shaft increases to six turns, while the corkscrew spiral of the free part becomes much more pronounced. During coitus, a slow process that may last for as long as 30 minutes, the boar is said to "soak" because of the absence of obvious activity on his part. However, forward and backward twisting movements of the penis do occur under the influence of the retractor muscle. There is no substance to the persistent belief that the prominences of the cervical mucosa form a canal with a left-hand thread matching that of the spiraled end of the penis. The end of the penis is considered to almost enter the uterus.

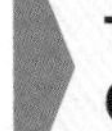

THE LYMPHATIC STRUCTURES OF THE PELVIS

The *medial iliac lymph nodes* grouped about the terminal branches of the aorta have been shown in Fig. 34.18. They are continued into the pelvic cavity by *sacral nodes* below the sacrum and anorectal nodes below the tailhead. The latter nodes drain the rectum, anus, and tail; their efferents pass to the medial iliac nodes. *Ischial nodes* receiving lymph from the perineum, caudal thigh, and *popliteal nodes and gluteal nodes* draining the gluteal region lie lateral to the sacrosciatic ligament. Both sets also drain to the medial iliac nodes.

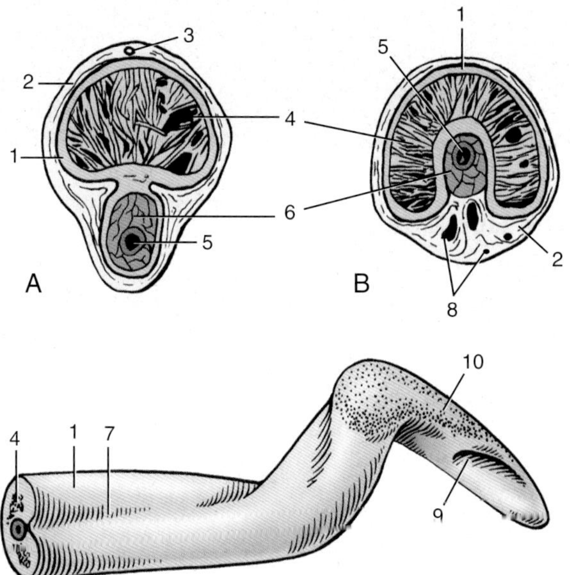

Fig. 35.9 Transverse sections of the penis. (A) Proximal to the sigmoid flexure. (B) Distal to the sigmoid flexure. (C) Free end of penis. *1,* Tunica albuginea; *2,* connective tissue surrounding penis; *3,* dorsal artery of penis; *4,* corpus cavernosum; *5,* urethra; *6,* corpus spongiosum; *7,* urethral groove; *8,* blood vessels; *9,* external urethral orifice; *10,* thin glans penis.

THE ANATOMY OF RECTAL EXPLORATION

Rectal palpation is possible in sows weighing 150 kg or more without great difficulty or ill effects on the animal. It is generally found that the small diameter and short suspension of the descending colon are greater impediments to these examinations than constriction of the pelvic canal. With ample lubrication and sufficient cooperation, the arm can be introduced almost to the elbow; however, because the forearm is solidly wedged in the pelvic canal, the scope for exploration depends entirely on the length of and the mobility that may be exercised by the hand. The procedure allows examination of the pelvic inlet and bladder and, more important, the ovaries, cervix, and uterine artery for pregnancy diagnosis. The right kidney and the spiral colon—recognized through its coarse, granular content—may also be identified; the colon prevents access to the left kidney. Examination of the more confined pelvic cavity of boars is not feasible; the intrusion causes obvious pain.

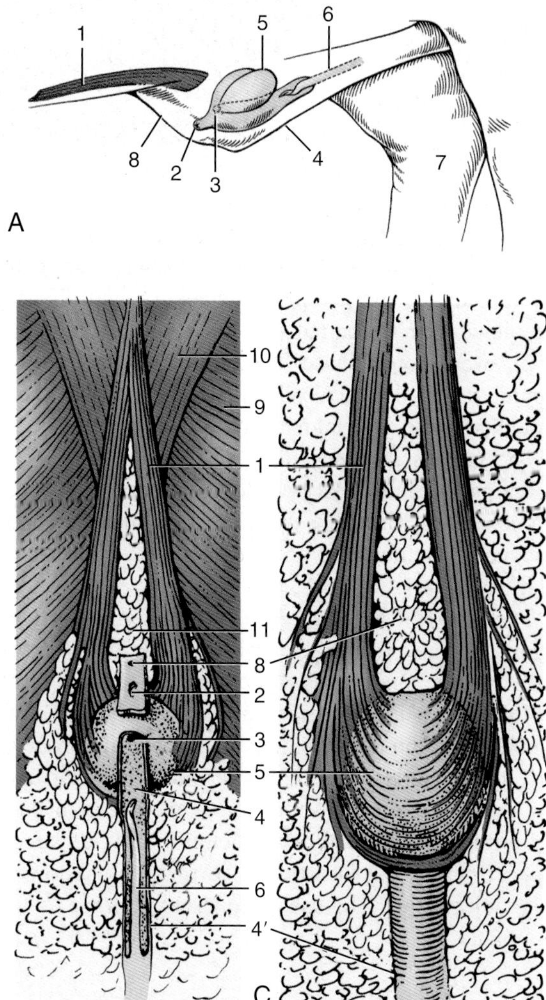

Fig. 35.10 Prepuce and preputial diverticulum. (A) In situ, craniolateral view (schematic). (B) Ventral view. (C) Dorsal view. *1,* Cranial preputial muscle, in (A) cut at both ends; *2,* preputial orifice; *3,* orifice between prepuce and diverticulum; *4* and *4′,* wide cranial and narrow caudal parts of preputial cavity, respectively; *5,* preputial diverticulum; *6,* penis; *7,* medial surface of right hock; *8,* umbilicus; *9,* cutaneous trunci; *10,* pectoralis profundus; *11,* preputial fat.

COMPREHENSION CHECK

Compare the anatomic features of the male and female reproductive systems of the pig with those of the horse.

Review the blood and nerve supply to the pelvic viscera of the pig.

36 The Limbs of the Pig

The principal distinguishing features of the limb skeleton of the pig are the well-developed, weight-bearing ulnae and fibulae and the complete metapodial and phalangeal complements in the paired accessory digits (Figs. 36.1 and 36.2), even though these fail to make contact with firm ground. It will also be recalled that very few pigs live long enough to attain skeletal maturity.

The hooves resemble those of cattle and have a soft digital pad, or bulb, that is well demarcated from the wall and sole (Fig. 36.3). The short life span and the common practice of running pigs on concrete make hoof trimming rarely necessary.

The limbs of pigs received little veterinary attention before it was recognized that articular disease (especially osteochondrosis) was relatively common. This stimulated a belated interest in the anatomy of the major joints and in the development of appropriate procedures for their injection. The causes of much articular pathology are uncertain. However, rapid weight gain beyond the ability of the immature skeleton to provide adequate support may result in articular cartilage breakdown and bone deformities. The use of concrete flooring may also be a factor.

THE FORELIMB

Skeletal features that may be identified on palpation include the cranial and caudal angles and the tubercle on the spine of the scapula; the caudal part of the greater tubercle of the humerus; the medial and lateral condyles of the humerus and the olecranon at the elbow; and the accessory carpal, revealing the level of the proximal row of carpal bones (see Fig. 32.1). Soft tissue structures that may be identified include the cephalic vein on the cranial aspect of the arm (not always visible but possibly available for puncture) and the skin glands at the caudomedial aspect of the carpus (Fig. 36.4).

The Shoulder Joint

The large cranial part of the greater tubercle deflects the intertubercular groove medially and, with it, the biceps tendon. Even so, it is the smaller caudal part of the tubercle that is palpable, together with the infraspinatus tendon approaching it. Intra-articular injection is made at the cranial border of the tendon, immediately proximal to the bone.

The Elbow Joint

The lateral epicondyle of the humerus is accentuated by the sharp crest presented by its caudal border. Insertion of the needle for puncture is made just caudal to this crest, between it and the ulna. In an alternative method that uses the same landmark, the needle is entered at a site 2 or 3 cm proximal to the previous one and is directed mediodistally to pierce the capsule within the olecranon fossa.

The Carpal Joint

This exceptionally movable joint (Fig. 36.1) permits almost 180 degrees of flexion. The accessory carpal bone reveals the locations of the two more proximal compartments of the joint, which are in communication with each other and thus allow a single injection to reach both. Entry is made to either side of the extensor carpi radialis tendon, which is readily identified.

No features of the limb arteries demand notice. Lymph originating from superficial structures of the arm and forearm passes to the ventral superficial cervical nodes. That from deeper structures and from the entire distal part of the limb goes to the axillary lymph nodes of the first rib (cranial to the first rib and ventral to the axillary vessels).

THE HINDLIMB

Palpable skeletal features of this limb include the coxal tuber (a slight enlargement at the ventral end of the iliac crest) and the ischial tuber (lateral to the vulva in the female); the greater trochanter of the femur (less readily palpated as it is more deeply placed); the patella, the single patellar ligament, the crest and extensor groove of the tibia, and the collateral ligaments, at the stifle; the entire medial surface of the tibia in the leg; and the calcaneus and calcaneal tendon and the medial and lateral malleoli (and adjacent part of the fibula) at the hock (see Fig. 32.1). The use of the hamstring muscles for intramuscular injection is contraindicated because of the risks of an adverse effect on the quality of the ham and because of injury to the sciatic nerve.

It is usually impossible to find the subiliac lymph nodes (Fig. 36.5/5), located at the cranial border of the thigh, but the popliteal nodes (Fig. 36.5/7) may often be palpated, depending on how deeply they lie within the popliteal fossa.

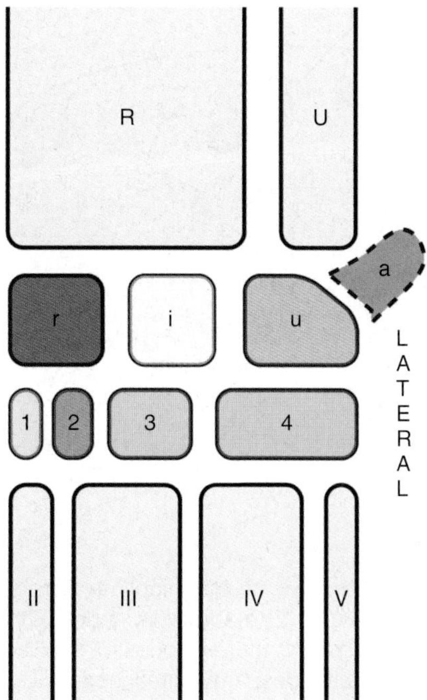

Fig. 36.1 The bones of the carpal skeleton in the pig. *Roman numerals* identify the metacarpal bones, *Arabic numerals* the distal carpal bones. *a,* Accessory carpal bone; *i,* intermediate carpal bone; *r,* radial carpal bone; *R,* radius; *U,* ulna; *u,* ulnar carpal bone.

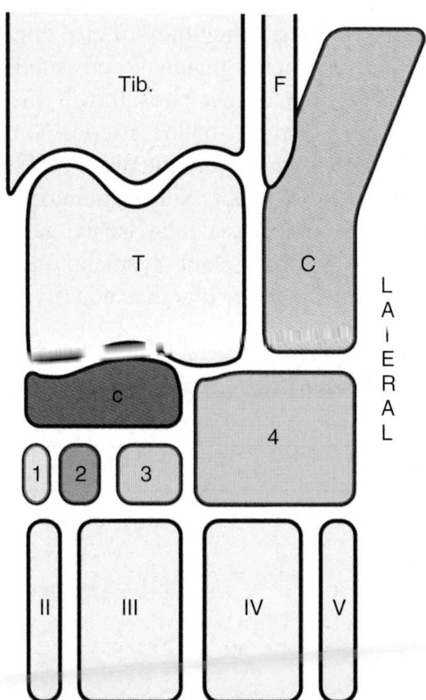

Fig. 36.2 The bones of the tarsal skeleton in the pig, schematic. *Roman numerals* identify the metatarsal bones, *Arabic numerals* the distal tarsal bones. *C,* Calcaneus; *c,* central tarsal bone; *F,* fibula; *T,* talus; *Tib.,* tibia.

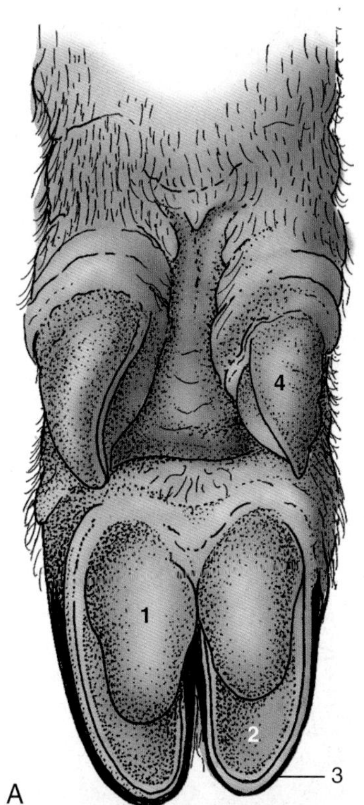

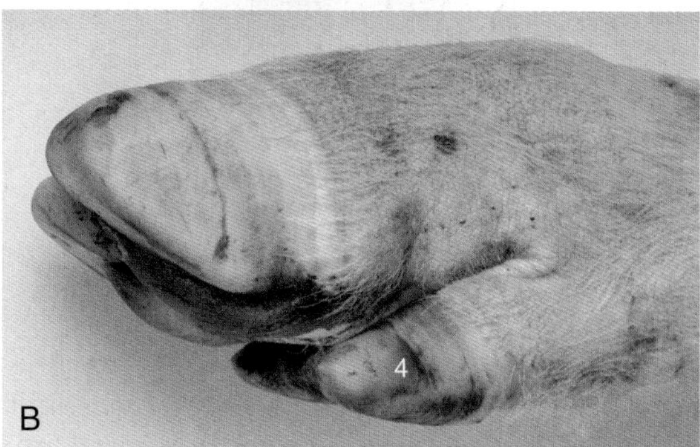

Fig. 36.3 (A) Palmar surface of the foot of a pig. *1,* Bulb (digital pad) of hoof; *2,* sole of hoof; *3,* wall of hoof; *4,* hoof of accessory digit. (B) Lateral view of foot of a pig.

The Hip Joint

Because of its deep situation, the available landmarks are at some distance from this joint. Depending on the size of the pig, the greater trochanter is located from 2 to 4 cm ventral to the line joining the coxal with the lateral part of the ischial tuber. The needle is inserted at the same distance cranial to the trochanter and passed, at right angles to the skin, through the gluteal muscles to enter the dorsal part of the joint. The greater resistance offered by the fibrous tissue of the deep gluteal muscle and the joint capsule warns that the cavity is close.

The Stifle Joint

The three compartments of this joint communicate, which allows a single injection to reach all parts

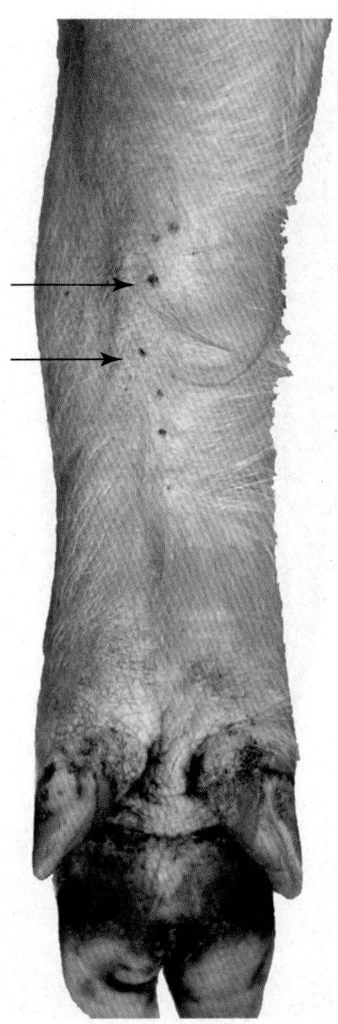

Fig. 36.4 Carpal glands *(arrows)* of a pig, palmar view.

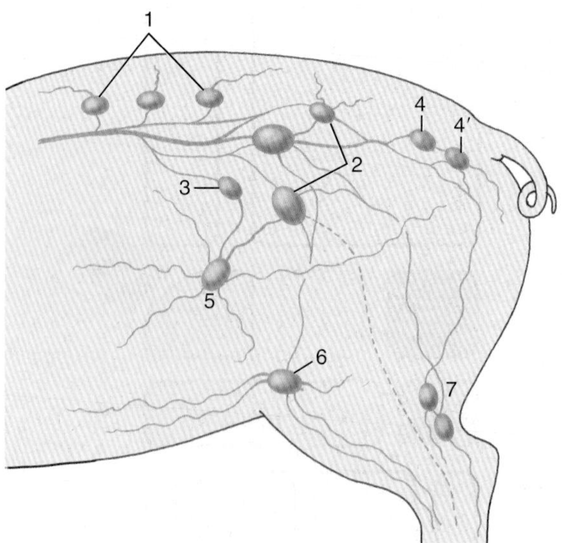

Fig. 36.5 Lymph flow of the hindlimb, lateral view. *1,* Lumbar aortic nodes; *2,* medial iliac nodes; *3,* lateral iliac node; *4,* ischial node; *4′,* gluteal nodes; *5,* subiliac nodes; *6,* superficial inguinal nodes; *7,* popliteal nodes.

(see the dog in Fig. 2.63 for the general idea). The puncture is made lateral to the patellar ligament, about one-third of the distance down from the patella to the tibial tuberosity.

The Hock Joint

The tarsocrural and proximal intertarsal joints, the only joint compartments at the hock accessible for injection, do not communicate. Two sites are available for injection of the tarsocrural joint, both on the lateral side: one is dorsal and the other is plantar to the collateral ligament. The proximal intertarsal joint is entered from the medial side, plantar to the collateral ligament. There are two independent joint spaces at the tarsometatarsal level: one is proximal to metatarsals II and III, and the other is proximal to metatarsals IV and V. The first of these communicates with the distal intertarsal joint (Fig. 36.2).

No account will be given of the arteries of the limb. Lymph from superficial structures of the thigh and leg drains to the superficial inguinal and subiliac nodes (Fig. 36.5); that from deeper parts travels in lymphatic vessels that run with the major arteries to reach the medial iliac nodes. Lymph from the distal part of the limb drains to the popliteal nodes. Some efferents from these nodes proceed to the gluteal and ischial nodes on the lateral surface of the sacrosciatic ligament; others join the lymphatics running to the medial iliac nodes.

COMPREHENSION CHECK

Compare the anatomy of the distal limb of the pig, including nerve supply, with that of the horse.

Part VI

Birds and Camelids

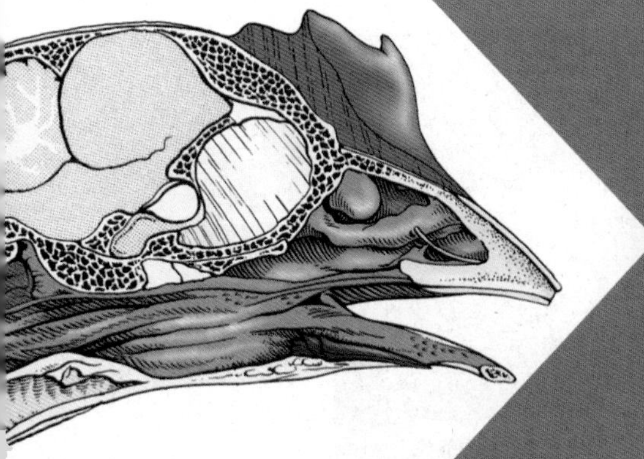

The Anatomy of Birds

37

Avian medicine is an important interest of the veterinary profession. It comprises two significantly different branches, one concerned with disease control in commercial flocks of the half-dozen species of domestic poultry and the other with the treatment of the much larger variety of cage, aviary, and zoo birds; frequently, some of the latter group are treated as individual patients. In addition, rehabilitation of wild birds, most notably oiled seabirds and injured raptors, is rapidly increasing. This chapter seeks to supply practitioners working in poultry medicine with a basic knowledge of anatomy sufficient for the understanding of the special features of poultry physiology and pathology, including that required for the conduct of postmortem examinations. This chapter is based on the chicken, and most of the data and illustrations refer to that species. Some details relevant to the examination and treatment of companion and exotic birds are included.

The evolution of birds from reptiles is indicated by reptilian features such as scales on their beaks, legs, and feet; a single occipital condyle; a single middle ear bone (columella); and a complex construction of the jaws. Birds have nucleated erythrocytes and a renal portal system that excretes uric acid. They range in size from the ostrich, weighing more than 100 kg, to tiny species such as the wren. They owe their extreme evolutionary success to the acquisition of the power of flight, which has enabled them to disperse ubiquitously and adapt to more niches than any other class of vertebrate. However, the imposition of rigid anatomic requirements for flight has limited the variation in morphology among all species. The high metabolic demands of flight have resulted in anatomic or physiologic modifications or both in nearly every body system. These modifications increase energy output and stability while decreasing body weight and wind resistance. They range from the grossly visible, as in the loss of heavy teeth and masticatory musculature, to the microscopic, as in the airways of the lung and the arrangement of conduction fibers in the heart. Together, these specializations render birds at once singularly uniform and strikingly diverse.

EXTERNAL FEATURES AND INTEGUMENT

Feathers provide the principal characteristic that distinguishes birds from mammals. They streamline the body and assist in transforming the forelimbs into wings. The feathers are among the features (others are mentioned later) that lighten birds relative to their size and thus enhance their efficiency in the air. Feathers have many functions that in mammals are performed by hairy skin: thermoregulation, communication, and protection against mechanical, radiological, thermal, chemical, and biological influences.

The *skin* is thin and loose and tears easily. Because of poor vascular and nerve supply, the skin wounds do not bleed as much as in mammals, and birds seem relatively insensitive to manipulation of their skin. The skin in chickens is yellowish over the body but may be more

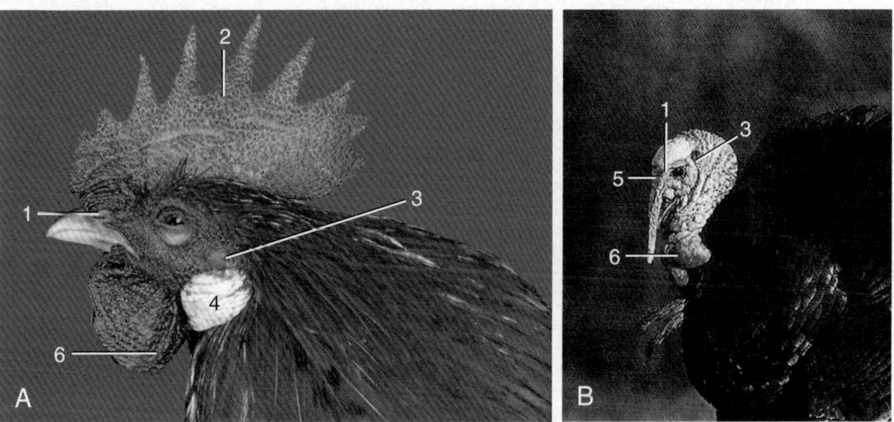

Fig. 37.1 Head of the chicken (A) and the turkey (B). *1,* Nostril; *2,* comb; *3,* ear opening; *4,* earlobes; *5,* snood; *6,* wattles.

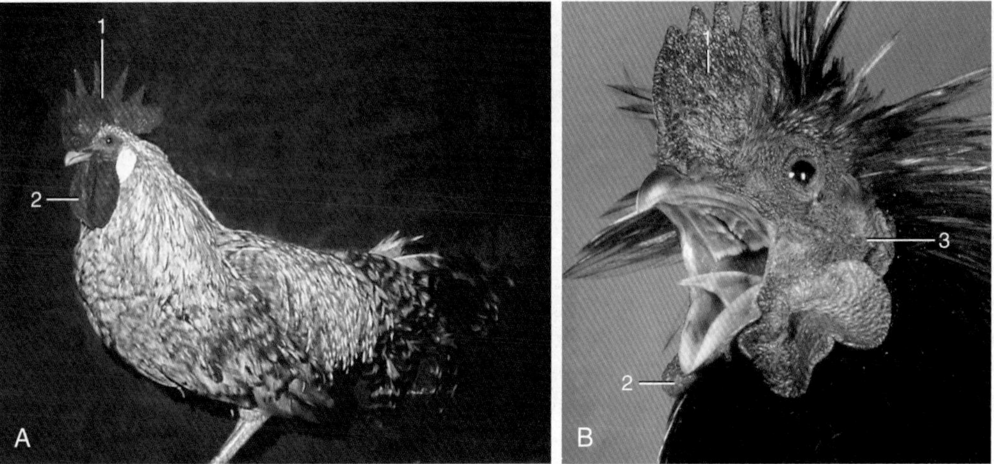

Fig. 37.2 (A) and (B), Two chickens with ornaments. *1,* Comb; *2,* wattles; *3,* earlobe.

deeply pigmented on the shanks and feet. It is paler in productive laying hens, in which the pigment is withdrawn and incorporated in the yolk. The dorsal surface of the neck–trunk junction, the cranial skinfold of the knee, and the lateral side of the thorax are recommended for subcutaneous injections. In most species, including the domestic chicken, localized changes in the skin occur during the brooding period for the more efficient incubation of the eggs. Brooding (incubation) patches that develop on the breast are characterized by feather loss and by thickening, edema, and increased vascularity. The subcutaneous layer is mainly composed of loose connective tissue. It also contains fat, most copiously present in aquatic and arctic species such as penguins, ducks, geese, and swans, and in migratory species before migration.

The *comb, wattles,* and *earlobes* (and the snood of turkeys) are soft ornamental outgrowths of the skin about the head (Figs. 37.1 and 37.2). Their dermis is thick and vascular, but the covering epidermis is thin. They are thus easily injured and provide potential portals for infection. In nearly all commercially reared chicks, the comb (and snood) are snipped off (dubbing, desnooding) to prevent their traumatization in the confined spaces in which these birds are held. The edges of the wattles are used for intradermal injections.

The *beak* (bill) is the functional skin-derived counterpart of the lips and teeth of mammals. It provides a horny cover *(rhamphotheca)* for the rostral parts of both upper *(rhinotheca)* and lower *(gnathotheca)* jawa and grows continuously to compensate for natural wear. The beak varies tremendously in form among species, according to diet (Fig. 37.3). A rich innervation causes it to be quite sensitive. Most commercially raised chickens and turkeys are debeaked when young (cutting off the upper beak in front of the nostrils) to prevent cannibalism. In psittacines, pigeons, and raptors, the base of the maxillary rhamphotheca, called the *cere,* may enclose the nostrils (Fig. 37.3C and D).

The beak is composed of softer keratin than the rest and is particularly prominent and fleshy in waterfowl as well as in budgerigars, in which it is used as a guide to their sex. The cere of the cock is blue, and that of the hen is light brownish pink.

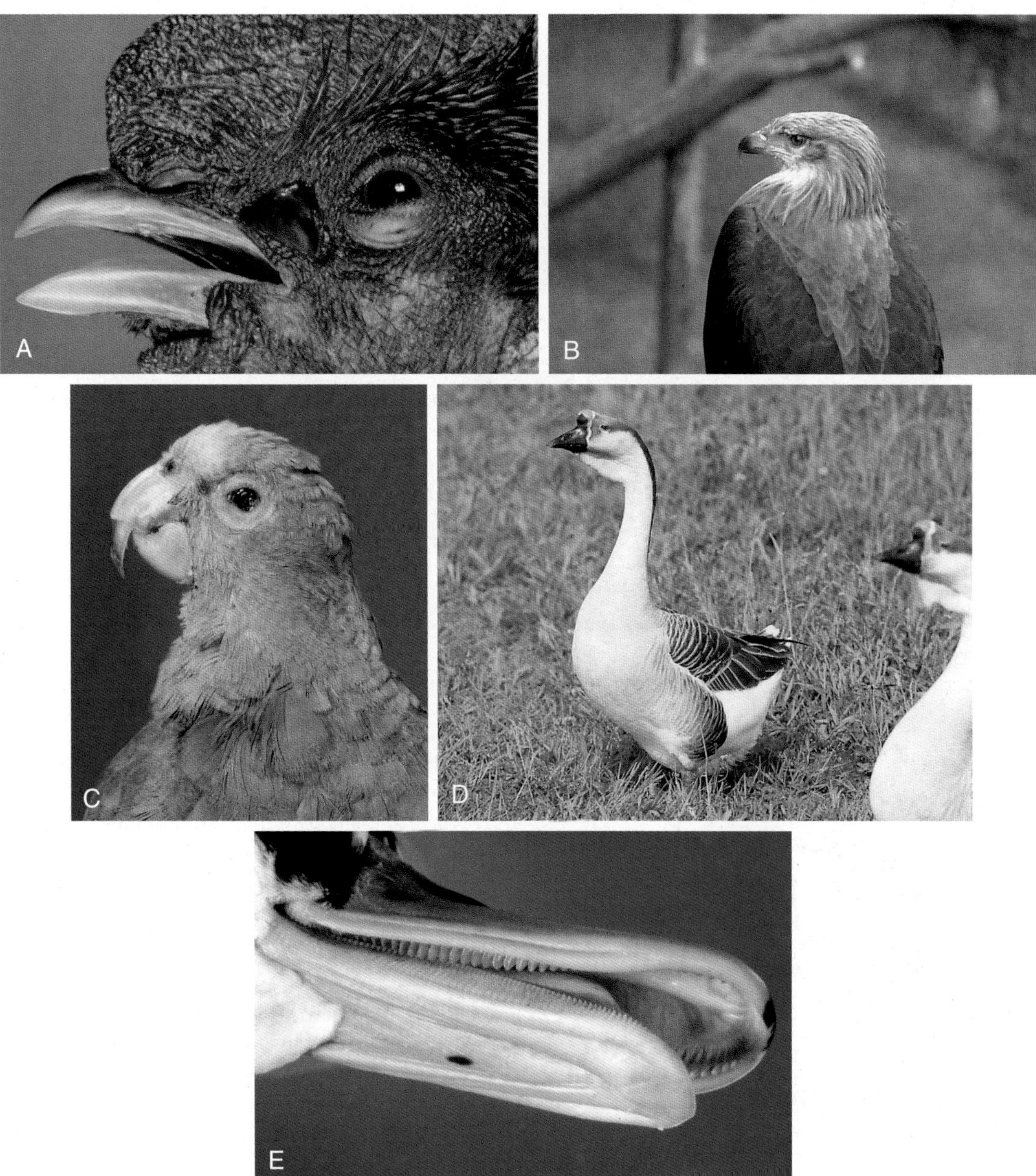

Fig. 37.3 (A to D) Differences in the form of the avian head. (E) The filter mechanism in the beak of a duck.

The scales on the shanks and feet are cornified epidermal patches similar to those of reptiles (Fig. 37.4). The feet of most birds are adapted for perching or holding prey and have one toe facing backward and three facing forward *(anisodactyl)*. In waterfowl the three forward-pointing toes are webbed to make more efficient sculls *(palmate)*. Some species, such as psittacines, have two (first and fourth) toes facing backward and two (second and third) facing forward *(zygodactyl)* to enable grasping and climbing. The *spur* with an osseous core within a cone of horn, on the caudomedial surface of the rooster's shank is used as a weapon. The length of the spur and the growth rings at its base may be used for determining age. Removal of the spur papilla in the chick inhibits its growth, much as the removal of the horn bud prevents horn growth in ruminants.

There are *only three discrete skin glands*: the sebaceous uropygial gland (preen or oil gland; Fig. 37.5), the aural gland, and the vent gland. The absence of sweat glands means that the birds have to lose heat through their skin and by evaporation from the respiratory system. The epidermis has a unique feature that allows it to act like a holocrine sebaceous gland, secreting a thin lipid film that helps in the maintenances of the plumage.

The *uropygial gland* in chickens is bilobed, about 2 cm in diameter, and located dorsal to the vertebrae that form the short tail. Its fatty secretion that emerges from

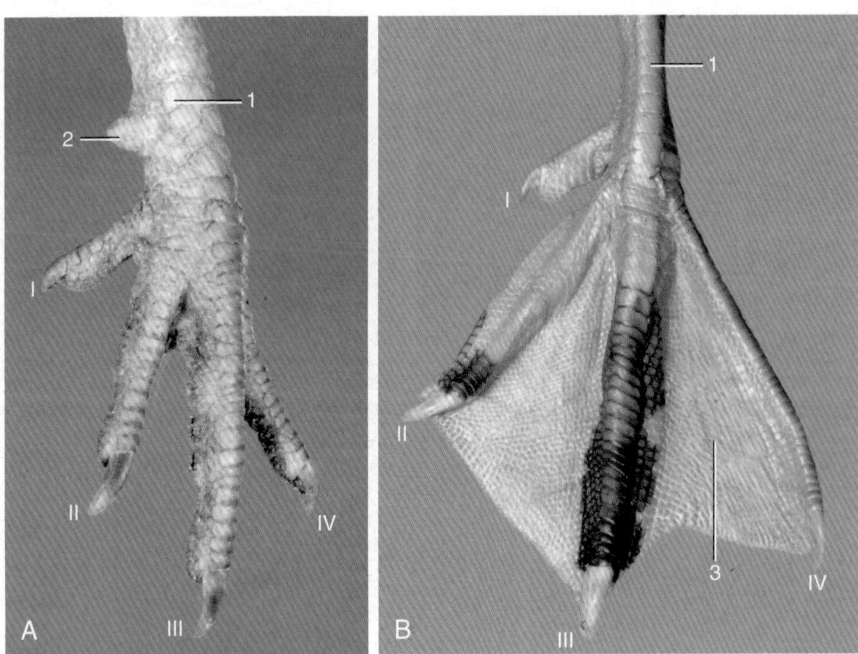

Fig. 37.4 Left foot of a cockerel (A) and a goose (B). *1,* Shank (metatarsus); *2,* spur; *3,* web between toes; *I to IV,* toes.

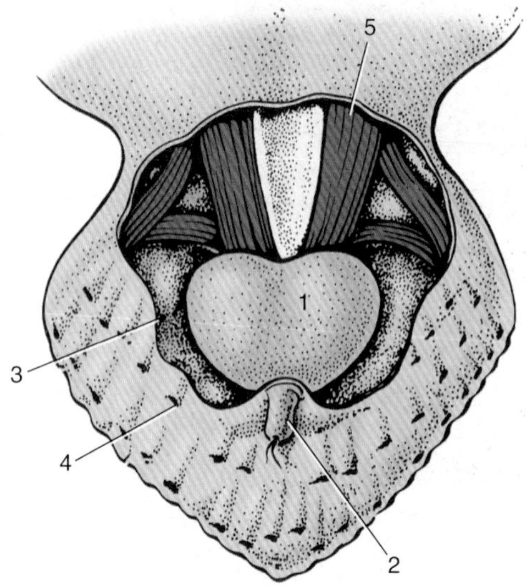

Fig. 37.5 Uropygial (preen) gland, dorsal view (schematic). *1,* Uropygial gland; *2,* papilla of uropygial gland through which the secretion is extruded; *3,* cut edge of skin; *4,* feather follicle; *5,* caudal vertebrae and associated muscles.

paired openings atop a small cutaneous papilla is carried to the body and wing feathers during preening. In waterfowl the secretion is important for waterproofing the feathers and insulating the submerged part of the body. This bacteriostatic lipid layer may be the reason why birds are little prone to skin infections. The uropygial gland is prominent in budgerigars and African grey parrots *(Psittacus erithacus)* but absent from many other parrots (e.g., Amazon parrots), ostriches, and many pigeons.

Aural sebaceous glands around the external ear secrete a waxy substance. *Vent glands* secrete mucus; their function is uncertain but may be linked to internal fertilization.

The Feathers

Feathers are highly specialized epidermal structures that have evolved from the scales of reptiles. Although light in relation to their size, they are of sturdy construction. Six types are recognized (*contour feathers, semiplumes, filoplumes, down feathers, afterfeathers,* and *bristles*), but only the contour and down feathers are described here. The contour are the externally visible feathers of flight that modify the body contours, the wings, and the tail. The contour feathers (tectrices) conceal the down feathers, which create an effective dead air space that insulates the body. The wing feathers (remiges) are made of approximately 10 primaries or hand feathers (Fig. 37.6) and 10 to 20 secondaries or arm feathers. The tail feathers (rectrices) are attached to the pygostyle and are used for steering and braking during flight. There are usually 6 pairs, but numbers can vary from 4 to 10 pairs depending on the species. Feathers are concentrated in tracts (pterylae), leaving bare areas (apteria) that are preferred surgical sites. Feathers hide emaciation.

The exposed portion of a typical *contour feather* consists of a main shaft extended on each side by the vane (Fig. 37.7). The vanes in wing feathers are asymmetrical;

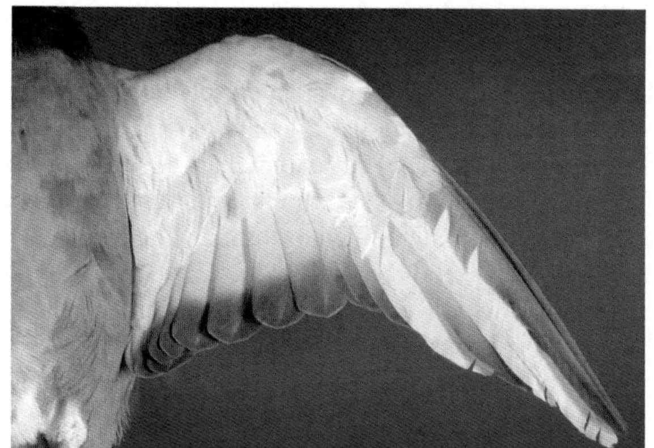

Fig. 37.6 Wing feathers of a pigeon. There are 10 primary or hand feathers and 10 secondary or arm feathers.

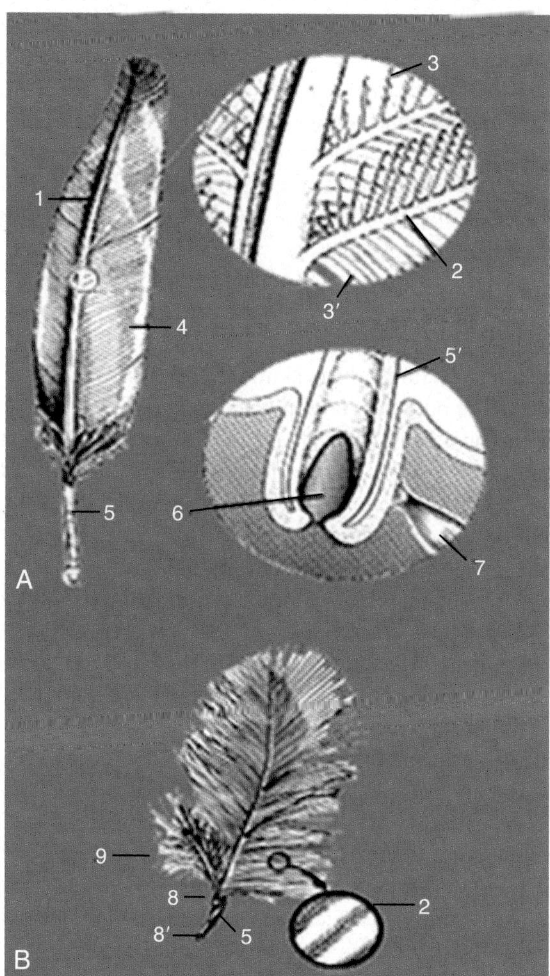

Fig. 37.7 (A) Contour feather (with enlargements). (B) Down feather (with enlargement). *1,* Main shaft; *2,* barb with barbules; *3,* distal barbules with microscopic hooks; *3′,* proximal barbules; *4,* vane formed by the barbs; *5,* quill; *5′,* quill in feather follicle; *6,* dermal papilla; *7,* feather muscle; *8,* distal umbilicus; *8′,* proximal umbilicus; *9,* afterfeather.

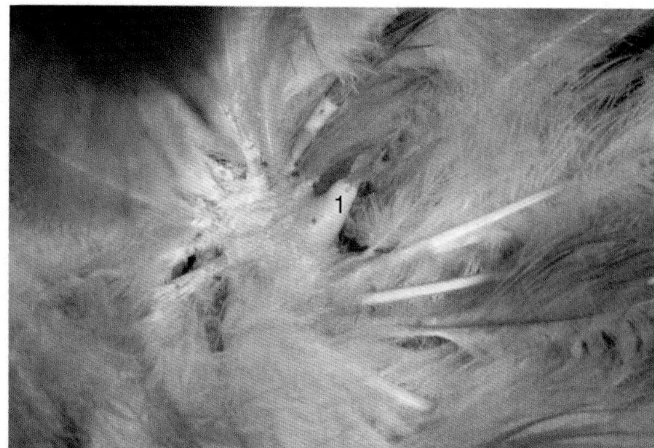

Fig. 37.8 Dermal papilla *(1).*

the external side of the vane is narrower than the internal for aerodynamic flight. The vane consists of numerous closely ranked branches (barbs; Fig. 37.7/*2*) that leave the shaft at angles of about 45 degrees. Adjacent barbs are connected by large numbers of minute barbules to form the level surfaces of the vane. This connection is effected by microscopic hooks on the distal ranks of barbules that loosely engage the proximal barbules crossing under them (Fig. 37.7/*3′*). Neighboring barbs are easily disconnected but reattach if brought together, as in preening or grooming the feathers.

The main shaft on the undersurface of the feather presents a longitudinal groove that ends in a depression (distal umbilicus; Fig. 37.7B/*8*) opposite the fluffy proximal part of the vane. A small downy afterfeather (*hyopenna;* Fig. 37.7/*9*) may emerge from the umbilicus and contribute to the fluffiness.

The embedded part (quill, calamus) of the feather occupies the feather follicle, an oblique tubular invagination of the skin (Fig. 37.7/*5′*). The small dermal papilla at the bottom of the follicle extends into the opening (proximal umbilicus) at the proximal end of the quill (Fig. 37.8). The quill itself is hollow and contains air and cellular debris (pulp caps) derived from the papilla. Feather muscles (Fig. 37.7/*7*), similar to the mammalian arrector pili muscles, attach to the sides of the follicles; they often form extensive networks that elevate or lower whole groups of feathers.

The barbs of the *down feathers* (Fig. 37.8) do not interlock to form a closed vane. Their haphazard arrangement gives these feather their fluffy appearance. In pigeons and many psittacines, such as cockatoos and African grey parrots, specialized down feathers produce a fine powder keratin dust from the barbs. This talclike powder is then coated over the plumage during preening; its absence is often the first sign of psittacine beak and feather disease. In pigeons the production of powder down (bloom) has been associated with human allergic alveolitis or pigeon fancier's lung.

Feather color plays a major role in camouflage, courtship, and protection from heat and light. Color, produced by pigments and by the intersection of light with feather structure, may complement other features of the feathers or feather tracts in indicating sex. Other species are monomorphic, and in them sex determination is dependent on endoscopy or molecular techniques (DNA analysis).

Colors of Feathers: The black tyrosine-derived pigment melanin, which also produces grays and browns, is the most commonly found in birds. The red, orange, and yellow carotenoid pigments that produce such colors as cardinal red and flamingo pink are obtained from the diet. Blue pigments are not found in birds, but the color may appear when white light is scattered by feathers that absorb the red (short-wavelength) end of the spectrum while the blue end is reflected (Tyndall effect). More green is produced by the combination of this effect with a yellow carotenoid pigment than is produced by porphyrins. Porphyrins, nitrogenous pigments also synthesized by birds, provide green, red, and some browns. They occur in gallinaceous birds, pigeons, and owls and may fluoresce when exposed to ultraviolet light. The iridescence seen in starlings and peacocks is produced by a combination of melanin with the structural breakdown of light striking the feather barbules. The color varies with the angle from which it is viewed.

At set times birds replace their feathers (*molt* or *ecdysis*) to discard worn ones or to change their plumage for display or camouflage. This occurs usually once a year after the breeding season (postnuptial or winter plumage) and is regulated through the actions of the thyroid hormone. Other factors influencing molting are nutrition, time of year, temperature, and light. It also depends on habitat and whether the species is migratory. Young birds molt their juvenile feathers before they become adults and often go through a series of subadult plumages. During molt, which is a slow and gradual process, birds should be provided rest and a diet rich in protein (especially the amino acids lysine, cystine, and arginine) and minerals (calcium and iron) to support the higher metabolic demands (increases of 15%–25%) made by the rapid epidermal proliferation and loss of insulation. Birds in poor condition often produce misshapen feathers. In most species, replacement of the large contour (flight) feathers is sequential (inside primaries first) and symmetrical so that flight always remains possible. Ducks and geese, however, lose all of these feathers at once, leaving them temporarily flightless. The old feather is pushed out by epidermal growth at the base of the follicle, and as it vacates the follicle, its replacement begins to grow. Before the barbs are released, they are encased in a sheath called a *bloodfeather* or *pinfeather*. The loss of a feather by plucking initiates a similar sequence of events. Clipping feathers is therefore unlikely to permanently disable birds for flight.

THE MUSCULOSKELETAL SYSTEM

The avian *skeleton* is highly adapted for flight: it is light, compact, and strong and has a greater content of calcium phosphate than is found in mammalian bone. It is characterized by a prominent sternum, a pelvis that is open ventrally, a forelimb modified to form a wing, and considerable fusion of vertebrae (Fig. 37.9).

A peculiar avian feature is the pneumatization of bones by air sacs, which are extensions of the lungs. The sacs are principally found in the body cavity, where they mingle with the viscera. However, they extend diverticula through pneumatic foramina into the medullary cavities of neighboring bones, which causes a considerable part of the skeleton to be filled with air. Pneumatization, a gradual process achieved at the expense of the bone marrow, is most advanced in the best fliers, which thus obtain a large and strong but not correspondingly heavy skeleton. Much of the adult skull is also pneumatized, but the spaces there connect with airways in the head and not with the system of sacs. Another peculiarity is the appearance of (trabecular) medullary bone, the most important calcium reserve for egg production, before the laying season; the extra bone (polyostotic hyperostosis) may be mistaken for pathologic processes on radiographs.

The Skull

The salient features of the skull are the large orbits placed between the bulbous cranium and the pyramidal face (Fig. 37.10). The mandible is flat and adds only marginally to the height of the head. The enormous eyes have displaced the bones found between the orbits in most mammalian skulls and have reduced others to a thin median plate (interorbital septum; Fig. 37.10/*11*). Several cranial bones consist of two plates separated by spongy bone, making them thicker than they would otherwise be and also making the cranial cavity appear bigger than it actually is. The occipital bone encloses the foramen magnum. The single occipital condyle forms an articulation with the atlas to enable birds to rotate the head on the vertebral column to a much greater extent than is allowed to mammals. The semispherical depression in the lower part of the lateral cranial wall is the tympanic cavity (Fig. 37.10/*19*). Its rim bounds the external acoustic meatus, which is closed by the tympanic membrane in life. Cochlear and vestibular windows in the depth of the depression lead into the inner ear.

The *facial part of the skull* is formed principally by the nasal and premaxillary bones that surround the large nasal aperture (Fig. 37.10/*2*). The nasal bone is dorsal, and in many birds—for example, in the psittacine species—it makes a flexible cartilaginous connection with the frontal bone, which permits the upper jaw to be raised as the mandible is depressed. The maxilla below the nasal aperture is small and is connected to the mandibular joint by the

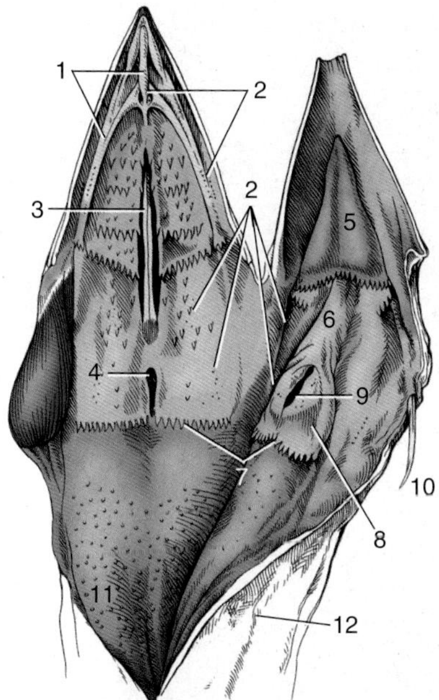

Fig. 37.14 Oropharynx opened by the reflection of the lower jaw. *1,* Median and lateral palatine ridges; *2,* openings of salivary glands; *3,* choana; *4,* infundibular cleft; *5,* body of tongue; *6,* root of tongue; *7,* "mechanical" papillae; *8,* laryngeal mound; *9,* glottis; *10,* branchial cornu of hyobranchial apparatus; *11,* esophagus; *12,* position of trachea.

the auditory tubes. The two clefts open together in the budgerigar. Numerous caudally directed "mechanical" *papillae* populate the oropharyngeal wall, either scattered singly or arranged in transverse rows, to aid in moving the bolus toward the esophagus. Generous amounts of saliva, discharged through the barely visible openings (Fig. 37.14/*2*) of several sets of salivary glands, moisten the food. The triangular nonprotrusible *tongue* (Fig. 37.14) is supported by a delicate hyoid apparatus. It moves the bolus within the oropharynx and, when the bird swallows, propels it into the esophagus while the choanal cleft is closed. Ducks and geese have tongues fringed with papillae that fit loosely into grooves in the edges of the beak, which provides a means of sifting food particles from water (Fig. 37.3E). In some bird species the tongue is more actively used for collecting, manipulating, and swallowing food. Psittacines are unique in having paired entoglossal bones and a large muscular tongue capable of amazing dexterity.

Birds appear to have a poorly developed sense of taste. The *laryngeal mound* (Fig. 37.14/*8*) caudal to the base of the tongue presents a median slit (glottis), which is not guarded by an epiglottis. A row of papillae marks the level of origin of the esophagus.

The Esophagus

The esophagus at first lies between the trachea and the cervical muscles but soon deviates to the right, a position it maintains throughout the remainder of the neck, although both it and the trachea are quite movable (Fig. 37.15). This topography makes it essential that a crop needle be introduced into the esophagus for gavage feeding or oral medication from the left side of the beak. Approach from the right side contains a high risk of perforating this thin-walled tube. At the thoracic inlet the ventral wall of the chicken's esophagus is greatly expanded to form the *crop* (Fig. 37.15/*8*), which bulges farther to the right and lies against the breast muscles. In most birds, including ducks and geese, the crop is merely a fusiform enlargement of the esophagus, and stores food for short periods when the muscular stomach is full. Both the cervical esophagus and the crop are subcutaneous and palpable, ideally placed for surgery (foreign bodies, impaction) but vulnerable to laceration. In species such as owls, gulls, and penguins, which have no crop, food enters directly into the proventriculus. In piscivorous birds, fish can often be seen stretching from the proventriculus and projecting out of the beak without causing any choking or discomfort. Within the body cavity the esophagus passes over the bifurcation of the trachea, between the ventral surface of the lungs and the base of the heart (Fig. 37.16). It merges into the proventriculus directly to the left of the median plane. Much lymphoid tissue (esophageal tonsil) is present in the caudal segment of the esophagus of the duck.

The esophagus is capable of great distention; its lamina propria contains mucous glands whose secretion lubricates the passage of the bolus. There is little chemical activity in the esophagus and crop, although salivary amylase may initiate carbohydrate digestion.

During brooding, the large symmetrical crop of both male and female pigeons elaborates a crumbly material (crop milk) consisting of desquamated lipid-laden epithelial cells; mixed with ingested food, it is regurgitated and fed to the nestlings in the first days after hatching.

The Stomach

Species variation in the gastrointestinal tract is most marked where the stomach is concerned. The stomach of fish- and flesh-eating species (raptors, hawks, ospreys, vultures, and owls) is primarily a storage organ appropriate for the chemical digestion of a soft diet. In contrast, the stomach of birds with a herbivorous diet is adapted to the mechanical reduction of tougher material through powerful muscular development. Domestic poultry (chicken, geese, and others that are similar) possess stomachs of the second category and exhibit only minor interspecific variation.

The stomach of these birds is divided by a constriction (isthmus) into a predominantly glandular proventriculus and a predominantly muscular ventriculus (gizzard) placed one behind the other close to the median plane. The proventriculus is ventrally in contact with the left lobe of the liver. The larger, more caudal gizzard has more extensive contact with the sternum and the lower part of the left lateral abdominal wall. It is exposed when the sternum and abdominal muscles are removed during necropsy (Fig. 37.17).

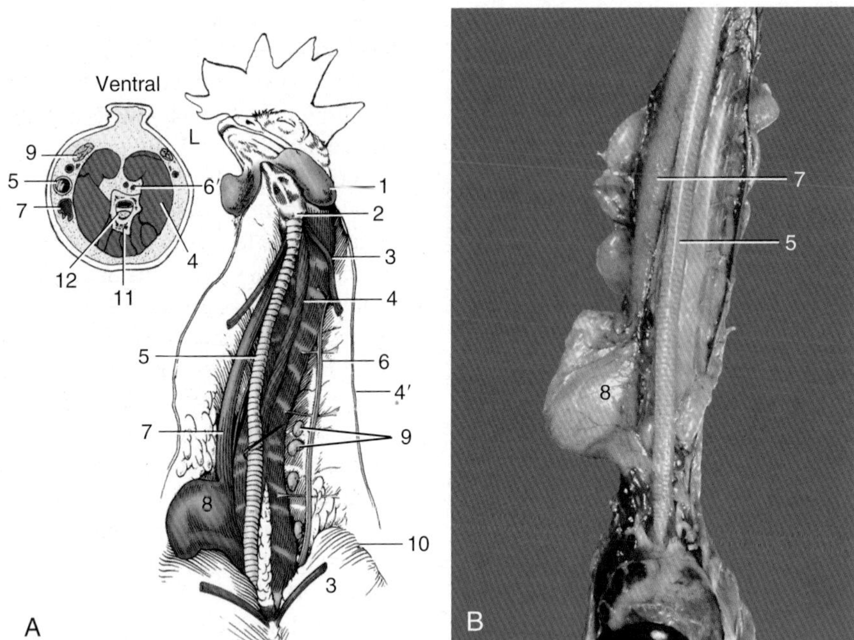

Fig. 37.15 Ventral view of the dissected neck. (A) Schematic; the *inset* shows a transverse section through the middle of the neck. (B) Detail of neck with crop. *L,* Left side of the transverse sect; *1,* wattle; *2,* larynx; *3,* sternothyroideus, cut; *4,* cervical muscles; *4′,* cervical nerve; *5,* trachea; *6,* jugular vein and vagus nerve; *6′,* internal carotid arteries; *7,* esophagus; *8,* crop; *9,* thymus; Left side of the transverse section *10,* pectoralis; *11,* vertebra; *12,* spinal cord.

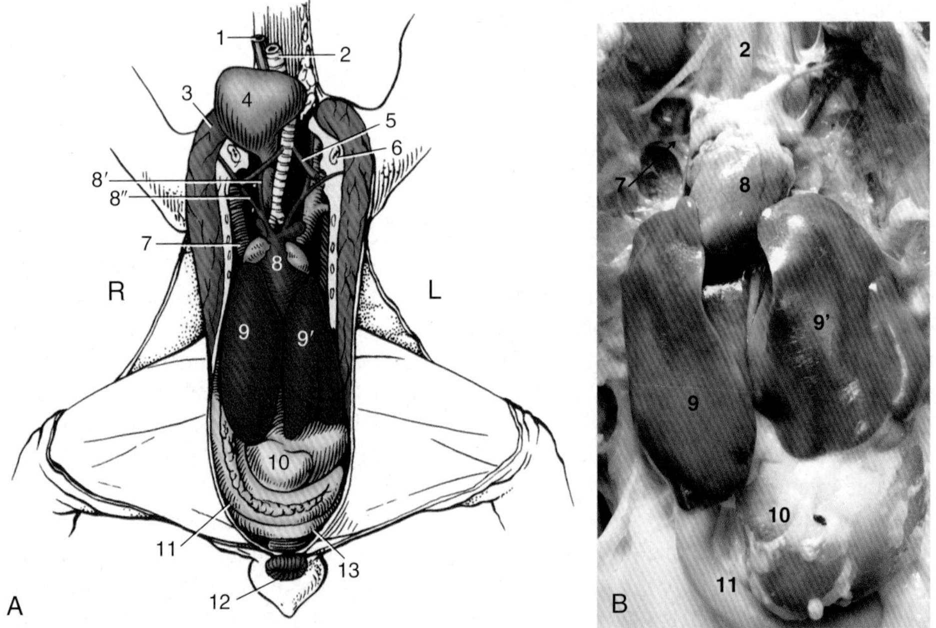

Fig. 37.16 Ventral view of the viscera. (A) Schematic. (B) Viscera after removal of ventral body wall, ventral view. *L,* Left; *R,* right; *1,* esophagus; *2,* trachea; *3,* pectoralis, cut; *4,* crop; *5,* sternotrachealis; *6,* coracoid bone, cut; *7,* right cranial vena cava; *8,* heart; *8′,* common carotid artery; *8″,* subclavian artery; *9* and *9′,* right and left lobes of liver, respectively; *10,* gizzard (its caudal blind sac); *11,* duodenal loop, enclosing pancreas; *12,* vent; *13,* one of the ceca.

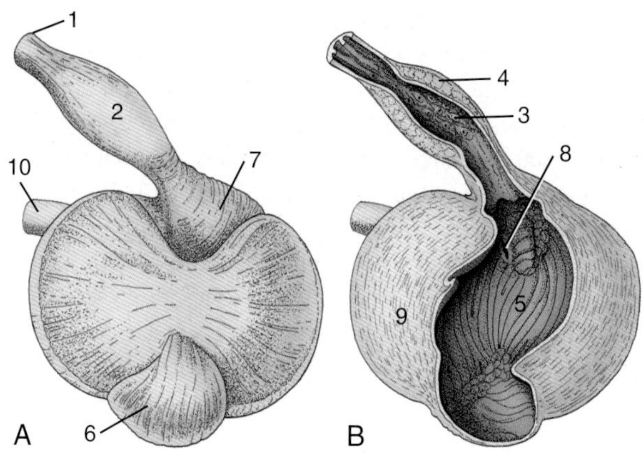

Fig. 37.17 Stomach, ventral surface (A) and opened ventrally (B). *1,* Esophagus; *2,* proventriculus; *3,* papillae; *4,* deep proventricular glands, visible on cut surface; *5,* lumen of gizzard; *6,* caudal blind sac; *7,* cranial blind sac; *8,* pyloric orifice; *9,* cranioventral muscle mass; *10,* duodenum.

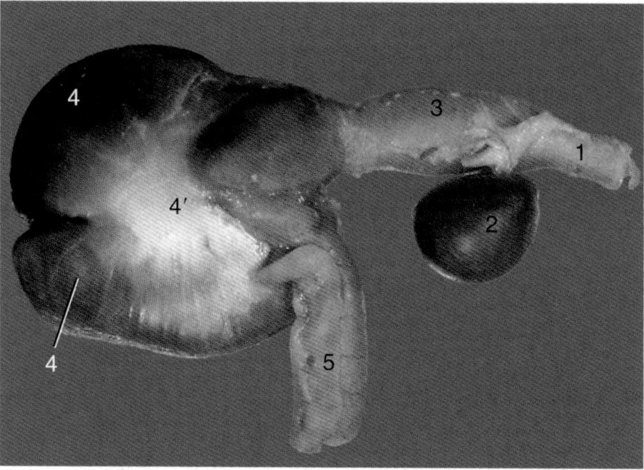

Fig. 37.18 Stomach of chicken. *1,* Esophagus; *2,* spleen; *3,* proventriculus; *4,* gizzard with aponeurosis *(4′)*; *5,* duodenum.

The *proventriculus* is spindle shaped and about 4 cm long. Its whitish mucosa, lined with a mucus-secreting, columnar epithelium, is clearly demarcated from the more reddish lining of the esophagus (Figs. 37.18 and 37.19). It presents numerous macroscopic elevations (papillae) through which pass the collecting ducts from a thick bed of glands, very visible on the cut surface of the wall. The papillae are so prominent that they may be mistaken for parasitic lesions. There are two kinds of epithelial cells in the glands: oxynticopeptic cells that produce both hydrochloric acid and pepsinogen and cells that produce mucus.

The *isthmus* is the transition from the glandular stomach to the muscular gizzard. It has no glands in its thinner, less rigid wall. In many parrots the koilin layer from the gizzard extends some way into it.

The *ventriculus* or *gizzard* is lens shaped in herbivores, poultry, and waterfowl and is positioned with its convex surfaces facing more or less to the right and left (Fig. 37.15). Its interior is elongated, enlarged by cranial and caudal blind sacs, of which the former connects with the proventriculus. The duodenum arises on the right surface, adjacent to the cranial blind sac. The bulk of the organ consists of two thick masses of muscle that insert on glistening tendinous centers, one on each surface. Thinner muscles cover the blind sacs. The mucous membrane is thin but very tough. It has a cuboidal epithelium and largely consists of tubular glands. Catalyzed by the low pH resulting from the hydrochloric acid from the proventriculus, the secretion of the glands forms a hard *cuticle* of koilin (a carbohydrate–protein complex). The koilin, a rough plicated layer, is replenished from the glands below as it is worn on the surface. It obtains a yellow-green color from the bile refluxed from the duodenum. In herbivorous and omnivorous birds, powerful contractions of the gizzard crush the food, assisted by ingested grit, which must be provided in the diet (Fig. 37.19). Being

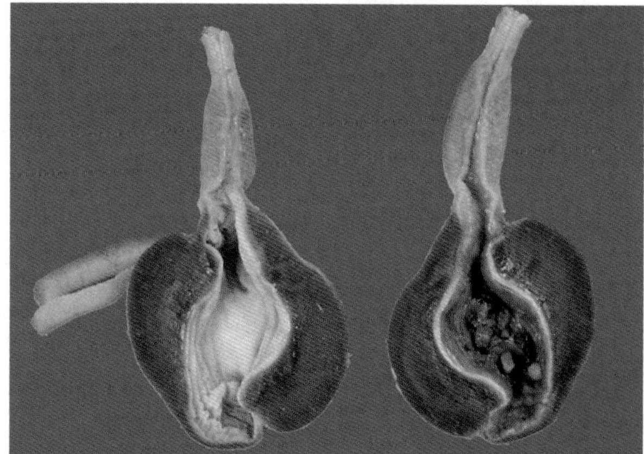

Fig. 37.19 Opened stomach. Note grit inside gizzard *(right).*

radiodense, the grit identifies the gizzard in radiographs. The gizzard is the site of protein digestion.

In granivores, psittacine species, and songbirds the gizzard is less muscular because these birds dehusk and crumble their seeds before swallowing. These birds do not always require grit.

Muscular activity moves food back and forth between the proventriculus and gizzard during digestion; the location of the pylorus then enables some of the food that does not require grinding to escape into the duodenum, bypassing the gizzard.

The Intestines

The intestines occupy the caudal part of the body cavity, making extensive contact with the gizzard and reproductive organs (Fig. 37.16). They consist of the duodenum, jejunum, ileum, and colon, which opens into the cloaca. In herbivorous birds two ceca arise from the ileocolic junction and accompany the ileum in retrograde fashion (Fig. 37.20).

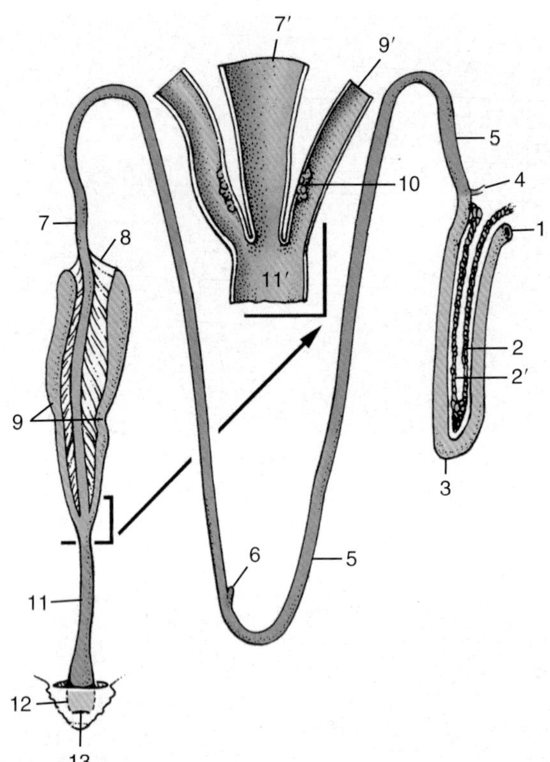

Fig. 37.20 Isolated intestinal tract with detail of ileocolic junction (top center). *1,* Pylorus; *2* and *2′,* dorsal and ventral lobes of pancreas, respectively; *3,* duodenal loop; *4,* bile and pancreatic ducts entering duodenum; *5,* jejunum; *6,* vitelline diverticulum; *7,* ileum; *7′,* ileum opened; *8,* ileocecal fold; *9,* ceca; *9′,* cecum opened; *10,* cecal tonsil; *11,* colon; *11′,* colon opened; *12,* cloaca; *13,* vent.

The *duodenum* passes caudally from the right surface of the gizzard. It forms a tight U-shaped loop that returns the duodenojejunal junction to the vicinity of the stomach. Most of the loop lies on the abdominal floor and follows the caudal curvature of the gizzard (Fig. 37.16). The pancreas lies between the limbs and empties into the distal end of the ascending duodenum; the bile ducts enter close by (Fig. 37.20/*4*).

The *jejunum* forms loose coils along the edge of the mesentery and is so thin walled that its content causes it to appear greenish (Fig. 37.21). A small outgrowth (vitelline or Meckel diverticulum; Fig. 37.21/*8*) marks the former connection with the yolk sac that persists within the body cavity to nourish the hatchling for a few days. Patches of aggregate lymph nodules are present. In the duck and goose, the jejunum is arranged in several U-shaped loops; in the pigeon, it forms a cone-shaped mass with outer centripetal and inner centrifugal turns. In insect- and fruit-eating birds the jejunum is very short and wide.

The *ileum* continues from the jejunum without demarcation. It is variably described as beginning at the vitelline diverticulum or opposite the apices of the ceca (Fig. 37.20).

The large intestine comprises the ceca and the colon (Fig. 37.20/*9* and *11*). The *ceca,* relatively long in the chicken and the turkey, arise at the ileocolic junction and pursue retrograde courses beside the ileum to which they are attached by ileocecal folds. They pass cranially at first, then double back so that their blind ends usually lie near the cloaca (Fig. 37.16/*13*). The proximal segment of each has a heavy muscle coat (cecal sphincter) and contains much lymphoid tissue (the so-called cecal tonsil; Fig. 37.20/*10*). The thin-walled middle part appears greenish because of its content. The blind end is thicker walled and bulbous. Bacterial breakdown of cellulose occurs in the ceca. Passerine birds and pigeons have very short lymphoid ceca; psittacines and some carnivorous birds have none.

The *(colo)rectum* is about 10 cm long in chickens and ends by a slight enlargement at the cloaca. The colorectum is no thicker than the small intestine and reabsorbs water and electrolytes by antiperistaltic movements. Urine is moved from the cloaca into the colorectum by antiperistalsis.

The Cloaca

The cloaca, common to the digestive and urogenital systems, opens to the exterior at the *vent* (Fig. 37.22/*5*). The colorectum, ureters, and deferent ducts (or the left oviduct) enter it at various levels. The cloaca is divided sequentially into coprodeum, urodeum, and proctodeum by two more or less complete annular folds. The bursa of Fabricius is located in the dorsal wall of the proctodeum (Figs. 37.22/*9* and 37.23).

The *coprodeum* is the ampulliform continuation of the colorectum in which feces are stored (Fig. 37.22/*2*). In some desert species (e.g., budgerigar) it is lined with villi and is a site of water absorption. It is bounded caudally by the coprourodeal fold (Fig. 37.22/*2′*), which may be stretched by the pressure of the feces so that its central opening is everted through the vent. The urodeum and proctodeum (Fig. 37.22/*3* and *4*) are described with the urogenital system (p. 792).

The Liver and Pancreas

The avian *liver* is dark brown (except in the first 2 weeks after hatching, when it obtains a yellow color from yolk pigments, which continue to be absorbed from the intestine before the yolk sac finally regresses). It consists of right and left lobes, connected cranially by a bridge dorsal to the heart (Fig. 37.16). Because there is no diaphragm, the lobes of the liver embrace the caudal portion of the heart. The larger right lobe carries the gallbladder on its visceral surface and is perforated by the caudal vena cava; the left lobe is divided (Fig. 37.24). The convex parietal surface lies against the sternal ribs and sternum and is exposed when the breast muscles and sternum are removed in postmortem

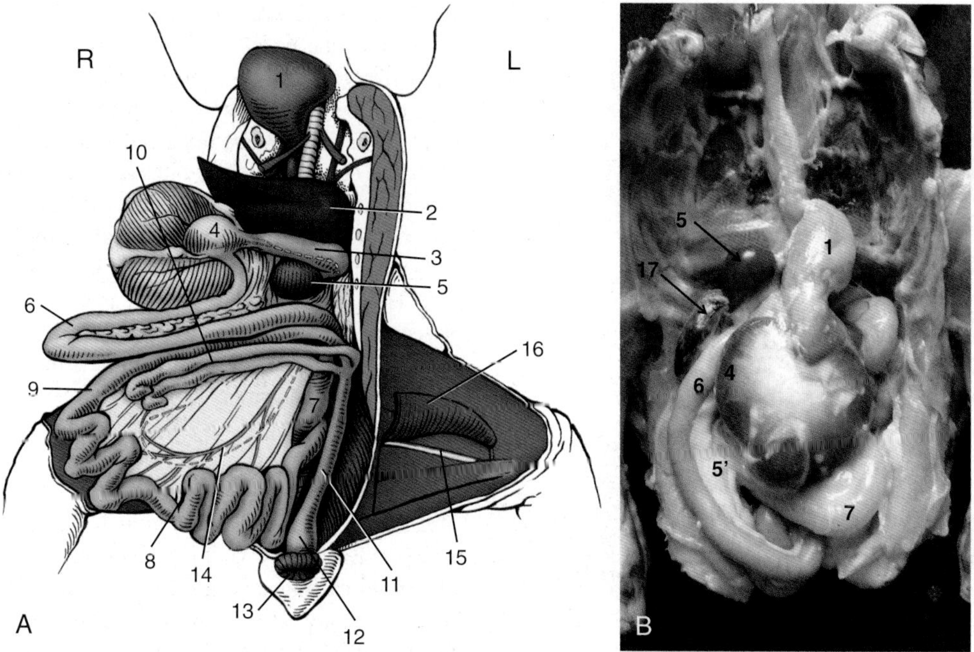

Fig. 37.21 (A) Gastrointestinal tract after reflection of liver, stomach, and small intestine craniodextrally, ventral view. *L,* Left; *R,* right. (B) Detail of stomach and duodenum loop with pancreas within the loop. *1,* Crop; *2,* left lobe of liver; *3,* proventriculus with vagus on dorsal surface; *4,* cranial blind sac on right side of reflected gizzard; *5,* spleen; *5′,* Pancreas; *6,* duodenal loop enclosing pancreas; *7,* jejunum; *8,* vitelline diverticulum; *9,* ileum; *10,* ceca; *11,* colon; *12,* cloaca; *13,* vent; *14,* cranial mesenteric vessels and intestinal nerve in mesentery; *15,* sciatic nerve and ischial artery; *16,* gracilis and adductor; *17,* Gall bladder.

examination. The liver is covered by a peritoneal sac *(cava peritonaei hepatis)* that can contain much fat, and fills with transudate in certain diseases. The concave visceral surface makes contact with the spleen, proventriculus, gizzard, duodenum, jejunum, and ovary (or right testis). Two bile ducts, one from each lobe, enter the distal end of the duodenum close to the pancreatic ducts; only the duct from the right lobe is connected to the gallbladder. Pigeons, most parrots, budgerigars, and Struthioniformes lack a gallbladder. Except near the hilus, the hepatic lobules are indistinct because of the lack of perilobular connective tissue.

The elongated *pancreas* lies between the limbs of the duodenal loop (Fig. 37.20/*2* and *2′*). It consists of dorsal and ventral lobes distally connected. Two or three ducts convey pancreatic juice into the distal end of the duodenum.

The Spleen

The spleen (see also p. 798) is mentioned here because of its relationship to the stomach and liver (Fig. 37.18). It is a brownish red sphere, about 2 cm in diameter, and lies in the median plane beside the proventriculus. It contacts the liver cranioventrally (Fig. 37.24/5). The spleen is best exposed during postmortem examination by reflecting the left lobe of the liver and the gizzard, duodenum, and jejunum craniodextrally (Fig. 37.21A). The spleen is triangular in the duck and goose, oval in the pigeon, round in psittacines, and elongated in Passeriformes.

THE RESPIRATORY SYSTEM

The indoor flocks of the modern poultry industry are particularly prone to respiratory infections, which may be very costly. Employed by birds for vocalization and thermoregulation in addition to gaseous exchange, the respiratory apparatus differs considerably from that of mammals. In particular, the lungs are small, undergo little change in volume during breathing, and are extended by air sacs that do not participate in gaseous exchange but act as bellows effecting the flow of air. The segregation of ventilation and exchange allows a continuous air flow as opposed to the "in-and-out" tidal flow in mammals. This explains how birds are able to extract up to 10 times the amount of oxygen from the air as is possible by mammals. The different manner of breathing is also related to the absence of a muscular diaphragm; its place is taken by a passive horizontal septum that merely holds the viscera in place.

Distinctions of lesser importance include the separation of a vocalization organ (syrinx) from the larynx and the possession of closed and possibly mineralized tracheal rings.

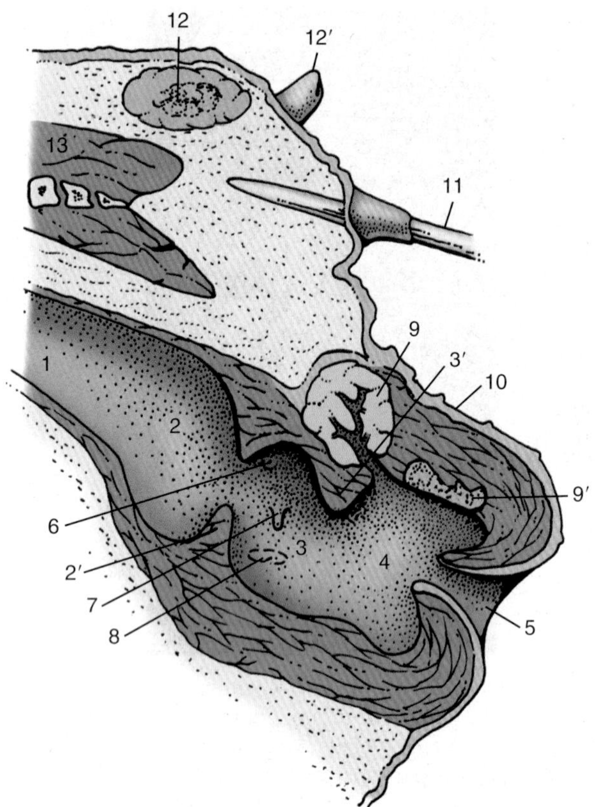

Fig. 37.22 Median section of the cloaca (semi-schematic). *1,* Colon; *2,* coprodeum; *2′,* coprourodeal fold; *3,* urodeum; *3′,* uroproctodeal fold; *4,* proctodeum; *5,* vent; *6,* ureteric orifice; *7,* papilla of deferent duct; *8,* position of oviduct orifice (only on left side); *9,* cloacal bursa; *9′,* dorsal proctodeal gland; *10,* skin; *11,* tail feather; *12,* uropygial gland; *12′,* papilla of uropygial gland; *13,* muscles surrounding caudal vertebrae.

The Nasal Cavity

The *nostrils* (Fig. 37.1/*1*) or nares at the base of the beak are overhung by a horny flap (operculum) or surrounded by a thick cere as in psittacines. They lead into the nasal cavity, which is divided, as in the mammal, by a median septum and is in wide communication with the oropharynx through the choana (Fig. 37.14/*3*).

The nasal cavities are laterally compressed and extend to the large orbits. Rostral, middle, and caudal *conchae* that arise from the lateral wall encroach on the space (Fig. 37.25/*2, 2′,* and *2″*). They play a major role in olfaction, filtering, and thermoregulation. The rostral and middle conchae enclose recesses that communicate with the nasal cavity; the caudal one encloses a diverticulum of the *infraorbital sinus.* This sinus lies lateral to the nasal cavity, into which it opens by a narrow duct so placed that natural drainage is impeded. The sinus wall is thin and directly subcutaneous rostral and ventral to the eye, where it may be identified by its yielding on palpation. It may be opened and any exudate, which accumulates in several diseases, may be flushed out. The relatively wide nasolacrimal duct opens into the nasal cavity ventral to the middle concha. The infraorbital sinus is particularly well developed in psittacines, in which it becomes superficial ventromedial to the orbit. It has numerous diverticula and also communicates with the cervicocephalic air sac at its caudal extent. The elongated *nasal gland* extends forward from the dorsal part of the orbit in the lateral wall of the nasal cavity. Its duct opens into the cavity at the level of the rostral concha. The gland is widely known as the salt gland, although it secretes a hypertonic sodium chloride solution only in marine (and a few other) species; it is this that enables seabirds to drink seawater.

The Larynx, Trachea, and Syrinx

The *larynx* occupies a mound on the floor of the oropharynx (see Fig. 37.14/*8*). It is supported by cricoid and paired arytenoid cartilages that differ markedly from their mammalian counterparts but occupy similar positions. The arytenoids articulate with the rostrodorsal part of the annular cricoid. The glottis, formed by the arytenoids, closes the entrance to the larynx by reflex muscular action, preventing food particles and other foreign matter from reaching the lower air passages. Despite the narrowness of the glottis, it is possible to intubate the trachea in larger cage birds. There are no vocal folds; voice production occurs in the syrinx, a specialization at the tracheal bifurcation.

The *trachea,* composed of tightly stacked, complete, and overlapping cartilaginous rings, accompanies the esophagus through the neck. It can be palpated on the right side (Fig. 37.15). In a long-necked species—for example, trumpeter swans and cranes—it is much longer than the neck and forms a loop that is accommodated in an excavation of the sternum at the thoracic inlet. The trachea bifurcates into two primary bronchi dorsal to the base of the heart. These enter the ventral surface of the lungs after a short course. In penguins, a median septum divides the trachea into left and right tubes, making it very easy to intubate a primary bronchus by mistake.

The *syrinx* is formed by the terminal part of the trachea and first parts of the primary bronchi (Fig. 37.26). The tracheal cartilages of the syrinx are sturdy, but the bronchial cartilages are largely lacking, although a short vertical bar (pessulus; Fig. 37.26/*3*) separates the bronchial openings. The lateral and medial walls of the initial segments of the bronchi are membranous and produce the voice when caused to flutter (Fig. 37.26/*2* and *2′*). The male duck and swan have an osseous bulla (believed to be a resonator) on the left side of the syrinx. In psittacines a median pessulus is missing. A small paired muscle, the sternotrachealis (Fig. 37.16/*5*), pulls the trachea toward the syrinx and aids in vocalization. An elaborate set of five pairs of syringeal muscles is present in Passeriformes (songbirds), and the surrounding interclavicular air sac gives the voice resonance by pushing against these membranes. Despite their great

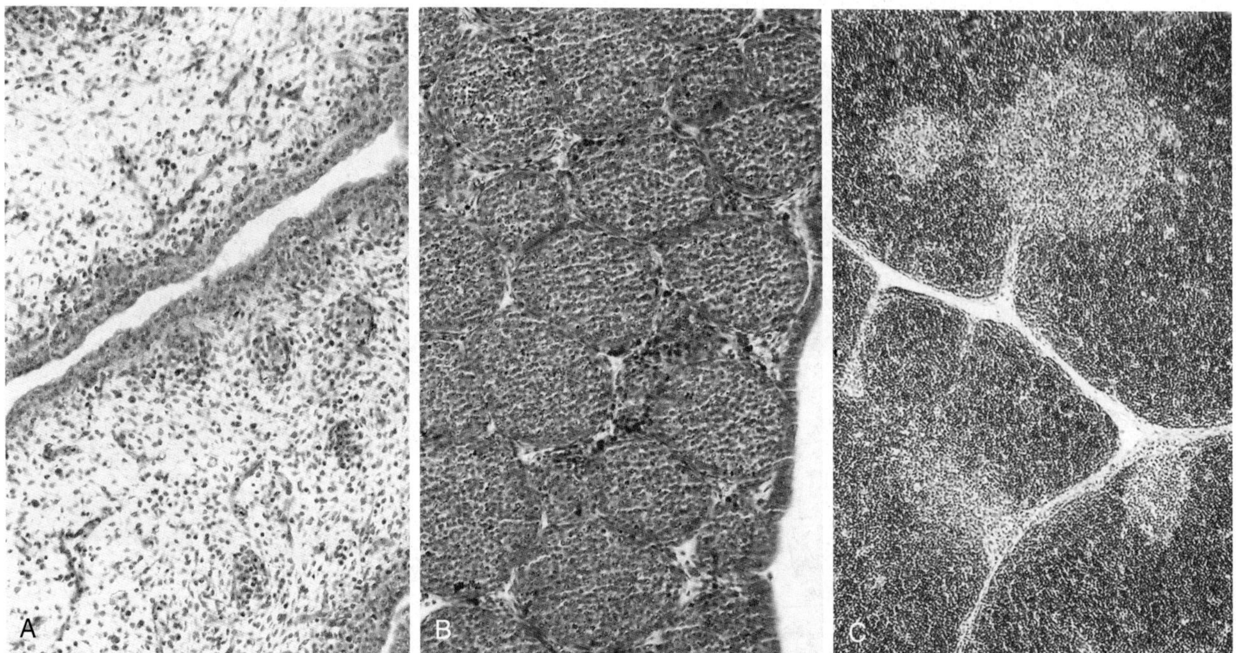

Fig. 37.23 (A) Bursa of 15-day-old embryo (hematoxylin and eosin [H&E] stain); some infiltrating lymphocytes are present (magnification ×70). (B) Bursa of 18-day-old embryo (Azan stain) showing developing epithelial buds (magnification ×70). (C) Bursa of 6-week-old chick (H&E stain) showing developed bursa follicles (magnification ×70).

speaking ability, parrots have a relatively simple syringeal apparatus with only three pairs of syringeal muscles.

Because the trachea is narrowed at the syrinx, this is a common site of obstruction by seeds or other foreign bodies or by fungal granulomas. Birds exhibiting voice changes should have the syrinx examined endoscopically. Other common causes of voice changes are a goiter pressing against the syrinx or an *Aspergillus* infection of the surrounding interclavicular air sac.

The Lungs

The lungs are relatively small, unlobed, bright pink, and nonexpansile. Although somewhat firmer than mammalian lungs because they contain far more cartilage, the lungs of birds are soft and velvety to the touch. They are confined to the craniodorsal part of the body cavity; their convex dorsal surface lies against and is deeply indented by the thoracic vertebrae and vertebral ribs. The lungs fail to cover the lateral surfaces of the heart as they do in mammals. The concave ventral (septal) surface lies against the horizontal septum (see further on) and faces the esophagus, heart, and liver (Fig. 37.27). The lungs are lightly attached to the body wall and to the horizontal septum that confines them from below. No pleural cavity corresponding to that of mammals is necessary because the capacity for expansion is negligible. The nonexpansile nature of the lungs, their abundant cartilage, and their confinement high within the body cavity surrounded by bone render them largely incompressible.

The *primary bronchus* (Fig. 37.28) enters the ventral surface, passes diagonally through the lung (as the *mesobronchus*), narrowing as it goes, and at the caudal border becomes continuous with the abdominal air sac (Fig. 37.28/*13*; see later). In the chicken it gives off 40 to 50 *secondary bronchi* classified as medioventral, mediodorsal, lateroventral, and laterodorsal according to the general areas of the lung they supply (Figs. 37.27/*a–d* and 37.28/*3–5*). These groups of secondary bronchi have various connections with the air sacs; these communications are essential to the passage of air through the lungs.

The *secondary bronchi* give off 400 to 500 *parabronchi,* which contain gas exchange sites in their relatively thick walls. The parabronchi arise from the medioventral and mediodorsal bronchi and connect with each other end-to-end to form loops of various lengths (Fig. 37.28/*6*). These loops, which are tightly packed and parallel, constitute about three-quarters of the lung tissue, forming the functional division known as the *paleopulmo*. The parabronchi from the smaller lateroventral and laterodorsal bronchi form the less regular and more caudal functional division known as the *neopulmo*.

The internal and external diameters of the parabronchi measure about 1 mm and 2 mm, respectively. The parabronchi anastomose with their neighbors, from which they are separated by fenestrated septa (Fig. 37.28/*f*). Numerous extensions (atria) of the parabronchial lumen give rise to the *air capillaries*. These form a dense network of interconnected loops (Fig. 37.28/*e*) that spread into the interparabronchial septa. Anastomoses with air capillaries of

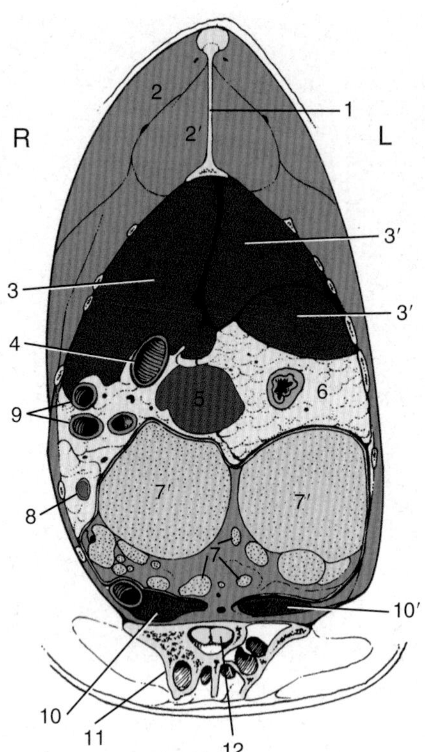

Fig. 37.24 Transverse section of the trunk at the cranial end of the ilium. *L,* Left; *R,* right; *1,* keel of sternum, *2,* pectoralis; *2′,* supracoracoideus; *3* and *3′,* right and left lobes of liver, respectively; *4,* gallbladder; *5,* spleen; *6,* constriction between proventriculus and gizzard; *7,* ovary; *7′,* follicle; *8,* cranial mesenteric vein in mesenteric fat; *9,* small intestine; *10* and *10′,* right and left kidneys, respectively; *11,* ilium; *12,* spinal cord.

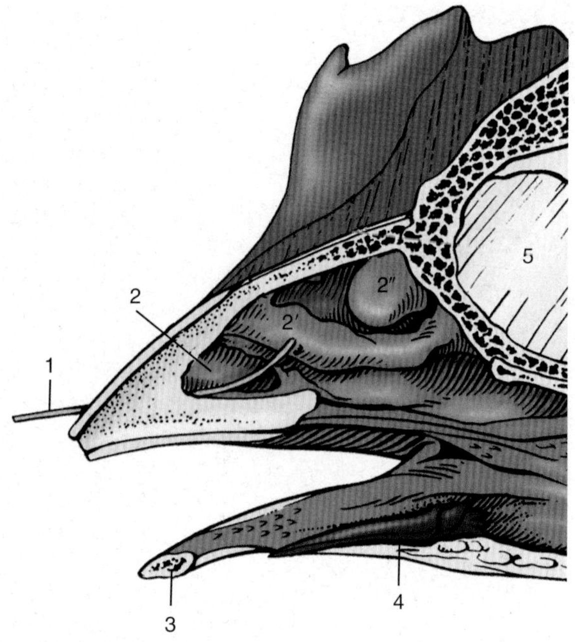

Fig. 37.25 Section through rostral part of the head of a chicken. *1,* Wire in nostril; *2, 2′,* and *2″,* rostral, middle, and caudal nasal conchae, respectively; *3,* mandible; *4,* tongue; *5,* interorbital septum.

adjacent parabronchi are found where the septa are deficient (Fig. 37.28/*g*). The air capillaries are closely intertwined with blood capillaries; the two networks constitute the bulk of the parabronchial wall. The arrangement of flow in the blood capillaries is crosscurrent, a feature contributing to the extreme efficiency of the avian lung. The air capillaries, about 5 μm in diameter, are lined by a single layer of epithelial cells resting on a basement membrane. The capillary endothelium is applied to the other side of the basement membrane. Gas exchange takes place across the barrier. The air capillaries are therefore comparable with the alveoli of the mammalian lung; the essential difference is that the air capillaries are not terminations of the respiratory tree but continuous channels that can receive oxygen-rich air from either direction.

Gas Exchange: Compared with mammals, the capture of oxygen in birds is much more efficient because of the following modifications: a thin blood–gas barrier, cross-current blood flow, one-way air flow, and pulmonary rigidity. However, the efficiency of gas exchange has its downside in that it makes birds much more susceptible to inhaled toxins and infections.

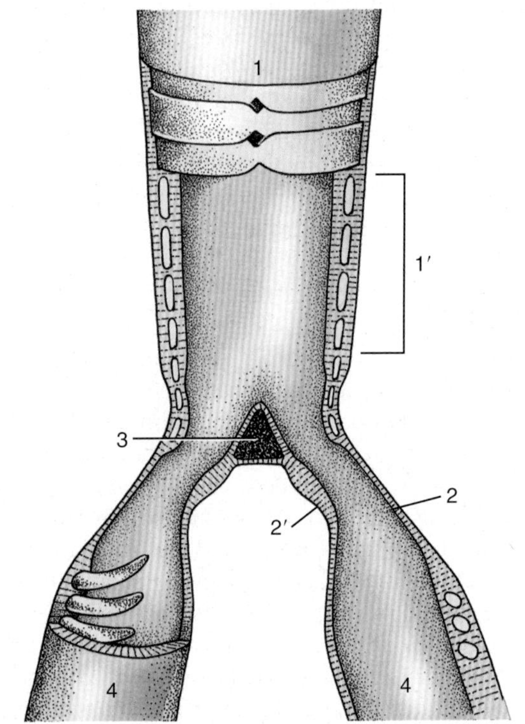

Fig. 37.26 Semi-schematic representation of the opened syrinx. *1,* Trachea; *1′,* tympanum; *2* and *2′,* lateral and medial tympaniform membranes; *3,* pessulus; *4,* primary bronchi.

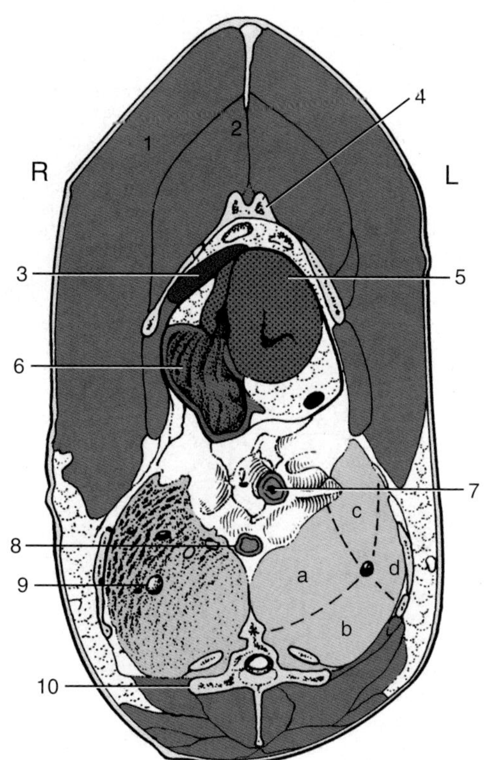

Fig. 37.27 Transverse section of the trunk at the level of the heart and lungs. *L,* Left; *R,* right; *1,* pectoralis; *2,* supracoracoideus; *3,* liver; *4,* sternum; *5,* left ventricle; *6,* right atrium; *7,* esophagus; *8,* descending aorta; *9,* primary bronchus in right lung; *10,* thoracic vertebra (notarium); *a, b, c,* and *d,* areas of left lung supplied by medioventral, mediodorsal, lateroventral, and laterodorsal secondary bronchi, respectively.

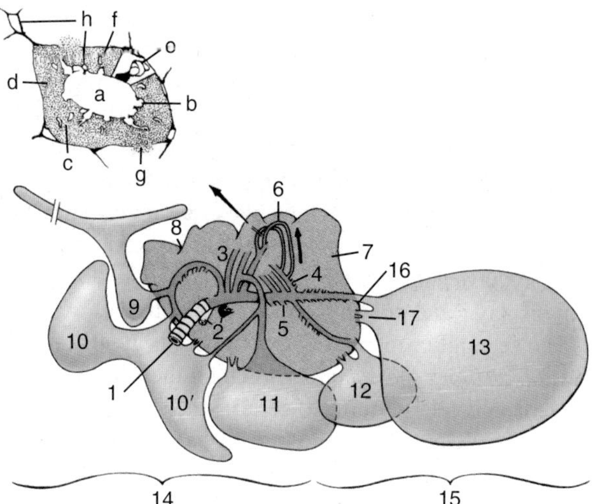

Fig. 37.28 Right lung (medioventral view) and related air sacs (schematic). The intrapulmonic structures have been simplified. *1,* Primary bronchus; *2,* pulmonary vessels at hilus; *3,* medioventral bronchi; *4,* mediodorsal bronchi; *5,* lateroventral bronchi; *6,* loops of parabronchi; *7,* lung; *8,* indentations caused by ribs; *9,* cervical air sac; *10* and *10′,* extrathoracic and intrathoracic parts of clavicular air sac, respectively; *11,* cranial thoracic air sac; *12,* caudal thoracic air sac; *13,* abdominal air sac; *14,* cranial air sacs, functionally related to paleopulmonic parabronchi; *15,* caudal air sacs, functionally related to neopulmonic parabronchi; *16,* direct (saccolobronchial) connection of air sac to lung; *17,* indirect (recurrent bronchial) connection of air sac to lung. *Inset,* Transverse section of a parabronchus. *a,* Lumen; *b,* atria; *c,* infundibula; *d,* network of air and blood capillaries; *e,* solidly drawn atrium and schematic air capillaries to show their continuity; *f,* interparabronchial septum; *g,* gas exchange tissue anastomosing through gap in interparabronchial septum; *h,* blood vessels.

The *air sacs* are blind, thin-walled (two cells thick) enlargements of the bronchial system that extend beyond the lung in close relationship to the thoracic and abdominal viscera. Diverticula from some sacs enter various bones and even reach between muscles.

The chicken has *eight air sacs:* single cervical and clavicular, and paired cranial thoracic, caudal thoracic, and abdominal sacs. The *cervical sac* (Fig. 37.28/*9*) consists of a small central chamber ventral to the lungs from which long diverticula extend into and alongside the cervical and thoracic vertebrae. The much larger *clavicular sac* lies in the thoracic inlet. Its thoracic part (Fig. 37.28/*10′*) fills the space cranial to and around the heart and extends into the sternum; extrathoracic diverticula (Fig. 37.28/*10*) pass between the muscles and bones of the shoulder girdle to pneumatize the humerus. Compound fractures of the humerus may therefore introduce infection to the air sacs and lungs. The paired *cranial thoracic sacs* (Fig. 37.28/*11*) lie ventral to the lungs between the sternal ribs and the heart and liver. The paired *caudal thoracic sacs* (Fig. 37.28/*12*) lie more caudally between the body wall and the abdominal sacs. The paired *abdominal sacs* (Fig. 37.28/*13*) are the largest. They occupy the caudodorsal parts of the abdominal cavity, where they are in broad contact with the intestines, gizzard, genital organs, and kidneys. Their diverticula enter recesses of the synsacrum and the acetabulum.

The air sacs function primarily in respiration, although their poorly vascularized walls deny them any role in gas exchange. Nonetheless, healthy air sacs are requisite to normal lung function. Indeed, their general arrangement is such that, in stark contrast to the process in mammals, fresh air is moved through the lung on expiration as well as inspiration. This feature is an obvious contribution to the remarkable efficiency of the avian lung and the truly prodigious athletic capabilities it can support. The air sacs also lighten the body and, being largely dorsal, lower the center of gravity, presumably for improved stability in flight. Those in the body cavity sharply delineate certain organs in radiographs.

The cervical, clavicular, and cranial thoracic sacs form one (cranial) functional group connected to the ventral bronchi, and the caudal thoracic and abdominal sacs form a second (caudal) group connected to the primary bronchus. The cranial air sacs are thus related to the paleopulmo, the caudal to the neopulmo.

In summary, the air sacs function to create a unidirectional flow of air through the lungs, which is important for maximizing oxygen extraction. By evaporation, they also help to reduce the amount of heat produced during flight and may have subsidiary roles in sound production, courtship displays, and possibly cooling of the testes.

The account of respiration given here is greatly simplified. *Inspiratory movements* (in which the ribs are drawn forward and the sternum lowered) draw air through the lungs into the air sacs; the caudal sacs (Fig. 37.28/*15*) receive relatively fresh air, and the cranial sacs (Fig. 37.28/*14*) receive air that has already lost much oxygen by passing through the paleopulmonic parabronchi. On expiration the air sacs are compressed; most air from the caudal sacs now passes through the neopulmonic parabronchi, while most of that from the cranial sacs leaves through the trachea. The air sacs thus act like bellows, moving air through largely passive lungs. The flow is circular, with air passing through the paleopulmonic parabronchial loops in the same direction. The feature is unique among vertebrates and in sharp contrast to the tidal flow in mammals.

Respiration is effected by the *intercostal and abdominal muscles*. For inspiration there are six muscles, but the principal ones are the external intercostals and the costosternalis. On expiration the rib cage moves outward and the sternum moves downward. This negative pressure causes air to be sucked in via the nares to the air sacs. There are nine muscles of expiration, but the internal intercostal and the abdominal musculature are the main ones. On expiration the rib cage moves upward, which reduces the chest size and compresses air from the air sacs back through the lungs.

The avian flow-through system means that artificial ventilation can be achieved by passing fresh oxygen down the trachea or via an air sac cannula if the trachea is obstructed. Manual ventilation by compressing and lifting the sternum can also be undertaken.

THE UROGENITAL APPARATUS

The Kidneys and Ureters

The *kidneys* are brown and elongated (Figs. 37.29 and 37.30). They fill the recesses in the ventral surfaces of the hip bones and lie against the synsacrum, reaching almost to its caudal limit, while contacting the lungs cranially. The abdominal air sacs that lie against their ventral surfaces extend diverticula that penetrate the dorsal renal surfaces. Several vessels and nerves pass through the kidneys, which makes it impossible to remove them without resulting

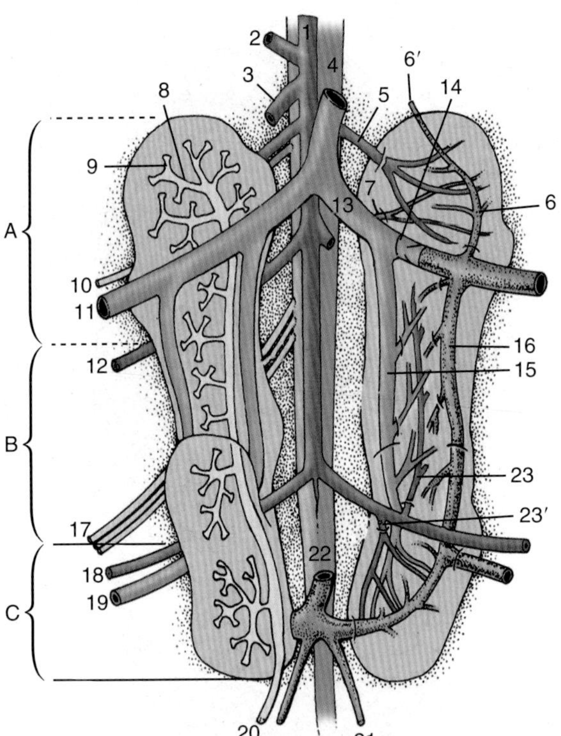

Fig. 37.29 Ventral view of the kidneys and vessels and nerves in their vicinity (schematic). The right kidney shows the branches of the ureter; the left, the renal vessels. Cranial (A), middle (B), and caudal (C) divisions of kidney. *1,* Aorta; *2,* celiac artery (a.); *3,* cranial mesenteric a.; *4,* caudal vena cava; *5,* cranial renal a.; *6,* cranial renal portal vein (v.); *6′,* anastomosis with vertebral venous sinus; *7,* cranial renal v.; *8,* primary branch of ureter; *9,* secondary branch of ureter; *10,* femoral nerve; *11,* external iliac v.; *12,* external iliac a.; *13,* common iliac v.; *14,* portal valve; *15,* caudal renal v.; *16,* caudal renal portal v.; *17,* sciatic nerve; *18,* ischial a.; *19,* ischial v.; *20,* ureter; *21,* internal iliac v.; *22,* caudal mesenteric v.; *23* and *23′,* middle and caudal renal arteries, respectively.

injury. Birds suffering from renal gout (not uncommon in commercial flocks) or tumors (common in budgerigars) may therefore have lameness as the presenting sign.

Each kidney is arbitrarily divided into cranial, middle, and caudal divisions by the external iliac and ischial arteries (Fig. 37.29/*12* and *18*). In some species, but not the chicken, the right and left caudal divisions are fused.

The cortex and medulla are not clearly demarcated, and there is no renal pelvis. The ureter (Fig. 37.29/*20*) arises in the cranial division by the confluence of several primary branches and passes over the medioventral surface of the kidney, receiving further branches from the middle and caudal divisions in its passage. The ureter then continues caudally alongside the genital duct to end in the dorsal wall of the urodeum (see later). It obtains a whitish tinge from the concentrated urine within it. Neither a bladder nor a urethra is present.

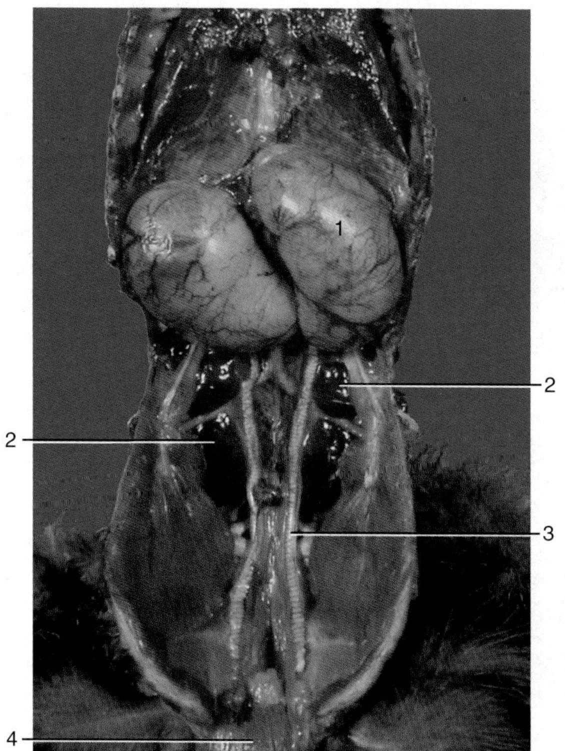

Fig. 37.30 Ventral view of the male reproductive organs. *1*, Testis; *2*, kidney; *3*, deferent duct; *4*, cloaca.

Each branch of the ureter (Fig. 37.29/*8* and *9*) results from the confluence of several secondary branches that receive urine from a small group (five or six) of cone-shaped *renal lobules,* each 1 to 2 mm in diameter. Those near the surface bulge slightly, providing a visible pattern. Each lobule contains nephrons of two types: medullary nephrons resembling the mammalian type (with the loop of Henle) and cortical nephrons resembling the reptilian type together with the vascular networks responsible for extracting urine from the blood. The collecting tubules lie in the periphery of the cone and become confluent at the apex.

The Blood Vessels of the Kidneys

The kidney is supplied by three *renal arteries,* one for each division (Fig. 37.29/*5, 23,* and *23'*). The cranial artery arises from the aorta, while the others arise from the ischial artery, and together they form the interlobular arteries. Intralobular arteries branch from the interlobular arteries and give rise in turn to two or more afferent arterioles that supply the renal corpuscles (i.e., glomeruli and tubules). However, it is not uncommon for interlobular arteries to give rise to afferent arterioles directly, especially to those supplying nearby glomeruli. The smaller veins are satellite to the arteries, but the several renal veins (Fig. 37.29/*7* and *15*) leaving the organ join the common iliac vein (Fig. 37.29/*13*) and, via this, the caudal vena cava. Superimposed on this is a portal system comprising cranial and caudal renal portal veins (Fig. 37.29/*6* and *16*). These receive blood from caudal parts of the body (through the external iliac vein) and channel it to the intralobular capillary beds that also receive arterial blood from the renal arteries. Thus, blood that has already passed one capillary bed (in the hindlimb or the pelvis) passes through a second bed within the kidneys. A portal valve (Fig. 37.29/*14*) (situated peripheral to the union of the external iliac and caudal renal veins to form the caudal iliac vein) regulates the flow of blood from the external iliac vein to the kidney; when it is narrowed, more blood enters the kidney, although some always escapes via connections with the vertebral sinuses and caudal mesenteric vein (Fig. 37.29/*6'* and *22*) at the cranial and caudal ends of the system. Most blood in the caudal mesenteric vein passes through the right hepatic portal vein and the liver before arriving at the heart. (Because of this, it has been suggested that antibiotics should not be injected into the muscles of the hindlimb, because some of the drug would then be excreted by the kidneys before reaching the heart for general distribution.)

The Male Reproductive Organs

These consist of paired testes, epididymides, and deferent ducts and a single phallus that in some species, including chickens, ducks, and ostriches, is the copulatory organ. The testes remain at their sites of origin; spermatic cord, tunica vaginalis, and scrotum are therefore lacking. Neither accessory reproductive glands nor a urethra exists.

The Testis

The bean-shaped testes are relatively large (about 5 cm long) and white during the breeding season (Fig. 37.30/*1*); however, they shrink to about half that size and become yellowish during the quiescent period (during molt). In some birds, especially Passeriformes, the difference in size is even more dramatic. Attached by short mesorchia, the testes are placed symmetrically against the cranial ends of the kidneys, just caudal to the adrenals, related ventrally to the abdominal sacs, proventriculus, liver, and intestines (Fig. 37.31/*3*). Removal of the testes (caponizing) to promote fattening may be performed through an incision near the last rib. Before the advent of simpler and safer tests to determine the sex of a bird of a monomorphic species, sexing, at least in larger cage birds, could be performed by introducing an endoscope through a small incision.

The serosa covers a thin tunica albuginea from which a scanty stroma is derived; no mediastinum testis exists. The seminiferous tubules pass to the dorsomedial surface, where they open into the rete testis. The *epididymis* is not divided into head, body, and tail and appears as a slight bulge on the testis. It is formed by tightly packed efferent ductules that join to form the epididymal duct that transports the spermatozoa to the deferent duct (Figs.

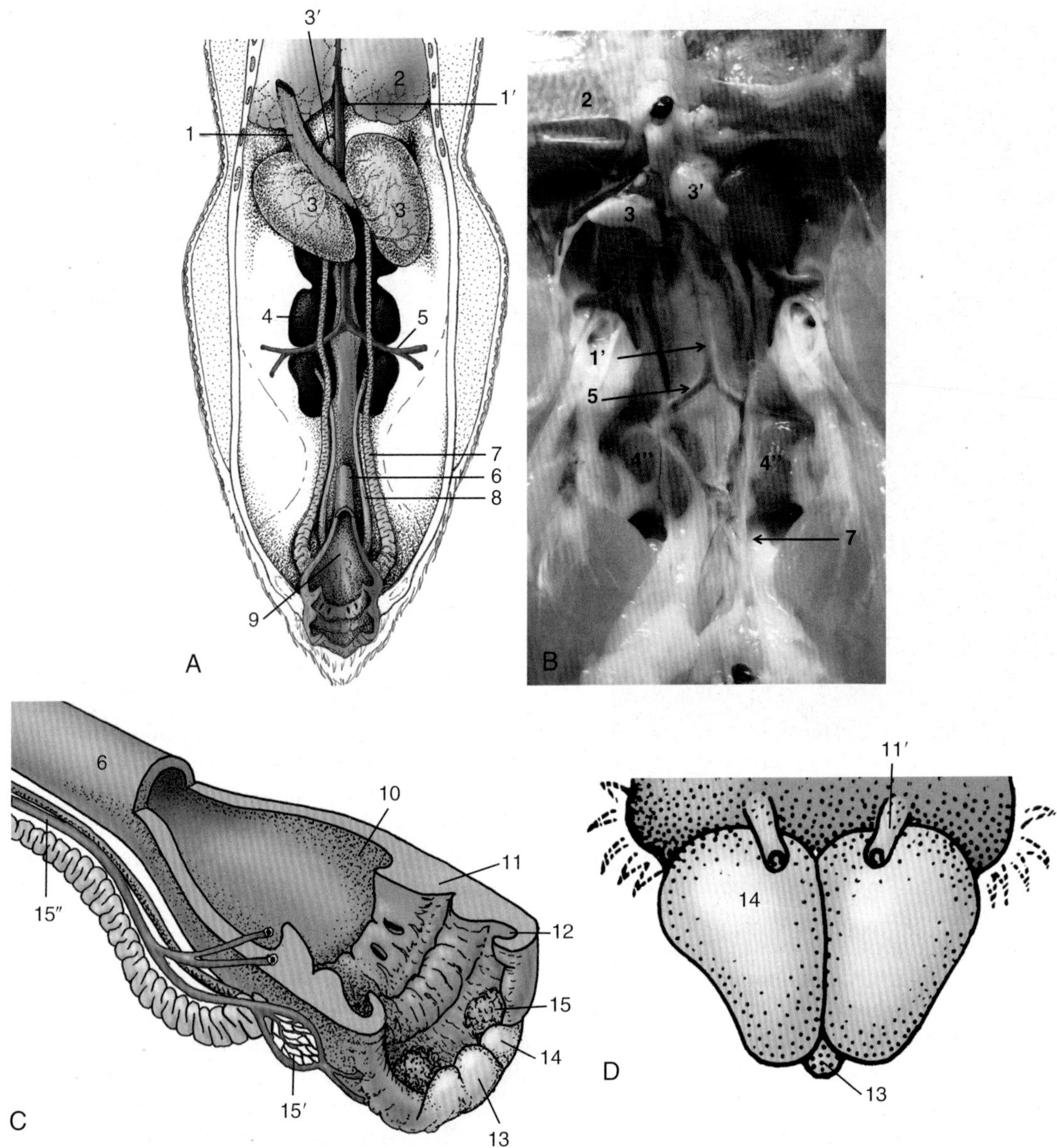

Fig. 37.31 (A) Ventral view of the male reproductive organs (schematic). (B) Ventral view of the male reproductive organs. (C) The floor of the cloaca has been removed and is shown turned over. (D) Caudal view of the tumescent phallus. *1,* Caudal vena cava; *1′,* aorta; *2,* lung; *3,* right testis; *3′,* left testis; *4,* kidney-Cranial lobe; *4′,* Kidney-Middle lobe; *4″,* Kidney-Caudal lobe; *5,* ischial artery; *6,* rectum; *7,* deferent duct; *8,* ureter; *9,* cloaca; *10,* coprodeum; *11,* urodeum; *11′,* papilla of right deferent duct; *12,* proctodeum; *13,* median phallic tubercle; *14,* lateral phallic body; *15,* lymphatic folds; *15′,* paracloacal vascular body; *15″,* pudendal artery.

37.30/*3* and 37.31/*7*). The tightly coiled deferent duct arises from the caudal end of the epididymis and accompanies the ureter to the cloaca, where it opens on a low papilla on the lateral wall of the urodeum (Fig. 37.22). The duct shows a slight terminal enlargement (receptacle). During the reproductive period the duct, packed with spermatozoa, appears white. The ejaculate of the cockerel is generally not quite 1 mL. The seminal fluid is elaborated in the testes and by the epithelial cells lining the extratesticular ducts.

The Cloaca and Phallus

The *coprodeum,* the most cranial division of the cloaca, has been described (p. 784). The urodeum (Fig. 37.22/*3*), caudal to the coprourodeal fold, is indistinctly demarcated from the proctodeum by a shallow, ventrally incomplete uroproctodeal fold (Fig. 37.22/*3′*). The ureteric orifice is in the dorsolateral wall, above the papilla of the deferent duct. In the female, the slitlike opening of the oviduct (Fig. 37.22/*8*) occupies a similar position on the left side (see further on). A small patch of vascular tissue (paracloacal vascular body;

Fig. 37.31/*15'*) in the lateral wall of the urodeum is thought to supply lymph for the tumescence of the phallus.

The *proctodeum*—the short, most caudal segment of the cloaca—ends at the vent. A small opening in its dorsal wall leads to the cloacal bursa (bursa of Fabricius; Fig. 37.22/*9*), an accumulation of lymphatic tissue that is the differentiation site of B lymphocytes (Fig. 37.23). The cloacal bursa is thus an immunologic organ analogous to the thymus (see pp. 797–798). A small (dorsal proctodeal) gland is found caudal to the bursa (Fig. 37.22/*9'*).

The vent is a horizontal slit. The ventral lip is of interest because in the male chicken it bears the nonprotrusible *phallus*, the analogue of the mammalian penis, on its internal surface. The phallus consists of a small median tubercle flanked by a pair of larger lateral phallic bodies (Fig 37.31/*13* and *14*). These enlarge in the tumescent state and together form a channel that receives the ejaculate from the deferent ducts (Fig. 37.31C). During insemination, the vent is everted and the phallus is pressed against the cloacal mucosa of the female (cloacal "kiss"). The phallus of the tom turkey is similar. The gander and the drake have a protrusible phallus, several centimeters long and capable of intromission. It is shaped like a thin cone and exhibits a spiral groove that conveys the semen to the tip (Fig. 37.32/*8*). A protrusible phallus, also seen in ratites, is capable of true intromission into the female cloaca.

Psittacines, passerines, pigeons, and birds of prey all have no phallus. These species copulate by transferring semen from the everted cloaca directly into the female oviduct.

Day-old chicks of both sexes of chickens present a minute genital protuberance at the future location of the phallus. A slight visible difference in form (which is rounded in males and conical in females) is distinguishable by the experienced eye and enables almost all male chicks to be discarded when selecting a laying flock.

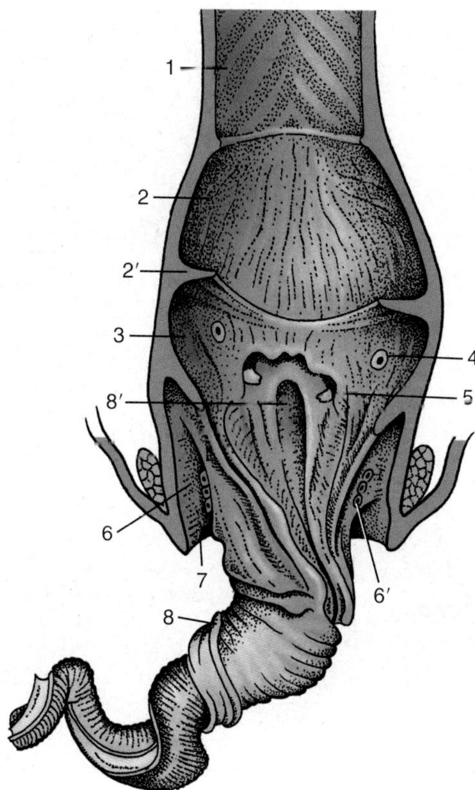

Fig. 37.32 Cloaca of a drake with protruded phallus whose tip has been cut off, dorsal view. *1*, Colon; *2*, coprodeum; *2'*, coprourodeal fold; *3*, urodeum; *4*, ureteric orifice; *5*, papilla of deferent duct; *6*, proctodeum; *6'*, proctodeal glands; *7*, lip of vent; *8*, spiral groove of phallus; *8'*, beginning of spiral groove.

The Female Reproductive Organs

These consist of the ovary and oviduct. Generally only the left organs are functional in birds, and the right set regresses after development. The avian oviduct represents the entire genital tract and extends from the ovary to the cloaca. The gonad and tubular tracts of both male and female fill much of the body cavity while productive but, when inactive outside of the breeding season, regress to such an extent that they may be difficult to locate.

The Ovary

In the first 5 months after hatching, the ovary gradually develops from a small irregular structure with a finely granular surface to one in which individual *follicles* can be distinguished. These then rapidly increase in number and size until some are several centimeters in diameter (the size of an egg yolk (Figs. 37.33 and 37.34 and see Fig. 37.24/*7*). The mature ovary resembles a truss of grapes, of various sizes, that is broadly attached to the cranial division of the left kidney. It contains several thousand follicles—far more than the number of eggs (about 1500) laid by even the most productive hen. The larger follicles are pendulous and make contact with the stomach, spleen, and intestines. Each consists of a large, yolk-filled oocyte surrounded by a highly vascular follicular wall. Shortly before ovulation, a devascularized white band (stigma) appears opposite the stalk, indicating where the wall will rupture at ovulation (Fig. 37.35/*2* and see Fig. 37.34). The empty follicle (calix) regresses after ovulation and disappears in a few days. No corpus luteum is required because there is no embryo to maintain within the bird's body.

The Oviduct

The oviduct conducts the fertilized ovum to the cloaca, adds substantial amounts of nutrients (including the albumen), and encloses it with membranes and a shell to protect the developing embryo. It conveys spermatozoa to the ovum for immediate fertilization and may store them for a time for future use. In the chicken, one insemination is sufficient to fertilize the ova released during the following 10 days or so.

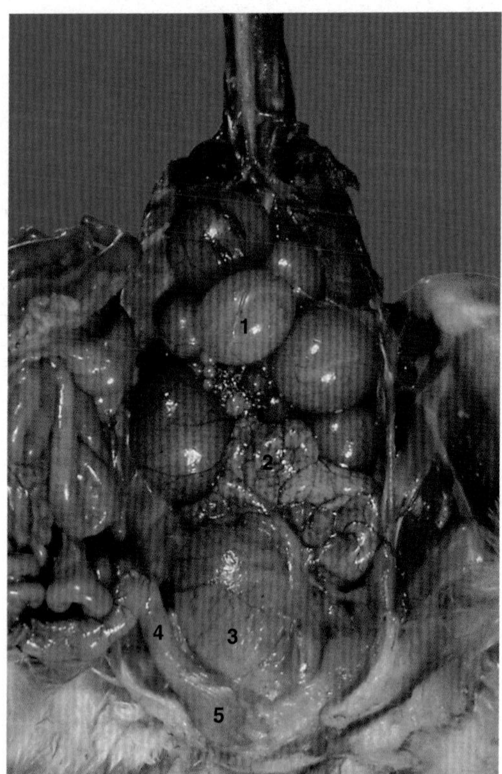

Fig. 37.33 Ventral view of reproductive organs of a hen. *1,* Ovary with follicles in different stages of development; *2,* oviduct; *3,* uterus; *4,* rectum; *5,* cloaca.

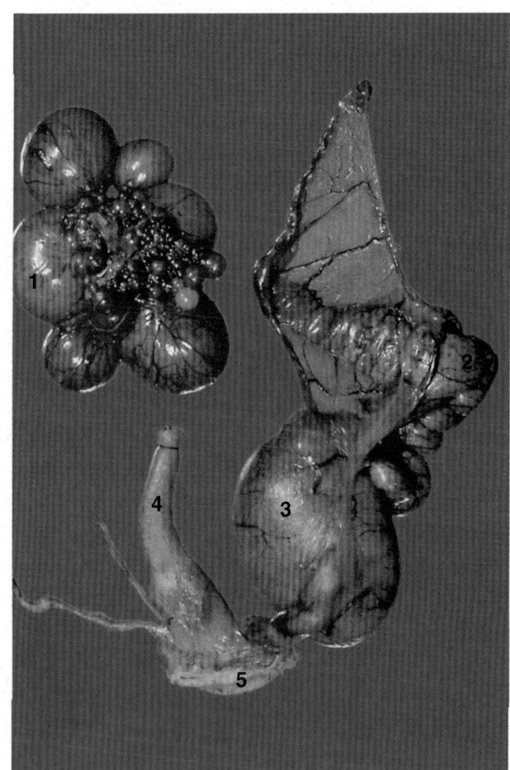

Fig. 37.34 Isolated female reproductive organs. *1,* Ovary with follicles in different stages of development; *2,* oviduct; *3,* uterus; *4,* rectum; *5,* cloaca.

The *oviduct* (Fig. 37.35/*3–7* and see Figs. 37.33 and 37.34) may be divided into infundibulum, magnum, isthmus, uterus, and vagina according to the function of its parts; the uterus and vagina are, of course, not analogous to the like-named organs of mammals. The oviduct occupies the left dorsal part of the body cavity, where it is related to the kidney, intestines, and gizzard. It is a massive coil, approximately 60 cm long (i.e., about twice the body length) when fully functional but much smaller in juveniles and during the nonlaying period. It is suspended from the roof of the body cavity by a peritoneal fold (mesoviductus), and some coils are connected by a continuation that forms the prominent muscular ventral ligament (Fig. 37.35/*12*). The wall of the oviduct consists of the usual layers: serosa, tunica muscularis (consisting of outer spiral and inner circular layers), a scanty submucosa, and a tunica mucosa containing many glands.

The cranial end is formed by the 7-cm-long infundibulum (Fig. 37.35/*3*), consisting of fluted and tubular parts. The thin-walled fluted part is stretched to form a slit (infundibular ostium) several centimeters long. Its lateral end is attached to the body wall near the last rib. The ostium is positioned by the left abdominal air sac in such a way that it can grasp newly released oocytes. The oocyte passes through the infundibulum in about 15 minutes. Fertilization must take place before the infundibular glands provide the chalaziferous layer, the thin coat of dense albumen directly around the yolk. The chalazae—the coiled strands that suspend the yolk and allow it to rotate so that the germinal disk remains uppermost, although part of this layer—develop farther along the genital tract (Fig. 37.36/*3'*). Some species have an infundibular sperm host gland in which sperm may be stored.

The highly coiled *magnum* (Figs. 37.33, 37.34, and 37.35/*4*) measures about 30 cm and is the longest segment of the duct. Its walls carry massive mucosal folds and are thickened by the glands that contribute about half the total albumen to the egg. Calcium, sodium, and magnesium are also added here. The mucosal folds are lower and the secretion more mucous in the distal end of the magnum. The egg takes about 3 hours to pass through this part.

The *isthmus* (Fig. 37.35/*5*), about 8 cm long, is demarcated from the magnum by a narrow, translucent glandular zone. The isthmus, thinner and with lower mucosal folds than the magnum, secretes more albumen and also a material that rapidly congeals to form the two homogeneous membranes found between the albumen and the shell. The egg takes upward of 1 hour to traverse the isthmus. The isthmus is lacking in psittacines.

The *uterus* (shell gland; Fig. 37.35/*6*) that follows the isthmus is about 8 cm long; it is a thinner walled and

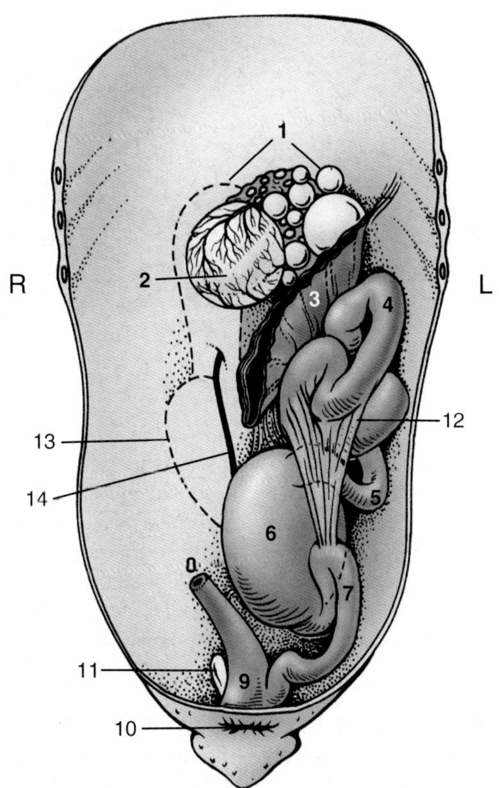

Fig. 37.35 Ventral view of the reproductive organs of a laying hen (semi-schematic). *L*, Left; *R*, right; *1*, ovary; *2*, stigma on mature follicle; *3*, infundibulum; *4*, magnum; *5*, isthmus; *6*, uterus containing egg; *7*, vagina; *8*, rectum; *9*, cloaca; *10*, vent; *11*, vestigial right oviduct; *12*, free border of ventral ligament of oviduct; *13*, outline of right kidney; *14*, right ureter.

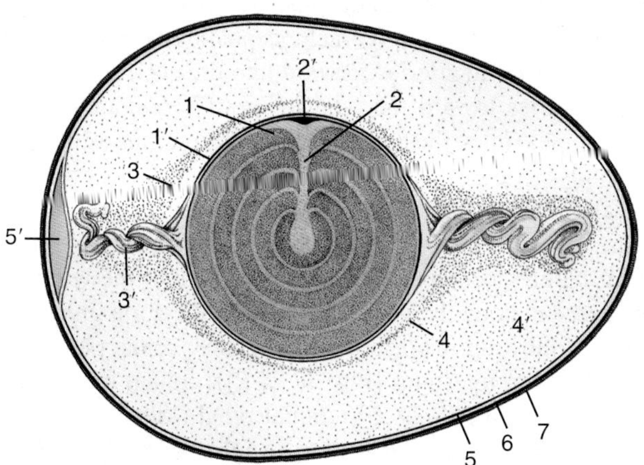

Fig. 37.36 A semi-schematic section of a fertilized egg. *1*, Yolk; *1'*, yolk membrane; *2*, latebra; *2'*, germinal disk; *3*, chalaziferous layer; *3'*, chalaza; *4* and *4'*, thin and dense albumen, respectively; *5*, internal and external shell membranes; *5'*, air cell; *6*, shell; *7*, cuticle.

slightly enlarged chamber. Its mucosa bears many low folds and ridges that flatten themselves against the egg, which remains here for about 20 hours. Passing through the permeable membranes, some watery albumen is added to the egg. This secretion is then followed by the deposition of the shell and shell pigments and an outer glazing or cuticle.

The final part, the *vagina* (Fig. 37.35/*7*), is a muscular, S-shaped tube through which the completed egg passes in seconds when it is laid. Its junction with the uterus is marked by a sphincter. Glandular crypts in the region of the sphincter have been found to store sperm. The vagina ends at a slitlike opening in the lateral wall of the urodeum. When the egg is laid (blunt end first), the vaginal opening protrudes through the vent, which minimizes contamination by the feces. Sperm host glands, where sperm can be stored for many months, may also be found at the uterovaginal junction. A remnant of the right oviduct (Fig. 37.35/*11*) is found on the right side of the cloaca; it may become cystic and enlarged.

THE BODY CAVITY

Now that the organs and air sacs have been described, a brief account of how the body cavity (celom) is subdivided may be helpful. In birds no diaphragm separates thoracic from abdominal organs. However, the body cavity is divided into three parts by horizontal and oblique septa, which are mostly thin and translucent but may contain some fibrous tissue. The horizontal septum has some muscle toward the periphery. The oblique septum is usually destroyed when the viscera are handled during dissection.

The *horizontal septum* is attached laterally to the ribs and medially to the bodies of the thoracic vertebrae; caudally it makes contact with the oblique septum. It forms the ventral surface of paired cavities that are bounded laterally and dorsally by the ribs and thoracic vertebrae. These spaces contain the lungs.

The larger *oblique septum* is attached to the sternum ventrally, the sixth and seventh ribs laterally, and the horizontal septum and thoracic vertebrae dorsally. It forms the caudoventral surface of paired cavities that are bounded dorsally by the horizontal septum and laterally by the thoracic and abdominal wall. This part of the body cavity contains the thoracic air sacs and the thoracic parts of the cervical and clavicular air sacs.

The largest of the three parts is caudal to the oblique septum. It is bounded dorsally by the pelvis, dorsocranially by the oblique septum, and ventrally by the caudal portion of the sternum and abdominal muscles. It contains the heart, liver, spleen, gastrointestinal and urogenital tracts, and abdominal air sacs. It is further divided by mesenteries and peritoneal folds, resulting in a complex set of compartments.

THE ENDOCRINE GLANDS

The paired *thyroid glands* (Fig. 37.37/*5*) of the chicken are reddish brown, oval, and about 10 mm long and 5 mm wide. In the budgerigar, in which thyroid disease is a major problem in iodine-deficient areas, they are paler and only 2 to 3 mm long and 1 to 2 mm wide. The thyroid glands are located in the thoracic inlet, caudal to the crop and closely related to the common carotid artery, trachea, jugular vein, and vagus nerve (which accompanies the vein)—indeed, they lie just cranial to where these vessels are joined by the subclavian vessels (Fig. 37.37/*16*). Their color distinguishes them from the neighboring rather similar but pale thymic lobes.

The *parathyroid glands* (Fig. 37.37/*7*), two or three on each side, are minute (1- to 3-mm) yellowish brown structures immediately caudal to the thyroid gland, to which one may be attached. They become enlarged (increased parathyroid hormone production) when the diet is deficient in calcium, which leads to decalcification of the bones. In African grey parrots there is a specific problem in which calcium fails to be mobilized from the skeleton despite a dietary deficiency. In this situation the bird will die of hypocalcemia, and much enlarged parathyroid glands will be found at necropsy.

The even more minute pink *ultimobranchial glands* (Fig. 37.37/*8*) lie next to the parathyroids.

The *adrenal glands* (Fig. 37.31/*3′*) are yellowish brown, oval or triangular, and about 13 mm long and 8 mm wide. Each lies at the cranial pole of the corresponding kidney, related ventrally to the ovary (or epididymis). There is no distinct separation of cortex and medulla.

The *hypophysis* (or pituitary gland) (Fig. 37.38/*7*) is attached below the diencephalon and occupies the hypophyseal fossa in the base of the skull. It resembles that of mammals in its division and formation.

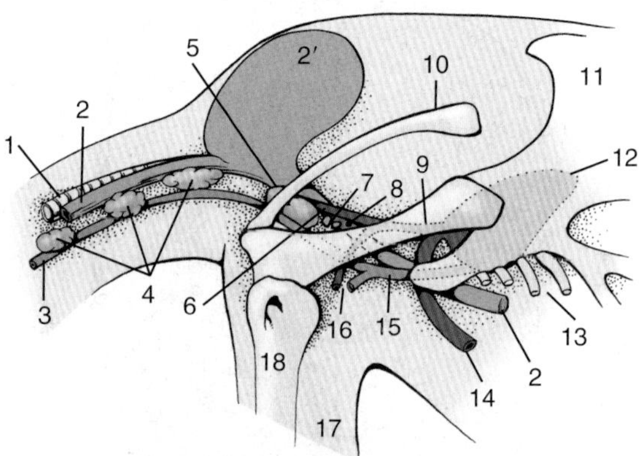

Fig. 37.37 Junction of neck and trunk as viewed from the right (semi-schematic). Cranial is to the left. *1,* Trachea; *2,* esophagus; *2′,* crop; *3,* right jugular vein; *4,* thymus; *5,* thyroid gland; *6,* right common carotid artery; *7,* parathyroid glands; *8,* ultimobranchial gland; *9,* right brachiocephalic artery; *10,* clavicle; *11,* sternum; *12,* position of heart; *13,* sternal ribs; *14,* descending aorta; *15,* right cranial vena cava; *16,* subclavian artery and vein; *17,* wing; *18,* humerus.

THE CIRCULATORY SYSTEM

The Heart

The avian heart is four chambered and broadly similar to that of mammals. It is, however, relatively much larger, and its rate of contraction is much faster—up to 1000 times per minute in certain small birds! It is conical, with the apex formed solely by the left ventricle. The heart lies within the thorax both between and in front of the lobes of the liver (Fig. 37.16/*8*). It is attached to the sternum by the fibrous pericardium.

The right atrium receives paired cranial venae cavae and a single caudal vena cava. The right atrioventricular valve is formed by a single muscular flap without chordae tendineae. The thin-walled right ventricle lays itself around the left ventricle so that its lumen on cross section is shaped like a crescent. The pulmonary veins combine to form a single trunk before entering the left atrium at an entrance provided with a valve capable of preventing reflux. The left atrioventricular valve has three cusps attached to chordae tendineae. The thick-walled left ventricle (Fig. 37.27/*5*) is conical. Internally, muscular bars give the cross section a rosette-like form. Cardiac puncture, performed for blood sampling, is dangerous in small birds.

The Arteries

The first part of the *aorta* gives rise to right and left coronary arteries and a brachiocephalic trunk that immediately divides into right and left brachiocephalic arteries that send common carotid arteries forward into the neck and subclavian arteries toward the wings (Fig. 37.16/*8′* and *8″*). In the thoracic inlet, the common carotids continue as internal carotids lying side by side on the ventral surface of the cervical vertebrae (Fig. 37.15/*6′*). The subclavian artery gives off a large pectoral trunk for the breast muscles and sternum before accompanying the humerus into the wing. In its descent along the vertebral column, the aorta gives rise to the following major arterial branches: celiac (stomach, spleen, liver, intestines [Fig. 37.29/*2*]), cranial mesenteric (intestines [Fig. 37.29/*3*]), cranial renal (kidneys, gonads [Fig. 37.29/*5*]), external iliac (thighs [Fig. 37.29/*12*]), ischial (kidneys, oviduct, hindlimbs [Fig. 37.29/*18*]), and caudal mesenteric (intestines, cloaca). It ends by supplying the end of the oviduct, pelvic structures, and tail.

The Veins

The two *cranial venae cavae* (Fig. 37.16/*7*) are satellite to the brachiocephalic arteries and receive tributaries (jugular

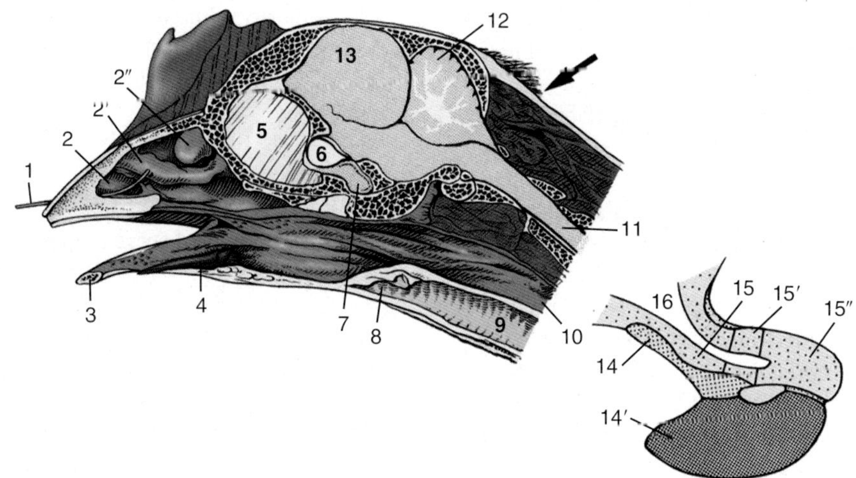

Fig. 37.38 Median section of the head with an enlargement of the hypophysis *(inset)*. The *arrow* indicates the approach to the foramen magnum through which euthanasia may be performed by injection into the brain. *1,* Wire in nostril; *2, 2',* and *2",* rostral, middle, and caudal nasal conchae, respectively; *3,* mandible; *4,* tongue; *5,* interorbital septum; *6,* optic chiasm; *7,* hypophysis (see also *inset*); *8,* larynx; *9,* trachea; *10,* esophagus; *11,* spinal cord; *12,* cerebellum; *13,* cerebrum; *14* and *14',* pars tuberalis and pars distalis of the adenohypophysis, respectively; *15, 15',* and *15",* median eminence, infundibulum, and neural lobe of the neurohypophysis, respectively; *16,* third ventricle.

and subclavian veins) from the neck and head and the breast and wing.

Venipuncture: The right jugular vein, always larger than the left, is visible through the skin and available for venipuncture (Fig. 37.15/*6*). However, this is not possible in pigeons, in which the skin is very thick in this area. Venipuncture in these birds is done from the medial metatarsal vein. In many small cage birds the left jugular is very small. The cutaneous ulnar vein (wing vein), subcutaneous on the ventral surface of the extended wing, may also be used for the administration of fluids or collection of very small volumes of blood (Fig. 37.13/*9*). The habit of clipping a claw for a small amount of blood is now condemned: it is much better to puncture the medial metatarsal vein.

The *caudal vena cava* drains the liver, kidneys, gonads, and oviduct. It forms ventral to the kidneys from the union of the common iliac veins that drain the pelvis and hindlimbs (Fig. 37.29/*13*). As described on page 791, some blood from the pelvis and hindlimbs passes through the kidneys (renal portal system) before reaching the caudal vena cava. Blood from the gastrointestinal tract reaches the liver by separate right and left *hepatic portal veins* that enter the respective lobes. The left vein drains the left and ventral parts of the stomach. The much larger right vein drains the right and dorsal parts of the stomach, the spleen, and the remainder of the gastrointestinal tract through cranial and caudal mesenteric veins. The *caudal mesenteric* vein, connected to the caudal end of the renal portal system (Fig. 37.29/*22*), also conveys a considerable amount of blood toward the kidneys. Thus, some blood from the gastrointestinal tract may return to the heart without passing through the liver.

The Lymphatic Structures

Only the goose and duck (among domestic poultry) have lymphoid tissue encapsulated as true lymph nodes—a pair of cervicothoracic nodes in the thoracic inlet and a pair of lumbar nodes close to the kidneys. However, lymphatic tissue, present in all species, exists as relatively unorganized aggregates in most of the species.

Lymphatics are less numerous than in mammals. They accompany (and wind around) the blood vessels, are valved, and present microscopic lymph nodules scattered at intervals in their walls. They conduct the lymph to the thoracic inlet, where it is discharged into the cranial venae cavae.

Although true lymph nodes are absent, much lymphatic tissue occurs in various organs (liver, pancreas, lungs, and kidneys) in the form of *solitary lymph nodules,* especially prominent in pathologic conditions, and in the oropharynx and intestine as patches of *aggregate lymph nodules.* These lymphoid aggregates are called gut-associated lymphoid tissue (GALT) and bronchiolar-associated lymphoid tissue (BALT). Cecal patches (cecal tonsils; Fig. 37.20/*10*) are particularly evident.

The *thymus* consists of several separate lobes that accompany the jugular veins (Fig. 37.15/*9*). The lobes are divided into lobules, each of which consists of a dark cortex and a pale medulla. The thymus, best developed in the young, regresses with the onset of sexual maturity.

The *cloacal bursa,* which has been described earlier (Fig. 37.22/*9*), is a lymphoepithelial organ and has a thin wall made uneven by the enclosed lobules that surround an irregular lumen. In the second week of embryonic development (in the chicken), lymphoid precursor cells migrate into the developing organ (Fig. 37.23B), and longitudinal plicae form and protrude into the lumen. Nodular epithelial formations, originating from the plicae, now begin to penetrate the lamina propria. With the initiation of lymphopoiesis, lymphoid cells invade these buds from the lamina propria. The buds increase considerably by day 18 through active proliferation of lymphoid cells. The bursa reaches its greatest size approximately 6 weeks after hatching, when the plicae are completely filled by large epithelial accumulations (or bursa follicles), which results in the histology of the organ showing many similarities with that of the thymus (Fig. 37.23C). The bursa is the site of antigen-independent differentiation of B lymphocytes and antibody production. The bursa gradually regresses from the age of 2 to 3 months, but a small nodule remains in the adult. In young birds the bursa is an important organ for investigating and diagnosing several viral infections (e.g., circovirus infections).

The location and shape of the *spleen* have been described (p. 785; Fig. 37.24/*5*). Its structure resembles that of the mammal, although the distinction between the red and white pulp is less marked.

THE NERVOUS SYSTEM AND SENSE ORGANS

The Brain and Spinal Cord

The brain is small, indeed, barely larger than one of the eyes (Fig. 37.38). The cerebral *hemispheres* are pear shaped; their pointed rostral ends (olfactory bulbs) are wedged between the large orbits. Compared with their mammalian counterparts, the hemispheres are small and relatively smooth. The right and left hemispheres are separated from each other by a median fissure and from the cerebellum by a transverse fissure. The tip of the epiphysis can be seen at the intersection of those fissures. The *optic lobes,* homologous with the rostral colliculi of the mammal, are located caudoventral to the hemispheres. They are exceedingly large—corresponding to the development of the eyes—and are visible from both dorsal and ventral aspects. The *optic chiasm* (Fig. 37.38/*6*) is also correspondingly large. The small olfactory bulbs point to an underdeveloped sense of smell. The *cerebellum* (Fig. 37.38/*12*), also relatively large, consists essentially of a central body (the homologue of the mammalian vermis) with small lateral appendages (flocculi).

A peculiarity of the *spinal cord* is a glycogen-rich gelatinous body at the dorsal surface of the lumbosacral enlargement; it is 3 to 5 mm in size and should not be mistaken for a lesion.

Some Peripheral Nerves

The normal peripheral nerve is white, faintly cross-striated, and uniformly wide. In Marek disease (neural lymphomatosis) this appearance is altered, especially in the nerves of the limbs. The following nerves are usually examined at necropsy. The cervical nerves emerge from the cervical muscles and pass to the skin at right angles to the neck (Fig. 37.15/*4'*). The vagus nerve (Fig. 37.15/*6*) accompanies the jugular vein. The cervical sympathetic trunk lies deep to the muscles. The vagus is seen again on the dorsal surface of the proventriculus (Fig. 37.21A/*3*). The brachial plexus is exposed on each side of the cervical muscles when the esophagus, trachea, and major vessels cranial to the heart are reflected. Most branches pass into the wing ventral to the scapula and caudal to the humerus. The intercostal nerves are exposed by the removal of the lungs. The intestinal nerve (Fig. 37.21/*14*) accompanies the cranial mesenteric vessels in the mesentery. Nerves of the lumbar and synsacral plexuses pass through the kidney, which must be removed to expose them (Fig. 37.29/*10* and *17*). Finally, the sciatic nerve can be examined on the medial surface of the thigh by reflecting two thin muscles (Fig. 37.21A/*15*).

The Eye

The *eyeball* resembles that of the globular mammalian one. The general structure is globular, although the shape may differ, especially in its anterior part, which may be flat, globose, or tubular depending on the species (Fig. 37.39). The eyeball almost fills the orbit, leaving little room for movement; however, the long neck and mobile occipitoatlantal joint compensate for this.

The lower lid is the larger and more movable. The third eyelid has a stiffened edge; being translucent, it does not seem to impair vision when drawn across the cornea. The secretions of the lacrimal gland and the deep gland of the third eyelid leave the conjunctival sac through two puncta that lead to a spacious nasolacrimal duct. The upper punctum is surprisingly large.

The cornea is thin and strongly curved. Its small diameter belies the enormous eyeball to which it belongs. The sclera is reinforced by a layer of cartilage transformed into a ring of ossicles near the cornea (Fig. 37.39/*1'*). No tapetum lucidum is present. The iris of the chicken is yellow-brown but turns slightly paler during the laying period. It surrounds a round pupil that can rapidly change in size through the action of the *striated* sphincter and dilator muscles. Even so, the avian iris is surprisingly unresponsive to light. In most other species the iris is

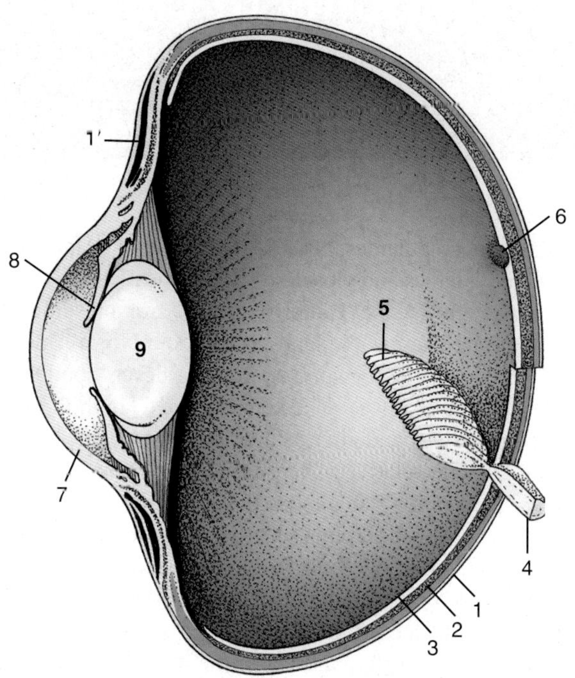

Fig. 37.39 Section through the eyeball (schematic). *1,* Sclera; *1',* ring of scleral ossicles; *2,* choroid; *3,* retina; *4,* optic nerve; *5,* pecten; *6,* fovea centralis; *7,* cornea; *8,* iris; *9,* lens.

darker, ranging from brown to black, although it can be bright yellow in owls. In African grey parrots the grey iris of the juvenile becomes yellow at maturity. In cockatoos the female has a red to brown iris, and the male has dark brown to black. The *retina* is devoid of blood vessels. It displays a remarkable outgrowth (pecten; Fig. 37.39/*5*) over the optic disk. This is a black, pleated ridge that projects into the vitreous; rich in blood vessels, it is thought to play a role in the nutrition of the retina. The extraocular muscles are similar to those of mammals, although a retractor bulbi is lacking.

The Ear

There is no auricle; the *external ear* consists only of the external acoustic meatus, which opens on the side of the head under cover of a patch of small feathers. The meatus is short and straight, so the relatively large tympanic membrane can easily be examined (and as easily injured). A lobe, similar in structure to the comb and wattle, is present ventral to the opening (Fig. 37.1/*4*). Among domestic chickens, the color of the earlobe matches the color of the shell of the eggs the hen lays.

The *middle ear* resembles that of mammals, except for the modification of the ossicles. The tympanic membrane is connected to the vestibule window by the columella and the homologue of the mammalian stapes, a tiny osseous rod expanded at each end.

The structure and subdivision of the *inner ear* follow the mammalian pattern. The cochlea does not form a spiral and is only slightly curved, although it is significantly shorter than its mammalian counterpart; a relatively thick layer of sensory cells seems to compensate for brevity.

COMPREHENSION CHECK

Because of the importance of the following in poultry diseases, review the structure of the following organs: lungs, heart, kidneys, liver, and lymphoid organs.

Of the 27 orders among which birds are divided, those likely to be of the most frequent veterinary concern are Galliformes, Anseriformes, Columbiformes, Psittaciformes, Falconiformes, and Passeriformes—or, in more familiar terms, the domestic chicken and its relatives, ducks and geese, pigeons, parrots and budgerigars, hawks and eagles, and the so-called songbirds, respectively. This list is less limited than it might initially appear because, by itself, the Passeriformes order includes some 5700 of the nearly 9700 species of birds currently recognized.

38 The Clinical Anatomy of Llamas and Alpacas

> "Among the living selenodont Artiodactyla the Camels and Llamas of the Old and New World represent a very aberrant group. Even if one were not familiar with the wonderful record of their past history as revealed in the Tertiary deposits of this country he would be quite justified, from the number of anatomical peculiarities which they exhibit, in placing their origin far back in the Tertiary, at a time when the primitive divergence of the various lines of the Selenodonts was taking place."
>
> ***J. L. Wortman, 1898***

This chapter is intended to introduce veterinary students and veterinarians to the clinically relevant anatomic differences between domesticated South American camelids and domestic ungulates, particularly ruminants and horses. In many instances their anatomy is somewhat unique, but the specific anatomy of llamas and alpacas has not been reported extensively, especially with regard to the muscular, nervous, and vascular system differences that may exist in these animals. Because of the relative paucity of anatomic studies on the llama and alpaca, this chapter is not intended to be a complete treatise on anatomy of South American camelids but a summary of the documented anatomic differences that need to be taken into account in handling and treating llamas and alpacas. Unless otherwise mentioned, as far as the authors know camelid anatomy conforms to the general mammalian pattern exemplified by the other domestic species commonly studied.

Major information sources used for this chapter include *Medicine and Surgery of Camelids, Llama and Alpaca Care,* and *Veterinary Techniques for Llamas and Alpacas.*[1] In addition, a literature search was conducted of the major databases for veterinary medicine to identify papers and other sources of information specific to the llama or alpaca, and these are referenced as appropriate. Original sketches were done from photographs.

Camelids evolved in North America in the early Epocene epoch but were extinct in North America by the end of the last Ice Age. Modern camelids belong to one of two general groups: "old-world" camelids include the dromedary and the Bactrian camels, and "new-world," or South American, camelids include llamas, alpacas, vicuñas, and guanacos, of which only llamas and alpacas are domesticated.

African and Asian camel ancestors are presumed to have migrated across the land bridge from North America to Asia, where they became adapted to desert conditions, while llama and alpaca ancestors migrated south to South America. Llamas and alpacas are thought to be descended from their wild relatives, the guanaco and vicuña, respectively. These animals adapted to the high altitudes and harsh conditions of the high puna of the South American Andes. Llamas are among the longest domesticated species in the world and were first used primarily as pack animals, while alpacas were raised for their finer fleece quality. They were first brought to North America in the late 1800s but were kept mainly in zoos and private collections until the 1970s.

Today they are increasing in popularity as companion and farm animals in the United States. According to U.S. Department of Agriculture livestock census data, between 2007 and 2012 the number of alpacas in the United States increased from 121,904 to 140,601, although the numbers of llamas in the United States decreased from 122,880 to 76,086 in the same time period. Alpacas commanded an exorbitant price at the height of their popularity, but prices have declined considerably; females sold for up to $70,000 in 2005 versus $1000 in 2014, and males brought up to $30,000 in 2005 and as little as $200 in 2014. Domesticated South American camelids are used for food, fiber, packing (Fig. 38.1), agility (Fig. 38.2), showing, as pets, and as projects for Scouts or 4-H groups, and llamas are also used as guard animals for sheep and other smaller livestock. The life span of llamas and alpacas is about 20 to 25 years.

South American camelids are most similar to ruminants among domestic animals, being herbivorous and having a three-chambered stomach. Camelids chew and regurgitate food during a normal gastric cycle. However, they are not small ruminants, as they have sometimes been characterized in the past.

SIZE AND CONFORMATION

Alpacas weigh between 120 and 200 pounds and stand 30 to 38 inches at the withers. Fig. 38.3 shows alpacas with a handler. The llama was developed into a pack animal in addition to its use for food and fiber and is the largest of the South American camelids, roughly twice the size of alpacas. Adult llamas weigh between 250 and 550 pounds and stand 40 to 47 inches at the withers.

[1] Fowler ME: Medicine and surgery of camelids, 3rd ed, Ames, IA, 2010, Wiley-Blackwell; Cebra C, Anderson DE, Tibary A, et al: Llama and alpaca care: medicine, surgery, reproduction, nutrition, and herd health, St. Louis, 2014, Elsevier; and Anderson DE, Jones, ML, Miesner MD: Veterinary techniques for llamas and alpacas, Ames, IA, 2013, Wiley-Blackwell.

There are no breed standards for conformation of camelids, but general principles of balance and symmetry as applied to other livestock will work well in evaluating llamas and alpacas. The large amount of fleece can obscure details about body condition and conformation, however, as can be seen in Fig. 38.4, comparing unshorn and shorn alpacas.

In llamas, the fiber rarely extends distal to the carpus or tarsus, while it does extend onto the distal leg in the alpaca. Llamas have more variety of coat colors than do alpacas and tend to have a longer face that is not covered by fiber, whereas alpacas have a short face that typically is covered by fiber (Fig. 38.5). Alpaca ears are shorter and more rounded, while llamas have typically a banana-shaped ear that points inward.

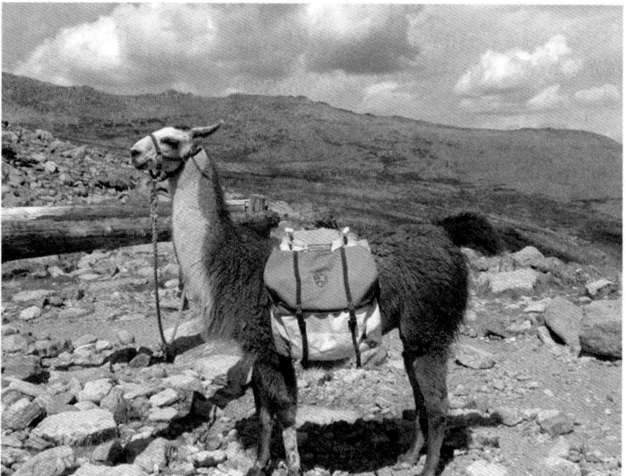

Fig. 38.1 Lloyd the llama. (Image by Richard Masoner; unmodified from original. Available at: https://commons.wikimedia.org/w/index.php?curid=3131886. This work is licensed under the Creative Commons Attribution-Share Alike 2.0 Generic license.)

Fig. 38.6 is a comparison of the general conformation of adult and newborn llamas and alpacas. The distribution of weight in camelids is 63% on the forelimbs and 37% on the pelvic limbs. The legs of the llama are longer than those of the alpaca, the topline is relatively straight, and the rump squarer than in the alpaca. Alpacas tend to have a slightly sickle-hocked conformation, and the pelvic structure is rotated under relative to that of the llama, giving them a "camped under" stance. The pastern is nearly vertical in the alpaca, and it is more sloped in the llama.

Camelids have a tendency to "toe out" in the forelimb. In general, however, evaluation of conformation of the trunk and limbs is similar to principles used for the horse. Llamas and alpacas should have straight legs when viewed from either the front or back; a line from the point of the shoulder should bisect the forelimb. The stance of the foot differs markedly from that of other domestic quadrupeds, in that the middle and distal phalanges are normally parallel to the ground in the camelid. For a more detailed description of the normal and abnormal conformation of the South American camelids, the reader is referred to *Medicine and Surgery of Camelids,* by Fowler. Angular limb deformities, especially of the carpus, occur in camelids as they do in horses. In evaluating neonatal animals, it should be noted that many animals will outgrow conformation faults such as tendon laxity if given a few weeks.

The usual gait of llamas and alpacas is a slightly broken pace. Other gaits include the walk, trot, pace, gallop, and "pronk" or "prong" (a springing hop).

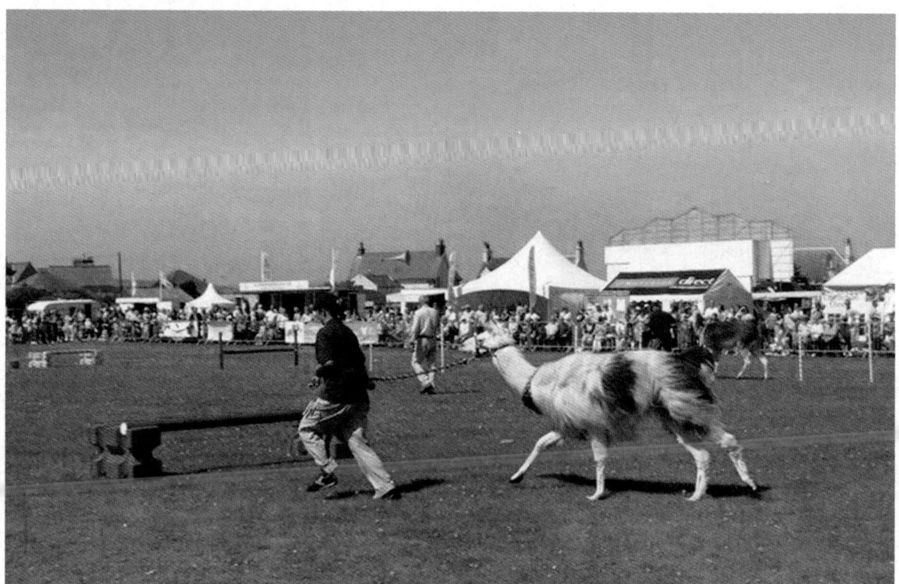

Fig. 38.2 Llama agility class, Blackrock Llama Agility Display Team. (Image by Andy Farrington; modified from original [cropped]. Available at: http://www.geograph.org.uk/reuse.php?id=2525996 This work is licensed under the Creative Commons Attribution-Share Alike 2.0 Generic license.)

EXTERNAL FEATURES AND INTEGUMENT

Alpacas come in two varieties with different fleece types. Huacaya alpacas have a short fiber (giving them a teddy bear appearance), which is in contrast to the long crimped dreadlock-like fibers of the Suri variety.

The skin thickness of the camelid varies, with the skin of the neck being very thick in both intact and late-castrated male alpacas and llamas. This increases the difficulty of venipuncture in the neck. The thickest skin is found on the lateral and dorsal sides of the neck and the dorsal thorax. Camelids develop a large callus over the sternum, and also develop calluses over the carpus and stifle, as a result of sternal recumbency being the preferred resting position. The skin is the thinnest in the concave surface of the pinnae, perineal region, axillae, and caudal ventral abdomen. Fiber density also varies on the body, with relatively sparse fiber in the perineal, sternal, ventral, axillary, and inguinal areas, making these areas convenient to observe the skin. The coat can also be parted to observe the character of the skin. Some llamas may shed from the neck and shoulder region twice yearly.

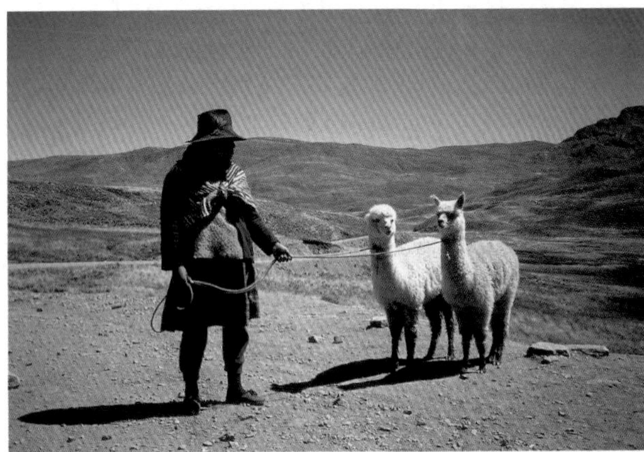

Fig. 38.3 Andean woman with alpacas in Huascarán National Park (Perù). (Image by Jaxxon; unmodified from original. Available at: https://commons.wikimedia.org/wiki/File:Andean_woman_with_alpaca.jpg. This work is licensed under the Creative Commons Attribution-Share Alike 3.0 Unported, 2.5 Generic, 2.0 Generic and 1.0 Generic license.)

Camelid Skin: The relatively hairless axilla and inguinal regions are important for dissipation of heat because these areas contain the highest concentrations of sweat glands and also high concentrations of blood vessels. Camelids often rest in sternal recumbency with the hocks elevated behind them for air circulation over these areas for cooling. The preferred place for intradermal tuberculin skin testing is in the axillary region.

Llamas have the normal sebaceous glands and sweat glands seen in other species, but the sebaceous glands are less active than those of sheep, and the fleece is not

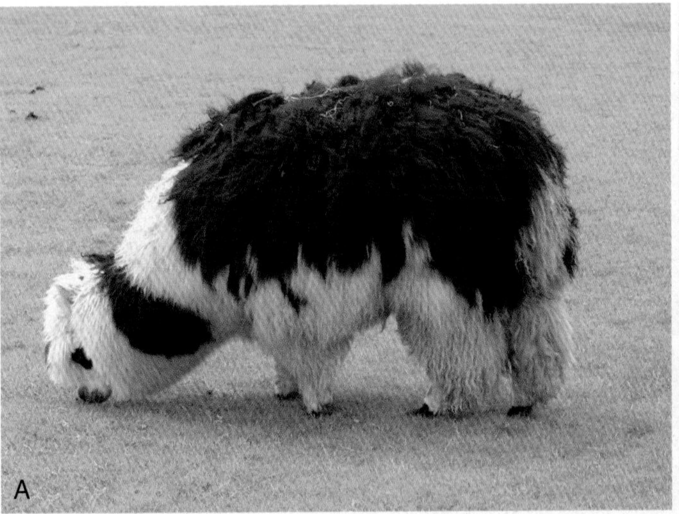

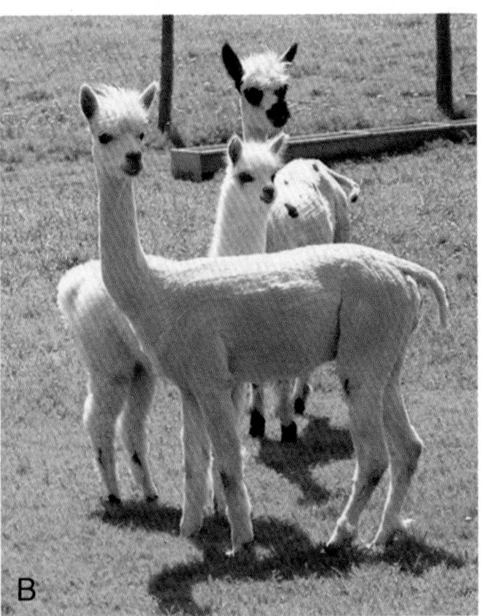

Fig. 38.4 (A) Unshorn alpaca. (B) Shorn alpaca. (A, Image by Johann Dréo, Wikimedia Commons. Unmodified from original. Available at: https://en.wikipedia.org/wiki/File:Unshorn_alpaca_grazing.jpg. This work is licensed under the Creative Commons Attribution-Share Alike 2.0 Generic license. B, Alpaca at Little Durnford Manor, by Trish Steel; modified from original [cropped]. Available at: https://commons.wikimedia.org/wiki/File:Alpaca_-_geograph.org.uk_-_511843.jpg. This work is licensed under the Creative Commons Attribution-Share Alike 2.0 Generic license.)

as oily. Llamas also lack modified sebaceous glands found in other species, in specialized areas such as the perianal region, prepuce, glans penis, vulva, anus, and eyelid. The sebaceous glands that are present have non-keratinized ducts, in contrast to most species. South American camelids appear to have a concentration of sweat glands similar to those of other species, whereas camels are reported to have fewer sweat glands to help prevent water loss. A study of the microanatomy of healthy alpaca skin found it to be very similar to that of the llama.

Oblong skin thickenings are located on the dorsolateral and dorsomedial aspect of each metatarsal region, referred to as metatarsal glands (*arrows* in Figs. 38.6B and D). Some authors believe them to be associated with pheromone release as an alarm mechanism, but their histologic structure is very similar to that of the eccrine sweat glands found in the llama and carnivore foot pad, and the overlying epidermis is very similar to that of the equine chestnut. Both of these ultrastructural aspects would argue for the metatarsal glands being vestigial digits. They are most easily seen on animals with light-colored legs and actually contain very little glandular tissue. There are also interdigital glands in the dorsal interdigital space. Histologically, the glands seen in the metatarsal glands, the interdigital glands, and the glands of the footpad all resemble eccrine sweat glands.

Whereas other domestic animals usually have either simple or compound hair follicles, llamas have both simple and compound hair follicles. Another peculiarity of the llama skin is the presence of vascular plexuses similar to ones described in guanacos and alpacas and thought to be involved in thermoregulation or water conservation.

SKULL

The skulls of the llama and the alpaca are compared in Fig. 38.7. The skull of camelids is similar to that of a small ruminant, with a few distinct features. The nasal bone of camelids is shortened compared to other species, and it is shorter in the alpaca than in the llama. The relatively short nasal bone has implications for handling and restraint, as discussed later. The bony orbit is complete, with a prominent palpable notch on the dorsomedial orbit margin in the llama. Llamas and alpacas have an opening rostral to the orbit that is similar to an opening found in cervids, and variously referred to as the rostral foramen, rostral fenestra, prelacrimal vacuity, lacrimal vacuity, lacrimal fenestra, antorbital vacuity, or ethmoidal vacuity (Fig. 38.7). This foramen is reported to be absent in the vicuña, and it is absent in the camel as well. The function of this foramen is unknown. Although one source speculated that this is associated with a scent gland, species with scent glands in this location, such as the deer and sheep, have a lacrimal fossa rostroventral to the orbit to house the scent gland, which the camelids do not have.

There is no facial tuberosity, and the facial crest is inconspicuous. The tympanic bulla is flattened in the rostrocaudal plane and extends ventrally to the level of the occipital condyles. Other features are typical of other herbivores and are unremarkable.

The mandible has a reduced angular process, a very rounded angle, and a tall and narrow coronoid process but is otherwise typical of herbivores. The rami of the mandibles are narrowly spaced. The mental foramen is slightly caudal to the mandibular canine tooth.

The frontal and maxillary paranasal sinuses of a llama are outlined in Fig. 38.8. The maxillary sinus is associated with the roots of the upper cheek teeth, as is common in most species.

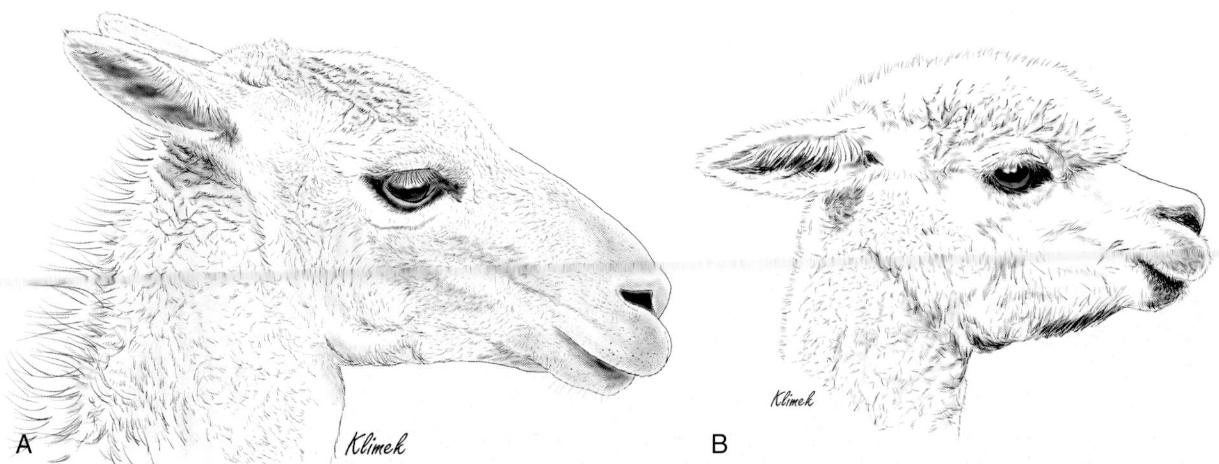

Fig. 38.5 Face structure of (A) llama and (B) alpaca. Llamas have a longer and less hairy face than do alpacas.

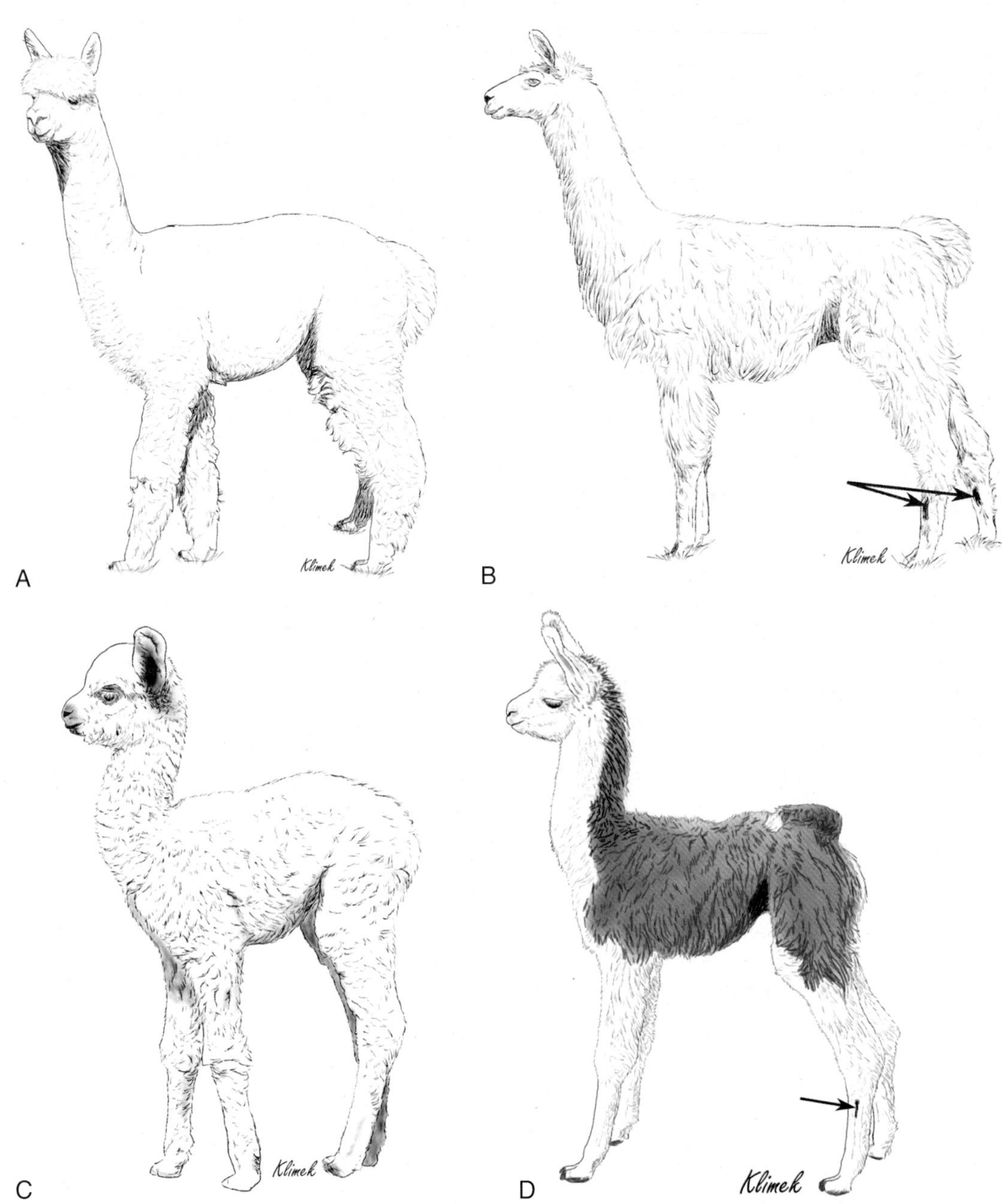

Fig. 38.6 Adult and juvenile South American camelids. (A) Adult alpaca. (B) Adult llama. (C) Alpaca cria. (D) Llama cria. *Arrows* in B and D indicate the position of the metatarsal glands. In addition to the larger size of llamas, they have a straighter topline than do alpacas. Alpacas tend to stand with pelvic limbs more tucked under the pelvis.

EXTERNAL AND SUPERFICIAL FEATURES OF THE HEAD

The upper lip of the llama and alpaca should protrude slightly. It is split in a manner similar to that of small ruminants, which improves prehension. The nostrils do not have rigid support because the nasal bones are relatively short, and there are no alar cartilages. Camels can in fact completely close their nostrils with muscle contraction to protect against blowing sand (Fig. 38.9), but llamas and alpacas lack this ability.

Specific information about superficial structures of the head is very limited in the literature. The muscles of facial expression are assumed to follow the typical mammalian pattern. The facial nerve is superficial and vulnerable. Camelids have salivary glands typical of other species. The parotid, mandibular, and sublingual salivary glands are the

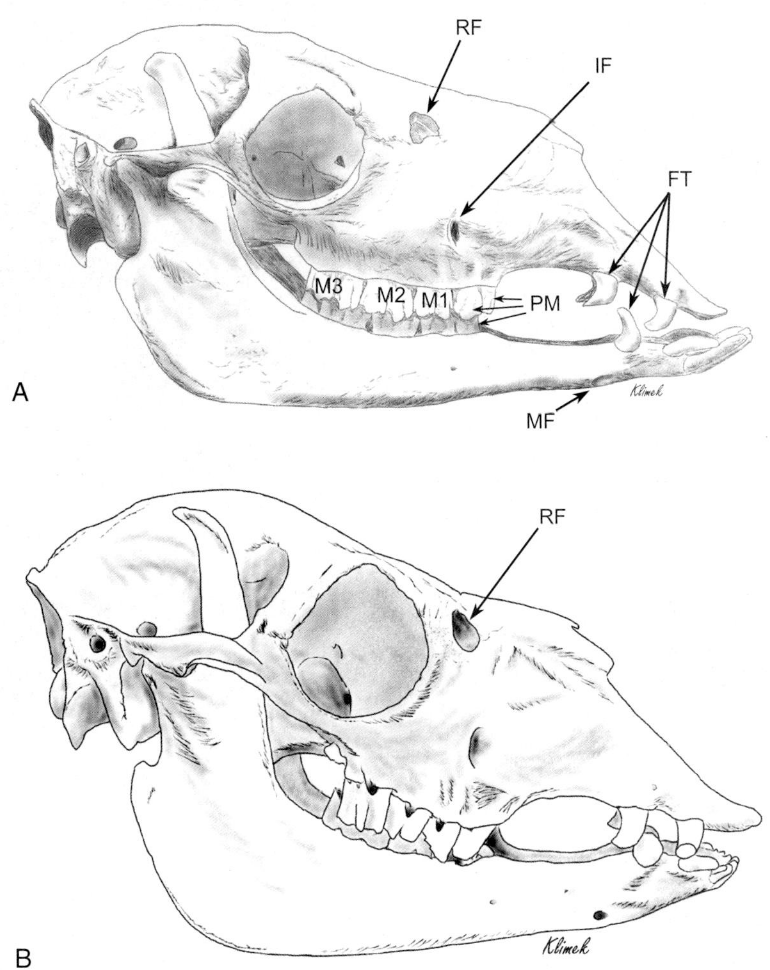

Fig. 38.7 (A) Llama skull. (B) Alpaca skull. *FT,* "Fighting teeth"; *IF,* infraorbital foramen; *M1* to *M3,* molars 1 to 3; *MF,* mental foramen; *PM,* premolars; *RF,* "rostral foramen." Premolars in the upper arcade are rostral to the infraorbital foramen and are smaller than the molars. Molars increase in size from rostral to caudal.

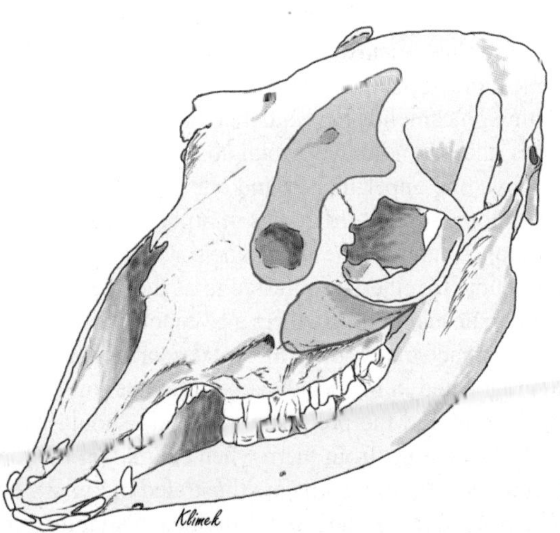

Fig. 38.8 Llama skull with frontal (upper) and maxillary (lower) sinuses shaded in *blue.*

major glands, and they also have minor salivary glands in the oral cavity. The parotid duct also runs across the surface of the masseter, 1 to 1.5 cm dorsal to the facial vein, and opens opposite the rostral end of the upper first molar. Lymph nodes are generally not palpable.

Oral Cavity

The mouth is long and narrow, and it does not open widely. The tongue is not as mobile as other large animals and usually does not extend beyond the lips, so it is not used for prehension of food. The rostral two-thirds of the tongue is about 2 cm thick in the llama. The tongue has a prominent dome-shaped projection in the root that is 5 cm in depth, similar to the torus linguae of ruminants. There are several kinds of mechanical and gustatory papillae on the tongue and buccal mucosa. Foliate papillae are lacking, and the vallate papillae are large and oval in shape.

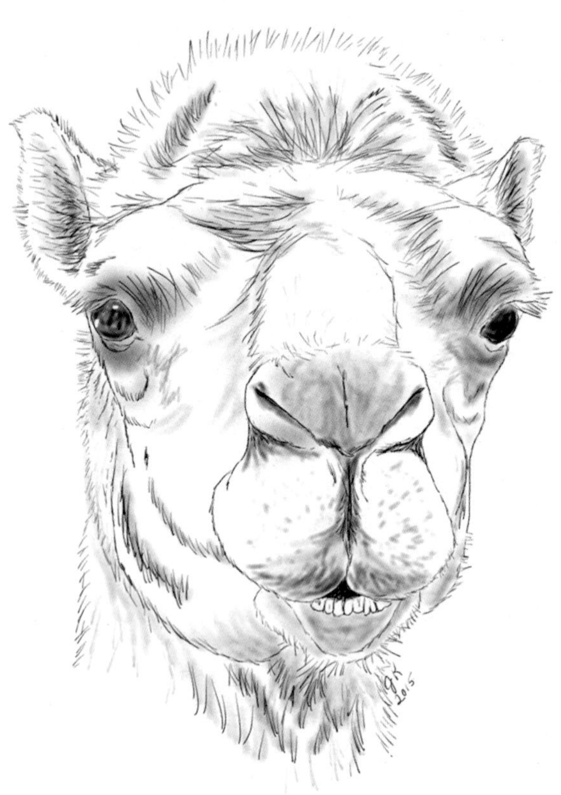

Fig. 38.9 Camels have the ability to completely close the nostril via muscular depression of the alae of the nostril, whereas llamas and alpacas lack this ability.

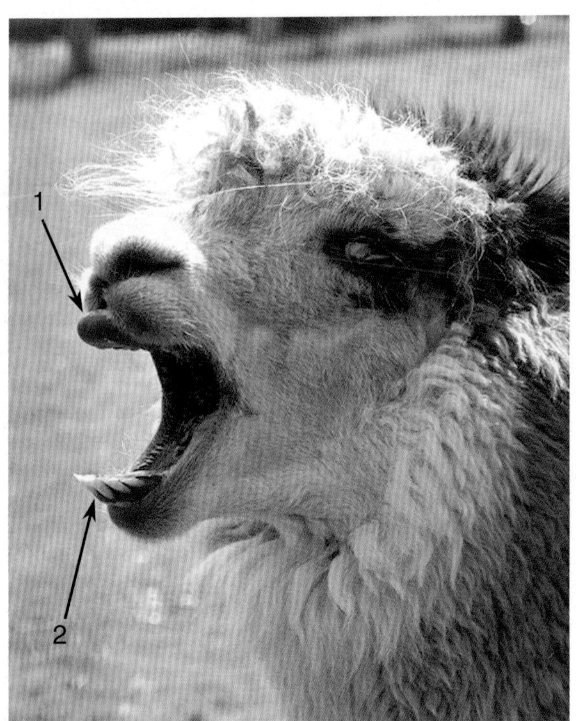

Fig. 38.10 Alpaca. *1,* Dental pad; *2,* lower incisors. (Image by Arbutus Photography. Available at: https://www.flickr.com/photos/arbutusridge/8672528601/in/pool-1087584@n20. This work is licensed under the Creative Commons Attribution-Share Alike 2.0 Generic license.)

The dentition of camelids is complex compared to ruminants and horses, and dental disease is common in llamas and alpacas. Similar to ruminants, camelids have a dental pad, shown in Fig. 38.10, and a reduced number of upper incisors. The deciduous dental formula of llamas and alpacas (incisors, canine, premolars) is:

$$\frac{1-1-2(3)}{3-1-1(2)}$$

Note that one source indicates there may be 1 or 2 upper deciduous incisors. The permanent dental formula (incisors, canine, premolars, molars) is:

$$\frac{1-1-1(2)-3}{3-1-1(2)-3}$$

Fig. 38.7A is an illustration of an individual with two upper premolars and one lower premolar. Eruption dates are discussed later.

Deciduous incisors of both llamas and alpacas are spatula shaped. They are slightly smaller than permanent incisors and have a chalky color; permanent incisors are more translucent.

Fig. 38.11 is a schematic illustration of the radiographic appearance of llama and alpaca permanent incisors, demonstrating some differences in their shape. Llama permanent incisors are spatula shaped with tapered roots, do not grow continuously, and have enamel over the entire crown. Alpaca permanent incisors are long and narrow and rectangular in cross section and erupt throughout life. The occlusal surface of the alpaca incisor is chisel shaped. Although alpacas have been reported to lack enamel on the lingual surface of the permanent incisors, similar to the vicuña, one histologic study demonstrated that there is enamel on both surfaces of the alpaca incisor. The tips of the incisors should meet the dental pad; incisors are oriented somewhat vertically early in life and become more horizontally oriented as the animal ages.

Although camelids have a dental pad opposing the lower incisors, they do not have a total absence of upper incisors. They have one upper incisor and one upper canine on each side, and the upper incisor is morphologically identical to the upper canine. The upper incisor and canine and the lower canine together are referred to as the "fighting teeth," because male camelids use them as weapons. They are much larger in intact males than in females or geldings. These teeth are located in the diastema between the lower incisors or dental pad and the premolars, and care should be taken to avoid lacerations from them when examining the mouth. The fighting teeth of a llama are illustrated in Fig. 38.7A.

There is some gender and individual variability in the deciduous and permanent premolars, and premolars can be difficult to tell apart from molars, but premolars are much smaller than molars when present. The premolars on the upper

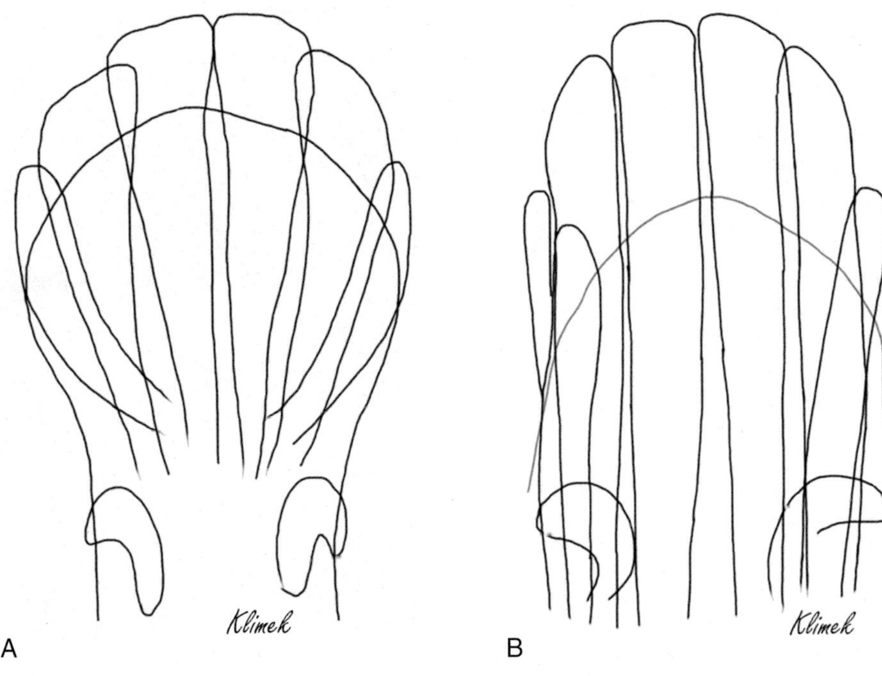

Fig. 38.11 Schematic illustration of the permanent lower incisors of the llama (A) and alpaca (B), as viewed on ventrodorsal intraoral radiographs. Alpaca incisors have straight, parallel outlines, whereas llama incisors taper at the roots.

arcade are rostral to the infraorbital foramen. The deciduous upper premolars 3 and 4 are usually present, but deciduous upper premolar 2 is present in only 65% of males and 45% of females. Deciduous lower premolar 4 is consistent; lower premolar 3 is present in 91% of males and 82% of females.

The lower permanent premolar 3 is absent in the male and sometimes present in the female (15%). The upper permanent premolar 3 is consistently present in males and usually present in females. There are consistently three upper and three lower permanent molars in all individuals. Fig. 38.7A shows permanent premolars and molars in a llama. Molars increase in size from rostral to caudal.

The form of the cheek teeth is similar to that of cattle and horses. Although camelid cheek teeth do not erupt throughout life, they are subject to wear, and new bone formation below the teeth does force them out gradually to compensate for this wear.

Cheek Teeth of Camelids: The upper arcade is wider than the lower arcade, and the upper cheek teeth themselves are wider than the lower cheek teeth. Thus, similar to the cheek teeth of horses, the premolars and molars of camelids develop normal points on the labial side of the upper teeth and the lingual side of the lower teeth. These should not be floated in the camelid, however, in the absence of any evidence of trauma resulting from the points or in the absence of abnormal mastication.

Upper premolars have three roots, and upper molars have four roots. The lower cheek teeth all have two roots, but in the last lower molar the caudal root is a fusion of two roots.

It is challenging to observe the teeth of camelids because of the restriction to opening the mouth widely and the long and narrow oral cavity. Cheek teeth can be observed with the use of a speculum or mouth gag. The cheek teeth may also be palpated through the cheek tissue. In one study of tooth eruption in [illegible] alpacas, alpaca-vicuña crosses, and llamas of known ages, the investigator found very little variation between llamas and alpacas, so alpacas and llamas can be assumed to follow the same pattern of eruption.

At birth in full-term crias (the term describing neonatal camelids), all of the deciduous mandibular incisors are erupted. The deciduous fighting teeth are present in all animals but often not erupted. It is possible to estimate the age of the animal by eruption of the incisors up to about age 5; beyond that it is difficult. Permanent incisors erupt caudal to the deciduous incisors, at ages 2 to 2.5 years for incisor 1, 3 to 3.25 years for incisor 2, and 3 and 6 years for incisor 3. Retained deciduous incisors can occur and may need to be removed.

The first two permanent molars can be a reliable estimate of age; the lower molar 1 erupts at age 6 to 9 months; the lower molar 2 erupts between 17 and 24 months of age. The lower molar 3 can erupt anywhere between 2 years 9 months and 3 years 8 months.

Trimming Camelid Teeth: Some of the teeth may require trimming. Lower incisors should meet the tip of the dental pad. If these teeth do not meet the dental pad properly they can become overgrown and will need to be trimmed to restore appropriate function; Fig. 38.12 shows an alpaca with incisor teeth that are overgrown. There are various methods to accomplish trimming, but care should be taken with power tools to avoid overheating or cracking the tooth. The fighting teeth, if present, need to be trimmed to prevent injury to herd mates and handlers. The teeth should be trimmed annually during their active growth period, generally between ages 3 and 8. They can be trimmed to 2 to 4 mm from the gum line to avoid damage to the gums or formation of a recess where food can accumulate. The use of cutters for these teeth is not advised because of the possibility of fracture of the tooth. In addition, the mandibular canine is immediately adjacent to the mental foramen and to the root of the third incisor, and care must be taken to protect these structures.

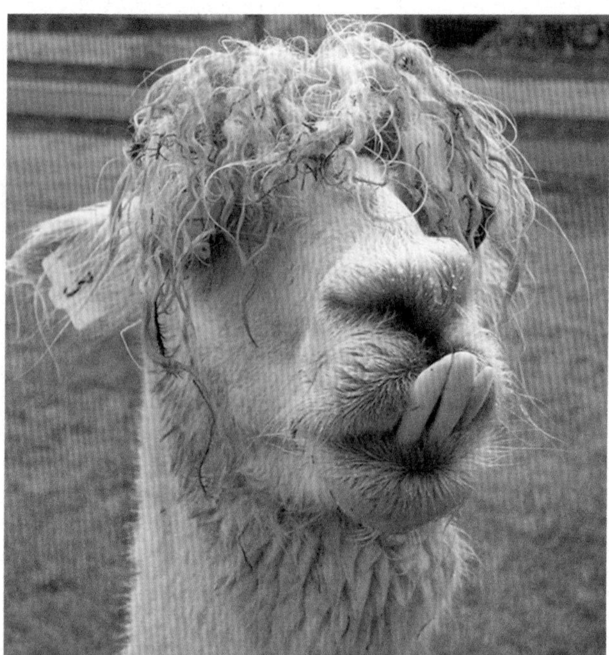

Fig. 38.12 Mucho the alpaca, demonstrating teeth that are overgrown as a result of malocclusion. (Unmodified from original. Available at: https://www.flickr.com/photos/justinlindsay/91878991. This work is licensed under the Creative Commons Attribution-Share Alike 2.0 Generic license.)

Camelids have a high incidence of tooth root abscesses, especially on the lower arcade, and especially between the ages of 4 and 8 years. When examining the head, the jaws and the lymph nodes should be examined for swellings. The upper cheek teeth roots can be accessed, and the teeth repulsed, if necessary, through the maxillary sinus, dorsal to the facial crest, and ventral to a line drawn from the medial canthus to the infraorbital foramen. One should be aware that the infraorbital canal is in this area and lies between the medial and lateral roots of the molars. Because its roots are ventral to the orbit, the last upper molar is not accessible unless approached through the zygomatic bone, after reflecting the masseter muscle from the facial crest.

Nerve blocks for the teeth similar to those used for ruminants can be used for anesthesia of teeth that can be removed orally under sedation. The infraorbital nerve can be blocked through the infraorbital foramen, which is palpable dorsal to the premolars. The mental nerve can be blocked at its termination by inserting the needle into the mental foramen, located just caudal to the lower canine tooth (or 2–3 cm caudal to the incisors). Alternately, the inferior alveolar nerve can be blocked as it enters the mandibular foramen on the medial side of the ramus of the mandible. This foramen is located rostral and dorsal to the ventral curvature of the ramus of the mandible.

The locations of foramina associated with nerve blocks for the teeth are illustrated in Fig. 38.13.

Ear

The external ear canal has a vertical and a horizontal portion. On the medial side of the pinna there is a conchal eminence that may interfere with advancing an otoscope into the vertical ear canal. The vertical portion continues to the external opening of the osseous ear canal, with the beginning of the turn to the horizontal portion immediately before reaching the opening. The horizontal portion of the ear canal is narrow and surrounded by the petrous temporal bone. To further complicate viewing the deepest part of the osseous horizontal ear canal using standard otoscopic equipment, the canal is very narrow and makes a medial and ventral turn before reaching the tympanic membrane. To visualize the deepest part of the external ear canal, flexible equipment may be necessary. The position of the external acoustic meatus, and its relationship to the tympanic bulla, is shown in Fig. 38.14.

Upper Airway

The soft palate is relatively long in the camelid. Llamas, alpacas, and Bactrian camels lack the dulaa (the diverticulum of the soft palate) present in dromedary camels. Camelids are obligate (or nearly obligate) nasal breathers because of the relatively long length of the soft palate and the arrangement of the intrapharyngeal ostium to the glottis in a manner similar to horses. The caudal end of the

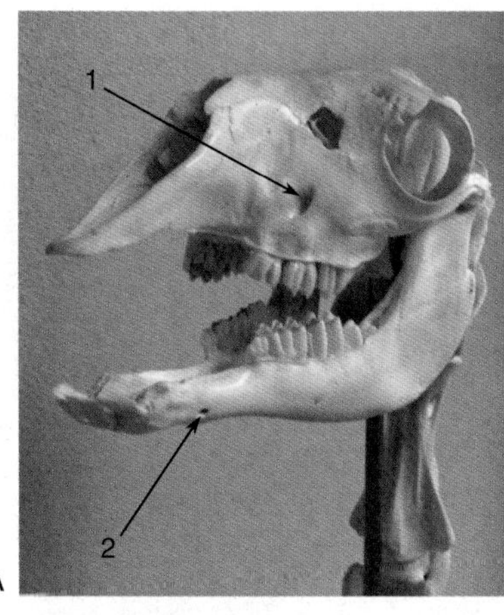

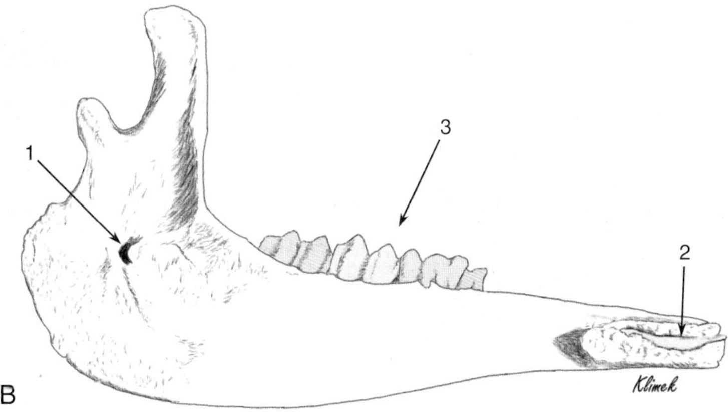

Fig. 38.13 (A) Rostrolateral view of a llama skull. *1,* Infraorbital foramen; *2,* mental foramen. (B) Medial view of a llama mandible. *1,* Mandibular foramen; *2,* incisor tooth; *3,* one premolar and three molars (color added for contrast of individual teeth).

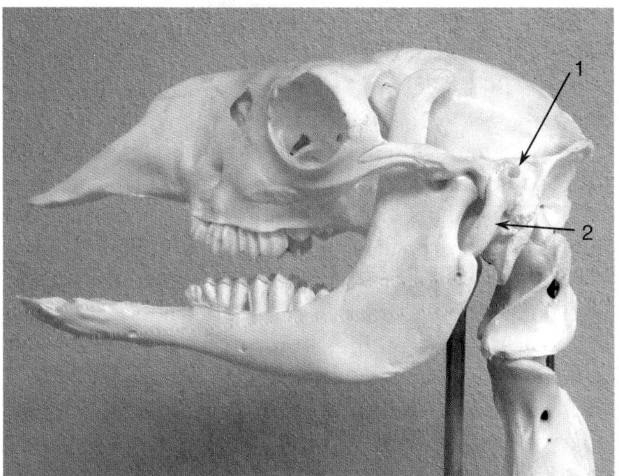

Fig. 38.14 Llama skull. *1,* External acoustic meatus; *2,* tympanic bulla.

soft palate is usually ventral to the epiglottis. The nasal cavity also has less rigid support than most other species, because the nasal septum is mainly cartilaginous and the nasal bones do not extend as far rostrally.

Fitting a Halter: The less rigid support of the nasal cavity is important to remember when restraining the animal and when fitting a halter because pressure on the top of the nose can easily collapse and block the nasal passage, causing discomfort and distress to the animal and possibly making handling more difficult. For this reason, the nosepiece of the halter must fit close to the eyes and must not be allowed to slip forward. This also needs to be balanced against the need to allow movement of the jaws for mastication, so there must be slack in the nosepiece. Fig. 38.15 illustrates an appropriately fitted halter.

About 8 cm caudal to the nares, the nasal septum ends, and a common meatus is formed. This allows observation of the caudal portion of the entire nasal cavity via an endoscope passed through the ventral nasal meatus on either side. The anatomy of the larynx is typical, although the larynx is relatively narrow.

Endotracheal, Orotracheal, and Nasotracheal Intubation: The anatomy of the oral cavity and oropharynx complicates endotracheal intubation for inhalation anesthesia. Visualization of the glottis for orotracheal intubation is difficult or impossible without the use of a laryngoscope. Nasotracheal intubation is possible, especially when access to the oral cavity is necessary during anesthesia, but llamas and alpacas have a pharyngeal diverticulum that must be avoided if this method is chosen. The opening is approximately 1 cm in diameter and the diverticulum extends caudally for approximately 2 cm between the longus capitis muscles. In adult llamas, when the tube is passed in the ventral meatus, the ethmoid conchae are about 10 cm from the nares and may be contacted by the tube. The pharyngeal diverticulum is about 25 cm from the nares and can also prevent further passage if it is entered. Camelids are at risk of dorsal displacement of the soft palate following extubation from the orotracheal route because of relaxation of the pharynx after the tube is removed.

Eye

Camelids have eyes almost as large as horses and cattle, despite having a proportionately smaller head, and eye injuries are common because of the prominent and protruding eyes. Very little of the sclera is visible in a normal camelid, and what can be seen is often highly pigmented. Camelids have long eyelashes, and they lack meibomian

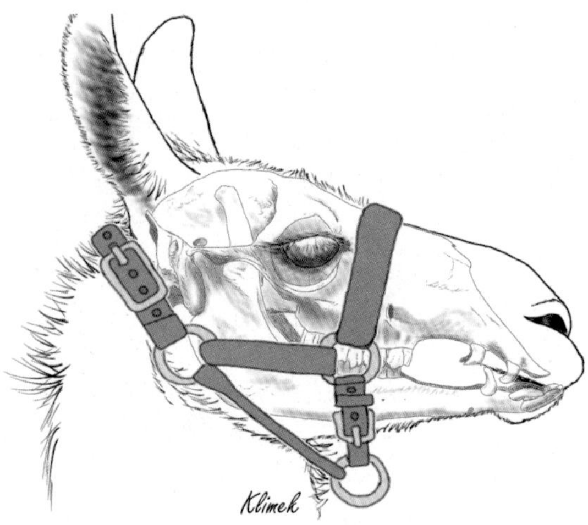

Fig. 38.15 Semi-schematic illustration of llama head with properly fitted halter. The noseband should fit very close to the eye to avoid compressing the nose.

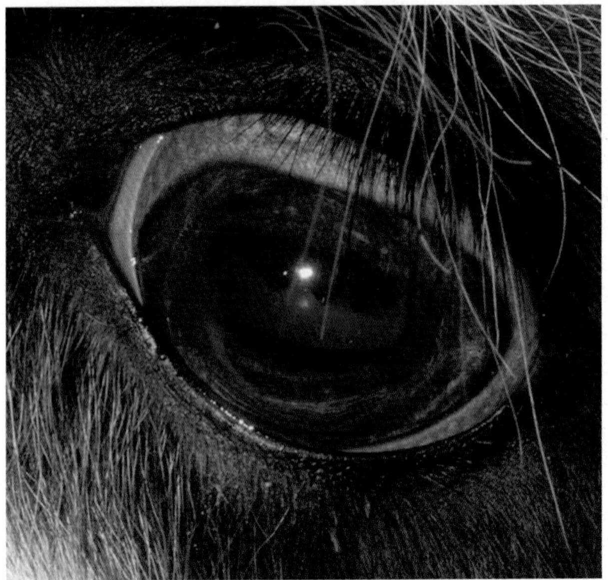

Fig. 38.16 The normal appearance of the globe and adnexa of an alpaca eye. The cornea and pupil are oblong in a horizontal plane, and the pupillary margins contain prominent iridal folds that are larger on the upper margin. The bulbar conjunctiva is usually pigmented, as in this individual. (From Cebra C, Anderson DE, Tibary A, et al: Llama and alpaca care: medicine, surgery, reproduction, nutrition, and herd health, St. Louis, 2014, Elsevier, Fig. 38.11.)

glands within the eyelids. They do, however, have sebaceous glands on the nictitating membrane and the caruncle of the eye. The lacrimal caruncle normally has hair. Fig. 38.16 illustrates features of the normal llama eye.

The lacrimal glands are in the typical location and are about 31 mm × 0.9 mm × 0.5 mm in size. The superficial gland of the third eyelid is also in a typical position. It surrounds the crossbar portion of the cartilage of the third eyelid,

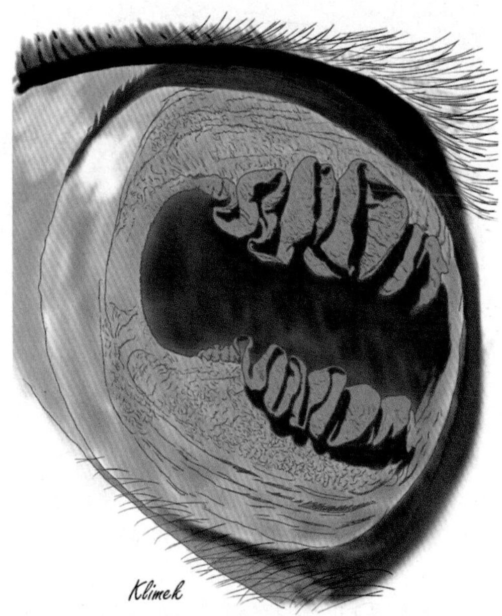

Fig. 38.17 Illustration of the iris of a llama showing the folded corpora nigra.

and it is 25 mm × 1.6 mm × 0.8 mm in size, on the ventral aspect of the orbit. The lacrimal glands and superficial glands of the third eyelid are seromucous, and there are numerous lymphoid nodules on the bulbar surface of the third eyelid.

Camelid eyes have structures analogous to the corpora nigra on the pupillary margin of cattle and horses. In llamas and alpacas, these proliferations of the iridic pigmented epithelium are elaborately folded vertically and are called *pupillary ruffs, iridic granules,* or *corpora nigra.* They are larger and very prominent on the upper pupillary margin, and the folds interdigitate with each other when the pupil is constricted. Fig. 38.17 is a drawing illustrating these folds on the pupillary margin.

The pigmentation of the iris varies with coat color. Animals with dark coats tend to have a brown iris, and those with light coats have combinations of gray, blue, and brown iris pigmentation. There is no tapetum lucidum or fovea, but the fundus is reflective, and the pigmentation of the fundus also varies with coat color, from nonpigmented to red-brown to brown, with dark-coated animals having heavier pigmentation. The vascular pattern normally has three to five pairs of prominent vessels originating at the optic disk.

Characteristics of the Alpaca Eyes: There are several characteristics of the eyes with which practitioners should be familiar, based on a study of alpaca eyes. The eyes of the neonate may have visible hyaloid arteries coming from the area of the optic disk and coursing toward the lens, and remnants of these are sometimes visible in older animals. As in other species, there is an association among white coat, blue eyes, and deafness, although deafness does not occur in all animals with a white coat and blue eyes. Finally, out of the 50 animals in the study, only one had a clear lens with no opacities of any kind; the most common finding was a ring or rings of opacity in the lens. Three animals with large focal dense opacities had no indication of visual deficits; thus lens opacities may be an incidental finding in the alpaca. However, this frequency of lens opacities was not noted in another study of 29 alpacas; in this study 2 animals had focal incipient primary cataracts. The eyelids may exhibit a slight ectropion when the animal is excited.

The nasolacrimal duct system follows the usual pattern. The lacrimal puncta are easily visible about 5 to 7 mm from the medial canthus and accessible to cannulate. The nasal opening of the nasolacrimal duct is laterally placed in the ventrocaudal aspect of the vestibule, about 1.5 to 2 cm proximal to the wing of the nostril, near the mucocutaneous junction.

NECK AND TRUNK

Fig. 38.18 shows the skeleton of a llama. The vertebral formula of the llama and alpaca (cervical, thoracic, lumbar, sacral, and caudal) is $C_7T_{12}L_7S_5Cd_{10-15}$. The neck is long and very flexible in all directions and has sparse musculature and prominent cervical vertebrae. The normal neck carriage is vertical in the llama and about a 70-degree angle in the alpaca.

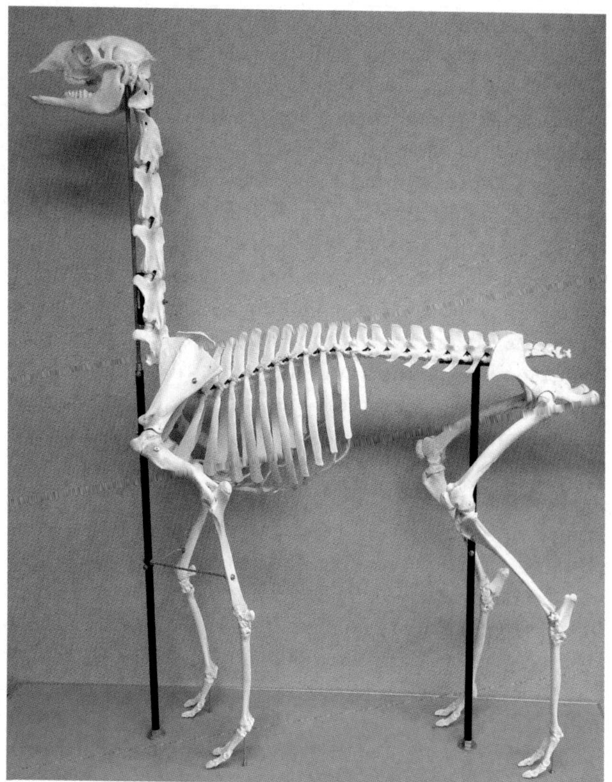

Fig. 38.18 Llama skeleton.

The length and flexibility of the neck, along with the relative lack of supporting musculature, make cervical subluxations and fractures more common in camelids. In fact, bone tissue in general in camelids is relatively thin and easily fractured.

No description of the nuchal ligament is available for the llama or alpaca. The nuchal ligament is illustrated in one source as only consisting of the funicular part, similar to the nuchal ligament of the dog; however, the camel has both funicular and laminar parts of the nuchal ligament.

Fig. 38.19 shows the skull and cervical vertebrae of a llama. In the cervical region the bodies of the vertebrae are relatively long with the exception of C1 and C7, and the dorsal spinous processes are much reduced compared to other species. Cervical vertebrae 3 through 7 have downward-projecting transverse processes that protect structures in the visceral space of the neck. These are very well developed cranially and caudally on the sixth cervical vertebra and are easily identified on a radiograph.

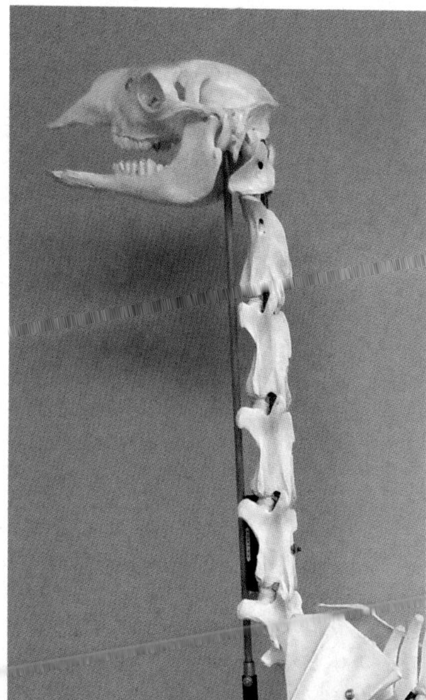

Fig. 38.19 Llama skull and cervical vertebrae. Llamas carry their head and neck in a nearly vertical orientation.

The cervical vertebrae of camelids lack transverse foramina. The vertebral artery in the llama, and presumably in the alpaca as well, travels mostly within the vertebral canal, passing through osseous canals within the cranial portion of the vertebral canals of the second through the sixth cervical vertebrae. According to one source, the seventh cervical vertebra may or may not have a transverse foramen. The authors could find no information on the vertebral nerve in llamas and alpacas, but in the camel this nerve is inside this osseous channel; presumably it is in the same location in llamas and alpacas. This could have implications for the location of the communicating branches that normally leave the vertebral nerve to join the cervical spinal nerves.

There are some interesting differences from the usual mammalian pattern with some of the nerves of the neck in llamas and alpacas. Both the recurrent laryngeal nerve and the external branches of the accessory nerve have been reported to be lacking in the alpaca. In one study the recurrent laryngeal nerve was absent, with both branches of the vagus to the extrinsic muscles of the larynx arising from the vagus nerve just outside the jugular foramen. In addition, the trapezius was innervated by branches of cervical nerves in the absence of the cervical branch of the accessory nerve. The external branch of the accessory nerve has also been found to be absent in the camel and the llama. The dromedary camel has cranial and caudal laryngeal nerves that originate from the vagus near its origin but also a small recurrent laryngeal nerve that follows the conventional route and travels cranially to the larynx to anastomose with the caudal laryngeal nerve.

The paired thyroid glands are on the dorsolateral aspect of the trachea. They are 4 cm long and 2 cm wide and extend from the cricoid cartilage to the third or fourth tracheal ring.

Jugular Venipuncture: Several features of cervical anatomy combine to make jugular venipuncture a particular challenge. There is only one jugular vein present in the llama, the internal jugular vein, and it is therefore relatively deep in the neck. The skin on the neck is up to 1 cm thick, which is a protective mechanism against fighting but makes venipuncture more challenging and, in the case of catheterization, necessitates making a small stab incision through the skin over the vein to avoid damaging the tip of the catheter. There is no jugular groove in camelids because of the sparse musculature, and the jugular vein and carotid artery are in close proximity for much of their course through the neck. The jugular vein is relatively superficial only in the cranial part of the neck near the mandible and is separated from the carotid artery by a small omohyoideus muscle for only a short distance.

The general rule for jugular venipuncture is to stay in either the rostral or the caudal third of the neck. Both the high and low locations have advantages and disadvantages. In either location, valves in the jugular vein may interfere with venipuncture. It is not always necessary to clip the fleece to locate the vein, and owners may resent the veterinarian clipping fleece because it can take 12 to 18 months to regrow. The fibers can be parted and taped out of the way to access the site for venipuncture or catheterization. The right side of the neck is preferred because a hematoma on the left side, from either jugular or carotid puncture, may compress the esophagus or cause choking.

The high jugular venipuncture location is near the ramus of the mandible, where the jugular vein is most superficial and there is more separation between it and the common carotid artery, and the skin is thinner, but landmarks are harder to palpate. To estimate the correct location for jugular venipuncture in this area, the needle is inserted dorsal to the intersection of a line drawn at the ventral border of the mandible and the tendon of the sternomandibularis muscle. The jugular vein in this location is lateral to the tendon as it inserts on the mandible but then moves dorsal, and then medial, to the tendon as it moves down the neck. Also in this location, the omohyoideus, much smaller than that in cattle or horses, is positioned deep to the jugular vein, between it and the common carotid artery. The omohyoideus only extends for a distance of about 14 cm caudal to the ramus of the mandible. There is one set of valves approximately 1 cm caudal to the origin of the jugular vein and angle of the mandible and another set 5 cm caudal to that.

As the jugular vein moves caudally in the neck, it becomes surrounded by the same fascial sheath as the common carotid artery and the vagosympathetic trunk. These structures are located between the trachea medially and the ventral projections of the transverse processes of cervical vertebrae laterally. The low position for venipuncture is medial to the ventral projections of the transverse processes of the fifth or sixth cervical vertebrae, with the advantage that here the vein is larger and landmarks are easy to palpate. The disadvantage of this location is a heavier fiber coat here and closer proximity of the carotid artery to the vein in this position. To find the jugular vein in this location, the ventral projection of the sixth cervical vertebra is located, and the thumb or fingers of the occluding hand are wrapped medial to this projection, between it and the trachea. The jugular vein should be medial to this projection. The carotid artery should be close, and pulsations may be felt. The needle is advanced slightly medial to the projection and toward the center of the neck. There may be a set of valves in this location as well.

THORAX

The ribs and the thoracic vertebrae are typical. In llamas and alpacas there are seven sternal ribs and five asternal ribs. The anatomy of the thorax with regard to auscultation and thoracic imaging is very similar to that of other species. In llamas and alpacas, the long axis of the heart in a standing animal is approximately perpendicular to the vertebrae and parallel to the ribs, and on radiographs the heart extends from about the third rib to the fifth intercostal space. The axis of the heart will be tilted more cranially in a lateral radiograph. A heart that is wider than 3 intercostal spaces or taller than three-fourths of the depth of the thorax is considered enlarged.

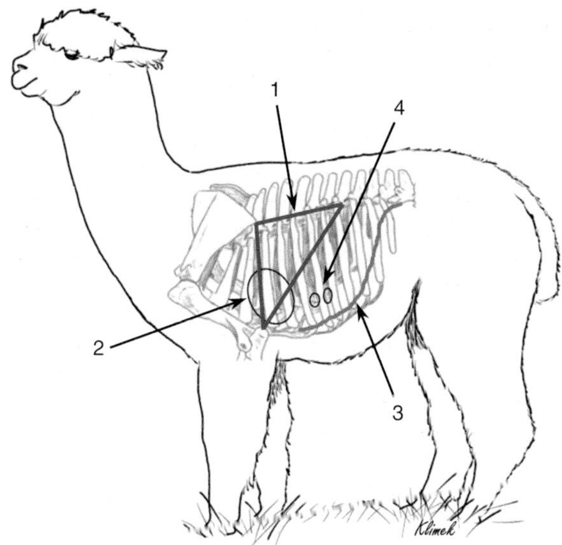

Fig. 38.20 Alpaca thorax showing auscultation landmarks (schematic). *1,* Area for auscultation of the lungs *(red triangle); 2,* position of the heart *(large black circle); 3,* diaphragmatic line of pleural reflection *(purple line); 4,* locations to obtain pleural fluid in the seventh or sixth intercostal space *(small black circles).*

The carina of the trachea is usually at the fourth rib or fourth intercostal space. The angle of the thoracic trachea with the vertebral bodies is 10 to 19 degrees in normal adult llamas and 9 to 22 degrees in normal alpaca crias. This angle may be diminished with heart enlargement.

The boundaries for auscultation of the lungs are typical: the caudal border of the triceps brachii, the lateral border of the epaxial muscles, and a line from the olecranon to the dorsal part of the eighth or ninth intercostal space. The diaphragmatic line of pleural reflections extends dorsally from caudal to the last rib, through the middle of the 11th rib, to the costochondral junction of the 10th rib, and finally follows the costal arch to about the 7th rib. These landmarks are shown schematically in Fig. 38.20.

The lungs of the camelid do not have obvious lobation. There is a tracheal bronchus similar to that found in ruminants that supplies the cranial portion of the right lung. The trachea is often focally enlarged at that point. The right lung extends farther cranially and caudally than does the left.

ABDOMINAL TOPOGRAPHY

Similar to other quadrupeds, the diaphragm extends forward to about the fifth intercostal space or sixth rib, meaning that a good portion of the abdomen is under the cover of the rib cage. Similar to the ruminant, a good portion of the left side of the abdomen is occupied by the stomach. The liver is entirely on the right side of the abdomen, deep to the diaphragm, extending from the last rib caudodorsally to the fifth or sixth rib cranioventrally. The spleen is located on the left side, caudal to the last rib. The small intestines occupy the right ventral portion of the abdomen, and the transition from ileum to colon is in a central location of the caudal abdomen, with the cecum pointing toward the pelvis. The spiral colon is in the caudal to ventrocaudal abdomen. The kidneys are relatively farther caudal than in most species, being ventral to the fourth to seventh lumbar transverse processes. The right kidney is more cranially placed than the left kidney, which is in the area of the wing of the ileum.

Laparotomy can be performed from a lateral approach on either side, or a ventral approach. The particular structure of interest dictates the specific approach; dorsal structures such as the spleen, kidneys, and duodenum are more easily accessed through a lateral approach, but most abdominal viscera can be exteriorized through either a right paralumbar or a ventral midline approach. When making an incision in the lateral abdomen, the standard layers will be encountered, from superficial to deep: skin, thin subcutaneous layer, external abdominal oblique muscle, internal abdominal oblique muscle, transversus abdominis muscle, and peritoneum.

DIGESTIVE SYSTEM

The esophagus is located on the left side of the neck and is unremarkable, except that it is relatively more deeply placed than in other species and the position of the circular and longitudinal muscle layers are reversed from the typical mammalian pattern; in the camelid there is an inner longitudinal layer and an outer circular layer.

South American camelids have a three-chambered stomach with the chambers identified as C1, C2, and C3. There is no stratification of stomach contents as in ruminants; the ingesta has a consistent composition throughout the chambers and is relatively dry. Figs. 38.21 and 38.22 illustrate the external and internal appearance of the stomach chambers.

All three stomach chambers have glandular saccules, which can develop gastroliths visible on radiographs, and ulcerations can develop in any of the chambers. The most common site for ulceration is at the junction of the nonglandular and true glandular portion of C3. Chambers C1, C2, and the cranial four-fifths of C3 are the sites of anaerobic fermentation of forage. There is a groove that allows milk to bypass the first two chambers when the neonate suckles, although it is not as well defined as the groove found in ruminants.

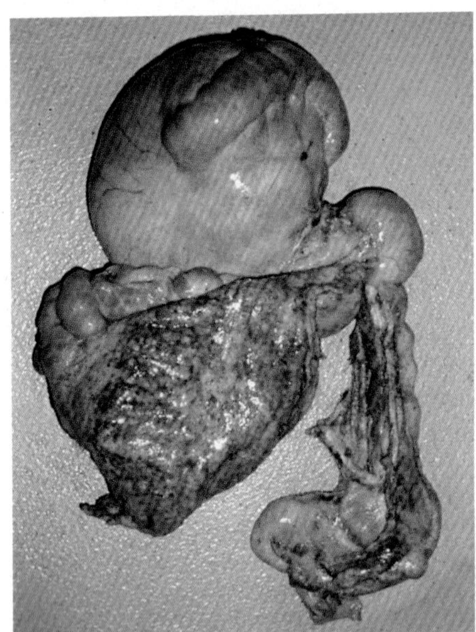

Fig. 38.21 Comparison of the sizes of the large cranial *(top left)* and caudal *(bottom left)* sacs of C1 and the smaller, narrower C3 *(bottom right)*. The small C2 makes up the rounded canal in the *upper right*. The two *large dark areas* on C1 are the saccular regions. (From Cebra C, Anderson DE, Tibary A, et al: Llama and alpaca care: medicine, surgery, reproduction, nutrition, and herd health, St. Louis, 2014, Elsevier, Fig. 40-5.)

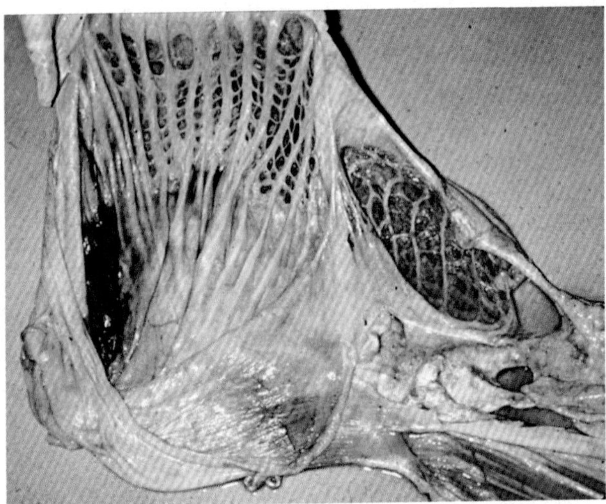

Fig. 38.22 The internal surfaces of C1 *(left)* and C2 *(right)*. Note the lack of papillae and the presence of muscular septae dividing the glandular saccules or cells and the wider opening of the second chamber cells. (From Cebra C, Anderson DE, Tibary A, et al: Llama and alpaca care: medicine, surgery, reproduction, nutrition, and herd health, St. Louis, 2014, Elsevier, Fig. 40-6).

The first chamber is by far the largest, holding 83% of the volume, and it is divided into a cranial and caudal sac by a transversely oriented pillar. Most of the surface area of C1 has glandular saccules arranged in rows on the ventral aspect, and only a small portion is covered by stratified squamous epithelium in llamas and alpacas. The glandular saccules contain folds of simple columnar cells that have ultrastructural features indicating both secretory and absorptive function. C1 occupies much of the left side of the abdomen.

Stomach Chamber 1: Distention of C1 causes obvious left-sided abdominal distention. C1 stomach contents are drier than in ruminants, making collection of a fluid sample more challenging. C1 fluid can be obtained through the left flank, midway between the last rib and the stifle. The contractions (three to four per minute; faster if recently fed) cannot be palpated but can be auscultated through the left ventral inguinal area; sounds on the right side are minimal.

The small second chamber holds only 6% of the stomach volume. Its surface contains glandular cells separated by muscular septae, except in the lower curvature where the epithelium is stratified squamous. The mucosa in the glandular cells may be papillated. Despite being referred to as "glandular" saccules and cells, they are not typical stomach glands, and there is little evidence of glandular function of the saccules or cells of C1 and C2, beyond secretion of a thin protective mucous coat. They seem to function by retaining a small volume of stomach contents adjacent to the absorptive cells, with constant turnover from frequent contractions.

The third chamber is long and tubular and contains typical gastric and pyloric glands in its caudal one-fifth. It is located mainly on the right, and its caudal portion curves upward in the area of the umbilicus. Fig. 38.23 shows the right and left views of the stomach schematically, and Fig. 38.24 illustrates their approximate location within the animal.

Passage of a stomach tube should be done via the oral route, because the nasal cavity diameter is usually too small to accommodate a stomach tube. To avoid laceration of the tube by the sharp cheek teeth, a speculum is used. The tube can be palpated in the esophagus on the left side of the neck; if it is not palpable as the tube is advanced, the tube may be in the trachea.

In the camelid neonate the fermentative chambers of the stomach are relatively more developed than those of ruminant neonates. C1 is about 45% of stomach volume at birth and increases to 60% by 6 weeks of age, while the second chamber starts out at about 10% of the stomach volume and gradually declines.

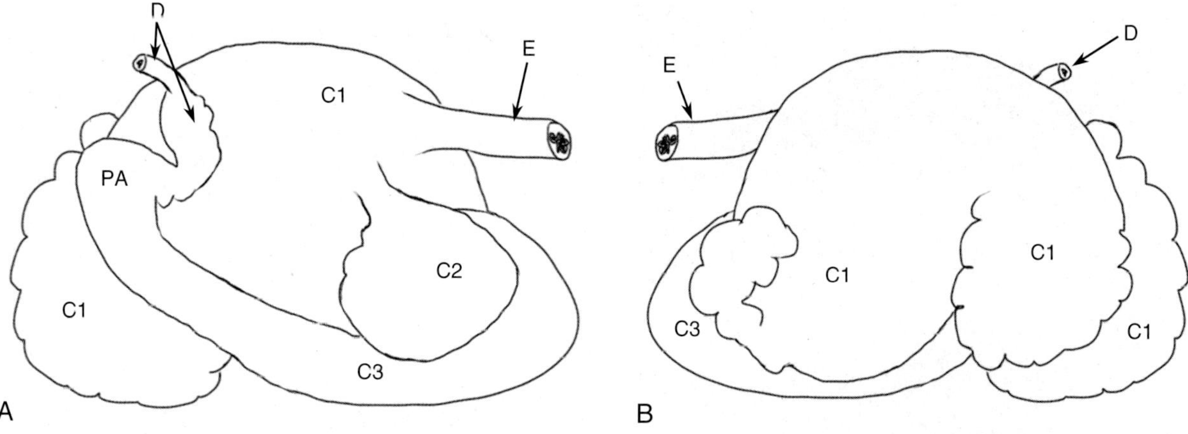

Fig. 38.23 Camelid stomach chamber (schematic). (A) Right side view. (B) Left side view. *C1,* First chamber; *C2,* second chamber; *C3,* third chamber. *D,* duodenum; *E,* esophagus; *PA,* pyloric antrum.

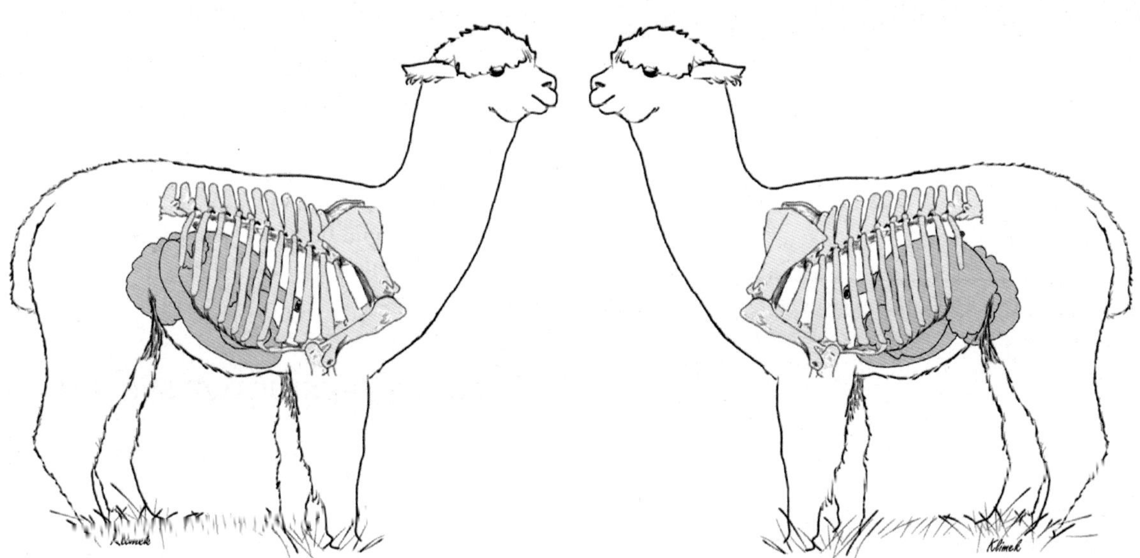

Fig. 38.24 Right and left views of the alpaca illustrating the approximate position of the stomach.

The greater omentum is often translucent because it lacks the extensive fat deposits of the ruminant. It is relatively smaller than that of the ruminant, and there is no omental sling.

The proximal portion of the duodenum has a normal dilatation, referred to as the *ampulla,* where it connects with and wraps partially around the pylorus in an M-shaped flexure, and then it narrows considerably, making the duodenum one of the common sites for obstruction. The descending duodenum is accessible through the right flank. The mass of the jejunum occupies the right dorsal abdomen. Most of the jejunum is coiled tightly, with a short mesentery that prevents exteriorization, but the distal one-third has a looser mesentery that allows more mobility. The small intestine in llamas, except for the ampulla of the duodenum, is about 2 cm in diameter in the adult, and in the adult alpaca it is about 1 cm in diameter.

The cecum is relatively small, and its base is centrally located in the abdomen with the apex pointing caudally. The spiral colon is similar to that of the ruminant but with more coils and a large, circular proximal loop. The spiral colon is usually caudal to the stomach chambers in the ventral abdomen, but it may be found in the right lateral abdomen. Fig. 38.25 shows the small and large intestine of a llama. Normal feces are formed into pellets that either are separate or are clumped but easily separated.

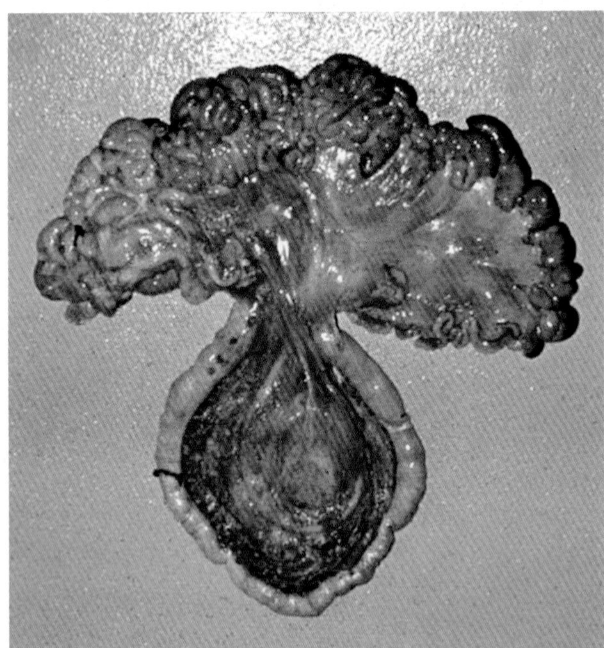

Fig. 38.25 Small intestine *(top)* and ascending colon *(bottom)*. The mesentery of the ascending colon is long and pendulous; this section of the intestines can most easily become torsed or entrapped. (From Cebra C, Anderson DE, Tibary A, et al: Llama and alpaca care: medicine, surgery, reproduction, nutrition, and herd health, St. Louis, 2014, Elsevier, Fig. 40-8.)

In the spiral colon, camelids have an increased chance of obstruction from a foreign body compared to ruminants, because the diameter of the colon decreases from about 5 cm at the beginning of the loops to about 2 cm at the first centripetal coil. Hairballs are not uncommon in young camelids. Because the spiral colon has a relatively loose mesenteric attachment, it can be entirely exteriorized from either a midventral or right paralumbar incision.

The descending colon has a short mesentery; this needs to be noted when performing rectal palpations, which are possible in adult llamas if the examiner has small hands and arms.

The shape and right-sided position of the liver of camelids is very similar to that of ruminants, although camelids usually lack a gallbladder. The liver covers C2 and most of C3, except for a small portion ventrally. Camelids have right, left, caudate, and quadrate lobes of the liver and a fimbriated caudal border.

The preferred site for a liver biopsy is at the right ninth intercostal space, about 20 to 22 cm below the topline.

The pancreas is long and Y-shaped and runs from the area of the common bile duct caudodorsally along the mesentery of the duodenum.

URINARY SYSTEM

The kidneys are not lobated and resemble those of the small ruminant, with a traditional bean shape and a smooth exterior. They are of equal size and relatively slightly more caudal than in other species; the right one is ventral to the transverse processes of the fourth to sixth lumbar vertebrae, and the left one is ventral to the transverse processes of the fifth to seventh lumbar vertebrae. The kidneys are easily accessible for ultrasound. The ureter and bladder are similar to those in other species.

In the male camelid there is a urethral recess at the level of the ischial arch, presenting the same difficulty in catheterization of the urinary bladder in camelids as in ruminants, although it theoretically may be possible to guide the catheter past the urethral diverticulum by digital palpation through the rectum. There is a suburethral diverticulum in the female where the urethra enters the vestibule; this can also cause difficulty when catheterizing a female if it is not actively avoided.

Male camelids may be affected by urethral calculi, either at the distal end of the penis where the urethra narrows as it enters the glans or a similar site of narrowing of the urethra as it leaves the pelvis and travels into the penis, just cranial to the opening of the urethral recess. Camelids are not commonly affected with urethral obstruction in the sigmoid flexure of the penis, as often occurs in cattle. The female urethra is relatively wide and not prone to obstruction.

MALE REPRODUCTIVE SYSTEM

The scrotum is positioned high in the perineal region, in a position similar to that in the cat or the pig. The testes are relatively small, and although present at birth, they are soft and may be difficult to palpate in the newborn. In adult male llamas the size of the testis is 5 to 7 cm in length, 3 to 4 cm in depth, and 2.5 to 3.5 cm wide. Adult male alpacas have slightly smaller testes, at 4 to 5 cm long and 2.5 to 3 cm wide. Their orientation in the scrotum can be vertical or horizontal; the tail of the epididymis is usually directed dorsocaudally, and the body of the epididymis runs dorsally on the testis and faces laterally. The scrotum is not pendulous in camelids, although it becomes somewhat pendulous in the summer months.

Male Reproductive Organ Disorders: The spermatic cord is not as accessible for vasectomy as it is in ruminants. Cryptorchidism is rare in llamas and alpacas, but testicular hypoplasia, sometimes unilateral, occurs in an estimated 10% of individuals. Absence of one testicle has also been reported and is associated with absence of the kidney of the same side.

Male camelids lack seminal vesicles. The ductus deferens has a small ampulla at the junction with the pelvic urethra. The prostate is small (1.5–2.7 cm in length and 1–2.1 cm in width; larger in older animals) and H-shaped or bilobed, sitting dorsal to the urethra near the trigone of the bladder. It can occasionally be palpated per rectum, but usually it is evaluated via ultrasound. The bulbourethral glands are about 2 cm in diameter in the llama and are situated dorsolateral to the urethra at the level of the ischial arch. They can be digitally palpated per rectum.

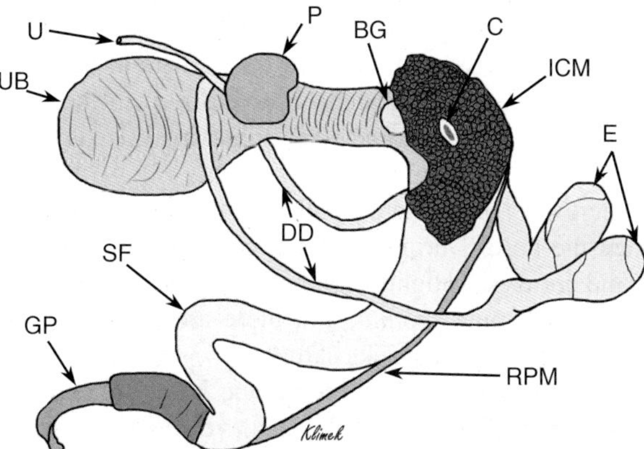

Fig. 38.26 Male llama reproductive tract (schematic). *BG,* Bulbourethral gland; *C,* transected crus of the penis; *DD,* ductus deferens; *E,* tail of the epididymis; *GP,* glans penis; *ICM,* ischiocavernosus muscle; *P,* prostate; *RPM,* retractor penis muscle, *SF,* sigmoid flexure; *U,* ureter; *UB,* urinary bladder. (Drawn from Tibary A, Vaughan J: Reproductive physiology and infertility in male South American camelids: a review and clinical observations, *Small Ruminant Res* 61:283–298, 2006.)

Male camelids have a low volume of ejaculate (3 mL or less), probably as a result of the relatively small size of the testis as well as the relatively small accessory sex glands and the lack of the seminal vesicle. In addition, the diameter of the penile urethra is small. All of these factors contribute to the "dribbling" character of ejaculation in llamas and alpacas.

Camelids have a typical fibroelastic penis with a prescrotal sigmoid flexure. The retractor penis attaches to the distal part of the sigmoid flexure. The penis is about 35 to 45 cm in length in adult llamas and alpacas, with 18 to 25 cm exposed beyond the prepuce in the erect state. Fig. 38.26 is a schematic of the entire male reproductive tract.

The distal end of the penis of camelids possesses a cartilaginous tip that may be confused with the urethral process of the small ruminant, but that does not communicate with the urethra. This corkscrew-shaped cartilaginous tip has a slight clockwise twist; this matches the clockwise spiral course of the lumen of the cervix of the female and serves to dilate the cervix so that semen is deposited in the uterus. The urethral process is small and located at the base of the cartilaginous tip. The distal end of the penis is shown in Fig. 38.27. There is an adhesion of the penis to the prepuce that prevents protrusion of the penis before 2 to 3 years of age. Sexual maturity in the male llama is at 2.5 to 3 years of age; in the male alpaca it is 5 years of age.

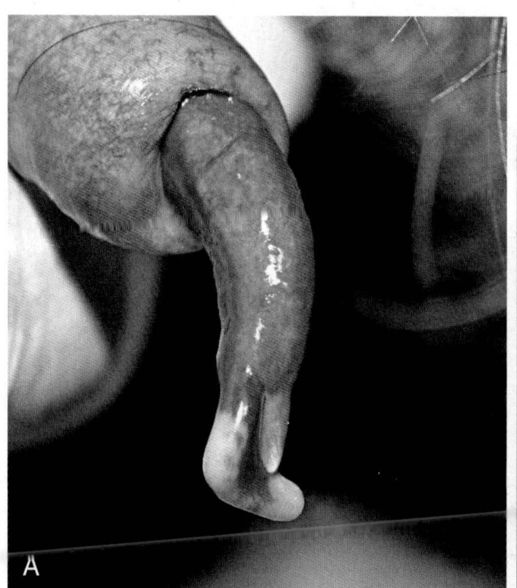

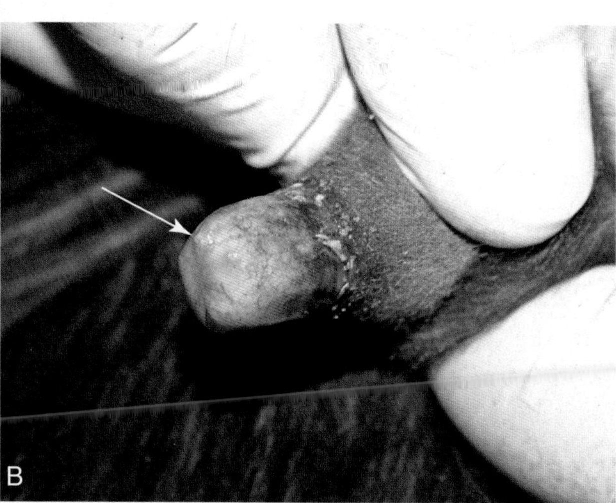

Fig. 38.27 (A) Distal end of the penis of a breeding male (age 3 years). The penis has a corkscrew orientation on its long axis and a blunt cartilaginous tip that spirals around the smaller urethral process. (B) Distal end of the penis of an immature male (age 4 months). Note that the prepuce is adhered to the distal penis. *Arrow* indicates the distal urethra. (From Cebra C, Anderson DE, Tibary A, et al: Llama and alpaca care: medicine, surgery, reproduction, nutrition, and herd health, St. Louis, 2014, Elsevier, Fig. 18-3.)

The triangular-shaped prepuce is in the inguinal region, and its opening is directed caudally in the absence of sexual stimulation. There are well-developed cranial, lateral, and caudal preputial muscles that help direct the opening of the prepuce ventrally and cranially for mating. Fig. 38.28 illustrates schematically the position of the reproductive tract of the male llama.

Semen Collection: Copulation takes place in the sitting (or "cush") position (Fig. 38.29), which presents some logistic challenges for semen collection beyond the low volume of ejaculate. Semen can be collected using an artificial vagina on a dummy, or it can be aspirated from a mated female.

FEMALE REPRODUCTIVE SYSTEM

Camelid Gestation: Sexual maturity occurs in female camelids at about 1 year of age, although ovarian activity begins at 10 months. Camelids are induced ovulators, with ovulation occurring 26 to 30 hours after a single mating on average. The right and left ovaries ovulate with equal frequency, but the conceptus usually implants in the left horn. The gestation period is 11 months. Birth generally takes place between 6:00 AM and 2:00 PM, with the dam in a standing position.

The female llama reproductive tract most closely resembles that of the mare, but the uterine body and the straight uterine horns are short and blunt ended. The blood supply to the uterus more closely resembles that of the carnivore than other large domestic animals and is discussed more fully later.

Inactive ovaries measure approximately 1.5 × 1 × 0.5 cm but may be double that size when active. Corpora lutea normally project from the surface but may be found internally. The ovarian bursa is large and completely surrounds the ovary. Active ovaries can vary in size depending on the number of follicles and corpora lutea present but are generally 1.5 to 2.5 × 1.2 × 1 cm. Most growing follicles and corpora lutea protrude from the surface of the ovary, but corpora lutea have been observed deep in the ovary. Follicles are between 5 and 12 mm; maximal size is 14 mm in llamas and 12 mm in alpacas.

There is a prominent papilla where the uterine tube enters the horn. During the luteal phase of the cycle, the uterine horns curl slightly and become more flaccid. There is an intercornual septum, and there are no intercornual ligaments. The uterus lacks caruncles.

In a nulliparous animal the uterine horns are similar in size (2 × 6 cm), but in animals that have given birth the left horn is usually larger (3 × 10 cm) because 90% to 95% of pregnancies implant in the left horn. The blood supply is also asymmetrical, as is discussed later. The body of the uterus is about 2.5 to 3 cm long and 2.5 to 3 cm wide in the nonpregnant animal. The cervix is 2 to 4 cm long and contains two or three clockwise spiral rings. The vagina is about 15 to 25 cm long, with the cervix protruding slightly into the vagina. The vulvar opening is normally 2.5 to 3 cm in length. The clitoris is located at the ventral edge of the vulvar opening. Fig. 38.30 shows the normal conformation of the female perineal region. The perineal body is relatively small in the camelid.

From the perspective of the caudal end of the animal, the uterine horns of a nonpregnant animal are normally placed at the 3 o'clock and 9 o'clock position. The gravid horn in a pregnant animal will usually move ventrally, producing a slight twist in the opposite horn.

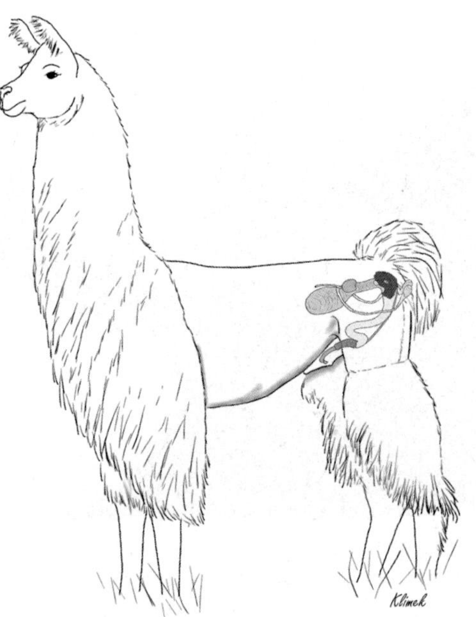

Fig. 38.28 Topographic position of reproductive tract in male llama.

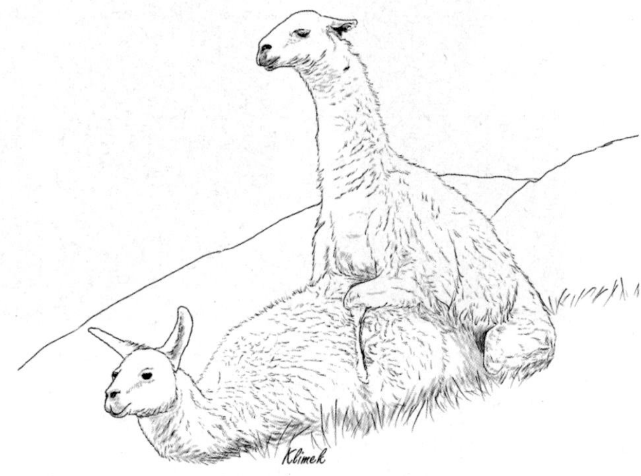

Fig. 38.29 Mating position of the llama and alpaca.

Uterine Torsion: The uterus can become torsed during gestation; if the left horn rotates up and over the right horn, the torsion is said to be clockwise. Alternatively, if the right horn rotates up and over the left horn, the torsion is counterclockwise.

Although rectal palpation of female (and male) reproductive tracts is possible in llamas, evaluation of the female reproductive tract for pregnancy determination is usually done via either transrectal ultrasound for early pregnancies or transabdominal ultrasound in later stages.

The structure of the teat and udder, and their blood supply, is very similar to that of the cow. Although it is much less conspicuous than that of the cow, the camelid udder is divided and supported by a similar suspensory apparatus. Fig. 38.31 shows the normal udder and teats of an alpaca. The teats are small, and the two teats on each side are relatively close together. Each of the four quarters of the udder has two separate lactiferous systems.

Separation of Teats/Supernumerary Teats: Because there are two lactiferous systems per quarter, there is sometimes complete or partial separation of teats associated with the lactiferous systems, and supernumerary teats do occur; these do not always communicate with a lactiferous system.

Placenta

The camelid placenta is chorioallantoic, diffuse, and epitheliochorial, with densely folded papillae on the chorionic surface. The ultrastructure of the papillae has been compared to the shape of a morel mushroom, with a constricted base and an expanded folded apex. Other sources describe the chorionic surface as simply folded. The allantoic sac does not fill the space in the pregnant horn but extends into the full area of the nonpregnant horn. The amnion fills the space of the pregnant horn that is not occupied by the allantoic sac and is adhered to the inner surface of the chorion as well as to the allantois, which generally remains intact in unassisted deliveries. There is a normal 3-cm-wide nonvilliated area of the chorion along the lesser curvature, corresponding to the position of the main chorionic vessels. Hippomanes can be found in the allantoic cavity and are generally tan to dark brown in color, and amniotic plaques are normal. There is generally no remnant of the yolk sac. The umbilical cord of camelids has two umbilical arteries and, unlike most domestic animals, two umbilical veins and also contains the remnant of the allantoic stalk. The umbilical arteries and veins are similar in structure.

Camelids have an extra fetal membrane derived from the epidermis and referred to as the *epidermal membrane.* It develops from the outer epidermis and adheres to the surface of the fetus until hair begins to form and pushes it away, after which some keratinization develops. In camels this separation from the surface of the fetus occurs in the latter fourth of gestation. The epidermal membrane covers the body of the fetus, being joined to it at mucocutaneous junctions and at the junction of the footpads and nails with the skin. It usually breaks down and wears off with little friction following birth. In camelids the amniotic fluid remains watery, lacking the mucus component that develops in the mare and cow, and the epidermal membrane may facilitate lubrication of the fetus. Camelids do not lick their newborn or remove any fetal membranes.

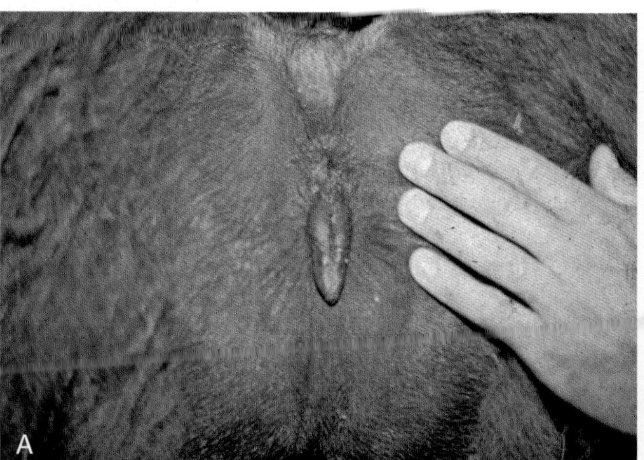

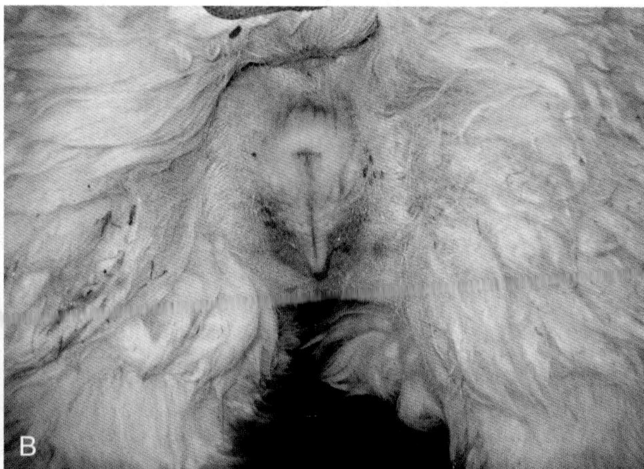

Fig. 38.30 Normal conformation of the vulva of the llama (A) and alpaca (B). Note the small perineal body and the prominent clitoris. (From Cebra C, Anderson DE, Tibary A, et al: Llama and alpaca care: medicine, surgery, reproduction, nutrition, and herd health, St. Louis, 2014, Elsevier, Fig. 17-1.)

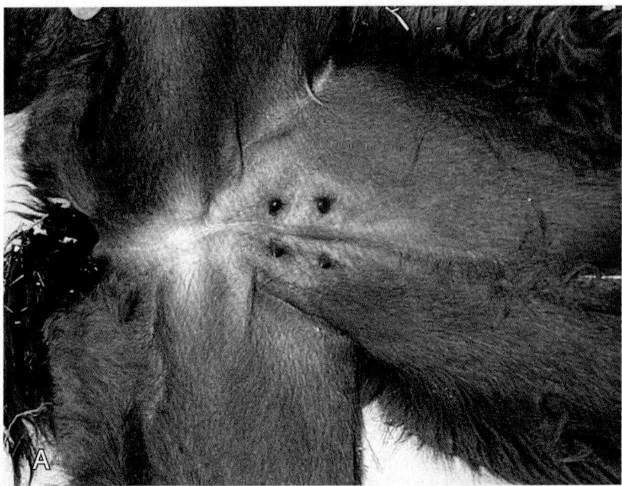

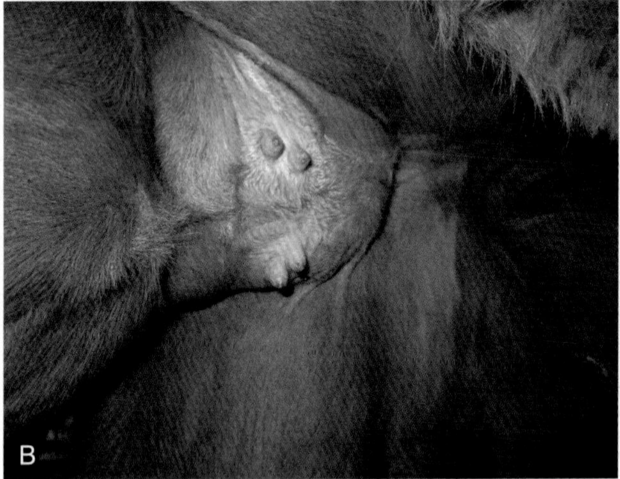

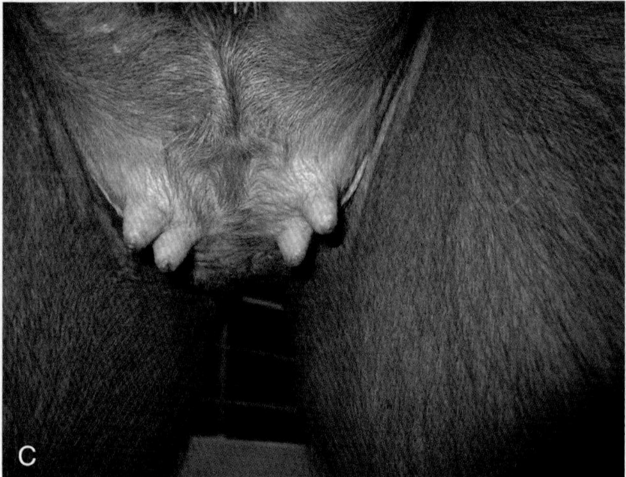

Fig. 38.31 Normal conformation of the udder in the nonlactating (A) and lactating (B and C) alpaca. (From Cebra C, Anderson DE, Tibary A, et al: Llama and alpaca care: medicine, surgery, reproduction, nutrition, and herd health, St. Louis, 2014, Elsevier, Fig. 25-10.)

Delivered or Retained Placenta: The placenta is normally delivered within 1 h after birth. Parturitions that take place outside the normal parturition window are more likely to result in a retained placenta.

BLOOD SUPPLY TO PELVIC WALL AND VISCERA

The ovarian artery is similar to that of other animals in that it is tortuous and has branches to the uterine tube and to the tip of the horn of the uterus. The uterine branch of the ovarian vein is not as prominent in camelids as in some other animals, such as the sheep.

Despite llamas and alpacas being Artiodactyla, the blood supply to rest of their pelvic viscera and perineum has some interesting differences from that of other Artiodactyla. The internal iliac artery is of intermediate length in the llama, with a relatively caudal termination, similar to ruminants and pigs, but despite this, the distribution and origination of the intrapelvic vessels in the llama is more similar to that of the carnivore than to that of ruminants or other Artiodactyla.

The cranial gluteal artery is a branch of the internal iliac artery caudal to the body of the ilium and exits the pelvis through the greater sciatic foramen. The obturator artery and the iliolumbar artery arise via a common trunk about 1 cm caudal to the cranial gluteal artery. The internal iliac artery then terminates at the level of the third sacral vertebra as the caudal gluteal and internal pudendal arteries.

The vaginal or prostatic artery is a branch of the internal pudendal artery right after the internal iliac artery divides into internal pudendal and caudal gluteal branches. This pattern is like the carnivores and the mare and is in contrast to the usual artiodactyl pattern of a long internal iliac artery that gives rise to the vaginal or prostatic artery before it terminates as the caudal gluteal and internal pudendal arteries. The caudal gluteal artery exits the pelvis through its own foramen, cranial to the lesser ischiatic foramen.

The urethral artery is a branch of the internal pudendal artery, cranial to its termination. The middle rectal artery is usually absent in the llama, and the cranial rectal artery (from the caudal mesenteric artery) is prominent and serves the area usually supplied by the middle rectal artery. The dorsal perineal artery is also absent in the llama.

The artery of the penis or clitoris, and the ventral perineal arteries, are the terminal branches of the internal pudendal artery. The ventral perineal artery is the source of arteries supplying several perineal structures, including the ischiocavernosus muscle and bulb of the penis in the male and vestibular bulb in the female, before supplying the caudal rectal artery in both genders. The ventral perineal artery ends in the ventral perineal region; it continues as the dorsal labial artery in the female. The blood supply to the penis (or clitoris) follows the branching pattern of the carnivore, with the artery of the penis dividing into the deep artery of the penis, the artery of the bulb of the penis, and the dorsal artery of the penis.

In the llama there is no branch to the uterus or ductus deferens arising from the umbilical artery. In the female, the main blood supply to the uterus is via a uterine artery originating from the vaginal artery, and in the male the artery of the ductus deferens is a branch of the prostatic artery. This follows the carnivore pattern rather than that of the horse or ruminant.

The blood supply to the uterus is asymmetrical, with the right uterine artery being larger than the left in 90% to 95% of animals in one study. Also in the llamas and alpacas in this study, there was a large crossover vein from the left horn of the uterus to the right uterine vein, and a parallel branch of the right uterine artery to the left horn of the uterus, so that much of the left horn is supplied by vessels from the right side. (In the other 5%–10% of animals, the asymmetry was present but was reversed in direction.) There was also an additional venous anastomosis connecting the right and left sides ventral to the cervix, as is seen in other domestic species. The authors of this study noted that this vascular pattern in camelids is interesting in light of the observation that the left uterine horn causes luteolysis in the right or the left ovary, while the right uterine horn causes luteolysis in the right ovary only; however, the study did not identify a place where blood from the left horn could drain to the right ovarian vein, and thus participate in a countercurrent mechanism with right-side ovarian arterial blood.

PELVIC LIMB

The pelvic bones have few remarkable features. Fig. 38.32 shows the skeleton of the pelvic limb of a llama. The obturator foramen is very large and extends laterally to near the acetabulum. The femur, tibia, and metatarsal bones are all long and slender. The femur lacks a third trochanter.

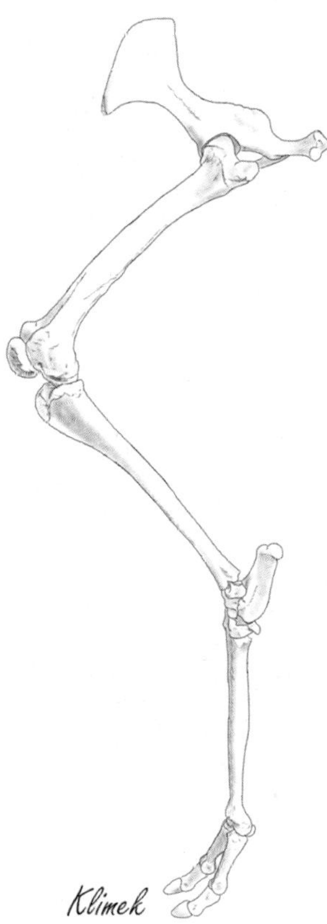

Fig. 38.32 Llama rear limb.

The medial and lateral trochlear ridges of the femur are nearly the same size. The stifle is freer of the trunk than in other species. The stifle is described as having three synovial joint compartments that all communicate, or as having one single compartment, depending on the author. There is one patellar ligament; however, the ligament is broad. The menisci and cruciate ligaments are typical. The lateral collateral ligament has been reported to be absent, with the tendons of origin of the long digital extensor and peroneus tertius acting as support for the joint. The patella is held in place in the trochlear groove by typical femoropatellar ligaments.

Damage to the femoropatellar ligaments can allow medial or lateral patellar luxation, and upward fixation of the patella can also occur, with the patella catching on the proximal portion of either the medial or the lateral trochlear ridge. Straight-legged ("post-legged") conformation may also cause the patella to ride more proximally, predisposing to upward fixation.

The fibula is reduced to a small projection distal to the lateral condyle of the tibia that is not present in all individuals. The tarsus consists of the talus and calcaneus in the proximal row, the central tarsal bone in the middle row, and the first, fused second and third, and fourth tarsal bones in the distal row. The lateral malleolus of the tibia is a separate

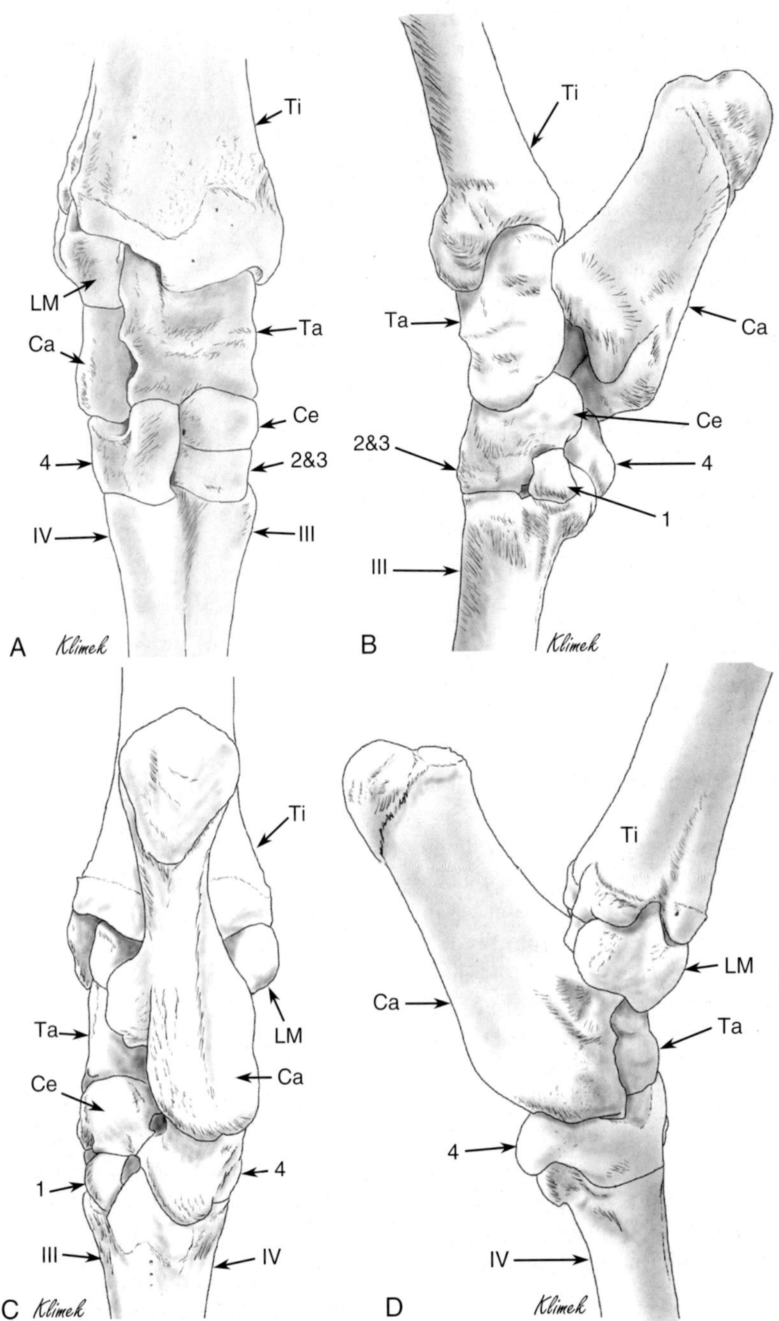

Fig. 38.33 Right tarsus of a llama. (A) Dorsal view. (B) Medial view. (C) Plantar view. (D) Lateral view. In this specimen, the central tarsal bone was partially fused with tarsal bone 2&3. *Ca,* Calcaneus; *Ce,* central tarsal bone; *LM,* lateral malleolus; *Ta,* talus; *Ti,* tibia; *1,* first tarsal bone; *2&3,* fused second and third tarsal bones; *4,* fourth tarsal bone; *III,* third metatarsal bone; *IV,* fourth metatarsal bone.

bone as in ruminants. The tarsal bones are illustrated in Fig. 38.33. Radiographs of the tarsus are shown in Fig. 38.34.

There is wide individual variability in the extent that synovial joints communicate in the compound joints of the tarsus and carpus in the camelid. There are four separate synovial joints in the tarsus. The tibiotarsal and proximal intertarsal joints always communicate; the proximal and distal intertarsal joints communicate at a rate of 34%; the distal intertarsal and tarsometatarsal joints communicate in 64% of cases; and in 26% of tarsi, all of the synovial joints communicate. There are differences between the right and left tarsus in 23% of animals.

The third and fourth metatarsal bones are fused as they are in other artiodactyls, with separate marrow cavities

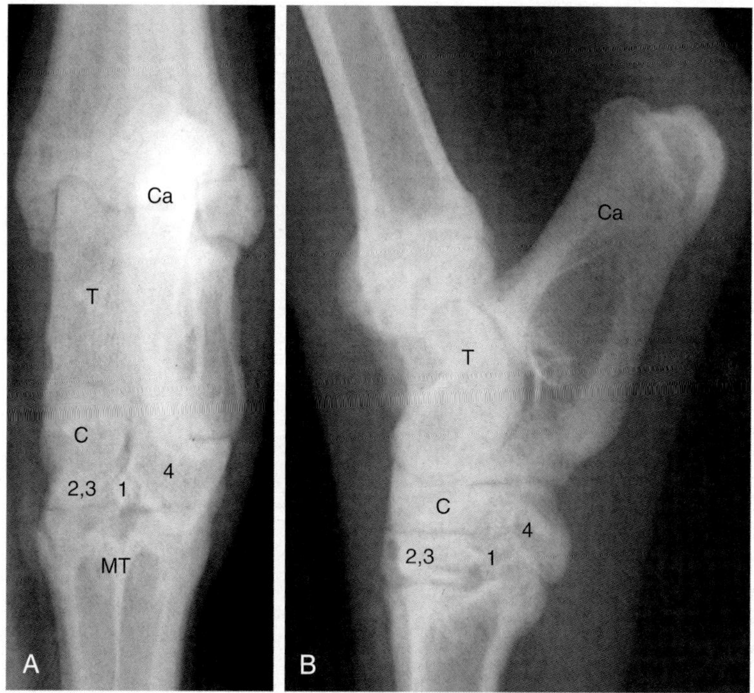

Fig. 38.34 Dorsopalmar (A) and lateral (B) radiographs of the llama tarsus. *C,* Central tarsal bone; *Ca,* calcaneus; *MT,* fused third and fourth metatarsal bones; *T,* talus; *1,* first tarsal bone; *2,3,* fused second and third tarsal bones; *4,* fourth tarsal bone. (From Cebra C, Anderson DE, Tibary A, et al: Llama and alpaca care: medicine, surgery, reproduction, nutrition, and herd health, St. Louis, 2014, Elsevier, Fig. 58-10.)

and separate articular surfaces at the distal end for each digit. The sagittal crest on each of these articular surfaces is only present on the plantar aspect of the articular surface. Each digit has two proximal sesamoids and the usual three phalanges, but there are no distal sesamoids in either the forelimb or the hindlimb digits. The bones of the digit are described more fully with the foot.

Although there is not much specific information about the musculature of the llama or alpaca in the literature, the hindlimb digital flexor muscles and suspensory apparatus of the llama have been studied. Alpacas can be presumed to be similar. Proximal to the tarsus these muscles as well as the gastrocnemius are similar to those of ruminants. In the llama the soleus is absent. The deep digital flexor has three heads; lateral head, medial head, and caudal head. The tendons of the lateral head and the small caudal head join to travel together across the sustentaculum tali. The medial head crosses the medial malleolus and joins the main tendon distal to the sustentaculum tali. A small muscle not found in ruminants, the quadratus plantae, arises from the medioplantar aspect of the calcaneus, is deep to the flexor retinaculum, and inserts at the level of the fusion of the tendons of the deep digital flexor. There is no reciprocal apparatus, accessory ligament of the deep digital flexor tendon, or stay apparatus in the hindlimb of llamas.

Llamas have a pair of lumbricalis pedis muscles in the distal plantar aspect of the metatarsus, at the level of the bifurcation of the deep digital flexor tendon. The tendons of these muscles pass through the interdigital space and attach dorsally to the axial tendons arising from the lateral branch of the long digital extensor. Similar muscles are also present in the forelimb. Axial or abaxial extensor branches of the interosseus muscles are not present in llamas and alpacas. However, these lumbricalis pedis muscles (or lumbricalis manus muscles in the forelimb) have attachments similar to the axial extensor branches of the interosseus in ruminants.

The fetlock joints of the llama have ligaments that share characteristics with both the horse and the ruminants. There is an interdigital metatarsointersesamoid ligament, which is present in the horse (as the metatarsointersesamoid ligament) but not in the ruminant. However, there is no straight sesamoidean ligament, a ligament found in horses. Llamas have oblique sesamoid ligaments, which are present in horses but not ruminants. However, instead of taking the equine form of the ligament, that of a solid sheet, llamas have separate axial and abaxial branches of this ligament. Interdigital phalangosesamoid ligaments of ruminants are replaced with interdigital metatarsophalangosesamoid ligaments, described for the first time in llamas. The axial proximal sesamoid bones are connected to each other via an interdigital intersesamoid ligament and to the distal end of the metatarsal bone via the interdigital metatarsointersesamoid ligament. Llamas additionally have short and cruciate sesamoid ligaments.

Very little has been published in the English language regarding the vasculature and nerve supply of the pelvic limb of the llama or alpaca. The arteries and nonsatellite veins of the hindlimb in the llama have been described. In llamas there is a greater development and importance of the saphenous artery to the blood supply of the distal hindlimb than is typical of other domestic animals.

The main artery to the distal hindlimb in the llama is the caudal branch of the saphenous artery. This artery is accessible to take the pulse. It divides at the tuber calcanei into the medial and lateral plantar arteries, of which the medial is the larger and is the main source of blood to the distal limb. The cranial tibial and dorsal pedal arteries are small and not important to the blood supply of the hindfoot, and there is no perforating tarsal artery.

Among the more notable findings of the blood supply of the alpaca rear limb was the absence of a deep femoral artery in this species. Branches of the femoral artery generally follow the typical pattern, but the descending genicular artery originates from the popliteal artery rather than the femoral artery. The branches of the cranial and caudal tibial and saphenous arteries distal to the tarsus are similar to those described in the llama.

The distribution of the plantar arteries resembles that of the horse, but the medial vessels are much larger. The medial plantar artery gives off a deep branch at the base of the metatarsus and continues as the superficial branch between the deep digital flexor tendon and the medial plantar nerve. The superficial branch of the medial plantar artery moves axially at the level of the distal third of the metatarsus and, after anastomosing with plantar metatarsal artery III, gives rise to plantar common digital arteries II, III, and IV and distal perforating metatarsal artery III.

Plantar common digital artery III is much larger than the other two. It divides into axial plantar proper digital arteries III and IV; each of these gives off a plantar branch to the proximal phalanx that moves abaxially under the flexor tendons and then continues as the axial branch, supplying the dorsal artery of the middle phalanx, the coronal artery, and a branch to the digital pad, and ends in the dermal laminae. The plantar branch to the proximal phalanx continues as the abaxial plantar proper digital artery (III or IV), with branches similar to the axial plantar proper digital arteries. A terminal arch can be seen with contrast angiography.

One study found a superficial set and a deep set of veins in the pelvic limb of the llama. The medial saphenous vein is present. The deep set of veins generally follows the arteries, with some notable exceptions. There is a femoral vein and a medial circumflex femoral vein in the thigh, but the absence of the deep femoral artery as mentioned previously would imply that there is no medial circumflex femoral artery. There is also an extra vein in the thigh without a companion artery. This vein joins the femoral vein at the junction of the medial circumflex femoral and the femoral veins and appears to serve the area supplied by the lateral saphenous vein in other species. It anastomoses with the popliteal vein distally. The popliteal vein is in the typical location. Coming off the caudal side of the popliteal vein is an expansion located between

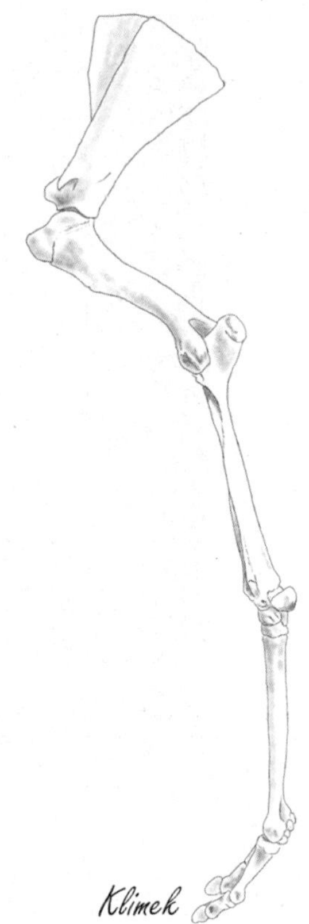

Fig. 38.35 Llama foreleg.

the heads of the gastrocnemius muscle, which may serve as a pump with contraction of the gastrocnemius muscle. This expansion is continued by a vein that ultimately anastomoses with the medial saphenous vein and may be analogous to the caudal branch of the medial saphenous vein of the horse. The medial saphenous vein connects to either the caudal tibial vein or the femoral vein directly. Although the lateral saphenous vein was reported to be absent in this investigation, other authors mention its use for venipuncture.

The nerve supply of the pelvic limb of the llama or alpaca has not been reported in the literature.

THORACIC LIMB

There is nothing remarkably different about the thoracic limb skeleton of the camelid compared to other livestock species. Fig. 38.35 is a drawing of the forelimb skeleton of the llama. The spine of the scapula is unremarkable. It is offset such that the infraspinous fossa is larger than the supraspinous fossa. The coracoid process has a lip that angles medially. The humerus has an intermediate tubercle similar to that of the horse, with the greater and lesser tubercles being of equal size and both projecting proximal to the head of the humerus. The deltoid tuberosity is prominent. The ulna is partially fused to the radius, with its distal end visible as a distinct but fused portion and with remnants of the interosseus space both proximally and distally. The fused radius and ulna and the third and fourth metacarpal bones are very long and slender.

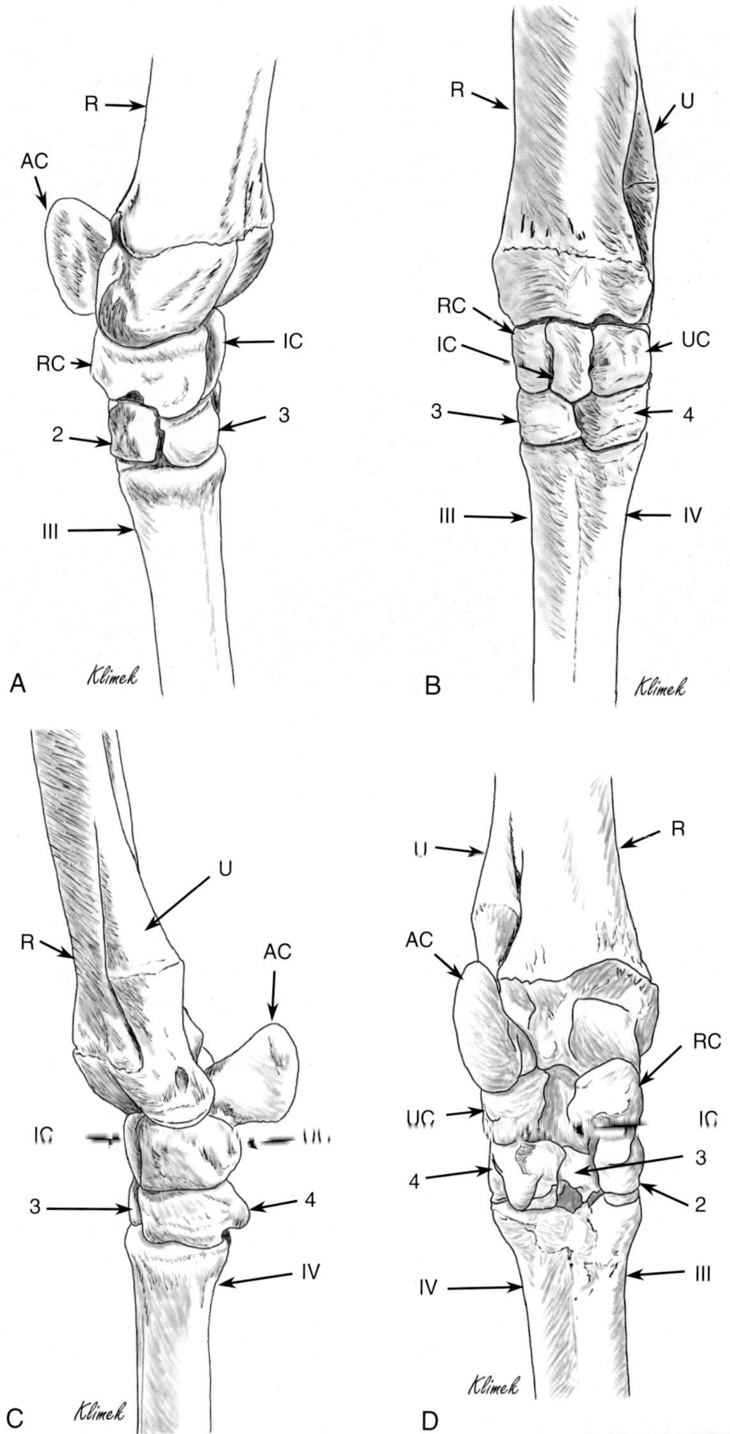

Fig. 38.36 Left carpus of a llama. (A) Dorsomedial view. (B) Dorsal view. (C) Lateral view. (D) Palmar view. *AC*, Accessory carpal bone; *IC*, intermediate carpal bone; *R*, radius; *RC*, radial carpal bone; *U*, ulna; *UC*, ulnar carpal bone; *2*, second carpal bone; *3*, third carpal bone; *4*, fourth carpal bone; *III*, third metacarpal bone; *IV*, fourth metacarpal bone.

The carpus has the accessory, radial, intermediate, and ulnar carpal bones in the proximal row and a small second carpal bone and larger and separate third and fourth carpal bones in the distal row. There are no sesamoids or first carpal bone in the llama. The individual joints can be palpated with the joint flexed, but there is a callus on the dorsal surface of the carpus that may make palpation more difficult. Fig. 38.36 shows the bones of the llama carpus, and Fig. 38.37 shows radiographs of the carpus of a llama.

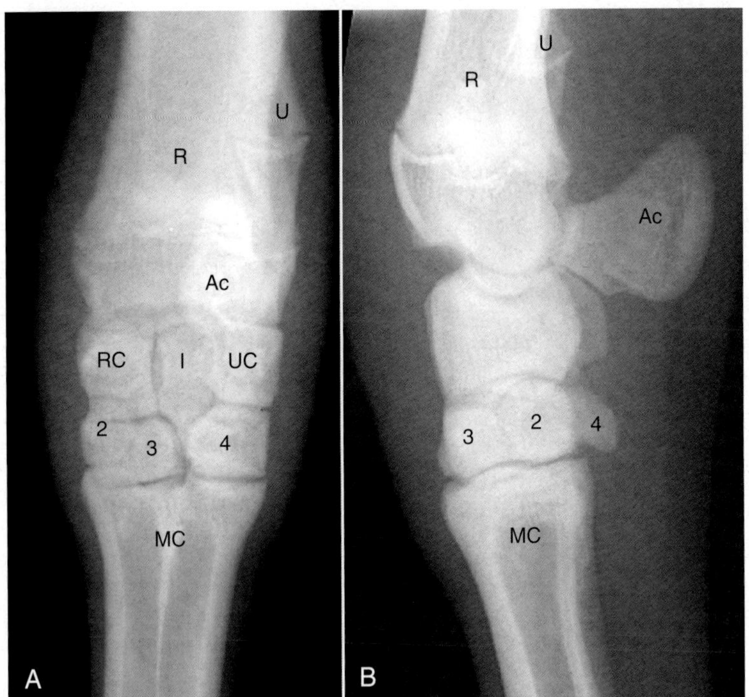

Fig. 38.37 Dorsopalmar (A) and lateral (B) radiographs of the llama carpus. *Ac,* Accessory carpal bone; *I,* intermediate carpal bone; *MC,* fused third and fourth metacarpal bones; *R,* radius; *RC,* radiocarpal bone; *U,* ulna; *UC,* ulnar carpal bone; *2,* second carpal bone; *3,* third carpal bone; *4,* fourth carpal bone. (From Cebra C, Anderson DE, Tibary A, et al: Llama and alpaca care: medicine, surgery, reproduction, nutrition, and herd health, St Louis, 2014, Elsevier, Fig. 58-9.)

The carpal synovial joints communicate with each other with higher frequency than reported in horses and cattle. The radiocarpal joint communicates with the middle carpal joint in about one in three individuals, and the middle carpal joint always communicates with the carpometacarpal joint. The tendon sheaths for the carpus are typical of those in other species, but there is frequently (64%) communication between the carpal sheath (the tendon sheath for the superficial and deep digital flexors) and the radiocarpal joint in the llama.

The two metacarpal bones are fused, with features similar to those described for the hindlimb. The skeletal structures of the foot are described later.

The suspensory apparatus and digital flexor muscles of the forelimb have been described. The flexor carpi ulnaris was found to have a strong humeral head and a reduced ulnar head in the llama. In llamas there is only one belly of the superficial digital flexor muscle, in contrast to the two bellies that are found in ruminants. The superficial digital flexor tendon is relatively small and crosses the carpal canal in the superficial compartment. Distal to the carpus, the tendon of the superficial digital flexor joins the much larger palmar fascia; this is analogous to the accessory ligament of the superficial digital flexor as seen in the horse. This combined structure bifurcates at the fetlock into the two tendons serving the digits. The superficial digital flexor forms a manica flexoria in each digit, as in other species, and inserts on the middle phalanx via the middle scutum.

The deep digital flexor has the usual three heads—radial, ulnar, and humeral—and the humeral head additionally has a superficial and a deep portion. The tendons of all of these portions unite at the level of the carpus and are also joined by a small branch from the flexor carpi ulnaris muscle. The deep digital flexor bifurcates above the fetlock in the usual manner to pass to the distal phalanx of each digit. It is described in more detail later with the foot.

The interosseus muscle is mainly tendinous, as in the horse. It inserts via two symmetrical branches on the four proximal sesamoids, but it lacks the extensor branches found in horses and ruminants. The palmar fascia fuses on the lateral aspect with the origin of interosseous muscles III and IV (analogous to the suspensory ligament of the horse).

As is the case in ruminants, the common digital extensor (and the long digital extensor in the rear limb) has two tendons referred to as the *medial* and *lateral tendons,* and the lateral tendon divides to serve both digits. There is also a lateral digital extensor in both the forelimb and hindlimb. As described for the hindlimb, either one or two lumbricalis manus muscles are present on the palmar aspect of the metacarpus, at the level of the bifurcation of the deep digital flexor muscle; the number varies between individuals. These muscles, when present, each have a tendon that

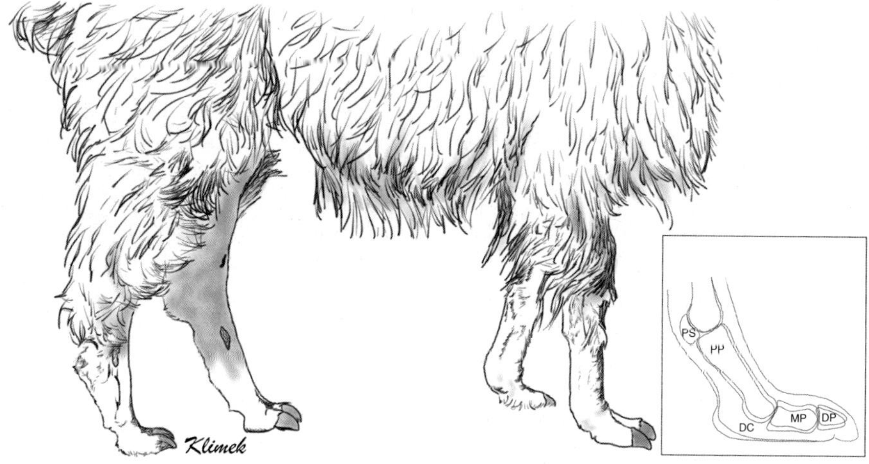

Fig. 38.38 Llama feet. *Inset* shows that camelids stand with the middle and distal phalanges parallel to the ground. There is no distal sesamoid. *DC,* Digital cushion; *DP,* distal phalanx; *MP,* middle phalanx; *PP,* proximal phalanx; *PS,* proximal sesamoid.

joins the axial extensor tendon of digit 3 or digit 4, a tendon that originates from the lateral head of the common digital extensor to serve either digit 3 or digit 4.

Little information about the specific pattern of vessel or nerve supply of the forelimb exists in the literature.

FOOT

Camelids have a skeletal structure of the foot similar to that of domestic ungulates; however, there are some differences of note. Because camelids do not have hooves, but instead have nails and a soft pad (sole, or "slipper"), they are not ungulates, even though they are sometimes referred to as such. They are considered to be tylopods (having padded, rather than hoofed, digits), and they have a modified digitigrade stance. The weight is borne entirely on the pad, which is similar to the bulb of the heel of small ruminants. Deep to the pad is a digital cushion.

The nails possess primary and secondary laminae, although they are not as well developed as those in the horse. Fig. 38.38 shows the feet of a llama, and Fig. 38.39 shows the palmar and dorsal aspects of the llama foot.

Camelid Nails: The nails need to be trimmed regularly, and they are non–weight bearing.

The fused metacarpal and metatarsal bones have separate articular surfaces for each digit, as in ruminants, and similar to ruminants, they also have two proximal sesamoids per digit. However, in contrast to ruminants, the two synovial compartments of the metacarpophalangeal or metatarsophalangeal joints usually do not communicate in the camelid. There are no vestigial digits or associated skeletal structures. Each digit has an ergot at the level of the fetlock joint, and a ligament of the ergot descends on the abaxial side of each digit from the ergot to the digital cushion.

Within the foot, there are proximal, middle, and distal phalanges, but camelids lack a distal sesamoid bone. Because of the stance of the camelid, the proximal interphalangeal joint is hyperextended. The angle of the first phalanx with the ground is normally 52 degrees. The bones of the hindfoot of a camel, which are similar to those in llamas and alpacas, are shown in Fig. 38.40.

Each digit has a combined palmar annular ligament and proximal interdigital ligament to hold the digital flexor tendons in place. The digital flexors share a tendon sheath at the level of the fetlock joint. The deep digital flexor tendon connects to the middle phalanx; this connection is termed the *vinculum,* and it carries vasculature to the bone. The deep digital flexor tendon also has fibers that enter the digital cushion.

The deep digital flexor is reinforced by a cartilage plate as it passes over the middle scutum (a flat plate where the superficial digital flexor tendon inserts on the middle phalanx) at this level. Also at this level, a distal digital annular ligament is present over the deep digital flexor tendon, and an interdigital ligament passes between the two digits. The distal scutum is a thick cartilage plate in the location of the distal sesamoid bone of other species, attached to the distal phalanx and the digital cushion, and over which the deep digital flexor tendon passes. Some of these features are shown in Fig. 38.41.

NERVOUS SYSTEM

The brain and spinal cord do not differ appreciably from the usual pattern. The difference in the spinal accessory nerve has been previously noted. Few other studies on specific cranial nerves of the llama or alpaca are available, and function of the cranial nerves can be assessed in the traditional manner. As in other species, the facial nerve is relatively superficial and can be damaged from trauma peripherally, or from inflammation in its passage through the skull.

The spinal cord ends at the second sacral vertebra. The basic distribution of the peripheral nerves is presumed to be similar to other species as well, although specific anatomic studies on the peripheral nerves of the llama and alpaca are lacking, and evidence suggests that the nerves to the distal limb differ somewhat from the symmetrical medial/lateral pattern of the horse and ruminant. In contrast to the situation in horses and ruminants, the major nerve supply to the foot of the South American camelid is on only the medial aspect of the metatarsus or metacarpus.

Epidural Anesthesia and Collection of Cerebrospinal Fluid: Regional nerve blocks for the limbs are used less in llamas and alpacas than in other species because the path of individual nerves is not well described. Epidural anesthesia can be performed in camelids. The caudal location for perineal procedures is determined by moving the tail and palpating for the first movable joint. In most individuals, the five sacral vertebrae are fused, and the first freely movable joint is S5–C1. However, in some animals, S5 is free but the joint space between S4 and S5 is small enough that injection is usually difficult. If difficulty is encountered, one should move to the next most caudal movable joint. Because camelids have little negative pressure in the epidural space, the method of inserting only the needle and watching for a drop of anesthetic to be pulled in, is unreliable in these species, and instead the syringe should be left attached to the needle and anesthetic injected when resistance to pressure on the plunger is detected. One must be aware of the fact that the anesthetic may travel cranially enough to involve the lumbosacral nerve roots and cause recumbency. Lumbosacral epidural anesthesia is also possible for abdominal and orthopedic procedures; one must again avoid cranial spread of the anesthetic agent to the level of the brachial plexus and phrenic nerve.

Collection of cerebrospinal fluid is similar to procedures used for cattle and horses, and either the atlanto-occipital space or the lumbosacral space may be used.

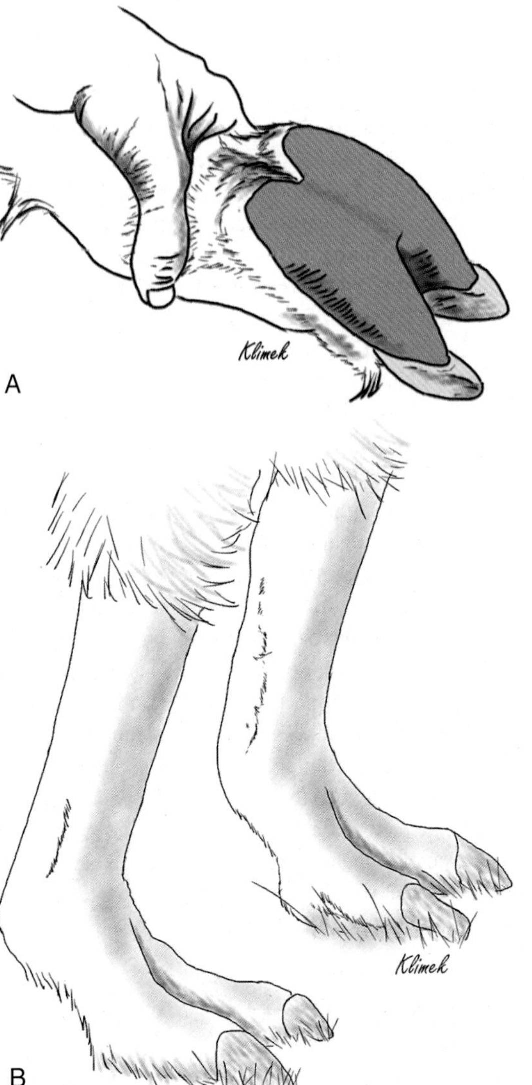

Fig. 38.39 Palmar (A) and dorsal (B) views of the front foot of a llama.

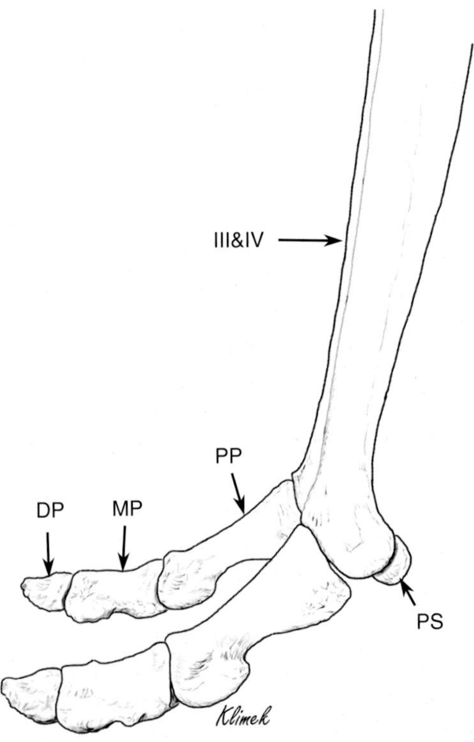

Fig. 38.40 Hindfoot of a camel. *DP,* Distal phalanx; *MP,* middle phalanx; *PP,* proximal phalanx; *PS,* proximal sesamoid. *III&IV,* Fused third and fourth metatarsals.

LYMPHATIC SYSTEM

Little information about the lymphatics of the llama or alpaca is available in the literature. The distribution of the lymph nodes is reported to be similar to that of cattle and sheep. Lymph nodes are small and not readily palpable in a normal adult llama or alpaca but may be palpable in a neonate or an emaciated animal. Similar to the horse, multiple lymph nodes may be observed rather than a single node. The antimesenteric border of the large intestine has aggregations of lymphoid tissue. Mediastinal and mesenteric lymph nodes are present but small.

MISCELLANEOUS CLINICAL NOTES

Congenital developmental problems are fairly common in camelids. Readers interested in a complete discussion of congenital defects seen in llamas and alpacas, especially as they relate to heritability, are referred to Fowler's *Medicine and Surgery of Camelids*.

- The most common congenital disorder of llamas and alpacas involves the development of the mandible, which can either be too long or too short, causing the incisor teeth to not meet the dental pad properly. Cleft palate, or complete palatal agenesis, can both occur.
- A potential impediment to airflow in the newborn is congenital choanal atresia, usually identified when the cria (baby llama or alpaca) exhibits dyspnea or inability to nurse. Affected animals will often stand with the head extended, nostrils flared, and mouth open. In affected animals, a soft rubber catheter passed through the ventral meatus will not advance farther than the medial canthus.
- Several congenital eye abnormalities are reported in llamas and alpacas.
- Atresia of any part of the gastrointestinal tract can occur in any species, but crias are more frequently affected with congenital atresia ani than are neonates of other species.
- Aplasia or atresia of portions of the female reproductive tract is not uncommon. Pseudohermaphroditism, with female external genitalia but an enlarged clitoris, can occur but is infrequent. Supernumerary teats occur in 17% of llamas and 6% of alpacas.
- Camelids can also be afflicted with ligament laxity, flexural deformities, and angular limb deformities.

The normal temperature of llamas and alpacas is between 99.5° and 102°F but can be as high as 104°F in extreme heat, in which case exertion may cause heat stress. The heart rate varies between 60 and 90 beats/min, and respiratory rates are in the range of 10 to 30 breaths/min. The pulse can be taken using the saphenous artery in the middle of the thigh, being careful to approach gradually and to avoid contact with the lower leg, as these animals usually resent handling of the lower limbs.

The preferred sites for intramuscular injections are the caudal neck, semimembranosus, semitendinosus, or triceps brachii muscles. The practitioner should keep in mind that the musculature of the neck is sparse and the vertebral

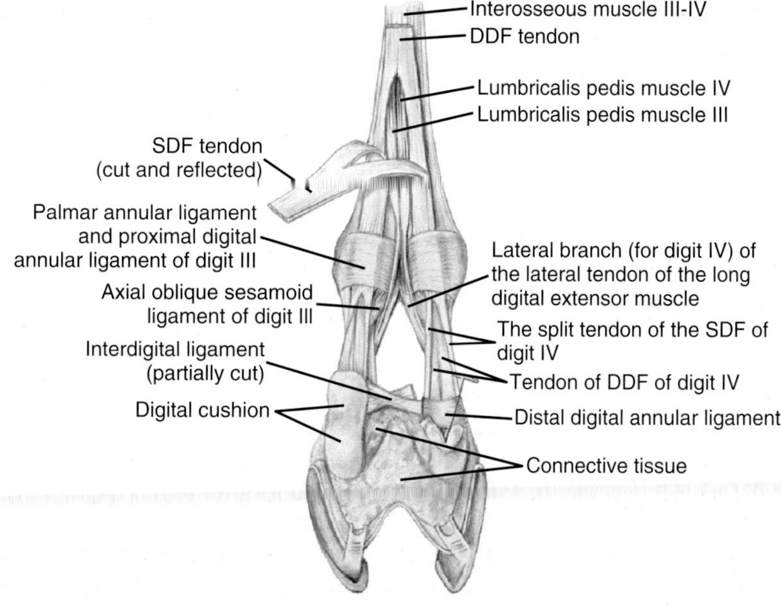

Fig. 38.41 Distal left pelvic limb of the llama with the superficial digital flexor (SDF) tendon reflected to reveal the emergence of the lumbricalis muscles at the bifurcation of the deep digital flexor (DDF) tendon. (From Cebra C, Anderson DE, Tibary A, et al: Llama and alpaca care: medicine, surgery, reproduction, nutrition, and herd health, St. Louis, 2014, Elsevier, Fig. 58-8.)

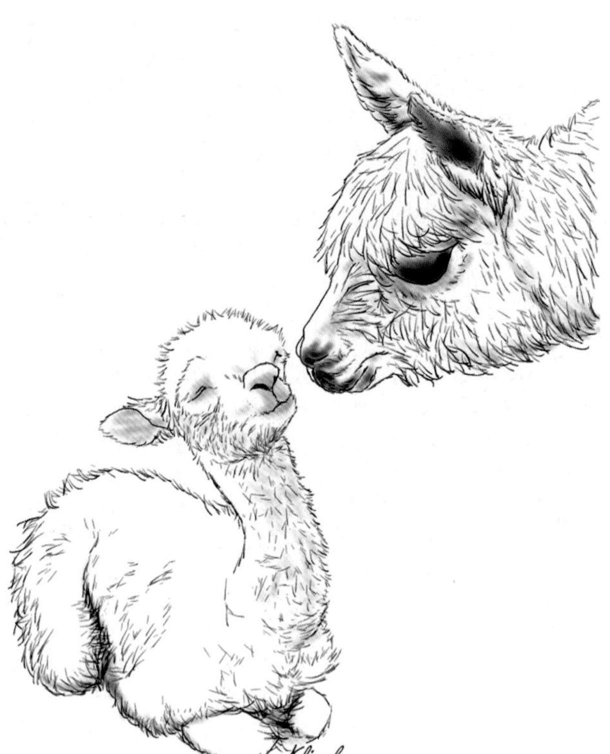

Fig. 38.42 Alpaca cria in the "cush" position.

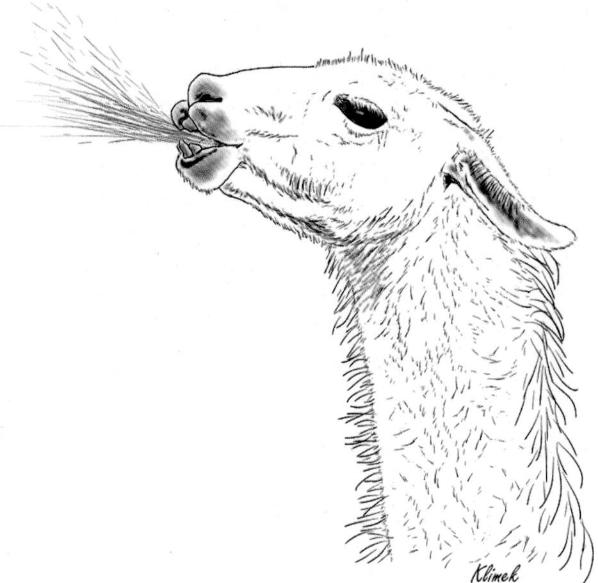

Fig. 38.43 Illustration of the aggressive posture of the head and neck that accompany spitting in the camelid.

column is relatively close to the surface of the neck as compared to other species.

Sites for venipuncture include the jugular vein, the medial saphenous vein at the stifle in laterally recumbent patients, the middle coccygeal vein on the ventral surface of the tail, and veins on the pinna of the ear. The right jugular vein is preferred to avoid damage to the esophagus.

Intravenous catheterization can be done using the jugular, cephalic, lateral saphenous, lateral thoracic, or auricular veins. Of note, one report based on dissections indicated that the lateral saphenous vein is absent in the llama, but this contradicts clinical sources. The femoral artery can be catheterized for arterial blood sampling and blood pressure monitoring. It is also possible to place a cannula in the medullary cavity of the femur.

The veins of the distal limb can be used for regional intravenous anesthesia. After application of a tourniquet, any palpable vein can be catheterized for this procedure, with the dorsal common digital being commonly used. The lateral saphenous vein or the cephalic vein in the forelimb may also be used. Some clinicians note that the thick skin on the distal limbs makes placement of a catheter difficult in the veins of the distal limb.

Camelids rest in the "cush" position, as seen in the cria in Fig. 38.42, with forelimbs and hindlimbs tucked under them in a sternal position. The cush position is an effective position for restraint and handling for certain procedures. They will also lie down in lateral recumbency for deep sleep.

The red blood cell of the camelid is oval shaped and relatively small, and the packed cell volume is higher than for other species. White blood cells are not significantly morphologically different from those of other species, but the leukocyte count is higher than in other species. The neutrophil–lymphocyte ratio is similar to that of the horse, and most of the cells are neutrophils. Llamas and alpacas have been reported to have a higher eosinophil count than other species, but this has not been correlated to parasite counts. Fowler's *Medicine and Surgery of Camelids* contains reference values for blood parameters of llamas and alpacas.

BEHAVIORAL CONSIDERATIONS

Camelids create communal dung piles and often visit them upon waking in the morning. This creates an opportunity to collect fresh fecal samples or urine samples. Males and females both have the same basic stance for urination and for defecation—a semisquatting position—with urine directed caudally.

The ears and the tail can be useful indicators of the mood of a camelid. Relaxed animals usually have ears pointed forward or relaxed to the back or out to the side of the head, and the tail is hanging straight. Alert animals may have erect ears and a slight elevation of the tail. Mildly annoyed camelids will have more elevation of the tail, but it will still be below horizontal; the head is elevated and the ears will be held back and horizontal or below horizontal. Intense aggression is signaled by pointing the nose in the air, pinning the ears back against the neck, and elevating the tail above horizontal. This position is illustrated in Fig. 38.43. Camelids can spit stomach contents when they are intensely displeased. People handling them should be aware of behavioral signals indicating the animal may spit, although this is uncommon in interactions with people if the animals are used to being handled and are appropriately socialized.

COMPREHENSION CHECK

The anatomy of the cervical region in camelids is unique when compared to other species. What features of the camelid cervical region make jugular venipuncture challenging?

What is the clinical significance of the fiberless region on the ventral abdomen of all camelids?

Compare and contrast the camelid stomachs to a ruminant stomach. Which stomach chamber is most closely related to the ruminant true stomach? Compared to rumen contractions in a ruminant, how many C1 contractions should be auscultated per minute in a camelid? Why are there more C1 contractions in a minute compared to rumen contractions in a minute?

What is the clinical significance of the unique camelid dentition?

Index

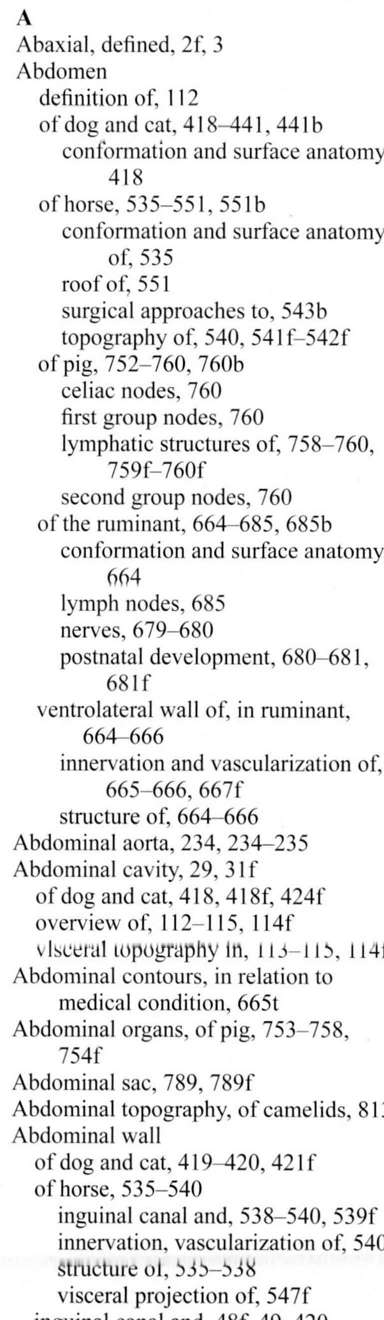

Page numbers followed by *"b"* indicate boxes; *"f"* figures; *"t"* tables.

D